CAMPBELL-WALSH
UROLOGY

ELEVENTH EDITION

Editor-in-Chief

ALAN J. WEIN, MD, PhD (HON), FACS
Founders Professor of Urology
Division of Urology
Penn Medicine, Perelman School of Medicine;
Chief of Urology
Division of Urology
Penn Medicine, Hospital of the University of Pennsylvania;
Program Director, Residency in Urology
Division of Urology
Penn Medicine, University of Pennsylvania Health System
Philadelphia, Pennsylvania

LOUIS R. KAVOUSSI, MD, MBA
Waldbaum-Gardner Distinguished
Professor of Urology
Department of Urology
Hofstra North Shore-LIJ School of Medicine
Hampstead, New York;
Chairman of Urology
The Arthur Smith Institute for Urology
Lake Success, New York

ALAN W. PARTIN, MD, PhD
Professor and Director of Urology
Department of Urology
The Johns Hopkins School of Medicine
Baltimore, Maryland

CRAIG A. PETERS, MD
Professor of Urology
University of Texas Southwestern
Medical Center;
Chief, Section of Pediatric Urology
Children's Health System
Dallas, Texas

ELSEVIER

ELSEVIER

1600 John F. Kennedy Blvd.
Ste 1800
Philadelphia, PA 19103-2899

CAMPBELL-WALSH UROLOGY, ELEVENTH EDITION   ISBN: 978-1-4557-7567-5
INTERNATIONAL EDITION   ISBN: 978-0-323-34148-6
Copyright © 2016 by Elsevier, Inc. All rights reserved.

Previous editions copyrighted 2012, 2007, 2002, 1998, 1992, 1986, 1978, 1970, 1963, and 1954.

Exceptions as follows:
1. Chapter 35: Surgery of Testicular Tumors—IUSM retains copyright for all original illustrations created by IUSM. The following copyright notice shall be used under said illustrations in the Work: © 2016 Section of Medical Illustration in the Office of Visual Media at the Indiana University School of Medicine. Published by Elsevier Inc. All rights reserved.
2. Chapter 63: Treatment of Advanced Renal Cell Carcinoma by W. Marston Linehan and Ramaprasad Srinivasan— Chapter is in public domain.
3. Chapter 85: Complications Related to the Use of Mesh and Their Repair—Shlomo Raz retains copyright for his original videos. © 2016 Shlomo Raz. All rights reserved.

Library of Congress Cataloging-in-Publication Data

Campbell-Walsh urology / editor-in-chief, Alan J. Wein ; editors, Louis R. Kavoussi, Alan W. Partin, Craig A. Peters.—Eleventh edition.
      p. ; cm.
  Urology
  Preceded by Campbell-Walsh urology / editor-in-chief, Alan J. Wein ; editors, Louis R. Kavoussi ... [et al.]. 10th ed. c2012.
  Includes bibliographical references and index.
  ISBN 978-1-4557-7567-5 (4 vol. set; hardcover : alk. paper)—ISBN 978-0-323-34148-6 (international edition)
  I. Wein, Alan J., editor.   II. Kavoussi, Louis R., editor.   III. Partin, Alan W., editor.   IV. Peters, Craig (Craig Andrew), editor.   V. Title: Urology.
  [DNLM: 1. Female Urogenital Diseases.   2. Male Urogenital Diseases.   3. Urology–methods. WJ 140]
  RC871
  616.6—dc23

                                                                                    2015032028

Senior Content Strategist: Charlotta Kryhl
Senior Content Development Specialist: Deidre Simpson
Publishing Services Manager: Catherine Jackson
Book Production Specialist: Kristine Feeherty
Design Direction: Amy Buxton

Printed in China

Last digit is the print number: 9 8 7 6 5 4 3 2 1

Every 4 years or so, a small group of crazed individuals are privileged to convene and embark on a seemingly near impossible task—to improve upon what, a relatively short time ago, they had created as the gold standard textbook in urology. A week or so later, they emerge with a plan, each with their assignments for what they now are convinced is the best ever repository of total urologic knowledge. This group and this edition are no exceptions to this routine.

The four of us feel very honored and privileged to be a part of this tradition that began in 1954 with the publication of the first Campbell's Urology (then titled simply "Urology"), which consisted of 3 volumes in which 51 individuals contributed 2356 pages and 1148 illustrations. We are grateful to our current colleagues and friends who accepted the responsibility of producing anew the 156 chapters that comprise our text and acknowledge their expertise and the unselfish contribution of their time and effort.

Our gratitude to the chapter authors notwithstanding, we would like ultimately to dedicate this edition to two sets of individuals: One group includes our mentors in urology—those whom each of us separately admired and learned from, and whose educational and clinical achievements in various aspects of our field we have sought to imitate. Hopefully, they would or will be proud of our part in this 11th edition of the gold standard textbook. The greatest debt and thanks, however, are owed to our families, specifically our wives and children who were in the "line of fire" during the preparation of this edition. They deserve more than a medal or a copy of the book. So, to Noele and Nolan; to Julianne, Nick, Rebecca and Dree; to Vicky, Topper, David, Dane and Michael; and to Kathy, Jessica, Lauren, and Ryan, our thanks for your patience, understanding, and continued support. The good news is that you have a few years until the cycle begins again.

For myself and my fellow editors,
Alan J. Wein

Louis R. Kavoussi
Alan W. Partin
Craig A. Peters

CONTRIBUTORS

Paul Abrams, MD, FRCS
Professor of Urology
Bristol Urological Institute
Southmead Hospital
Bristol, United Kingdom

Mark C. Adams, MD, FAAP
Professor of Urologic Surgery
Department of Urology
Division of Pediatric Urology
Monroe Carell Jr. Children's Hospital at
Vanderbilt
Nashville, Tennessee

**Hashim U. Ahmed, PhD, FRCS (Urol),
BM, BCh, BA (Hons)**
MRC Clinician Scientist and Reader in
Urology
Division of Surgery and Interventional
Science
University College London;
Honorary Consultant Urological Surgeon
University College London Hospitals NHS
Foundation Trust
London, United Kingdom

Mohamad E. Allaf, MD
Buerger Family Scholar
Associate Professor of Urology, Oncology,
and Biomedical Engineering
Director of Minimally Invasive and
Robotic Surgery
Department of Urology
James Buchanan Brady Urological Institute
Johns Hopkins University School of
Medicine
Baltimore, Maryland

Karl-Erik Andersson, MD, PhD
Professor
Aarhus Institute for Advanced Studies
Aarhus University
Aarhus, Jutland, Denmark;
Professor
Wake Forest Institute for Regenerative
Medicine
Wake Forest University School of Medicine
Winston-Salem, North Carolina

**Sero Andonian, MD, MSc, FRCS(C),
FACS**
Associate Professor
Division of Urology
Department of Surgery
McGill University
Montreal, Quebec, Canada

Jennifer Tash Anger, MD, MPH
Associate Professor
Department of Surgery
Cedars-Sinai Medical Center;
Adjunct Assistant Professor
Urology
University of California, Los Angeles
Los Angeles, California

Kenneth W. Angermeier, MD
Associate Professor
Glickman Urological and Kidney Institute
Cleveland Clinic
Cleveland, Ohio

Emmanuel S. Antonarakis, MD
Associate Professor of Oncology
Sidney Kimmel Comprehensive Cancer
Center
Johns Hopkins University
Baltimore, Maryland

Jodi A. Antonelli, MD
Assistant Professor
Department of Urology
University of Texas Southwestern Medical
Center
Dallas, Texas

Anthony Atala, MD
Director, Wake Forest Institute for
Regenerative Medicine
William H. Boyce Professor and Chair
Department of Urology
Wake Forest School of Medicine
Winston-Salem, North Carolina

Paul F. Austin, MD
Professor
Division of Urologic Surgery
Washington University School of Medicine
in St. Louis
St. Louis, Missouri

Gopal H. Badlani, MD, FACS
Professor and Vice Chair
Department of Urology
Wake Forest University Baptist Medical
Center
Winston-Salem, North Carolina

**Darius J. Bägli, MDCM, FRCSC, FAAP,
FACS**
Professor of Surgery and Physiology
Division of Urology, Departments of
Surgery and Physiology
University of Toronto;
Senior Attending Urologist, Associate
Surgeon-in-Chief, Senior Associate
Scientist
Division of Urology, Department of
Surgery, Division of Developmental and
Stem Cell Biology
Sick Kids Hospital and Research Institute
Toronto, Ontario, Canada

Daniel A. Barocas, MD, MPH, FACS
Assistant Professor
Department of Urologic Surgery
Vanderbilt University Medical Center
Nashville, Tennessee

Julia Spencer Barthold, MD
Associate Chief
Surgery/Urology
Nemours/Alfred I. duPont Hospital for
Children
Wilmington, Delaware;
Professor
Departments of Urology and Pediatrics
Sidney Kimmel Medical College of
Thomas Jefferson University
Philadelphia, Pennsylvania

Stuart B. Bauer, MD
Professor of Surgery (Urology)
Harvard Medical School;
Senior Associate in Urology
Department of Urology
Boston Children's Hospital
Boston, Massachusetts

Mitchell C. Benson, MD
Department of Urology
New York-Presbyterian Hospital/Columbia
University Medical Center
New York, New York;

Brian M. Benway, MD
Director, Comprehensive Kidney Stone
Program
Urology Academic Practice
Cedars-Sinai Medical Center
Los Angeles, California

Jonathan Bergman, MD, MPH
Assistant Professor
Departments of Urology and Family
    Medicine
David Geffen School of Medicine at UCLA;
Veterans Health Affairs, Greater Los
    Angeles
Los Angeles, California

Sara L. Best, MD
Assistant Professor
Department of Urology
University of Wisconsin School of
    Medicine and Public Health
Madison, Wisconsin

Sam B. Bhayani, MD, MS
Professor of Surgery, Urology
Department of Surgery
Washington University School of Medicine
    in St. Louis;
Vice President, Chief Medical Officer
Barnes West Hospital
St. Louis, Missouri

Lori A. Birder, PhD
Professor of Medicine and Pharmacology
Medicine-Renal Electrolyte Division
University of Pittsburgh School of
    Medicine
Pittsburgh, Pennsylvania

Jay T. Bishoff, MD, FACS
Director, Intermountain Urological
    Institute
Intermountain Health Care
Salt Lake City, Utah

Brian G. Blackburn, MD
Clinical Associate Professor
Department of Internal Medicine/
    Infectious Diseases and Geographic
    Medicine
Stanford University School of Medicine
Stanford, California

Jeremy Matthew Blumberg, MD
Chief of Urology
Harbor-UCLA Medical Center;
Assistant Professor of Urology
David Geffen School of Medicine at UCLA
Los Angeles, California

Michael L. Blute, Sr., MD
Chief, Department of Urology
Walter S. Kerr, Jr., Professor of Urology
Massachusetts General Hospital/Harvard
    Medical School
Boston, Massachusetts

Timothy B. Boone, MD, PhD
Professor and Chair
Department of Urology
Houston Methodist Hospital and Research
    Institute
Houston, Texas;
Professor
Department of Urology
Weill Medical College of Cornell
    University
New York, New York

Stephen A. Boorjian, MD
Professor of Urology
Department of Urology
Mayo Clinic
Rochester, Minnesota

Joseph G. Borer, MD
Associate Professor of Surgery (Urology)
Harvard Medical School;
Reconstructive Urologic Surgery Chair
Director, Neurourology and Urodynamics
Director, Bladder Exstrophy Program
Department of Urology
Boston Children's Hospital
Boston, Massachusetts

Charles B. Brendler, MD
Co-Director, John and Carol Walter Center
    for Urological Health
Department of Surgery
Division of Urology
NorthShore University HealthSystem
Evanston, Illinois;
Senior Clinician Educator
Department of Surgery
Division of Urology
University of Chicago Pritzker School of
    Medicine
Chicago, Illinois

Gregory A. Broderick, MD
Professor of Urology
Mayo Clinic College of Medicine
Program Director, Urology Residency
    Program
Mayo Clinic
Jacksonville, Florida

James D. Brooks, MD
Keith and Jan Hurlbut Professor
Chief of Urologic Oncology
Department of Urology
Stanford University
Stanford, California

Benjamin M. Brucker, MD
Assistant Professor
Urology and Obstetrics & Gynecology
NYU Langone Medical Center
New York, New York

Kathryn L. Burgio, PhD
Professor of Medicine
Department of Medicine
Division of Gerontology, Geriatrics, and
    Palliative Care
University of Alabama at Birmingham;
Associate Director for Research
Birmingham/Atlanta Geriatric Research,
    Education, and Clinical Center
Birmingham VA Medical Center
Birmingham, Alabama

Arthur L. Burnett II, MD, MBA, FACS
Patrick C. Walsh Distinguished Professor
    of Urology
Department of Urology
Johns Hopkins University School of
    Medicine
Baltimore, Maryland

Nicol Corbin Bush, MD, MSCS
Co-Director, PARC Urology
Dallas, Texas

Jeffrey A. Cadeddu, MD
Professor of Urology and Radiology
Department of Urology
University of Texas Southwestern Medical
    Center
Dallas, Texas

**Anthony A. Caldamone, MD, MMS, FAAP,
FACS**
Professor of Surgery (Urology)
Division of Urology
Section of Pediatric Urology
Warren Alpert Medical School of Brown
    University;
Chief of Pediatric Urology
Division of Pediatric Urology
Hasbro Children's Hospital
Providence, Rhode Island

Steven C. Campbell, MD, PhD
Professor of Surgery
Department of Urology
Glickman Urological and Kidney Institute
Cleveland Clinic
Cleveland, Ohio

Douglas A. Canning, MD
Professor of Urology (Surgery)
Perelman School of Medicine
University of Pennsylvania;
Chief, Division of Urology
The Children's Hospital of Philadelphia
Philadelphia, Pennsylvania

Michael A. Carducci, MD
AEGON Professor in Prostate Cancer
    Research
Sidney Kimmel Comprehensive Cancer
    Center
Johns Hopkins University
Baltimore, Maryland

Peter R. Carroll, MD, MPH
Professor and Chair
Ken and Donna Derr–Chevron
    Distinguished Professor
Department of Urology
University of California, San Francisco
San Francisco, California

Herbert Ballentine Carter, MD
Professor of Urology and Oncology
Department of Urology
James Buchanan Brady Urological Institute
Johns Hopkins School of Medicine
Baltimore, Maryland

Clint K. Cary, MD, MPH
Assistant Professor
Department of Urology
Indiana University
Indianapolis, Indiana

Pasquale Casale, MD
Professor
Department of Urology
Columbia University Medical Center;
Chief, Pediatric Urology
Morgan Stanley Children's Hospital of
New York-Presbyterian
New York, New York

William J. Catalona, MD
Professor
Department of Urology
Northwestern University Feinberg School
of Medicine
Chicago, Illinois

Frank A. Celigoj, MD
Male Infertility/Andrology Fellow
Department of Urology
University of Virginia
Charlottesville, Virginia

Toby C. Chai, MD
Vice Chair of Research
Department of Urology
Yale School of Medicine;
Co-Director of Female Pelvic Medicine and
Reconstructive Surgery Program
Department of Urology
Yale New Haven Hospital
New Haven, Connecticut

Alicia H. Chang, MD, MS
Instructor
Department of Internal Medicine/
Infectious Diseases and Geographic
Medicine
Stanford University School of Medicine
Stanford, California;
Medical Consultant
Los Angeles County Tuberculosis Control
Program
Los Angeles County Department of Public
Health
Los Angeles, California

**Christopher R. Chapple, MD, FRCS
(Urol)**
Professor and Consultant Urologist
Department of Urology
The Royal Hallamshire Hospital
Sheffield Teaching Hospitals
Sheffield, South Yorkshire, United
Kingdom

Mang L. Chen, MD
Assistant Professor
Department of Urology
University of Pittsburgh
Pittsburgh, Pennsylvania

Ronald C. Chen, MD, MPH
Associate Professor
Department of Radiation Oncology
University of North Carolina at Chapel
Hill
Chapel Hill, North Carolina

Benjamin I. Chung, MD
Assistant Professor
Department of Urology
Stanford University School of Medicine
Stanford, California

Michael J. Conlin, MD, MCR
Associate Professor of Urology
Portland VA Medical Center
Portland, Oregon

Christopher S. Cooper, MD, FAAP, FACS
Professor
Department of Urology
University of Iowa;
Associate Dean, Student Affairs and
Curriculum
University of Iowa Carver College of
Medicine
Iowa City, Iowa

Raymond A. Costabile, MD
Jay Y. Gillenwater Professor of Urology
Department of Urology
University of Virginia
Charlottesville, Virginia

Paul L. Crispen, MD
Assistant Professor
Department of Urology
University of Florida
Gainesville, Florida

Juanita M. Crook, MD, FRCPC
Professor
Division of Radiation Oncology
University of British Columbia, Okanagan;
Radiation Oncologist
Center for the Southern Interior
British Columbia Cancer Agency
Kelowna, British Columbia, Canada

Douglas M. Dahl, MD, FACS
Associate Professor of Surgery
Harvard Medical School;
Chief, Division of Urologic Oncology
Department of Urology
Massachusetts General Hospital
Boston, Massachusetts

Marc Arnaldo Dall'Era, MD
Associate Professor
Department of Urology
University of California, Davis
Sacramento, California

Anthony V. D'Amico, MD, PhD
Eleanor Theresa Walters Distinguished
Professor and Chief of Genitourinary
Radiation Oncology
Department of Radiation Oncology
Brigham and Women's Hospital and
Dana-Farber Cancer Institute
Boston, Massachusetts

Siamak Daneshmand, MD
Professor of Urology (Clinical Scholar)
Institute of Urology
University of Southern California
Los Angeles, California

Shubha De, MD, FRCPC
Assistant Professor
University of Alberta
Edmonton, Alberta, Canada

Jean J. M. C. H. de la Rosette, MD, PhD
Professor and Chairman
Department of Urology
AMC University Hospital
Amsterdam, Netherlands

Dirk J. M. K. De Ridder, MD, PhD
Professor
Department of Urology
University Hospitals KU Leuven
Leuven, Belgium

G. Joel DeCastro, MD, MPH
Assistant Professor of Urology
Department of Urology
New York-Presbyterian Hospital/Columbia
University Medical Center
New York, New York

Michael C. Degen, MD, MA
Clinical Assistant
Department of Urology
Hackensack University Medical Center
Hackensack, New Jersey

Sevag Demirjian, MD
Assistant Professor
Cleveland Clinic Lerner College of
Medicine
Department of Nephrology and
Hypertension
Cleveland Clinic
Cleveland, Ohio

Francisco Tibor Dénes, MD, PhD
Associate Professor
Division of Urology
Chief, Pediatric Urology
University of São Paulo Medical School
Hospital das Clínicas
São Paulo, Brazil

John D. Denstedt, MD, FRCSC, FACS
Professor of Urology
Chairman of the Department of Surgery
Western University
London, Ontario, Canada

Theodore L. DeWeese, MD, MPH
Professor and Chair
Radiation Oncology and Molecular
Radiation Sciences
Johns Hopkins University School of
Medicine
Baltimore, Maryland

David Andrew Diamond, MD
Urologist-in-Chief
Department of Urology
Boston Children's Hospital;
Professor of Surgery (Urology)
Department of Surgery
Harvard Medical School
Boston, Massachusetts

Colin P. N. Dinney, MD
Chairman and Professor
Department of Urology
The University of Texas MD Anderson
  Cancer Center
Houston, Texas

Roger R. Dmochowski, MD, MMHC, FACS
Professor of Urology and Gynecology
Vanderbilt University Medical School
Nashville, Tennessee

Charles G. Drake, MD, PhD
Associate Professor of Oncology,
  Immunology, and Urology
James Buchanan Brady Urological Institute
Johns Hopkins University;
Attending Physician
Department of Oncology
Johns Hopkins Kimmel Cancer Center
Baltimore, Maryland

Marcus John Drake, DM, MA, FRCS (Urol)
Senior Lecturer in Urology
School of Clinical Sciences
University of Bristol;
Consultant Urologist
Bristol Urological Institute
Southmead Hospital
Bristol, United Kingdom

Brian D. Duty, MD
Assistant Professor of Urology
Oregon Health & Science University
Portland, Oregon

James A. Eastham, MD
Chief, Urology Service
Surgery
Memorial Sloan Kettering Cancer Center;
Professor
Department of Urology
Weill Cornell Medical Center
New York, New York

Louis Eichel, MD
Chief, Division of Urology
Rochester General Hospital;
Director, Minimally Invasive Surgery
Center for Urology
Rochester, New York

J. Francois Eid, MD
Attending Physician
Department of Urology
Lenox Hill Hospital
North Shore-LIJ Health System
New York, New York

Mario A. Eisenberger, MD
R. Dale Hughes Professor of Oncology and
  Urology
Sidney Kimmel Comprehensive Cancer
  Center;
Johns Hopkins University
Baltimore, Maryland

Mohamed Aly Elkoushy, MD, MSc, PhD
Associate Professor
Department of Urology
Faculty of Medicine
Suez Canal University
Ismailia, Egypt

Mark Emberton, MD, MBBS, FRCS (Urol), BSc
Dean, Faculty of Medical Sciences
University College London
Honorary Consultant Urological Surgeon
University College London Hospitals NHS
  Foundation Trust
London, United Kingdom

Jonathan I. Epstein, MD
Professor of Pathology, Urology, and
  Oncology
Reinhard Professor of Urological Pathology
Director of Surgical Pathology
Johns Hopkins Medical Institutions
Baltimore, Maryland

Carlos R. Estrada, Jr., MD
Associate Professor of Surgery
Harvard Medical School;
Director, Center for Spina Bifida and
  Spinal Cord Conditions
Co-Director, Urodynamics and
  Neuro-Urology
Boston Children's Hospital
Boston, Massachusetts

Michael N. Ferrandino, MD
Assistant Professor
Division of Urologic Surgery
Duke University Medical Center
Durham, North Carolina

Lynne R. Ferrari, MD
Associate Professor of Anesthesiology
Department of Anaesthesia
Harvard Medical School;
Medical Director, Perioperative Services
  and Operating Rooms
Chief, Division of Perioperative Anesthesia
Robert M. Smith Chair in Pediatric
  Anesthesia
Department of Anesthesiology,
  Perioperative and Pain Medicine
Boston Children's Hospital
Boston, Massachusetts

Fernando A. Ferrer, MD
Peter J. Deckers, MD, Endowed Chair of
  Pediatric Surgery
Surgeon-in-Chief
Director, Division of Urology
Connecticut Children's Medical Center
Hartford, Connecticut;
Vice Chair
Department of Surgery
Professor of Surgery, Pediatrics, and Cell
  Biology
University of Connecticut School of
  Medicine
Farmington, Connecticut

Richard S. Foster, MD
Professor
Department of Urology
Indiana University
Indianapolis, Indiana

Dominic Frimberger, MD
Professor of Urology
Department of Urology
University of Oklahoma
Oklahoma City, Oklahoma

Pat F. Fulgham, MD
Director of Surgical Oncology
Texas Health Presbyterian Dallas
Dallas, Texas

John P. Gearhart, MD
Professor of Pediatric Urology
Department of Urology
Johns Hopkins University School of
  Medicine
Baltimore, Maryland

Glenn S. Gerber, MD
Professor
Department of Surgery
University of Chicago Pritzker School of
  Medicine
Chicago, Illinois

Bruce R. Gilbert, MD, PhD
Professor of Urology
Hofstra North Shore-LIJ School of
  Medicine
New Hyde Park, New York

Scott M. Gilbert, MD
Associate Member
Department of Genitourinary Oncology
H. Lee Moffitt Cancer Center and Research
  Institute
Tampa, Florida

Timothy D. Gilligan, MD, MS
Associate Professor of Medicine
Department of Solid Tumor Oncology
Cleveland Clinic Lerner College of
  Medicine;
Co-Director, Center for Excellence in
  Healthcare Communication
Program Director, Hematology/Oncology
  Fellowship
Medical Director, Inpatient Solid Tumor
  Oncology
Taussig Cancer Institute
Cleveland Clinic
Cleveland, Ohio

David A. Goldfarb, MD
Professor of Surgery
Cleveland Clinic Lerner College of
  Medicine;
Surgical Director, Renal Transplant
  Program
Glickman Urological and Kidney Institute
Cleveland Clinic
Cleveland, Ohio

Irwin Goldstein, MD
Director of Sexual Medicine
Alvarado Hospital;
Clinical Professor of Surgery
University of California, San Diego;
Director, San Diego Sexual Medicine
San Diego, California

Marc Goldstein, MD, DSc (Hon), FACS
Matthew P. Hardy Distinguished Professor
  of Urology and Male Reproductive
  Medicine
Department of Urology and Institute for
  Reproductive Medicine
Weill Medical College of Cornell
  University;
Surgeon-in-Chief, Male Reproductive
  Medicine and Surgery
New York-Presbyterian Hospital/Weill
  Cornell Medical Center;
Adjunct Senior Scientist
Population Council
Center for Biomedical Research at
  Rockefeller University
New York, New York

Leonard G. Gomella, MD, FACS
Bernard Godwin Professor of Prostate
  Cancer and Chair
Department of Urology
Associate Director, Sidney Kimmel Cancer
  Center
Thomas Jefferson University
Philadelphia, Pennsylvania

Mark L. Gonzalgo, MD, PhD
Professor of Urology
University of Miami Miller School of
  Medicine
Miami, Florida

Tomas L. Griebling, MD, MPH
John P. Wolf 33-Degree Masonic
  Distinguished Professor of Urology
Department of Urology and the Landon
  Center on Aging
The University of Kansas
Kansas City, Kansas

Hans Albin Gritsch, MD
Surgical Director, Kidney Transplant
Department of Urology
University of California, Los Angeles
Los Angeles, California

Frederick A. Gulmi, MD
Chairman and Residency Program Director
Chief, Division of Minimally Invasive and
  Robotic Surgery
Department of Urology
Brookdale University Hospital and Medical
  Center
Brooklyn, New York;
Clinical Associate Professor of Urology
New York Medical College
Valhalla, New York

Khurshid A. Guru, MD
Robert P. Huben Endowed Professor of
  Urologic Oncology
Director, Robotic Surgery
Department of Urology
Roswell Park Cancer Institute
Buffalo, New York

Thomas J. Guzzo, MD, MPH
Associate Professor of Urology
Penn Medicine, Perelman School of
  Medicine
Division of Urology
Hospital of the University of Pennsylvania
University of Pennsylvania Health System
Philadelphia, Pennsylvania

Jennifer A. Hagerty, DO
Attending Physician
Surgery/Urology
Nemours/Alfred I. duPont Hospital for
  Children
Wilmington, Delaware;
Assistant Professor
Departments of Urology and Pediatrics
Sidney Kimmel Medical College of
  Thomas Jefferson University
Philadelphia, Pennsylvania

Ethan J. Halpern, MD, MSCE
Professor of Radiology and Urology
Department of Radiology
Thomas Jefferson University
Philadelphia, Pennsylvania

Misop Han, MD, MS
David Hall McConnell Associate Professor
  in Urology and Oncology
Johns Hopkins Medicine
Baltimore, Maryland

Philip M. Hanno, MD, MPH
Professor of Urology
Department of Surgery
University of Pennsylvania
Philadelphia, Pennsylvania

Hashim Hashim, MBBS, MRCS (Eng), MD, FEBU, FRCS (Urol)
Consultant Urological Surgeon and
  Director of the Urodynamics Unit
Continence and Urodynamics Unit
Bristol Urological Institute
Bristol, United Kingdom

Sender Herschorn, MD, FRCSC
Professor
Division of Urology
University of Toronto;
Urologist
Division of Urology
Sunnybrook Health Sciences Centre
Toronto, Ontario, Canada

Piet Hoebeke, MD, PhD
Full Professor
Ghent University;
Chief of Department of Urology and
  Pediatric Urology
Ghent University Hospital
Ghent, Belgium

David M. Hoenig, MD
Professor and Chief
LIJ Medical Center
The Arthur Smith Institute for Urology
North Shore-LIJ-Hofstra University
Lake Success, New York

Michael H. Hsieh, MD, PhD
Associate Professor
Departments of Urology (primary),
  Pediatrics (secondary), and
  Microbiology, Immunology, and
  Tropical Medicine (secondary)
George Washington University;
Attending Physician
Division of Urology
Children's National Health System
Washington, DC;
Stirewalt Endowed Director
Biomedical Research Institute
Rockville, Maryland

Tung-Chin Hsieh, MD
Assistant Professor of Surgery
Department of Urology
University of California, San Diego
La Jolla, California

Douglas A. Husmann, MD
Professor
Department of Urology
Mayo Clinic
Rochester, Minnesota

Thomas W. Jarrett, MD
Professor and Chairman
Department of Urology
George Washington University
Washington, DC

J. Stephen Jones, MD, MBA, FACS
President, Regional Hospitals and Family
  Health Centers
Cleveland Clinic
Cleveland, Ohio

Gerald H. Jordan, MD, FACS, FAAP (Hon), FRCS (Hon)
Professor
Department of Urology
Eastern Virginia Medical School
Norfolk, Virginia

David B. Joseph, MD, FACS, FAAP
Chief of Pediatric Urology
Children's Hospital at Alabama;
Professor of Urology
Department of Urology
University of Alabama at Birmingham
Birmingham, Alabama

Martin Kaefer, MD
Professor
Department of Urology
Indiana University School of Medicine
Indianapolis, Indiana

Jose A. Karam, MD
Assistant Professor
Department of Urology
The University of Texas MD Anderson
 Cancer Center
Houston, Texas

Louis R. Kavoussi, MD, MBA
Waldbaum-Gardner Distinguished
 Professor of Urology
Department of Urology
Hofstra North Shore-LIJ School of
 Medicine
Hampstead, New York;
Chairman of Urology
The Arthur Smith Institute for Urology
Lake Success, New York

Parviz K. Kavoussi, MD, FACS
Reproductive Urologist
Austin Fertility & Reproductive Medicine;
Adjunct Assistant Professor
Neuroendocrinology and Motivation
 Laboratory
Department of Psychology
The University of Texas at Austin
Austin, Texas

Antoine E. Khoury, MD, FRCSC, FAAP
Walter R. Schmid Professor of Urology
University of California, Irvine;
Head of Pediatric Urology
CHOC Children's Urology Center
Children's Hospital of Orange County
Orange, California

Roger S. Kirby, MD, FRCS
Medical Director
The Prostate Center
London, United Kingdom

Eric A. Klein, MD
Chairman
Glickman Urological and Kidney Institute
Cleveland Clinic;
Professor of Surgery
Cleveland Clinic Lerner College of
 Medicine
Cleveland, Ohio

David James Klumpp, PhD
Associate Professor
Department of Urology
Northwestern University Feinberg School
 of Medicine
Chicago, Illinois

Bodo E. Knudsen, MD, FRCSC
Associate Professor and Interim Chair,
 Clinical Operations
Department of Urology
Wexner Medical Center
The Ohio State University
Columbus, Ohio

Kathleen C. Kobashi, MD, FACS
Section Head
Urology and Renal Transplantation
Virginia Mason Medical Center
Seattle, Washington

Thomas F. Kolon, MD, MS
Associate Professor of Urology (Surgery)
Perelman School of Medicine
University of Pennsylvania;
Director, Pediatric Urology Fellowship
 Program
The Children's Hospital of Philadelphia
Philadelphia, Pennsylvania

Bridget F. Koontz, MD
Butler-Harris Assistant Professor
Department of Radiation Oncology
Duke University Medical Center
Durham, North Carolina

**Martin Allan Koyle, MD, FAAP, FACS,
FRCSC, FRCS (Eng)**
Division Head, Pediatric Urology
Women's Auxiliary Chair in Urology and
 Regenerative Medicine
Hospital for Sick Children;
Professor
Department of Surgery
Division of Urology
Institute of Health Policy, Management
 and Evaluation
University of Toronto
Toronto, Ontario, Canada

Amy E. Krambeck, MD
Associate Professor
Department of Urology
Mayo Clinic
Rochester, Minnesota

Ryan M. Krlin, MD
Assistant Professor of Urology
Department of Urology
Louisiana State University Health Science
 Center
New Orleans, Louisiana

Bradley P. Kropp, MD, FAAP, FACS
Professor of Pediatric Urology
Department of Urology
University of Oklahoma Health Sciences
 Center
Oklahoma City, Oklahoma

Alexander Kutikov, MD, FACS
Associate Professor of Urologic Oncology
Department of Surgery
Fox Chase Cancer Center
Philadelphia, Pennsylvania

Jaime Landman, MD
Professor of Urology and Radiology
Chairman, Department of Urology
University of California, Irvine
Orange, California

Brian R. Lane, MD, PhD
Betz Family Endowed Chair for Cancer
 Research
Spectrum Health Regional Cancer Center;
Chief of Urology
Spectrum Health Medical Group;
Associate Professor of Surgery
Michigan State University;
Grand Rapids, Michigan

Stephen Larsen, MD
Chief Resident
Department of Urology
Rush University Medical Center
Chicago, Illinois

David A. Leavitt, MD
Assistant Professor
Vattikuti Urology Institute
Henry Ford Health System
Detroit, Michigan

Eugene Kang Lee, MD
Assistant Professor
Department of Urology
University of Kansas Medical Center
Kansas City, Kansas

Richard S. Lee, MD
Assistant Professor of Surgery (Urology)
Harvard Medical School;
Department of Urology
Boston Children's Hospital
Boston, Massachusetts

W. Robert Lee, MD, MEd, MS
Professor
Department of Radiation Oncology
Duke University School of Medicine
Durham, North Carolina

Dan Leibovici, MD
Chairman of Urology
Kaplan Hospital
Rehovot, Israel

Gary E. Lemack, MD
Professor of Urology and Neurology
Department of Urology
University of Texas Southwestern Medical
 Center
Dallas, Texas

Herbert Lepor, MD
Professor and Martin Spatz Chairman
Department of Urology
NYU Langone Medical Center
New York, New York

Laurence A. Levine, MD, FACS
Professor
Department of Urology
Rush University Medical Center
Chicago, Illinois

**Sey Kiat Lim, MBBS, MRCS (Edinburgh),
MMed (Surgery), FAMS (Urology)**
Consultant
Department of Urology
Changi General Hospital
Singapore

W. Marston Linehan, MD
Chief, Urologic Oncology Branch
Physician-in-Chief, Urologic Surgery
National Cancer Institute
National Institutes of Health Clinical
    Center
Bethesda, Maryland

James E. Lingeman, MD
Professor
Department of Urology
Indiana University School of Medicine
Indianapolis, Indiana

Richard Edward Link, MD, PhD
Associate Professor of Urology
Director, Division of Endourology and
    Minimally Invasive Surgery
Scott Department of Urology
Baylor College of Medicine
Houston, Texas

Michael E. Lipkin, MD
Associate Professor
Division of Urologic Surgery
Duke University Medical Center
Durham, North Carolina

Mark S. Litwin, MD, MPH
The Fran and Ray Stark Foundation Chair
    in Urology
Professor of Urology and Health Policy &
    Management
David Geffen School of Medicine at UCLA
UCLA Fielding School of Public Health
Los Angeles, California

Stacy Loeb, MD, MSc
Assistant Professor
Urology, Population Health, and Laura
    and Isaac Perlmutter Cancer Center
New York University and Manhattan
    Veterans Affairs
New York, New York

**Armando J. Lorenzo, MD, MSc, FRCSC,
FAAP, FACS**
Staff Paediatric Urologist
Hospital for Sick Children
Associate Scientist
Research Institute, Child Health Evaluative
    Sciences;
Associate Professor
Department of Surgery
Division of Urology
University of Toronto
Toronto, Ontario, Canada

Yair Lotan, MD
Professor
Department of Urology
University of Texas Southwestern Medical
    Center
Dallas, Texas

Tom F. Lue, MD, ScD (Hon), FACS
Professor
Department of Urology
University of California, San Francisco
San Francisco, California

Dawn Lee MacLellan, MD, FRCSC
Associate Professor
Departments of Urology and Pathology
Dalhousie University
Halifax, Nova Scotia, Canada

Vitaly Margulis, MD
Associate Professor
Department of Urology
University of Texas Southwestern Medical
    Center
Dallas, Texas

Stephen David Marshall, MD
Chief Resident
Department of Urology
SUNY Downstate College of Medicine
Brooklyn, New York

Aaron D. Martin, MD, MPH
Assistant Professor
Department of Urology
Louisiana State University Health Sciences
    Center;
Pediatric Urology
Children's Hospital New Orleans
New Orleans, Louisiana

Darryl T. Martin, PhD
Associate Research Scientist
Department of Urology
Yale University School of Medicine
New Haven, Connecticut

Neil Martin, MD, MPH
Assistant Professor
Department of Radiation Oncology
Brigham and Women's Hospital and
    Dana-Farber Cancer Institute
Boston, Massachusetts

Timothy A. Masterson, MD
Associate Professor
Department of Urology
Indiana University Medical Center
Indianapolis, Indiana

Ranjiv Mathews, MD
Professor of Urology and Pediatrics
Director of Pediatric Urology
Southern Illinois University School of
    Medicine
Springfield, Illinois

Surena F. Matin, MD
Professor
Department of Urology;
Medical Director
Minimally Invasive New Technology in
    Oncologic Surgery (MINTOS)
The University of Texas MD Anderson
    Cancer Center
Houston, Texas

Brian R. Matlaga, MD, MPH
Professor
James Buchanan Brady Urological Institute
Johns Hopkins Medical Institutions
Baltimore, Maryland

Richard S. Matulewicz, MS, MD
Department of Urology
Northwestern University Feinberg School
    of Medicine
Chicago, Illinois

Kurt A. McCammon, MD, FACS
Devine Chair in Genitourinary
    Reconstructive Surgery
Chairman and Program Director
Professor
Department of Urology
Eastern Virginia Medical School;
Sentara Norfolk General Hospital
Urology
Norfolk, Virginia;
Devine-Jordan Center for Reconstructive
    Surgery and Pelvic Health
Urology of Virginia, PLLC
Virginia Beach, Virginia

James M. McKiernan, MD
Chairman
Department of Urology
New York-Presbyterian Hospital/Columbia
    University Medical Center
New York, New York

Alan W. McMahon, MD
Associate Professor
Department of Medicine
University of Alberta
Edmonton, Alberta, Canada

Chris G. McMahon, MBBS, FAChSHM
Director, Australian Centre for Sexual
    Health
Sydney, New South Wales, Australia

**Thomas A. McNicholas, MB, BS, FRCS,
FEBU**
Consultant Urologist and Visiting
    Professor
Department of Urology
Lister Hospital and University of
    Hertfordshire
Stevenage, United Kingdom

Kevin T. McVary, MD, FACS
Professor and Chairman, Division of
    Urology
Department of Surgery
Southern Illinois University School of
    Medicine
Springfield, Illinois

Alan K. Meeker, PhD
Assistant Professor of Pathology
Assistant Professor of Urology
Assistant Professor of Oncology
Johns Hopkins University School of
    Medicine
Baltimore, Maryland

Kirstan K. Meldrum, MD
Chief, Division of Pediatric Urology
Professor of Surgery
Michigan State University
Helen DeVos Children's Hospital
Grand Rapids, Michigan

Cathy Mendelsohn, PhD
Professor
Departments of Urology, Pathology, and
    Genetics & Development
Columbia University College of Physicians
    and Surgeons
New York, New York

Maxwell V. Meng, MD
Professor
Chief, Urologic Oncology
Department of Urology
University of California, San Francisco
San Francisco, California

Jayadev Reddy Mettu, MD, MBBS
Department of Urology
Wake Forest School of Medicine
Winston-Salem, North Carolina

Alireza Moinzadeh, MD
Director of Robotic Surgery
Institute of Urology
Lahey Hospital & Medical Center
Burlington, Massachusetts;
Assistant Professor
Department of Urology
Tufts University School of Medicine
Boston, Massachusetts

Manoj Monga, MD, FACS
Director, Stevan B. Streem Center for
    Endourology and Stone Disease
Glickman Urological and Kidney Institute
Cleveland Clinic
Cleveland, Ohio

Allen F. Morey, MD, FACS
Professor
Department of Urology
University of Texas Southwestern Medical
    Center
Dallas, Texas

Todd M. Morgan, MD
Assistant Professor
Department of Urology
University of Michigan
Ann Arbor, Michigan

Ravi Munver, MD, FACS
Vice Chairman
Chief of Minimally Invasive and Robotic
    Urologic Surgery
Department of Urology
Hackensack University Medical Center
Hackensack, New Jersey;
Associate Professor of Surgery (Urology)
Department of Surgery
Division of Urology
Rutgers New Jersey Medical School
Newark, New Jersey

Stephen Y. Nakada, MD, FACS
Professor and Chairman
The David T. Uehling Chair of Urology
Department of Urology
University of Wisconsin School of
    Medicine and Public Health;
Chief of Service
Department of Urology
University of Wisconsin Hospital and
    Clinics
Madison, Wisconsin

Leah Yukie Nakamura, MD
Associate in Urology
Orange County Urology Associates
Laguna Hills, California

Neema Navai, MD
Assistant Professor
Department of Urology
The University of Texas MD Anderson
    Cancer Center
Houston, Texas

Joel B. Nelson, MD
Frederic N. Schwentker Professor and
    Chairman
Department of Urology
University of Pittsburgh School of
    Medicine
Pittsburgh, Pennsylvania

Diane K. Newman, DNP, ANP-BC, FAAN
Adjunct Associate Professor of Urology in
    Surgery
Division of Urology
Research Investigator Senior
Perelman School of Medicine
University of Pennsylvania;
Co-Director, Penn Center for Continence
    and Pelvic Health
Division of Urology
Penn Medicine
Philadelphia, Pennsylvania

Paul L. Nguyen, MD
Associate Professor
Department of Radiation Oncology
Harvard Medical School;
Director of Prostate Brachytherapy
Department of Radiation Oncology
Brigham and Women's Hospital and
    Dana-Farber Cancer Institute
Boston, Massachusetts

J. Curtis Nickel, MD, FRCSC
Professor and Canada Research Chair
Department of Urology
Queen's University
Kingston, Ontario, Canada

Craig Stuart Niederberger, MD, FACS
Clarence C. Saelhof Professor and Head
Department of Urology
University of Illinois at Chicago College of
    Medicine
Professor of Bioengineering
University of Illinois at Chicago College of
    Engineering
Chicago, Illinois

Victor W. Nitti, MD
Professor
Urology and Obstetrics & Gynecology
NYU Langone Medical Center
New York, New York

Victoria F. Norwood, MD
Robert J. Roberts Professor of Pediatrics
Chief of Pediatric Nephrology
Department of Pediatrics
University of Virginia
Charlottesville, Virginia

**L. Henning Olsen, MD, DMSc, FEAPU,
FEBU**
Professor
Department of Urology & Institute of
    Clinical Medicine
Section of Pediatric Urology
Aarhus University Hospital & Aarhus
    University
Aarhus, Denmark

Aria F. Olumi, MD
Associate Professor of Surgery/Urology
Department of Urology
Massachusetts General Hospital/Harvard
    Medical School
Boston, Massachusetts

Michael Ordon, MD, MSc, FRCSC
Assistant Professor
Division of Urology
University of Toronto
Toronto, Ontario, Canada

David James Osborn, MD
Assistant Professor
Division of Urology
Walter Reed National Military Medical
    Center
Uniformed Services University
Bethesda, Maryland

Nadir I. Osman, PhD, MRCS
Department of Urology
The Royal Hallmashire Hospital Sheffield
    Teaching Hospitals
Sheffield, South Yorkshire, United
    Kingdom

Michael C. Ost, MD
Associate Professor and Vice Chairman
Department of Urology
University of Pittsburgh Medical Center;
Chief, Division of Pediatric Urology
Children's Hospital of Pittsburgh at the
    University of Pittsburgh Medical Center
Pittsburgh, Pennsylvania

Lance C. Pagliaro, MD
Professor
Department of Genitourinary Medical
    Oncology
The University of Texas MD Anderson
    Cancer Center
Houston, Texas

Ganesh S. Palapattu, MD
Chief of Urologic Oncology
Associate Professor
Department of Urology
University of Michigan
Ann Arbor, Michigan

Drew A. Palmer, MD
Institute of Urology
Lahey Hospital & Medical Center
Burlington, Massachusetts;
Clinical Associate
Tufts University School of Medicine
Boston, Massachusetts

Jeffrey S. Palmer, MD, FACS, FAAP
Director
Pediatric and Adolescent Urology Institute
Cleveland, Ohio

Lane S. Palmer, MD, FACS, FAAP
Professor and Chief
Pediatric Urology
Cohen Children's Medical Center of New
    York/Hofstra North Shore-LIJ School of
    Medicine
Long Island, New York

John M. Park, MD
Cheng Yang Chang Professor of Pediatric
    Urology
Department of Urology
University of Michigan Medical School
Ann Arbor, Michigan

J. Kellogg Parsons, MD, MHS, FACS
Associate Professor
Department of Urology
Moores Comprehensive Cancer Center
University of California, San Diego
La Jolla, California

Alan W. Partin, MD, PhD
Professor and Director of Urology
Department of Urology
Johns Hopkins School of Medicine
Baltimore, Maryland

Margaret S. Pearle, MD, PhD
Professor
Departments of Urology and Internal
    Medicine
University of Texas Southwestern Medical
    Center
Dallas, Texas

Craig A. Peters, MD
Professor of Urology
University of Texas Southwestern Medical
    Center;
Chief, Section of Pediatric Urology
Children's Health System
Dallas, Texas

Andrew Peterson, MD, FACS
Associate Professor
Urology Residency Program Director
Surgery
Duke University
Durham, North Carolina

Curtis A. Pettaway, MD
Professor
Department of Urology
The University of Texas MD Anderson
    Cancer Center
Houston, Texas

Louis L. Pisters, MD
Professor
Department of Urology
The University of Texas MD Anderson
    Cancer Center
Houston, Texas

Emilio D. Poggio, MD
Associate Professor of Medicine
Cleveland Clinic Learner College of
    Medicine;
Medical Director, Kidney and Pancreas
    Transplant Program
Department of Nephrology and
    Hypertension
Cleveland Clinic
Cleveland, Ohio

Hans G. Pohl, MD, FAAP
Associate Professor of Urology and
    Pediatrics
Children's National Medical Center
Washington, DC

Michel Arthur Pontari, MD
Professor
Department of Urology
Temple University School of Medicine
Philadelphia, Pennsylvania

John C. Pope IV, MD
Professor
Departments of Urologic Surgery and
    Pediatrics
Vanderbilt University Medical Center
Nashville, Tennessee

Glenn M. Preminger, MD
Professor and Chief
Division of Urology
Duke University Medical Center
Durham, North Carolina

Mark A. Preston, MD, MPH
Instructor in Surgery
Division of Urology
Brigham and Women's Hospital/Harvard
    Medical School
Boston, Massachusetts

Raymond R. Rackley, MD
Professor of Surgery
Glickman Urological and Kidney Institute
Cleveland Clinic
Cleveland, Ohio

Soroush Rais-Bahrami, MD
Assistant Professor of Urology and
    Radiology
Department of Urology
University of Alabama at Birmingham
Birmingham, Alabama

Jay D. Raman, MD
Associate Professor
Surgery (Urology)
Penn State Milton S. Hershey Medical
    Center
Hershey, Pennsylvania

Art R. Rastinehad, DO
Director of Interventional Urologic
    Oncology
Assistant Professor of Radiology and
    Urology
The Arthur Smith Institute for Urology and
    Interventional Radiology
Hofstra North Shore-LIJ School of
    Medicine
New York, New York

Yazan F. H. Rawashdeh, MD, PhD, FEAPU
Consultant Pediatric Urologist
Department of Urology
Section of Pediatric Urology
Aarhus University Hospital
Aarhus, Denmark

Shlomo Raz, MD
Professor of Urology
Department of Urology
Division of Pelvic Medicine and
    Reconstructive Surgery
UCLA School of Medicine
Los Angeles, California

Ira W. Reiser, MD
Clinical Associate Professor of Medicine
State University of New York Health
    Science Center at Brooklyn;
Attending Physician and Chairman
    Emeritus
Department of Medicine
Division of Nephrology and Hypertension
Brookdale University Hospital and Medical
    Center
Brooklyn, New York

W. Stuart Reynolds, MD, MPH
Assistant Professor
Department of Urologic Surgery
Vanderbilt University
Nashville, Tennessee

Koon Ho Rha, MD, PhD, FACS
Professor
Department of Urology
Urological Science Institute
Yonsei University College of Medicine
Seoul, South Korea

Kevin R. Rice, MD
Urologic Oncologist
Urology Service, Department of Surgery
Walter Reed National Military Medical
    Center
Bethesda, Maryland

Lee Richstone, MD
System Vice Chairman
Department of Urology
Associate Professor
Hofstra North Shore-LIJ School of
  Medicine
Lake Success, New York;
Chief
Urology
The North Shore University Hospital
Manhasset, New York

Richard C. Rink, MD, FAAP, FACS
Robert A. Garret Professor
Pediatric Urology
Riley Hospital for Children
Indiana University School of Medicine;
Faculty
Pediatric Urology
Peyton Manning Children's Hospital at St.
  Vincent
Indianapolis, Indiana

Michael L. Ritchey, MD
Professor
Department of Urology
Mayo Clinic College of Medicine
Phoenix, Arizona

Larissa V. Rodriguez, MD
Professor
Vice Chair, Academics
Director, Female Pelvic Medicine and
  Reconstructive Surgery (FPMRS)
Director, FPMRS Fellowship
University of Southern California Institute
  of Urology
Beverly Hills, California

Ronald Rodriguez, MD, PhD
Professor and Chairman
Department of Urology
University of Texas Health Science Center
  at San Antonio
San Antonio, Texas;
Adjunct Professor
Department of Urology
Johns Hopkins University School of
  Medicine
Baltimore, Maryland

Claus G. Roehrborn, MD
Professor and Chairman
Department of Urology
University of Texas Southwestern Medical
  Center
Dallas, Texas

Lisa Rogo-Gupta, MD
Assistant Professor
Urogynecology and Pelvic Reconstructive
  Surgery
Urology
Stanford University
Palo Alto, California

Theodore Rosen, MD
Professor of Dermatology
Baylor College of Medicine;
Chief of Dermatology
Department of Medicine
Michael E. DeBakey VA Medical Center
Houston, Texas

Ashley Evan Ross, MD, PhD
Assistant Professor of Urology, Oncology,
  and Pathology
James Buchanan Brady Urological Institute
Johns Hopkins Medicine
Baltimore, Maryland

Eric S. Rovner, MD
Professor of Urology
Department of Urology
Medical University of South Carolina
Charleston, South Carolina

Richard A. Santucci, MD, FACS
Specialist-in-Chief
Department of Urology
Detroit Medical Center;
Clinical Professor
Department of Osteopathic Surgical
  Specialties
Michigan State College of Osteopathic
  Medicine
Detroit, Michigan

Anthony J. Schaeffer, MD
Herman L. Kretschmer Professor of
  Urology
Department of Urology
Northwestern University Feinberg School
  of Medicine
Chicago, Illinois

Edward M. Schaeffer, MD, PhD
Associate Professor of Urology and
  Oncology
Johns Hopkins Medicine
Baltimore, Maryland

Douglas S. Scherr, MD
Associate Professor of Urology
Clinical Director of Urologic Oncology
Department of Urology
Weill Medical College of Cornell
  University
New York, New York

Francis X. Schneck, MD
Associate Professor of Urology
Division of Pediatric Urology
Children's Hospital of Pittsburgh at the
  University of Pittsburgh Medical Center
Pittsburgh, Pennsylvania

Michael J. Schwartz, MD, FACS
Assistant Professor of Urology
Hofstra North Shore-LIJ School of
  Medicine
New Hyde Park, New York

Karen S. Sfanos, PhD
Assistant Professor of Pathology
Assistant Professor of Oncology
Johns Hopkins University School of
  Medicine
Baltimore, Maryland

Robert C. Shamberger, MD
Chief of Surgery
Department of Surgery
Boston Children's Hospital;
Robert E. Gross Professor of Surgery
Department of Surgery
Harvard Medical School
Boston, Massachusetts

Ellen Shapiro, MD
Professor of Urology
Director, Pediatric Urology
Department of Urology
New York University School of Medicine
New York, New York

David S. Sharp, MD
Assistant Professor
Department of Urology
Ohio State University Wexner Medical
  Center
Columbus, Ohio

Alan W. Shindel, MD, MAS
Associate Professor
Department of Urology
University of California, Davis
Sacramento, California

Daniel A. Shoskes, MD, MSc, FRCSC
Professor of Surgery (Urology)
Glickman Urological and Kidney Institute
Department of Urology
Cleveland Clinic
Cleveland, Ohio

Aseem Ravindra Shukla, MD
Director of Minimally Invasive Surgery
Pediatric Urology
The Children's Hospital of Philadelphia
Philadelphia, Pennsylvania

Eila C. Skinner, MD
Professor and Chair
Department of Urology
Stanford University
Stanford, California

Ariana L. Smith, MD
Associate Professor of Urology
Penn Medicine, Perelman School of
  Medicine
Division of Urology
Hospital of the University of Pennsylvania
University of Pennsylvania Health System
Philadelphia, Pennsylvania

Armine K. Smith, MD
Assistant Professor of Urology and
    Director of Urologic Oncology at Sibley
    Hospital
James Buchanan Brady Urological Institute
Johns Hopkins University;
Assistant Professor of Urology
Department of Urology
George Washington University
Washington, DC

Joseph A. Smith, Jr., MD
William L. Bray Professor of Urology
Department of Urologic Surgery
Vanderbilt University School of Medicine
Nashville, Tennessee

Warren T. Snodgrass, MD
Co-Director, PARC Urology
Dallas, Texas

Graham Sommer, MD
Professor of Radiology
Division of Diagnostic Radiology
Stanford University School of Medicine
Stanford, California

Rene Sotelo, MD
Chairman, Department of Urology
Minimally Invasive and Robotic Surgery
    Center
Instituto Médico La Floresta
Caracas, Miranda, Venezuela

Mark J. Speakman, MBBS, MS, FRCS
Consultant Urological Surgeon
Department of Urology
Musgrove Park Hospital;
Consultant Urologist
Nuffield Hospital
Taunton, Somerset, United Kingdom

Philippe E. Spiess, MD, MS, FRCS(C)
Associate Member
Department of Genitourinary Oncology
Moffitt Cancer Center;
Associate Professor
Department of Urology
University of South Florida
Tampa, Florida

Samuel Spitalewitz, MD
Associate Professor of Clinical Medicine
State University of New York Health
    Science Center at Brooklyn;
Attending Physician
Division of Nephrology and Hypertension
Supervising Physician of Nephrology and
    Hypertension, Outpatient Services
Brookdale University Hospital and Medical
    Center
Brooklyn, New York

Ramaprasad Srinivasan, MD, PhD
Head, Molecular Cancer Section
Urologic Oncology Branch
Center for Cancer Research
National Cancer Institute
National Institutes of Health
Bethesda, Maryland

Joph Steckel, MD, FACS
Department of Urology
North Shore-LIJ Health System
New Hyde Park, New York;
Vice Chairman, Department of Urology
North Shore University Hospital
Manhasset, New York

**Andrew J. Stephenson, MD, MBA, FACS,
FRCS(C)**
Associate Professor of Surgery
Department of Urology
Cleveland Clinic Lerner College of
    Medicine
Case Western Reserve University;
Director, Urologic Oncology
Glickman Urological and Kidney Institute
Cleveland Clinic
Cleveland, Ohio

Julie N. Stewart, MD
Assistant Professor
Department of Urology
Houston Methodist Hospital
Houston, Texas

Douglas W. Storm, MD, FAAP
Assistant Professor
Department of Urology
University of Iowa Hospitals and Clinics
Iowa City, Iowa

Li-Ming Su, MD
David A. Cofrin Professor of Urology
Chief, Division of Robotic and Minimally
    Invasive Urologic Surgery
Department of Urology
University of Florida College of Medicine
Gainesville, Florida

Thomas Tailly, MD, MSc
Fellow in Endourology
Department of Surgery
Division of Urology
Schulich School of Medicine and Dentistry
Western University
London, Ontario, Canada

Shpetim Telegrafi, MD
Associate Professor (Research) of Urology
Senior Research Scientist
Director, Diagnostic Ultrasound
Department of Urology
New York University School of Medicine
New York, New York

John C. Thomas, MD, FAAP, FACS
Associate Professor of Urologic Surgery
Department of Urology
Division of Pediatric Urology
Monroe Carell Jr. Children's Hospital at
    Vanderbilt
Nashville, Tennessee

J. Brantley Thrasher, MD
Professor and William L. Valk Chair of
    Urology
Department of Urology
University of Kansas Medical Center
Kansas City, Kansas

Edouard J. Trabulsi, MD, FACS
Associate Professor
Department of Urology
Kimmel Cancer Center
Thomas Jefferson University
Philadelphia, Pennsylvania

Chad R. Tracy, MD
Assistant Professor
Department of Urology
University of Iowa
Iowa City, Iowa

Paul J. Turek, MD, FACS, FRSM
Director, the Turek Clinic
Beverly Hills and San Francisco, California

Robert G. Uzzo, MD, FACS
Chairman
G. Willing "Wing" Pepper Professor of
    Cancer Research
Department of Surgery
Deputy Chief Clinical Officer
Fox Chase Cancer Center
Philadelphia, Pennsylvania

Sandip P. Vasavada, MD
Professor of Surgery (Urology)
Glickman Urological and Kidney Institute
Cleveland Clinic
Cleveland, Ohio

David J. Vaughn, MD
Professor of Medicine
Division of Hematology/Oncology
Department of Medicine
Abramson Cancer Center at the University
    of Pennsylvania
Philadelphia, Pennsylvania

Manish A. Vira, MD
Assistant Professor of Urology
Vice Chair for Urologic Research
The Arthur Smith Institute for Urology
Hofstra North Shore-LIJ School of
    Medicine
Lake Success, New York

Gino J. Vricella, MD
Assistant Professor of Urologic Surgery
Urology Division
Washington University School of Medicine
    in St. Louis
St. Louis, Missouri

John T. Wei, MD, MS
Professor
Department of Urology
University of Michigan
Ann Arbor, Michigan

Alan J. Wein, MD, PhD (Hon), FACS
Founders Professor of Urology
Division of Urology
Penn Medicine, Perelman School of
    Medicine;
Chief of Urology
Division of Urology
Penn Medicine, Hospital of the University
    of Pennsylvania;
Program Director, Residency in Urology
Division of Urology
Penn Medicine, University of Pennsylvania
    Health System
Philadelphia, Pennsylvania

Jeffrey Paul Weiss, MD
Professor and Chair
Department of Urology
SUNY Downstate College of Medicine
Brooklyn, New York

Robert M. Weiss, MD
Donald Guthrie Professor of Surgery/
    Urology
Department of Urology
Yale University School of Medicine
New Haven, Connecticut

Charles Welliver, MD
Assistant Professor of Surgery
Division of Urology
Albany Medical College
Albany, New York

Hunter Wessells, MD, FACS
Professor and Nelson Chair
Department of Urology
University of Washington
Seattle, Washington

J. Christian Winters, MD, FACS
Professor and Chairman
Department of Urology
Louisiana State University Health Sciences
    Center
New Orleans, Louisiana

J. Stuart Wolf, Jr., MD, FACS
David A. Bloom Professor of Urology
Associate Chair for Urologic Surgical
    Services
Department of Urology
University of Michigan
Ann Arbor, Michigan

Christopher G. Wood, MD
Professor and Deputy Chairman
Douglas E. Johnson, M.D. Endowed
    Professorship in Urology
Department of Urology
The University of Texas MD Anderson
    Cancer Center
Houston, Texas

David P. Wood, Jr., MD
Chief Medical Officer
Beaumont Health;
Professor of Urology
Department of Urology
Oakland University William Beaumont
    School of Medicine
Royal Oak, Michigan

**Christopher R. J. Woodhouse, MB, FRCS,
FEBU**
Emeritus Professor
Adolescent Urology
University College
London, United Kingdom

Stephen Shei-Dei Yang, MD, PhD
Professor
Department of Urology
Buddhist Tzu Chi University
Hualien, Taiwan;
Chief of Surgery
Taipei Tzu Chi Hospital
New Taipei, Taiwan

Jennifer K. Yates, MD
Assistant Professor
Department of Urology
University of Massachusetts Medical
    School
Worcester, Massachusetts

**Chung Kwong Yeung, MBBS, MD, PhD,
FRCS, FRACS, FACS**
Honorary Clinical Professor in Pediatric
    Surgery and Pediatric Urology
Department of Surgery
University of Hong Kong;
Chief of Pediatric Surgery and Pediatric
    Urology
Union Hospital
Hong Kong, China

Richard Nithiphaisal Yu, MD, PhD
Instructor in Surgery
Harvard Medical School;
Associate in Urology
Department of Urology
Boston Children's Hospital
Boston, Massachusetts

Lee C. Zhao, MD, MS
Assistant Professor
Department of Urology
New York University
New York, New York

Jack M. Zuckerman, MD
Fellow in Reconstructive Surgery
Department of Urology
Eastern Virginia Medical School
Norfolk, Virginia

PREFACE

Since it was first published in 1954, Campbell-Walsh Urology (born Urology) has been the gold standard for a comprehensive review of our specialty. We are proud and pleased to present the 11th edition of this text as a worthy successor to the 10 editions that have preceded it. The four volumes remain essentially a series of comprehensive mini-textbooks on every major subject in urology. There are significant changes for this edition in organization, content, and authorship, and these reflect the ever-changing nature of our field, and, for many subjects, the passing of the baton from one generation to the next. Twenty-two totally new chapters have been added, along with 61 new first authors. All other chapters have been revised, new and revised guidelines incorporated, and the well-accepted format of the use of extensive boldface and Key Points boxes and algorithms retained. Ownership of the 11th edition includes the print product, access to the full text online, and a downloadable eBook version through ExpertConsult.com. The online and eBook version of the 11th edition will have updates by key opinion leaders added periodically to reflect important changes and controversies in the field.

Content changes include restructuring of the chapter on basic principles of radiologic imaging in adult urology, a new chapter on pediatric urologic imaging, and separate new chapters on the surgical, radiographic, and endoscopic anatomy of the male reproductive system, the retroperitoneum, the kidney and ureter, the adrenals, and the male and female pelvis. The chapter on androgen deficiency has been expanded to encompass integrated men's health, including cardiovascular risks and metabolic syndrome. There are totally new added chapters on basic energy modalities in urologic surgery, management of urinary tract hemorrhage, strategies for medical management of upper urinary tract calculi, inguinal lymph node dissection, overview of the evaluation and management of urinary incontinence in men, the underactive detrusor, complications related to the use of mesh in the treatment of urinary incontinence and prolapse and their repair, and minimally invasive urinary diversion. Additionally, in the pediatric volume, totally new chapters have been added on the principles of laparoscopic and robotic surgery, functional disorders of the lower urinary tract, management of defecation disorders, and adolescent and transitional urology. Totally new content has been provided for existing chapters on sexually transmitted infections, tuberculosis and other opportunistic infections, the basics of male infertility, disorders of male orgasm and ejaculation, surgery for erectile dysfunction, Peyronie disease, female sexual function and dysfunction, renovascular hypertension and ischemic neuropathy, renal trans-

plantation, and nonmedical management of upper urinary tract calculi. Within the section on urine transport, storage, and emptying, totally new content has been provided for the chapters on physiology and pharmacology of the bladder and urethra, epidemiology and pathophysiology of urinary incontinence and pelvic prolapse, nocturia, conservative management of urinary incontinence, urinary fistulae, geriatric lower urinary tract dysfunction and incontinence, and additional therapies for storage and emptying failure. Reflecting all the latest changes in the field, the chapter on minimally invasive and endoscopic management of benign prostatic hyperplasia has been totally redone. In the area of cancer, many chapters have been totally rewritten to reflect contemporary data and thought: Basic Principles of Immunology and Immunotherapy in Urologic Oncology, Neoplasms of the Testis, Retroperitoneal Tumors, Open Surgery of the Kidney, Nonsurgical Focal Therapy for Renal Tumors, Surgery of the Adrenal Glands, Management of Metastatic and Invasive Bladder Cancer, Transurethral and Open Surgery for Bladder Cancer, Prostate Biopsy: Techniques and Imaging (including fusion techniques), Diagnosis and Staging of Prostate Cancer, Active Surveillance of Prostate Cancer, Focal Therapy for Prostate Cancer, Radiation Therapy for Prostate Cancer, Management of Biochemical Recurrence after Definitive Therapy for Prostate Cancer, and Tumors of the Urethra. In the pediatric volume, a number of existing chapters have been totally rewritten as well: Disorders of Renal Functional Development in Children, Infection and Inflammation of the Pediatric Genitourinary Tract, Surgery of the Ureter in Children, Posterior Urethral Valves, and separate chapters on Management of Abnormalities of the External Genitalia in boys and girls.

We editors are grateful for the support of Elsevier, and special thanks are due to our extraordinary editorial and support staff: Charlotta Kryhl and Stefanie Jewel-Thomas (Senior Content Strategists), Dee Simpson (Senior Content Development Specialist), and Kristine Feeherty (Book Production Specialist). Without their expertise, patience, and gentle pushing, this edition would not have been brought to press on time.

We hope your experience in reading this 11th edition of the gold standard textbook of urology will be as pleasurable as ours has been in watching it develop.

Alan J. Wein, MD, PhD (Hon), FACS

for the editors Louis R. Kavoussi, MD, MBA,
Alan W. Partin, MD, PhD, and Craig A. Peters, MD

CONTENTS

VIDEOS

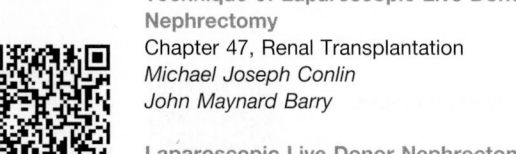

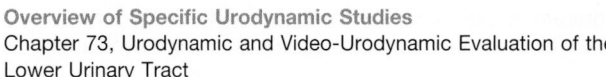

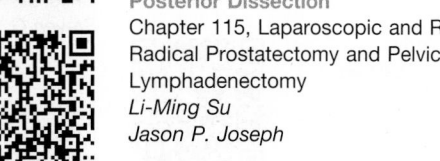
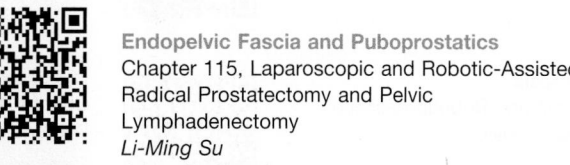

1

Evaluation of the Urologic Patient: History, Physical Examination, and Urinalysis

Glenn S. Gerber, MD, and Charles B. Brendler, MD

History

Physical Examination

Urinalysis

Summary

Urologists have a unique position in medicine because their patients encompass all age groups, including prenatal, pediatric, adolescent, adult, and geriatric. Because there is no medical subspecialist with similar interests, **the urologist has the ability to make the initial evaluation and diagnosis and to provide medical and surgical therapy for all diseases of the genitourinary (GU) system.** Historically, the diagnostic armamentarium included urinalysis, endoscopy, and intravenous (IV) pyelography. Recent advances in ultrasonography, computed tomography (CT), magnetic resonance imaging (MRI), and endourology have expanded our diagnostic capabilities. Despite these advances, however, the basic approach to the patient is still dependent on taking a complete history, executing a thorough physical examination, and performing a urinalysis. These basics dictate and guide the subsequent diagnostic evaluation.

HISTORY

Overview

The medical history is the cornerstone of the evaluation of the urologic patient, and a well-taken history will frequently elucidate the probable diagnosis. However, many pitfalls can inhibit the urologist from obtaining an accurate history. The patient may be unable to describe or communicate symptoms because of anxiety, language barrier, or educational background. Therefore the urologist must be a detective and lead the patient through detailed and appropriate questioning to obtain accurate information. There are practical considerations in the art of history-taking that can help to alleviate some of these difficulties. In the initial meeting, an attempt should be made to help the patient feel comfortable. During this time, the physician should project a calm, caring, and competent image that can help foster two-way communication. Impaired hearing, mental capacity, and facility with English can be assessed promptly. These difficulties are frequently overcome by having a family member present during the interview or, alternatively, by having an interpreter present.

Patients need to have sufficient time to express their problems and the reasons for seeking urologic care; the physician, however, should focus the discussion to make it as productive and informative as possible. Direct questioning can then proceed logically. The physician needs to listen carefully without distractions to obtain and interpret the clinical information provided by the patient. **A complete history can be divided into the chief complaint and history of the present illness, the patient's past medical history, and a family history.** Each segment can provide significant positive and negative findings that will contribute to the overall evaluation and treatment of the patient.

Chief Complaint and Present Illness

Most urologic patients identify their symptoms as arising from the urinary tract and frequently present to the urologist for the initial evaluation. For this reason, the urologist frequently has the opportunity to act as both the primary physician and the specialist. The chief complaint must be clearly defined because it provides the initial information and clues to begin formulating the differential diagnosis. Most importantly, **the chief complaint is a constant reminder to the urologist as to why the patient initially sought care.** This issue must be addressed even if subsequent evaluation reveals a more serious or significant condition that requires more urgent attention. In our personal experience, a young woman presented with a chief complaint of recurrent urinary tract infections (UTIs). In the course of her evaluation, she was found to have a right adrenal mass. We subsequently focused on this problem and performed a right adrenalectomy for a benign cortical adenoma. We forgot about the woman's original symptoms until she presented for her subsequent postoperative examination. She reminded us of her original symptoms at that time, and subsequent evaluation revealed that she had a nylon suture that had eroded into the anterior wall of her bladder from a previous abdominal vesicourethropexy performed 2 years earlier for stress urinary incontinence. Her UTIs resolved after surgical removal of the suture.

In obtaining the history of the present illness, **the duration, severity, chronicity, periodicity, and degree of disability are important considerations.** The patient's symptoms need to be clarified for details and quantified for severity. Listed next are a variety of typical initial complaints. Specific questions that focus on the differential diagnosis are provided.

Pain

Pain arising from the GU tract may be quite severe and is usually associated with either urinary tract obstruction or inflammation. Urinary calculi cause severe pain when they obstruct the upper urinary tract. Conversely, large, nonobstructing stones may be totally asymptomatic. Thus a 2-mm-diameter stone lodged at the ureterovesical junction may cause excruciating pain, whereas a large staghorn calculus in the renal pelvis or a bladder stone may be totally asymptomatic. Urinary retention from prostatic obstruction is also quite painful, but the diagnosis is usually obvious to the patient.

Inflammation of the GU tract is most severe when it involves the parenchyma of a GU organ. This is due to edema and distention of the capsule surrounding the organ. Thus pyelonephritis, prostatitis, and epididymitis are typically quite painful. Inflammation of the mucosa of a hollow viscus such as the bladder or urethra usually produces discomfort, but the pain is not nearly as severe.

Tumors in the GU tract usually do not cause pain unless they produce obstruction or extend beyond the primary organ to involve adjacent nerves. Thus pain associated with GU malignancies is usually a late manifestation and a sign of advanced disease.

Renal Pain. Pain of renal origin is usually located in the ipsilateral costovertebral angle just lateral to the sacrospinalis muscle and beneath the 12th rib. **Pain is usually caused by acute distention of the renal capsule, generally from inflammation or obstruction.** The pain may radiate across the flank anteriorly toward the upper abdomen and umbilicus and may be referred to the testis or labium. A corollary to this observation is that renal or retroperitoneal disease should be considered in the differential diagnosis of any man who complains of testicular discomfort but has a normal scrotal examination. Pain due to inflammation is usually steady, whereas pain due to obstruction fluctuates in intensity. Thus the pain produced by ureteral obstruction is typically colicky in nature and intensifies with ureteral peristalsis, at which time the pressure in the renal pelvis rises as the ureter contracts in an attempt to force urine past the point of obstruction.

Pain of renal origin may be associated with gastrointestinal symptoms because of reflex stimulation of the celiac ganglion and because of the proximity of adjacent organs (liver, pancreas, duodenum, gallbladder, and colon). Thus renal pain may be confused with pain of intraperitoneal origin; it can usually be distinguished, however, by a careful history and physical examination. Pain that is due to a perforated duodenal ulcer or pancreatitis may radiate into the back, but the site of greatest pain and tenderness is in the epigastrium. Pain of intraperitoneal origin is seldom colicky, as with obstructive renal pain. Furthermore, pain of intraperitoneal origin frequently radiates into the shoulder because of irritation of the diaphragm and phrenic nerve; this does not occur with renal pain. Typically, patients with intraperitoneal pathology prefer to lie motionless to minimize pain, whereas patients with renal pain usually are more comfortable moving around and holding the flank.

Renal pain may also be confused with pain resulting from irritation of the costal nerves, most commonly T10-T12. Such pain has a similar distribution from the costovertebral angle across the flank toward the umbilicus. However, the pain is not colicky in nature. Furthermore, the intensity of radicular pain may be altered by changing position; this is not the case with renal pain.

Ureteral Pain. Ureteral pain is usually acute and secondary to obstruction. The pain results from acute distention of the ureter and by hyperperistalsis and spasm of the smooth muscle of the ureter as it attempts to relieve the obstruction, usually produced by a stone or blood clot. The site of ureteral obstruction can often be determined by the location of the referred pain. With obstruction of the midureter, pain on the right side is referred to the right lower quadrant of the abdomen (McBurney point) and thus may simulate appendicitis; pain on the left side is referred over the left lower quadrant and resembles diverticulitis. Also, the pain may be referred to the scrotum in the male or the labium in the female. Lower ureteral obstruction frequently produces symptoms of vesical irritability, including frequency, urgency, and suprapubic discomfort that may radiate along the urethra in men to the tip of the penis. Often, by taking a careful history, the astute clinician can predict the location of the obstruction. Ureteral pathology that arises slowly or produces only mild obstruction rarely causes pain. Therefore ureteral tumors and stones that cause minimal obstruction are seldom painful.

Vesical Pain. Vesical pain is usually produced either by overdistention of the bladder as a result of acute urinary retention or by inflammation. **Constant suprapubic pain that is unrelated to**

urinary retention is seldom of urologic origin. Furthermore, patients with slowly progressive urinary obstruction and bladder distention (e.g., diabetics with a flaccid neurogenic bladder) frequently have no pain at all despite residual urine volumes over 1 L.

Inflammatory conditions of the bladder usually produce intermittent suprapubic discomfort. Thus the pain in conditions such as bacterial cystitis or interstitial cystitis is usually most severe when the bladder is full and is relieved at least partially by voiding. Patients with cystitis sometimes experience sharp, stabbing suprapubic pain at the end of micturition, and this is termed *strangury*. Furthermore, patients with cystitis frequently experience pain referred to the distal urethra that is associated with irritative voiding symptoms such as urinary frequency and dysuria.

Prostatic Pain. Prostatic pain is usually secondary to inflammation with secondary edema and distention of the prostatic capsule. Pain of prostatic origin is poorly localized, and the patient may complain of lower abdominal, inguinal, perineal, lumbosacral, penile, and/or rectal pain. Prostatic pain is frequently associated with irritative urinary symptoms such as frequency and dysuria, and, in severe cases, marked prostatic edema may produce acute urinary retention.

Penile Pain. Pain in the flaccid penis is usually secondary to inflammation in the bladder or urethra, with referred pain that is experienced maximally at the urethral meatus. Alternatively, penile pain may be produced by *paraphimosis*, a condition in which the uncircumcised penile foreskin is trapped behind the glans penis, resulting in venous obstruction and painful engorgement of the glans penis (see later). Pain in the erect penis is usually due to Peyronie disease or priapism (see later).

Testicular Pain. Scrotal pain may be either primary or referred. **Primary pain arises from within the scrotum and is usually secondary to acute epididymitis or torsion of the testis or testicular appendices.** Because of the edema and pain associated with both acute epididymitis and testicular torsion, it is frequently difficult to distinguish these two conditions. Alternatively, scrotal pain may result from inflammation of the scrotal wall itself. This may result from a simple infected hair follicle or sebaceous cyst, but it may also be secondary to Fournier gangrene, a severe, necrotizing infection arising in the scrotum that can rapidly progress and be fatal unless promptly recognized and treated.

Chronic scrotal pain is usually related to noninflammatory conditions such as a hydrocele or a varicocele, and the pain is generally characterized as a dull, heavy sensation that does not radiate. Because the testes arise embryologically in close proximity to the kidneys, pain arising in the kidneys or retroperitoneum may be referred to the testes. Similarly, the dull pain associated with an inguinal hernia may be referred to the scrotum.

Hematuria

Hematuria is the presence of blood in the urine; **greater than three red blood cells (RBCs) per high-power microscopic field (HPF) is significant.** Patients with gross hematuria are usually frightened by the sudden onset of blood in the urine and frequently present to the emergency department for evaluation, fearing that they may be bleeding excessively. Hematuria of any degree should never be ignored and, in adults, should be regarded as a symptom of urologic malignancy until proved otherwise. In evaluating hematuria, several questions should always be asked, and the answers will enable the urologist to target the subsequent diagnostic evaluation efficiently:

Is the hematuria gross or microscopic?
At what time during urination does the hematuria occur (beginning or end of stream or during entire stream)?
Is the hematuria associated with pain?
Is the patient passing clots?
If the patient is passing clots, do the clots have a specific shape?

Gross versus Microscopic Hematuria. The significance of gross versus microscopic hematuria is simply that **the chances of**

identifying significant pathology increase with the degree of hematuria. Thus patients with gross hematuria usually have identifiable underlying pathology, whereas it is quite common for patients with minimal degrees of microscopic hematuria to have a negative urologic evaluation.

Timing of Hematuria. The timing of hematuria during urination frequently indicates the site of origin. **Initial hematuria usually arises from the urethra;** it occurs least commonly and is usually secondary to inflammation. Total hematuria is most common and indicates that the bleeding is most likely coming from the bladder or upper urinary tracts. Terminal hematuria occurs at the end of micturition and is usually secondary to inflammation in the area of the bladder neck or prostatic urethra. It occurs at the end of micturition as the bladder neck contracts, squeezing out the last amount of urine.

Association with Pain. Hematuria, although frightening, is usually not painful unless it is associated with inflammation or obstruction. Thus patients with cystitis and secondary hematuria may experience painful urinary irritative symptoms, but the pain is usually not worsened with passage of clots. More commonly, **pain in association with hematuria usually results from upper urinary tract hematuria with obstruction of the ureters with clots.** Passage of these clots may be associated with severe, colicky flank pain similar to that produced by a ureteral calculus, and this helps identify the source of the hematuria.

The American Urological Association (AUA) has published guidelines regarding patients with asymptomatic microhematuria (AMH), which is defined as three or more RBCs per HPF in the absence of an obvious benign cause. A determination of AMH should be based on microscopic, not dipstick, examination of the urine. Careful history, physical examination, and laboratory examination should be done to rule out benign causes of AMH, such as infection, medical renal disease, and others. Once these causes are ruled out, urologic evaluation that includes a measurement of renal function is recommended. If factors such as dysmorphic RBCs, proteinuria, casts, or renal insufficiency are present, nephrologic workup should be considered in addition to the urologic evaluation. AMH that occurs in patients who are anticoagulated still warrants urologic evaluation.

The evaluation of patients over 35 years of age with AMH should include cystoscopy, which is optional in younger patients. However, all patients should have cystoscopy if risk factors such as irritative voiding symptoms, tobacco use, or chemical exposures are present. Radiologic evaluation should be performed in the initial evaluation, and the procedure of choice is multiphasic CT urography with and without IV contrast. Magnetic resonance urography, with or without IV contrast, is an acceptable alternative in patients who cannot undergo multiphasic CT scan. In cases where collecting system detail is needed, noncontrast CT, MRI, or renal ultrasonography with retrograde pyelograms is an acceptable alternative if there is a contraindication to the use of IV contrast.

Among the modalities not recommended in the routine evaluation of patients with AMH are urine cytology, urine markers, and blue light cystoscopy. However, cytology may be useful in those patients with persistent AMH following a negative workup or those with other risk factors for carcinoma in situ, such as irritative voiding symptoms, use of tobacco, or chemical exposures. For patients with persistent AMH, yearly urinalysis should be performed. The presence of two consecutive annual negative urinalyses indicates that no further urinalyses are needed for this purpose. For patients with persistent or recurrent AMH, repeat evaluation within 3 to 5 years should be considered.

Presence of Clots. The presence of clots usually indicates a more significant degree of hematuria, and, accordingly, the probability of identifying significant urologic pathology increases.

Shape of Clots. Usually, if the patient is passing clots, they are amorphous and of bladder or prostatic urethral origin. However, **the presence of vermiform (wormlike) clots, particularly if associated with flank pain, identifies the hematuria as coming from the upper urinary tract** with formation of vermiform clots within the ureter.

It cannot be emphasized strongly enough that **hematuria, particularly in the adult, should be regarded as a symptom of malignancy until proved otherwise and demands immediate urologic examination.** In a patient who presents with gross hematuria, cystoscopy should be performed as soon as possible because frequently the source of bleeding can be readily identified. Cystoscopy will determine whether the hematuria is coming from the urethra, bladder, or upper urinary tract. In patients with gross hematuria secondary to an upper tract source, it is easy to see the jet of red urine pulsing from the involved ureteral orifice.

Although inflammatory conditions may result in hematuria, all patients with hematuria, except perhaps young women with acute bacterial hemorrhagic cystitis, should undergo urologic evaluation. Older women and men who present with hematuria and irritative voiding symptoms may have cystitis secondary to infection arising in a necrotic bladder tumor or, more commonly, flat carcinoma in situ of the bladder. **The most common cause of gross hematuria in a patient older than age 50 years is bladder cancer.**

Lower Urinary Tract Symptoms

Irritative Symptoms. *Frequency* is one of the most common urologic symptoms. The normal adult voids five or six times per day, with a volume of approximately 300 mL with each void. **Urinary frequency is due to either increased urinary output (polyuria) or decreased bladder capacity.** If voiding is noted to occur in large amounts frequently, the patient has polyuria and should be evaluated for diabetes mellitus, diabetes insipidus, or excessive fluid ingestion. Causes of decreased bladder capacity include bladder outlet obstruction with decreased compliance, increased residual urine, and/or decreased functional capacity due to irritation, neurogenic bladder with increased sensitivity and decreased compliance, pressure from extrinsic sources, or anxiety. By separating irritative from obstructive symptoms, the astute clinician should be able to arrive at a proper differential diagnosis.

Nocturia is nocturnal frequency. Normally, adults arise no more than twice at night to void. As with frequency, nocturia may be secondary to increased urine output or decreased bladder capacity. **Frequency during the day without nocturia is usually of psychogenic origin and related to anxiety. Nocturia without frequency may occur in the patient with congestive heart failure and peripheral edema in whom the intravascular volume and urine output increase when the patient is supine. Renal concentrating ability decreases with age; therefore urine production in the geriatric patient is increased at night, when renal blood flow is increased as a result of recumbency.** In general, nocturia may be attributed to nocturnal polyuria (nocturnal urine overproduction) and/or diminished nocturnal bladder capacity (Weiss and Blaivas, 2000). Nocturia may also occur in people who drink large amounts of liquid in the evening, particularly caffeinated and alcoholic beverages, which have strong diuretic effects. In the absence of these factors, nocturia signifies a problem with bladder function secondary to urinary outlet obstruction and/or decreased bladder compliance.

Dysuria is painful urination that is usually caused by inflammation. **This pain is usually not felt over the bladder but is commonly referred to the urethral meatus.** Pain occurring at the start of urination may indicate urethral pathology, whereas pain occurring at the end of micturition (strangury) is usually of bladder origin. Dysuria is frequently accompanied by frequency and urgency.

Obstructive Symptoms. *Decreased force of urination* is usually secondary to bladder outlet obstruction and commonly results from benign prostatic hyperplasia (BPH) or a urethral stricture. In fact, except for severe degrees of obstruction, **most patients are unaware of a change in the force and caliber of their urinary stream.** These changes usually occur gradually and go generally unrecognized by most patients. The other obstructive symptoms noted later are more commonly recognized and are usually secondary to bladder outlet obstruction in men due to either BPH or a urethral stricture.

Urinary hesitancy refers to a delay in the start of micturition. Normally, urination begins within a second after relaxing the urinary sphincter, but it may be delayed in men with bladder outlet obstruction.

Intermittency refers to involuntary start-stopping of the urinary stream. It most commonly results from prostatic obstruction with intermittent occlusion of the urinary stream by the lateral prostatic lobes.

Postvoid dribbling refers to the terminal release of drops of urine at the end of micturition. **This is secondary to a small amount of residual urine in either the bulbar or the prostatic urethra that is normally "milked back" into the bladder at the end of micturition** (Stephenson and Farrar, 1977). In men with bladder outlet obstruction, this urine escapes into the bulbar urethra and leaks out at the end of micturition. Men will frequently attempt to avoid wetting their clothing by shaking the penis at the end of micturition. In fact, this is ineffective, and the problem is more readily solved by manual compression of the bulbar urethra in the perineum and blotting the urethral meatus with a tissue. Postvoid dribbling is often an early symptom of urethral obstruction related to BPH, but, in itself, seldom necessitates any further treatment.

Straining refers to the use of abdominal musculature to urinate. Normally, it is unnecessary for a man to perform a Valsalva maneuver except at the end of urination. Increased straining during micturition is a symptom of bladder outlet obstruction.

It is important for the urologist to distinguish irritative from obstructive lower urinary tract symptoms. This most frequently occurs in evaluating men with BPH. Although BPH is primarily obstructive, it produces changes in bladder compliance that result in increased irritative symptoms. In fact, men with BPH more commonly present with irritative than obstructive symptoms, and the most common presenting symptom is nocturia. **The urologist must be careful not to attribute irritative symptoms to BPH unless there is documented evidence of obstruction.** In general, lower urinary tract symptoms are nonspecific and may occur secondary to a wide variety of neurologic conditions, as well as to prostatic enlargement (Lepor and Machi, 1993). In this regard, two important examples are mentioned. Patients with high-grade flat carcinoma in situ of the bladder may present with urinary irritative symptoms. The urologist should be particularly aware of the diagnosis of carcinoma in situ in men who present with irritative symptoms, a history of cigarette smoking, and microscopic hematuria. In our personal experience, we cared for a 54-year-old man who presented with this history and was treated for BPH for 2 years before the diagnosis of bladder cancer was established. Once the correct diagnosis was made, the patient had developed muscle-invasive disease and required a cystectomy for cure.

The second important example is irritative symptoms resulting from neurologic disease such as cerebrovascular accidents, diabetes mellitus, and Parkinson disease. Most neurologic diseases encountered by the urologist are upper motor neuron in etiology and result in a loss of cortical inhibition of voiding with resultant decreased bladder compliance and irritative voiding symptoms. The urologist must be extremely careful to rule out underlying neurologic disease before performing surgery to relieve bladder outlet obstruction. Such surgery not only may fail to relieve the patient's irritative symptoms but also may result in permanent urinary incontinence.

Since its introduction in 1992, **the AUA symptom index has been widely used and validated as an important means of assessing men with lower urinary tract symptoms** (Barry et al, 1992). The original AUA symptom score is based on the answers to seven questions concerning frequency, nocturia, weak urinary stream, hesitancy, intermittency, incomplete bladder emptying, and urgency. The International Prostate Symptom Score (I-PSS) includes these seven questions, as well as a global quality-of-life question (Table 1-1). The total symptom score ranges from 0 to 35 with scores of 0 to 7, 8 to 19, and 20 to 35 indicating mild, moderate, and severe

TABLE 1-1 International Prostate Symptom Score

SYMPTOM	NOT AT ALL	<1 TIME IN 5	LESS THAN HALF THE TIME	ABOUT HALF THE TIME	MORE THAN HALF THE TIME	ALMOST ALWAYS	YOUR SCORE
1. INCOMPLETE EMPTYING Over the past month, how often have you had a sensation of not emptying your bladder completely after you finished urinating?	0	1	2	3	4	5	
2. FREQUENCY Over the past month, how often have you had to urinate again less than 2 hours after you finished urinating?	0	1	2	3	4	5	
3. INTERMITTENCY Over the past month, how often have you found you stopped and started again several times when you urinated?	0	1	2	3	4	5	
4. URGENCY Over the past month, how often have you found it difficult to postpone urination?	0	1	2	3	4	5	

TABLE 1-1 International Prostate Symptom Score—cont'd

SYMPTOM	NOT AT ALL	<1 TIME IN 5	LESS THAN HALF THE TIME	ABOUT HALF THE TIME	MORE THAN HALF THE TIME	ALMOST ALWAYS	YOUR SCORE
5. WEAK STREAM Over the past month, how often have you had a weak urinary stream?	0	1	2	3	4	5	
6. STRAINING Over the past month, how often have you had to push or strain to begin urination?	0	1	2	3	4	5	
	NONE	**1 TIME**	**2 TIMES**	**3 TIMES**	**4 TIMES**	**≥5 TIMES**	
7. NOCTURIA Over the past month, how many times did you most typically get up to urinate from the time you went to bed at night until the time you got up in the morning?	0	1	2	3	4	5	
TOTAL INTERNATIONAL PROSTATE SYMPTOM SCORE							

QUALITY OF LIFE DUE TO URINARY SYMPTOMS	DELIGHTED	PLEASED	MOSTLY SATISFIED	MIXED—ABOUT EQUALLY SATISFIED AND DISSATISFIED	MOSTLY DISSATISFIED	UNHAPPY	TERRIBLE
If you were to spend the rest of your life with your urinary condition just the way it is now, how would you feel about that?	0	1	2	3	4	5	6

From Cockett A, Aso Y, Denis L. Prostate symptom score and quality of life assessment. In: Cockett ATK, Khoury S, Aso Y, et al, editors. Proceedings of the Second International Consultation on Benign Prostatic Hyperplasia (BPH); 27-30 June 1993; Paris. Channel Island, Jersey: Scientific Communication International; 1994. p. 553–5.

lower urinary tract symptoms, respectively. The I-PSS is a helpful tool both in the clinical management of men with lower urinary tract symptoms and in research studies regarding the medical and surgical treatment of men with voiding dysfunction.

The use of symptom indices has limitations, and it is important for the physician to discuss the patient's responses with him. It has been demonstrated that a grade 6 reading level is necessary to understand the I-PSS, and some patients with neurologic disorders and dementia may also have difficulty completing the symptom score (MacDiarmid et al, 1998). In addition, the symptom score and obstructive and irritative voiding symptoms are nonspecific, and the symptoms may be caused by a variety of conditions other than BPH. Similar symptom scores have been demonstrated to be present in age-matched men and women between 55 and 79 years of age (Lepor and Machi, 1993). **Despite these limitations, the I-PSS is a simple adjunct in assessing men with lower urinary tract symptoms and may be used in the initial evaluation of men with lower urinary tract symptoms, as well as in the assessment of treatment response.**

Incontinence. *Urinary incontinence* is the involuntary loss of urine. A careful history of the incontinent patient will often determine the etiology. Urinary incontinence can be subdivided into four categories.

Continuous Incontinence. **Continuous incontinence is most commonly due to a urinary tract fistula that bypasses the urethral sphincter.** The most common type of fistula that results in urinary incontinence is a vesicovaginal fistula usually secondary to gynecologic surgery, radiation, or obstetric trauma. Less commonly, ureterovaginal fistulae may occur from similar causes.

A second major cause of continuous incontinence is an ectopic ureter that enters either the urethra or the female genital tract. An ectopic ureter usually drains a small, dysplastic upper pole segment of kidney, and the amount of urinary leakage may be quite small. Such patients may void most of their urine normally but have a continuous amount of small urinary leakage that may be misdiagnosed for many years as a chronic vaginal discharge. In our experience, we cared for a 30-year-old woman—who had been misdiagnosed with enuresis in childhood and as having a chronic vaginal discharge in adult life—whose urinary leakage was totally corrected by surgical removal of the dysplastic, upper pole segment of her right kidney. Ectopic ureters never produce urinary incontinence in males because they always enter the bladder neck or prostatic urethra proximal to the external urethral sphincter.

Stress Incontinence. Stress incontinence refers to the sudden leakage of urine with coughing, sneezing, exercise, or other activities that increase intra-abdominal pressure. During these activities, intra-abdominal pressure rises transiently above urethral resistance, resulting in a sudden, usually small amount of urinary leakage. Stress incontinence is most common in women after childbearing or menopause and is related to a loss of anterior vaginal support and weakening of pelvic tissues. Stress incontinence is also observed in men after prostatic surgery, most commonly radical prostatectomy, in which there may be injury to the external urethral sphincter. **Stress urinary incontinence is difficult to manage pharmacologically, and patients with significant stress incontinence are usually best treated surgically.**

Urgency Incontinence. Urgency incontinence is the precipitous loss of urine preceded by a strong urge to void. This symptom is commonly observed in patients with cystitis, neurogenic bladder, and advanced bladder outlet obstruction with secondary loss of bladder compliance. It is important to distinguish urgency incontinence from stress incontinence for two reasons. First, **urgency incontinence may result from a secondary underlying pathologic process, which should be identified;** treatment of this primary problem such as infection or bladder outlet obstruction may result in resolution of urgency incontinence. Second, patients with urgency incontinence are usually not amenable to surgical correction but, rather, are more appropriately treated with pharmacologic agents that increase bladder compliance and/or increase urethral resistance.

Overflow Urinary Incontinence. Overflow urinary incontinence, often called *paradoxical incontinence,* is secondary to advanced urinary retention and high residual urine volumes. In these patients, the bladder is chronically distended and never empties completely. Urine may dribble out in small amounts as the bladder overflows. This is particularly likely to occur at night when the patient is less likely to inhibit urinary leakage. **Overflow incontinence has been termed *paradoxical incontinence* because it can often be cured by relief of bladder outlet obstruction.** It is, however, often difficult to make the diagnosis of overflow incontinence by history and physical examination alone, particularly in the obese patient, in whom percussion of the distended bladder may be difficult. Overflow incontinence usually develops over a considerable length of time, and patients may be totally unaware of incomplete bladder emptying. Thus any patient with significant incontinence should undergo measurement of postvoid residual urine.

Enuresis. *Enuresis* refers to urinary incontinence that occurs during sleep. It occurs normally in children up to 3 years of age **but persists in about 15% of children at age 5 and about 1% of children at age 15** (Forsythe and Redmond, 1974). Enuresis must be distinguished from continuous incontinence, which occurs in the day and night and which, in a young girl, usually indicates the presence of an ectopic ureter. All children older than age 6 years with enuresis should undergo a urologic evaluation, although the vast majority will be found to have no significant urologic abnormality.

Sexual Dysfunction

Male sexual dysfunction is frequently used synonymously with *impotence* or erectile dysfunction, although impotence refers specifically to the inability to achieve and maintain an erection adequate for intercourse. Patients presenting with "impotence" should be questioned carefully to rule out other male sexual disorders, including loss of libido, absence of emission, absence of orgasm, and, most commonly, premature ejaculation. It is important to identify the precise problem before proceeding with further evaluation and treatment.

Loss of Libido. Because androgens have a major influence on sexual desire, a decrease in libido may indicate androgen deficiency arising from either pituitary or testicular dysfunction. This can be evaluated directly by **measurement of serum testosterone that, if abnormal, should be further evaluated by measurement of serum gonadotropins and prolactin.** Because the amount of testosterone required to maintain libido is usually less than that required for full stimulation of the prostate and seminal vesicles, patients with hypogonadism may also note decreased or absent ejaculation. Conversely, if semen volume is normal, it is unlikely that endocrine factors are responsible for loss of libido. A decrease in libido may also result from depression and a variety of medical illnesses that affect general health and well-being.

Impotence. *Impotence* refers specifically to the inability to achieve and maintain an erection sufficient for intercourse. **A careful history will often determine whether the problem is primarily psychogenic or organic.** In men with psychogenic impotence, the condition frequently develops rather quickly secondary to a precipitating event such as marital stress or change or loss of a sexual partner. In men with organic impotence, the condition usually develops more insidiously and frequently can be linked to advancing age or other underlying risk factors.

In evaluating men with impotence, it is important to determine whether the problem exists in all situations. Many men who report impotence may not be able to have intercourse with one partner but will with another. Similarly, it is important to determine whether men are able to achieve normal erections with alternative forms of sexual stimulation (e.g., masturbation, erotic videos). Finally, the patient should be asked whether he ever notes nocturnal or early morning erections. In general, **patients who are able to achieve adequate erections in some situations but not others have primarily psychogenic rather than organic impotence.**

Failure to Ejaculate. **A failure to ejaculate may result from several causes: (1) androgen deficiency, (2) sympathetic denervation, (3) pharmacologic agents, and (4) bladder neck and prostatic surgery.** Androgen deficiency results in decreased secretions from the prostate and seminal vesicles, causing a reduction or loss of seminal volume. Sympathectomy or extensive retroperitoneal surgery, most notably retroperitoneal lymphadenectomy for testicular cancer, may interfere with autonomic innervation of the prostate and seminal vesicles, resulting in absence of smooth muscle contraction and absence of seminal emission at time of orgasm. Pharmacologic agents, particularly α-adrenergic antagonists, may interfere with bladder neck closure at time of orgasm and result in retrograde ejaculation. Similarly, previous bladder neck or prostatic urethral surgery, most commonly transurethral resection of the prostate, may interfere with bladder neck closure, resulting in retrograde ejaculation. Finally, retrograde ejaculation may develop spontaneously in diabetic men.

Patients who complain of absence of ejaculation should be questioned regarding loss of libido or other symptoms of androgen deficiency, present medications, diabetes, and previous surgery. A careful history will usually determine the cause of this problem.

Absence of Orgasm. **Anorgasmia is usually psychogenic or caused by certain medications used to treat psychiatric diseases.** Sometimes, however, anorgasmia may be due to decreased penile sensation owing to impaired pudendal nerve function. Most commonly, this occurs in diabetics with peripheral neuropathy. Men who experience anorgasmia in association with decreased penile sensation should undergo vibratory testing of the penis and further neurologic evaluation as indicated.

Premature Ejaculation. Men who complain of premature ejaculation should be questioned carefully because this is obviously a subjective symptom. It is common for men to ejaculate within 2 minutes after initiation of intercourse, and many men who complain of premature ejaculation in actuality have normal sexual function with abnormal sexual expectations. However, there are men with true premature ejaculation who reach orgasm within less than 1 minute after initiation of intercourse. **This problem is almost always psychogenic** and best treated by a clinical psychologist or psychiatrist who specializes in treatment of this problem and other psychological aspects of male sexual dysfunction. With counseling and appropriate modifications in sexual technique, this problem can usually be overcome. Alternatively, treatment with serotonin reuptake inhibitors such as sertraline and fluoxetine has been demonstrated to be helpful in men with premature ejaculation (Murat Basar et al, 1999).

Hematospermia

Hematospermia refers to the presence of blood in the seminal fluid. **It almost always results from nonspecific inflammation of the prostate and/or seminal vesicles and resolves spontaneously, usually within several weeks.** It frequently occurs after a prolonged period of sexual abstinence, and we have observed it several times in men whose wives are in the final weeks of pregnancy. Patients with hematospermia that persists beyond several weeks should undergo further urologic evaluation because, rarely, an underlying etiology will be identified. A genital and rectal examination should be done to exclude the presence of tuberculosis; a prostate-specific antigen (PSA) and a rectal examination done to exclude prostatic carcinoma; and a urinary cytology done to exclude the possibility of transitional cell carcinoma of the prostate. It should be emphasized, however, that hematospermia almost always resolves spontaneously and rarely is associated with any significant urologic pathology.

Pneumaturia

Pneumaturia is the passage of gas in the urine. In patients who have not recently had urinary tract instrumentation or a urethral catheter placed, this is almost always **due to a fistula between the intestine and the bladder. Common causes include diverticulitis, carcinoma of the sigmoid colon, and regional enteritis (Crohn disease).** In rare instances, patients with diabetes mellitus may have gas-forming infections, with carbon dioxide formation from the fermentation of high concentrations of sugar in the urine.

Urethral Discharge

Urethral discharge is the most common symptom of venereal infection. A purulent discharge that is thick, profuse, and yellow to gray is typical of gonococcal urethritis; the discharge in patients with nonspecific urethritis is usually scant and watery. A bloody discharge is suggestive of carcinoma of the urethra.

Fever and Chills

Fever and chills may occur with infection anywhere in the GU tract but are most commonly observed in patients with pyelonephritis, prostatitis, or epididymitis. **When associated with urinary obstruction, fever and chills may portend septicemia and necessitate emergency treatment to relieve obstruction.**

Medical History

The past medical history is extremely important because it frequently provides clues to the patient's current diagnosis. The past medical history should be obtained in an orderly and sequential manner.

Previous Medical Illnesses with Urologic Sequelae

Many diseases may affect the GU system, and it is important to listen to the patient and record previous medical illnesses. **Patients with diabetes mellitus frequently develop autonomic dysfunction that may result in impaired urinary and sexual function.** A previous history of tuberculosis may be important in a patient presenting with impaired renal function, ureteral obstruction, or chronic, unexplained UTIs. Patients with hypertension have an increased risk of sexual dysfunction because they are more likely to have peripheral vascular disease and because many of the medications that are used to treat hypertension frequently cause impotence. Patients with neurologic diseases such as multiple sclerosis are also more likely to develop urinary and sexual dysfunction. In fact, 5% of patients with previously undiagnosed multiple sclerosis present with urinary symptoms as the first manifestation of the disease (Blaivas and Kaplan, 1988). As mentioned earlier, in men with bladder outlet obstruction, it is important to be aware of preexisting neurologic conditions. Surgical treatment of bladder outlet obstruction in the presence of detrusor hyperreflexia may result in increased urinary incontinence postoperatively. Finally, patients with sickle cell anemia are prone to a number of urologic conditions, including papillary necrosis and erectile dysfunction secondary to recurrent priapism. There are many other diseases with urologic sequelae, and it is important for the urologist to take a careful history in this regard.

Family History

It is similarly important to obtain a detailed family history because many diseases are genetic and/or familial. Examples of genetic diseases include adult polycystic kidney disease, tuberous sclerosis, von Hippel-Lindau disease, renal tubular acidosis, and cystinuria; these are but a few common and well-recognized examples.

In addition to these diseases of known genetic predisposition, there are other conditions in which the precise pattern of inheritance has not been elucidated but that clearly have a familial tendency. It is well known that individuals with a family history of urolithiasis are at increased risk for stone formation. More recently, it has been recognized that **8% to 10% of men with prostate cancer have a familial form of the disease that tends to develop about a decade earlier than the more common type of prostate cancer** (Bratt, 2000). Other familial conditions are mentioned elsewhere in the text, but suffice it to state again that obtaining a careful history of previous illnesses and a family history of urologic disease can be extremely valuable in establishing the correct diagnosis.

Medications

It is similarly important to obtain an accurate and complete list of present medications because many drugs interfere with urinary and sexual function. For example, **most of the antihypertensive medications interfere with erectile function, and changing antihypertensive medications can sometimes improve sexual function.** Similarly, many of the psychotropic agents interfere with emission and orgasm. In our own recent experience, we cared for a man who presented with anorgasmia. He had been to several physicians without improvement in this problem. When we obtained his past medical history, he mentioned that he had been taking a psychotropic agent for transient depression for several years, and his anorgasmia resolved when this no-longer-needed medication was discontinued. The list of medications affecting urinary and sexual function is exhaustive, but, once again, each medication should be recorded and its side effects investigated to be sure that the patient's problem is not drug related. A listing of common medications that may cause urologic side effects is presented in Table 1-2.

Previous Surgical Procedures

It is important to be aware of previous operations, particularly in a patient who may have surgery, because previous operations may make subsequent ones more difficult. If the previous surgery was in a similar anatomic region, it is worthwhile to try to obtain the previous operative report. In our own experience, this small additional effort has been rewarded on numerous occasions by providing a clear explanation of the patient's previous surgery that greatly simplified the subsequent operation. In general, **it is worthwhile to obtain as much information as possible** *before* **any intended surgery** because most surprises that occur in the operating room are unhappy ones.

Smoking and Alcohol Use

Cigarette smoking and consumption of alcohol are clearly linked to a number of urologic conditions. **Cigarette smoking is associated with an increased risk of urothelial carcinoma, most notably bladder cancer, and it is also associated with increased peripheral vascular disease and erectile dysfunction. Chronic alcoholism may result in autonomic and peripheral neuropathy**

TABLE 1-2   Drugs Associated with Urologic Side Effects

UROLOGIC SIDE EFFECTS	CLASS OF DRUGS	SPECIFIC EXAMPLES
Decreased libido	Antihypertensives	Hydrochlorothiazide
Erectile dysfunction	Psychotropic drugs	Propranolol Benzodiazepines
Ejaculatory dysfunction	α-Adrenergic antagonists	Prazosin Tamsulosin α-Methyldopa
	Psychotropic drugs	Phenothiazines Antidepressants
Priapism	Antipsychotics Antidepressants Antihypertensives	Phenothiazines Trazodone Hydralazine Prazosin
Decreased spermatogenesis	Chemotherapeutic agents Drugs with abuse potential	Alkylating agents Marijuana Alcohol Nicotine
	Drugs affecting endocrine function	Antiandrogens Prostaglandins
Incontinence or impaired voiding	Direct smooth muscle stimulants	Histamine Vasopressin
	Others	Furosemide Valproic acid
	Smooth muscle relaxants	Diazepam
	Striated muscle relaxants	Baclofen
Urinary retention or obstructive voiding symptoms	Anticholinergic agents or musculotropic relaxants	Oxybutynin Diazepam Flavoxate
	Calcium channel blockers Antiparkinsonian drugs	Nifedipine Carbidopa Levodopa
	α-Adrenergic agonists	Pseudoephedrine Phenylephrine
	Antihistamines	Loratadine Diphenhydramine
Acute renal failure	Antimicrobials	Aminoglycosides Penicillins Cephalosporins Amphotericin
	Chemotherapeutic drugs Others	Cisplatin Nonsteroidal anti-inflammatory drugs Phenytoin
Gynecomastia	Antihypertensives Cardiac drugs Gastrointestinal drugs	Verapamil Digoxin Cimetidine Metoclopramide
	Psychotropic drugs Tricyclic antidepressants	Phenothiazines Amitriptyline Imipramine

with resultant impaired urinary and sexual function. Chronic alcoholism may also impair hepatic metabolism of estrogens, resulting in decreased serum testosterone, testicular atrophy, and decreased libido.

In addition to the direct urologic effects of cigarette smoking and alcohol consumption, patients who are actively smoking or drinking up to the time of surgery are at increased risk for perioperative complications. Smokers are at increased risk for both pulmonary and cardiac complications. If possible, they should **discontinue smoking at least 8 weeks before surgery to optimize their** pulmonary function (Warner et al, 1989). If they are unable to do this, they should at least quit smoking for 48 hours before surgery because this will result in a significant improvement in cardiovascular function. Similarly, chronic alcoholics are at increased risk for hepatic toxicity and subsequent coagulation problems postoperatively. Furthermore, alcoholics who continue drinking up to the time of surgery may experience acute alcohol withdrawal during the postoperative period that can be life threatening. Prophylactic administration of lorazepam (Ativan) greatly reduces the potential risk of this significant complication.

Allergies

Finally, medicinal allergies should be questioned because these medications should be avoided in future treatment of the patient. **All medicinal allergies should be marked boldly on the front of the patient's chart** to avoid potential complications from inadvertent exposure to the same medications.

In summary, a careful and thorough medical history including the chief complaint and history of present illness, past medical history, and family history should be obtained for every patient. Unfortunately, time constraints often make it difficult for the physician to spend the necessary time to obtain a full history. A reasonable substitute is to have a trained nurse or other health professional see the patient first. By using a standard history form, much of the information discussed previously can be obtained in a preliminary interview. It then remains for the urologist to only fill in the blanks, have the patient elaborate on potentially relevant aspects of the past medical history, and then perform a complete physical examination.

PHYSICAL EXAMINATION

KEY POINTS

- The urologist can undertake the initial evaluation and establish a diagnosis for almost all patients with diseases of the GU system.
- A complete history and appropriate physical examination is critical in the assessment of urologic patients.
- A complete urinalysis including chemical and microscopic analyses should be performed because this may provide important information critical to the diagnosis and treatment of urologic patients.

A complete and thorough physical examination is an essential component of the evaluation of patients who present with urologic disease. Although it is tempting to become dependent on results of laboratory and radiologic tests, **the physical examination often simplifies the process and allows the urologist to select the most appropriate diagnostic studies.** Along with the history, the physical examination remains a key component of the diagnostic evaluation and should be performed conscientiously.

General Observations

The visual inspection of the patient provides a general overview. The skin should be inspected for evidence of jaundice or pallor. The nutritional status of the patient should be noted. **Cachexia is a frequent sign of malignancy, and obesity may be a sign of underlying endocrinologic abnormalities.** In this instance, one should search for the presence of truncal obesity, a "buffalo hump," and abdominal skin striae, which are stigmata of hyperadrenocorticism. In contrast, debility and hyperpigmentation may be signs of hypoadrenocorticism. Gynecomastia may be a sign of endocrinologic disease and a possible indicator of alcoholism or previous hormonal therapy for prostate cancer. Edema of the genitalia and lower extremities may be associated with cardiac decompensation, renal failure, nephrotic syndrome, or pelvic and/or retroperitoneal lymphatic obstruction. Supraclavicular lymphadenopathy may be seen with any GU neoplasm, most commonly prostate and testis cancer; inguinal lymphadenopathy may occur secondary to carcinoma of the penis or urethra.

Kidneys

The kidneys are fist-sized organs located high in the retroperitoneum bilaterally. In the adult, the kidneys are normally difficult to palpate because of their position under the diaphragm and ribs with abundant musculature both anteriorly and posteriorly. Because of the position of the liver, the right kidney is somewhat lower than the left. **In children and thin women, it may be possible to palpate the lower pole of the right kidney with deep inspiration.** However, it is usually not possible to palpate either kidney in men, and the left kidney is almost always impalpable unless it is abnormally enlarged.

The best way to palpate the kidneys is with the patient in the supine position. **The kidney is lifted from behind with one hand in the costovertebral angle** (Fig. 1-1). On deep inspiration, the examiner's hand is advanced firmly into the anterior abdomen just below the costal margin. At the point of maximal inspiration, the kidney may be felt as it moves downward with the diaphragm. With each inspiration, the examiner's hand may be advanced deeper into the abdomen. Once again, it is more difficult to palpate kidneys in men because the kidneys tend to move downward less with inspiration and because they are surrounded with thicker muscular layers. In children, it is easier to palpate the kidneys because of decreased body thickness. In neonates, the kidneys can be felt quite easily by palpating the flank between the thumb anteriorly and the fingers over the costovertebral angle posteriorly.

Transillumination of the kidneys may be helpful in children younger than 1 year of age with a palpable flank mass. Such masses are frequently of renal origin. A flashlight or fiberoptic light source is positioned posteriorly against the costovertebral angle. Fluid-filled masses such as cysts or hydronephrosis produce a dull reddish glow in the anterior abdomen. Solid masses such as tumors do not transilluminate. Other diagnostic maneuvers that may be helpful in examining the kidneys are percussion and auscultation. Although renal inflammation may cause pain that is poorly localized, percussion of the costovertebral angle posteriorly more often localizes the pain and tenderness more accurately. Percussion should be done gently because in a patient with significant renal inflammation, this may be quite painful. Auscultation of the upper abdomen during deep inspiration may occasionally reveal a systolic bruit associated with renal artery stenosis or an aneurysm. A bruit may also be detected in association with a large renal arteriovenous fistula.

Every patient with flank pain should also be examined for possible nerve root irritation. The ribs should be palpated carefully to rule out a bone spur or other skeletal abnormality and to determine the point of maximal tenderness. Unlike renal pain, radiculitis usually causes hyperesthesia of the overlying skin innervated by the irritated peripheral nerve. This hypersensitivity can be elicited with a pin or by pinching the skin and fat overlying the involved area. Finally, the pain experienced during the pre-eruptive phase of herpes zoster involving any of the segments between T11 and L2 may also simulate pain of renal origin.

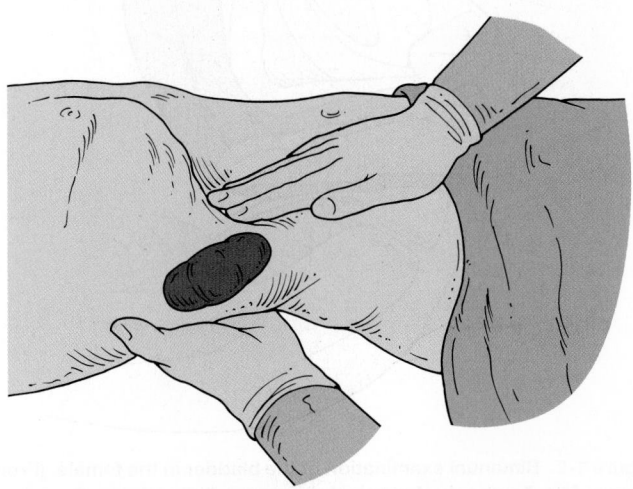

Figure 1-1. **Bimanual examination of the kidney.**

Bladder

A normal bladder in the adult cannot be palpated or percussed until there is at least 150 mL of urine in it. At a volume of about 500 mL, the distended bladder becomes visible in thin patients as a lower midline abdominal mass.

Percussion is better than palpation for diagnosing a distended bladder. The examiner begins by percussing immediately above the symphysis pubis and continuing cephalad until there is a change in pitch from dull to resonant. Alternatively, it may be possible in thin patients and in children to palpate the bladder by lifting the lumbar spine with one hand and pressing the other hand into the midline of the lower abdomen.

A careful bimanual examination, best done with the patient under anesthesia, is invaluable in assessing the regional extent of a bladder tumor or other pelvic mass. The bladder is palpated between the abdomen and the vagina in the female (Fig. 1-2) or the rectum in the male (Fig. 1-3). In addition to defining areas of induration, the bimanual examination allows the examiner to assess the mobility of the bladder; such information cannot be obtained by radiologic techniques such as CT and MRI, which convey static images.

Penis

If the patient has not been circumcised, the foreskin should be retracted to examine for tumor or balanoposthitis (inflammation of the prepuce and glans penis). **Most penile cancers occur in uncircumcised men and arise on the prepuce or glans penis.** Therefore in a patient with a bloody penile discharge in whom the foreskin cannot be withdrawn, a dorsal slit or circumcision must be performed to adequately evaluate the glans penis and urethra.

The position of the urethral meatus should be noted. It may be located proximal to the tip of the glans on the ventral surface (hypospadias) or, much less commonly, on the dorsal surface (epispadias). The penile skin should be examined for the presence of superficial vesicles compatible with herpes simplex and for ulcers that may indicate either venereal infection or tumor. The presence of venereal warts (condylomata acuminata), which appear as irregular, papillary, velvety lesions on the male genitalia, should also be noted.

The urethral meatus should be separated between the thumb and the forefinger to inspect for neoplastic or inflammatory lesions within the fossa navicularis. The dorsal shaft of the penis should be palpated for the presence of fibrotic plaques or ridges typical of Peyronie disease. Tenderness along the ventral aspect of the penis is suggestive of periurethritis, often secondary to a urethral stricture.

Scrotum and Contents

The scrotum is a loose sac containing the testes and spermatic cord structures. The scrotal wall is made up of skin and an underlying thin muscular layer. The testes are normally oval, firm, and smooth; in adults, they measure about 6 cm in length and 4 cm in width. They are suspended in the scrotum, with the right testis normally anterior to the left. The epididymis lies posterior to the testis and is palpable as a distinct ridge of tissue. The vas deferens can be palpated above each testis and feels like a piece of heavy twine.

The scrotum should be examined for dermatologic abnormalities. **Because the scrotum, unlike the penis, contains both hair and sweat glands, it is a frequent site of local infection and sebaceous cysts.** Hair follicles can become infected and may present as small pustules on the surface of the scrotum. These usually resolve spontaneously, but they can give rise to more significant infection, particularly in patients with reduced immunity and diabetes. Patients often become concerned about these lesions, mistaking them for testicular tumors.

The testes should be palpated gently between the fingertips of both hands. The testes normally have a firm, rubbery consistency with a smooth surface. Abnormally small testes suggest hypogonadism or an endocrinopathy such as Klinefelter disease. **A firm or hard area within the testis should be considered a malignant tumor until proved otherwise.** The epididymis should be palpable as a ridge posterior to each testis. Masses in the epididymis (spermatocele, cyst, and epididymitis) are almost always benign.

To examine for a hernia, the physician's index finger should be inserted gently into the scrotum and invaginated into the external inguinal ring (Fig. 1-4). The scrotum should be

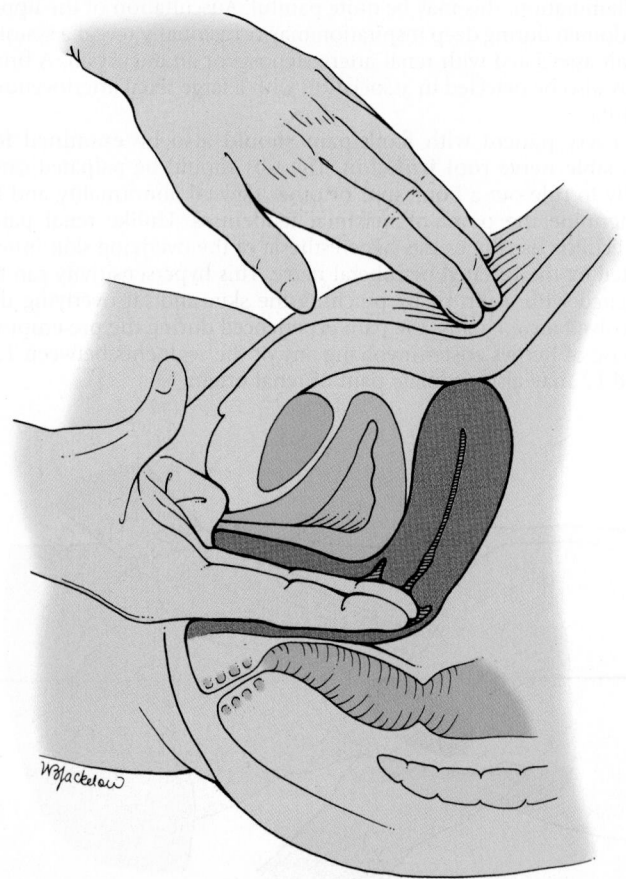

Figure 1-2. **Bimanual examination of the bladder in the female. (From Swartz MH. Textbook of physical diagnosis. Philadelphia: Saunders; 1989. p. 405.)**

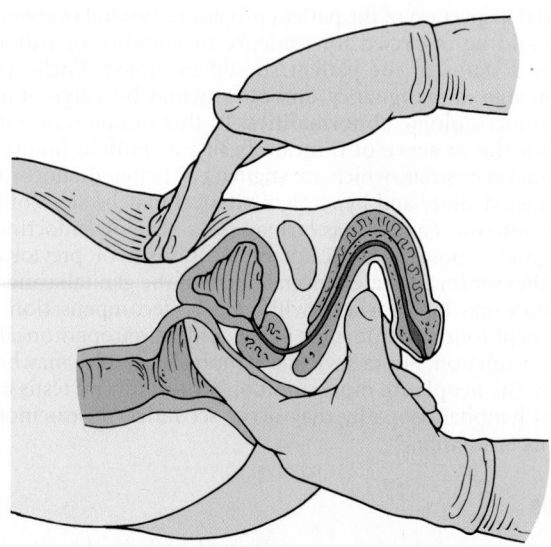

Figure 1-3. **Bimanual examination of the bladder in the male.**

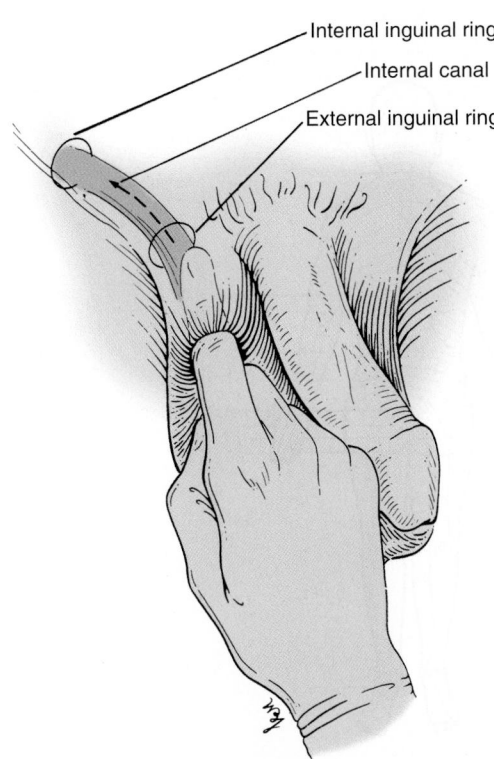

Internal inguinal ring
Internal canal
External inguinal ring

Figure 1-4. **Examination of the inguinal canal. (From Swartz MH. Textbook of physical diagnosis. Philadelphia: Saunders; 1989. p. 376.)**

invaginated in front of the testis, and care should be taken not to elevate the testis itself, which is quite painful. Once the external ring has been located, the physician should place the fingertips of his or her other hand over the internal inguinal ring and ask the patient to bear down (Valsalva maneuver). A hernia will be felt as a distinct bulge that descends against the tip of the index finger in the external inguinal ring as the patient bears down. Although it may be possible to distinguish a direct inguinal hernia arising through the floor of the inguinal canal from an indirect inguinal hernia prolapsing through the internal inguinal ring, this is seldom possible and of little clinical significance because the surgical approach is essentially identical for both conditions.

The spermatic cord is also examined with the patient in the standing position. A varicocele is a dilated, tortuous spermatic vein that becomes more obvious as the patient performs a Valsalva maneuver. The epididymis can again be palpated as a ridge of tissue running longitudinally, posterior to each testis. The testis should be palpated again between the fingers of both hands, once again taking care not to exert any pressure on the testis itself so as to avoid pain.

Transillumination is helpful in determining whether scrotal masses are solid (tumor) or cystic (hydrocele, spermatocele). A small flashlight or fiberoptic light cord is placed behind the mass. A cystic mass transilluminates easily, whereas light is not transmitted through a solid tumor.

Rectal and Prostate Examination in the Male

Digital rectal examination (DRE) should be performed in every male after age 40 years and in men of any age who present for urologic evaluation. Prostate cancer is the second most common cause of male cancer deaths after age 55 years and the most common cause of cancer deaths in men older than 70 years. Many prostate cancers can be detected in an early curable stage by DRE, and about 25% of colorectal cancers can be detected by DRE in combination with a stool guaiac test.

DRE should be performed at the end of the physical examination. It is done best with the patient standing and bent over the examining table or with the patient in the knee-chest position. In the standing position, the patient should stand with his thighs close to the examining table. The feet should be about 18 inches apart, with the knees flexed slightly. The patient should bend at the waist 90 degrees until his chest is resting on his forearms. The physician should give the patient adequate time to get in the proper position and relax as much as possible. A few reassuring words before the examination are helpful. The physician should place a glove on the examining hand and should lubricate the index finger thoroughly.

Before performing the DRE, the physician should place the palm of his other hand against the patient's lower abdomen. This provides subtle reassurance to the patient by allowing the physician to make gentle contact with the patient before touching the anus. It also allows the physician to steady the patient and provide gentle counterpressure if the patient tries to move away as the DRE is being performed. The DRE itself begins by separating the buttocks and inspecting the anus for pathology, usually hemorrhoids, but, occasionally, an anal carcinoma or melanoma may be detected. The gloved, lubricated index finger is then inserted gently into the anus. Only one phalanx should be inserted initially to give the anus time to relax and to easily accommodate the finger. Estimation of anal sphincter tone is of great importance; a flaccid or spastic anal sphincter suggests similar changes in the urinary sphincter and may be a clue to the diagnosis of neurogenic disease. If the physician waits only a few seconds, the anal sphincter will normally relax to the degree that the finger can be advanced to the knuckle without causing pain. The index finger then sweeps over the prostate; the entire posterior surface of the gland can usually be examined if the patient is in the proper position. **Normally, the prostate is about the size of a chestnut and has a consistency similar to that of the contracted thenar eminence of the thumb (with the thumb opposed to the little finger).**

The index finger is extended as far as possible into the rectum, and the entire circumference is examined to detect an early rectal carcinoma. The index finger is then withdrawn gently, and the stool on the glove is transferred to a guaiac-impregnated (Hemoccult) card for determination of occult blood. Although there may be a significant incidence of false-positive and false-negative results associated with fecal occult blood testing, particularly without dietary and drug restrictions, **the guaiac test is simple and inexpensive and may lead to the detection of significant gastrointestinal abnormalities** (Bond, 1999). Adequate tissues, soap, and towels should be available for the patient to cleanse himself after the examination. The physician should then leave the room and allow the patient adequate time to wash and dress before concluding the consultation.

Pelvic Examination in the Female

Male urologists should always perform the female pelvic examination with a female nurse or other health care professional present. The patient should be allowed to undress in privacy and be fully draped for the procedure before the physician enters the room. The examination itself should be performed in standard lithotomy position with the patient's legs abducted. Initially, the external genitalia and introitus should be examined, with particular attention paid to atrophic changes, erosions, ulcers, discharge, or warts, all of which may cause dysuria and pelvic discomfort. The urethral meatus should be inspected for caruncles, mucosal hyperplasia, cysts, and mucosal prolapse. The patient is then asked to perform a Valsalva maneuver and is carefully examined for a cystocele (prolapse of the bladder) or rectocele (prolapse of the rectum). The patient is then asked to cough, which may precipitate stress urinary incontinence. Palpation of the urethra is done to detect induration, which may be a sign of chronic inflammation or malignancy. Palpation may also disclose a urethral diverticulum, and palpation of a diverticulum may cause a purulent discharge from the urethra. Bimanual examination of the bladder, uterus, and adnexa should then be performed with two fingers in the vagina and the other hand on the lower abdomen. Any abnormality of the pelvic organs should be evaluated further with a pelvic ultrasound or CT scan.

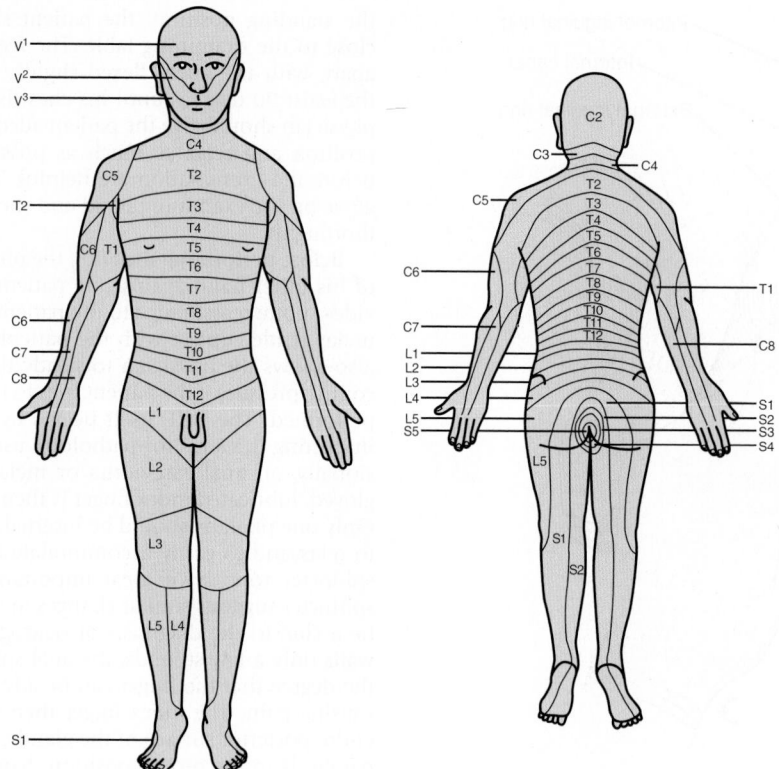

Figure 1-5. Sensory dermatome maps used to help localize the level of neurologic deficit.

Neurologic Examination

There are various clinical situations in which the neurologic examination may be helpful in evaluating urologic patients. In some cases, the level of neurologic abnormalities can be localized by the pattern of sensory deficit noted during physical examination using a dermatome map (Fig. 1-5). Sensory deficits in the penis, labia, scrotum, vagina, and perianal area generally indicate damage or injury to sacral roots or nerves. In addition to sensory examination, testing of reflexes in the genital area may also be performed. The most important of these is the bulbocavernosus reflex (BCR), which is a reflex contraction of the striated muscle of the pelvic floor that occurs in response to various stimuli in the perineum or genitalia. This reflex is most commonly tested by placing a finger in the rectum and then squeezing the glans penis or clitoris. If a Foley catheter is in place, the BCR can also be elicited by gently pulling on the catheter. If the BCR is intact, tightening of the anal sphincter should be felt and/or observed. The BCR tests the integrity of the spinal cord–mediated reflex arc involving S2-S4 and may be absent in the presence of sacral cord or peripheral nerve abnormalities.

The cremasteric reflex can be elicited by lightly stroking the superior and medial thigh in a downward direction. The normal response in males is contraction of the cremasteric muscle that results in immediate elevation of the ipsilateral scrotum and testis. There is limited clinical utility for testing superficial reflexes such as the cremasteric when investigating neurologic dysfunction. However, there may be a role for testing this reflex when assessing patients with suspected testicular torsion or epididymitis. Finally, an overly active cremasteric reflex in children can lead to the mistaken diagnosis of an undescended testis in some cases.

URINALYSIS

The urinalysis is a fundamental test that should be performed in all urologic patients. Although in many instances a simple dipstick urinalysis will provide the necessary information, **a complete urinalysis includes both chemical and microscopic analyses.**

Collection of Urinary Specimens

Males

In the male patient, a midstream urine sample is obtained. The uncircumcised male should retract the foreskin, cleanse the glans penis with antiseptic solution, and continue to retract the foreskin during voiding. The male patient begins urinating into the toilet and then places a wide-mouth sterile container under his penis to collect a midstream sample. This avoids contamination of the urine specimen with skin and urethral organisms.

In men with chronic UTIs, four aliquots of urine are obtained. **These aliquots have been designated Voided Bladder 1, Voided Bladder 2, Expressed Prostatic Secretions, and Voided Bladder 3 (VB1, VB2, EPS, and VB3).** The VB1 is the initial 5 to 10 mL of urine voided, whereas the VB2 is the midstream urine. The EPS is the secretions obtained after gentle prostatic massage, and the VB3 specimen is the initial 2 to 3 mL of urine obtained after prostatic massage. The value of these cultures for localization of UTIs is that the VB1 sample represents urethral flora; the VB2, bladder flora; and the EPS and VB3 samples, prostatic flora. The VB3 sample is particularly helpful when little or no prostatic fluid is obtained by massage. To better obtain prostatic secretions, patients should be instructed to attempt to void during prostatic massage and to avoid tightening the anal sphincter and pelvic floor muscles. The four-part urine sample is particularly useful in evaluating men with suspected bacterial prostatitis (Meares and Stamey, 1968).

Females

In the female, it is more difficult to obtain a clean-catch midstream specimen. The female patient should cleanse the vulva, separate the labia, and collect a midstream specimen as described for the male patient. If infection is suspected, however, the midstream specimen is unreliable and should never be sent for culture and sensitivity. **To evaluate for a possible infection in a female, a catheterized urine sample should always be obtained.**

Neonates and Infants

The usual way to obtain a urine sample in a neonate or infant is to place a sterile plastic bag with an adhesive collar over the infant's genitalia. However, these devices may not be able to distinguish contamination from true UTI. Whenever possible, **all urine samples should be examined within 1 hour of collection and plated for culture and sensitivity if indicated.** If urine is allowed to stand at room temperature for longer periods of time, bacterial overgrowth may occur, the pH may change, and red and white blood cell casts may disintegrate. If it is not possible to examine the urine promptly, it should be refrigerated at 5° C.

Physical Examination of Urine

The physical examination of the urine includes an evaluation of color, turbidity, specific gravity and osmolality, and pH.

Color

The normal pale yellow color of urine is due to the presence of the pigment urochrome. **Urine color varies most commonly because of concentration, but many foods, medications, metabolic products, and infection may produce abnormal urine color.** This is important because many patients will seek consultation primarily because of a change in their urine color. Thus it is important for the urologist to be aware of the common causes of abnormal urine color, and these are listed in Table 1-3.

Turbidity

Freshly voided urine is clear. **Cloudy urine is most commonly due to phosphaturia,** a benign process in which excess phosphate crystals precipitate in an alkaline urine. Phosphaturia is intermittent and usually occurs after meals or ingestion of a large quantity of milk. Patients are otherwise asymptomatic. The diagnosis of phosphaturia can be accomplished either by acidifying the urine with acetic acid, which will result in immediate clearing, or by performing a microscopic analysis, which will reveal large amounts of amorphous phosphate crystals.

Pyuria, usually associated with a UTI, is another common cause of cloudy urine. The large numbers of white blood cells cause the urine to become turbid. **Pyuria is readily distinguished from phosphaturia either by smelling the urine** (infected urine has a characteristic pungent odor) or by microscopic examination, which readily distinguishes amorphous phosphate crystals from leukocytes.

Rare causes of cloudy urine include chyluria (in which there is an abnormal communication between the lymphatic system and the urinary tract resulting in lymph fluid being mixed with urine), lipiduria, hyperoxaluria, and hyperuricosuria.

Specific Gravity and Osmolality

Specific gravity of urine is easily determined from a urinary dipstick and usually varies from 1.001 to 1.035. Specific gravity usually reflects the patient's state of hydration but may also be affected by abnormal renal function, the amount of material dissolved in the urine, and a variety of other causes mentioned later. A specific gravity less than 1.008 is regarded as dilute, and a specific gravity greater than 1.020 is considered concentrated. A fixed specific gravity of 1.010 is a sign of renal insufficiency, either acute or chronic.

In general, specific gravity reflects the state of hydration but also affords some idea of renal concentrating ability. Conditions that decrease specific gravity include (1) increased fluid intake,

TABLE 1-3   Common Causes of Abnormal Urine Color

COLOR	CAUSE
Colorless	Very dilute urine Overhydration
Cloudy/milky	Phosphaturia Pyuria Chyluria
Red	Hematuria Hemoglobinuria/myoglobinuria Anthocyanin in beets and blackberries Chronic lead and mercury poisoning Phenolphthalein (in bowel evacuants) Phenothiazines (e.g., Compazine) Rifampin
Orange	Dehydration Phenazopyridine (Pyridium) Sulfasalazine (Azulfidine)
Yellow	Normal Phenacetin Riboflavin
Green-blue	Biliverdin Indicanuria (tryptophan indole metabolites) Amitriptyline (Elavil) Indigo carmine Methylene blue Phenols (e.g., IV cimetidine [Tagamet], IV promethazine [Phenergan]) Resorcinol Triamterene (Dyrenium)
Brown	Urobilinogen Porphyria Aloe, fava beans, and rhubarb Chloroquine and primaquine Furazolidone (Furoxone) Metronidazole (Flagyl) Nitrofurantoin (Furadantin)
Brown-black	Alcaptonuria (homogentisic acid) Hemorrhage Melanin Tyrosinosis (hydroxyphenylpyruvic acid) Cascara, senna (laxatives) Methocarbamol (Robaxin) Methyldopa (Aldomet) Sorbitol

IV, intravenous.
From Hanno PM, Wein AJ. A clinical manual of urology. Norwalk (CT): Appleton-Century-Crofts; 1987. p. 67.

(2) diuretics, (3) decreased renal concentrating ability, and (4) diabetes insipidus. Conditions that increase specific gravity include (1) decreased fluid intake; (2) dehydration owing to fever, sweating, vomiting, and diarrhea; (3) diabetes mellitus (glucosuria); and (4) inappropriate secretion of antidiuretic hormone. Specific gravity will also be increased above 1.035 after IV injection of iodinated contrast and in patients taking dextran.

Osmolality is a measure of the amount of material dissolved in the urine and usually varies between 50 and 1200 mOsm/L. Urine osmolality most commonly varies with hydration, and the same factors that affect specific gravity will also affect osmolality. Urine osmolality is a better indicator of renal function, but it cannot be measured from a dipstick and must be determined using standard laboratory techniques.

pH

Urinary pH is measured with a dipstick test strip that incorporates two colorimetric indicators, methyl red and bromothymol blue, which yield clearly distinguishable colors over the pH range from 5 to 9. Urinary pH may vary from 4.5 to 8; the average pH varies between 5.5 and 6.5. A urinary pH between 4.5 and 5.5 is considered acidic, whereas a pH between 6.5 and 8 is considered alkaline.

In general, the urinary pH reflects the pH in the serum. In patients with metabolic or respiratory acidosis, the urine is usually acidic; conversely, in patients with metabolic or respiratory alkalosis, the urine is alkaline. Renal tubular acidosis (RTA) presents an exception to this rule. In patients with both type I and II RTA, the serum is acidemic, but the urine is alkalotic because of continued loss of bicarbonate in the urine. In severe metabolic acidosis in type II RTA, the urine may become acidic, but in type I RTA, the urine is always alkaline, even with severe metabolic acidosis (Morris and Ives, 1991). Urinary pH determination is used to establish the diagnosis of RTA; inability to acidify the urine below a pH of 5.5 after administration of an acid load is diagnostic of RTA.

Urine pH determinations are also useful in the diagnosis and treatment of UTIs and urinary calculus disease. **In patients with a presumed UTI, an alkaline urine with a pH greater than 7.5 suggests infection with a urea-splitting organism, most commonly** *Proteus.* Urease-producing bacteria convert ammonia to ammonium ions, markedly elevating the urinary pH and causing precipitation of calcium magnesium ammonium phosphate crystals. The massive amount of crystallization may result in staghorn calculi.

Urinary pH is usually acidic in patients with uric acid and cystine lithiasis. Alkalinization of the urine is an important feature of therapy in both of these conditions, and frequent monitoring of urinary pH is necessary to ascertain adequacy of therapy.

Chemical Examination of Urine

Urine Dipsticks

Urine dipsticks provide a quick and inexpensive method for detecting abnormal substances within the urine. Dipsticks are short, plastic strips with small marker pads that are impregnated with different chemical reagents that react with abnormal substances in the urine to produce a colorimetric change. **The abnormal substances commonly tested for with a dipstick include (1) blood, (2) protein, (3) glucose, (4) ketones, (5) urobilinogen and bilirubin, and (6) white blood cells.**

Substances listed in Table 1-3 that produce an abnormal urine color may interfere with appropriate color development on the dipstick. In our experience, this most commonly occurs in patients taking phenazopyridine (Pyridium) for a UTI. Phenazopyridine turns the urine bright orange and makes dipstick evaluation of the urine unreliable.

Appropriate technique must be used to obtain an accurate dipstick determination. The reagent areas on the dipstick must be completely immersed in a fresh uncentrifuged urine specimen and then must be withdrawn immediately to prevent dissolution of the reagents into the urine. As the dipstick is removed from the urine specimen container, the edge of the dipstick is drawn along the rim of the container to remove excess urine. The dipstick should be held horizontally until the appropriate time for reading and then compared with the color chart. **Excess urine on the dipstick or holding the dipstick in a vertical position will allow mixing of chemicals from adjacent reagent pads on the dipstick, resulting in a faulty diagnosis.** False-negative results for glucose and bilirubin may be seen in the presence of elevated ascorbic acid concentrations in the urine. However, increased levels of ascorbic acid in the urine do not interfere with dipstick testing for hematuria. Highly buffered alkaline urine may cause falsely low readings for specific gravity and may lead to false-negative results for urinary protein. Other common causes of false results with dipstick testing are outdated test strips and exposure of the sticks, leading to damage to the reagents. In general, when the sticks are damaged, there will be color changes on the pads before their immersion in urine. If such color changes are noted, results with the dipstick may be inaccurate.

Hematuria

Normal urine should contain fewer than three RBCs per HPF. A positive dipstick for blood in the urine indicates either hematuria, hemoglobinuria, or myoglobinuria. **The chemical detection of blood in the urine is based on the peroxidase-like activity of hemoglobin.** When in contact with an organic peroxidase substrate, hemoglobin catalyzes the reaction and causes subsequent oxidation of a chromogen indicator, which changes color according to the degree and amount of oxidation. The degree of color change is directly related to the amount of hemoglobin present in the urine specimen. Dipsticks frequently demonstrate both colored dots and field color change. If present, free hemoglobin and myoglobin in the urine are absorbed into the reagent pad and catalyze the reaction within the test paper, thereby producing a field change effect in color. Intact erythrocytes in the urine undergo hemolysis when they come in contact with the reagent test pad, and the localized free hemoglobin on the pad produces a corresponding dot of color change. The greater the number of intact erythrocytes in the urine specimen, the greater the number of dots that will appear on the test paper, and a coalescence of the dots occurs when there are more than 250 erythrocytes/mL.

Hematuria can be distinguished from hemoglobinuria and myoglobinuria by microscopic examination of the centrifuged urine; the presence of a large number of erythrocytes establishes the diagnosis of hematuria. If erythrocytes are absent, examination of the serum will distinguish hemoglobinuria and myoglobinuria. A sample of blood is obtained and centrifuged. In hemoglobinuria, the supernatant will be pink. This is because free hemoglobin in the serum binds to haptoglobin, which is water insoluble and has a high molecular weight. This complex remains in the serum, causing a pink color. Free hemoglobin will appear in the urine only when all of the haptoglobin-binding sites have been saturated. In myoglobinuria, the myoglobin released from muscle is of low molecular weight and water soluble. It does not bind to haptoglobin and is therefore excreted immediately into the urine. Therefore in myoglobinuria the serum remains clear.

The sensitivity of urinary dipsticks in identifying hematuria, defined as greater than three erythrocytes/HPF of centrifuged sediment examined microscopically, is higher than 90%. Conversely, the specificity of the dipstick for hematuria compared with microscopy is somewhat lower, reflecting a higher false-positive rate with the dipstick (Shaw et al, 1985).

False-positive dipstick readings are most often due to contamination of the urine specimen with menstrual blood. Dehydration with resultant urine of high specific gravity can also yield false-positive results owing to the increased concentration of erythrocytes and hemoglobin. The normal individual excretes about 1000 erythrocytes/mL of urine, with the upper limits of normal varying from 5000 to 8000 erythrocytes/mL (Kincaid-Smith, 1982). Therefore examining urine of high specific gravity such as the first morning voided specimen increases the likelihood of a false-positive result. In addition to dehydration, another cause of false-positive results is exercise, which can increase the number of erythrocytes in the urine.

The efficacy of hematuria screening using the dipstick to identify patients with significant urologic disease is somewhat controversial. Studies in children and young adults have shown a low rate of significant disease (Woolhandler et al, 1989). In older adults, one study from the Mayo Clinic of 2000 patients with asymptomatic hematuria showed that only 0.5% had a urologic malignancy and only 1.8% developed other serious urologic diseases within 3 years after identification of the hematuria (Mohr et al, 1986). Conversely, investigators at the University of Wisconsin found that 26% of adults who had at least one positive dipstick reading for hematuria were subsequently found to have significant urologic pathology (Messing et al, 1987). The age of the population, the completeness of the subsequent urologic evaluation, and the definition of significant disease all influence the disease rate in the group of patients with asymptomatic hematuria identified by dipstick screening. It is important to remember that, before proceeding to more complicated studies, the dipstick result should be confirmed with a microscopic examination of the centrifuged urinary sediment.

Differential Diagnosis and Evaluation of Hematuria. Hematuria may reflect either significant nephrologic or urologic disease. **Hematuria of nephrologic origin is frequently associated with casts in the urine and almost always associated with significant proteinuria. Even significant hematuria of urologic origin will not elevate the protein concentration in the urine into the 100 to 300 mg/dL or 2+ to 3+ range on dipstick,** and proteinuria of this magnitude almost always indicates glomerular or tubulointerstitial renal disease.

Morphologic evaluation of erythrocytes in the centrifuged urinary sediment also helps localize their site of origin. **Erythrocytes arising from glomerular disease are typically dysmorphic and show a wide range of morphologic alterations. Conversely, erythrocytes arising from tubulointerstitial renal disease and of urologic origin have a uniformly round shape;** these erythrocytes may or may not retain their hemoglobin ("ghost cells"), but the individual cell shape is consistently round. In individuals without significant pathology with minimal amounts of hematuria, the erythrocytes are characteristically dysmorphic but the number of cells observed is far fewer than that observed in patients with nephrologic disease. Erythrocyte morphology is more easily determined using phase contrast microscopy, but with practice this can be accomplished using a conventional light microscope (Schramek et al, 1989).

Glomerular Hematuria. **Glomerular hematuria is suggested by the presence of dysmorphic erythrocytes, RBC casts, and proteinuria.** Of those patients with glomerulonephritis proven by renal biopsy, however, about 20% will have hematuria alone without RBC casts or proteinuria (Fassett et al, 1982).

The glomerular disorders associated with hematuria are listed in Table 1-4. Further evaluation of patients with glomerular hematuria should begin with a thorough history. Hematuria in children and young adults, usually males, associated with low-grade fever and an erythematous rash suggests a diagnosis of immunoglobulin A (IgA) nephropathy (Berger disease). A family history of renal disease and deafness suggests familial nephritis or Alport syndrome. Hemoptysis and abnormal bleeding associated with microcytic anemia are characteristic of Goodpasture syndrome, and the presence of a rash and arthritis suggest systemic lupus erythematosus. Finally, poststreptococcal glomerulonephritis should be suspected in a child with a recent streptococcal upper respiratory tract or skin infection.

Further laboratory evaluation should include measurement of serum creatinine, creatinine clearance, and, when proteinuria in the urine is 2+ or greater, a 24-hour urine protein determination. Although these tests will quantitate the specific degree of renal dysfunction, further tests are usually required to establish the specific diagnosis and particularly to determine whether the disease is due to an immune or a nonimmune etiology. **Frequently, a renal biopsy is necessary to establish the precise diagnosis, and biopsies are particularly important if the result will influence subsequent treatment of the patient.** Renal biopsies are extremely informative when examined by an experienced pathologist using light, immunofluorescent, and electron microscopy.

An algorithm for the evaluation of glomerular hematuria is provided in Figure 1-6.

IgA Nephropathy (Berger Disease). IgA nephropathy, or Berger disease, is the most common cause of glomerular hematuria, accounting for about 30% of cases (Fassett et al, 1982). Therefore it is described in greater detail in this section. IgA nephropathy occurs most commonly in children and young adults, with a male predominance (Berger and Hinglais, 1968). Patients typically present with hematuria after an upper respiratory tract infection or exercise. Hematuria may be associated with a low-grade fever or rash, but most patients have no associated systemic symptoms. Gross hematuria occurs intermittently, but microscopic hematuria is a constant finding in some patients. The disease is chronic, but the prognosis in most patients is excellent. Renal function remains normal in the majority, but about 25% will subsequently develop renal insufficiency. An older age at onset, initial abnormal renal function, consistent proteinuria, and hypertension are indicators of a poor prognosis (D'Amico, 1988).

The pathologic findings in Berger disease are limited to either focal glomeruli or lobular segments of a glomerulus. The changes are proliferative and usually confined to mesangial cells (Berger and Hinglais, 1968). Renal biopsy reveals deposits of IgA, IgG, and β_{1c}-globulin, although IgA and IgG mesangial deposits are found in other forms of glomerulonephritis as well. The role of IgA in the disease remains uncertain, although the deposits may trigger an inflammatory reaction within the glomerulus (van den Wall Bake et al, 1989). Because gross hematuria frequently follows an upper respiratory tract infection, a viral etiology has been suspected but not established. The frequent association between hematuria and exercise in this condition remains unexplained.

The clinical presentation of IgA glomerulonephritis is alarming and similar to certain systemic diseases, including Schönlein-Henoch purpura, systemic lupus erythematosus, bacterial endocarditis, and Goodpasture syndrome. Therefore a careful clinical and laboratory evaluation is indicated to establish the correct diagnosis. The presence of RBC casts establishes the glomerular origin of the hematuria. In the absence of casts, a urologic evaluation is indicated to exclude the urinary tract as a source of bleeding and to confirm that the hematuria is arising from both kidneys. The diagnosis of IgA nephropathy is confirmed by renal biopsy demonstrating the classic deposits of immunoglobulins in mesangial cells, as described previously. Once the diagnosis has been established, repeat evaluations for hematuria are generally not indicated. Although there is no effective treatment for this condition, renal function remains stable in most patients and there are no other known long-term complications.

TABLE 1-4 Glomerular Disorders in Patients with Glomerular Hematuria

DISORDER	PATIENTS
IgA nephropathy (Berger disease)	30
Mesangioproliferative GN	14
Focal segmental proliferative GN	13
Familial nephritis (e.g., Alport syndrome)	11
Membranous GN	7
Mesangiocapillary GN	6
Focal segmental sclerosis	4
Unclassifiable	4
Systemic lupus erythematosus	3
Postinfectious GN	2
Subacute bacterial endocarditis	2
Others	4
TOTAL	100

GN, glomerulonephritis; IgA, immunoglobulin A.
Modified from Fassett RG, Horgan BA, Mathew TH. Detection of glomerular bleeding by phase-contrast microscopy. Lancet 1982;1:1432.

Nonglomerular Hematuria

Medical. Except for renal tumors, nonglomerular hematuria of renal origin is secondary to either tubulointerstitial, renovascular,

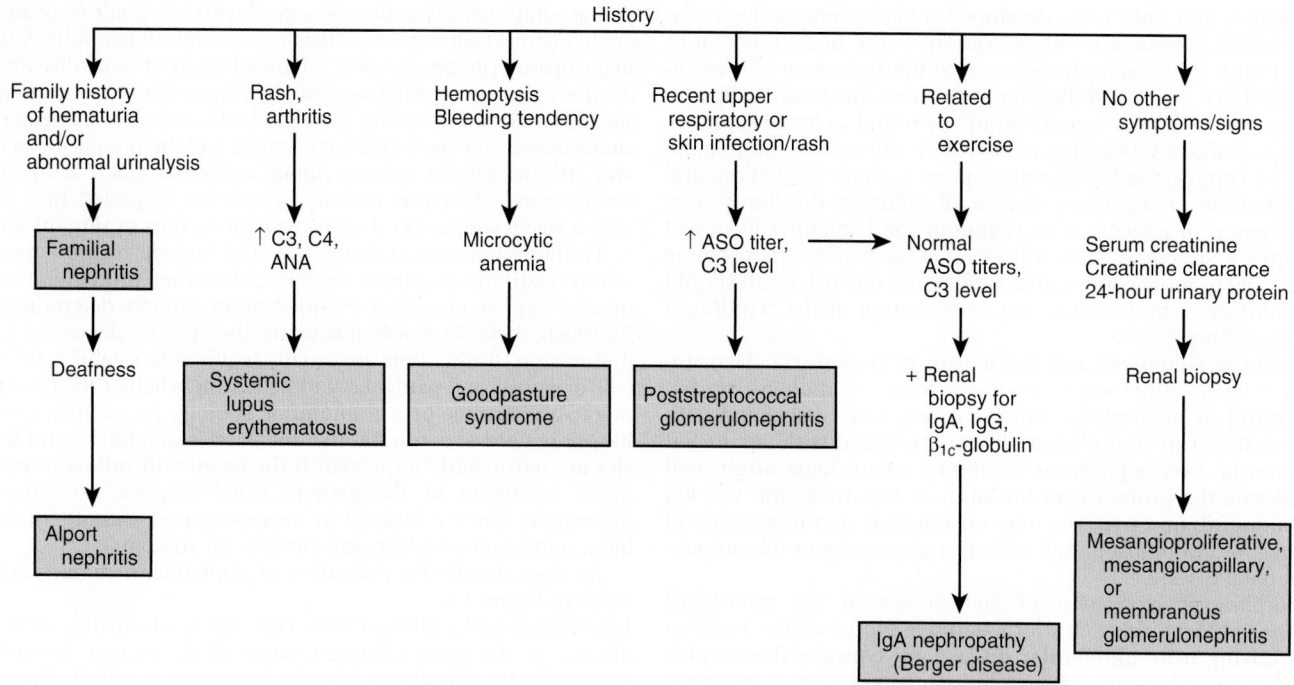

Figure 1-6. **Evaluation of glomerular hematuria (dysmorphic erythrocytes, erythrocyte casts, and proteinuria). ANA, antinuclear antibody; ASO, antistreptolysin O; Ig, immunoglobulin.**

or systemic disorders. **The urinalysis in nonglomerular hematuria is distinguished from that of glomerular hematuria by the presence of circular erythrocytes and the absence of erythrocyte casts.** Like glomerular hematuria, nonglomerular hematuria of renal origin is frequently associated with significant proteinuria, which distinguishes these nephrologic diseases from urologic diseases in which the degree of proteinuria is usually minimal, even with heavy bleeding.

As with glomerular hematuria, a careful history frequently helps establish the diagnosis. A family history of hematuria or bleeding tendency suggests the diagnosis of a blood dyscrasia, which should be investigated further. A family history of urolithiasis associated with intermittent hematuria may indicate stone disease, which should be investigated with serum and urine measurements of calcium and uric acid. A family history of renal cystic disease should prompt further radiologic evaluation for medullary sponge kidney and adult polycystic kidney disease. **Papillary necrosis as a cause of hematuria should be considered in diabetics, African-Americans (secondary to sickle cell disease or trait), and suspected analgesic abusers.**

Medications may induce hematuria, particularly anticoagulants. **Anticoagulation at normal therapeutic levels, however, does not predispose patients to hematuria.** In one study, the prevalence of hematuria was 3.2% in anticoagulated patients versus 4.8% in a control group. Urologic disease was identified in 81% of patients with more than one episode of microscopic hematuria, and the cause of hematuria did not vary between groups (Culclasure et al, 1994). Thus anticoagulant therapy per se does not appear to increase the risk of hematuria unless the patient is excessively anticoagulated.

Exercise-induced hematuria is being observed with increasing frequency. It typically occurs in long-distance runners (>10 km), is usually noted at the conclusion of the run, and rapidly disappears with rest. The hematuria may be of renal or bladder origin. An increased number of dysmorphic erythrocytes have been noted in some patients, suggesting a glomerular origin. Exercise-induced hematuria may be the first sign of underlying glomerular disease such as IgA nephropathy. Conversely, cystoscopy in patients with

exercise-induced hematuria frequently reveals punctate hemorrhagic lesions in the bladder, suggesting that the hematuria is of bladder origin.

Vascular disease may also result in nonglomerular hematuria. Renal artery embolism and thrombosis, arteriovenous fistulae, and renal vein thrombosis may all result in hematuria. Physical examination may reveal severe hypertension, a flank or abdominal bruit, or atrial fibrillation. In such patients, further evaluation for renal vascular disease should be undertaken.

An algorithm for the evaluation of nonglomerular hematuria is provided in Figure 1-7.

Surgical. Nonglomerular hematuria or essential hematuria includes primarily urologic rather than nephrologic diseases. Common causes of essential hematuria include urologic tumors, stones, and UTIs.

The urinalysis in both nonglomerular medical and surgical hematuria is similar in that both are characterized by circular erythrocytes and the absence of erythrocyte casts. Essential hematuria is suggested, however, by the absence of significant proteinuria usually found in nonglomerular hematuria of renal parenchymal origin. It should be remembered, however, that proteinuria is not always present in glomerular or nonglomerular renal disease.

The AUA Best Practice Policy Panel on Microscopic Hematuria has formulated practice recommendations for the detection and evaluation of asymptomatic microscopic hematuria (Grossfeld et al, 2001a, 2001b). The panel concluded that, due to the lack of specificity of urinary dipstick examination, as well as the risk and expense of evaluation, patients with a positive dipstick test should only undergo complete evaluation for hematuria if this is confirmed by the finding of 3 or more RBCs/HPF on subsequent microscopic evaluation. The mainstays of evaluation, according to the panel, are voided urinary cytology, cystoscopy, and urinary tract imaging using ultrasonography, CT, and/or intravenous urography (IVU). The use of these tests in an individual patient should be based in most cases on the relative risk of significant urinary tract pathology.

An algorithm for the evaluation of essential hematuria is provided in Figure 1-8.

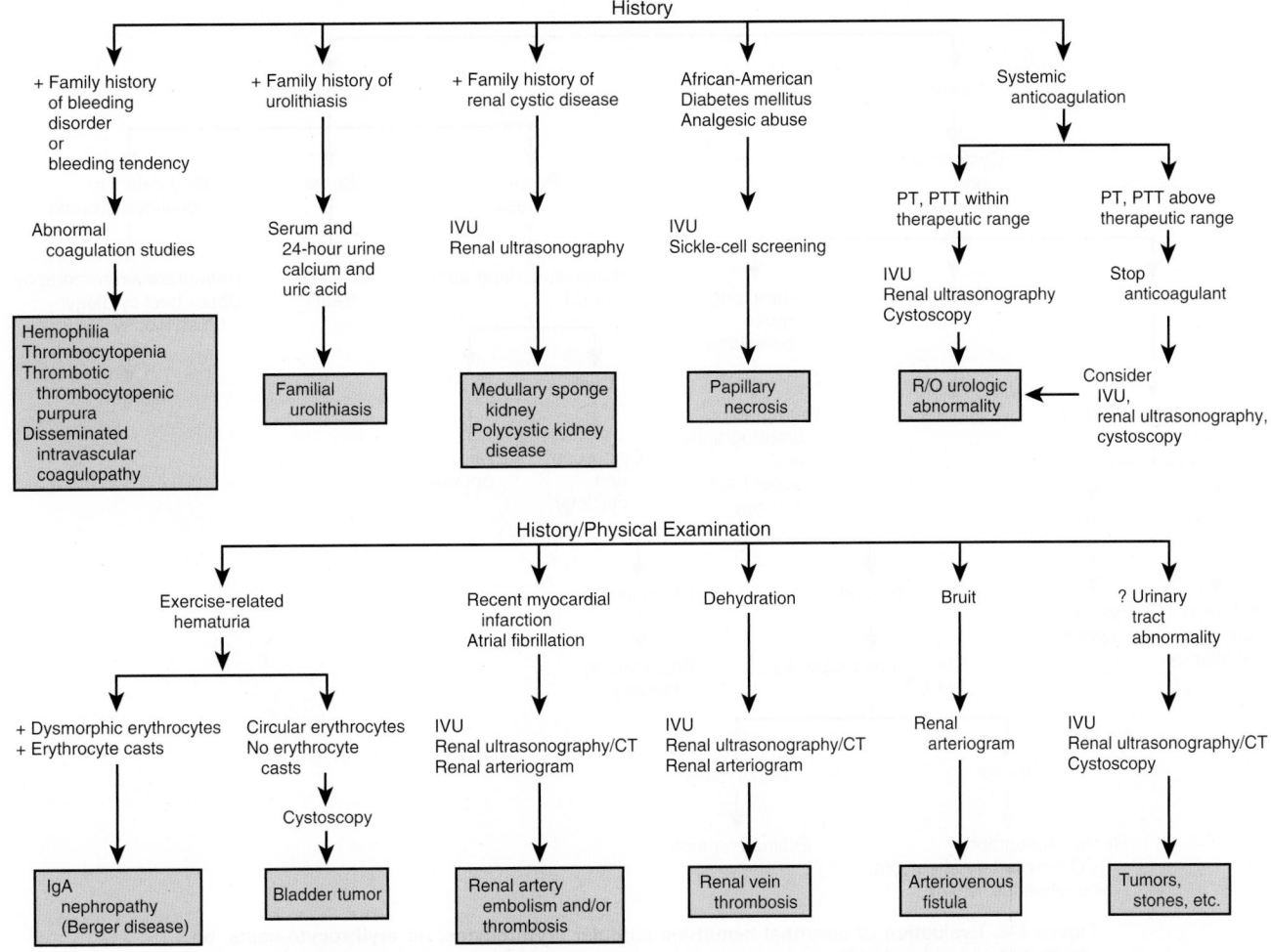

Figure 1-7. Evaluation of nonglomerular renal hematuria (circular erythrocytes, no erythrocyte casts, and proteinuria). CT, computed tomography; IgA, immunoglobulin A; IVU, intravenous urography; PT, prothrombin time; PTT, partial thromboplastin time; R/O, rule out.

Proteinuria

Although healthy adults excrete 80 to 150 mg of protein in the urine daily, the qualitative detection of proteinuria in the urinalysis should raise the suspicion of underlying renal disease. **Proteinuria may be the first indication of renovascular, glomerular, or tubulointerstitial renal disease, or it may represent the overflow of abnormal proteins into the urine in conditions such as multiple myeloma.** Proteinuria can also occur secondary to nonrenal disorders and in response to various physiologic conditions such as strenuous exercise.

The protein concentration in the urine depends on the state of hydration, but it seldom exceeds 20 mg/dL. In patients with dilute urine, however, significant proteinuria may be present at concentrations less than 20 mg/dL. **Normally, urine protein is about 30% albumin, 30% serum globulins, and 40% tissue proteins, of which the major component is Tamm-Horsfall protein.** This profile may be altered by conditions that affect glomerular filtration, tubular reabsorption, or excretion of urine protein. Determination of the urine protein profile by such techniques as protein electrophoresis may help determine the etiology of proteinuria.

Pathophysiology. **Most causes of proteinuria can be categorized into one of three categories: glomerular, tubular, or overflow. Glomerular proteinuria is the most common type of proteinuria and results from increased glomerular capillary permeability to protein, especially albumin.** Glomerular proteinuria occurs in any of the primary glomerular diseases such as IgA nephropathy or in glomerulopathy associated with systemic illness such as diabetes

mellitus. Glomerular disease should be suspected when the 24-hour urine protein excretion exceeds 1 g and is almost certain to exist when the total protein excretion exceeds 3 g.

Tubular proteinuria results from failure to reabsorb normally filtered proteins of low molecular weight such as immunoglobulins. In tubular proteinuria, the 24-hour urine protein loss seldom exceeds 2 to 3 g and the excreted proteins are of low molecular weight rather than albumin. Disorders that lead to tubular proteinuria are commonly associated with other defects of proximal tubular function such as glucosuria, aminoaciduria, phosphaturia, and uricosuria (Fanconi syndrome).

Overflow proteinuria occurs in the absence of any underlying renal disease and is due to an increased plasma concentration of abnormal immunoglobulins and other low-molecular-weight proteins. The increased serum levels of abnormal proteins result in excess glomerular filtration that exceeds tubular reabsorptive capacity. The most common cause of overflow proteinuria is multiple myeloma, in which large amounts of immunoglobulin light chains are produced and appear in the urine (Bence Jones protein).

Detection. Qualitative detection of abnormal proteinuria is most easily accomplished with a dipstick impregnated with tetrabromophenol blue dye. The color of the dye changes in response to a pH shift related to the protein content of the urine, mainly albumin, leading to the development of a blue color. Because the background of the dipstick is yellow, various shades of green will develop, and the darker the green, the greater the concentration of protein in the urine. The minimal detectable protein concentration by this method is 20 to 30 mg/dL. **False-negative results can occur in alkaline**

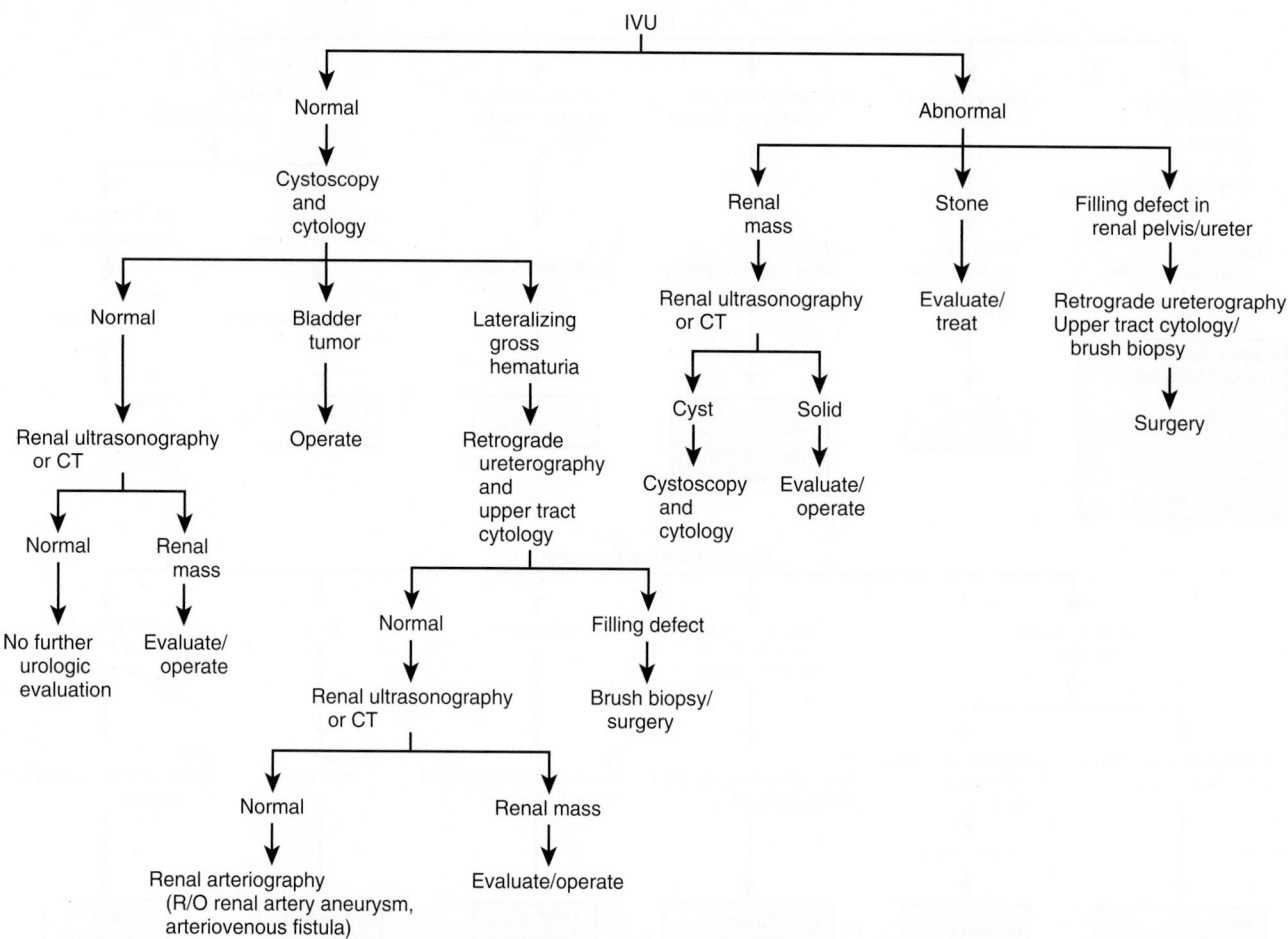

Figure 1-8. **Evaluation of essential hematuria (circular erythrocytes, no erythrocyte casts, no significant proteinuria). CT, computed tomography; IVU, intravenous urography; R/O, rule out.**

urine, dilute urine, or when the primary protein present is not albumin. Nephrotic range proteinuria in excess of 1 g/24 hr, however, is seldom missed on qualitative screening. Precipitation of urinary proteins with strong acids such as 3% sulfosalicylic acid will detect proteinuria at concentrations as low as 15 mg/dL and is more sensitive at detecting other proteins and albumin. Patients whose urine is negative on dipstick but strongly positive with sulfosalicylic acid should be suspected of having multiple myeloma, and the urine should be tested further for Bence Jones protein.

If qualitative testing reveals proteinuria, this should be quantitated with a 24-hour urinary collection. Further qualitative assessment of abnormal urinary proteins can be accomplished by either protein electrophoresis or immunoassay for specific proteins. **Protein electrophoresis is particularly helpful in distinguishing glomerular from tubular proteinuria. In glomerular proteinuria, albumin makes up about 70% of the total protein excreted, whereas in tubular proteinuria, the major proteins excreted are immunoglobulins with albumin making up only 10% to 20%. Immunoassay is the method of choice for detecting specific proteins such as Bence Jones protein in multiple myeloma.**

Evaluation. Proteinuria should first be classified by its timing into transient, intermittent, or persistent. Transient proteinuria occurs commonly, especially in the pediatric population, and usually resolves spontaneously within a few days (Wagner et al, 1968). It may result from fever, exercise, or emotional stress. In older patients, transient proteinuria may be due to congestive heart failure. If a nonrenal cause is identified and a subsequent urinalysis is negative, no further evaluation is necessary. If proteinuria persists, it should be evaluated further.

Proteinuria may also occur intermittently, and this is frequently related to postural change (Robinson, 1985). Proteinuria

that occurs only in the upright position is a frequent cause of mild, intermittent proteinuria in young males. Total daily protein excretion seldom exceeds 1 g, and urinary protein excretion returns to normal when the patient is recumbent. Orthostatic proteinuria is thought to be secondary to increased pressure on the renal vein while standing. It resolves spontaneously in about 50% of patients and is not associated with any morbidity. Therefore if renal function is normal in patients with orthostatic proteinuria, no further evaluation is indicated.

Persistent proteinuria requires further evaluation, and most cases have a glomerular etiology. A quantitative measurement of urinary protein should be obtained through a 24-hour urine collection, and a qualitative evaluation should be obtained to determine the major proteins excreted. The findings of greater than 2 g of protein excreted per 24 hours, of which the major components are high-molecular-weight proteins such as albumin, establish the diagnosis of glomerular proteinuria. Glomerular proteinuria is the most common cause of abnormal proteinuria, especially in patients presenting with persistent proteinuria. If glomerular proteinuria is associated with hematuria characterized by dysmorphic erythrocytes and erythrocyte casts, the patient should be evaluated as outlined previously for glomerular hematuria (see Fig. 1-6). Patients with glomerular proteinuria who have no or little associated hematuria should be evaluated for other conditions, of which the most common is diabetes mellitus. Other possibilities include amyloidosis and arteriolar nephrosclerosis.

In patients in whom total protein excretion is 300 to 2000 mg/day, of which the major components are low-molecular-weight globulins, further qualitative evaluation with immunoelectrophoresis is indicated. This will determine whether the excess proteins are normal or abnormal. Identification of normal proteins establishes a diagnosis of tubular proteinuria, and further evaluation for a specific cause of tubular dysfunction is indicated.

If qualitative evaluation reveals abnormal proteins in the urine, this establishes a diagnosis of overflow proteinuria. Further evaluation should be directed to identify the specific protein abnormality. The finding of large quantities of light-chain immunoglobulins or Bence Jones protein establishes a diagnosis of multiple myeloma. Similarly, the finding of large amounts of hemoglobin or myoglobin establishes the diagnosis of hemoglobinuria or myoglobinuria.

An algorithm for the evaluation of proteinuria is provided in Figure 1-9.

Glucose and Ketones

Urine testing for glucose and ketones is useful in screening patients for diabetes mellitus. Normally, almost all the glucose filtered by the glomeruli is reabsorbed in the proximal tubules. Although small amounts of glucose may normally be excreted in the urine, these amounts are not clinically significant and are below the level of detectability with the dipstick. If, however, the amount of glucose filtered exceeds the capacity of tubular reabsorption, glucose will be excreted in the urine and detected on the dipstick. **This so-called renal threshold corresponds to serum glucose of about 180 mg/dL; above this level, glucose will be detected in the urine.**

Glucose detection with the urinary dipstick is based on a double sequential enzymatic reaction yielding a colorimetric change. In the first reaction, glucose in the urine reacts with glucose oxidase on the dipstick to form gluconic acid and hydrogen peroxide. In the second reaction, hydrogen peroxide reacts with peroxidase, causing oxidation of the chromogen on the dipstick, producing a color change. **This double-oxidative reaction is specific for glucose, and there is no cross-reactivity with other sugars.** The dipstick test becomes less sensitive as the urine increases in specific gravity and temperature.

Ketones are not normally found in the urine but will appear when the carbohydrate supplies in the body are depleted and body fat breakdown occurs. This happens most commonly in diabetic ketoacidosis but may also occur during pregnancy and after periods of starvation or rapid weight reduction. **Ketones excreted include acetoacetic acid, acetone, and β-hydroxybutyric acid. With abnormal fat breakdown, ketones will appear in the urine before the serum.**

Dipstick testing for ketones involves a colorimetric reaction: Sodium nitroprusside on the dipstick reacts with acetoacetic acid to produce a purple color. **Dipstick testing will identify acetoacetic acid at concentrations of 5 to 10 mg/dL but will not detect acetone or β-hydroxybutyric acid.** A dipstick that tests positively for glucose should also be tested for ketones, and diabetes mellitus is suggested. False-positive results, however, can occur in acidic urine of high specific gravity, in abnormally colored urine, and in urine containing levodopa metabolites, 2-mercaptoethane sulfonate sodium, and other sulfhydryl-containing compounds (Csako, 1987).

Bilirubin and Urobilinogen

Normal urine contains no bilirubin and only small amounts of urobilinogen. There are two types of bilirubin: direct (conjugated) and indirect. Direct bilirubin is made in the hepatocyte, where bilirubin is conjugated with glucuronic acid. **Conjugated bilirubin has a low molecular weight, is water soluble, and normally passes from the liver into the small intestine through the bile ducts, where it is converted to urobilinogen. Therefore conjugated bilirubin does not appear in the urine except in pathologic conditions in which there is intrinsic hepatic disease or obstruction of the bile ducts.**

Indirect bilirubin is of high molecular weight and bound in the serum to albumin. It is water insoluble and therefore does not appear in the urine even in pathologic conditions.

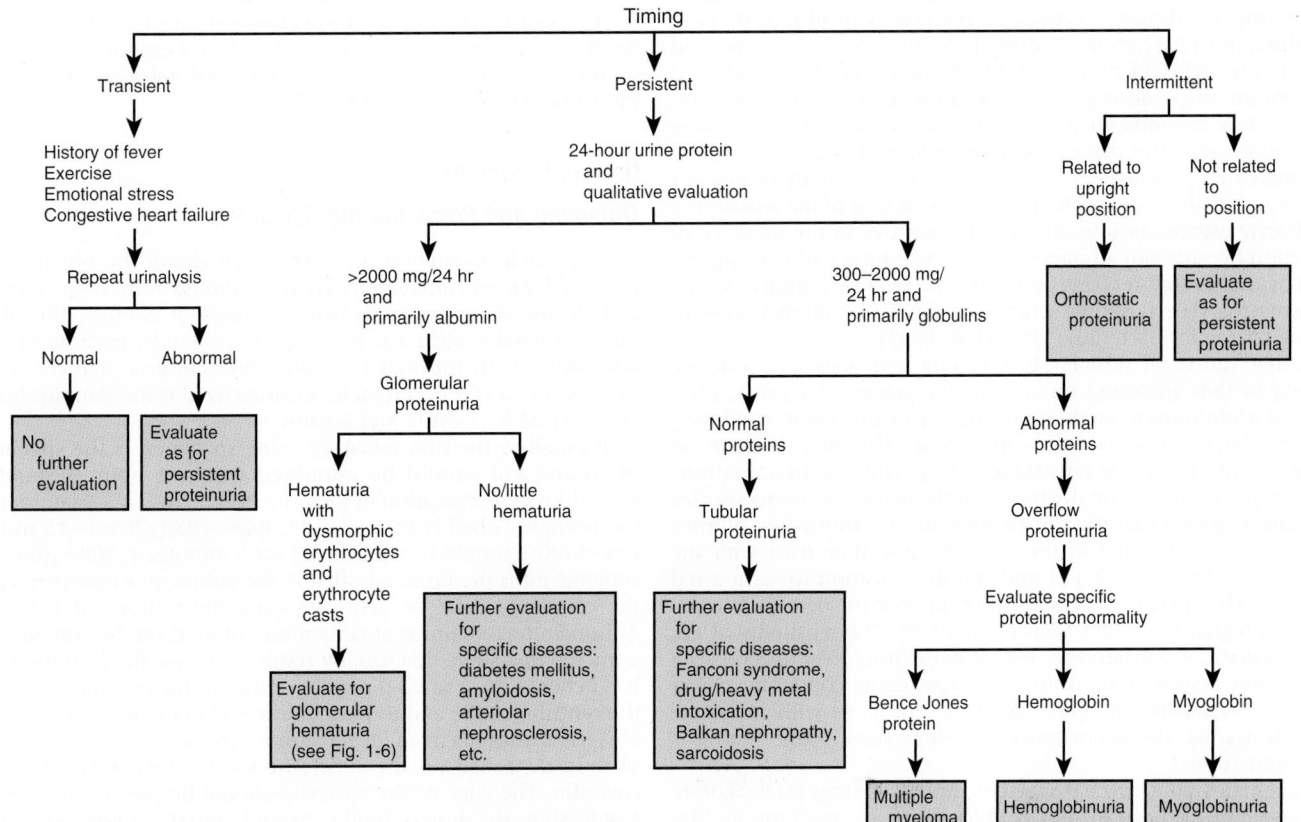

Figure 1-9. **Evaluation of proteinuria.**

Urobilinogen is the end product of conjugated bilirubin metabolism. Conjugated bilirubin passes through the bile ducts, where it is metabolized by normal intestinal bacteria to urobilinogen. Normally, about 50% of the urobilinogen is excreted in the stool and 50% is reabsorbed into the enterohepatic circulation. A small amount of absorbed urobilinogen, about 1 to 4 mg/day, will escape hepatic uptake and be excreted in the urine. Hemolysis and hepatocellular diseases that lead to increased bile pigments can result in increased urinary urobilinogen. Conversely, obstruction of the bile duct or antibiotic usage that alters intestinal flora, thereby interfering with the conversion of conjugated bilirubin to urobilinogen, will decrease urobilinogen levels in the urine. In these conditions, serum levels of conjugated bilirubin rise.

There are different dipstick reagents and methods to test for both bilirubin and urobilinogen, but the basic physiologic principle involves the binding of bilirubin or urobilinogen to a diazonium salt to produce a colorimetric reaction. False-negative results can occur in the presence of ascorbic acid, which decreases the sensitivity for detection of bilirubin. False-positive results can occur in the presence of phenazopyridine because it colors the urine orange and, similar to the colorimetric reaction for bilirubin, turns red in an acid medium.

Leukocyte Esterase and Nitrite Tests

Leukocyte esterase activity indicates the presence of white blood cells in the urine. The presence of nitrites in the urine is strongly suggestive of bacteriuria. Thus both of these tests have been used to screen patients for UTIs. Although these tests may have application in nonurologic medical practice, the most accurate method to diagnose infection is by microscopic examination of the urinary sediment to identify pyuria and subsequent urine culture. All urologists should be capable of performing and interpreting the microscopic examination of the urinary sediment. Therefore leukocyte esterase and nitrite testing are less important in a urologic practice. For purposes of completion, however, both techniques are described briefly herein.

Leukocyte esterase and nitrite testing are performed using the Chemstrip LN dipstick. Leukocyte esterase is produced by neutrophils and catalyzes the hydrolysis of an indoxyl carbonic acid ester to indoxyl (Gillenwater, 1981). The indoxyl formed oxidizes a diazonium salt chromogen on the dipstick to produce a color change. It is recommended that leukocyte esterase testing be done 5 minutes after the dipstick is immersed in the urine to allow adequate incubation (Shaw et al, 1985). The sensitivity of this test subsequently decreases with time because of lysis of the leukocytes. Leukocyte esterase testing may also be negative in the presence of infection because not all patients with bacteriuria will have significant pyuria. Therefore if one uses leukocyte esterase testing to screen patients for UTI, it should always be done in conjunction with nitrite testing for bacteriuria (Pels et al, 1989).

Other causes of false-negative results with leukocyte esterase testing include increased urinary specific gravity, glycosuria, presence of urobilinogen, medications that alter urine color, and ingestion of large amounts of ascorbic acid. **The major cause of false-positive leukocyte esterase tests is specimen contamination.**

Nitrites are not normally found in the urine, but many species of gram-negative bacteria can convert nitrates to nitrites. Nitrites can readily be detected in the urine because they react with the reagents on the dipstick and undergo diazotization to form a red azo dye. The specificity of the nitrite dipstick for detecting bacteriuria is higher than 90% (Pels et al, 1989). The sensitivity of the test, however, is considerably less, varying from 35% to 85%. The nitrite test is less accurate in urine specimens containing fewer than 10^5 organisms/mL (Kellogg et al, 1987). As with leukocyte esterase testing, the major cause of false-positive nitrite testing is contamination.

It remains controversial whether dipstick testing for leukocyte esterase and nitrites can replace microscopy in screening for significant UTIs. This issue is less important to urologists, who usually have access to a microscope and who should be trained and

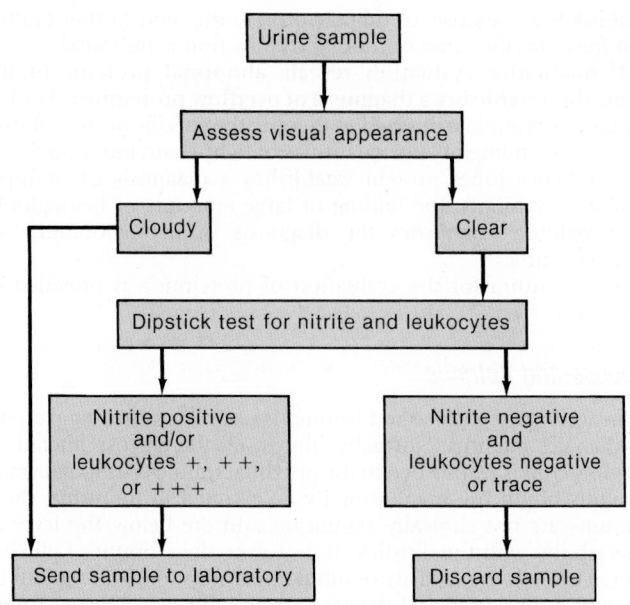

Figure 1-10. Protocol for determining the need for urine sediment microscopy in an asymptomatic population. (From Flanagan PG, Rooney PG, Davies EA, et al. Evaluation of four screening tests for bacteriuria in elderly people. Lancet 1989;1:1117. © by The Lancet Ltd., 1989.)

encouraged to examine the urinary sediment. **A protocol combining the visual appearance of the urine with leukocyte esterase and nitrite testing has been proposed** (Fig. 1-10). It reportedly detects 95% of infected urine specimens and decreases the need for microscopy by as much as 30% (Flanagan et al, 1989). Other studies, however, have shown that dipstick testing is not an adequate replacement for microscopy (Propp et al, 1989). In summary, it has not been demonstrated conclusively that dipstick testing for UTI can replace microscopic examination of the urinary sediment. In our personal experience, we always examine the urinary sediment whenever we suspect a UTI and subsequently culture the urine when pyuria is identified.

Urinary Sediment

Obtaining and Preparing the Specimen

A clean-catch midstream urine specimen should be obtained. As described earlier, uncircumcised men should retract the prepuce and cleanse the glans penis before voiding. It is more difficult to obtain a reliable clean-catch specimen in females because of contamination with introital leukocytes and bacteria. If there is any suspicion of a UTI in a female, a catheterized urine sample should be obtained for culture and sensitivity.

If possible, **the first morning urine specimen is the specimen of choice and should be examined within 1 hour.** A standard procedure for preparation of the urine for microscopic examination has been described (Cushner and Copley, 1989). Ten to 15 milliliters of urine should be centrifuged for 5 minutes at 3000 rpm. The supernatant is then poured off, and the sediment is resuspended in the centrifuge tube by gently tapping the bottom of the tube. Although the remaining small amount of fluid can be poured onto a microscope slide, this usually results in excess fluid on the slide. It is better to use a small pipette to withdraw the residual fluid from the centrifuge tube and to place it directly on the microscope slide. This usually results in an ideal volume of between 0.01 and 0.02 mL of fluid deposited on the slide. The slide is then covered with a coverslip. The edge of the coverslip should be placed on the slide first to allow the drop of fluid to ascend onto the coverslip by capillary action. The coverslip is then gently placed over the drop of fluid, and this technique allows for most of the air between the drop of fluid and the coverslip to be expelled. If one simply drops the coverslip over the urine, the urine will disperse over the slide and there will be a considerable number of air bubbles that may distort the subsequent microscopic examination.

Microscopy Technique

Microscopic analysis of the urinary sediment should be performed with both low-power (×100 magnification) and high-power (×400 magnification) lenses. The use of an oil immersion lens for higher magnification is seldom, if ever, necessary. Under low power, the entire area under the coverslip should be scanned. **Particular attention should be given to the edges of the coverslip, where casts and other elements tend to be concentrated.** Low-power magnification is sufficient to identify erythrocytes, leukocytes, casts, cystine crystals, oval fat macrophages, and parasites such as *Trichomonas vaginalis* and *Schistosoma hematobium*.

High-power magnification is necessary to distinguish circular from dysmorphic erythrocytes, to identify other types of crystals, and, particularly, to identify bacteria and yeast. In summary, **the urinary sediment should be examined microscopically for (1) cells, (2) casts, (3) crystals, (4) bacteria, (5) yeast, and (6) parasites.**

Cells

Erythrocyte morphology may be determined under high-power magnification. Although phase contrast microscopy has been used for this purpose, circular (nonglomerular) erythrocytes can generally be distinguished from dysmorphic (glomerular) erythrocytes under routine brightfield high-power magnification (Figs. 1-11 to 1-15). **This is assisted by adjusting the microscope condenser to** its lowest aperture, thus reducing the intensity of background light. This allows one to see fine detail not evident otherwise and also creates the effect of phase microscopy because cell membranes and other sedimentary components stand out against the darkened background.**

Circular erythrocytes generally have an even distribution of hemoglobin with either a round or crenated contour, whereas dysmorphic erythrocytes are irregularly shaped with minimal hemoglobin and irregular distribution of cytoplasm. Automated techniques for performing microscopic analysis to distinguish the two types of erythrocytes have been investigated but have not yet been accepted into general urologic practice and are probably unnecessary. In one study using a standard Coulter counter, microscopic analysis was found to be 97% accurate in differentiating between the two types of erythrocytes (Sayer et al, 1990). **Erythrocytes may be confused with yeast or fat droplets** (Fig. 1-16). Erythrocytes can be distinguished, however, because yeast will show budding and oil droplets are highly refractile.

Leukocytes can generally be identified under low power and definitively diagnosed under high-power magnification (Figs. 1-17 and 1-18; see also Fig. 1-16). It is normal to find 1 or 2 leukocytes/HPF in men and up to 5/HPF in women in whom the urine sample may be contaminated with vaginal secretions. A greater number of leukocytes generally indicates infection or inflammation in the urinary tract. It may be possible to distinguish **old leukocytes, which have a characteristic small and wrinkled appearance** and which are commonly found in the vaginal secretions of normal women, from fresh leukocytes, which are generally indicative of urinary tract pathology. Fresh leukocytes are generally larger and

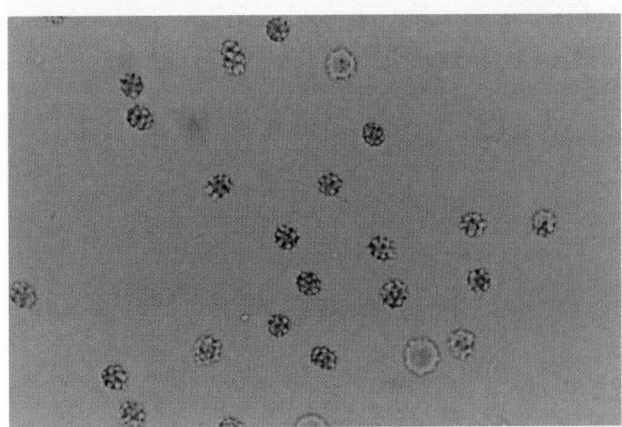

Figure 1-13. **Red blood cells from a patient with interstitial cystitis. Cells were collected at cystoscopy.**

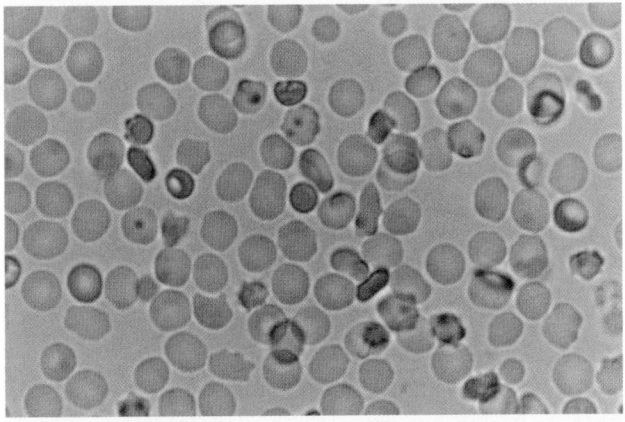

Figure 1-11. **Red blood cells, both smoothly rounded and mildly crenated, typical of epithelial erythrocytes.**

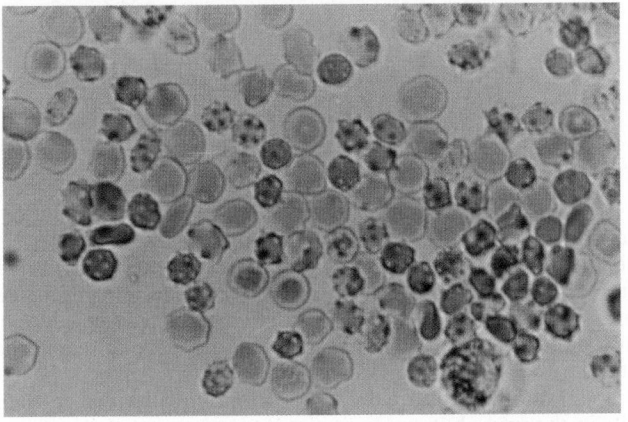

Figure 1-12. **Red blood cells from a patient with a bladder tumor.**

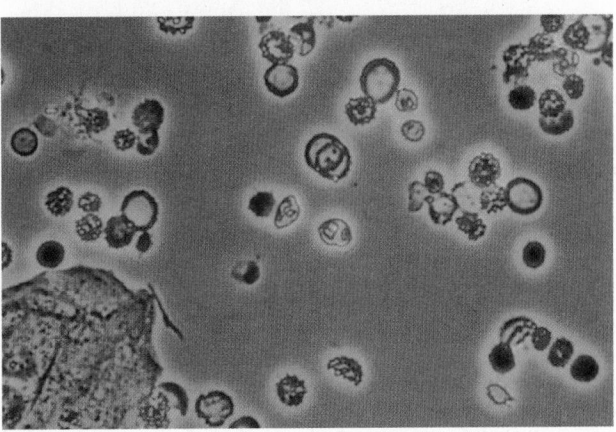

Figure 1-14. **Red blood cells from a patient with Berger disease. Note variations in membranes characteristic of dysmorphic red blood cells.**

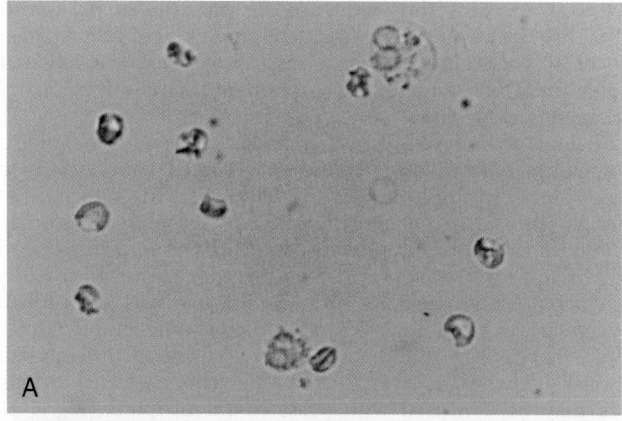

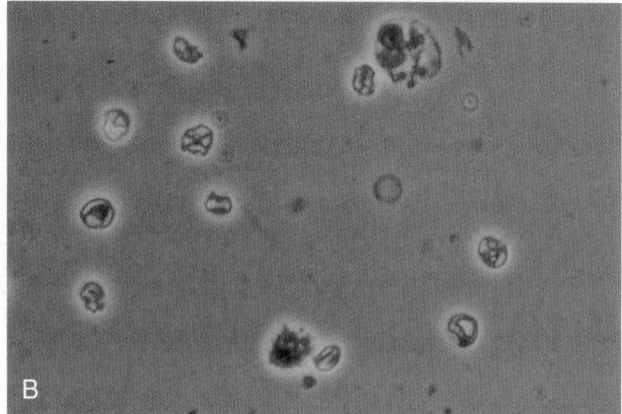

Figure 1-15. Dysmorphic red blood cells from a patient with Wegener granulomatosis. A, Brightfield illumination. B, Phase illumination. Note irregular deposits of dense cytoplasmic material around the cell membrane.

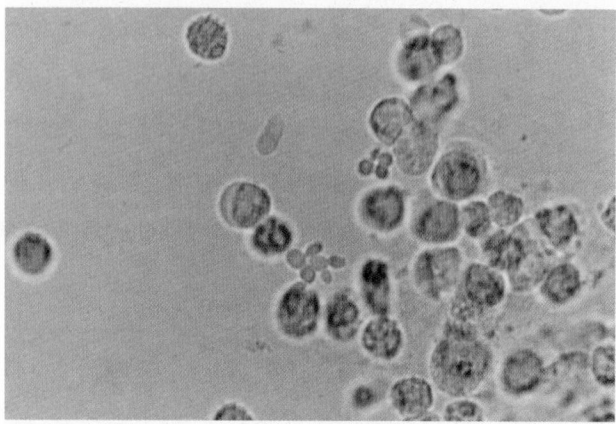

Figure 1-16. *Candida albicans*. Budding forms surrounded by leukocytes.

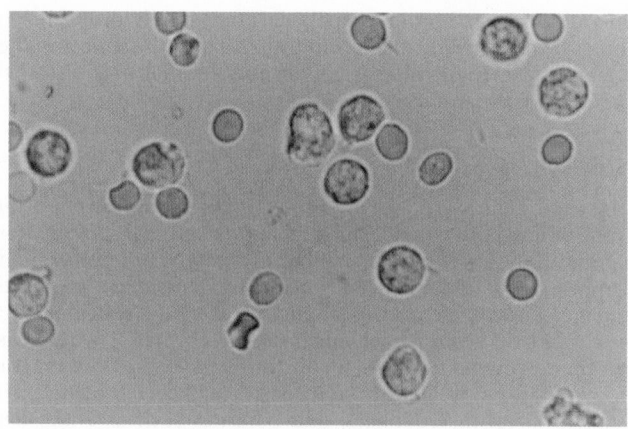

Figure 1-17. **Old leukocytes. Staghorn calculi with *Proteus* infection.**

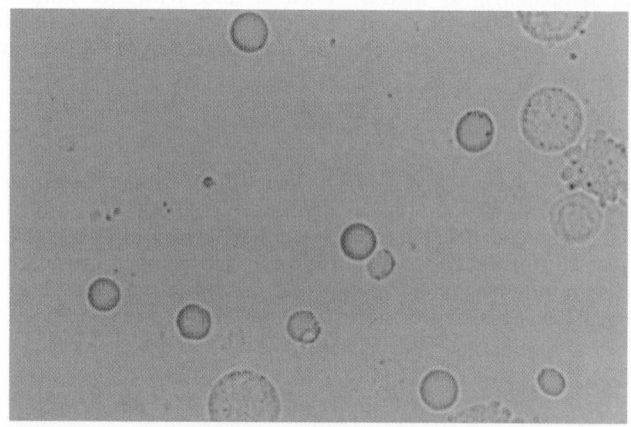

Figure 1-18. **Fresh "glitter cells" with erythrocytes in background.**

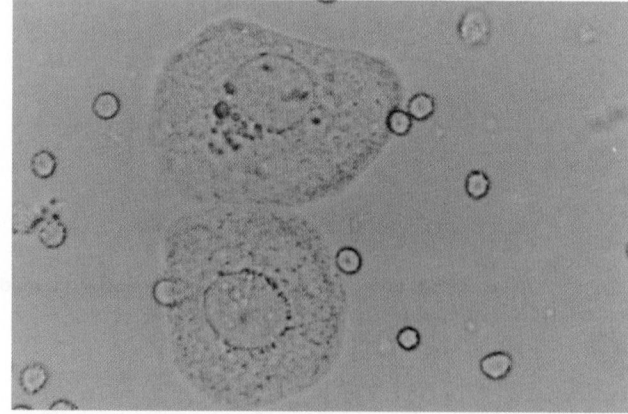

Figure 1-19. Transitional epithelial cells from bladder lavage.

rounder, and, when the specific gravity is less than 1.019, the granules in the cytoplasm demonstrate glitterlike movement, so-called glitter cells.

Epithelial cells are commonly observed in the urinary sediment. Squamous cells are frequently detected in female urine specimens and are derived from the lower portion of the urethra, the trigone of postpubertal females, and the vagina. **Squamous epithelial cells are large, have a central small nucleus about the size of an erythrocyte, and have an irregular cytoplasm with fine granularity.**

Transitional epithelial cells may arise from the remainder of the urinary tract (Fig. 1-19). Transitional cells are smaller than squamous cells, have a larger nucleus, and demonstrate prominent cytoplasmic granules near the nucleus. Malignant transitional cells have altered nuclear size and morphology and can be identified with either routine Papanicolaou staining or automated flow cytometry.

Renal tubular cells are the least commonly observed epithelial cells in the urine but are most significant because their presence in the urine is always indicative of renal pathology. Renal tubular

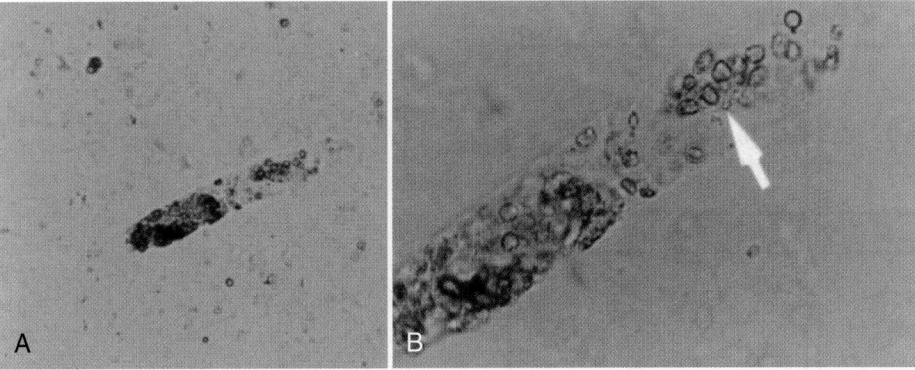

Figure 1-20. **Red blood cell cast. A, Low-power view demonstrates distinct border of hyaline matrix. B, High-power view demonstrates the sharply defined red blood cell membranes** *(arrow).* **Berger disease.**

cells may be difficult to distinguish from leukocytes, but they are slightly larger.

Casts

A cast is a protein coagulum that is formed in the renal tubule and traps any tubular luminal contents within the matrix. **Tamm-Horsfall mucoprotein is the basic matrix of all renal casts; it originates from tubular epithelial cells and is always present in the urine.** When the casts contain only mucoproteins, they are called *hyaline casts* and may not have any pathologic significance. Hyaline casts may be seen in the urine after exercise or heat exposure but may also be observed in pyelonephritis or chronic renal disease.

RBC casts contain entrapped erythrocytes and are diagnostic of glomerular bleeding, most likely secondary to glomerulonephritis (Figs. 1-20 and 1-21). White blood cell casts are observed in acute glomerulonephritis, acute pyelonephritis, and acute tubulointerstitial nephritis. Casts with other cellular elements, usually sloughed renal tubular epithelial cells, are indicative of nonspecific renal damage (Fig. 1-22). Granular and waxy casts result from further degeneration of cellular elements. Fatty casts are seen in nephrotic syndrome, lipiduria, and hypothyroidism.

Crystals

Identification of crystals in the urine is particularly important in patients with stone disease because it may help determine the etiology (Fig. 1-23). Although other types of crystals may be seen in normal patients, **the identification of cystine crystals establishes the diagnosis of cystinuria.** Crystals precipitated in acidic urine include calcium oxalate, uric acid, and cystine. Crystals precipitated in an alkaline urine include calcium phosphate and triple-phosphate (struvite) crystals. Cholesterol crystals are rarely seen in the urine and are not related to urinary pH. They occur in lipiduria and remain in droplet form.

Bacteria

Normal urine should not contain bacteria; in a fresh uncontaminated specimen, the finding of bacteria is indicative of a UTI. Because each HPF views between 1/20,000 and 1/50,000 mL, each bacterium seen per HPF signifies a bacterial count of more than 30,000/mL. Therefore, **5 bacteria/HPF reflects colony counts of about 100,000/mL.** This is the standard concentration used to establish the diagnosis of a UTI in a clean-catch specimen. This level should apply only to women, however, in whom a clean-catch specimen is frequently contaminated. The finding of any bacteria in a properly collected midstream specimen from a male should be further evaluated with a urine culture.

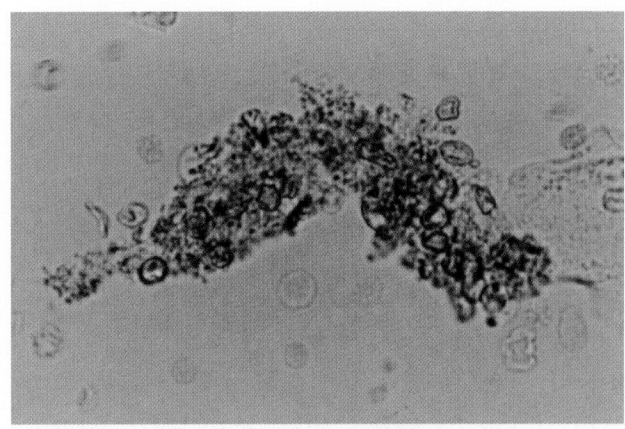

Figure 1-21. **Red blood cell cast.**

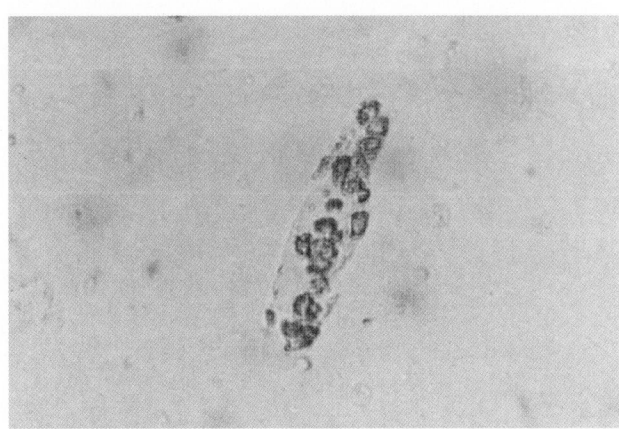

Figure 1-22. **Cellular cast. Cells entrapped in a hyaline matrix.**

Under high power, it is possible to distinguish various bacteria. Gram-negative rods have a characteristic bacillary shape (Fig. 1-24), whereas streptococci can be identified by their characteristic beaded chains (Figs. 1-25 and 1-26) and staphylococci can be identified when the organisms are found in clumps (Fig. 1-27).

Yeast

The most common yeast cells found in urine are *Candida albicans.* The biconcave oval shape of yeast can be confused with

Crystals

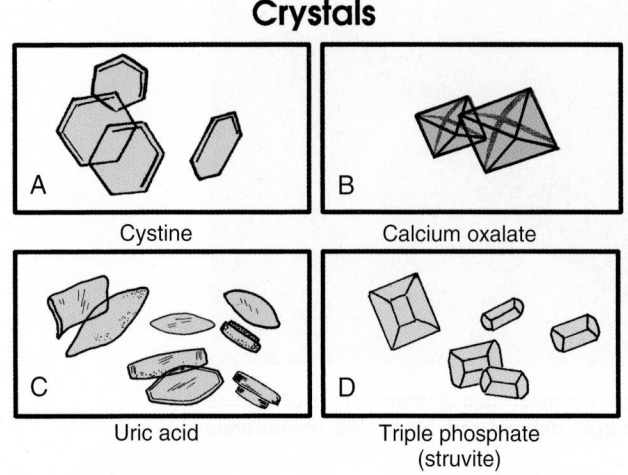

Figure 1-23. Urinary crystals. A, Cystine. B, Calcium oxalate. C, Uric acid. D, Triple phosphate (struvite).

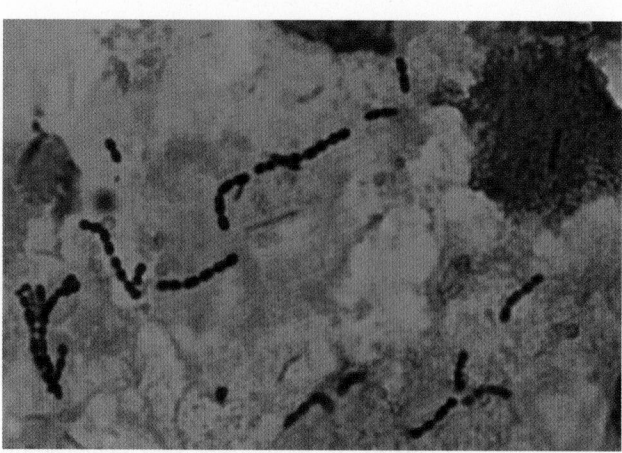

Figure 1-26. Streptococcal urinary tract infection (Gram stain).

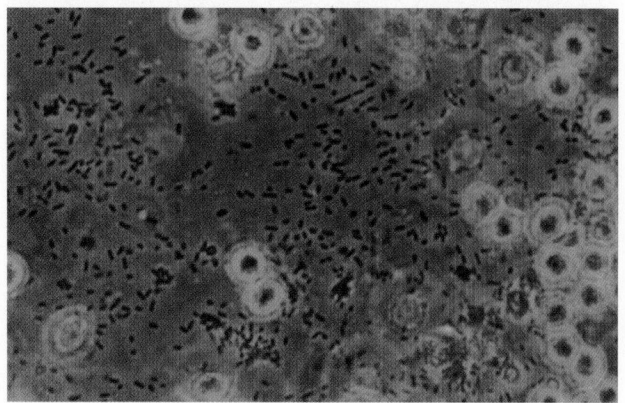

Figure 1-24. Gram-negative bacilli. Phase microscopy of *Escherichia coli*.

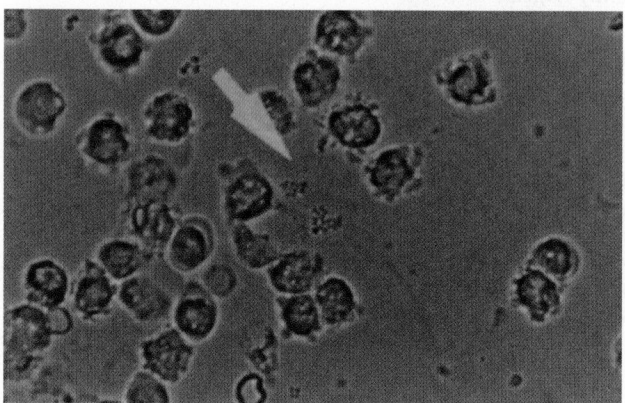

Figure 1-27. *Staphylococcus aureus* in typical clumps *(arrow)*.

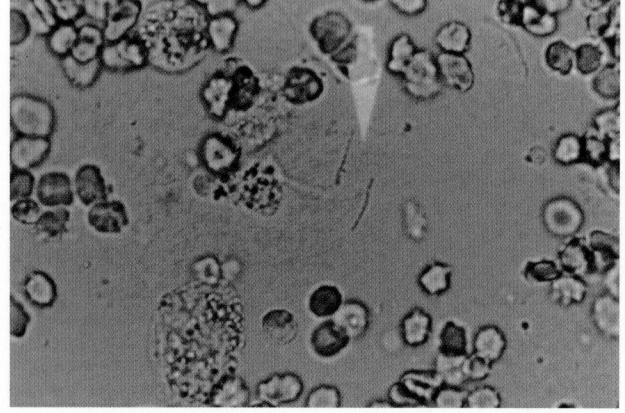

Figure 1-25. Streptococcal urinary tract infection with typical chain formation *(arrow)*.

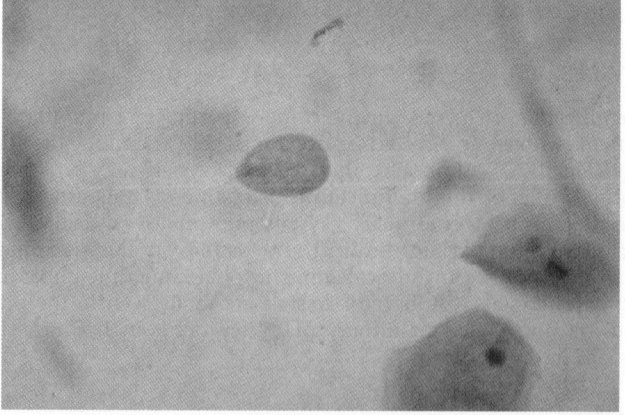

Figure 1-28. Trichomonad with ovoid shape and motile flagella.

Parasites

***Trichomonas vaginalis* is a frequent cause of vaginitis in women and occasionally of urethritis in men.** Trichomonads can be readily identified in a clean-catch specimen under low power (Fig. 1-28). Trichomonads are large cells with rapidly moving flagella that quickly propel the organism across the microscopic field.

erythrocytes and calcium oxalate crystals, but **yeasts can be distinguished by their characteristic budding and hyphae** (see Fig. 1-16). Yeasts are most commonly seen in the urine of patients with diabetes mellitus or as contaminants in women with vaginal candidiasis.

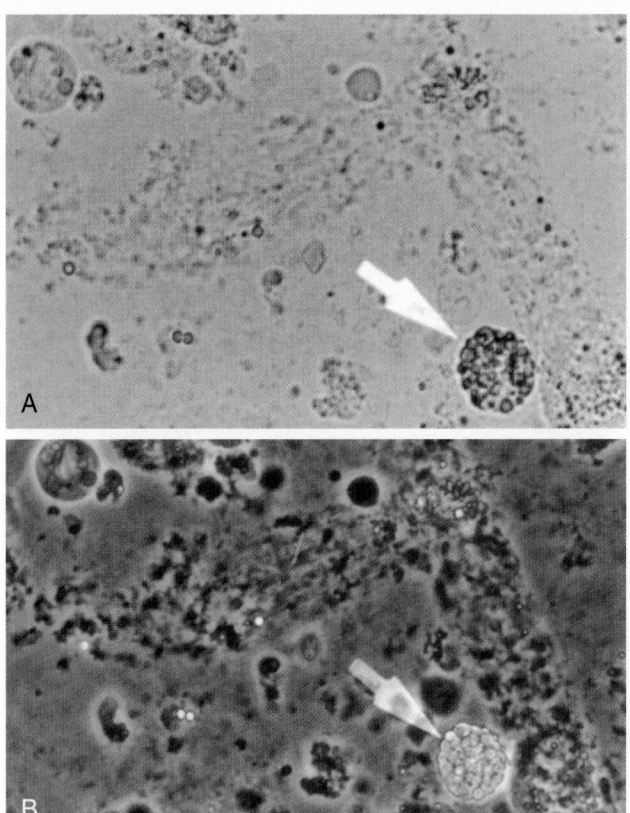

Figure 1-29. Oval fat macrophage. A, High-power view showing doubly refractile fat particles *(arrow)*. **B, Phase microscopy of the same specimen** *(arrow)*.

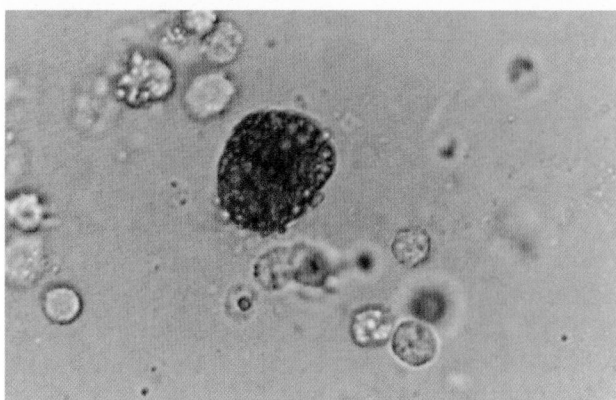

Figure 1-30. Oval fat macrophage, high-power view. Note the fine secretory granules in the prostatic fluid.

SUMMARY

This chapter has detailed the basic evaluation of the urologic patient, which should include a careful history, physical examination, and urinalysis. These three basic components form the cornerstone of the urologic evaluation and should precede any subsequent diagnostic procedures. After completion of the history, physical examination, and urinalysis, the urologist should be able to establish at least a differential, if not specific, diagnosis that will allow the subsequent diagnostic evaluation and treatment to be carried out in a direct and efficient manner.

REFERENCES

The complete reference list is available online at www.expertconsult.com.

SUGGESTED READINGS

Barry MJ, Fowler FJ Jr, O'Leary MP, et al. The American Urological Association symptom index for benign prostatic hyperplasia. J Urol 1992;148:1549.

Grossfeld GD, Litwin MS, Wolf JS Jr, et al. Evaluation of asymptomatic microscopic hematuria in adults: the American Urological Association best practice policy—part I: definition, prevalence, and etiology. Urology 2001a;57:599.

Grossfeld GD, Litwin MS, Wolf JS Jr, et al. Evaluation of asymptomatic microscopic hematuria in adults: the American Urological Association best practice policy—part II: patient evaluation, cytology, voided markers, imaging, cystoscopy, nephrology evaluation, and follow-up. Urology 2001b;57:604.

Mohr DN, Offord KP, Owen RA, et al. Asymptomatic microhematuria and urologic disease. A population-based study. JAMA 1986;256:224.

Pels RJ, Bor DH, Woolhandler S, et al. Dipstick urinalysis screening of asymptomatic adults for urinary tract disorders. II: Bacteriuria. JAMA 1989;262:1221.

Schramek P, Schuster FX, Georgopoulos M, et al. Value of urinary erythrocyte morphology in assessment of symptomless microhaematuria. Lancet 1989;2:1316.

Schistosoma hematobium is a urinary tract pathogen that is not found in the United States but is extremely common in countries of the Middle East and North Africa. Examination of the urine shows the characteristic parasitic ova with a terminal spike.

Expressed Prostatic Secretions

Although not strictly a component of the urinary sediment, the expressed prostatic secretions should be examined in any man suspected of having prostatitis. Normal prostatic fluid should contain few, if any, leukocytes, and the presence of a larger number or clumps of leukocytes is indicative of prostatitis. **Oval fat macrophages are found in postinfection prostatic fluid** (Figs. 1-29 and 1-30). Normal prostatic fluid contains numerous secretory granules that resemble but can be distinguished from leukocytes under high power because they do not have nuclei.

2

Urinary Tract Imaging: Basic Principles of Computed Tomography, Magnetic Resonance Imaging, and Plain Film

Jay T. Bishoff, MD, FACS, and Art R. Rastinehad, DO

Imaging continues to play an indispensable role in the diagnosis and management of urologic diseases. Because many urologic conditions cannot be assessed by physical examination, conventional radiography has long been critical to the diagnosis of conditions of the adrenals, kidneys, ureters, and bladder. The development of computed tomography (CT) imaging and the use of intravenous contrast agents have provided detailed anatomic, functional, and physiologic information about urologic conditions. In this chapter we will discuss the indications for imaging in urology with an emphasis on the underlying physical principles of the imaging modalities. The strengths and limitations of each modality, as well as the techniques necessary to maximize image quality and minimize the risks and harms to urologic patients, are discussed.

CONVENTIONAL RADIOGRAPHY

Conventional radiography, although eclipsed by CT and magnetic resonance imaging (MRI) for certain indications, remains useful for preoperative diagnosis and postoperative evaluation in a variety of different urologic conditions. Conventional radiography includes abdominal plain radiography, intravenous excretory urography, retrograde pyelography, loopography, retrograde urethrography, and cystography. Urologists frequently perform and interpret conventional radiography examinations, including fluoroscopic examinations, in the office and operating room environments.

Physics

It is important for urologists to understand the physics of conventional radiography and fluoroscopy, as well as the implications and dangers of radiation exposure to the patient and the operator. The underlying physical principles of conventional radiography involve emitting a stream of photons from an x-ray source. These photons travel through the air and strike tissue, imparting energy to that tissue. Some of the photons emerge from the patient with varying amounts of energy attenuation and strike an image recorder such as a film cassette or the input phosphor of an image-intensifier tube, thus producing an image (Fig. 2-1).

RADIATION MANAGEMENT IN URORADIOLOGY

When diagnostic radiation passes through tissue, it creates ion pairs. The resultant charge per unit mass of air is referred to as the **radiation exposure**. The current unit of radiation exposure is coulombs(C)/kg. **Absorbed dose** is the energy absorbed from the radiation exposure and is measured in units called gray (Gy). The older unit of absorbed dose was called the rad (1 rad =100 Gy).

Because different types of radiation have different types of interaction with tissue, a conversion factor is applied to better express the amount of energy absorbed by a given tissue. The application of this conversion factor to the **absorbed dose** yields the **equivalent dose** measured in sieverts (Sv). For diagnostic x-rays the conversion factor is 1, so the absorbed dose is the same as the equivalent dose. When discussing the amount of radiation energy absorbed by patients during therapeutic radiation, the dose is given in gray. When discussing exposure to patients or medical personnel because of diagnostic ionizing radiation procedures, the dose is given in sieverts.

The distribution of energy absorption in the human body will be different based on the body part being imaged and a variety of other factors. The most important risk of radiation exposure from diagnostic imaging is the development of cancer. The **effective dose** is a quantity used to denote the radiation risk (expressed in **sieverts**) to a population of patients from an imaging study. See Table 2-1 for a description of the relationship between these measures of radiation exposure.

The average person living in the United States is exposed to 6.2 mSv of radiation per year from ambient sources, such as radon and cosmic rays, and medical procedures, which account for 36% of the annual radiation exposure (National Council on Radiation Protection and Measurements, 2012). The recommended occupational exposure limit to medical personnel is 50 mSv per year (National Council on Radiation Protection and Measurements, 2012). Exposure to the eyes and gonads has a more significant biologic impact than exposure to the extremities, so recommended exposure limits vary according to the body part. The linear no-threshold model (LNT) used in radiation protection to quantify exposition and to set regulatory limits assumes that the long-term, biologic damage caused by ionizing radiation is directly proportional to the dose. **Based on the LNT, there is no safe dose of radiation.** An effective radiation dose of as little as 10 mSv may result in the development of a malignancy in 1 of 1000 individuals exposed (National Research Council of the National Academies, 2006).

Relative Radiation Levels

The assessment of biologic risk from radiation exposure is complex. By estimating the range of effective doses for various imaging modalities, they can be assigned a **relative radiation level (RRL)** (Table 2-2). The effective dose from a 3-phase CT of the abdomen and pelvis without and with contrast may be as high as 25 to 40 mSv. Another often overlooked source of significant radiation exposure is fluoroscopy. Fluoroscopy for 1 minute results in a radiation dose to the skin equivalent to 10 times that of a single radiograph of the same anatomic area (Geise and Morin, 2000).

Radiation Protection

The cumulative dose of radiation to patients increases relatively rapidly with repeated CT imaging studies or procedures guided by fluoroscopy. Certain patient populations such as those with recurrent renal calculus disease or those with a urologic malignancy may be at increased risk of developing cancer because of repeated exposures to ionizing radiation. Attempts should be made to limit axial imaging studies to the anatomic area of interest and to substitute imaging studies not requiring ionizing radiation when feasible. The cumulative dose of radiation to medical personnel, including physicians, may increase relatively rapidly when fluoroscopy is used.

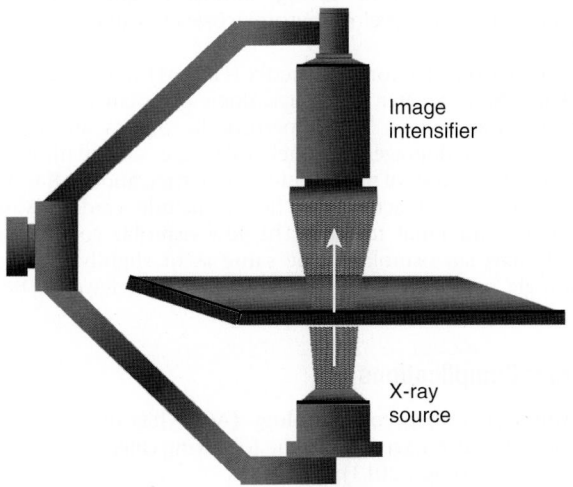

Figure 2-1. Equipment setup for fluoroscopy. The x-ray source located beneath the table reduces the radiation exposure to the surgeon. Locating the image intensifier as close to the patient as feasible reduces scatter radiation. Equipment setup will vary based on application.

Reduction in radiation exposure to medical personnel is achieved by three major mechanisms: (1) limiting the time of exposure; (2) maximizing distance from the radiation source; and (3) shielding. Radiation dose during fluoroscopy is directly proportional to the **time of exposure** and the **number of exposures**. The exposure time during fluoroscopy should be minimized by using short bursts of fluoroscopy and using the "last image hold" feature of the fluoroscopy unit. Radiation beams diverge with distance, and therefore radiation exposure diminishes as the square of the distance from the radiation source. Maintaining the maximum practical distance from an active radiation source significantly decreases exposure to medical personnel. Positioning the image intensifier as close as feasible to the patient substantially reduces scatter radiation. Standard aprons, thyroid shields, proper eye protection, and leaded gloves provide significant shielding for medical personnel and should be worn by all personnel involved in the use of fluoroscopy. **A practice of routinely collimating to the minimum required visual fluoroscopy field results in significant reductions in radiation exposure, compared with a usual approach to collimation. This may have important implications for decreasing the risk of malignancy in patients and operators.**

KEY POINTS: CONVENTIONAL RADIOGRAPHY/ RADIATION MANAGEMENT IN URORADIOLOGY

- The effective radiation dose describes the potential for adverse health effects from ionizing radiation.
- The effective dose is a quantity used to denote the radiation risk (expressed in sieverts) to a population of patients from an imaging study. See Table 2-1 for a description of the relationship between these measures of radiation exposure.
- Based on the LNT model, there is no safe dose of radiation.
- Relative radiation levels (RRL) categorize diagnostic imaging studies by their estimated effective dose of radiation.
- Radiation protection for medical personnel includes (1) limiting time of exposure; (2) maximizing distance from radiation source; and (3) shielding.
- Collimating to the minimum required visual fluoroscopy field reduces exposure to the patient and operator.

CONTRAST MEDIA

The urologist ordering a radiographic evaluation on a patient must consider the risks and benefits associated with a contrast-enhanced imaging study, as well as alternative imaging modalities that could provide the same information without the need for contrast exposure.

Many different types of contrast media have been used to enhance medical imaging and thus improve diagnostic and therapeutic decisions made by urologists. These agents are used on a daily basis throughout the world with great safety and efficacy. However, there are inherent risks associated with the use of contrast

---

TABLE 2-1 Units of Radiation Exposure and Clinical Relevance of the Measures

RADIATION QUANTITY	TRADITIONAL UNIT	SI UNIT	CONVERSION	CLINICAL RELEVANCE
Exposure	Roentgen (R)	Coulomb (C)/kg	1 C/kg = 3876 R	Charge per unit mass
Absorbed dose	Rad	Gray (Gy)	1 Gy = 100 rad	Energy absorbed by tissue
Equivalent dose	Rem	Sievert (Sv)	1 Sv = 100 rem	Absorbed energy based on tissue type
Effective dose	Rem	Sievert (Sv)		Biologic risk associated with absorbed energy

Modified from Geise RA, Morin RL. Radiation management in uroradiology. In: Pollack HM, McClennan BL, editors. Clinical urography. 2nd ed. Philadelphia: Saunders; 2000. p. 13.

TABLE 2-2 Radiation Exposure from Common Urologic Imaging Procedures

RELATIVE RADIATION LEVEL (RRL)	EFFECTIVE DOSE ESTIMATED RANGE	EXAMPLE EXAMINATIONS
None	0	Ultrasonography, MRI
Minimal	<0.1 mSv	Chest radiographs
Low	0.1-1.0 mSv	Lumbar spine radiographs, pelvic radiographs
Medium	1-10 mSv	Abdomen CT without contrast, nuclear medicine, bone scan, ^{99m}Tc-DMSA renal scan, IVP, retrograde pyelograms, KUB, CT chest with contrast
High	10 mSv-100 mSv	Abdomen CT without and with contrast, whole-body PET

CT, computed tomography; IVP, intravenous pyelogram; KUB, kidneys, ureters, bladder; MRI, magnetic resonance imaging; ^{99m}Tc-DMSA, technetium 99m-dimercaptosuccinic acid; PET, positron emission tomography. Modified from American College of Radiology. ACR appropriateness criteria radiation dose assessment introduction, <http://www.acr .org/SecondaryMainMenuCategories/quality_safety/app_criteria/ RRLInformation.aspx>; 2008.

media, as with other pharmaceuticals. Adverse side effects and adverse drug reactions (ADRs) can directly result from the use of contrast media and vary from minor disturbances to severe, life-threatening situations. Imaging centers must be prepared with trained personnel, readily available medications, equipment, and an ongoing system to educate clinic personnel on the recognition and treatment of ADRs associated with contrast media.

Intravascular Iodinated Contrast Media

Iodine is the most common element in general use as an intravascular radiologic contrast medium (IRCM). With an atomic weight of 127, iodine has radiopacity, whereas other elements included in IRCM have no radiopacity and act only as carriers of the iodine elements, increasing solubility, and reducing toxicity. Four basic types of iodinated IRCM are available for clinical use: ionic monomer, nonionic monomer, ionic dimer, and nonionic dimer. They can be further characterized as being iso-, hyper-, or low-osmolar compared to physiologic osmolality of 300 mOsm/kg water.

All are derived from a 2,4,6 tri-iodinated benzene ring compound with three atoms of iodine in the case of monomers and six atoms of iodine in the case of dimers. The chemical composition of these agents makes them highly hydrophilic, low in lipid solubility, and of low binding affinity for protein receptors or membranes. Because they do not enter red blood cells or tissue cells and are rapidly excreted, they are designed for use in imaging and are not therapeutic. Approximately 90% will be eliminated by the kidneys within 12 hours of administration.

Relative to the body's iodine stores, large quantities of iodine are required for imaging enhancement. The total body iodine content, found mainly in the thyroid gland is 0.01 g and the average daily turnover of iodine is only 0.0001 g. For renal CT imaging a common dose of IRCM will expose the patient to between 25 and 50 g of iodine, which is approximately 400,000 times the daily turnover rate in the human body, but this dose will rarely cause any toxicity or lasting effects (Morris, 1993).

Adverse Reactions to Intravascular Iodinated Contrast Media

ADRs associated with intravenous (IV) contrast media can be divided into two broad categories: idiosyncratic anaphylactoid (IA) and nonidiosyncratic (NI) reactions. The IA reactions are most concerning because they are potentially fatal and can occur without any predictable or predisposing factors. Approximately 85% of IA reactions occur during or immediately after injection of IRCM and are more common in patients who have a prior ADR to contrast media, have impaired renal function or diminished cardiac function, are on β-adrenergic blockers, or have asthma or diabetes (Spring et al, 1997).

The exact mechanism of IA reactions is unknown but thought to be a combination of systemic effects. IA reactions have not been shown to result from a true immunoglobulin E (IgE) antibody immunologic reaction to the contrast media (Dawson et al, 1999). At least four mechanisms may play a role in IA reactions: (1) release of vasoactive substances including histamine, (2) activation of physiologic cascades including complement, kinin, coagulation, and fibrinolytic systems, (3) inhibition of enzymes including cholinesterase, which may cause prolonged vagal stimulation, (4) the patient's own anxiety and fear of the actual procedure. IA reactions are not dose dependent. Severe reactions have been reported after an injection of only 1 mL at the beginning of a procedure and have also occurred after completion of a full dose despite no reaction to the initial test dose (Nelson et al, 1988; Thomsen et al, 1999; American College of Radiology, 2013).

NI reactions are dose dependent and consequently related to the osmolality, concentration, volume, and injection rate of the IRCM. Because the concentration of absorbed or free iodine is very low, only patients with an underlying iodine deficiency are at risk for increased intake of iodine during contrast imaging. Patients with endemic goiter may develop thyrotoxicosis after injection of IRCM agents.

The hyperosmolar contrast media (HOCM) have an osmolality that is five times greater than physiologic osmolality of body cells (300 mOsm/kg water). The hyperosmolar agents are associated with erythrocyte damage, endothelial damage, vasodilation, hypervolemia, interruption of the blood-brain barrier, and cardiac depression. Chemotoxic reactions to IRCM include cardiac, vascular, neurologic, and renal toxicity. The low osmolar contrast media (LOCM) have an osmolality the same as or slightly higher than physiologic osmolality and are associated with fewer ADRs and toxic events (Dawson et al, 1999).

Contrast Complications

The American College of Radiology (ACR) has divided these NI reactions to contrast agents into the following categories (American College of Radiology, 2013):

Mild Nonidiosyncratic Reactions

Fortunately, most NI reactions are classified as mild. Signs and symptoms appear self-limited without evidence of progression. These include the following:

Nausea, vomiting	Flushing
Cough	Chills, shaking
Warmth (heat)	Sweats
Headache	Rash, hives
Dizziness	Nasal stuffiness
Altered taste	Swelling: eyes, face
Itching	Anxiety
Pallor	

Treatment. Treatment consists of observation and reassurance; usually no intervention or medication is required. If needed, an H_1 receptor blocker such as diphenhydramine (Benadryl) orally (PO), intramuscularly (IM), or IV 1 to 2 mg/kg (up to 50 mg) may be helpful. Be careful because these reactions may progress into a more severe category. If necessary, administer chlorphenamine, 4 to 10 mg PO/IM/IV, or diazepam 5 mg for anxiety.

Moderate Nonidiosyncratic Reactions

The following reactions occur in 0.5% to 2% of patients and require treatment but are not immediately life threatening.

Tachycardia/bradycardia	Dyspnea
Hypertension	Pronounced skin reaction
Pulmonary edema	Bronchospasm, wheezing
Hypotension	Laryngeal edema

Treatment. These reactions are usually transient and will need treatment with close observation. Appropriate treatments are hydrocortisone 100 to 500 mg IM or IV, or β-agonist inhalation for bronchospasm in addition to bronchiolar dilators (metaproterenol [Alupent], terbutaline [Brethaire], or albuterol [Proventil or Ventolin]) 2 to 3 puffs; repeat as necessary.

Severe Nonidiosyncratic Reactions

Life-threatening reactions occur in approximately 1 in 1000 uses for high osmolar agents and are far less frequent for low osmolar contrast media, with both types of agents resulting in mortality rates of 1 in 170,000 uses (Spring et al, 1997). Life-threatening events with more severe signs or symptoms include the following:

Laryngeal edema (severe or progressive)	Hypotension
	Convulsions
Unresponsiveness	Clinically manifest arrhythmias
Cardiopulmonary arrest	

Treatment. Immediate treatment is required. The patient will usually require emergency care involving particular attention to the respiratory and cardiovascular systems. If bronchospasm is severe and not responsive to inhalers, or if an upper airway edema (including laryngospasm) is present, epinephrine should be used promptly. **Rapid administration of epinephrine is the treatment of choice for severe contrast reactions. Epinephrine can be administered in the dose of 0.01 mg/kg of 1:10,000 dilution or 0.1 mL/kg slowly into a running IV infusion of saline and can be repeated every 5 to 15 minutes as needed. If no IV access is available, the recommended IM dose of epinephrine is 0.01 mg/kg of 1:1000 dilution (or 0.01 mL/kg to a maximum of 0.15 mg of 1:1000 if less than 30 kg; 0.3 mg if weight is more than 30 kg) injected in the lateral thigh.** Subcutaneous injection is much less effective (Lightfoot et al, 2009; American College of Radiology, 2013). Epinephrine must be administered with care to patients who have cardiac disease or those who are taking β-blockers because the unopposed alpha effects of epinephrine in these patients may cause severe hypertension or angina.

Antihistamines do not have a major role in the treatment of severe reactions. Careful monitoring of patient vital signs is paramount; the presence of both hypotension and tachycardia indicates a higher likelihood of anaphylactic reaction. Bradycardia is a sign of vasovagal reaction, and therefore the use of β-blockers is to be avoided. Hypotension resulting from an anaphylactic reaction can be treated with IV iso-osmolar fluids (e.g., 0.9% normal saline or Ringer lactate solution); several liters of fluid may be needed before obtaining a significant hemodynamic response. If fluid and oxygen are unsuccessful in reversing the patient's hypotension, the use of vasopressors is indicated. The most effective vasopressor is dopamine. Dopamine should be used at infusion rates between 2 and 10 μg/kg/min.

Premedication Strategies

There is no known premedication strategy that will eliminate the risk of a severe adverse reaction to IRCM. The regimens suggested in the literature include the use of corticosteroids, antihistamines, H$_1$ and H$_2$ antagonists, and ephedrine. Patients at high risk should be premedicated with corticosteroids and possibly antihistamines 12 to 24 hours before and after use of IRCM. LOCM should be used in these patients. Several premedication regimens have been proposed to reduce the frequency and/or severity of reactions to contrast media. Two frequently used regimens are outlined in Box 2-1.

It has been demonstrated that the use of nonionic contrast media combined with a premedication strategy including corticosteroids results in a reduction in reaction rates compared to other protocols for patients who have experienced a prior contrast media–induced reaction. However, no controlled studies are available to determine whether pretreatment alters the incidence of serious reactions. Oral administration of steroids seems preferable to intravascular administration, and prednisone and methylprednisolone are equally effective. If the patient is unable to take oral medication, 200 mg of hydrocortisone IV may be substituted for oral prednisone. **One consistent finding is that steroids should be given at least 6 hours before the injection of contrast media regardless of the route of steroid administration. It is clear that administration for 3 hours or less before contrast does not decrease adverse reactions** (Lasser, 1988).

Supplemental administration of an H$_1$ antihistamine (e.g., diphenhydramine), PO or IV, may reduce the frequency of urticaria, angioedema, and respiratory symptoms. In emergency situations, IV corticosteroid (e.g., 200 mg hydrocortisone) every 4 hours plus an H$_1$ antihistamine (e.g., 50 mg diphenhydramine) 1 hour before the procedure has been used. In patients who have a prior, documented contrast reaction, the use of a different contrast agent has been advocated and may be protective. Switching to a different agent should be in combination with a premedication regimen.

Although rare, ADRs are reported after extravascular instillation of IRCM (e.g., retrograde pyelography). **In patients with a positive history of previous severe IA or IN reactions to IRCM undergoing a nonvascular study, premedication with corticosteroids should be considered.**

Delayed Contrast Reactions

Delayed contrast reactions can occur from 3 hours to 7 days following the administration of contrast. These reactions are identified in as many as 14% to 30% of patients after the injection of ionic monomers and in 8% to 10% of patients after the injection of nonionic monomers. Cutaneous reactions are the most frequent

---

BOX 2-1 Premedication Strategies to Reduce Severity of Reactions to Contrast Media

1. Prednisone—50 mg PO at 13 hr, 7 hr, and 1 hr before contrast media injection
   Plus diphenhydramine (Benadryl)—50 mg IV, IM, or PO 1 hr before contrast medium injection
2. Methylprednisolone (Medrol)—32 mg PO 12 hr and 2 hr before contrast media injection
   Plus diphenhydramine (Benadryl)—50 mg IV, IM, or PO 1 hr before contrast medium injection

From ACR Committee on Drugs and Contrast Media. ACR manual on contrast media: version 9, <http://www.acr.org/quality-safety/resources/~/media/37D84428BF1D4E1B9A3A2918DA9E27A3.pdf/>; 2013 [accessed 06.10.14].

form of delayed contrast reaction with a reported incidence of 0.5% to 9%. The most common reactions include a cutaneous exanthem or pruritus without urticaria. Nausea, vomiting, drowsiness, headache and flulike symptoms can also occur. These signs and symptoms almost always resolve spontaneously.

Specific Contrast Consideration

Cardiac Abnormalities. Patients with underlying cardiac disease, including chest pain and cardiac arrest, have an increased incidence and/or severity of cardiovascular side effects. Pulmonary angiography and intracardiac and coronary artery injections carry the highest degree of risk. Possible reactions include hypotension, tachycardia, and arrhythmias. More severe but uncommon reactions include congestive heart failure, pulmonary edema, and cardiac arrest.

Extravasation of Contrast Material. Large-volume extravasation can be seen with power injections not monitored with electrical skin impedance devices that detect extravasation and arrest the injection process. When large-volume extravasation of IRCM occurs, the result can be swelling, edema, erythema, pain, and cellulitis. The most severe consequences may not be manifest immediately, and the inflammatory reaction usually reaches a maximum in 24 to 48 hours. The primary underlying mechanism is believed to be the hyperosmolality of the contrast agent. Mechanical compression caused by a compartment syndrome may also occur, leading to tissue necrosis. Management steps are immediate cessation of injection, notification of responsible and referring physicians, and elevation of the affected extremity above the level of the heart. If a large volume of extravasate occurs, manual massage is recommended to promote drainage. If the patient becomes symptomatic, plastic surgery consultation may also be needed. Admission to the hospital for observation or frequent follow-up in clinic may be necessary in some cases of large-volume extravasation.

Metformin. Metformin, an oral antihyperglycemic drug used to treat diabetes, is eliminated unchanged through the kidneys, most likely by glomerular filtration and tubular excretion. As a biguanide, it stimulates intestinal production of lactic acid. Some conditions can reduce metformin excretion or increase serum lactate, such as renal disease (decreases metformin excretion), liver disease (decreases lactic acid metabolism), and cardiac disease (increases anaerobic metabolism). **Patients with type 2 diabetes mellitus receiving metformin may have an accumulation of the drug after administering IRCM, resulting in biguanide lactic acidosis with symptoms of vomiting, diarrhea, and somnolence. This condition is fatal in approximately 50% of cases** (Wiholm and Myrhed, 1993). **Biguanide lactic acidosis is rare in patients with normal renal function. Consequently in patients with normal renal function and no known comorbidities there is no need to discontinue metformin before IRCM use, nor is there a need to check creatinine following the imaging study. However, in patients with renal insufficiency metformin should be discontinued the day of the study and withheld for 48 hours. Postprocedure creatinine should be measured at 48 hours and metformin started once kidney function is normal** (Bailey and Turner, 1996). **It is not necessary to discontinue metformin before gadolinium-enhanced MRI studies when the amount of gadolinium administered is in the usual dosage range of 0.1 to 0.3 mmol per kilogram of body weight.**

Contrast-Induced Nephropathy. While there are no standard criteria for contrast-induced nephropathy (CIN), the diagnosis can be made if one of the following occurs within 48 hours after administration of iodinated contrast medium: increase in serum creatinine of greater than 0.3 mg/dL, more than a 50% increase in serum creatinine from baseline, or urine output reduced to less than 0.5 mL/kg/hr for at least 6 hours (Mehta et al, 2007). The precise cause of CIN is still unknown but is believed to be a combination of tubular toxicity, tubular obstruction, and renal ischemia by vasoconstriction (Katholi et al, 1998; Heinrich et al, 2005). High doses of IRCM can impair renal function in some patients for 3 to 5 days, and the creatinine level usually returns to baseline in 10 to 14 days.

The incidence of contrast agent–related nephropathy is estimated to be 2% to 5%, and up to 25% of those with CIN will have persistent renal dysfunction. Clinical manifestations are highly variable and may be absent or proceed to oliguria. CIN in patients with normal kidney function is rare (Pannu et al, 2006; Kelly et al, 2008). CIN is the third most common cause of acute kidney failure in hospitalized patients (Nash et al, 2002). **The most common patient-related risk factors for CIN are chronic kidney disease (creatinine clearance <60 mL/min), diabetes mellitus, dehydration, diuretic use, advanced age, congestive heart failure, hypertension, low hematocrit, and ventricular ejection fraction less than 40%. The patients at highest risk for developing CIN are those with both diabetes *and* pre-existing renal insufficiency. Other risk factors are concomitant exposure to** chemotherapy, aminoglycoside or nonsteroidal anti-inflammatory agents, hyperuricemia, and diseases that affect renal hemodynamics, such as end-stage liver disease and nephrotic syndrome. Patients with a diagnosis of a paraproteinemia syndrome/disease (e.g., multiple myeloma), history of a kidney transplant, renal tumor, renal surgery, or single kidney may also be at higher risk of CIN.

The most common nonpatient-related causes are high osmolar contrast agents, ionic contrast, increased contrast viscosity, multiple contrast-enhanced studies performed within a short period, and large contrast volume infused (Pannu et al, 2006).

Despite significant discussion among radiologists and urologists, the literature does not support an absolute serum creatinine level that prohibits the use of contrast media. Prevention of CIN has been the subject of many research studies, and the results have been summarized by several different meta-analyses. In these meta-analyses the baseline serum creatinine of study participants ranged from 0.9 to 2.5 mg/dL. **In one survey the policies regarding the cutoff value for serum creatinine varied widely among radiology practices. Thirty-five percent of respondents used 1.5 mg/dL, 27% used 1.7 mg/dL, and 31% used 2.0 mg/dL (mean, 1.78 mg/dL) as a cutoff value in patients with no risk factors other than elevated creatinine; threshold values were slightly lower in diabetic patients (mean, 1.68 mg/dL). Patients in end-stage renal disease who have no remaining natural renal function are no longer at risk for CIN and may receive LOCM or iso-osmolar contrast media** (Elicker et al, 2006).

Prevention of CIN is of great concern and has been a subject of many different studies. Hydration is the major preventative action against CIN. Periprocedural IV hydration with 0.9% saline at 100 mL/hr 12 hours before to 12 hours after has been shown to decrease the incidence of CIN after IV contrast use (Solomon et al, 2007). **The use of sodium bicarbonate has not been definitively shown to prevent CIN in patients receiving IV iodinated contrast material. (The use of *N*-acetylcysteine for the prevention of CIN is controversial)** (Safirstein et al, 2000). **Currently there is insufficient evidence to make a definitive recommendation for its use, and therefore it should not be considered a substitute for appropriate screening and hydration** (Zoungas et al, 2009; Newhouse and RoyChoudhury, 2013). Furosemide was found to increase the risk of developing CIN (Pannu et al, 2006; Kelly et al, 2008).

Magnetic Resonance Imaging Contrast Agents

Because MRI offers previously unseen detailed soft tissue imaging compared with CT, it was initially believed that MRI would not require contrast enhancement. However, by 2005, almost 50% of MRI studies were being performed with contrast media. Extracellular MRI contrast agents contain paramagnetic metal ions. Copper, manganese, and gadolinium (Gd) were the potential paramagnetic ions for use with MRI. Gadolinium, however, is the most powerful with 7 unpaired electrons, but its toxicity required encapsulation by a chelate. Paramagnetic agents such as Gd are positive enhancers reducing the T1 and T2 relaxation times and increasing tissue signal intensity (SI) on T1-weighted images, while having little effect on T2-weighted images.

Gadolinium

Acute adverse reactions are encountered less frequently with Gd-based contrast media (GBCM) than after administration of iodinated contrast media. The frequency, of all acute adverse events after an injection of 0.1 or 0.2 mmol/kg of gadolinium chelate, ranges from 0.07% to 2.4%. The vast majority of these reactions are mild, including coldness at the injection site, nausea, emesis, headache, warmth or pain at the injection site, paresthesias, dizziness, and itching. Reactions resembling an "allergic" response occur with a frequency of 0.004% to 0.7%. Reactions consisting of rash, hives, or urticaria are most frequent; the patient rarely develops bronchospasm. Severe, life-threatening anaphylactoid or nonallergic anaphylactic reactions are exceedingly rare (0.0001% to 0.001%). In a meta-analysis of 687,000 Gd doses for MRI, only five reactions were severe. In another survey based on 20 million administered doses, 55 patients (0.0003%) had severe reactions. Fatal reactions to gadolinium chelate agents have been reported, but they are extremely rare (Murphy et al, 1999). There have been no documented vaso-occlusive or hemolytic complications when administering GBCM to patients with sickle cell disease (Elicker et al, 2006; Dillman et al, 2011). Gd agents are considered to have no nephrotoxicity at approved doses for MRI. However, because of the risk of nephrogenic systemic fibrosis (NSF) in patients with severe renal dysfunction, the use of Gd agents in this patient population requires some precaution and a review of the current recommendations.

Extracellular MRI agents are known to interfere with some serum chemistry assays. For example, serum calcium tests will often be measured as a false reading of hypocalcemia for 24 hours after MRI with Gd enhancement, even though serum calcium is actually in the normal range. Other tests including iron, magnesium, iron-binding capacity, and zinc may also have spurious results. Biochemical assessment is more reliable when performed 24 hours after exposure to Gd contrast media.

Nephrogenic Systemic Fibrosis

NSF is a fibrosing disease of the skin, subcutaneous tissues, lungs, esophagus, heart, and skeletal muscles. Initial symptoms typically include skin thickening and/or pruritus. Symptoms and signs may develop and progress rapidly, with some affected patients developing contractures and joint immobility within days of exposure. Death may result in some patients, presumably as a result of visceral organ involvement.

In 1997 NSF was described in dialysis patients who had not been exposed to GBCM. The condition was previously known as *nephrogenic fibrosing dermopathy*. In 2006 independent reports surfaced defining a strong association with GBCM in patients with advanced renal disease (Cowper et al, 2000; Grobner, 2006; Marckmann et al, 2006). It is now currently accepted that GBCM exposure is a necessary factor in the development of NSF. Onset of NSF varies between 2 days and 3 months, with rare cases appearing years after exposure (Shabana et al, 2008). Early manifestations include subacute swelling of distal extremities, followed by severe skin induration and later even organ involvement. In a 2007 survey performed by the ACR, 156 cases of NSF were reported by 27 responding institutions; 140 of these 156 patients were known to have received GBCM. In 78 patients, the specific GBCM was known. Forty-five of them received gadodiamide, 17 gadopentetate dimeglumine, 13 gadoversetamide, and three gadobenate dimeglumine. NSF following gadoteridol administration has also been reported. Many of the cases in which agents other than gadodiamide and gadopentetate dimeglumine were used are confounded by the fact that affected patients were injected with other agents as well (American College of Radiology, 2013). Between 12% and 20% of confirmed cases of NSF occurred in patients with acute kidney injury. Patients with chronic kidney disease have a 1% to 7% chance of developing NSF after MRI with Gd agents (Todd et al, 2007).

Patients with a glomerular filtration rate (GFR) less than 30 mL/min/1.73 m^2 not on chronic dialysis are the most difficult patient population in terms of choosing imaging modality. They are at risk for CIN if exposed to iodinated contrast media for CT imaging and are also at significant risk of developing NSF if exposed to GBCM during MRI. Recent data suggest that the risk of NSF may be greatest in patients with a GFR of less than 15 mL/min/1.73 m^2. These patients have a 1% to 7% chance of developing NSF after exposure to GBCM during MRI, with the incidence being much less in patients with GFRs that are higher (Kanal et al, 2008). In patients with chronic kidney disease, it is recommended that contrast media be avoided if possible. If MRI contrast media is absolutely essential, use of the lowest possible doses (needed to obtain a diagnostic study) of selected GBCM is recommended. In this setting, patients should be informed of the risks of GBCM administration and must give their consent to proceed. There is no proof that any GBCM is completely safe in this patient group; however, some have suggested avoiding gadodiamide and considering use of macrocyclic agents (Kanal et al, 2008). Patients with chronic kidney disease but GFR more than 30 mL/min/1.73 m^2 are considered to be at extremely low or no risk for developing NSF if a dose of GBCM of 0.1 mmol/kg or less is used. Patients with GFR more than 60 mL/min/1.73 m^2 do not appear to be at increased risk of developing NSF, and the current consensus is that all GBCM can be administered safely to these patients. In their publications, the ACR stresses that the current information on NSF and its relationship to GBCM administration is very preliminary and further research is needed to better understand this potentially devastating complication.

KEY POINTS: CONTRAST MEDIA

- Type 2 diabetic patients with renal insufficiency who are receiving oral metformin biguanide hyperglycemic therapy are at risk for developing biguanide lactic acidosis after exposure to intravascular radiologic contrast media; they should stop metformin the day before the procedure and restart 48 hours after if they have a normal or baseline serum creatinine.
- Patients at risk for adverse reaction to contrast include those with previous adverse reactions, history of asthma, severe cardiac disease, renal insufficiency, dehydration, sickle cell anemia, anxiety, apprehension, hyperthyroidism, and presence of adrenal pheochromocytoma.
- Epinephrine can be administered IV in the dose of 0.01 mg/kg of 1:10,000 dilution or 0.1 mL/kg slowly into a running infusion of saline and can be repeated every 5 to 15 minutes as needed. If no IV access is available, the recommended IM dose of epinephrine is 0.01 mg/kg of 1:1000 dilution (or 0.01 mL/kg to a maximum of 0.15 mg of 1:1000 if less than 30 kg; 0.3 mg if weight is greater than 30 kg) injected in the lateral thigh.
- Patients at greatest risk for contrast-induced nephropathy are those with diabetes mellitus and dehydration.
- Steroids given to prevent adverse contrast agents should be given at least 6 hours before injection.

INTRAVENOUS UROGRAPHY

Once the mainstay of urologic imaging, the intravenous excretory urographic (IVU) study has essentially been replaced by CT and MRI. With the ability of new scanners to perform axial, sagittal, and coronal reconstruction of the upper tract urinary system, essentially all of the data and information obtained by traditional IVU can be realized with CT imaging. In addition, some parenchymal defects, cysts, and tumors can be better delineated with CT than with IVU.

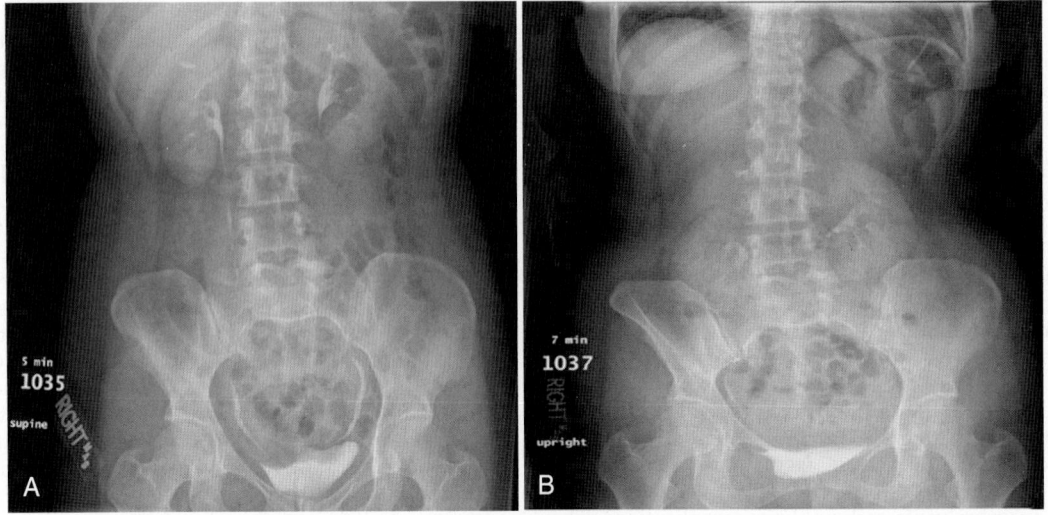

Figure 2-2. Intravenous excretory urogram (IVU) in a 40-year-old woman with the complaint of a mobile mass in the right lower quadrant with standing associated with bilateral flank and back pain that resolved in the supine position. A, Supine IVU shows kidneys in the normal position with normal ureters and proximal collecting systems. B, Standing film shows significant displacement of both kidneys, with the right kidney moving onto the pelvis as described by the patient.

Technique

Bowel prep may help to visualize the entire ureters and upper collecting systems. Patients with chronic constipation may benefit most from complete bowel prep with clear liquids for 12 to 24 hours and an enema 2 hours before the procedure.

Before injection of contrast, a scout radiograph or KUB (kidney-ureter-bladder) film is taken demonstrating the top of the kidneys and the entire pelvis to the pubic symphysis. This allows determination of adequate bowel prep, confirms correct positioning, and exposes kidney stones or bladder stones.

Contrast is injected as a bolus of 50 to 100 mL of contrast. The nephrogenic phase is captured with a radiograph immediately after injection. In the past, tomograms were used to look for parenchymal defects, but now CT or MRI is preferred. A film is taken at 5 minutes and then additional films at 5-minute intervals until the question that prompted the IVU is answered. Abdominal compression may be used to better visualize the ureters. Occasionally, oblique films will be used to better define the course of the ureter in the bony pelvis and to precisely differentiate ureteral stones from pelvic calcifications.

Upright films may be helpful in certain situations. In the rare case of suspected symptomatic renal ptosis, IVU can be particularly helpful (Fig. 2-2). Supine films are compared with upright films to measure the degree of ptosis. Such a comparison cannot be made with MRI or CT imaging. In the case of calyceal stones or milk of calcium stones, layering of the contrast can be helpful to evaluate the anatomy of the calyx harboring the stones.

Postvoid films are obtained to evaluate the presence of outlet obstruction, prostate enlargement, and bladder filling defects, including stones and urothelial cancers.

Indications

1. Demonstration of renal collecting systems and ureters
2. Investigation of level of ureteral obstruction
3. Demonstration of intraoperative opacification of collecting system during extracorporeal shock wave lithotripsy or percutaneous access to the collecting system
4. Demonstration of renal function during emergent evaluation of unstable patients

5. Demonstrate renal and ureteral anatomy in special circumstances (e.g., ptosis, after transureteroureterostomy, and after urinary diversion)

PLAIN ABDOMINAL RADIOGRAPHY

The plain abdominal radiograph is a conventional radiography study, which is intended to display the kidneys, ureters, and bladder. The plain abdominal radiograph may be employed as a primary study or a scout film in anticipation of contrast media. Plain films are widely used in the management of renal calculus disease. Plain radiography is also useful in evaluation of the trauma patient because it can be performed as a portable study in the trauma unit. Secondary findings on plain radiography, such as rib fractures, fractures of the transverse processes of the vertebral bodies, and pelvic fractures, may indicate serious associated urologic injuries.

Technique

An abdominal plain radiograph is obtained with the patient in the supine position, using an anterior to posterior exposure. The study typically includes that portion of the anatomy from the level of the diaphragm to the inferior pubic symphysis. It may occasionally be necessary to make two exposures to cover the desired anatomic field. Depending on the indication for the study, oblique films are obtained to clarify the position of structures in relation to the urinary tract. If small bowel obstruction or free peritoneal air is suspected, upright films will be obtained.

Indications

1. Used as a preliminary film in anticipation of contrast administration
2. Assessment of presence of residual contrast from a previous imaging procedure
3. Assessment of renal calculus disease before and after treatment
4. Assessment of the position of drains and stents
5. Used as an adjunct to the investigation of blunt or penetrating trauma to the urinary tract

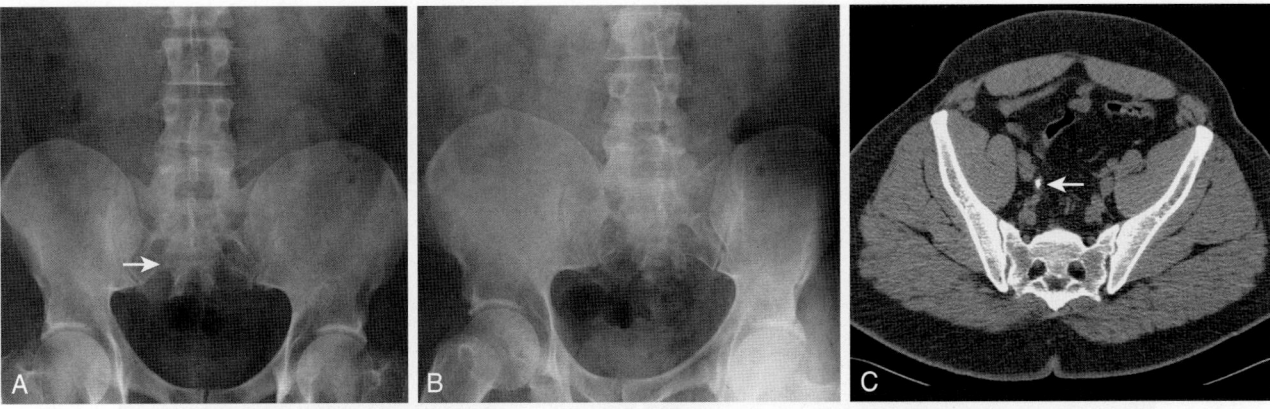

Figure 2-3. **A, Right ureteral calculus** *(arrow)* **overlying the sacrum is difficult to visualize on the plain film. B, The right posterior oblique study fails to confirm the location of the ureteral calculus. C, Computed tomography confirms this 6-mm calculus in the right ureter at the level of the third sacral segment** *(arrow).*

Limitations

Although plain film radiography is often used in the evaluation of renal colic, it is unreliable in the demonstration of calculus disease for a variety of reasons: (1) overlying stool and bowel gas may obscure small calculi; (2) stones may be obscured by other structures such as bones or ribs (Fig. 2-3); (3) calcifications in pelvic veins or vascular structures may be confused with ureteral calculi; and (4) stones that are poorly calcified or composed of uric acid may be radiolucent. Nevertheless, plain film radiography is very valuable in assessing the suitability of a patient for extracorporeal shock wave lithotripsy because the ability to identify the stone on fluoroscopy is critical to targeting. Furthermore, a KUB is very cost-effective for monitoring residual stone burden after treatment (Fig. 2-4). For complex pathology of the urinary tract, plain abdominal radiography has been supplanted by axial imaging. Plain radiography has a very limited role in evaluating soft tissue abnormalities of the urinary tract.

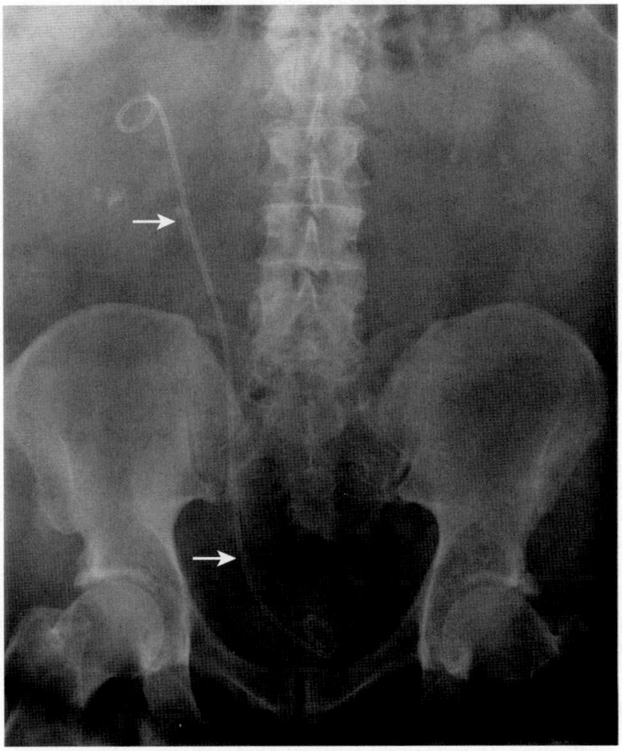

RETROGRADE PYELOGRAPHY

Retrograde pyelograms are performed to opacify the ureters and intrarenal collecting system by the retrograde injection of contrast media. Any contrast media that can be used for excretory urography is also acceptable for retrograde pyelography. Attempts should be made to sterilize the urine before retrograde pyelography because there is a risk of introducing bacteria into the upper urinary tracts or into the bloodstream. Although many studies are able to document the presence or absence of dilation of the ureter, retrograde pyelography has the unique ability to document the normalcy of the ureter distal to the level of obstruction and to better define the extent of the ureteral abnormality.

Technique

Retrograde pyelography is usually performed with the patient in the dorsal lithotomy position. An abdominal plain radiograph (scout film) is obtained to ensure that the patient is in the appropriate position to evaluate the entire ureter and intrarenal collecting system. Cystoscopy is performed and the ureteral orifice is identified.

Contrast may be injected through either a nonobstructing catheter or an obstructing catheter. Nonobstructing catheters include whistle tip, spiral tip, or open-ended catheters. Use of nonobstructing catheters allows passage of the catheter into the ureter and up to the collecting system, over a guidewire if necessary. Contrast can then be introduced directly into the upper collecting system and the

Figure 2-4. **KUB (kidney-ureter-bladder) film demonstrating residual stone fragments** *(arrows)* **adjacent to a right ureteral stent 1 week following right extracorporeal shock wave lithotripsy.**

ureters visualized by injection of contrast as the catheter is withdrawn.

The other commonly employed method is the use of an obstructing ureteral catheter such as a bulb-tip, cone-tip, or wedge-tip catheter. These catheters are inserted into the ureteral orifice and then pulled back against the orifice to effectively obstruct the ureter. Contrast is then injected to opacify the ureter and intrarenal collecting system. Depending on the indication for the study, it is useful to dilute the contrast material (to 50% or less) with sterile fluid. This prevents subtle filling defects in the collecting system or ureter from being obscured. Care should be taken to evacuate air bubbles from the syringe and catheter before injection. Such air bubble artifacts could be mistaken for stones or tumors.

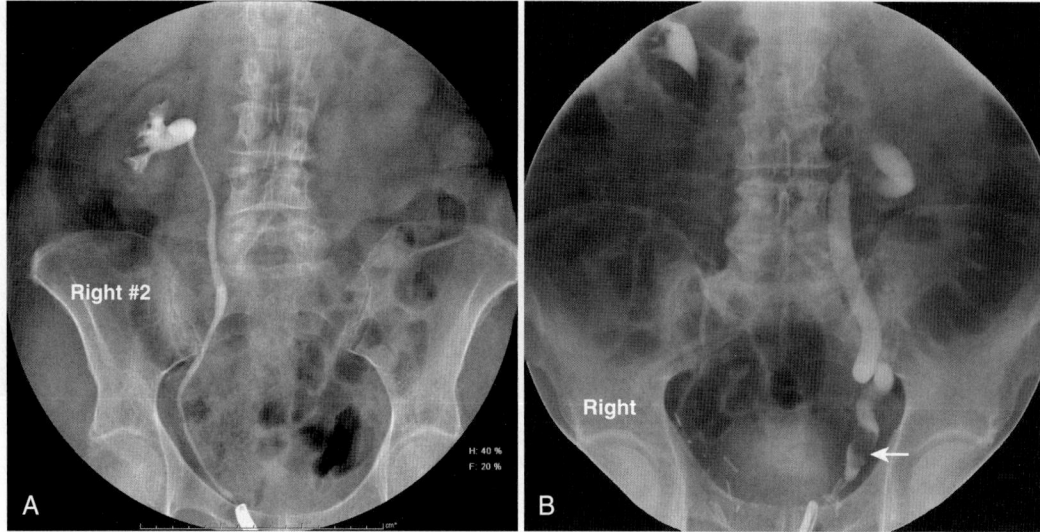

Figure 2-5. **A,** Right retrograde pyelogram performed using an 8-Fr cone-tipped ureteral catheter and dilute contrast material. The ureter and intrarenal collecting system are normal. **B,** Left retrograde pyelogram using an 8-Fr cone-tipped ureteral catheter. A filling defect in the left distal ureter *(arrow)* is a low-grade transitional cell carcinoma. The ureter demonstrates dilation, elongation, and tortuosity, the hallmarks of chronic obstruction.

After air is expelled from the catheter into the bladder, the ureteral orifice is intubated. Contrast is injected slowly, usually requiring 5 to 8 mL to completely opacify the ureter and intrarenal collecting system in adults (Fig. 2-5). More or less contrast may be required, depending on the size of the patient and the capaciousness of the collecting system. Limited use of fluoroscopy while injecting will help prevent overdistention of the collecting system and reduce the risk of extravasation of contrast.

Historically, when a retrograde pyelogram consisted of a series of radiographs taken at intervals, it was important to document various stages of filling and emptying of the ureter and collecting systems. Because of peristalsis the entire ureter will often not be seen on any given static exposure or view. With current equipment, including tables which incorporate fluoroscopy, it is possible to evaluate the ureter during peristalsis in real time, thus reducing the need for static image documentation. Documentary still images or "spot films" may be saved for future comparison. Urologists interpret retrograde pyelograms in real time as they are performed.

Indications

1. Evaluation of congenital ureteral obstruction
2. Evaluation of acquired ureteral obstruction
3. Elucidation of filling defects and deformities of the ureters or intrarenal collecting systems
4. Opacification or distention of collecting system to facilitate percutaneous access
5. In conjunction with ureteroscopy or stent placement
6. Evaluation of hematuria
7. Surveillance of transitional cell carcinoma
8. Evaluation of traumatic or iatrogenic injury to the ureter or collecting system

Limitations

Retrograde pyelography may be difficult in cases where the bladder is involved with diffuse inflammation or neoplastic changes, especially when bleeding is present. Identification of the ureteral orifices may be facilitated in such cases by the IV injection of indigotindisulfonate sodium or methylene blue. Changes associated with bladder outlet obstruction may result in angulation of the intramural ureters. This may make cannulation with an obstructing catheter quite difficult. Attempts to cannulate the ureteral orifice may result in trauma to the ureteral orifice and extravasation of contrast material into the bladder wall. The potential for damage to the intramural ureter must be weighed against the potential information to be obtained by the retrograde pyelogram.

Complications

Backflow occurs during retrograde pyelography when contrast is injected under pressure and escapes the collecting system. Contrast may escape the collecting system by one of four routes: **Pyelotubular** backflow occurs when contrast fills the distal collecting ducts producing opacification of the medullary pyramids (Fig. 2-6A). **Pyelosinus** backflow occurs when a tear in the calyces at the fornix allows contrast to leak into the renal sinus (Fig. 2-6B). **Pyelolymphatic** backflow is characterized by opacification of the renal lymphatic channels (Fig. 2-6C). **Pyelovenous** backflow is seen when contrast enters the venous system, resulting in visualization of the renal vein.

Although backflow does not usually cause measurable clinical harm, the potential implications of backflow include (1) introduction of bacteria from infected urine into the vascular system and (2) the absorption of contrast media, which could result in adverse reactions in susceptible patients. It has been demonstrated that the risk of significant urinary tract infection is only about 10% and the risk of sepsis is low when antibiotic prophylaxis therapy is administered before endoscopic procedures (including retrograde pyelography) (Christiano et al, 2000). Although contrast reactions are rare with retrograde pyelography, they have been reported (Johenning, 1980; Weese et al, 1993). In patients with documented severe contrast allergy, prophylactic pretreatment may be appropriate. In those patients considered at risk, care should be taken to inject under low pressures to minimize the probability of backflow and absorption of the contrast into the vasculature system.

LOOPOGRAPHY

Loopography is a diagnostic procedure performed in patients who have undergone urinary diversion. Historically the term

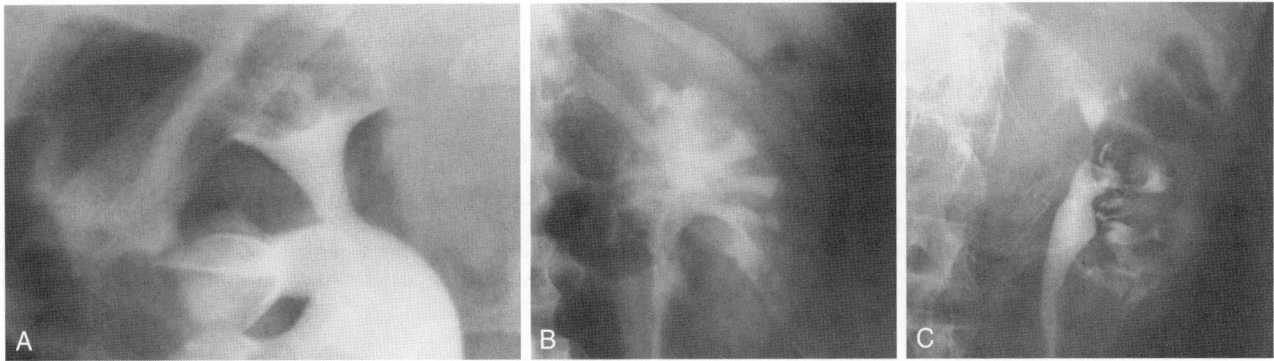

Figure 2-6. Patterns of backflow during retrograde pyelography. A, Pyelotubular backflow. B, Pyelosinus backflow. C, Pyelolymphatic backflow.

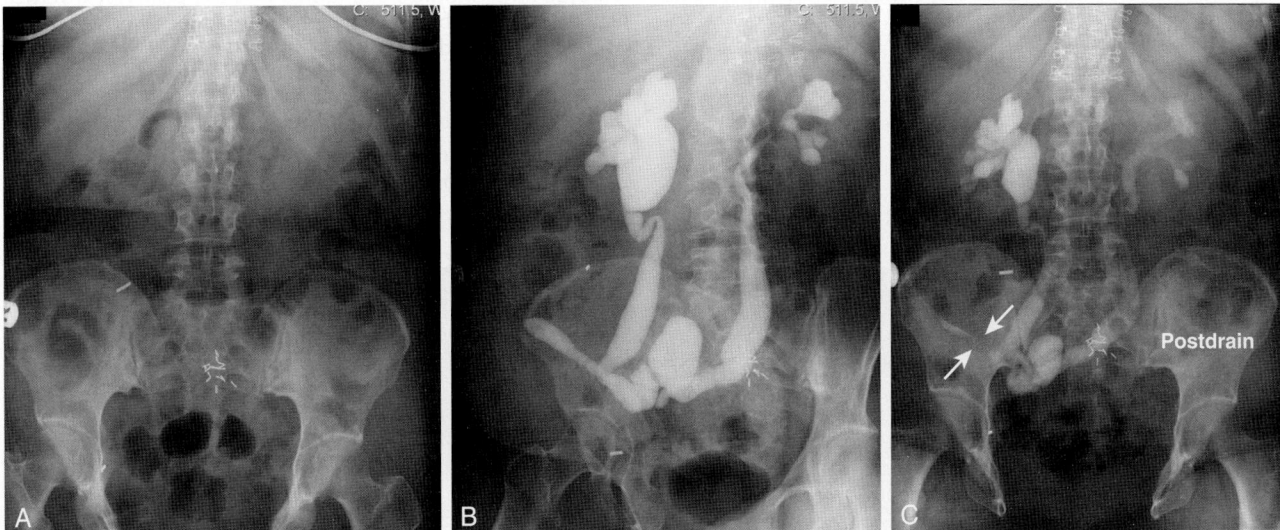

Figure 2-7. Loopogram in a patient with epispadias/exstrophy and ileal conduit urinary diversion. The plain film (A) shows wide diastasis of the pubic symphysis. After contrast administration via a catheter placed in the ileal conduit, free reflux of both ureterointestinal anastomoses is demonstrated (B). A postdrain radiograph (C) demonstrates persistent dilation of the proximal loop, indicating mechanical obstruction of the conduit *(arrows)*.

"loopogram" has been associated with ileal conduit diversion but may be used in reference to any bowel segment serving as a urinary conduit. When imaging patients with a continent diversion involving a reservoir or neobladder, "pouch-o-gram" would be more accurately descriptive. Because an ileal conduit urinary diversion usually has freely refluxing ureterointestinal anastomoses, the ureters and upper collecting systems may be visualized. In other forms of diversion, the ureterointestinal anastomoses may be purposely nonrefluxing. In such circumstances, when opacification of the upper urinary tract is desirable, antegrade ureteral imaging such as IVU, CT or MRI urography, or antegrade nephrostography may be required. When the patient has compromised renal function or is allergic to iodinated contrast material, loopogram can be performed with a low risk of systemic absorption (Hudson et al, 1981).

Technique

The patient is positioned supine. An abdominal plain radiograph is obtained before the introduction of contrast material (Fig. 2-7A). A commonly employed technique is to insert a small-gauge catheter

into the ostomy of the loop, advancing it just proximal to the abdominal wall fascia. The balloon on such a catheter can then be inflated to 5 to 10 mL with sterile water. By gently introducing contrast through the catheter, the loop can be distended, usually producing bilateral reflux into the upper tracts. Oblique films should be obtained in order to evaluate the entire length of the loop (Fig. 2-7B). Because of the angle at which many loops are constructed, a traditional anteroposterior (AP) view will often show a foreshortened loop and could miss a substantial pathology. A drain film should be obtained (Fig. 2-7C). This may demonstrate whether there is obstruction of the conduit.

Indications

1. Evaluation of infection, hematuria, renal insufficiency, or pain after urinary diversion
2. Surveillance of upper urinary tract for obstruction
3. Surveillance of upper urinary tract for urothelial neoplasia
4. Evaluation of the integrity of the intestinal segment or reservoir

RETROGRADE URETHROGRAPHY

A retrograde urethrogram is a study to evaluate the anterior and posterior urethra. Retrograde urethrography may be particularly beneficial in demonstrating the total length of a urethral stricture that cannot be negotiated by cystoscopy. Retrograde urethrography also demonstrates the anatomy of the urethra distal to a stricture that may not be assessable by voiding cystourethrography. Retrograde urethrography may be performed in the office or in the operating room before performing visual internal urethrotomy or formal urethroplasty.

Technique

A plain film radiograph is obtained before injection of contrast. The patient is usually positioned slightly obliquely to allow evaluation of the full length of urethra. The penis is placed on slight tension. A small catheter may be inserted into the fossa navicularis with the balloon inflated to 2 mL with sterile water. Contrast is then introduced via a catheter-tipped syringe. Alternatively, a penile clamp (e.g., Brodney clamp) may be used to occlude the urethra around the catheter (Fig. 2-8).

Indications

1. Evaluation of urethral stricture disease
   a. Location of stricture
   b. Length of stricture

2. Assessment for foreign bodies
3. Evaluation of penile or urethral penetrating trauma
4. Evaluation of traumatic gross hematuria

STATIC CYSTOGRAPHY

Static cystography is used primarily to evaluate the structural integrity of the bladder. The shape and contour of the bladder may give information about neurogenic dysfunction or bladder outlet obstruction. Filling defects such as tumors and stones may be appreciated.

Technique

The patient is positioned supine. A plain radiograph is performed to evaluate for stones and residual contrast and to confirm position and technique. The bladder is filled with 200 to 400 mL of contrast, depending on bladder size and patient comfort. Adequate filling is important to demonstrate intravesical pathology or bladder rupture. Oblique films should be obtained because posterior diverticula or fistulae may be obscured by the full bladder. A postdrainage film completes the study (Fig. 2-9).

Indications

1. Evaluation of intravesical pathology
2. Evaluation of bladder diverticula

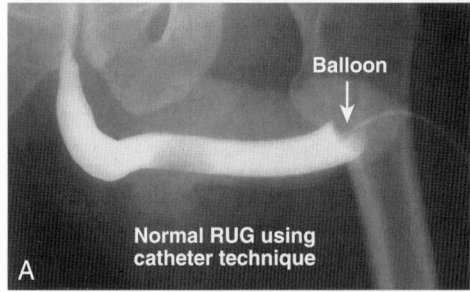
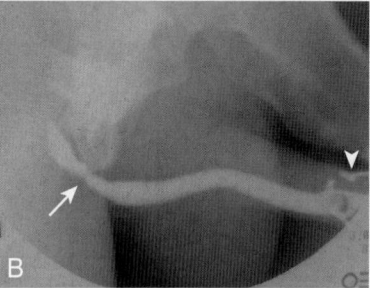
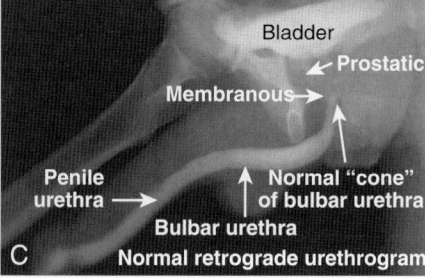

Figure 2-8. Normal retrograde urethrogram demonstrating **(A)** the balloon technique for retrograde urethrography and **(B)** Brodney clamp *(arrowhead)* technique; note the bulbar urethral stricture *(arrow)*. **C,** Normal structures of the male urethra as seen on retrograde urethrogram.

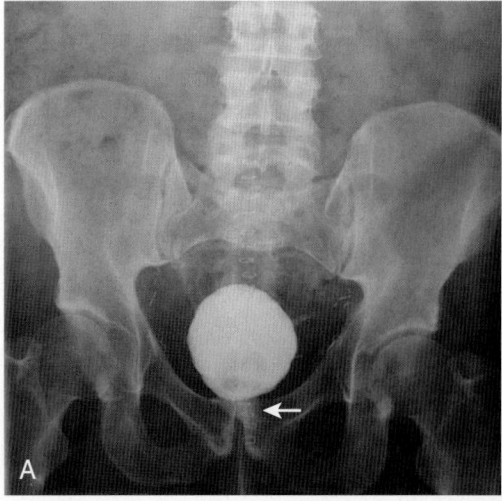
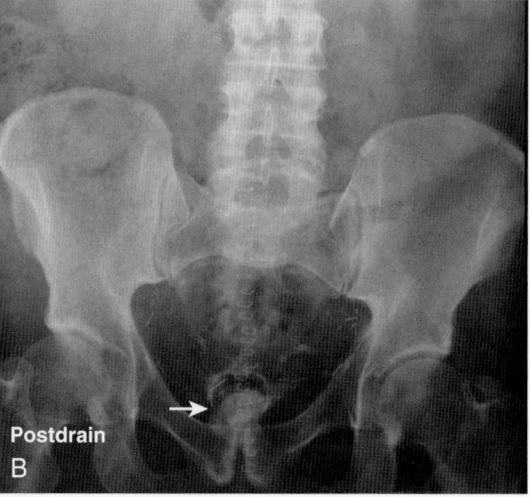

Figure 2-9. The patient has undergone radical retropubic prostatectomy. **A,** During bladder filling, contrast is seen adjacent to the vesicoureteral anastomoses *(arrow)*. **B,** The postdrain film clearly demonstrates a collection of extravasated contrast *(arrow)*.

3. Evaluation of inguinal hernia involving the bladder
4. Evaluation of colovesical or vesicovaginal fistulae
5. Evaluation of bladder or anastomotic integrity after surgical procedure
6. Evaluation of blunt or penetrating trauma to the bladder

Limitations

Abdominal and pelvic CT is so commonly used in the evaluation of blunt or penetrating trauma to the abdomen that CT cystography is often performed in conjunction with the trauma evaluation. However, studies have shown that conventional static cystography is as sensitive as CT cystography in detecting bladder rupture (Quagliano et al, 2006; Broghammer and Wessells, 2008).

VOIDING CYSTOURETHROGRAM

A voiding cystourethrogram (VCUG) is performed to evaluate the anatomy and physiology of the bladder and urethra. The study provides valuable information regarding the posterior urethra in pediatric patients. VCUG has long been used to demonstrate vesicoureteral reflux.

Technique

The study may be performed with the patient supine or in a semiupright position using a table capable of bringing the patient into the full upright position. A preliminary pelvic plain radiograph is obtained. In children, a 5- to 8-Fr feeding tube is used to fill the bladder to the appropriate volume. Patient comfort should be taken into account when determining the appropriate volume. In the adult population a standard catheter may be placed and the bladder filled to 200 to 400 mL. The catheter is removed and a film is obtained. During voiding, AP and oblique films are obtained. The bladder neck and urethra may be evaluated by fluoroscopy during voiding. Bilateral oblique views may demonstrate low-grade reflux, which is not able to be appreciated on the AP film. In addition, oblique films will demonstrate bladder or urethral diverticula, which are not always visible in the straight AP projection. Postvoiding films should be performed (Fig. 2-10).

Indications

1. Evaluation of structural and functional bladder outlet obstruction
2. Evaluation of reflux
3. Evaluation of the urethra in males and females

Limitations

This study requires bladder filling using a catheter. This may be traumatic in children and difficult in some patients with anatomic abnormalities of the urethra or bladder neck. Filling of the bladder may stimulate bladder spasms at low volumes and some patients are unable to hold adequate volumes for investigation. **Bladder filling in patients with spinal cord injuries higher than T6 may precipitate autonomic dysreflexia** (Barbaric, 1976; Fleischman and Shah, 1977; Linsenmeyer et al, 1996).

NUCLEAR SCINTIGRAPHY

Radionuclide imaging is the procedure of choice to evaluate renal obstruction and function. It is very sensitive to changes that induce focal or global changes in kidney function. Because neither Gd nor iodinated IV contrast agents are used, scintigraphy does not damage the kidney, has no lingering toxicity, results in minimal absorbed radiation, and is free from allergic reactions. Compared to other diagnostic imaging studies such as retrograde pyelogram, renal scintigraphy is noninvasive, has minimal risk and minimal discomfort, and allows determination of the function of the kidney.

Once the agent is injected IV, gamma scintillation cameras measure radiation emitted from the radioisotope, and digital work stations gather, process, and display the information. There is an extensive list of radiopharmaceuticals used for renal scintigraphy. This section will be limited to those agents most commonly used in urologic practice.

Technetium 99m-diethylenetriamine pentaacetic acid (^{99m}Tc-DTPA) is primarily a glomerular filtration agent (Peters, 1998; Gates, 2004). It is most useful for evaluation of obstruction and renal function. Because it is excreted through the kidney and dependent on GFR, it is less useful in patients with renal failure because impaired GFR may limit adequate evaluation of the collecting

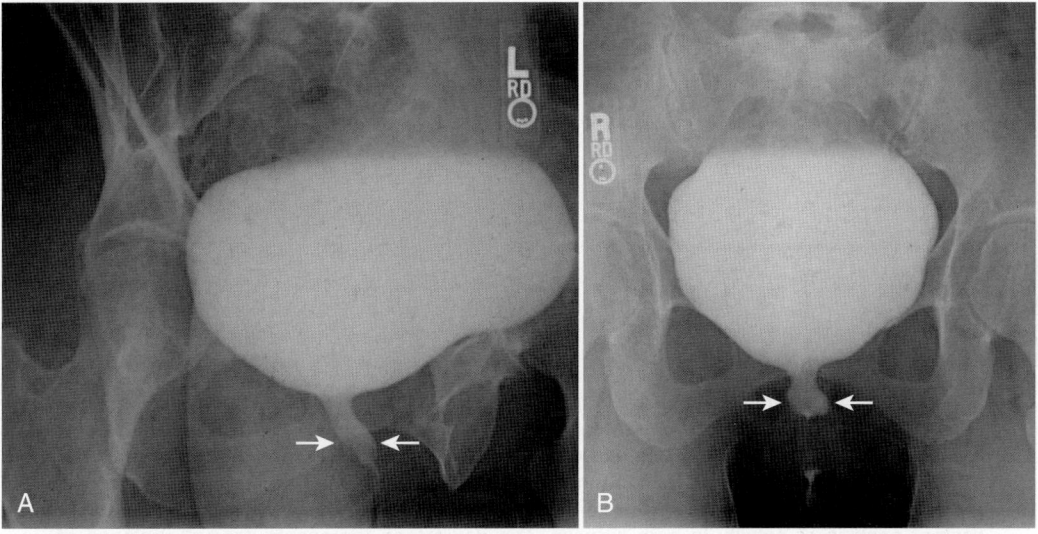

Figure 2-10. **A voiding cystourethrography performed for the evaluation of recurrent urinary tract infection in this female patient. A, An oblique film during voiding demonstrates thickening of the midureteral profile** (arrows). **B, After interruption of voiding, a ureteral diverticulum is clearly visible extending posteriorly and to the left of the midline** (arrows).

system and ureters. It is readily available and relatively inexpensive (Klopper et al, 1972).

Technetium 99m-dimercaptosuccinic acid (^{99m}Tc-DMSA) is cleared by both filtration and secretion. It localizes to the renal cortex with very little accumulation in the renal papilla and medulla (Lin et al, 1974). Therefore it is most useful for identifying cortical defects and ectopic or aberrant kidneys. With these properties, ^{99m}Tc-DMSA can distinguish a benign functioning abnormality in the kidney from a space-occupying malignant lesion, which would not have normal renal function. No valuable information on the ureter or collecting system can be obtained with ^{99m}Tc-DMSA, but it remains a standard for renal cortical imaging.

Technetium 99m-mercaptoacetyl triglycine (^{99m}Tc-MAG3) is an excellent agent for imaging because of its photon emission, 6-hour half-life, and ease of preparation. It is cleared mainly by tubular secretion (Fritzberg et al, 1986). A small amount, approximately 10%, of ^{99m}Tc-MAG3, is excreted by extrarenal means, and most of this is hepatobiliary excretion (Eshima et al, 1990; Itoh, 2001). Because it is extensively bound to protein in plasma, it is limited in its ability to measure GFR, but it is an excellent choice for patients with renal insufficiency and urinary obstruction. The tracer is well suited for evaluation of renal function and diuretic scintigraphy. Also, it is an excellent tracer to evaluate renal plasma flow.

Diuretic Scintigraphy

Nuclear medicine imaging plays a crucial role unmet by CT, MRI, or ultrasonography in the diagnosis of upper tract obstruction, and its unique characteristics provide noninvasive information regarding dynamic renal function. The diuretic renal scan using ^{99m}Tc-MAG3 is able to provide differential renal function and clearance time comparing right and left kidneys, which is pivotal in patient management. The initial phase is the flow phase where 2-second images are gathered for 2 minutes and then 1-second images for 60 seconds. The flow phase shows renal uptake, background clearance, and abnormal vascular lesions, which may indicate arteriovenous malformations, tumors, or active bleeding. In the second phase, the renal phase, time-to-peak uptake is typically between 2 and 4 minutes. The renal phase is the most sensitive indicator of renal dysfunction. One-minute images are taken for 30 minutes. In the final phase, the excretory phase, 1-minute images are taken for 30 minutes. **A diuretic (usually furosemide 0.5 mg/kg) is administered when maximum collecting system activity is visualized. The $T_{1/2}$ is the time it takes for collecting system activity to decrease by 50% from that at the time of diuretic administration. This is highly technician dependent because the diuretic must be given when the collecting system is displaying maximum activity. Transit time through the collecting system in less than 10 minutes is consistent with a normal, nonobstructed collecting system. $T_{1/2}$ of 10 to 20 minutes shows mild to moderate delay and may be a mechanical obstruction. The patient's perception of pain after diuretic administration can be helpful for the treating urologist to consider when planning surgery in the patient with mild to moderate obstruction. A $T_{1/2}$ of greater than 20 minutes is consistent with a high-grade obstruction. The level of obstruction can usually be determined, as can abnormalities such as ureteral duplication** (Ell and Gambhir, 2004). A normal renal scan is shown in Figure 2-11.

Hepatobiliary excretion can cause false-positive readings if the area of intestinal activity or gallbladder activity is included in the area of interrogations during the study (Fig. 2-12).

The diuretic renal scan is another imaging study where communication with the interpreting physician is vital for correct performance of the test, as well as appropriate interpretation. For example, there are times when patients with unilateral or bilateral ureteral stents are sent for diuretic scintigraphy to determine differential renal function. If a bladder catheter is not placed and open to drainage during the diuretic renal scan, the radiopharmaceutical excreted from the healthy kidney may wash up into or back flow via the ureteral stent into the stented kidney, giving the false-positive appearance to have more function than is physiologically present. This false-positive test may lead to inappropriately reconstructing a kidney that in reality has little or insufficient function.

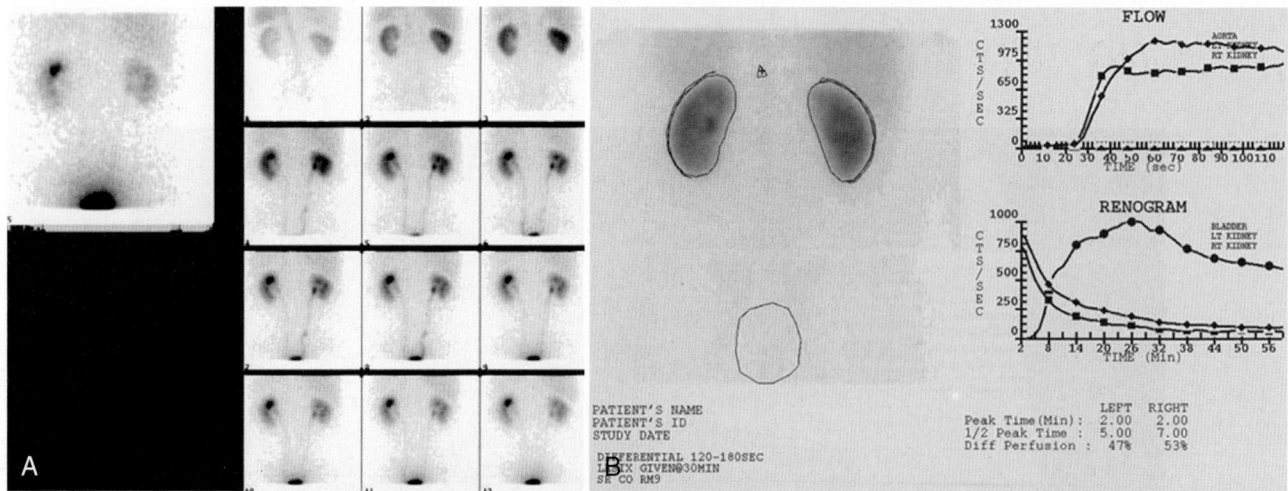

Figure 2-11. A, Technetium 99m-mercaptoacetyl triglycine (^{99m}Tc-MAG3) perfusion images demonstrate normal, prompt, symmetrical blood flow to both kidneys. **B,** Perfusion time-activity curves demonstrate essentially symmetrical flow to both kidneys. Note the rising curve typical of ^{99m}Tc-MAG3 flow studies. Dynamic function images demonstrate good uptake of tracer by both kidneys and prompt visualization of the collecting systems. This renogram demonstrates prompt peaking of activity in both kidneys. The downslope represents prompt drainage of activity from the kidneys. The printout of quantitative data shows the differential renal function to be 47% on the left, 53% on the right. The normal half-life for drainage is less than 20 minutes when ^{99m}Tc-MAG3 is used. The $T_{1/2}$ is 5 minutes on the left and 7 minutes on the right consistent with both kidneys being unobstructed.

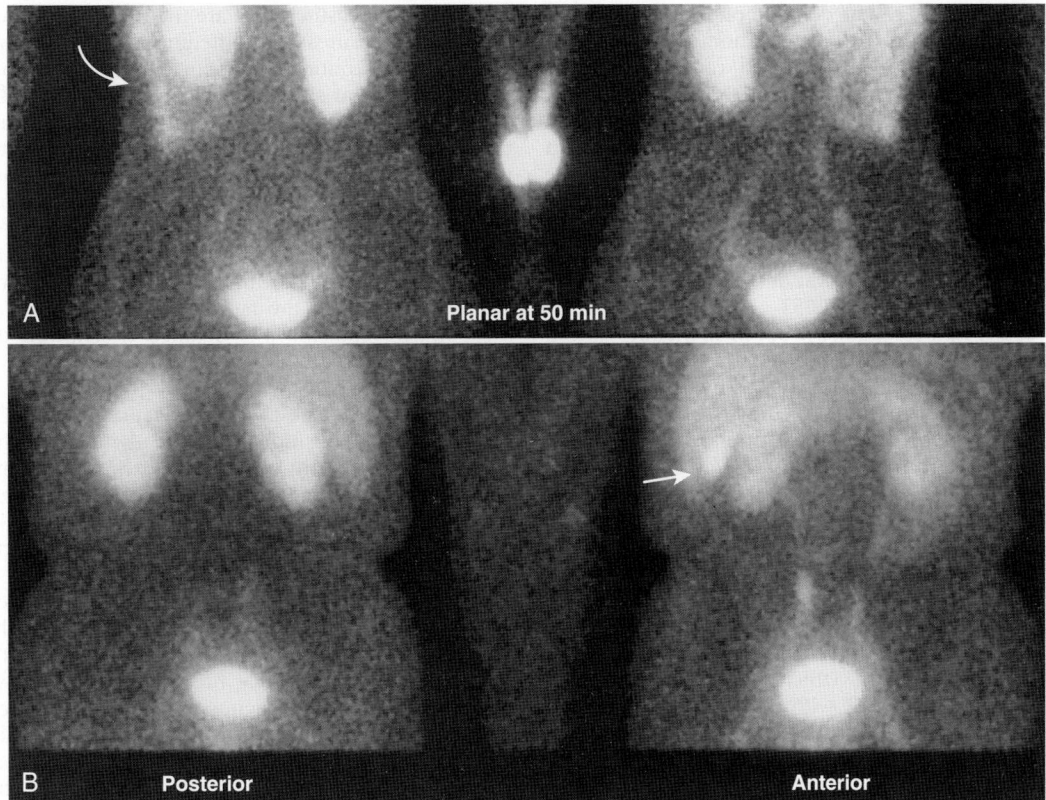

Figure 2-12. Delayed static images in the posterior and anterior projections demonstrate intestinal activity (*arrow* in A) and gallbladder activity (*arrow* in B), reflecting a normal mode of excretion of technetium 99m-mercaptoacetyl triglycine (^{99m}Tc-MAG3). Gallbladder activity, in particular, can cause false-positive interpretation when it overlies activity in the renal collecting system or is inappropriately included in the area of interrogation. Liver activity is variable and tends to be more pronounced in children and patients with renal insufficiency.

Nuclear Medicine in Urologic Oncology

Whole-Body Bone Scan

Conventional radionuclide imaging in urologic malignancy has long been the standard for detecting bone metastasis. The whole-body bone scan or skeletal scintigraphy is the most sensitive method for detecting bone metastasis (Narayan et al, 1988). A "positive" bone scan is not specific for cancer and may require plain film radiography, CT, or MRI to confirm, as well as correlation with prior history of bone fractures, trauma, surgery, or arthritis. In patients with diffuse metastatic bone involvement, the bone scan can be mistaken for normal because there is uniformly increased uptake in the bony structures (Kim et al, 1991).

Positron Emission Tomography

The most recent advance in nuclear scintigraphy is in the detection of primary and metastatic cancer using positron emission tomography (PET). Depending on the radiotracer used, PET offers diagnostic information based on glucose, choline, or amino acid metabolism and has also been applied to imaging tumor cell proliferation and tissue hypoxia in urologic malignancies. The diagnostic performance of fluorodeoxyglucose (FDG)-PET is hampered by the renal excretion of FDG and by the low metabolic activity often seen in tumors such as prostate cancer. However, new PET tracers including radiolabeled choline and acetate may offer an alternative approach. There is consistent evidence that FDG-PET provides important diagnostic information in detecting metastatic and recurrent germ cell tumors, and it might offer additional information in the staging and restaging of bladder and renal cancer (Powles et al, 2007; Rioja et al, 2010).

Molecular imaging with PET may help individualize the surgical and medical care of urologic oncology patients. PET is certainly having an impact in general oncology and is being actively investigated for use in urologic malignancies. PET provides unique insights into molecular pathways of diseases. PET using ^{18}F-FDG has gained increasing acceptance for the diagnosis, staging, and treatment monitoring of various tumor types.

There are data on the use of PET/CT in testis cancer, where PET/CT was found to have a higher diagnostic accuracy than CT for staging and restaging in the assessment of a CT-visualized residual mass following chemotherapy for seminoma and non-seminomatous germ cell tumors (Albers et al, 1999; Hain et al, 2000). There may be a role for detection of recurrent nonteratoma disease and the assessment of residual masses after chemotherapy. In a series of seminoma patients who were evaluated after chemotherapy for residual retroperitoneal masses, PET was accurate in 14 of 14 patients with tumors greater than 3 cm and in 22 of 23 patients with lesions less than 3 cm. Overall the sensitivity and specificity was 89% and 100%, respectively (De Santis et al, 2004). The accuracy of PET seems to be compromised if performed within 2 weeks of completion of chemotherapy, likely because of decreased metabolism and increased macrophage activity (Eary, 1999). It is recommended that PET/CT be delayed for 4 to 12 weeks following completion of chemotherapy (Shvarts et al, 2002).

PET/CT may have a promising role in clear cell renal cell carcinoma. An antibody (cG250) recognizing carbonic anhydrase IX has been developed. Carbonic anhydrase IX is a protein related to the unrestrained growth of clear cell renal cancers. A positron-emitting radionuclide (iodine 124) has been attached to the cG250 antibody and injected into renal cell cancer patients. The radionuclide antibody complex attaches to the carbonic anhydrase IX protein from clear cell renal cancer cells and can be detected on PET/CT imaging. Using this scheme in 26 patients with renal tumors, there was 94% sensitivity and 100% specificity in renal cell carcinoma before surgery (Larson and Schöder, 2008).

There are at least seven tracers being investigated for detection of metastatic prostate cancer. Each tracer is directed at a different part of cell function such as glycolysis, amino acid transport, choline kinase activity, fatty acid synthesis, androgen receptor, and bone mineralization. FDG as a PET tracer was investigated in 91 patients with prostate-specific antigen (PSA) recurrence after radical prostatectomy. FDG-PET was able to detect local or systemic recurrence in only 34% of patients (Schöder et al, 2005).

Very few studies have addressed the use of PET in bladder cancer. FDG is renal excreted and not useful in bladder cancer. Only 78% of bladder cancer could be visualized using ^{11}C-methionine tracer and PET did not improve local staging of the disease. ^{11}C-choline was also found to be a poor predictor of primary or metastatic urothelial carcinoma (Ahlstrom et al, 1996; de Jong et al, 2002).

PET is still in the early stages of investigation for urologic tumors. The exact role in the practice of urology has yet to be determined but will certainly have a great role in the future as more tracers specific to urologic cancers are discovered. Using the combination of nuclear imaging and ever-increasing knowledge about cancer cell biology, radiotracers have been developed to be incorporated into dividing cells or cellular mechanisms involved in the increased metabolic activity of malignancies, which can then be detected using PET imaging. Combining PET with high-resolution CT has the ability to increase our detection of recurrent or metastatic urologic cancers. Many different isotopes are being investigated for the detection of metastatic disease.

KEY POINTS: NUCLEAR SCINTIGRAPHY

- During diuretic renal scan, the diuretic must be given when maximum activity is seen in the kidney.
- An elimination $T_{1/2}$ less than 10 minutes is an unobstructed system, and a $T_{1/2}$ greater than 20 minutes is consistent with high-grade obstruction.
- If ureteral stents are in place, patients undergoing diuretic renal scan should have an unclamped bladder catheter in place during the study.
- ^{99m}Tc-MAG3 is the agent of choice for diuretic renal scan to determine differential renal function and obstruction.

COMPUTED TOMOGRAPHY

The 1979 Nobel Prize in Medicine and Physiology was awarded to Allan M. Cormack and Sir Godfrey N. Hounsfield for the development of computer-assisted tomography. While basic principles remain the same, significant advances over the past 35 years have resulted in the development of multidetector CT devices, improving soft tissue detail and allow the possibility of rapid three-dimensional (3D) reconstruction of the entire genitourinary system.

CT has become one of the most integral parts of urologic practice, and the CT urogram (CTU) has replaced IVU as the imaging modality of choice in modern urology for the workup of hematuria, urologic malignancies, detection of kidney stones, and preoperative planning. As in the case of conventional radiographic imaging, the basis for CT imaging is the attenuation of x-ray photons as they pass through the patient. Tomography is an imaging method that produces 3D images of internal structures by recording the passage of x-rays as they pass through different body tissues. In the case of CT, a computer reconstructs cross-sectional images of the body based on measurements of x-ray transmission through thin slices of the body tissue (Brant, 1999). A collimated x-ray beam is generated on one side of the patient, and the amount of transmitted radiation is measured by a detector placed on the opposite side of the x-ray

beam. These measurements are then repeated systematically, while a series of exposures from different projections is made as the x-ray beam rotates around the patient. The result is production of a 3D image of internal structures in the human body by recording the passage of different energy waves through various internal structures. Data collected by the detectors are reconstructed by computerized algorithms to result in a viewable tomographic display.

There are several different imaging variables that are adjusted to allow adequate, detailed image resolution while minimizing the time on the scanner and limiting exposure to radiation. The variable application of pitch, beam collimation, detector size, and tube voltage are used by the radiologist and imaging technologist for ideal image requisition. A detailed description of each of these variables is beyond the scope of this chapter (see Suggested Readings).

Perhaps the greatest recent advancement in CT is the use of helical image acquisition techniques with multichannel or multidetectors (MDCT). In a helical CT the patient moves through a continuously rotating gantry. The helical raw images are processed using interpolation algorithms in order to visualize the internal structures as sagittal, coronal, or axial reconstructed images. The "single slice spiral CT," introduced in 1988, had a single row of detectors and required multiple passes to visualize a small area of interrogation. The standard scanners in use today have between 64 and 320 rows of detectors, which allow the patient's entire body to be imaged during a single breath hold, with few or no motion artifacts, more precise diagnostic accuracy, increased concentration of contrast material, shorter scanning time, less radiation exposure, and significant increase in anatomic coverage with a single scan. CT scanners with 750 rows of detectors are currently being developed. For example, in one second, a 320-slice CT scanner can image slices as large as 16 cm (6.3 inches), capturing all of the body's organs in a single rotation of the central x-ray-emitting gantry (Wang et al, 1994; Mahesh, 2002) (Fig. 2-13).

Readily available software is capable of 3D processing of CT images to recreate the urinary system. These 3D images offer improved preoperative planning, appreciation of proximity to adjacent organs, the ability to define vasculature, and improved communication with patients, who can now easily see their particular pathology and better appreciate the challenges faced by their surgeon (Fig. 2-14).

Dual-source CT (DSCT) is a relatively new technique used for diagnostic imaging, using two rotating tubes to acquire both high- and low-voltage images allowing tissue differentiation, visualization of tendons and ligaments, improved CT angiography, and differentiation of kidney stones based on stone composition (Coursey et al, 2010). Using DSCT, a reliable distinction can be made between uric acid and calcium oxalate and between brushite and uric acid stones (Ferrandino et al, 2010; Botsikas et al, 2013).

Real-time CT fluoroscopy is now available as an option on new CT imaging equipment. CT fluoroscopy gives a 3D CT image that is much more detailed and offers greater soft tissue contrast and resolution than conventional CT. The most common use in urology is for biopsy of the kidney. CT fluoroscopy helps to overcome movement of the kidney during respiratory variation. It also has been used for fluid aspiration, drain placement, catheter placement, percutaneous cryoablation, and radiofrequency (RF) ablation of renal tumors. **One significant disadvantage of CT fluoroscopy is the increased radiation exposure to the patient and radiologist or surgeon performing the procedure** (Daly et al, 1999; Keat, 2001; Gupta et al, 2006).

The CTU is an excretory urography in which the MDCT is used for imaging of the urinary tract. It is indicated in the workup of hematuria, kidney stones, renal masses, renal colic, and urothelial tumors. The CT scan examination starts with the physician's request for imaging. Radiologists around the world appreciate a brief description from the urologist of the question to be answered by the CT scan. Equipped with a better understanding of why the CT was ordered, the radiologist and the CT technician can adjust different CT variables and choose the appropriate contrast media needed to deliver a valuable report back to the ordering urologist.

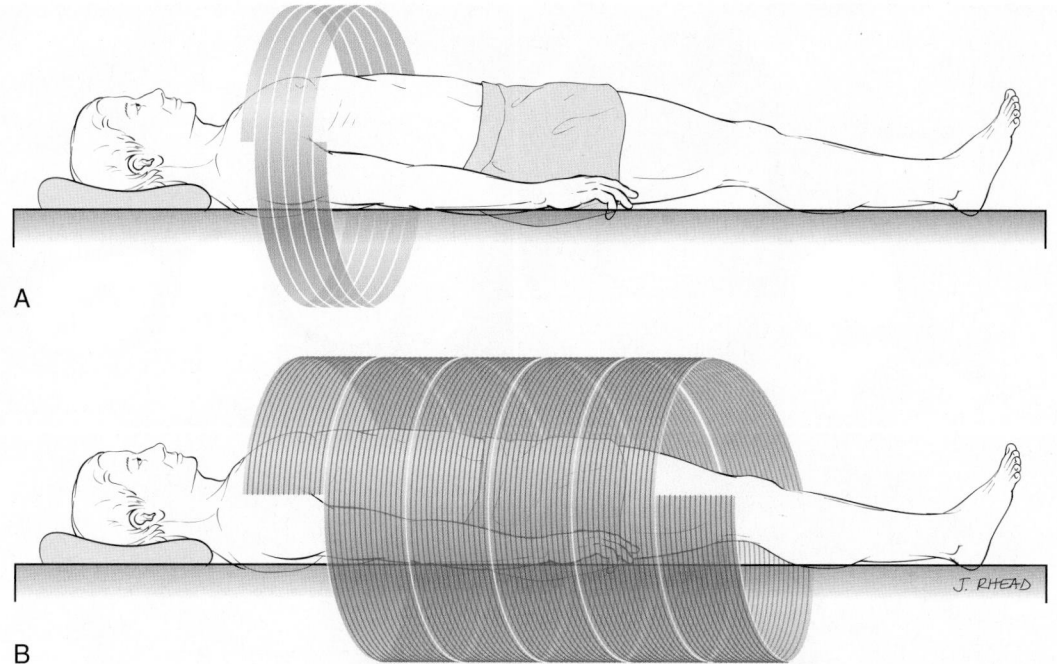

Figure 2-13. A, A computed tomography scanner with a single-row detector requires five circular passes around the patient to image a small area of the patient's body. **B,** With a 16-slice, multirow detector, the chest, abdomen, and pelvis can be imaged with five circular passes, easily obtained during a single breath hold. The thin slices offered by the 16-slice detector offer much greater detail of internal structures.

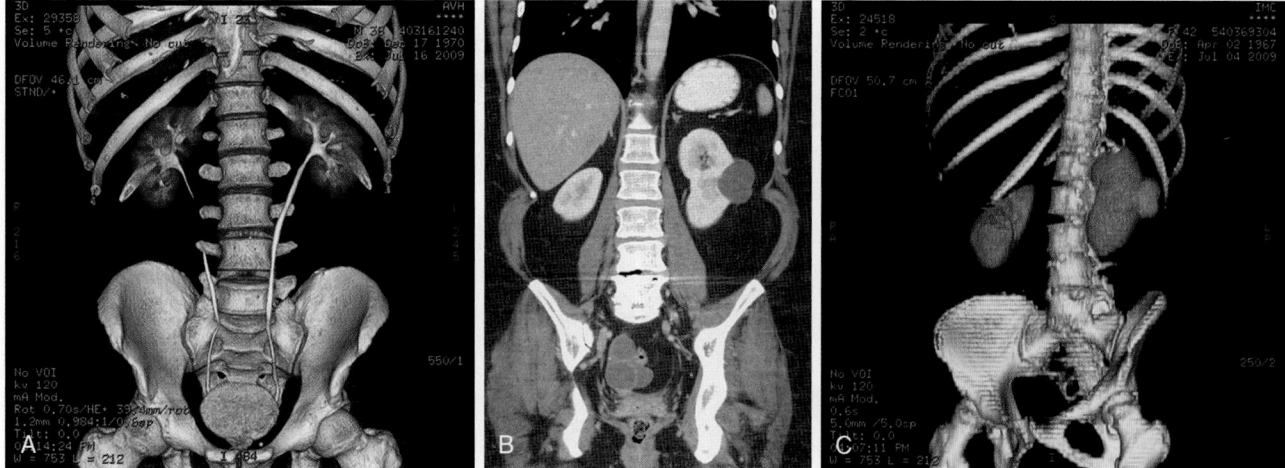

Figure 2-14. A, Three-dimensional (3D) colored reconstruction of the kidneys, ureters, and bladder from computed tomography urogram. **B,** Coronal reconstruction in a patient with a clear cell renal cell carcinoma in a complex renal cystic mass and enhancing mural nodule. **C,** 3D reconstruction of the same patient with slight posterior rotation.

Urologists often request a CT evaluation of the abdomen and pelvis. An abdominal CT starts at the diaphragm and ends at the iliac crest. If the pelvis is to be imaged, a separate request is usually required. The pelvic CT begins at the iliac crest and terminates at the pubis symphysis. Intravenous contrast may be required for better delineation of soft tissue. Oral contrast is not commonly used in urology but may be helpful in certain patients to differentiate bowel from lymph nodes, scar, or tumor (Fig. 2-15).

Hounsfield Units

A single CT image generated by the scanner is divided into many tiny blocks of different shades of black and white called pixels. The actual gray scale of each pixel on a CT depends on the amount of radiation absorbed at that point, which is termed an attenuation value. **Attenuation values are expressed in Hounsfield units (HU). The HU scale, or attenuation value, is based on a reference scale in which air is assigned a value of −1000 HU and dense bone is assigned the value of +1000 HU. Water is assigned 0 HU.**

Urolithiasis

Patients coming to the emergency department with abdominal pain or renal colic are frequently evaluated with CT imaging. The use of unenhanced CT imaging to identify urolithiasis was first reported in 1995 (Smith et al, 1995) and has now become the standard

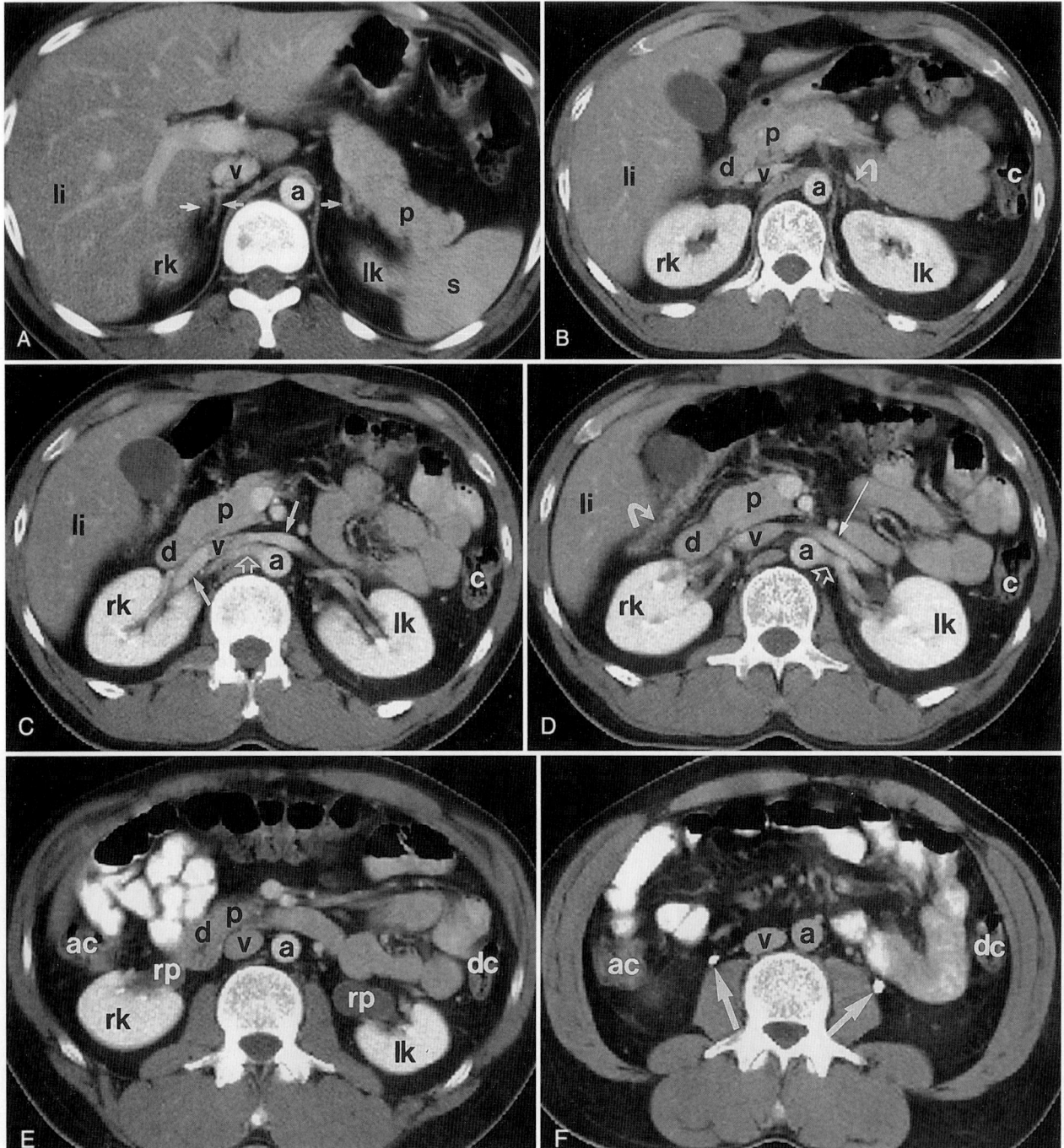

Figure 2-15. Computed tomography of the abdomen and pelvis demonstrating normal genitourinary anatomy. A, The adrenal glands are indicated with *arrows.* The upper poles of the right and left kidneys are indicated with rk and lk, respectively. a, aorta; li, liver; p, pancreas; s, spleen; v, inferior vena cava. B, Scan through the upper pole of the kidneys. The left adrenal gland is indicated with an *arrow.* a, aorta; c, colon; d, duodenum; li, liver; lk, left kidney; p, pancreas; rk, right kidney; v, inferior vena cava. C, Scan through the hilum of the kidneys. The main renal veins are indicated with *solid arrows*, and the right main renal artery is indicated with an *open arrow.* a, aorta; c, colon; d, duodenum; li, liver; lk, left kidney; p, pancreas; rk, right kidney; v, inferior vena cava. D, Scan through the hilum of the kidneys slightly caudal to C. The left main renal vein is indicated with a *solid straight arrow*, and the left main renal artery is indicated with an *open arrow.* The hepatic flexure of the colon is indicated with a *curved arrow.* a, aorta; c, colon; d, duodenum; li, liver; lk, left kidney; p, pancreas; rk, right kidney; v, inferior vena cava. E, Scan through the mid to lower polar region of the kidneys. a, aorta; ac, ascending colon; d, duodenum; dc, descending colon; lk, left kidney; p, pancreas; rk, right kidney; rp, renal pelvis; v, inferior vena cava. F, CT scan obtained below the kidneys reveals filling of the upper ureters *(arrows).* The wall of the normal ureter is usually paper thin or not visible on CT. a, aorta; ac, ascending colon; dc, descending colon; v, inferior vena cava.

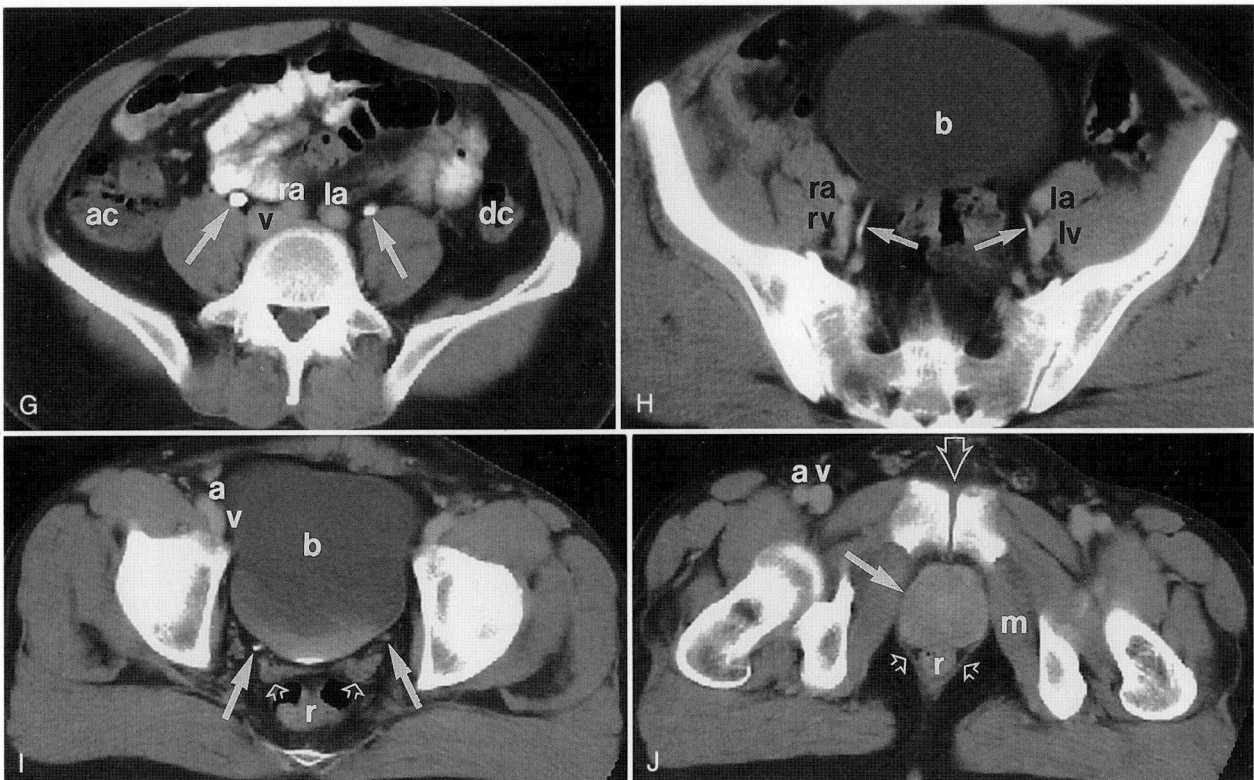

Figure 2-15, cont'd   G, Contrast filling of the midureters *(arrows)* on a scan obtained at the level of the iliac crest and below the aortic bifurcation. ac, ascending colon; dc, descending colon; la, left common iliac artery; ra, right common iliac artery; v, inferior vena cava. **H,** The distal ureters *(arrows)* course medial to the iliac vessels on a scan obtained below the promontory of the sacrum. b, urinary bladder; la, left external iliac artery; lv, left external iliac vein; ra, right external iliac artery; rv, right external iliac vein. **I,** Scan through the roof of the acetabulum reveals distal ureters *(solid arrows)* near the ureterovesical junction. The bladder (b) is filled with urine and partially opacified with contrast material. The normal seminal vesicle *(open arrows)* usually has a paired bow-tie structure with slightly lobulated contour. a, right external iliac artery; r, rectum; v, right external iliac vein. **J,** Scan at the level of the pubic symphysis *(large open arrow)* reveals the prostate gland *(solid arrow)*. a, right external iliac artery; m, obturator internus muscle; r, rectum; v, right external iliac vein; *small open arrows,* seminal vesicle.

diagnostic tool to evaluate renal colic. It offers the advantage over IVU of avoiding contrast and being able to diagnose other abdominal abnormalities that can also cause abdominal pain. MDCT can readily diagnose radiolucent stones which may not have been seen on IVU, as well as small stones even in the distal ureter (Federle et al, 1981). **With the exception of some indinavir stones, all renal and ureteral stones can be detected on helical CT scan** (Schwartz et al, 1999). In the workup of urolithiasis, the unenhanced CT has a sensitivity ranging between 96% and 100% and specificity ranging between 92% and 100% (Memarsadeghi et al, 2005). **Stones in the distal ureter can be difficult to differentiate from pelvic calcifications. In these cases, the urologist needs to look for other signs of obstruction which indicate the presence of a stone, including ureteral dilation, inflammatory changes in the perinephric fat, hydronephrosis, and a soft tissue rim surrounding the calcification within the ureter. The soft tissue rim around a stone represents irritation and edema in the ureteral wall** (Heneghan et al, 1997; Dalrymple et al, 2000) (Fig. 2-16).

Stone patients are frequently subjected to radiation exposure as part of diagnosis, treatment, and follow-up. Increasing awareness of the potential long-term adverse effects of radiation exposure has encouraged urologists and radiologists to discover means to decrease the amount of radiation exposure. The low-dose, unenhanced helical CT scan is gaining increasing popularity for initial diagnosis of renal colic suspected to be due to urolithiasis and for follow-up

in stone patients. Using low-dose CT protocols, the specificity and sensitivity of unenhanced low-dose helical CT scan is approximately 96% and 97%, respectively. Low-dose techniques offer a 99% positive predictive value and a 90% negative predictive value for urolithiasis. The end result is a 50% to 75% decrease in the patient's total radiation exposure for each CT obtained (Liu et al, 2000; Hamm et al, 2002; Kalra et al, 2005).

Cystic and Solid Renal Masses

The frequent CT imaging of patients in the emergency department has resulted in an increase in the detection of incidental renal masses. Using CT imaging the mass can be characterized as a simple or complex cyst, or a solid mass. Based on the HU attenuation scale, we would expect simple cysts to have HU near zero (Fig. 2-17).

When the unenhanced CT images of a renal mass are compared to the enhanced images obtained in the cortical medullary or nephrogenic phase, an increase in HU (measured in the area of the renal mass) by 15 to 20 HU confirms the presence of a solid enhancing mass, which is usually renal cancer. Pseudoenhancement is maximal when small (≤1.5 cm) intrarenal cysts are scanned during maximal levels of renal parenchymal enhancement. The magnitude of this effect varies with scanner type but may be large enough to prevent accurate lesion characterization, despite use of a thin-section helical CT data acquisition technique (Birnbaum

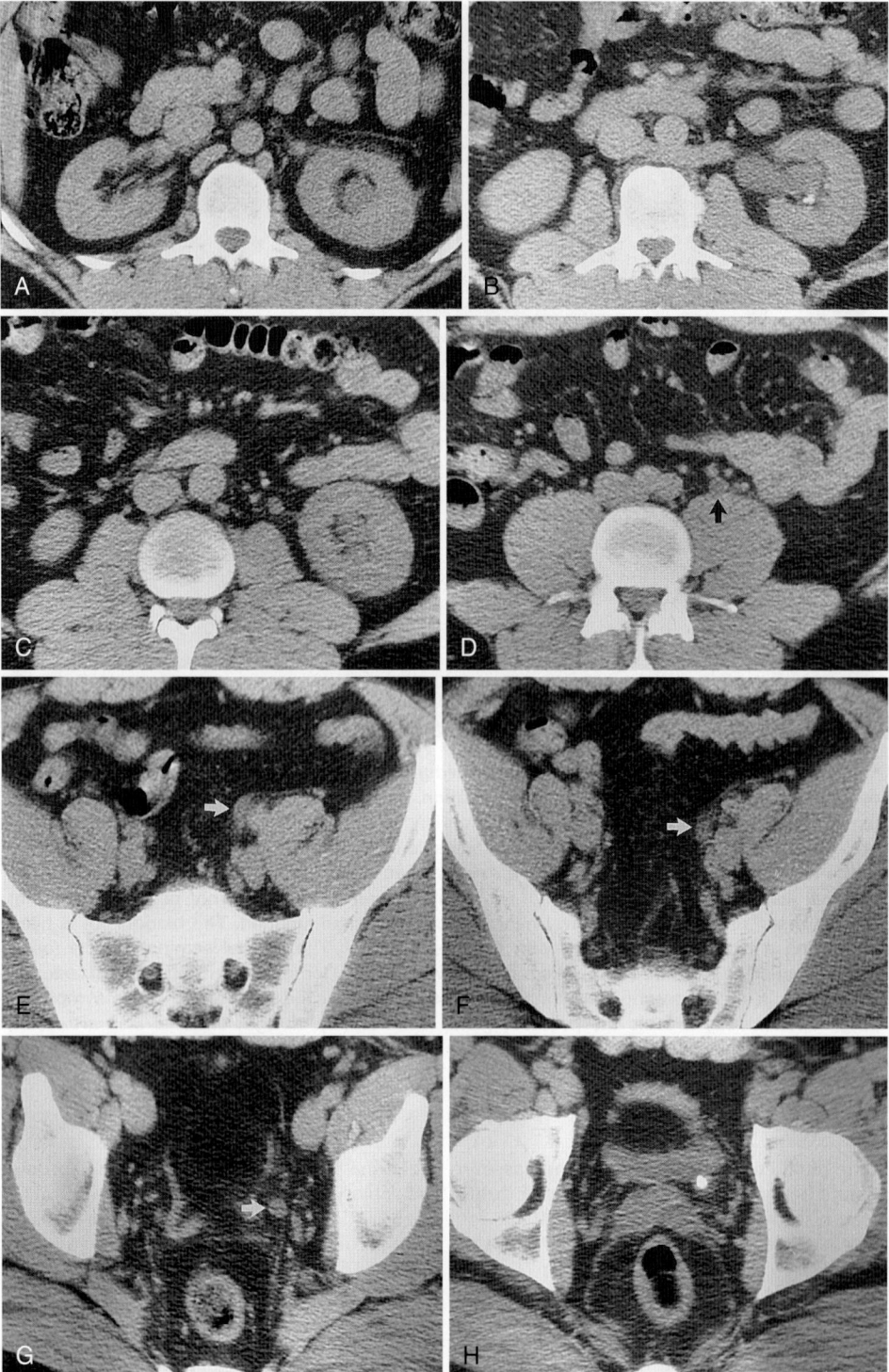

Figure 2-16. Computed tomography of the abdomen and pelvis in patient with an obstructing ureteral stone at the level of the ureterovesical junction (UVJ). A, Level of the left upper pole. Mild renal enlargement, caliectasis, and perinephric stranding are apparent. B, Level of the left renal hilum. Left pyelectasis with a dependent stone, mild peripelvic and perinephric stranding, and a retroaortic left renal vein are shown. C, Level of the left lower pole. Left caliectasis, proximal ureterectasis, and mild periureteral stranding are present. D, Level of the aortic bifurcation. The dilated left ureter *(arrow)* has lower attenuation than do nearby vessels. E, Level of the upper portion of the sacrum. A dilated left ureter *(arrow)* crosses anteromedial to the common iliac artery. F, Level of the midsacrum. A dilated left ureter *(arrow)* is accompanied by periureteral stranding. G, Level of the top of the acetabulum showing a dilated pelvic portion of the left ureter *(arrow)*. H, Level of the UVJ. The impacted stone with a "cuff" or "tissue rim" sign that represents the edematous wall of the ureter. (From Talner LB, O'Reilly PH, Wasserman NF. Specific causes of obstruction. In: Pollack HM, McClennan BL, Dyer R, et al, editors. Clinical urography. 2nd ed. Philadelphia: Saunders; 2000.)

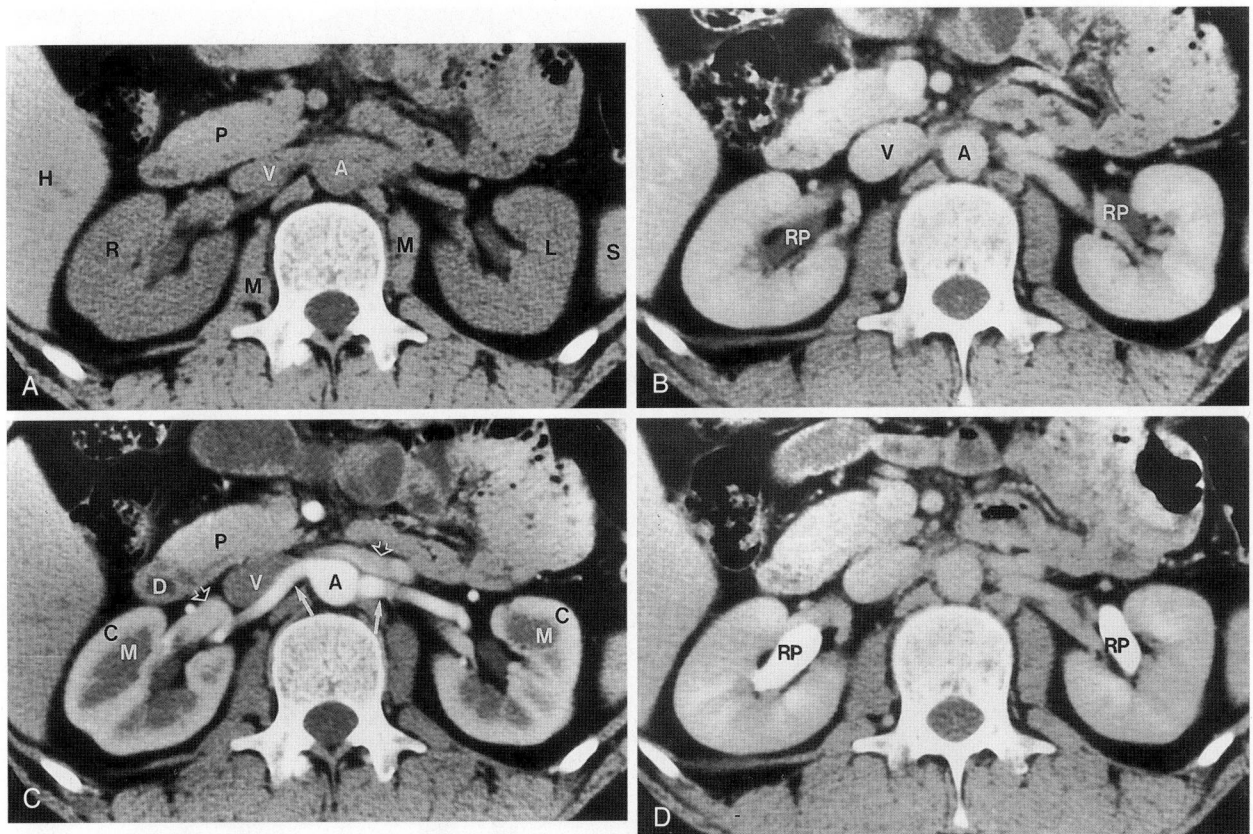

Figure 2-17. **Renal computed tomography (CT) demonstrating normal nephrogenic progression. A, Unenhanced CT scan obtained at the level of the renal hilum shows right (R) and left (L) kidneys of CT attenuation values slightly less than those of the liver (H) and pancreas (P). A, abdominal aorta; M, psoas muscle; S, spleen; V, inferior vena cava. B, Enhanced CT scan obtained during a cortical nephrographic phase, generally 25 to 80 seconds after contrast medium injection, reveals increased enhancement of the renal cortex (C) relative to the medulla (M). The main renal artery is indicated with *solid arrows* bilaterally. Main renal veins *(open arrows)* are less opacified with respect to the aorta (A) and arteries. D, duodenum; P, pancreas; V, inferior vena cava. C, CT scan obtained during the homogeneous nephrographic phase, generally between 85 and 120 seconds after contrast medium administration, reveals a homogeneous, uniform, increased attenuation of the renal parenchyma. The wall of the normal renal pelvis (RP) is paper thin or not visible on the CT scan. A, abdominal aorta; V, inferior vena cava. D, CT scan obtained during the excretory phase shows contrast medium in the renal pelvis (RP) bilaterally; this starts to appear approximately 3 minutes after contrast medium administration.**

et al, 2002). **The presence of fat, which should enhance less than 10 HU, is diagnostic for angiomyolipoma.** A hyperdense cyst shows no change in density between the postcontrast and delayed phase images (Fig. 2-18).

Complex cystic masses are usually characterized based on the Bosniak classification system. The most important criteria used to differentiate a lesion that should be considered for surgery versus a nonsurgical lesion is the presence or absence of tissue vascularity or enhancement. Bosniak category I, II, and IIF lesions do not enhance to any measurable degree. Category I lesions are simple cysts and considered to be benign. Category II lesions are more complicated and may have calcifications, high attenuation fluid, and several thin septae. Category III lesions are more complex, have small areas of calcification, and may also have irregular walls or septate where there is measurable enhancement. Cystic lesions discovered on CT scan that are difficult to categorize as either II or III are categorized as IIF. **Bosniak III lesions have been reported to be malignant renal cell carcinoma in 60% of cases and require close follow-up or surgical extirpation. Bosniak category IV lesions are cystic masses that meet all the criteria of category**

III, but also have enhancing soft tissue components adjacent to or independent of the wall or septum of the cyst; they have been reported to be malignant renal cell carcinoma in 100% of cases (Bosniak, 1997; Curry et al, 2000; Israel and Bosniak, 2005).

Hematuria

The CTU is one of the most common studies ordered for the workup of gross or microscopic hematuria. With MDCT it is possible to perform a comprehensive evaluation of the patient with one single examination (Chai et al, 2001). The study images the abdomen and pelvis and typically includes four different phases. The first scan is an unenhanced CT to distinguish between different masses that can be present in the kidney and uncover kidney stones that would later be obscured by the excretion of contrast into the renal collecting system. At 30 to 70 seconds after contrast injection, the corticomedullary phase is captured with another pass through the MDCT, helping to define vasculature and perfusion. The nephrogenic phase occurs between 90 to 180 seconds after injection of contrast

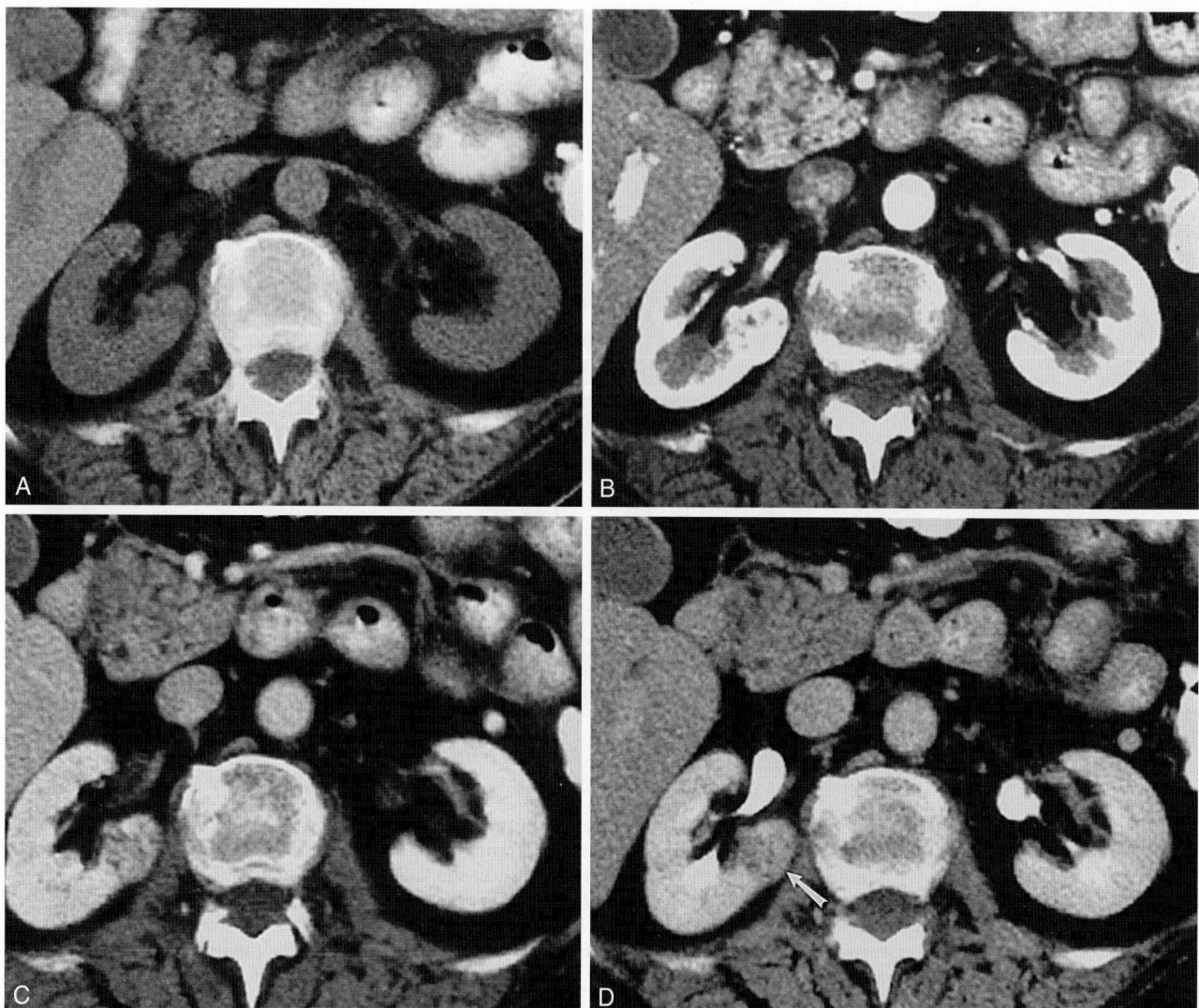

Figure 2-18. Small renal cell carcinoma in the infrahilar lip of the right kidney is not easily seen on unenhanced image (A). On corticomedullary phase image (B), the lesion is subtly visible as a hyperenhancing focus within the renal medulla. On nephrographic (C) and pyelographic phase (D) images, the full extent of the lesion *(arrow)* within the medulla and cortex is depicted. (From Brink JA, Siegel CL. Computed tomography of the upper urinary tract. In: Pollack HM, McClennan BL, Dyer R, et al, editors. Clinical urography. 2nd ed. Philadelphia: Saunders; 2000.)

and, when compared to the unenhanced images, allows sensitive detection and characterization of renal masses. The final phase is the excretory phase, imaged approximately 3 to 5 minutes after injection of contrast. This phase allows complete filling of the collecting system and usually allows visualization of the ureter (Joudi et al, 2006) (see Fig. 2-18).

CTU has been shown to be sensitive in detecting upper tract urothelial cancers. In one series of 57 patients with hematuria, 38 were found to have urothelial carcinoma. CT urography detected 37 of 38 urothelial cancers for a sensitivity of 97%, compared to retrograde pyelogram which detected 31 of 38 lesions and had a sensitivity of 82%. Approximately 90% of malignant upper tract lesions can be detected with CT urography (McCarthy and Cowan, 2002; Lang et al, 2003; Caoili et al, 2005). CT urography is not as sensitive as cystoscopy for the detection of urothelial tumors in the bladder. Only large bladder tumors are visualized with CT imaging studies as filling defects in the lumen of the bladder. Carcinoma in situ cannot be visualized on CT scanning, and therefore cystoscopy is still an important part of a comprehensive hematuria workup.

> **KEY POINTS: CT IMAGING**
>
> - The CTU is an excellent imaging choice to evaluate the kidney, upper tract collecting system, and ureter.
> - The CTU is highly sensitive and specific for upper tract urothelial carcinoma.
> - A renal mass in the kidney seen on CTU that enhances more than 15 to 20 HU is most likely a renal cancer.
> - With the exception of indinavir stones, all urinary stones are visible on unenhanced CT of the abdomen and pelvis.

MAGNETIC RESONANCE IMAGING

CT imaging remains the mainstay of urologic cross-sectional body imaging; however, MRI is increasingly being applied to the genitourinary system. With constant improvements in technology, MRI is gradually narrowing the overall resolution quality gap between the two techniques. A significant advantage of MRI is the excellent signal contrast resolution of soft tissue, without the need for IV contrast in many situations.

To obtain MR images, the patient is placed on a gantry that passes through the bore of the magnet. When exposed to a magnet field of sufficient strength, the free water protons in the patient orient themselves along the magnetic field's z-axis. This is the head-to-toe axis, straight through the bore of the magnet. An RF antenna or "coil" is placed over the body part to be imaged. It is the coil that transmits the RF pulses through the patient. When the RF pulse stops, protons release their energy, which is detected and processed to obtain the MR image. Currently, some coils can transmit and receive a signal, which is referred to dual channel RF. An MR sequence exploits the body's different tissue characteristics and the particular manner that each type of tissue absorbs and then releases this energy.

Weighting of the image depends on how the energy is imparted through the physics of the pulse sequence and whether the energy is released quickly or slowly. Images are described as being T1 or T2 weighted. The T1-weighted images are generated by the time required to return to equilibrium in the z-axis. The T2-weighted images are generated by the time to return to equilibrium in the xy-axis. **On T1-weighted MR images, fluid has a low SI and appears dark. T2-weighted MR images have a high SI and appear bright. In the kidney this translates into the cortex having a higher SI or being brighter than the medulla, which gives off a lower signal and is darker.**

MRI has significant advantages over other imaging modalities. First, and most importantly, no risks are associated with secondary malignancies from radiation exposure (Berrington de González and Darby, 2004). It is the modality of choice in patients who are pregnant, suffer from renal insufficiency, and/or have an iodine contrast allergy.

The contrast agents in MRI are noniodinated compounds. Iodinated compounds as used in CT imaging function by absorbing x-rays. **Gd-based contrast agents function on MRI secondary to shortening the relaxation times of water.** This results in an increase in SI (enhancement), most commonly assessed in a T1 sequence. Gd is a toxic heavy metal that is chelated to prevent cellular absorption and any associated toxicities (Lin and Brown, 2007). The dose of Gd is nontoxic for almost all patients except ones with *severe* renal insufficiency. **NSF occurs in patients with acute or chronic renal insufficiency with a GFR less than 30 mL/min/1.73 m^2** (see Contrast Media). Gd is deposited in skin and muscle as an insoluble precipitate that leads to the systemic fibrosis (Grobner, 2006). In response, the FDA has issued warnings regarding the association between NSF and Gd-based contrast agents because no effective treatment is available (U.S. Food and Drug Administration, 2006). The current guidelines are available at the FDA.gov official website (U.S. Food and Drug Administration, 2010).

Adrenal Magnetic Resonance Imaging

One of the key differences between MRI and other imaging modalities is its ability to characterize soft tissues without the use of IV contrast. In the adrenal gland, minute quantities of lipids can help differentiate between malignancies or benign adenomas. Most adrenal masses are identified incidentally and are nonfunctioning. **Adrenal adenomas are usually less than 3 cm in size and nonfunctional** (Boland et al, 2008). Adrenal adenomas have a high lipid content (74%), which makes them more readily differentiated from malignant processes (Dunnick and Korobkin, 2002).

Inversion-recovery imaging, chemical shift imaging (CSI), and fat saturation imaging are three approaches to assess lipid content on masses. These approaches use the differences in the behavior of fat protons and water protons within the magnetic field. CSI is the most commonly used technique for urologic patients.

Adrenal Adenoma

Adrenal adenomas are characterized by assessing the lipid content within cells. CSI uses the difference in the behavior of water protons

(H_2O) versus fat protons (-CH2-). The oxygen atom in water pulls on the electron cloud surrounding the hydrogen atom, whereas the carbon atom in fat is less electronegative and has a decreased effect on the hydrogen electron cloud (Pokharel et al, 2013). This difference in the magnetic field (shielding) for these two types of protons is the precessional frequencies or the chemical shift (Pokharel et al, 2013).

CSI obtains images "in-phase" (IP) and "out-of-phase" (OP) with regard to the water and fat protons. The signals detected for a given voxel can be additive or cancelled out. The IP imaging refers to the contribution of both fat and water, or additive to the signal at a given voxel. This occurs when the echo time (TE) is set to align the fat and water protons.

In the OP imaging, the TE is set to cancel the signals obtained, thus the subtraction of the protons results in a decrease, or cancelling, in signal at that given voxel and produces a lower SI if both fat and water are present.

The next step is to compare the two data sets (IP and OP) obtained to determine if there is a loss of signal (decrease) on the OP images, which is indicative of intracytoplasmic fat (Fig. 2-19). If there is no change between the two data sets, then there is a lower probability that fat is present within the mass. This was initially determined on a qualitative basis by visually comparing signal intensities between the two sequences (Korobkin et al, 1996). The loss of signal on CSI is 92% sensitive and has a limited specificity of 17% for adrenal adenoma (Boland et al, 2008).

Other investigators have attempted to determine SI index by quantitatively comparing the IP and OP images. Nakamura reported that using a 5% SI yielded an accuracy of 100% (3 tesla) in determining if intracytoplasmic lipid was present and thus a diagnosis of an adenoma (Nakamura et al, 2012). Although there are currently no set thresholds, cutoff ranges are reported to be between 1.7% and 20% (Nakamura et al, 2012). The limited specificity reported by the qualitative approach (17%) was increased to 100% specificity using quantitative SI index (Boland et al, 2008).

$$SI\ index\ (\%) = (SI\ in\ phase - SI\ out\ of\ phase)/SI\ in\ phase \times 100$$

In some clinical situations, lipid poor adenomas (10% to 30% incidence) can result in an indeterminate study (Elsayes et al, 2004). The typical washout of an adrenal cortical carcinoma is slow. Therefore an enhanced CT with washout may be a better study to differentiate lipid-poor adrenal adenomas from other adrenal masses (Park et al, 2007).

Adrenal Cortical Carcinoma

An adrenal cortical carcinoma (ACC) diagnosis is usually made using a combination of clinical factors and imaging characteristics (Fig. 2-20). In a review by Ng and Libertino (2003), ACC is hormonally active in 62% of cases. **The incidence of ACC is related to size, and adrenal lesions equal to or less than 4 cm represented 2% of all ACC diagnosed. The incidence of ACC increased to 6% for lesions 4 to 6 cm and to 25% for lesions greater than 6 cm** (Mansmann et al, 2004). T2- and T1-weighted images with Gd usually are heterogeneous with a high SI and a heterogeneous enhancement, respectively. CSI exhibits a low signal (Bharwani et al, 2011). **ACC is also associated with local vascular thrombosis, which can be detected on MRI** (Mezhir et al, 2008). ACC has an increased metabolic activity and can be visualized on FDG-PET imaging, and this can differentiate ACC from adenomas with 100% sensitivity and 88% specificity (Groussin et al, 2009).

Myelolipoma

Myelolipoma is a benign adrenal mass that consists of mature fatty tissues and bone marrow elements. Myelolipoma occurs in approximately 6.5% of patients with incidentally detected adrenal masses (Song et al, 2008). The complicating issue with myelolipomas is that the size of the mass can be greater than 4 cm, and this carries significant overlap with malignant adrenal lesions (Meyer

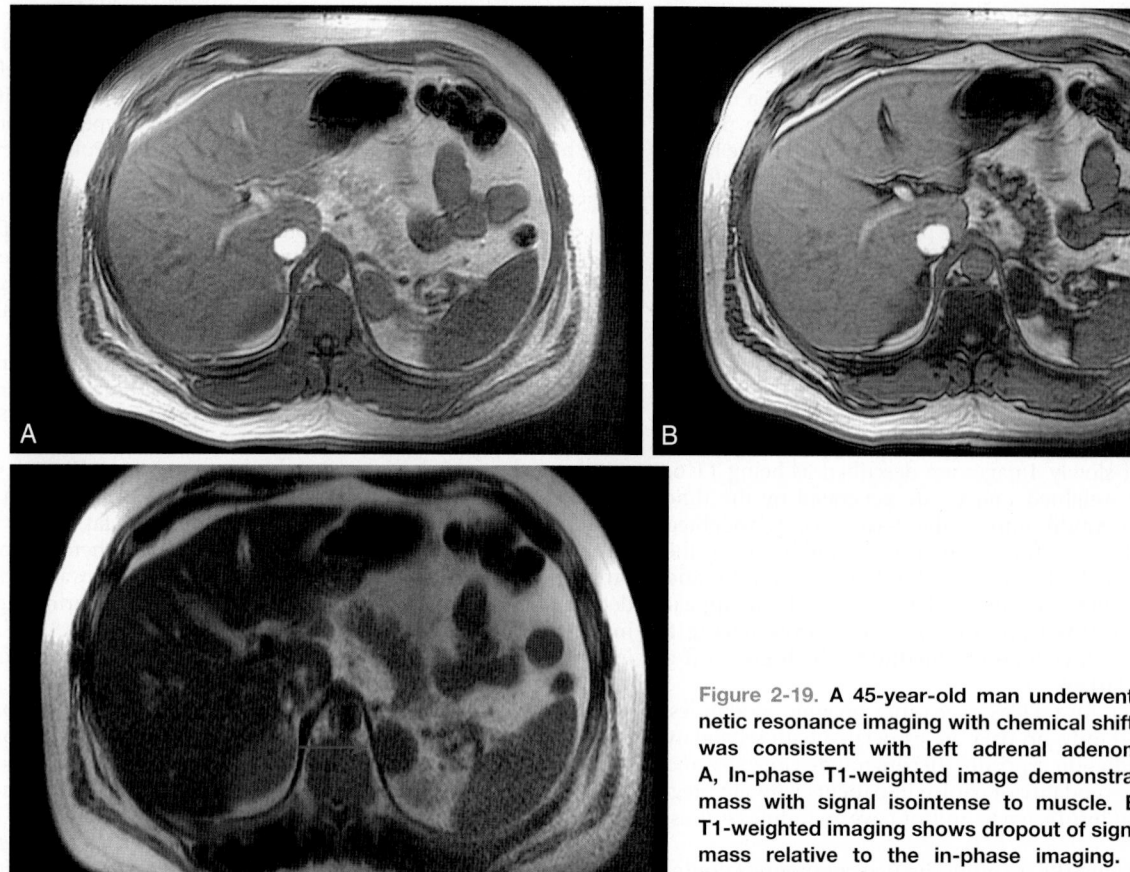

Figure 2-19. **A 45-year-old man underwent 1.5-tesla magnetic resonance imaging with chemical shift imaging, which was consistent with left adrenal adenoma *(red arrow)*. A, In-phase T1-weighted image demonstrates left adrenal mass with signal isointense to muscle. B, Out-of-phase T1-weighted imaging shows dropout of signal in left adrenal mass relative to the in-phase imaging. C, Single-shot, T2-weighted spin echo image reveals left adrenal nodule with low signal intensity.**

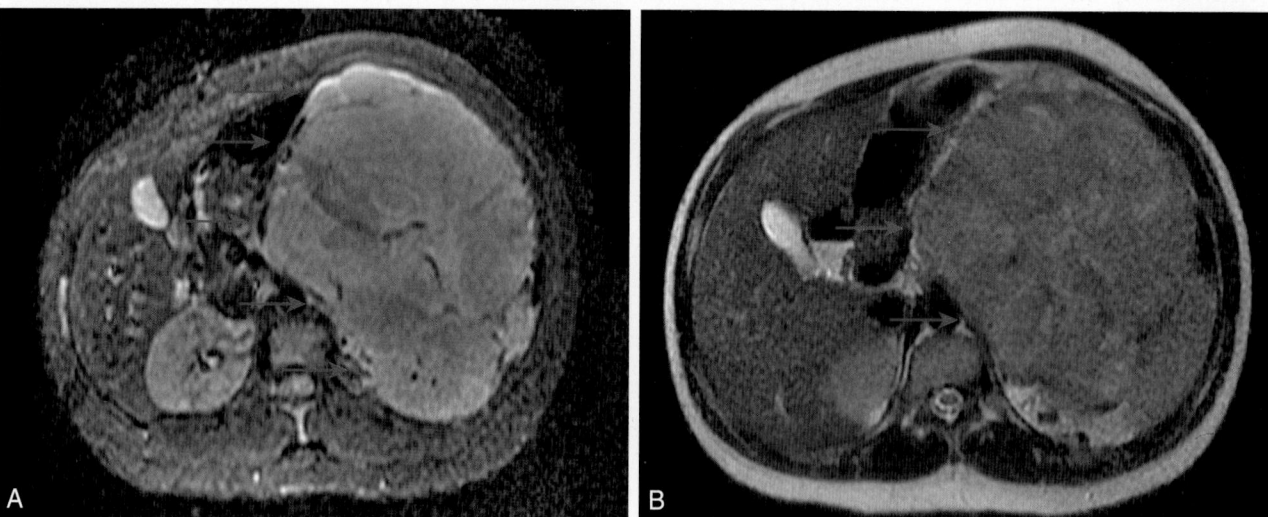

Figure 2-20. **A 65-year-old woman with left side heterogeneous enhancing suprarenal lesion (adrenal cortical carcinoma) with select images from a 1.5-tesla abdominal magnetic resonance image. A, Moderately weighted T2 STIR (short-tau inversion recovery) images with a hyperintense signal *(red arrows)*. B, Heavily weighted T2 single-shot, fast spin echo isointense signal. These findings are all dependent on the degree of T2 weighting.**

and Behrend, 2005). On MRI a myelolipoma has a high SI on T1-weighted imaging, suppressed signal on frequency selective fat suppression, and an India ink artifact (Taffel et al, 2012) (Fig. 2-21). India ink artifact appears as a dark line around the lesion and/or organs and is the result of a voxel containing both fat and water on chemical shift OP images.

Metastasis

An adrenal mass is considered to be metastatic in the setting of a known primary malignancy. The MRI findings are consistent with a large, irregular, heterogeneous mass with occasional necrosis present on imaging. Metastases have a high signal on T2-weighted

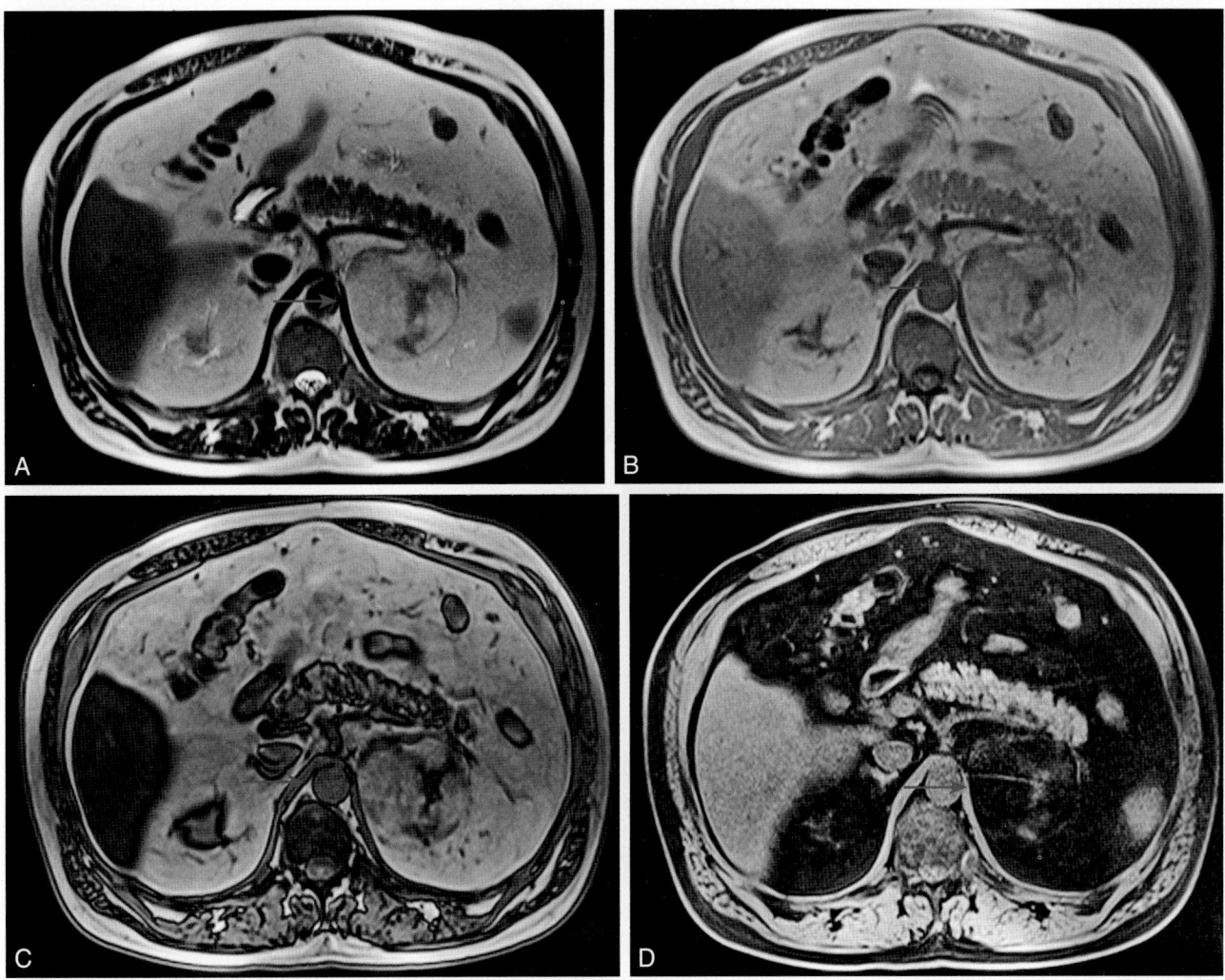

Figure 2-21. **A 44-year-old man, with prior abdominal ultrasonography detecting an indeterminate renal mass, underwent 1.5-tesla magnetic resonance imaging with chemical shift imaging, which was consistent with left adrenal myelolipoma *(red arrow)*. A, T2 single-shot spin echo demonstrates a large left adrenal mass with signal isointense to abdominal fat. B, T1 in-phase imaging demonstrates a left adrenal mass with signal similar to the abdominal fat. C, T1 out-of-phase imaging shows no drop of signal compared with in-phase imaging. D, T1 fat-suppressed precontrast imaging shows loss of signal within the mass consistent with gross fat.**

images secondary to higher fluid content, compared with adrenal adenoma (Sahdev et al, 2010). Gd enhancement on T1-weighted images demonstrates heterogeneous enhancement with a delayed peak enhancement (65 seconds) when compared with adrenal adenomas (40 seconds). Using a time to peak enhancement cutoff of 53 seconds or greater resulted in 87.5% sensitivity and 80% specificity in characterizing metastatic adrenal lesions (Inan et al, 2008).

Patients with primary lesions that are known to contain intracytoplasmic fat may require additional imaging to better differentiate an adrenal gland lesion. The metastatic sites often carry the same histologic features as the primary tumor. This can result in a false-positive for adrenal adenomas if the primary contains intracytoplasmic lipid content (CSI positive) (Krebs and Wagner, 1998) (Fig. 2-22). This has been reported in liposarcoma, renal cell carcinoma, and hepatocellular carcinoma (Krebs and Wagner, 1998; Sydow et al, 2006).

Pheochromocytoma was traditionally considered to be diagnostic if on T2-weighted images the lesion demonstrated an increased SI (Fig. 2-23). However, Varghese and colleagues (1997) reported that 35% of pheochromocytomas demonstrated low T2 signal,

contrary to conventional teaching. **Pheochromocytoma, ACC, and metastatic lesions to the adrenal gland can exhibit a hyperintense SI or appear bright on T2-weighted images.** It is important to understand that the SI can vary because of degree of weighting of the T2 signal and not have the traditional findings of being bright on T2-weighted images (see Figs. 2-20, 2-22, and 2-23). The pheochromocytoma can be characterized on MRI without the need for contrast enhancement, avoiding a potential hypertensive crisis that has been associated with iodine contrast media in these patients (Raisanen et al, 1984).

Lymphoma, neuroblastoma, ganglioneuroma, hemangioma, and granulomatous diseases of the adrenal gland have an intermediate SI index on CSI and other imaging findings (Table 2-3).

Adrenal hematomas have variable imaging characteristics on MRI because of changes in the hematoma from initial acute bleeding to breakdown products of red blood cells with deposition of hemosiderin within the hematoma. This progresses from an isointense to hypointense signal on T1 and low signal on T2 to hyperintense on T1 fat-suppressed sequences and T2 sequences at 1 to 7 weeks. A low signal rim is present on both T1 and T2 sequences because of hemosiderin deposits (Taffel et al, 2012).

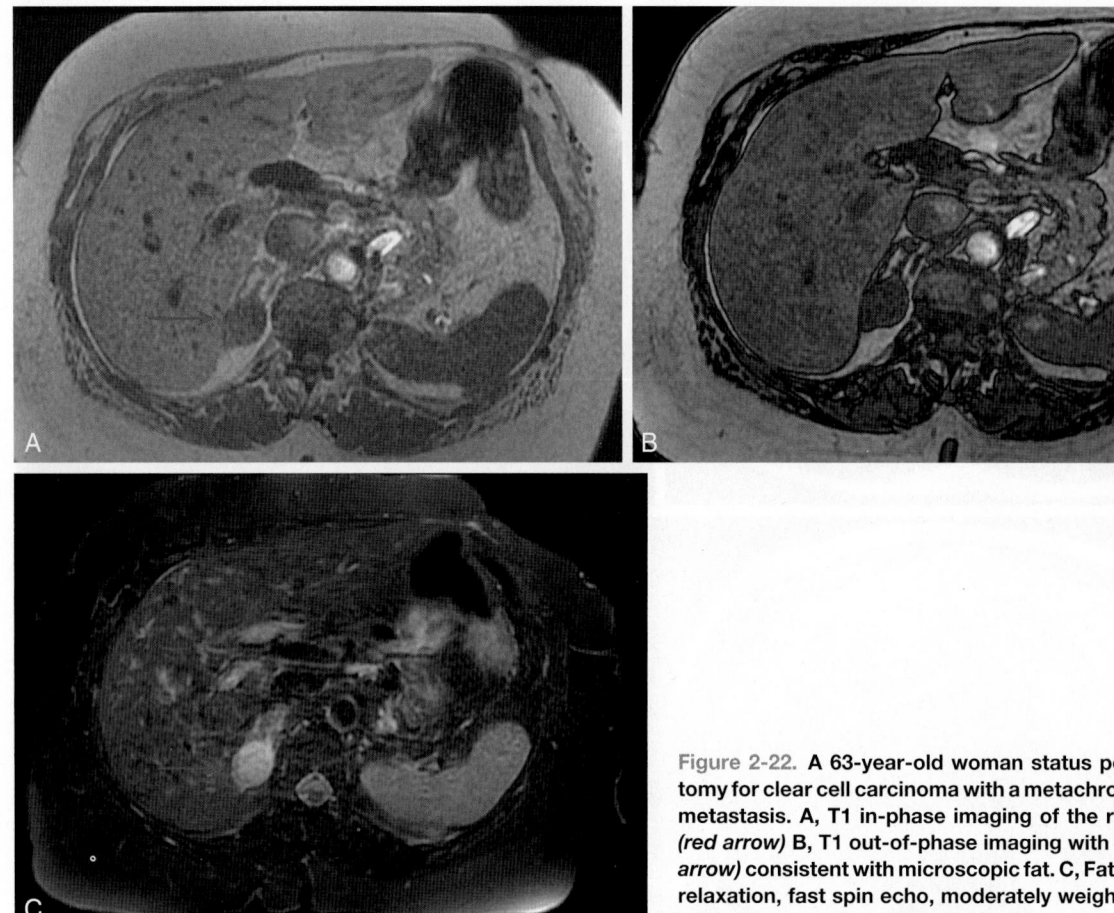

Figure 2-22. A 63-year-old woman status post right nephrectomy for clear cell carcinoma with a metachronous right adrenal metastasis. A, T1 in-phase imaging of the right adrenal mass *(red arrow)* **B, T1 out-of-phase imaging with drop in signal** *(red arrow)* **consistent with microscopic fat. C, Fat-suppressed, fast-relaxation, fast spin echo, moderately weighted T2 image with hyperintense signal** *(red arrow).*

Renal Magnetic Resonance Imaging

Simple cysts have similar characteristics on ultrasonography, CT, and MRI. Complex cysts can also be differentiated or characterized using MRI. Hemorrhage within the cyst results in a high signal on T1-weighted images because of the paramagnetic effects of blood breakdown products (hemosiderin) (Roubidoux, 1994) (Fig. 2-24).

Proteinaceous contents within a cyst can also demonstrate high signal on T1-weighted images. Chronic hemorrhage results in a black ring along the cyst wall on T2-weighted images. **For benign, complex cysts there should be no enhancement of any component of the cysts** (Israel et al, 2004).

Because MRI is insensitive to calcifications, any calcifications present on the lining of a complex cyst are not well visualized. When evaluating independent risk factors for renal cell carcinoma, enhancement of the cyst wall had higher sensitivity and specificity than calcifications on the cyst wall. Calcifications can cause artifacts that may decrease the ability to appreciate enhancement of small nodules within the wall of a complex cyst on CT imaging. MRI has the advantage of not being influenced by calcifications within the wall of a complex cyst. Therefore MRI is more likely to detect enhancement of a renal cell carcinoma in the wall of a complex cyst, compared with CT imaging when mural calcifications are present (Israel and Bosniak, 2003).

MRI offers a distinct advantage over CT imaging with regard to detection and evaluation of the pseudocapsule that appears on T1- and T2-weighted images as a low signal surrounding the lesion. The lack of pseudocapsule surrounding a renal mass had an accuracy of 91% in predicting pT3a disease (Roy et al, 2005).

MRI allows differentiation of different subtypes of renal cell carcinoma by using a multiparametric approach. These sequences can include: T1-weighted images; multiplanar T2-weighted sequences with and without fat suppression; dynamic contrast enhanced

(DCE) sequences with arterial, corticomedullary, and nephrogenic and excretory phases; diffusion-weighted images (DWI) with corresponding apparent diffusion coefficient (ADC) maps; and CSI. Using these unique features we are better able to differentiate the subtypes of renal masses compared with CT imaging.

Renal cell carcinoma clear cell type (cRCC) is the most common type of renal cell carcinoma. It is characterized by a heterogeneous high signal on T2-weighted sequences because of the presence of hemorrhage, necrosis, and/or cysts (see Fig. 2-24). Papillary renal cell carcinoma (pRCC), when compared to cRCC, exhibits a homogenous lower SI on T2-weighted images, which is secondary to hemosiderin deposition (histiocytes) within the tumor (Fig. 2-25). Hemorrhagic cysts with an enhancing peripheral wall growth and/or a solid hypoenhancing mass with low SI on T2-weighted images resulted in 80% sensitivity and 94% specificity in differentiating pRCC from other types of RCCs (Fig. 2-26) (Pedrosa et al, 2008).

Like adrenal MR imaging, CSI can detect intracytoplasmic lipids and aid in the differentiation of cRCC from other RCC subtypes (see Fig. 2-24). Microscopic intracytoplasmic lipids have been found in 59% of clear cell carcinomas (Outwater et al, 1997). Karlo and colleagues (2013) reported that once angiomyolipoma (AML) has been ruled out using standard MRI techniques (Fig. 2-27) in which macroscopic fat has been detected, CSI sequences with a 25% decrease in SI can be considered diagnostic for cRCC from other renal tumors. Pedrosa and colleagues (2008) reported the sensitivity and specificity of CSI for cRCC was 42% and 100%, respectively. There are rare cases of RCC with macroscopic fat; however, if calcifications are also present, this would favor the diagnosis of RCC over AML (Wasser et al, 2013).

Gd-enhanced T1-weighted images with a relative SI increase of 15% is considered to be positive enhancement, which results in a 100% sensitivity in differentiation of cysts from renal cell carcinoma

Text continued on p. 56

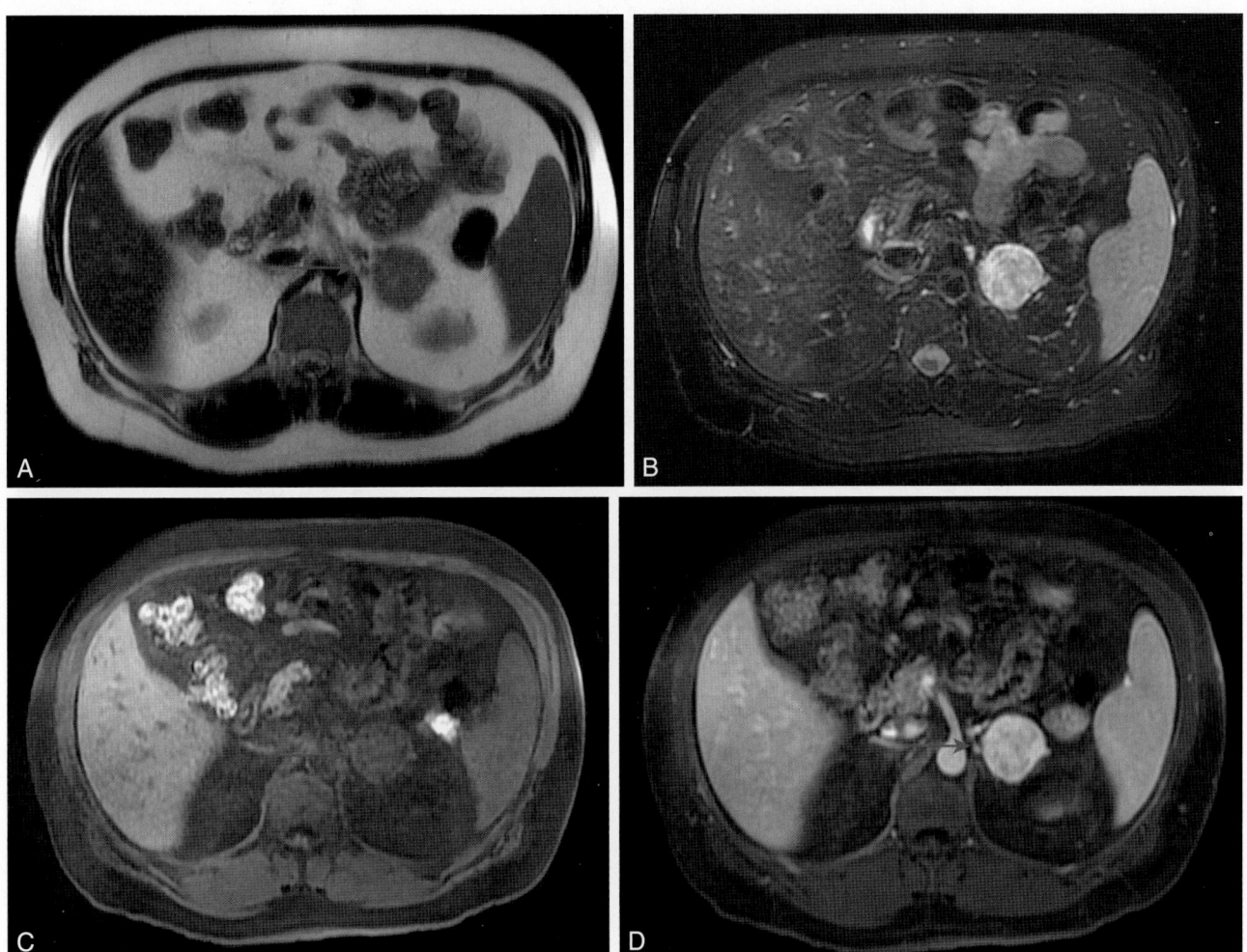

Figure 2-23. **A 50-year-old man with a left side pheochromocytoma (as shown by *arrows*) and select images from 1.5-tesla magnetic resonance imaging. A, Heavily weighted T2 single-shot fast spin echo with an isointense signal (not bright). B, Moderately weighted T2 fat-suppressed, fast-recovery, fast spin echo with hyperintense signal (bright). C, T1-weighted precontrast image. D, T1-weighted postcontrast image with marked early enhancement.**

TABLE 2-3 Morphologic and Imaging Characteristics of Incidental Adrenal Lesions

IAL	SIZE (cm)	SHAPE	TEXTURE	UNENHANCED CT ATTENUATION (HU)	15-MINUTE CT WASHOUT (%)	MRI SIGNAL CHARACTERISITCS	NUCLEAR MEDICINE CHARACTERISTICS
Adrenal metastasis	Variable	Variable	Heterogeneous when larger	>10	RPW <40	High T2 signal	Positive on PET images
Adrenal cortical carcinoma	>4	Variable	Variable	>10	RPW <40	Intermediate to high T2 signal	Positive on PET images
Pheochromocytoma	Variable	Variable	Variable	>10, rarely <10	RPW <40	High T2 signal	Positive on MIBG
Cyst	Variable	Smooth, round	Smooth	<10	Does not enhance	High T2 signal	Negative
Adenoma	1-4	Smooth, round	Homogeneous	<10 in 70%	RPW >40; APW >60	SI dropoff on OP images	Variable on PET images
Myelolipoma	1-5	Smooth, round	Variable with macroscopic fat	<0, often ≤50	No data	High T1 signal, India ink, variable SI dropoff on OP images	Negative on PET images
Lymphoma	Variable	Variable	Variable	>10	RPW <40	Intermediate SI	Variable positivity on PET images
Hematoma	Variable	Smooth	Variable	>10, sometimes >50	No data	Variable signal	Negative
Neuroblastoma	Variable	Variable	Smooth, round	>10	RPW <40	Variable if necrotic	Positive
Ganglioneuroma	Variable	Variable	Variable	>10	No data	Usually intermediate SI	Usually negative
Hemangioma	Variable	Variable	Variable	>10	No data	Usually intermediate SI	Usually negative
Granulomatous	1-5	Smooth	Usually homogeneous	>10	No data	Usually intermediate SI	Positive on PET images if active

APW, absolute percentage washout; CT, computed tomography; HU, Hounsfield unit; IAL, incidental adrenal lesion; MIBG, m-iodobenzylguanidine; MRI, magnetic resonance imaging; OP, out-of-phase; PET, positron emission tomography; RPW, relative percentage washout; SI, signal intensity.

From Boland GW, Blake MA, Hahn PF, et al. Incidental adrenal lesions: principles, techniques, and algorithms for imaging characterization. Radiology 2008;249:756–75; and Taffel M, Haji-Momenian S, Nikolaidis P, et al. Adrenal imaging: a comprehensive review. Radiol Clin North Am 2012;50:219–43.

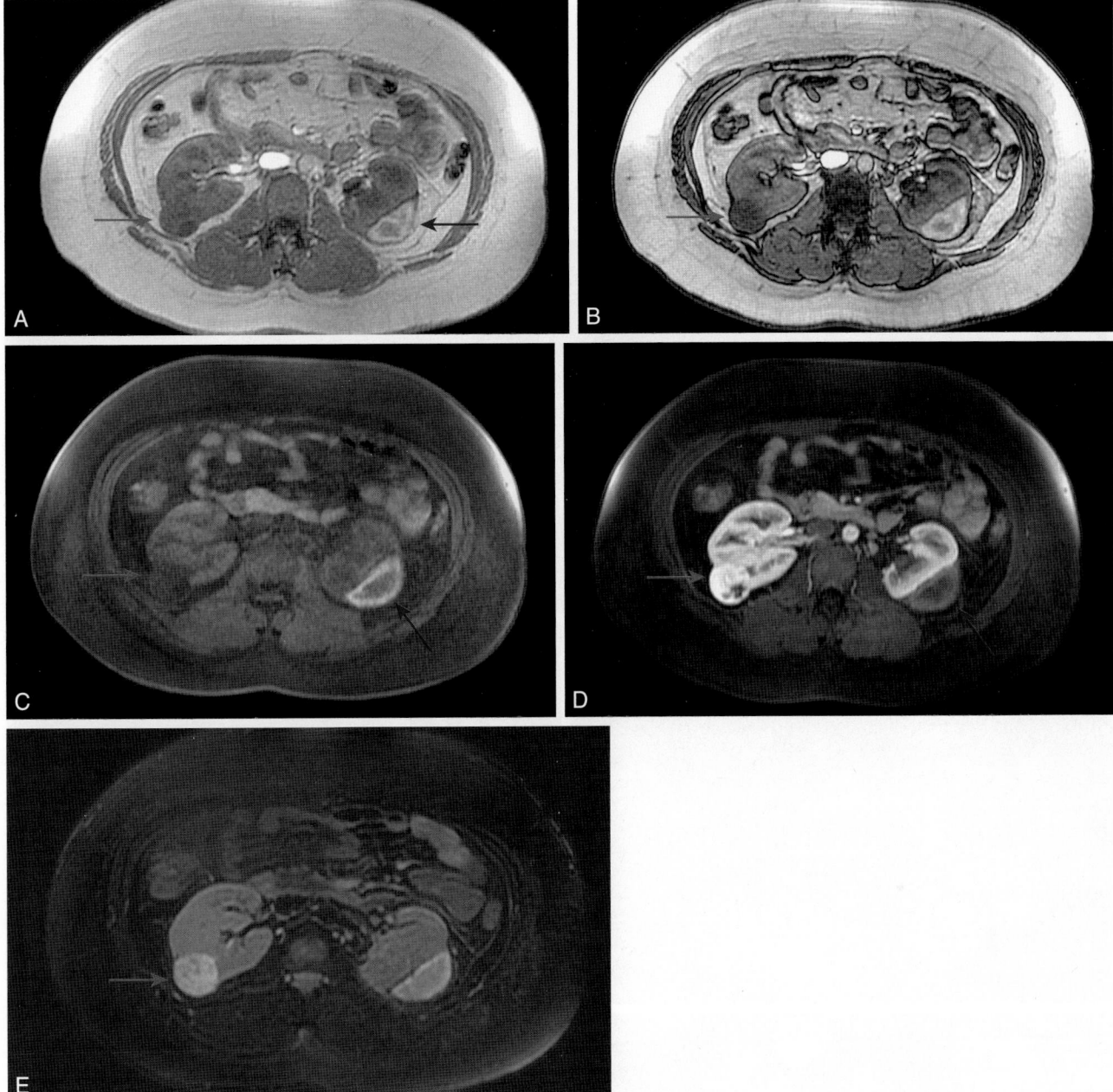

Figure 2-24. A 31-year-old woman, after left extracorporeal shock wave lithotripsy with a subcapsular hematoma and right side pathology confirmed 3.5-cm clear cell carcinoma, underwent 1.5-tesla magnetic resonance imaging of the abdomen. A, T1-weighted in-phase imaging of a right renal nodule with mild heterogeneity *(red arrow)* but primarily isointense signal intensity (SI). Left kidney subcapsular hematoma with a rim of high SI *(blue arrow).* **B,** T1-weighted out-of-phase image shows diffuse signal dropout within the renal nodule consistent with microscopic fat. **C,** T1-weighted fat-suppressed precontrast image with a low SI of the right renal nodule *(red arrow)* and high SI of the left subcapsular hematoma *(blue arrow).* Blood is high SI on precontrast T1-weighted images. **D,** T1 fat-suppressed postcontrast images of the right renal nodule with avid heterogeneous enhancement. Unenhancing left subcapsular hematoma *(blue arrow).* **E,** Diffusion-weighted imaging b-1000 shows high SI throughout the right renal nodule.

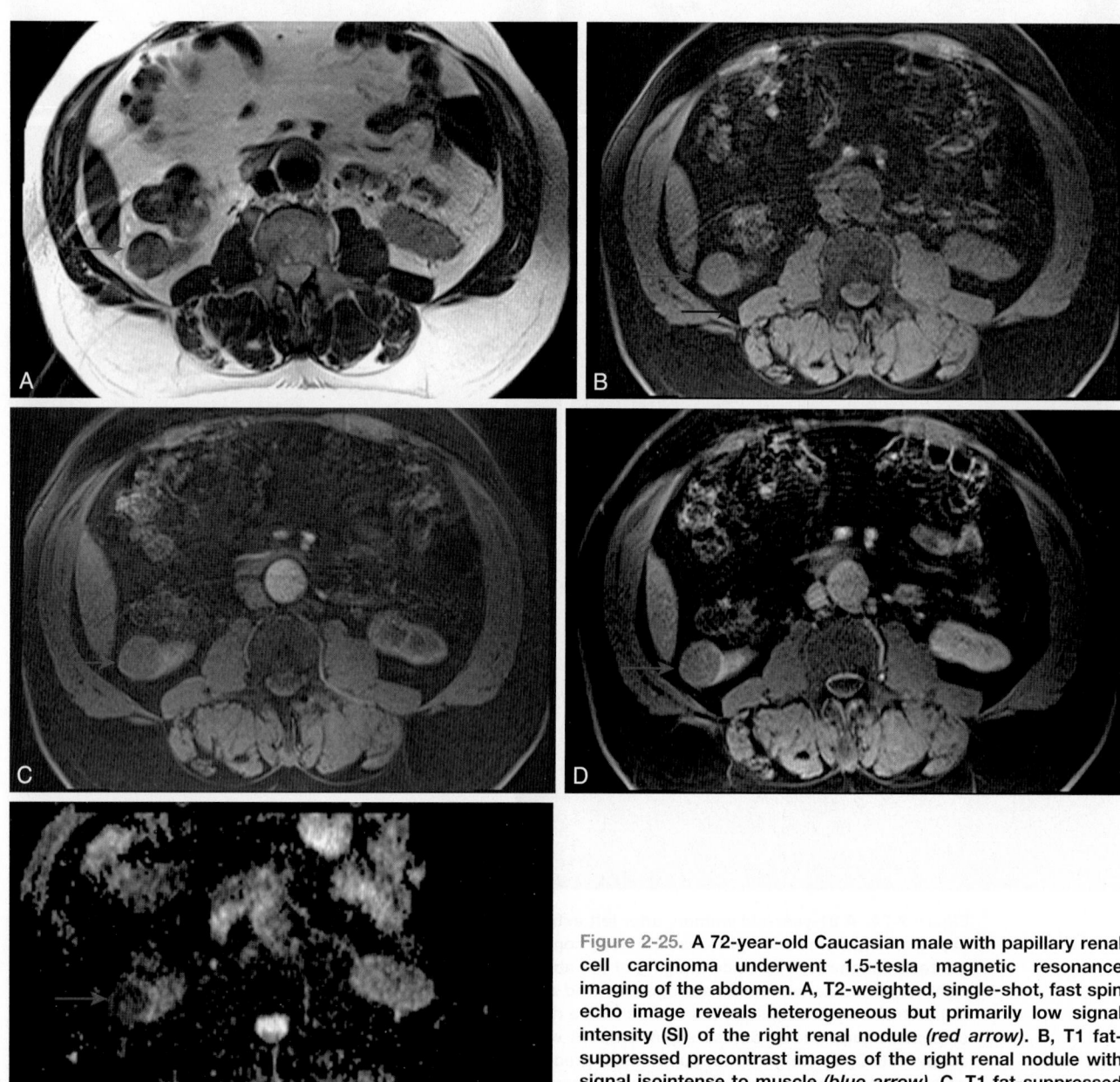

Figure 2-25. **A 72-year-old Caucasian male with papillary renal cell carcinoma underwent 1.5-tesla magnetic resonance imaging of the abdomen. A, T2-weighted, single-shot, fast spin echo image reveals heterogeneous but primarily low signal intensity (SI) of the right renal nodule *(red arrow)*. B, T1 fat-suppressed precontrast images of the right renal nodule with signal isointense to muscle *(blue arrow)*. C, T1 fat-suppressed postcontrast cortical medullary phase with no significant enhancement. D, T1 fat-suppressed postcontrast nephrogenic phase demonstrates minimal central enhancement. E, Apparent diffusion coefficient map with low SI of the renal nodule.**

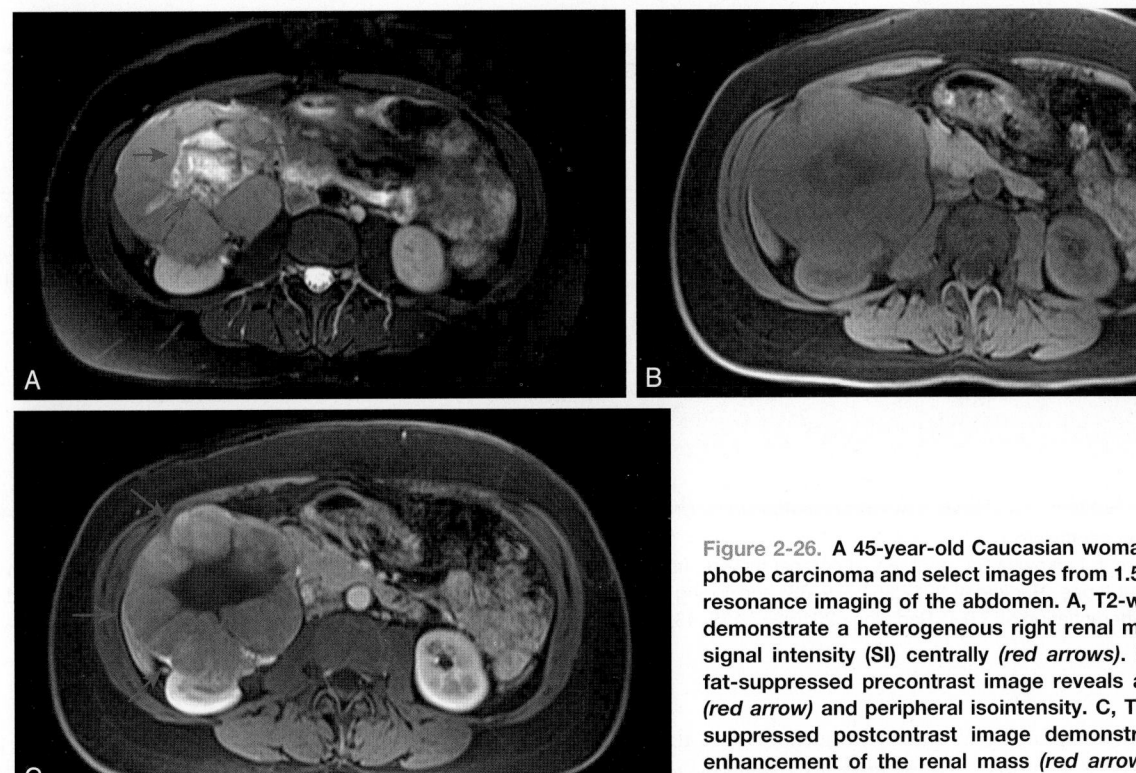

Figure 2-26. **A 45-year-old Caucasian woman with chromo-phobe carcinoma and select images from 1.5-tesla magnetic resonance imaging of the abdomen. A, T2-weighted images demonstrate a heterogeneous right renal mass with a high signal intensity (SI) centrally *(red arrows)*. B, T1-weighted, fat-suppressed precontrast image reveals a central low SI *(red arrow)* and peripheral isointensity. C, T1-weighted, fat-suppressed postcontrast image demonstrates peripheral enhancement of the renal mass *(red arrows)* with lack of enhancement centrally.**

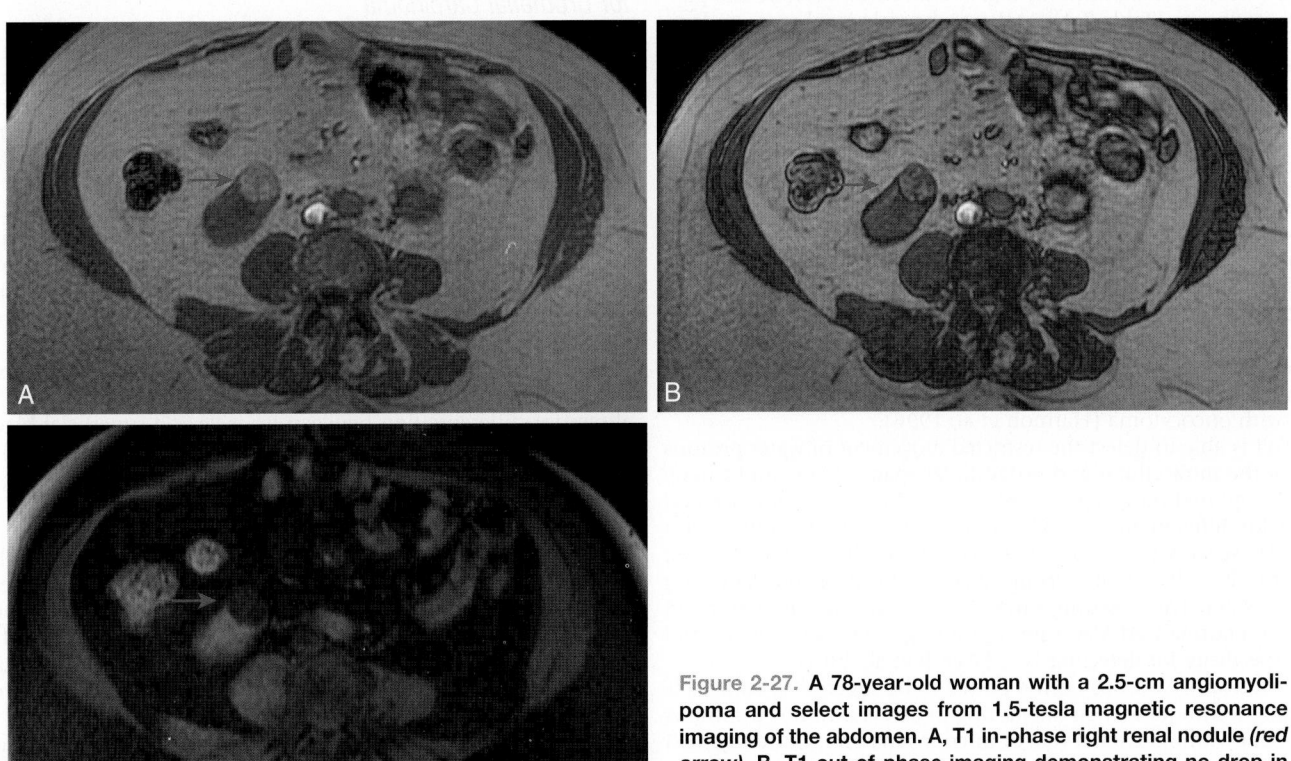

Figure 2-27. **A 78-year-old woman with a 2.5-cm angiomyoli-poma and select images from 1.5-tesla magnetic resonance imaging of the abdomen. A, T1 in-phase right renal nodule *(red arrow)*. B, T1 out-of-phase imaging demonstrating no drop in signal intensity (SI) *(red arrow)*. C, T1 fat-suppressed precontrast demonstrates drop in SI within the lesion consistent with macroscopic fat.**

TABLE 2-4 Magnetic Resonance Imaging Characteristics of Renal Masses

	SIGNAL INTENSITY (SI) % CHANGE				
	CORTICOMEDULLARY PHASE	NEPHROGENIC PHASE	EXCRETORY PHASE	ADC AT B VALUES 0 AND 800 sec/mm^2 ($\times 10^{-6}$ mm^2/sec)	T2-WEIGHTED IMAGES SI
Clear cell	230%	250%	227%	1698	High SI heterogeneous
Papillary carcinoma	49%	92%	88%	884	Low SI homogeneous
Chromophobe carcinoma	98%	183%	159%	1135	High T2-weighted SI for central scar
Oncocytoma	208%	265%	237%		High T2-weighted SI for central scar
Angiomyolipoma	353%	285%	222%		Variable
Renal parenchyma				2303	
Transitional cell carcinoma				<450	High signal

ADC, apparent diffusion coefficient.
From Vargas HA, Chaim J, Lefkowitz RA, et al. Renal cortical tumors: use of multiphasic contrast-enhanced MR imaging to differentiate benign and malignant histologic subtypes. Radiology 2012;264:779–88; and Wang H, Cheng L, Zhang X, et al. Renal cell carcinoma: diffusion-weighted MR imaging for subtype differentiation at 3.0 T. Radiology 2010;257:135–43.

with peak enhancement occurring at 2 to 4 minutes (Ho et al, 2002) Using the specific characteristics of DCE MR sequences, Vargas and colleagues (2012) assessed the enhancement characteristics of cRCC, pRCC, AML, and chromophobe carcinoma in the corticomedullary, nephrogenic, and excretory phases. Clear cell demonstrated greater than 200% SI increase in all three contrast phases, which was significantly higher than chromophobe and papillary carcinoma (Table 2-4). AML was the only renal mass to demonstrate a decrease in SI from the corticomedullary phase to the nephrogenic phase (see Fig. 2-27). Because of a high degree of overlap, it is difficult to assign cutoff points. It was not possible to find characteristics to differentiate oncocytoma from cRCC (Israel and Bosniak, 2003).

Oncocytoma is typically described with a central scar that is observed as a high SI on T2-weighted images. However, this is present only in 54% to 80% of cases (Cornelis et al, 2013). Unfortunately, a central scar has also been reported in 37% of chromophobe carcinomas (Rosenkrantz et al, 2010) (see Fig. 2-26). Both oncocytoma and chromophobe carcinomas are usually peripheral and are hypovascular compared with the renal cortex (Ho et al, 2002). Necrosis has a high SI on T2-weighted images and low SI on T1-weighted images, which is the same for the central scar associated with oncocytoma (Harmon et al, 1996).

DWI is able to detect the restricted movement of water protons within the intracellular and extracellular spaces. Wang and Cheng (2010) reported on using a threshold of 1281×10^{-6} mm^2/sec and above for differentiating cRCC from non–clear cell carcinomas with a 95.9% sensitivity and 94.4% specificity (see Table 2-4). Central RCC can be differentiated from transitional cell carcinoma (TCC) of the renal pelvis by setting a threshold of 451×10^{-6} mm^2/sec and below on normalized ADC values, resulting in a 83% sensitivity and 71% specificity for detecting TCC (Wehrli et al, 2013).

Historically, MRI has been reported to be superior to earlier CT imaging techniques when attempting to assess if tumor thrombus is present within the renal vein or inferior vena cava. Currently, MRI and CT have the same performance when evaluating for tumor thrombus (Hallscheidt et al, 2005). **Gd-contrast agent is used to differentiate tumor thrombus, which exhibits enhancement, compared with a bland thrombus (clot), which exhibits no enhancement.**

The size of the lymph nodes observed via MRI and CT is used to detect lymphadenopathy. Several investigators have been evaluating the use of nanoparticles that are composed of supraparamagnetic iron oxide in the evaluation of lymphadenopathy (Eisner and Feldman, 2009). Normal lymph nodes take up the iron oxide particles via phagocytosis, which results in a signal loss on T2-weighted sequences.

Upper Tract and Lower Tract Imaging for Urothelial Carcinoma

Urothelial carcinoma of the upper tract can be assessed by an MR urogram (MRU) in addition to the standard renal mass MRI techniques. MRU can be used in patients for whom other imaging modalities are contraindicated. MRU is accomplished by using heavily weighted T2 sequences in which fluid/urine have a high SI on T1-weighted images with Gd (Chahal et al, 2005). MRU and CTU have the same accuracy in assessing renal obstruction (Silverman et al, 2009). Nephrolithiasis/calcification on MRI has no signal characteristics; therefore it appears as a void on imaging. Urothelial tumors, blood clots, gas, or sloughed renal papilla may exhibit a low signal or signal voids on T2-weighted images secondary to the high signal of urine (Kawashima et al, 2003).

MRI is advantageous over CT imaging of the bladder because of the increased signal contrast between the layers of the bladder. This allows for differentiation between invasive and superficial bladder cancer with an accuracy of 85% (Tekes et al, 2005) (Fig. 2-28).

Prostate

Prostate cancer is one of the few solid organ malignancies that have not had reliable imaging. Over the past 10 years several developments have led to the increased use of MRI for the detection of prostate cancer. The increase in the field strength of magnets from 1 to 3 tesla improved techniques and surface coils have increased the signal contrast (differentiation of normal prostate versus cancer) leading to improved visualization within the gland.

Several authors have reported on varying standards that should be used for prostate imaging. The currency in MRI is signal. Signal detection is optimized by using external surface coils and/or an endorectal coil (ERC) and therefore leads to improved image quality. The National Institutes of Health (NIH) recently completed a study comparing the diagnostic accuracy at 3 tesla with and without ERC in the same patients and compared findings to whole mount histopathology. Results indicated a 36% decrease in sensitivity in detecting prostate cancer when the ERC was not used (Turkbey et al, 2014).

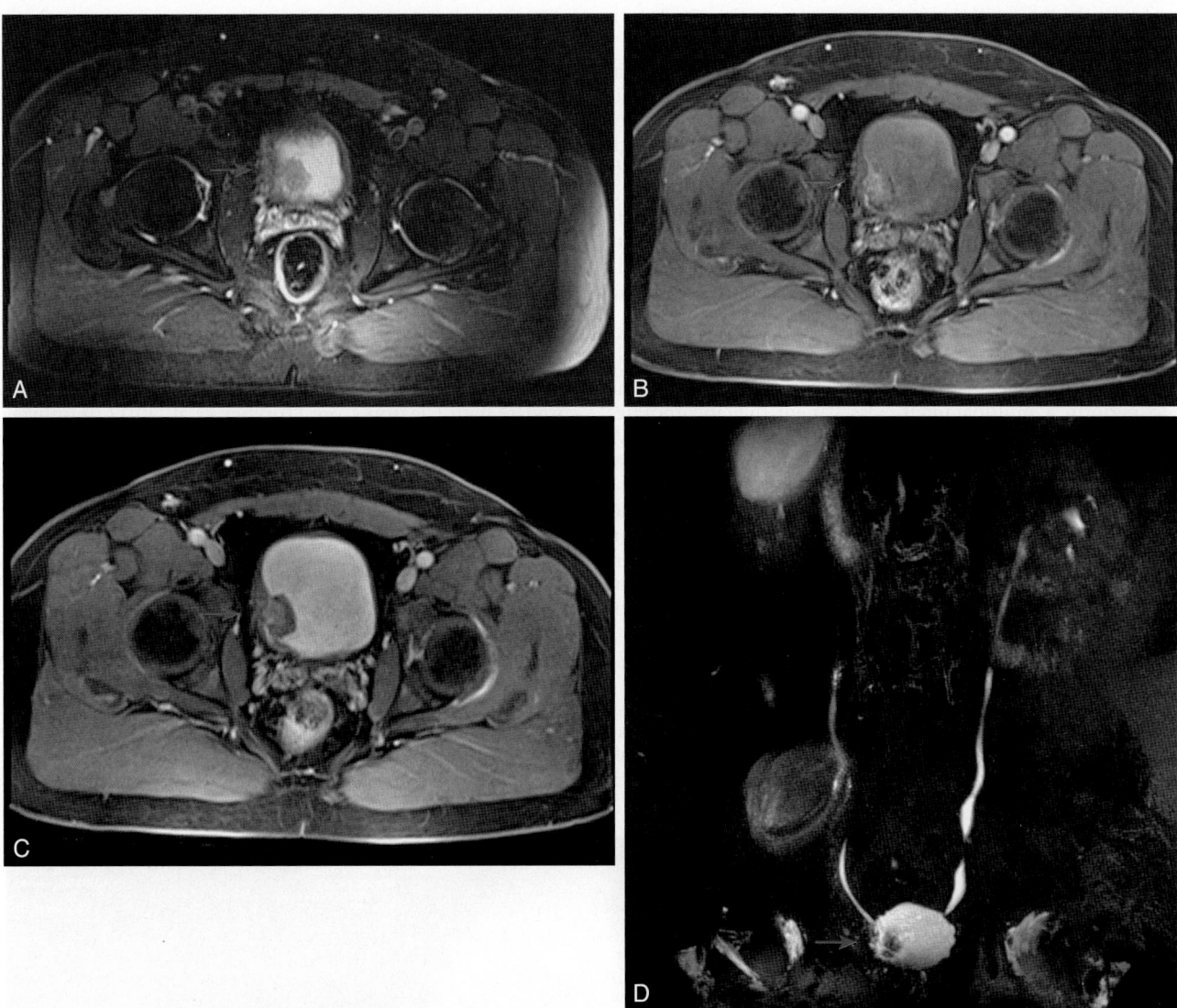

Figure 2-28. **A 51-year-old man with a history of gross hematuria underwent a 1.5-tesla magnetic resonance urogram. A, T2 fat-saturated sequence with high T2 signal in bladder (urine). Right bladder wall low signal intensity filling defect** *(red arrow).* **B, Fat-suppressed T1 postcontrast arterial phase shows enhancing right bladder wall polypoid mass and is without bladder wall invasion. C, Fat-suppressed T1 delayed contrast imaging shows high signal in bladder consistent with intravenous contrast excretion. Mild persistent signal in right bladder wall mass. D, Heavily weighted T2 urogram selectively demonstrates high signal of fluid within the ureters and bladder. Right wall bladder filling defect** *(red arrow)* **is evident. Transurethral resection of bladder tumor confirmed no bladder wall invasion of a high-grade papillary urothelial carcinoma.**

Prostate MRI is usually referred to as a multiparametric (MP) MRI. This consists of anatomic and functional imaging techniques. Anatomic imaging should include T1- and T2-weighted images. Functional imaging includes DWI with ADC maps, DCE sequences, and possibly spectroscopy. MR spectroscopy is not always included in the standard MP-MRI. MR spectroscopy takes approximately 15 minutes to perform, is labor intensive, and may not add additional information to affect the clinical interpretation of the study.

Initial T1-weighted sequences are obtained to determine if hemorrhage is present within the prostate; this may limit the diagnostic interpretation of the study. If there is hemorrhage, it can lead to false positives on T2 sequences, DWI/ADC, and DCE images, although some authors report no difference in diagnostic accuracy with or without hemorrhage present (Rosenkrantz et al, 2010). There is debate regarding the time between biopsy and the MP-MRI, which can be performed 3 to 8 weeks after a biopsy to optimize

intraprostatic anatomy (Ikonen et al, 2001; Qayyum et al, 2004; Muller et al, 2014). The wait period is not required for presurgical staging to determine if there is extraprostatic extension (EPE) and/or seminal vesicle invasion (SVI).

The most recent consensus meeting reported that the minimum examination should be a 1.5-tesla MRI with an ERC or a 3 tesla with or without an ERC and a multiparametric approach (Muller et al, 2014). Use of external phased array coils increases signal detection and therefore improves image quality. A 3-tesla MP-MRI with a minimum of 16-channel phased array coil with an ERC detects the highest signal and therefore provides the highest quality images. However, it is unclear if a radiologist needs this level of quality to make a diagnostic impression. It is important that an ERC should never be filled with air or water (Rosen et al, 2007). The result is a decrease in the performance of the T2, DWI, and MR spectroscopy. The most optimal fluids are diamagnetic and proton neutral (Rosen et al, 2007).

T2-Weighted Imaging

T2-weighted sequences of the prostate provide anatomic information and should include triplanar (axial, coronal, and sagittal) sequences. These images provide a detailed anatomic assessment of the gland. The normal peripheral zone appears as an area of high SI. The central gland with benign prostatic hyperplasia (BPH) appears as areas of well-demarcated nodules with heterogeneous SIs. Areas of low SI on T2-weighted sequences can represent prostate cancer or prostatitis, atrophy, scars, hemorrhage after prostate biopsy, and/or BPH nodules (Barentsz et al, 2012). Rarely, BPH nodules can be observed within the peripheral zone and can lead to a false-positive MRI for cancer (Fig. 2-29).

T2-weighted imaging alone results in 58% sensitivity and 93% specificity for detecting prostate cancer within the gland at 3 tesla with an ERC (Turkbey et al, 2011). These limitations reinforce the need to perform a multiparametric assessment that incorporates functional imaging and increases the positive predictive value (PPV) and negative predictive value (NPV) of the examination to greater than 90% (Turkbey et al, 2011). T2-weighted sequences are used to assess EPE and SVI. These areas are represented by low SI. MP-MRI at 3 tesla with an ERC has an approximate 90% accuracy when assessing EPE on a per lesion analysis. At the patient level, comparing the accuracy of staging, including microscopic EPE, overall accuracy decreased to 78.5%. The use of ERC improves the accuracy of detecting EPE and SVI (Heijmink et al, 2007).

Diffusion-Weighted Imaging/Apparent Diffusion Coefficient

DWI assesses the diffusion of water (Brownian motion) within the magnetic field. The MR magnet is able to detect the phase shift changes in the motion of the water protons. The more cellular a tissue is, the closer the cells are together, resulting in a limited motion of water, which is reflected as a high signal on DWI (Manenti et al, 2006).

As with all MR sequences, there are several details that one should observe. Most important is the b-values associated with DWI. B-values represent a threshold for detecting restriction. As a b-value is increased, less restricted tissues do not exhibit a high signal on DWI. DWI can include multiple b-values, and it is recommended to include at least one b-value greater than 1000 (Rosenkrantz et al, 2010). The ADC is a quantitative assessment of the DWI. This is represented by an area of low signal on the images (dark spot) (Fig. 2-30D). Some authors recommend including a b-2000 sequence on DWI; it has been shown that prostate cancer exhibits a high SI compared with the rest of the gland (Ueno et al, 2013) (Fig. 2-30F).

The ADC value computed from DWI has been shown to directly correlate with Gleason score (Turkbey et al, 2011). Intuitively this makes sense because an increase in cellularity results in an increase in Gleason score. The extracellular/intracellular spaces between the cells are decreased and therefore are reflected as areas of increased restriction.

Dynamic Contrast Enhanced Magnetic Resonance Imaging

DCE-MRI refers to T1-weighted imaging with Gd-based contrast agents. DCE-MRI is not a simple assessment of enhancement versus no enhancement. It assesses vascular permeability and perfusion of the prostate by obtaining multiple image acquisitions over 5 to 10 minutes at a temporal resolution of less than or equal to 5 seconds (Verma et al, 2012). The 5-second temporal resolution requires a decrease in the size of the imaging matrix, therefore resulting in a lower resolution image. DCE-MRI is not meant to obtain clear

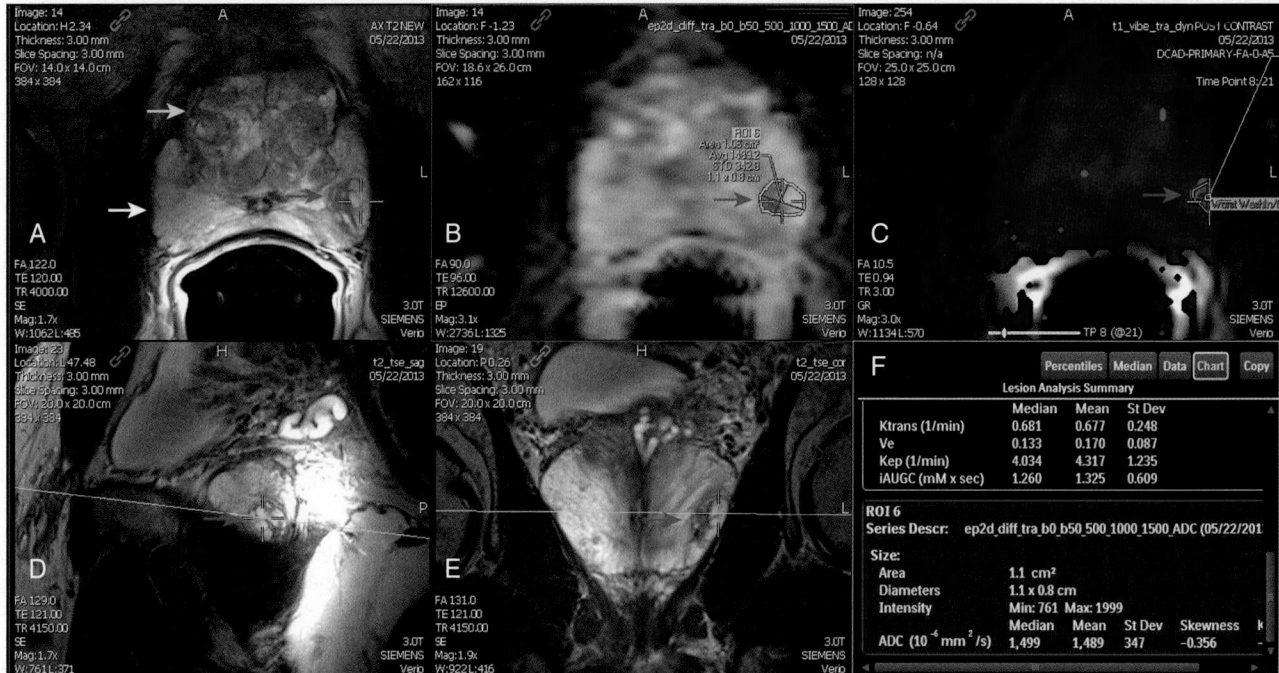

Figure 2-29. A 66-year-old man with a prostate-specific antigen of 7.0 and two prior negative biopsies. A 3-tesla multiparametric magnetic resonance imaging (MP-MRI) with an endorectal coil of the prostate was obtained. There were two suspicious areas. **A, D,** and **E,** Triplanar images in axial, sagittal, and coronal planes. The peripheral zone *(white arrow)* and the central gland *(yellow arrow)* are well visualized. The red arrow represents a well-circumscribed heterogeneous benign prostatic hypertrophy nodule (11 mm × 11 mm × 14 mm) within the peripheral zone with no communication to the central gland. The corresponding apparent diffusion coefficient map **(B)** demonstrates areas of heterogeneous restriction (761 × 10⁻⁶ mm²/sec). The lesion on the dynamic contrast enhanced MRI (DCE-MRI) **(C)** exhibits focal type 2 and 3 enhancement curves. The DCE-MRI quantitative analysis is listed **(F).** The patient underwent a fusion biopsy. The lesion was also appreciated on ultrasonography, and no cancer was detected.

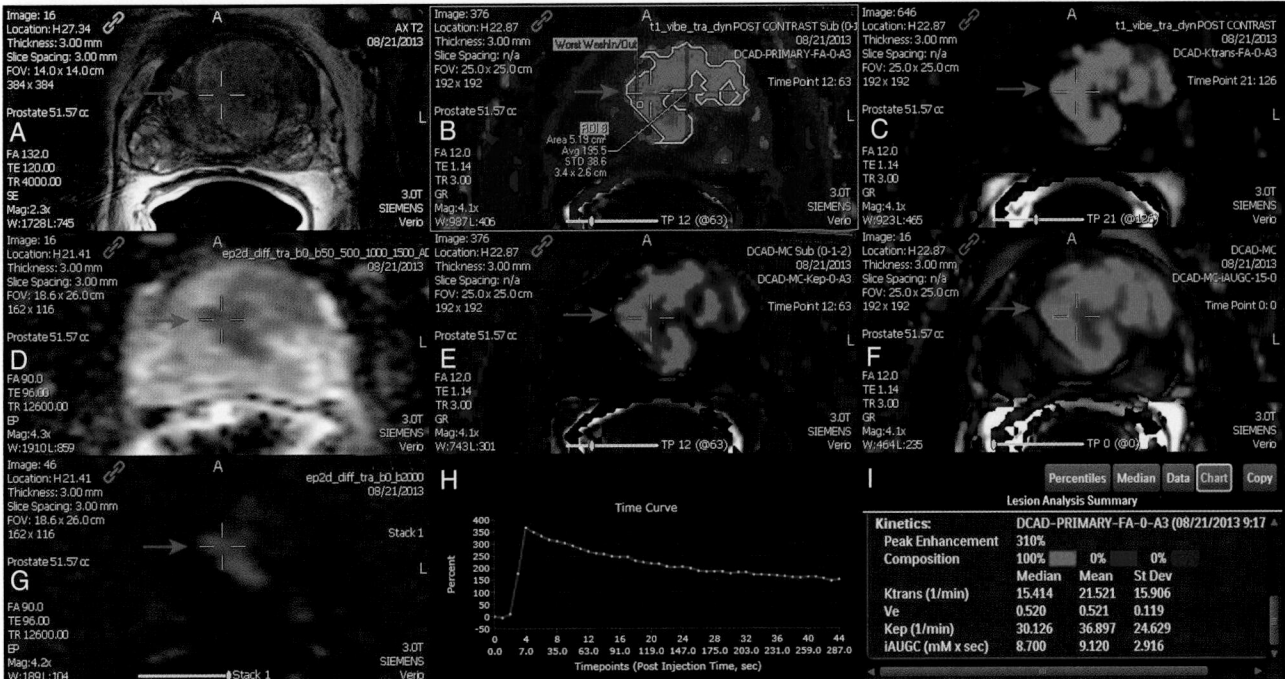

Figure 2-30. A 65-year-old man with a prostate-specific antigen of 38.9 and 16 prior negative biopsies with magnetic resonance (MR) ultrasound fusion biopsy proven Gleason 4 + 4 prostate cancer. A, T2-weighted image with an anterior lesion within the central gland, 3.5 cm × 2.7 cm × 3.5 cm *(red arrow)*. B and H, Dynamic contrast enhanced MRI (DCE-MRI) with color mapping exhibiting a focal type 3 enhancement curve. C, Elevated K^{trans} (transfer constant). D, Apparent diffusion coefficient map with low signal. E, Elevated K^{ep} (rate constant). F, Area under the curve. G, B-2000 diffusion-weighted sequence with an area of high signal intensity. I, Quantitative summary of the large anterior central gland lesion.

anatomic images; it is used to assess the blood flow and vascular permeability throughout the gland over time.

DCE-MRI provides qualitative, semiquantitative, and quantitative information regarding enhancement within the prostate. A qualitative approach consists of visually assessing early enhancement and early washout within the prostate. The use of computer-aided diagnostic systems allows one to obtain specific information with regard to enhancement characteristics. A semiquantitative approach assesses enhancement over time (Tofts et al, 1991). There are three distinct curves associated with prostate imaging (Fig. 2-31). Because of the overlap of all three curve types with benign conditions, it is useful to combine these approaches in a MP-MRI. A quantitative assessment for cancer was first proposed by Tofts and colleagues (1991), observing the pharmacokinetics of the contrast within the gland. K^{trans} (transfer constant) represents the transfer rate (permeability) of contrast between the intravascular space and the extracellular space (or blood flow) to the tissues depending on the hemodynamics at the time of the study. K^{ep} (rate constant) is the rate of efflux of contrast back into the vascular space (Tofts et al, 1999). These quantitative metrics have not been incorporated in the daily work flow of most radiologists; however, they are currently being evaluated for possible decision analysis software (see Fig. 2-30C, D, E, H).

DCE-MRI has a reported 46% to 96% sensitivity and a 74% to 96% specificity for detecting prostate cancer. These large ranges can be the result of the high variability related to patient selection, MRI technique, pathology correlation, and reader experience (Tofts et al, 1991).

Magnetic Resonance Spectroscopy

Proton MR spectroscopic imaging (MRSI) is able to detect the concentration of citrate, choline, and creatine within the prostate. As cells go through malignant transformation, citrate decreases and creatine and choline levels increase secondary to increased cellular turnover (Choi et al, 2007). An increase of two standard deviations of choline-to-citrate ratio is indicative of cancer (Kurhanewicz et al, 1996). This process is time consuming (15 minutes and has fallen out of favor when used in a nonresearch setting. Turkbey and colleagues (2011) reported only a 7% increase in PPV and NPV using MRSI. Therefore the additional time may not clinically impact cancer detection rates. There is still a significant research potential associated with MRSI. Some authors are using MRSI assessment of cellular metabolism (choline, creatine, and citrate) to evaluate recurrence after radiation therapy (Zhang et al, 2014).

Multiparametric Magnetic Resonance Imaging

The combination of T2, DCE, and DWI has yielded both NPV and PPV greater than 90% (Turkbey et al, 2011; Abd-Alazeez et al, 2014). It is important to understand that high-quality MRI requires tuning of the MR magnets, a dedicated staff to perform the studies, and pathology correlation for the radiologists. There are thousands of settings one can adjust to obtain high-quality images. It is important to start with the basics, which are outlined in European Society of Urogenital Urology (ESUR) 2012 guidelines (Barentsz et al, 2012). If an ERC is used during the study, an antispasmodic agent should be used to decrease the artifact created by rectal spasms. Also, to get the highest quality images, the MR technologist should actively review images during the study and make adjustments or repeat sequences as needed. The goal is to have a prostate MRI scanning time of 30 minutes or less to maintain economical feasibility. Using new magnets with higher field strength, external coils, and an ERC can decrease image acquisition time and may also improve image quality (Heijmink et al, 2007) (Fig. 2-32).

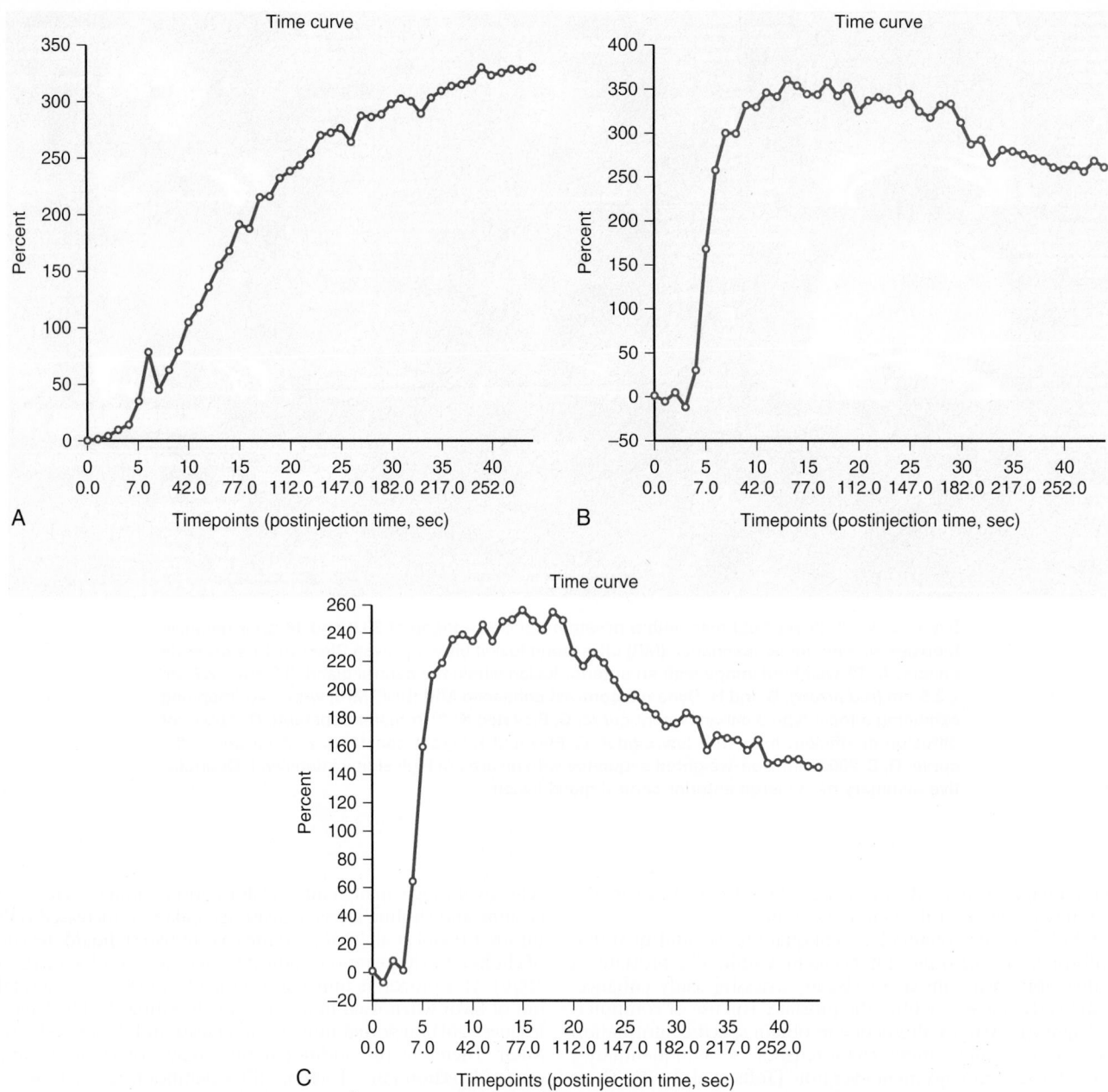

Figure 2-31. **A, Type 1 curve is normal enhancement with persistent increase in enhancement over time. B, Type 2 curve is early enhancement with a plateau (no washout). C, Type 3 curve, which is the most indicative of prostate cancer, can overlap with inflammation; this is characterized by early enhancement with an early washout of contrast.**

As more physicians begin to use MP-MRI of the prostate, maintaining quality and improving interpretation is extremely important. Each center should have designated readers. Prostate MRI is like no other study in radiology; it benefits from consensus reading and pathology correlation (Muller et al, 2014). Currently, there is no consensus on how a prostate MRI report should be completed. An international working group attempted to standardize reporting for MR targeted biopsies (Moore et al, 2013). The group used predefined prostate zones dividing the prostate into apex, mid, and base (Fig. 2-33A). Unfortunately, these zones do not always correlate well with end-fire images in the United States. However, if slices are used instead of the predefined zones, urologists can use the information regarding sequence, slice number, and primary zones to find the suspicious area within the prostate to aid in targeting during biopsy and possible surgical planning (Fig. 2-33B). In addition to location and 3D size, the radiologist's report should include a score for clinical

suspicion of disease. Multiple scoring systems exist; objective criteria for each sequence can be reported using the Prostate Imaging Reporting and Data System (PI-RADS) and the NIH scoring systems, as well as a subjective assessment using a five-point Likert scale for each lesion and the overall clinical suspicion for the patient (Barentsz et al, 2012; Moore et al, 2013; Turkbey et al, 2014) (Box 2-2).

In summary, MP-MRI of the prostate is a potential new tool that is able to detect, quantify, stage, and influence treatment planning for patients with prostate cancer. MP-MRI has also been shown to correctly select patients with low-grade/low-volume disease for active surveillance with an accuracy of 92% (Turkbey et al, 2014). MP-MRI of the prostate also provides information on possible bone involvement or lymphadenopathy at the time of diagnosis. The accuracy of MRI detecting lymphadenopathy has a sensitivity up to 86% and specificity of 78% to 90% (Talab et al, 2012).

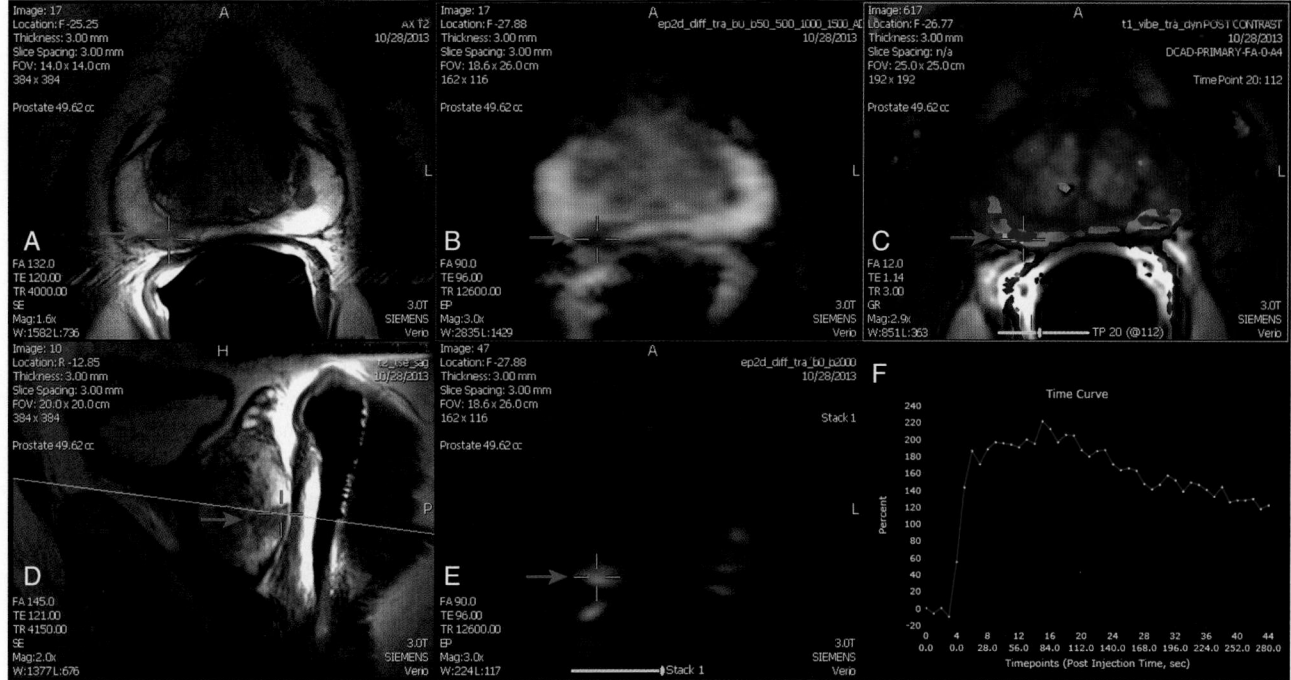

Figure 2-32. **A 61-year-old Caucasian man with an increasing prostate-specific antigen (4.65 ng/mL) after a prior negative biopsy 1 year ago. Three-tesla multiparametric magnetic resonance imaging (MP-MRI) of the prostate with an endorectal coil was obtained. A, T2-weighted image with a homogeneous low signal intensity (SI) lesion within the right posterior peripheral zone *(red arrow)*. B, Apparent diffusion coefficient (ADC) map with a corresponding low SI to the T2 sequence. C, Dynamic contrast enhanced MRI (DCE-MRI) with color mapping exhibiting a focal type 3 enhancement curve. D, Sagittal T2 sequence with a low-signal lesion within the peripheral zone. E, B-2000 diffusion-weighted imaging with high signal corresponding to T2, ADC, DCE abnormalities. F, Type 3 enhancement curve. The pathology was Gleason 3+4 prostate cancer, zone 3L, volume 0.3 mL (9 mm × 8 mm × 9 mm).**

Magnetic Resonance Ultrasound Fusion-Guided Prostate Biopsy

MR ultrasound fusion-guided prostate biopsy is the next step in the integration of high-quality intraprostatic imaging for screening and diagnosing prostate cancer. There are multiple fusion biopsy systems on the market. The performance of these systems differs slightly from one vendor to the other. However, the most important factor is the quality of the MP-MRI and abilities of the imaging team. These two factors have been shown to result in increased cancer detection rates in patients undergoing targeted biopsies (Pinto et al, 2011; Sonn et al, 2013).

Currently, a targeted biopsy or MP-MRI alone is not an alternative to the standard of care in screening men for prostate cancer. MP-MRI offers a distinct advantage when selecting men to undergo a biopsy with an elevated PSA. PSA is not prostate cancer specific and can be elevated for numerous reasons, including inflammation/infection, BPH, and physical manipulation. The MRI is able to assess BPH and inflammation before biopsy, and this may allow men who have persistently elevated PSA and an initial negative 12-core biopsy to avoid undergoing a second biopsy. Additionally, MP-MRI of the prostate can detect intermediate- and high-risk disease, but it has difficulty detecting low-grade/low-volume cancers, which may decrease overdiagnosis and overtreatment of clinically insignificant disease. Moore and colleagues (2013) reported that 38% of men with an elevated PSA did not have any visible lesions on MP-MRI. In this study, a 12-core biopsy detected only clinically significant cancer for 2.3% of the patients (Gleason score ≥7 or a core length of >5 mm).

The MR ultrasound fusion-guided biopsy has the advantage of using the MRI to target specific areas (i.e., anterior or central gland lesions) within the prostate that may be missed on a standard systematic 12-core biopsy. In addition, the 12-core biopsy may miss many lesions within the peripheral zone.

The cancer detection rates for targeted biopsies are superior to using the information from the MRI and then attempting to cognitively find the same area on ultrasonography to perform the biopsy (Wysock et al, 2014). The cancer detection rates for these types of targeted biopsies in patients with moderate to high suspicion on MRI are approximately 50% to 72% (Pinto et al, 2011; Sonn et al, 2013; Rastinehad et al, 2014).

All these new technologies do come at a cost. However, if one is able to select specific areas of the prostate to be targeted, instead of performing a 12-core biopsy, the savings from the decrease in number of pathology specimens collected could offset the cost of the MRI (Rastinehad et al, 2014). There is mounting evidence that a negative MP-MRI may effectively rule out a patient having clinically significant disease. The group from the University College London reported that a MP-MRI has an 89% to 100% NPV for ruling out clinically significant prostate cancer in patients with a negative MP-MR (Abd-Alazeez et al, 2014). This may result in patients foregoing a prostate biopsy and avoiding associated side effects.

ACKNOWLEDGMENTS

Thank you to the Drs. Ben-Levi, Villani, and Friedman for their help acquiring and reviewing images.

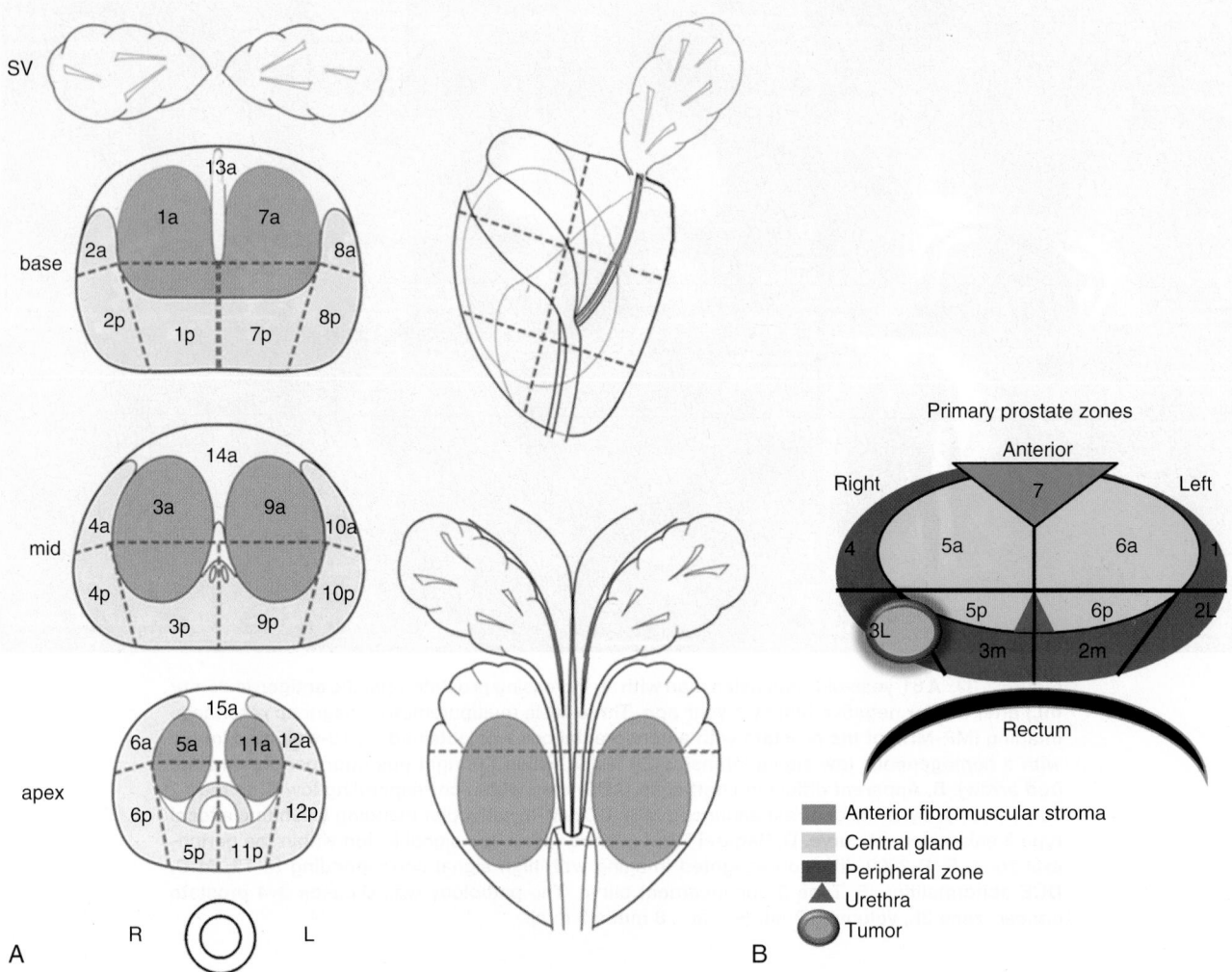

Figure 2-33. **A, Standards of reporting for MRI-targeted biopsy studies (START) reporting zones. SV, seminal vesicle. B, Primary prostate zones for reporting. The lesion is marked in the T2-weighted sequence because this is typically the sequence used for fusion-guided biopsies. This would be a Zone 3L (lateral) lesion on slice 17 (see Fig. 2-32). The slice levels for base and apex of the prostate are also reported. This allows one to convert the information to the START criteria zones for publication; however, this approach allows the urologist to locate the lesion on the multiparametric magnetic resonance image with ease (sequence, slice number, and zone number).**

BOX 2-2 Five-Point Likert Scale for Prostate Imaging

1. Clinically significant disease is highly unlikely to be present.
2. Clinically significant disease is unlikely to be present.
3. Clinically significant disease is equivocal.
4. Clinically significant disease is likely to be present.
5. Clinically significant disease is highly likely to be present.

From Moore CM, Kasivisvanathan V, Eggener S, et al; START Consortium. Standards of reporting for MRI-targeted biopsy studies (START) of the prostate: recommendations from an International Working Group. Eur Urol 2013;64:544–52.

KEY POINTS: MRI

• When a renal mass is seen on MRI, the most important characteristic indicating the presence of a malignancy is enhancement of the mass.
• NSF is seen in patients with severe renal insufficiency who are exposed to Gd contrast media.
• Pheochromocytoma, metastatic lesion to the adrenal gland, and primary ACC are all bright on T2-weighted images.

REFERENCES

The complete reference list is available online at www.expertconsult.com.

SUGGESTED READINGS

Gomella LG, Halpern EJ, Trabulsi EJ. Prostate biopsy: techniques and imaging. In: Wein AJ, Kavoussi LR, Partin AW, et al., editors. Campbell-Walsh urology. 11th ed. Philadelphia: Saunders; 2016 [chapter 109].
Siegelman E. Body MRI. Philadelphia: Saunders; 2004.

3 Urinary Tract Imaging: Basic Principles of Urologic Ultrasonography

Bruce R. Gilbert, MD, PhD, and Pat F. Fulgham, MD

Ultrasonography has often been referred to as the "urologist's stethoscope" because much of the genitourinary system is not easily evaluated by physical examination and requires imaging for diagnosis. Therein lies one of the unique aspects of ultrasound studies performed and interpreted by urologists. The mandate to examine the patient coupled with the urologist's experience in both surgical and medical treatment engenders an unparalleled ability to meld the healer's art with advanced imaging technology. In addition, ultrasonography is a versatile and relatively inexpensive imaging modality that has the unique feature of being the only imaging modality to provide real-time evaluation of urologic organs and structures without the need for ionizing radiation. To use this technology best on behalf of their patients, urologists must have a mature understanding of the underlying physical principles of ultrasonography. They must also understand how the manipulation of ultrasound equipment can affect the quality of ultrasound images. The technical skills required to perform and interpret urologic ultrasonography represent a combination of practical scanning ability and knowledge of the underlying disease process in organs being imaged. To communicate the findings appropriately, urologists should understand the nomenclature of ultrasonography and have a specific plan for documentation of each type of study. Understanding how ultrasonography interacts with human tissues allows urologists to use this modality effectively, appropriately, and safely. The aim of this chapter is to encourage urologists to embrace the art and science of ultrasonography in their mission to provide excellence in patient care.

BRIEF HISTORY OF ULTRASONOGRAPHY IN UROLOGY

In 1963, Japanese urologists Takahashi and Ouchi became the first to attempt ultrasonic examination of the prostate. However, the image quality that resulted was not interpretable and carried little medical utility (Takahashi and Ouchi, 1963). Wild and Reid (1952) also attempted transrectal ultrasonography (TRUS) but were met with the same result. Progress was not made until Watanabe and colleagues (1974) demonstrated radial scanning that could adequately identify prostate and bladder pathology. Using a purpose-built device modeled after a museum sculpture entitled "Magician's Chair," Watanabe seated his patients on a chair with a hole cut in the center such that the transducer tube could be passed through the hole and into the rectum of the seated patient (Watanabe et al, 1974). Images from Watanabe's seated probe are shown in Figure 3-1. As is evident in Figures 3-1B (demonstrating an area of circumscribed symmetric echogenicity, representing benign prostatic hyperplasia), and 3-1C (demonstrating an asymmetric area of hyperechogenicity, representing prostate cancer), resolution was poor, and images displayed extreme contrast. Subsequent development of biplanar, high-frequency probes created increased resolution and allowed for TRUS to become the standard for diagnosis of prostatic disease.

In 1971 Goldberg and Pollack, frustrated with the inability of intravenous pyelography to differentiate benign from malignant lesions, employed A-mode ultrasonography to evaluate the kidney. In their report on "nephrosonography," they demonstrated in a series of 150 patients the capability of ultrasonography to discern solid, cystic, and complex masses with an accuracy of 96%. Diagrammatic representations of the three ultrasound patterns they found are depicted in Figure 3-2 (Goldberg and Pollack, 2002). In cystic lesions, the first spike represents the striking of the front wall of the cyst and the second spike represents the striking of the back wall. More complex lesions have return of more spikes.

In 1974 Holm and Northeved introduced a transurethral ultrasonic device that would be interchangeable with conventional optics during cystoscopy for the purpose of imaging the prostate and bladder. Their other goals for this device included the ability to determine depth of bladder tumor penetration, to determine prostatic volume, to evaluate prostatic tumor progression, and to assist with transurethral resection of the prostate (Holm and Northeved, 1974).

Perri and colleagues were the first to use Doppler as a sonic "stethoscope" in their work-up of patients with an acute scrotum in 1976. Although they were able to identify patients with epididymitis and torsion of the appendix testis as having increased flow and patients with spermatic cord torsion as having no blood flow, they also reported that false-negative images in cases of torsion could result from increased flow secondary to reactive hyperemia (Perri et al, 1976).

Watanabe and colleagues (1976), pioneers in the use of ultrasonography in urology, demonstrated that Doppler could be used to identify the renal arteries in a noninvasive way in 1976, and Greene and colleagues (1981) documented 5 years later that Doppler could adequately differentiate stenotic from normal renal arteries. In 1982 Arima and associates used Doppler to differentiate acute from chronic rejection in patients with renal transplants, noting that acute rejection is characterized by the disappearance of diastolic phase, with reappearance being indicative of recovery from rejection. These authors concluded that Doppler could guide the management of rejection as an index for steroid therapy (Arima et al, 1982).

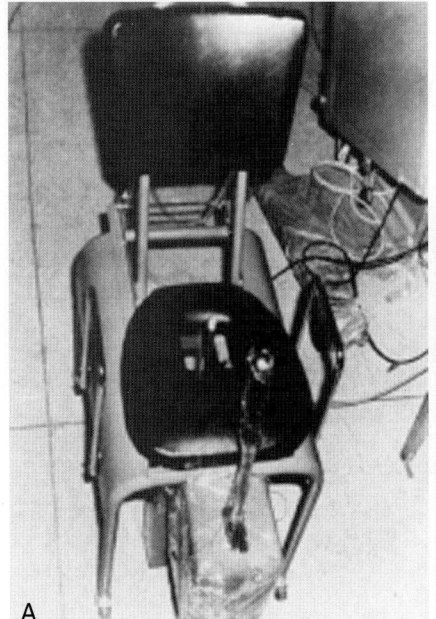

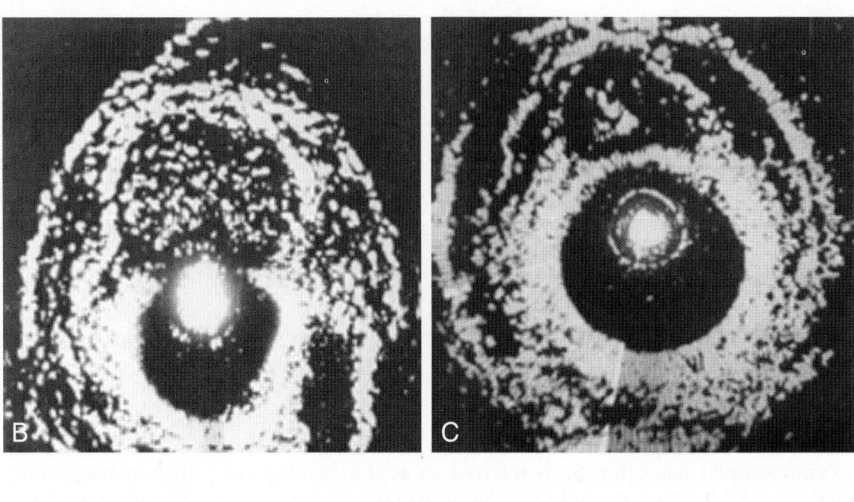

Figure 3-1. **A,** Watanabe's chair. **B,** Display of patient with benign prostatic hyperplasia. **C,** Display of prostate cancer. (From Watanabe H, Igari D, Tanahasi Y, et al. Development and application of new equipment for transrectal ultrasonography. J Clin Ultrasound 1974;2:91–8.)

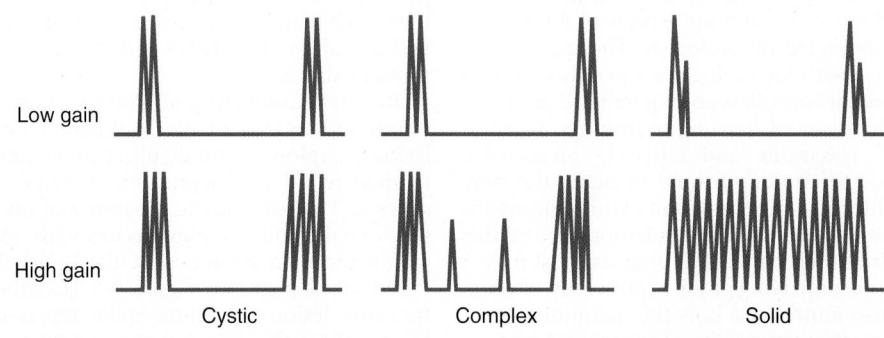

Figure 3-2. **Goldberg and Pollack were the first to differentiate between solid, complex, and cystic masses by ultrasonography. In cystic lesions, the first spike represents the striking of the front wall of the cyst, and the second spike represents the striking of the back wall. More complex lesions have return of more spikes. (From Goldberg B, Pollack H. Differentiation of renal masses using A-mode ultrasound. J Urol 2002;167:1022–6.)**

In the early 1990s numerous authors investigated the therapeutic uses of high-intensity focused ultrasonography (HIFU). Following prior reports of histologic changes after HIFU (Burgess et al, 1987), Madersbacher and colleagues (1993) were the first to report the safety and efficacy of HIFU in patients with symptomatic benign prostatic hyperplasia. The utility of HIFU in the treatment of testicular cancer (Madersbacher et al, 1998), early prostate cancer (Chapelon et al, 1999), recurrent prostate cancer (Berge et al, 2010), and renal cell cancer transcutaneously (Köhrmann et al, 2002) and laparoscopically (Margreiter and Marberger, 2010) was soon explored as well.

The field of urology continues to demand and discover novel uses for ultrasound technology. Chen and coworkers (2010) used TRUS guidance to inject botulinum toxin into the external urethral sphincters of a series of patients with detrusor external sphincter dyssynergia. Ozawa and colleagues (2010) used perineal ultrasound video-urodynamics to diagnose bladder outlet obstruction accurately in a noninvasive manner. The possibilities for application of ultrasonography in diagnosing or treating urologic conditions are endless.

Urologic ultrasonography continues to evolve with the use of contrast agents and new modalities such as sonoelastography that include groundbreaking discoveries and new applications of basic

physical principles. This homage to the innovators of the past serves both to recognize prior achievements and to acknowledge that future work in the development of new applications for ultrasonography will always be needed.

PHYSICAL PRINCIPLES

All ultrasound imaging is the result of the interaction of sound waves with tissues and structures within the human body. Ultrasound waves are produced by applying short bursts of alternating electrical current to a series of crystals housed in the transducer. Alternating expansion and contraction of the crystals via the piezoelectric effect creates a mechanical wave that is transmitted through a coupling medium to the skin and then into the body. The waves that are produced are longitudinal waves. In a longitudinal wave, the particle motion is in the same direction as the propagation of the wave (Fig. 3-3). This motion produces areas of rarefaction and compression of tissue in the direction of travel of the ultrasound wave (Fig. 3-4). A portion of the wave is reflected toward the transducer. The transducer serves as a receiver and "listens" for the returning sound wave reconverting the mechanical wave to electrical energy. The transducer must be in direct,

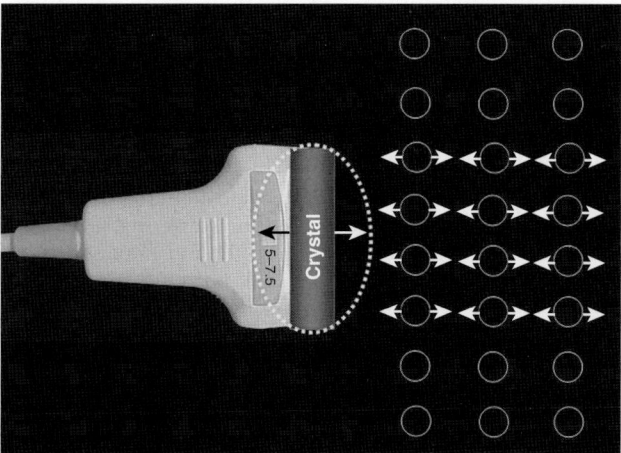

Figure 3-3. The alternating expansion and contraction of the crystal produces longitudinal mechanical waves. In this simplified schematic drawing, the individual molecules (depicted as circles) are displaced in the direction of the propagated wave.

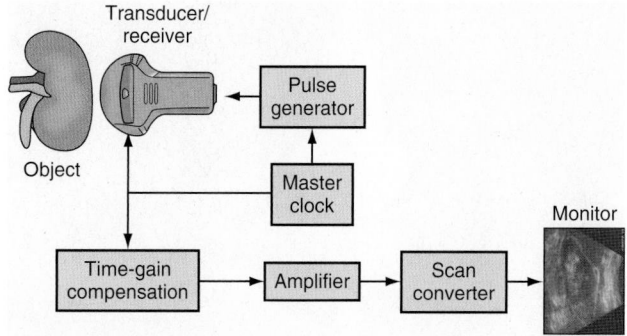

Figure 3-5. In this simplified schematic diagram of ultrasound imaging, the ultrasound wave is produced by means of a pulse generator controlled by a master clock. The reflected waves received by the transducer are analyzed for amplitude and transit time within the body. The scan converter produces the familiar picture seen on the monitor. The actual image is a series of vertical lines that are continuously refreshed to produce the familiar real-time, gray-scale image.

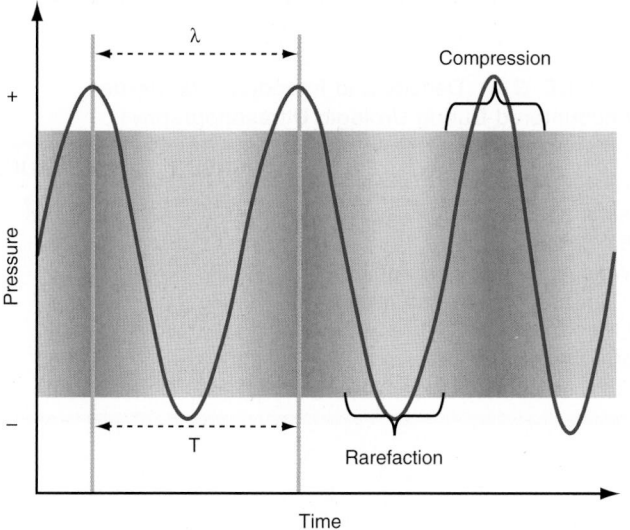

Figure 3-4. Areas of compression alternating with areas of rarefaction are depicted as a sine wave. The wavelength (λ) is the length from peak compression to peak compression in this drawing. This graphic depiction is critical to understanding the behavior of sound waves in the human body and how ultrasound images are generated. (From Merritt CRB. Physics of ultrasound. In: Rumack CM, Wilson SR, Charboneau JW, Johnson J, editors. Diagnostic ultrasound. 3rd ed. St. Louis: Mosby; 2005. p. 3–34.)

next peak. The complete path traveled by the wave from one peak to the next is called a *cycle*. One cycle per second is known as *1 hertz* (Hz). The "period" is the time it takes for one complete cycle of the wave.

The "amplitude" of a wave is the maximal excursion in the positive or negative direction from the baseline. Amplitude corresponds to the mechanical energy associated with the sound wave and is a key property in assigning pixel brightness to a gray-scale ultrasound image. The greater the amplitude, the brighter is the corresponding pixel.

Ultrasound Image Generation

The image produced by an ultrasound machine begins with the transducer. In ultrasound imaging, the transducer has a dual function as a sender and a receiver. Sound waves are created in short pulses and transmitted into the body and are then at least partially reflected. Reflected mechanical sound waves are received by the transducer and converted back into electrical energy. The transducer acts as a receiver more than 99% of the time. The electrical energy is converted by the ultrasound machine to an image displayed on a monitor (Fig. 3-5).

Resolution

The resolution of an ultrasound image refers to the ability to discriminate two objects in close proximity to one another. **Axial resolution** refers to the ability to identify as separate two objects in the direction of the traveling sound wave. Axial resolution is directly dependent on the frequency of sound waves. The higher the frequency of the sound wave, the better the axial resolution. **Lateral resolution** refers to the ability to identify separately objects that are equidistant from the transducer. Lateral resolution is a function of the focused width of the ultrasound beam and is a characteristic of the transducer. The location of the narrowest beam width can be adjusted by the user. The more focused the beam, the better the lateral resolution at that location. Image quality can be enhanced by locating the narrowest beam width (focus or focal zone) at the depth of the object or tissue of interest (Fig. 3-6).

The velocity with which a sound wave travels through tissue is a product of its frequency and wavelength (Fig. 3-7). The **average velocity of sound in human tissues is 1540 m/sec.** Because the average velocity of sound in tissue is a constant, changes in frequency result in changes in wavelength.

The optimal ultrasound image requires tradeoffs between resolution and depth of penetration. High-frequency transducers of 6 to 10 MHz may be used to image structures near the surface of the

secure contact with the subject to transmit and receive the reflected sound waves.

The appearance of the image produced by ultrasonography is the result of the interaction of mechanical ultrasound waves with biologic tissues and materials. Because ultrasound waves are transmitted and received at frequent intervals, the images can be rapidly reconstructed and refreshed, providing a real-time image. The frequencies of the sound waves used for urologic ultrasound imaging are in the range of 3.5 to 12 MHz.

Mechanical waves are represented graphically as a sine wave alternating between a positive and negative direction from the baseline. In the case of ultrasonography, the amplitude of the sine wave describes differences in pressure. Ultrasound waves are described using the standard nomenclature for sine waves. A wavelength (λ) is described as the distance between one peak of the wave and the

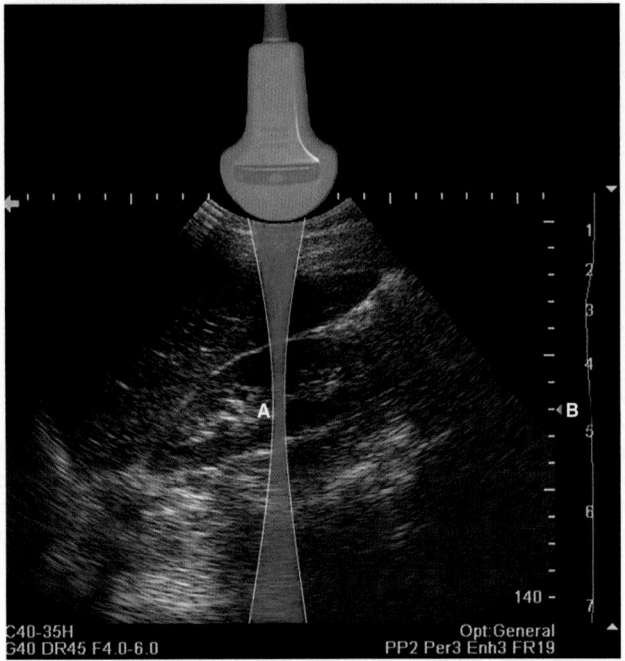

Figure 3-6. The shape of the ultrasound beam is simulated in this drawing *(purple)*. The focal zone (A) is located to produce the best lateral resolution of the medial renal cortex. The location of the focal zone is designated by the caret (B). The location of the focal zone can be adjusted by the operator.

$$v = f \times \lambda$$
$$velocity = frequency \times wavelength$$

Figure 3-7. The relationship between velocity, frequency, and wavelength of sound waves in tissue. Wavelength and frequency vary in an inverse relationship.

body (e.g., testis, pediatric kidney) with excellent resolution. However, deeper structures (e.g., right kidney, bladder) require lower frequencies of 3.5 to 5 MHz to penetrate. Such images have poorer axial resolution.

Mechanisms of Attenuation

As sound waves transit tissues, energy is lost or attenuated. Mechanisms of attenuation include **reflection, scattering, interference, and absorption.** Reflection is the key physical phenomenon that allows for information to return to the transducer as mechanical energy. Reflection occurs when ultrasound waves strike an object, a surface, or a boundary (called an **interface**) between unlike tissues. The shape and size of the object and the angle at which the advancing wave strikes the object are critical determinants of the amount of energy reflected. The amount of energy reflected from an interface is also influenced by the **impedance** of the two tissues at the interface. Impedance is a property that is influenced by tissue stiffness and density. The difference in impedance allows an appreciation of interfaces between different types of tissue (Table 3-1).

The impedance difference between perinephric fat and the kidney allows a sharp visual distinction at the interface. If the impedance difference between tissues is small (e.g., between liver and kidney), the interface between the tissues is more difficult to see (Fig. 3-8A). If impedance differences are large, there is

TABLE 3-1   Density and Impedance of Tissues Encountered During Urologic Ultrasonography

	DENSITY	IMPEDANCE
Air and other gases	1.2	0.0004
Fat tissue	952	1.38
Water and other clear liquids	1000	1.48
Kidney (average of soft tissue)	1060	1.63
Liver	1060	1.64
Muscle	1080	1.70
Bone and other calcified objects	1912	7.8

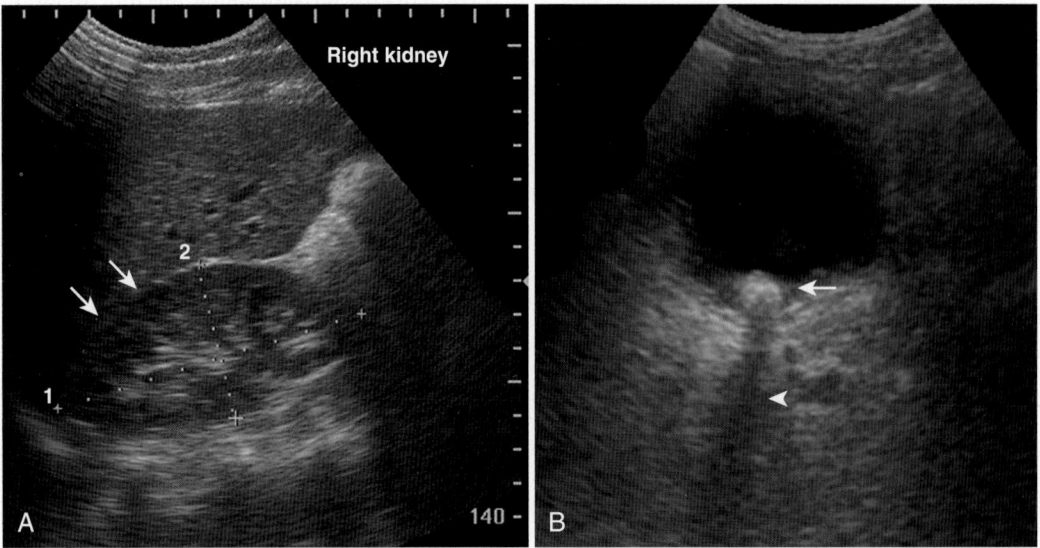

Figure 3-8. A, In this sagittal view of the right kidney, the paucity of perinephric fat and the small impedance difference make it difficult to distinguish the interface between the kidney and the liver *(arrows)*. **B,** The large impedance difference at the interface between urine and a bladder stone *(arrow)* results in significant reflection and attenuation of the sound wave. An acoustic shadow is seen distal to the stone *(arrowhead)*.

significant reflection of the sound wave producing an acoustical shadow distal to the interface (Fig. 3-8B).

Scattering occurs when sound waves strike a small or irregular object. The resulting spherical wave overlaps waves of surrounding scattering objects (Fig. 3-9).

When interacting sound waves are in phase or out of phase, their amplitude is enhanced or diminished. This **pattern of interference** is partially responsible for the echo architecture or texture of organs. One pattern of interference, commonly called **"speckling"** (Fig. 3-10), is seen in organs with fine, internal histology (i.e., reflectors such as the testis).

Absorption occurs when the mechanical energy of the ultrasound waves is converted to heat. Absorption is directly proportional to frequency. The higher the frequency of the incident wave, the greater the absorption of energy, and more tissue heating results. It follows that higher frequency waves are more rapidly attenuated and have a limited depth of penetration (Fig. 3-11).

Artifacts

The interaction of ultrasound waves with tissues may produce images that do not reflect the true underlying anatomy. These misrepresentations are called "artifacts." Artifacts may be misleading but, if recognized, may also assist diagnosis. **Acoustical shadowing** occurs when there is significant attenuation or reflection of sound waves at a tissue interface. Echo information posterior to the interface may be obscured or lost. An anechoic or hypoechoic "shadow" is produced. Under these conditions, three-dimensional (3D) objects such as stones may appear as crescentic objects, making it difficult to obtain accurate measurements (Fig. 3-12). Important pathology posterior to such an interface may be missed. This problem may often be overcome or mitigated by changing the angle of insonation, changing the frequency of the transducer, or changing the focal zone of the transducer.

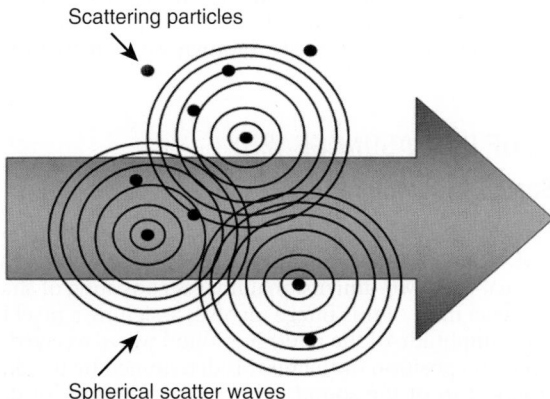

Figure 3-9. **Scattering is a phenomenon that occurs when sound waves strike small objects. The resulting pattern of energy dispersal often results in interference.**

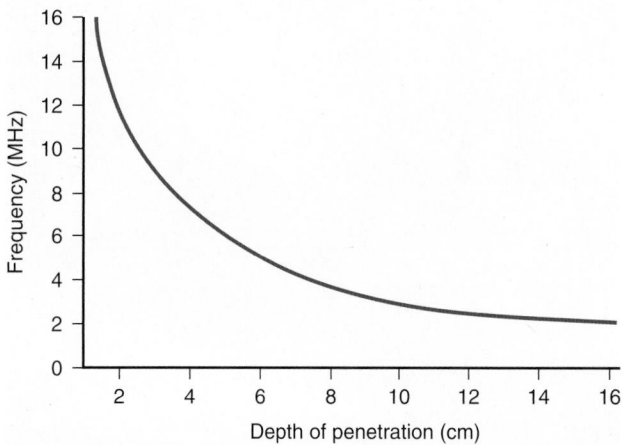

Figure 3-11. **Relationship between frequency and tissue penetration. High-frequency sound waves are rapidly attenuated and are unable to penetrate deeply. Conversely, low-frequency waves are less attenuated and able to penetrate deeply to internal structures.**

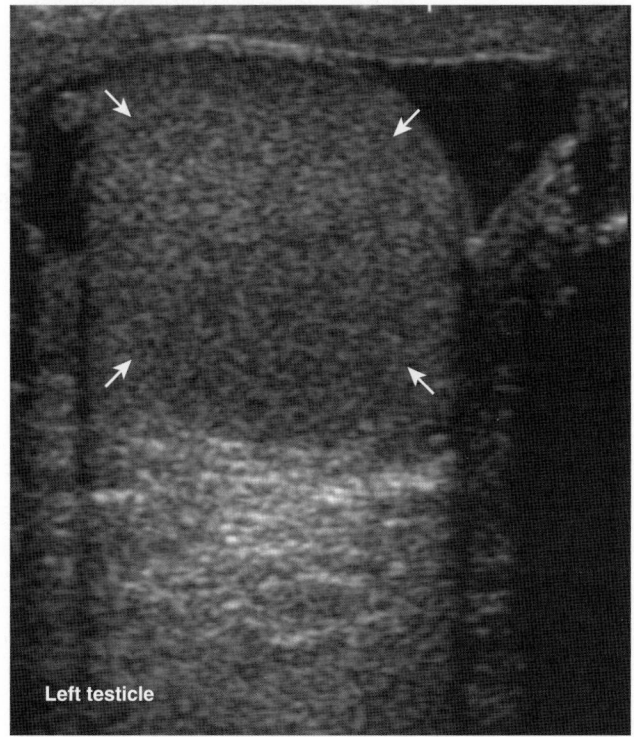

Figure 3-10. **Fine internal echogenicity called "speckle" is caused by scattering of sound waves, resulting in a pattern of interference. Note the resulting finely granular, homogeneous echogenicity *(arrows)* of the testicular parenchyma.**

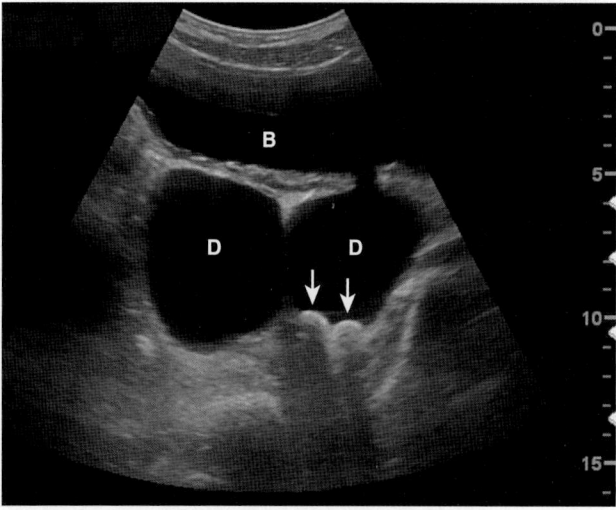

Figure 3-12. **In this transverse view of the urinary bladder (B), there are two large bladder diverticula (D). Two stones *(arrows)* strongly reflect and attenuate the incident sound wave, producing an acoustical shadow. The stones appear crescentic even though they are ovoid in shape.**

Increased through-transmission is observed when sound waves are less attenuated while passing through a given structure or tissue than by the surrounding tissues. For example, when imaging a simple cyst of the kidney, sound waves passing through the cyst are less attenuated than sound waves passing through the surrounding renal cortex and renal sinus. When the waves transiting the cyst strike the back wall of the cyst and posterior renal tissue, the waves are more energetic on arrival to these tissues. The reflected sound waves are also more energetic and less attenuated as they return to the transducer. The result is that tissue posterior to the cyst appears hyperechoic compared with the surrounding renal tissue, even though the tissues are histologically identical (Fig. 3-13). The effect of this artifact can be mitigated by changing the angle of insonation or adjusting the time-gain compensation settings.

An **edging artifact** occurs when sound waves strike a curved surface or interface at an incident angle, resulting in refraction of the wave along the plane of the interface (Fig. 3-14). An incident wave at this angle (the critical angle) is not directly reflected to the transducer, resulting in a hypoechoic "shadow." This artifact is commonly seen in testicular ultrasonography and TRUS (Fig. 3-15). It can be overcome by changing the angle of insonation.

A **reverberation artifact** results when there are large differences in impedance between two adjacent tissues or surfaces with a strong reflection of the incident wave. The ultrasound wave bounces back and forth (reverberates) between the reflective interfaces. With the second transit of the sound wave, the ultrasound equipment interprets a second object that is twice as far away as the first. There is ongoing attenuation of the sound wave with each successive reverberation, resulting in a slightly less intense image displayed on the screen. Echoes are produced, spaced at equal intervals from the transducer but progressively less intense (Fig. 3-16).

The reverberation artifact can also be seen in cases where the incident sound wave strikes a series of smaller reflective objects (e.g., the gas-fluid mixture in the small bowel), which results in multiple reflected sound waves of various angles and intensity (Fig. 3-17). The resultant echo pattern is a collection of hyperechoic artifactual reflections distal to the structure with progressive attenuation of the sound wave.

MODES OF ULTRASONOGRAPHY
Gray-Scale Ultrasonography

Gray-scale B-mode ultrasonography is the most commonly employed mode of ultrasonography. This pulsed-wave technique produces real-time two-dimensional images consisting of shades of gray. The generation of this image involves assigning a pixel brightness to the amplitude of the returning sound waves received by the transducer. The position of the pixel is determined by the duration of the round trip of the sound wave. Individual lines of data are displayed sequentially on the monitor to produce a continuous or real-time image. Evaluation of gray-scale imaging requires the ability to recognize normal patterns of echogenicity from anatomic

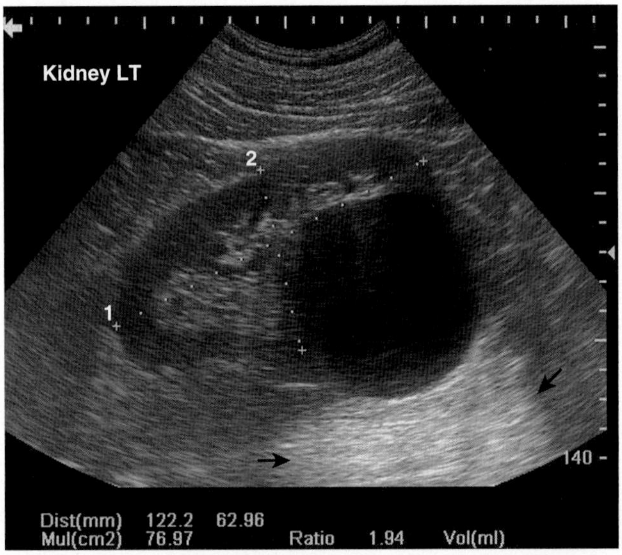

Figure 3-13. Increased through-transmission (also called "distal enhancement") is demonstrated in this longitudinal view of the left kidney. The tissue distal to the cyst appears hyperechoic *(arrows)* compared with adjacent tissue.

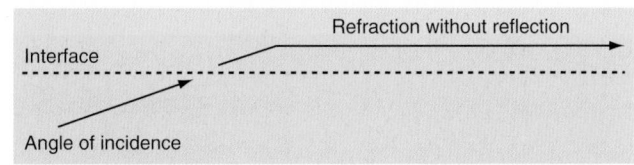

Figure 3-14. When sound waves strike a surface or interface at a "critical angle," the wave is refracted without significant reflection.

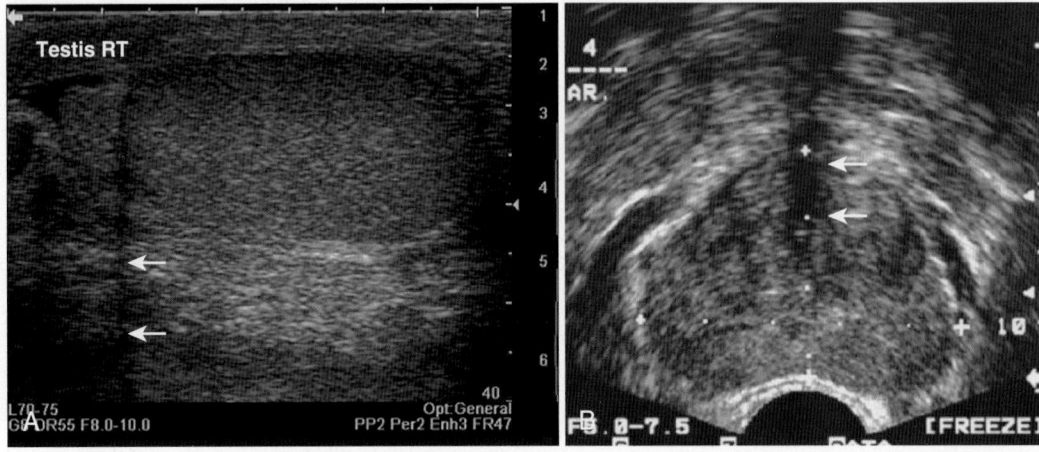

Figure 3-15. **A,** The curved surface of the tunica albuginea of the upper pole of the testis creates a critical angle edging artifact *(arrows)*. **B,** The rounded surfaces of the lateral lobes of the prostate as they meet in the prostatic urethra create an edging artifact *(arrows)* in this transverse image of the prostate.

structures. Variations from these expected patterns of echogenicity indicate disorders of anatomy or physiology.

Doppler Ultrasonography

Doppler ultrasonography depends on the physical principle of frequency shift when sound waves strike a moving object. The basic principle of Doppler ultrasonography is that sound waves of a certain frequency are shifted or changed on the basis of the direction and velocity of the moving object as well as the angle of insonation. This phenomenon allows for the characterization of motion, most commonly the motion of blood through vessels, but it may also be useful for detecting the flow of urine.

Color Doppler ultrasonography allows for evaluation of the velocity and direction of motion. A color map may be applied to direction with the most common assignation of the color blue to

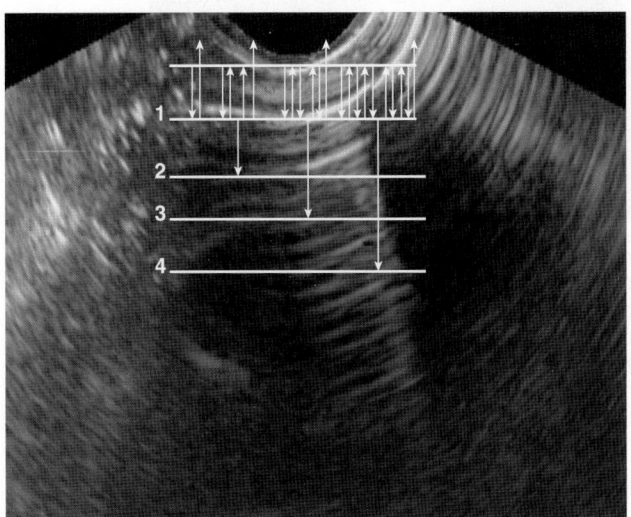

Figure 3-16. Reverberation artifact. A virtual representation of the strongly reflective interface is projected with decreasing amplitude as the incident sound wave makes multiple round trips.

motion away from the transducer and red to motion toward the transducer. The velocity of motion is designated by the intensity of the color: The brighter the color, the greater the velocity. Color Doppler may be used to evaluate the presence or absence of blood flow in the kidney, testes, penis, and prostate. It also may be useful in the detection of ureteral "jets" of urine emerging from the ureteral orifices.

Color flow with spectral display allows the interrogation of particular areas within an ultrasound field for flow and displays the flow as a continuous waveform. This mode is commonly used to evaluate the pattern and velocity of blood flow in the intrarenal or penile vasculature. The waveform provides information about peripheral vascular resistance in the tissues. The most commonly used index of these velocities is the resistive index. The **resistive index** is peak systolic velocity (PSV) minus the end-diastolic velocity over the PSV. This index is helpful in characterizing many clinical conditions including renal artery stenosis, ureteral obstruction, and penile arterial insufficiency.

Power Doppler ultrasonography assigns the amplitude of frequency change to a color map. This mode does not permit evaluation of velocity or direction of flow but is less affected by backscatter waves and is a more sensitive mode for detecting blood flow. Power Doppler is less angle dependent than color Doppler and is three to five times as sensitive as color Doppler ultrasonography for detecting flow. It may be useful for evaluating testicular torsion.

Harmonic Scanning

Harmonic scanning uses aberrations related to the nonlinear propagation of sound waves within tissue. These asymmetrically propagated waves generate fewer harmonics, but those that are generated have greater amplitudes. Because these harmonics are not subject to scattering at the frequency associated with the incident wave, there is less noise associated with the signal. By concentrating on the harmonic frequencies produced within the body and reflected to the transducer, it is possible to produce an image with less artifact and greater resolution (Fig. 3-18).

Spatial Compounding

Spatial compounding is a scanning mode whereby the direction of insonation is electronically altered, and a composite image is

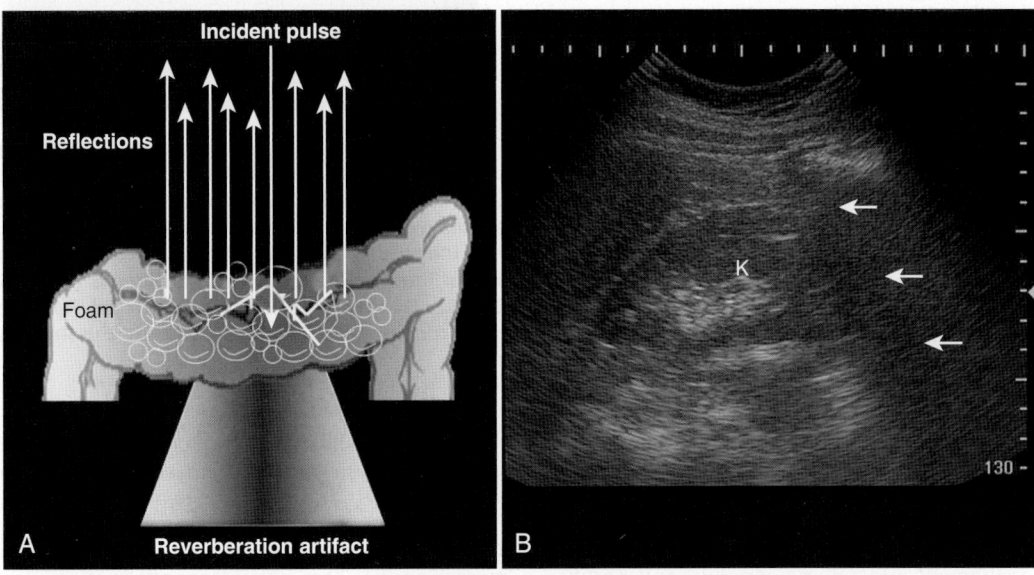

Figure 3-17. When an ultrasound wave strikes a structure such as bowel, which contains gas bubbles (A), the resultant reverberation artifact has a characteristic appearance sometimes called a "comet tail." B, A comet tail artifact produced by bowel gas (arrows) obscures the lower pole of the kidney (K).

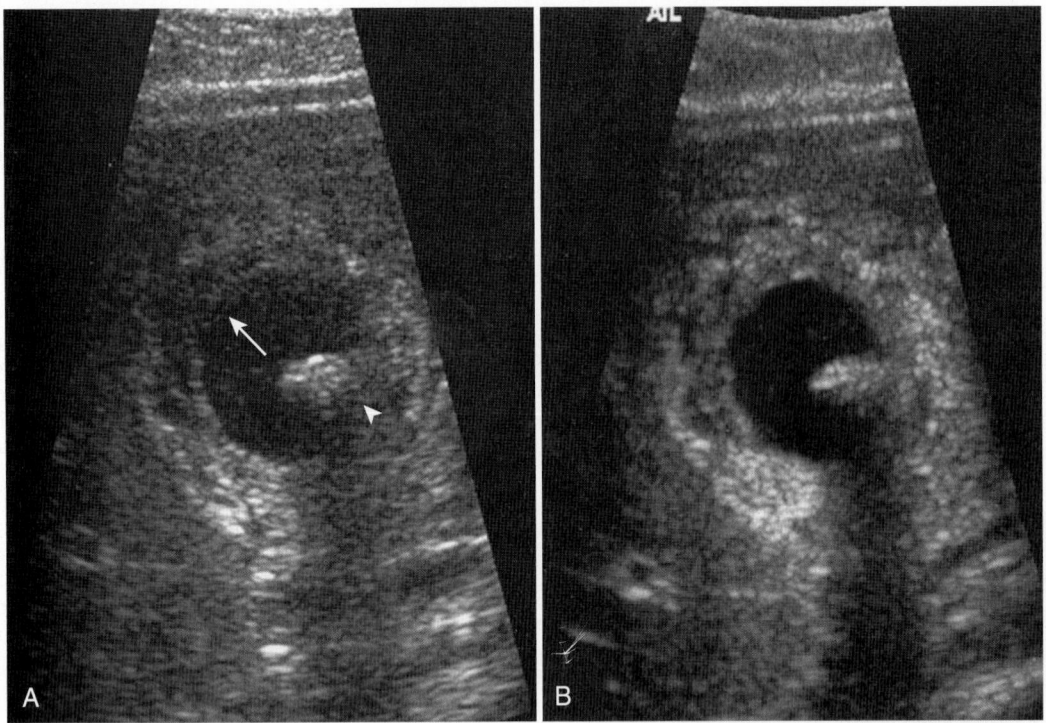

Figure 3-18. **A, Standard gray-scale image of a cyst containing a mural nodule *(arrowhead)*. Note the artifactual echogenicity within the cyst *(arrow)*. B, The same structure on harmonic scanning is seen more clearly. There is less artifact within and distal to the cyst. (From Merritt CRB. Physics of ultrasound. In: Rumack CM, Wilson SR, Charboneau JW, Johnson J, editors. Diagnostic ultrasound. 3rd ed. St. Louis: Mosby; 2005. p. 3–34.)**

generated. This technique reduces the amount of artifact and noise, producing a scan of better clarity.

Sonoelastography

The ability to access pathology by palpation has long been a key part of a physician's physical examination. Hard lesions are often a sign of pathology. Sonoelastography (tissue elasticity imaging) is an evolving ultrasound modality that adds the ability to evaluate the elasticity (compressibility and displacement) of biologic tissues. Essentially, it gives a representation, using color, of the softness or hardness of the tissue of interest. To use ultrasonography to "palpate" an organ requires a compressing mechanical wave to be produced in the tissue of interest. Presently, there are two ways to produce this mechanical wave: real-time elastography (RTE) and shear wave elastography (SWE).

In RTE, as in standard diagnostic ultrasonography, an external, nonquantifiable mechanically produced compression wave travels in tissue (1540 m/sec). These waves successively compress tissue layers producing backscatter reflected waves that are received and processed by the ultrasound equipment producing an image. Because the stress producing the mechanical compression wave cannot be directly measured, only a relative elasticity can be determined.

With RTE (Fig. 3-19), deformation is induced by manually pressing on the anatomy with the transducer and is measured using ultrasonography. RTE is a qualitative technique and highly user-dependent. Because of the requirement of manual displacement, RTE is unable to measure absolute tissue stiffness as currently employed. Its major benefits are that it has a high spatial resolution, it is a real-time measurement, and it does not require any modifications to conventional ultrasound hardware. Spatial resolution is the ability to distinguish two separate objects that are close together and encompasses both axial resolution and lateral resolution as defined previously.

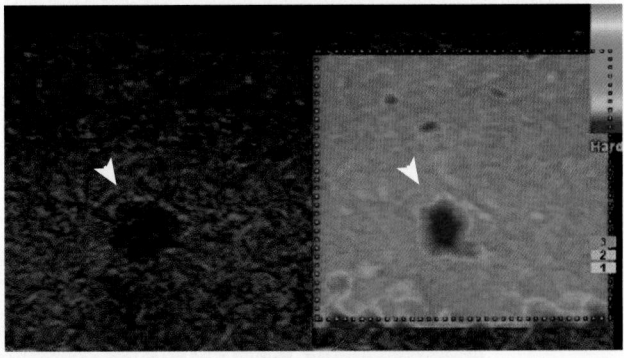

Figure 3-19. **Real-time elastography. A 4-mm hypoechoic nodule *(arrow, left panel)* was found with Doppler ultrasonography with vascular flow internally. Real-time sonoelastography suggested a hard nodule (with this equipment blue is hard, not soft). Close follow-up with ultrasound examinations every 3 months found no increase in size of the nodule, and it was considered "probably" benign. (From Goddi A, Sacchi A, Magistretti G, Almolla J. Real-time tissue elastography for testicular lesion assessment. Eur Radiol 2012;22:721–30.)**

In SWE, the shear wave produced can be precisely measured and travels more slowly (1 to 10 m/sec). The shear wave is propagated by a tangential "sliding" force between tissue layers. The elasticity (E), density of the tissue (p, kg/m^2), and shear wave propagation speed (c) are directly related through the equation $E = 3pc^2$. By measuring the shear wave propagation speed, the elasticity of the tissue can be directly determined.

With SWE (Fig. 3-20), low-frequency (approximately 100 Hz) pulses are rapidly transmitted into the tissue to induce a vibration in the tissue. Depending on the manufacturer's implementation, the

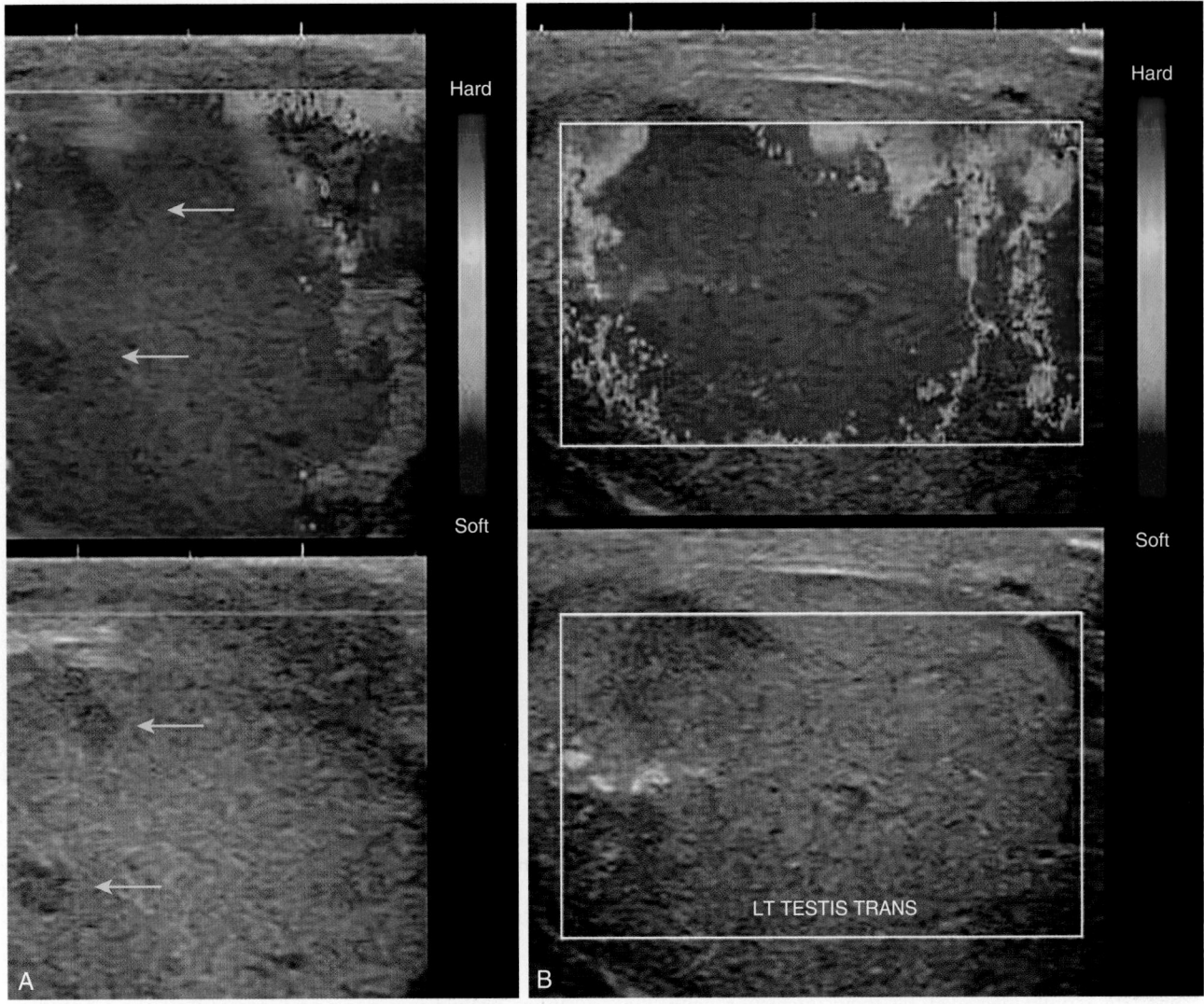

Figure 3-20. **Shear wave elastography (SWE). A,** Two small hypoechoic vascular lesions *(arrows, lower panel)* found with B-mode ultrasonography are shown in the upper panel to be soft *(blue)* lesions with SWE ultrasonography. Biopsy confirmed a Sertoli cell nodule. **B,** A larger lesion with heterogeneous echogenicity on B-mode ultrasonography *(lower panel)* demonstrates diffuse "hardness" on SWE *(upper panel).* Pathology demonstrated a nonseminomatous germ cell tumor.

vibrations can be induced in a single area or in a vertical plane by rapidly altering focal depth. Subsequently, the observation of the propagation velocity of the resultant transient shear waves determines the viscoelastic properties of the tissues. Two typical limitations of generated shear waves are as follows: (1) They are very weak resulting in only a few millimeters of propagation, and (2) detection of shear wave propagation requires very rapid acquisition speeds (pulse repetition frequency is >5000 Hz), which may limit the area of detection. However, some new-generation ultrasound systems have overcome these obstacles and allow large areas of interest to be displayed at near real-time imaging frame rates.

Several approaches for elastography have been introduced. All of them have three common steps, as follows:

1. The sonographer manually compresses (RTE) or the machine automatically generates (SWE) a low-frequency vibration in tissue to induce stress.
2. The tissue is imaged with the goal of analyzing the resulting strain.
3. Parameters are defined related to tissue stiffness.

The principle of elastography is based on the concept that a given force applied to softer tissue results in a larger displacement than the same force applied to harder tissue. By measuring the tissue displacement induced by compression, it is possible to estimate the tissue hardness and to differentiate benign (soft) from malignant (hard) lesions. This relationship between stress (s) and strain (e) is given by Young's modulus or elasticity (E):

$$E = s/e$$

E is larger in hard tissues and lower in soft tissues.

Visually, the elasticity of a tissue is represented by color spectrum. The color given to hard lesions is determined by the manufacturer of the equipment and can be set by the user. Just as in using color Doppler, the user needs to look at the color bar (see Figs. 3-19 and 3-20) to know what colors represent "hard" and "soft" lesions.

Three-Dimensional Scanning

3D scanning has been used extensively in obstetrics and gynecology but so far has limited application in urology. 3D scanning produces a composite of images (data set), which can be manipulated to generate additional views of the anatomy in question (Fig. 3-21).

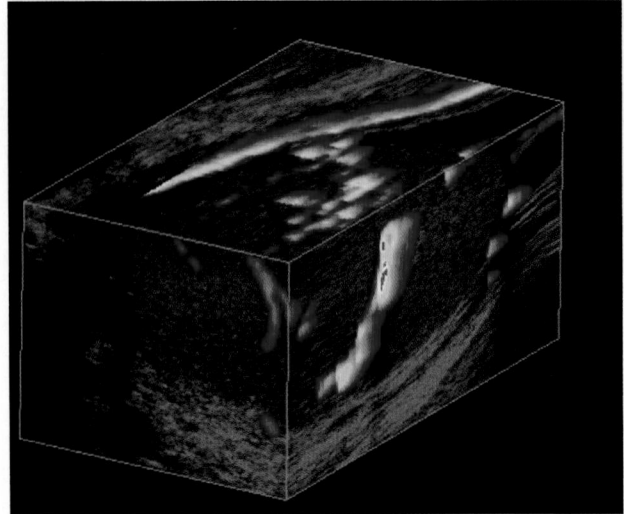

Figure 3-21. Three-dimensional image of the testis demonstrating intratesticular blood flow on power Doppler. The image can be virtually rotated and manipulated to produce unique anatomic perspectives. (Used with permission by BK Medical, Peabody, MA.)

3D rendering may be important in procedural planning and precise volumetric assessments (Ghani et al, 2008a, 2008b). 3D scanning may allow the recognition of some tissue patterns that would otherwise be unapparent on two-dimensional scanning (Mitterberger et al, 2007b; Onik and Barzell, 2008).

CONTRAST AGENTS IN ULTRASONOGRAPHY

Intravenous compounds that contain microbubbles have been used for enhancing the echogenicity of blood and tissue. Microbubbles are distributed in the vascular system and create strong echoes with harmonics when struck by sound waves. The bubbles themselves are rapidly degraded by their interaction with the sound waves. Contrast agents may be useful in ultrasonography of the prostate by enhancing the ability to recognize areas of increased vasculature. The use of intravenous ultrasound contrast agents is considered investigational but has shown promise in numerous urologic scanning situations (Mitterberger et al, 2007a; Wink et al, 2008).

DOCUMENTATION AND IMAGE STORAGE

Documentation is essential for insuring high-quality patient care. Proper documentation includes the production of a permanent record of the ultrasound examination and interpretation of the examination. This documentation is inclusive of the report and acquired images (American Institute of Ultrasound in Medicine, 2009). All documentation must be retrievable and comply with local, state, and federal requirements.

Report

The report should include specific information, including patient identification details, the date of the examination, and the measurement parameters and a description of findings of the examination. Ideally, the report should also include specifics on how the evaluation was performed, including the transducer used, machine used, and settings employed. Most of these details should be on the recorded image that is also stored with the report. The report must be signed by the physician who performed the ultrasound examination, and the indications for performing the examination should be prominently displayed at the top of the report.

Description of ultrasound images

The liver is used as a benchmark for echogenicity:

- Hypoechoic = darker
- Hyperechoic = brighter and white
- Isoechoic = similar to reference point of liver
- Anechoic = black, without echoes

Figure 3-22. **Nomenclature for describing the appearance of ultrasound images.**

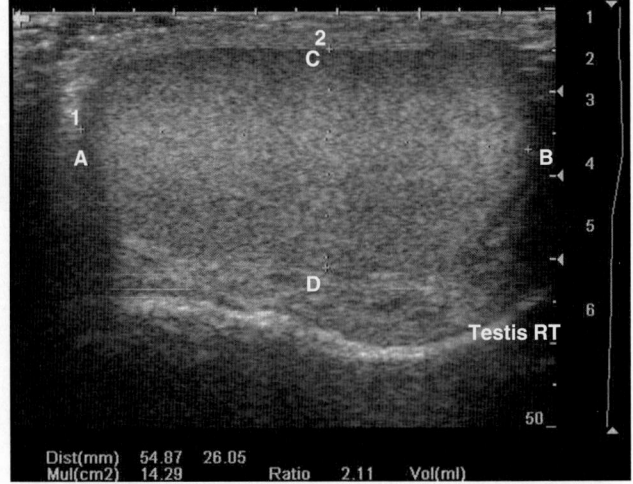

Figure 3-23. **In this sagittal image of the right testis, the superior pole of the testis (A) is to the left, the inferior pole of the testis (B) is to the right. The anterior aspect of the testis (C) is at the top of the image, and the posterior aspect (D) is at the bottom. Without the label, there would be no way to distinguish the right from the left testis.**

When urologists perform and interpret ultrasound studies, it is important that appropriate nomenclature be used to describe the objects imaged (Fig. 3-22). By convention, the liver is used as a benchmark for echogenicity. If a structure is hypoechoic, it means it is darker than the surrounding tissues. If it is hyperechoic, it means it is brighter than the surrounding tissues. If a structure is isoechoic, it is similar to the surrounding tissues. Structures that do not generate echoes are called *anechoic*. A simple cyst is an example of a structure with an anechoic interior. In general, a high water content causes tissue to appear hypoechoic, and a high fat content causes tissue to appear hyperechoic.

Images

Images should include patient identification details, the date and time of each image, and clear image orientation. Measurements should also be clearly identified with labeling of anatomy and any abnormalities. The image should be able to be interpreted by any appropriately trained sonographer and demonstrate a clear, unimpeded ultrasound image of the anatomy of interest. Images should always be attached to the report or be easily accessible from the report.

By convention, structures imaged by ultrasonography should be oriented so that the superior aspect of the structure is to the left as the image is viewed and the inferior aspect of the structure to the right. With paired structures, it is critical to document right or left. It is useful to use equipment-generated icons to illustrate patient position and the orientation of insonation (Fig. 3-23).

The appropriate number of images to be captured for documentation is the number necessary to document a systematic and complete examination and to document relevant pathology.

Report and Image Storage

The use of electronic medical records has made the documentation of ultrasound examinations easier. However, it has also created challenges in the archiving of images for easy reviewing. These images can occupy large portions of digital storage, and because they are part of the medical record and contain protected health information, they must comply with local, state, and federal regulations. Many validated systems are available for both small and large practices that meet current regulatory requirements.

PATIENT SAFETY

Diagnostic ultrasonography transmits energy into the patient that has the potential to produce biologic effects. The two main categories of biologic effects are **mechanical effects** and **thermal effects.**

The mechanical effects of ultrasonography are torque and streaming. The mechanical effects of an acoustic field may produce a phenomenon called *cavitation.* **Cavitation** occurs when small gas-filled bubbles form and then collapse. These collapsing bubbles liberate a large amount of energy, which may cause damage to tissue in certain circumstances. Mechanical effects are most likely to be observed around gas-containing structures such as lung and bowel.

The thermal effects of ultrasonography are primarily the result of tissue heating resulting from the absorption of energy. The amount of tissue heating is influenced by several factors, including beam focusing, transducer frequency, exposure time, scanning mode, and tissue density.

To assist the sonographer in monitoring the biologic effects of ultrasonography, the **output display standard (ODS)** has been adopted. Two values are typically displayed: the **mechanical index (MI)** and the **thermal index (TI).** These indices are calculated **estimates** of the potential for biologic effects of ultrasonography based on the mode of ultrasonography being used, frequency, power output, and time of insonation. The MI indicates the probability that cavitation will occur. For tissues not containing stabilized gas bodies (lung and intestine), the risk of cavitation is low as long as the MI is less than or equal to 0.7. For structures adjacent to lung or intestine, scanning time should be limited if the MI exceeds 0.4. The TI indicates the probability that tissue temperature within the sonographic field will be increased by 1° C. Although the precise consequences of tissue heating are not completely understood, tissue temperature elevations of up to 6° C are not likely to be dangerous unless exposure time exceeds 60 seconds. TI values should be less than 2 for most urologic ultrasound studies (Nelson et al, 2009). The MI and TI are typically displayed on the monitor during ultrasound examinations, and all practitioners should be familiar with the location. **These indices are not safety limits.**

Ultrasonography performed by urologists generally has a low risk for patient harm as long as standard protocols are followed (Rumack et al, 2005). Although tissue heating may occur, there are no confirmed biologic effects of tissue heating in nonfetal scanning except when heating is sustained for extended periods. Users should be aware that for soft tissues not known to contain gas bodies, there is no basis in present knowledge to suggest an adverse nonthermal biologic effect from current diagnostic instruments not exceeding the U.S. Food and Drug Administration output limits (Rumack et al, 2005). Nevertheless, all urologists should endeavor to follow the principles of **ALARA,** which stands for **"As Low As Reasonably Achievable."** The ALARA principle is intended to limit the total energy imparted to the patient during an examination. This limitation can be accomplished by (1) keeping power outputs low, (2) using appropriate scanning modes, (3) limiting examination times, (4) adjusting focus and frequency, and (5) using the sine function during documentation.

Ultrasound scanning offers an excellent, cost-effective modality for diagnosing and treating urologic conditions. **The most important factor in ultrasound safety is an informed operator.**

Urologists should endeavor to perform limited examinations using consistent technique for specific indications. Patient safety and equipment maintenance should be emphasized in all environments where ultrasound technology is used.

CLINICAL UROLOGIC ULTRASONOGRAPHY

The use of ultrasonography in urology has expanded dramatically because of its profound utility in the clinic and operating room. Long the mainstay of the diagnosis of prostatic disease, ultrasonography is increasingly being used by urologists in the clinical environment for initial diagnosis, interventional management, and longitudinal follow-up of urologic diseases.

Renal Ultrasonography

Urologists, by virtue of their intimate knowledge of surgical anatomy of the kidneys and retroperitoneum, are uniquely qualified to perform and interpret selected ultrasound examinations of the abdomen. These skills are relevant in both the office and the operating room environment. Urologists generally perform abdominal ultrasonography for a specific clinical indication and less often for general screening of the abdominal contents. In most clinical situations, a limited retroperitoneal examination is used in urologic practice.

Technique

The transducer normally used for renal ultrasonography is a curved array transducer of 3.5 to 5.0 MHz. Transducers of a higher frequency may be used for pediatric patients. For intraoperative and laparoscopic renal ultrasonography, a linear array transducer of 6 to 10 MHz is typically employed.

Scanning of the right kidney is performed with the patient supine. The kidney is located by beginning in the midclavicular line in the right upper quadrant. In the sagittal plane, the transducer is moved laterally until the midsagittal plane of the kidney is imaged. After the kidney has been imaged anteriorly and posteriorly in the sagittal plane, the probe is rotated 90 degrees counterclockwise. The midtransverse plane demonstrates the renal hilum containing the renal vein. The kidney is scanned from upper pole to lower pole.

The technique and documentation for left renal ultrasonography are identical to right renal ultrasonography. However, the left kidney is slightly more cephalad than the right kidney. Bowel gas is more problematic on the left because of the position of the splenic flexure of the colon. Visualization of the left kidney often requires the patient to be turned into a lateral position. Ultrasound imaging of the left kidney lacks the liver as an acoustic window, and it is sometimes more difficult to image the left kidney in a true sagittal plane.

Indications

1. Assessment of renal and perirenal masses
2. Assessment of the dilated upper urinary tract
3. Assessment of flank pain during pregnancy
4. Evaluation of hematuria in patients who are not candidates for intravenous pyelography, computed tomography, or magnetic resonance imaging because of renal insufficiency, allergy to contrast media, or physical impediment
5. Assessment of the effects of voiding on the upper urinary tract
6. Evaluation for and monitoring of urolithiasis
7. Intraoperative renal parenchyma and vascular imaging for ablation of renal masses
8. Percutaneous access to the renal collecting system
9. Guidance for transcutaneous renal biopsies, cyst aspiration, or ablation of renal masses
10. Postoperative evaluation of patients after renal and ureteral surgery
11. Postoperative evaluation of patients with renal transplants

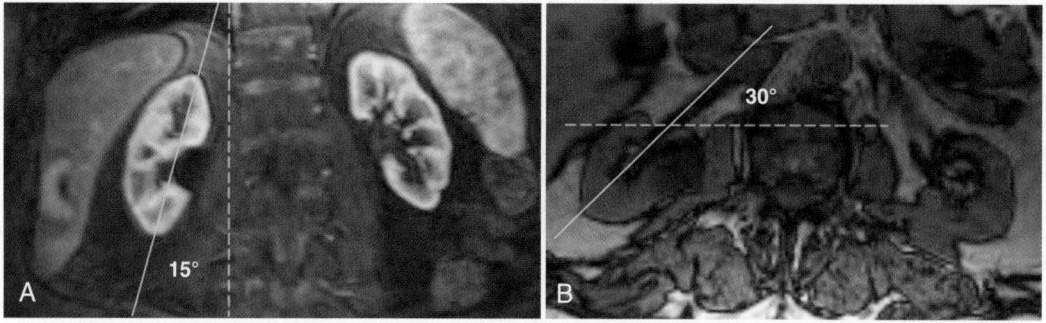

Figure 3-24. **A,** The lower pole of the kidney is displaced 15 degrees laterally compared with the upper pole. **B,** The kidney is rotated 30 degrees posterior to the true coronal plane. The lower pole of the kidney is slightly anterior compared with the upper pole.

Normal Findings

It is helpful during scanning of the kidney to understand its anatomic position within the retroperitoneum. This understanding assists identifying the midsagittal plane, which serves as a reference point for a complete examination (Fig. 3-24).

The adult right kidney in the sagittal view demonstrates a cortex that is usually hypoechoic with respect to the liver. The central band of echoes in the kidney is a hyperechoic area that contains the renal hilar adipose tissue, blood vessels, and collecting system. Acoustic shadowing from ribs overlying the inferior pole can be eliminated by moving the probe to a more lateral position or into the intercostal space. By having the patient take a deep breath, the kidney can be moved inferiorly to assist complete imaging (Fig. 3-25).

The echogenicity of the kidney varies with age. The renal cortex of an infant is relatively hyperechoic compared with that of an adult. In addition, there is a smaller and less apparent central band of echoes in the infant. In the adult, the echogenicity of the renal cortex is usually hypoechoic with respect to the liver (Emamian et al, 1993). In patients with chronic renal diseases, the renal cortex is often thinned and isoechoic or hyperechoic with respect to the liver (O'Neill, 2001).

Renal size changes over the lifetime of an individual. Nomograms for pediatric renal size should be consulted; these are based on age, height, and weight of the patient. The average adult kidney measures 10 to 12 cm in length and 4 to 5 cm in width. Measurements of renal volume may be appropriate in cases of severe renal impairment. Renal measurements should be obtained in the midsagittal plane and midtransverse plane. Measurements taken in other than the midsagittal plane and midtransverse plane may be spuriously low. The thickness of the parenchyma is the average distance between the renal capsule and the central band of echoes. The precise location for making this measurement is subjective. The midlateral renal parenchyma in the sagittal view is a common choice for obtaining this measurement (Fig. 3-26). Although there is no universal standard, the renal cortical thickness should be greater than 7 mm (Roger et al, 1994), and the renal parenchymal thickness should be greater than 15 mm in adults (Emamian et al, 1993).

Doppler ultrasound may be helpful in evaluating the renal artery and renal vein and assessing the vascular resistance in the kidney. Doppler modes may also be useful in evaluating neovascularity associated with renal tumors and in correctly characterizing hypoechoic structures in the renal pelvis, such as a parapelvic cyst, the renal vein, or the dilated collecting system.

Procedural Applications

Percutaneous renal biopsy has been performed as an office procedure by several groups for the past 2 decades and found to be a safe and effective procedure (Christensen et al, 1995; Fraser and Fairley, 1995; Hergesell, 1998). In a series of 131 ultrasound-guided

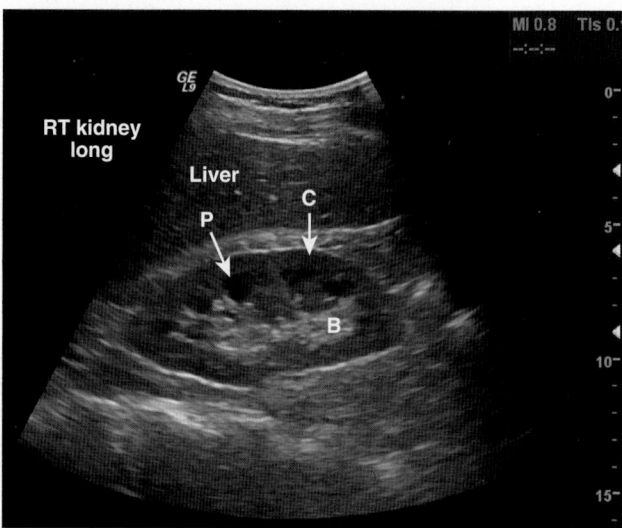

Figure 3-25. **Midsagittal plane of the kidney.** Note the relative hypoechogenicity of the renal pyramids (P) compared with the cortex (C). The central band of echoes (B) is hyperechoic compared with the cortex. The midsagittal plane has the greatest length measurement pole to pole. A perfectly sagittal plane results in a horizontal long axis of the kidney.

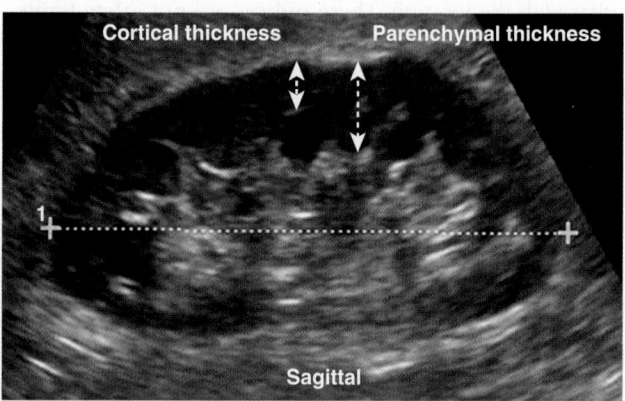

Figure 3-26. **The distinction between renal cortical thickness and renal parenchymal thickness is that the renal parenchyma is measured from the central band of echoes to the renal capsule. The renal cortex is measured from the outer margin of the medullary pyramid to the renal capsule.**

biopsies by Christensen and colleagues (1995), complications occurred in 21% of patients (18% minor complications and 3% major complications). In their series, increasing the number of biopsy passes did not increase the complication rate, whereas the presence of severe hypertension did. Fraser and Fairley (1995) compared 118 outpatient ultrasound-guided biopsies with 232 inpatient procedures and found no difference in complication rate. Hergesell (1998) reviewed a series of 1090 percutaneous biopsies performed with local anesthesia and ultrasound guidance. Only one case required interventional radiology for persistent blood loss, 2.2% (25 of 1090) of cases had minor hematoma that was conservatively treated, and self-limited macrohematuria was found in 0.8% (9 of 1090) of cases. In a subset of the population evaluated by Doppler ultrasonography, hemodynamically irrelevant arteriovenous fistula was found in 9% (48 of 533) of cases. Sufficient tissue was obtained in 98.8% of cases.

Al-Hweish and Abdul-Rehaman (2007) followed two groups. Patients in group I (n = 22) had a 24-hour hospital admission after the biopsy, and patients in group II (n = 22) were observed for 6 hours after the biopsy and then discharged. A small perinephric hematoma that resolved spontaneously was observed in a single patient in group II. Gross hematuria (13.6% in group I and 9.1% in group II) was the only significant complication observed and occurred in all cases within 6 hours.

The safety and efficacy of outpatient percutaneous renal biopsy have also been reported for pediatric patients (Davis et al, 1998; Kamitsuji et al, 1999; Hussain et al, 2003) and elderly patients (Kohli et al, 2006; Stratta et al, 2007; Moutzouris et al, 2009).

Limitations

Some patients are not favorable candidates for renal ultrasonography. Obesity, intestinal gas, and physical deformity may be impediments to complete renal evaluation. Renal ultrasonography has poor sensitivity for renal masses less than 2 cm (Warshauer et al, 1988). There is a lack of specificity for renal tumor type except for angiomyolipoma. Angiomyolipoma has characteristics that are distinctive on ultrasonography (highly echoic), but some small renal cell carcinomas have been shown to be indistinguishable from angiomyolipoma by ultrasound criteria (Yamashita et al, 1992; Forman et al, 1993).

Transabdominal Pelvic Ultrasonography

Transabdominal pelvic ultrasonography is a tremendously versatile tool for the urologist. It is a noninvasive method for evaluating the lower urinary tract and prostate in men and the bladder in women. A curved array transducer of 3.5 to 5 MHz is most commonly employed to perform transabdominal ultrasonography. In pediatric

patients, a higher frequency transducer may be used. In cases in which only a residual urine or bladder volume is to be determined, an automated bladder scanner is often employed.

Technique

Bladder ultrasonography is most commonly performed with the patient supine and the sonographer on the patient's right side. The scan should be performed in a warm room, and the patient should be draped to provide for comfort and privacy. If necessary, a roll may be placed beneath the patient's hips. The scanning technique depends on the circumstances and the reason for the examination, but in general the scan should be performed with a moderately filled bladder. The bladder should be scanned in a sagittal and transverse manner angling the probe into the pelvis so that the bladder can be visualized beneath the pubic bone. Although the prostate cannot be imaged with the same resolution achieved during transrectal scanning, the size and morphology of the prostate can be demonstrated. Although transabdominal scanning is the most common means of evaluating the bladder, the bladder may also be assessed using transvaginal and transrectal approaches. These approaches are useful in patients who are obese or who are not suitable candidates for transabdominal scanning.

Indications

1. Measurement of bladder volume or postvoid residual urine
2. Assessment of prostate size and morphology
3. Demonstration of secondary signs of bladder outlet obstruction
4. Evaluation of bladder wall configuration and thickness
5. Evaluation of hematuria of lower urinary tract origin
6. Detection of ureteroceles
7. Assessment for ureteral obstruction
8. Detection of perivesical fluid collections
9. Evaluation of clot retention
10. Confirmation of catheter position
11. Removal of retained catheter
12. Guidance of suprapubic tube placement
13. Establishment of bladder volume before and after flow rate determination

Normal Findings

Transabdominal pelvic ultrasonography should include evaluation of the lumen of the bladder and bladder wall configuration and thickness. The presence of specific lesions such as stones or tumors should be documented. The structures immediately surrounding the bladder may also be evaluated, including the distal ureters, the prostate in men, and the uterus and ovaries in women (Fig. 3-27).

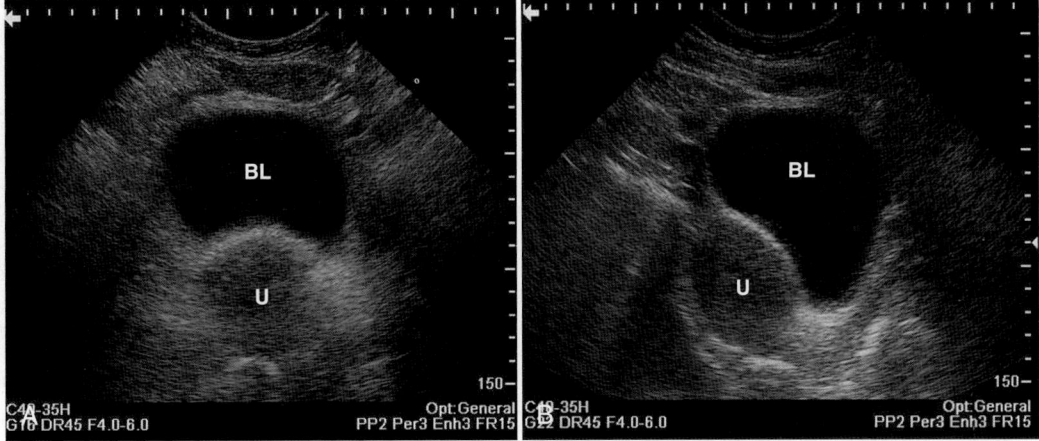

Figure 3-27. **A,** Transverse view of the bladder (BL) in a female patient demonstrates the uterus (U). **B,** Sagittal view of the bladder shows the uterus posterior to the bladder.

The emergence of urine from the ureteral orifices (ureteral jets) can be demonstrated. The clinical value of demonstrating ureteral jets has been questioned. To verify the absence of a ureteral jet, 10 minutes of continuous observation may be required (Fig. 3-28) (Delair and Kurzrock, 2006).

Bladder volume can be calculated manually by obtaining measurements in the midtransverse plane and midsagittal plane (Fig. 3-29). Numerous studies have shown that for bladder volumes of 100 to 500 mL, such calculated volumes are within 10% to 20% of the actual bladder volume (Simforoosh et al, 1997; Ghani et al, 2008b; Park et al, 2011). Measuring bladder wall thickness may assist the clinician in understanding the degree of bladder outlet obstruction (Fig. 3-30). Bladder wall thickness varies depending on the volume of urine in the bladder and on which part of the bladder wall is measured. It has been shown that measuring bladder wall thickness may predict bladder outlet obstruction with greater accuracy than free uroflowmetry, postvoid residual urine, and prostate volume (Oelke et al, 2007).

Transabdominal ultrasonography of the prostate requires angling the probe beneath the pubic bone. In the transverse plane, the transducer is fanned inferiorly until the largest transverse diameter of the prostate is identified. Measurements of the transverse width and height are obtained (Fig. 3-31A). The transducer is then rotated 90 degrees clockwise to produce a true sagittal image of the prostate. The transducer is fanned until the midline is identified; this is recognized by a V-shaped indention at the bladder neck (Fig. 3-31B). Depending on the degree of prostatic hypertrophy and the presence or absence of a middle lobe, this V may be more or less apparent and more or less anterior or posterior in its position. A sagittal measurement is made from the bladder neck to the apex of the prostate. The apex of the prostate may be identified by using the hypoechoic urethra as a guide.

The degree of protrusion of the prostate into the bladder may have some predictive value for bladder outlet obstruction. It has been shown that intravesical prostatic protrusion correlates well with formal urodynamic evaluation of bladder outlet obstruction (Chia et al, 2003; Keqin et al, 2007). The measurement is obtained by drawing a line corresponding to the bladder base on a sagittal scan and measuring the perpendicular distance from bladder base to greatest protrusion of the prostate into the bladder (Fig. 3-32).

Transabdominal ultrasonography of the prostate is useful in characterizing prostatic urethral length, the size and configuration of the middle lobe of the prostate, and some secondary information about the physiology of bladder outlet obstruction. This information is valuable in treatment planning for bladder outlet obstruction.

Procedural Applications

Transabdominal ultrasound-guided percutaneous bladder aspiration with or without catheter placement has been successfully used in neonates, children, and adults (Gochman et al, 1991; Wilson and Johnson, 2003). It has also been employed for treatment of bladder stones (Ikari et al, 1993; Sofer et al, 2004). Ultrasound-guided aspiration has also been used for peritoneal drainage after bladder perforation (Manikandan et al, 2003).

Limitations

Transabdominal pelvic ultrasonography yields limited information in patients with an empty bladder. The ability to identify distal

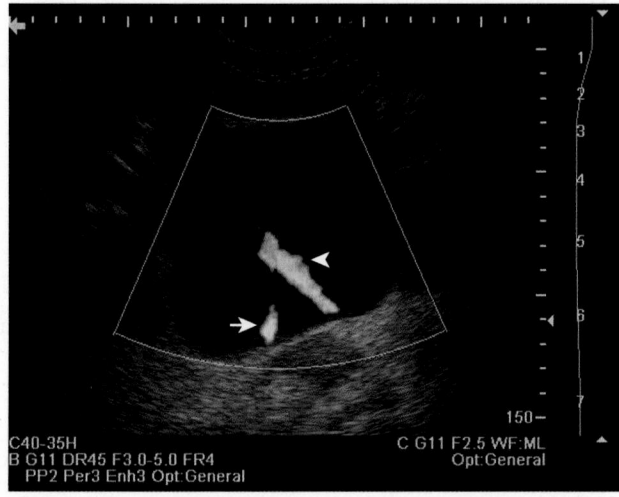

Figure 3-28. In this transverse view of the bladder, urine "jets" emerging from the left *(arrow)* and right *(arrowhead)* ureteral orifices are demonstrated by power Doppler.

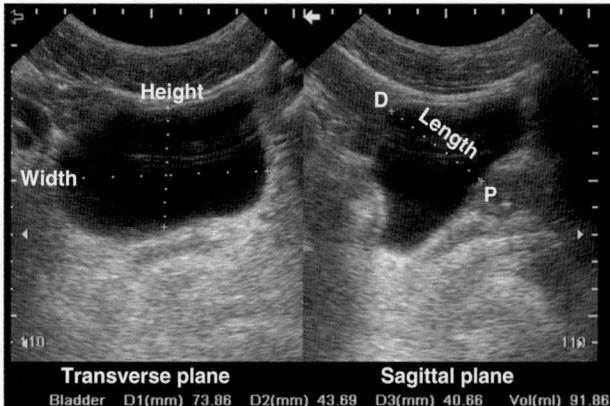

Figure 3-29. Measurement of bladder volume using the formula: bladder volume = width (transverse plane) × height (transverse plane) × length (midsagittal plane) × 0.625. In the sagittal plane, the dome (D) of the bladder is to the left, and the prostate (P) is to the right.

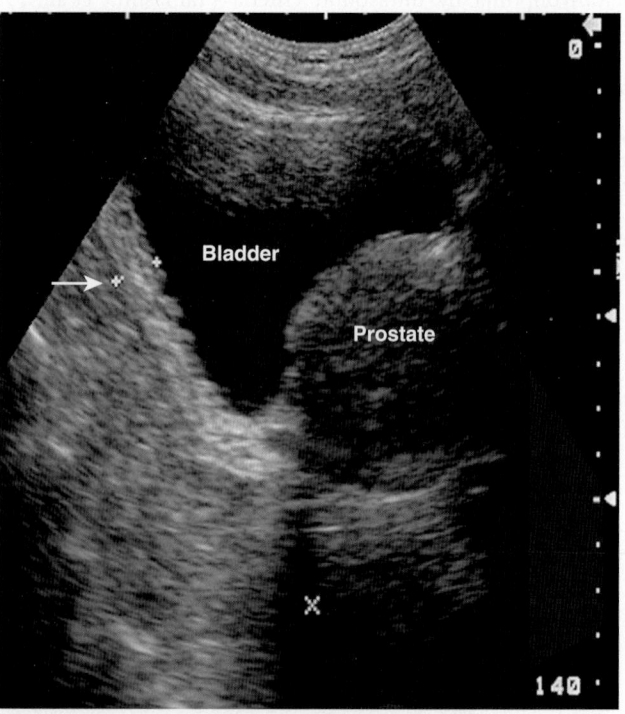

Figure 3-30. Bladder wall thickness may provide information about bladder outlet obstruction. In this sagittal view, bladder wall thickness is measured posteriorly *(arrow)* near the midline. Note the trabeculation of the relatively hyperechoic bladder wall.

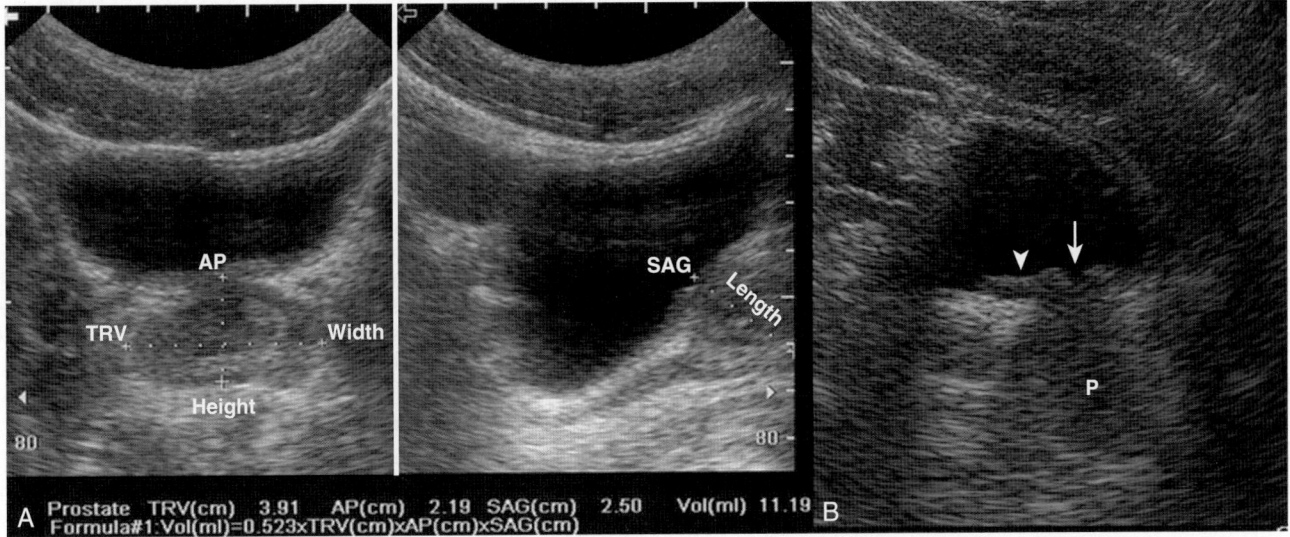

Figure 3-31. **A,** Transabdominal ultrasonography is extremely useful for measuring prostatic volume and evaluating prostatic morphology. The volume of the prostate can be calculated using the formula: prostate volume (mL) = width (cm) × height (cm) × length (cm) × 0.523. **B,** In this midsagittal view of the prostate (P), the bladder neck is identified as a V-shaped indentation *(arrow).* Note the characteristically hyperechoic trigone *(arrowhead).*

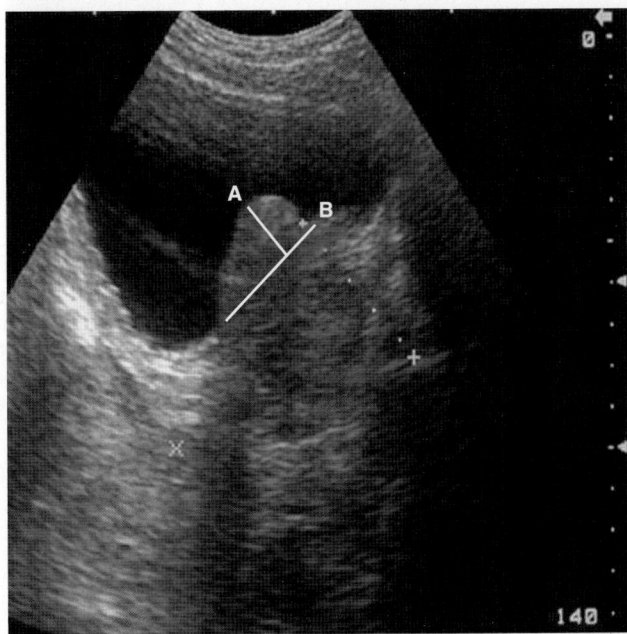

Figure 3-32. **In this sagittal view of the prostate, the middle lobe extends into the bladder (A). The bladder base is defined by the line B. The length of line A is the intravesical prostatic protrusion.**

ureteral obstruction, bladder stones, and bladder tumors requires a full bladder. Although prostatic morphology and volume can be assessed with an empty bladder, it is much easier when the bladder is full. Pelvic structures may be difficult to evaluate in patients with a protuberant abdomen or panniculus. **Although ultrasonography is used, automated measurement of bladder volume or residual urine is not an imaging study.** Lack of imaging confirmation can lead to inaccurate residual urine determinations in patients with obesity, clot retention, ascites, bladder diverticulum, or perivesical fluid collection (e.g., urinoma, lymphocele).

Ultrasonography of the Scrotum

No aspect of urologic care is better suited to the use of ultrasonography than evaluation of the scrotum. Urologists have a surgical understanding of the anatomy and extensive experience with the diagnosis and treatment of disorders that affect the scrotum. Because the scrotum and its contents are superficial, high-frequency transducers may be employed to yield excellent and detailed anatomic and physiologic information. Imaging information can be correlated with findings on direct physical examination.

Technique

Sound technique is critical to performing adequate ultrasonography of the scrotum. In general, the examination should be carried out in a quiet room that is adequately warm for patient comfort. The patient should be supine with the scrotum supported on a towel or on the anterior thighs. The patient should be draped in such a way as to hold the penis out of the way and to ensure patient privacy. Copious amounts of conducting gel should be used to provide a good interface between the transducer and the scrotal skin because air trapping by scrotal hair results in unwanted artifacts. Complete but gentle contact between skin and transducer is essential because excessive pressure results in movement of testis or compression of the testis. Compression may change echogenicity and obscure fine anatomic detail. In addition, compression may significantly alter volume measurements.

Scrotal ultrasonography is performed with a high-frequency linear array transducer, generally in the range of 7 to 18 MHz. Transducers may be 4 to 7.5 cm in width. Some sonographers prefer the maneuverability of a 4-cm transducer, whereas others prefer the longer 7.5-cm transducer for its ability to image the entire testis simultaneously in the sagittal plane. Imaging should be done in a systematic fashion and should include sagittal and transverse views of the testis. The sagittal view should proceed from the midline medially and then laterally and from the midtransverse section of the testis to the upper pole and the lower pole of the testis. In addition to the testis, the epididymis and entire scrotal contents should be imaged.

Indications

1. Assessment of scrotal and testicular mass
2. Assessment of scrotal and testicular pain
3. Evaluation of scrotal trauma
4. Evaluation of infertility
5. Follow-up of scrotal surgery
6. Evaluation of empty or abnormal scrotum

Normal Findings

It is important to document the size and, if appropriate, the volume of the testes. The echo architecture of the testis should be described (Fig. 3-33). It is important to compare the testes for echogenicity because some infiltrative processes may result in diffuse changes in a testis that would be noticed only when that testis is compared with its contralateral mate (Fig. 3-34). For example, lymphomatous or leukemic involvement of the testis may result in a diffusely hypoechoic and homogeneous appearance, which may be unilateral (Mazzu et al, 1995). If paratesticular fluid is present, the epididymis and the testicular and epididymal appendages are more easily identified (Fig. 3-35).

Normal testicular blood flow may be demonstrated with color or power Doppler (Fig. 3-36) (Barth and Shortliffe, 1997). Intratesticular blood flow is low velocity with the average PSV of less than 10 cm/sec (Middleton et al, 1989). Intratesticular blood flow is primarily supplied by the testicular artery, which ultimately divides to supply the individual testicular septa. The fibrous septa coalesce to form the mediastinum testis, which is a hyperechoic linear structure seen in the sagittal plane (Fig. 3-37).

Spectral Doppler is useful in evaluating the intratesticular blood flow with elevated resistive index greater than 0.6 suggestive of impaired spermatogenesis (Fig. 3-38) (Biagiotti et al, 2002; Pinggera et al, 2008; Hillelsohn et al, 2013).

Procedural Applications

The testis lends itself to easy access for ultrasound localization of internal structures and for percutaneous access. In particular, small nonpalpable lesions can be localized by ultrasonography, guiding

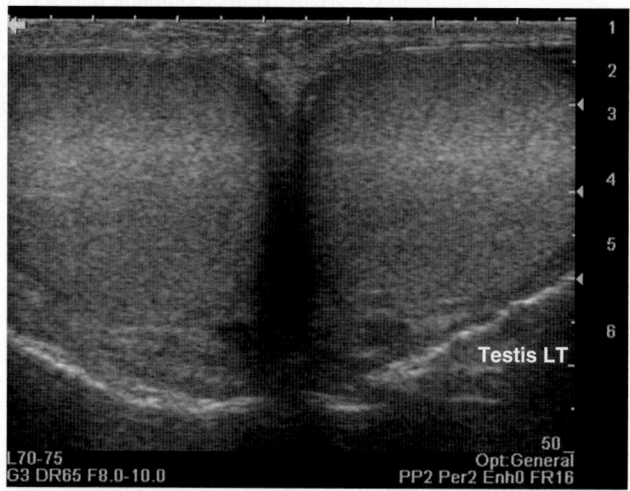

Figure 3-33. In this longitudinal view, the head of the epididymis (E) is seen to the left, and the lower pole of the testis is to the right. Normal testicular sonographic anatomy is characterized by a homogeneous, finely granular appearance of the testis.

Figure 3-34. Simultaneous bilateral views are important to rule out a diffuse infiltrative process such as lymphoma. A diffuse and homogeneous change in echogenicity in one testis could otherwise be unappreciated. In this example, the testes are symmetric and normal. This view is also required to document the presence of two testes.

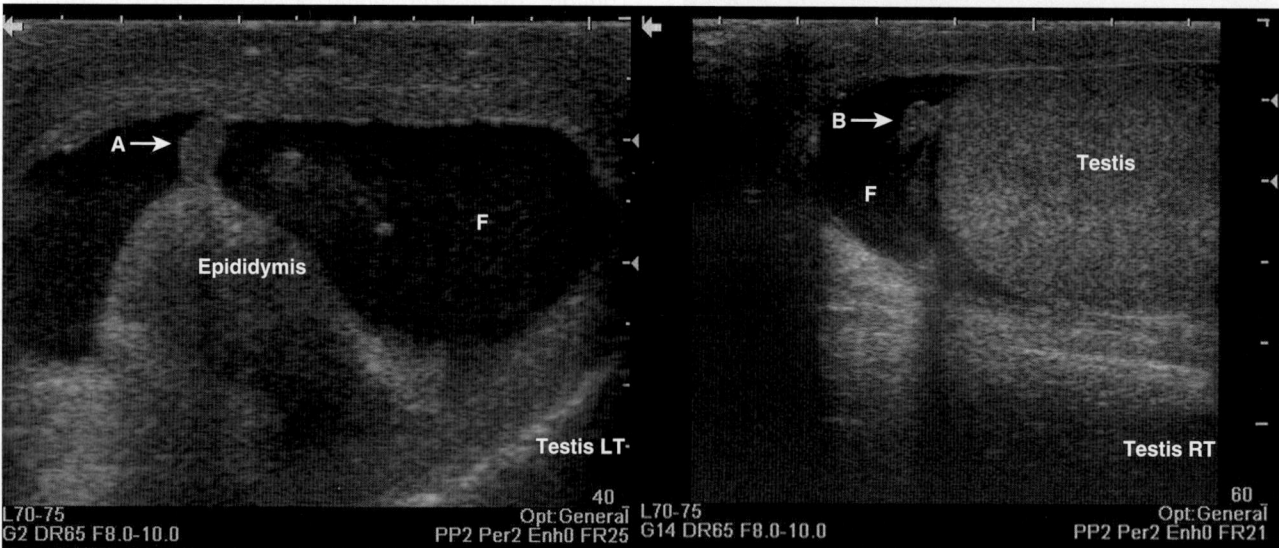

Figure 3-35. The presence of paratesticular fluid (F) permits the identification of the appendix epididymis (A) and the appendix testis (B).

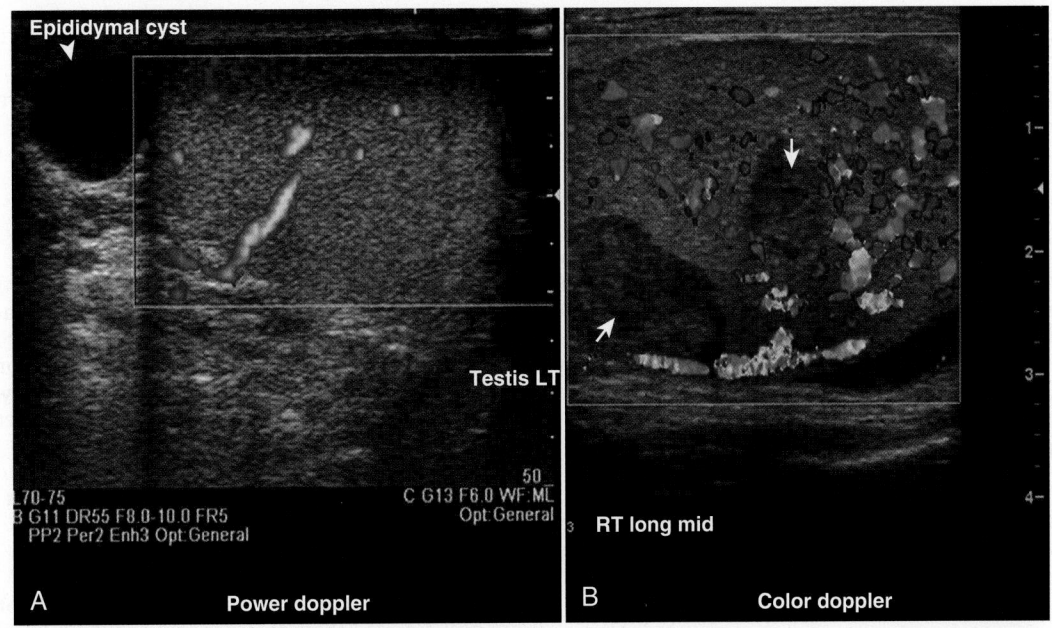

Figure 3-36. A, Normal intratesticular blood flow by power Doppler; note the epididymal cyst *(arrowhead)*. **B,** Increased blood flow in an irregular pattern demonstrated by color Doppler was associated with necrotizing vasculitis; note the relatively hypoechoic areas of decreased vascularity *(arrows)*.

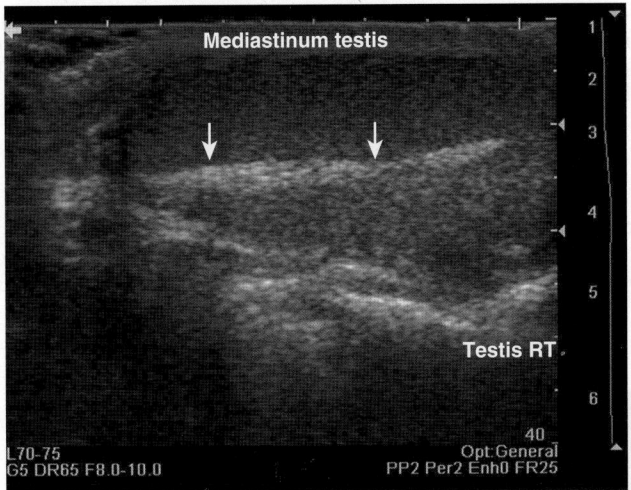

Figure 3-37. Sagittal image of this testis demonstrates a common anatomic finding, the hyperechoic mediastinum testis *(arrows)*. The mediastinum testis is a normal structure resulting from the coalescence of the fibrous septa of the testis.

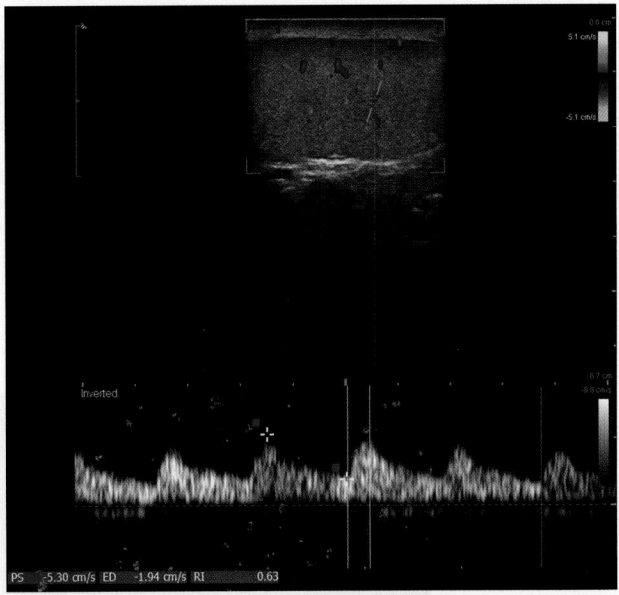

Figure 3-38. Spectral Doppler analysis of an intratesticular artery demonstrating a peak systolic velocity of 5.3 cm/sec, an end-diastolic velocity of 1.94 cm/sec, and a calculated resistive index of 0.63 in a patient with dyspermia.

placement of a needle for percutaneous biopsy or injection of a dye for localization during open biopsy (Buckspan et al, 1989).

Current therapeutic applications using ultrasound guidance include percutaneous testicular sperm aspiration (Friedler et al, 1997; Belker et al, 1998; Khadra et al, 2003) and percutaneous epididymal sperm aspiration (Craft et al, 1995; Belker et al, 1998; Levine and Lisek, 1998; Meniru et al, 1998; Rosenlund et al, 1998; Lin et al, 2000; Pasqualotto et al, 2003). Future ultrasound-guided applications might include spermatogonia stem cell transfer to testes devoid of germ cells after gonadotoxic therapies.

Sonoelastography

Two more recent studies used real-time elastography to differentiate benign from malignant testicular lesions because it is postulated that malignant lesions have an increased stiffness secondary to a higher concentration of vessels and cells compared with surrounding tissues. Goddi and colleagues (2012) assessed 88 testes with 144 lesions and found a 93% positive predictive value, 96% negative predictive value, and 96% accuracy (see Fig. 3-19). Aigner and associates (2012) assessed 50 lesions and found a 92% positive predictive value, 100% negative predictive value, and 94% accuracy in differentiating malignant from benign lesions. Additionally, Li and coworkers (2012) found that men with non-obstructive azoospermia had significantly different testicular elasticity compared with patients with obstructive azoospermia and healthy controls with a normal semen analysis. Real-time tissue elastography (see Fig. 3-20) is an exciting new innovation in assessing abnormalities on scrotal examination; however, more data are necessary before surgical intervention can be safely avoided based on the findings.

Limitations

Caution should be used when interpreting Doppler flow studies in the evaluation of suspected testicular torsion. The hallmark of testicular torsion is the absence of **intratesticular** blood flow (Fig. 3-39). Paratesticular flow in epididymal collaterals may appear within hours of torsion. Comparison with the contralateral testis should be performed to ensure that the technical attributes of the study are adequate to demonstrate intratesticular blood flow.

Ultrasonography of the Penis and Male Urethra

Ultrasonography of the penis and male urethra provides exquisite anatomic detail and may be used in many cases in lieu of studies requiring ionizing radiation.

Technique

Penile and urethral ultrasonography is best performed with a 12- to 18-MHz linear array transducer for optimal resolution. The technique for penile and urethral ultrasonography includes imaging the phallus in the longitudinal and transverse planes. Both ventral and dorsal surfaces of the phallus can be interrogated. Similar to scrotal ultrasonography, the examination is best carried out in a quiet room that is adequately warm for patient comfort. Draping is done to ensure patient privacy. The examination is performed in a systematic fashion beginning at the base of the penis and proceeding distally to the glans. It is possible to obtain an image of the proximal urethra and corporeal bodies by scanning through the scrotum or the perineum.

It may be helpful when evaluating the penile urethra, especially for stricture disease, to inject a sterile gel into the urethra in a retrograde fashion. The gel distends the urethra and allows better identification of urethral anatomy and the anatomy of the corpus spongiosum.

Indications

1. Evaluation of penile vascular dysfunction
2. Documentation of fibrosis of the corpora cavernosa
3. Localization of foreign body
4. Evaluation of urethral stricture
5. Evaluation of urethral diverticulum
6. Assessment of penile trauma or pain

Normal Findings

Scanning of the external portion of the phallus can be performed either from the dorsal or from the ventral surface (Fig. 3-40). Transverse scanning of the phallus reveals the two corpora cavernosa dorsally and the urethra ventrally. The sagittal view of the phallus demonstrates the corpora cavernosa with a hyperechoic, double linear structure representing the cavernosal artery (Fig. 3-41). The corpus spongiosum is isoechoic to slightly hypoechoic and contains the coapted urethra. The urethra is collapsed except during voiding.

Perineal Ultrasonography

The more proximal aspects of the urethra and corpora cavernosa are best assessed through a perineal approach by placement of the transducer on the perineum. The bulbar urethra with the bulbar branch of the pudendal artery and the proximal cavernosal bodies and the cavernosal branch of the pudendal artery can be visualized (Fig. 3-42).

Transperineal and translabial ultrasonography has also been used for evaluation of the pelvic floor for both diagnostic purposes and postprocedural follow-up. The anterior, central, and posterior compartments are well visualized. In contrast to a transvaginal approach, this approach is noninvasive and does not distort the pelvic anatomy (Baxter and Firoozi, 2013).

Procedural Applications

The most common application of penile ultrasonography is in the evaluation of erectile dysfunction and penile curvature. Pharmacostimulation provides quantification of cavernosal artery blood flow velocity (Fig. 3-43). Primary criteria for arteriogenic erectile

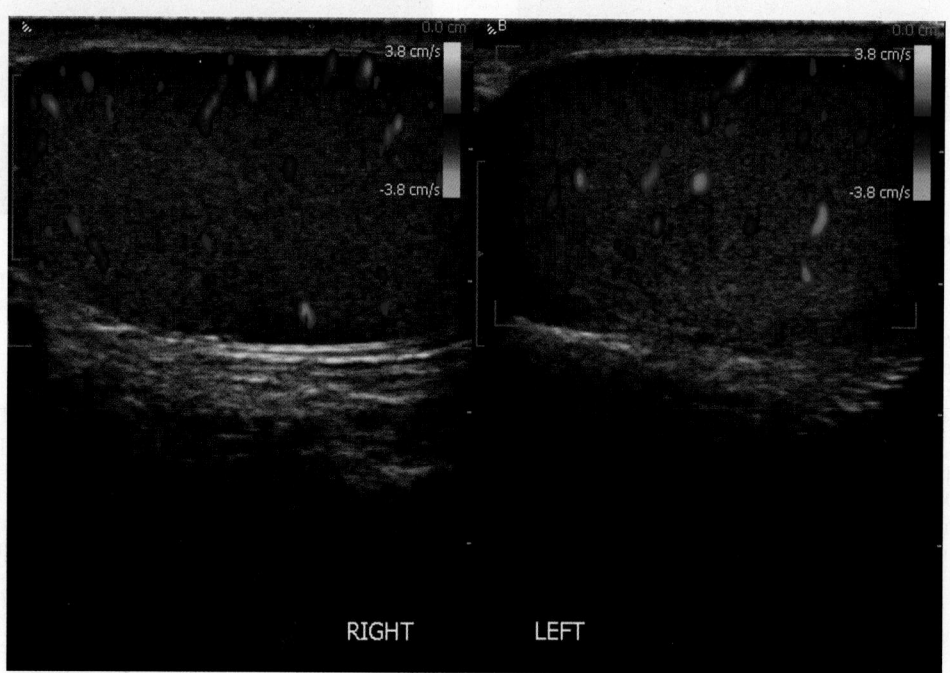

Figure 3-39. Demonstration of normal bilateral intratesticular blood flow by color Doppler.

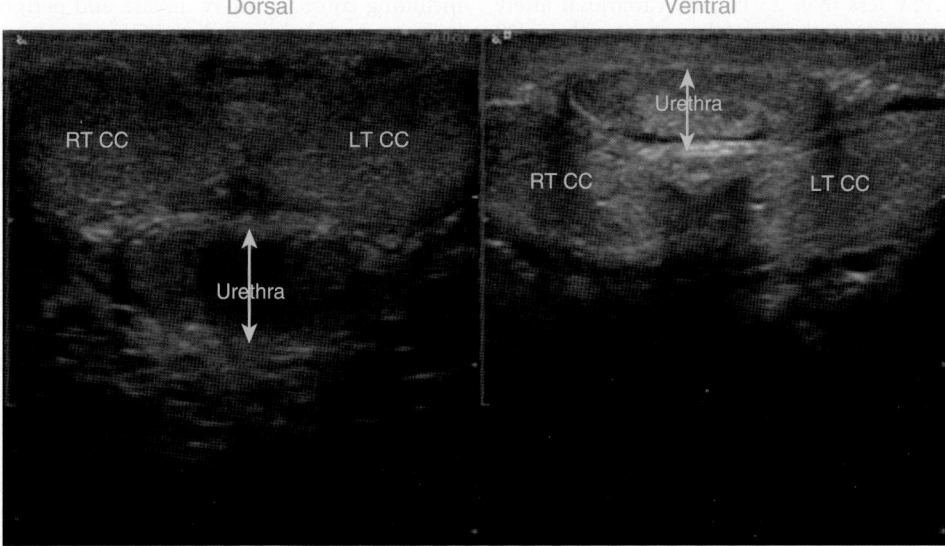

Figure 3-40. Transverse view of the phallus with the transducer placed either on the dorsal or the ventral surface. Note the compression of the urethra and corporal spongiosum compression in the ventral projection with minimal pressure applied to the phallus. CC, corpora cavernosa.

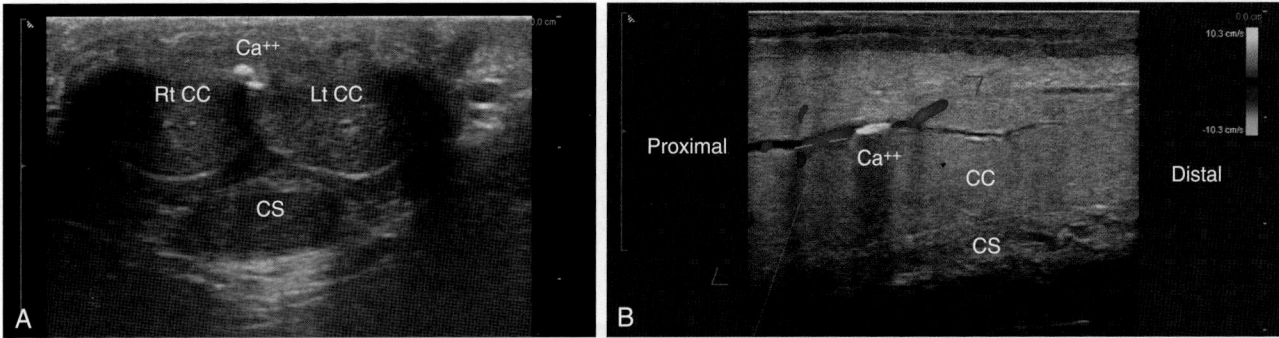

Figure 3-41. A, In the transverse plane scanning from the dorsal surface of the midshaft of the penis, the corpora cavernosa (CC) are paired structures seen dorsally, whereas the corpus spongiosum (CS) is seen ventrally in the midline. A calcification (Ca++) is seen between the two CC with posterior shadowing. B, In the parasagittal plane, the corporus cavernosum (CC) is dorsal with the relatively hypoechoic CS seen ventrally. Within the CC, the cavernosal artery is shown with a calcification (Ca++) in the wall of the artery and posterior shadowing.

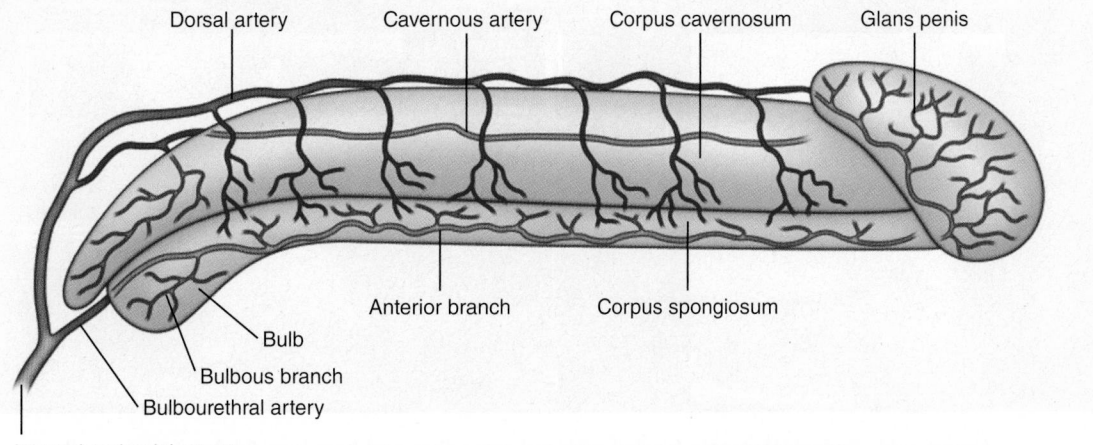

Figure 3-42. The internal pudendal artery gives rise to the bulbourethral artery, dorsal artery, and cavernosal artery. The most proximal aspect of the cavernosal artery is best imaged through the perineum. (From Gilbert BR. Ultrasound of the male genitalia. New York: Springer. In press.)

dysfunction include a PSV less than 25 cm/sec, cavernosal artery dilation less than 75%, and acceleration time greater than 110 msec. In cases of equivocal PSV measurements, particularly when PSV is between 25 cm/sec and 35 cm/sec, additional criteria are asymmetry of greater than 10 cm/sec in PSV comparing the two cavernosal arteries, focal stenosis of the cavernosal artery, and cavernosal-spongiosal flow reversal (Benson et al, 1993).

In addition, arteriogenic erectile dysfunction has been found to correlate directly with other systemic cardiovascular diseases,

including coronary artery disease and peripheral vascular disease, in many population studies. PSV is the most accurate measure of arterial disease as the cause of erectile dysfunction. The average PSV after intracavernosal injection of vasoactive agents in healthy volunteers without erectile dysfunction ranges from 35 to 47 cm/sec, with a PSV of 35 cm/sec or greater signifying arterial sufficiency after pharmacostimulation (Lue et al, 1985; Mueller and Lue, 1988; Benson and Vickers, 1989; Shabsigh et al, 1990; Broderick and Lue, 1991; Pescatori et al, 1994; Schaeffer et al, 2006). The first indication of vascular disease often can be the penile cavernosal artery being less than 1 mm. The finding of arteriogenic dysfunction can often provide a window of opportunity (Miner, 2011) to identify and potentially to alter the progressive nature of systemic vascular disease (Montorsi et al, 2006; Gazzaruso et al, 2008; Seftel, 2011).

Assessment of penile curvature most often involves palpation and ultrasound interrogation of the phallus after pharmacostimulation. However, a palpable plaque is not easily identified (Prando, 2009; Kalokairinou et al, 2012). In many cases, standard B-mode and color Doppler ultrasound modalities often do not localize pathology. Sonoelastography (tissue elasticity imaging) evaluates the stiffness of biologic tissues and localizes these nonpalpable lesions not visualized on ultrasonography for potential treatment (Fig. 3-44) (Richards et al, 2014).

Limitations

The complete evaluation of the penile urethra, corpora cavernosa, and corpus spongiosum requires a dorsal or ventral interrogation of the exposed phallus and a perineal approach to the nonexposed portions of the phallus; this is particularly important in evaluation of the bulbourethra and proximal corpora. In addition, the evaluation of erectile dysfunction requires qualitative and quantitative measurements of blood flow in the penile arteries. Such evaluation requires blood flow measurements before and after intracavernosal injection of vasoactive substances.

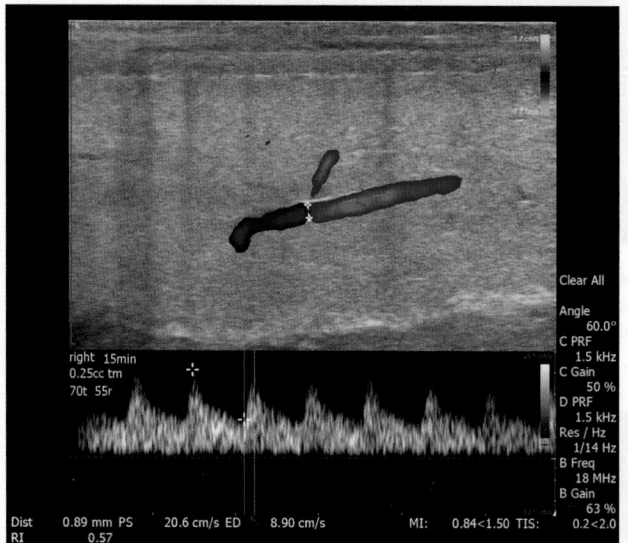

Figure 3-43. Longitudinal view of the right corpora cavernosa demonstrating peak systolic and end-diastolic flow velocity in the right cavernosal artery, which measures 0.89 mm in diameter.

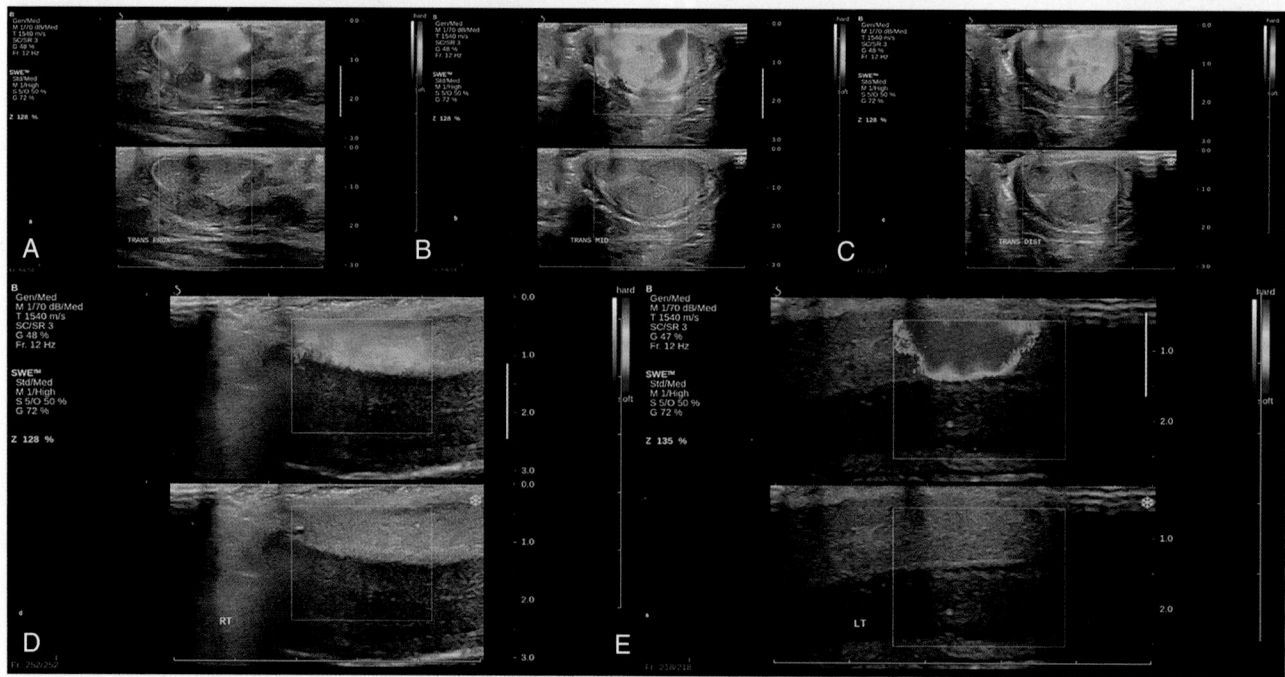

Figure 3-44. Sonoelastograms (scaled with red more firm and blue less firm) superimposed over transverse B-mode ultrasound images of the **(A)** proximal, **(B)** mid and **(C)** distal phallus. Sonoelastograms superimposed over parasagittal views of the **(D)** right and **(E)** left cavernosal bodies. (From Richards G, Goldenberg E, Pek H, Gilbert BR. Penile sonoelastography for the localization of a non-palpable, non-sonographically visualized lesion in a patient with penile curvature from Peyronie's disease. J Sex Med 2014;11:516–20.)

Transrectal Ultrasonography of the Prostate

TRUS of the prostate is the sonographic imaging procedure most commonly performed by urologists (Trabulsi et al, 2013). It is minimally invasive and provides exquisite anatomic detail of the prostate and periprostatic tissues. An overview is presented here of transrectal prostate imaging. A comprehensive discussion is provided in Chapter 109. TRUS performed by the urologist enhances patient care by providing a minimally invasive procedure that gives real-time information for a rapid and accurate diagnosis.

Technique

A systematic scan insures that a comprehensive examination is performed and appropriately documented. A high-frequency 7.5- to 10-MHz transducer is usually used. This can be a biplanar or single-plane transducer (i.e., "end fire" or "side fire").

It is essential to perform a digital rectal examination **before** inserting the ultrasound probe. Pain or tenderness, rectal stricture, mass, lesion, or bleeding that is encountered when performing the rectal examination or when inserting the probe might preclude TRUS.

After probe insertion, a "survey" scan is performed of the prostate from base to apex including the seminal vesicles and rectal wall. The seminal vesicles are then examined in the transverse plane for comparative evaluation of echogenicity and measurements of seminal vesicle height and ampulla (vas deferens) diameter. Next, the midsagittal transverse and longitudinal image of the prostate is examined, and anteroposterior, height, and length measurements are taken. Prostate volume, predicted prostate-specific antigen (PSA), and PSA density can be calculated usually by formulas already programmed in the ultrasound machine. As in many urologic applications of sonography, color Doppler can add valuable information.

The rectal wall thickness must be evaluated and documented as well as any other notable findings (Trabulsi et al, 2013). Rectal cancer, polyps, and inflammatory processes require further evaluation. The appearance of rectal abnormalities should be documented, and a referral may need to be made.

Indications

1. Measurement of prostate volume for determination of PSA density
2. Abnormal digital rectal examination
3. Prostatic assessment with sonographic controlled biopsy
4. Cysts
5. Evaluation for and aspiration of prostate abscess
6. Assessment for suspected congenital abnormality
7. Lower urinary tract symptoms
8. Pelvic pain
9. Prostatitis or prostadynia
10. Hematospermia
11. Infertility (e.g., azoospermia)
    a. Low volume or poorly motile specimen
    b. Cysts
    c. Hypoplastic or dilated seminal vesicle
    d. Impaired motility
    e. Antisperm antibodies

Normal Findings

Echogenicity is best evaluated by comparing the left and right sides of the prostate (Fig. 3-45). In a young man, TRUS is often indicated in the evaluation of subfertility. The young male prostate is homogeneous with zones often difficult to visualize. The "sonographic capsule" can be identified because of the impedance difference between the prostate and surrounding fat. The prominence of the urethra ("u" in Fig. 3-45) is related to the surrounding low reflectivity of urethral muscles. In the young male prostate,

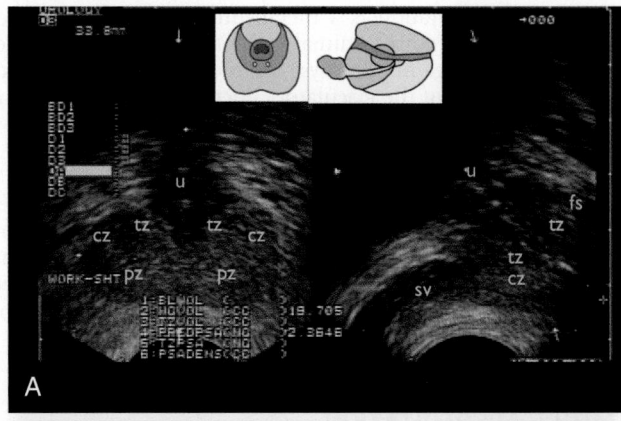

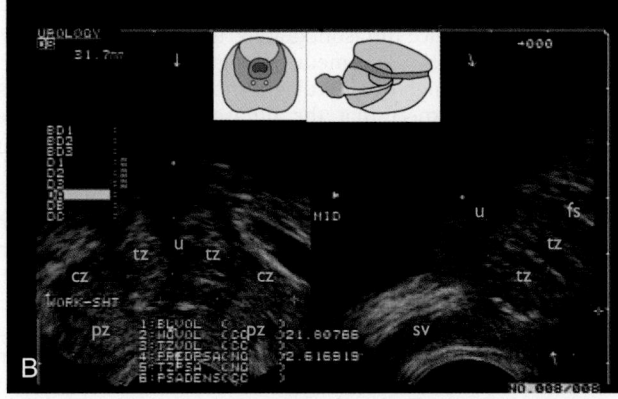

Figure 3-45. A, Young male prostate. The peripheral zone (pz) is often hyperreflective to the central (cz) and transition (tz) zones. The cz and tz are difficult to differentiate from each other, and the fibromuscular stroma (fs) is positioned anterior to the urethra. B, Older male prostate. The glandular and stromal elements enlarge increasing the size of the tz and occasionally pz. The tz is seen independent of other zones, and the cz is difficult to visualize.

the peripheral zone ("pz" in Fig. 3-45) is often hyperreflective to the central and transition zones ("cz" and "tz" in Fig. 3-45). The central and transition zones are difficult to differentiate from each other, and the fibromuscular stroma ("fs" in Fig. 3-45) is positioned anterior to the urethra. In an older man, the glandular and stromal elements enlarge increasing the size of the transition zone and occasionally the peripheral zone. The transition zone is seen independent of other zones, and the central zone is difficult to visualize.

The base of the prostate is located at the superior aspect of the prostate contiguous with the base of the bladder. The apex of the prostate is located at the inferior aspect of the prostate continuous with the striated muscles of the urethral sphincter.

Procedural Applications

Biopsy of the prostate guided by TRUS is most often initially performed for a specific clinical indication, such as an elevation or change in the PSA or an abnormal digital rectal examination (Porter, 2013). High-grade prostatic intraepithelial neoplasia and atypical small acinar proliferation on an initial biopsy specimen are considered by some clinicians to be indications for immediate or planned repeat biopsy. TRUS biopsy may be performed for an increasing PSA after initial therapy. In the case of a patient with an increasing PSA after radical retropubic prostatectomy, ultrasonography and biopsy of the prostatic fossa and vesicourethral anastomosis may be performed to aid in diagnosis of local recurrence. TRUS biopsy is performed after radiation therapy or cryotherapy to aid in diagnosis of local treatment failure.

Prostatic cyst aspiration is a therapeutic procedure easily performed in the office with minimal patient discomfort. It is often indicated when a large midline cyst obstructs the ejaculatory ducts resulting in dilation of the ejaculatory ducts or seminal vesicles or both. Refilling of the cyst is common.

Limitations

Bowel preparation is sometimes necessary for imaging. In addition, the patient's body habitus might make it difficult to image the base of the prostate, seminal vesicles, and bladder adequately. Current technology limits the diagnostic capabilities of TRUS to anatomic anomalies.

PRACTICE ACCREDITATION

When performing office ultrasonography, urologists must be committed to ensure that equipment, sonographers, and protocols are able to provide high-quality diagnostic information. Likewise, patients rightfully expect that the ultrasound examination performed uses equipment that is safe and can effectively image the organ of interest. In addition, third-party payers have instituted requirements for practices, including urology practices, to follow to be compensated for their work in providing ultrasound imaging services. One way the urologist sonographer ensures that his or her ultrasound examination is compliant with current standards and protocols is through practice accreditation. There are presently two acknowledged accrediting agencies: the American College of Radiology (ACR) and the American Institute for Ultrasound in Medicine (AIUM). The AUA and the AIUM have partnered to develop a pathway whereby urology practices can obtain accreditation that is recognized by regulatory authorities and third-party payers.

There are few laws regulating the performance and interpretation of ultrasound examinations. Any licensed physician may purchase an ultrasound machine and begin performing and interpreting sonograms. To ensure quality of an ultrasound examination, the ACR and the AIUM began to develop programs in 1995 to accredit ultrasound practices, and the two organizations accredited the first ultrasound practices in 1996. As of this writing, there are 4401 practices (each site applies as a single practice) with ACR ultrasound accreditation and 1210 (a total of 2039 sites) with AIUM ultrasound accreditation.

The ACR offers ultrasound practice accreditation in breast, general, gynecologic, obstetric, and vascular ultrasonography. The AIUM offers ultrasound practice accreditation in abdominal/general, breast, dedicated musculoskeletal, dedicated thyroid/parathyroid, gynecologic, fetal echocardiography, obstetric, and more recently urologic ultrasonography.

How does ultrasound practice accreditation differ from AUA board certification? Certification is granted to an individual who has demonstrated a level of knowledge and who continues to meet the requirements necessary to maintain the certification. The individual remains certified regardless of where he or she works. Accreditation is granted to a practice (which may be the practice of a solo practitioner) that demonstrates that all of the individuals in the practice, all the relevant policies and procedures, and equipment and maintenance meet certain requirements. Practices must continue to demonstrate compliance at regular intervals, regardless of whether there are changes in personnel, policies, or equipment. An individual who works in an accredited practice cannot go to another practice and claim that the services provided at the second facility are accredited.

The process of practice accreditation is not without challenges to both the urologists and the urology practice. Urologists have traditionally viewed imaging as a tool, similar to a stethoscope, that assists them in providing care for their patients. The process of accreditation changes this traditional view by requiring both the urologist and the urology practice to expend resources to meet the requirements of accreditation. However, the accreditation process

helps organize the approach to the ultrasound examination and markedly improves quality. This translates into improved diagnostic ultrasound examinations and improved patient care (Abuhamad and Benacerraf, 2004).

KEY POINTS

- An ultrasound wave is a mechanical wave that creates alternating areas of compression and rarefaction in tissue.
- Axial resolution improves with increasing frequency of the ultrasound wave.
- Depth of ultrasound penetration decreases with increasing frequency.
- Optimal ultrasound imaging requires tradeoffs between resolution and depth of penetration.
- Artifacts may be helpful in the diagnosis of certain conditions.
- The appropriate number of images to be captured for documentation is the number necessary to document a systematic and complete examination and to document relevant pathology.
- The mechanical index and the thermal index are not safety limits.
- The ALARA principle is intended to limit the total energy imparted to the patient during an examination.
- The most important factor in ultrasound safety is the informed operator.
- Angiomyolipoma has a characteristic hyperechoic appearance, but some renal cell carcinomas are also hyperechoic.
- Although ultrasonography is used in automated measurement of bladder volume or residual urine, this is not an imaging study.
- Sonoelastography extends the ability of ultrasonography to detect "hardness" of a lesion.
- The hallmark of testicular torsion is the absence of intratesticular blood flow. However, ultrasonography cannot diagnose torsion—only the surgeon or the pathologist can.

Please visit the accompanying website at www.expertconsult.com to view videos associated with this chapter.

REFERENCES

The complete reference list is available online at www.expertconsult.com.

SUGGESTED READINGS

Fulgham PF. Basic ultrasound DVD. In: Linthicum MD, editor. Urologic Ultrasound DVD Series. American Urological Association; 2007.

Fulgham PF. Abdominal ultrasound DVD. In: Linthicum MD, editor. Urologic Ultrasound DVD Series. American Urological Association; 2008.

Fulgham PF, Gilbert BR. Practical urological ultrasound. New York: Springer; 2013.

Gilbert BR. Ultrasound of the male genitalia DVD. In: Linthicum MD, editor. Urologic Ultrasound DVD Series. American Urological Association; 2008.

Holland CK, Fowlkes JB. Biologic effects and safety. In: Rumack CM, Wilson SR, Charboneau JW, et al, editors. Diagnostic ultrasound. 3rd ed. St. Louis: Mosby; 2005. p. 35–53.

Merritt CRB. Physics of ultrasound. In: Rumack CM, Wilson SR, Charboneau JW, et al, editors. Diagnostic ultrasound. 3rd ed. St. Louis: Mosby; 2005. p. 3–34.

O'Neill WC. Atlas of renal ultrasonography. Philadelphia: Saunders; 2001.

Rifkin MD, Cochlin MD, Goldberg BB. Imaging of the scrotum and contents. London: Martin Dunitz Ltd; 2002.

Scoutt LM, Burns P, Brown JL, et al. Ultrasound evaluation of the urinary tract. In: Pollack HM, McClennan BL, editors. Clinical urography. 2nd ed. Philadelphia: Saunders; 2000. p. 388–472.

Thurston W, Wilson SR. The urinary tract. In: Rumack CM, Wilson SR, Charboneau JW, et al, editors. Diagnostic ultrasound. 3rd ed. St. Louis: Mosby; 2005. p. 321–93.

Outcomes Research

Mark S. Litwin, MD, MPH, and Jonathan Bergman, MD, MPH

Health services research, often loosely described as *outcomes research*, is the study of the end results of health services, taking into account patient preferences, values, and experiences (Ware, 1984; Clancy and Eisenberg, 1998). It focuses on access to care, cost of care, quality of care, health systems, and population health (Epstein and Sherwood, 1996; Israel et al, 1998; Kane, 2006; Minkler and Wallerstein, 2008).

ACCESS TO CARE

Access to care includes the "actual use of personal health services and everything that facilitates or impedes their use. It is the link between health services systems and the populations they serve" (Aday and Andersen, 1974; Andersen et al, 2002; Andersen and Davidson, 2007). Improving access can reduce mortality, increase self-reported health, and decrease delays in care (Zweifler et al, 2011; Sabik, 2012; Sommers et al, 2012). Variations in access correlate with variable quality, including receipt of preventive care (Radley and Schoen, 2012). As certain aspects of urologic care become centralized, access to care is an increasingly important issue in urology (Stitzenberg et al, 2012).

Andersen presented a behavioral model for considering health care access in which three categories of factors determine how and whether individuals use medical services (Andersen and Davidson, 2007). These include predisposing factors (e.g., health beliefs, attitudes); enabling factors (e.g., health insurance, geographic proximity); and need factors (e.g., the presence of symptoms or diseases) (Northam, 1996; Shaw, 2012). Barriers to health care access often result from financial determinants such as the lack of health insurance or adequate income; logistic challenges in coordinating child care, public transportation, and work schedules; clinic waiting times; and difficulties with the geographic proximity of clinics and hospitals (DeVoe et al, 2007; Carrillo et al, 2011; Parikh et al, 2012). Adequate access requires more than a guarantee of payment for services; even with generous benefits, individuals must navigate nonfinancial barriers. Among these are minority status (Mandelblatt et al, 1999; Rosenbaum et al, 2000; Lurie and Dubowitz, 2007; Barocas et al, 2013a; Dickson et al, 2013; Flores and Lin, 2013); gender (Li et al, 2007; Kullgren et al, 2012; Ghani et al, 2013; Kates et al, 2013); sexual orientation (Buchmueller and Carpenter, 2010; Ponce et al, 2010; Mattocks et al, 2014; McKirnan et al, 2013); environmental factors (Davidson et al, 2004; Capezuti et al, 2012); health behaviors (Andersen, 1995; Lasser et al, 2006; Stringhini et al, 2010); acculturation, language, and citizenship (Derose et al, 2009; Kinsler et al, 2009; Zambrana and Carter-Pokras, 2010; Wright et al, 2013); provider proximity (Cordasco et al, 2011; Paquette et al, 2011); available safety-net services (Katz, 2010; Cordasco et al, 2011; Katz and Brigham, 2011; Ku et al, 2011; Chatterjee et al, 2012; Spatz et al, 2012); and the absence of a usual source of care (Phillips et al, 2009; Bodenheimer and Pham, 2010). Even in health care systems that are considered to provide "equal access," such as the U.S. Department of Veterans Affairs hospitals, different patient groups use outpatient and inpatient care at markedly different rates, leading to variations in outcomes (Jha et al, 2001; Kizer and Dudley, 2009; Frayne et al, 2013).

In this context, differential access to care has been proposed as an important determinant of racial and ethnic disparities in prostate cancer screening, treatment, morbidity, and mortality (Moul et al, 1995; Optenberg et al, 1995; Klabunde et al, 1998; Stitzenberg et al, 2012; Barocas et al, 2013a). Discrepancies in accessibility and continuity of medical care may explain the lower use and awareness of prostate-specific antigen (PSA) testing among Hispanic men in the United States (McFall, 2006; Spencer et al, 2006; McFall, 2007); it remains unknown whether access or continuity issues mediate the greater dissatisfaction with prostate cancer treatment decisions among Hispanic men (Hoffman et al, 2003; Resnick et al, 2013a). Access to health care reflects not only the potential for entry into the health care system, but also the actual consumption of services. In one public-assistance program for low-income, uninsured men with prostate cancer, special attention to overcoming the financial and nonfinancial barriers has eliminated racial and ethnic disparities in health services use (Miller et al, 2008a). Nonetheless, because men from historically disadvantaged groups often do not access adequate and timely care, they continue to suffer a disproportionate burden (Miller et al, 2009a).

COSTS OF CARE

The cost of medical care may be measured in many ways. Although it is difficult to put a price tag on the toll of human suffering, physicians today are asked to reduce costs, improve quality, and provide services for greater numbers of patients in an increasingly austere environment. This often requires rationing of resources, though it is seldom explicitly labeled as such. In the present era of sweeping change in health care financing and health services delivery, increasing emphasis has been placed on efficiency in the allocation of scarce medical resources. The field of medical economics is well beyond its nascence, and broad public interest has emerged in studying the costs of medical and surgical therapies. As we spend more administrative dollars on cost containment, scrutiny is reaching all potential areas for conservation, including oncology—a province once considered sacred and off limits to cost-cutting efforts.

Health policy decisions today must be based not only on biomedical research but also on sound evaluations of health care costs. The use of oral erectogenic medications, beginning in the late 1990s, provides a perfect illustration of the tension between therapeutic advances and economic forces. The scientific discoveries that led to the advent of sildenafil and similar agents (Rajfer et al, 1992) were rewarded with a Nobel Prize, yet insurers initially fervently resisted paying for them (McGarvey, 2000; Smith and Roberts, 2000). This led to widespread controversy, generated numerous studies, and even raised questions of constitutional law (Finley, 1999; Julka, 1999; Connolly, 2001; Haff, 2006; Ki and Kim, 2008). **As a surgical subspecialty whose practitioners have discovered and use several exciting but expensive new drugs** (Kantoff et al, 2010; de Bono et al, 2011; Fizazi et al, 2011; Cabot et al, 2012; Parker et al, 2013), **urology is at the forefront of helping patients make rational health care choices and balance competing priorities.** Urologists must be especially conscientious and evidence based in advocating for new and expensive therapies, given the human toll (Gore et al, 2009a; Huang et al, 2010; Johansson et al, 2011; Song et al, 2011; Holmberg et al, 2012; Harden et al, 2013) and economic ramifications (Bolenz et al, 2010; Krahn et al, 2010; Andersson et al, 2011; Nguyen et al, 2011; Lowrance et al, 2012b) of overtreatment of indolent prostate cancer (Daskivich et al, 2010a, 2010b, 2011a, 2011c; Chamie et al, 2012a) over the past two decades.

Terms and Methods of Analysis

In its purest form, research on health care costs involves counting the amount of money that is spent on facilities, equipment, supplies, and personnel during the provision of medical care. But many costs are hidden. A more extensive approach would also include the opportunity cost of the time patients spend receiving care. For example, when estimating the cost of an interval cystoscopy after resection of a bladder tumor, a thorough assessment would include not only the cost of overhead, supplies, lidocaine jelly, urine cytology, and professional fees, but also the cost to the patient in lost wages—or to his or her employer in lost productivity—during the time away from work for the procedure, travel, or any complications. This component is not insignificant. Employee absence from work has been estimated to cost U.S. businesses tens of millions of dollars annually (Loeppke et al, 2009; Volpp et al, 2011; Zhang et al, 2011).

Because true costs are difficult to quantify at the individual, institutional, or population level, researchers instead often report data on charges. *Charges* represent the amount that is billed for a service, whereas *costs* reflect what the provider spent to supply that service. Most of the available administrative databases in health care are based on either financial discharge abstracts from hospitals or claims data from large payers, insurance companies, or government agencies such as the Centers for Medicare and Medicaid Services. These data sets primarily include information on charges and payments, but not costs. The major advantage of using charge data is that they are much easier to obtain. The primary disadvantage is that they may not accurately reflect the true underlying costs of individual medical services. For example, a hospital that is losing money on magnetic resonance imaging may make up the deficit by increasing its charges for urine cytology procedures. This practice may help balance the annual budget, but it corrupts the quality of the charge data. An economic analysis using charges for bladder cancer follow-up in such a hospital will err by incorporating the inflated amounts charged for interval urine cytology procedures. Some analysts attempt to circumvent this problem by calculating a ratio of costs to charges for entire facilities, individual medical services, or diagnosis-based categories of care. Charges are frequently used to estimate the amount of money spent on health care, although such calculations are imperfect. To avoid the inherent problems in calculating costs and charges, some researchers instead measure *resource utilization* in terms of duration, frequency, and intensity of services (Washburn et al, 2006; Unroe et al, 2010).

One of the most commonly reported units of comparative analysis is length of stay (LOS). After 1983, when the prospective payment system was instituted to reimburse hospitals a predetermined amount of money on the basis of the diagnosis-related group (DRG) into which each Medicare inpatient is classified (Vladeck, 1984; Hsia et al, 1988; Goldfield, 2010), attention to LOS as an outcome variable in cost analyses greatly increased. In the United States, inpatient LOSs are now believed to have reached their floor, and effort has shifted from this measure. Costs of care may be measured as intensity or numbers of services provided. For example, rather than calculating the costs or charges for a 3-day hospitalization for radical nephrectomy, analysis may be based on the total number of complete blood counts, chest radiographs, bags of intravenous fluid, doses of antibiotic, and doses of narcotic and antibiotic ordered on any given day of the hospital stay or during the entire stay. By examining duration or frequency of medical services when studying costs, researchers can avoid the biases involved in using financial data. **Although the overall costs of diseases such as bladder cancer are high** (James and Gore, 2013), **opportunities for quality improvement often go hand in hand with cost reduction when pharmacoeconomics are considered** (Gore and Gilbert, 2013).

Cost-effectiveness analysis is another popular technique used to evaluate new or established medical therapies. **Ideally, preventive care can obviate the need to treat a disease by preventing its onset, and the cost of prevention can be compared with the cost of disease treatment** (Maciosek et al, 2010). Alternatively, a cost-effectiveness analysis is performed by developing a probability model of the possible medical outcomes of one intervention compared with another, such as sacral neuromodulation versus medication for storage symptoms (Anger et al, 2014), or with a nonintervention such as watchful waiting for benign prostatic hyperplasia (Saigal and Joyce, 2005; Bellinger et al, 2012; Strope et al, 2012), identifying the expenses associated with each outcome, and comparing the results, typically reported as cost per year of life saved (Lee et al, 2009; Binagwaho et al, 2010; MacKenzie et al, 2010; Wheeler et al, 2010; Ciaranello et al, 2013). Years of life saved, or *life years (LYs)*, are calculated for a population, not for individuals. Ten LYs might represent two patients, each of whom survives for 5 additional years, or 120 patients, each of whom survives for 1 additional month (Baker et al, 2010; Jia and Lubetkin, 2010; Soerjomataram et al, 2012). LYs are usually adjusted to account for different health states that may result from various treatments. These are called *quality-adjusted life years (QALYs)*. For example, when comparing two treatments for localized prostate cancer, if both options are determined to cost $10,000 per year of life saved, then the two may seem equivalent. However, if one treatment yields years that are compromised by bothersome sexual dysfunction (Le et al, 2010), whereas the other yields years that are free of such problems, then the difference in quality of the years saved must be factored into the equation. Analyses that rely on QALYs are facilitated by the estimation of patient utilities, or preferences, for various health states (Albertsen et al, 1998; Saigal et al, 2001, 2002; Owens and Shekelle, 2013). If patients appraise an impotent year as being worth less than a potent year, then quality adjustments may make the first treatment more expensive per QALY saved. Couples approached 1 year after treatment for prostate cancer were found to be willing to pay approximately $800 per month for a hypothetical new treatment that cures prostate cancer without side effects (Zeliadt et al, 2010, 2011; Ramsey et al, 2011; Li et al, 2012).

Cost-benefit analysis differs by including not only the costs but also the equivalent monetary value of any benefits garnered during the extra years of life. Often, this refers to wages earned or income accrued during that time. In more sophisticated analyses, future income and expenses related to a particular health state are discounted to present value by incorporating projected interest and inflation rates over time. Reducing cost in the treatment of one disease liberates resources to invest in exciting new projects (Behesnilian and Yel, 2005; Chu et al, 2012). Cost studies may be undertaken as descriptive analyses that chronicle the economic burden of one disease in a group of patients, such as the cost of care for interstitial cystitis in a managed care plan (Clemens et al, 2009; Anger et al, 2011; Beckett et al, 2014). They may examine the financial impact on the general population such as national annual expenditures for urolithiasis (Raman et al, 2010; Lotan and Pearle, 2011; Lotan et al, 2012; Sutherland et al, 2013). They may also track cumulative costs over time, such as for different prostate cancer treatments (Krahn et al, 2010; Snyder et al, 2010; Krahn et al, 2014). Alternatively, they may present economic models comparing different approaches to managing an illness, such as whether it is more costly to correct cryptorchidism in infants or in older boys (Hsieh et al, 2009), or to manage small renal tumors with laparoscopic or percutaneous cryoablation (Bensalah et al, 2008; Hui et al, 2008; Pandharipande et al, 2008; Panumatrassamee et al, 2013).

Value of Care

The cost of health care should be considered in the context of the outcomes it produces. **The "value" of a health care service or intervention is defined as quality divided by cost** (Porter, 2010; Weinberger, 2011). Outcomes are more relevant than services rendered, or health care inputs, because significant health inputs without good outcomes do not produce value (Kaplan and Porter, 2011; Berwick and Hackbarth, 2012). Considering cost in the context of value can help policy makers decide which interventions should be amplified and which may be reduced (Orszag and Emanuel, 2010). The ultimate reflection of value is life expectancy divided by cost. The Organisation for Economic Co-operation and Development (www.oecd.org) reports these outcomes. Among 34 participating countries, the United States ranks first in total health expenditures per capita and 26th in life expectancy (Auerbach and Kellermann, 2011; Fuchs, 2013; van Baal et al, 2013). Among 28 participating countries reporting public expenditure on education and 24 describing tertiary education rates, the United States ranks 16th and 15th, respectively (Hudson and Kühner, 2009; Mahon, 2013).

Patterns of Care

Variations in patterns of care are vast, and incompletely understood. The Dartmouth Atlas Project has studied practice patterns most broadly, and for over 20 years has documented glaring variations in distribution and use of medical resources in the United States (Hudson, 1996; Wennberg, 1998). The project uses Medicare data to provide information and analysis about national, regional, and local markets, as well as hospitals and their affiliated physicians. Data from the project demonstrate significant variation among different regions of the country (Weinstein et al, 2006; Wennberg et al, 2008; Wennberg, 2011), especially at the end of life (Morden et al, 2012; Prigerson and Maciejewski, 2012) and often incongruously with patient preferences (Keating et al, 2010; Mitchell, 2010; Patel and Schulman, 2012). That variation in health care spending does not correlate with outcomes suggests that good outcomes can be achieved with lowered cost, and that current spending can be targeted more thoughtfully. In urology, significant hospital-level variation exists in outcomes and readmission after surgery (Gore et al, 2012).

Performance of appropriate and inappropriate procedures often varies concomitantly, as is the case with imaging of men with prostate cancer. Regions with higher rates of indicated imaging also have higher rates of extraneous imaging, and those with lower rates of unnecessary scans have lower rates of appropriate utilization (Lavery et al, 2011; Makarov et al, 2012a, 2012b). National efforts to decrease inappropriate imaging by disseminating utilization data and imaging guidelines to urologists can lead to meaningful decreases in unsupported imaging, but may also reduce appropriate use among high-risk patients (Makarov et al, 2013). Meaningfully improving practice patterns requires fastidious collaboration (Miller et al, 2010, 2011).

Regional variation in bladder cancer cost and outcomes has been noted, with higher-spending regions using more services and interventions, but lower-spending regions demonstrating superior cancer-specific survival (Skolarus et al, 2010). Significant regional variation also exists in the cost of radical prostatectomy (Makarov et al, 2010). Clearly, practice patterns are not always driven by data. For instance, acquisition of a surgical robot increases the number of both robotic and open prostatectomies performed in a hospital referral region (Makarov et al, 2011; Stitzenberg et al, 2012), and increases in surgical treatment of prostate cancer are both geographically and temporally related to acquisition of robotic surgical systems (Makarov et al, 2011; Lowrance et al, 2012a; Stitzenberg

et al, 2012). The increase in the overall number of surgical prostatectomies performed raises concern of overtreatment of men who would otherwise die with, rather than of, their disease (Burgess et al, 2006; Tewari et al, 2006; Steinberg et al, 2008; Andriole et al, 2009; Hu et al, 2009; Hugosson et al, 2010; Andriole et al, 2012; Carter et al, 2012a, 2013b; Huang et al, 2013; Laviana and Hu, 2013; Bolenz et al, 2014). Concerning patterns abound beyond cancer care. Opening of ambulatory surgery centers is associated with increased use of discretionary surgery (Strope et al, 2009; Hollingsworth et al, 2010, 2011; Schroeck et al, 2012), and introduction of physician ownership of lithotripter units influences treatment selection (Tan et al, 2011).

Conversely, some evidence-based advances have diffused much more slowly. Adoption of laparoscopic approaches to radical nephrectomy is variable, as is quality of kidney cancer care (Harper et al, 2012). Diffusion of evidence-based technologies and practices is limited by physician preferences, as is the case with partial or laparoscopic nephrectomy for small renal masses (Miller et al, 2006; Morris et al, 2007; Miller et al, 2008b) or continent reconstruction after cystectomy (Gore et al, 2006). Patient age and physician variables do affect practice patterns (Quinn et al, 2009; Cooperberg et al, 2010; Dulabon et al, 2010; Bleich et al, 2011; Klabunde et al, 2013).

The National Institute of Diabetes and Digestive and Kidney Diseases funds the Urologic Diseases in America project (www.udaonline.net), which seeks to define the burden of urologic disease on the American public by quantifying trends in resource usage, practice patterns, costs, outcomes, and epidemiology across the spectrum of urologic conditions (Litwin et al, 2005a, 2005b; Miller et al, 2009b). Documenting these trends has broad implications for quality of health care, access to care, and the equitable allocation of scarce resources, in terms of both medical services and research budgets. Among the most financially burdensome urologic conditions are urolithiasis (Scales et al, 2011), urinary tract infection (Griebling, 2005a, 2005b; Carter et al, 2012b), urinary incontinence (Anger et al, 2006a, 2006b, 2006c; Rogo-Gupta et al, 2013), and benign prostatic hyperplasia (Nickel, 2006; Roehrborn et al, 2011b; Stewart et al, 2012). Urologic diseases exert a substantial impact on resource usage within the U.S. Veterans Affairs health system (Anger et al, 2008).

Analyses from the Urologic Diseases in America project have revealed not only disturbing trends and variations in care, but also avenues for potential improvements for both benign and malignant disease. Surgical quality among Medicare beneficiaries undergoing outpatient urologic surgery varies by location of care delivery (Hollingsworth et al, 2012a). The prevalence of kidney stones has increased sharply, particularly in black, non-Hispanic and Hispanic individuals, and now affects 1 in 11 people in the United States (Scales et al, 2012). Once an individual has been diagnosed with a kidney stone, treatment varies significantly, often driven by nonclinical factors associated with provider and/or patient preferences or experience (Scales et al, 2011). In bladder cancer, delays before radical cystectomy can increase mortality (Gore et al, 2009b), and use of radical cystectomy varies by clinical and sociodemographic factors (Gore et al, 2010b). Adherence to guideline-recommended bladder cancer care is poor (Chamie and Litwin, 2011; Chamie et al, 2011; Chamie et al, 2012b). One exciting positive avenue for expansion is smoking cessation: smokers newly diagnosed with bladder cancer are five times as likely as the general population to quit smoking, especially if counseled appropriately by their urologist (Bassett et al, 2012). For men with prostate cancer, patterns of care after failure of primary prostate cancer treatment depended on use of standardized clinical algorithms, initial therapy, and geographic region (Krupski et al, 2006). Patients with kidney cancer who are treated with partial rather than radical nephrectomy have fewer adverse renal outcomes, including less frequent receipt of dialysis services, dialysis access surgery, or renal transplantation (Miller et al, 2008c). These findings are consistent with a subsequent population-based study using instrumental variable analysis to assess outcomes after partial versus radical nephrectomy, which showed that for individuals with early-stage kidney cancer, treatment with partial nephrectomy was associated with improved survival (Tan et al, 2012).

Case Mix

In studying patterns of care or medical costs, it is critical to adjust for case mix. *Case mix* refers to the severity of illness and degree of comorbidity in a group of patients (Iezzoni, 1989; Covinsky et al, 1997b; Birkmeyer et al, 2012; Maas et al, 2013). These characteristics may influence treatment outcomes. For example, because they typically have a greater burden of comorbidity, older patients are more likely to experience complications after surgery. This comorbidity must be accounted for in evaluations of clinical outcomes (Hong et al, 2010; Zelefsky et al, 2010; Epstein et al, 2011). Kidneys from donors older than 50 years may provide fewer years of service to their recipient (Ng et al, 2012). If these facts are not considered when comparing surgical complication rates across hospitals, evaluators may erroneously conclude that a hospital with an older patient population is providing poorer care. To use outcomes to measure quality of care, we need to adjust for these other factors including baseline patient characteristics and intervening treatments. This adjustment (referred to as *case-mix adjustment* or *risk adjustment*) can be extremely complex, and the selection of factors must be carried out carefully so that outcomes can be interpreted accurately. For a variety of reasons, sicker patients cost more, and it is important to control for this difference in comparative analyses. In examining the factors that lead to higher hospital charges for more ill patients, two forces must be considered: duration and intensity of care. Duration is usually quantified as inpatient LOS, whereas intensity of care may be assessed as numbers of services or charges per day. Patients with greater comorbidity may remain hospitalized longer even if they do not receive more intense care during their stays. Duration and not intensity appears to be the primary force driving up hospital charges for sicker urology patients (Litwin et al, 1993). Various comorbidity measures (Kaplan and Feinstein, 1974; Charlson et al, 1987; Stier et al, 1999; Crabtree et al, 2000; Di Gangi Herms et al, 2003; Daskivich et al, 2011b, 2011c, 2013a) have been used by researchers to adjust for case mix and predict mortality from competing causes in clinical studies.

The impact of case mix on urologic disease outcomes has been studied most broadly in men treated for prostate cancer. Comorbidity is more important than age in predicting perioperative mortality after radical prostatectomy (Alibhai et al, 2004, 2005; Chamie et al, 2012a; Daskivich et al, 2013b). Among men with high comorbidity, low- and intermediate-risk prostate cancer is overtreated (Daskivich et al, 2010a, 2011a, 2011b, 2011c, 2013a; Chamie et al, 2012a), and often with advanced treatment technologies that have not been shown to be superior to prior standards (Jacobs et al, 2013). Conversely, men with high-risk prostate cancer are undertreated across all levels of comorbidity (Chamie et al, 2012a; Daskivich et al, 2011a, 2013a, 2013b). A revised index that reweighs Charlson comorbidities can more accurately identify men at highest risk for non–prostate cancer mortality, and aid in medical decision making (Daskivich et al, 2011b, 2011c, 2013a).

Comorbidities such as obesity also affect the incidence and severity of benign urologic conditions, including urinary incontinence (Richter et al, 2010), chronic prostatitis and chronic pelvic pain syndrome (Anothaisintawee et al, 2011), benign prostatic hyperplasia and lower urinary tract symptoms (Schenk et al, 2010; Parsons et al, 2013), and erectile dysfunction (Chitaley et al, 2009; Tsai and Sarwer, 2009). Weight loss meaningfully reduces incontinence in overweight and obese women (Subak et al, 2009; Smith et al, 2010), and lengthens life expectancy as well (Keating et al, 2009; Stewart et al, 2009; Majer et al, 2011).

Cost Savings in Urology

As the cost of health care expands (Sutherland et al, 2009; Kellermann and Weinick, 2012) **and crowds out other societal priorities** (Auerbach and Kellermann, 2011), **urologists have continued their central role in the ongoing struggle to balance the** sometimes-competing **priorities of minimizing costs and maximizing quality** (Botteman et al, 2003; Lotan, 2009; Lotan and Pearle, 2011; Staskin et al, 2012). For common procedures, such as transurethral resection of the prostate, urologists standardized care and cut costs long before it was mandated by the government (Sage et al, 1988). They made similar improvements for radical prostatectomy (Kramolowsky et al, 1995a, 1995b; Konety et al, 1996) and nephrectomy (Wilson et al, 1995; Uzzo et al, 1999). Unfortunately, such initiatives were insufficiently broad and sustained (in urology and beyond) to achieve high-quality care at sustainable cost throughout health systems, and the government intervened to buttress efforts to minimize cost and maximize quality. Medicare's pay-for-performance program differentially reimburses hospitals, medical groups, and clinicians based on adherence to quality metrics and elimination of medical errors (Rosenthal et al, 2004; Kindig, 2006). The need to realign incentives was reinforced by the Institute of Medicine's report, *Rewarding Provider Performance: Aligning Incentives in Medicare*, which stated, "The existing systems do not reflect the relative value of health care services in important aspects of quality, such as clinical quality, patient-centeredness, and efficiency" (Fisher, 2006). It recommended pay-for-performance as an immediate opportunity to better align incentives for improved performance. Methods of standardizing care and improving quality include clinical pathways, which have maximized value for hematuria (Vasdev et al, 2012), incontinence (Romeyke and Stummer, 2012; Rotter et al, 2012), and prostatitis (Shoskes, 2008), among others.

As an extension of this concept, under the Patient Protection and Affordable Care Act of 2010 (which was almost fully implemented in 2014), Medicare fee-for-service is being restructured into "bundled payments." A bundled payment is a single payment for an episode of care, such as a radical prostatectomy, rather than reimbursement to individual entities or providers based on services rendered. An interesting historical footnote is that the first self-imposed bundled payment was taken on by the father of American urology, Hugh Hampton Young. In his autobiography, Dr. Young described a patient on whom he agreed to perform a prostatectomy in the 1920s for a fixed fee of $500 with a promise of only 3 weeks in the hospital. Because the patient developed complications and remained hospitalized for much longer than planned, Young had to spend his entire professional fee plus an additional $350 to pay off the hospital bill (Young and Didusch, 1940).

The Affordable Care Act also includes several incentive programs that should affect individuals with urologic diseases. For instance, the act supports participatory wellness programs, which would reimburse for the cost of membership in a fitness center, potentially mitigating the noxious effect of obesity on prostate cancer (Freedland et al, 2008a, 2008b; Jayachandran et al, 2008, 2009; De Nunzio et al, 2012; Gollapudi et al, 2012; Keto et al, 2012; Byrd et al, 2013; Wu et al, 2013). Likewise, it supports employees attending no-cost health education seminars, including smoking cessation classes, which has significant consequences for individuals with bladder cancer (Bassett et al, 2012).

QUALITY OF CARE

Quality of care research evaluates "the degree to which health services for individuals and populations increase the likelihood of desired health outcomes and are consistent with current professional knowledge" (Brook and Lohr, 1981, 1985; Lohr, 1988; Lohr et al, 1988; Donabedian et al, 1989). The Institute of Medicine's landmark report *Crossing the Quality Chasm* outlined six principles that define high-quality health care: care that is safe, effective, efficient, patient-centered, timely, and equitable (Institute of Medicine, 2001). More recently, greater emphasis has been placed on efficiency, or value-based care, with value defined as patient-centered health outcomes divided by cost (Porter, 2010; Swensen et al, 2010; James and Savitz, 2011).

To reach a desired patient-centered health outcome, provided services must satisfy both content quality and delivery quality.

Content quality involves the technical component of health care and includes quality processes and metrics (James, 1989; Washington and Lipstein, 2011). It is defined and evaluated by health care providers. Delivery quality addresses interpersonal relationships on which delivery of health services are based, and is evaluated by patients and caregivers. Continuous quality improvement is the guiding principle for establishing a high-quality health care delivery system, and relies on an electronic health record system as well as on quality improvement oversight (Pham et al, 2007; Gabow et al, 2012; Cosgrove et al, 2013). An electronic health record system can improve quality on the front end with electronic order entry, built-in order sets, and standardized clinical care pathways, and on the back end with facile data abstraction and reports built around broad sets of quality outcomes (Gabow and Mehler, 2011; Cosgrove et al, 2012). Electronic systems are easily modifiable for changing metrics over time, and cloud-based systems allow sharing of information between inpatient and outpatient facilities, as well as with other institutions (Schweitzer, 2012). Compared with other industries, information technology has been less aggressively adopted in health care (Menachemi et al, 2006; Simon et al, 2007). As of 2008, fewer than 20% of physicians used an electronic health record (DesRoches et al, 2008; Jha et al, 2009). The Health Information Technology for Economic and Clinical Health Act of 2009, part of the government's stimulus package, provided funding for adoption and meaningful use of electronic health records, to achieve improvements in care (Blumenthal, 2009; Jha et al, 2009). Hospitals and physicians not using electronic health records by 2015 are subject to financial penalties under Medicare. Quality improvement oversight is typically undertaken by a quality improvement department, and involves data collection and monitoring systems, confidential reporting, and dashboards (Gabow et al, 2012). Such quality improvement projects have been piloted in urology but have not yet been implemented broadly (Gambone and Broder, 2007; Lee et al, 2011).

Descriptive quality measures abound, but for quality metrics to affect outcomes, they must be based on solid evidence, be feasible, and have resources devoted to tracking and improvement. In 2005, the U.S. Congress passed the Patient Safety and Quality Improvement Act, which helped reinforce ongoing quality improvement initiatives and also launched several new initiatives to collect and disseminate performance information about medical care (Patient Safety and Quality Improvement Act, 2005). For example, the ECRI Institute (www.ecri.org) collects and analyzes data about adverse events as well as near misses. The National Committee for Quality Assurance (www.ncqa.org) provides information to health care purchasers about the comparative performance of health plans in the United States. The Joint Commission (TJC, www.jointcommission.org) applies outcomes-based quality measures to accredit hospitals, and TJC accreditation is mandatory for participation in Medicare. Hundreds of performance indicators have been collected in its National Library of Healthcare Indicators, and a root cause analysis system was developed to understand the causes of sentinel events. The National Quality Forum (www.qualityforum.org/home.aspx) has focused on patient safety and endorsed six sets of "never events." The Leapfrog Group (www.leapfroggroup.org) includes almost 200 large private and public health care purchasers that attempt to leverage their purchasing power to influence quality and affordability. The Leapfrog Safe Practices Score assesses computer physician order entry, evidence-based hospital referral, and appropriate intensive care unit staffing. Leapfrog volume thresholds suggest that individuals undergoing radical prostatectomy at high-volume institutions have shorter LOSs and receive fewer blood transfusions compared with those treated at low-volume institutions (Penson, 2013). The Institute for Healthcare Improvement (www.ihi.org) is a nonprofit organization seeking to optimize health care performance by improving quality and patient satisfaction, improving the health of populations, and reducing the per capita cost of health care. The National Patient Safety Foundation (www.npsf.org) was formed in partnership between the American Medical Association and private industry to provide research support, education, and leadership training in

patient safety. It holds an annual Patient Safety Congress and publishes the *Journal of Patient Safety*. The Institute for Safe Medication Practices (www.ismp.org) aims to reduce medication error and operates an anonymous practitioner reporting program to understand the causes of medication errors and to eliminate them.

One of the most widely used performance measures, maintained by the National Committee for Quality Assurance, is the Healthcare Effectiveness Data and Information Set (HEDIS, www.ncqa.org/hedisqualitymeasurement). HEDIS's 75 measures are divided into eight domains: effectiveness, access/availability, experience, health plan stability, utilization and relative resource use, cost, informed health care choices, and health plan descriptive information. Consumers can use these data to compare the performance of health plans; the Centers for Medicare and Medicaid Services uses HEDIS to determine reimbursement for enrollees in Medicare Advantage. The broadest set of measures specific to surgery is the American College of Surgeon's National Surgical Quality Improvement Program (NSQIP) (Birkmeyer et al, 2008). The measures quantify risk-adjusted 30-day surgical outcomes, including mortality and morbidity in 21 categories. Collection and reporting of NSQIP measures have been shown to improve outcomes (Hall et al, 2009). Another often-used set of indicators is the Patient Safety Indicators (www.qualityindicators.ahrq.gov) published by the U.S. Department of Health and Human Services' Agency for Healthcare Research and Quality (AHRQ). The indicators focus on hospital and postoperative complications. On the basis of extensive reviews of available evidence, AHRQ developed four categories of quality indicators (prevention, patient safety, inpatient, and pediatric), which are now being used to modulate hospital and physician reimbursement.

Several consumer groups also publish health care performance metrics. The Foundation for Accountability (www.facct.org), a consumer organization, creates tools that help people understand and use quality information, develops consumer-focused quality measures, supports efforts to gather and provide quality information, and encourages health policy to empower and inform consumers. Consumer Reports uses Medicare billing data to rate surgical performance (www.consumerreportshealth.org); such approaches have been criticized for lacking critical clinical data (Conaboy, 2013). Families USA (www.familiesusa.org) is a nonprofit organization that produces health policy reports outlining problems from a consumer perspective and describing steps to solve them.

Quality Conceptual Framework

The conceptual framework for the measurement of quality of care in medicine was established almost 50 years ago by Donabedian (Donabedian, 1966). **In this model, quality-of-care measures are categorized into three domains—structure, process, and outcome.**

Structure of Care

Structure encompasses the fixed aspect of health care delivery and includes the space, equipment, human resources, and provider experience necessary to provide care. Examples include clinician characteristics (e.g., percentage of physicians who have board certification, average years of experience, distribution of specialties); organizational characteristics (e.g., staffing patterns, reimbursement method); patient characteristics (e.g., insurance type, illness profile); and community characteristics (e.g., per capita hospital beds, transportation system, environmental risks). Structural measures specific to prostate cancer quality could include the presence of a multidisciplinary cancer center or psychological support services (Spencer et al, 2003).

Although certain structural characteristics may be necessary to provide good care, they are usually insufficient to ensure high-quality care. Therefore the best structural measures are those that can be shown to have a positive influence on the process of care and on patient outcomes (Brook and McGlynn, 1996). One structural measure that is positively associated with outcomes is the number of patients treated by a particular physician or institution, especially for major procedures such as radical cystectomy

(Hollenbeck et al, 2007a, 2007b; Porter et al, 2011; Morgan et al, 2012) or radical prostatectomy (Siu et al, 2008; Trinh et al, 2013). Surgeon volume is also associated with structural covariates such as lymph node count at the time of robotic cystectomy (Marshall et al, 2013). Hospitals with higher lymph node counts have been shown to have higher survival rates after radical cystectomy (Hollenbeck et al, 2008). Patients with renal trauma are more likely to be offered conservative management and have a lower chance of requiring multiple procedures if they are treated at a level 1 trauma center (Hotaling et al, 2012).

Process of Care

Process of care is the set of activities that goes on between patients and practitioners and is often divided into interpersonal process and technical process. Examples include antibiotic prophylaxis and discussion of treatment options (Wolf et al, 2008). Process measures are often considered to be the best measure of quality (Brook and McGlynn, 1996; Brook et al, 2000), and the most fertile area for improvement in value (Schneider et al, 2004; Malin et al, 2006). *Interpersonal process* refers to how the clinician relates to the patient and includes issues such as whether the clinician supplies sufficient information in a clear enough manner for the patient to make an informed treatment choice. Patient survey data are generally used to assess quality of interpersonal process. *Technical process* refers to whether medically appropriate decisions are made when diagnosing and treating the patient and whether care is provided in an effective and skillful manner—for instance, selecting the correct operative repair for female urethral stricture disease (Ackerman et al, 2010). One way to evaluate the appropriateness of medical treatment is to determine if the care provided is consistent with current medical knowledge and adheres to the professional standard. This assessment can be done by developing *quality indicators,* such as those delineated earlier, that describe a process of care that should occur for a particular type of patient in a specific clinical circumstance. To be valid, these quality indicators should be based on the evidence in the medical literature and on current professional standards of care. Determining the latter often requires an expert panel to achieve consensus. The performance of physicians and health plans is then assessed by calculating rates of adherence to the indicators for a sample of patients. Using quality indicators to evaluate appropriateness of care is relatively straightforward. However, assessing the effectiveness or skill of technical process of care is much more difficult. Indeed, direct observation may be necessary to assess the quality of technical process of care. Alternatively, it may be necessary to rely on measuring outcomes to evaluate whether care was provided in a skillful manner. For example, measurement of surgical blood loss or number of specimens with positive margins, both surgical outcomes, may be indicators of the quality of surgical technical process. Conversely, operative time may represent the surgeon's manual dexterity or the technical complexity of a case. Hence celerity is not generally considered an accurate indicator of operative quality.

Outcomes of Care

Outcomes include changes in patients' current and future health status including health-related quality of life (HRQOL) and satisfaction. Cancer researchers generally use survival or progression-free survival as the main outcome measure in clinical studies. Sometimes proxy measures (also called *surrogate end points* or *intermediate outcomes*) that do not measure the outcome directly but are thought to be correlated with it are used. When a proxy measure is used as a quality indicator, there must be evidence that the proxy measure is truly a substitute for the outcome of interest. For example, the presence of unfavorable PSA kinetics after treatment for localized prostate cancer appears to be associated with cause-specific mortality (Freedland et al, 2005; Roach et al, 2006; Stephenson et al, 2009; Eggener et al, 2011), so this may be a reasonable proxy outcome. Although the ultimate outcome may be mortality, many conditions in urology such as prostate cancer take an indolent course, making mortality impractical (and often irrelevant). In such conditions, more proximal outcomes such as LOS, complications, and the need for salvage therapy provide a useful proxy (Bastide et al, 2010; Eggener et al, 2011). For proxy measures to be useful as quality measures, intervention should affect both the measure and the underlying disease (Guyatt et al, 1993; Girling et al, 2012).

The most important patient-reported outcome is HRQOL, a multidimensional construct that includes somatic symptoms, functional ability, emotional well-being, social functioning, and body image, as well as overall well-being (Guyatt et al, 1993; Wilson and Cleary, 1995). Quality-of-life assessment, typically by patient survey, provides a comprehensive evaluation of how the illness and its treatment affect patients.

Quality Metrics Applied to Urology

General quality metrics applied to urology have shown that patients undergoing cystectomy, nephrectomy, and prostatectomy are at significant risk of developing deep venous thromboses or pulmonary emboli (Gore et al, 2012). Readmission and mortality are highest after cystectomy, with readmission rates of over 35% and mortality over 6% after 90 days. Measurable variation in surgical quality exists by location of surgery for a range of outpatient urologic procedures (Hollingsworth et al, 2012a).

Urology-specific quality indicators and covariates have been developed, validated, and applied for localized prostate cancer (Spencer et al, 2003; Miller et al, 2007; Spencer et al, 2008; Ritchey et al, 2012). The 48 quality-of-care indicators include 5 structure, 23 process, and 20 outcome variables, plus 15 covariates (such as patient age). Quality metrics specific to bladder cancer have been proposed but have yet to be developed and validated (Montgomery et al, 2013). Candidate structure indicators include use of multidisciplinary teams, operating room facilities, and surgical volume (Cooperberg et al, 2009); process measures include adequate staging, complication rates, chemotherapy at transurethral resection, neoadjuvant or adjuvant chemotherapy use, time to cystectomy, adequate lymphadenectomy, and discussion of continent diversion if appropriate (Cooperberg et al, 2009; Gore et al, 2009b; Chamie et al, 2012b); and outcome measures include morbidity, mortality (overall and disease specific), and HRQOL, which would be best evaluated with bladder cancer–specific instruments (Gore et al, 2012).

Quality metrics for kidney cancer also have not been formalized, but use of partial versus radical nephrectomy in individuals with early-stage cancer may be a good candidate. All-cause and kidney cancer–specific mortality are lower when partial nephrectomy is employed when feasible (Tan et al, 2012). Clinical pathways for patients undergoing radical nephrectomy hold promise in shortening hospital stay and reducing cost (Chang et al, 2000). Disease-specific metrics have been developed and validated for urinary incontinence (Anger et al, 2013a) and prolapse (Anger et al, 2013b), but they still need to be tested for feasibility.

Advanced cancer and benign diseases have been left behind in urologic quality monitoring. Disease-specific metrics are needed for nephrolithiasis (Donnally et al, 2011), benign prostatic hyperplasia (McVary et al, 2011), stricture disease (Jackson et al, 2012), and erectile dysfunction (Avasthi et al, 2011), among others (Clavijo et al, 2010; Kaplan and Hu, 2013). For end-of-life care, the National Quality Forum has endorsed the need to improve quality (Lorenz et al, 2006, 2007; Seow et al, 2009a, 2009b). Although knowledge about interventions to improve supportive care is abundant (McNiff et al, 2008; Wright et al, 2008; Zhang et al, 2009; Engelberg et al, 2010; Temel et al, 2010; Walling et al, 2010; Curtis et al, 2011; Malin et al, 2011; Meyer, 2011; Teno et al, 2013), tools to evaluate whether patients receive effective supportive care are lacking, limiting provider ability to improve over time. The Cancer Quality-ASSIST Project used the VA Health Services Research and Development appropriateness method to identify quality indicators in six categories: pain, depression, dyspnea, nausea and vomiting, fatigue and anorexia, and other treatment-related toxicities (Lorenz et al, 2009;

Dy et al, 2010). These metrics are specific neither to urology nor to life's final days. Moving forward, quality-of-care indicators need to be defined, validated, and used for individuals with kidney cancer, bladder cancer, locally invasive and metastatic prostate cancer, benign disease, and advanced urologic malignancies.

Quality Improvement Frameworks

Several health systems have committed to institution-wide quality improvement frameworks. The Lean model of continuous quality improvement was used by most of these systems, although each adapted Lean principles to suit the specific needs of its organization (Mazzocato et al, 2010; Blackmore et al, 2013). The method was originally used by the Toyota Production System, which sought to eliminate waste in production and maximize value for the customer. **The process empowers all stakeholders in an institution to identify waste (defined as anything that does not add value or serve the patient's needs), suggest improvement, measure results, and pursue continuous improvement.** Several health care systems, including Virginia Mason, ThedaCare, Intermountain, and Denver Health, have employed Toyota's Lean methodology to improve value (Mazzocato et al, 2010; Gabow and Mehler, 2011; James and Savitz, 2011; Gabow et al, 2012; Blackmore et al, 2013; Cosgrove et al, 2013). Nursing always plays a critical role in quality improvement initiatives. Return on investment is high, with savings of up to $160 million over a 5-year period (Cosgrove et al, 2013; Gabow and Mehler, 2011).

Quality improvement frameworks have been created specifically for and implemented in urology. The Urological Surgery Quality Collaborative and the Michigan Urologic Surgery Improvement Collaborative connect urologists from different practices and feed back data for individual and group quality improvement (Miller et al, 2010, 2011; Burks et al, 2012; Barocas et al, 2013b). The collaboration has succeeded in improving the appropriate use of bone scan and computed tomography imaging for men with localized prostate cancer by lowering overuse when imaging is not indicated and increasing use when it is needed (Miller et al, 2010). It has also improved use of intravesical chemotherapy after transurethral resection of bladder tumors (Barocas et al, 2013b) and reduced variations in practice patterns and improved adherence to recommended staging practices (Miller et al, 2010). Another paradigm shift led by urology involves graphic representation of quality-of-life outcomes, to make measures more actionable for individuals with urologic malignancies. This user-centered design improves patient comprehension and enhances the clinical experiences of men with prostate cancer (Izard et al, 2012).

Integrated patient-centered medical homes also hold promise in improving value and quality in urology (Fisher, 2008). Such a model, with each patient empanelled to a unique primary care physician overseeing his or her medical care, improves care integration and quality (Coleman et al, 2010; Marx et al, 2011; Driscoll et al, 2013; Sarfaty et al, 2013) Nearly three quarters of urology practices currently meet the National Committee for Quality Assurance's standard for a medical home (Sakshaug et al, 2013), and primary care providers devote significant time to care for survivors of urologic malignancies. In contrast, only 54% of all physician practices have sufficient medical home infrastructure (Hollingsworth et al, 2012b). However, in safety-net and other systems, specialty resources are scarce, and successful strategies have placed the face-to-face onus on primary care providers, buttressed by specialist support (Chen et al, 2010; Neuhausen et al, 2012; Chen et al, 2013). Whether the optimal medical neighborhood will be built by employing urologists at the center of a medical home (Sakshaug et al, 2013) or in a supportive role (Chen et al, 2010, 2013) remains an open question (Hollingsworth et al, 2012b; Sakshaug et al, 2013).

Challenges to Using Outcomes to Evaluate Quality of Care

Adverse outcomes may be uncommon events, so large samples of patients may be necessary when using outcome measures to detect differences in quality among health systems or hospitals. For example, to detect a 2% difference in the rate of postoperative wound infections between two hospitals (e.g., 5% for 1 and 7% for the other), each hospital would need to have at least 1900 patients who had undergone the surgery. In addition, a single outcome may be affected by many different factors, making it difficult to establish accountability. When comparing differences in surgical outcomes across hospitals, one does not know if the differences in outcomes are related to the skill of the surgeon, the competence of the surgical team, the postoperative care, the case mix, or some unmeasured factor. And the more time that elapses between the intervention and the outcome, the more difficult this problem becomes. For example, in comparing 10-year outcomes in women treated for incontinence at different facilities, what is more important, the quality of the initial treatment or the quality of care for recurrent symptoms?

Using patient satisfaction as an outcome is also fraught with limitations (Neuhausen and Katz, 2012). Although higher patient satisfaction is associated with increased overall health care expenditures and drug prescription (Fenton et al, 2012), a relationship between patient experience and quality of care does not necessarily exist (Chang et al, 2006; Rao et al, 2006). In one study, high satisfaction correlated with increased mortality (Fenton et al, 2012). Factors other than quality appear to affect patient satisfaction, and incentives based on satisfaction scores may unintentionally lead to worse outcomes and higher cost. Medicare's Value-Based Purchasing program will penalize hospitals that score poorly on patient satisfaction surveys (Chatterjee et al, 2012; Shoemaker, 2012; VanLare and Conway, 2012; Weston et al, 2013).

Levels of Evidence

Ranking systems to classify levels of evidence were first described by the Canadian Task Force on the Periodic Health Examination in the late 1970s (Delbanco and Taylor, 1980). These have since been adapted to reflect the strength of a study or clinical trial. Evidence levels range from I to IV, as follows:

- Level Ia: Meta-analysis of randomized controlled trials
- Level Ib: At least one randomized controlled trial
- Level IIa: At least one well designed, controlled trial, not randomized
- Level IIb: At least one well designed experimental trial
- Level III: Case, correlation, or comparative study
- Level IV: Expert opinion

Level I evidence is considered most strongly when policy recommendations are being constructed (Moyer, 2012).

HEALTH-RELATED QUALITY OF LIFE

Health-related quality of life encompasses a wide range of human experience including the daily necessities of life such as food and shelter, intrapersonal and interpersonal responses to illness, and activities associated with professional fulfillment and personal happiness (Barofsky, 2012). Contemporary interpretations of HRQOL are based on the World Health Organization's long-standing definition of health as a "state of complete physical, mental, and social well-being and not merely the absence of disease" (Sharp, 1947; World Health Organization, 1948). HRQOL involves patients' own perceptions of their health and ability to function in life. In light of evidence that survival and clinical outcomes may be similar across treatments for many conditions, quality-of-life considerations may be the critical factor in medical decision making in some instances. Data are collected with HRQOL surveys, called *instruments*. Instruments typically contain questions, or items, that are organized into scales. Each scale measures a different aspect, or domain, of HRQOL. Instruments are best when they are self-administered by the patient, but if interviewer assistance is required, it must be from a neutral third party in a standardized fashion (Chang et al, 2011).

Health-Related Quality-of-Life Instruments

HRQOL instruments may be general or disease specific. General HRQOL domains address the components of overall well-being, whereas disease-specific domains focus on the impact of particular organic dysfunctions that may affect HRQOL. Numerous HRQOL instruments have been validated for use in urologic and other conditions. In urology, HRQOL research has been broad, but much has focused on individuals with prostate cancer (Litwin et al, 1995; Litwin et al, 1998; Huang et al, 2010; Mehnert et al, 2010; Ramsey et al, 2010; Szymanski et al, 2010; Resnick and Penson, 2012; Resnick et al, 2013a, 2013b; Resnick and Penson, 2013), urinary incontinence (Richter et al, 2010; Smith et al, 2010; Chong et al,

2011; Coyne et al, 2012; Liebergall-Wischnitzer et al, 2012), benign prostatic hyperplasia (McConnell et al, 2003; Coyne et al, 2009; Montorsi et al, 2010; Roehrborn et al, 2011a; Chokkalingam et al, 2012; Roehrborn et al, 2013), end-stage renal disease (Abdel-Kader et al, 2009; Goldstein et al, 2009; Griva et al, 2009), and bladder cancer (Nagele et al, 2006; Gilbert et al, 2010; Hedgepeth et al, 2010; Large et al, 2010; Nagele et al, 2012). A comprehensive resource for validated HRQOL instruments is available at www.proqolid.org. The National Cancer Institute has been particularly active in establishing interest in outcomes measurement for patients with malignant disease (www.outcomes.cancer.gov). Table 4-1 presents many of the validated HRQOL instruments available for the assessment of patients with urologic conditions. For each

TABLE 4-1 Characteristics of Health-Related Quality-of-Life (HRQOL) Instruments in Urologic Diseases

INSTRUMENT NAME	ITEMS	TIME RECALL, WEEKS	READING GRADE LEVEL OF ITEMS, MEDIAN (RANGE)	REFERENCE
GENERAL HRQOL				
Medical Outcomes Study 36-Item Health Survey (SF-36)	36	4	5.9 (2.2-12.0)	Ware and Sherbourne, 1992
Medical Outcomes Study 12-Item Health Survey (SF-12)	12	4	5.2 (2.2-12.0)	Ware et al, 1996
Quality of Well-Being Scale (QWB)	24	1	6.3 (0.9-12.0)	Kaplan et al, 1976
Sickness Impact Profile (SIP)	136	1 and 7	7.4 (0.5-12.0)	Bergner et al, 1981
Nottingham Health Profile (NHP)	38	At present	4.5 (2.1-12.0)	Hunt et al, 1985
Profile of Mood States (POMS)	65	1	7.2 (0.6-12.0)	Norcross et al, 1984
Mental Health Inventory (MHI)	38	4	5.8 (0.6-12.0)	Berwick et al, 1991
McGill-Melzack Pain Questionnaire	20	At present	N/A	Melzack, 1975
GENERAL HRQOL IN CANCER				
Functional Assessment of Cancer Therapy–General (FACT-G)	28	1	3.4 (1.1-12.0)	Cella et al, 1993
Cancer Rehabilitation Evaluation System Short Form (CARES-SF)	59	4	8.2 (1.0-12.0)	Schag et al, 1991
European Organization for Research and Treatment of Cancer Quality of Life Questionnaire C30 (EORTC-QLQ-C30)	30	1	2.6 (1.8-12.0)	Aaronson et al, 1993
Rotterdam Symptom Checklist	27	1	4.6 (0.7-12.0)	de Haes et al, 1990
Prostate Cancer Treatment Outcome Questionnaire (PCTO-Q)	41	1	6.2 (2.1-12.0)	Shrader-Bogen et al, 1997
PROSTATE CANCER				
University of California, Los Angeles Prostate Cancer Index (UCLA-PCI)	20	4	5.2 (1.2-12.0)	Litwin et al, 1998
UCLA-PCI Short Form (UCLA-PCI-SF)	15	4	4.9 (1.2-12.0)	Litwin and McGuigan, 1999
Expanded Prostate Cancer Index-50 (EPIC-50)	50	4	5.8 (2.5-11.9)	Wei et al, 2000
Functional Assessment of Cancer Therapy–Prostate (FACT-P)	47	1	2.8 (0.5-12.0)	Esper et al, 1997
Prostate Cancer Specific Quality of Life Instrument (PROS-QOLI)	10	1 and 7	6.4 (2.8-10.4)	Stockler et al, 1998
European Organization for Research and Treatment of Cancer Quality of Life Questionnaire Prostate Module (EORTC-QLQ-PR25)	25	1	6.7 (0.5-12.0)	Borghede and Sullivan, 1996
Total Illness Burden Index–Prostate Cancer (TIBI-CaP)	25	26	7.6 (2.4-11.3)	Litwin et al, 2007
The Prostate Cancer Radiation Late Toxicity Questionnaire (PCRT)	29	4	9.2 (3.6-12.0)	Rodrigues et al, 2007
Quality of Life Module-Prostate 14 (QOLM-P14)	14	1	3.2 (0.6-9.0)	Osoba et al, 1999
Memorial Anxiety Index–Prostate Cancer (MAX-PC)	18	1	6.2 (3.7-12.0)	Roth et al, 2003
Clark and Talcott	20	1	5.8 (2.4-10.4)	Clark and Talcott, 2001

TABLE 4-1   Characteristics of Health-Related Quality-of-Life (HRQOL) Instruments in Urologic Diseases—cont'd

INSTRUMENT NAME	ITEMS	TIME RECALL, WEEKS	READING GRADE LEVEL OF ITEMS, MEDIAN (RANGE)	REFERENCE
Clark et al	35	4	5.2 (1.0-10.7)	Clark et al, 2003
Dale et al	35	1	7.1 (2.8-11.8)	Dale et al, 1999
Borghede et al	19	1	6.7 (2.3-12.0)	Borghede et al, 1997
Giesler et al	52	4	8.8 (3.6-12.0)	Giesler et al, 2000
BLADDER CANCER				
Functional Assessment of Cancer Therapy–Bladder (FACT-BL)	40	1	3.6 (0.7-12.0)	Mansson et al, 2002
Functional Assessment of Cancer Therapy Vanderbilt Cystectomy Index (FACT-VCI)	19	1	3.7 (0.6-10.2)	Cookson et al, 2003
European Organization for Research and Treatment for Cancer Quality of Life Questionnaire Bladder Module (EORTC-QLQ-BLS24)	24	1	5.5 (0.5-12.0)	Pavone-Macaluso et al, 1997
BENIGN PROSTATIC HYPERPLASIA AND LOWER URINARY TRACT SYMPTOMS				
American Urological Association Symptom Index (AUASI) (i.e., IPSS)	7	4	9.3 (2.2-12.0)	Barry et al, 1992a, 1992b
Benign Prostatic Hyperplasia Health-Related Quality of Life Survey (BPH-HRQOL)	49	4	7.3 (1.8-12.0)	Lukacs et al, 1997
Benign Prostatic Hyperplasia Impact Index (BPHII)	4	4	9.8 (5.9-11.8)	Barry et al, 1995b
Danish Prostatic Symptom Score-1 (DAN-PSS-1)	15	4	8.1 (2.2-12.0)	Meyhoff et al, 1993
International Continence Society–Male Questionnaire (ICSmale)	34	4	5.4 (1.2-12.0)	Donovan et al, 2000
International Continence Society–Quality of Life questionnaire (ICSQoL)	8	4	6.9 (3.6-9.0)	Donovan et al, 1997
Nocturia Quality of Life Questionnaire (NQOL)	13	2	5.3 (2.3-9.3)	Mock et al, 2008
Overactive Bladder Symptom and Health-Related Quality of Life Questionnaire (OAB-q)	33	4	4.7 (0.6-12.0)	Coyne et al, 2005
Urgency Questionnaire (UQ)	19	1	4.2 (1.0-12.0)	Coyne et al, 2004
Primary Overactive Bladder Symptom Questionnaire (POSQ)	5	2	6.2 (2.4-12.0)	Matza et al, 2005
Patient Perception of Bladder Condition (PPBC)	1	At present	8.8 (8.1-9.4)	Matza et al, 2005
PROSTATITIS				
National Institutes of Health Chronic Prostatitis Symptom Index (NIH-CPSI)	9	1	7.7 (3.8-11.7)	Litwin et al, 1999
Giessen Prostatitis Symptom Score (GPSS)	12	Not specified	8.8 (1.2-12.0)	Brahler et al, 1997
Nickel and Sorensen	20	1	8.7 (5.0-12.0)	Nickel and Sorensen, 1996
Neal and Moon	4	Not specified	12.0 (12.0-12.0)	Neal and Moon, 1994
ERECTILE DYSFUNCTION				
International Index of Erectile Function (IIEF)	15	4	7.7 (4.7-12.0)	Rosen et al, 1997
Self-Esteem and Relationship Questionnaire (SEAR)	14	4	4.8 (2.1-12.0)	Cappelleri et al, 2004
Male Sexual Health Questionnaire (MSHQ)	25	4	9.0 (5.2-12.0)	Rosen et al, 2004
Brief Sexual Function Inventory (BSFI)	11	4	6.9 (5.0-12.0)	Mykletun et al, 2006
Erectile Dysfunction Inventory of Treatment Satisfaction Questionnaire (EDITS)	11	4	6.7 (4.4-12.0)	Althof et al, 1999
Erection Distress Scale (EDS)	5	Not specified	6.7 (3.6-9.0)	Seftel et al, 2007
URINARY INCONTINENCE				
Incontinence Impact Questionnaire (IIQ)	30	Not specified	7.0 (2.3-12.0)	Shumaker et al, 1994
Incontinence Impact Questionnaire Short Form (IIQ-7)	7	Not specified	12.0 (4.4-12.0)	Uebersax et al, 1995
Urological Distress Inventory (UDI)	19	Not specified	5.8 (0.8-12.0)	Shumaker et al, 1994

Continued

TABLE 4-1 Characteristics of Health-Related Quality-of-Life (HRQOL) Instruments in Urologic Diseases—cont'd

INSTRUMENT NAME	ITEMS	TIME RECALL, WEEKS	READING GRADE LEVEL OF ITEMS, MEDIAN (RANGE)	REFERENCE
Urogenital Distress Inventory Short Form (UDI-6)	6	Not specified	8.4 (4.8-12.0)	Uebersax et al, 1995
International Consultation on Incontinence Questionnaire–Female Lower Urinary Tract Symptoms (ICIQ-FLUTS)	12	4	1.0 (0.5-9.3)	Brookes et al, 2004
International Consultation on Incontinence Questionnaire (ICIQ)	4	4	4.6 (0.7-8.7)	Avery et al, 2004
Symptoms of Incontinence Questionnaire (i.e., PRAFAB-Q)	20	Not specified	6.7 (2.2-11.9)	Hendriks et al, 2008
Urinary Incontinence Quality of Life Questionnaire (I-QOL)	22	Not specified	8.9 (4.3-12.0)	Wagner et al, 1996
Stress-Related Leak, Emptying Ability, Anatomy, Protection, Inhibition, Quality of Life, Mobility and Mental Status (SEAPI-QMM)	15	Not specified	9.4 (3.6-12.0)	Raz and Erickson, 1992
King's Health Questionnaire (KHQ)	21	At present	4.5 (0.7-12.0)	Kelleher et al, 1997
Bristol Female Lower Urinary Tract Symptoms Questionnaire (BFLUTS)	33	Not specified	7.1 (2.2-12.0)	Jackson et al, 1996
Bristol Female Lower Urinary Tract Symptoms Questionnaire Short Form (BFLUTS-SF)	19	Not specified	6.3 (3.2-12.0)	Brookes et al, 2004
Urge-Incontinence Impact Questionnaire (U-IIQ)	32	4	4.1 (0.5-12.0)	Lubeck et al, 1999
Urge-Urinary Distress Inventory (U-UDI)	10	4	4.9 (1.8-12.0)	Lubeck et al, 1999
Symptom Severity Index (SSI)	13	1 and 52	3.6 (2.2-6.2)	Black et al, 1996
Symptom Impact Index (SII)	3	Not specified	7.3 (4.9-10.8)	Black et al, 1996
Stress and Urge Incontinence and Quality of Life Questionnaire	9	1 and 26	5.8 (0.8-12.0)	Kulseng-Hanssen and Borstad, 2003
Urinary Incontinence Severity Score (UISS)	10	Not specified	9.2 (2.8-12.0)	Stach-Lempinen et al, 2001
CONTILIFE	28	2 and 4	5.6 (0.8-12.0)	Amarenco et al, 2003
Female Incontinence Severity Index (ISI)	2	Not specified	5.8 (0.8-10.7)	Sandvik et al, 1993
INTERSTITIAL CYSTITIS				
O'Leary-Sant Interstitial Cystitis Symptom Index and Problem Index (OSICSI-PI)	23	4	7.1 (2.3-11.0)	O'Leary et al, 1997
Pelvic Pain and Urgency/Frequency Questionnaire (PUF)	8	Not specified	4.9 (0.5-12.0)	Parsons et al, 2002
Female Genitourinary Pain Index (FGUPI)	9	1	7.7 (3.8-11.7)	Parsons et al, 2002
KIDNEY CANCER				
Functional Assessment of Cancer Therapy–Kidney Symptom Index (FKSI-15)	15	1	1.3 (0.3-8.2)	Cella et al, 2006
RENAL TRANSPLANT				
End-Stage Renal Disease Symptom Checklist–Transplantation Module (ESRD-SCL)	43	4	6.2 (1.8-12.0)	Franke et al, 1999
Kidney Disease and Quality of Life Questionnaire (KDQOL-36)	36	4	4.9 (0.8-12.0)	Hays et al, 1997
URINARY TRACT INFECTION				
Activity Impairment Assessment (AIA)	5	1 and 7	9.7 (3.6-12.0)	Wild et al, 2005
SEXUALITY				
Index of Premature Ejaculation (IPE)	10	4	9.1 (1.3-12.0)	Althof et al, 2006
Sexual Quality of Life (Male) Instrument (SQOL-M)	11	Not specified	8.6 (2.6-12.0)	Abraham et al, 2008
Profile of Female Sexual Function (PFSF)	38	Not specified	4.3 (0.5-12.0)	Derogatis et al, 2004
Brief Profile of Female Sexual Function (B-PFSF)	7	Not specified	3.9 (0.9-9.2)	Rust et al, 2007
Male Sexual Quotient Questionnaire (MSQ)	10	6	7.0 (1.4-12.0)	Abdo, 2007

instrument, the table includes the number of items, recall time, and Flesch-Kinkaid reading grade level (Flesch, 1948; Kincaid et al, 1975).

General Health-Related Quality-of-Life Instruments

General quality-of-life instruments have been extensively studied and validated in many types of patients, sick and well. Examples include the RAND Medical Outcomes Study 36-Item Health Survey, also known as the SF-36 (Ware and Sherbourne, 1992; Hays et al, 1993; McHorney et al, 1994), the Quality of Well-Being scale (Kaplan et al, 1979; Bush et al, 1982; Anderson et al, 1989), the Sickness Impact Profile (Bergner et al, 1976a, 1976b; Carter et al, 1976; Martin et al, 1976; Pollard et al, 1976; Gilson et al, 1980; Bergner et al, 1981), and the Nottingham Health Profile (Martini and McDowell, 1976; Hunt et al, 1981). Each assesses various components of HRQOL including physical and emotional functioning, social functioning, and symptoms. Each has been thoroughly validated and tested for reliability, validity, and responsiveness. Another approach to quantifying general HRQOL is to blend a self-assessment of physical, emotional, and social functioning and well-being with a self-report of preferences, or utilities, for those health states. Developed by the Euroqol Group, a measurement collaborative, the EQ-5D is such an instrument (Brooks et al, 1991; Johnson et al, 1998; Johnson and Coons, 1998; Johnson et al, 2005; Shaw et al, 2005; Nan et al, 2007; Pickard et al, 2012).

Benign Disease–Targeted Health-Related Quality-of-Life Instruments

The best-known outcomes instrument in urology is no doubt the American Urological Association Symptom Index (AUASI) (Barry et al, 1992a, 1992b; O'Leary et al, 1992; Barry et al, 1995a). Its simplicity belies its elegance and utility. It includes seven items, each self-rated on a scale of 0 to 5, yielding a summary score that ranges from 0 to 35. Symptom scores are considered mild (0 to 7), moderate (8 to 19), or severe (20 to 35). It has been used to longitudinally assess symptoms in men treated for prostate cancer (Gore et al, 2010a). With the addition of a separate quality-of-life item, the worldwide urology community embraced the AUASI as the International Prostate Symptom Score (IPSS) (Plante et al, 1996; Badia et al, 1997, 1998; Garcia-Losa et al, 2001).

Modeled after the AUASI, and in an attempt to standardize assessment of urinary incontinence and allow cross-cultural comparisons, the Scientific Committee of the International Consultation on Incontinence (ICIQ) supported the development and validation of a universally applicable questionnaire for research as well as clinical practice (Abrams et al, 2010). The ICIQ–Urinary Incontinence Short Form has now been translated into 30 languages (Abrams et al, 2006; Hashim et al, 2006; Klovning et al, 2009; Timmermans et al, 2013). Other high-quality questionnaires were included under the ICIQ umbrella and are available at www.iciq.net. Table 4-2 details some of the validated and published ICIQ modules endorsed by the Fourth International Consultation on Incontinence (Abrams et al, 2010).

Cancer-Specific Health-Related Quality-of-Life Instruments

Because of the well-documented impact of malignancies and their treatment on HRQOL, cancer-specific domains have also been investigated extensively. Numerous instruments have been developed and tested that measure the special impact of cancer (regardless of primary site) on patients' routine activities. Readers are directed to the Quality of Life Instruments Database (www.proqolid.org) for guidance when selecting an instrument for quality-of-life measurement in studies of prostate or other cancers.

Selecting a Health-Related Quality-of-Life Instrument

Investigators or clinicians considering measuring HRQOL in a clinical study or in clinical practice should base their choice of instrument(s) on the particular population being studied and the clinical questions being asked. Using previously validated instruments, to the extent to which they are applicable and appropriate, obviates the need for an arduous process of instrument development and validation. Use of a general and a disease-specific module in combination is suitable for most studies. However, if a particular domain (e.g., pain) is the focus of the study, specific, expanded questionnaires focusing on the area of interest should be sought. Respondent burden needs to be considered, particularly for longitudinal studies in which subjects will complete the same instruments multiple times. Pretesting of instruments that will be used in clinical studies is advisable.

TABLE 4-2 International Consultation on Incontinence Questionnaire (ICIQ) Modules

MODULE	QUESTIONNAIRE FROM WHICH DERIVED	SYMPTOMS ASSESSED	REFERENCE
ICIQ-FLUTS	BFLUTS Short Form (Brookes et al, 2004)	Female urinary	Brookes et al, 2004
ICIQ-FLUTS Long Form	BFLUTS (Jackson et al, 1996)	Female urinary	Jackson et al, 1996
ICIQ-MLUTS	ICSmale Short Form (Donovan et al, 2000)	Male urinary	Donovan et al, 2000
ICIQ-MLUTS Long Form	ICSmale (Donovan et al, 1996)	Male urinary	Donovan et al, 1996
ICIQ-LUTSqol	KHQ (Kelleher et al, 1997)	Urinary quality of life	Kelleher et al, 1997
ICIQ-N	ICSmale (Donovan et al, 1996) BFLUTS (Jackson et al, 1996)	Nocturia	Donovan et al, 1996 Jackson et al, 1996
ICIQ-Nqol	N-QOL (Abraham et al, 2004)	Nocturia quality of life	Abraham et al, 2004
ICIQ-VS		Vaginal	Abrams et al, 2006
ICIQ-B		Bowel	Abrams et al, 2006
ICIQ-FLUTSsex	BFLUTS (Jackson et al, 1996)	Female sexual related to urinary symptoms	Jackson et al, 1996
ICIQ-MLUTSsex	ICSmale (Donovan et al, 1996)	Male sexual related to urinary symptoms	Donovan et al, 1996
ICIQ-OAB	ICSmale (Donovan et al, 1996) BFLUTS (Jackson et al, 1996)	Overactive bladder	Donovan et al, 1996 Jackson et al, 1996
ICIQ-OABqol	OABq (Coyne et al, 2002)	Overactive bladder quality of life	Coyne et al, 2002
ICIQ-UI Short Form		Urinary incontinence	Abrams et al, 2006

Psychometric Validation of New Health-Related Quality-of-Life Instruments

The development and validation of new instruments and scales is a long and arduous process. When scales and instruments are developed, they are first pilot tested to ensure that the target population can understand and complete them with ease. Pilot testing is usually preceded by work with focus groups, and includes formal cognitive testing. Pilot testing can reveal problems that might otherwise go unrecognized by researchers. For example, many terms that are commonly used by medical professionals are poorly understood by patients. In fact, because the average adult reads at the fifth- to eighth-grade level, items should be drafted at no higher than an eighth-grade reading level (Paasche-Orlow et al, 2003; Osborn et al, 2007; Paasche-Orlow and Wolf, 2007, 2010; Osborn et al, 2011; Waite et al, 2013). In addition, the digital divide between those of low and high socioeconomic status should be considered (Levy et al, 2013).

Scales and instruments are also evaluated for three fundamental statistical properties—reliability, validity, and responsiveness (Litwin, 1995; Ware et al, 1996; Resnick and Nahm, 2001; DeVellis, 2011).

Reliability

Reliability (Table 4-3) refers to how free the scale is of measurement error—that is, what proportion of a patient's test score is true and what proportion is the result of chance variation. Two of the most commonly used metrics are test-retest and internal consistency reliability. *Test-retest reliability* is the most commonly used indicator of survey instrument reliability. It is measured by having the same respondents complete a survey at two different points in time to see how stable their responses are. It is a measure of how reproducible a set of results is. When measuring test-retest reliability, one must be careful not to select items or scales that measure variables likely to change over short periods of time. Variables that are likely to change over a given period of time will produce low test-retest reliability in measurement instruments. This does not mean that the survey instrument is performing poorly but simply that the attribute itself has changed.

When measuring test-retest reliability, one must also consider that individuals may become familiar with the items and answer partly on the basis of their memory of what they answered the last time. Called the *practice effect*, this presents a challenging problem to address in measures of test-retest reliability over short periods of time. As a result of the practice effect, test-retest reliability figures can be falsely inflated. *Alternate-form reliability* provides one way to escape the problem of the practice effect. It involves using differently worded items to measure the same attribute. Questions and responses are reworded or their order is changed to produce two items that are similar but not identical. One way to test alternate-form reliability is to change the wording of the response sets without changing the meaning. Another common method to test alternate-form reliability is to change the actual wording of the items themselves.

The correlation between two data sets from the same individual is commonly known as *intraobserver reliability*. It measures the stability of responses from the same respondent and is a form of test-retest reliability. *Interobserver (inter-rater) reliability* provides a measure of how well two or more evaluators agree in their assessment of a variable. When survey instruments are self-administered and designed to measure the respondent's own behaviors or attitudes, interobserver reliability is not used. *Internal consistency reliability* is a measure of the similarity of an individual's responses across several items, indicating the homogeneity of a scale (Henson, 2001). It is applied not to single items but to groups of items that are thought to measure different aspects of the same concept.

Validity

Validity (Table 4-4) refers to how well the item, scale, or instrument measures the attribute it is intended to measure. Validity has three general forms: content, criterion, and construct. *Content validity*, sometimes referred to as *face validity*, involves a subjective assessment of the scope and completeness of a scale and is usually measured in the early stages of an instrument's development by experts and through use of patient focus groups. The assessment of content validity typically involves an organized review of an instrument's contents to ensure that it includes everything it should and does not include anything it should not. *Criterion validity* is a more quantitative approach to assessing the performance of scales and instruments. It requires the correlation of scale scores with results from other established tests (concurrent validity) or with future measurable outcomes (predictive validity). *Concurrent validity* requires that the survey instrument in question be judged against some other method that is acknowledged as a gold standard for assessing the same variable. It may be a published psychometric index, a scientific measurement of some factor, or another generally accepted test. *Predictive validity* is the ability of a survey instrument to forecast future events, behaviors, attitudes, or outcomes. It may be used during the course of a study to predict response to a stimulus, success of an intervention, or time to a medical end point. *Construct*

TABLE 4-3   Reliability Assessments for Health-Related Quality-of-Life Instruments

TYPE OF RELIABILITY	CHARACTERISTICS	COMMENTS
Test-retest	Measures the stability of responses over time, typically in the same group of respondents	Requires administration of survey to a sample at two different and appropriate points in time. Time points that are too far apart may produce diminished reliability estimates that reflect actual change over time in the variable of interest.
Intraobserver	Measures the stability of responses over time, in the same individual respondent	Requires completion of a survey by an individual at two different and appropriate points in time. Time points that are too far apart may produce diminished reliability estimates that reflect actual change over time in the variable of interest.
Alternate-form	Uses differently worded stems or response sets to obtain the same information about a specific topic	Requires two items in which the wording is different but aimed at the same specific variable and at the same vocabulary level.
Internal consistency	Measures how well several items in a scale vary together in a sample	Usually requires a computer and statistician to carry out calculations.
Interobserver	Measures how well two or more different respondents rate the same phenomenon	May be used to demonstrate reliability of a survey or may itself be the variable of interest in a study.

TABLE 4-4 Validity Assessments for Health-Related Quality-of-Life Instruments

TYPE OF VALIDITY	CHARACTERISTICS	COMMENTS
Content	Formal expert review of how good an item or series of items appear	Usually assessed by individuals with expertise in some aspect of the subject under study
Criterion: Concurrent	Measures how well the item or scale correlates with gold-standard measures of the same variable	Requires the identification of an established, generally accepted gold standard
Criterion: Predictive	Measures how well the item or scale predicts expected future observations	Used to predict outcomes or events of significance that the item or scale might subsequently be used to predict
Construct	A theoretic measure of how meaningful a survey instrument is, usually after years of experience by numerous investigators	Not easily quantifiable

validity is the most valuable yet most difficult way of assessing a survey instrument. It is a measure of how meaningful the scale or survey instrument is when in practical use.

Responsiveness

Responsiveness of an HRQOL instrument refers to how sensitive the scales are to change over time (Murawski and Miederhoff, 1997; Terwee et al, 2003). That is, a survey may be reliable and valid when used at a single point in time, but in some circumstances it must also be able to detect meaningful improvements or decrements in quality of life during longitudinal studies. The instrument must "react" in a time frame that is relevant for patients over time. Because HRQOL may change over time, longitudinal measurement of these outcomes is important. In urology, widely used instruments such as the University of California–Los Angeles Prostate Cancer Index and the National Institutes of Health Chronic Prostatitis Symptom Index are highly responsive to clinical changes.

Comparison Groups

Prospective, longitudinal data collection beginning at baseline before treatment is always best because this approach may reveal time-dependent evolution of HRQOL domains (Litwin et al, 2001; Malcolm et al, 2010; Reeve et al, 2012). Patients may then serve as their own controls. Assessing HRQOL at baseline before treatment allows for the inclusion of baseline age- or comorbidity-related changes that should not be attributed to treatment. This approach facilitates the stratification of discriminants from determinants of HRQOL.

Caveats on the Collection of Health-Related Quality-of-Life Data

The overarching goals of HRQOL research are summarized in Box 4-1. Although there are some single instruments that are multidimensional, many quality-of-life researchers have endorsed a "battery approach," in which the various components of HRQOL are measured with different scales to ensure that each domain receives adequate attention. Longer instruments can provide greater precision, but they also increase the chance that patients will tire of the exercise and not provide reliable or valid answers. Hence, shorter instruments are usually preferable when one is performing HRQOL measurements in such circumstances. In general, it is easier and more efficient to use established instruments that have already undergone psychometric validation. Use of HRQOL data collected using published instruments allows the researcher to compare the study results with data from other samples or diverse populations with various chronic diseases. Nevertheless, sometimes it is necessary to develop new questionnaire items to ensure that a particular concept is adequately evaluated. Under such circumstances new

BOX 4-1 Quality-of-Life Objectives in Research and Practice

- To assess overall treatment efficacy including subjective morbidity
- To help determine whether the goals of treatment have been met
- To educate patients and clinicians about the full spectrum of treatment outcomes
- To facilitate medical decision making
- To provide the defining issue if treatments are otherwise equivalent

scales can be tested for reliability and validity during the course of data collection.

HEALTH SERVICES RESEARCH METHODOLOGIES

Retrospective Review of the Medical Record

The image of an "outcomes" researcher retrospectively reviewing charts to understand variations in an outcome of interest originated in the Crimean War, when Florence Nightingale documented high death rates among injured soldiers treated at overcrowded facilities with poor hygiene (Cook, 1914; Kopf, 1916). Although retrospective chart review is only one arrow in a health services researcher's quiver, it can unearth important health systems failings, such as poor follow-up of positive fecal occult blood testing results at the time of hospital admission (Scales et al, 2006). Such failings can then be targeted for quality improvement interventions.

Secondary Data Analysis

Secondary data involve an analysis of information collected by someone other than the researcher. Examples include hospital and outpatient claims, censuses, and pharmaceutical records, as well as qualitative data obtained by a third party. One of the main benefits of secondary data analyses is that the data have already been collected; a corollary downfall is that the researcher is limited to those data. In selecting an optimal data set, criteria to consider include availability of information regarding the data collection process, issues related to study design, the need for adjustment for sample design characteristics, the relative robustness of the data set, and the time required to procure and analyze the data (Litwin et al, 2005b). If several different data sets are chosen for a common venture, selecting complementary rather than overlapping data sets affords a view through the broadest possible lens. One limitation of secondary data analysis is the reliance of accurate coding, without which overestimation or underestimation is possible.

Community-Partnered Participatory Research

Community-partnered participatory research involves a collaborative process among researchers, communities, and others; all partners collaborate and are valued equally (Humphreys et al, 2008; Chung et al, 2009; Khodyakov et al, 2009; Wells and Jones, 2009; Chung et al, 2010, 2011; Lizaola et al, 2011; Hunt et al, 2012; Wells et al, 2013a, 2013b). **Its goal is to develop, implement, and disseminate work that will benefit a community.** Community strengths can then be celebrated, and community needs not only identified, but also addressed from within. For example, interventions in which urologists partner with barbershops help promote prostate cancer knowledge and, when appropriate, screening (Releford et al, 2010). Results are then shared with the community to promote ongoing partnerships and build trust and capacity. Interventions do not need to focus on disadvantaged communities; when researchers collaborate with physician practices and feed findings back to those groups, substantial improvement can be made in clinical care, including use of immediate intravesical therapy after resection for non–muscle invasive bladder cancer and appropriate metastatic workup for men with prostate cancer (Miller et al, 2010; Barocas et al, 2013b).

Implementation Science

In medicine, translating good evidence into broadly implemented practice takes, on average, 17 years (Pfeffer and Sutton, 2006). Delays in uptake exist in medical treatment to facilitate passage of urinary stones (Hollingsworth et al, 2006; Scales et al, 2007), chemoprevention of prostate cancer (Hamilton et al, 2010), and weight loss for urinary incontinence (Bland et al, 2003; Subak et al, 2009; Wing et al, 2010; Holroyd-Leduc et al, 2011; St Sauver et al, 2011; Phelan et al, 2012). Implementation science seeks to compress the timeline. Implementation research studies methods for systematically adopting evidence-based practices into routine care, to improve quality and effectiveness (Stetler et al, 2008; Proctor et al, 2009; Eccles et al, 2012; Methodology Committee of the Patient-Centered Outcomes Research Institute, 2012; Yano et al, 2012; Meissner et al, 2013). It encompasses field research, clinical work, communities, and health policy. In surgery, implementation of evidence-based infection control processes using comprehensive unit-based safety programs reduces rates of surgical site infections (Wick et al, 2012). For urologists, evidence-based guidelines abound (Davis et al, 2012; Sharlip et al, 2012; Carter et al, 2013a; Cookson et al, 2013; Donat et al, 2013), but broad implementation remains an unmet challenge (Chamie et al, 2011; Chamie and Litwin, 2011; Chamie et al, 2012b; Strope et al, 2011, 2012). Implementation strategies may focus on small-group continuing education with urologists and primary care providers, lectures, patient education materials, and public endorsement by national figures (Puech et al, 1998). Engagement of all stakeholders during guideline development and dissemination is key (Smith and Hillner, 2001).

Qualitative Research

Qualitative research involves interviews, group discussions, field notes, and observations. It allows exploration of aspects of care that may not be accessible from other data sources, and issues may be unearthed that were not readily apparent at the beginning of data collection. Qualitative methods can also be used to explore options for overcoming obstacles, such as renegotiating masculine identity after treatment for prostate cancer (Maliski et al, 2008). Methodologic rigor must be applied to data collection and analysis, and data analysis options include coding, recursive abstraction, interpretive techniques, and mechanical techniques (Erickson, 2012).

FUTURE IMPLICATIONS

Balancing Analysis of Current Shortcomings with Interventions for Change

That current urologic care leaves significant space for improvement has now been well documented. Likewise, disparities in quality of care often overshadow the more salient understanding that care is often mediocre, even in the best circumstances, and must be improved for all individuals. **Although further analyses of shortcomings and disparities are important, the most pressing need is development and broad implementation of interventions that can improve care.** For example, a novel method of patient preference elicitation using conjoint analysis improves decision-making quality in men with prostate cancer (Saigal et al, 2012). Developing similar interventions and identifying strategies to broadly implement them will allow urology to remain at the forefront of health care innovation and value.

Patient-Centeredness and Comparative Effectiveness

Comparative effectiveness research uses outcomes data to guide health care policy. The American Recovery and Reinvestment Act of 2009 invested $1.1 billion to fund comparative effectiveness research (American Recovery and Reinvestment Act, 2009), and the recently enacted Patient Protection and Affordable Care Act formalized a private, nonprofit Patient-Centered Outcomes Research Institute (www.pcori.org) to equitably distribute funding (Selby et al, 2012). The allocated funds target not only reviews of existing evidence, but also new prospective, randomized trials.

Evidence-Based Health Care Policy

To maintain control over treatment decisions, urologists must work fastidiously to improve value and ensure broad implementation of evidence-based practices. For instance, if PSA screening is to continue, more nuanced strategies must be implemented to minimize overdiagnosis and overtreatment (Gulati et al, 2013) Policy makers can use several levers to encourage evidence-based care. For example, when reimbursement levels were high, androgen deprivation therapy was overused in treatment of localized prostate cancer (Cooperberg et al, 2003; Shahinian et al, 2005a; Sharifi et al, 2005; Badiozamani et al, 2009), despite well documented noxious effects (Potosky et al, 2002; Shahinian et al, 2005b; Saigal et al, 2007) Inappropriate use of androgen deprivation fell significantly after the Medicare Modernization Act lowered reimbursement (Elliott et al, 2010; Shahinian et al, 2010; Gilbert et al, 2011).

Maximizing Value

Ultimately, a urologist cares for an individual, not merely that individual's urologic needs. Whereas organizations such as the U.S. Food and Drug Administration (FDA) may approve a medication or device if it is "safe and effective" (Meadows, 2002; Institute of Medicine, 2011), physicians are held to a higher standard. We must consider not only whether a drug extends life by 3 to 5 months (Kantoff et al, 2010; de Bono et al, 2011; Fizazi et al, 2011; Cabot et al, 2012; Parker et al, 2013), but whether use of the drug is sensible in the context of competing priorities. Examples of alternative investments include early childhood and depression: each dollar invested in a child yields $7 in return (Campbell and Ramey, 1994; Clarke and Campbell, 1998; Campbell et al, 2012), and of all socioeconomic and clinical variables, depression is singly linked with health (Covinsky et al, 1997a; Jackson-Triche et al, 2000) and wealth (Wells et al, 2000; Beddington et al, 2008). **As our population ages (Vincent and Velkoff, 2010), urologists are uniquely empowered to continue to lead the effort to maximize value and shape rational policies that will make each person as healthy and happy as possible.**

KEY POINTS

- Health services research focuses on access to care, cost of care, quality of care, health systems, and population health.
- The "value" of a health care service or intervention is defined as patient-centered health outcomes divided by cost. Considering cost in the context of value can help policy makers decide which interventions should be amplified and which may be reduced.
- That variation in health care spending does not correlate with outcomes suggests that good outcomes can be achieved with lowered cost, and that current spending can be targeted more thoughtfully. In urology, significant hospital-level variation exists in outcomes and readmission after surgery.
- Quality of care research evaluates "the degree to which health services for individuals and populations increase the likelihood of desired health outcomes and are consistent with current professional knowledge." Descriptive quality measures abound, but for quality metrics to affect outcomes, they must be based on solid evidence, be measurable, and have resources devoted to tracking and improving them.
- Health-related quality of life (HRQOL) encompasses a wide range of human experience including the daily necessities of life such as food and shelter, intrapersonal and interpersonal responses to illness, and activities associated with professional fulfillment and personal happiness.
- To maintain control over treatment decisions, urologists must work fastidiously to improve value and ensure broad implementation of evidence-based practices.

REFERENCES

The complete reference list is available online at www.expertconsult.com.

SUGGESTED READINGS

Andersen RM, Davidson PL. Improving access to care in America. Changing the U.S. health care system: key issues in health services policy and management. 3rd ed. San Francisco: Jossey-Bass; 2007. p. 3–31.

Barry MJ, Fowler FJ Jr, O'Leary MP, et al. The American Urological Association symptom index for benign prostatic hyperplasia. The Measurement Committee of the American Urological Association. J Urol 1992b;148: 1549–57, discussion 1564.

Litwin MS, Hays RD, Fink A, et al. Quality-of-life outcomes in men treated for localized prostate cancer. JAMA 1995;273:129–35.

Miller DC, Murtagh DS, Suh RS, et al. Establishment of a urological surgery quality collaborative. J Urol 2010;184:2485–90.

Orszag PR, Emanuel EJ. Health care reform and cost control. N Engl J Med 2010;363:601–3.

5 Core Principles of Perioperative Care

Manish A. Vira, MD, and Joph Steckel, MD, FACS

While the practice of urology continues to move toward office-based and nonsurgical treatments, the diversity of genitourinary disease requires that the practicing urologist be familiar with perioperative surgical principles to improve clinical care. This chapter provides the reader with basic tools to understand the preoperative assessment, intraoperative techniques, and postoperative management necessary to promote a culture of patient safety and optimal surgical outcomes.

PREOPERATIVE EVALUATION

The perioperative management of patients undergoing urologic surgery continues to evolve. Over the past two decades, the economics of health care has added increasing pressure for more outpatient surgery, decreased hospital stays, and decreased complication rates. Furthermore, the acuity of surgical patients is increasing in that patients are older with more significant comorbidities. It has become standard for patients undergoing even the most sophisticated and complex urologic procedures in the hospital to be admitted on the same day as the surgery. **Therefore the urologic surgeon is responsible for ensuring that the patient has been thoroughly evaluated by the other physicians on the health care team and arrives in the operating room in the most optimized medical condition.** The preoperative use of appropriate medical specialist consultations will result in improved patient safety and obviate the need for unnecessary cancelled surgeries resulting from the inadequacy of medical optimization.

PRESURGICAL TESTING

The goal of presurgical testing is to identify an undiagnosed comorbidity, an undertreated medical problem, or a significant exacerbation of existing comorbid illness that may affect the operative outcome (Townsend et al, 2008). Ideally, the preoperative evaluation should be individualized on the basis of age, history, physical examination findings, and the surgical procedure to be performed. Although most hospitals or ambulatory surgery centers have requirements for baseline evaluation, routine testing has never been shown to be cost-effective. In fact, the results of routine testing are less predictive of perioperative morbidity than the American Society of Anesthesiologists (ASA) status or the American Heart Association (AHA) and American College of Cardiology (ACC) guidelines for surgical risk. A recent systematic review found no evidence to support routine preoperative testing in patients undergoing noncardiac elective surgery (Johansson et al, 2013). Most commonly, presurgical testing includes complete blood count (CBC); basic metabolic panel (BMP); prothrombin time (PT), partial thromboplastin time (PTT), and international normalized ratio (INR) (controversial); electrocardiogram (ECG); and chest radiograph. The routine ordering of a PT/PTT in a patient not currently on warfarin or in a patient without a prior history of increased bleeding with other surgical procedures is controversial, and these tests can be omitted in the majority of patients. **Any woman of childbearing age, unless the ovaries or uterus have been previously surgically removed, must undergo a urine pregnancy test on the morning of surgery** (Halaszynski et al, 2004). The value of a preoperative ECG in identification of underlying acute cardiac disease and prediction of perioperative cardiac morbidity is also controversial. Some studies have shown that ECG abnormalities have no significant predictive value (Goldman et al, 1978), whereas others found that an abnormal ECG was the best diagnostic predictor of an adverse cardiac event (Carliner et al, 1985). Nonetheless, current recommendations, in general, suggest that a preoperative ECG be obtained from patients older than 40 years or those with a history of any cardiac disease. Similarly, the routine preoperative use of a chest radiograph, in the absence of preexisting cardiopulmonary disease, is not indicated. Overall, even an ASA Task Force on Preanesthesia Evaluation could not make firm recommendations other than "preoperative tests may be ordered, required, or performed on a selective basis for purposes of guiding or optimizing perioperative management" (Practice advisory for preanesthesia evaluation, 2002).

SURGICAL RISK EVALUATION

American Society of Anesthesiologists Classification and Risk Stratification

Approximately 27 million patients undergo surgery each year in the United States, and 8 million (30%) have significant coronary artery disease or other cardiac comorbidities. Appropriately, the cardiovascular system is targeted during the preoperative assessment of patients. The ASA classification was first developed in 1961 and has been revised to categorize risk into six stratifications (Box 5-1).

The goal of the classification system is to assess the overall physical status of the patient before surgery (not to assess surgical risk), and although quite subjective, it remains a significant independent predictor of mortality (Davenport et al, 2006). Other tools to assess the preoperative risks were developed by multivariate statistical analysis of patient-related factors correlated with surgical outcomes. One such scoring system, Goldman's criteria (Table 5-1), assigns points to easily reproducible characteristics. The points are then added to compute the perioperative risk of cardiac-related complications. Another system, the Cardiac Risk Index, simplified this concept; it uses only six predictors to estimate cardiac complication risk in noncardiac surgical patients (Table 5-2) (Akhtar and Silverman, 2004).

Cardiac Evaluation

The preoperative cardiac evaluation, which consists of an initial history and physical examination and ECG, attempts to identify potential serious cardiac disorders such as coronary artery disease, heart failure, symptomatic arrhythmias, the presence of a pacemaker or implantable defibrillator, or a history of orthostatic hypotension (Eagle et al, 1996). Furthermore, it is essential

---

BOX 5-1 American Society of Anesthesiologists (ASA) Classification

ASA Class I—Normal healthy patient

ASA Class II—Patient with mild systemic disease

ASA Class III—Patient with severe systemic disease that limits activity but is not incapacitating

ASA Class IV—Patient who has incapacitating disease that is a constant threat to life

ASA Class V—Moribund patient not expected to survive 24 hours with or without an operation

ASA Class VI—A declared brain-dead patient whose organs are being removed for donor purposes

ASA Class E—In the event of emergency surgery, an E is added after the Roman numeral (in I through V classes)

TABLE 5-1 Goldman's Cardiac Risk Index

PATIENT RISK FACTORS	POINTS
Third heart sound or jugular venous distention	11
Recent myocardial infarction	10
Nonsinus rhythm or premature atrial contraction on electrocardiogram	7
More than five premature ventricular contractions	7
Age older than 70 yr	5
Emergency operations	4
Poor general medical condition	3
Intrathoracic, intraperitoneal, or aortic surgery	3
Significant valvular aortic stenosis	3
For noncardiac surgery, the risk of cardiac complications is: • 6-12 points = 7% risk • 13-25 points = 14% risk • >26 points = 78% risk	

Modified from Akhtar S, Silverman DG. Assessment and management of patients with ischemic heart disease. Crit Care Med 2004;32:S126–36.

---

to define the severity and stability of existing cardiac disease before surgery. Cardiac-specific risk is also altered by the patient's functional capacity, age, and other comorbid conditions such as diabetes, peripheral vascular disease, renal dysfunction, and chronic obstructive pulmonary disease (COPD). The ACC and AHA recently collaborated to develop guidelines regarding perioperative cardiac evaluation before surgery (Fleisher et al, 2007a). In general, the guidelines use three categories of clinical risk predictors: clinical markers, functional capacity, and type of surgical procedure (Eagle et al, 2002).

Clinical Markers

The major clinical predictors of increased perioperative cardiovascular risk are a documented acute myocardial infarction less than 7 days previously, a recent myocardial infarction (defined as at least 7 days but less than 1 month before surgery), unstable angina, evidence of any ischemic burden by clinical symptoms or noninvasive testing, decompensated heart failure, significant arrhythmias, and severe valvular disease. Intermediate predictors include mild angina, previous myocardial infarction by history or pathologic Q waves, compensated heart failure, diabetes, or renal insufficiency (creatinine >2 mg/dL). Minor predictors of risk are advanced age, abnormal ECG, rhythms other than sinus (i.e., atrial fibrillation), history of stroke, or uncontrolled systemic hypertension. The historical dictum suggesting that elective surgery after a myocardial infarction be performed after a 3- to 6-month interval is now currently avoided (Tarhan et al, 1972). **The ACC cardiovascular database committee stratifies risk on the basis of the severity of the myocardial infarction and the likelihood of reinfarction based on a recent exercise stress test.** However, in the absence of adequate clinical trials on which to base firm recommendations, it is reasonable to wait 4 to 6 weeks after myocardial infarction to perform elective surgery.

Functional Capacity

Functional capacity, or one's ability to meet aerobic demands for a specific activity, is quantified as metabolic equivalents (METs). For example, a 4-MET demand is comparable with a patient's ability to climb two flights of stairs. This simple measurement continues to be an easy and inexpensive method to determine a patient's cardiopulmonary functional capacity (Biccard, 2005). **The Duke Activity Status Index (Table 5-3) allows the physician to easily determine a patient's functional capacity** (Hlatky et al, 1989). **In general, a capacity of 4 METs indicates no further need for invasive cardiac evaluation.**

Surgery-Specific Cardiac Risk

Two important factors determine the surgery-specific cardiac risk: the type of surgery and the degree of hemodynamic stress.

TABLE 5-2 Modified Cardiac Risk Index

PATIENT RISK FACTORS	POINTS
Ischemic heart disease	1
Congestive heart failure	1
Cerebral vascular disease	1
High-risk surgery	1
Preoperative insulin treatment for diabetes	1
Preoperative creatinine ≥2 mg/dL	1
Each increment in point increases risk of perioperative cardiovascular morbidity.	

Modified from Akhtar S, Silverman DG. Assessment and management of patients with ischemic heart disease. Crit Care Med 2004;32:S126–36.

TABLE 5-3 Duke Activity Status Index*

ACTIVITY	YES	NO
Can you take care of yourself (eating, dressing, bathing, or using the toilet)?	2.75	0
Can you walk indoors such as around your house?	1.75	0
Can you walk a block or two on level ground?	2.75	0
Can you climb a flight of stairs or walk up a hill?	5.50	0
Can you run a short distance?	8.00	0
Can you do light work around the house such as dusting or washing dishes?	2.70	0
Can you do moderate work around the house such as vacuuming, sweeping floors, or carrying in groceries?	3.50	0
Can you do heavy work around the house such as scrubbing floors or lifting and moving heavy furniture?	8.00	0
Can you do yardwork such as raking leaves, weeding, or pushing a power mower?	4.50	0
Can you have sexual relations?	5.25	0
Can you participate in moderate recreational activities such as golf, bowling, dancing, doubles tennis, or throwing a baseball or football?	6.00	0
Can you participate in strenuous sports such as swimming, singles tennis, football, basketball, or skiing?	7.50	0
Duke activity status index (DASI) = SUM (values for all 12 questions).		
Estimated peak oxygen uptake ($\dot{V}O_2$peak) in mL/min = 0.43 × (DASI) + 9.6.		
$\dot{V}O_2$peak mL/kg/min − 0.286 (mL/kg/min)$^{-1}$ = METs		

*The most widely recognized measure of cardiorespiratory fitness is maximal oxygen consumption ($\dot{V}O_2$peak) measured in mL/kg/min. The Index score correlates directly with $\dot{V}O_2$peak and therefore is an indirect measure of maximal METs.
Modified from Hlatky MA, Boineau RE, Higginbotham MB, et al. A brief self-administered questionnaire to determine functional capacity (the Duke Activity Status Index). Am J Cardiol 1989;64:651–4.

Surgery-specific risk is stratified into high-, intermediate-, and low-risk procedures. High-risk procedures include both major emergent surgery, particularly in the elderly, and surgery associated with increased operative time resulting in large fluid shifts or blood loss. Intermediate risk procedures include intraperitoneal surgery, laparoscopic procedures, and robotic-assisted laparoscopic surgeries. Low-risk procedures include endoscopic procedures or superficial surgeries (i.e., not involving entrance into a body cavity) (Eagle et al, 2002).

Pulmonary Evaluation

Preoperative pulmonary evaluation is important in all urologic procedures but critical in those surgeries involving the thoracic or abdominal cavities. These procedures, which include intra-abdominal, laparoscopic, or robotic surgeries, can decrease pulmonary function and predispose to pulmonary complications. Accordingly, it is wise to consider pulmonary functional assessment in patients who have significant underlying medical disease, significant smoking history, or overt pulmonary symptoms. Pulmonary function tests that include a forced expiratory volume in 1 second (FEV_1), forced vital capacity, and the diffusing capacity of carbon monoxide are quite easily performed and provide a preoperative baseline. **Patients with an FEV_1 of less than 0.8 L/sec or 30% of predicted are at high risk for complications**

(Arozullah et al, 2003). Specific pulmonary risk factors include COPD, smoking, preoperative sputum production, pneumonia, dyspnea, and obstructive sleep apnea. **It has been shown that smokers have a fourfold increased risk for postoperative pulmonary morbidity and as high as a 10-fold higher mortality rate** (Fowkes et al, 1982). In general, it is interesting to note that patients with restrictive pulmonary disease fare better than those with obstructive pulmonary disease because the former group maintains an adequate maximal expiratory flow rate, which allows for a more effective cough with less sputum production (Pearce and Jones, 1984). In addition to the specific pulmonary risk factors, general factors contribute to increased pulmonary complications such as increased age, lower serum albumin levels, obesity, impaired sensorium, previous stroke, immobility, acute renal failure, and chronic steroid use.

Hepatobiliary Evaluation

Because the survival of patients with advanced liver disease has improved over the past decade, surgery is being performed more frequently in these patients. Furthermore, patients with mild to moderate hepatic disease are often asymptomatic. These patients need to be identified and evaluated before surgery. Patients are usually aware of a prior diagnosis of hepatitis, and they should be questioned regarding the timing of diagnosis and the precipitating factors. This history is particularly important if a member of the health care team is inadvertently stuck with a needle or scalpel during the surgical procedure. A review of systems should include questions regarding pruritus, excessive bleeding, abnormal abdominal distention, and weight gain. On physical examination, jaundice and scleral icterus may be evident with serum bilirubin levels higher than 3 mg/dL. Skin changes such as caput medusae, palmar erythema, spider angiomas, and clubbing all indicate hepatic dysfunction. Severe manifestations include abdominal distention, encephalopathy, asterixis, or cachexia. Again, identification of underlying hepatic illness is important in the preoperative risk assessment of the patient. Although the estimation of perioperative mortality is limited by the lack of high-quality clinical studies, the use of the Child classification and Model for End-Stage Liver Disease (MELD) score offers a reasonable estimation.

The Child classification assesses perioperative morbidity and mortality in patients with cirrhosis and is based on the patient's serum markers (bilirubin, albumin, PT) and severity of clinical manifestations (i.e., encephalopathy and ascites). **Mortality risk for patients undergoing surgery stratified by Child class is as follows: Child Class A—10%, Child Class B—30%, and Child Class C—76% to 82%.** The Child classification also correlates with the frequency of complications such as liver failure, encephalopathy, bleeding, infection, renal failure, hypoxia, and intractable ascites. Independent risk factors other than the Child class that can increase the mortality rate in patients with liver disease include emergency surgery and COPD (Pearce and Jones, 1984; O'Leary et al, 2009).

The MELD score is perhaps a more accurate assessment of perioperative mortality in patients with hepatic dysfunction. The score is derived from a linear regression model based on serum bilirubin, creatinine levels, and the INR. It is more accurate than the Child classification in that it is objective, gives weights to each variable, and does not rely on arbitrary cutoff values (Teh et al, 2007). **Clinicians can use a website (http://mayoclinic.org/meld/mayomodel9.html) to calculate the 7-day, 30-day, 90-day, 1-year, and 5-year surgical mortality risk on the basis of the patient's age, ASA class, INR, serum bilirubin, and creatinine levels.** A recent study also found that MELD score was tightly correlated with 30-day mortality risk in all patients undergoing colorectal surgery regardless of the presence of liver disease (Hedrick et al, 2013). Taken together, the Child classification and the MELD score complement each other and provide an important assessment of the risk of surgery in cirrhotic patients (O'Leary and Friedman, 2007; O'Leary et al, 2009).

OPTIMIZATION OF COMORBID ILLNESS

Just as adequate preoperative evaluation is important, optimization of comorbid illness is critical in reducing perioperative morbidity and mortality. With regard to cardiac disease, many studies have evaluated the prophylactic use of nitrates, calcium-channel blockers, and β-blockers for patients who are at risk for perioperative myocardial ischemia. Only β-blockade has been shown to improve outcomes (Pearse et al, 2004). In a landmark study, Mangano and colleagues reported in the *New England Journal of Medicine* that there was an improvement in outcomes with the prophylactic use of atenolol in patients undergoing vascular surgery (Mangano et al, 1996). Similarly, a retrospective, cooperative group study of more than half a million patients showed that perioperative β-blockade is associated with a reduced risk of death among high-risk patients undergoing major noncardiac surgery (Lindenauer et al, 2005). In addition to β-blockade, the concept of goal-directed therapy, employing the judicious use of fluids, inotropes, and oxygen therapy to achieve therapeutic goals, may further reduce perioperative risk (Pearse et al, 2004). This concept was validated by Shoemaker, who reported an impressive reduction in mortality from 28% to 4% (*P* < .02) when goal-directed therapy was used (Shoemaker et al, 1988).

Specific preoperative interventions can decrease pulmonary complications. Smoking must be discontinued at least 8 weeks before surgery to achieve a risk reduction. Patients who discontinue smoking less than 8 weeks before surgery may actually have a higher risk of complication because the acute absence of the noxious effect of cigarette smoke decreases postoperative coughing and pulmonary toilet. **However, patients who stop smoking at least 8 weeks preoperatively will significantly lower their complication rate, and patients who have ceased smoking for more than 6 months have a pulmonary morbidity comparable with that of nonsmokers** (Warner et al, 1989). The use of preoperative bronchodilators in COPD patients can dramatically reduce postoperative pulmonary complications. Aggressive treatment of preexisting pulmonary infections with antibiotics, as well as the pretreatment of asthmatic patients with steroids, is essential in optimizing pulmonary performance. Likewise, the use of epidural and regional anesthetics, vigorous pulmonary toilet, rehabilitation, and continued bronchodilation therapy are all beneficial (Arozullah et al, 2003).

As with cardiopulmonary comorbidities, the preoperative management and optimization of diabetic patients are quite important. Perioperative hyperglycemia can lead to impaired wound healing and a higher incidence of infection (Golden et al, 1999). Hypoglycemia in an anesthetized or sedated diabetic patient may be unrecognized and carries its own significant risks. **Non–insulin-dependent diabetic patients may need to discontinue long-acting hypoglycemics because of this risk of intraoperative hypoglycemia. Shorter-acting agents or sliding scale insulin regimens are preferable, in general.** It is recommended that blood glucose levels be controlled between 80 and 250 mg/dL. Frequent fingerstick glucose checks and a sliding scale short-acting insulin regimen are used in the postoperative period. Once the patient is eating, the usual insulin regimen can be resumed. Patients who monitor their diabetes with the use of insulin pumps should continue their basal insulin infusions on the day of surgery. The pump is then used to correct the glucose level as it is measured. It is important to know the sensitivity factor that corrects the glucose so that the patient's sugars can be managed in the operating room (Townsend et al, 2008).

Patients with either hyperthyroidism or hypothyroidism should be evaluated by an endocrinologist, and surgery should be deferred until a euthyroid state has been achieved. **The greatest risk in the hypothyroid patient is thyrotoxicosis or thyroid storm, which can manifest with fevers, tachycardia, confusion, and cardiovascular collapse.** Atrial fibrillation may also be present in 20% of hyperthyroid patients (Klein and Ojamaa, 2001). With regard to hyperthyroidism, careful attention should be given to the airway because the trachea can be compressed or deviated by a large goiter. In general, antithyroid medications such as propylthiouracil or methimazole, as well as β-blockers, are continued on the day of surgery. In the event of thyroid storm, iodine and steroids may be necessary (Schiff and Welsh, 2003). Hypothyroidism is usually associated with an increased sensitivity to medications such as anesthetic agents and narcotics. Severe hypothyroidism can be associated with myocardial dysfunction, coagulopathy, electrolyte imbalance, and a decreased gastrointestinal (GI) motility. Symptoms include lethargy, cold intolerance, hoarseness, constipation, dry skin, and apathy. The decrease in metabolic rate produces periorbital edema, thinning of the eyebrows, brittle hair, dry skin, hyperthermia, bradycardia, and a prolonged relaxation of the deep tendon reflexes (Murkin, 1982). Once the diagnosis has been confirmed by a low thyroxine level and an elevated thyroid stimulating hormone level, thyroid replacement with levothyroxine can be initiated (Schiff and Welsh, 2003).

The evaluation of the patient either taking corticosteroids or suspected of having an abnormal response of the hypothalamic-pituitary-adrenal (HPA) axis is also important. There is a wide variability in HPA suppression in patients receiving exogenous steroids. Nonetheless, it seems clear that the administration of oral steroids equivalent to less than 5 mg of prednisone for any duration of time does not cause clinically significant suppression of the HPA axis. **By contrast, any patient taking more than 20 mg of prednisone or its equivalent per day for more than 3 weeks or who is clinically cushingoid has probable HPA axis suppression** (LaRochelle et al, 1993). HPA suppression can occur even in patients using potent topical steroids at doses of 2 g/day, as well as in patients using inhaled corticosteroids at doses of 0.8 mg/day. Although the duration of functional HPA axis suppression after glucocorticoids have been stopped is debatable, perioperative supplemental steroids are recommended for patients who have received HPA axis–suppressive doses within 1 year of surgery. A low-dose adrenocorticotropic hormone (ACTH) stimulation test can be used to assess the HPA axis and the need for stress steroids. For patients who take 5 mg of prednisone or the equivalent each day, no supplemental steroids are necessary and the usual daily glucocorticoid dose may be given in the perioperative period. **For those in whom the HPA axis is presumed to be suppressed or is documented to be suppressed, then 50 to 100 mg of intravenous hydrocortisone is given before the induction of anesthesia and 25 to 50 mg of hydrocortisone is given every 8 hours thereafter for 24 to 48 hours until the usual steroid dose can be resumed.** Minor procedures under local anesthesia do not require stress-dose steroids (Schiff and Welsh, 2003).

SPECIAL POPULATIONS

Elderly

It is estimated that by 2050 the number of Americans over the age of 65 will more than double to 89 million individuals, with more than 20% over the age of 85 (Jacobsen et al, 2011). Accordingly, octogenarians and nonagenarians are undergoing an increasing number of surgeries annually. Because of elderly patients' special physiologic, pharmacologic, and psychological needs, a unique set of health care challenges is encountered. It is still unclear whether advanced age independently predicts surgical risk or whether it is coexisting medical conditions that adversely affect surgical outcomes. However, in a large study published by Turrentine, it was shown that increased age independently predicted morbidity and mortality (Turrentine et al, 2006). This confirmed the study by Vemuri, who also found increased age to be an independent risk factor for morbidity and mortality in patients undergoing aneurysm surgery (Vemuri et al, 2004). Within the urologic literature, Liberman and colleagues reported 90-day mortality rates after radical cystectomy in patients younger than 70 years, 70 to 80 years, and older than 80 years of 2%, 5.4%, and 9.2%, respectively (Liberman et al, 2011). The studies suggest that independent of comorbidities, perhaps the elderly patient cannot meet the increased functional demand required during the perioperative and postoperative periods. Hypertension and dyspnea were the most frequently seen comorbid risk factors in patients older than 80 years, and preoperative transfusion history, emergency operation, and weight loss best predicted postoperative morbidity. Each 30-minute increment of operative time increased the odds of mortality by 17% in octogenarians (Turrentine et al, 2006). A unique and important factor in the perioperative care of the elderly is in the identification and prevention of delirium. Often overlooked as "sundowning," delirium can be the first clinical sign of metabolic and infectious complications (Townsend et al, 2008).

Morbid Obesity

With the rising incidence of obesity, as well as the vast experience gathered from bariatric surgery, the care of the morbidly obese patient has been extensively studied. One must carefully weigh the risk of any surgical procedure with the natural history of the disease when deciding the optimal time of the surgery in the morbidly obese. **It is estimated that patients with a body mass index (BMI) of 45 kg/m^2 or higher may lose anywhere from 8 to 13 years of life expectancy** (Fontaine et al, 2003). The careful selection of the morbidly obese patient for elective surgery is of paramount importance. Cardiac symptoms such as exertional dyspnea and lower extremity edema are nonspecific in morbidly obese patients, and many of these patients have poor functional capacity. The physical examination often underestimates cardiac dysfunction in the severely obese patient. Severely obese patients with more than three coronary heart disease risk factors may require noninvasive cardiac evaluation (Poirier et al, 2009). Obesity is associated with a vast array of comorbidities. Morbidly obese patients often have atherosclerotic cardiovascular disease, heart failure, systemic hypertension, pulmonary hypertension related to sleep apnea and obesity, hypoventilation, cardiac arrhythmias, deep vein thrombosis, history of pulmonary embolism, and poor exercise capacity. There are also numerous pulmonary abnormalities that result in a ventilation perfusion mismatch and alveolar hypoventilation. Obesity is a risk factor for postoperative wound infections, and, when appropriate, laparoscopic surgery should be considered.

Pregnancy

Urologic surgery in the pregnant woman is most commonly related to the management of renal colic and urinary tract stones. In the asymptomatic woman, the stones can be discovered during the sonographic evaluation of the fetus or during the evaluation of the pregnant woman who is experiencing renal colic. **The fetus is at the highest risk from radiation exposure from the preimplantation period to approximately 15 weeks' gestation.** Because the radiation dose that is associated with congenital malformations is 10 cGy, the evaluation of renal colic in a pregnant patient is performed usually with sonography (radiation dose with abdominal computed tomography [CT]—1 cGy; intravenous pyelogram—0.3 cGy). The indications for operative intervention in the pregnant patient are discussed elsewhere in this book. Anesthetic risks during pregnancy concern both the mother and the fetus. During the first trimester the fetus may be directly exposed to the teratogenic effects of certain anesthetic agents. Later in pregnancy, anesthesia places the mother at risk for preterm labor and the fetus at risk for hypoxemia secondary to changes in uterine blood flow and maternal acid base balance. These risks seem to be greatest during the first and third trimesters. **For semielective procedures, an attempt should be made to delay surgery until after the first trimester.** However, one must consider the continued exposure of the underlying condition in relation to the operative risks to both the mother and the fetus. **The second trimester is the safest time to perform surgery because organ system differentiation has occurred and there is almost no risk for anesthetic-induced malformation or spontaneous abortion.** When one is contemplating surgery on a pregnant patient, consultation with the obstetrician, perinatologist, and anesthesiologist is essential. These specialists will help determine the optimum technique to monitor the status of the fetus. Fetal heart rate monitors and tocometer monitoring for uterine activity are used before and after the procedure. Postoperative pain is best managed with narcotic analgesics because they have not been shown to cause birth defects in humans when used in normal dosages. Nonsteroidal anti-inflammatory medication should be avoided because of the risk for premature closure of the ductus arteriosus. Chronic use of narcotics during pregnancy may cause fetal dependency, and it is recommended that the pregnant postsurgical patient be weaned off narcotic use as soon as possible (Mikami et al, 2008).

Nutritional Status

Malnutrition compromises host defenses and increases the risk of perioperative morbidity and mortality. Adequate nutritional status is essential for proper wound healing, management of infections, return of GI activity, and maintenance of vital organ function (McDougal, 1983). The preoperative evaluation and classification of the patient's nutritional status typically consist of the assessment of any recent weight loss and the measurement of laboratory values, such as lymphocyte count and serum albumin. A 20-pound weight loss in the preceding 3 months before surgery is considered to be a reflection of severe malnutrition. The lymphocyte count and serum albumin level reflect visceral protein status, with lower levels indicating malnutrition (Reinhardt et al, 1980). Several assessment tools have been validated to quantitate nutritional status, including the Subjective Global Assessment (http://subjectiveglobalassessment.com).

There are two methods for nutritional support. Total parenteral nutrition (TPN) is used for patients who are severely malnourished and who have a nonfunctioning GI tract. Several studies have shown that 7 to 10 days of preoperative parenteral nutrition improves postoperative outcome in undernourished patients (Von Meyenfeldt et al, 1992). However, its use in well-nourished or mildly undernourished patients either is of no benefit or increases risk of sepsis (Perioperative total parenteral nutrition in surgical patients, 1991). On the other hand, enteral nutrition has fewer complications than TPN and can provide a more balanced physiologic diet. Elemental nutrition is accomplished via a feeding tube, gastrostomy, or feeding jejunostomy. Enteral nutrition maintains the gut-associated lymphoid tissue, enhances mucosal blood flow, and maintains the mucosal barrier. There are hundreds of enteral products on the market, and most have a caloric density of 1 to 2 kcal/mL. These formulas are also lactose free and provide the recommended daily allowances of vitamins and minerals in less than 2 L/day. The patients receiving enteral feedings must be monitored for improvement in nutritional status, GI intolerance, and fluid and electrolyte imbalance. **Preoperative enteral feedings can decrease postoperative complication rates by 10% to 15% when used for 5 to 20 days before surgery** (Guidelines for the use of parenteral and enteral nutrition, 2002). **The guidelines recommend postoperative parenteral nutrition in patients who are unable to meet their caloric requirements within 7 to 10 days.** Just as in the perioperative state, enteral feedings are preferred over parenteral nutrition when feasible. Moreover, the routine use of postoperative TPN has not proven useful in well-nourished patients or in those with adequate oral intake within 1 week after surgery (Byers and Hameed, 2008). Complications can occur with either enteral nutrition or parenteral nutrition. Dislodgement of nasoenteral tubes and percutaneous enteral catheters can result in pulmonary and peritoneal complications. Adynamic ileus may also occur because of decreased splanchnic perfusion, sympathetic tone, or opiate use. With regard to TPN, establishing central access is associated with a significant risk of complications. These include pneumothorax or hemothorax secondary to poor line placement and chylothorax secondary to thoracic duct injury. Line sepsis is the most common complication of indwelling central catheters and necessitates catheter removal. Venous thrombosis with associated thrombophlebitis and extremity edema has been reported. Catheter thrombosis has also been reported and can be treated with thrombolytic agents (Guidelines for the use of parenteral and enteral nutrition, 2002).

PREPARATION FOR SURGERY

Antibiotic Prophylaxis

In 1999 the Centers for Disease Control and Prevention (CDC) issued its third report on the prevention of surgical site infections (SSIs), highlighting the importance of standardization of prophylactic treatment to prevent this universal surgical complication (Mangram et al, 1999). **The report indicated that SSIs account for approximately 40% of nosocomial infections in surgical patients and potentially prolong hospital stay by 7 to 10 days.** A study of national SSIs from the 2005 Healthcare Cost and Utilization Project National Inpatient Sample (HCUP NIS) calculated an increase in hospital stay of 9.7 days and in per-patient cost of $20,892 (de Lissovoy et al, 2009). This translated nationally into an additional 1 million inpatient hospital days and additional health care cost of $1.6 billion. Bowater and colleagues published a systematic review of meta-analyses (level 1 evidence) and concluded that there was substantial evidence that antibiotic prophylaxis was an effective prevention for SSI over a wide variety of surgical procedures (Bowater et al, 2009). **Given both the ethical responsibility of the surgeon to decrease surgical morbidity and the recent policy shift by the Centers for Medicare and Medicaid Services to withhold reimbursement for hospital admissions secondary to specific SSI, it is mandatory for urologists to understand the principles behind and to practice SSI prevention.**

Along with antibiotic prophylaxis, proper hand washing and scrubbing and sterile preparation of the operative field have always been central to the prevention of SSI. For procedures involving the GI tract, mechanical and oral antibiotic bowel preparation had been standard practice until more recent literature, calling into question its usefulness (discussed later). Preoperative hair removal has not been associated with a decrease in SSI, but if performed, use of mechanical clippers or depilatory creams as opposed to razors is associated with a decreased risk of SSI (Wolf et al, 2008).

The risk of SSI and therefore the recommendation for antibiotic prophylaxis is composed of three risk factors: the patient's susceptibility to and ability to respond to localized and systemic infection, the procedural risk of infection, and the potential morbidity of infection. Patient-related factors, listed in Box 5-2, increase risk by decreasing natural defenses, increasing the local bacterial concentration, and/or altering the spectrum of bacterial flora. Second, surgical procedure–specific factors can affect the route of entry, site of infection, and pathogen involved. This idea was first described in the landmark study from the National Research Council and later formalized by the CDC; specifically, surgical wounds are now classified by degree of contamination (i.e., the inoculum of potential

pathogen) (Box 5-3; Hart et al, 1968). To predict the risk of SSI, several scoring systems have been developed incorporating patient-related factors with wound classification. Finally, the risk to the patient from SSI is an important consideration in determining the need for prophylaxis. For example, routine cystoscopy in the evaluation of microhematuria in an otherwise young, healthy patient may not warrant prophylaxis; however, the same procedure in an elderly, insulin-dependent diabetic (immunocompromised) does warrant prophylaxis given the high likelihood that a postprocedural urinary tract infection would result in a significant deterioration in the patient's overall health. Understanding the three factors together then allows the urologist to make a rational decision regarding the risks and benefits of antibiotic prophylaxis.

Once the decision for antibiotic prophylaxis has been made, the keys to successful prevention are proper timing and administration of the antibiotic and the proper choice of antibiotic for the particular procedure. Since the pivotal study by Classen and colleagues, particular emphasis has been placed on the timing of prophylaxis to be given within 2 hours of incision (Classen et al, 1992). This emphasis was exemplified by the Joint Commission's Surgical Care Improvement Project (SCIP) guideline for administration of antibiotic prophylaxis 60 minutes before incision in a broader effort to decrease overall surgical complications by 25% by 2010. A multi-institutional trial involving more than 4400 patients at 29 institutions reported results of their analysis on the optimal timing of antibiotic prophylaxis (Steinberg et al, 2009). **The results suggested an improvement in prevention of SSI when antibiotics were administered within 30 minutes of incision as compared with 31 to 60 minutes (adjusted odds ratio [OR] 1.48, $P = .06$).** More important, this larger study confirmed the significantly increased risk of SSI when antibiotics were administered at the time of or following incision, with an adjusted OR of 2.20, $P = .02$. The duration of antibiotic prophylaxis is more controversial; however, most recommendations advocate no more than 24 hours in a patient without an established infection. Routine antibiotic use beyond 24 hours increases the risk of *Clostridium difficile* colitis, increases the development of antibiotic resistance, and increases costs. Along with timing and duration, proper administration of

---

> **BOX 5-2 Patient Factors That Increase the Risk of Infection**
>
> Advanced age
> Anatomic anomalies
> Poor nutritional status
> Smoking
> Chronic corticosteroid use
> Immunodeficiency
> Chronic indwelling hardware
> Infected endogenous or exogenous material
> Distant coexistent infection
> Prolonged hospitalization

Data from Cruse PJ. Surgical wound infection. In: Wonsiewicz MJ, editor. Infectious disease. Philadelphia: Saunders; 1992. p. 758–64; and Mangram AJ, Horan TC, Pearson ML, et al. Guideline for prevention of surgical site infection, 1999. Hospital Infection Control Practices Advisory Committee. Infect Control Hosp Epidemiol 1999;20:250–78; quiz 279–80.

> **BOX 5-3 Surgical Wound Classification**
>
> **CLEAN**
> - Uninfected wound without inflammation or entry into the genital, urinary, or alimentary tract
> - Primary wound closure, closed drainage
>
> **CLEAN CONTAMINATED**
> - Uninfected wound with controlled entry into the genital, urinary, or alimentary tract
> - Primary wound closure, closed drainage
>
> **CONTAMINATED**
> - Uninfected wound with major break in sterile technique (gross spillage from gastrointestinal tract or nonpurulent inflammation)
> - Open fresh accidental wounds
>
> **DIRTY INFECTED**
> - Wound with preexisting clinical infection or perforated viscera
> - Old traumatic wounds with devitalized tissue

Data from Garner JS. CDC guideline for prevention of surgical wound infections, 1985. Supersedes guideline for prevention of surgical wound infections published in 1982. (Originally published in 1995.) Revised. Infect Control 1986;7(3):193–200; and Simmons BP. Guideline for prevention of surgical wound infections. Infect Control 1982;2:185–96.

antibiotics implies proper dosage. Antibiotic dose is dependent on the patient's body weight, renal function and hepatic function, and duration of procedure (readministration is required if longer than 4 hours). The second key to successful prevention is the proper choice of antibiotic for the procedure in question. As mentioned earlier, surgery-specific factors affect the type of pathogen, route of entry, and likelihood of systemic infection. For example, the choice of antibiotic is different for transurethral resection of the prostate (TURP; need coverage for common urinary tract pathogens) than for a cystectomy with planned sigmoid colon urinary diversion (need coverage for anaerobic bacteria). Another important consideration is the rate of antibiotic resistance in the community. **Although there is level 1 evidence for the use of fluoroquinolones as prophylaxis for urologic endoscopic procedures, the emerging *Escherichia coli* resistance in the community is changing practice patterns in many practices and high-resistance hospitals.** One resource that is particularly useful is the hospital antibiogram. These reports are published monthly at most major hospitals and quantify the susceptibility and resistance of common organisms to a wide variety of antibiotics. A summary of the recent American Urological Association (AUA) best practice statement on antibiotic prophylaxis

is shown in Table 5-4. In 2012 the AUA issued an amendment to the best practice statement with regard to prostate biopsy, acknowledging the emerging resistance to fluoroquinolones and recommending cephalosporins and/or aminoglycosides in certain communities.

Bowel Preparation

Since antibiotics were first shown to reduce infectious complications in GI surgery, mechanical and antibiotic bowel preparation has been a mainstay of urologic surgery employing intestinal segments. The rationale for bowel preparation before intestinal surgery is to decrease intraluminal feces and decrease bacterial colony counts to decrease the rate of anastomotic leak, intra-abdominal abscesses, and wound infections. The bacterial flora in the bowel consists of aerobic organisms, the most common of which are *E. coli* and *Enterococcus faecalis,* and anaerobic organisms, the most common of which are *Bacteroides* species and *Clostridium* species. **The bacterial concentration ranges from 10 to 10^5 organisms per gram of fecal content in the jejunum, 10^5 to 10^7 in the distal ileum, 10^6 to 10^8 in the ascending colon, and 10^{10} to 10^{12} in the**

TABLE 5-4 American Urological Association Best Practice Statement on Recommended Antimicrobial Prophylaxis for Urologic Procedures

PROCEDURE	ORGANISMS*	PROPHYLAXIS INDICATED?	ANTIMICROBIALS OF CHOICE	ALTERNATIVE ANTIMICROBIALS	DURATION
LOWER TRACT INSTRUMENTATION					
Removal of external urinary catheter	GU tract	If risk factors	Fluoroquinolone TMP-SMX	Aminoglycoside ± ampicillin First- or second-generation cephalosporin Amoxicillin/clavulanate	≤24 hr
Cystography, urodynamic study, or simple cystoscopy	GU tract	If risk factors	Fluoroquinolone TMP-SMX	Aminoglycoside ± ampicillin First- or second-generation cephalosporin Amoxicillin/clavulanate	≤24 hr
Cystoscopy with manipulation	GU tract	All	Fluoroquinolone TMP-SMX	Aminoglycoside ± ampicillin First- or second-generation cephalosporin Amoxicillin/clavulanate	≤24 hr
Prostate brachytherapy or cryotherapy	Skin	Uncertain	First-generation cephalosporin	Clindamycin	≤24 hr
Transrectal prostate needle biopsy	Intestine	All	Fluoroquinolone Second- or third-generation cephalosporin	Aminoglycoside + metronidazole or clindamycin	≤24 hr
UPPER TRACT INSTRUMENTATION					
Shock-wave lithotripsy	GU tract	All	Fluoroquinolone TMP-SMX	Aminoglycoside ± ampicillin First- or second-generation cephalosporin Amoxicillin/clavulanate	≤24 hr
Percutaneous renal surgery	GU tract Skin	All	First- or second-generation cephalosporin Aminoglycoside + metronidazole or clindamycin	Ampicillin/sulbactam Fluoroquinolone	≤24 hr
Ureteroscopy	GU tract	All	Fluoroquinolone TMP-SMX	Aminoglycoside ± ampicillin First- or second-generation cephalosporin Amoxicillin/clavulanate	≤24 hr

TABLE 5-4 American Urological Association Best Practice Statement on Recommended Antimicrobial Prophylaxis for Urologic Procedures—cont'd

PROCEDURE	ORGANISMS*	PROPHYLAXIS INDICATED?	ANTIMICROBIALS OF CHOICE	ALTERNATIVE ANTIMICROBIALS	DURATION
OPEN OR LAPAROSCOPIC SURGERY					
Vaginal surgery (including urethral sling procedures)	GU tract Skin Group B *Streptococcus*	All	First- or second-generation cephalosporin Aminoglycoside + metronidazole or clindamycin	Ampicillin/sulbactam Fluoroquinolone	≤24 hr
Open or laparoscopic surgery without entering GU tract	Skin	If risk factors	First-generation cephalosporin	Clindamycin	Single dose
Surgery involving entry into GU tract	GU tract Skin	All	First- or second-generation cephalosporin Aminoglycoside + metronidazole or clindamycin	Ampicillin/sulbactam Fluoroquinolone	≤24 hr
Intestinal surgery	GU tract Skin Intestinal flora	All	Second- or third-generation cephalosporin Aminoglycoside + metronidazole or clindamycin	Ampicillin/sulbactam Ticarcillin/clavulanate Piperacillin/tazobactam Fluoroquinolone	≤24 hr
Implanted prosthesis	GU tract Skin	All	Aminoglycoside + first- or second-generation cephalosporin or vancomycin	Ampicillin/sulbactam Ticarcillin/clavulanate Piperacillin/tazobactam	≤24 hr

*Common pathogens include the following: GU tract—*Escherichia coli, Proteus, Klebsiella, Enterococcus;* skin—*Staphylococcus aureus,* coagulase-negative *Staphylococcus* species, group A *Streptococcus;* and intestine—*E. coli, Klebsiella, Enterobacter, Serratia, Proteus, Enterococcus,* and anaerobes.
GU, genitourinary; TMP-SMX, trimethoprim-sulfamethoxazole.
Modified from Wolf JS Jr, Bennett CJ, Dmochowski RR, et al. Best practice policy statement on urologic surgery antimicrobial prophylaxis. J Urol 2008;179:1379–90.

descending colon. The preparation itself consists of two components: antibiotic preparation and mechanical preparation. Because there are only a few small series in the urologic literature, the rationale for each must be inferred from the general surgery literature—specifically, from colorectal surgery literature.

Although preoperative parenteral antibiotic prophylaxis before intestinal surgery is well established and widely used, oral antibiotic preparation is still somewhat controversial. Several oral antibiotic regimens are used today. The most commonly used regimen, oral neomycin and erythromycin, first became established with the landmark study by Nichols and Condon in 1977 (Clarke et al, 1977). In a double-blind, placebo-controlled study, 167 patients undergoing elective colonic surgery were randomized to receive mechanical bowel preparation with or without oral neomycin and erythromycin. The overall rates of septic complications were 43% with mechanical-only preparation and 9% with antibiotic plus mechanical preparation ($P = .001$). However, with current standards of the use of preoperative *parenteral* antibiotics, the benefit of oral antibiotic preparation was debated. Several older studies reported decreased infectious complications; however, these studies were small and there have been no randomized controlled trials (RCTs) to document the benefit. **The disadvantage of oral antibiotic preparation is primarily related to increased incidence of pseudomembranous colitis secondary to *C. difficile* infection.** In a retrospective analysis of 304 patients, Wren and colleagues reported a significantly decreased incidence of *C. difficile* colitis in patients who did not receive oral antibiotics before elective colorectal surgery (2.6% vs. 7.2%, $P = .03$) (Wren et al, 2005). Inferring from the colorectal literature, most current guidelines and a 2009 Cochrane review recommend both intravenous and oral antibiotic prophylaxis before elective colorectal surgery (Nelson et al, 2009). Despite the lack of level 1 evidence in the literature, a recent survey of colorectal surgeons revealed that up to 87% of surgeons continue to administer oral antibiotic bowel preparation before elective surgery (Zmora et al, 2003).

Mechanical bowel preparation predates the use of antibiotics in intestinal surgery and was thought to decrease the rate of anastomotic complications. Before the development of nonabsorbable liquids, patients underwent several days of oral laxatives, bowel irrigations via nasogastric tubes, and repeat enemas. These regimens were associated with significant patient discomfort and clinical morbidity caused by electrolyte imbalances. The development of polyethylene glycol solution (GoLYTELY) and sodium phosphate solution (Fleet Phospho-soda) reduced much of the electrolyte disturbance and allowed for mechanical bowel preparation to be done in the outpatient setting. **Both regimens are suitable for most patients; however, polyethylene glycol is preferred in the elderly and in patients with renal insufficiency, congestive heart failure, existing electrolyte disturbances, and cirrhosis because it is completely nonabsorbable.**

The benefit of mechanical bowel preparation has been assumed for decades as evidenced by 99% positive response by colorectal surgeons when asked if mechanical preparation is routinely used (Zmora et al, 2003). However, RCTs have called into doubt the true benefit. Slim and colleagues published a meta-analysis of RCTs including a total of 4859 patients (Slim et al, 2009). The analysis included 14 trials including two large trials from the Netherlands and Sweden (Contant et al, 2007; Jung et al, 2007). **Overall, the analysis revealed that mechanical bowel preparation provided no benefit for anastomotic leak (OR 1.12, 95% confidence interval [CI] 0.82 to 1.53, *P* = .46); abdominal or pelvic abscess (OR 0.90, 95% CI 0.47 to 1.72, *P* = .75); or mortality (OR 0.91, 95% CI 0.57 to 1.45, *P* = .70).** In fact, when overall SSI was considered, mechanical bowel preparation was associated with a significantly increased risk (OR 1.40, 95% CI 1.05 to 1.87, *P* = .02). These results were reiterated in an updated Cochrane review, which found no significant differences in anastomotic leak rate or wound infection, need for reoperation, and mortality rates (Guenaga et al, 2011). The authors concluded that there was no evidence that mechanical bowel preparation improves patient outcome after elective colorectal surgery. Although similar studies have not been done in patients undergoing elective urologic surgery, urologists can make inferences from the colorectal literature and should reevaluate the common practice of mechanical bowel preparation before urologic intestinal surgery. To date there have been multiple single institution reports suggesting equivalent SSI outcomes with or without bowel preparation before radical cystectomy and urinary diversion (Zaid et al, 2013). Two specific exceptions are transrectal ultrasound-guided prostate needle biopsy and laparoscopic urologic surgery. Given the portal of entry and subsequent risk of bacteremia, most urologists have advocated for mechanical rectal cleansing with an enema before transrectal ultrasound-guided prostate needle biopsy. With regard to laparoscopy, surgeons who perform minimally invasive procedures have long believed that preoperative bowel preparation improves operative exposure because of bowel decompression and decreases the incidence of postoperative ileus. However, to date there have been no trials to support this assertion.

In the early postoperative period, most patients experience some degree of primary ileus and delayed GI activity. Any patient with ileus lasting more than 72 to 96 hours after surgery should be evaluated for a mechanical bowel obstruction secondary to adhesions, an intra-abdominal pathologic process, or retroperitoneal hemorrhage. Given that return of GI function is often the rate-limiting factor for hospital discharge, efforts to reduce ileus including minimization of parenteral or oral opioid use, selective use of nasogastric tubes, and correction of electrolyte imbalances should be employed. More recently, methods to accelerate GI recovery have been investigated. Gum chewing—that is, sham feeding—was evaluated and reported to be associated with improvements in GI recovery and reduction in length of stay in patients undergoing colorectal surgery (Ho et al, 2014). Alvimopan (Entereg) is a peripherally acting opioid antagonist that was approved by the U.S. Food and Drug Administration (FDA) in 2008 to help restore bowel function after surgery. With the validation of alvimopan established in the colorectal literature, there have been several studies performed in patients undergoing cystectomy including a phase 4 trial whose findings were recently published. Use of alvimopan compared with placebo resulted in decreased length of stay of 2.6 days in patients undergoing radical cystectomy (Kauf et al, 2014). Many high-volume centers are now incorporating both strategies into enhanced recovery after surgery (ERAS) clinical pathways to reduce postoperative ileus and reduce hospital stays.

Venous Thromboembolic Prophylaxis

Venous thromboembolic complications are a major cause of potentially preventable morbidity and mortality among surgical patients in the United States. A recent study from the Center for Quality Improvement and Patient Safety and the Agency for Healthcare Research and Quality found postoperative venous thromboembolism (VTE) to be the second most common cause of excess length of stay, charges, and mortality among surgical patients discharged from acute care hospitals (Zhan and Miller, 2003). Urology patients in particular have an increased incidence, estimated to be 10% to 40% in patients without any prophylaxis (Geerts et al, 2008). Although these estimates are based on historical studies conducted before the routine use of mechanical prophylaxis and the recognition of the benefits of early ambulation, the increased risk persists, with more recent studies reporting incidences of 1% to 5%. Urologic patients followed prospectively in the European @RISTOS study developed VTE in 1.9% undergoing open surgery despite a high rate of prophylaxis (Scarpa et al, 2007). For patients in the United Kingdom undergoing urologic procedures, Dyer and colleagues reported an overall incidence of 0.66% including a 2.8% incidence among patients undergoing radical cystectomy (Dyer et al, 2013). Overall, VTE is the most important cause of nonsurgical mortality among urology patients (Forrest et al, 2009).

Although the use of perioperative mechanical prophylaxis (pneumatic compression stockings) is fairly universal, pharmacologic prophylaxis is administered only after weighing the risk of VTE versus risk of perioperative bleeding complications (Table 5-5). Leonardi and colleagues reviewed and analyzed 33 RCTs to assess the incidence of bleeding complications in general surgery patients receiving pharmacologic prophylaxis (Leonardi et al, 2006). **Although there was a significantly higher rate of minor complications (injection site bruising and wound hematoma), there was no significant difference in major complications (i.e., GI tract bleeding [0.2%] or retroperitoneal bleeding [<0.1%]).** Although these results are applicable in general to urology patients, certain urologic procedures, such as TURP and partial nephrectomy, have a specifically higher rate of bleeding complications. Regarding an individual's risk of VTE, both surgery-related risk factors and patient-related risk factors must be considered. Surgical factors specific to urologic surgery to be weighed include general versus

TABLE 5-5 Mechanical and Pharmacologic Venous Thromboembolism Prophylaxis

PROPHYLAXIS	DOSE	ADVANTAGES	DISADVANTAGES
Pneumatic compression stockings	—	Can be used in patients with high bleeding risk Easily standardized for all patients Studied in multiple patient groups	No standards for size, pressure Individual models not specifically studied Less effective than pharmacologic prophylaxis in high-risk groups
Low-molecular-weight heparin	40 mg SC once daily	Once-daily administration Less risk of heparin-induced thrombocytopenia No blood monitoring necessary	Not reversible High cost Relative contraindication in patients with renal insufficiency
Low-dose unfractionated heparin	5000 U SC q8h	Reversible Can be used safely in patients with renal insufficiency Relatively inexpensive	Needs readministration q8-12h Heparin-induced thrombocytopenia

BOX 5-4 Patient-Related Factors Increasing Risk for Venous Thromboembolism

Surgery
Trauma (major trauma or lower extremity injury)
Immobility, lower extremity paresis
Cancer (active or occult)
Cancer therapy (hormonal, chemotherapy, angiogenesis inhibitors, radiotherapy)
Venous compression (tumor, hematoma, arterial abnormality)
Previous venous thromboembolism
Increasing age
Pregnancy and the postpartum period
Estrogen-containing oral contraceptives or hormone replacement therapy
Selective estrogen receptor modulators
Erythropoiesis-stimulating agents
Acute medical illness
Inflammatory bowel disease
Nephrotic syndrome
Myeloproliferative disorders
Paroxysmal nocturnal hemoglobinuria
Obesity
Central venous catheterization
Inherited or acquired thrombophilia

Modified from Geerts WH, Bergqvist D, Pineo GF, et al. Prevention of venous thromboembolism: American College of Chest Physicians evidence-based clinical practice guidelines (8th edition). Chest 2008;133: 381S–453S.

TABLE 5-6 Patient Risk Assessment Model and American Urological Association Best Practice Recommendations

PATIENT RISK STRATIFICATION	
Low risk	Minor surgery in patients younger than 40 yr with no additional risk factors
Moderate risk	Minor surgery in patients with additional risk factors Surgery in patients aged 40-60 yr with no additional risk factors
High risk	Surgery in patients older than 60 yr Surgery in patients aged 40-60 yr with additional risk factors (see Box 5-4)
Highest risk	Surgery in patients with multiple risk factors (e.g., age older than 40 yr, cancer, prior venous thromboembolism)

LEVEL OF RISK	RECOMMENDATIONS
Low risk	No prophylaxis other than early ambulation
Moderate risk	Heparin 5000 units q12h SC starting after surgery or Enoxaparin 40 mg (for CrCl <30 mL/min, use 30 mg) SC daily or Pneumatic compression device if risk of bleeding is high
High risk	Heparin 5000 units q12h SC starting after surgery or Enoxaparin 40 mg (for CrCl <30 mL/min, use 30 mg) SC daily or Pneumatic compression device if risk of bleeding is high
Highest risk	Enoxaparin 40 mg (for CrCl <30 mL/min, use 30 mg) SC daily and adjuvant pneumatic compression device or Heparin 5000 units q8h SC starting after surgery and adjuvant pneumatic compression device

CrCl, creatinine clearance.
Modified from Forrest JB, Clemens JQ, Finamore P, et al. AUA best practice statement for the prevention of deep vein thrombosis in patients undergoing urologic surgery. J Urol 2009;181:1170–7.

neuraxial anesthesia, supine versus dorsal lithotomy position, abdominal versus pelvic surgery with or without lymphadenectomy, and open versus laparoscopic approach. Patient-related risk factors are listed in Box 5-4, with increasing age, malignancy, history of cancer therapy, and others being fairly common among urology patients. In fact, both the @RISTOS study and a recent report on minimally invasive radical prostatectomy confirmed several of these factors as being associated with increased risk of VTE in urologic patients (Scarpa et al, 2007; Secin et al, 2008). In 2008 the American College of Chest Physicians (ACCP) issued guidelines on the prevention of VTE with a strong recommendation that hospitals develop a formal, active strategy to address VTE prevention. **Although prior recommendations from the ACCP advocated individualized risk assessment models to guide therapy, the current recommendations advocate implementation of group-specific thromboprophylaxis routinely for all patients who belong to each of the major surgical groups (e.g., urologic surgery)** (Geerts et al, 2008). The AUA has published a best practice statement on the use of VTE prophylaxis in urologic patients (Forrest et al, 2009). These recommendations combine an individualized risk assessment model with each type of urologic surgery. For example, a high-risk patient (multiple patient risk factors) undergoing low-risk surgery may require pharmacologic prophylaxis, as might a low-risk patient undergoing high-risk surgery. The recommendations are summarized in Table 5-6.

Antithrombotic Therapy

Most urologic patients have medical comorbidities; urologists frequently encounter patients on chronic vitamin K antagonist therapy (e.g., warfarin) or antiplatelet therapy for the management of atrial fibrillation, mechanical heart valves, or coronary artery disease. Perioperative management including interruption of this antithrombotic therapy can be a challenging problem. Unlike VTE pharmacologic prophylaxis, warfarin and antiplatelet

therapies have been shown to be associated with significant bleeding complications after surgery. Therefore urologists must carefully consider the risk of interruption of chronic anticoagulation to determine the best course of perioperative management of these medications.

Chronic anticoagulation with warfarin is most frequently encountered in patients with atrial fibrillation, mechanical heart valves, or prior VTE. **The pharmacologic half-life of warfarin is 36 to 42 hours, and therefore most guidelines recommend cessation of therapy 5 days before surgery to ensure an INR less than 1.5.** Recently, several new oral anticoagulants (e.g., apixaban, dabigatran, and rivaroxaban), have been introduced to improve efficacy, decrease patient variability, and improve patient convenience. Each of the new medications has different pharmacologic properties, and therefore it is imperative for the surgeon to be familiar with these medications to properly advise the patient (Douketis, 2010). The larger issue is whether patients require a bridge with short-term anticoagulation between the time of subtherapeutic INR and

TABLE 5-7 Risk Stratification for Arterial or Venous Thromboembolism Events during Perioperative Period in Patients on Chronic Anticoagulant Therapy

	INDICATIONS FOR ANTICOAGULANT THERAPY		
	MECHANICAL HEART VALVE	ATRIAL FIBRILLATION	RECENT VTE
Low	Bileaflet aortic valve prosthesis without atrial fibrillation and no other risk factors for stroke	CHADS$_2$ score of 0-2 (and no prior stroke or transient ischemic attack)	Single VTE occurred >12 mo ago and no other risk factors
Moderate*	Bileaflet aortic valve prosthesis plus one of the following: atrial fibrillation, prior stroke or transient ischemic attack, hypertension, diabetes, congestive heart failure, age above 75 yr	CHADS$_2$ score of 3-4	VTE within the past 3-12 mo Nonsevere thrombophilic conditions (e.g., heterozygous factor V Leiden mutation, heterozygous factor II mutation) Recurrent VTE Active cancer (treated within 6 mo or palliative)
High*	Any mitral valve prosthesis Recent (within 6 mo) stroke or transient ischemic attack	CHADS$_2$ score of 5 or 6 Recent (within 3 mo) stroke or transient ischemic attack Rheumatic valvular heart disease	Recent (within 3 mo) VTE Severe thrombophilia (e.g., deficiency of protein C, protein S, or antithrombin; presence of antiphospholipid antibodies; multiple abnormalities)

*Patients at moderate or high risk are recommended to undergo bridging anticoagulation with therapeutic-dose subcutaneous low-molecular-weight heparin or intravenous unfractionated heparin.
CHADS$_2$, congestive heart failure–hypertension–age–diabetes–stroke; VTE, venous thromboembolism.
Modified from Douketis JD, Berger PB, Dunn AS, et al. The perioperative management of antithrombotic therapy: American College of Chest Physicians evidence-based clinical practice guidelines (8th edition). Chest 2008;133:299S–339S.

surgery. The decision is based on risk of a thrombotic event. Regarding atrial fibrillation, clinical scoring systems such as congestive heart failure–hypertension–age–diabetes–stroke (CHADS2), stratify patients into risk groups that predict risk of stroke while patients are not undergoing anticoagulation therapy. Patients with mechanical heart valves can also be stratified into risk groups according to the location (mitral versus aortic) and type of valve used. Similarly, patients with a prior history of VTE are stratified according to duration since last VTE and the patient's risk of recurrent VTE (Table 5-7). **In general, the ACCP, which released its guidelines in 2008, recommends that patients in the moderate- and high-risk groups undergo bridging anticoagulation with therapeutic-dose subcutaneous low-molecular-weight heparin or intravenous unfractionated heparin** (Douketis et al, 2008).

An increasing number of patients are receiving chronic antiplatelet therapy in the prevention of cardiovascular events and, more important, in the prevention of coronary stent thrombosis. Although the former indication poses little controversy for the urologist, the latter indication presents a significant and complex clinical question in which the urologist must weigh the risk of bleeding with the potentially devastating risk of perioperative stent thrombosis. Aspirin and clopidogrel are the two most commonly used antiplatelet drugs and are frequently used together. Both are irreversible inhibitors of platelet function and therefore need to be stopped 7 to 10 days before surgery to minimize bleeding risk. **Current recommendations require dual antiplatelet therapy for 6 weeks after bare metal coronary stents and 12 months for drug-eluting stents. Premature interruption of antiplatelet therapy has been associated with a 25% to 50% risk of significant myocardial infarction with resultant increased perioperative mortality** (O'Riordan et al, 2009). In most patients, urologists should defer elective surgery until after antiplatelet therapy can be safely interrupted. In a review of the literature, Gupta and colleagues recommend delay of elective urologic surgery for at least 30 days for bare metal stents and, if possible, longer than 1 year for drug-eluting stents (Gupta et al, 2012). Even then, because acute stent thrombosis has been described with drug-eluting stents after 12 months, urologists should strongly consider at least single-agent antiplatelet therapy in these patients. Given the current lack of

clinically useful alternatives to antiplatelet therapy, when surgery cannot be delayed (e.g., because of malignancy), the ACCP strongly recommends continuing aspirin and clopidogrel during the perioperative period in patients with drug-eluting stents (Douketis et al, 2012). Obviously, communication between the urologist and the cardiologist throughout the perioperative period is essential to minimize complications.

ANESTHETIC CONSIDERATIONS

The basic tenet of anesthesia is to deliver hypnosis, amnesia, and analgesia while maintaining satisfactory operating conditions. An understanding of the basic pharmacologic principles, anesthetic equipment and monitoring, and patient analgesia is important to any surgeon including the urologist for successful operative outcomes and avoidance of surgical complications. Although urologists are performing increasingly more procedures in the office, the bulk of urologic surgery occurs in the operating room under monitored anesthesia care, regional anesthesia, or general anesthesia. Current practice in operative anesthesia employs a combination of inhalational agents and intravenous medications along with analgesics (for pain control) and benzodiazepines (for anxiolysis and amnesia). Of course, improved presurgical evaluation, pharmacologic drugs, and perioperative monitoring have dramatically decreased the risks of anesthesia. A recent study of New York hospital-based and freestanding ambulatory surgical centers reported the risk of all-cause mortality to be 1 in 49,012 and the rate of immediate admission to an inpatient facility to be 0.6% (Fleisher et al, 2007b).

Selection of Mode of Anesthesia

An important role of the urologist in the anesthetic evaluation is to determine what mode of anesthesia is best for the particular patient and surgical procedure. The choice depends on patient-related factors including comorbidities, airway, and patient preference and procedural factors including complexity, duration, anatomic location, and expected fluid and blood loss. A basic understanding of each method of anesthesia and the pharmacologic principles will aid the urologist in making recommendations to the anesthesiologist.

Monitored Anesthesia Care

Although *monitored anesthesia care* is defined as conscious sedation under the care of an anesthesiologist in a monitored situation, it encompasses a wide range of levels of anesthesia from minimal sedation to brief intervals of unconscious general anesthesia. Most commonly, anesthesiologists combine intravenous opioid analgesics and benzodiazepines to maintain a sufficient level of patient comfort and anxiolysis. Monitored anesthesia care is widely used in urology in the ambulatory setting and is suitable for short-duration endoscopic procedures, transrectal ultrasound-based procedures, and, when combined with a local anesthetic, superficial procedures of the external genitalia. Conscious sedation can be administered in the office setting but only with proper monitoring of the patient during and after the procedure. **The Joint Commission has strict guidelines to ensure that the patients receive the same level of monitoring as if under the care of an anesthesiologist including a requirement for a trained monitoring assistant, immediate access to airway and resuscitation equipment, and specific preprocedure and postprocedure evaluations.**

Regional Anesthesia

Regional anesthesia incorporates different levels of anesthesia directed toward the surgical site, including local anesthesia, spinal anesthesia, and epidural anesthesia. The use of local anesthetics is typically combined with monitored anesthesia care for superficial procedures in an isolated anatomic location. The keys to proper local anesthetic administration are avoidance of intravascular injection and knowledge of pharmacology. The two most commonly used drugs are lidocaine and bupivacaine, with the primary differences being the onset and duration of action. Infiltration of local anesthetics before surgical incision decreases nociceptor sensitization and conduction and results in decreased postoperative pain and analgesic requirements.

Spinal and epidural anesthesia involves injection of anesthetic (most commonly lidocaine or bupivacaine) into the subarachnoid space or epidural space with direct effect on the spinal cord, resulting in sensory, motor, and sympathetic blockade. In urologic procedures, epidural anesthesia is most useful for postoperative pain management for major abdominal procedures, thereby avoiding the adverse effects of high doses of intravenous opioids (i.e., respiratory depression, GI dysfunction). Spinal anesthesia is suitable for most urologic endoscopic procedures and lower abdominal surgical procedures and is limited only by the duration of anesthesia required. Spinal anesthesia avoids the cardiopulmonary effects and complications of general anesthesia. Several factors affect the spinal level and efficacy of administration. In general, larger volume and increased doses result in longer duration and increased cephalad migration. The addition of low-dose opioids and/or vasoconstrictors prolongs the duration of analgesia while reducing the dose of anesthetic. The anesthetic-related adverse effect is hypotension as a result of sympathetic blockade and occurs in 10% to 40% of patients (Di Cianni et al, 2008). **The primary technique-related complication is post–dural puncture headache (results from cerebrospinal fluid leak) with an incidence of less than 2% with currently used 29-gauge pencil-tipped needles** (Turnbull and Shepherd, 2003). **Overall, spinal anesthesia has become safe, with the incidence of serious neurologic deficits being 0.05%.**

General Anesthesia

Inhalational General Anesthesia. Inhalational drug development has emphasized inhalational agents that facilitate rapid induction and emergence and are nontoxic. **Two of the most important characteristics of inhalational anesthetics are the blood/gas solubility coefficient (B/G) and the minimum alveolar concentration (MAC). The B/G refers to the serum uptake of the inhaled agent, and the MAC is a measure of the potency of a volatile anesthetic (i.e., the serum level required to prevent movement in response to a skin incision in 50% of patients).** The various inhalational agents differ not only in the B/G and MAC but also in their cardiopulmonary effects. Obviously, a basic understanding of these properties is important for the urologic surgeon, especially during instances of surgical complication.

Nitrous oxide (NO) is one of the most commonly used agents because of its propensity for rapid induction and emergence; however, because of its low potency, it is often combined with other agents. Because of NO's high B/G and tendency to increase the volume and pressure of closed spaces, its use is contraindicated in certain clinical situations such as small bowel obstruction and pneumothorax. During laparoscopic abdominal procedures, surgeons often prefer to avoid the use of NO because of resultant bowel distention and subsequent interference in the operative field. Although this effect is debated in the surgical literature, El-Galley and colleagues reported significantly increased bowel distention and surgical interference with NO use in patients undergoing laparoscopic donor nephrectomy (El-Galley et al, 2007).

Once introduced in the 1950s, halothane rapidly became one of the most commonly used anesthetic agents because of its high potency. **However, halothane has several important risks that have since limited its use. It has significant cardiac effects and can precipitate failure in patients with left ventricular dysfunction. Furthermore, it sensitizes the myocardium to the effects of catecholamines (relevant for local anesthetics injected into the surgical site).** Finally, there is a 1 in 35,000 incidence of fulminant hepatitis, which can be lethal as a result of overaccumulation of toxic metabolites. More recent advancements in inhalational agents have focused on reduction in toxicity while maintaining the potency and rapidity of halothane. Three of the most commonly used current agents are isoflurane, sevoflurane, and desflurane. Isoflurane, less expensive than the other agents because of the availability of generic equivalents, is widely used as a result of its low cardiac depression, lower myocardial sensitization to catecholamines, and minimal metabolism. The primary unique toxicity is variable response tachycardia, which can lead to significantly increased myocardial oxygen consumption. Unlike isoflurane, which has a putrid odor, sevoflurane is often used for inhalation induction (odorless) because of its rapid induction and emergence, decreased incidence of postoperative nausea (important in outpatient surgery), and minimal cardiac toxicity. It is, in general, the preferred agent for difficult airways requiring mask induction and in patients with severe bronchospastic disease. Desflurane, like isoflurane, has a pungent odor and is not used for inhalational induction. Its primary advantage over isoflurane is a more rapid recovery in patients requiring anesthesia over 3 hours.

Intravenous General Anesthesia. Intravenous anesthesia consists of a combination of induction agent, opioid, and neuromuscular relaxant. Anesthesiologists often prefer intravenous induction with a combination of inhalational and intravenous agents for maintenance of anesthesia. Intravenous induction offers several advantages in that it is rapid, minimizes patient discomfort, and is preferred by children and most adults. Thiopental, the oldest and least expensive agent, is a suitable choice for uncomplicated situations but is limited in more complex cases because of its significant vasodilation, cardiac depression, and risk of bronchospasm, especially in patients with reactive airway disease. Ketamine is a preferred choice for procedures that are brief and superficial because of its profound amnesia and somatic analgesia. It is associated with increased arteriolar and bronchomotor tone and is advantageous during induction for hypovolemic and asthmatic patients. **Propofol is among the most commonly used anesthetic agents, especially in outpatient surgery. It has a rapid onset, produces excellent bronchodilation in patients with reactive airway disease, and, perhaps most important, is associated with smooth, nausea-free emergence from anesthesia.** Its primary adverse effect is significant blood pressure reduction. Midazolam, never used as a single agent, produces profound amnesia and anxiolysis while having a rapid onset and short duration and producing minimal cardiac side effects.

Although these agents induce unconsciousness and amnesia, opioids have become an integral component to all forms of anesthesia. Opioids result in significant analgesia without an increase in cardiac side effects. Several studies have documented the decreased requirements of other agents when used in combination with opioids, thus reducing the overall cardiopulmonary side effects of anesthesia (Fukuda, 2009). Opioids themselves are differentiated in their potency, onset of action, duration of action, and metabolism and excretion. **Fentanyl (synthetic opioid) is probably the most widely used because of its potency (100 to 150 times that of morphine), rapid onset, and short duration of action.** Newer synthetics are geared toward shorter duration and more rapid metabolism.

For major operative cases, complete neuromuscular relaxation is required for sufficient exposure and successful outcome. Although full relaxation can be achieved with intravenous and inhalational agents, the dose required is extremely high. The use of intravenous neuromuscular blockers allows for neuromuscular relaxation and minimization of inhalational and intravenous drugs. **There are two types of neuromuscular blockers: depolarizing drugs, which depolarize the plasma membrane of skeletal muscle fibers, making the fibers resistant to further stimulation by acetylcholine; and nondepolarizing drugs, which block the binding of acetylcholine to cholinergic receptors on the presynaptic and postsynaptic membrane.** Succinylcholine, the only depolarizing drug on the market, is chosen for its rapid onset (used in rapid induction sequences), relatively short duration (around 5 minutes), and rapid metabolism. Its use is limited because of the risk of malignant hyperthermia (when used in combination with volatile inhalational agents), hyperkalemia, and bradycardia in children. When succinylcholine is contraindicated, nondepolarizing agents are used. Several nondepolarizing drugs are available and differ in routes of metabolism and adverse effects. Furthermore, multiple medications including desflurane can alter the metabolism of these drugs and potentiate their actions. The most important consideration in the use of neuromuscular blockers is the assessment of adequate return of neuromuscular function after withdrawal of the drug. The most common complication of neuromuscular-blocking drugs is inadequate reversal resulting in respiratory failure and reintubation. Numerous reports in the literature correlate residual neuromuscular blockade with increased postoperative pulmonary complications in the postanesthesia care unit (PACU) and in the postoperative period. **The concept of train-of-four fade ratio (TOF) was developed to devise an objective measure of adequate neuromuscular function. This concept refers to the magnitude of the fourth of four twitches in response to maximal stimuli to the ulnar nerve delivered at 0.5-second intervals. Historically, a TOF of 0.7 (meaning that the fourth twitch was 70% the magnitude of the first twitch) correlated with adequate return of neuromuscular function; however, more recent standards have raised the threshold to 0.9 as an indicator of complete return of neuromuscular function** (Kopman et al, 1997). Currently, anesthesiologists use several clinical assessments including head lift, tongue depressor test, and hand grip to estimate a TOF of 0.9. A recent study revealed that with use of clinical assessments alone, 16% and 45% of patients 2 hours after a single intubating dose of neuromuscular blocker had a TOF of less than 0.7 and less than 0.9, respectively, in the PACU (Debaene et al, 2003). As such, current recommendations are that quantitative TOF measurement (acceleromyography) be combined with clinical assessments before extubation in the operating room (Viby-Mogensen, 2009).

Pain Management

Equally important to intraoperative anesthetic considerations, proper pain management after surgery is crucial to minimizing postoperative complications and delayed recovery. **Untreated acute pain not only is unacceptable for the patient, but also may increase the risk of complications by causing increased physiologic stress in the recovery period.** The neural process, referred to as *nociception*, involves signal transduction from noxious stimuli via sensory afferent nerves to the spinal cord and cerebral cortex, resulting in the perception of pain. Analgesia aims to block the pain sensation along various points of this signal transduction pathway.

Opioids are perhaps the most commonly used analgesic medications in the immediate postoperative period. These drugs primarily act in the CNS at both the dorsal root ganglion and the cerebral cortex to modulate the perception of pain. Administration can be oral, intravenous, neuraxial, or transdermal. In general, the choice of route of administration is dependent on patient's severity of pain and ability to take oral medications. Although typically very effective for providing analgesia, opioids can cause decreased GI activity, respiratory suppression, sedation, and mental confusion. Weaker (less potent) opioids, such as hydrocodone and codeine, may minimize these adverse effects but are often combined with acetaminophen and should be used with caution in patients with hepatic insufficiency.

Nonsteroidal anti-inflammatory drugs (NSAIDs) are being employed in the postoperative setting more frequently now to avoid the unwanted effects of opioids. These medications act by inhibition of cyclooxygenase enzyme activity, resulting in decreased prostaglandin production. Prostaglandins are the primary mediators of nociceptor activation at the tissue level. **Multiple studies have demonstrated that the appropriate use of NSAIDs can result in decreased use of opioid analgesics and decreased nausea and vomiting after anesthesia** (Rawlinson et al, 2012). In a randomized study of patients undergoing laparoscopic colon surgery, the use of intravenous ketorolac was associated with improved pain scores and reduced postoperative ileus (Schlachta et al, 2007). NSAIDs are usually very well tolerated but should be avoided in patients with renal insufficiency and used with caution in patients with a history of esophageal reflux or peptic ulcer disease.

For major abdominal surgery in which prolonged opioid use is expected, neuraxial analgesia (i.e., epidural) can provide significant patient benefits. Epidural analgesia is administered and monitored by the anesthesia or pain management team. Both opioids and local anesthetic medications are infused in the epidural space via catheter and are given as a continuous infusion and/or patient-controlled infusion. Epidural analgesia has the advantage of improved pain control while minimizing the central nervous and GI adverse effects of intravenous opioid medications. Block and colleagues performed a meta-analysis of randomized trials to review the efficacy and concluded that epidural analgesia, regardless of agent or location of catheter placement, provided better pain control than parenteral opioids (Block et al, 2003). **In fact, a recent review of RCTs found that in patients undergoing general anesthesia, the use of concomitant epidural analgesia resulted in decreased perioperative mortality and improved comorbidity end points across multiple organ systems** (Pöpping et al, 2014).

BLOOD PRODUCTS

Given the vascular nature of urologic organs, the urologist often confronts the issue of indication and necessity of transfusion in the perioperative period. Therefore it is important that the urologist understand the indications, implications, and risks associated with blood product transfusion. Before the acquired immunodeficiency syndrome (AIDS) epidemic, blood transfusion was liberally administered, often for any patient with a hematocrit less than 30%. However, fear and concern about the infectious risk led to the convening of a National Institutes of Health (NIH) panel to develop consensus recommendations for the indication of blood product transfusion (NIH Consensus Statement, 1988). The principles in these guidelines largely hold true today as reflected by the ASA practice guidelines issued in 2006 (Practice guidelines for perioperative blood transfusion and adjuvant therapies, 2006). **To summarize, the guidelines indicate that transfusion is rarely indicated with hematocrit greater than 30% and often indicated** for hematocrit less than 21%. **For levels between 21% and 30%, clinical factors such as risk of complications from inadequate oxygenation should guide the need for transfusion, balancing the risks and benefits.** In general, patients with relatively minor comorbidities can tolerate hematocrit of greater than 21% before transfusion is indicated. Patients with moderate to severe comorbidity (e.g., significant pulmonary compromise, coronary artery disease, or vascular insufficiency, or with signs or symptoms of hypovolemic, hemorrhagic shock) warrant transfusion to achieve hematocrit greater than 30%. Ultimately, until technology is available to directly measure inadequate oxygen-carrying capacity, the urologist should individualize the decision to transfuse for each patient and clinical situation.

A major advance in blood banking and product transfusion has been the development of component therapy allowing for administration for specific fractions of whole blood. Packed red blood cells (PRBCs) are equivalent to whole blood minus the plasma component. Whereas the hematocrit in whole blood is 40%, it is 70% in PRBC units. These units are reconstituted and administered with crystalloid. Given the lack of the remaining components, in instances of massive PRBC transfusions and associated bleeding, platelets and occasionally fresh frozen plasma (FFP) should be given to avoid dilutional coagulopathy. Platelet transfusion is rarely indicated empirically except in patients with significant thrombocytopenia ($<50,000/mm^3$) and a planned surgical procedure or with moderate thrombocytopenia (50,000 to $100,000/mm^3$) and either a high-risk procedure or evidence of platelet dysfunction. Similarly, empirical transfusion with FFP for massive transfusion is not indicated. With the development of component therapy, the use of FFP increased dramatically, leading to consensus statements from the NIH and the ASA to guide practitioners (Consensus conference, 1985; Practice guidelines for perioperative blood transfusion and adjuvant therapies, 2006). **The current indications for FFP transfusion are immediate reversal of warfarin-induced coagulopathy, replacement in patients with specific clotting factor deficiencies, and evidence of bleeding and INR greater than 1.5. According to the ASA guidelines, in patients with massive transfusion and no INR readily available, FFP should be given after replacement of 1 blood volume.**

There are well-documented risks of transfusion, and these risks should always be discussed with the patient before administration. Hemolytic transfusion reactions occur as a result of incompatibility between donor and recipient (either ABO or non-ABO incompatibility). According to the 2007 FDA Annual Summary, from 2005 to 2007 transfusion reactions accounted for 22% of transfusion-related fatalities in the United States (U.S. Food and Drug Administration, 2007). Transfusion reactions occur relatively frequently and, if identified early, can be treated with rare catastrophic events. The early signs and symptoms include fever, chills, chest pain, hypotension, and bleeding diathesis occurring during or immediately after transfusion. Reactions may also occur in a delayed fashion, which is characterized by significant intravascular hemolysis secondary to recipient antibodies. The treatment of transfusion reaction is centered on fluid resuscitation, cessation of the transfusion, and alkalinization of the urine to prevent renal failure. **The most common cause of transfusion-related fatality is transfusion-related acute lung injury (TRALI). This entity accounted for 55% of transfusion mortality from 2005-2007. The injury is characterized by noncardiogenic pulmonary edema injury and manifests 1 to 2 hours after transfusion.** Although no specific treatment other than supportive measures is indicated, most patients recover without significant sequelae. Finally, one of the most feared complications (at least in the public eye) is the transmission of bacterial or viral infection. Although the risk of hepatitis virus and human immunodeficiency virus (HIV) transmission was unacceptably high in the 1970s and 1980s, the initiation of more stringent screening procedures for high-risk populations and the development of nucleic acid amplification technology (polymerase chain reaction [PCR] and transcription-mediated amplification) have resulted in dramatically reduced risk and incidence of viral transmission. **Currently, the risk of HIV and hepatitis C transmission is approximately 1 in 2**

million cases, whereas the risk of hepatitis B transmission is 1 in 200,000. The highest risk of infectivity occurs with platelet transfusion, in which bacterial contamination develops at a rate of 1 in 5000 units (Eder et al, 2007).

Although very high–blood loss procedures in urology are uncommon, given the proximity of major vascular structures to several genitourinary organs, occasionally the urologist is faced with a clinical situation in which a large-volume blood transfusion is necessary. Traditionally, component transfusion would not begin until more than 6 units of PRBCs had been given to the patient. More recently, evidence from the trauma literature supports the use of an increased ratio of platelets to fresh frozen plasma to red blood cells (RBCs)—that is, massive transfusion protocol. The protocol is triggered in the anticipation of greater than 10 units of PRBCs per 24 hours and mobilizes blood bank and hospital resources to provide an adequate supply of RBC and component transfusion. There are multiple reports of improved survival of trauma patients managed with massive transfusion protocols. A study from Ball and colleagues demonstrated improved abdominal wall closure rates among patients with high-grade liver injuries when a massive transfusion protocol was used (Ball et al, 2013).

PATIENT ENVIRONMENT

Patient Temperature

Although hypothermia can be therapeutic in certain situations of trauma and brain injury, for elective surgical procedures, hypothermia is associated with significantly increased morbidity to the patient. **There are two primary reasons for hypothermia to develop in the operating room. Anesthetic agents induce peripheral vasodilation, redistributing heat from the core (trunk, head) with a resultant drop in immediate core temperature after induction. Throughout the rest of the surgical procedure, radiation and conductive heat loss account for most of the heat loss.** *Normothermia* is defined as a core temperature between $36°C$ and $38°C$, and hypothermia of even $1°C$ to $2°C$ results in adverse effects. **Rajagopalan and colleagues performed a meta-analysis of RCTs and reported that mild hypothermia (decrease of $1°C$) resulted in a 16% increase in estimated blood loss and 22% increase in transfusion requirements** (Rajagopalan et al, 2008). The increased bleeding risk is thought to result from a hypothermia-associated decrease in clotting cascade enzymatic function and platelet aggregation. Even more significant is the increase in the risk of SSIs associated with mild hypothermia ($34°C$ to $36°C$). Hypothermia increases the risk of SSI by impairing immune mechanisms and vasoconstriction, resulting in regional tissue hypoxia. In a landmark study, Kurz and colleagues with the Study of Wound Infection and Temperature Group tested in 200 patients undergoing elective colorectal surgery the hypothesis that hypothermia increases the rate of wound infection and hospital stay (Kurz et al, 1996). **Hypothermia was associated with a three times increased risk of wound infection and a 2.6-day increase in hospitalization.** More recent studies have confirmed these findings in general in other series of surgical patients (Mauermann and Nemergut, 2006). In its overall goal of reducing SSI, the SCIP has also included perioperative normothermia as one of its guidelines. Strategies to improve maintenance of normothermia include regular use of warming blankets, warmed intravenous fluids, warmed irrigation fluids (especially during TURP and other prolonged endoscopic procedures), warmed humidified CO_2 gas during laparoscopy, and increase in ambient operating room temperature. Although there have been few studies in the urologic literature, the findings can be generalized to all surgical patients.

Skin Preparation

Sterile skin preparation is fundamental in the prevention of SSI for any procedure. Currently the most commonly used skin antiseptics are alcohol, povidone-iodine, or chlorhexidine based. Whichever antiseptic is chosen, the solution should be applied in concentric circles from the center of the surgical site and allowed to dry before incision. **The Cochrane Wound Study group recently published their updated second analysis on various preoperative skin preparations. The authors again were unable to report conclusive evidence of superior efficacy of one particular skin preparation** (Dumville et al, 2013). Furthermore, although the CDC clearly recommends preoperative showering or bathing to reduce SSI, there is no evidence that bathing with an antiseptic solution reduces the rate of infection (Webster and Osborne, 2007). Regarding hair removal, the CDC recommends that if hair removal is performed, it should be performed immediately before the surgical procedure and performed with clippers (rather than shaving) (Mangram et al, 1999).

Patient Safety

In 1991 Brennan and colleagues published their seminal work describing adverse events, defined as injuries caused by medical management in hospitalized patients, revealing that 48% of the events accompanied a surgical operation (Brennan et al, 1991; Leape et al, 1991). This important study inspired the publication of "To Err Is Human: Building a Safer Health System," a comprehensive study by the Institute of Medicine on medical errors. Regarding surgical patients, the most frequent venue of preventable injuries is the operating room. **Although the surgeon is the "captain of the ship" and ultimately responsible, it takes cognizance and attention to detail from each member of the operating room team to prevent iatrogenic injuries to the patient.** Three causes of immediately preventable injuries are retractor-associated injuries, thermal injuries, and patient position–related injuries. There are several reports in the literature documenting an increased rate of neuropathy (especially femoral nerve) after laparotomy with self-retaining retractors versus without self-retaining retractors (Irvin et al, 2004). Careful attention to be certain that the lateral blades do not directly compress the psoas muscle and only cradle the rectus abdominal muscles will ensure avoidance of femoral neuropathy. Furthermore, periodic reinspection of the retractor blades is also warranted. Many devices used in urologic surgery employ thermal energy for desired effect and therefore can result in thermal injury to the patient. These include Bovie cautery, the argon beam coagulator, bipolar devices, and lasers. In both endoscopic and laparoscopic surgery, high-wattage light sources are used to illuminate the operative field. While it is illuminated, the ends of the light cords can result in burns when in direct contact with the patient (even through draping). These light sources should be turned off at all times when not in use. Special mention is deserved for the morbidly obese patient. The operating room should be equipped with a hydraulic table, extra-long instruments, additional padding, wide venous compression devices, and side extensions to ensure a safe operating room environment for the patient.

Patient Positioning

Although often given only a cursory evaluation, proper patient positioning in the operating room can prevent potentially devastating complications. Ultimately, proper positioning is the shared responsibility of each member of the operating room team. Much of the knowledge and guidelines for avoidance of position-related injury are drawn from the anesthesia literature. In fact, in response to a 1999 study of the ASA Closed Claims Database, which found neuropathy as second-leading cause of liability, the ASA published a practice advisory for the prevention of perioperative peripheral neuropathies (Practice advisory for the prevention of perioperative peripheral neuropathies, 2000). The recommendations are listed in Box 5-5. **Although the exact mechanisms of peripheral neuropathy are not always known, the cause of position-related neuropathy is usually secondary to excessive stretch, prolonged compression, or ischemia.** Given the variety of different patient

---

BOX 5-5   American Society of Anesthesiologists Task Force Recommendations on the Prevention of Perioperative Peripheral Neuropathies

PREOPERATIVE ASSESSMENT

- When judged appropriate, it is helpful to ascertain that patients can comfortably tolerate the anticipated operative position.

UPPER EXTREMITY POSITIONING

- Arm abduction should be limited to 90 degrees in supine patients; patients who are positioned prone may comfortably tolerate arm abduction greater than 90 degrees.
- Arms should be positioned to decrease pressure on the postcondylar groove of the humerus (ulnar groove). When arms are tucked at the side, a neutral forearm position is recommended. When arms are abducted on armboards, either supination or a neutral forearm position is acceptable.
- Prolonged pressure on the radial nerve in the spiral groove of the humerus should be avoided.
- Extension of the elbow beyond a comfortable range may stretch the median nerve.

LOWER EXTREMITY POSITIONING

- Lithotomy positions that stretch the hamstring muscle group beyond a comfortable range may stretch the sciatic nerve.
- Prolonged pressure on the peroneal nerve at the fibular head should be avoided.
- Neither extension nor flexion of the hip increases the risk of femoral neuropathy.

PROTECTIVE PADDING

- Padded armboards may decrease the risk of upper extremity neuropathy.
- The use of chest rolls in laterally positioned patients may decrease the risk of upper extremity neuropathies.
- Padding at the elbow and at the fibular head may decrease the risk of upper and lower extremity neuropathies, respectively.

EQUIPMENT

- Properly functioning automated blood pressure cuffs on the upper arms do not affect the risk of upper extremity neuropathies.
- Shoulder braces in steep head-down positions may increase the risk of brachial plexus neuropathies.

POSTOPERATIVE ASSESSMENT

- A simple postoperative assessment of extremity nerve function may lead to early recognition of peripheral neuropathies.

DOCUMENTATION

- Charting specific positioning actions during the care of patients may result in improvements of care by (1) helping practitioners focus attention on relevant aspects of patient positioning and (2) providing information that continuous improvement processes can use to effect refinements in patient care.

Modified from Practice advisory for the prevention of perioperative peripheral neuropathies: a report by the American Society of Anesthesiologists Task Force on Prevention of Perioperative Peripheral Neuropathies. Anesthesiology 2000;92:1168–82.

positions used in urologic surgery, it is critical for the urologist to be an active participant in the positioning of the patient and to understand the potential patient compromise that accompanies each position.

The supine position, used in abdominal, pelvic, and penile procedures, is in general considered the safest patient position. However, several specific issues should be considered. **Excessive upper extremity abduction (>90 degrees) can lead to tension on the brachial plexus, leading to upper extremity neuropathy.** The armboard should be padded to avoid excessive pressure on the ulnar groove and spiral groove of the humerus (radial nerve injury). In cases in which the arms are tucked at the patient's side, care must be taken to avoid excessive pressure on the hand and forearm. Moreover, peripheral intravenous catheter infiltration must be identified quickly because forearm compartment syndrome may develop.

One of the most frequent positions used in urology is the lithotomy position. Improper positioning can lead to transient and occasionally prolonged lower extremity neuropathy. In a retrospective evaluation of more than 190,000 cases from 1957 to 1991 involving the lithotomy position, persistent neuropathy was found in 0.03%; however, the same group in a prospective study of 991 patients reported an incidence of 1.5% (15 patients) with resolution of symptoms by 6 months in all but one patient (Warner et al, 1994, 2000). **The basic principle of position involves manipulation of both lower extremities simultaneously with flexion of the hips at 80 to 100 degrees with 30- to 45-degree abduction.** The legs should be padded to avoid excessive compression against the stirrup. Particular caution should be given to the patient's hands to avoid entrapment within the moving parts of the stirrups.

For most open and laparoscopic upper urothelial tract and renal procedures, the patient is placed in some degree of lateral decubitus position. Proper padding of the patient is important, with appropriate anterior and posterior support to maintain the decubitus position. The most frequent focus of compromise involves positioning of the arms and the potential for brachial plexus injury. The ipsilateral arm should be placed on an elevated arm rest or gel pad, avoiding abduction of more than 90 degrees and excessive stretch on the shoulder. The contralateral arm should be placed on an armboard with ulnar padding. Furthermore, in patients in full flank position, an axillary roll should be placed just caudal to the axilla (not in the axilla) to avoid compression of the contralateral brachial plexus. Finally, after the patient has been positioned and before sterile draping, the operating table should be fully rotated to ensure that the patient is adequately secured in all positions.

Two patient positions used in specific urologic cases deserve attention: the prone position for percutaneous nephroscopy and the full Trendelenburg position for robotic-assisted laparoscopic procedures in the pelvis. In the prone position, special care should be taken to pad the torso, elbows, hips, and legs. The anesthesiologist should ensure that the endotracheal tube and all vascular accesses are properly secured. Coordination of the entire team is required during transfer from the supine position on the stretcher to the prone position on the operating room table. A stretcher should always be available immediately in case of airway compromise and the need for rapid transfer to the supine position. Regarding the full Trendelenburg position for minimally invasive pelvic procedures, the primary issues involve the physiologic changes in respiratory function, cardiovascular function, and increases in central venous and intracranial pressures. **Patient positioning should focus on properly padding and securing the patient to the operating table to prevent cephalad sliding. Although fixed shoulder braces will undoubtedly prevent patient movement, these braces should be avoided because of the risk of brachial plexus compression and resultant neuropathy.**

ABDOMINAL INCISIONS AND WOUND CLOSURE

Abdominal Incisions

Urologic surgery can encompass a large area of the trunk, and therefore the urologist should be familiar with all type of incisions of the abdomen. The most commonly used incision in surgery including urology is the midline abdominal incision. This incision can provide access to the entire peritoneum and retroperitoneum. For procedures focused on particular areas of the abdomen, alternative incisions provide more focused exposure with certain benefits. A Pfannenstiel incision (transverse lower abdominal incision) can be used for virtually all pelvic procedures and results in improved cosmesis and possibly decreased pain. For access to the lower third of the ureter, a Gibson incision (i.e., an oblique incision in the lower quadrant) can be used. With a Gibson incision, entry into the retroperitoneum is gained by splitting the external and internal oblique muscles in the direction of its fibers. Access to the upper abdomen and retroperitoneum for renal and adrenal surgery can be gained using various kinds of incisions. An extraperitoneal approach is best performed via a flank incision over the 11th or 12th rib, with or without partial rib removal. An extraperitoneal approach avoids the complications of transperitoneal surgery such as bowel injury, postoperative ileus, and adhesion formation. Transperitoneal access can be obtained via an anterior subcostal incision (two fingerbreadths below the costal margin). This incision provides better access to the midline vascular structures by allowing for complete medial mobilization of the posterior peritoneum. For large or locally advanced (vena cava thrombus) tumors, a thoracoabdominal or chevron incision provides the best exposure in general. A thoracoabdominal approach is preferred for large upper retroperitoneal tumors or tumors with extension into the thoracic cavity (supradiaphragmatic vena cava tumor thrombus). On the other hand, a chevron incision is preferred for access to both the right and left abdomen (e.g., bilateral renal tumors). In summary, proper choice of incision is often critical to successful surgical outcome, especially for complex operative cases.

Wound Healing

Knowledge of the basic principles of wound healing is important to properly assess incision closure and its associated complications. All cutaneous wounds progress stepwise through a series of events toward complete wound repair; in a particular wound, different phases of events may occur simultaneously. **The series of steps can be divided broadly into three stages: reactive phase, proliferative phase, and maturational phase.** The reactive phase occurs immediately with the two primary responses of hemostasis and inflammation. Disruption of vascular membranes results in platelet activation and aggregation, which in turn initiate the inflammatory response. During this stage of wound healing, inflammatory cells including polymorphonuclear cells, macrophages, and lymphocytes migrate into the wound and become activated, leading to cytokine activation and secretion of various growth factors. The second stage, proliferative, results in the formation of granulation tissue. The stage is characterized by proliferation of endothelial cells and fibroblasts leading to angiogenesis and epithelialization, which eventually results in growth of immature blood vessels and deposition of extracellular matrix and early collagen scaffolding. Finally, the maturation stage occurs with further deposition of collagen and wound contraction. **The maturational phase begins approximately 1 week after injury and progresses rapidly over 6 weeks, with increasing wound strength over the next 12 months. The scar regains approximately 3% strength after 1 week, 20% after 3 weeks, and 80% after 3 months** (Witte and Barbul, 1997).

Wound Closure

Along with choice of incision, proper closure is necessary to avoid certain surgical complications including wound infection and fascial dehiscence. In general there are three types of wound closure: primary, secondary, and tertiary (or delayed primary closure). In the vast majority of elective procedures, the urologist should attempt a permanent closure after the operation (primary closure). Secondary closure is reserved for heavily contaminated wounds for which the fascia is closed primarily but the skin and subcutaneous tissues are allowed to heal via re-epithelialization and contraction. Tertiary closures are reserved for patients with abdominal compartment syndrome or patients requiring re-explorations, in whom temporary closure is initially performed with intention of future permanent closure. Unless the procedure involves heavy contamination, incision closure involves reapproximation of the fascia (in one or multiple layers) and the skin. Choice of suture type by the surgeon depends on preferences of braided versus nonbraided, monofilament versus multifilament, and absorbable versus nonabsorbable. A full description of different suture types and their properties is listed in Table 5-8 (Hochberg et al, 2009). Although the method of fascial closure has been studied extensively, a definitive, superior method is not universally agreed upon. van 't Riet and colleagues performed a meta-analysis of available RCTs (van 't Riet et al, 2002). **In all, 6566 patients from 15 studies were included; the primary outcome measure was incidence of incisional hernia. The analysis indicated that between slowly absorbable and nonabsorbable sutures there was no difference in risk of incisional hernia in continuous versus interrupted fascial closures, although nonabsorbable closure was associated with increased wound pain and sinus formation. For rapidly absorbable suture types, continuous fascial closure was significantly associated with increased rate of incisional hernias.** Because of the limited number of patients, a definitive conclusion could not be made for interrupted rapidly absorbable suture closure versus continuous slowly nonabsorbable suture closure. The authors, however, concluded that mass closure with slowly absorbable suture in a continuous fashion is the optimal method. To address the limitation found in previous meta-analyses, Seiler and colleagues completed an RCT of 625 patients (Seiler et al, 2009). Patients were randomized to one of three arms: interrupted closure with rapidly absorbable suture or continuous closure with one of two different slowly absorbable sutures. They found no significant difference in incisional hernia (15.9% vs. 8.4% vs.

12.2%, $P = .09$), fascial dehiscence, wound infection, or serious adverse events. In conclusion, although incisions may be closed either with interrupted, rapidly absorbable suture closure or with continuous slowly absorbable suture closure, careful attention should be paid to the technique, given the relatively high incidence of incisional hernia. A subsequent meta-analysis of existing literature again could not find a significant difference between continuous closure with slowly absorbable suture versus interrupted closure with rapidly absorbable suture (Diener et al, 2010).

Perhaps the most frequently encountered complication of abdominal wounds is the SSI. Because of different reporting methods and descriptions in the literature, the National Health Care Safety Network of the CDC published definitions of SSIs with clearly defined, objective criteria (Kirby and Mazuski, 2009). The infections are classified as follows:

- Superficial incisional infection: involves only skin and subcutaneous tissue and occurs within 30 days of surgery
- Deep incisional infection: involves deep soft tissues (muscle or fascial planes) and occurs within 30 days of surgery (or within 1 year if implant is in place)
- Organ or space infection: involves any part of the body that is opened or manipulated during the operative procedure and has purulent drainage from a drain placed in the wound or evidence of infection on radiographic imaging

Specific risk factors predisposing to SSIs were previously listed in Box 5-2. The mainstay of treatment centers on adequate drainage of the infected area. **Superficial infections and some deep incisional infections can usually be managed with opening of the skin incision and packing of the wound. Care should be taken to open the incision widely to ensure complete drainage of underlying purulent fluid. The use of oral or intravenous antibiotics is not necessary unless the infection is associated with significant skin cellulitis (erythema extending >2 cm from**

TABLE 5-8 Properties of Suture Materials

SUTURE	ORIGIN	TISSUE ABSORPTION	PHYSICAL CONFIGURATION	TENSILE STRENGTH	COMMENTS
Vicryl	Synthetic	Absorbable	Braided	65% 2 wk 40% 4 wk	Slower loss of function and higher knot-breaking strength compared with polyglycolic acid (Dexon).
Dexon	Synthetic	Absorbable	Braided	63% 2 wk 17% 3 wk	Lubricant coating decreases coefficient of friction.
Monocryl	Synthetic	Absorbable	Monofilament	30%-40% 2 wk (dyed) 25% 2 wk (undyed)	Excellent tensile strength allows use of smaller sutures for skin closure.
PDS	Synthetic	Delayed absorbable	Monofilament	74% 2 wk 50% 4 wk 25% 6 wk	No absorption until after 90 days; low reactivity, tends to maintain strength in presence of infection; newer barbed version is knotless.
Maxon	Synthetic	Delayed absorbable	Monofilament	81% 2 wk 59% 4 wk 30% 6 wk	
Chromic gut	Natural	Absorbable	Monofilament	0% 3 wk	Can also be found as plain gut (untreated) for faster absorption.
Nylon	Synthetic	Nonabsorbable	Monofilament	50% 1-2 yr	Very low tissue reactivity.
Prolene	Synthetic	Nonabsorbable	Monofilament	No significant loss over time	High plasticity, extremely smooth surface (requires extra knot throws).
Silk	Natural	Nonabsorbable	Braided	Degraded over time	Braided for easier handling; can be prone to infection.
Mersilene	Synthetic	Nonabsorbable	Braided or monofilament	No significant loss over time	Braided should not be used in infection.

incision edge or systemic signs of toxicity, e.g., fever, sepsis) (Barie and Eachempati, 2005). Once opened, the wound should be allowed to heal by secondary intention. Many deeper incisional infections are too extensive for bedside incision and require operative debridement under anesthesia. It is critical to carefully examine any infected wound for signs of necrotizing infection, most commonly secondary to *Clostridium perfringens*. Signs include drainage of grayish, dishwater-colored fluid, frank necrosis of the fascial layer, and wound crepitus. A necrotizing infection requires immediate return to the operating room for wide debridement and washout. In contrast to incisional infections, deeper organ and space infections may cause no superficial signs at the level of the incision. Rather, patients often show systemic signs of infection, pain, or sepsis; cross-sectional imaging is used to reveal the putative source. Again, the principle of adequate drainage applies, and management involves percutaneous or operative drainage of the abscess fluid. A controversial issue in the prevention of organ and space infections is the routine placement of drainage systems at the time of the initial operative procedure. A wide variety of surgical drains is available. Drains are broadly categorized as open nonsuction, closed nonsuction, and closed suction drains. Open nonsuction drains are employed when accurate quantification of drainage amount is not necessary. These drains are associated with less patient discomfort and are the easiest to remove. Closed drains are chosen if quantification of drainage amounts or characterization of drainage fluid is necessary. The use of suction in closed drain systems is in general preferred if immediate recognition of small amounts of drainage is important (e.g., a drain around a ureterointestinal anastomosis). Although drains continue to be widely used in various urologic procedures, several prospective studies in the general surgical literature have failed to show significant benefit; therefore most experts caution against their routine use (unless strong indication exists) (Barie, 2002).

Perhaps the most dreaded complication of surgical incisions is acute wound failure (or fascial dehiscence). Overall the incidence of fascial dehiscence is 1% to 2%, and the complication usually occurs 1 week after surgery, although it may occur up to 30 days postoperatively. Risk factors for dehiscence include patient-related factors (advanced age, malnutrition, corticosteroid use, obesity, and prior history of radiotherapy); SSI; and technical errors at the time of wound closure. The most common technical errors associated with wound failure are placing the suture too close to the fascial edge, knot slippage, and excessive suture tension. **Multiple studies have investigated the type of closure, and there is no difference in dehiscence risk between interrupted and continuous closures as long as rapidly absorbable sutures are not used with the latter.** Historically, in high-risk patients retention sutures were strongly advocated and widely used as a preventive measure for wound dehiscence. Literature evidence, however, was primarily retrospective, and subsequent prospective trials have failed to show evidence of benefit (Carlson, 1997). One recent trial by Rink and colleagues randomized 95 high-risk patients to retention sutures versus standard closure; the researchers reported that although no difference in wound failure rates was seen, retention sutures were associated with a significantly increased rate of patient morbidity, primarily pain (Rink et al, 2000). Accordingly, recent surgical trends suggest a movement away from the use of retention sutures and, alternatively, toward the increased use of grafts and synthetic mesh in wounds thought to be at increased risk of fascial dehiscence. **When acute wound failure does occur, it is usually immediately preceded by a sudden gush of serosanguineous fluid from the wound. Some small fascial disruptions can be managed conservatively with wound packing and close observation, but the majority of disruptions, particularly in the setting of bowel evisceration, mandate urgent return to the operating room. At the bedside, a sterile, saline-moistened towel should be placed over the eviscerated components while the patient is being prepared for the operating room.** At the time of reoperation, the fascial edges are inspected for the cause of the disruption. In cases of technical errors or fascial tearing in which the fascial edges are healthy and can be brought together without tension, a primary closure is appropriate. In all other cases, the fascial edges are debrided and the wound is closed with absorbable mesh or biologic prosthetic grafts. A full discussion of the different materials is beyond the scope of this chapter, but strong consideration should be given to an intraoperative general surgical consultation.

Whether because of a deep abdominal infection or an acute wound failure, the urologist is often faced with decisions regarding temporary versus permanent closure and primary versus secondary permanent abdominal wall closure. In general, a temporary abdominal closure is considered in situations of significant deep abdominal infection (e.g., bacterial peritonitis secondary to bowel anastomosis breakdown, ischemic bowel) or significant abdominal wall failure (e.g., necrotizing fasciitis). **Perhaps the biggest recent advance in temporary abdominal wall closure was the development of the negative-pressure vacuum pack. This technique allows safe, inexpensive temporary closure, facilitates wound healing by reducing chronic bowel edema and improving local blood flow, and can result in relatively high delayed primary abdominal wall closure rates.** To determine the effectiveness of temporary closure, Bhangu and colleagues performed a meta-analysis of the existing literature on whether temporary closure of contaminated abdominal wounds reduces the rate of deep SSI (Bhangu et al, 2013). **Although the currently available literature is not substantial, they concluded that delayed primary closure of the abdomen was a reliable and potentially cost-saving method to prevent SSI in contaminated wounds.** When delayed primary fascial closure is not feasible, newer biologic prosthetic mesh can be used to close the abdomen and the remaining wound can close secondarily (in conjunction with use of a negative-pressure vacuum-assisted device). These mesh prosthetics are derived from human, porcine, or bovine sources and in general are synthesized at acellular collagen matrices. Although the long-term durability of these materials is not known, they are usually safer in contaminated wounds.

KEY POINTS

- Proper preoperative evaluation of the patient will prevent unanticipated cancellations and decrease the risk of postoperative complications.
- The indications for preoperative cardiac testing depend on three groups of factors: the functional capacity of the patient, cardiac risk factors, and surgery-specific risk factors.
- SSIs are one of the leading causes of perioperative complications and increased hospital stay. Antibiotic prophylaxis is indicated in virtually all surgical procedures.
- VTE is a common complication of urologic procedures, and the AUA recommends either mechanical or pharmacologic prophylaxis (or both for patients at highest risk) for all urologic procedures.
- Proper understanding of the pharmacologic principles of anesthesia will allow the urologist to actively participate in the decision process of choosing which mode of anesthesia will be appropriate for a particular patient and procedure.
- Current guidelines advocate blood product transfusion for hematocrit less than 21% in most patients unless there are specific cardiopulmonary risk factors.
- Perioperative hypothermia of even 1° C to 2° C is associated with increased estimated blood loss and increased risk of SSI.
- Proper choice of surgical incision results in optimal surgical exposure and therefore improved outcomes.
- Current literature suggests that closure with continuous, slowly absorbing suture results in the lowest risk of incision-related complications.

REFERENCES

The complete reference list is available online at www.expertconsult.com.

SUGGESTED READINGS

Brennan TA, Leape LL, Laird NM, et al. Incidence of adverse events and negligence in hospitalized patients. Results of the Harvard Medical Practice Study I. N Engl J Med 1991;324:370–6.

Douketis JD, Berger PB, Dunn AS, et al. The perioperative management of antithrombotic therapy: American College of Chest Physicians evidence-based clinical practice guidelines (8th edition). Chest 2008;133: 299S–339S.

Eagle KA, Berger PB, Calkins H, et al. ACC/AHA guideline update for perioperative cardiovascular evaluation for noncardiac surgery—executive summary: a report of the American College of Cardiology/American Heart Association Task Force on Practice Guidelines (Committee to Update the 1996 Guidelines on Perioperative Cardiovascular Evaluation for Noncardiac Surgery). J Am Coll Cardiol 2002;39:542–53.

Geerts WH, Bergqvist D, Pineo GF, et al. Prevention of venous thromboembolism: American College of Chest Physicians evidence-based clinical practice guidelines (8th edition). Chest 2008;133:381S–453S.

Practice guidelines for perioperative blood transfusion and adjuvant therapies: an updated report by the American Society of Anesthesiologists Task Force on Perioperative Blood Transfusion and Adjuvant Therapies. Anesthesiology 2006;105:198–208.

van 't Riet M, Steyerberg EW, Nellensteyn J, et al. Meta-analysis of techniques for closure of midline abdominal incisions. Br J Surg 2002;89:1350–6.

Wolf JS Jr, Bennett CJ, Dmochowski RR, et al. Best practice policy statement on urologic surgery antimicrobial prophylaxis. J Urol 2008;179:1379–90.

6 Fundamentals of Urinary Tract Drainage

Thomas Tailly, MD, MSc, and John D. Denstedt, MD, FRCSC, FACS

Understanding the fundamentals of urinary tract drainage is essential to every practicing urologist and urology trainee. This chapter covers basic aspects of the indications, devices, and descriptions of the various techniques of urinary tract drainage.

LOWER URINARY TRACT: HISTORIC NOTE

Descriptions of draining bladder urinary retention predate the ancient Egyptian civilization and have surfaced from Asian, Chinese, Egyptian, Roman, Byzantine, and Greek civilizations, emphasizing the long-standing importance of this clinical problem. Reports from ancient times describe catheterization with straws, reeds, polished or waxed rolled-up leaves, and hollow twigs (Mattelaer and Billiet, 1995).

In the Hippocratic writings *On Diseases* (around 400 BCE), the use of a bladder catheter for urinary drainage was considered a basic skill of any physician (Moog et al, 2005a). In the 7th century AD, Paulus Aegineta described bladder drainage with use of a slender silver catheter, a technique that became very popular in medieval times. Remarkably, even in that scientifically naive era, the concept of silver having an antiseptic function was postulated (Mattelaer and Billiet, 1995). The use of silver catheters remained popular until the introduction of natural rubber for the manufacture of urinary catheters. Galen (2nd century AD), Paulus Aegineta (7th century AD), and Avicenna (11th century AD) also describe the use of a catheter to deliver a substance into the bladder to treat several ailments including pyocystis, hematuria, and inflammation (Moog et al, 2005a, 2005b; Madineh, 2009).

The 19th century was pivotal in the evolution of the catheter to the devices we use to this day. Joseph F. B. Charrière introduced the Charrière unit to measure the size of a catheter, a scale which has been adopted worldwide. One French unit equals 0.33 mm in the external diameter (Mattelaer and Billiet, 1995). Mercier invented the coudé-tipped catheter in 1836 (*coudé* means "elbow" in French) (Mattelaer and Billiet, 1995). In 1860 Auguste Nelaton created the Nelaton catheter, a soft tubular rubber bladder catheter with a solid straight tip and one side hole, made of vulcanized rubber (Mattelaer and Billiet, 1995). In the 1930s, Frederick E. B. Foley invented a catheter with an inflatable balloon attached to the catheter tip as a retainment mechanism (Tatem et al, 2013). This represented a foundational development that forms the basis for most lower urinary tract catheters used today.

ANATOMIC CONSIDERATIONS

Thorough knowledge of the relevant anatomy is a prerequisite to performing urinary tract drainage.

Male Urethra

The average length of the male urethra is 17.5 to 20 cm from bladder neck to external urethral meatus from postmortem studies as reported in *Gray's Anatomy* (Standring, 2008). More recent literature, measuring the urethra in vivo with a bladder catheter, confirms these lengths to be quite accurate (Kohler et al, 2008; Krishnamoorthy and Joshi, 2012).

In general, the male urethra is divided into segments: bladder neck or preprostatic urethra, prostatic urethra, membranous urethra, and penile or spongy urethra, which in turn can be subdivided into the bulbous urethra, pendulous urethra, and fossa navicularis. An alternative classification for urethral segments is anterior and posterior urethra; the posterior segment consists of the prostatic and membranous urethra, and the anterior segment equates to the penile urethra.

The caliber of the urethra varies throughout its course. The normal healthy external meatus should allow a 24-F catheter to pass. More proximal portions of the adult urethra have a larger caliber, the largest being the prostatic urethra with a caliber of approximately 32 F. The normal bladder neck is usually of a caliber to allow passage of a 28-F instrument (Davis, 1913).

Female Urethra

In nulliparous, continent women, the urethra and bladder neck reside in the connective tissue of the anterior vaginal wall. The urethra measures approximately 4 cm and can be divided into three segments: the distal segment, mid-urethra, and proximal segment (Wieczorek et al, 2012). In a supine position, the urethra has a downward inclination with a slight angle more horizontally approximately midway, and the mean caliber is approximately 22 F (Uehling, 1978).

INDICATIONS FOR LOWER URINARY TRACT DRAINAGE

The indications for inserting a bladder catheter can conveniently be divided into two categories: therapeutic or diagnostic catheterization.

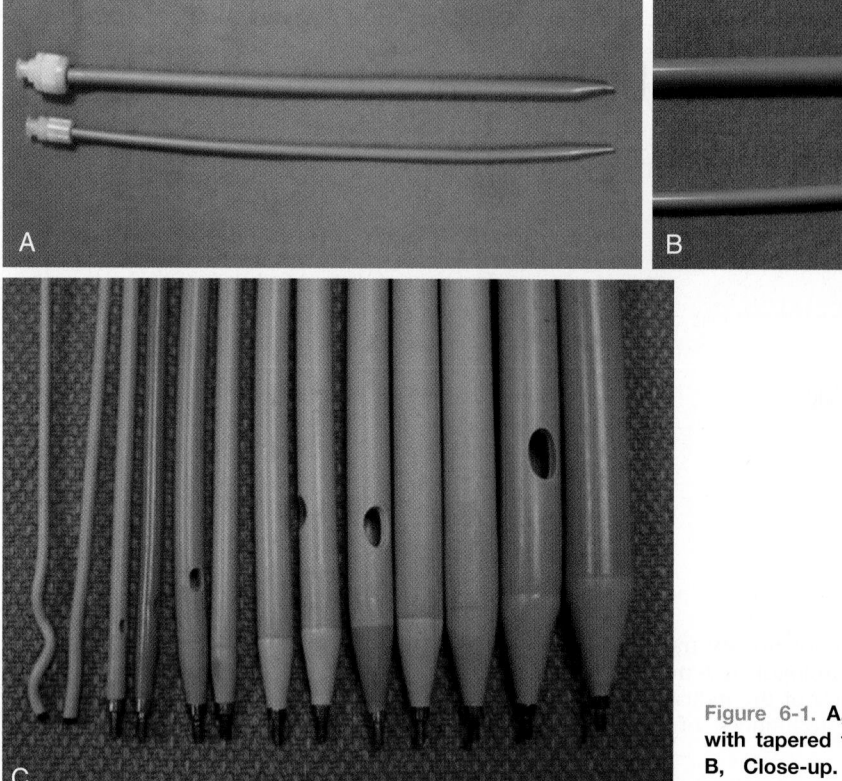

Figure 6-1. **A, Urethral dilators with tapered tip (12 and 18 Fr). B, Close-up. C, Filiform and followers.**

The most common indication for transurethral bladder catheterization is for drainage of an acute or chronic urinary retention or postvoid residual volume. Drainage can be accomplished by an indwelling catheter or by intermittent catheterization, depending on the pathology, the recurring need for drainage, and the dexterity of the patient or caregivers. Although ultrasound-based bladder scanners are widely used to estimate postvoid residual urine volume, the most accurate method of measurement is by emptying the bladder with transurethral catheterization. The second most common indication for bladder catheterization is to monitor urinary output. Patients with gross hematuria, regardless of its cause, will often require a catheter for bladder irrigation and drainage of bloody urine and blood clots.

Dilation with urethral catheters is the most commonly used primary treatment in the management of urethral strictures (Bullock and Brandes, 2007). Simple urethral dilation can be performed by blind insertion of a filiform leader followed by coaxial followers of increasing diameter or by passing Councill catheters of increasing diameter over a cystoscopically placed guidewire (Fig. 6-1). A recent Cochrane meta-analysis comparing simple dilation with endoscopic urethrotomy and open urethroplasty for urethral stricture was not definitive in providing recommendations surrounding preferred treatment of urethral stricture (Wong et al, 2012). The only randomized trial comparing dilation with urethrotomy reported no significant difference in efficacy and stricture-free rates (Steenkamp et al, 1997; Heyns et al, 1998).

In patients unable to provide a clean urine sample with repeated contamination of a midstream urine sample, single catheterization may be used to obtain an uncontaminated urine sample.

Manometer-tipped catheters are used in urodynamic studies to measure the intravesical and urethral pressure. Thermometer-tipped catheters are occasionally used during prolonged surgeries providing both continuous thermometry and adequate drainage for urinary output measurement.

Intravesical therapy with, for instance, dimethyl sulfoxide for interstitial cystitis (Colaco and Evans, 2013), alum for intractable hematuria (Abt et al, 2013), or Mitomycin C or bacille

TABLE 6-1 Catheter Size Based on Age

AGE IN YEARS	CATHETER SIZE (Fr)
<5	5-8
5-10	8-10
10-14	10
>14	10-14

Calmette-Guérin (BCG) solution for nonmuscle invasive bladder cancer (van Lingen and Witjes, 2013) is also administered through a transurethral catheter.

In performing retrograde cystography, radiographic contrast material is administered by bladder catheterization to opacify the urinary tract for diagnostic purposes.

In urogenital trauma, which is covered elsewhere in this text, insertion of a bladder catheter is, depending on the extent of the trauma, often the first choice of treatment. This should be considered only after diagnostic workup of the possible urethral trauma has been completed so that the feasibility and appropriateness of transurethral catheter placement can be defined.

CATHETER SELECTION

A wide variety of catheters are available for transurethral catheterization. Differences in materials used in manufacture; variations in length, circumference, shape of the catheter tip, and number of channels; and varieties of coatings contribute to this vast array of such devices.

The choice of catheter design and size depends on the indication for use, expected fluid requiring drainage, anticipated indwelling time, age, gender, previous history, and patient anatomy. One should choose the smallest size available based on these variables (Table 6-1). The use of feeding tubes as urethral catheters should be discouraged because their stiffness and length can be a source of complications (ischemic ulcers, urethral strictures, and knotting in the bladder) (Smith, 2003; Sarin, 2011).

The optimal catheter for an initial attempt at transurethral bladder catheterization in adult patients with no past urologic history, no risk of urinary tract abnormality, and no known allergies, is a 16-Fr latex straight-tipped catheter.

CATHETER DESIGN

The most basic catheter design is constructed with a single lumen to allow for drainage or instillation. The most frequently used retention mechanism is the retention balloon, which is inflated through a dedicated channel. The three-way catheter allows for simultaneous instillation and drainage of fluids and is especially useful in patients with hematuria, clot retention, and pyuria. Continuous bladder irrigation is most commonly used postoperatively after urologic surgery, when hematuria and possible clot formation are to be expected. The three-way catheter is designed with a larger-than-average balloon to allow for instillation of 30 mL or more, which can be helpful in achieving hemostasis after transurethral resection of the prostate by applying traction on the catheter, thus compressing vessels at the bladder neck (Fig. 6-2).

The addition of channels to the initial single catheter design comes with potentially negative design requirements. The extra lumens occupy space in the internal lumen of the catheter, reducing the internal diameter. The inner diameter of a 24-Fr single-lumen catheter is larger than the inner lumen of a 24-Fr two-way catheter, which in its turn is larger than the inner lumen of a 24-Fr three-way catheter.

There are basically two available tip shapes, the Nelaton blind-ending straight tip and the coudé tip, or elbowed or Tiemann tip. Both versions exist in a Councill catheter version, which can be passed into the bladder over a guidewire if necessary. Multiple variations such as tapered tips or multiple side holes exist throughout the wide array of available catheters.

Materials and Coatings

Most catheters for everyday use are composed of latex, rubber, silicone, or polyvinylchloride (PVC). For short-term catheterization, latex or rubber catheters are preferred because of their availability and low cost. Silicone is relatively inert, and randomized controlled trials (RCTs) have demonstrated silicone to induce significantly less tissue inflammation than latex catheters (Nacey et al, 1985; Talja et al, 1990; Schumm and Lam, 2008). Silicone is preferred over latex catheters for long-term catheterization. Silicone catheters are

stiffer and less prone to buckling when encountering resistance (Villanueva et al, 2011).

Several coatings have been studied in an attempt to reduce trauma, urethritis, and catheter-associated urinary tract infection (CAUTI). The use of hydrophilic-coated catheters is of interest for intermittent catheterization. Such catheters have been associated with less discomfort, fewer traumatic catheterizations, and decreased incidence of symptomatic urinary tract infections (UTIs) and urethral strictures (Wyndaele, 2002; De Ridder et al, 2005; Cardenas et al, 2011). A recent meta-analysis by Bermingham was unable to identify a significant difference in the incidence of symptomatic UTIs when comparing different catheter types used for clean intermittent catheterization (CIC). Li and colleagues, on the other hand, in a meta-analysis focusing on the spinal cord injury population, demonstrated that the use of hydrophilic-coated catheters in CIC significantly reduced the UTI and hematuria rates (Bermingham et al, 2013; Li et al, 2013). Because the use of clean uncoated catheters for CIC was most cost-effective and the use of gel-reservoir was second most cost-effective in the Bermingham analysis (Bermingham et al, 2013), **the routine use of hydrophilic catheters for CIC in non–spinal cord injury patients is not recommended.**

Antibiotic-impregnated catheters may delay bacteriuria in short-term catheterization (<1 week). Such benefit has not been substantiated in patients requiring longer-term catheterization (Schumm and Lam, 2008; Hooton et al, 2010).

Bacterial-coated catheters have the theoretic benefit of colonizing the urine with a nonvirulent strain of *Escherichia coli* and have shown promising results in small pilot trials. Studies on the feasibility and efficacy of clinical use of such catheters are ongoing (Trautner et al, 2007; Prasad et al, 2009; Darouiche and Hull, 2012).

A 2008 Cochrane meta-analysis demonstrated that the use of silver-alloy–coated catheters significantly reduced the incidence of asymptomatic bacteriuria in short- and long-term (>1 week) use of such catheters (Schumm and Lam, 2008). In a more recent multicenter RCT including more than 6000 patients, antimicrobial-coated catheters demonstrated a statistically significant benefit in reducing CAUTI compared with polytetrafluoroethylene (PTFE)–coated catheters, whereas silver-alloy catheters demonstrated no beneficial effect. **Because no clinically significant benefit was noted for short-term catheterization with either catheter, the routine use of these catheters cannot be recommended** (Pickard et al, 2012).

New coatings to enhance biocompatibility are still being developed and investigated, with the desired outcome being coatings that prevent encrustation and UTIs (Siddiq and Darouiche, 2012).

TECHNIQUE OF URETHRAL CATHETERIZATION

After establishing the indication for catheterization, a medical and surgical history, including allergies, focusing on previous urologic history, surgeries, and catheterization attempts should be obtained. This information is necessary for optimal catheter choice and complication risk assessment.

When performing urethral catheterization, the physician assumes a position at the side of the patient corresponding to the physician's dominant hand (if the physician is right handed, the position is on the right-hand side of the patient). All materials expected to be required should be readily available on the sterile drape. The patient should be in supine position at a comfortable height for the individual performing the catheterization. A frog-leg position is preferred for female patients. Catheterization should be carried out in a sterile fashion and should start with sterile draping of the patient. When an indwelling catheter is being placed, the balloon should be checked for integrity before catheterization.

The most recent American Heart Association guidelines no longer recommend routine use of infective endocarditis prophylaxis for any genitourinary procedure, even in patients with the highest-risk cardiac conditions (Wilson et al, 2007).

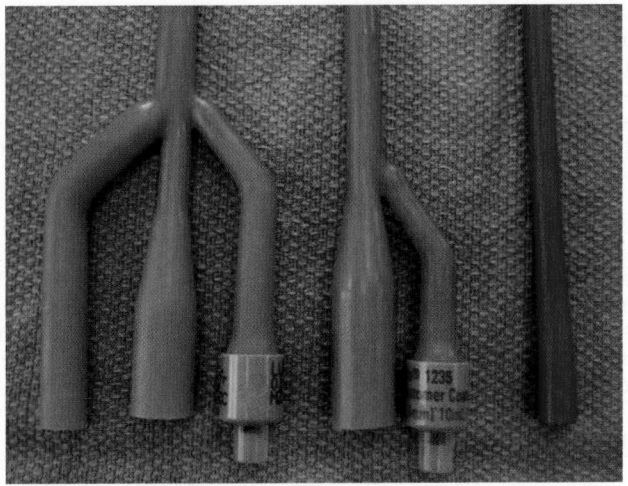

Figure 6-2. **Three-way, two-way, and single-lumen catheters.**

Lubrication of the catheter is advised for smooth catheterization and minimization of risk of urethral trauma. Four categories of lubricants exist: plain lubricant, lubricant-anesthetic, lubricant-disinfectant, and lubricant-anesthetic-disinfectant.

The use of 2% lidocaine urethral instillation before instrumentation was first reported safe and efficacious in the mid-20th century (Haines and Grabstald, 1949; Persky and Davis, 1953) and is still widely practiced; however, evidence of benefit has been a topic of conflicting literature.

The safety of urethral lidocaine use has been well established in situations in which the urethra is intact. The systemic uptake of lidocaine through intact mucosa after instillation of doses of up to 550 mg (approximately 27 mL of 2% lidocaine lubricant) reaches a very low peak concentration that never reaches a toxic level (Ouellette et al, 1985; Eardley et al, 1989; Birch and Miller, 1994). However, toxicity has been reported in patients in whom lidocaine gel was used in the presence of a disrupted mucosal barrier, leading to a high peak serum concentration within minutes. Reported symptoms are confusion, lethargy, seizures, disorientation, and anaphylactic shock (Sundaram, 1987; Clapp et al, 1999; Priya et al, 2005; Sinha and Sinha, 2008).

Chitale and McFarlane showed no difference in pain experience during flexible cystoscopy after plain or anesthetic lubricant (McFarlane et al, 2001; Chitale et al, 2008). Ho and coworkers concluded that insertion of an anesthetic lubricant is paradoxically more painful than plain lubricant (Ho et al, 2003). Cooling the lubricant to 4° C has been shown to significantly decrease pain perception compared with lubricant at room or body temperature, possibly because of a cryoanalgesic effect (Thompson et al, 1999; Goel and Aron, 2003).

The anesthetic lubricant should be indwelling in the urethra longer than 15 minutes to provide a beneficial effect (Choong et al, 1997; Siderias, 2004). A short delay (<15 minutes) does not seem to have any benefit compared with no delay (Birch et al, 1994; Garbutt et al, 2008; Losco et al, 2011). In female catheterization, the use of an anesthetic lubricant has been shown to be effective even after only several minutes of indwelling time (Chan et al, 2013; Chung et al, 2007).

Two available meta-analyses on the use of anesthetic versus non-anesthetic lubricant report conflicting results and recommendations, possibly because of different inclusion criteria and a high grade of heterogeneity in included studies. Patel and colleagues demonstrated no difference in use of anesthetic versus plain lubricant; in contradistinction, Aaronson and colleagues reported a statistical beneficial effect (Patel et al, 2008; Aaronson et al, 2009).

Considering the conflicting data available, **the routine use of anesthetic lubricant cannot be recommended. If anesthetic lubricant is to be used, the limited evidence available suggests slowly instilling (3 to 10 seconds) a minimum amount of 20 mL of cooled lubricant and allowing a minimum of 15 minutes of exposure to maximize benefit to the patient** (Schede and Thüroff, 2006; Tzortzis et al, 2009).

Catheterization in Male Patients

The true external urethral meatus is exposed by retracting the foreskin if present. In the presence of phimosis, catheterization can be attempted blindly with a smaller-gauge flexible catheter. Hypospadias is not uncommon, and some hypospadiac patients have a blind-ending navicular fossa, which should not be catheterized.

If a meatal stricture or stenosis is apparent, passing a catheter of a smaller size should be attempted first. Gentle dilation of the stenosis with sounds can be attempted if catheterization is unsuccessful.

After skin and meatus preparation and sterile draping, the initial maneuver is to grasp the penis with the nondominant hand, which is from then on regarded as no longer sterile. The pendulous curvature of the penis is eliminated by pulling the shaft upward. The catheter is inserted into the meatus after lubrication and advanced approximately 7 to 12 cm. The penis should be brought into a horizontal position, parallel to the patient. Some slight resistance can be appreciated at the membranous urethra, the most fragile

segment. The entire catheter is introduced into the penis, up to the bifurcation of the catheter and balloon valve. Spontaneous drainage of urine should occur if the bladder is not empty. If no spontaneous urine drainage appears, gently pushing down on the suprapubic region or instilling a small amount of clear sterile fluid and aspirating the catheter with a syringe should result in drainage. The lumen of the catheter can be obstructed with lubricant jelly, pus, or blood. If after such maneuvers no drainage occurs, the bladder is empty or the catheter is malpositioned.

After verifying the correct position of the catheter in the bladder, inflate the balloon with sterile water, which has been demonstrated to be the optimal filling solution, especially if the catheter is to be in place for several days or longer (Sharpe et al, 2011). Although not conclusively proven, saline or glucose-based solutions can theoretically occlude the tubing by precipitation (Hui et al, 2004; Huang et al, 2009). In uncircumcised patients, the foreskin is reduced to its normal position to avoid paraphimosis.

The penis and catheter should be taped in an upright position to prevent pressure ulceration from occurring at the curve in the pendulous urethra and iatrogenic hypospadias at the urethral meatus. Iatrogenic hypospadias, when missed or untreated, can evolve into severe deformations (Andrews et al, 1998; Gokhan et al, 2006; Cipa-Tatum et al, 2011).

Ideally, a closed circuit should be maintained with the catheter connected to a sterile closed bag system, positioned lower than the bladder to allow gravity to assist in bladder emptying.

Although it is believed that rapid complete emptying of a urinary retention results more frequently in possible complications such as hematuria, hypotension, or pain, **efficient complete emptying has been demonstrated to be safe and is recommended** (Nyman et al, 1997; Muhammed and Abubakar, 2012).

Catheterization in Female Patients

With the patient in a frog-leg position and adequately draped, the nondominant hand is used to spread the inner labia to reveal the external urethral meatus. This hand is now considered contaminated. The urethral meatus should be found 1 to 2.5 cm inferior to the clitoris. After the meatus has been cleaned and lubricated, the catheter is inserted into the meatus and gently advanced until approximately half the catheter has been inserted. It is not necessary to advance the catheter up to the valve bifurcation. The balloon is inflated after confirming the correct position of the catheter in the bladder.

Catheterization in Children

Catheter use in children is predominantly for diagnostic purposes or postoperative drainage. In infants, suprapubic puncture for obtaining a urine sample is often preferred over a bag sample because it is more likely to be sterile. Bladder catheterization, however, is preferred over suprapubic aspiration because it is less painful and has a higher success rate in obtaining a satisfactory urine sample (Pollack et al, 1994; Kozer et al, 2006; El-Naggar et al, 2010). Portable bedside bladder ultrasound is useful to identify a sufficient amount of urine in the bladder before attempted catheterization (Chen et al, 2005; Robson et al, 2006; Baumann et al, 2008).

Children are presented with a phimosis more frequently than men. As in adults, it is useful to align the preputial opening with the meatus to facilitate catheterization. Compared with women, the urethral orifice in young girls may be partly obscured behind the hymen. To reveal the meatus, it is useful to apply some downward pressure on the hymen. If the meatus cannot be visualized, the same maneuver as in women should be applied: the tip of the catheter is slid down from the clitoris toward the introitus, above the hymen.

Difficult Catheterization

The most commonly encountered cause of difficult catheterization in men without previous relevant history is inability to pass the catheter beyond the prostate. This is commonly the result of an enlarged prostate or a closed striated sphincter. The attempted catheter is retracted, and the catheter tip evaluated for the presence of blood. If the catheter tip is clean, the next option is a 14-Fr or 16-Fr silicone catheter because it is somewhat stiffer and may pass the slight resistance more effectively. If blood is present at the catheter tip, there is a possibility of a false passage and a coudé-tipped catheter should be used for the next attempt. A false passage is most commonly created in the membranous urethra, the most fragile segment of the urethra, which can be palpated transrectally at the apex of the prostate. One can try guiding the catheter past the false passage transrectally with the index finger. If transrectal guidance does not facilitate passage and if the caliber of the urethra allows, placement of a small-caliber catheter (10 or 12 Fr) in the false passage may be attempted. This may close off the false passage and allow for passage of a second transurethral catheter into the bladder. If passage of a catheter is still not possible, a flexible cystoscope is used to assess the urethra for size, strictures, false passage, or bladder neck stenosis. If the bladder is successfully accessed, a guidewire can be passed and used to pass a Councill catheter. If a stricture is apparent and cannot be catheterized with a smaller catheter, a guidewire is cystoscopically passed through the stricture into the bladder, and the urethra dilated to allow for a catheter of adequate size to be placed. If the urethral stricture is a new diagnosis, this should be documented with a view toward follow-up and treatment if necessary. The use of stylets is recommended only in experienced hands and only if cystoscopic guidance is unavailable. If all attempts at urethral catheterization including with flexible cystoscopy guidance are unsuccessful and there are no absolute contraindications, one should consider placing a suprapubic catheter (Fig. 6-3).

Although the female urethra is short, catheterization can be challenging because of inability to find the urethral meatus. In obese patients or in patients unable to assume the frog-leg position, the use of stirrups and assistance for retraction to optimize visualization is advised and may be useful.

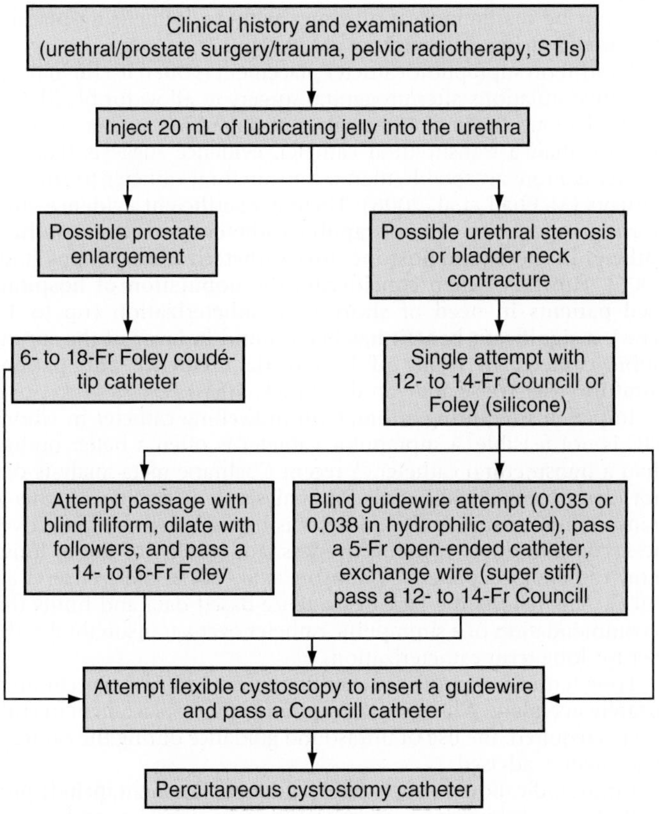

In rare instances such as extreme labial adhesions, introital stenosis, or stricture or stenosis of the female urethra, urethral catheter placement is sometimes not feasible. The same approach as described for male urethral stricture should be applied.

COMPLICATIONS

Catheterization of the urethra is an everyday practice on almost every hospital ward. It is an intervention of significance, however, that may be associated with short- and long-term complications.

From 15% to 25% of hospitalized patients undergo a urethral catheter placement at some point during their stay (Glynn et al, 1997). UTIs account for approximately 35% of hospital-acquired infections, with almost 95% of UTIs in the intensive care unit setting resulting from bladder catheters (Richards et al, 2000; Klevens et al, 2007). Overuse of bladder catheterization has been reported to range from 15% to 40% of cases and is correlated with prolonged hospital stay (Apisarnthanarak et al, 2007; Tiwari et al, 2012). In the United States, the economic impact associated with CAUTI accumulates to an annual cost of about $300 million (Zimlichman et al, 2013). Implementation of quality improvement and awareness projects has contributed to significantly reducing the incidence and duration of catheterization, and ultimately CAUTI rates (Janzen et al, 2013; Parry et al, 2013; Saint et al, 2013).

As of 2009, the definition for CAUTI was modified to exclude asymptomatic bacteriuria (Dudeck et al, 2011). In current guidelines, a **CAUTI is defined as significant bacteriuria in a patient with symptoms or signs indicating a UTI,** whereas *asymptomatic bacteriuria* refers to significant bacteriuria in asymptomatic patients. **Asymptomatic bacteriuria does not require antibiotic treatment.** Because there is no evidence supporting that treatment of asymptomatic bacteriuria provides any benefit in reducing morbidity or mortality, the European Association of Urology (EAU) and Infectious Diseases Society of America (IDSA) guidelines specifically recommend against screening and treatment of asymptomatic bacteriuria (Tenke et al, 2008; Hooton et al, 2010). The most important risk factor for developing CAUTI is prolonged catheterization (longer than 6 days). Other risk factors include catheterization outside of the operating room, female sex, body mass index (BMI) greater than 30, diabetes, and other active site of infection (Maki and Tambyah, 2001; Stenzelius et al, 2011).

Universal recommendations in guidelines for preventing CAUTI are avoidance of catheter use, maintenance of a closed drainage system, and removal of a catheter as soon as deemed possible. Catheters should be placed under antiseptic conditions, placing the smallest possible catheter with adequate lubrication. Routine irrigation should be avoided (Gould et al, 2010; Hooton et al, 2010; Tambyah and Oon, 2012).

A recent Cochrane meta-analysis showed no difference in urinary infection rates in long-term catheterized patients when different catheter types were compared (Jahn et al, 2012). There is insufficient evidence to reliably recommend the use of one catheter type over another.

Short-term antibiotic treatment (5 days) with catheter exchange has been proven to be equally as effective as long-term treatment (10 days) without catheter exchange in treating CAUTI (Darouiche et al, 2014).

Long-term antibiotic prophylaxis has not been demonstrated to significantly reduce symptomatic CAUTI in patients performing CIC. Interrupting long-term prophylaxis in spina bifida patients results in a nonsignificant increase in UTIs, without clinical significance (Wolf et al, 2008; Hooton et al, 2010; Zegers et al, 2011). Use of prophylactic antibiotics on removal of a bladder catheter, even after short-term catheterization, has been both recommended and discouraged (Wolf et al, 2008; Hooton et al, 2010). American Urological Association (AUA) guidelines published in 2008 recommended the use of antibiotic prophylaxis after catheter removal if bacteriuria is present, particularly in patients with risk factors such as advanced age, immunodeficiency, or corticosteroid use (Wolf et al, 2008). In 2010 the IDSA discouraged the use of prophylactic

Figure 6-3. **Flowchart for managing difficult catheterization. STIs, sexually transmitted infections.**

antibiotics before catheter removal or catheter change (Hooton et al, 2010). The most recent meta-analysis attempting to answer this question reports a reduction in UTI incidence when antibiotic prophylaxis is administered on removal of a bladder catheter in surgical patients (Marschall et al, 2013). Taking into consideration that up to 25% of hospitalized patients are catheterized at some point during their stay, recommending the **routine use of antibiotics after catheter removal** would entail an enormous usage of antibiotics with the associated risks of bacterial resistance and other drug-related side effects. Therefore, prophylaxis **should be considered a recommendation only in patients with risk factors**, as previously stated by the AUA guidelines panel.

A comprehensive overview and meta-analysis of all possible complications of urethral catheterization reports that noninfectious complications are at least as frequent as CAUTI in short-term catheterizations and up to four times more prevalent in long-term catheterizations. Complications include pericatheter urine leakage, accidental removal, catheter blockage, hematuria, bladder stones, and bladder cancer. The subgroup of patients with spinal cord injuries is at greater risk of complications (Hollingsworth et al, 2013).

Inability to remove a transurethral bladder catheter can be a challenging complication. Entrapment of the catheter by anastomotic sutures after urethroplasty or radical prostatectomy poses a unique postoperative complication. When sutures are known to be degradable, one can retry catheter removal 1 or 2 weeks after the initial attempt. If the sutures are nondegradable, the urethra can be accessed with a semirigid ureteroscope to visualize and divide the suture with laser energy (Nagarajan et al, 2005; Nagele et al, 2006). Cuffing of the balloon after deflation can cause the catheter to bind at the bladder neck. This phenomenon is dependent on the catheter used (material and manufacturer), indwelling time, urinary infection, and deflation method, with indwelling time being the most significant predictor. Slow deflation of the balloon and the use of hydrogel-coated or PTFE catheters reduce the chance of balloon cuffing (Chung and So, 2012). Gonzalgo proposed a technique of instillation of 0.5 to 1 mL of fluid in the balloon to smooth out the cuff for easier catheter removal (Gonzalgo and Walsh, 2003).

Inability to deflate the Foley balloon is not uncommon. Resolution of this problem may be achieved by instilling an extra 1 or 2 mL of fluid in the balloon and trying to repeat aspiration. Overinflation of the balloon with the intention of having it burst should be avoided because this may be painful and possibly result in retained fragments of the catheter balloon in the bladder. Cutting off the inflation valve may assist if the valve is not functioning correctly. If the balloon still does not deflate, one can pass a guidewire through the inflation channel to try and perforate the balloon. If all else fails, ultrasound-guided needle puncture of the balloon is typically the final approach. Inability to remove a catheter with a fully deflated balloon can also be caused by catheter encrustation, especially if the catheter has been indwelling for an extended time. There is strong evidence that the main causal factor of catheter encrustation is infection with *Proteus mirabilis*. Especially in patients with long-term bladder catheterization, this circumstance can cause recurrent blockage of the catheter (Stickler and Feneley, 2010). Applying gentle traction to the catheter can cause the encrustation to dislodge, facilitating catheter removal. If this does not solve the problem and encrustation is suspected, ultrasound or x-ray imaging can be used for confirmation. For more significant encrustations, one can consider using a semirigid ureteroscope and the holmium:YAG laser to remove the encrustation material. Increasing patient fluid intake and ingestion of citrate could delay or control this problem in known stone formers and chronic catheter blockers (Stickler and Feneley, 2010).

Urethral stricture is not an uncommon complication after catheterization. Lumen and colleagues reported that 11.2% of urethral stricture disease requiring urethroplasty is causally related to urethral catheterization. When site of stricture was taken into account, history of urethral catheterization was the most important causal factor of multifocal or panurethral strictures (Lumen et al, 2009).

Fenton and associates reported 32% of urethral strictures as being caused by iatrogenic trauma; 36.5% of these were the result of prolonged catheterization. The authors proposed that prolonged catheterization leads to urethral inflammation and ischemia, and ultimately to urethral stricture (Fenton et al, 2005).

Inflation of the balloon in the prostatic urethra or in a false passage can cause severe hematuria, urethral rupture, and subsequent stricture (Lang et al, 2012).

Prevention of Iatrogenic Trauma

The pressure in the catheter balloon when an incorrectly placed catheter is being inflated is much higher than when the catheter is in a correct position. Forces of extraction of a catheter are much lower with 5 mL in the balloon than with 10 mL in the balloon (Wu et al, 2012). When high pressure is perceived when inflating the balloon, one should reassess and ensure that the catheter is in the bladder. In patients at risk of inadvertent traumatic catheter extraction, the balloon is filled with 5 mL instead of 10 mL to decrease the chance of significant urethral trauma.

When prolonged catheterization is required, a smaller catheter, such as 16 Fr, should be used. There should be a lower threshold for placing a suprapubic catheter when prolonged catheterization is anticipated (Fenton et al, 2005). With training and education, trauma from urethral catheterization can be reduced fivefold (Kashefi et al, 2008; Thomas et al, 2009).

LOWER URINARY TRACT: SUPRAPUBIC CATHETER DRAINAGE

Indications

If bladder drainage is necessary but access to the bladder cannot or should not be obtained transurethrally, the placement of a suprapubic catheter should be considered.

During transurethral resection of the prostate, suprapubic catheter placement is preferred by some urologists because a continuous flow can be maintained at all times without influencing bladder pressure (Sánchez Zalabardo et al, 2003).

Short-term suprapubic catheter placement is often useful in postoperative situations after urogenital surgery to allow for bladder or urethral tissue healing. Although a suprapubic catheter is more invasive than a transurethral catheter, evidence suggests that the former is more acceptable than a transurethral catheter to surgical patients (McPhail et al, 2006). There is **insufficient evidence supporting superiority of a suprapubic catheter over a transurethral catheter in short-term postoperative catheterization** (Phipps et al, 2006). **However, when considering the population of hospitalized patients in need of short-term catheterization (up to 14 days), a significant benefit has been found in favor of the suprapubic catheter in terms of bacteriuria incidence and patient comfort** (Niël-Weise and van den Broek, 2005).

In patients requiring a long-term indwelling catheter in whom CIC is not feasible, a suprapubic catheter is often a better option than a transurethral catheter. A recent Cochrane meta-analysis did not identify any eligible trials for analysis to determine whether a transurethral or suprapubic catheter is better in terms of effectiveness, complications, cost-effectiveness, and quality of life in long-term catheterized patients (Jamison et al, 2011; Niël-Weise et al, 2012). This reflects the lack of evidence-based data and limits the recommendation of a suprapubic catheter over a transurethral catheter for long-term catheterization.

Long-term suprapubic catheter placement in infants or children is rarely necessary. Whenever suprapubic catheter placement in children is required, the use of ultrasound guidance during the catheter placement is advised.

Contraindications to suprapubic catheter placement include previous lower abdominal surgery resulting in unsafe percutaneous passage to the bladder, bladder cancer, uncorrected coagulopathies or anticoagulation, abdominal wall infection at the desired puncture site, and the presence of vascular grafts near the preferred tract (Harrison et al, 2011).

In patients in whom one may suspect the presence of ascites, ultrasound is always used to confirm a large postvoid residual urine volume because ascites can sometimes be mistaken for a large post-micturitional volume on ultrasound bladder scan.

Advantages of a suprapubic catheter include elimination of risk of urethral stricture and penile erosion. A trial to void can be attempted without the need for recatheterization if unsuccessful. Wound care for a suprapubic catheter is often easier, especially in chair-bound patients.

In patients requiring long-term catheter drainage, the placement of a suprapubic catheter as an alternative to a transurethral catheter can be considered, and advantages and disadvantages should be discussed with the patient.

Technique of Suprapubic Catheter Placement: Percutaneous

For suprapubic catheter placement, the patient should be placed in supine position at a comfortable height for the physician.

In most patients the distended bladder displaces the intraperitoneal bowel loops out of the pelvis and away from the pubic symphysis. A minimum bladder volume of 300 mL on bladder scan is advised before suprapubic catheter placement is attempted (Albrecht et al, 2004).

The patient's infraumbilical abdomen should be prepared and draped in a sterile fashion. In performing blind puncture, the symphysis should be palpated and the access site should be chosen approximately one to two fingerbreadths above the symphysis. In obese patients with an abdominal pannus, placement of the tract in a skin fold is avoided to prevent dermatitis (Harrison et al, 2011). Local anesthetic is injected into the skin and along the preferred trajectory using a 10- to 20-mL syringe and an 18-gauge needle. The tract should be almost perpendicular to the skin. Aspirating urine will confirm access to the bladder. A midline 5- to 10-mm transverse incision is made at the injection site.

The safest technique for catheterization is the **Seldinger technique.** A floppy-tip guidewire is advanced into the bladder through an 18-Fr access needle. The percutaneous tract is dilated with coaxial dilators. A Cope loop or Councill catheter can be placed over the guidewire into the bladder after the tract is dilated (Fig. 6-4).

The **trocar technique** employs a peel-away trocar that envelops the catheter. The trocar should be advanced firmly but under steady control of the trocar. Once entry into the bladder has been confirmed by urine flashback or aspiration, the catheter is advanced completely into the bladder, and the trocar is retracted and peeled away. If the suprapubic catheter does not have a retention mechanism, the catheter is sutured to the skin.

Obesity, previous lower abdominal or pelvic surgery or radiation therapy, and a nondistended bladder that cannot be palpated should prompt the physician to use ultrasound guidance. It is preferable to have an assistant operate the ultrasound probe, thus allowing both hands to be available for catheter placement. When the bladder is being punctured, the needle tip will appear as a hyperechoic structure on the ultrasound image (Jacob et al, 2012). The use of ultrasound-guided suprapubic catheter placement has a high success ratio, and the procedure is safe and has a low complication rate (Cronin et al, 2011). Cystoscopic visual guidance can be of additional help in performing percutaneous suprapubic catheter placement.

Technique of Suprapubic Catheter Placement: Open

Open suprapubic catheter placement should be undertaken when a percutaneous technique cannot be performed safely. After the infraumbilical abdomen is prepared and draped, a small incision is made about one to two fingerbreadths above the pubic symphysis, providing access to the retroperitoneal space of Retzius. Two stay sutures are placed to stabilize the bladder, and a small incision is

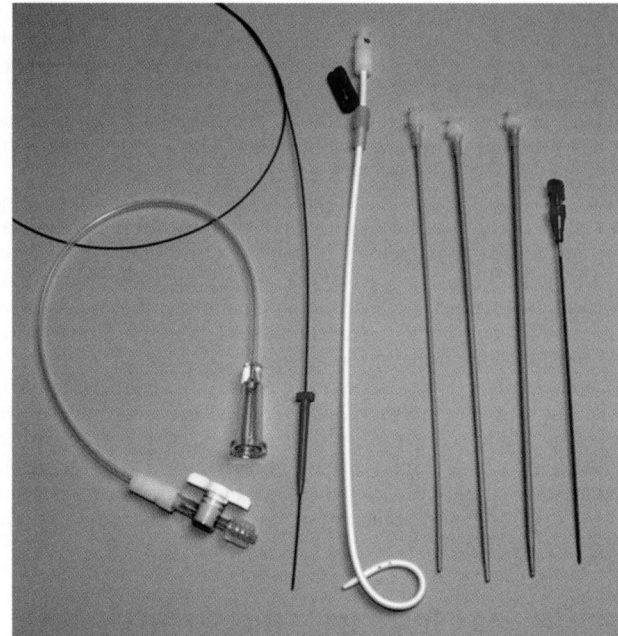

Figure 6-4. Percutaneous suprapubic catheter kit. *Left to right,* **Guidewire, drainage bag connection tubing, Cope loop catheter, Amplatz dilators, and cystostomy needle. (Courtesy Cook Medical, Bloomington, IN.)**

made through the bladder wall between the sutures, allowing for easy passage of a 16- to 18-Fr catheter. The catheter should be introduced through the skin in line with the bladder incision to prevent kinking and should be secured in the bladder with a purse suture to prevent urine extravasation.

Because of the invasiveness of suprapubic catheter placement and its transcutaneous character, it is subject to complications such as wound infection, hematoma, and perivesical fluid collection. **Surrounding organ injury is the most severe complication and has been reported to occur in less than 1% to 2.7% of procedures** (Sheriff et al, 1998; Ahluwalia et al, 2006; Cronin et al, 2011).

Catheter Exchange

Before exchanging a suprapubic catheter, it should be left in place for at least 2 to 4 weeks to allow for tract maturation. After the patient has been prepared and all required materials are readily available, the physician deflates the balloon and extracts the catheter. Some lubricant gel is instilled in the tract, and the new catheter is placed into the bladder. A small amount of fluid in the bladder adds safety by providing the possibility of aspirating the catheter to ensure correct placement. Catheter exchange over a guidewire can be performed in patients with difficult tracts.

Complications

Complications from the presence of the suprapubic catheter are similar to those of a transurethral catheter. A meta-analysis comparing suprapubic to transurethral drainage after gynecologic surgery concluded that suprapubic catheterization significantly reduces the rate of UTI but, on the other hand, was significantly correlated with a higher rate of minor complications such as hematuria, leakage, blockage, or accidental catheter loss. Superiority of one over the other could not be determined (Healy et al, 2012, 2013).

Frequent blockage of a suprapubic catheter can be caused by encrustation or bladder stones. Frequent catheter blockage should prompt consideration of cystoscopy to evaluate for the presence of bladder stones. Excessive granulation tissue at the suprapubic tract can be treated by silver nitrate application.

Catheter placement technique with a trocar or Seldinger technique, catheter type, and catheter size do not seem to influence the complication rate of ultrasound-guided suprapubic catheterization (Cronin et al, 2011).

Bowel perforation during catheter exchange has been reported and has been associated with difficult exchange and use of stiffer catheters (Mongiu et al, 2009; Kass-Iliyya et al, 2012).

An accidentally removed suprapubic catheter is a unique, sometimes challenging complication. Pigtail or Cope loop catheters are more prone to dislodgement than balloon retained catheters (Cronin et al, 2011). The tract of the suprapubic catheter can close in a short period of time, encouraging prompt tube replacement. Smaller catheters, guidewire placement, and dilation of the tract can be of assistance for catheter replacement.

Although there is no available literature on learning curve in suprapubic catheter placement, practice and experience are expected to translate to a lower complication rate. Hossack recently proposed the first design of a simple, useful, and cheap training model for percutaneous suprapubic catheter placement for practitioners to gain experience before placing suprapubic catheters in patients (Hossack et al, 2013).

UPPER URINARY TRACT: URETERAL STENTS AND CATHETERS

Historic Note

The use of ureteral stents in surgery was described as early as the 19th century (Shoemaker, 1895). The first urologist to access the ureter endoscopically was Dr. James Brown at Johns Hopkins Hospital in 1893 (Arcadi, 1999). Zimskind, however, in 1967 was the first to describe the cystoscopic placement of indwelling ureteral stents for obstructed ureters (Zimskind et al, 1967). At that time, stents were very prone to migration and device expulsion, which deterred widespread adoption. Gibbons was the first to patent a barbed stent as a self-retaining mechanism (Gibbons et al, 1976). The first "double-J" (DJ) or double pigtail stent was developed

almost simultaneously by Finney and Hepperlen (Finney, 1978; Hepperlen et al, 1978). After this novel advance, the use of DJ stents increased dramatically in urology departments worldwide, which had a tremendous positive impact on endourologic surgery and patient care. Today, ureteral stents are of fundamental importance to any urologic practice.

Stent Technology

The ideal stent is easy to insert, has the ability to relieve intraluminal and extraluminal obstruction, has excellent flow characteristics, is resistant to encrustation and infection, is chemically stable after implantation in a urinary environment, and does not induce patient symptoms. Stents should therefore have high tensile strength, a low friction coefficient, memory, and a self-retainment mechanism and should be both biocompatible and affordable. The number of new patents filed annually related to ureteral stents is shown in Figure 6-5 and demonstrates that development of new designs, biomaterials, and coatings for ureteral stents has increased dramatically over the past decade. This effort reflects the many initiatives in stent design aligned to achieve the ideal characteristics.

Biomaterials

Early ureteral stents were manufactured from silicone (Zimskind et al, 1967). Although **silicone is the most biocompatible material tested to date** (Beiko et al, 2003; Watterson et al, 2003b), the high friction coefficient and flexibility that are characteristic of silicone make silicone stents more difficult to navigate through a tortuous or obstructed ureter. Polyethylene was introduced as the first plastic polymer in the commonly used DJ stents (Mardis et al, 1979). Polyethylene stents become brittle after prolonged exposure to the urinary environment and are prone to encrustation, blockage, and fragmentation, leading to the discontinuation of use of this material in stent manufacture and the development of newer polymers. Currently used stents are commonly composed of polyurethane, silicone, or proprietary copolymers such as Silitek (Surgitek, Medical Engineering Company, Racine, WI), C-Flex (Cook Medical,

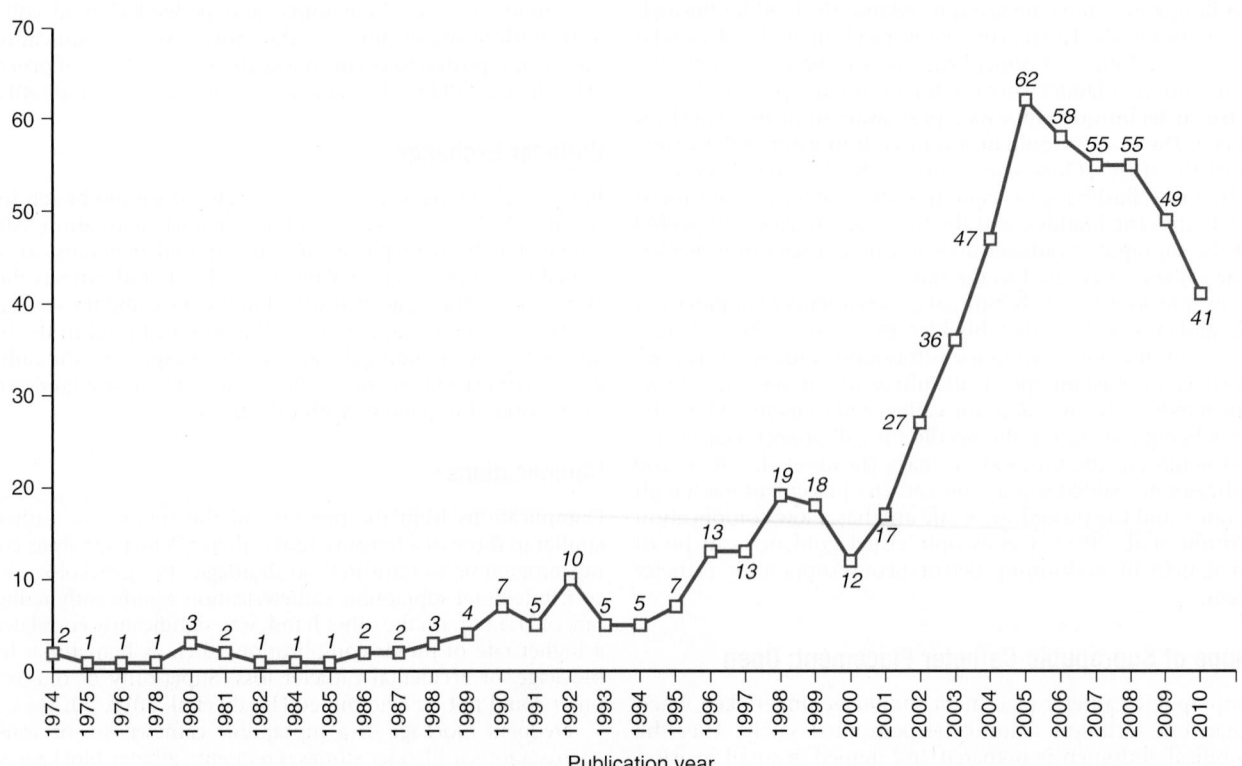

Figure 6-5. Graph showing annual number of patents filed related to ureteral stents. (Courtesy Dolcera Patent and Market Research Services.)

Bloomington, IN), Percuflex (Boston Scientific, Marlborough, MA), or Tecoflex (PNN Medical, Kvistgaard, Denmark).

Ureteric obstruction caused by extrinsic, usually malignant, compression requires stents that can withstand these radial compressive forces. Mechanical tests on nonmetal stents evaluating resistance to radial compression demonstrated the C-Flex (Cook Medical, Bloomington, IN) stent to resist extrinsic compressive forces best (Hendlin et al, 2006). **Although it is common practice to use a larger-lumen stent to achieve adequate drainage, stents with a smaller lumen have been shown to be more resistant to radial compressive forces** in experimental studies (Hendlin et al, 2006).

The **self-expanding metallic Wallstent** has been used to treat ureteric obstruction since 1992 (Pauer and Lugmayr, 1992). Although the stent is reported to be safe and effective, its primary patency rates are low, ranging from 29% to 54% at 3 to 12 months, mainly because of hyperplastic tissue ingrowth. With additional endoscopic interventions, secondary patency can be maintained in up to 100% of stents in short- and long-term follow-up (Flueckiger et al, 1993; Lugmayr and Pauer, 1996; Lang et al, 1998, 2013).

The **Resonance metallic ureteral stent** (Cook Medical, Bloomington, IN) is constructed from tightly coiled spirals of a corrosion-resistant nickel-cobalt-chromium-molybdenum alloy wire and is designed to resist encrustation and tissue overgrowth. Although the overall flow was inferior compared with conventional stents in an in vivo porcine study, the Resonance stent can easily withstand compression forces that completely obstruct conventional stents (Blaschko et al, 2007; Pedro et al, 2007). Long-term results and follow-up in larger cohorts demonstrate a failure rate of 28% to 35%, which is comparable to conventional stents (Liatsikos et al, 2010; Goldsmith et al, 2012; Kadlec et al, 2013). Because the Resonance stent can be safely retained in the ureter for extended periods, the reduced hospital and procedure costs may mitigate the higher cost of the stent itself (López-Huertas et al, 2010; Polcari et al, 2010; Taylor et al, 2012).

Newer metal stents have been designed and tested in vitro and are awaiting clinical trials. The **Silhouette stent** (Applied Medical Resources Corporation, Rancho Santa Margarita, CA) is a soft, coil-reinforced stent with a hydrophilic coating. It is less prone to kinking than other stents and can resist higher compressional forces than the Resonance stent, theoretically resulting in a lower chance of stent failure (Pedro et al, 2007; Christman et al, 2010; Miyaoka et al, 2010). The **Passage and Snake stents** (ProSurg, San Jose, CA) are open-ended and less tightly coiled than the Resonance and Silhouette stents, allowing for more flexibility. Both stents sustain higher extrinsic radial compression forces than the Silhouette stent and have lower tensile strength (Hendlin et al, 2012).

The **Memokath 051 ureteral stent** (PNN Medical, Kvistgaard, Denmark) is a nickel-titanium alloy (nitinol) stent with a thermo-expandable anchoring mechanism. The initial report on the use of the Memokath stent in obstructed ureters demonstrated a high patency rate of the lumen after 10.6 months of follow-up (Kulkarni and Bellamy, 1999). In addition to having long-term patency in ureteral obstruction, the Memokath 051 is better tolerated than conventional ureteral stents in terms of urinary symptoms, pain, and general health (Maan et al, 2010). Late complications include stent migration in 15% to 18% and encrustation in 3% to 5%. Stent manipulation or reinsertion has been reported to be necessary in 20% to 25% of patients (Agrawal et al, 2009; Papatsoris and Buchholz, 2010).

The **Uventa stent** (Taewoong Medical, Gimpo, South Korea) is also a nickel-titanium alloy, segmental, thermally expandable stent. A PTFE coating is positioned between the outer and inner mesh. The outer mesh provides extra friction to prevent stent migration, and the PTFE coating prevents hyperplastic stent ingrowth (Chung et al, 2008). Kim reported a 100% primary patency in 20 stents with an average follow-up of 7.3 months (Kim et al, 2012). After a 10-month follow-up period, primary patency rates decrease to 64.8% and secondary patency rates to 81.7%. Stent failure is predominantly a result of tumor progression at an adjacent ureteral segment. Migration has not been reported (Chung et al, 2013).

The **Allium stent** (Allium Medical Solutions, Israel) is a large-caliber (24 Fr or 30 Fr) nickel-titanium alloy, expandable mesh stent coated with a biocompatible polymer to prevent stent ingrowth. The Allium stent was specifically developed for use in the distal ureter and has an intravesical anchor to facilitate removal. Limited data are available in the published literature, reporting patency rates of greater than 95% and migration in 14% of stents, necessitating removal. No encrustation was documented at an average of 17-months' follow-up (Moskovitz et al, 2012; Leonardo et al, 2013) (Fig. 6-6).

A common problem among metal mesh stents is reduced patency in long-term follow-up and late complications such as migration, encrustation, and erosion. Coatings to prevent hyperplasia and stent ingrowth in metal mesh stents have been adopted from the endovascular stent realm. In comparison to uncoated metal mesh stents, a paclitaxel drug-eluting metal mesh stent was shown to generate less inflammation and hyperplasia of the surrounding tissue in a porcine model (Liatsikos et al, 2007). The zotarolimus-eluting metal stent induced a significantly lower hyperplastic reaction without influencing inflammation rates in a porcine and rabbit model (Kallidonis et al, 2011). These coatings have the potential to improve patency and reduce complication rates.

The development of **a biodegradable stent could theoretically eliminate the need for cystoscopic stent removal and could help prevent the occurrence of forgotten stents.** Biodegradable materials are composed of high-molecular-weight polymers such as

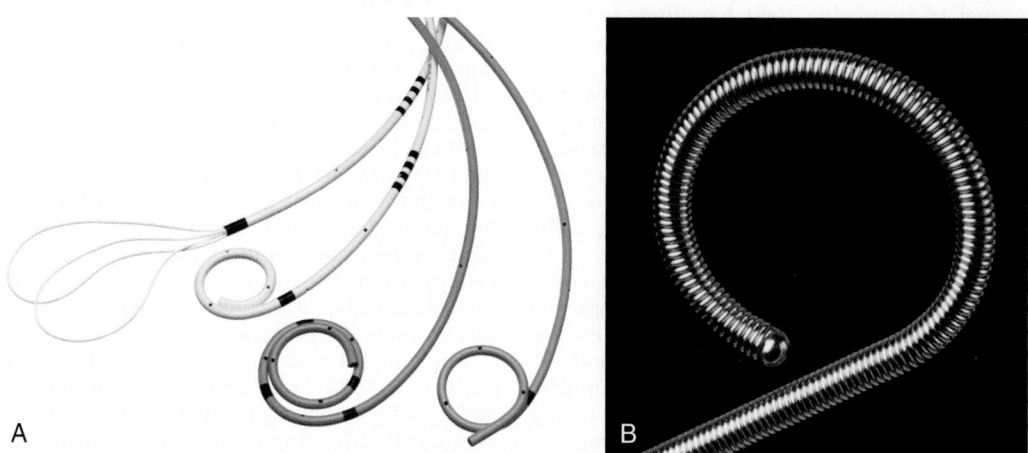

Figure 6-6. **Different stent designs. A, Polaris Loop stent, Polaris Ultra stent, Percuflex Plus stent, and Contour VL stent. B, Resonance metal stent. (A, Courtesy Boston Scientific, Marlborough, MA; B, courtesy Cook Medical, Bloomington, IN.)**

polylactide or polyglycolide. Surface modification of bioresorbable polymers with, for instance, hydroxyethylmethacrylate (HEMA), oligo(ethyleneoxide)-monomethacrylate (OEOMA), or acrylic acid (AAc) results in improved biocompatibility without toxicity of these polymers and thus allows use in a urinary environment (Brauers et al, 1998). The main challenge of biodegradable materials is controlling the rate of degradation. In vivo tests with a poly-L,D-lactide polymer in a canine model demonstrated promising results with complete degradation of all stents within 24 weeks without induction of ureteral histologic changes (Lumiaho et al, 1999, 2000).

In vivo tests in a porcine model with Uriprene, a biodegradable copolymer composed of L-glycolic acid, polyethylene glycol, and barium sulfate, show promising preliminary results. With the current chemical formulation, Uriprene stents reliably achieve degradation after 4 weeks. The Uriprene stents induced a lower degree of ureteral inflammatory change when compared with conventional stents in a porcine model (Hadaschik et al, 2008; Chew et al, 2010, 2013). Olweny and colleagues established that use of a degradable poly-L-lactide–co-glycolide polymer stent in a porcine ureter after endopyelotomy was feasible but induced more tissue inflammation than a conventional stent (Olweny et al, 2002).

Newer polymer components are currently under investigation for future stent development. Magnesium-yttrium alloy potentially offers many benefits over currently existing stents because the alloy is biodegradable and seems to inhibit bacterial viability in vitro. The rate and mode of degradation can be controlled through alloy design and surface modification (Lock et al, 2012, 2014). Degradable polyfilament, fibrous stents composed of polyglycolic acid (PGA) and polylactic acid (PLA) demonstrated complete degradation after 8 weeks. The resistance to compression of the stent was comparable to that of conventional stents during the first 2 weeks after insertion (Shang et al, 2011).

The feasibility of a natural, tissue-engineered ureteral stent has been investigated in vitro with the goal of achieving optimal biocompatibility. Amiel demonstrated that seeding chondrocytes on a polylactic–co-glycolic acid enforced PGA polymer scaffold was feasible in vitro and that the tissue-engineered stents were readily elastic and could withstand compression (Amiel et al, 2001). No in vivo trials have yet been reported.

The first and to date only trial studying the use of biodegradable stents in human subjects demonstrated adequate drainage while maintaining a high patient tolerance. After 90 days, 96.6% of patients were stent free. Three patients, however, required shockwave lithotripsy (SWL) and one patient subsequently required ureteroscopy (URS) to clear retained stent fragments (Lingeman et al, 2003).

Coatings

Drug-eluting and antiadhesive stent coatings are under investigation with the goal of improving stent handling, reducing biofilm formation, preventing encrustation, and improving patient comfort.

Hydrogel is a commonly applied stent coating composed of hydrophilic polymers that absorb water. This added surface water reduces friction and increases elasticity, rendering the stent easier to insert and theoretically more biocompatible. In vitro tests, however, have demonstrated hydrogel-coated stents to both reduce and increase encrustation and biofilm formation (Tunney et al, 1996; Desgrandchamps et al, 1997; Gorman et al, 1998).

Pentosan polysulfate (PPS), phosphorylcholine (PC) copolymer, and polyvinylpyrrolidone (PVP) are newer coatings that have been demonstrated to reduce inflammatory response, encrustation, and biofilm formation. **Polyvinylpyrrolidone-iodine (PVP-I) complex** modified polyurethane Tecoflex stents (Lubrizol, Wickliffe, OH) appear to be highly hydrophilic and to reduce encrustation deposits and adherence of *Pseudomonas aeruginosa* and *Staphylococcus aureus* by 80% to 86% in in vitro tests (Khandwekar and Doble, 2011). A **diamond-like carbon (DLC) coating** has been noted to render the stent surface ultrasmooth, thereby decreasing friction and improving biocompatibility. DLC-coated

polyurethane demonstrated significant resistance to biofilm formation and microbial adherence in in vitro and in vivo studies (Jones et al, 2006; Laube et al, 2007). Silicone coated with *Oxalobacter formigenes*–derived oxalate degrading enzymes demonstrated a modest reduction in encrustation in vivo compared with uncoated controls (Watterson et al, 2003a). **Triclosan-eluting stents (Triumph** [Boston Scientific, Marlborough, MA]) initially demonstrated a significant decrease in growth and survival of *P. mirabilis* in a rabbit study (Cadieux et al, 2006). The Triumph stent significantly reduced stent-related pain and urinary symptoms in short-term stented patients and reduced symptomatic UTI rate in long-term stented patients without, however, influencing biofilm formation, encrustation, or urine cultures (Cadieux et al, 2009; Mendez-Probst et al, 2012). A **ketorolac-eluting stent (Lexington** [Boston Scientific, Marlborough, MA]) was developed with the goal of reducing stent-induced pain symptoms. A prospective multicenter double-blind RCT evaluating the effect of Lexington stents reported no statistical difference in unplanned postoperative medical visits or pain perception. The authors did, however, demonstrate a significant reduction in the need for analgesia in the ketorolac-eluting stent group on post-URS day 2. Benefits of the stent were most evident in a subgroup of men and patients younger than 45 years (Krambeck et al, 2010). Although in vitro tests with **heparin-coated stents** did not show a significant benefit, in vivo tests demonstrated a significantly reduced encrustation rate. Tenke and Cauda noted that heparin-coated stents may remain indwelling for longer than 6 months and potentially up to 12 months, translating into an economic benefit (Riedl et al, 2002; Tenke et al, 2004; Cauda et al, 2008; Lange et al, 2009). Polyethylene glycol conjugated with 3,4-dihydroxyphenylalanine polymer, **mPEG-DOPA$_3$**, is a novel antifouling coating that demonstrated in vitro and in vivo resistance to bacterial attachment and biofilm formation. A cross-linked DOPA-anchored antifouling polymer was identified as the most resistant to *E. coli* adherence (Ko et al, 2008; Pechey et al, 2009). **Sustained-release varnish containing chlorhexidine (CHX-SRV)–coated stents** significantly reduce bacterial growth in vitro and in vivo with the initial 1% chlorhexidine concentration. The newly tested 2% concentration prolonged the inhibitory effect on bacterial growth up to 2 weeks (Shapur et al, 2012; Segev et al, 2013; Zelichenko et al, 2013).

Development of **antibiotic coatings** is still in a preliminary phase. Tests on rat models show promising results for rifampin-coated stents in combination with tigecycline and clarithromycin-coated stents in combination with systemic amikacin (Cirioni et al, 2011; Minardi et al, 2012).

Applying **silver coatings** on ureteral stents appears to be an effective strategy in reducing biofilm adherence without the risk of inducing resistance (Schierholz et al, 2002).

Stent Design

Simple variations to the initial DJ stent developed by Finney (Finney, 1978) include different biomaterials as discussed previously, different diameters and lengths, more or fewer side holes, and an open or closed tip.

The newly developed 3F Microstent (Percutaneous Systems, Palo Alto, CA) uses a film anchor as a proximal retaining mechanism. Once above the obstruction, the film anchor is deployed by retracting the integrated guidewire. Flow characteristics of the 3F Microstent are equivalent to those of a 4.7-Fr DJ stent and significantly better than those of a 3-Fr DJ stent (Lange et al, 2011). Because a smaller-caliber stent occupies less space in the ureter, stone passage may theoretically improve.

The grooved stent, initially invented by Finney in 1980 (U.S. patent 4,307,723), was demonstrated to have better extraluminal and total flow compared with a regular stent of equal size (Koleski et al, 2000). The Towers stent (Cook Medical, Bloomington, IN) and the LithoStent (Boston Scientific, Marlborough, MA) are two grooved stents still manufactured today.

The dual-lumen stent, developed with the goal of optimizing urinary drainage, significantly improved the flow in an ex vivo obstructed ureter model compared with a single 7-Fr stent and had similar flow rates compared with two ipsilateral 7-Fr stents (Hafron et al, 2006). Insertion of a dual-lumen stent has a practical advantage over insertion of two ipsilateral stents because it can be inserted in one pass.

The Spirastent (Urosurge Medical, Coralville, IA), a DJ stent with helical metal ridges, was designed to obtain better flow and easier stone fragment passage by theoretically increasing the distance between ureter wall and stent. Although an in vitro study showed promising results, the stent appeared to allow less flow than the conventional DJ stent in an in vivo porcine model and was not successful in promoting enhanced stone clearance (Olweny et al, 2000; Stoller et al, 2000; Gerber et al, 2004).

The **Open-Pass ureteral stent** (Fossa Medical, Sandy Hook, CT) has 15 to 17 radially expanding baskets along its length and was developed for dilation of the ureter up to 20 Fr and stone fragment entrapment after SWL. Entrapped stone fragments are subsequently removed with the removal of the stent (L'Esperance et al, 2007).

Animal studies with a novel helical-cut Percuflex stent demonstrate the device to have flow characteristics and biocompatibility comparable to those of a conventional Percuflex stent. The touted advantage of the stent and its possible benefit in reducing stent-related symptoms depends on improved conformity to the ureter (Mucksavage et al, 2012).

Stents equipped with an antireflux valve mechanism at the intravesical portion of the stent demonstrate a significant decrease in reflux rate compared with a conventional DJ stent, resulting in less flank and bladder pain and thus improved patient comfort (Ecke et al, 2010; Ritter et al, 2012). Lumiaho reported that a 4-cm-long double-helix spiral stent made from biodegradable material allowed for adequate or improved flow compared with a conventional DJ stent in an vivo porcine study. The absence of an intravesical coil prevented vesicoureteral reflux (Lumiaho et al, 2011).

The hypothesis that less or softer material in the bladder would result in fewer symptoms has influenced stent design toward variable diameter, dual durometer, and softer stents. Stents developed for use after endopyelotomy have a conventional 7-Fr proximal and distal coil and a broader body of 10 Fr or more. Tail stents or buoy stents were developed to prevent stent-related lower urinary tract symptoms and are composed of a 7-Fr or 10-Fr upper body that tapers down to a 3-Fr distal tail rather than a coil. Tail stents and buoy stents (10 Fr to 3 Fr) are reported to have significantly better drainage, reduced bladder inflammation, and reduced irritative bladder symptoms (Dunn et al, 2000; Krebs et al, 2009).

Reports on **dual durometer stents,** composed of a conventional upper body and a softer biomaterial at the distal segment, have not been proven to be consistently beneficial. Whereas Lingeman and colleagues reported significant reduction of stent-related symptoms with dual durometer stents, Davenport and Joshi could not identify significant differences between dual durometer and conventional DJ stents (Lennon et al, 1995; Joshi et al, 2005; Davenport et al, 2011; Kawahara et al, 2012a).

The **Magnetip stent** (Surgitek, Medical Engineering Company, Racine, WI) has been developed to avoid cystoscopic removal of the stent. It has a metallic bead at the distal tip and can be removed with a magnetic-tipped urethral catheter. Studies have demonstrated up to 100% successful retrieval in women and 75% to 97% in men (Macaluso et al, 1989; Taylor and McDougall, 2002).

Indications

Ureteral stent placement is most commonly performed to relieve ureteral obstruction. Intrinsic obstruction is typically caused by stones, tumors, or strictures, whereas extrinsic obstruction is often caused by compression by tumor, overlying vessels, retroperitoneal fibrosis, or lymphadenopathies. This relief of obstruction by stent placement can be temporary until more definitive treatment is performed or permanent if further definitive treatment is not feasible or desired.

Absolute and usually emergent indications for drainage of the kidney(s) are bilateral obstruction, unilateral obstruction in the absence of a functional contralateral kidney, and ureteral obstruction with hydronephrosis and urinary infection or sepsis. Intractable renal colic that cannot be controlled by analgesia also requires urinary drainage by either a ureteral stent or nephrostomy placement.

Stent placement before or after treatment of urolithiasis has been a subject of controversy. A meta-analysis of the available literature demonstrated that **stenting before SWL of upper urinary tract calculi may have a beneficial effect on the incidence of Steinstrasse after SWL. This result was, however, heavily influenced by one RCT with 400 participants with stones between 1.5 and 3.5 cm** (Al-Awadi et al, 1999). **There was no difference in need for auxiliary treatments between the two groups in the meta-analysis. Stenting has not conclusively demonstrated a beneficial effect on stone-free rates,** and patients with a stent had more lower urinary tract symptoms (Ather et al, 2009; Shen et al, 2011a).

Current stone treatment guidelines from both the EAU and the AUA indicate that **routine use of DJ stenting before SWL for kidney or ureteral stones does not improve stone-free rates.** Although the guidelines advise against stent placement before an SWL-treatment regardless of stone size, it is still common practice and considered by many safer to place a ureteral stent in combination with SWL for a stone larger than 1.5 to 2 cm.

The requirement for routine stent placement **after ureteroscopic lithotripsy (URSL) for stone treatment** has also been widely debated. Findings from RCTs illustrating that stenting after uncomplicated URSL is not routinely required were published as early as 2001 (Denstedt et al, 2001). Three meta-analyses over the following decade all confirmed that **routine stenting has no beneficial effect on stone-free rate or ureteral stricture formation. The procedure takes longer and costs more, especially combined with the cost of subsequent cystoscopic stent extraction. Quality of life appears to be better in the non-stented group** (Shen et al, 2011b; Tang et al, 2011; Song et al, 2012a). The 2013 EAU stone guidelines advise that stenting is not routinely required after uncomplicated URSL (Türk et al, 2013). Stenting a ureter post-URSL is, on the other hand, still advised if there are sizeable residual fragments, in the presence of an anatomically or functionally solitary kidney, if the ureter has been balloon dilated, if the patient has a UTI, or if a complication such as bleeding or perforation has occurred. Even these commonly accepted indications for stent placement have been challenged in recent studies. A multicenter RCT demonstrated no benefit from stent placement after ureteric balloon-dilatation in an otherwise uncomplicated URSL. Stented patients had more discomfort, and there was no beneficial effect on postoperative pain, stone-free rate, or short- or long-term complication rates (Başeskioğlu et al, 2011).

A single retrospective study has evaluated the recommended indwelling time of ureteral stents post-URSL. The authors suggest that **indwelling time shorter than 14 days was associated with fewer adverse effects compared with having the stent in for 15 days or longer** (Shigemura et al, 2012). Because there are no RCTs in the current literature, there is not sufficient evidence to make conclusive recommendations on the indwelling time of a ureteral stent post-URSL. Common clinical practice is to remove a stent 1 to 2 weeks post-URSL if the patient is stone free or has small passable fragments on postoperative follow-up imaging.

Stenting as a preemptive maneuver before URS was first described and found beneficial as early as 1990 (Jones et al, 1990). Cetti and colleagues reported presenting to be useful in 8% of patients in a tertiary referral center (Cetti et al, 2011). Although no prospective RCTs have been performed to date, **current literature suggests that placing a ureteral stent for 1 to 2 weeks after initial unsuccessful URSL leads to a higher success rate of secondary URSL** (Rubenstein et al, 2007; Shields et al, 2009; Ji et al, 2012; Netsch et al, 2012). This passive dilative effect of an indwelling stent has also been demonstrated in the pediatric population (Hubert and Palmer, 2005; Corcoran et al, 2008). In addition, placement of a ureteral access sheath is easier in presented patients (Kawahara et al, 2012b).

Chu and coworkers demonstrated that stenting before a first attempt at URSL did not significantly improve stone-free rates; the authors reported, however, that preoperative stenting for stones larger than 1 cm was associated with decreased operative time, lower reoperative rates, and lower cost (Chu et al, 2011a, 2011b). **Whether or not a priori stenting before initial URSL should be routinely recommended for large impacted stones remains unclear because of a lack of qualitative trials.**

Routine placement of an internal stent after uncomplicated percutaneous nephrolithotomy (PCNL) with a low tract is not necessarily required. Stenting is, however, advised in the presence of residual stone burden in the kidney, migration of residual fragments to the ureter, extensive edema, perforation of the collecting system, or high tract placement with risk of hydrothorax; for performance of tubeless PCNL; or in the presence of persistent urinary leakage after nephrostomy tube removal.

The first RCT comparing **drainage modalities for pyonephrosis** was reported by Pearle and colleagues in 1998 and did not demonstrate superiority of stenting versus nephrostomy tube placement (Pearle et al, 1998). Mokhmalji concluded nephrostomy tube placement to be superior compared with internal stents, based mainly on more discomfort and pain in the stented group (Mokhmalji et al, 2001). Although Joshi reported significantly more irritative symptoms in stented patients compared with those with nephrostomy tubes, a patient preference for either could not be demonstrated (Joshi et al, 2001). The proportion of patients treated with percutaneous nephrostomy (PCN) for pyonephrosis in the United States decreased from 16% in 1999 to 11% in 2009. Recent literature suggests a preference for PCN tube for patients who have larger stones and are more acutely ill. These patients are also more likely to be admitted to an intensive care unit (Goldsmith et al, 2013; Sammon et al, 2013). **When considering the training and skill sets of most urologists, a "stent first where possible" policy has been suggested by Ramsey and associates** (Ramsey et al, 2010).

Stents are widely used in urologic reconstructive surgery for splinting the ureter. Stents have a dual role in this setting, the first being scaffolding the tissue to improve organized healing, and the second being to allow urine to flow unhindered past the operated field. Stents have shown usefulness in ureteral trauma treatment, ureteral realignment, pyeloplasty, ureteral reimplantation, ureteroureterostomy, and other reconstructive procedures. A particularly important and well-studied postoperative use of ureteral stents is **after renal transplantation.** A recent meta-analysis in the renal transplant population demonstrated that **routine prophylactic stenting significantly reduces the incidence of major urologic complications** (Wilson et al, 2013). Removing the stent after 8 days as opposed to after 15 days reduces UTI rate (40% vs. 73%) and is more cost-effective (Parapiboon et al, 2012).

Stents are often placed **prophylactically before gynecologic, urologic, or abdominal surgery.** This facilitates identification of the ureter during surgery and theoretically may reduce iatrogenic ureteral trauma. Although such benefit has been suggested in gynecologic surgery, especially in patients with risk factors such as previous pelvic radiation or surgery, endometriosis, or pelvic inflammatory disease, a single-center RCT in a cohort of over 3000 patients showed **no significant difference in ureteral injury rate with or without prophylactic stenting** (1.09% vs. 1.2%, $P = .774$). It is, however, **easier to identify ureteric trauma with a stent in situ** (Chou et al, 2009; Park et al, 2012).

Several authors have reported on the use of stents in the **treatment of malignant pathology of the upper urinary tract** with, for instance, BCG or Mitomycin C. After intravesical instillation of the agent, vesicoureteral reflux may permit the substance to reach the upper urinary tract (Nonomura et al, 2000; Irie et al, 2002; Hayashida et al, 2004). Audenet suggests that BCG instillation in the upper urinary tract by single-J ureteral catheter, via reflux through DJ stent, or antegrade via a nephrostomy tube should be considered a first-line treatment for upper tract carcinoma in situ in patients who are not candidates for surgery (Audenet et al, 2013).

When a single ureteric stent is insufficient in relieving benign or malignant extrinsic ureteral compression, placing an additional ipsilateral stent has been reported to be successful in achieving adequate kidney drainage (Liu and Hrebinko, 1998; Rotariu et al, 2001; Elsamra et al, 2013). This technique has also been successfully applied in ureteral anastomotic strictures in renal transplant patients (Miyaoka et al, 2011).

Persistent urinary extravasation after blunt renal trauma can be treated by ureteral stent placement with high success rates (Matthews et al, 1997; Haas et al, 1998; Alsikafi et al, 2006; Long et al, 2013). Simultaneous bladder drainage is advised to maintain low intrarenal pressure and optimal drainage.

Technique

Stents can be placed using various techniques including endoscopic retrograde or antegrade placement or during open or laparoscopic surgery of the urinary tract. The following procedure describes a commonly used technique for retrograde endoscopic placement of a simple 7-Fr DJ stent of appropriate length without special design or coating and with a regular pusher, under cystoscopic and fluoroscopic guidance.

Antibiotic prophylaxis before endoscopic stent placement by means of oral fluoroquinolones is deemed appropriate and is recommended in AUA guidelines with level 1B evidence (Wolf et al, 2008).

Stent placement in males can be performed with the patient in a supine position with flexible cystoscopy or in lithotomy position when a rigid cystoscope is used. In females one can attempt flexible cystoscopy with the patient in a frog-leg position or perform rigid cystoscopy using the lithotomy position. Fluoroscopic guidance during the procedure to confirm the correct position of the guidewire and subsequently placed stent is advised. Ultrasound guidance can be used instead of fluoroscopy when placing a stent in a pregnant woman.

Ureteral stents are most commonly placed over a guidewire, and there is a vast array of available guidewires for this purpose. Hydrophilic nitinol guidewires have the optimal characteristics to easily overcome obstruction or follow the course of a tortuous ureter with a minimal risk of perforation. Stiffer wires such as Teflon-containing Benson wires provide higher resistance against bending when placing ureteral stents (Clayman et al, 2004; Liguori et al, 2008; Sarkissian et al, 2012; Torricelli et al, 2013).

Because stent diameter does not seem to influence stent symptoms, one should choose the largest fitting stent available for optimal drainage (Candela and Bellman, 1997; Erturk et al, 2003). In general, a 6-Fr or 7-Fr diameter stent is preferred.

After fluoroscopically confirming the position of the guidewire in the renal pelvis, the stent is advanced over the guidewire with a pusher under cystoscopic guidance. When the tip of the pusher is visualized at the bladder neck, the guidewire is retracted while the stent coils are fluoroscopically confirmed in the renal pelvis and the distal stent coil is cystoscopically confirmed in the bladder.

Alternatively, one can place a stent by primarily relying on fluoroscopic guidance. After placement of the guidewire in the renal pelvis, the cystoscope is removed and an 8-Fr to 10-Fr coaxial Amplatz dilator is advanced over the guidewire under fluoroscopic guidance until the 10-Fr component is at the urethral meatus. After removal of the 8-Fr component, the 10-Fr sheath will allow a 7-Fr stent to be passed through it over the guidewire while the stent is prevented from coiling in the bladder. Under fluoroscopic guidance, the stent is advanced with a pusher that has a radiopaque marker at the tip. The distal end of the stent is positioned by advancing the radiopaque marker under fluoroscopic guidance at the middle of the pubic symphysis in male patients and the lower border of the pubic symphysis in female patients. The 10-Fr sheath is removed and subsequently the guidewire, with fluoroscopic confirmation of the proximal stent coils in the renal pelvis and the distal loop coils in the bladder (Fig. 6-7).

Although usually performed with the patient under general anesthesia, stent placement with local anesthesia using lidocaine

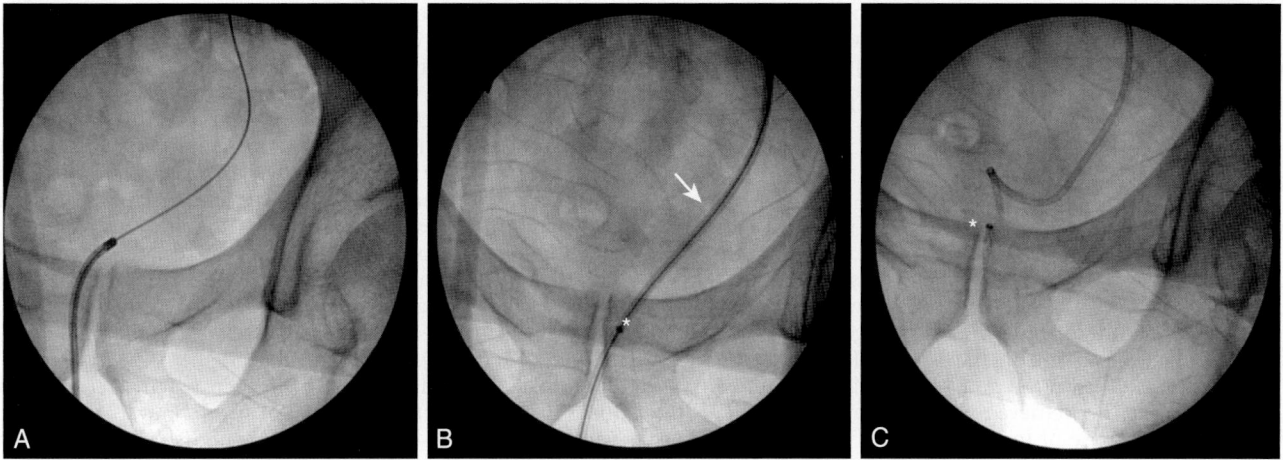

Figure 6-7. A, Cystoscope in bladder plus guidewire in ureter. **B,** Stent placed in ureter through 10-Fr sheath (*asterisk* indicates radiopaque marker of pusher; *arrow* indicates 10-Fr sheath). **C,** Guidewire and 10-Fr sheath removed, distal stent section coiled in bladder.

jelly is feasible (Mark and Montgomery, 1996). Sivalingam describes that in compliant patients in whom difficult stent placement is not expected, in-office stent placement is feasible, is less costly, and has a low failure rate of approximately 9% (Sivalingam et al, 2013).

Complications

Stent Symptoms

Stent-associated symptoms can have a significant impact on patient quality of life. Hematuria, urgency, frequency, dysuria, and both bladder and flank pain are the most prevalent symptoms related to indwelling ureteral stents. Joshi and colleagues developed the ureteral stent symptom questionnaire (USSQ) to evaluate symptoms and impact on quality of life of ureteral stents. The authors reported quality of life to be influenced in 80% of stented patients. From an economic perspective, 58% of patients had reduced work capacity because of stent discomfort, and approximately half of the patients had sought medical professional help for stent-related symptoms (Joshi et al, 2003a, 2003b). Leibovici reported that 45% of patients had been unable to work for at least 2 days for a total of 435 workdays lost in 135 stented patients (Leibovici et al, 2005). A prospective cohort study reported that approximately one third of patients required early removal of ureteral stents because of stent discomfort (Ringel et al, 2000). Sexual dysfunction has been reported in 42% to 82% of male patients and 30% to 86% of female patients with an indwelling ureteral stent (Joshi et al, 2003b; Leibovici et al, 2005; Sighinolfi et al, 2007).

The pathophysiologic explanation for such stent-related symptoms is not yet fully understood. Irritation of the bladder mucosa and especially the trigone by the distal portion of the stent, reflux of urine, and smooth muscle spasm are thought to contribute to stent-related symptoms (Miyaoka and Monga, 2009; Regan et al, 2009). Vesicoureteral reflux as measured on cystoureterogram has been reported in 56% to 62% of stented patients (Mosli et al, 1991; Yossepowitch et al, 2005). Fluoroscopic imaging in patients with an indwelling stent revealed positional changes of the stent in relation to standing, sitting, and bending, which may explain why physical activity can influence stent discomfort (Chew et al, 2007).

Positioning the proximal coil in the upper pole of the kidney in contrast to in the renal pelvis appears to be better tolerated by stented patients (Liatsikos et al, 2001). Several authors have reported that stents crossing the midline of the bladder have a significant and deleterious influence on associated discomfort. Choosing the appropriate stent length may therefore aid in ameliorating stent symptoms (Rane et al, 2001; Al-Kandari et al, 2007; Ho et al, 2009, 2010; Giannarini et al, 2011a). Predictive parameters for ideal stent length have been studied extensively. The in vivo measurement of the ureter with a 5-Fr ureteric catheter is often assumed as the true ureteral length. Pilcher and Patel suggested a predictive model for ideal stent length based on patient height: shorter than 5 feet 10 inches, 22-cm stent; 5 feet 10 inches to 6 feet 4 inches, 24-cm stent; and taller than 6 feet 4 inches, 26-cm stent (Pilcher and Patel, 2002). This model has been adopted widely and has been both confirmed by many (Hruby et al, 2007; Ho et al, 2009) and also contested (Paick et al, 2005; Kawahara et al, 2012d; Novaes et al, 2013; Shrewsberry et al, 2013). Paick and colleagues suggested that straight linear measurement from ureteropelvic junction to vesicoureteric junction on preoperative intravenous pyelography correlated better with the actual ureteric length than the patient's height (Paick et al, 2005). Postmortem measurement of ureteric length could not identify a significant correlation with any anthropomorphic measurement (Novaes et al, 2013). Recent reports demonstrate actual ureteric length to correlate better with computed tomography (CT)–measured length than with any other imaging-based or anthropomorphic measurement (Kawahara et al, 2012d; Shrewsberry et al, 2013). Ideal stent length for children has been formulated as "child's age + 10" cm (Resnick et al, 2007).

Pharmacologic treatment and altered stent design have been extensively studied in attempts to reduce stent-related symptoms. Meta-analysis of four RCTs with a total of 341 patients that assessed the efficacy of α-blockers with the USSQ has demonstrated that the use of α-blockers significantly reduces urinary symptoms and pain and significantly improves general health (Yakoubi et al, 2011). **The use of α-blocker medications to mitigate stent discomfort has been recommended by EAU guidelines (Türk et al, 2013). Solifenacin and tolterodine can significantly reduce irritative urinary tract symptoms and pain symptoms with a very low complication rate (Park et al, 2009; Lee et al, 2013). The combination of tamsulosin and solifenacin appears to significantly improve stent-related irritative and obstructive symptoms compared with monotherapy with either agent alone (Lim et al, 2011).** Intravesical instillation with ketorolac seems to have a short-lived but significant beneficial effect on postoperative stent-related pain (Beiko et al, 2004). Periureteral injection of botulinum toxin A has been demonstrated to safely reduce stent-related pain and need for narcotic pain medication up to 1 week after stent placement (Gupta et al, 2010). Injection of ropivacaine in proximity to the ureteric orifice and at the bladder neck demonstrated a trend toward decreased postoperative pain and voiding symptoms when assessed in a small RCT (Sur et al, 2008). Appropriate stent position with the distal coil not crossing over the midline of the bladder appeared to have more effect on stent-related symptoms than α-blockers or anticholinergics in a prospective RCT (Lee et al, 2010).

Stent Migration

Despite the self-retaining design of DJ ureteral stents, distal migration into the bladder or proximal into the ureter is possible. Proximal stent migration into the ureter has been reported to occur in 1% to 8% of patients. This can largely be prevented by choosing a sufficiently long stent and having an adequate loop both in the renal pelvis and in the bladder (Slaton and Kropp, 1996; Richter et al, 2000; Breau and Norman, 2001). A proximally migrated stent can be retrieved ureteroscopically (Bagley and Huffman, 1991). The use of toothed graspers, grasping or coaxial cannulation of the stent with a basket, and a dilation balloon have been reported to aid in the retrieval of proximally migrated stents (Chin and Denstedt, 1992; Livadas et al, 2007; Meeks et al, 2008). Migration of the stent into the bladder can be treated by stent exchange.

Urinary Tract Infection

Ureteral stents are inherently subject to bacterial colonization and therefore represent a source of UTI. Short-term ureteral stent placement (3 weeks) in a cohort of 209 children after ureteral reimplantation eventuated in UTI in only 4.8% of patients. Asymptomatic bacteriuria was reported in an additional 6.5% of patients, whereas almost half of the stents were colonized with bacteria (Uvin et al, 2011). **In chronically stented patients, bacterial colonization reaches 100%** (Riedl et al, 1999). Indwelling time, female sex, diabetes, and chronic kidney disease are factors influencing colonization of ureteral stents (Kehinde et al, 2002). A negative urine culture has low predictive value for stent bacterial colonization (Kehinde et al, 2004; Rahman et al, 2012). Routine screening for bacteriuria and treatment of asymptomatic bacteriuria is not recommended. **Antibiotics are recommended only in instances of symptomatic UTI and appear not to have a role in long-term prophylaxis.** A small RCT with 95 patients demonstrated that continuous low-dose antibiotic treatment during the indwelling time of ureteral stents does not influence the incidence or severity of stent-related symptoms or UTIs (Moltzahn et al, 2013).

Encrustation

Minor encrustation on stent surfaces is often present and usually does not result in stent blockage or resistance at stent removal. More extensive and clinically significant encrustation can be a very challenging complication and often arises from a forgotten or retained stent. Removal of encrusted stents requires endourologic experience and, depending on the extent of encrustations, may include multiple interventions. Failure to acknowledge the presence of and render treatment for an encrusted stent can lead to significant renal functional impairment including renal unit loss and in rare instances mortality (Singh et al, 2005; Aron et al, 2006).

The duration of indwelling time of ureteral stents is the most important risk factor for development of encrustation. Encrustation has been reported to occur in 9.2% to 26.8% of stents indwelling for less than 6 weeks, in 47.5% to 56.9% of stents indwelling 6 to 12 weeks, and in approximately 75% of stents indwelling longer than 12 weeks (el-Faqih et al, 1991; Kawahara et al, 2012c). Kawahara and coworkers observed that **stents smaller than 6 Fr were significantly more likely to encrust than stents 7 Fr or larger.** The authors reported complete obstruction in 8.6% of stents after more than 12 weeks, and 1% of stents required additional treatments to facilitate stent removal (Kawahara et al, 2012c). Additional risk factors for stent encrustation include pregnancy, UTI or urosepsis, history of stone disease, metabolic or congenital abnormalities,

urinary diversions, and chronic renal failure (Robert et al, 1997; Vanderbrink et al, 2008; Ahallal et al, 2010). Calcium oxalate appears to be the major component of stent encrustation in the absence of UTI, pH values below 5.5, and hyperuricosuria (Robert et al, 1997; Grases et al, 2001).

Because indwelling time is the most important risk factor for encrustation, **timely stent removal or exchange is the most important preventive measure**. Most stent manufacturers recommend stent removal or exchange within 4 months of placement. In patients with additional risk factors for encrustation, a 6- to 8-week interval is recommended (Aravantinos et al, 2006). Pregnant patients are especially prone to stent encrustation, and stent exchange is suggested every 4 to 6 weeks in this population (Denstedt and Razvi, 1992).

Encrustation and inability to extract a stent are usually diagnosed in an office setting at a trial of stent removal. Applying excessive force to achieve stent extraction is not recommended, to avoid the risk of inflicting ureteral damage, avulsion, or stent fragmentation. Adequate cross-sectional imaging to assess the extent of encrustation is assistive in developing a treatment strategy because conventional x-ray examination may underestimate the extent of encrustation. Mistry and coworkers reported on the placement of an additional stent for 1 to 2 weeks adjacent to mildly encrusted stents, facilitating a second extraction attempt. The authors hypothesize that friction between the two stents might disrupt the encrustation in addition to the beneficial effect of ureteral dilation (Mistry et al, 2013).

Several authors have created an algorithm for the treatment of encrusted stents involving SWL, URS, cystolitholapaxy, and PCNL. One to six multiple sequential procedures are often necessary to successfully remove the encrusted stent (Borboroglu and Kane, 2000; Singh et al, 2001; Lam and Gupta, 2002; Bultitude et al, 2003; Aravantinos et al, 2006; Weedin et al, 2011). The multitude of different algorithms reflects the lack of consensus on optimal treatment. In general, the site and level of encrustation burden guide the specific approach.

Forgotten or Neglected Stents

The forgotten or neglected stent is a multifactorial problem that originates from both poor patient compliance and health system issues related to patient follow-up. The surgeon responsible for stent insertion is also accountable for its timely removal.

The cost of forgetting a stent, including radiologic investigations, medical treatment, invasive and noninvasive interventions, and hospital stay is on average sevenfold higher than the cost of cystoscopic timely removal (Sancaktutar et al, 2012).

Divakaruni and colleagues identified male patients and uninsured patients to be at higher risk of noncompliance with planned stent removal. When relying only on patient information and education, the authors reported a 16% forgotten stent rate (Divakaruni et al, 2013). In addition to patient education, several reminder mechanisms incorporated into patient follow-up protocols such as log books, card- or Web-based registries, computerized logs, and software that arranges stent change or removal and sends reminder e-mails to patient and physician have been proposed to prevent the forgotten stent scenario from occurring, with variable effectiveness. None of these preventive mechanisms can completely eliminate the retained stent issue (Monga et al, 1995; McCahy and Ramsden, 1996; Ather et al, 2000; Lynch et al, 2007; Thomas et al, 2007; Tang et al, 2008; Withington et al, 2013).

Forgotten stents can develop severe encrustation, as previously described. In the presence of a large encrustation burden, nuclear imaging to quantify the renal function of the affected kidney is advised for planning stent removal. If split renal function shows insufficient contribution of the stented kidney, nephrectomy may be the most appropriate course of action.

Forgotten ureteral stents account for the highest number of postoperative-related claims pertaining to urology that are closed with indemnity payment in the United Kingdom (Osman and Collins, 2011).

UPPER URINARY TRACT: NEPHROSTOMY TUBE

Historic Note

Thomas Hillier reported on the first PCN for the drainage of a hydronephrotic kidney in a 4-year old boy in 1865 (Hillier, 1865). Goodwin described PCN to drain an obstructed kidney in 16 patients almost a century later (Goodwin et al, 1955). Fernström's report on the first percutaneous stone extraction in 1976 initiated the PCNL era, enhancing popularity of the percutaneous access and drainage of the kidney (Fernström and Johansson, 1976). The early literature review, pooling data of 516 PCN insertions, reported a success rate of 90%, major complication rate of 4%, and minor complication rate of 15% (Stables et al, 1978).

Available Materials and Nephrostomy Tube Design

Similar to ureteral stents, an ideal nephrostomy tube is biocompatible; has excellent flow characteristics; is easy to insert; resists infection, encrustation, and dislodgement; and does not induce symptoms.

The pigtail and balloon catheter are probably the most commonly used tube designs. In general, pigtail catheters are smaller than other nephrostomy tubes and are very useful for drainage of clear fluids but are often insufficient in the presence of gross hematuria or thick pus. Councill catheters are particularly useful because they can be inserted or exchanged over a guidewire without losing access to the kidney. Malecot and Pezzer nephrostomies have the advantage of a larger lumen because of their lack of retention balloon tubing. Re-entry catheters are designed to permit nephrostomy drainage while ensuring access to the ureter, should this be necessary. A tamponade (Kaye) catheter can be of specific use in instances of postoperative bleeding (Paul et al, 2003). Although small-bore catheters (smaller than 18 Fr) are less painful and better tolerated than large-bore catheters (larger than 18 Fr) (Maheshwari et al, 2000; Pietrow et al, 2003; Desai et al, 2004), overall complication rate and bleeding incidence after PCNL may be lower with a large-bore catheter (Cormio et al, 2013). Currently the placement of a 16-Fr to 18-Fr nephrostomy tube is common practice in nontubeless PCNL.

Canales and colleagues compared a pigtail stent, a Malecot catheter, a catheter with a symmetrical balloon, and a catheter with an eccentric balloon in an artificial kidney model in an effort to identify the best tube design for nephrostomy placement after PCNL. The catheter with a symmetrical balloon had significantly better flow with water and higher-viscosity fluid and better retention strength compared with the other catheters (Canales et al, 2005) (Fig. 6-8).

Indications

When upper urinary tract drainage is desired and retrograde ureteral stent placement is not successful or feasible, PCN tube placement is considered the procedure of choice. Advantages of PCN drainage include the placement and exchange of the tube under local anesthesia and the belief that a nephrostomy tube offers better flow characteristics. Anesthesia may not be an option in ill patients with acute renal failure or sepsis with hemodynamic instability. Because stent placement under local anesthesia appears to be feasible even in an office setting, this relative advantage may decline in the future (Sivalingam et al, 2013). In contrast to a DJ stent, the external drainage nephrostomy tube can be easily unblocked by gentle irrigation in the event of blockage.

Whereas patients with a stent have more discomfort from stent-related symptoms, the presence of a PCN tube has a negative influence on quality of life because of the external drainage characteristics. Overall quality of life, however, has not been demonstrated to be statistically different between the two groups (Joshi et al, 2001; Monsky et al, 2013). Although Monsky reported more minor complications and dislodgement in the PCN group resulting in more frequent exchanges, Song and colleagues reported a shorter interval of exchanges in the DJ stent group than in the PCN group (respectively, every 2.7 vs. 4.2 months). DJ stent placement was, however, less costly, and the procedure time was shorter (Song et al, 2012b; Monsky et al, 2013). Exchange frequency may have an economic and quality-of-life impact.

Acute decompression of obstructed pyonephrosis is a urologic emergency, and failure to achieve prompt drainage is related to a higher mortality risk (Borofsky et al, 2013). As previously discussed, there is not enough evidence from the current literature to demonstrate superiority of either nephrostomy or stent drainage in centers where both are readily available (Pearle et al, 1998; Mokhmalji et al, 2001).

Multiple meta-analyses have consistently reported that **tubeless PCNL is feasible and considered safe after an uncomplicated procedure without residual fragments, infection, bleeding, or collecting system perforation.** In addition, a tubeless procedure reduces hospital stay, analgesia requirement, and time to return to normal activity (Yuan et al, 2011; Shen et al, 2012; Wang et al, 2012; Zhong et al, 2013).

Nephrostomy tubes may also be used to administer therapeutic drugs to the upper urinary tract. BCG or Mitomycin C for the treatment of upper urinary tract urothelial cancer as well as chemolytic agents to achieve stone dissolution are examples. Giannarini identified patients with carcinoma in situ of the upper urinary tract to benefit the most from upper tract BCG instillations (Giannarini et al, 2011b). If a nephrostomy tube is in place, it can be used to obtain a nephrostogram for diagnostic imaging.

In the treatment of malignant ureteric obstruction, drainage failure is significantly more prevalent in patients with ureteral stents compared with patients with a nephrostomy tube (Ku et al, 2004). Song suggested that patients with an obstruction larger than 3 cm are more likely to benefit from PCN than from DJ stent placement (Song et al, 2012b).

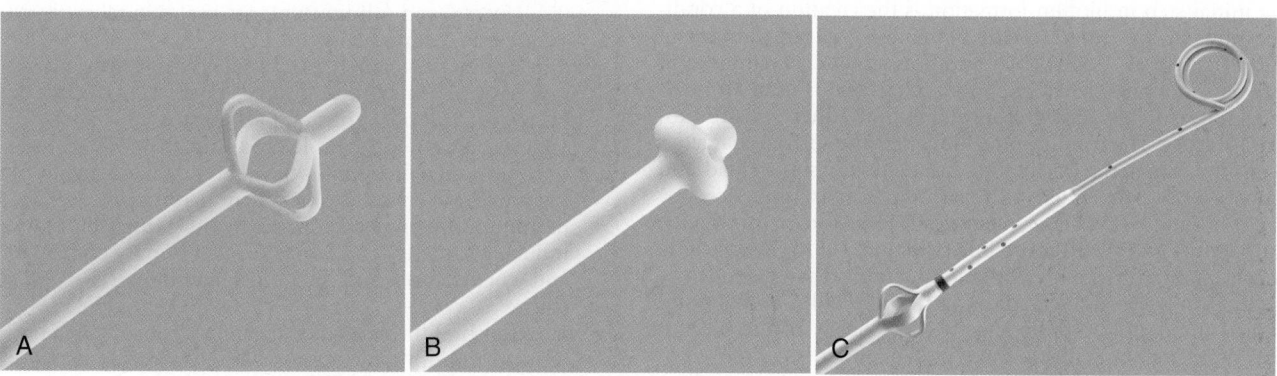

Figure 6-8. Nephrostomy tubes: types of nephrostomy catheters. A to C, Malecot, Pezzer, and Hulbert re-entry catheter. (Permission for use granted by Cook Medical, Bloomington, IN.)

How to obtain percutaneous access to the kidney is described in Chapter 8.

Complications

Hemorrhage, hematuria, clot colic, and UTIs are frequently reported minor complications of nephrostomy tube insertion. Sepsis occurs in 1.3% to 7% of patients, and trauma to adjacent organs caused by the procedure is uncommon. Transfusion rates of 2% to 4% have been reported as a result of venous or arterial bleeding. Venous bleeding is usually self-limiting. Persistent arterial bleeding or arteriovenous fistula is an uncommon but more severe complication that requires adequate imaging assessment and, if necessary, treatment with angioembolization. Thoracic complications (pneumothorax, hemothorax, hydrothorax, empyema) occur in 0.1% to 0.2% of nephrostomy tube placements. Late complications include tube dislodgement and blockage. Nephrostomy tube dislodgement is reported to occur in 2.5% of patients; this requires urgent assessment and, if necessary, tube replacement. A self-retaining catheter or retainment suture fixation to the skin can aid in preventing tube dislodgement (Lewis and Patel, 2004; Wah et al, 2004; Hausegger and Portugaller, 2006; Rana et al, 2007; Ali et al, 2013).

Major complications are more common when procedures are performed during on-call hours, with lack of experienced staff implicated as a contributing factor (Lewis and Patel, 2004). Performing 10 to 20 PCNs per year improves success rate of the procedure (Lee et al, 1994).

Biofilm Formation on Urinary Tract Biomaterials

A *biofilm* is defined as a structured community of bacterial cells enclosed in a self-produced polymeric matrix and adherent to an inert or living surface.

Bacteria attempt to control their immediate environment by limiting exposure to harmful factors (waste products, antimicrobial agents, the host's immune response) while enhancing the exposure to trophic factors.

Despite continuing developmental efforts to achieve more biocompatible materials and surface coatings, indwelling catheters, stents, and nephrostomy tubes completely resistant to biofilm formation are as yet unavailable.

Biofilm-producing bacteria are the most important factor in inducing catheter- or stent-associated UTI and encrustation and the most common cause of stent failure (Ando et al, 2004; Chew et al, 2006; Ferrières et al, 2007).

Biofilm structures consist of three layers: (1) **the innermost layer,** attached to the surface of the biomaterial, which **functions as a linking film** for subsequent layers; (2) **the base film,** composed of microorganisms attached to the linking film; and (3) **an outer layer or surface film,** where microorganisms can be released (Tenke et al, 2012). The thickness of a biofilm can range from 3 to 490 μm and is composed of a few cell layers ranging to up to 400 cells deep (Ganderton et al, 1992).

The initial step in biofilm formation is the creation of a conditioning film on the surface of the biomaterial within minutes of insertion (Reid et al, 1995). This conditioning film is composed of **urinary components such as polysaccharides, Tamm-Horsfall proteins, electrolytes, and glycoproteins that adhere to the biomaterial surface.** The conditioning film alters the surface characteristics of the biomaterial, facilitating bacterial adhesions (Reid and Busscher, 1992). The initial bacterial adhesion is influenced by hydrophobic and electrostatic interactions, ionic forces, osmolality, and urinary pH and is **still reversible** (Gristina, 1987). The bacteria produce a matrix of exopolysaccharides and glycocalyx, rendering their adhesion irreversible. Eradication of the biofilm at this point is deemed impossible. Approximately 5% to 35% of the biofilm consists of bacterial microcolonies. The remainder is composed of interstitial spaces filled with fluid and water channels that allow transportation of nutrients and oxygen to the colonies (Tenke et al, 2012).

Resistance to antimicrobial treatment of bacterial biofilm infections is multifactorial:

1. **Quorum sensing** is a bacterial communication process depending on population density. Diffusible signaling molecules allow bacterial colonies to react to their environment in a synchronized manner, regulating biofilm formation, virulence, and antibiotic resistance (Li and Nair, 2012; Bhardwaj et al, 2013).
2. **The polymicrobial nature of biofilm** increases antibacterial resistance. Bacteria contained in biofilm actively recruit other bacterial strains, resulting in biofilm consisting of up to six different strains. *E. coli, P. aeruginosa,* and *Enterococcus faecalis* are most frequently found in biofilm in the urinary tract. *P. mirabilis, E. faecalis,* and *S. aureus* have a stronger biofilm forming capacity (Holá et al, 2010).
3. **Persister cells,** contributing up to 1% to the entire biofilm, reside in a dormant state and do not grow, which enhances resistance to the usual antibiotic mechanism of action. They are often the cause of chronic infections (Wood et al, 2013).
4. Although antimicrobial agents may have the ability to penetrate into a biofilm, antimicrobial action is compromised by **waste accumulation and an altered microenvironment** (low pH, low PO_2, high PCO_2, low divalent cation and pyrimidine concentration, low hydration level) (del Pozo and Patel, 2007).

Urease-producing bacteria in biofilm, such as *P. mirabilis, Proteus vulgaris,* and *Providencia rettgeri,* are able to raise the urinary pH to an alkaline level at which calcium and magnesium phosphates (hydroxyapatite and struvite) crystallize, deposit onto catheter or stent surfaces, and are incorporated into the organic matrix, creating encrustation (Broomfield et al, 2009). Canales and colleagues demonstrated that components of the conditioning film, α_1-antitrypsin, Ig kappa, IgH G_1, and histone H2B and H3A, were highly associated with stent encrustation (Canales et al, 2009).

The difficulty in preventing and treating biofilm and biofilm-induced infections is the consequence of the complexity of biofilm

---

KEY POINTS

- The routine use of coated catheters for short-term catheterization is not recommended.
- Screening for asymptomatic bacteriuria in patients with an indwelling catheter or ureteral stent should not be performed.
- Surrounding organ injury is the most significant complication of suprapubic catheter placement and has been reported to occur in less than 1% to 2.7% of procedures.
- Stent symptoms influence the quality of life in 80% of stented patients and reduce work capacity in 58%.
- α-Blockers and anticholinergic medications may be useful for modifying irritative and obstructive symptoms related to indwelling double-J stents.
- The indwelling time of a ureteral stent is the most important risk factor for encrustation.
- Metal and segmental stents such as Resonance, Memokath 051, Uventa, and Allium stents are useful in relieving extrinsic ureteric compression.
- Innovations in stent design and coatings are undergoing investigation with the desired goal of reducing stent-associated complications and symptoms.
- Tubeless PCNL is feasible and considered safe after an uncomplicated procedure without residual fragments, bleeding, infection, or collecting system perforation.
- Biofilm-producing bacteria are the most important factor in inducing catheter- or stent-associated urinary tract infection and encrustation and the most common cause of stent failure.
- Bacterial biofilm resistance to antimicrobial treatment is a result of multiple factors including quorum sensing, polymicrobial nature of biofilm, the presence of persister cells, and an altered microenvironment in the biofilm.

structure and the different mechanisms that compromise antibacterial mechanisms of action. Better understanding of basic processes and insights into biofilm formation and resistance mechanisms will guide the next generation of catheter and stent development and design in search of the ideal biomaterial and coating.

REFERENCES

The complete reference list is available online at www.expertconsult.com.

SUGGESTED READINGS

Dellis A, Joshi HB, Timoney AG, et al. Relief of stent related symptoms: review of engineering and pharmacological solutions. J Urol 2010;184: 1267–72.

Feneley MR, Allen DJ, Longhorn SE, et al. Percutaneous urinary drainage and ureteric stenting in malignant disease. Clin Oncol 2010;22:733–9.

Ghaffary C, Yohannes A, Villanueva C, et al. A practical approach to difficult urinary catheterizations. Curr Urol Rep 2013;14:565–79.

Hooton TM, Bradley SF, Cardenas DD, et al. Diagnosis, prevention, and treatment of catheter-associated urinary tract infection in adults: 2009 international clinical practice guidelines from the Infectious Diseases Society of America. Clin Infect Dis 2010;50:625–63.

Mangera A, Osman NI, Chapple CR. Anatomy of the lower urinary tract. Surg 2013;31:319–25.

Tenke P, Köves B, Nagy K, et al. Update on biofilm infections in the urinary tract. World J Urol 2012;30:51–7.

Türk C, Knoll T, Petrik A, et al. Guidelines on urolithiasis. <www.uroweb.org/gls/pdf/21_Urolithiasis_LR.pdf>; 2013 [accessed 03.09.14].

Tzortzis V, Gravas S, Melekos MM, et al. Intraurethral lubricants: a critical literature review and recommendations. J Endourol 2009;23:821–6.

Venkatesan N, Shroff S, Jayachandran K, et al. Polymers as ureteral stents. J Endourol 2010;24:191–8.

7 Principles of Urologic Endoscopy

Brian D. Duty, MD, and Michael J. Conlin, MD, MCR

The development of rigid and flexible endoscopes in combination with their myriad ancillary equipment transformed many of the surgical specialties including urology. Management of bladder outlet obstruction, urothelial tumors, ureteral obstruction, and nephrolithiasis have all been revolutionized by endoscopic procedures. This chapter highlights major events in the development of modern endoscopes and indications for cystourethrography and ureteropyeloscopy along with patient preparation; techniques are then described in detail. Many of these principles are greatly expanded on in other sections of this book.

HISTORY OF ENDOSCOPY

The term *endoscope* is credited to the French urologist Antonin Jean Desormeaux in 1853; however, attempts to look inside the human body date back to antiquity (Natalin and Landman, 2009). Major progress occurred in 1806 when Philipp Bozzini developed the first "modern" endoscope (Engel, 2003). The Lichtleiter or "Light Conductor" used angled mirrors to conduct candlelight from a sharkskin-covered box into the body through aluminum tubing. The instrument was too large to be used on the genitourinary system. In 1853 Desormeaux introduced a similarly designed but smaller-profile endoscope with improved mirrors that used a kerosene lamp for illumination (Shah, 2002). Through this instrument he excised a urethral papilloma, becoming the first individual to perform a therapeutic endoscopic procedure.

Both Bozzini's and Desormeaux's endoscopes were severely hampered by their poor illumination and limited field of view. In 1877 Max Nitze designed a cystoscope that helped overcome both obstacles (Herr, 2006). He moved the source of illumination (water-cooled electric platinum filament) to the end of the instrument and used a series of optical lenses placed at precise distances along the length of a hollow, air-filled scope to conduct and magnify the image. In 1887 Nitze abandoned the platinum filament for Edison's light bulb.

The development of the Amici prism in 1906 allowed cystoscopic images to be offset 90 degrees while maintaining correct image orientation, (Gow, 1998). No major developments occurred in cystoscope design until 1966, when Harold Hopkins introduced glass rods with only short gaps of air between. Hopkins was able to greatly improve light transmission while decreasing scope size, paving the way for contemporary rigid cystoscopes and the first rigid ureteroscope in 1979 (Lyon et al, 1979).

The development of flexible endoscopes was made possible by the advent of fiberoptics. In 1854 John Tyndall demonstrated that light could travel through a curved stream of water by internal reflection (Whewell et al, 1854). This finding led to molten glass being drawn into flexible, small-diameter fibers for light transmission. Further refinements in this process eventually led to the development of fiberoptics for medical use.

Although still widely used, fiberoptics are fragile and have limited optical resolution. In 1970 Boyle and Smith developed the charge-coupled device (CCD), a sensor with the ability to convert photons to an electrical charge and ultimately a digital image (Samplaski and Jones, 2009). Traditionally these chips were housed within cameras attached to existing scopes. Over the last three decades, advancements in endoscope design led to the incorporation of the CCD chip within the distal tip. Introduced in 2005, the ACMI DCN-2010 flexible cystoscope was the first commercially available digital endoscope (Natalin et al, 2009). **Compared with rod-lens and fiberoptic bundle systems, digital sensor technology offers improved image resolution and durability without the need for a separate light cable and camera** (Quayle et al, 2005).

BASIC EQUIPMENT AND VIDEO-ENDOSCOPIC SYSTEMS

At minimum, cystourethroscopy requires irrigation fluid, a light source, and an endoscope. Typical irrigation fluids include sterile water, glycine, and normal saline. If electrocautery is needed, a solution free of electrolytes should be used.

A high-intensity xenon or halogen external light source is used to deliver white light to the endoscope through a fiberoptic cable. Some units include an automatic light-sensing feature that provides constant illumination by adjusting light output.

First introduced into urologic practice in 2007, narrow band imaging uses only blue (415 nm) and green (540 nm) wavelengths to image the urothelium (Bryan et al, 2008). These two wavelengths are strongly absorbed by hemoglobin, improving visibility of urothelial capillaries, small papillary lesions, and carcinoma in situ. A meta-analysis of eight studies including 1022 patients found that narrow band imaging improves accuracy of detection of noninvasive lesions, including carcinoma in situ (Zheng et al, 2012). The impact of narrow band imaging on tumor recurrence has not been prospectively evaluated.

In the absence of an endoscope camera the practitioner views the image directly through the optical eyepiece at the proximal end of the instrument. However, in most instances the image will be viewed on a monitor that is part of a dedicated video-endoscopic unit arranged in a fixed or mobile tower (Fig. 7-1). Video-endoscopic units have several advantages, including better visualization, enhanced patient safety and surgical training, decreased risk of bodily fluid exposure to the urologist, and improved operative ergonomics.

Traditional video-endoscopic systems consist of a light source, endoscope camera, image processor and recorder, and monitor. Newer digital units have eliminated the need for an external camera, allowing the light source and video cable to be incorporated into a single, built-in housing (Fig. 7-2). In the traditional system the endoscopic image is conveyed to the camera via a series of glass pyelography, upper tract washes for cytology, and brush biopsies for histologic evaluation.

Lower urinary tract complaints such as recurrent infections, obstructive and irritative voiding symptoms, and chronic pelvic pain may be worked up cystoscopically. In select patients, urethral strictures, bladder stones, and foreign bodies may be treated in the office. Ureteral stents can also be placed or exchanged in clinic with fluoroscopic assistance.

Equipment

Cystourethroscopes are manufactured in a variety of sizes expressed in French (Fr) gauge. **In the system devised by French instrument designer Joseph-Frédéric-Benoît Charrière (1803-1876), a 1-Fr instrument has a circumference of $\frac{1}{3}$ mm** (Osborn and Baron, 2006).

Cystourethroscopes are available in rigid and flexible models. Each has its own advantages and disadvantages. Rigid cystoscopes use the Hopkins rod-lens optical system, which provides improved optical clarity compared with the fiberoptic bundles used in flexible endoscopes. This is becoming less noticeable because of the increasing adoption of digital flexible cystourethroscopes. Visualization is also enhanced by the greater irrigant flow rate of rigid endoscopes. Rigid cystourethroscopes have larger working channels, allowing a wider array of instruments to be used. Their rigid design also makes them easier to control with one hand, freeing the surgeon's second hand to manipulate ancillary instruments.

In contrast, the smaller size of flexible cystourethroscopes improves patient comfort, making them ideal for office-based procedures. Endoscope passage does not require the patient to be in the frog-leg or lithotomy position. Their active tip deflection makes it easier to completely inspect the bladder and negotiate an elevated bladder neck or median lobe of the prostate.

Rigid Cystourethroscopes

Rigid cystourethroscopes are manufactured in sets consisting of an optical lens, bridge, sheath, and obturator (Fig. 7-3). Configurations differ by vendor (Table 7-1). Optical lenses come with tip angles ranging from 0 to 120 degrees. Visualization of the urethra is best performed with a 0- or 12-degree lens. A 25- or 30-degree lens is commonly used for therapeutic purposes. A 70- or 120-degree lens may be required to completely inspect the anterior and inferolateral walls, dome, and neck of the bladder.

The bridge connects the optical lens to the sheath. Diagnostic bridges do not have a working channel. Therapeutic bridges have one or two working channels. Patients with an elevated bladder neck, large median lobe of the prostate, or ureteroneocystostomy may require use of an Albarran bridge. This specialized bridge contains a lever that deflects wires and catheters passed through the working channel to facilitate ureteral orifice canalization (Fig. 7-4).

Cystourethroscope sheaths come in a variety of sizes. Most have markings indicating the size of the sheath and associated working channels (Fig. 7-5). Smaller sheaths (15 and 17 Fr) are ideal for diagnostic cystoscopy; the larger models are used for therapeutic procedures requiring improved irrigant flow and larger working channels. Each sheath has an associated obturator that blunts the distal end of the sheath for passage into the bladder without visual assistance. In most instances blind endoscope passage should be performed only in women.

Flexible Cystourethroscopes

Flexible cystourethroscopes range between 16 and 17 Fr. Models differ with regard to tip deflection, direction of view, field of view, working channel size, illumination, and optics (Table 7-2). Most models do not have an offset lens and provide a field of view of approximately 120 degrees. Tip deflection ranges from 120 to 210 degrees and is either intuitive (same direction as lever deflection) or counterintuitive (opposite direction of lever deflection). Irrigation and instrument passage occur through the same working

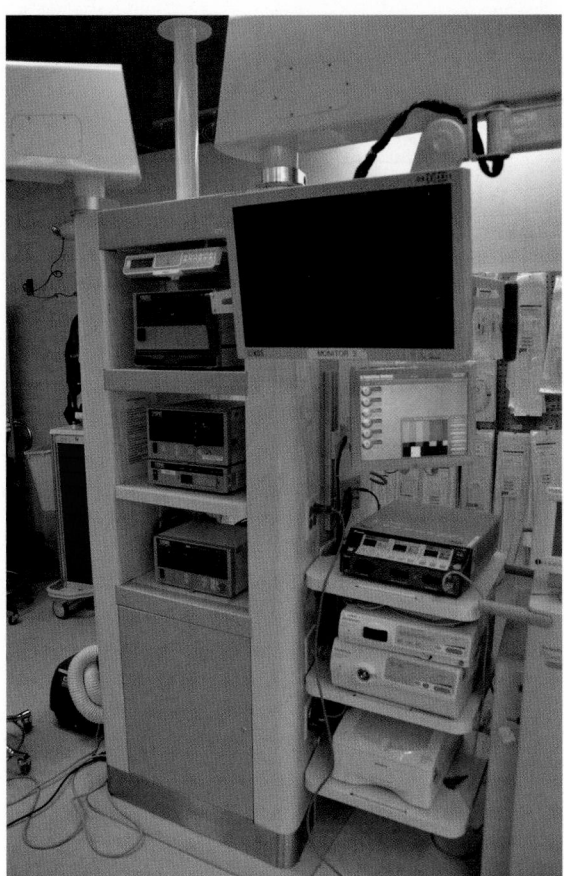

Figure 7-1. Video-endoscopic unit consisting of a fixed tower, monitor, light source, image processor, video-recording device, and printer.

rods or fiberoptic bundles. The optical image is then converted to an electrical charge (voltage waveform) by the camera's CCD chip. The unit's video processor then converts the analog voltage waveform into a digital video signal that is sent to the monitor. In contrast, digital video-endoscopic systems have the CCD chip located at the distal end of the endoscope. The image is immediately converted into an electrical signal that is once again managed by the video processor without the need for internal optics and a CCD camera.

CYSTOURETHROSCOPY

Indications

Cystourethroscopy is one of the most common procedures in urology. Routinely performed in both the office and operating room setting, cystourethroscopy provides direct visualization of the urethra and bladder. The upper urinary tract may be evaluated fluoroscopically by ureteral catheterization with retrograde instillation of contrast material.

Indications for office-based cystourethroscopy are summarized in Box 7-1. Most are for diagnostic purposes, but a limited number of therapeutic procedures may also be performed. One of the most frequent reasons to perform cystourethroscopy is for microscopic and gross hematuria. In addition to directly visualizing the lower urinary tract, cystourethroscopy permits collection of cytologic specimens and retrograde pyelography in patients who are not candidates for intravenous contrast.

Urothelial carcinoma surveillance is another routine indication for cystourethroscopy. Small urothelial lesions may be biopsied and fulgurated in the clinic. Upper tract surveillance may be accomplished by selective ureteral catheterization with retrograde

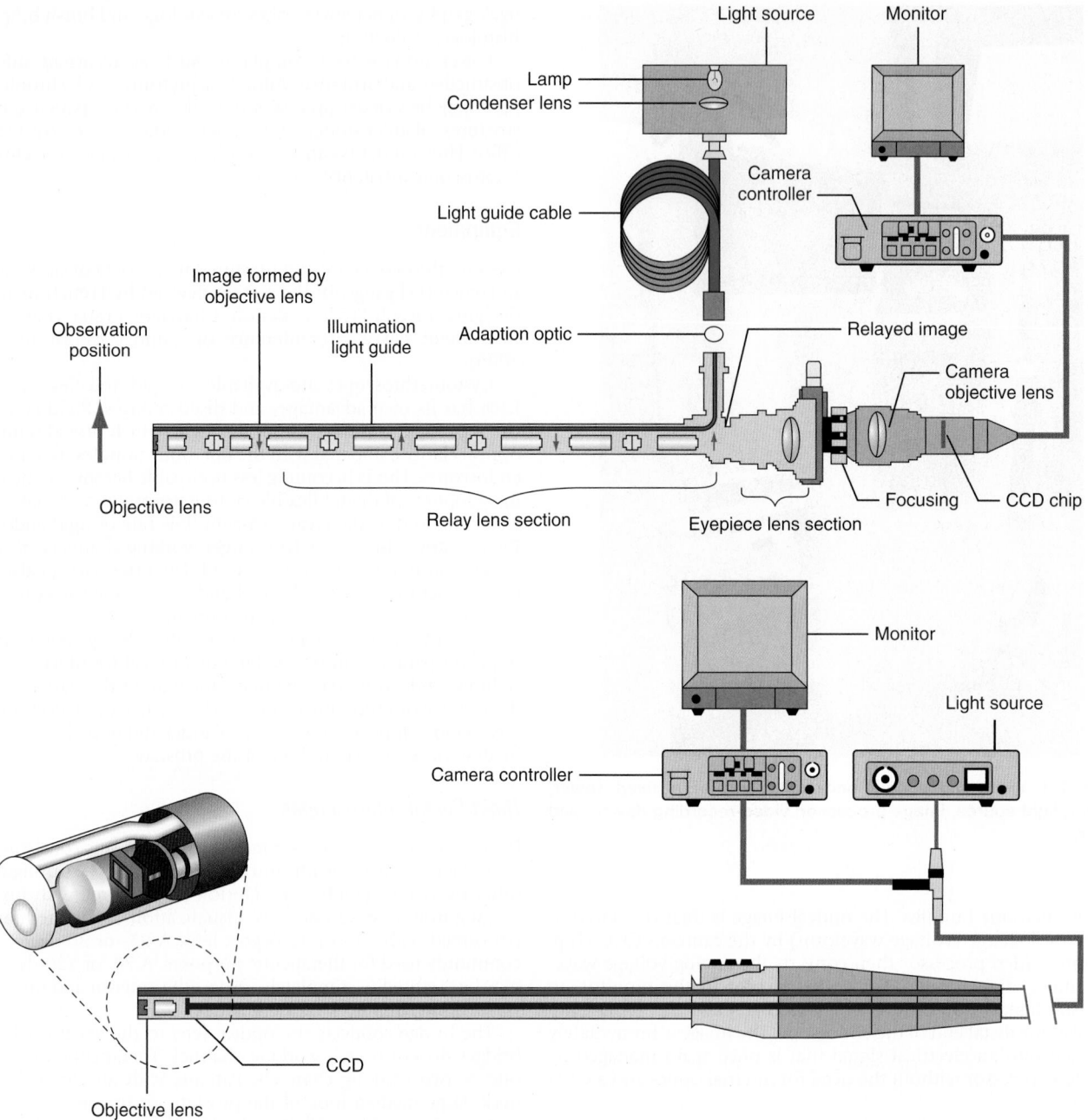

Figure 7-2. Traditional rod-lens optical system compared with digital sensor video-endoscopes. CCD, charge-coupled device. (Courtesy Olympus, Center Valley, PA.)

channel. Photodynamic and narrow band imaging capabilities are available in some models.

Flexible cystourethroscopes are available in fiberoptic and digital models. Digital scopes do not require focusing or white balancing. They are now available in high-definition (1920×1080 pixels) and standard-definition (720×480 pixels) models. An in vitro study compared the resolution, contrast evaluation, depth of field, color representation, and illumination of fiberoptic, standard-definition, and high-definition flexible cystoscopes (Lusch et al, 2013). All three scopes were manufactured by Olympus (Olympus, Center Valley, PA). Compared with the fiberoptic and standard-definition models, the high-definition scope had a significantly higher resolution and depth of field. The high-definition scope's resolution was five times greater and it had a 37% larger image than the standard-definition model. Color representation was only slightly better, and there was no difference in contrast evaluation among the three

models. Illumination was significantly better in the fiberoptic model compared with both digital cystoscopes.

A randomized study of 1022 flexible cystoscopy cases compared optics, performance, and durability of fiberoptic and standard-definition digital scopes (Okhunov et al, 2009). There was a trend toward improved mean surgeon optical ranking in favor of the digital scopes ($P = .076$). There was no difference in durability between the models. Only two cystoscopes required repair (0.2% incidence rate), and both were damaged when the endoscope was placed in a storage case rather than during use.

Data from an independent endoscope repair company found that flexible cystoscopes require less than one repair every 2 years (Canales et al, 2007). The most common repair was to the rubber overlying the distal flexible segment. Unlike flexible ureteroscopes, flexible cystourethroscopes are robust, likely making the optical mechanism a lesser determinant of scope durability.

BOX 7-1 Indications for Office-Based Cystourethroscopy

HEMATURIA
Gross
Microscopic

MALIGNANCY
Urethral cancer
Bladder cancer
Atypical cytology
Upper tract transitional cell carcinoma surveillance

LOWER URINARY TRACT SYMPTOMS
Recurrent urinary tract infections
Obstructive voiding symptoms
Irritative voiding symptoms
Urinary incontinence
Chronic pelvic pain syndrome
Urethral stricture disease

MISCELLANEOUS
Trauma
Bladder abnormalities seen on imaging
Removal of foreign bodies and small bladder stones
Hematospermia
Obstructive azoospermia

Patient Preparation

Informed consent must be obtained before any cystoscopic procedure is performed. A urinalysis and urine culture, if indicated, should be completed before cystoscopy. All urinary tract infections must be treated, given the risk of bacteremia and sepsis after lower urinary tract manipulation.

The American Urological Association (AUA) Best Practice Policy Statement on antimicrobial prophylaxis does not recommend antibiotic administration for routine diagnostic

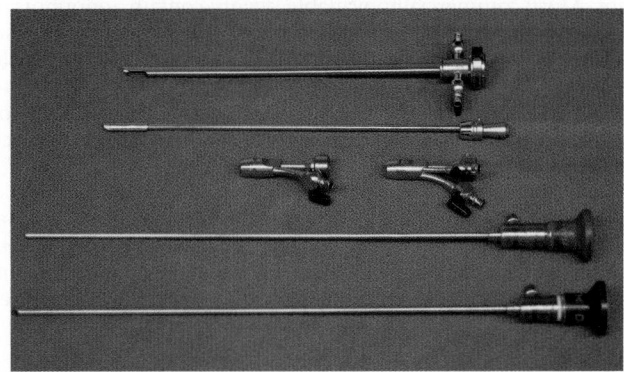

Figure 7-3. Rigid cystourethroscope set consisting of sheath, obturator, bridges, and lenses (from *top* to *bottom*).

TABLE 7-1 Rigid Cystoscopes (Information Supplied by Manufacturers)

	KARL STORZ	OLYMPUS	GYRUS/ACMI	WOLF
Lenses	0, 12, 30, 70, 120	0, 12, 30, 70, 110	0, 12, 30, 70, 110	0, 12, 30, 70
	Diameter: 4 mm	Diameter: 4 mm	Diameter: 4 mm	Diameter: 4 mm
	Length: 30 cm	Length: 28 cm	Length: 28 cm	Length: 29.5 cm
Bridges	Telescopic	Telescopic	Telescopic	Telescopic
	• Diagnostic	• Diagnostic	• Diagnostic	• Diagnostic
	• Single and dual channel	• Single and dual channel	• Single and dual channel	• Single and dual channel
	Deflecting (Albarran lever)	Deflecting (Albarran lever)	Deflecting (Albarran lever)	Deflecting (Albarran lever)
	• Single and dual channel	• Single and dual channel	• Single and dual channel	• Single and dual channel
Sheaths and working channels		15 Fr		16 Fr
		SB: none		SB: 5 Fr
		DB: none		DB: none
	17 Fr	17 Fr	17 Fr	17.5 Fr
	SB: 5 Fr	SB: none	SB: 5 Fr	SB: 5 Fr
	DB: 5 Fr × 1	DB: none	DB: 4 Fr × 2	DB: 4 Fr × 2
	19 Fr	19.8 Fr		19.5 Fr
	SB: 6 Fr	SB: 6 Fr		SB: 7 Fr
	DB: 5 Fr × 2	DB: 5 Fr, 6 Fr		DB: 5 Fr x 2
	20 Fr	21 Fr	21 Fr	21 Fr
	SB: 7 Fr	SB: 8 Fr	SB: 9 Fr	SB: 10 Fr
	DB: 6 Fr × 2	DB: 6 Fr, 7 Fr	DB: 6 Fr × 2	DB: 6 Fr × 2
	22 Fr	22.5 Fr	23 Fr	23 Fr
	SB: 10 Fr	SB: 10 Fr	SB: 10 Fr	SB: 12 Fr
	DB: 7 Fr × 2	DB: 8 Fr x 2	DB: 8 Fr × 2	DB: 7 Fr × 2
	25 Fr	25 Fr	25 Fr	25 Fr
	SB: 12 Fr	SB: 12 Fr	SB: 12 Fr	SB: 15 Fr
	DB: 8 Fr × 2	DB: 8 Fr × 2	DB: 8 Fr × 2	DB: none

DB, dual bridge; Fr, French; SB, single bridge.

cystoscopy in the absence of patient-related risk factors (Box 7-2) (Wolf et al, 2008). Prophylaxis lasting less than 24 hours with either a fluoroquinolone or trimethoprim-sulfamethoxazole is recommended for therapeutic procedures. Second-line alternatives include an aminoglycoside with or without ampicillin, a first- or second-generation cephalosporin, or amoxicillin/clavulanate. This recommendation is largely based on a meta-analysis of 32 randomized controlled trials evaluating antimicrobial prophylaxis before transurethral resection of the prostate (TURP), which showed a decrease in bacteriuria, bacteremia, symptomatic urinary tract infection, and high-grade fever (Berry and Barratt, 2002). Similar trials have not been performed for minor cystoscopic procedures.

Before cystourethroscopy the skin is prepared with an antiseptic agent. Most commercially available agents contain iodophors or chlorhexidine gluconate in either an aqueous or alcohol-based solution. **Both chlorhexidine gluconate and alcohol-based solutions can damage mucous membranes and therefore are not recommended for use on the genitalia.** Aqueous-based iodophor-containing products such as Betadine are safe on all skin surfaces regardless of patient age.

After application of an antiseptic agent a lubricating gel is injected into the urethra of patients undergoing flexible cystourethroscopy. Either a plain or lidocaine gel may be used. **A meta-analysis of four randomized trials involving 411 patients found that patients who received lidocaine gel were 1.7 times less likely** to experience moderate to severe pain during the procedure (Aaronson et al, 2009). However, only one of the four trials showed a statistical benefit to lidocaine gel, which is consistent with a larger meta-analysis involving 817 patients from nine randomized trials that showed no difference in procedure tolerance (Patel et al, 2008b).

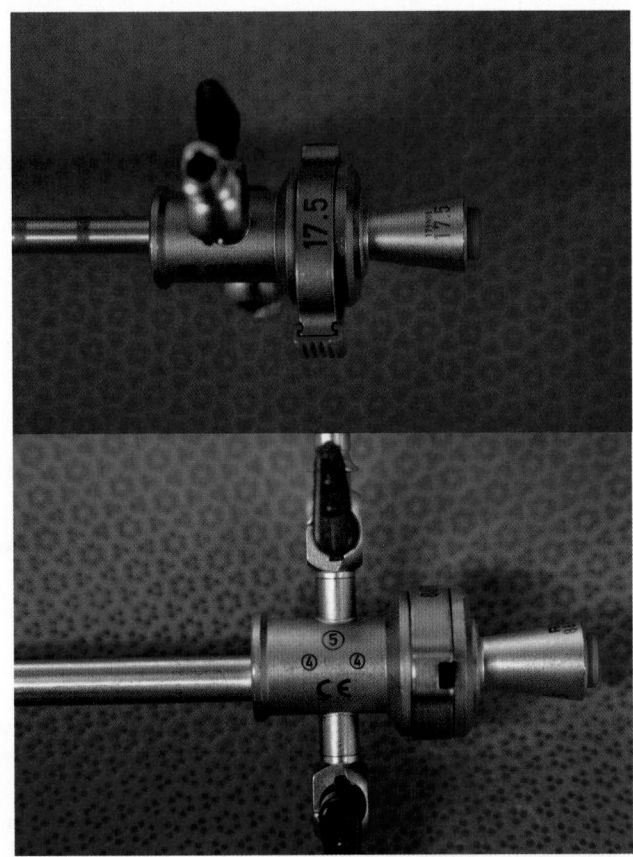

Figure 7-5. **Markings on rigid cystoscope sheath. The largest number on the base of the scope indicates the outer diameter (17.5 Fr). The numbers on the side of the sheath indicate the maximum working channel size when a dual bridge is used (4 Fr for both lumens) or when a single bridge is employed (5 Fr).**

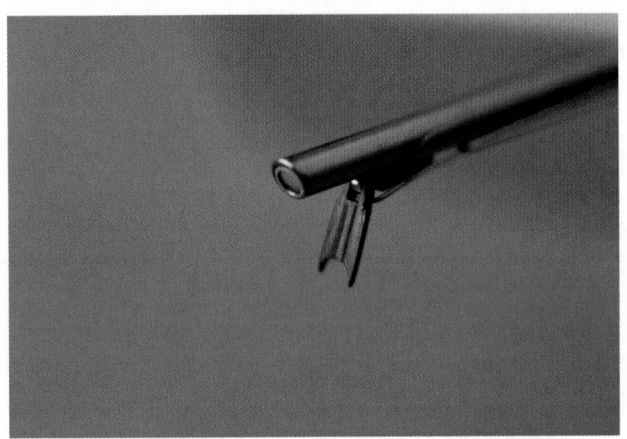

Figure 7-4. **Albarran bridge, which is used to deflect wires and catheters passed through the rigid cystoscope working channel.**

TABLE 7-2 Flexible Cystoscopes (information Supplied by Manufacturers)

MANUFACTURER	OPTICS	DEFLECTION (DEGREES)	DIRECTION OF VIEW (DEGREES)	ANGLE OF VIEW (DEGREES)	WORKING LENGTH	WORKING CHANNEL	SHEATH SIZE
Karl Storz	Fiberoptic	Up: 210	0	110	37 cm	7.0 Fr	15.5 Fr
	• Multiple models	Down: 140					
	Digital (standard definition)	Up: 210	0	120	37 cm	6.5 Fr	16.0 Fr
	• Multiple models	Down: 140					
Olympus	Fiberoptic	Up: 210	0	120	38 cm	7.2 Fr	16.5 Fr
	• Model CYF-5	Down: 120					
	Digital (standard definition)	Up: 210	0	120	38 cm	6.6 Fr	16.2 Fr
	• Model CYF-V2	Down: 120					
	Digital (high definition)	Up: 210	0	120	38 cm	6.6 Fr	16.5 Fr
	• Model CYF-VH	Down: 120					
Wolf	Fiberoptic	Up: 180	0	105	37 cm	6.4 Fr	15.9 Fr
	• Model CAN-2	Down: 170					

BOX 7-2 Patient Risk Factors Requiring Antimicrobial Prophylaxis

Advanced age
Anatomic anomalies of the urinary tract
Chronic corticosteroid use
Colonized endogenous or exogenous material
Distant coexistent infection
Immunodeficiency
Poor nutritional status
Prolonged coexistent infection
Smoking

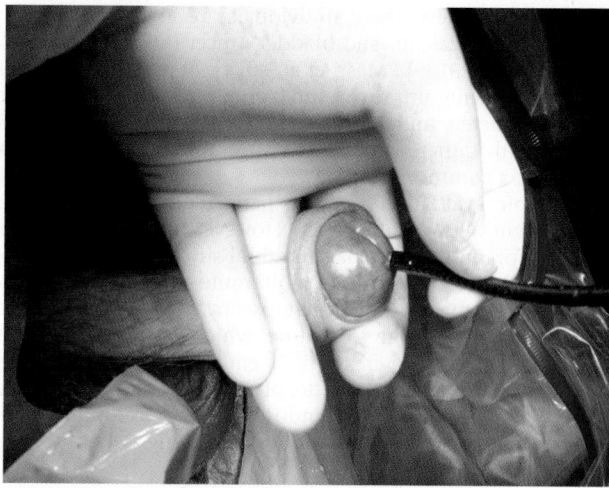

Figure 7-6. During flexible cystoscopy the distal penis is grasped between the surgeon's third and fourth fingers and placed on stretch while the thumb and index finger advance the cystoscope into the urethral meatus.

Other techniques have been employed to improve patient comfort during flexible cystourethroscopy. For the majority of men, the most uncomfortable part of the procedure is when the scope passes through the membranous urethra (Taghizadeh et al, 2006). A randomized trial was performed on 151 men undergoing flexible cystourethroscopy (Gunendran et al, 2008). Half of the subjects had the hydrostatic pressure of the irrigation solution increased by manual compression of the irrigation bag during passage of the scope through the membranous urethra. Gravity irrigation alone was used for the remaining patient. A significant improvement on an analog pain scale score was noted (1.38 vs. 3.00, $P < .001$) in the manual compression group.

The impact of being allowed to observe the procedure has also been evaluated. One hundred male patients undergoing flexible cystourethroscopy were randomized; half the subjects were allowed to observe the procedure on a video monitor whereas the remaining patients were not (Patel et al, 2007). **Men who watched the procedure had significantly less pain on a 100-mm visual analog pain scale (14 vs. 23, $P = .02$). These findings were confirmed by another randomized study of 76 male patients (Soomro et al, 2011). Men in the observation group had less pain and lower postprocedure pulse rates.** In contrast, a randomized study of 100 women undergoing office-based cystoscopy with a 17-Fr rigid scope found no difference in procedural pain (Patel et al, 2008a).

The potentially calming effect of music has also been examined. Seventy men undergoing flexible cystoscopy were randomized to either no music or classical music played during the procedure (Yeo et al, 2013). Patients listening to classical music had significantly less pain, greater satisfaction, lower postprocedure pulse rates, and lower systolic blood pressures.

Technique

Before insertion of the cystourethroscope, the external genitalia is inspected for cutaneous lesions and anatomic abnormalities. Mild meatal stenosis may be addressed with sequential metal dilators. Dilation should be performed to at least 2 Fr wider than the intended endoscope.

In women, rigid cystourethroscope insertion is safest using the sheath obturator. The scope will often need to be directed anteriorly as it is advanced into the bladder. Flexible cystourethroscopes can often be inserted into the bladder like a Foley catheter, with active deflection being used as needed.

In men, the penis is placed on maximal stretch to straighten the urethra. When a rigid cystourethroscope is being passed, the penis is typically grasped with all five digits of the surgeon's nondominant hand. With flexible cystourethroscopy the penis is pinched between the fourth and fifth digits of the nondominant hand at the corona while the thumb and index finger help advance and direct the scope into the urethra (Fig. 7-6). In morbidly obese

patients it is often easier to lay the scope down, retract the pannus with the nondominant hand, and direct the tip of the flexible scope into urethra like a Foley catheter. Once in the mid-penile urethra the scope is placed in the dominant hand and advanced as usual.

The penis should be angled 45 to 90 degrees relative to the abdominal wall while the scope is passed through the anterior urethra. Once beyond the membranous urethra the cystoscope is directed anteriorly to enter the bladder. With flexible cystoscopes this is accomplished by active upward deflection and with rigid cystoscopes by dropping the distal end of the scope toward the operative table.

The lower urinary tract is systematically evaluated under maximal irrigation as the scope is advanced. The penile and bulbar urethra are inspected for strictures. The periurethral glands of Littre should be noted as they drain into the urethra dorsally. Patients, in particular young men, should be encouraged to relax as much as possible as the scope is advanced through the membranous urethra. Once the scope is in the prostatic urethra, the verumontanum and utricle are identified posteriorly. The length of the posterior urethra is measured and the size of the prostatic lobes is evaluated.

Once the scope is in the bladder, the mucosa is carefully inspected. Rigid cystoscopy is usually begun with a 25- or 30-degree lens. The floor of the bladder and trigone are surveyed. The number, location, and configuration of the ureteral orifices are noted. Efflux from each ureter should be observed for the presence of gross blood. The remainder of the bladder is inspected for stones, trabeculation, cellules, diverticula, erythematous patches, and papillary and sessile lesions. Visualization of the lateral walls is accomplished by rotating the cystoscope while keeping the camera orientation fixed. The dome and anterior and posterolateral walls are inspected with a 70- or 120-degree lens. After completion of the procedure, the bladder is emptied and the endoscope withdrawn. If a Foley catheter is to be placed after the procedure, it is best to leave the bladder at least partially full before removing the cystoscope.

Special Circumstances

Suprapubic Cystostomy

The indications for cystoscopy in patients with suprapubic cystostomy tubes are the same as for those without chronic indwelling catheters. Nevertheless, these individuals are at increased risk of infection, bladder calculi, and bladder cancer (Subramonian et al, 2004; Welk et al, 2013; El Masri et al, 2014). At present there are no level 1 data showing improved survival in patients with long-term indwelling catheters undergoing surveillance cystoscopy. However, in patients with catheters for more than 5 to 10 years, surveillance cystoscopy is a common practice.

Cystoscopic evaluation may be performed transurethrally or via the patient's suprapubic tract. However, many patients with long-term suprapubic tubes have urethral stricture disease, making the suprapubic tract the only feasible route to the bladder. Every effort should be made to avoid endoscopy through a suprapubic tract until it has had time to mature, which usually takes several weeks from the time of creation. If endoscopy of an immature tract is required, it is advisable to place a wire through the tract into the bladder to guide the endoscope. This technique is also helpful in morbidly obese patients with long, often tortuous tracts.

Ureteral access is often challenging during rigid cystoscopy because of the acute angle required to cannulate the ureteral orifice via the cystostomy tract. Use of angled catheters such as the Kumpe Catheter (Cook Medical, Bloomington, IN) or an Albarran deflector may facilitate ureteral access. Use of a flexible cystoscope will often overcome these problems. Alternatively, patients with low-grade urethral strictures may be able to accommodate transurethral passage of a semirigid ureteroscope facilitating standard ureteral access. Lastly, the ureteral orifices may be difficult to identify because of edema caused by the chronic suprapubic tube. Administering intravenous indigo carmine or methylene blue early in the procedure may help visualize the ureteral orifices.

Continent Urinary Diversions

There are two general classes of continent urinary diversions after cystectomy. Orthotopic urinary diversions are anastomosed to the urethra and rely on the striated urinary sphincter to maintain continence. Continent cutaneous reservoirs use a catheterizable channel anastomosed to the diversion and anterior abdominal wall. The catheterizable channel may be composed of the appendix (Mitrofanoff), tapered or imbricated terminal ileum and ileocecal valve, or an intussuscepted nipple valve.

Before any endoscopic procedure involving a continent urinary diversion, it is imperative to obtain the operative note. It is important to know the bowel segment used, type and location of the ureteroenteric anastomoses, continence mechanism employed, and whether an afferent limb was created.

Transurethral access to orthotopic diversions is often straightforward and can be accomplished using a rigid cystoscope. If a contracture is noted at the urethral anastomosis and the patient does not have outlet obstruction, then it is advisable to use the smallest scope possible rather than dilate or incise the stricture because of the risk of worsening urinary incontinence.

Diagnostic procedures on continent cutaneous reservoirs are best accomplished with a flexible cystoscope through the catheterizable channel. Therapeutic procedures should be performed percutaneously, given that continence mechanisms are often fragile and excess manipulation may result in either stomal stenosis or urinary incontinence (L'Esperance et al, 2004). Preoperative computed tomography (CT) or intraoperative ultrasound should be used to minimize the risk of bowel injury during percutaneous access.

Once within the diversion, visualization is often challenging because of mucus, mucosal folds, bowel peristalsis, and, if present, tortuous afferent limb. Begin by irrigating out all of the mucus. Irrigation should then be used judiciously. Too little irrigation will make mucosal folds more prominent and impair visualization, but overdistending the diversion will prevent access to the afferent limb. Once again, ancillary techniques such as use of angled catheters and indigo carmine or methylene blue may be required.

UPPER TRACT ENDOSCOPY

Indications

Urolithiasis

The treatment of stones is the most common indication for ureteroscopy. Rigid ureteroscopy has long been the preferred treatment for distal ureteral stones. Shock wave lithotripsy (SWL) was favored for stones above the iliac vessels, because early results using rigid ureteroscopy for mid-ureteral and proximal ureteral calculi were discouraging. However, improvements in ureteroscopes and working instruments, the use of the holmium laser, and greater use of the flexible ureteroscope have significantly improved stone-free rates after ureteroscopic treatment of stones above the iliac vessels.

Although SWL remains a valuable treatment option for renal and ureteral stones, there are certain clinical situations in which, because of SWL limitations, ureteroscopy is preferred. Frequent causes of shock wave lithotripsy failure include radiolucent or difficult-to-visualize calculi, concomitant obstruction distal to the calculus, poor passage of lower pole fragments, and failure to fragment dense calculi. In addition, morbidly obese patients who exceed the weight limit or focal length of many shock wave lithotripters can be successfully treated ureteroscopically.

Percutaneous nephrostolithotomy is the treatment of choice for large (>2 cm) intrarenal calculi. **However, in patients with significant comorbidities that would make percutaneous nephrostolithotomy dangerous, flexible ureteroscopy has been successfully used. Two studies have reported stone-free rates of 91% and 93% for ureteroscopic treatment of patients with stones larger than 2 cm** (Grasso et al, 1997; Breda et al, 2008).

Upper Urinary Tract Transitional Cell Carcinoma

The standard treatment for upper urinary tract transitional cell carcinoma is nephroureterectomy. However, with improvements in flexible ureteroscopic instrumentation and technique, there is increased use of endoscopic treatment of well-selected patients with upper urinary tract transitional cell carcinoma. Accordingly, **the principles of endoscopic management of transitional cell carcinoma have been extended from the bladder to the upper urinary tract. With expansion of ureteroscopy for the diagnosis, ablation, and subsequent surveillance phases of upper tract transitional cell carcinoma management, this is becoming a frequent indication for ureteroscopy.**

Many patients treated ureteroscopically for upper urinary tract transitional cell carcinoma are those in whom nephroureterectomy would be dangerous: patients with a solitary kidney, renal insufficiency, bilateral upper tract transitional cell carcinoma, or significant medical comorbidities. There is also increasing use of ureteroscopic treatment for patients with low-grade, low-volume disease. Endoscopic management of these patients has proven to be a reasonable option, without compromise of patient survival (Cutress et al, 2012b; Grasso et al, 2012). Larger tumors can be difficult to fully ablate in one session. Percutaneous nephroscopy and electroresection have been used and permit resection of large amounts of tumor (Irwin et al, 2010; Cutress et al, 2012a). However, the ureteroscopic approach may be preferred because it avoids the risk of seeding the percutaneous tract and retroperitoneum with tumor. The risk of tract seeding is small, but it has been reported (Sharma et al, 1994; Sengupta and Harewood, 1998).

Ureteropelvic Junction Obstruction and Ureteral Stricture

Despite the growing and successful use of laparoscopic ureteropyeloplasty, endopyelotomy is still a reasonable choice for the management of select patients with ureteropelvic junction (UPJ) obstruction. This can be performed percutaneously, ureteroscopically, or with the Acucise (Applied Medical Resources, Laguna Hills, CA) cutting balloon catheter device. The advantages of the ureteroscopic approach include the ability to control the length and depth of the incision under direct vision, the avoidance of percutaneous renal access, and the ability to perform the procedure in an outpatient setting.

There are two situations in which ureteroscopic endopyelotomy may not be the preferred approach. Patients with concomitant renal calculi should be treated via a percutaneous approach to allow simultaneous removal of the calculi and endopyelotomy. Also, several studies have demonstrated a decreased success rate with endopyelotomy in patients who have vessels crossing at the UPJ (Van Cangh et al, 1994; Bagley et al, 1995; Conlin et al, 1998; Tawfiek et al, 1999). **It may be best to limit ureteroscopic endopyelotomy to those patients without known crossing vessels, and treat those with crossing vessels with laparoscopic ureteropyeloplasty.**

Patients with ureteral strictures can also be managed from a ureteroscopic approach. The technique is nearly identical to the ureteroscopic endopyelotomy technique. Endoureterotomy will be less successful in patients with ureteral strictures longer than 1.5 cm, allograft ureters, previously irradiated ureters, ureters draining poorly functioning kidneys, and ureteral-enteral anastomotic strictures (Wolf et al, 1997). Ureteroscopic incision of short ureteral strictures in otherwise healthy ureters is a reasonably successful treatment option.

Other Indications for Ureteroscopy

Diagnostic flexible ureteroscopy can be performed in patients with persistent positive cytology, filling defects, hematuria, and recurrent urinary tract infections localized to a single renal unit. With the miniaturization of flexible ureteroscopes, the safety of flexible ureteroscopy has increased significantly. Rather than relying on ureteropyelography alone, we can now safely and easily perform diagnostic ureteroscopy.

Ureteroscopy has also been used for removal of foreign bodies including suture, proximally migrated ureteral stents, balloon catheters, and other fractured working instruments. The three-pronged grasping forceps are ideally suited for grasping and removing these foreign bodies.

Benign essential hematuria can be diagnosed and treated with flexible ureteroscopy. This condition is defined as unilateral gross hematuria for which there is no radiographically defined cause (Lano et al, 1979; Bagley et al, 1987). These patients frequently have had studies including excretory urography, renal sonography, and/or arteriography. Flexible ureteroscopic inspection of the kidney involved usually results in diagnosis and successful treatment. The most common finding in patients with benign essential hematuria is a small hemangioma, which can often be fulgurated. Other endoscopic findings in patients with benign essential hematuria include small venous ruptures, papillary tumors, varices, and calculi (Dooley and Pietrow, 2004).

Equipment

Semirigid Ureteroscopes

Performance of successful ureteroscopy requires a variety of instrumentation—most important, appropriate and modern ureteroscopes. Although larger rod-lens rigid ureteroscopes are still available in some operating rooms, the smaller-diameter fiberoptic ureteroscopes are less traumatic, less often require ureteral dilation, and are equally effective.

Semirigid ureteroscopes are smaller in diameter because of the incorporation of fiberoptics into their construction. Fiberoptic bundles are created from molten glass that has been pulled into small-diameter fibers. Each individual glass fiber is "cladded" with a second layer of glass of a different refractive index. This cladding improves the internal reflection, light transmission, and durability of the fiberoptic bundle. The meshlike appearance of the image from fiberoptic image bundles is caused by the lack of light transmission through this cladding. These fibers uniformly transmit light from one end of the fiber to the other proportional to the light input. The glass fibers of a fiberoptic bundle can be arranged randomly or in a precise orientation with identical location at each end of the fiber (i.e., coherent). When the fibers are grouped randomly, such as those within the light bundle, they provide excellent light transmission for illumination, but no image. When the fibers are arranged in a coherent fashion, the light from each fiber within the bundle will coalesce to transmit images.

Small lenses are attached to the proximal and distal ends of the image bundle to create a telescope. By controlling the number of fibers in the bundle, and the type and orientation of the lenses, the manufacturers can determine the degree of image magnification, field of view, and focusing ability for different fiberoptic endoscopes. For example, by changing the axis of the lens at the distal tip of the image bundle, the angle of view of the ureteroscope can be changed to improve visibility of any working instruments passed out the working channel (Higashihara et al, 1990).

Improvements in image bundle construction have allowed closer packing of more fibers, resulting in improved images, smaller outer diameters, and larger working channels in both rigid and flexible ureteroscopes. Another design modification is the splitting of the light bundle distally into two points of light transmission (Conlin et al, 1997). This makes possible a more centrally placed working channel as well as better distribution of the light within the working field of view.

Current semirigid ureteroscopes typically have tip diameters of 7 Fr or smaller and working channels larger than 3 Fr. Semirigid ureteroscopes have either large single or two smaller individual working channels. **An advantage of the separate working channels is the ability to irrigate through one unrestricted channel while a working instrument occupies the other. Separate working channels also permit passage of a lithotripsy device through the separate channel to fracture a stone that cannot be disengaged from a basket in the other channel.** With a single channel, this can be difficult because of entanglement between the two working instruments.

Eyepieces are commonly "in line" with the ureteroscope, which allows easy introduction of the scope (Fig. 7-7). Offset eyepiece design makes possible a straight working channel for the use of more rigid working instruments such as rigid biopsy forceps or a pneumatic lithotripsy probe (Fig. 7-8). Increased availability and use of the holmium laser for ureteroscopic lithotripsy has decreased the need for ureteroscopes with offset eyepieces.

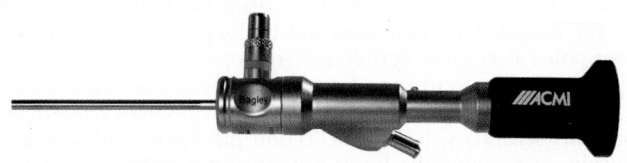

Figure 7-7. **Semirigid ureteroscope with "in-line" eyepiece.**

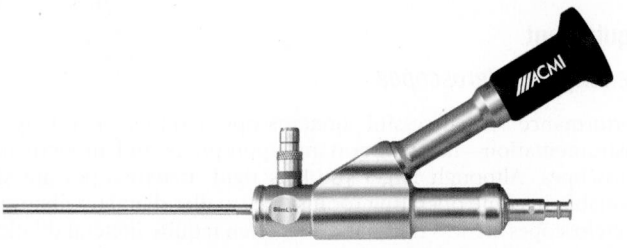

Figure 7-8. **Semirigid ureteroscope with an offset eyepiece, which has a straight working channel permitting passage of rigid instruments.**

Larger ureteroresectoscopes (11.5 Fr) can be useful for large distal ureteral tumor resection. Some surgeons also preferred using this instrument for ureteroscopic endopyelotomies (Thomas et al, 1996). Preoperative ureteral stenting will be necessary in this setting to allow passage of the larger-diameter ureteroresectoscope, especially to the UPJ.

Currently available semirigid ureteroscopes and their characteristics are listed in Table 7-3.

Flexible Ureteroscopes

The fundamental components of flexible ureteroscopes include the optical system, deflection mechanism, and working channel. The nondigital optical system consists of flexible fiberoptic image and light bundles. Improvements in the fiberoptic image bundles are discussed in the preceding section and are similar to those used in semirigid ureteroscopes.

The deflection mechanism is an integral part of every flexible ureteroscope. It permits complete maneuverability within the intrarenal collecting system (Bagley, 1989). The deflecting mechanism consists of control wires running down the length of the ureteroscope that are attached proximally to a manually operated lever mechanism. The control wires pass through movable metal rings to the distal end of the scope where they are fixed. Moving the lever up or down pulls the control wire through these rings and deflects the tip. When the tip moves in the same direction as the lever, the deflection is said to be "intuitive" (i.e., down is down and up is up). Most modern flexible ureteroscopes allow both up and down deflection in a single plane (Grasso and Bagley, 1994). **The plane of deflection is designated by the reticle, seen as a notch within the field of view of the ureteroscope (Fig. 7-9). When the flexible ureteroscope is maneuvered, it must be rotated to align the plane of deflection with the intended target.** The active deflection mechanism eventually wears out with repeated use, necessitating repair or replacement of the ureteroscope. Improvements in the construction of the deflecting mechanism with each new generation of flexible ureteroscopes continue to improve durability.

Most current flexible ureteroscopes permit deflection of 180 degrees or more. The amount of deflection necessary to reach the lower pole of the kidney varies among patients. One group of investigators measured ureteroinfundibular angle (between the major axis of the ureter and the lower pole infundibulum) in 30 patients. They determined an average angle of 140 degrees with a maximum of 175 degrees (Bagley and Rittenberg, 1987). Active deflection of the ureteroscope of 180 degrees should allow visualization of the lower pole in most patients. However, reaching into the lower pole calyx with the tip of the ureteroscope in a fashion that allows endoscopic work to be done can still be challenging.

Active deflection occurs only at the distal tip of the ureteroscope, and the deflected segment may not be long enough to reach the lower pole calyx. Most flexible ureteroscopes have a more flexible segment of the ureteroscope because of a weakness in the durometer of the sheath, located just proximal to the point of active deflection. This secondary, passive deflection mechanism addresses the difficulty of reaching the lower pole in some patients. By passive bending of the tip of the ureteroscope off the superior margin of

the renal pelvis, the point of deflection is effectively moved more proximally on the ureteroscope, thereby extending the tip of the ureteroscope. When passive deflection is used, the lower pole calyx can be reached in the majority of patients. Many of the failures to reach the lower pole will occur in patients with significant hydronephrosis, which can limit the ability to engage passive secondary deflection.

To address the difficulties with ureteroscopic access to the lower pole, two innovations in ureteroscope deflection have been developed. These are active secondary deflection and exaggerated deflection. The first ureteroscope incorporating active secondary deflection, the DUR-8 Elite, was developed by Circon-ACMI, now part of Olympus (Center Valley, PA). In addition to active primary deflection of 185 degrees down and 175 degrees up, there is a second control lever for active secondary deflection of 165 degrees, which can be locked in place. Combining both primary and secondary deflection resulted in a maximum deflected angle of 234 degrees (Shvarts et al, 2004). This ureteroscope can assist the urologist to reach the lower pole even under conditions in which access with passive secondary deflection is not possible (Fig. 7-10). Locking the secondary deflection in place simplifies manipulation of the primary deflection within the lower pole calyx. The usefulness of active secondary deflection has been evaluated by Ankem and coworkers (Ankem et al, 2004). In a series of 54 patients, they found the dual deflecting DUR-8 Elite ureteroscope helpful in cases in which the single-deflection flexible instruments failed in accessing and treating upper urinary tract pathology. Despite these advantages, the DUR-8 Elite is no longer manufactured by Olympus, and there is currently no available flexible ureteroscope with active secondary deflection.

Karl Storz Endoscopy (Tuttlingen, Germany) introduced exaggerated deflection with their Flex-X model flexible ureteroscope (Johnson and Grasso, 2004). This modification of the deflection mechanism permits active primary deflection of greater than 300 degrees (Fig. 7-11). When approaching the lower pole calyx, the deflected segment of the ureteroscope will effectively lengthen as it is deflected against the lower pole infundibulum. This improvement of the deflection mechanism results in easier lower pole access and improved deflection when working instruments are used.

All currently available flexible ureteroscopes have working channels of 3.6 Fr diameter. This allows use of instruments up to 3 Fr while still permitting adequate irrigation. When working instruments are used, higher pressure irrigation will be necessary to compensate for the effectively smaller irrigation channel (Bach et al, 2011). This higher pressure irrigation can be delivered using a pressurized irrigation bag, roller pump, or hand-held devices. The development of a dual channel flexible ureteroscope, the Cobra from Richard Wolf (Vernon Hills, IL), is an innovation that can improve irrigation through the ureteroscope. The dual 3.3 Fr channels will permit unimpeded irrigation through one channel while the working instrument occupies the other (Haberman et al, 2011). One may also use both channels for working instruments, such as a laser and a basket, but this is rarely necessary.

Digital Ureteroscopes

Digital flexible ureteroscopes have been developed and released by each of the three primary endoscope manufacturers. Like digital flexible cystoscopes described earlier in this chapter, these ureteroscopes integrate the endoscope, the digital camera, and the light source. A separate camera head is not needed because the scope has a digital camera chip (CCD or complementary metal-oxide semiconductor [CMOS]) mounted on its tip. Because these devices do not require a separate light cord or camera head, they are potentially less prone to damage and may have a prolonged life span.

Currently the digital flexible ureteroscopes available are larger diameter. One group of investigators performed a prospective comparison between digital and fiberoptic ureteroscopes to determine the influence of these larger-diameter digital scopes on patient outcomes. They found a higher use of ureteral access sheaths and related complications in those patients who underwent

TABLE 7-3 Semirigid Ureteroscopes (Information Supplied by Manufacturers)

MODEL	EYEPIECE	DIAMETER (Fr)	WORKING LENGTH (cm)	NO. OF CHANNELS	SIZE OF CHANNELS (Fr)	FIELD OF VIEW (DEGREES)	ANGLE OF VIEW (DEGREES)	AUTOCLAVABLE
OLYMPUS (WHITE PLAINS, NY)								
MR-6A	Straight	6.9/8.2/10.2	33	2	2.3; 3.4	61	5	Yes
MR-6AL	Straight	6.9/8.2/10.2	43	2	2.3; 3.4	61	5	Yes
MRO-733A	Angled offset	7.7/9.2/10.8	33	1	5.4	65	5	Yes
MRO-742A	Angled offset	7.7/9.2/10.8	42	1	5.4	65	5	Yes
WA29040A WA29041A	Angled	6.4/7.8/12	43 (WA29040A); 33 (WA29041A)	1	4.2	90	7	Yes
WA29042A	Angled	8.6/9.8/13.5	43	1	6.4	95.1	7	Yes
WA29048A; WA29049A	Straight	6.4/7.8/12	43 (WA29048A) 33 (WA29049A)	1	4.2	90	7	Yes
WA02943A	Angled	7.5	43	2	2.5; 3.6	90	7	Yes
WA02944A	Straight	7.5	43	2	2.5; 3.6	90	7	Yes
WA02946A	Straight	7.5	33	2	2.5; 3.6	90	7	Yes
KARL STORZ ENDOSCOPY (CULVER CITY, CA)								
27001KA/LA	Angled	7/8/12	34 (KA)/43(LA)	1	5		6	Yes
27002KA/LA	Angled	8/9.5/12	34 (KA)/43(LA)	1	6		6	Yes
27003KA/LA	Angled	9/9.5/12	34 (KA)/43(LA)	2	3.8; 5		6	Yes
27000KA/LA	Angled	6/7/9.9	34 (KA)/43(LA)	1	4.8		6	Yes
27010KA/LA	Straight	7/8.4/9.9	34 (KA)/43(LA)	2	2.4; 3.4		6	Yes
RICHARD WOLF MEDICAL INSTRUMENTS (VERNON HILLS, IL)								
8701.517 8701.518	Straight	4.5/6	33 (517) 43 (518)	2	2.5; 3	75	5	Yes
8701.533 8701.534	Angled	4.5/6	31.5 (533) 43 (534)	2	2.5;3	75	5	Yes
8702.517 8702.518	Straight	6/7.5	33 (517) 43(518)	1	4.2 × 4.6 (oval)	75	5	Yes
8702.523 8702.524	Offset	6/7.5	31.5 (523) 43 (524)	1	4.2 × 4.6 (oval)	75	5	Yes
8702.533 8702.534	Angled	6/7.5	31.5 (533) 43 (534)	1	4.2 × 4.6 (oval)	75	5	Yes
8703.517 8703.518	Straight	8/9.8	33 (517) 43 (518)	1	5.2 × 6.2 (oval)	75	12	Yes
8704.523 8704.524	Offset	8.5/11.5	31.5 (523) 43 (524)	1	Accepts 6.0	75	12	Yes
8708.517 8708.518	Straight	6.5/8.5	33 (517) 43 (518)	2	2.55; 4.2	75	5	Yes
8708.533 8708.534	Angled	6.5/8.5	31.5 (517) 43 (518)	2	2.55; 4.2	75	5	Yes

ureteroscopy performed with a digital ureteroscope (Bach et al, 2012). In another analysis of the efficacy of digital and flexible ureteroscopes, investigators determined a statistically equivalent stone-free rate but a significantly shorter operative time in the digital group (Somani et al, 2013). This is presumed to be a result of the improved visibility of the digital ureteroscopes (Fig. 7-12). These digital ureteroscopes may advance future miniaturization, optimize digital resolution, and improve durability.

The specifications of currently available flexible ureteroscopes are detailed in Table 7-4.

Care and Sterilization

Rigid and especially flexible ureteroscopes are very delicate instruments and need to be handled accordingly. Any damage to the working channel, deflecting mechanism, or fibers within the image bundle can render the ureteroscope useless. One series reported that repairs of flexible ureteroscopes were necessary after only 3 to 13 hours of use (Afane et al, 2000). The repairs were usually caused by deterioration of the deflecting mechanism.

The working channels of flexible ureteroscopes are also easily damaged. This primarily occurs during passage of the small (200 µ) holmium laser fiber. **When the fiber is introduced into a flexible ureteroscope that is even minimally deflected, the tip of the fiber may scrape the inner working channel. This can raise a small irregular area of the channel that will be more prone to damage.**

With each future pass of a laser fiber, the working channel can be increasingly damaged and ultimately perforated by the fiber. Once perforated, sterilization of the flexible ureteroscope will result in fluid damage to the imaging system of the scope, making the scope unusable. **Firing the fiber within the working channel will also result in damage. The holmium laser may damage the working channel when the tip is very near the end of the working channel** (Fig. 7-13). To prevent this, the tip of the fiber must be seen in the central portion of the field of view. **The golden rule of safe holmium laser lithotripsy is "Do not step on the pedal if you cannot see the tip of the fiber in contact with the stone." This will prevent injury to the ureter, as well as damage to the ureteroscope.**

A recent development in flexible ureteroscope design is the ability of the video system to prevent laser activation when the laser fiber is too close to the tip of the endoscope (Xavier et al, 2009). This "endoscope protection system" is activated in response to the video imaging system not "seeing" the blue color of the outer cladding of the laser fiber. When this "proximity alert" is activated, the laser will automatically pause firing to prevent damage to the scope.

Ureteroscopes, including the working channel, should be cleansed with warm water and a nonabrasive detergent after each use. Sterilization of ureteroscopes can be performed by gas (ethylene oxide), by soaking in a glutaraldehyde solution, or by use of the STERIS system (STERIS, Mentor, OH) (Gregory et al, 1988). The STERIS system provides automated washing and rinsing of the endoscopes in a peracetic acid solution.

Guidewires

Guidewires are essential to endourologic procedures. They are used for many portions of these procedures including establishment of percutaneous and ureteroscopic access, for straightening of the ureter, as a guide for dilation of the ureter or percutaneous tract, and for stent placement. There are many guidewires available differing in diameter, rigidity, tip design, materials, and coating. The choice of the most appropriate wire depends on the task involved and the patient's anatomy and upper urinary tract problem being confronted.

The most common design is a solid stainless steel core around which an outer wire is wrapped. Nitinol (nickel-titanium) can be used for inner core construction, and this gives guidewires a kink-resistant, slightly stiffer character. Many newer wires (Zebra wire, Boston Scientific, Natick, MA; Roadrunner wire, Cook Medical, Bloomington, IN) have a nitinol core wire and polyurethane outer layer. These wires are well suited for passage of the ureteroscope because there is less friction of the ureteroscope over the polyurethane, and the stiffer core allows more reliable transmission of the "push" from the urologist to the tip of the ureteroscope. Angling of the tip is also possible because of the "memory" quality of the

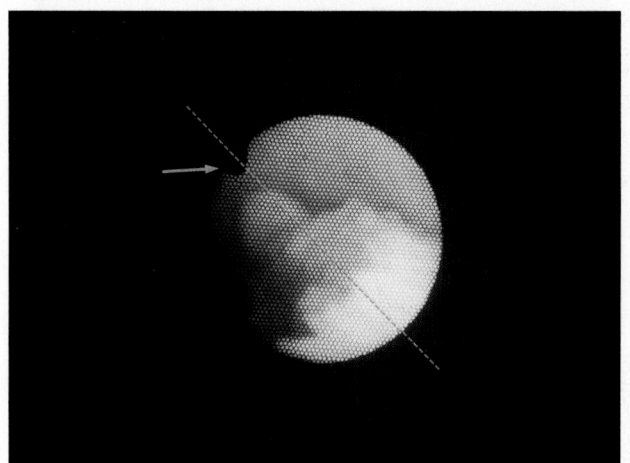

Figure 7-9. Flexible ureteroscopic image showing the reticle *(arrow)*, which designates the plane of deflection *(dotted line)*.

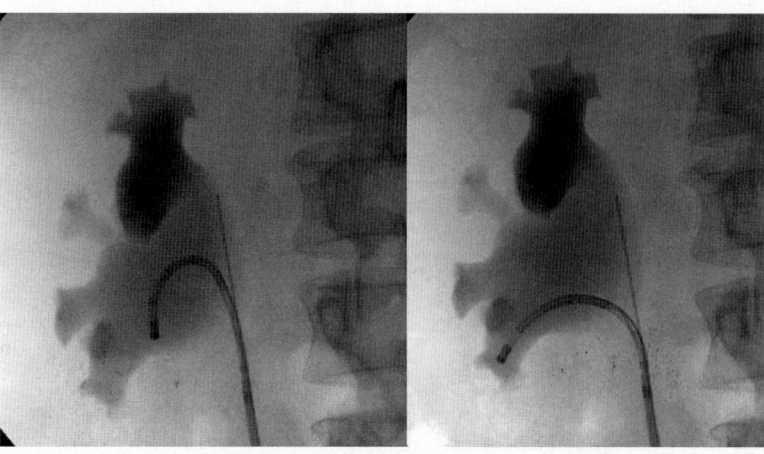

Figure 7-10. **Inability to access the lower pole calyx with typical primary deflection *(left)*. Successful access of the lower pole using active secondary deflection *(right)*.**

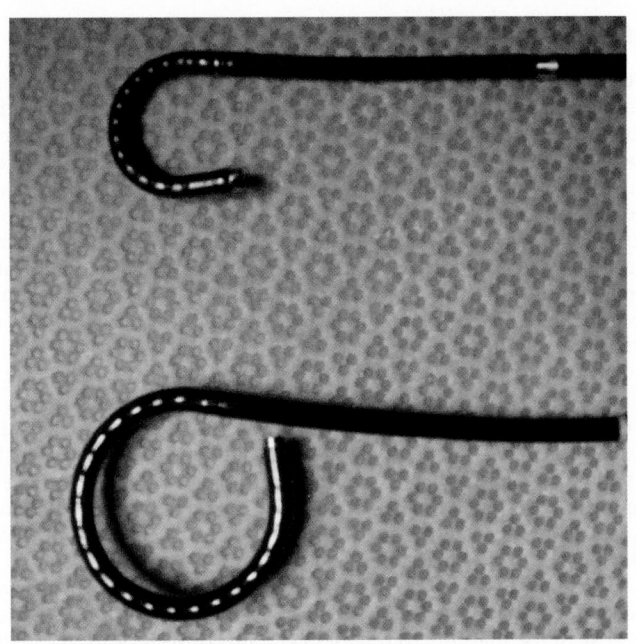

Figure 7-11. Flexible ureteroscopes with standard primary deflection *(top)* and exaggerated primary deflection *(bottom).*

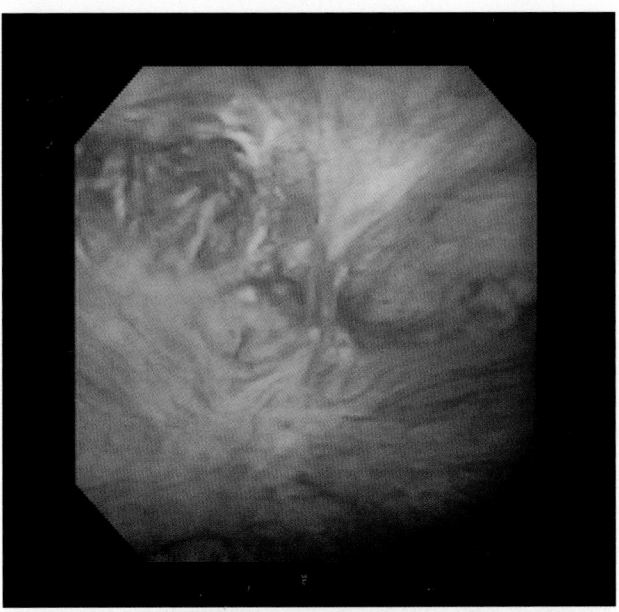

Figure 7-12. Excellent optical clarity of a digital ureteroscope image of a compound calyx.

TABLE 7-4 Flexible Ureteroscopes (Information Supplied by Manufacturers)

CHARACTERISTIC	OLYMPUS				KARL STORZ		RICHARD WOLF	
	URF-V	DUR-D	URF-P5	URF-P6	FLEX-XC	FLEX-X2	VIPER	COBRA
Digital or fiberoptic?	Digital	Digital	Fiberoptic	Fiberoptic	Digital	Fiberoptic	Fiberoptic	Fiberoptic
Tip diameter (Fr)	8.5	8.7	5.3	4.9	8.5	7.5	6.0	6.0
Shaft diameter (Fr)	9.9	9.3	8.4	7.9	8.5	8.4	8.8	9.9
Working length (cm)	67	65	70	67	67.5	70	68	68
Channel size (Fr)	3.6	3.6	3.6	3.6	3.6	3.6	3.6	3.3 (×2)
Up deflection (degrees)	180	250	180	275	270	270	270	270
Down deflection (degrees)	275	250	275	275	270	270	270	270
Angle of view (degrees)	0	9	0	0	0	0	0	0
Field of view (degrees)	90	80	90	90	90	85	85	85
Depth of field (mm)	2-50	2-40	2-50	2-50	Focal length = 15 mm	2-40	2-40	2-40
Magnification (×)	Digital zoom	Digital zoom	52	52	Digital zoom	50	50	50
Comments							Digital model soon	Dual channels; digital model soon

nitinol material. When the outer polyurethane layer is coated with a hydrophilic polymer, these wires become exceptionally slippery. These "glide wires" are useful for negotiating around impacted ureteral calculi, tortuous ureters, and ureteral strictures. **Hydrophilic-coated wires are too slippery to be reliable safety wires, because of their tendency to slide out of the patient. When these wires are used for initial access, they are exchanged for a standard safety wire through an open-ended catheter.** A new hybrid designed wire (Sensor, Boston Scientific, Natick, MA) incorporating

a hydrophilic tip with a standard polytetrafluoroethylene (PTFE)-coated shaft may serve as both an access and safety wire for procedures in which access is difficult.

Guidewires for urology range in diameter from 0.018 to 0.038 inch, the most commonly used being 0.038 inch. Lengths vary from 80 to 260 cm. The most useful length for endourology is 145 cm. The tips of these wires are typically "floppy" for 1 to 3 cm. Bentson and Newton wire designs have flexible tips of up to 15 cm and are seldom used today. Some wires have a movable core that can be

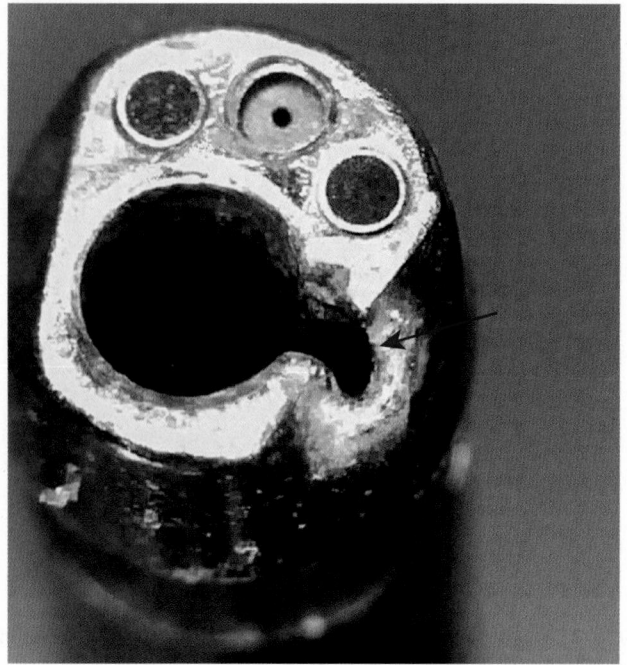

Figure 7-13. Image of the tip of a flexible ureteroscope that has been damaged by firing of the holmium laser within the working channel *(arrow)*.

partially withdrawn to increase the length of the flexible tip. Other variable characteristics in guidewire construction include the distal tip design and the wire stiffness. The distal tip can be straight, angled, or J tipped. The rigidity of the wires can be varied by changing the diameter and design of the inner core wire. Stiffer wires can be useful for straightening out tortuous ureters or displacing a large prostatic lobe.

The choice of the most appropriate guidewire for the endourologic task at hand can mean the difference between success and failure. Despite all of these advances in wire design and construction, a 0.038-inch diameter, straight, flexible-tip, Teflon-coated, stainless steel wire is still a good choice for most cases.

Dilation Devices

Ureteral dilation is less necessary for ureteroscopy with the advent of newer, smaller-diameter ureteroscopes. Hudson and colleagues determined that the need for dilation was directly related to the diameter of the ureteroscope and was as low as 0.9% for 7.4-Fr diameter scopes (Hudson et al, 2005). When needed, ureteral dilation can be accomplished passively with indwelling stent placement or actively with dilating catheters or balloons. Ureteral dilating catheters are hydrophilic-coated polyurethane catheters tapered from a 6-Fr tip to a 12-Fr shaft and are passed over a wire to dilate the ureter (Gaylis et al, 2000). Ureteral balloon dilators are also passed over a wire, have a low profile of 3 to 8 Fr, and have dilation diameters of 12 to 30 Fr. **Dilation of the ureter beyond 15 Fr is rarely necessary for routine ureteroscopy.** Balloons can have maximum inflation pressures of 8 to 20 atmospheres depending on the design and the balloon material. Zero-tipped design ureteral balloon dilators are useful for dilating immediately adjacent to an impacted ureteral calculus. Ureteroscopic balloon dilators are 3 Fr in size, can be inflated to 12 Fr, and are passed directly through the ureteroscope. They are used to dilate under direct vision such as dilation of stenotic infundibula or calyceal diverticular necks. Once inflated, these ureteroscopic balloons cannot be removed through the ureteroscope but must be removed together with the ureteroscope.

Intraluminal Lithotripsy Devices

Intraluminal lithotripsy can be performed with several different modalities. Electrohydraulic lithotripsy (EHL) is widely available worldwide and is cost effective. Fragmentation of calculi is produced by shock waves generated from an electric spark produced on the tip of the electrode (Denstedt and Clayman, 1990). Fragmentation of most calculi is good but can be less effective for more dense calculus compositions such as cystine or calcium oxalate monohydrate. The small flexible EHL probes can be used with both rigid and flexible ureteroscopes. EHL can cause ureteral trauma because the energy is poorly focused. Although this rarely results in stricture formation, it can hinder visibility.

Pneumatic lithotripsy devices fragment calculi using mechanical ("jackhammer") energy (Schulze et al, 1993). Fragmentation is very good, and the potential for ureteral injury is low. Unfortunately, the mechanical energy can produce significant stone retropulsion. In general, the rigid probes are limited to use with rigid scopes. There are flexible probes available that can be used with flexible ureteroscopes, but they significantly limit scope deflection (Zhu et al, 2000).

The first laser successfully used for intraluminal lithotripsy was the pulsed dye laser. This laser energy is essentially no longer used because of the inability to fragment certain compositions of calculi, and the high cost of purchase and maintenance. **The holmium:YAG laser has become the intraluminal lithotripsy energy of choice. It has a wavelength of 2100 nm, which is absorbed in 3 mm of water, making it very safe for use in urology** (Blomley et al, 1995). Fragmentation is produced by a photothermal reaction with the crystalline matrix of calculi and produces stone dust rather than fragments, effectively removing a moderate volume of the stone (Zagone et al, 2002). The flexible quartz fibers can be used with both rigid and flexible ureteroscopes and are reusable. The holmium laser is effective for any composition of calculi (Bagley and Erhard, 1995; Denstedt et al, 1995; Erhard and Bagley, 1995; Grasso, 1996).

The thulium fiber laser (TFL) has been investigated as a potential alternative to the holmium laser for endoscopic lithotripsy. The TFL has a higher absorption coefficient and shorter optical penetration in water, which results in a 4-times lower ablation threshold for the TFL compared with the holmium laser. It is also a diode-pumped laser (holmium is flashlamp pumped), allowing greater control over the pulse length and duration (Hutchens et al, 2013). Most important, the TFL has been shown in vitro to have 5- to 10-times higher rates of stone vaporization than the holmium laser (Blackmon et al, 2010). There are still some practical fiber issues that need to improve before this laser can become commercially available, but it is a promising new development in endoscopic lithotripsy.

Stone Retrieval Devices

The components of stone retrieval devices include the control handle, the control wire, the sheath, and the device itself. Stone retrieval devices have shaft diameters that vary in size from 1.9 to 7.0 Fr. Devices for ureteroscopy are 3.0 Fr, and larger sizes can be used for cystoscopic or percutaneous procedures.

Three-pronged stone-grasping forceps are the safest instruments for removing calculi with the flexible ureteroscope. They permit disengagement of calculi that have been found to be too large to be safely removed from the ureter. In addition, the weak grasp will release the stone if too much force is applied, preventing damage to the ureter. This is critical when performing flexible ureteroscopy because there is no second channel to permit fragmentation of an unyielding stone trapped within a basket. Rigid ureteroscopes with two working channels have this additional degree of safety, permitting more routine use of baskets for removal of ureteral calculi. Although three-pronged graspers are the safest devices for ureteroscopic stone removal, they are seldom used because of improvements in the design and safety of stone baskets.

Stone baskets are available in helical, flat-wire, and other shapes. Baskets can also vary in the number and type of wires used. Two sheathing materials, PTFE and polyimide, are commonly used for working instruments including stone baskets. A sheath made of polyimide is very durable but stiff and limits deflection of the flexible ureteroscope. PTFE does not limit deflection as much as polyimide but is less durable and prone to stretching. Hybrid sheath designs incorporate Teflon at the tip and polyimide in the shaft, maximizing the advantages of each material. Helical baskets can be made with three-, four-, or double-wire designs with six or more wires. The double-wire designs have improved opening strength, which may facilitate removal of impacted calculi. Other basket designs such as the Parachute and LithoCatch from Boston Scientific (Natick, MA), the NCompass and NTrap from Cook Medical (Bloomington, IN), and the Sur-Catch basket from Olympus (Center Valley, PA) have more wires exposed on the distal end of the basket, making them effective for removing multiple small fragments. Helical baskets have round wires and, unlike flat-wire baskets, are safe to rotate within the ureter. They are opened above the stone and pulled down while rotating the basket to engage the stone.

Flat-wire baskets are nonhelical and are designed to have larger spaces among the four wires to allow engagement of larger stones. They were originally designed for percutaneous use, where, by filling the calyx when opened, they could more easily engage calyceal stones. They are also useful for biopsy of papillary ureteral tumors (Bagley, 1998).

There are two basket designs that attempt to combine the safety of three-prong graspers with the reliable grasp of baskets, the Graspit from Boston Scientific (Natick, MA) and NGage from Cook Medical (Bloomington, IN). These tipless devices open like three-pronged graspers and are advanced onto the stone, permitting easier disengagement of a calculus that is too large to be safely withdrawn from the ureter.

The latest material innovation is the use of nitinol for the basket wires. **The soft nitinol wires have memory, maintain their shape, resist kinking, and therefore open more safely and allow disengagement of stones more reliably than stainless steel baskets. The unique qualities of nitinol also allow basket construction in a tipless fashion.** These tipless baskets are soft and safe for use in the ureter and can be more fully deployed in a calyx without the interference from the tip, unlike stainless steel baskets.

Retropulsion Prevention Devices

Any type of intraluminal lithotripsy within the ureter will risk propelling the stone upward ("retropulsion"). The amount of retropulsion depends on the size and location of the stone, the degree of ureteral dilation, and the lithotripsy energy being used. If the stone is pushed back into the kidney, passing the flexible ureteroscope into the kidney and treating the stone there is usually not a problem. However, prevention of retropulsion may be more time efficient and is particularly important when no flexible ureteroscope is available.

Several devices are designed to prevent retropulsion of ureteral stones (Fig. 7-14). The Stone Cone and BackStop (Boston Scientific, Natick, MA), the NTrap (Cook Medical, Bloomington, IN), and the Accordion and CoAx (Accordion Medical, Indianapolis, IN) (Eisner et al, 2009; Wang et al, 2011; Wu et al, 2013). The Stone Cone is a 3-Fr device with a distal coil that can be deployed above the stone before fragmentation to help prevent stone migration. After fragmentation of the stone, it can be withdrawn to remove fragments. Any fragments too large to safely remove will be left behind because the coil simply unravels around the stone. The NTrap device is similar, 3 Fr, and is deployed above the ureteral stone. It is a meshlike wire basket that deploys perpendicular to the shaft, preventing migration of all but the smallest stone fragments. A recent devlopment in the prevention of stone retropulsion is the BackStop device (Rane et al, 2010). This is a reverse-thermosensitive gel that is injected above the stone, conforming to and completely occluding the ureter. The deployment catheter can then be removed from the ureter, preventing hindrance of the ureteroscopic procedure. The gel is then dissolved by irrigating with cold saline solution.

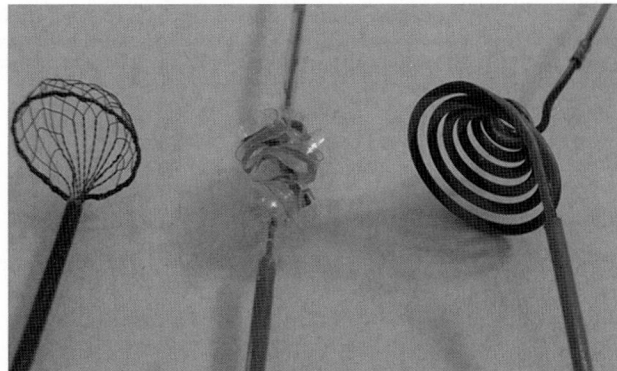

Figure 7-14. **Stone migration devices designed to prevent stone retropulsion during lithotripsy.** *Left to right,* **NTrap (Cook Medical, Bloomington, IN), Accordion (PercSys, Palo Alto, CA), and Stone Cone (Boston Scientific, Natick, MA).**

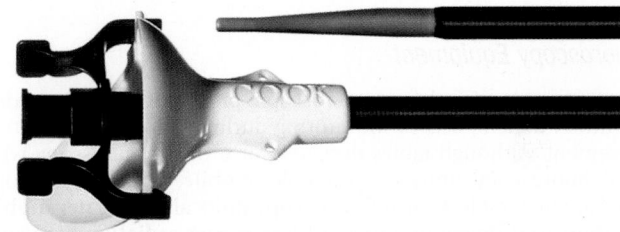

Figure 7-15. **The distal** *(top)* **and proximal** *(bottom)* **portions of a typical ureteral access sheath. The distal portion of the internal obturator** *(blue)* **is tapered. The access sheath is placed over a super-stiff guidewire, and the internal obturator is removed before ureteroscope insertion. The proximal end of the obturator accepts a Luer-Lock syringe, facilitating retrograde pyelography.**

Miscellaneous Devices

Other devices are available for ureteroscope use. Small 3-Fr cup biopsy forceps can be used to perform biopsy of sessile tumors. A larger biopsy forceps, the BIGopsy (Cook Medical, Bloomington, IN) provides a much larger biopsy specimen, which may improve diagnostic yield (Wason et al, 2012). The large forceps requires backloading of the device into the ureteroscope, and after the biopsy it must be removed together with the ureteroscope. Electrodes are available in various shape including pencil point, ball point, and angled and straight tips. These can be used for fulguration and incision procedures such as endoureterotomy and endopyelotomy.

Ureteral Access Sheaths

Ureteral access sheaths allow repeated access to the intrarenal collecting system without having to replace the working guidewire with each passage of the endoscope (Fig. 7-15). They are available in 11- to 16-Fr sheath outer diameters. Currently available ureteral access sheaths are listed in Table 7-5.

In addition to facilitating stone fragment retrieval, access sheaths have been shown to decrease the intrapelvic pressure during ureteroscopy, which may decrease the risk of infectious complications from pyelovenous backflow (Auge et al, 2004). Their primary disadvantage is related to their size and their (small) potential for ureteral injury (Delvecchio et al, 2003; Traxer et al, 2013). Furthermore, the majority of intrarenal stones require only a single passage of the ureteroscope to access and fully fragment the calculi. For these patients, an access sheath is usually unnecessary.

TABLE 7-5 Access Sheaths (Information Supplied by Manufacturers)

MANUFACTURER	SHEAT NAME	DILATOR/SHEATH (Fr)	LENGTHS (cm)	UNIQUE FEATURES
Boston Scientific	Navigator	11/13 13/15	28, 36, 46	
	Navigator HD	11/13 12/14 13/15	28, 36, 46	
Applied	Forte (AxP and HD)	10/12-16; 12/14-18; 14/16-18	20, 28, 35, 45, 55	
	Forte Plus	10/14	35, 55	Active deflecting mechanism
Bard	AquaGuide	10/12-14; 11/13-15	25, 35, 45, 55	Dual-lumen design
Cook	Flexor	9.5/11; 12/13.7; 14/16	13, 20, 28, 35, 45, 55	
	Flexor DL	9.5/14; 12/16.7	13, 20, 28, 35, 45, 55	Dual-lumen design
	Flexor Parallel	9.5/11; 12/13.7; 14/16	13, 20, 28, 35, 45, 55	Rapid release design for single wire external to sheath
Olympus	UroPass	12/14	24, 28, 54	

Fluoroscopy Equipment

Fluoroscopy is critical for ureteroscopic procedures and is needed for initial ureteral access, monitoring during endoscopy, and stent placement. Although tables designed for urologic endoscopy with fixed fluoroscopy units are available, mobile C-arm fluoroscopy units are preferable. **C-arm fluoroscopy units allow greater mobility, improved image quality, and less scatter radiation exposure to the surgeon because the x-ray source is below the patient.** Modern C-arm fluoroscopy units incorporate digital enhancement of the image and "last image hold" technology to minimize radiation exposure. Exposure can also be decreased by using image collimation and pulsed fluoroscopy. The urologist should control the fluoroscopy unit with foot pedal control, which will facilitate the speed of the procedure and minimize excessive fluoroscopy time. When possible, collimation and pulsed fluoroscopy should be employed to further limit exposure.

Ureteroscopy Technique

Preparation for Ureteroscopy

Upper tract imaging is performed to fully delineate the pathologic process being treated and to define the collecting system anatomy. This can be accomplished via intravenous pyelography or, more commonly, helical CT scan. Urinary tract infections are treated preoperatively, and infections above an obstruction are drained. **According to the AUA Best Practice Policy Statement, a routine preoperative antibiotic (first line, a fluoroquinolone) is given to all patients unless a culture provides antibiotic sensitivities for more targeted therapy** (Wolf et al, 2008). Anesthesia can be general (endotracheal or laryngeal mask), regional, or local with sedation (Vögeli et al, 1993; Hosking et al, 1996). It is important to communicate to the anesthesiologist the need for the patient to remain still throughout the procedure. Significant patient movement during rigid ureteroscopy can result in ureteral injury or perforation.

Endourologic procedures should be performed in a fully equipped operating room. The urologist should be prepared for any unanticipated problem encountered. In addition to routine Teflon-coated stainless steel guidewires, angled hydrophilic, nitinol core, and extra-stiff guidewires should be readily available. Dilation devices including dilating catheters, high-pressure balloon catheters, and zero-tipped balloon catheters are standard. Angled catheters that can be reliably rotated or "torqued" are very useful for gaining access around impacted calculi, strictures, or tortuous ureters. These include the Imager II catheter (Boston Scientific, Natick, MA) and the Kumpe catheter (Cook Medical, Bloomington, IN). The urologist should be very familiar with the endoscopes available and the size of their working channels to choose appropriately sized working instruments when needed (see Tables 7-3 and 7-4). The largest working channels of most of the fiberoptic rigid ureteroscopes are just over 3 Fr, so instruments 3 Fr or smaller are appropriate. Backup flexible and semirigid ureteroscopes should also be available to ensure availability of appropriately functioning endoscopic equipment to treat pathology regardless of location in the upper urinary tract. A list of common items needed for successful ureteroscopy is provided in Box 7-3.

Accessing the Ureter

The patient is placed in the cystolithotomy position. If a longer rigid ureteroscope is being used, the contralateral leg is elevated to allow for easier introduction of the ureteroscope. With the advent of improved flexible ureteroscopes, most rigid ureteroscopy is confined to below the iliac vessels, and shorter rigid ureteroscopes can be routinely used, decreasing interference from the contralateral leg.

Cystoscopy is performed, primarily to place a safety guidewire but also to fully inspect the bladder. Usually a simple 0.038-inch diameter flexible-tip Teflon-coated guidewire is sufficient. A safety guide is critical during rigid ureteroscopy to maintain access and allow placement of a ureteral stent if any problems are encountered. Care must be taken when trying to gain access around an impacted stone because the ureter can easily be perforated. Manipulation of the guidewire around the stone may require use of an angled hydrophilic-coated wire, an angled torqueable catheter, or both. If a guidewire cannot be safely passed beyond the stone, direct inspection of the ureter up to the stone with the rigid ureteroscope will permit passage of the wire under direct vision. Once access above the stone has been achieved, the hydrophilic wire is exchanged for a more secure standard 0.038-inch diameter Teflon-coated guidewire. If there is any suspicion about possible infection above the stone, an open-ended catheter should be passed over the wire to aspirate the renal pelvis. The hydronephrosis can be decompressed to permit irrigation; if the fluid appears very cloudy, a stent is placed and the ureteroscopy is canceled until the infection has been treated. Before the ureteroscopy proceeds, the bladder is drained to permit accumulation of irrigation fluid during ureteroscopy and minimize buckling of the flexible ureteroscope into the bladder (Fig. 7-16).

Semirigid Ureteroscopy Technique

Because flexible ureteroscopes better accommodate the natural tortuosity of the ureter and with deflection provide better access to the intrarenal collecting system, semirigid ureteroscopy is usually limited to the ureter distal to the iliac vessels. The rigid ureteroscope is passed through the urethra and into the bladder

URETEROSCOPES
Rigid
7-Fr or smaller semirigid ureteroscope
Larger ureteroscope with straight working channel (optional)

Flexible
7.5 Fr
8.6 Fr or larger
Secondary deflection or exaggerated deflection capable ureteroscope

DISPOSABLE SUPPLIES
Guidewires
0.038 Angled hydrophilic
0.038 Straight Teflon coated
0.038 Nitinol core, polyurethane coated
0.038 Extra stiff

Irrigation
Power irrigation device
High-pressure working port seal

Stone Retrieval Devices (3.0 Fr or smaller)
Helical basket
Tipless basket
Three-pronged grasping forceps or equivalent

Catheters
Dual-lumen catheter
6- to 12-Fr dilating catheter
5-Fr open-ended catheter
5-Fr angled-tip torqueable catheter

Dilation Devices
High-pressure ureteral dilating balloons (5 to 7 mm)
Zero-tipped ureteral dilating balloon

Biopsy Devices
3-Fr cup biopsy device
Flat-wire basket
BIGopsy (optional)

Ureteral Stents
5- to 7-Fr, 20- to 28-cm double pigtail

INTRALUMINAL LITHOTRIPSY DEVICES
Holmium laser
Pneumatic (optional)
Electrohydraulic (optional)

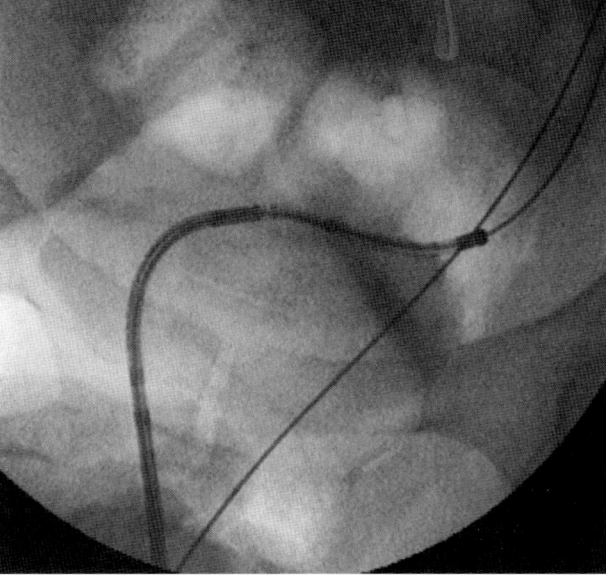

Figure 7-16. The bladder should be emptied before flexible ureteroscope passage to prevent buckling of the instrument within the bladder if resistance is met at the ureteral orifice.

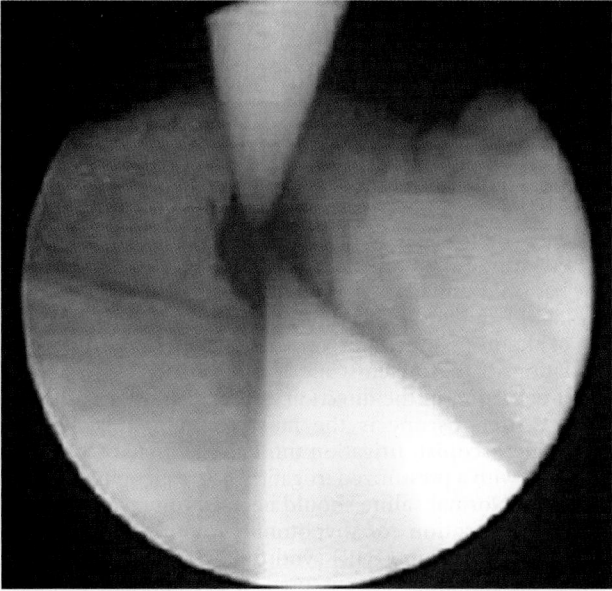

Figure 7-17. Semirigid ureteroscope passage between two wires ("railroad" technique). After safety wire placement *(bottom wire)*, a second wire *(top wire)* is passed through the working channel and up the ureter under fluoroscopic guidance and used to "tent open" the ureteral orifice. The ureteroscope is then gently advanced between the wires until ureteral access has been achieved.

under direct vision, usually with the aid of the video camera. Following the guidewire permits easy identification of the ureteral orifice.

By maneuvering the tip of the ureteroscope next to the guidewire posterolaterally, the physician can elevate the wire, thereby propping the ureteral orifice open to allow scope passage. If necessary, an additional guidewire can be passed through the ureteroscope just proximal to the intramural ureter. The ureteroscope is then rotated until it is directly between the two wires, which will hold the orifice wide open for entry of the scope (Fig. 7-17). Once the ureteroscope is through the intramural ureter, the additional guidewire can be

removed. This technique can also be useful for negotiating through tortuous segments of ureter and above the iliac vessels.

If the intramural ureter is too tight to allow safe passage of the ureteroscope, a dilating balloon catheter can be used to expand the orifice. In general, a 4-mm diameter balloon is sufficient. If there is a stricture beneath the stone that prevents safe visualization and lithotripsy, dilation beneath the stone is performed with a zero-tipped dilating balloon catheter. This balloon catheter can be passed over the safety wire immediately below the stone so dilation of the stenotic segment can be performed. The ureteroscope can then be safely introduced and the stone visualized. If the stone is impacted, it can be helpful to gently manipulate it with the tip of the ureteroscope proximally out of the traumatized area of ureter for improved visibility and safer lithotripsy. If this is not possible, the holmium laser energy can be used in a "drill and core" technique. This will ablate the central portion of the stone, and the outer shell of the stone will protect the ureteral wall. The outer shell can then be safely fragmented. The stone can be fragmented until no fragments are greater than 2 mm, or alternatively it can be cleaved until the fragments are small enough to be easily removed with a helical basket. A stent is placed and in general is left for 3 to 7 days.

Flexible Ureteroscopy Technique

The cystoscope is removed and a dual-lumen catheter is passed over the initial guidewire. This dual lumen catheter is 10 Fr, which will gently dilate the ureteral orifice and allow placement of a second, working wire. The flexible ureteroscope is then passed in a monorail fashion over the taut working wire to the point of the pathology being treated. Dilation of the ureteral orifice with the dual-lumen catheter is usually sufficient to permit passage of the flexible ureteroscope. The working channel of flexible ureteroscopes is not centrally located, so the tip of the ureteroscope will be eccentrically positioned in relation to the guidewire. If the flexible ureteroscope does not pass the ureteral orifice, the scope should be rotated 90 to 180 degrees on the guidewire to better position the tip of the ureteroscope relative to the ureteral orifice. If difficulty passing the flexible ureteroscope through the ureteral orifice is still encountered, a dilating catheter (Nottingham) or a dilating balloon catheter can be used to dilate the ureteral orifice. **Formal ureteral dilation is reported in most ureteroscopy series to be needed in 8% to 25% of patients; this incidence has obviously decreased with the advent of smaller-diameter flexible ureteroscopes** (Elashry et al, 1997; Grasso and Bagley, 1998; Tawfiek and Bagley, 1999).

If passing the flexible ureteroscope up the ureter is difficult in the absence of any significant ureteral stricture or other source of obstruction, the use of a nitinol core polyurethane-coated guidewire may be helpful. As previously discussed, these stiffer, smoother wires enable more efficient transmission of the push from the urologist to the tip of the ureteroscope.

The basic movements of the flexible ureteroscope include deflecting, rotating, and advancing and retreating the ureteroscope. The reticle of the flexible ureteroscope marks the plane of deflection, and rotation of the ureteroscope is often necessary to align this plane of deflection in the direction desired. **Failure to adequately rotate the ureteroscope is the most common mistake of the novice ureteroscopist.** Irrigation through the ureteroscope should be provided with a pressurized irrigation bag, roller pump, or handheld syringe. **Normal saline should be used to prevent accumulation and absorption of hypotonic solution and resultant transurethral resection (TUR) syndrome.**

When the holmium laser is used, it is important to pass the laser fiber through a straightened flexible ureteroscope (confirmed fluoroscopically) to prevent damage to the working channel. Once the fiber has been passed beyond the tip, the ureteroscope can be deflected appropriately. The most commonly used sizes of holmium laser fibers include the 365-micron fiber and the 200-micron fiber. When significant deflection of the ureteroscope is needed, the 200-micron fiber is preferred because it does not limit the deflection of the ureteroscope as much as the larger fibers. The tip of the fiber must be in contact with the stone during treatment because the holmium laser energy is absorbed in 3 mm of water. **The holmium laser can damage the ureteroscope, the guidewire, and the ureteral wall. These problems can be avoided by not activating the laser unless the tip of the fiber is seen to be in contact with the stone** (Beaghler et al, 1998). In addition, if the helium-neon aiming beam is not seen, the laser should not be activated because this may be an indication of fiber damage. Firing the holmium laser through a broken fiber can cause significant damage to the ureteroscope.

Once the pathology has been adequately addressed, a ureteral stent is typically placed and left indwelling for 3 to 5 days.

Postoperative pain management can be facilitated with the use of a cyclooxygenase-2 (COX-2) inhibitor and/or an α-adrenergic blocker (Nazim and Ather, 2012).

KEY POINTS: URETEROSCOPY

- Semirigid ureteroscopy is used below the iliac vessels and flexible ureteroscopy above.
- Semirigid ureteroscopes with two working channels permit better irrigation and offer the added safety of being able to pass a lithotripsy device through one channel when needing to fragment a stone engaged in a basket in the other channel.
- Flexible ureteroscopes must be straight during passage of a laser fiber or the working channel will be damaged.
- The golden rule of safe laser lithotripsy is "Do not step on the pedal if you cannot see the tip of the fiber in contact with the stone."
- Stone baskets made of nitinol maintain their shape, resist kinking, and allow disengagement of stones more reliably than stainless steel baskets.
- Ureteral access sheaths facilitate repeated passage of flexible ureteroscopes and decrease the intrapelvic pressure during ureteroscopy.
- Mobile C-arm fluoroscopy is preferred because of greater mobility, improved image quality, and less scatter radiation exposure to the surgeon compared with urology tables with fixed fluoroscopy units.
- A routine preoperative antibiotic should be given to all patients undergoing ureteroscopy.
- Normal saline should be used for irrigation during ureteroscopy to prevent absorption of a hypotonic solution.

CONCLUSIONS

Over the past 150 years tremendous advances have been made in endoscope design, revolutionizing urologic surgery. Visualization of both the upper and lower urinary tracts is now routinely performed with rigid and flexible endoscopes. A variety of urologic conditions can be evaluated efficiently with minimal discomfort in the office by flexible cystoscopy. A wide array of benign and malignant conditions affecting the bladder and urethra can be managed transurethrally with rigid cystourethroscopes in the operating room with limited morbidity. Improvements in flexible ureteroscopes, working instruments, and endoscopic techniques have significantly improved our ability to effectively treat upper urinary tract problems as well. With continued innovation and refinement, the role of ureteroscopy in the treatment of complex intrarenal calculi, ureteral obstruction, and upper tract tumors should continue to expand.

Please visit the accompanying website at www.expertconsult.com to view *videos associated with this chapter.*

REFERENCES

The complete reference list is available online at www.expertconsult.com.

SUGGESTED READINGS

Natalin RA, Landman J. Where next for the endoscope? Nat Rev Urol 2009;6:622–8.
Patel AR, Jones JS, Babineau D. Lidocaine 2% gel versus plain lubricating gel for pain reduction during flexible cystoscopy: a meta-analysis of prospective, randomized, controlled trials. J Urol 2008;179:986–90.
Somani BK, Al-Qahtani SM, de Medina SD, et al. Outcomes of flexible ureterorenoscopy and laser fragmentation for renal stones: comparison between digital and conventional ureteroscope. Urology 2013;82:1017–9.
Wolf JS Jr, Bennett CJ, Dmochowski RR, et al. Best practice policy statement on urologic surgery antimicrobial prophylaxis. J Urol 2008;179:1379–90.

8 Percutaneous Approaches to the Upper Urinary Tract Collecting System

J. Stuart Wolf, Jr., MD, FACS

HISTORY AND INTRODUCTION

Commonly ascribed to Goodwin and colleagues (1955), the first therapeutic percutaneous nephrostomy was actually performed by Thomas Hillier in 1865 (Bloom et al, 1989). Hillier, at the Hospital for Sick Children at Great Ormond Street, repeatedly aspirated the hydronephrotic kidney of a young boy for symptom relief throughout a 4-year period until his death at 8 years of age. Subsequently there were a few reports of diagnostic percutaneous renal aspirations, but it was not until Goodwin and colleagues published their landmark report in 1955 that therapeutic percutaneous nephrostomy was rediscovered. Even then, the use of percutaneous access to the upper urinary tract collecting system was limited to drainage of obstructed kidneys until Fernström and Johansson (1976) described the percutaneous removal of renal calculi, termed "percutaneous pyelolithotomy."

In the years since that report appeared, a number of procedures have been performed using the convenient and safe percutaneous route to access the upper urinary tract collecting system, including drainage of an obstructed kidney, nephrolithotomy, endopyelotomy, and resection of urothelial tumors. More recently, percutaneous access to portions of the kidney other than the collecting system has expanded the diagnostic and therapeutic choices for patients with renal diseases. Other chapters in this book address these indications, including Chapters 57 and 62. This chapter addresses only percutaneous access to the upper urinary tract collecting system, focusing on the creation, maintenance, and postprocedure management of the percutaneous tract. The final section of the chapter reviews the general complications of percutaneous access to the upper urinary tract collecting system. Specific aspects of the procedures performed through the percutaneous access are covered in Chapters 6, 49, 54, and 58.

INDICATIONS FOR PERCUTANEOUS ACCESS

Simple Drainage or Access

Percutaneous drainage of the upper urinary tract collecting system can be for diagnostic or therapeutic indications. **The only remaining popular indication for diagnostic percutaneous nephrostomy is to perform a Whitaker test,** which requires placement of a small-caliber nephrostomy tube through which contrast material is instilled at specific flow rates while pressures are measured to assess for ureteral obstruction (see a more detailed description in Chapter 49). In other cases, diagnostic nephrostography is performed as an adjunct to therapeutic percutaneous nephrostomy.

Therapeutic percutaneous nephrostomy tubes can be placed to drain the kidney (see Chapter 6) to access the upper urinary tract for direct instillation of therapeutic agents (see Chapter 58) or to perform a surgical procedure. **Percutaneous nephrostomy is indicated to drain the upper urinary tract collecting system in cases of obstruction at an intrarenal location, at the ureteropelvic junction, or anywhere in the ureter.** Obstruction of the lower urinary tract is best treated by drainage of the bladder rather than the kidney, unless secondary obstruction of the upper tract has developed that is refractory to vesicle drainage. An alternative to percutaneous drainage is drainage through a ureteral catheter or stent placed in a retrograde fashion (cephalad from the bladder to the kidney, as opposed to antegrade, which is placement from the kidney toward the bladder). **The choice of antegrade or retrograde drainage of the upper urinary tract collecting system depends on the indication for the procedure, patient's medical condition, particular anatomy of the patient, and preferences of both the patient and the physician.**

All things being equal, a retrograde route to drainage is preferred instead of the antegrade route. This includes most cases of acute and chronic ureteral obstruction without infection (Rosevear et al, 2007; Wenzler et al, 2008). **In the setting of upper urinary tract collecting system obstruction complicated by infection, however, drainage is an emergency and in many such cases percutaneous rather than retrograde drainage may be best** (Ng et al, 2002), **unless retrograde drainage can be obtained expeditiously and assuredly. Percutaneous nephrostomy tubes and retrograde ureteral stents are generally equivalent in their capacity to resolve fever in patients with upper urinary tract obstruction and fever** (Pearle et al, 1998; Goldsmith et al, 2013), **but in a given patient, circumstances may dictate a preference for one access instead of the other.** Retrograde placement of a ureteral stent generally requires regional or general anesthesia, whereas a percutaneous nephrostomy tube can be inserted under local anesthesia; this is an important consideration for an ill patient. Because the percutaneous route includes a greater initial success rate than the retrograde route in cases in which the collecting system is dilated, it might be preferred in a patient who needs rapid intervention. This is especially true when the ureteral obstruction is long, severe, or involving the ureteral orifice—all of which can make retrograde stent placement more difficult. Conversely, untreated coagulopathy is a contraindication to percutaneous access, but internal ureteral stents can be placed safely in an anticoagulated patient. A final consideration is patient preference. Although the health-related quality of life for patients with percutaneous nephrostomy tubes and for those with internal ureteral stents is similar, a given patient may prefer one route instead of the other (Joshi et al, 2001). For additional discussion of percutaneous nephrostomy versus internal ureteral stent for drainage of the upper urinary tract, see Chapter 6.

Percutaneous Surgery

Access into the upper urinary tract collecting system may be indicated to instill therapeutic agents directly. This includes chemolysis of urinary calculi and intracavitary topical therapy for urothelial carcinoma. In most cases, the access elected for the instillation will already be present after the preceding surgical procedure.

An important indication for percutaneous access into the upper urinary tract collecting system is the need for intrarenal or intraureteral surgery. This includes percutaneous endopyelotomy and endoureterotomy (see Chapter 49), nephrolithotomy, treatment of calyceal diverticula and hydrocalyces, and antegrade ureteroscopic treatment of large ureteral stones (see Chapter 54); it also includes percutaneous resection of urothelial tumors (see Chapter 58) and less-common procedures such as management of fungal bezoars. For all of these procedures, skillfully attaining access, properly managing postoperative drainage, and preventing and treating complications related to the percutaneous access are major procedural components. The remainder of this chapter centers on these topics.

ANATOMIC CONSIDERATIONS

Given that the visualization of the kidney and surrounding structures during standard percutaneous entry guided by fluoroscopy or ultrasonography is limited, understanding of the renal and perirenal anatomy is critical for obtaining access that is both effective and safe. Even armed with this knowledge, variations in anatomy can make access challenging for the experienced surgeon and prohibitive for the inexperienced one.

Perirenal Anatomy

The kidneys are well-protected organs, situated retroperitoneally and surrounded by adipose tissue. The short renal hilar vessels limit the mobility of the kidneys, although nephroptosis ("falling kidney") can occur, especially in thin women with a paucity of perirenal fat. In such cases the kidney not only descends but also rotates anteriorly. This can be troublesome during percutaneous punctures with the patient in a prone position.

The kidneys lie adjacent to the vertebral bodies, usually extending from the 11th or 12th thoracic to the 2nd or 3rd lumbar vertebrae (Fig. 8-1). The right kidney is displaced a few centimeters inferior to the left kidney. The longitudinal axis of the kidneys parallels the lateral edges of the psoas muscles, about 30 degrees from vertical, with the lower poles lateral to the upper poles. The kidneys are also tilted 30 degrees off the frontal plane, with the lower poles

anterior to the upper poles. Finally, the kidneys are rotated out of the frontal plane as well, with the lateral aspect of the kidney posterior to the medial aspect, such that each kidney is rotated 30 degrees posteriorly from the renal hilum.

Immediately posterior to the kidneys are the quadratus lumborum and psoas muscles, except at the upper poles where the diaphragm is posterior (Fig. 8-2). **The pleura can be violated during percutaneous entry into the upper pole of the kidney. This risk is greater as the access to the kidney is moved cephalad.** The lung itself lies above the 11th rib, so direct lung injury is unlikely unless the 10th intercostal space (superior to the 11th rib) is used as the entry site. The ribs curve inferiorly from medial to lateral, such that more portions of the kidney can be approached subcostally with a medial as opposed to a lateral access site.

The lateral, anterior, and medial perirenal relationships are more varied than the posterior ones (Fig. 8-3). On the right side, the liver is anterior to the upper pole of the kidney and can extend in some individuals to cover the entire anterior surface. On the left, the spleen covers less of the kidney anteriorly. Both the liver and spleen can extend lateral to the kidneys and are therefore at risk of injury with a lateral puncture into the kidney. **The ascending and descending colon can be lateral or even posterior to the right and left kidneys, respectively. The apposition of the colon to the kidney varies with location; it is greatest on the left side and at the lower pole.** In one study of computed tomograms, the left colon was posterior in 16.1% of cases, and the right colon was posterior in 9% of cases at the level of the lower pole. At the midaspect of the kidney the colon was posterior in 5.2% and 2.8%, respectively, and at the upper pole 1.1% and 0.4%, respectively (Boon et al, 2001).

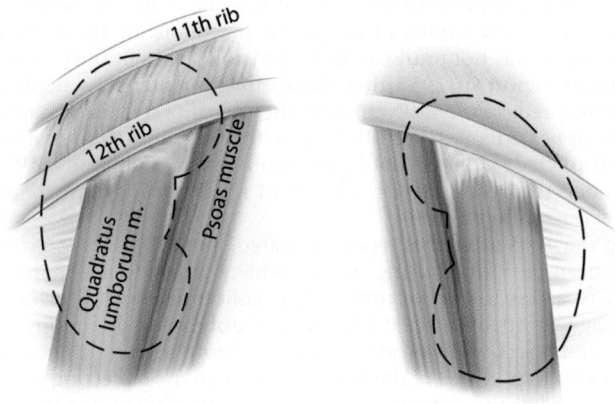

Figure 8-2. **Muscles and ribs posterior to the kidneys.**

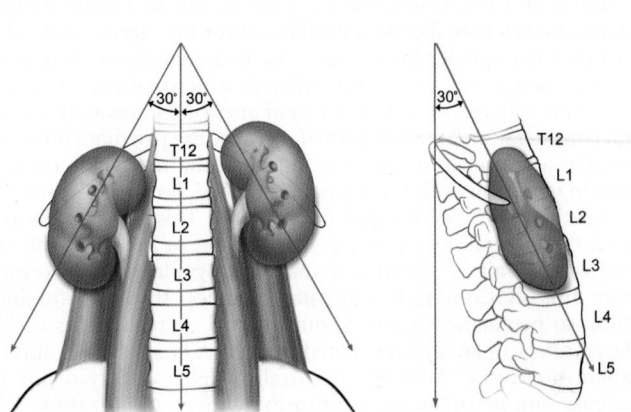

Figure 8-1. **Location of kidneys in the retroperitoneum.**

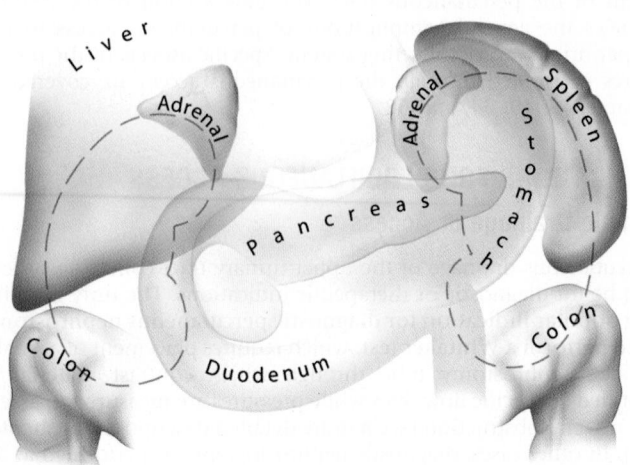

Figure 8-3. **Viscera lateral, anterior, and medial to the kidneys.**

Additional visceral relations to the kidney include the adrenal glands (medial to the upper pole of both kidneys), the duodenum and gallbladder (anterior and medial to the right kidney), and the tail of the pancreas (anterior and medial to the left kidney). These structures can be injured with a misdirected or excessively deep puncture.

Renal Parenchyma and Collecting System

The renal parenchyma is composed of cortical and medullary tissue. The renal cortex is the outermost layer. It contains the glomeruli and proximal and distal convoluted tubules. The more interior medulla contains the renal pyramids. These are inverted cones (the base of which is superficial and the apex of which is deep) that comprise the loops of Henle and the collecting ducts, which coalesce at the apex of the pyramid into papillary ducts that open on the surface of the renal papillae. There are approximately 20 papillary ducts draining into each papilla. The columns of Bertin are invaginations of cortical tissue that surround the renal pyramids except at their apices.

The renal papillae drain into the minor calyces, which are the most peripheral portions of the intrarenal collecting system. If only one papilla drains into a minor calyx, it is described as a simple calyx. When there are two or more papillae entering the calyx, it is termed a *compound calyx*. The outermost wall of the calyx, into which the papilla is set, is the calyceal fornix. **There are 5 to 14 minor calyces in each kidney (mean of 8, with 70% of kidneys having 7 to 9 minor calyces)** (Sampaio and Mandarim-de-Lacerda, 1988). **There are three calyceal groups: the upper, middle, and lower. Compound calyces are the rule in the upper calyceal group, are common in the lower calyceal group, and are rare in the middle calyceal group.** The minor calyces, either directly or after coalescing into major calyces, drain by infundibula into the renal pelvis (Fig. 8-4). Occasionally a minor calyx will open directly

into the renal pelvis without an intervening infundibulum. Some infundibula are unusually narrow, even if they drain adequately, and they can present an obstacle to endoscopy, especially with the relatively large rigid nephroscope.

The compound calyces of the poles of the kidney are oriented facing their respective poles. The simple calyces usually come in pairs, with one facing anteriorly and one facing posteriorly (Fig. 8-5). The upper pole calyceal system almost always contains at least one compound calyx, and in some cases this is the only calyx in the system. Drainage of the upper pole into the renal pelvis is by a single midline infundibulum in the majority of kidneys. The lower pole system often contains a compound calyx as well. The calyceal drainage from the lower pole is via a single infundibulum in about half of human kidneys and through a series of paired anterior and posterior calyces in approximately half of kidneys. With compound calyces rare in the middle calyceal system, the middle calyces are typically arranged in a series of paired anterior and posterior calyces. In about two thirds of kidneys, there are two major calyceal systems—an upper one and lower one—and the middle calyces drain into either or both systems. In the other third of kidneys, the middle calyceal system is distinct from the upper and lower systems, either coalescing into a middle major calyx before emptying into the renal pelvis or with drainage of the middle minor calyces directly into the renal pelvis through short infundibula.

An important consideration for percutaneous renal surgery is the determination of the anteroposterior orientation of the calyces, because access (from the typical posterior or posterolateral approach) into a posterior calyx allows relatively straight entry into the rest of the kidney, whereas percutaneous puncture of an anterior calyx requires an acute angulation to enter the renal pelvis, which may not be possible with rigid instrumentation (Fig. 8-6). Efforts have been made to determine which calyces are likely to be anterior and which are likely to be posterior, solely on the basis of their mediolateral position on anteroposterior radiography. The distinction pertains to the middle and lower calyceal system, which contains (in almost all middle systems and approximately half of the lower system) paired anterior and posterior minor calyces. The upper pole system, with its almost uniformly compound calyceal system, is less problematic in this regard. Paired anterior and posterior calyces usually enter at about 90 degrees from each other. As such, the relative mediolateral orientation (on anteroposterior radiography) is determined by the relationship of this 90-degree unit to the frontal plane of the kidney. In a Brödel-type kidney, this unit is rotated anteriorly, such that the posterior calyces are about 20 degrees behind the frontal plane and the anterior calyces are 70 degrees in front of the frontal plane. The posterior calyces are lateral, and the anterior calyces are medial in this case. The Hodson-type kidney is the opposite; the calyceal pairs are

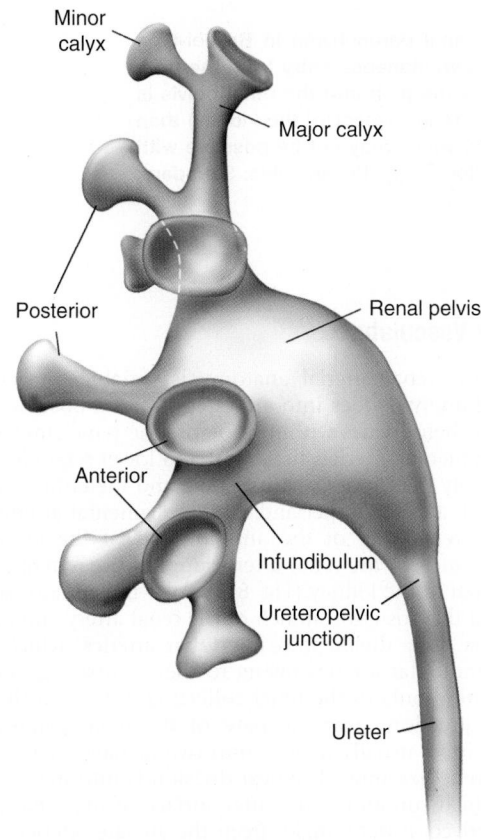

Figure 8-4. **Upper urinary tract collecting system.**

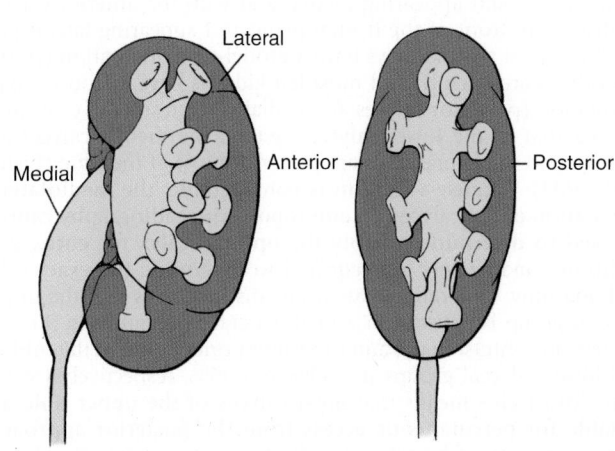

Figure 8-5. **Calyceal orientation of polar and middle calyces. (From Smith AD. Controversies in endourology. Philadelphia: Saunders; 1995.)**

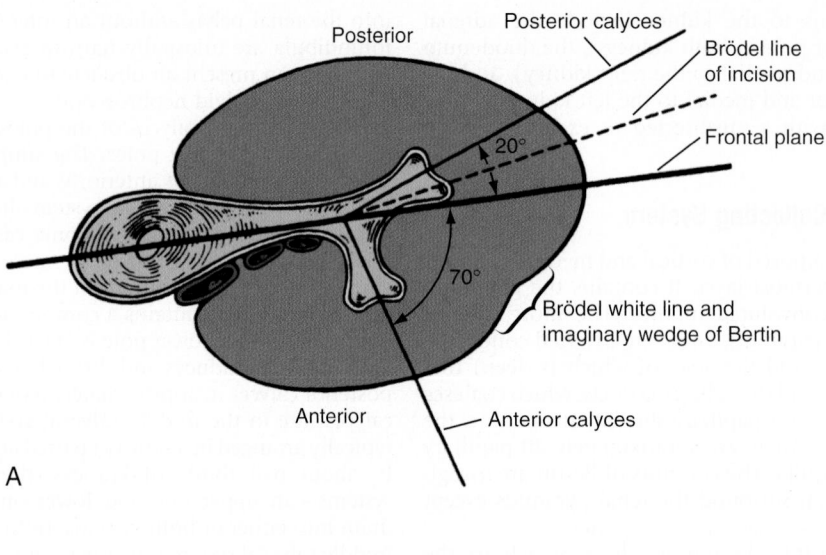

A

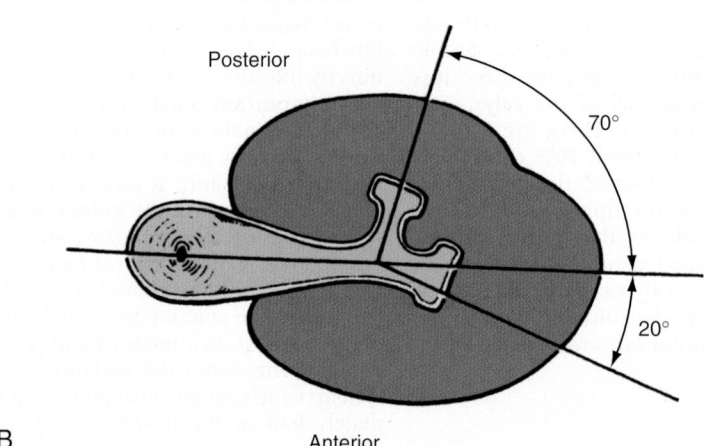

B

Figure 8-6. **Relation of anterior and posterior calyces to renal parenchyma in Brödel-type kidney (A) and Hodson-type kidney (B). The optimal site of percutaneous entry from the posterior aspect of the kidney is into a posterior calyx because the path into the renal pelvis is fairly straight. If entry is into an anterior calyx (from the posterior aspect of the kidney) then an acute angulation must be made to enter the renal pelvis, which may not be possible with rigid instrumentation. (From Smith AD. Controversies in endourology. Philadelphia: Saunders; 1995.)**

rotated posteriorly, with the posterior calyces 70 degrees behind the frontal plane and appearing medial and with the anterior calyces 20 degrees in front of the frontal plane and appearing lateral (see Fig. 8-6). Most right kidneys have a Brödel-type orientation (posterior calyces are lateral), and most left kidneys have a Hodson-type orientation (posterior calyces are medial). The results of one study showed that in the lower calyceal system, the medial calyces are anterior and the lateral ones are posterior most of the time (Eisner et al, 2009). **Because variation is considerable, the mediolateral orientation of the calyces on anteroposterior radiography cannot be used to determine reliably the optimal calyx for entry, and additional maneuvers are required to determine the exact calyceal anatomy.** One reliable anatomic distinction is that the upper calyceal group is situated in a mediolateral orientation in 95% of kidneys, in contrast to the anteroposterior orientation of the middle and lower calyceal groups in 100% and 95%, respectively (Miller et al, 2013.) This means that **most calyces of the upper pole are suitable for percutaneous access from the posterior approach, whereas care must be taken to select a posterior minor calyx in the middle and lower groups.** Within the lower calyceal group, the most inferior calyx is usually anterior, but the next most cephalad calyx is usually posterior (Miller et al, 2013).

Intrarenal Vasculature

Although the renal arterial anatomy is variable, in general the main renal artery divides into an anterior and a posterior branch. The former then divides within or before the renal sinus into four anterior segmental arteries: the apical and lower segmental arteries (which supply the tip of the upper pole and the entire lower pole, respectively), and the upper and middle segmental arteries (which supply the remainder of the anterior half of the kidney). The posterior branch of the renal artery supplies the remainder of the posterior half of the kidney (Fig. 8-7). After the anterior segmental arteries and the posterior branch of the renal artery enter the renal parenchyma, they divide into interlobar arteries, which are also called infundibular arteries owing to their course adjacent to the calyceal infundibula of the renal collecting system. At the corticomedullary junction, near the base of the renal pyramids, each interlobar artery usually divides into two arcuate arteries that run along the renal pyramid. The next division is into the interlobular arteries, which run along the outer surface of the renal pyramids and are derived at right angles from the arcuate arteries. The final divisions, the afferent arterioles of the glomeruli, come off the interlobular arteries in the peripheral renal cortex. Each renal

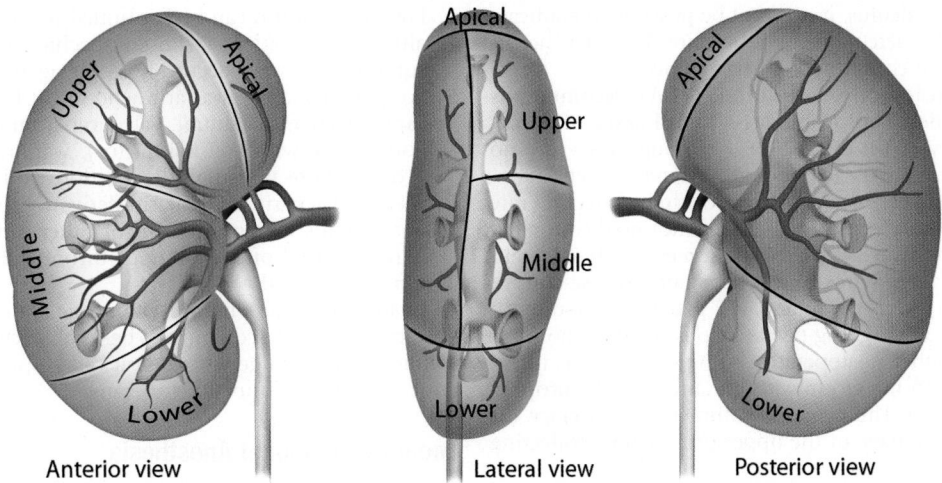

Figure 8-7. **Arterial supply to the kidney. The kidney is supplied by the anterior and posterior branches of the main renal artery. The anterior branch supplies both the anterior half of the kidney and the polar regions via four segmental branches. The posterior branch of the renal artery supplies the posterior aspect of the kidney (represented by the shaded region). An avascular plane, known as Brödel line, separates the anterior and posterior circulations.**

arteriole is an "end-artery," meaning that each cell in the kidney derives its blood supply from one arteriole. For this reason renal arterial vascular injury must be avoided to prevent loss of renal function. The potential for arterial injury is least in the Brödel line, which is an avascular plane approximately at the lateral margin of the kidney, extending from the superior apex of the kidney (limited by the circulation of the apical anterior segmental artery) to the lower pole of the kidney (limited by the circulation of the lower anterior segmental artery). **Additionally, the safest place to access percutaneously the collecting system is directly into the calyceal fornix, because this will avoid the interlobar (infundibular) arteries adjacent to the calyceal infundibula and the arcuate arteries that skirt the renal pyramid** (Sampaio et al, 1992).

The venous anatomy of the kidney does not have the same defined structure as the arteries. Moreover, there is free cross-circulation among the intrarenal veins via arcades. This enhances vascular outflow from the kidneys, reduces the risk of venous congestion, and makes renal venous injury less damaging to renal function than arterial injury.

KEY POINTS: ANATOMIC CONSIDERATIONS

- Both the diaphragm and pleura can be violated during percutaneous entry into the upper pole of the kidney.
- The ascending and descending colon can be lateral or even posterior to the right and left kidneys, respectively. The apposition of the colon to the kidney varies with location; it is greatest on the left side and at the lower pole.
- An important consideration for percutaneous renal surgery is the determination of the anteroposterior orientation of the calyces.
- The mediolateral orientation of the calyces on anteroposterior radiography cannot be reliably used to determine the optimal calyx for entry.
- Most calyces of the upper pole are suitable for percutaneous access from the posterior approach, whereas care must be taken to select a posterior minor calyx in the middle and lower groups
- The safest place to access percutaneously the collecting system is directly into the calyceal fornix.

OBTAINING PERCUTANEOUS ACCESS

Adequate percutaneous access to the upper urinary tract collecting system is a critical part of the percutaneous procedure. As time passes, more urologists are being trained to attain percutaneous access (Spann et al, 2011), but only a minority of urologists in the United States maintains this skill in practice (Bird et al, 2003; Lee et al, 2004a). Survey data from the United Kingdom suggest that the attainment of access for percutaneous surgery is almost equal between urologists and radiologists, with a combined urologist-radiologist team used in the most complex cases (Aslam et al, 2011). Although there is some controversy regarding the success and complications associated with access for percutaneous renal surgery attained by urologists versus radiologists (Watterson et al, 2006; El-Assmy et al, 2007; Tomaszewski et al, 2010a), the critical distinction in ensuring effective access for a subsequent percutaneous procedure is not who obtains access but rather that the access for urologic surgery is directed by a urologist. **The optimal situation is for the urologist to be present at the time access is attained, either performing the access procedure or actively directing the radiologist.** When access is gained without input of the urologist (whether present in person or directed beforehand), the access site is not acceptable for the subsequent percutaneous procedure in a large portion of cases (Tomaszewski et al, 2010a).

Periprocedural Antimicrobials

Prevention of infectious complications is a major consideration when considering percutaneous access into the upper urinary tract collecting system. **In an elective setting, confirmation that urine is sterile is optimal. In cases of anatomic abnormality, recent hospitalization, distant coexistent infection, recent catheterization, or other situations that suggest increased likelihood of bacteriuria, a urine culture is recommended. In the setting of an externalized catheter or staghorn renal calculus, bacteriuria is likely and a preoperative urine culture should be considered standard practice. In other cases, a screening urinalysis may be adequate, with subsequent culture if the urinalysis is suspicious for infection.** When there is bacteriuria, a therapeutic course of culture-directed antimicrobials should be administered to sterilize the urine. Optimally, a repeat urine culture should be obtained to confirm urine sterility, although this might not be practical. In cases with colonized exogenous material such as an externalized urinary catheter or an infected calculus, it may not be possible to eradicate the infection before the percutaneous procedure. The goal then is to suppress the bacterial count before intervention.

The American Urological Association (AUA) recommends periprocedural antimicrobial prophylaxis for all cases of percutaneous renal surgery (Wolf et al, 2008). Although there are no randomized, controlled trials to support this recommendation, nonrandomized data suggest a postprocedure urinary infection rate of 35% to 40% if antimicrobial prophylaxis is not used compared with 0% to 17% if prophylaxis is used (Charton et al, 1986; Darenkov et al, 1994). In a large retrospective but matched case-control study, comparing 162 patients with and 162 patients without antimicrobial prophylaxis undergoing percutaneous nephrolithotomy, the rate of fever and other postoperative complications was threefold to tenfold greater in the group without antimicrobial prophylaxis (Gravas et al, 2012). The need for antimicrobial coverage for simple percutaneous drainage of the upper urinary tract collecting system is not certain.

Antimicrobial coverage should include organisms common to the urinary tract (*Escherichia coli, Proteus* sp., *Klebsiella* sp., *Enterococcus* sp.) and the skin (*Staphylococcus aureus,* coagulase-negative *Staphylococcus* sp., group A *Streptococcus* sp.). Recommended agents include first- and second-generation cephalosporins; aminoglycosides (or aztreonam in patients with renal insufficiency) plus either metronidazole or clindamycin; ampicillin/sulbactam; or a fluoroquinolone. Although there are some series that suggest that the administration of antimicrobials for the week before percutaneous nephrolithotomy reduces the risk of infectious complications (Mariappan et al, 2006; Bag et al, 2011), the preponderance of evidence suggests that **when the antimicrobial is being administered only for prophylaxis (i.e., not treatment of known or presumed infection), immediate perioperative treatment for percutaneous nephrolithotomy (≤24 hours) is just as effective as a longer course and is therefore preferred** (Dogan et al, 2002; Demirtas et al, 2012; Seyrek et al, 2012; Tuzel et al, 2013). A short (≤24 hours) course of antimicrobials at the time of nephrostomy tube removal also can be considered (Wolf et al, 2008).

Management of Anticoagulation

With the increasing use of antiplatelet and anticoagulant medications in the general population, the urologist is faced more frequently with planning percutaneous renal surgery for patients taking such medications (Riley and Averch, 2012). In addition, other medications—such as nonsteroidal anti-inflammatory agents and some nutritional supplements—include anticoagulant or antiplatelet activity. Except as outlined in the following, these medications should generally be discontinued before percutaneous renal surgery. The preoperative cessation periods vary: herbal medicines, 1 week; aspirin, 1 week; warfarin, 5 days; clopidogrel, 5 days; nonsteroidal anti-inflammatory agents, 3 to 7 days. In their consensus document, the International Consultation on Urological Diseases and AUA (Culkin et al, 2014) recommend the following as related to percutaneous renal surgery:

1. Oral anticoagulant or antiplatelet activity medications should be discontinued before percutaneous renal surgery (except as noted in the following). Bridging with heparin derivatives may be required with resumption of oral anticoagulant or antiplatelet agents as soon as the risk of periprocedural hemorrhage has lessened. Expert multidisciplinary management may be required for those at high thromboembolic risk.
2. Because withdrawal of duel antiplatelet therapy (i.e., aspirin plus clopidogrel) should never occur within 12 months of drug-eluting stent placement or within 3 months of bare metal stent placement, elective percutaneous renal surgery should not be performed within these time periods.
3. For patients on clopidogrel or aspirin for secondary stroke prevention, especially after a recent stroke, cessation of the agent may be ill advised, and neurologic consultation is recommended if percutaneous renal surgery is being considered.

4. Low-dose aspirin can be continued in the perioperative period, although in patients without specific medical indications the surgical team may elect to hold the agent perioperatively.
5. For patients taking warfarin who are at high risk of thrombosis (any mechanical mitral valve replacement or a mechanical aortic valve with any risk factor), warfarin should be stopped 5 days before the surgical procedure and appropriate bridging therapy (heparin or heparin-derivative) should be instituted. For patients taking warfarin for other indications (atrial fibrillation, history of deep venous thrombosis, etc.), bridging may not be required.

In some patients who must continue anticoagulant or antiplatelet therapy, ureteroscopy might be a satisfactory alternative to percutaneous renal surgery because it can be performed with ongoing anticoagulant or antiplatelet therapy.

Local and Regional Anesthesia

Regardless of the type of primary anesthesia that is used for percutaneous renal surgery, the addition of local and regional anesthesia may be beneficial. Of eight randomized controlled trials assessing the impact of tract infiltration with various local anesthetics versus placebo on early postoperative pain and narcotic use, all but one demonstrated a benefit (Haleblian et al, 2007; Ugras et al, 2007; Jonnavithula et al, 2009; Gokten et al, 2011; Akbay et al, 2012; Shah et al, 2012; Kirac et al, 2013; Parikh et al, 2013). Additionally, intercostal nerve blocks and thoracic paravertebral block with long-acting local anesthetics have provided a similar benefit in randomized controlled trials (Ak et al, 2013; Honey et al, 2013; Ozkan et al, 2013).

Patient Positioning

Goodwin and colleagues (1955) described the prone position for percutaneous access to the upper urinary tract collecting system, and with time this position became standard. A "prone-flexed" position has also been described (Ray et al, 2009). The prone position has the advantage of presenting a large surface area (the patient's back) that provides many choices of access sites and a stable horizontal working surface. The posterior or posterolateral approach is the most direct one to the desirable posterior calyces and comes closest to approaching the kidney through the Brödel avascular line. Prone positioning does have some disadvantages, however. It is associated with a decrease in cardiac index (Hatada et al, 1991), and in cases where inadequate padding is provided it is associated with decreased pulmonary capacity, although if enough padded support ensures free abdominal and chest wall movement, then pulmonary capacity is greater in the prone compared with the supine position (Edgcombe et al, 2008). The anesthesiologist has poor access to the airway with the patient in the prone position. Prone positioning might not be possible in patients with morbid obesity and/or spinal concavity, and the prone position can be associated with neuromusculoskeletal complications such as nerve compression or stretch injury, ocular or facial injury, and rhabdomyolysis. Finally, the prone position requires that the surgeon stand, often holding instruments at a distance using outstretched arms, which leads to surgeon fatigue. To address these deficiencies, urologists have introduced supine and lateral decubitus positioning for percutaneous renal surgery.

Valdivia Uria and colleagues (1987) first reported the supine approach to percutaneous nephrolithotomy, culminating in their 1998 review of 557 patients with percutaneous nephrolithotomy performed in this position (Valdivia Uria et al, 1998). They reported few complications; there were no hydrothoraces or pneumothoraces, no colon injuries, and only a 0.5% rate of major hemorrhage (see later for further discussion of complications). Variations of this position include completely supine, supine with the ipsilateral side elevated, and supine combined with varying degrees of ipsilateral flank elevation (in some with 90-degree rotation) and asymmetric lithotomy position (Falahatkar et al, 2008; Papatsoris et al, 2008; Scoffone et al, 2008; Zhou et al, 2008; Moraitis et al, 2012). In the prone position, with a posterior or posterolateral skin entry, the posterior calyces are the best to enter because they allow access to the renal pelvis and the rest of the kidney. In the supine position, the skin entry site is lateral or anterolateral, so the best calyces to enter are often the anterior ones. For a procedure such as percutaneous nephrolithotomy with the patient in the supine position, the access sheath is angled toward horizontal (compared with vertical during percutaneous nephrolithotomy in the prone position), which reduces the pressure in the collecting system and facilitates stone fragments to wash out through the sheath. Supine positioning does not require repositioning after induction of anesthesia, and the urethra is more easily accessed than in the prone position. The supine position is a safer position with regard to neuromusculoskeletal complications, and the anesthesia team may prefer this position (Atkinson et al, 2011). Finally, because the percutaneous entry is more lateral than during a prone procedure, the instruments are closer to the surgeon, which results in less physical strain on the surgeon and the opportunity for the surgeon to sit during the procedure.

There are some disadvantages to the supine position for percutaneous renal surgery, however. First, it is not familiar to most urologists because the prone position is used in most training programs. Second, the reduced pressure in the collecting system results in a lower volume and thus less room for visualization and manipulation. Third, upper pole calyceal access is more difficult in the supine compared with prone position, and percutaneous tract length is longer than in the prone position (Azhar et al, 2011; Duty et al, 2012). Finally, with optimal placement of pads and bolsters, the prone position may provide better ventilation than the supine position (Edgcombe et al, 2008, Atkinson et al, 2011).

In a large, multi-institutional and retrospective study of percutaneous nephrolithotomy, including 4637 patients and 1138 patients with prone and supine positioning, respectively, operative time and stone-free rates favored the prone position, but some patient safety parameters favored the supine position (Valdivia et al, 2011). Two meta-analyses of supine versus prone positioning for percutaneous nephrolithotomy, 1 incorporating two randomized controlled trials and 2 case-control studies (Liu et al, 2010) and 1 including the same 4 studies plus 27 case series (Wu et al, 2011), both documented conclusions that operative time is shorter in the supine position but that there are no differences in other parameters.

The flank (lateral decubitus) position, which first was described by Kerbl and colleagues (1994), is less commonly used for percutaneous renal surgery. This position allows simultaneous access to the anterior and posterior aspects of the kidney and appears to be particularly useful for morbidly obese patients or those with spinal deformities in whom both supine and prone positioning are difficult (Gofrit et al, 2002; Basiri et al, 2008b; El-Husseiny et al, 2009). Randomized trials comparing flank to prone position (Karami et al, 2010) and flank to supine to prone positions (Karami et al, 2013) showed no difference in outcomes.

Although both the supine and flank positions offer some potential benefits over prone positioning in certain settings, particularly morbid obesity and spinal deformities, the evidence suggests no overwhelming differences, so surgeon preference can determine the choice of position for percutaneous renal surgery. As such, the remainder of this chapter concerns access into a posterior calyx from a posterior or posterolateral direction with the patient in the prone position, which remains the standard.

The initial step in a percutaneous procedure is often cystoscopic retrograde placement of a ureteral catheter. This can be performed with the patient in prone position (using a flexible cystoscope) or in lithotomy with subsequent prone repositioning. In the "upside-down" bladder, the bubble of air from initial introduction of the cystoscope often approximates the location of the ureteral orifices. Prone cystoscopy can be performed on a standard operating or fluoroscopy table but is simplified by the use of "spreader bars" on the foot of the table (also called a "split-leg table"). Abducting the legs with the knees straight spreads the legs. This provides better access to the external urethral meatus.

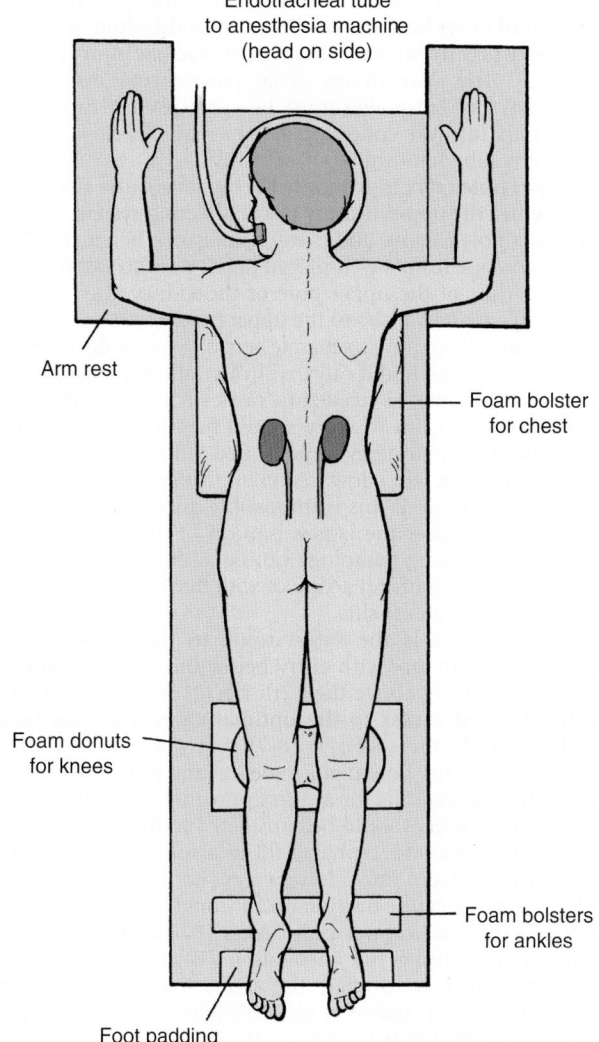

Figure 8-8. Padding for prone positioning.

Careful placement of padding is important in the prone position (Fig. 8-8). Support of the head with padding in a neutral position allows access to the mouth. Make sure there is not undue pressure on the facial bones, nose, and ears. Place the ipsilateral arm above the head to move it from the operative field, with the shoulder and elbow at right angles, and pad generously. Position the contralateral arm in the same way, or leave it straight and tucked at the side. Rest the lateral aspects of the chest on rolled blankets or other bulky foam or gel bolsters to allow for chest and abdominal wall expansion. Alternatively, purpose-made pads and supports provide more assured patient positioning (Papatsoris et al, 2009). Provide support under the ankles to take pressure off the feet, and pad the knees and feet. Prepare the perineum and ipsilateral flank sterilely, and cover unsterile areas with drapes. Cover the flank with an adherent drape that incorporates a fluid collection pouch.

Choice of Access Site to the Collecting System

The access site into the upper urinary tract collecting system is a critical determinant of the success of the subsequent procedure. **In the prone position, the preferred calyces are the posterior ones (or the posterior aspect of compound calyces), which allow better access to the remainder of the collecting system.** The anterior calyces can usually be approached through a posterior calyx. In cases that involve a calyceal diverticulum, narrow infundibulum, or pathology in an eccentric anterior calyx, direct puncture into an anterior location might be required. The ability to access the rest of the collecting system is limited with such access. **Percutaneous access should never be directly into an infundibulum or the renal pelvis, which greatly increases the risk of vascular injury** (Sampaio et al, 1992). The state of the renal parenchyma overlying the intended calyx of entry also must be considered because if it is thin, the tract into the collecting system may not close well after nephrostomy tube removal.

An upper pole calyx is generally the most versatile site through which to enter the upper urinary tract collecting system. The renal pelvis, lower pole calyces, and ureter usually can be entered with a rigid nephroscope from a well-placed upper pole access. Because of the posterior tilt of the upper pole of the kidney, the lower pole does not offer assured access to the upper pole. Access to the middle calyces will usually require a separate access or use of flexible instrumentation. Often a middle calyx will offer adequate access to the ureteropelvic junction, as needed in cases such as endopyelotomy. In other cases, the calyx of entry should be selected based on the distribution of the pathology to be treated. Efforts should be made to select a calyx that will allow treatment through a single site with rigid instrumentation. If this is impossible, then one should select the site that will allow the largest portion of the pathology to be treated. The remaining pathology can be addressed with a second (and rarely a third or more) access or with flexible instrumentation through the initial access site.

Subcostal access is the safest route to the kidney because pleural injuries are rare with entry below the 12th rib. Nonetheless, if entry directly above the 12th rib (11th intercostal space) provides the best access to the optimal calyx, then the benefit generally exceeds the risk (Fig. 8-9). Entry above the 11th rib, however, has a greater potential for pleural and even lung injury, so when the best access calls for a direct puncture above the 11th rib, additional maneuvers should be considered to displace the kidney inferiorly. These include: cephalad tilt of a subcostal access sheath or access needle placed into a lower calyx (Karlin and Smith, 1989; Lezrek et al, 2011); gentle traction on a through-and-through guidewire placed through a lower pole access (Goyal et al, 2012); and attaining access during full inspiration (Falahatkar et al, 2010). Another alternative is to angle the access tract cephalad from a subcostal entry site (Liatsikos et al, 2005; Rehman et al, 2008). This approach provides limited access to the rest of the kidney. All of these alternatives can result in damage if the kidney is moved caudally with excessive force. A multicenter retrospective study of patients undergoing percutaneous nephrolithotomy via upper pole access showed that patients with an intercostal approach experienced greater stone-free rates, fewer complications, and reduced

operating times compared to patients with a subcostal approach (Lang et al, 2009). Access above the 10th rib is associated with a high incidence of pleural violation and lung injury and should be avoided unless absolutely necessary. Thoracoscopically guided access superior to the 10th rib can be performed to reduce the risk of lung injury (Finelli and Honey, 2001).

Although standard preoperative ultrasonography or intravenous urography is sufficient in many cases for treatment planning, in complex cases cross-sectional imaging with computed tomography (CT) or magnetic resonance imaging (MRI) might be helpful. CT is a standard at many centers. For a more accurate representation of the renal collecting system, three-dimensional imaging reconstructions using CT or MRI are useful (Hubert et al, 1997; Buchholz, 2000; Ng et al, 2005; Thiruchelvam et al, 2005; Ghani et al, 2009; Kalogeropoulos et al, 2009; Patel et al, 2009). With specific timing of contrast injections and CT imaging, the vascular and collecting systems can be visualized simultaneously (Dalela et al, 2009).

Retrograde Assistance for Access into the Collecting System

One of the advantages of urologist participation in obtaining the initial percutaneous access is the opportunity to provide retrograde transurethral assistance. This assistance can take many forms, from placing a ureteral catheter, to inserting a flexible ureteroscope, to obtaining the percutaneous access using a retrograde-inserted device.

The simplest form of retrograde transurethral assistance is to place a 5- or 6-Fr straight ureteral catheter up into the renal pelvis (Fig. 8-10 on the Expert Consult website). Air and/or contrast material can be injected to delineate and dilate the intrarenal collecting system anatomy (Fig. 8-11 on the Expert Consult website), and a guidewire can be passed from below and grasped by the nephroscope to establish through-and-through access from the external urethral meatus to the percutaneous entry site. A dual-lumen catheter can be placed as well. The small caliber of either catheter, however, does not provide much outflow from the kidney and may not prevent stone or tumor fragments from passing into the ureter along the catheter. A ureteral occlusion balloon catheter, which incorporates an approximately 15-Fr spherical balloon on the distal tip, more consistently prevents material from migrating down the ureter. The balloon should be carefully inflated in the renal pelvis, making sure the balloon is not in the ureter—which could lead to ureteral rupture—and then gently pulled down to occlude the ureteropelvic junction (Fig. 8-12). Another alternative is to place a ureteral access sheath (usually 11 to 15 Fr) over a retrograde-inserted guidewire (Landman et al, 2003). The large outer diameter of the sheath effectively prevents particles from passing around the sheath into the ureter, and the large inner diameter affords excellent outflow of small stone particles. The disadvantages of using a ureteral access sheath include the potential ureteral trauma from passing such a large device into the ureter and the clogging of the catheter lumen by oversized stone fragments.

A ureteroscope passed retrograde can greatly facilitate percutaneous entry into the intrarenal collecting system (Grasso et al, 1995; Kidd and Conlin, 2003; Patel et al, 2008) by allowing the surgeon to observe and correct the percutaneous placement of a needle. A basket can then be passed through the ureteroscope to grasp the end of the percutaneous guidewire; pulling this out through the urethra provides through-and-through access (Fig. 8-13). Even if the pathology being addressed is so large that direct visualization of the percutaneous needle is obscured (e.g., complete staghorn calculus), one can still use the ureteroscope to rapidly attain through-and-through access. Moreover, the ureteroscope may have better access to some sites in the kidney than the nephroscope and can be used to assist in the procedure (e.g., fragment or relocate stones, fulgurate small tumors). Retrospective nonrandomized comparisons of ureteroscopic-assistance versus solely fluoroscopic guidance for access during percutaneous nephrolithotomy suggest

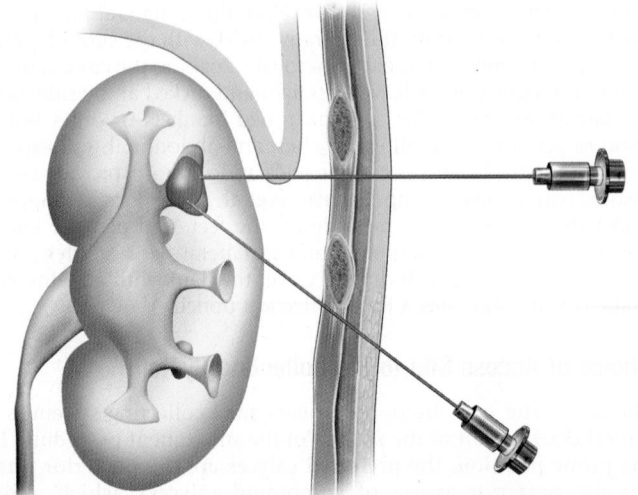

Figure 8-9. Subcostal and supracostal percutaneous access to an upper pole calyx. The supracostal approach provides more direct access and provides a better angle for endoscopy of the rest of the kidney.

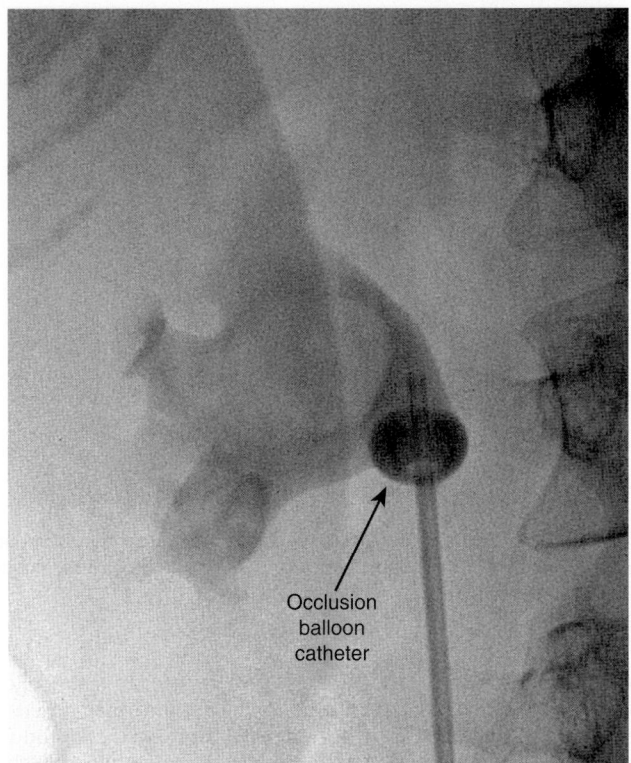

Figure 8-12. Occlusion balloon inflated and snugged down at ureteropelvic junction of contrast-filled upper tract collecting system.

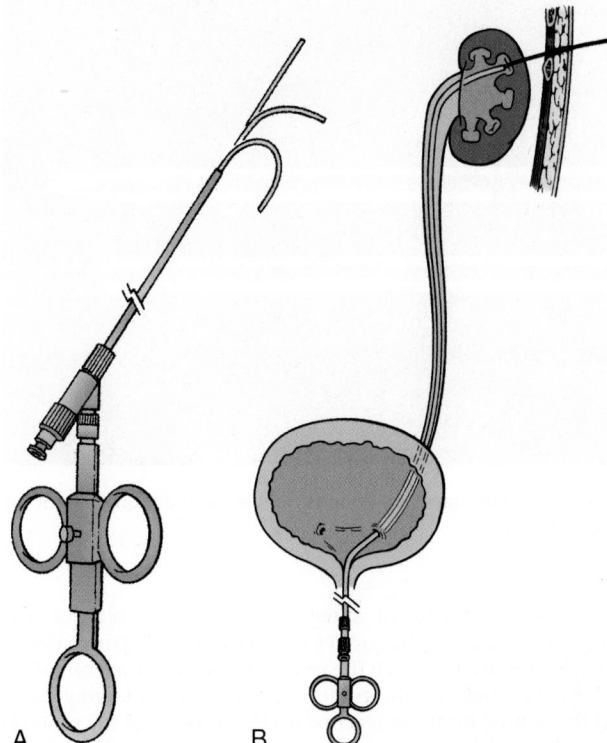

Figure 8-14. Retrograde percutaneous access. A, Torcon deflectable catheter. B, Assembled unit passing puncture needle out through the abdominal wall and skin.

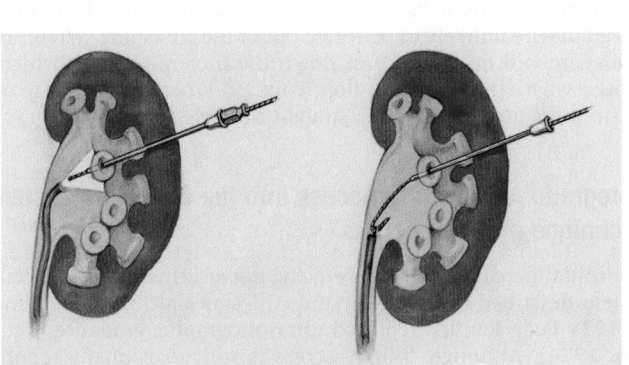

Figure 8-13. Ureteroscope retrograde assistance. The needle can be directly visualized entering the calyx, and a wire can be grasped and pulled down the ureter and out the urethra.

that the former may be associated with a lower transfusion rate (Sountoulides et al, 2009), decreased fluoroscopy time, reduced need for multiple accesses, and a reduction in the early termination of the procedure as a result of hemorrhage (Isac et al, 2013).

The "ultimate" retrograde assistance to percutaneous access into the upper urinary tract collecting system is the retrograde approach to percutaneous access. Although the antegrade approach is much more commonly performed, a retrograde approach may be selected when the surgeon has limited experience with antegrade percutaneous renal puncture or in situations where there might be a technical advantage to the retrograde approach, such as morbid obesity or a hypermobile or abnormally situated kidney (Mokulis and Peretsman, 1997). The Lawson Retrograde Nephrostomy Wire Puncture Set (Cook Urological, Spencer, IN) is the device commercially available for this approach. The fundamental maneuver of this procedure is to pass a stiff wire from inside the kidney toward and through the external body wall. This can be directed

fluoroscopically or under direct vision with ureteroscopy. For the former, pass a 7-Fr Torcon catheter (actively deflectable from 0 to 140 degrees; Fig. 8-14A) over a guidewire and direct it fluoroscopically into the targeted calyx. Insert the 3-Fr polytetrafluoroethylene (PTFE) sheath containing the 0.017-inch stainless steel puncture wire through the Torcon catheter. Advance the puncture wire through the kidney and body wall under fluoroscopic control, withdrawing and repositioning it if any obstacles such as a rib are encountered (Fig. 8-14B). Make a small skin incision and grasp the wire externally. Use the fascial dilators in an antegrade fashion until the Torcon catheter can be advanced through the tract. When the end of the catheter exits the skin, exchange the puncture wire for a standard 0.035-inch guidewire, thus attaining through-and-through access. This fluoroscopic technique is reported to be safe and effective (Sivalingam et al, 2013).

For the ureteroscopic approach to retrograde percutaneous access, direct the ureteroscope into the desired calyx and pass the 0.017-inch stainless steel puncture within the 3-Fr PTFE sheath though the working channel. First described in 1989 (Munch, 1989), in more recent reports it has been suggested that urologists without training in percutaneous antegrade access may be able to adopt this technique more readily (Wynberg et al, 2012) and that this approach may be associated with shorter operation time and fewer complications compared to antegrade access (Kawahara et al, 2012). Further experience is required before the role of retrograde percutaneous access (whether fluoroscopically or ureteroscopically directed) can be ascertained.

Antegrade Approach to Access into the Collecting System: Needles and Guidewires

The antegrade approach to percutaneous access into the upper urinary tract collecting system is the standard. It affords the most control of the skin entry site and can be guided by ureteroscopy or a variety of imaging modalities.

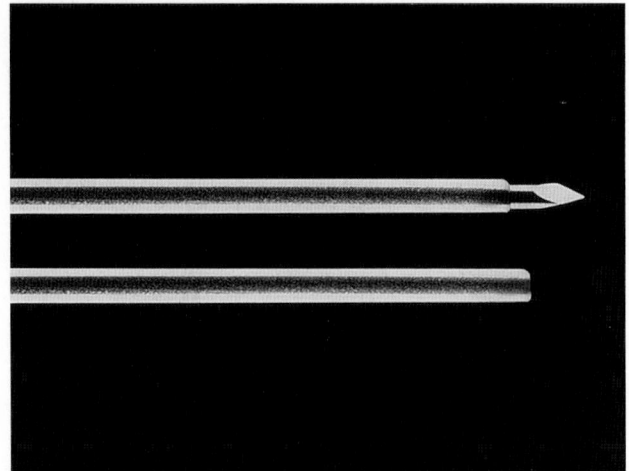

Figure 8-15. Percutaneous access needle, with a blunt sheath and a sharp obturator.

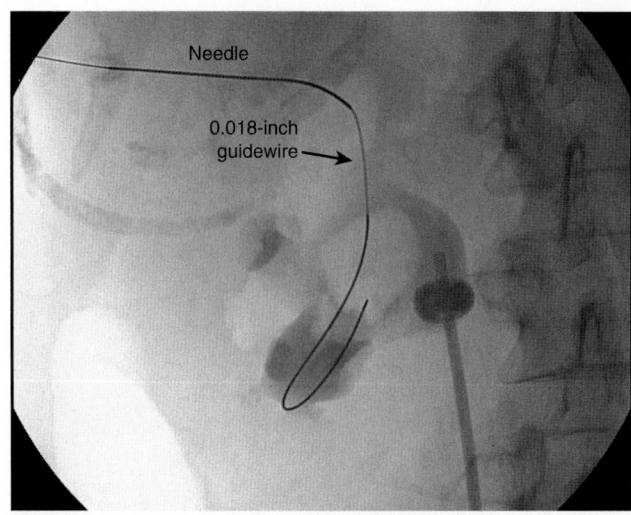

Figure 8-16. A 0.018-inch guidewire passed through percutaneous needle. This wire is exchanged for a 0.035-inch guidewire for subsequent manipulation.

The general scheme of antegrade access is to place a needle through the skin into the upper urinary tract collecting system. A guidewire is placed through the needle and then catheters and other devices are placed over the guidewire, eventually enlarging the tract until the desired lumen is reached for the purpose of the procedure. This is the Seldinger technique, described (for vascular access) by Sven-Ivar Seldinger (1953). The standard choices for the needle are a 21-gauge needle through which is passed a 0.018-inch guidewire or an 18-gauge needle through which is passed a standard 0.035-inch guidewire. Both needles have a blunt sheath and a sharp obturator (Fig. 8-15). The 21-gauge needle has the advantage of causing relatively minor injury as it is passed through tissue. Multiple passes can generally be made with little risk of hemorrhage from the needle itself; the option to place and replace the needle multiple times is advantageous because getting the tip of the needle into the right spot in the kidney is the most difficult aspect of percutaneous access into the upper urinary tract collecting system. The 18-gauge needle is more traumatic, and multiple passes should be avoided. The advantage of the 18-gauge needle is that it is stiffer. In a number of circumstances the 21-gauge needle does not adequately maintain trajectory (e.g., scarred kidney, obese patient) and the 18-gauge needle is more effective. In addition, the 0.018-inch guidewire that passes through the 21-gauge needle (Fig. 8-16) must be exchanged for a standard 0.035-inch guidewire for subsequent tract dilation or catheter placement. This requires an extra step, which adds to the complexity of the procedure and increases the risk of a loss of access. Balancing the reduced efficacy of the 21-gauge needle and its increased potential for loss of access, versus the increased risk of trauma with the 18-gauge needle, it is recommended that the 21-gauge needle be used when the operator is less experienced or if minimizing trauma is paramount. The 18-gauge needle should be used when an experienced operator is confident that the tip of the needle can be placed within the desired calyx with just a few attempts.

Two methods can be used to exchange the 0.018-inch for a 0.035-inch guidewire. A coaxial introducer incorporates a small catheter within a slightly larger catheter. After inserting the 0.018-inch guidewire and removing the needle, the coaxial introducer is advanced over the guidewire until the end is within the renal collecting system. The surgeon should remove the inner catheter and 0.018-inch guidewire and then should advance a 0.035-inch guidewire through the outer catheter into the collecting system. The second method uses a graduated introducer that fits over the 0.018-inch guidewire at its tip but then enlarges to a lumen that will accept the 0.035-inch guidewire. A few centimeters back from the tip is a hole through which the 0.035-inch guidewire can pass. After inserting the 0.018-inch guidewire and removing the needle, pass the graduated introducer over the guidewire until it is a few centimeters

inside the kidney, such that the side hole is within the renal collecting system. Remove the 0.018-inch guidewire and then insert an angled or J-tipped 0.035-inch guidewire through the introducer until the end of the wire exits the catheter within the collecting system. With either the coaxial or graduated introducer, a stiffener can be used to assist in passing the device over the relatively insecure 0.018-inch guidewire.

The safest initial 0.035-inch guidewire to use for upper urinary tract percutaneous access is a PTFE-coated J-wire. The "J" tip makes the guidewire unlikely to perforate out of the collecting system. This guidewire will not easily pass down the ureter, however, which is more easily handled with a floppy-tip PTFE-coated guidewire or a hydrophilic guidewire with a straight or angled tip.

Antegrade Approach to Access into the Collecting System: Technique of Initial Access

The initial percutaneous access to the upper urinary tract collecting system described by Goodwin and colleagues (1955) was "blind." In 1974 Pedersen first reported ultrasonographic guidance (Pedersen, 1974). Although "blind" access is still occasionally reported and in expert hands can be successful, in most cases the initial antegrade percutaneous access into the upper urinary tract collecting system is obtained with real-time imaging guidance. Ultrasonography and fluoroscopy are most commonly used, with the choice based on patient characteristics and physician preference (Basiri et al, 2008a). A large multi-institutional matched-case analysis did not show any differences between ultrasonographic and fluoroscopic guidance of percutaneous access for nephrolithotomy in terms of hemorrhage and treatment success (Andonian et al, 2013).

Ultrasonographic Guidance

Ultrasonography has the advantages of portability (the mobile ultrasound machine is easier to maneuver than a C-arm fluoroscopy unit and does not require a radiolucent operating table), the ability to assess intervening structures, and no delivery of ionizing radiation. In addition, retrograde injection of contrast material or air is not necessary because the collecting system can readily be distinguished within the kidney based on ultrasonographic appearance alone. **The disadvantages of ultrasonography include less clear visualization of the percutaneous needle (although etched needles created for enhanced sonographic appearance are available), a limited field of view compared with fluoroscopy, and difficulty monitoring the subsequent steps of**

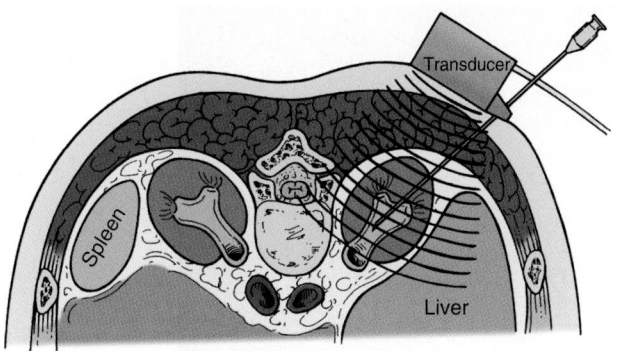

Figure 8-17. Ultrasonographic guidance of puncture needle.

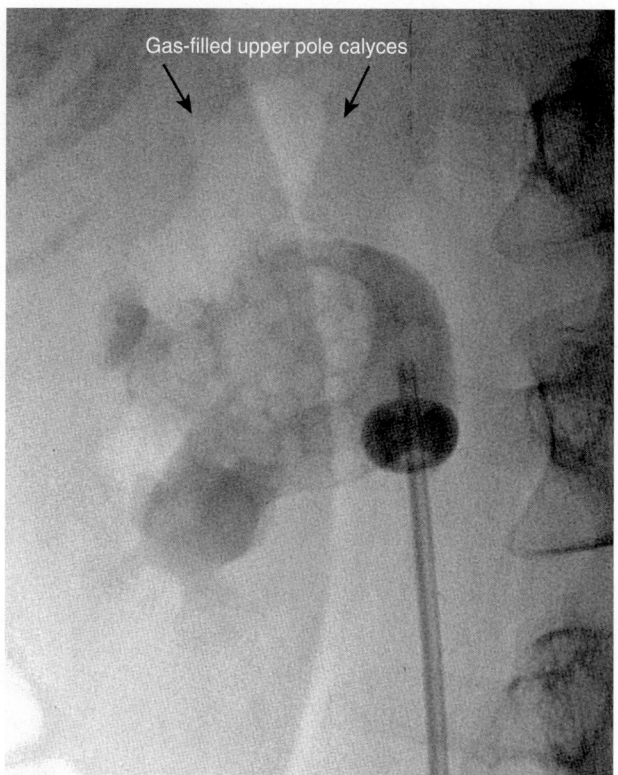

Figure 8-18. Injection of air into contrast-filled upper tract collecting system shows posterior calyces, in this case most clearly the upper pole calyces. Compare with Figure 8-12, before injection of air.

the procedure. Ultrasonography is the first choice in imaging when retrograde access cannot be attained or is difficult to attain, such as in kidneys above urinary diversions, transplanted kidneys, kidneys above a completely obstructed ureter, or when radiation exposure is a concern. Ultrasonography also may be useful in the setting of skeletal abnormalities or anomalous kidneys, when intervening anatomy may differ from the norm (Chen et al, 2013; Penbegul et al, 2013). When percutaneous access is necessary for simple drainage of the kidney, such that the exact site of access is not critical as long as puncture into the renal pelvis or an infundibulum is avoided, ultrasonography is more expedient and more convenient than fluoroscopy.

Using a handheld 3.5- or 5-MHz ultrasound transducer, inspect the kidney and select a calyx for percutaneous entry. Needle guides can be placed on the transducer to direct the needle in the plane of visualization of the probe. Some prefer to place the needle freehand instead, moving the transducer around to gain different views of the kidney and needle. Observe the needle as it is advanced until it appears that the tip is within the collecting system (Fig. 8-17). Removing the obturator and aspirating urine confirms entry. Saline infusion and furosemide administration may improve ultrasonographic visualization of a nondilated intrarenal collecting system (Yagci et al, 2013). In one nonrandomized comparison (Lu et al, 2010) and one randomized controlled trial (Tzeng et al, 2011), the addition of Doppler to ultrasound imaging (which facilitates visualization of blood vessels) was associated with less blood loss and/or lower transfusion rate than ultrasound alone.

Fluoroscopic Guidance

Fluoroscopic guidance is more commonly used for gaining antegrade access to the upper urinary tract collecting system for percutaneous renal surgery. **Although retrograde instillation of air and/or contrast material is not absolutely essential** (Tabibi et al, 2007), **most urologists find that it enhances fluoroscopically guided percutaneous access** (Fig. 8-18). **Fluoroscopy provides excellent delineation of the intrarenal collecting system anatomy and pathology (when contrast-enhanced), a wide field of view (that can be collimated down to reduce radiation exposure), and the ability to monitor all steps of the procedure. In some cases combining the techniques is an excellent approach, using ultrasonography to guide the initial needle placement and then using fluoroscopy (after injection of air and contrast through the sonographically guided needle) to confirm that the desired calyx has been accessed and to monitor the subsequent steps of the procedure** (Osman et al, 2005). If the entry site is incorrect, then fluoroscopy of the air-and-contrast–filled collecting system can be used to guide another needle into the desired calyx. With this combination, retrograde assistance is not necessary. A randomized controlled trial between percutaneous nephrolithotomy access directed only by fluoroscopy versus ultrasonography plus fluoroscopy showed fewer puncture attempts, shorter access time and reduced

fluoroscopy time in the ultrasonography-plus-fluoroscopy group, without differences in success rate or hemorrhage (Agarwal et al, 2011). This technique is especially useful in accessing nondilated systems without retrograde assistance (Patel and Hussain, 2004).

There are two well-described methods of fluoroscopic guidance for antegrade percutaneous access into the upper urinary tract collecting system: the "eye-of-the-needle" technique and the "triangulation" technique (Miller et al, 2007). Both have their proponents, and there is no clear advantage of one rather than the other, as confirmed by one randomized controlled trial (Tepeler et al, 2012). Through the retrograde device, inject contrast material to delineate the collecting system after first taking note of any radiopaque pathology for later reference. Comparing a spot film of the unopacified collecting system with the opacified view is useful in this regard. After the options for the calyces of entry are identified, inject air to define the calyces that are posterior. In the prone position, air rises up the posterior calyces. The "double-contrast" pyelogram (both contrast material and air) provides the best determination of the pertinent intrarenal anatomy.

To perform the "eye-of-the-needle" technique, first inspect the kidney with the fluoroscopy unit directly above the patient (directed vertically) and select the desired calyx. Next, rotate the top of the fluoroscopic unit 30 degrees toward the operator, which brings the fluoroscopic view more or less end-on with the posterior calyces. The unit can be additionally rotated slightly cephalad or caudad to line it up more exactly with the axis of the calyx. Place the tip of a hemostat on the skin and move it until it is directly over the desired calyx. Mark this site and make an incision large enough to accept the needle and initial dilators. Place the tip of the access needle into this incision, and then move the shaft of the needle while keeping the tip in place until the needle is directly in line with the axis of the fluoroscopy unit; doing so gives the appearance of a "bull's eye" with the hub of the needle (appearing as a circle) around the shaft (which appears as a dot). The fluoroscopic view is as if the operator is looking down the shaft of the needle at the targeted calyx—thus

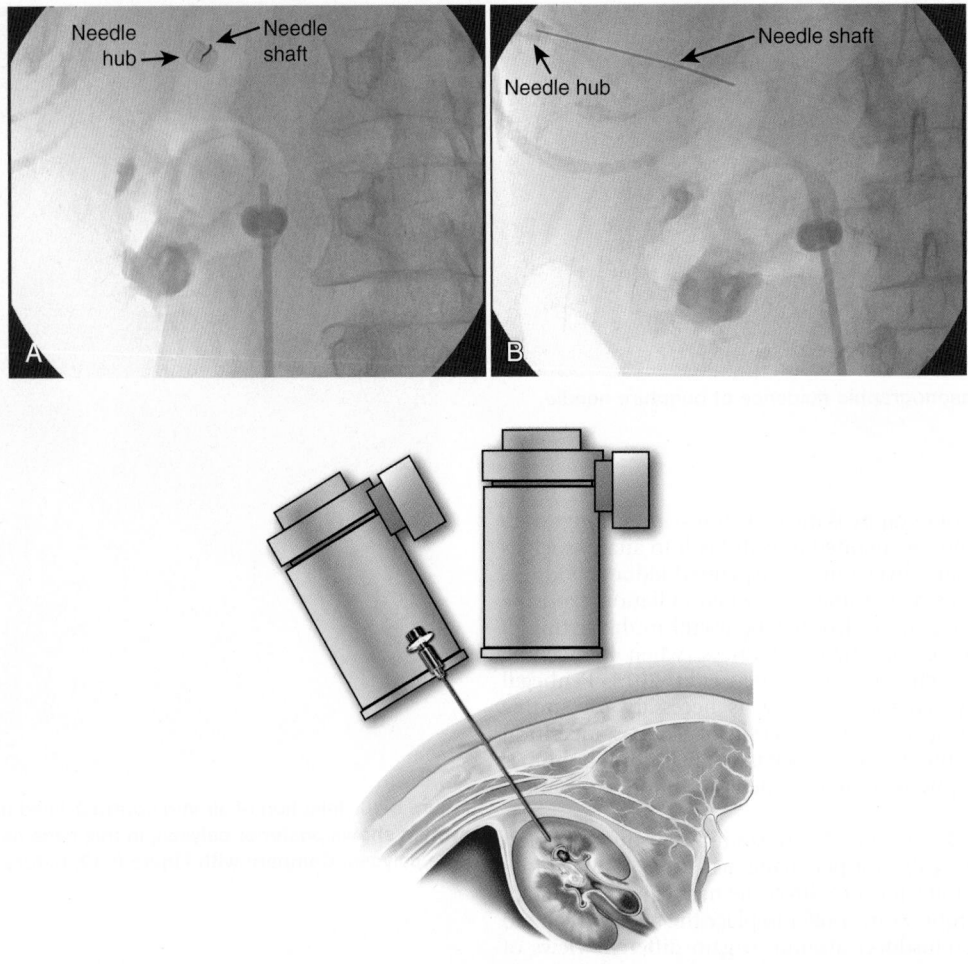

Figure 8-19. "Eye-of-the-needle" fluoroscopic guidance. A, With the top of the fluoroscopic unit rotated 30 degrees toward the operator, the needle is lined up directly over the intended calyx of entry. B, With the fluoroscopy unit rotated away from the operator, the needle is now seen in profile, and in the figure has already been advanced under fluoroscopic control to achieve collecting system entry.

the term "eye of the needle" (Fig. 8-19A). Advance the needle straight in, while checking with fluoroscopy and adjusting the angle of the needle as needed to maintain the "bull's-eye" appearance. If the needle is more than a few centimeters deep and readjustment is necessary, the needle may have to be withdrawn before a new trajectory can be followed. The 21-gauge needle can be difficult to control during this step. If difficulty occurs, substitute the more easily passed 18-gauge needle. After the needle's axis is fixed and it is thought that the needle is approaching or is in the kidney (typically a "pop" can be felt when the renal capsule is punctured), then rotate the fluoroscopy unit away from the operator, back to vertical or even 10 to 15 degrees beyond vertical. Now the needle appears "in profile" as a straight line. With the cephalo-caudad and mediolateral axes of the needle now fixed, advance or withdraw the needle to change its anteroposterior position (depth) to move the tip of the needle into the desired calyx (Fig. 8-19B). Aspiration of urine or air after removing the obturator confirms entry. Instillation of contrast material can be used to confirm entry as well, but if the needle is misplaced, the extravasated contrast material can obscure subsequent fluoroscopic visualization. If a gently passed guidewire stays within the contours of the collecting system, then this confirms proper entry without risking the troublesome extravasation of contrast material.

To use the "triangulation" technique, inspect the kidney with the fluoroscopy unit directly above the patient to select the desired calyx, and hold the needle in the approximate position of the

desired angle of entry. Rotate the top of the fluoroscopy unit cephalad and lateral, and widen the field of view with the collimator such that mediolateral (left-right) movements of the needle are apparent. Move the shaft of the needle while keeping its tip in place until the needle is aimed toward the desired calyx (Fig. 8-20A). Then rotate the top of the fluoroscopy unit medially 45 degrees. While keeping the mediolateral orientation of the needle constant, move the needle in the cephalo-caudad (up-down) plane until the needle is again aimed toward the desired calyx (Fig. 8-20B). Resting the forearm on the patient's back will help stabilize the needle in one plane while moving in the other. Move the fluoroscopy unit back and forth between these two positions until the needle remains aimed at the desired calyx on both views. Advance the needle under fluoroscopic guidance while monitoring the anteroposterior direction (depth) of the needle tip. If the needle position in the mediolateral and cephalo-caudad planes is maintained, the needle should enter the targeted calyx.

With the "eye-of-the-needle" technique, the proper cephalo-caudad and mediolateral axes of the needle are verified and maintained on a single fluoroscopic view, and the confirmatory view is necessary only to assure the depth of the needle tip. For the "triangulation" technique, one fluoroscopic view is used to assess the mediolateral axis and another is used to assess the cephalo-caudad axis, with the depth of the needle tip being assessed on both views (Miller et al, 2007). The advantage of the triangulation technique instead of the "eye-of-the-needle" technique is that the needle

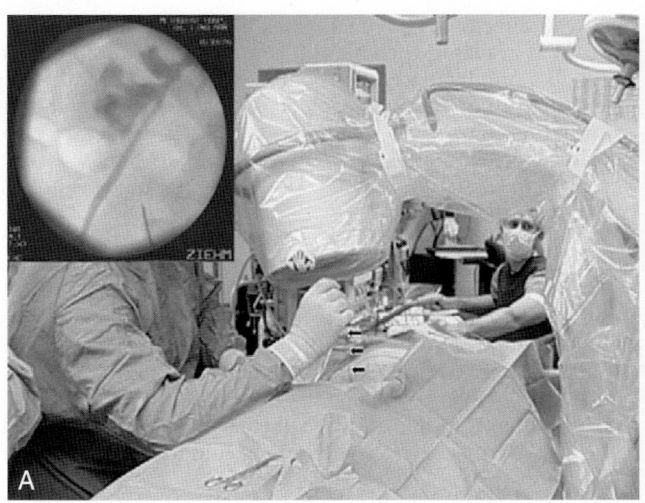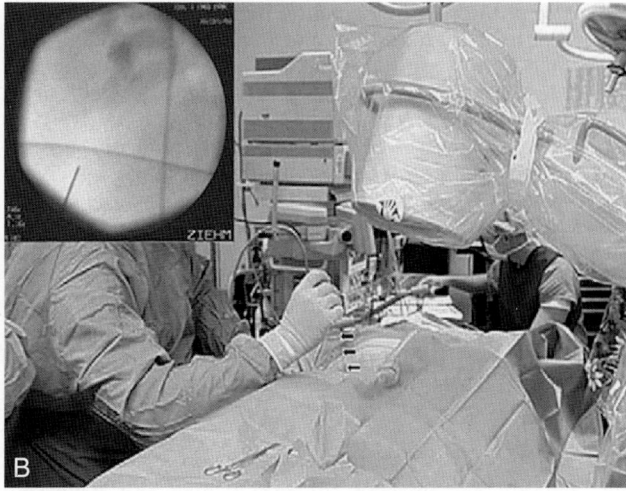

Figure 8-20. Triangulation fluoroscopic guidance. A, With the top of the fluoroscopy unit rotated laterally and cephalad, adjust the access needle *(arrows)* to a mediolateral orientation of the needle. B, After rotating the top of the fluoroscopy unit medially, and while keeping mediolateral orientation of the needle constant, move the needle in the cephalo-caudad plane until the needle is again aimed toward the desired calyx. (From Miller NL, Matlaga BR, Lingeman JE. Techniques for fluoroscopic percutaneous renal access. J Urol 2007;178:15–23.)

cannot be passed too deeply because the depth of advancement is monitored continuously. The disadvantage of the "triangulation" technique is that maintaining both the mediolateral and cephalo-caudad planes is difficult because both are not being monitored at the same time, as in the "eye-of-the-needle" technique. Use of the 18-gauge rather than a 21-gauge needle is recommended with the "triangulation" technique to help maintain the angle of entry. Mechanical devices that stabilize the needle during insertion might be helpful as well (Lazarus and Williams, 2011).

It should be remembered that the ionizing radiation presents a small but real risk. When the operator must grasp the access needle within the fluoroscopy field, it is best to hold the needle with a hemostat, sponge forceps, or purpose-built needle holder to reduce radiation exposure to the operator's hand. Collimating the field down as much as possible while still maintaining an adequate field of view reduces radiation exposure to the patient and all personnel in the room. Moving a collimated field around to maintain the object of interest in the field is preferable to maintaining a wide field that includes the operator's hands and unnecessary body parts of the patient. Increased body mass index, greater stone burden, nonbranched stones, a greater number of access sites, and the use of air rather than contrast during initial retrograde pyelography are associated with an increased radiation dose (Mancini et al, 2010; Lipkin et al, 2011). For additional information about radiation safety, see Chapter 2.

Advanced Guidance

In some complex cases, one might consider percutaneous access into the kidney guided by CT or MRI. The initial access is obtained into the desired calyx with the patient on the CT or MRI table, similar to the techniques used for needle biopsy (Barbaric et al, 1997; Hagspiel et al, 1998; Thanos et al, 2006). Bowel and other viscera can be imaged to protect against their injury, and this approach is especially useful in cases of anatomic abnormalities (LeMaitre et al, 2000; Matlaga et al, 2003; Srivastava et al, 2010) and for nondilated collecting systems (Merkle et al, 1999; Egilmez et al, 2007; Sommer et al, 2011).

A stereotactic fluoroscopy technique using three-dimensional coordinates for localization was reported as associated with greater accuracy and lower blood loss compared to standard fluoroscopy (Li et al, 2012a). The same principle can be computerized, as demonstrated in an experimental ex vivo model (Zarrabi et al, 2010).

An even more advanced modification of fluoroscopy is three-dimensional fluoroscopy, which provides images with a level of quality equivalent to CT. Application to percutaneous access of porcine kidneys appeared to be effective (Soria et al, 2009), and a clinical series has suggested potential benefits (Roy et al, 2012).

Three-dimensional ultrasonography accurately represents the renal collecting system (Ghani et al, 2008) and appears useful for renal imaging (Kim et al, 2008) and for teaching percutaneous access into an in vitro renal model (John et al, 2009). Given that three-dimensional ultrasonography has been applied to other therapeutic urologic applications (such as percutaneous drainage of prostatic abscesses) (Varkarakis et al, 2004), investigation of its use for clinical percutaneous access of the collecting system is anticipated.

Imaging modalities can also be combined. There has been one report of a novel image localization system that projects the ultrasonographic puncture tract onto the fluoroscopy screen (Mozer et al, 2007). Preoperative MRI data can be merged with intraoperative ultrasonography to improve puncture accuracy (Li et al, 2012b). More frequently reported is the integration of preoperative CT images with intraoperative ultrasonography (Leroy et al, 2004; Mozer et al, 2005; Wein et al, 2008).

In addition to advanced image guidance of percutaneous access to the intrarenal collecting system, technologic enhancements have been applied to the initial needle puncture. The URorobotics Laboratory at Johns Hopkins University has developed the robotic percutaneous access to the kidney with remote center of motion device (PAKY-RCM) (Cadeddu et al, 1997b). This is a robotic arm with 7 degrees of freedom that places a needle into the intrarenal collecting system as directed by the control device that pivots the tip of the needle about a fixed point on the skin. In a nonrandomized clinical trial, the PAKY-RCM system was equivalent to an expert physician in gaining access to the collecting system in terms of time and accuracy (Su et al, 2002). In a randomized trial in an in vitro kidney model, the PAKY-RCM took slightly more time but was more accurate than manual needle insertion (Challacombe et al, 2005b). This device can also be controlled at distance with telepresence technology (Bove et al, 2003; Netto et al, 2003). The same group subsequently developed a robot for percutaneous access that is MRI-compatible (Mozer et al, 2009). Percutaneous access needles incorporating advanced characteristics such as piezoelectric crystals that allow the needle to be adjusted for particular orientations (Yan et al, 2007), electromagnetic sensors that provide real-time information of position and orientation (Yaniv et al, 2009; Huber et al, 2011; Rodrigues et al, 2013), and impedance-based sensing systems to detect entry into the collecting system have also been developed (Hernandez et al, 2001; Roberts et al, 2002), but clinical use for percutaneous intrarenal surgery has not been reported. The "all-seeing needle" consists of a modified percutaneous access needle with 1.6-mm (4.85-Fr) outer diameter through which is inserted micro-optics (0.9-mm diameter) coupled to a zoom ocular that allows visualization of the needle access tract during initial entry (Bader et al, 2011). Clinical application has been reported and appears to be favorable. Finally, Rassweiler and associates (2012) have described an "augmented reality" application of an iPad combined with CT images obtained with markers, integrating radiographic and visual information, to direct percutaneous renal access.

"Blind" Access

The upper urinary tract collecting system can also be accessed "blindly," without any imaging guidance (Chien and Bellman, 2002). The only situation in which this should be considered is when sonography is not available and there is complete ureteral obstruction (precluding retrograde instillation of contrast material or opacification of the collecting system with intravenous contrast). The lumbar notch, also known as the *superior lumbar triangle* or *Grynfeltt lumbar triangle*, has been reported as a reliable landmark for blind percutaneous renal access (Fig. 8-21). The lumbar notch is an area of muscular insufficiency through which hernias can occur. It is located posteriorly below the 12th rib. The superior border is the 12th rib and the latissimus dorsi muscle, the lateral border is the transversus abdominis and external oblique muscles, the medial border is the quadratus lumborum and sacrospinalis muscles, and the inferior border is the internal oblique muscle. Insert a needle 3 to 4 cm deep into the notch at a 30-degree cephalad angle to enter the collecting system. Another blind approach to the collecting system is to insert a needle directly perpendicular to the body surface 1 to 1.5 cm lateral to the L1 vertebral body, which

will lead directly to the renal pelvis if anatomy is normal. If fluoroscopy is available, then air and contrast material can be injected through a blindly placed needle to assess fluoroscopically its position and to guide another needle if needed. In the only randomized clinical trial comparing "blind" access to image-guided access, entry into the collecting system was successful in 50% and 90% of cases, respectively (Basiri et al, 2007). Use of the technique is not recommended in most settings.

Working Access

After good access to the collecting system is attained, exchange the initial guidewire through a catheter for a different one as needed. Dilate the tract over the guidewire with stiff plastic dilators or a metal fascial cutter to enlarge the tract to 8 to 12 Fr. If the goal of the procedure is simple drainage, then a small-caliber nephrostomy tube can be placed over the single guidewire to complete the procedure.

Safety Wire

If ureteroscopic assistance is used, the first guidewire inserted into the kidney can be grasped with the ureteroscope and pulled down the ureter and out the external urethral meatus. With this through-and-through access, the guidewire cannot be lost. **In all other situations, the goal for a therapeutic percutaneous procedure is to move two guidewires down the ureter into the bladder, generally a super-stiff (working) guidewire and a floppy-tip or J-tipped PTFE-coated (safety) guidewire.** One important exception is in cases where a dependent lower pole has been accessed percutaneously. If there is extreme angulation to get from the lower pole calyx to the ureteropelvic junction and down the ureter, placing a super-stiff guidewire down the ureter may put undue force on the kidney and risk tearing the parenchyma. In such cases, the flexible safety guidewire should still be directed down the ureter if possible, but the stiff working wire over which the dilation is performed can

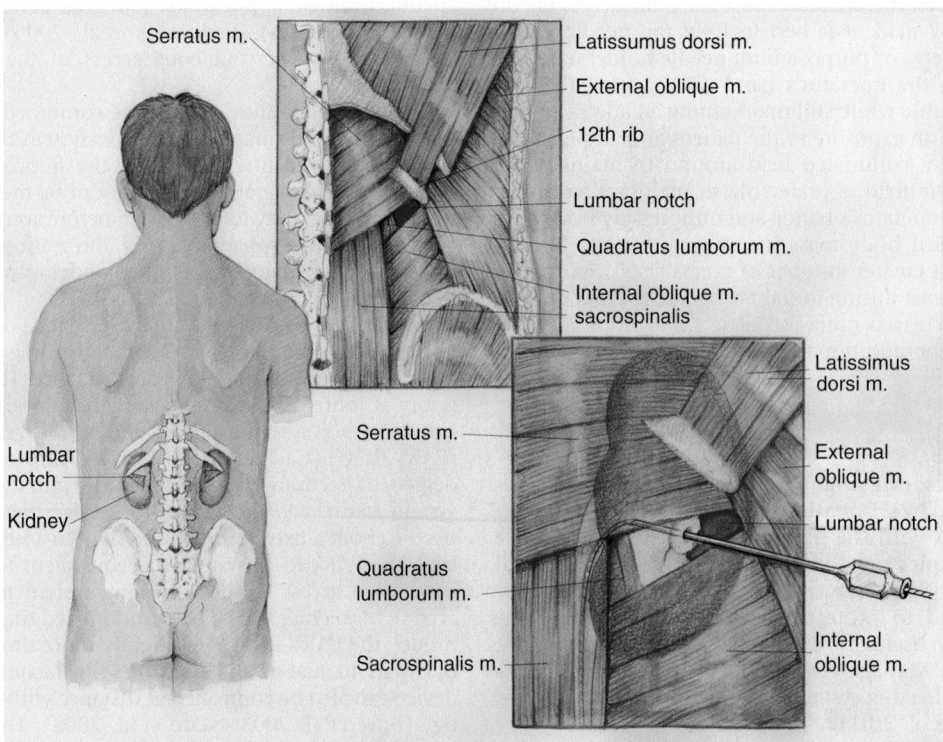

Figure 8-21. The lumbar notch is a useful anatomic landmark for blind percutaneous access to the renal collecting system. It is bounded superiorly by the latissimus dorsi muscle and the 12th rib, medially by the sacrospinalis and quadratus lumborum muscles, laterally by the transversus abdominis and external oblique muscles, and inferiorly by the internal oblique muscle.

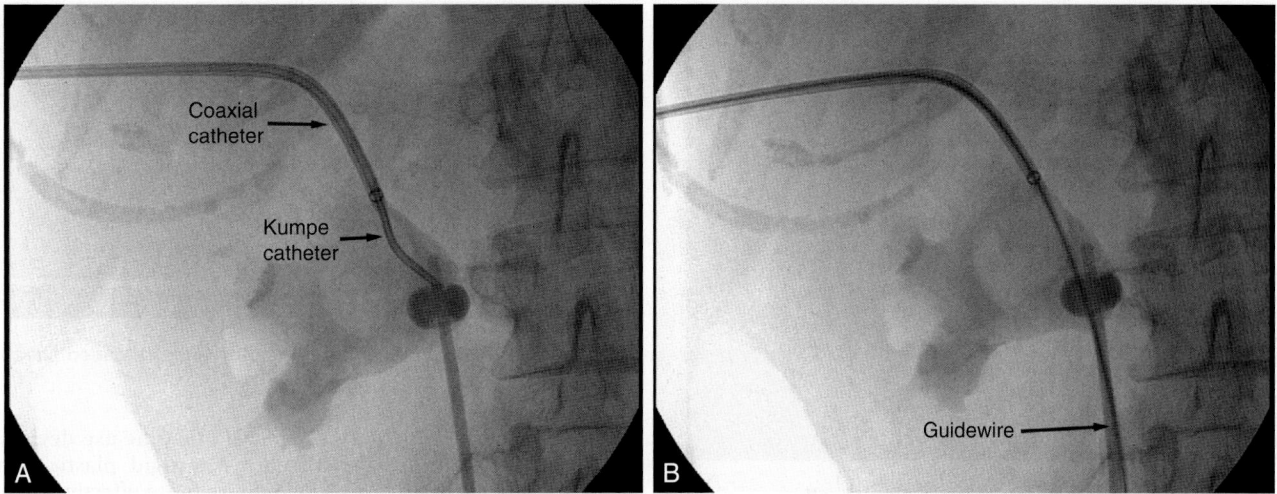

Figure 8-22. A, Kumpe catheter placed through the outer sheath of a coaxial catheter and manipulated toward the ureteropelvic junction helps direct a guidewire (B) down the ureter.

simply be directed toward the upper pole. Additionally, in some cases the pathology (e.g., calyceal obstruction, impacted ureteral stone, large staghorn stone) prevents the surgeon from getting a guidewire down the ureter or even into the remainder of the intra-renal collecting system. In such cases attempts should be made to move as much guidewire as possible into the upper urinary tract collecting system. A guidewire with a moveable core is useful in this setting because it can be coiled more tightly.

There are several techniques for inserting a guidewire down the ureter. The safest maneuver is to place a stiff angled-tip hydrophilic guidewire adjacent to the initial stiff angled-tip hydrophilic guide-wire using a coaxial or dual-lumen catheter. Remove the coaxial or dual-lumen catheter and place an angled-tip catheter (Kumpe, Cobra, or coudé tip) over the angled-tip hydrophilic guidewire to help direct it down the ureter. After the stiff angled-tip hydrophilic guidewire is down the ureter, optimally all the way into the bladder, use the coaxial or dual-lumen catheter to place a second guidewire down the ureter. In cases of secure access, the initial wire can be exchanged for a stiff angled-tip hydrophilic guidewire through an angled-tip catheter to pass down through the ureter quickly (Fig. 8-22); alternatively, the surgeon can use a stiff angled-tip hydro-philic guidewire as the initial wire.

Dilation of Tract

After there is adequate wire access into the upper urinary tract collecting system, dilate the tract to allow insertion of working instruments. In most cases the goal of dilation for percutaneous renal surgery is to place a 30-Fr inner-diameter/34-Fr outer-diameter plastic access sheath. In some cases a smaller sheath, with an inner diameter measuring 12- to 24-Fr, is adequate. Renal access sheaths generally have a beveled tip, such that one side of the sheath extends farther than the other part. This bevel is used to maintain access into part of the collecting system on one side of the sheath while allowing extra mobility on the other side. Sheath repositioning is facilitated by the bevel. In cases of pathology at the edge of the collecting system, however, the bevel presents a disadvantage because the entire tip of the sheath cannot be placed into the col-lecting system. Both opaque and clear sheaths are available; some prefer the clear sheaths because structures next to the sheath can be visualized.

In the early years of therapeutic percutaneous renal procedures, the tract was dilated gradually through the course of many days by placing sequentially larger tubes. Castañeda-Zúñiga and associates (1982) first reported acute dilation of the tract. There are several dilator systems available. **Regardless of the method used, it is imperative that the dilator does not pass too far into the**

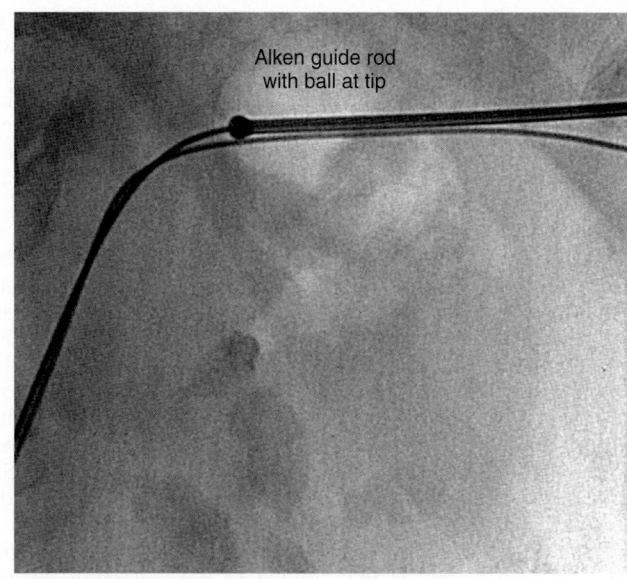

Figure 8-23. Alken guide rod is positioned with the ball at the tip of the rod positioned at the intended depth of the dilation.

collecting system. If this occurs, an infundibulum, the renal pelvis, or the ureteropelvic junction can be torn or perforated, either directly by the dilator or indirectly by a stone pushed aside by the dilator. The dilator should be passed just into the calyx. It is better to dilate a bit "short" of the targeted calyx than to dilate too far, which would create trauma. The initial inspection with the neph-roscope confirms entry of the sheath into the calyx. If the sheath is not deep enough, then simply replace the dilating device and redi-late after advancing the device. The dilators should not be used to dilate the skin; the skin should be incised to allow entry of the final sheath without pressure on the skin edges.

Sequential rigid metal dilators, introduced by Alken (1985), are a series of progressively enlarging coaxial stainless steel rods that pass over an 8-Fr guide rod. The first step in tract dilation is to pass the 8-Fr guide rod over a 0.035-inch guidewire. The end of the guide rod has a ball that prevents advancement of the first dilating rod beyond the tip. The ball is positioned at the intended depth of the dilation (Fig. 8-23). After passing the first rod, each successive metal rod is passed sequentially over the former until the desired tract is achieved, up to a 30-Fr rod over which is passed a 30/34-Fr plastic

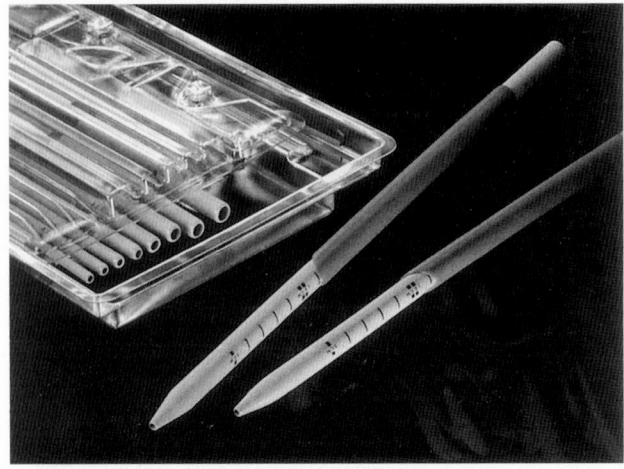

Figure 8-24. Amplatz dilators with sheaths.

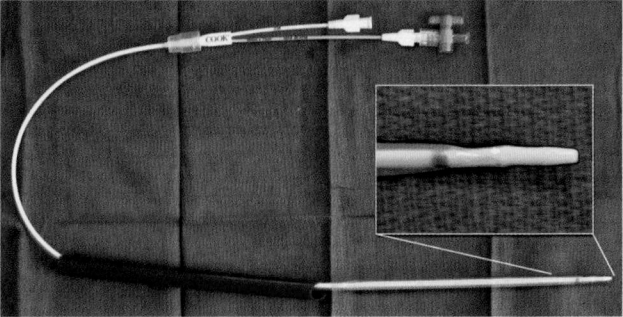

Figure 8-25. Balloon dilation catheter with preloaded sheath.

sheath. **The advantages of the rigid metal dilator system are that it is the most effective dilator, able to dilate even when there is dense perirenal scarring from previous procedures, and that it is inexpensive on a per-case basis because it is reusable. The disadvantage is that, for the same reason they are so effective, the rigid metal dilators can do considerable damage.** The depth of the dilation can be difficult to maintain accurately, especially when pushing against tough scar tissue. One group has modified the rigid metal rods, tapering the ends and adding centimeter markings (Shen et al, 2007).

Progressive semirigid plastic dilation sets (often referred to as "Amplatz" dilators after Kurt Amplatz, the senior author in the initial publication [Rusnak et al, 1982]) consist of progressively larger firm plastic (polyurethane) dilators that are passed over an 8-Fr PTFE guiding catheter that fits over a 0.035-inch guidewire (Fig. 8-24). The dilators are passed one after the other, not coaxially like the rigid metal dilators but progressively, advancing one dilator, removing it, advancing the next largest dilator, and so on until the final tract diameter is achieved. The working sheath is passed over the final dilator and then the dilator and 8-Fr catheter are removed, leaving the working wire and sheath in place. The dilators are made in increments of 2 Fr, but if the tissue being dilated is soft, then not every dilator needs to be used. **The advantage of the semirigid plastic dilation system is that trauma to the collecting system is theoretically less likely than with the rigid metal dilators (although experienced urologists have found no difference between the two systems in terms of safety), but the disadvantage is that hemorrhage can occur each time a dilator is withdrawn.** Current semirigid plastic dilators are sold as disposable devices, so they are more expensive on a per-case basis than rigid metal dilators. One retrospective comparison of the two techniques showed no other differences (Ozok et al, 2012).

Balloon dilators (Fig. 8-25) were developed to obviate the repetitive dilations of the rigid metal and semirigid plastic dilation systems, which are both time consuming and potentially dangerous. This is the most common dilation method for percutaneous renal surgery today (Benway and Nakada, 2008). The appropriate working sheath is back-loaded onto the balloon dilation catheter, which is passed over the working wire until the radiopaque marker is at the intended depth of dilation (Fig. 8-26A). The dilating balloon is inflated with a pressure syringe. A "waist" appears at the site(s) of greatest resistance, usually the abdominal wall fascia and the renal capsule (Fig. 8-26B). After the balloon is fully expanded (Fig. 8-26C), the working sheath is passed over the balloon (Fig. 8-26D) (Fig. 8-27 on the Expert Consult website). The balloon catheter has a "shoulder," which is the portion between the end of the balloon and the point at which the maximal diameter is achieved. The sheath should not be passed beyond the maximal diameter of the balloon because this can cause significant injury.

Balloon dilators, which are expensive one-time-use devices, are less effective than rigid metal and semirigid plastic dilation systems in densely scarred tissue but are more effective when the kidney is hypermobile (Kumar and Keeley, 2008). Most (Heggagi et al, 1991; Davidoff and Bellman, 1997; Safak et al, 2003; Kukreja et al, 2004), but not all (Gonen et al, 2008a; Wezel et al, 2009), single-series reports have suggested that hemorrhage and transfusion rates are less with the balloon dilators compared with rigid metal and semirigid plastic dilators. In a large multi-institutional study, however, balloon dilation was associated with longer operative time and greater bleeding and transfusion rates compared to rigid metal and semirigid plastic dilators (Lopes et al, 2011). Baseline differences between the groups, including more stones per kidney and more frequent treatment of staghorn calculi in the balloon dilation, may have created bias against balloon dilation.

In an effort to simplify dilation of the renal access tract further, a number of single-step techniques have been described. The simplest is passage of the final semirigid plastic dilator without previous dilation by the smaller dilators (Frattini et al, 2001). A meta-analysis of 4 randomized controlled trials comparing a single plastic dilator with sequential rigid metal dilators suggested that the former was associated with reduced access and fluoroscopy times without increased complications (Li et al, 2013b). Devices designed specifically for single-step dilation include a balloon dilator with an expandable sheath (Pathak and Bellman, 2005; Baldwin et al, 2006; Maynes et al, 2008; Kalpee et al, 2012) and a rigid dilator with an expandable sheath (Goharderakhshan et al, 2001). Preliminary results with these devices appear favorable.

The most common cause of difficult tract dilation is previous renal surgery (Joel et al, 2005). Densely scarred kidneys present a challenge. Even if semirigid plastic or rigid metal dilators fail, novel uses of devices such as Collings knives and atherotomy cutting balloons can be used (Davis et al, 1991; Williams et al, 2008). One group has reportedly used a bipolar resectoscope with a plasma vaporization electrode to enlarge the percutaneous tract, and in their randomized controlled trial there were some advantages over balloon dilation (Chiang et al, 2013).

Modifications in Special Situations

In cases of anomalous kidneys (malrotated, ptotic, ectopic, horseshoe, and other fused kidneys), alteration of the percutaneous approach to the upper urinary tract collecting system may be necessary. As noted earlier, in some situations real-time guidance of the needle puncture with CT or MRI might be considered, and ultrasonographic guidance may be useful, but in most cases preoperative CT or magnetic resonance suffices. Because the orientation of some organs might change with patient position, imaging in the intended position of surgery might be useful. **Preoperative cross-sectional imaging of anomalous kidneys helps plan patient position, choice of calyx, and orientation of the tract, taking into account distance of the kidney from the skin, calyceal orientation, vasculature, and the relative orientation of adjacent organs.**

Horseshoe kidneys frequently require percutaneous intervention. Although antegrade access into horseshoe kidneys is

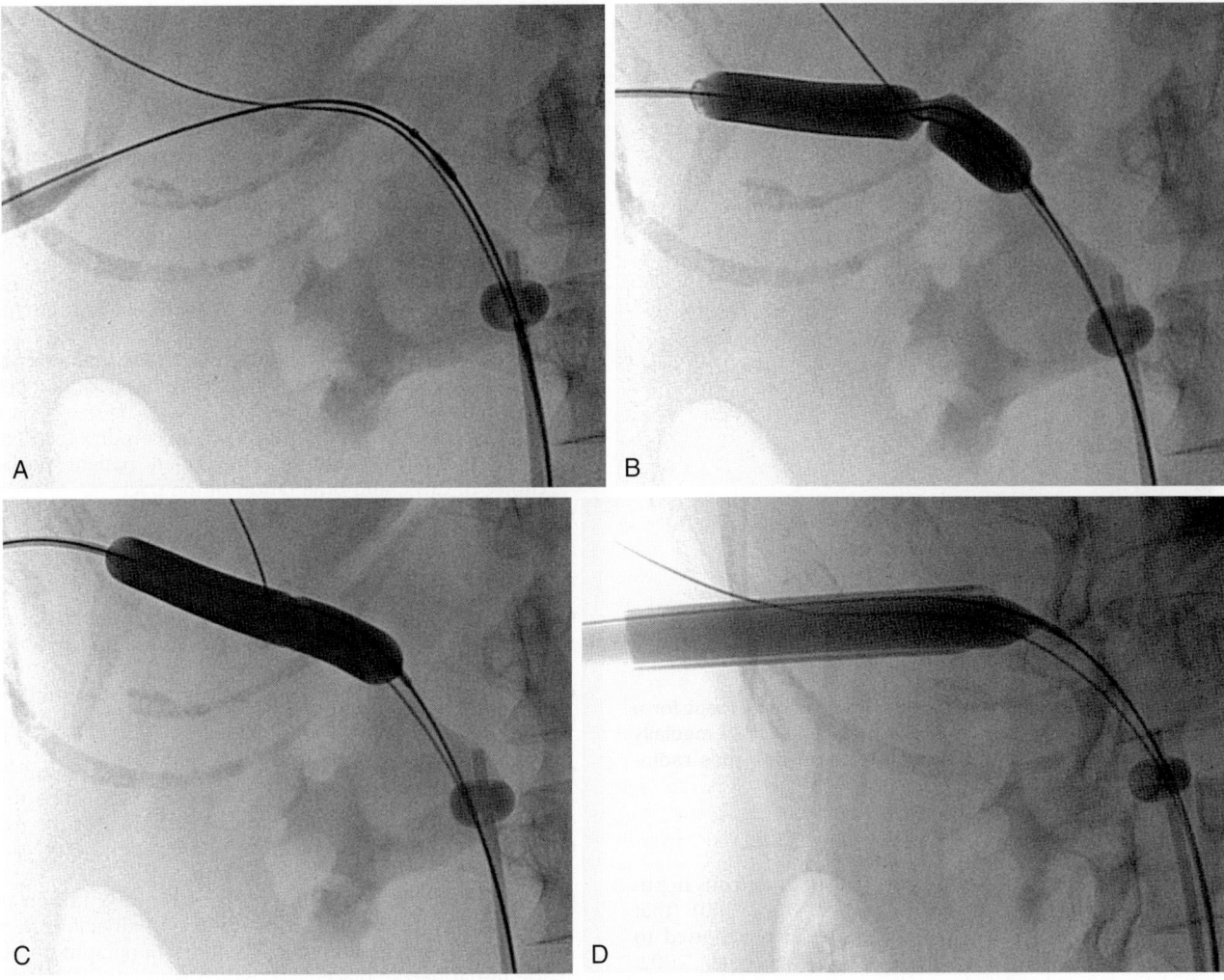

Figure 8-26. **Balloon dilation of tract and placement of working sheath. A, Balloon catheter is inserted over wire, with distal radiopaque marker at the intended depth of dilation. B, "Waist" appears as balloon is inflated. C, Balloon is fully expanded. D, Sheath is passed over balloon, taking care not to advance it beyond the point of maximal diameter of the balloon.**

somewhat different than into normal kidneys, standard techniques can generally still be used. CT or MRI should be considered for preoperative assessment of horseshoe kidneys, both to assess for the possibility of retrorenal colon (Skoog et al, 1985) and to assess the vasculature and relationship of the calyces to the anticipated puncture site. In a series of 12 patients undergoing percutaneous nephrolithotomy in horseshoe kidneys, 5 had bowel posterior to the kidney on CT (Al-Otaibi and Hosking, 1999). Horseshoe kidneys often have extra and eccentric calyces that can be difficult to access. In other ways, however, percutaneous access to a horseshoe kidney is more favorable than in normal kidneys. The anteroposterior tilt of the kidney is prominent, which makes the upper pole the most superficial and posterior aspect of the horseshoe kidney. In addition, the upper pole is usually inferior to the ribs. **Upper pole access is useful in horseshoe kidneys because this is the easiest calyx to enter, the puncture rarely needs to be supracostal, and it provides excellent access to most of the kidney and the ureter owing to the alignment of the long axis of the moiety** (Fig. 8-28). The initial entry into a horseshoe kidney is more medial than in normal kidneys and can pass through the paraspinous musculature. The distance to the lower pole and ureter can be great in an obese or muscular patient, such that extra-long rigid nephroscopes or flexible nephroscopy may be necessary. In some cases, middle calyceal access is preferred because the upper pole is so far away from the pathology, but lower pole calyces are usually not safely accessible with direct percutaneous puncture. The vasculature of

horseshoe kidneys is aberrant, but vessels enter and exit the kidney in an anteromedial location (except for some at the isthmus), so direct vessel injury is rare with well-planned access (Janetschek and Kunzel, 1988). Overall, among a total of 256 percutaneous procedures (primarily nephrolithotomy) recently reported in horseshoe kidneys, there were 11 (4.3%) major hemorrhagic complications and only 1 (<0.4%) colon injury (Al-Otaibi and Hosking, 1999; Shokeir et al, 2004; Lojanapiwat, 2005; Darabi Mahboub et al, 2007; Mosavi-Bahar et al, 2007; Viola et al, 2007; Majidpour and Yousefinejad, 2008; Miller et al, 2008; Symons et al, 2008; Gupta et al, 2009).

Another way to access anomalous kidneys is with an anterior approach using laparoscopic assistance. This is most applicable to pelvic ectopic kidneys because a posterior approach is often blocked by the bony pelvis, although laparoscopic assistance has been used for percutaneous nephrolithotomy of a large calculus in an anteriorly directed calyx in the isthmus of a horseshoe kidney (Maheshwari et al, 2004b) and a large calculus in an anterior diverticulum of a horseshoe kidney (Wong and Zimmerman, 2005). The bowels can be mobilized off the surface of the kidney laparoscopically, and the access needle is passed through the anterior abdominal wall into the kidney under vision from the laparoscope. Retrograde assistance is still desirable because opacifying the collecting system assists in simultaneous fluoroscopic confirmation of calyceal entry and wire passage. Dilation and sheath insertion can be assessed both laparoscopically and fluoroscopically. In a

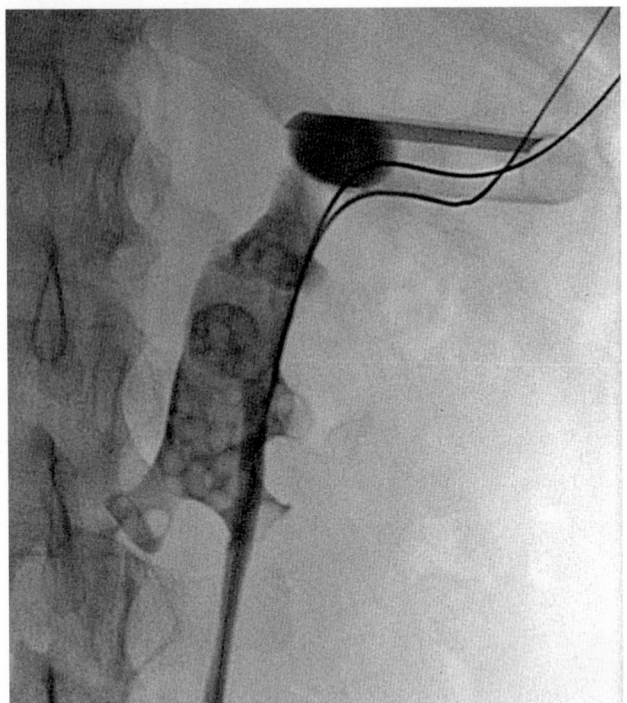

Figure 8-28. Percutaneous access sheath (radiolucent except for a radiopaque stripe) in upper pole of horseshoe kidney. Note medially directed lower pole calyx. Although not apparent from this radiograph, the access site is subcostal.

series of 12 laparoscopically directed antegrade percutaneous nephrolithotomies into pelvic kidneys published since 2001 that described a total of 35 patients, all procedures were reported to be successful and without complications (Troxel et al, 2002; Maheshwari et al, 2004a; Santos et al, 2004; Aron et al, 2005b; Aquil et al, 2006; Goel et al, 2006; Matlaga et al, 2006; El-Kappany et al, 2007; Mousavi-Bahar et al, 2008; Gupta et al, 2009; Tahmaz et al, 2009; Tepeler et al, 2013). As a simpler alternative to laparoscopic assistance, anterior percutaneous access into pelvic kidneys using a supine oblique position with a pad under the ipsilateral hemipelvis, as well as using ultrasonography to assess for intervening bowel, has been reported to be a safe technique in selected patients (Desai and Jasani, 2000; Mosavi-Bahar et al, 2007). If bone does not intervene between the appropriate calyx and the skin, then a posterior approach can be used just above the iliac bone (Atmaca et al, 2007) or through the greater sciatic foramen (Watterson et al, 2001).

Transplanted kidneys also mandate changes in the approach to percutaneous access of the upper urinary tract. The transplanted kidney, typically positioned extraperitoneally in the iliac fossa, has variable angles of the calyces depending on the placement of the kidney by the transplant surgeon. The usual approach is from the anterolateral direction, with the patient in the supine position. **Percutaneous nephrostomy is the preferred approach to obstruction and for endoscopy of the collecting system in the transplant kidney** (Mostafa et al, 2008). Ultrasonography is most convenient for initial access to the collecting system because retrograde assistance for fluoroscopy is difficult owing to the site and angle of the reimplanted ureter. Fluoroscopy can then be used as needed to facilitate subsequent steps. The dense fibrosis that often surrounds a transplant kidney can make dilation of the tract difficult, and semirigid plastic or rigid metal dilators may be necessary if balloon dilation fails. Of 75 percutaneous procedures in transplant kidneys reported in 10 recent series that used ultrasonographically and/or fluoroscopically directed percutaneous access, all but six were technically successful and there were no major complications (Francesca et al, 2002; Klingler et al, 2002; Challacombe et al, 2005a; He et al,

2007; Krambeck et al, 2008b; Rifaioglu et al, 2008; Wyatt et al, 2009; Oliveira et al, 2011; Stravodimos et al, 2012; Verrier et al, 2012).

KEY POINTS: OBTAINING PERCUTANEOUS ACCESS

- Optimally, the urologist is present at the time percutaneous access is attained, either performing the procedure or actively directing the radiologist.
- If there is increased likelihood of bacteriuria, preprocedure urine culture is recommended. Periprocedural antimicrobial prophylaxis is recommended in all cases.
- Except for aspirin in some cases, oral anticoagulant or antiplatelet activity medications should be discontinued before percutaneous renal surgery.
- Preoperative cross-sectional imaging of complex cases, especially anomalous kidneys, helps plan patient position, choice of calyx, and orientation of the tract.
- Supine and flank positions offer some potential benefits over prone positioning in certain settings, but surgeon preference generally can determine the choice of position for percutaneous renal surgery.
- In the prone position, the preferred calyces are the posterior ones. Percutaneous access should never be directly into an infundibulum or the renal pelvis.
- An upper pole calyx is generally the most versatile site through which to enter the upper urinary tract collecting system.
- Subcostal access is the safest route to the kidney, but if entry directly above the 12th rib provides the best access to the optimal calyx, then the benefit generally exceeds the risk.
- Retrograde assistance facilitates antegrade access to the upper urinary tract collecting system.
- Ultrasonography and fluoroscopy are both commonly used to guide percutaneous access to the intrarenal collecting system. A useful combination is ultrasonography to guide the initial needle placement, which is followed by fluoroscopy to confirm that the desired calyx has been accessed and to direct and monitor the subsequent steps of the procedure.

POSTPROCEDURAL NEPHROSTOMY DRAINAGE

The final surgical consideration after percutaneous renal surgery is deciding which drain(s), if any, to insert into the upper urinary tract collecting system. Options include an externalized nephrostomy tube or nephroureteral stent, an internal or externalized ureteral stent, or no drainage tube at all. Additional discussion of these options can be found in Chapter 6.

Nephrostomy Tube

For years, the standard drainage after percutaneous surgery of the upper urinary tract collecting system has been an externalized nephrostomy tube. There are a variety of choices for postoperative nephrostomy tubes.

Balloon Catheters

The Foley and Councill catheters used for transurethral drainage can be used as nephrostomy tubes as well (Fig. 8-29). These tubes come in a range of diameters; typically 16- to 24-Fr catheters are used for postoperative nephrostomy drainage. **The 5-mL retention balloon might be too large for some collecting systems and does not need to be completely inflated.** The balloon can cause calyceal obstruction if it is pulled into an infundibulum. **Saline or water should be used to inflate the balloon because viscous contrast material** might hinder emptying of the balloon when removal is attempted. An advantage of the Councill catheter is the ability to pass a small-caliber catheter through the end hole and down the ureter, providing more secure access to the upper urinary tract collecting system and maintaining ureteral patency. **All nephrostomy tubes, even ones with robust internal retention devices, should be fixed to the skin externally with a suture or other mechanism.** External fixation of a tube, however, does not necessarily prevent internal dislodgement of the tube. Especially in a large patient, the distance from the skin to the upper urinary tract collecting system can change with patient movement, and the tube (fixed at the skin) can pull out of the kidney. **The potential for tube dislodgement is one of the best arguments in favor of nephrostomy tubes that have some extension down the ureter to maintain a conduit to the upper urinary tract collecting system, even if the renal pelvic portion of the tube is pulled out of the kidney.**

Malecot Catheter

The wings of the Malecot catheter expand when the catheter is at rest, providing a modest but atraumatic and nonobstructive retention mechanism (Fig. 8-30A). When the catheter is being placed or removed, a stiffener is inserted through it to push on the distal end of the Malecot tip and straighten the wings. During removal this stiffener can misalign with the Malecot tip if the tube is not straight; pulling the catheter back until the tube is straight helps the stiffener line up properly. **The Malecot catheter is also available with an extension that is directed down the ureter. This modification is called a "re-entry" catheter, because it simplifies placing a guidewire through the Malecot catheter and down the ureter into the bladder** (Fig. 8-30B). The extension is long enough (18 cm) so that in most patients the Malecot tube can be withdrawn until the wings are externalized and a guidewire can be placed into the ureter. Malecot catheters for renal use are large-bore catheters, ranging from 16 to 30 Fr, although Malecot catheters as small as 8 Fr are available.

Cope Catheter

Cope nephrostomy tubes provide a more secure retention mechanism. **A string exits the catheter a few centimeters from the distal tip and then re-enters the catheter near the tip** (Fig. 8-31). **Pulling on the string forms a secure coil that is not easily dislodged from the renal pelvis.** The string is fixed at the external end of the tube with a locking mechanism or by wrapping it around the tube and fixing it in place with a rubber cuff. Cope catheters use the same coil shape used in pigtail ureteral stents. The active reinforcement of the coil strength by the string is thought to provide more secure retention than the passive coil of a pigtail, although one comparative study did not confirm this (Chuang et al, 2011), and as such Cope catheters have replaced pigtail catheters for most percutaneous uses. Cope nephrostomy tubes, ranging from 6 to 14 Fr in diameter, can be used for simple upper urinary tract drainage and instillation procedures, as well as after percutaneous surgery.

Nephroureteral Stent

The Cope retention mechanism is also used in nephroureteral stents. A nephroureteral stent has a renal coil like that of a Cope nephrostomy tube, but the tube continues on to a ureteral extension that travels down the ureter to end in a passive pigtail that rests in the bladder (Fig. 8-32). The ureteral portion can be the same diameter as the nephrostomy portion, or it can be narrower. A nephroureteral stent is passed percutaneously over a wire that ends in the bladder. After the end is coiled generously in the bladder, careful inspection of the fluoroscopy image shows the location of the side holes in the renal coil. By moving the catheter in and out while pulling on the string and rotating the external portion of the tube clockwise, the Cope retention coil is formed in the renal pelvis (Figs. 8-33 and 8-34 on the Expert Consult website) **A nephroureteral**

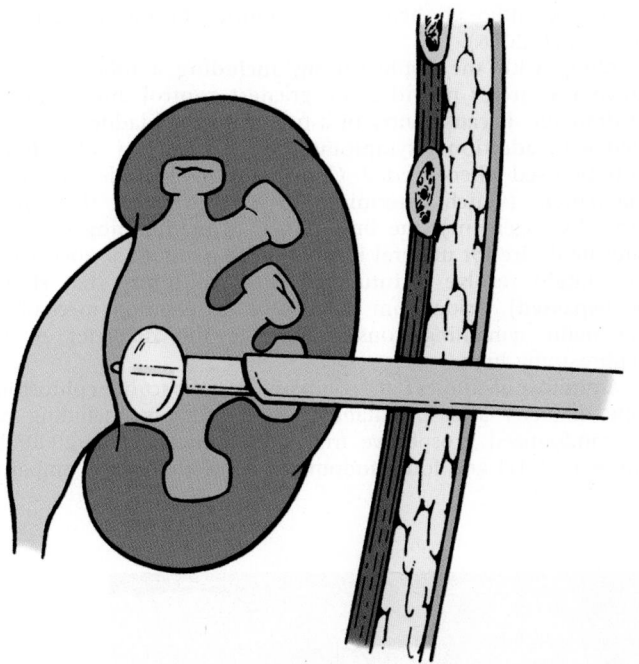

Figure 8-29. **Councill catheter.**

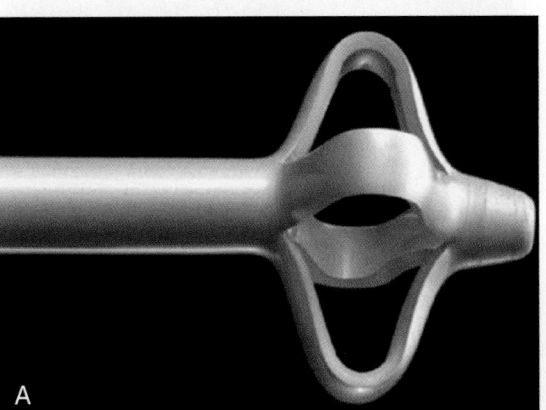

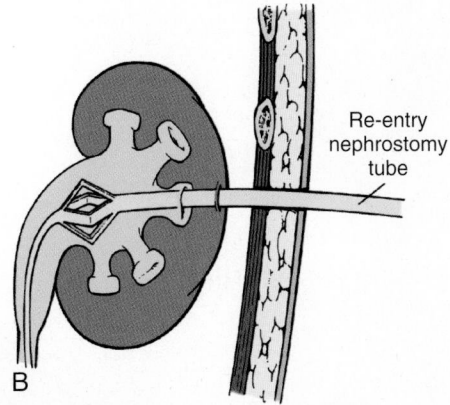

Re-entry nephrostomy tube

Figure 8-30. **A, Malecot catheter. B, Malecot catheter with ureteral extension ("re-entry" catheter).**

stent offers excellent control of the entire upper urinary tract, from renal pelvis to bladder, and is unlikely to become dislodged. Nephroureteral stents are available in diameters of 8.5 or 10.2 Fr, and the standard lengths (from renal to bladder coil) are 20 to 28 cm.

Circle Catheter

A final type of nephrostomy tube is the circle nephrostomy tube (Fig. 8-35), which is secure, easily exchanged, causes little trauma, rarely occludes, and provides excellent drainage and avenue for irrigation of the renal pelvis. The circle nephrostomy tube requires two percutaneous access sites to the kidney, and this tube is most useful when maintenance of two tracts is desired, such as for irrigation of the renal pelvis or if more than one access is necessary for second-look nephroscopy (Kim et al, 2005). After obtaining access at two distant calyces, a flexible nephroscope or flexible ureteroscope passed over one wire is used to grasp the wire coming from the other site. When the endoscope is withdrawn, the wire is now in position to guide placement of the circle nephrostomy tube. Radiopaque markers on the tube delineate the location of the

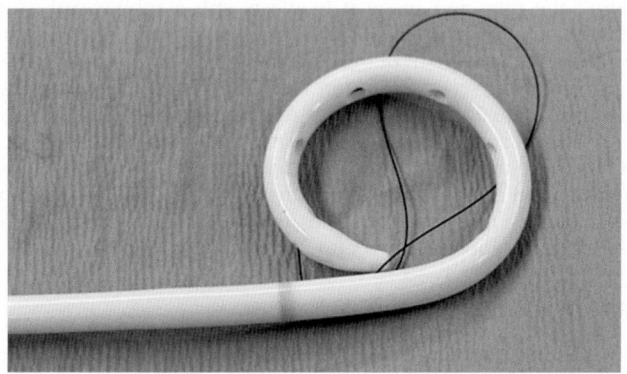

Figure 8-31. **Cope catheter, with the retention string loosened for demonstration.**

drainage holes, which should be maintained within the intrarenal collecting system. External drainage of the circle nephrostomy tube requires a Y-connector.

General Considerations

The advantages of a postoperative nephrostomy tube include good drainage and control of the upper urinary tract, and maintenance of percutaneous access for additional procedures. It was initially thought that a postoperative nephrostomy served to tamponade the nephrostomy tract and reduce hemorrhage, but subsequent studies have suggested that this is not the case. When hemorrhage does occur, however, the larger caliber of a nephrostomy tube provides better drainage of the upper urinary tract collecting system than does an internal ureteral stent. In addition, if a large perforation has occurred during the procedure, the additional diversion of urine away from the site might be advantageous. When a nephrostomy tube is left in place following percutaneous renal surgery, it is usually in the dilated access site. At least one group has attempted to reduce the discomfort associated with supracostal percutaneous renal surgery by placing a small-caliber postoperative nephrostomy tube in a new subcostal site and leaving the dilated supracostal access site without a nephrostomy tube (although there was no control cohort for comparison) (Kim et al, 2006).

Along with the nephrostomy, including a tube that goes down the ureter provides the greatest control and assurance of drainage. Because entry of a tube into the bladder is associated with additional symptoms, however, such a tube should only be used when needed. Considerations include the size of the patient (which determines to a large extent the risk of tube dislodgement), the importance of maintaining drainage, and the desire for ureteral intubation (e.g., ureteral obstruction that might resolve if intubated, ureteral injury that should be bypassed). Aside from the choice of retention mechanism, the main remaining consideration is the diameter of the nephrostomy tube.

A number of studies have compared the impact of nephrostomy tube diameter after percutaneous renal surgery, including two nonrandomized prospective trials (Maheshwari et al, 2000; De Sio et al, 2011) and four randomized controlled trials comparing

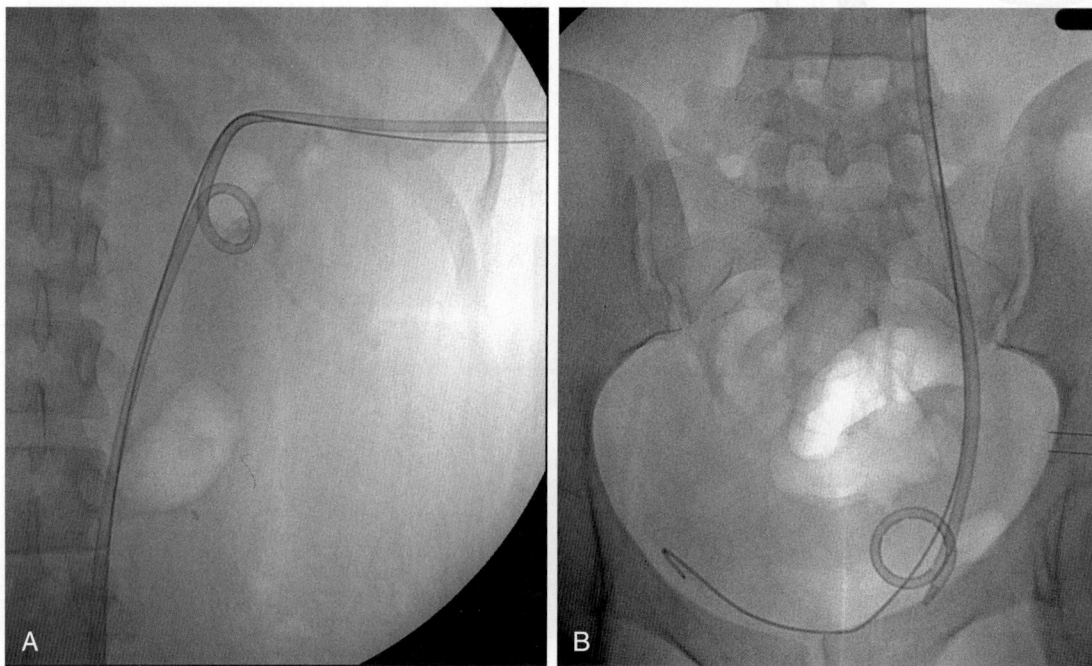

Figure 8-32. **Nephroureteral stent. A, Renal coil. B, Bladder coil.**

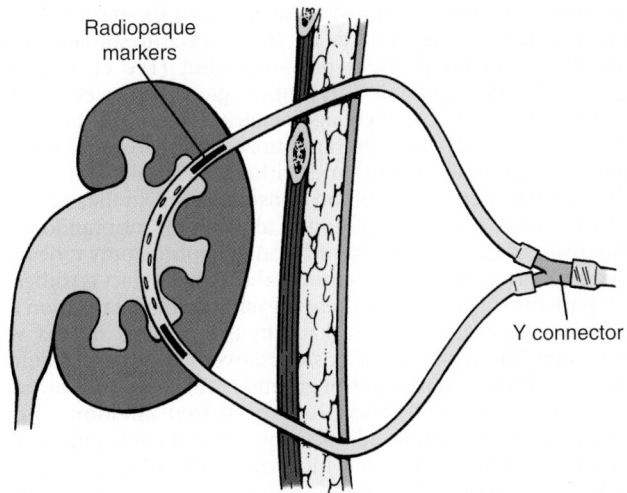

Radiopaque
markers

Y connector

Figure 8-35. Circle nephrostomy tube.

large-caliber tubes (20 to 24 Fr) to small-caliber tubes (8 to 18 Fr) (Liatsikos et al, 2002; Pietrow et al, 2003; Desai et al, 2004; Marcovich et al, 2004). **Among the six studies, comprising a total of 215 patients with nephrostomy tubes, five showed less pain and two reported less urinary leakage in the patients with smaller tubes. Bleeding did not increase in any of the studies for the groups with smaller tubes.** Only one study showed no benefit to the smaller tube (Marcovich et al, 2004). Although tube diameter is not related to bleeding overall, the removal of larger tubes occasionally can be followed by immediate hemorrhage; this is rare with smaller tubes. As such, large-caliber nephrostomy tubes should be removed in a radiology suite where there is the opportunity for immediate replacement of the tube. Small-caliber tubes can be removed safely at the bedside after a period of clamping to assess clinically for distal ureteral obstruction.

"Tubeless" with Ureteral Stent

Wickham and colleagues (1984) initially proposed a "tubeless" percutaneous procedure—one that omits the postoperative nephrostomy tube. This practice never met with widespread acceptance, especially after Winfield and colleagues (1986) reported disastrous outcomes with this technique. The concept was revived in 1997 by Bellman and colleagues (1997), with the addition of an internal ureteral stent left in place for a week or two. Since then, many studies have evaluated the practice of omitting the nephrostomy tube after percutaneous renal surgery. Although this technique is called "tubeless," most series employ a ureteral stent for a short period postoperatively.

Options for ureteral stenting without a nephrostomy tube after percutaneous renal surgery include an internal ureteral stent that is removed cystoscopically, an internal ureteral stent with an attached string that exits out the flank to allow removal of the ureteral stent without cystoscopy, and an externalized (out the urethra) ureteral stent that is removed along with the urethral catheter to which it is attached. The potential advantages of omitting the nephrostomy tube after percutaneous renal surgery include decreased pain and analgesic use, avoidance of an external drainage device, abbreviated hospital stay, and decreased health care costs (secondary to shortening the duration of hospitalization). Since the report of Bellman and colleagues (1997), many studies including several randomized controlled trials have evaluated the omission of a nephrostomy tube postoperatively with the placement of an internal ureteral stent. It is important to note that most of these studies excluded patients with significant bleeding or perforation or those for whom a second percutaneous procedure was anticipated.

A meta-analysis of tubeless percutaneous nephrolithotomies published in 2012 included 9 randomized controlled trials involving 547 patients (Shen et al, 2012). The results were stratified into 4 groups relative to the postprocedure drainage: tubeless with internal ureteral stent, small nephrostomy tube (8 to 9 Fr), medium nephrostomy tube (16 to 18 Fr), and large nephrostomy tube (20 to 24 Fr). The meta-analysis demonstrated that hospital stay and postoperative pain were reduced in the tubeless group compared to the medium and large tube groups, but were similar in the tubeless and small tube groups. There were no significant differences between the tubeless group and any of the nephrostomy tube groups with regard to fever/infection, transfusion, or operative time. In two earlier meta-analyses that combined the nephrostomy groups into two instead of three groups, 4 to 10 Fr versus 14 to 24 Fr (Yuan et al, 2011) and 8 to 9 Fr versus 14 to 26 Fr (Ni et al, 2011), shorter hospital stay and reduced postoperative pain were noted in the tubeless groups even in comparison to the small nephrostomy group. Thus the preponderance of evidence suggests that **tubeless percutaneous nephrolithotomy leads to shorter hospital stay and reduced postoperative pain in comparison to use of large postprocedure nephrostomy tubes, but that these benefits are less certain in comparison to small nephrostomy tubes.** Subsequent randomized controlled trials (Kara et al, 2010; Etemadian et al, 2011; Marchant et al, 2011; Shoma and Elshal, 2012; Lu et al, 2013) and one large multi-institutional matched case-control study involving 488 patients (Cormio et al, 2013) have yielded similar results with the exception of one study that indicated no benefit to the tubeless approach when the nephrostomy tube in the comparison group was removed the morning after the procedure (Mishra et al, 2010). This latter study was underpowered, however, with only 22 patients; all trends favored the tubeless group, but the differences did not reach statistical significance. In one randomized controlled trial, omission of the nephrostomy tube was associated with decreased cost (Feng et al, 2001). The tubeless approach appears to be safe even when supracostal access is used (Shah et al, 2006b; Jun-Ou and Lojanapiwat, 2010; Duty et al, 2013) and in the setting of bilateral simultaneous procedures (Gupta et al, 2003; Shah et al, 2005).

There are some disadvantages to using an internal ureteral stent as an alternative to a nephrostomy tube, however, including loss of the percutaneous tract for a secondary procedure and the cost, inconvenience, and discomfort associated with an internal ureteral stent that requires cystoscopic removal at a later date. To obviate the problems associated with the ureteral stent, several groups have offered alternatives including insertion of an externalized ureteral stent or insertion of an internal stent with an attached string that exits out the flank. In both cases the stent can then be removed before hospital discharge without an additional procedure. Goh and Wolf (1999) first reported the use of an externalized ureteral stent (single pigtail) as an alternative to a postoperative nephrostomy tube. Since then there have been a number of reports of this option (Lojanapiwat et al, 2001; Abou-Elela et al, 2007; Karami et al, 2007; Rana and Mithani, 2007; Al-Ba'adani et al, 2008) including three randomized controlled trials, one comparing an externalized ureteral stent to a large-caliber nephrostomy tube, which suggested a benefit in terms of reduced narcotic use and length of hospital stay (Tefekli et al, 2007), and two comparing internal and external ureteral stents, which showed no difference between the two techniques except for the association of the external stent with a lack of outpatient stent-related symptoms in one study (Gonen et al, 2009) and shorter hospital stay and less hematocrit drop in another study (Mercado et al, 2013). Shpall and colleagues (2007) described the modification of leaving the attached string on the stent and placing the stent "upside down" so that the string can exit the flank. They described removing the stent as an outpatient 3 and 12 days postoperatively, but since then others have reported removing the stent at the bedside on the first postoperative day (Berkman et al, 2008). Use of a Polaris Loop stent (Boston Scientific, Natick, MA) placed "upside down" offers less resistance at the time of removal (Fig. 8-36).

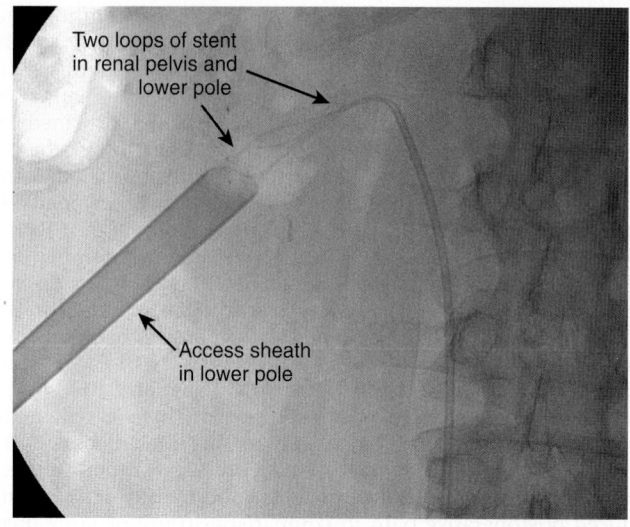

Two loops of stent in renal pelvis and lower pole

Access sheath in lower pole

Figure 8-36. Use of a Polaris Loop stent (Boston Scientific, Natick, MA) placed "upside down." An attached string is left exiting the flank, which allows removal of the stent without an additional procedure.

These modifications of nephrostomy tube omission avoid many of the disadvantages of an internal ureteral stent but still leave the problem of loss of access in case a secondary procedure is required. With improved endoscopes, better ancillary tools, and growing experience with percutaneous surgery, the need for secondary procedures is declining. In properly selected patients including those who do not for some other reason need external drainage (e.g., pyonephrosis, significant bleeding, significant collecting system injury) and those who are unlikely to need a secondary procedure, omission of the postoperative nephrostomy tube appears to be safe and effective.

No Drainage Tube

More recently, the idea of a "totally tubeless" percutaneous renal surgery, omitting both the nephrostomy tube and ureteral catheter, has been reintroduced. This can be considered in selected patients with low-volume stones, atraumatic single access, and no hemorrhage, perforation, or obstruction. A meta-analysis of five randomized controlled trials and four nonrandomized comparative studies comparing "totally tubeless" percutaneous nephrolithotomy to percutaneous nephrolithotomy with a postprocedure nephrostomy tube suggests that the "totally tubeless" approach reduces hospital stay, analgesic requirement, and time to return to normal activity without increasing complications (Zhong et al, 2013). A more pertinent comparison is "totally tubeless" versus internal stent without nephrostomy tube ("tubeless"); one retrospective nonrandomized comparison showed that the "totally tubeless" approach was associated with a longer hospital stay than the "tubeless" approach (Istanbulluoglu et al, 2010).

Adjuncts to Drainage without Nephrostomy Tubes

One of the concerns with any approach that omits the nephrostomy tube after percutaneous renal surgery is that of hemorrhage from the tract. **Although the evidence from randomized controlled trials suggests that the size or presence of the nephrostomy tube does not affect the degree of postoperative bleeding, there is still a potential for dramatic bleeding after any percutaneous procedure—and such bleeding would be more problematic without a nephrostomy tube in place.** Several groups have described adjuncts intended to enhance hemostasis of the percutaneous tract including placing a fascial suture (Li et al, 2011), direct monopolar cauterization of the tract (Mouracade et al, 2008; Chang et al, 2011), cryotreatment of the tract (Okeke et al, 2009), and

insertion/instillation of hemostatic agents into the tract including oxidized cellulose (Aghamir et al, 2006), gelatin sponge (Singh et al, 2008), gelatin granules plus thrombin (Lee et al, 2004b; Nagele et al, 2006; Li et al, 2011), fibrin glue (Noller et al, 2004; Gudeman et al, 2012), and collagen matrix coated with fibrin glue (Cormio et al, 2012). One nonrandomized comparison of percutaneous nephrolithotomy with and without electrode cauterization of the tract reported a lower blood transfusion rate in the first group (1.2% vs. 6.5%, respectively) (Jou et al, 2004). A nonrandomized comparison of tract cryotherapy without a nephrostomy tube in 30 patients versus a 24-Fr nephrostomy tube without tract cryotherapy in 30 patients suggested that there was shorter hospitalization and less hemorrhage and urine leakage in the patients treated with cryotherapy. The high rate of postoperative hemorrhage requiring angioembolization in the control group (13%) confounds the analysis (Okeke et al, 2009). There have been four randomized controlled trials of hemostatic adjuncts for percutaneous renal surgery without nephrostomy tubes, which compared patients managed without hemostatic adjuncts with those managed with gelatin sponge (Singh et al, 2008), oxidized cellulose (Aghamir et al, 2006), fibrin glue (Shah et al, 2006a), and collagen matrix coated with fibrin glue (Cormio et al, 2012). None of the three studies showed an impact of the adjunct on measures of hemostasis (postoperative hematocrit, hemorrhage, and/or blood transfusions). Narcotic use was less in the adjunct group in two of the three studies in which it was evaluated. Hospital stay and urinary leakage were each assessed in three studies, and each was improved in two studies. Some nonrandomized studies also have suggested a shortened hospitalization and/or reduced narcotic use after tract hemostatic maneuvers, but because improvements in hemostasis and urinary leakage are not consistently found, the mechanism for improvement in these secondary outcomes is not clear (Mikhail et al, 2003; Aron et al, 2004; Borin et al, 2005). Alternatives to local treatment of the tract include systemic enhancements to hemostasis. In one randomized trial, oral administration of the antifibrinolytic agent tranexamic acid was associated with less reduction in hematocrit and lower blood transfusion rate (Kumar et al, 2013). **Overall, the usefulness of any of the adjuncts for tract hemostasis is not certain and further study is necessary.**

> ### KEY POINTS: POSTPROCEDURAL NEPHROSTOMY DRAINAGE
>
> - The advantages of a postoperative nephrostomy tube include good drainage and control of the upper urinary tract, as well as maintenance of percutaneous access for additional procedures. Inclusion of an extension down the ureter provides the greatest control and assurance of drainage.
> - Small-caliber nephrostomy tubes are associated with less pain than large-caliber nephrostomy tubes and are not associated with any increased hemorrhage.
> - The use of a ureteral stent instead of a large-caliber nephrostomy tube is associated with reduced narcotic use and decreased length of hospitalization. The benefit of nephrostomy omission is less apparent when compared with a small-caliber nephrostomy. In properly selected patients, the use of a ureteral stent instead of a nephrostomy tube does not affect stone-free or complication rates.
> - Options for ureteral stenting without using a nephrostomy tube afterward include an internal ureteral stent that is removed cystoscopically, an internal ureteral stent removed by a string exiting out of the flank, and an externalized ureteral stent that is removed along with the urethral catheter to which it is taped.
> - Following straightforward procedures with atraumatic single access and no hemorrhage, perforation, or obstruction, some patients can be managed without a nephrostomy tube or a ureteral stent.
> - The usefulness of adjuncts for tract hemostasis is uncertain.

TRAINING IN PERCUTANEOUS ACCESS AND PROCEDURES

Efforts to enhance training for percutaneous surgery of the upper urinary tract have focused on obtaining percutaneous access. Summarizing their own experience and other reports (Allen et al, 2005; Tanriverdi et al, 2007), de la Rosette and colleagues (2008) estimated that a trainee must perform approximately 24 percutaneous nephrolithotomies to attain proficiency, whereas competence is not achieved until the experience includes 60 cases, and excellence is not obtained until more than 100 cases have been performed. The American College of Radiology's "Practice Guideline for the Performance of Percutaneous Nephrostomy" recommends that a physician must have performed at least 15 percutaneous nephrostomies as primary operator, with acceptable outcomes, to be considered qualified as a supervising physician (ACR, 2007). Training during residency is the most effective process for developing the skills, but maintenance of skills requires ongoing experience. In a survey of urologists who completed a single residency program, those trained in percutaneous access were more likely to perform percutaneous surgical procedures than those not trained in percutaneous access (92% vs. 33%). Of those who performed percutaneous surgery, urologists with training performed more procedures than those without training (14.0 vs. 3.3 procedures annually). However, only about one third of respondents in both groups continued to attain their own percutaneous access (27% vs. 11%) (Lee et al, 2004a).

Nonhuman models can also assist in training (Laguna et al, 2002). Inanimate trainers can be homemade using gelatin and a vinyl glove (Rock et al, 2010) and Limbs and Things (Savannah, GA) market a commercial model. Several biologic models using ex vivo porcine kidneys incorporate a body wall simulator composed of a chicken carcass (Hammond et al, 2004; Hacker et al, 2007) or full-thickness porcine skin including subcutaneous tissue and muscle, with or without ribs (Strohmaier and Giese, 2009; Imkamp et al, 2011; Qiu et al, 2011). The most advanced trainer is the PERC Mentor (Simbionix, Lod, Israel), a computer-assisted simulator for percutaneous access procedures guided by fluoroscopy (Fig. 8-37).

Some of the biologic models can be used to teach steps in the subsequent procedure (e.g., nephrolithotomy, endopyelotomy), but the main focus is on attaining percutaneous access. The PERC Mentor has undergone preclinical validation, confirming that training on the PERC Mentor improves performance on the PERC Mentor (Knudsen et al, 2006; Zhang et al, 2013), and that trained individuals more proficiently attain percutaneous renal access in a porcine in vivo model (Margulis et al, 2005), but validation of the impact on performance in the human operating room is lacking (Stern et al, 2007). At the least, these trainers can serve as an introduction for the trainee by orienting them to the necessary anatomic considerations and familiarizing them with the physical movements of the procedure. Whether these or other devices can be used to validate the skills of trainees and practitioners is unknown. Moreover, the most effective training will incorporate cognitive tasks as well as psychomotor ones (Tjiam et al, 2012; Mishra et al, 2013).

Taking simulation even farther, Bruyère and colleagues (2008) used computer-assisted design and rapid prototyping based on CT images to create a silicon model of a patient's kidney, complete with artificial flank and respiratory motion. After practicing percutaneous nephrolithotomy on the model several times, the percutaneous nephrolithotomy on the patient went smoothly using the practiced technique. Creating a specific renal model for each patient is too expensive and laborious for routine application currently, but with anticipated technical improvements, this iteration of "personalized medicine" might play a role in training and treatment planning.

COMPLICATIONS

Given enough time and access sites to the upper urinary tract collecting system, in most cases the primary goal of the percutaneous procedure can be achieved. The challenge with percutaneous surgery, then, is to do so while also avoiding complications. If complications do occur, then prompt recognition and management will usually prevent major morbidity. CT appears to be the most sensitive tool for determining postoperative complications (Semins et al, 2011; Gnessin et al, 2012). Some complications of percutaneous renal surgery are specific to the procedure, including migration of stone outside the kidney, retained foreign bodies such as tips of wires and probes, and tumor seeding of the percutaneous tract. In this section the general complications of percutaneous renal surgery are discussed.

Using the Dindo-modified Clavien system to categorize complications following percutaneous nephrolithotomy, 77% of patients in a systematic review of reports including a total of 11,929 patients experienced no complications (Clavien 0) (Seitz et al, 2012). An additional 11% of patients exhibited only minor deviations from the normal postoperative course (only minimal pharmacologic treatment, Clavien 1), and 7.0% showed Clavien 2 complications (includes additional pharmacologic treatment, blood transfusion, and parenteral nutrition). "Major" complications occurred in <5% of patients (4.1% Clavien 3, requiring surgical, endoscopic, or radiologic intervention; 0.6% Clavien 4, including life-threatening complications; 0.04% Clavien 5, mortality). Similar results were reported in a large multi-institutional study (including 5724 patients), which also used the Dindo-modified Clavien system (Labate et al, 2011). Of the patients, 79% had no complications, 16% had Clavien category 1 or 2 complications, and 4.2% had complications categorized as Clavien category 3 or greater.

Acute Hemorrhage

Acute hemorrhage is the most common significant complication of percutaneous access into the upper urinary tract collecting system. **Percutaneous nephrostomy alone results in hemorrhage requiring transfusion in 0.5% to 4% of procedures** (Radecka and Magnusson, 2004; Wah et al, 2004; ACR, 2007; Rana et al, 2007). **With the addition of percutaneous nephrolithotomy, likely owing to the larger caliber of the percutaneous tract and increased intrarenal manipulation, the incidence of hemorrhage requiring**

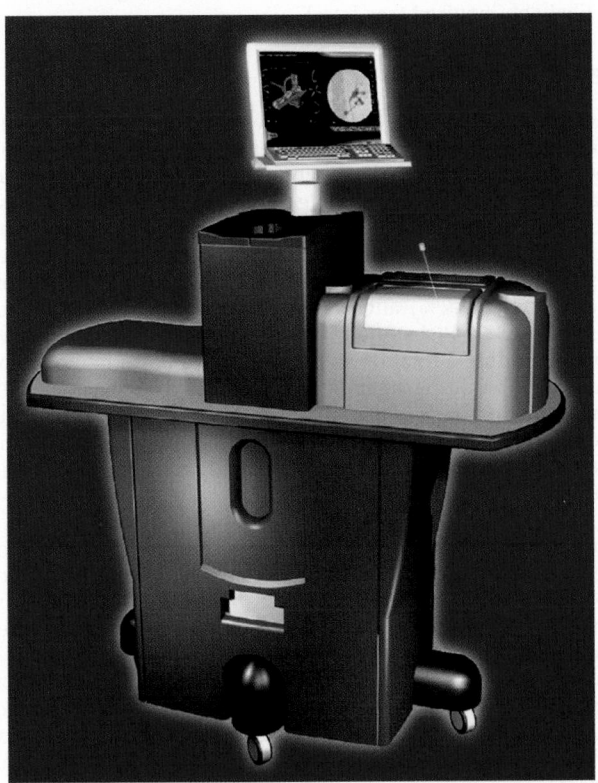

Figure 8-37. PERC Mentor (Simbionix, Lod, Israel).

blood transfusion rises to between 0.8% and 20% (Kukreja et al, 2004; Netto et al, 2005; Preminger et al, 2005; Muslumanoglu et al, 2006; Duvdevani et al, 2007; Chew et al, 2009; Tomaszewski et al, 2010b; Akman et al, 2011; Labate et al, 2011; Keoghane et al, 2012). This wide variation in transfusion rate, which likely is more variable than the rate of significant hemorrhage, reflects differences in the complexity of the procedure, patient factors, and physician triggers for the use of blood products. In a systematic review of reports including a total of 11,929 patients, a 7% blood transfusion rate was reported (Seitz et al, 2012). **Factors associated with hemorrhage during percutaneous renal surgery include patient characteristics, multiple access sites, supracostal access, increasing tract size, tract dilation with methods other than balloon dilation, prolonged operative time, and renal pelvic perforation** (Stoller et al, 1994; Martin et al, 1999; Kukreja et al, 2004; Netto et al, 2005; Hegarty and Desai, 2006; Chew et al, 2009; Rastinehad et al, 2009; Akman et al, 2011; Keoghane et al, 2012). In a large multi-institutional study including 5537 patients, the only factors associated with hemorrhage during percutaneous renal surgery were larger sheath size, prolonged operative time, and greater stone burden (Yamaguchi et al, 2011).

Technical errors predispose to hemorrhage as well. Infundibular entry risks injury to interlobar (infundibular) arteries. Access into an anterior calyx or any calyx that does not afford direct access to the pathology invites overly aggressive torquing of the sheath and rigid endoscope, which also can lead to hemorrhage. If direct access cannot be obtained, then flexible instrumentation should be considered. Additionally, misuse of any tool—lithotrites, resectoscopes, wires, sheaths, graspers, baskets, and so on—can cause hemorrhage.

Most hemorrhage occurs from the renal parenchyma, and in most cases this hemorrhage is not significant. Small arteries and veins are always injured to some degree by percutaneous entry into the kidney. Parenchymal bleeding is minimized by proper entry and dilation and by careful manipulation of the sheath, but it still can occur. **The access sheath provides intraoperative tamponade of parenchymal bleeding. Postoperatively, hemostasis is achieved by collapse of the parenchyma onto itself.** Unless the postoperative nephrostomy tube is as large as or larger than the sheath used during the procedure, it likely does not contribute to hemostasis. There is no difference in measures of postoperative bleeding between small (8- to 18-Fr) and large (20- to 28-Fr) tubes (Maheshwari et al, 2000; Liatsikos et al, 2002; Pietrow et al, 2003; Desai et al, 2004; Marcovich et al, 2004; De Sio et al, 2011), and randomized controlled trials suggest that hemorrhage is no greater when the nephrostomy tube is omitted altogether (Shen et al, 2012). **If there is noticeable bleeding from the tract after sheath removal following an otherwise unremarkable procedure, this suggests bleeding from intraparenchymal vessels.** Hemostatic maneuvers such as cauterization or placement of hemostatic material can be considered, **but in general the best management is to insert and occlude a nephrostomy tube, apply pressure to the incision, and allow the collecting system to clot off.** A tubeless approach is not advised in such cases because maintenance of percutaneous access to the upper tract might facilitate management. Nephrostomy tubes should not be irrigated on the day or evening of the procedure if they are not draining; it is best to allow the collecting system to remain occluded to tamponade bleeding. By the next morning, it is safe to irrigate the tube gently because hemostasis is more certain.

If the procedure was not complicated by bleeding, but severe hemorrhage occurs following sheath removal and is refractory to the hemostatic measures described earlier, then use of a Kaye Nephrostomy Tamponade Balloon (Cook Urological, Spencer, IN) should be considered. This is a nephrostomy tube surrounded by a balloon (Fig. 8-38) (Kaye and Clayman, 1986), which is inflated up to 36 Fr to tamponade the parenchymal bleeding just as the sheath did intraoperatively. This device should be removed under fluoroscopic guidance with guidewire access down the ureter in case tube reinsertion is required for recurrent bleeding.

Intraoperative hemorrhage from an injured vein or artery within the collecting system mandates cessation of the procedure

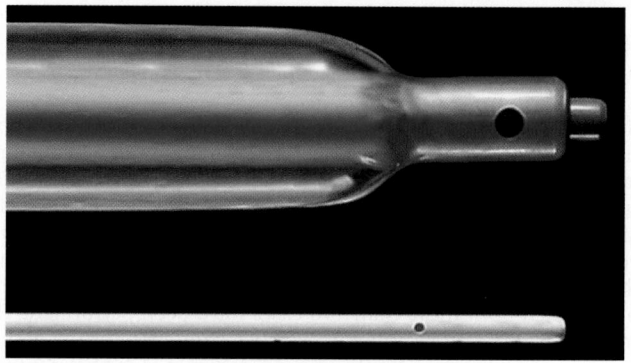

Figure 8-38. **Kaye Nephrostomy Tamponade Balloon.**

if vision is lost. **In most cases, especially if the injury appears to be venous, then placing a nephrostomy tube and letting the collecting system clot off is effective.** If this is not effective, however, Gupta and colleagues (1997) have described the insertion of a Councill catheter as a nephrostomy tube, with the balloon inflated slowly at the site where contrast material enters into the venous system until repeated nephrostography shows no more extravasation of contrast material (Fig. 8-39). A hole should be cut into the tube proximal to the balloon to provide drainage of calyces obstructed by the balloon (Fig. 8-40). Millard and associates (2010) have reported an addition to this technique, in which gelatin matrix hemostatic sealant is injected into the tract peripheral to the balloon occluding the renal injury and then a second catheter is inserted with the balloon placed just underneath the skin surface, such that the tract is occluded and the gelatin matrix hemostatic sealant contributes to hemostasis. Another alternative, described in one case of a large venous injury, is to place a large-bore catheter through the injury site into the main renal vein and then back it out several days later (Shaw et al, 2005). A small arterial injury can sometimes be addressed with fulguration under direct vision, but if this is not successful and bleeding does not cease with pressure, or in cases of significant arterial hemorrhage, then selective angioembolization will likely be required (see later).

Delayed Hemorrhage

Postoperative hemorrhage can occur with the nephrostomy tube in place, at time of tube removal, or after discharge from the hospital. **Approximately 1% of major percutaneous procedures are complicated by delayed hemorrhage requiring treatment** (Kessaris et al, 1995; Martin et al, 2000; Richstone et al, 2008; Tomaszewski et al, 2010b; Keoghane et al, 2012). In one large series, the incidence was greatest following percutaneous resection of upper tract urothelial carcinoma (3.2%) and least following percutaneous endopyelotomy (0.8%) (Richstone et al, 2008). In a systematic review of reports including a total of 11,929 patients, a 0.4% rate of delayed hemorrhage requiring treatment was reported (Seitz et al, 2012). **Delayed hemorrhage is usually a result of arteriovenous fistulas or arterial pseudoaneurysms, with the latter being more common.** Arteriovenous fistulas occur when a paired set of artery and vein is injured, and arterial blood enters directly into the vein (Fig. 8-41). The weak vein wall cannot sustain the high arterial pressure and ruptures. Bleeding into the collecting system is most commonly noted, but it can be outside the kidney as well. The latter should be suspected if the hematocrit falls but the urine remains relatively clear. It can be confirmed with CT or ultrasonography. An arterial pseudoaneurysm occurs when an artery is injured, clots off, and then intermittently ruptures, often clotting off again at variable intervals (Fig. 8-42A). Continuous bleeding suggests an arteriovenous fistula, and intermittent bleeding suggests arterial pseudoaneurysm, but the distinction is not critical because treatment is the same. In a large series conducted by Kessaris and colleagues (1995), of the 0.8% of 2200 patients requiring treatment for

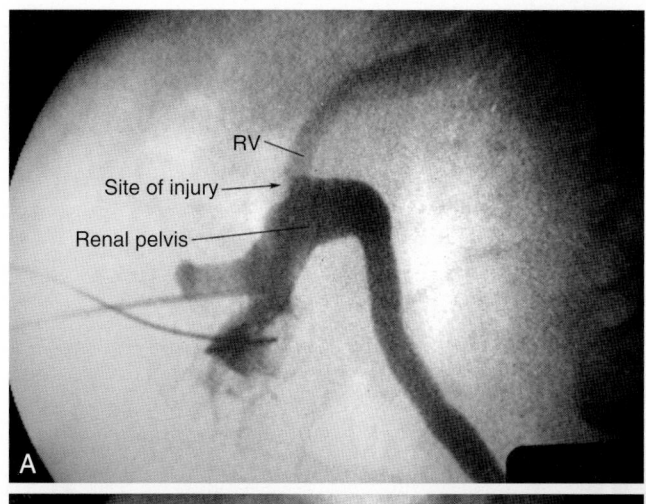

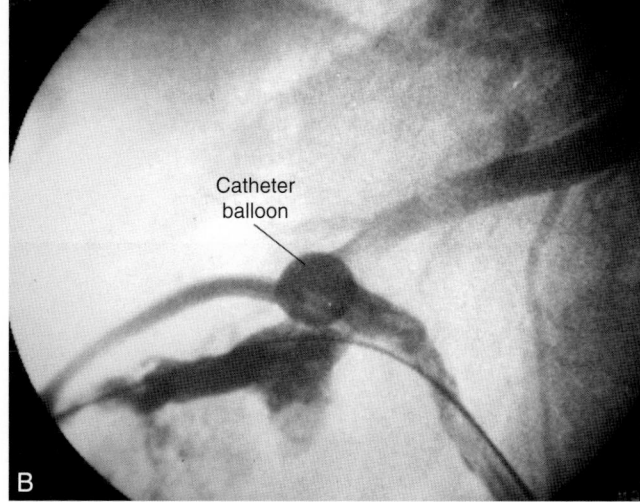

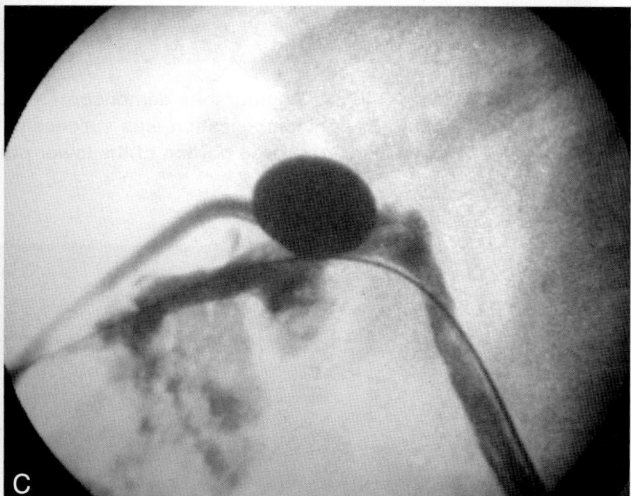

Figure 8-39. **A, Nephrostogram shows contrast material entering the renal vein (RV), indicating a large venous injury. B, The balloon of a Councill catheter nephrostomy tube is inflated at the site of injury (C) until contrast material no longer enters the RV.**

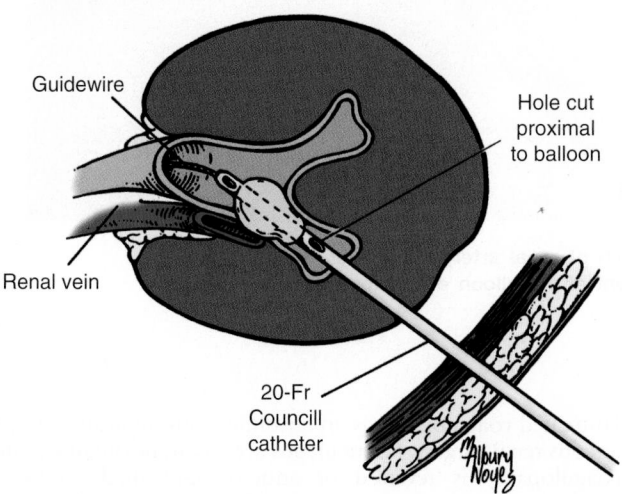

Figure 8-40. **An extra hole created proximal to the balloon of the Councill catheter allows for drainage of calyces obstructed by the balloon.**

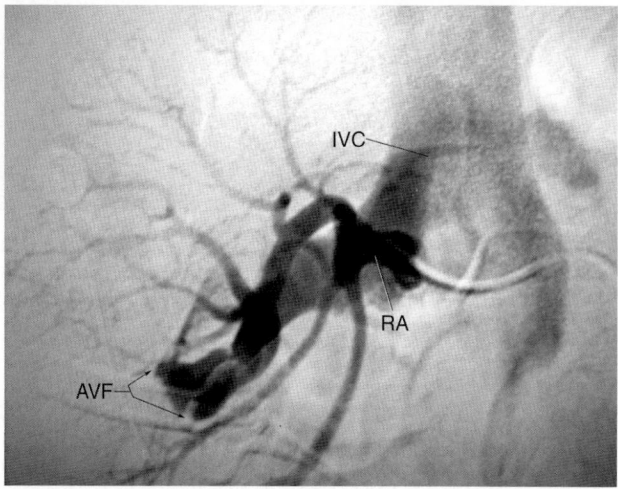

Figure 8-41. **Angiography of the renal artery (RA) is followed promptly by contrast material appearing in the inferior vena cava (IVC), suggesting the presence of an arteriovenous fistula (AVF).**

delayed hemorrhage after percutaneous renal surgery, 24% of the hemorrhages occurred within 24 hours of surgery, 41% between 2 and 7 days after surgery, and 35% more than 7 days later. **Any report of bright red blood in the urine after percutaneous renal surgery should prompt hospital admission and consideration of angiography, which is diagnostic in more than 90% of** cases (Richstone et al, 2008). **The standard treatment of renal arteriovenous fistulae and arterial pseudoaneurysms is selective angioembolization, which is highly effective.** Among five series reporting a total of 109 patients undergoing selective angioembolization after percutaneous renal surgery, there was success after a single treatment in 98 patients (90%) (Patterson et al, 1985; Martin

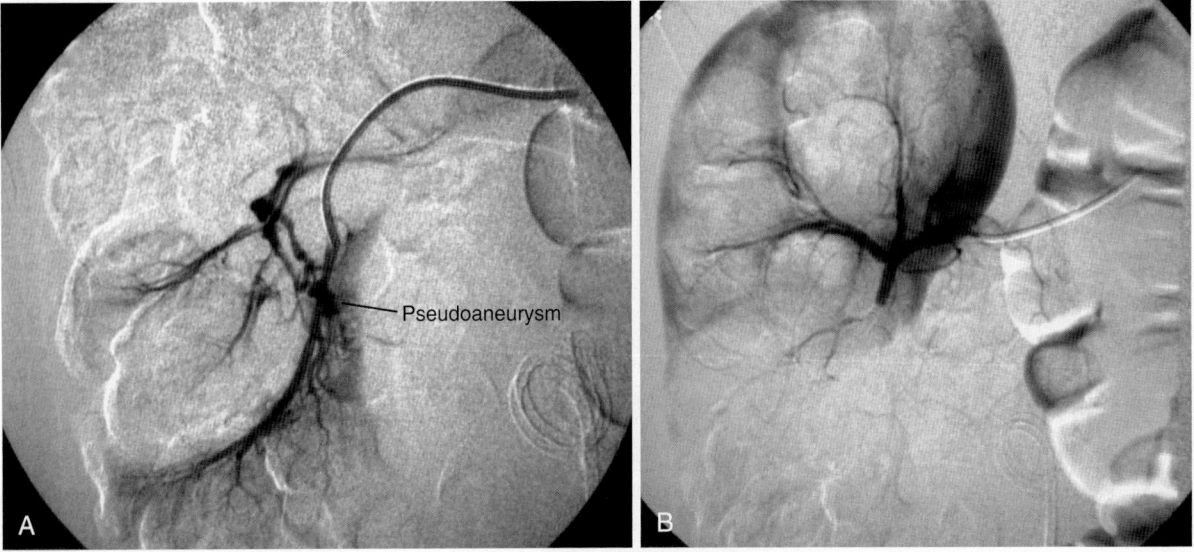

Figure 8-42. A, Angiography demonstrates a pseudoaneurysm in the lower pole of the right kidney. **B,** Angioembolization was successful at occluding the pseudoaneurysm, but it also devascularized a large portion of the lower pole.

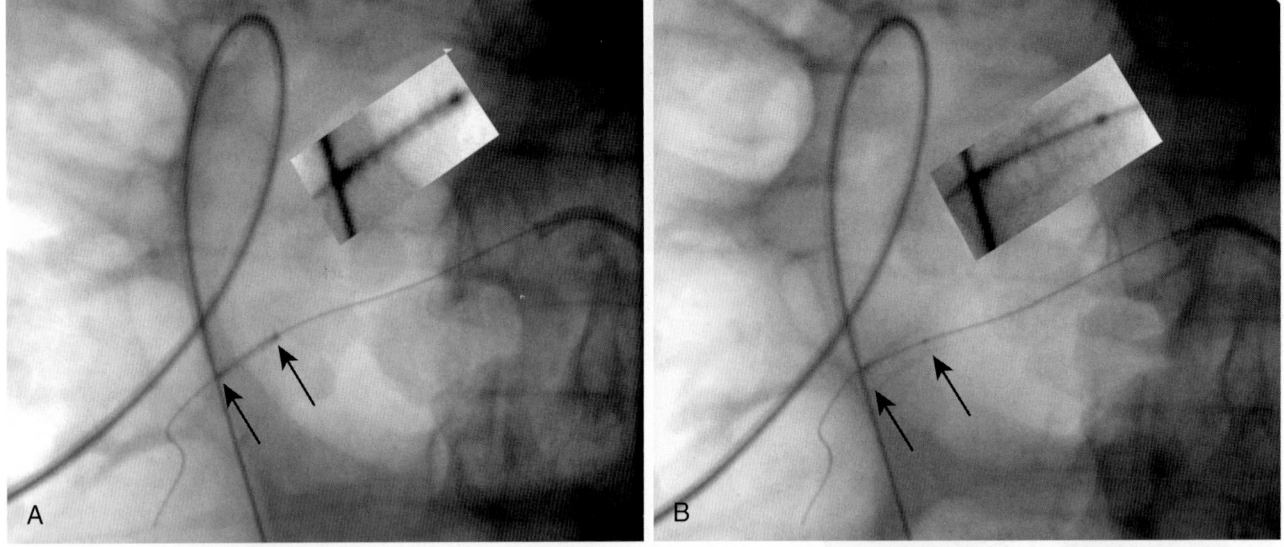

Figure 8-43. Covered arterial stent placed in branch of renal artery injured during endopyelotomy. **A,** Stent before balloon expansion. **B,** Stent after balloon expansion. Inset in each image is a 2× enlargement of stent *(arrows)*.

et al, 2000; Richstone et al, 2008; Jain et al, 2009; Ji et al, 2012). Nephrectomy may be required if selective angioembolization fails, and partial or total renal loss may occur if angioembolization is not selective enough (Fig. 8-42B). Additionally, the embolization coils can migrate to unwanted locations immediately or this migration might be delayed.

A recently introduced alternative to angioembolization is endovascular placement of a covered stent to occlude the site of arterial injury (Sprouse and Hamilton, 2002; Areste et al, 2005). This treatment maintains patency of the feeding artery, thereby preserving renal parenchyma, and obviates the risk of migration of embolization coils (Fig. 8-43). Another alternative is ultrasonographically guided percutaneous puncture of an arterial pseudoaneurysm, with injection of thrombin or fibrin tissue adhesive into the pseudoaneurysm (Benjaminov and Atri, 2002; Lagana et al, 2006; Sakr et al, 2009).

Untreated coagulopathy is an absolute contraindication to percutaneous renal surgery. Percutaneous access can be obtained safely if coagulopathy is reversed or anticoagulant medications are stopped. Anticoagulants can be restarted after the urine clears, preferably after nephrostomy tube removal, but the patient should be closely monitored.

Collecting System Injury

Tears in the infundibulum are not uncommon during percutaneous surgery of the upper urinary tract collecting system. They generally do not cause problems intraoperatively as long as there is no hemorrhage. Ureteral injuries are rare but can occur as a result of inflating the ureteral balloon occlusion catheter in the ureter or during other ureteral manipulation. These injuries generally will heal over a ureteral stent. Renal pelvic perforation can occur during initial

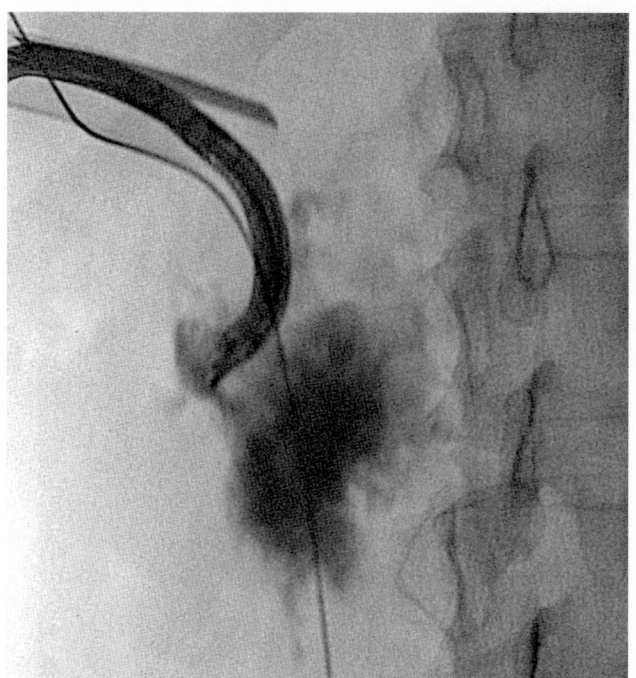

Figure 8-44. **Renal pelvic perforation confirmed with injection of contrast material through flexible nephroscope.**

access or during dilation. Pushing too hard on a renal pelvic stone during lithotripsy, or misusing a lithotripter or resectoscope, can also perforate the renal pelvis. **Renal pelvic perforation is usually recognized intraoperatively (Fig. 8-44). Collapse of a previously distended renal pelvis is a usual sign if the perforation is not visualized directly at first.** A perforation that has not been recognized intraoperatively might be heralded by postoperative abdominal distention, ileus, and/or fever. **If noted intraoperatively, abort the procedure unless it is near completion, in which case the task can be completed at lower irrigation pressure if the patient is doing well clinically. At the completion of a case in which renal pelvic perforation has been noted, insert a nephroureteral stent or a nephrostomy tube plus an internal ureteral stent to optimize drainage, and wait 2 to 7 days before nephrostography and tube removal, depending on the severity of the injury.** If renal pelvic perforation is detected postprocedure, despite adequate drainage of the collecting system, then placement of a percutaneous drain into the urinoma might be required. There have been reports of massive intra-abdominal collection of extravasated fluid after percutaneous renal surgery (Peterson et al, 1985; Pugach et al, 1999; Ghai et al, 2003; Etemadian et al, 2012).

Visceral Injury

Any abdominal organ close to the kidney can be injured during percutaneous renal surgery including the colon, duodenum, jejunum, spleen, liver, and biliary system.

Colon injury occurs during percutaneous renal surgery in the prone position at a rate of less than 1% (Segura et al, 1985; Lee et al, 1987; Gerspach et al, 1997; El-Nahas et al, 2006; Duvdevani et al, 2007; Michel et al, 2007; Kachrilas et al, 2012). **As one would expect based on the anatomy, with the apposition of the colon to the kidney being greatest on the left side and at the lower pole, the left colon is injured twice as often as the right colon, and the majority of colon injuries involve access to the lower pole** (El-Nahas et al, 2006). Additional risk factors include advanced patient age, dilated colon, previous colon surgery or disease, thin body habitus, and the presence of a horseshoe kidney (Goswami et al, 2001; El-Nahas et al, 2006; Michel et al, 2007; Korkes et al, 2009). Injury might be less likely with the patient in the supine position; one study reported a retrorenal colon on CT in 1.9% of

patients in the supine position versus 10% in prone patients (Hopper et al, 1987). The clinical incidence of colon injury, however, is much lower than this figure suggests.

Intraoperative detection of colonic injury confers easier management. If not determined intraoperatively, colon injury should be considered postoperatively if a patient develops unexplained fever, prolonged ileus, unexplained leukocytosis, rectal bleeding, evidence of peritoneal inflammation, or fecaluria or pneumaturia. Clinically apparent nephrocolonic fistula may be the presenting sign, or the injury may not be noted until the time of postoperative nephrostogram. **Most colon injuries are extraperitoneal and can be managed conservatively** (Gerspach et al, 1997; El-Nahas et al, 2006; Korkes et al, 2009; Traxer, 2009; Goger et al, 2012; Kachrilas et al, 2012). **The main principle of care is prompt and separate drainage of the colon and urinary collecting system.** The surgeon should back out the offending nephrostomy tube into the colon to serve as a colostomy tube, consider exchanging it for a larger tube to enhance colonic drainage, and obtain separate access to the upper urinary tract with either a new percutaneous access that does not traverse the colon or a retrograde-placed ureteral stent. Administer broad-spectrum antibiotics. Give nothing by mouth for a few days, and then start clear liquids. If there is no increase of colostomy output, then administer high-calorie protein supplementation and eventually a regular diet. Parenteral feeding is usually not required. Confirm lack of communication between the colon and collecting system with contrast injection of the tubes before removing them. If the injury is intraperitoneal, or if the patient develops peritonitis or sepsis, then open surgical repair may be required.

Small bowel injuries are even less common than colonic injury, described in only a few case reports (Culkin et al, 1985; Morris et al, 1991; Kumar et al, 1994; Ahmed and Reeve, 1995; Santiago et al, 1998; Lopes-Neto et al, 2000; Al-Assiri et al, 2005; Ricciardi et al, 2007; Traxer, 2009; Winer et al, 2009). Detection is by clinical signs and symptoms of peritonitis or by noting a nephroenteric fistula during postoperative nephrostography. Although open surgery may be required, conservative management using percutaneous intraduodenal catheterization or simple nasogastric or nasoduodenal drainage, combined with drainage of the upper urinary tract, fasting, and parenteral feeding, has been successful.

Studies based on CT and MRI have suggested that splenic and hepatic injuries should be unlikely unless the kidney is accessed above the 10th rib, although access above the 11th or 12th rib might traverse these organs in rare cases (Hopper and Yakes, 1990; Robert et al, 1999). If splenomegaly or hepatomegaly is present, these relationships change and access guided by CT is recommended. Splenic or hepatic injuries to orthotopic and normal-sized organs occur almost exclusively with supracostal upper pole renal access. Splenic injury might require laparotomy and potentially splenectomy owing to hemorrhage (Kondas et al, 1994; Shah et al, 2007), but conservative management has been successful as well (Goldberg et al, 1989; Santiago et al, 1998; Carey et al, 2006; Schaeffer et al, 2008; Thomas et al, 2009; Desai et al, 2010). Liver injury is less likely to be associated with significant hemorrhage—indeed the liver can be traversed percutaneously to obtain biliary access (Nadler et al, 2002), and purposeful transhepatic percutaneous renal surgery has been reported (Matlaga et al, 2006). As such, liver injuries during percutaneous renal surgery can be managed conservatively (El-Nahas et al, 2008).

There have been a few reported cases of biliary peritonitis resulting from injury of the gallbladder or biliary tree, which require exploratory laparotomy/laparoscopy and cholecystectomy owing to the high mortality rate of bile peritonitis (Martin et al, 1996; Saxby, 1996; Kontothanassis and Bissas, 1997; Fisher et al, 2004; Ricciardi et al, 2007; Patel and Nakada, 2010). Postoperative pancreatitis, without evidence of direct pancreatic injury, has been described as well (Chitale et al, 2005).

Pleural Injury

Hydrothorax, and occasionally pneumothorax, is a risk of percutaneous access to the upper urinary tract collecting system.

Supracostal access is the main risk factor; access below the 12th rib rarely results in hydrothorax or pneumothorax (<0.5%) (Munver et al, 2001; Radecka et al, 2003; Lojanapiwat and Prasopsuk, 2006; Maheshwari et al, 2009). The incidence of pleural complications with punctures above the 12th rib (the 11th intercostal space) is generally considered an acceptable risk if that approach provides optimal access to the upper urinary tract. Access above the 11th rib or higher carries a much greater risk of pleural injury. **Among 16 reports that distinguished between access above the 12th rib and access above the 11th rib, reporting a total of 1384 supracostal percutaneous accesses, the incidence of hydro/pneumothorax that required intervention varied from 0% to 18% for access superior to the 12th rib (weighted mean of 4.6%) and from 0% to 100% for access superior to the 11th rib (weighted mean of 24.6%)** (Young et al, 1985; Picus et al, 1986; Narasimham et al, 1991; Golijanin et al, 1998; Kekre et al, 2001; Munver et al, 2001; Gupta et al, 2002; Wong and Leveillee, 2002; Muzrakchi et al, 2003; Radecka et al, 2003; Aron et al, 2005c; Lojanapiwat and Prasopsuk, 2006; Yadav et al, 2006; Shaban et al, 2008; Sukumar et al, 2008; Yadav et al, 2008).

Nephropleural fistula (urinothorax) is a direct and persistent communication between the intrarenal collecting system and the intrathoracic cavity (Ray et al, 2003; Shleyfer et al, 2006; Handa et al, 2007). It can follow percutaneous renal access of the upper urinary tract in the setting of pleural transgression. Some degree of distal ureteral obstruction usually contributes to the problem. Most commonly, nephropleural fistula is diagnosed after the percutaneous tube is removed, but it can occur in the setting of a recognized hydrothorax when the persistent communication is documented on nephrostography at the time of intended tube removal. Lallas and colleagues (2004) reported that nephropleural fistula never occurred in association with subcostal access but did complicate 2.3% of punctures superior to the 12th rib and 6.3% of punctures superior to the 11th rib.

Pleural complications of supracostal percutaneous access can often be detected with chest fluoroscopy during or at the conclusion of the procedure. Fluid can be seen tracking along the lateral borders of the chest cavity and compressing the ipsilateral lung. Although postoperative chest radiography is more sensitive than intraoperative fluoroscopy, some authors report that thoracostomy was never required on the basis of postoperative chest radiography when intraoperative chest fluoroscopy was negative (Ogan et al, 2003; Bjurlin et al, 2012). **Nonetheless, formal chest radiography is recommended following all cases of supracostal percutaneous renal access.**

Thoracostomy is not necessary for all patients with hydrothorax. If hydrothorax is noted intraoperatively, then insert a small-caliber (8-Fr to 12-Fr) Cope nephrostomy tube as the thoracostomy (Fig. 8-45), using fluoroscopic guidance and the same general techniques as for antegrade percutaneous renal access (Ogan and Pearle, 2002). A Heimlich valve, rather than water seal drainage, is all that is necessary in the absence of lung injury. If a hydrothorax is noted on the postoperative chest radiograph, then place a small-caliber tube only if the effusion is large or if there is evidence of respiratory compromise or hemodynamic instability. A large-bore thoracostomy tube for lung injury is rarely required.

Metabolic and Physiologic Complications

Normal saline should be the irrigant for percutaneous renal surgery, with the exception of glycine or similar nonelectrolytic isotonic fluids when monopolar electrocautery is used. Irrigation with water during percutaneous renal surgery risks intravascular hemolysis, which can be fatal. At least one death associated with water irrigation during percutaneous nephrolithotomy has been described (Bennett et al, 1984), and the author is aware of an unreported case. Intravascular or extravascular extravasation of nonelectrolytic isotonic fluid from continued irrigation in the setting of a large venous injury or collecting system perforation, respectively, can result in hyponatremia and other electrolyte abnormalities, renal or hepatic dysfunction, and mental status changes. When

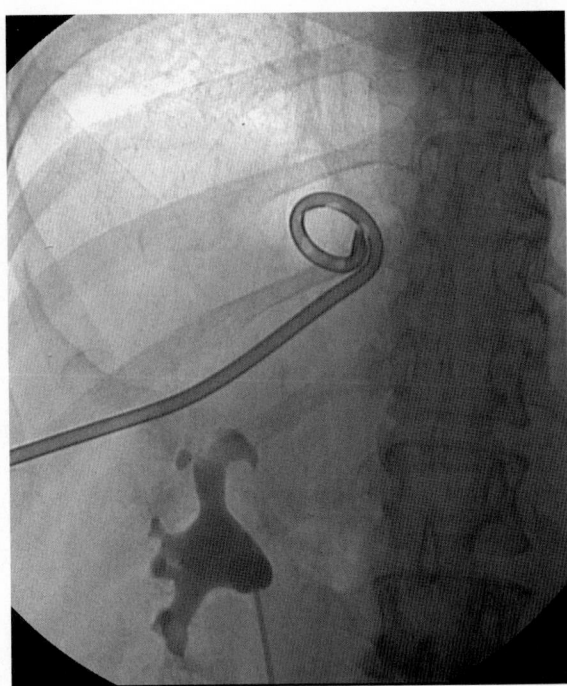

Figure 8-45. **A 12-Fr Cope catheter placed into the chest when a large hydrothorax was noted intraoperatively on fluoroscopy.**

normal saline is used in uncomplicated cases, the amount of fluid absorption is generally clinically insignificant (Kukreja et al, 2002; Koroglu et al, 2003), although in one study 28% of patients absorbed more than a liter (Malhotra et al, 2001). A large amount of saline extravasation can lead to clinically significant respiratory distress or cardiac failure resulting from volume overload.

Venous gas embolism is a rare but potentially fatal complication of percutaneous renal surgery. The gas (in this case, air) enters the venous system and passes through the right heart into the pulmonary circulation, blocking the output of the right heart, which results in hypoxemia, hypercapnia, and depressed cardiac output. Gas can also pass through a patent foramen ovale to enter the arterial system, which can result in neurologic deficits. Among six reported cases of venous gas embolism in association with percutaneous renal surgery, three were associated with air pyelography in combination with percutaneous access of the kidney (Miller et al, 1984; Cadeddu et al, 1997a; Droghetti et al, 2002), one involved percutaneous surgery without air pyelography (Turillazzi et al, 2009), and two occurred after retrograde injection of air into the renal pelvis but before percutaneous puncture (Varkarakis et al, 2003; Song et al, 2007). Venous gas embolism is indicated by hypoxemia, evidence of pulmonary edema, increased airway pressure, hypotension, jugular venous distention, facial plethora, dysrhythmias, and auscultation of a mill-wheel cardiac murmur and/or the appearance of a widened QRS complex with right heart strain patterns on electrocardiography. The most sensitive measure is a sudden decrease in capnometry reading of the $P(end\text{-}tidal)CO_2$. Swift response is required and includes rapid ventilation with 100% oxygen, positioning the patient head down with the right side up, and general resuscitative maneuvers.

Postoperative Fever and Sepsis

After percutaneous nephrolithotomy, 15% to 30% of patients develop a fever. Risk factors for fever/infectious complications following percutaneous nephrolithotomy include diabetes mellitus, paraplegia, indwelling ureteral stent or nephrostomy tube, previous percutaneous nephrolithotomy, multiple access tracts, infection stone, positive preoperative urine culture, larger stones, and hydronephrosis (Charton et al, 1986; Troxel and Low, 2002; Aghdas et al,

2006; Draga et al, 2009; Korets et al, 2011; Lojanapiwat and Kitirattrakarn, 2011; Kumar et al, 2012; Gutierrez et al, 2013). **Most patients with fever after percutaneous nephrolithotomy, assuming appropriate antimicrobial prophylaxis, do not have infection** (Cadeddu et al, 1998). **Sepsis occurs in 0.5% to 2.5% of patients after percutaneous nephrolithotomy** (Dogan et al, 2007; Duvdevani et al, 2007; Gonen et al, 2008b; Labate et al, 2011; Lojanapiwat and Kitirattrakarn, 2011; Seitz et al, 2012; Li et al, 2013a). Sepsis implies an infection, which is not always present; "systemic inflammatory response syndrome" is a more accurate description. Positive preoperative urine cultures should be treated. Even if bacteriologic cure is not possible (e.g., infectious stone, indwelling nephrostomy tube), bacterial counts should be suppressed as much as possible to reduce the risk of infectious complications. Nonetheless, a negative urine culture does not guarantee against sepsis because the voided urine culture may not reflect the intrarenal urine (Rao et al, 1991; Mariappan et al, 2005; Lojanapiwat and Kitirattrakarn, 2011; Korets et al, 2011). **Because the febrile patient who will progress to sepsis cannot be predicted, careful observation, appropriate diagnostic evaluation, and initiation of antimicrobial therapy and other supportive care are indicated if a postoperative fever does not resolve promptly.**

If pus is aspirated upon initial percutaneous entry to the upper urinary tract, the safest measure is to abort the procedure and leave a nephrostomy tube for drainage. Aron and associates (2005a), based on their experience in 19 patients with purulent fluid from the kidney at initial puncture for percutaneous nephrolithotomy, suggested that aborting the procedure might not always be necessary. They continued the procedure in 12 patients and delayed it in 7. Of the 12 patients in whom the procedure was continued, two (17%) experienced postprocedure sepsis. Among the seven patients in whom the procedure was delayed (for 3 to 7 days), two (29%) developed sepsis after the second procedure (both of whom had additional portions of the kidney containing undrained pus, which were discovered at the time of the delayed percutaneous nephrolithotomy). An important difference was in the quality of the aspirated material. One patient in whom percutaneous nephrolithotomy was continued and two in whom the procedure was delayed had "frank pus" as opposed to "purulent fluid" in the other cases. All three of these patients with frank pus were among the four who developed sepsis. The authors recommend that if frank pus is aspirated, then the procedure should be aborted. If the aspirate is a cloudy nonviscous liquid, it might be safe to proceed. This approach has not yet been validated in additional studies. This report also suggests that not all patients with "purulent fluid" are infected. Of the 19 patients, the culture of the aspirate showed bacteria in only 6. This suggests that infection may have been sterilized by previous antibiotic use. The turbid fluid may indicate a sterile inflammatory response to the stone, or the fluid may consist of debris related to the renal calculus. Another important point is that a single nephrostomy tube may not drain all areas of infection in the kidney, especially if there is intrarenal obstruction.

Neuromusculoskeletal Complications

Prone positioning for percutaneous renal surgery has the potential for a number of neuromusculoskeletal injuries (Shermak et al, 2006; Edgcombe et al, 2008). **Excessive pressure on neural and vascular structures, whether directly from the operative table or indirectly through the positioning of limbs, may lead to short- or long-term disability.** Most reported injuries associated with prone positioning are related to the head and neck region including ocular injury resulting in visual loss, facial nerve injury or necrosis over facial bones or the tip of the nose, and cerebrovascular accident resulting from carotid or vertebrobasilar artery dissection. Careful padding of the head, in a neutral and nonextended position, is important. Malpositioning of the extremities can lead to peripheral nerve injury (Winfree and Kline, 2005). The shoulder and elbow should not be abducted more than 90 degrees, so as to prevent brachial plexopathy, and generous padding at the elbow and forearm reduces the risk of nerve compression. Knees need to be padded. Ankles should be elevated to reduce pressure on the dorsum of the foot.

Venous Thromboembolism

The incidence of venous thromboembolism with percutaneous renal surgery is low (<3% in older series of percutaneous nephrolithotomy) (Segura et al, 1985; Lee et al, 1987), but there are no recent data. **The AUA's Best Practice Statement for the prevention of deep vein thrombosis in patients undergoing urologic surgery does not include percutaneous renal surgery among procedures for which prophylaxis against venous thromboembolism is recommended** (Forrest et al, 2009). Early ambulation is the best measure to reduce the already low risk of venous thromboembolism.

Tube Dislodgement

Whether the percutaneous nephrostomy tube is intended to be short term or long term, inadvertent tube dislodgement risks poor patient outcomes. The tube does not need to fall out of the patient completely; especially in a patient with a large subcutaneous layer, the tube can remain attached at the skin but pull out from within the kidney when the distance between the skin and kidney increases with patient movement. Nonetheless, **all tubes should be secured at the skin to reduce the risk of at least one mechanism of tube removal.** Tubes vary in their inherent ability to resist removal. **Malecot tubes are the easiest to pull out, and circle nephrostomy tubes are the most difficult. The Cope retention mechanism is more secure than Malecot wings but does not retain as well as a balloon** (Canales et al, 2005). For long-term indwelling, circle nephrostomy tubes and Cope nephrostomy tubes are most commonly used. Ironically, the Malecot tube is also the one most likely to become entrapped; tissue can grow over the wings, making removal difficult and traumatic (Sardina et al, 1995; Tasca and Cacciola, 2004).

If a nephrostomy tube has been in for only a short time, then complete dislodgement often leads to complete loss of percutaneous access. Using a nephrostomy tube with a ureteral extension, whether it is only partially down the ureter as in the Malecot re-entry tube or all the way into the bladder as in a nephroureteral stent, will increase the chance of having some access back into the kidney even if the renal retention device pulls out of the kidney. For tubes that have been in place for more than a few weeks, the tract is usually mature enough that carefully probing with an angled hydrophilic wire and judicious use of contrast material to outline the tract can allow restoration of the percutaneous access. Tube malposition can usually be corrected under fluoroscopic control, but guidance by CT might be helpful as well (Jones and McGahan, 1999).

Collecting System Obstruction

Transient ureteral obstruction owing to ureteral edema or blood clot occurs commonly. To assess for this, nephrostomy tubes should be removed after nephrostography or after a period of clamping to assess clinically for distal ureteral obstruction. Much more uncommon is stricture formation, which can occur in the ureter, at the ureteropelvic junction, or in an infundibulum. If the stricture occurs early in the postprocedure course, then a nephrocutaneous fistula will develop. If it develops late, then hydronephrosis or hydrocalyx will occur. **In one large series there was a 2% rate of infundibular stenosis after percutaneous nephrolithotomy** (Parsons et al, 2002). The obstructions developed in the areas that had been accessed percutaneously. Predisposing factors in this and other smaller reports (Ballanger et al, 1987; Weir and Honey, 1999; Buchholz, 2001) include large stone burden requiring multiple or long procedures and prolonged nephrostomy tube drainage, previous open stone surgery, diabetes mellitus, and obesity. The ureter (Culkin et al, 1987; Lopes-Neto et al, 2008) and the ureteropelvic junction (Green et al, 1987; Ben Slama et al, 2005) are smaller in caliber than the intrarenal collecting system and are therefore also susceptible to trauma.

Obstruction after percutaneous renal surgery should respond to endoscopic treatment in most cases, but open surgical reconstruction or excision with partial nephrectomy or total nephrectomy might be required.

Loss of Renal Function

Despite the direct puncture of renal parenchyma and enlargement of sometimes multiple tracts to as much as 34 Fr, the kidney suffers little permanent damage after uncomplicated percutaneous renal surgery. Renal function does decrease slightly immediately after percutaneous renal surgery, reaching a nadir 48 hours postprocedure (Nouralizadeh et al, 2011), but there is negligible long-term loss of function (Ekelund et al, 1986; Chen et al, 1992; Saxby, 1997; Kilic et al, 2006), and in one study there appeared to be less damage to the kidney after percutaneous nephrolithotomy than after shock wave lithotripsy (LeChevallier et al, 1993). In the setting of impaired function, especially because of obstructing calculi, percutaneous surgery will often improve renal function (Chandhoke et al, 1992; Chatham et al, 2002; Bilen et al, 2008). Percutaneous renal surgery also causes no significant change in function of solitary kidneys (Jones et al, 1991; Liou and Streem, 2001; Canes et al, 2009). In one study of patients who were surveyed a mean of 19 years after treatment, there was no difference between shock wave lithotripsy and percutaneous nephrolithotomy in the development of renal insufficiency or hypertension (Krambeck et al, 2008a).

When there is renal loss following percutaneous renal surgery, it usually is a result of disastrous vascular injury or the angioembolization used to treat hemorrhage. In the original AUA guideline on staghorn calculi (Segura et al, 1994), renal loss after percutaneous nephrolithotomy was estimated at 1.6%; data were insufficient to calculate a new figure in the 2005 update of the guidelines (Preminger et al, 2005).

Death

Death after percutaneous renal surgery is extremely rare, and when it occurs it is usually a result of underlying cardiovascular conditions (Labate et al, 2011; Seitz et al, 2012). In the current AUA guideline on the management of staghorn calculi, the median death estimate for percutaneous nephrolithotomy was zero, which reflects the paucity of data on the subject (Preminger et al, 2005).

Please visit the accompanying website at www.expertconsult.com to view videos associated with this chapter.

REFERENCES

The complete reference list is available online at www.expertconsult.com.

SUGGESTED READINGS

Basiri A, Ziaee AM, Kianian HR, et al. Ultrasonographic versus fluoroscopic access for percutaneous nephrolithotomy: a randomized clinical trial. J Endourol 2008;22:281–4.

Cadeddu JA, Chen R, Bishoff J, et al. Clinical significance of fever after percutaneous nephrolithotomy. Urology 1998;52:48–50.

Desai MR, Kukreja R, Desai MM, et al. A prospective randomized comparison of type of nephrostomy drainage following percutaneous nephrostolithotomy: large bore versus small bore versus tubeless. J Urol 2004; 172:565–7.

El-Nahas AR, Shokeir AA, El-Assmy AM, et al. Colonic perforation during percutaneous nephrolithotomy: study of risk factors. Urology 2006;67: 937–41.

Labate G, Modi P, Timoney A, et al. The percutaneous nephrolithotomy global study: classification of complications. J Endourol 2011;25: 1275–80.

Miller NL, Matlaga BR, Lingeman JE. Techniques for fluoroscopic percutaneous renal access. J Urol 2007;178:15–23.

Munver R, Delvecchio FC, Newman GE, et al. Critical analysis of supracostal access for percutaneous renal surgery. J Urol 2001;166:1242–6.

Netto NR Jr, Ikonomidis J, Ikari O, et al. Comparative study of percutaneous access for staghorn calculi. Urology 2005;65:659–62.

Ogan K, Corwin TS, Smith T, et al. Sensitivity of chest fluoroscopy compared with chest CT and chest radiography for diagnosing hydropneumothorax in association with percutaneous nephrostolithotomy. Urology 2003;62: 988–92.

Patel B, Mason BM, Hoenig DM. Retrograde endoscopic-assisted percutaneous renal access: a novel "lasso" technique to achieve rapid secure access to the collecting system. J Endourol 2008;22:591–6.

Preminger GM, Assimos DG, Lingeman JE, et al. Chapter 1: AUA guideline on management of staghorn calculi: diagnosis and treatment recommendations. J Urol 2005;173:1991–2000.

Rastinehad AR, Andonian S, Smith AD, et al. Management of hemorrhagic complications associated with percutaneous nephrolithotomy. J Endourol 2009;23:1763–7.

Richstone L, Reggio E, Ost MC, et al. Hemorrhage following percutaneous renal surgery: characterization of angiographic findings. J Endourol 2008; 22:1129–35.

Sampaio FJ, Zanier JF, Aragao AH, et al. Intrarenal access: 3-dimensional anatomical study. J Urol 1992;148:1769–73.

Seitz C, Desai M, Häcker A, et al. Incidence, prevention, and management of complications following percutaneous nephrolitholapaxy. Eur Urol 2012;61:146–58.

KEY POINTS: COMPLICATIONS

- Hemorrhage during percutaneous surgery is associated with inappropriate access site, multiple access sites, supracostal access, increasing tract size, tract dilation with methods other than balloon dilation, prolonged operative time, and renal pelvic perforation or other intraoperative technical errors.

- In most cases of hemorrhage during percutaneous surgery or at the time of sheath removal, placing a nephrostomy tube and letting the collecting system clot off is effective. If bleeding is more severe, additional measures may be required.

- Delayed hemorrhage is usually caused by arteriovenous fistulas or arterial pseudoaneurysms. Bright red blood in the urine after percutaneous renal surgery should prompt hospital admission and the consideration of angiography. Selective angioembolization is highly successful in treating this condition.

- If renal pelvic perforation is noted intraoperatively, abort the procedure unless it is near completion. Insert a nephroureteral stent or a nephrostomy tube plus a ureteral stent to optimize drainage.

- Most colon injuries from percutaneous renal surgery are extraperitoneal and can be managed conservatively by draining the colon and urinary collecting system separately.

- Hydrothorax or pneumothorax requiring intervention is related to the level of percutaneous access. Incidence estimates are less than 0.5% below the 12th rib, 4.6% above the 12th rib, and 24.6% above the 11th rib. Pleural complications can often be detected with chest fluoroscopy during the procedure, but a chest radiograph should also be obtained following all cases of supracostal percutaneous renal access.

- Normal saline should be the fluid used for irrigation during percutaneous renal surgery, with the exception of glycine or a similar nonconductive solution when monopolar electrocautery is used.

- If pus is aspirated on initial percutaneous entry to the upper urinary tract, the safest measure is to abort the procedure and leave a nephrostomy tube for drainage.

9

Evaluation and Management of Hematuria

Stephen A. Boorjian, MD, Jay D. Raman, MD, and Daniel A. Barocas, MD, MPH, FACS

Hematuria has been recognized as a sign of medical illness since antiquity (Ellis, 1979; Shokeir and Hussein, 1999; Armstrong, 2006). Yet it is only in the modern era that we have developed the technology to detect microscopic blood, the means to identify the source of hematuria, and the understanding of anatomy, physiology, and disease processes underlying this important sign. Today, hematuria is one of the most common indications for urologic evaluation (Mariani et al, 1989) and is recognized as a sign of potentially important illness. Therefore knowledge of the differential diagnosis, principles of evaluation, and strategies for management of hematuria is critical.

CLASSIFICATION AND TIMING OF HEMATURIA

Hematuria may be classified according to its visibility and timing during the urinary stream. That is, gross hematuria (GH), sometimes referred to as *frank hematuria, macrohematuria,* or *visible hematuria,* is hematuria that can be seen with the naked eye. GH may be further characterized as initial, terminal, or total, depending on the phase of the urinary stream in which it is visible. This characterization may give some indication of the source of hematuria, with initial hematuria most commonly emanating from a urethral source; terminal hematuria from the bladder trigone, bladder neck, or prostate; and total hematuria from the bladder or above (Sokolosky, 2001).

GH must be distinguished from pigmenturia, which may be due to endogenous sources (e.g., bilirubin, myoglobin, porphyrins), foods ingested (e.g., beets and rhubarb), drugs (e.g., phenazopyridine), and simple dehydration. This distinction can be made easily by urinalysis with microscopy. Notably, myoglobinuria and other factors can cause false-positive chemical tests for hemoglobin, so urine microscopy is required to confirm the diagnosis of hematuria. **GH also must be distinguished from vaginal bleeding in women,** which usually can be achieved by obtaining a careful menstrual history, collecting the specimen when the patient is not having menstrual or gynecologic bleeding, or, if necessary, obtaining a catheterized specimen. GH may also be detected by the presence of blood spotting on the undergarments of incontinent patients. After ruling out vaginal bleeding and mimics of hematuria, a urologic source must be suspected.

MICROSCOPIC HEMATURIA

In contrast to GH, microscopic hematuria, or microhematuria (MH), is a sign rather than a symptom; a laboratory diagnosis defined as the presence of red blood cells (RBCs) on microscopic examination of the urine not evident on visual inspection of the urine. **The prevalence of MH among healthy participants in screening studies is 6.5% (95% confidence interval [CI] 3.4 to 12.2),** with higher rates in studies with a predominance of males, older patients, and smokers (Davis et al, 2012). MH may be categorized by the presence or absence of associated symptoms and may be quantified according to number of RBCs per high-power field (HPF). The proper collection of a urine specimen and the details of urine dipstick testing and urinalysis are covered in Chapter 1.

Criteria for the Diagnosis of Microhematuria

A small number of RBCs may pass into the urine even under normal conditions, and normal processes (e.g., sexual activity, exercise) can result in minor amounts of MH (Kohanpour et al, 2012). **The American Urologic Association (AUA) guideline panel defined MH as three or more RBCs/HPF,** concluding that higher thresholds would lead to missed opportunities to diagnose treatable urologic conditions (Davis et al, 2012). Additionally, it has been shown that **MH caused by significant medical conditions, such as urinary tract malignancy, can be intermittent** (Davis et al, 2012). In fact, a meta-analysis reported that the rate of malignancy detected among patients evaluated for a single positive urinalysis was 3.6% (Davis et al, 2012). Thus the most recent AUA guideline panel has determined that **a single positive urinalysis is sufficient to prompt evaluation** (Davis et al, 2012).

Requirement for Microscopic Evaluation

The results of urine dipstick tests must be confirmed on urinalysis with microscopy and alone are considered insufficient to prompt an evaluation. Indeed, chemical tests for hematuria detect the peroxidase activity of hemoglobin using benzidine, and therefore conditions such as myoglobinuria can falsely activate the test (Mariani et al, 1984). Thus a positive dipstick test merits microscopic examination of the urinary sediment, but does not warrant full evaluation unless microscopy confirms the presence of three or more RBCs/HPF. If the urinalysis with microscopy is not confirmatory, but the clinician remains suspicious, repeat microscopic testing is reasonable with the frequency individualized based on provider judgment.

Specimens collected immediately after prolonged recumbency (first void in morning) or after vigorous physical or sexual activity may be falsely positive for hematuria (Addis, 1926; Kincaid-Smith, 1982). Additionally, dilute urine (osmolality <308 mOsm) may result in false-negative microscopic examination as a result of RBC lysis (Vaughan and Wyker, 1971).

Evaluation of Patients with Microhematuria

In most studies, **one third to two thirds of patients evaluated for MH have been found to have a demonstrable cause** (Mohr et al, 1986; Murakami et al, 1990), including calculus (6.0%), benign prostatic enlargement (12.9%), urethral stricture (1.4%), and various other conditions (Table 9-1) (Davis et al, 2012). Notably, **the evaluation of patients with MH yields a diagnosis of malignancy in 1.8% to 4.3% of cases**, depending on the characteristics of the population evaluated, the threshold for evaluation, and the completeness of the evaluation (Davis et al, 2012). **The likelihood of** identifying a malignancy is higher among patients with higher levels of microscopic hematuria (>25 RBCs/HPH), GH, or risk factors for malignancy (Sultana et al, 1996; Shephard et al, 2012; Loo et al, 2013). Risk factors for malignancy among patients with hematuria include male gender, older age, and tobacco use (Box 9-1).

Selecting Patients for Evaluation of Microhematuria

Recognizing that one third to two thirds of patients with MH will have a negative hematuria evaluation, interest is growing in an evidence-based selection of patients for hematuria evaluation to

TABLE 9-1 Differential Diagnosis of Asymptomatic Microhematuria*

CATEGORY	EXAMPLES	COMMON CLINICAL PRESENTATION AND RISK FACTORS
Neoplasm	Any	See Box 9-1
	Bladder cancer	Older age, male predominance, tobacco, occupational exposures, irritative voiding symptoms
	Ureteral or renal pelvis cancer	Family history of early colon cancers or upper tract tumors, flank pain
	Renal cortical tumor	Family history of early kidney tumors, flank pain, flank mass
	Prostate cancer	Older age, family history, African-American
	Urethral cancer	Obstructive symptoms, pain, bloody discharge
Infection/inflammation	Any	History of infection
	Cystitis	Female predominance, dysuria
	Pyelonephritis	Fever, flank pain, diabetes, female predominance
	Urethritis	Exposure to sexually transmitted infections, urethral discharge, dysuria
	Tuberculosis	Travel to endemic areas
	Schistosomiasis	Travel to endemic areas
	Hemorrhagic cystitis	See Box 9-2
Calculus	Any	
	Nephroureterolithiasis	Flank pain, family history, prior stone
	Bladder stones	Bladder outlet obstruction
Benign prostatic enlargement		Male, older age, obstructive symptoms
Medical renal disease†	Any	Hypertension, azotemia, dysmorphic erythrocytes, cellular casts, proteinuria
	Nephritis	
	IgA nephropathy	
Congenital or acquired anatomic abnormality	Polycystic kidney disease	Family history of renal cystic disease
	Ureteropelvic junction obstruction	History of UTI, stone, flank pain
	Ureteral stricture	History of surgery or radiation, flank pain, hydronephrosis;
	Urethral diverticulum	stranguria, spraying urine
	Fistula	Discharge, dribbling, dyspareunia, history of UTI, female predominance
		Pneumaturia, fecaluria, abdominal pain, recurrent UTI, history of diverticulitis or colon cancer
Other	Exercise-induced hematuria‡	Recent vigorous exercise
	Endometriosis	Cyclic hematuria in a menstruating woman
	Hematologic or thrombotic disease	Family history of personal history of bleeding or thrombosis
	Papillary necrosis	African-American, sickle cell disease, diabetes, analgesic abuse
	Arteriovenous malformation	
	Renal vein thrombosis	
	Interstitial cystitis	Voiding symptoms
	Trauma	History
	Recent genitourinary surgery or instrumentation	History

*Differential diagnosis, having ruled out obvious benign causes, such as menstruation, recent instrumentation, uncomplicated cystitis, etc.
†Presence of hematologic illness, medical renal illness or use of anticoagulants or antiplatelet agents does not preclude the need for a hematuria evaluation.
‡Exercise-induced hematuria is a diagnosis of exclusion. Absence of hematuria after abstinence from exercise must be confirmed.
IgA, immunoglobulin A; UTI, urinary tract infection.

minimize the financial burden and risks in evaluating all patients (Mohr et al, 1986; van der Molen and Hovius, 2012; Loo et al, 2013). For example, the Kaiser Permanente group demonstrated that, among patients undergoing a complete evaluation for hematuria, those at high risk for malignancy (age >50 years, history of GH, tobacco use, male gender, or >25 RBCs/HPF) had higher rates of malignancy (10.7% to 11.6%) than patients at intermediate (1.1% to 2.5%) or low (0 to 0.3%) risk (Loo et al, 2013). However, although the Kaiser study shows that we may be able to decide which patients referred to urologists can safely avoid complete evaluation, the reality is that **fewer than 25% of patients found to have hematuria are referred for evaluation and fewer than 10% undergo a complete evaluation with cystoscopy and imaging,** even among patients at high risk for malignancy (Elias et al, 2010; Buteau et al, 2012). Taken together, these studies suggest that ample room exists for improvement in developing evidence-based algorithms to guide the use of hematuria evaluation and in reducing nonclinical sources of variability in adherence to evidence-based practices.

The AUA guidelines recommend evaluating patients with MH "in the absence of an obvious benign cause" such as infection and menstruation. Therefore **it is imperative that patients who are found to have MH in the setting of a suspected benign cause have that benign cause substantiated by clinical evidence and be further evaluated once the suspected benign cause is resolved.** Unfortunately, uniform agreement does not exist on how to identify benign causes of hematuria. Perhaps, as a result, substantial delays in diagnosis and inferior bladder cancer outcomes have occurred related to repeated empirical treatment of urinary tract infection (UTI) and voiding symptoms, particularly among women (Henning et al, 2013; Lyratzopoulos et al, 2013; Tracey et al, 2014). Our recommendation is that the **presence of infection should be confirmed with a urine culture and the urinalysis should be repeated after treatment of the UTI to document resolution of the hematuria.** If hematuria persists, further evaluation is warranted.

In addition, recent vigorous exercise may be associated with MH, but this entity should be considered a diagnosis of exclusion (Kincaid-Smith, 1982; McInnis et al, 1998; Kohanpour et al, 2012). Thus it is necessary to confirm the absence of MH after a period of abstinence from exercise. In addition, **patients who develop hematuria (microscopic or gross) who are taking anticoagulation or antiplatelet medications (e.g., warfarin, enoxaparin, heparin, aspirin, clopidogrel, nonsteroidal anti-inflammatory agents) should undergo a complete evaluation in the same manner as patients not taking such medications,** because the prevalence of hematuria, as well as the likelihood of finding genitourinary

cancers, among patients with hematuria on anticoagulation has been reported to be no different from patients not taking such medications (Culclasure et al, 1994; Khadra et al, 2000; Davis et al, 2012; Jeong et al, 2013). In fact, it has been noted that these medications may unmask genitourinary lesions at an earlier stage (Antolak and Mellinger, 1969; Kraus et al, 1984; Schuster and Lewis, 1987; Mariani, 1989). In one series, 82% of anticoagulated male patients evaluated for GH were found to have significant urologic lesions (Antolak and Mellinger, 1969), and 13.9% of such lesions in another series were found to be malignant (Schuster and Lewis, 1987). Meanwhile, MH in the setting of trauma is detailed elsewhere (see Chapters 50 and 101) and will not be covered here.

The Question of Screening for Hematuria and Bladder Cancer

Bladder cancer is the sixth most commonly diagnosed cancer in the United States, and although no large-scale screening trials have been performed, **most believe that the harms and costs of mass screening for bladder cancer would prove to outweigh the potential benefits** (http://seer.cancer.gov/statfacts/html/urinb.html; Chou and Dana, 2010). Nonetheless, many primary care providers perform urinalysis as part of routine health examinations, creating numerous opportunistic screening events (Prochazka et al, 2005).

KEY POINTS: MICROSCOPIC HEMATURIA

- MH is defined as three or more RBCs/HPF, identified on one or more occasions on urine microscopy. Urine dipstick testing is insufficient for the diagnosis of MH.
- MH is quite common, with a prevalence of approximately 6.5% of adults, varying according to the characteristics of the population.
- Malignancy has been detected in approximately 4% of patients evaluated for asymptomatic MH. The proportion of malignancies detected is higher in patients with higher degrees of hematuria and/or risk factors for malignancy.

EVALUATION OF PATIENTS WITH MICROHEMATURIA

See Figure 9-1 for the evaluation algorithm of MH from the most recent AUA guidelines (Davis et al, 2012). Importantly, it is recommended that **patients meeting criteria for evaluation undergo a complete evaluation, even if one phase of the evaluation shows a suspected cause for the MH.** For example, a patient found to have a kidney tumor or stone disease during initial workup of MH should still undergo cystoscopy for clearance of bladder and urethral pathologic processes.

The evaluation of an appropriately selected patient with MH begins with a thorough history and physical examination. Specifically, one should aim to identify causes that would warrant variation from the standard evaluation, such as infection, menstruation, recent vigorous exercise, known medical renal disease, acute viral illness, trauma, and the presence of foreign bodies in the urinary tract or recent urologic instrumentation. The history also should include an assessment of associated symptoms, such as GH, voiding symptoms, or flank pain. Patients' risk factors for known causes of hematuria also should be queried. It is important to know the patient's urologic history, particularly any surgeries or febrile UTIs. It is also critical to ask about the patient's general medical history, to identify potentially contributory diagnoses, such as hypertension, renal insufficiency, bleeding disorders, or sickle cell disease. Current medication use, including anticoagulants and antiplatelet therapies, should be elicited, along with recent coagulation values and any concomitant medications that would potentiate the effects of blood thinners. Family history of nephritis, polycystic kidneys, and rare familial tumor syndromes of the kidney (e.g., von Hippel-Lindau) or urothelium (e.g., Lynch syndrome) also may

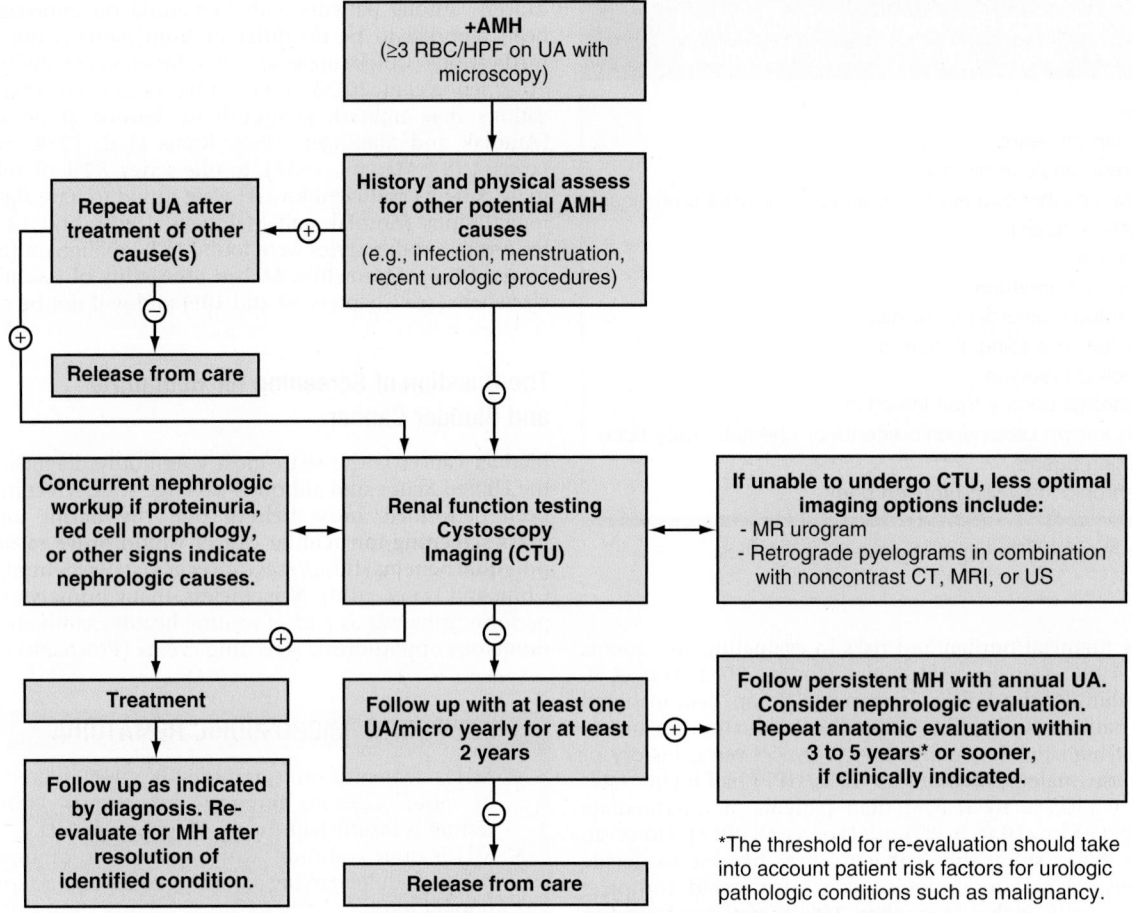

Figure 9-1. American Urological Association guideline algorithm for evaluation of adult patients with asymptomatic microhematuria. AMH, asymptomatic microhematuria; CT, computed tomography; CTU, computed tomography urogram; HPF, high-power field; MH, microhematuria; MR, magnetic resonance; MRI, magnetic resonance imaging; RBC, red blood cell; UA, urinalysis; US, ultrasound. (From the American Urological Association.)

be informative. In addition, the possibility of finding a tobacco-related illness, such as bladder cancer, makes this a potential "teachable moment" for tobacco users (Bassett et al, 2012; Fiore and Baker, 2013). Thus smoking cessation counseling should be a standard component of the hematuria evaluation discussion.

Physical examination should focus on the genitourinary system (e.g., flank tenderness; masses in the flank, abdomen, suprapubic area, or urethra; and enlarged, nodular, tender, or fluctuant prostate.) Physical examination also may identify signs of coagulopathy (bruising), infection (fever), or renal disease (hypertension, edema). If urethral stricture or benign prostatic hyperplasia (BPH) is suspected, a urine flow rate and postvoid residual measurement may be helpful as well.

Laboratory testing includes urinalysis (if not performed previously) to confirm the presence of hematuria and check for dysmorphic red cells, cellular casts, or proteinuria; a urine culture if the urinalysis or clinical presentation suggests infection; renal function testing (serum creatinine) to determine whether concomitant nephrologic evaluation is indicated and to guide the selection of appropriate upper tract imaging; and prostate-specific antigen in the appropriate setting.

If a benign cause of hematuria is discovered during the initial history and physical (e.g., UTI), that cause should be verified and treated and then the urine should be retested to ensure that the hematuria has resolved in the absence of the presumed benign cause. Moreover, **if a medical renal cause of hematuria is suspected based on the presence of renal insufficiency, hypertension, or abnormalities on urinalysis, nephrology evaluation is** recommended, but the patient should still undergo urologic evaluation.

Cystoscopy in the Diagnostic Evaluation of Hematuria

Cystoscopy is a key component of the hematuria evaluation because it is the most reliable way to evaluate the bladder for the presence of bladder cancer and provides the opportunity to evaluate the urethra. **Cystoscopy should be performed in all adults who meet criteria for hematuria evaluation who are 35 years of age or older and/or have risk factors for malignancy.** The potential risks include discomfort, injury to the urethra, infection, and the need for additional procedures, such as biopsy. At the population level, bladder cancer is quite rare (<1 per 100,000) among persons 35 years old or younger (van der Molen and Hovius, 2012; http://seer.cancer.gov/statfacts/html/urinb.html). That is, among 3762 individuals with asymptomatic MH from 17 screening studies, 98 (2.6%) were diagnosed with a urinary tract malignancy, of whom 95 (97%) were older than 35 years of age. For these reasons, **cystoscopy may be omitted in persons younger than age 35 years without risk factors or clinical suspicion for bladder cancer** or urethral pathology (see Box 9-1).

Of note, blue-light cystoscopy using 5-aminolevulinic acid (ALA) or hexyl-aminolevulinate (HAL) instillation is approved by the U.S Food and Drug Administration (FDA) for evaluation of patients with suspicion of papillary bladder cancer, but the studies supporting its use have been conducted in patients with known bladder cancer, thereby limiting generalizability to MH patients

(Davis et al, 2012; Malmstrom et al, 2012). In light of the small incremental risk associated with ALA or HAL and blue-light cystoscopy (rare anaphylactoid shock, hypersensitivity, pain, cystitis, dysuria, hematuria) and the risk for unnecessary biopsies compared to conventional white light cystoscopy, the **AUA guideline recommends against using blue-light cystoscopy for evaluation of MH** (Davis et al, 2012).

Upper Tract Imaging in the Diagnostic Evaluation of Hematuria

Multiphasic computed tomography (CT) urogram (i.e., CT with precontrast, nephrographic, and excretory series) is the imaging study of choice for the evaluation of asymptomatic MH (Vikram et al, 2009), because CT urography offers complete imaging of the urinary tract and has the highest sensitivity and specificity for detecting lesions of the renal parenchyma and the upper tracts. Nonetheless, CT urography does carry risks and may not be appropriate for all patients (e.g., pregnancy, iodinated contrast allergy, renal insufficiency). Indeed, in the setting of a contraindication to CT urogram, magnetic resonance urogram may be used as the upper tract study. Moreover, for patients with a contraindication to magnetic resonance imaging (e.g., pacemaker), as well as in the setting of significant renal function compromise (i.e., estimated glomerular filtration rate <30) when the administration of gadolinium risks nephrogenic systemic fibrosis, renal parenchymal imaging with noncontrast CT or ultrasound, in conjunction with retrograde pyelography to evaluate the calyces, renal pelvis, and ureters, may be most appropriate.

Urine Cytology and Urinary Biomarkers in the Diagnostic Evaluation of Hematuria

Urine cytologic examination is highly sensitive and specific for the detection of high-grade urothelial carcinoma, but sensitivity decreases significantly for low-grade urothelial carcinoma, resulting in an overall sensitivity of 15.8% to 54.5%, and specificity of 95.0% to 100% for bladder cancer detection (Miyanaga et al, 1999; Zippe et al, 1999; Chahal et al, 2001; Grossman et al, 2005; Steiner et al, 2008). Indeed, in a large study of patients with hematuria, the sensitivity and specificity of positive/suspicious/atypical cytology were 45.4% and 89.5%, respectively (Mishriki et al, 2013).

Meanwhile, although several urine biomarkers have been approved or cleared by the FDA for detection and surveillance of bladder cancer, few studies have been conducted to evaluate these markers in patients with MH who do not have a history of bladder cancer. Available assays include nuclear matrix protein-22 (NMP-22), bladder tumor antigen, fluorescence in situ hybridization (FISH) for abnormalities of chromosomes 3, 7, 17, and 9p21 (UroVysion [Abbott Molecular, Abbott Park, IL]) and immunocytology for carcinoembryonic antigen and mucin glycoproteins (ImmunoCyt [Scimedx, Denville, NJ] and CertNDx [PCLS, Rock Hill, SC]).

NMP-22 offers a potential advantage in management of patients with MH in that it is available as a point-of-care test. However, only two studies to date have focused on the asymptomatic patient with MH, with one finding a high sensitivity (90.9%), and the other, in a screening population, demonstrating very low sensitivity (6.0%). Specificity was moderate or high in both studies (76.3% and 82.5%, respectively) (Miyanaga et al, 1999; Steiner et al, 2008). Meanwhile, one study assessed FISH testing in patients with asymptomatic MH with a negative cytology and found that sensitivity and specificity may be high for upper tract tumors in this setting (Huang et al, 2012). A separate FISH study in asymptomatic MH patients (albeit without prior negative cytologic findings) showed sensitivity and specificity of 61% and 93%, respectively, for bladder tumors (Steiner et al, 2008). Immunocytology has been tested in the asymptomatic MH setting in one study of 189 patients (Schmitz-Drager et al, 2007). Here, eight bladder tumors were identified, of which seven were identified by

the ImmunoCyt test, for a sensitivity of 87%. However, studies in the urothelial carcinoma follow-up setting have found a far more modest sensitivity (68.1%) (Comploj et al, 2013). Finally, the multianalyte urine test CertNDx assesses several markers (mutant *FGFR3*, quantified matrix metalloproteinase-2 [MMP2], and hypermethylation of *TWIST1* and *NID2*). In a population of patients with hematuria (gross and microscopic) 50 years of age or older without diagnosis of bladder cancer, the sensitivity and specificity of this test were noted to be 87.9% and 56.3%, respectively (Karnes et al, 2012).

Together, because current evidence indicates that none of the available urinary biomarkers, including cytology, appear to be sufficiently sensitive or sufficiently validated to replace cystoscopy or imaging, **these studies are not recommended in the initial evaluation of patients with asymptomatic MH** (Davis et al, 2012). However, **cytologic examination may be considered in patients with a negative initial workup in whom urothelial carcinoma is still suspected, as well as in patients with symptomatic MH.**

Natural History of Microhematuria in Patients with a Negative Initial Evaluation

One of the most vexing questions in the management of MH is how to proceed in patients for whom the initial evaluation is negative. MH has been reported to resolve in approximately one third of these patients over a period of 3 months to several years (Yamagata et al, 1996; McGregor et al, 1998; Jaffe et al, 2001). Nevertheless, it is worth noting that these studies contained large proportions of younger patients, many of whom did not undergo a complete workup at any time, raising the possibility of persistent occult urologic disease. In a set of studies in which patients underwent further evaluation for MH after an initial negative evaluation, 41 malignancies were identified among 1475 patients (2.8%). However, the initial evaluations in these series were often incomplete, the follow-up evaluations were variable, and most of the malignancies were found in a study using CT urography in patients who were not evaluated by CT in the first evaluation (Davis et al, 2012).

In the absence of high-quality evidence, the AUA has issued three guidelines statements, based on expert opinion, pertaining to the follow-up of patients with an initial negative workup (Davis et al, 2012). The first two can be summarized as recommending **following up annual urinalysis for 2 years after a complete negative hematuria workup and releasing the patient from care if the urinalyses confirm resolution of hematuria.** The third statement recommends **repeating the hematuria evaluation within 3 to 5 years in cases of persistent or recurrent asymptomatic MH or for development of symptoms or GH. We would add that patients with persistent or recurrent MH in the setting of an incomplete initial evaluation should have the evaluation completed or repeated.**

KEY POINTS: EVALUATION OF PATIENTS WITH MICROHEMATURIA

- Evaluation of adults with microscopic hematuria includes a history and physical examination, renal function testing, and upper tract imaging for all patients.
- White light cystoscopy is recommended in the evaluation of asymptomatic MH for patients 35 years of age or older and/or those with risk factors for malignancy.
- CT urogram is the preferred imaging modality for the evaluation of hematuria.
- Urine cytologic examination and biomarkers are not indicated in the initial evaluation of asymptomatic MH.
- Patients with a negative complete evaluation can be released from care if subsequent urinalyses confirm resolution of MH. Re-evaluation should be considered in patients with persistent/recurrent MH and those with an incomplete initial evaluation.

SYMPTOMATIC MICROSCOPIC HEMATURIA

The differential diagnosis for symptomatic MH is equivalent to that for patients with asymptomatic MH. However, the risk for malignancy may be significantly higher than in asymptomatic MH (10.5% vs. 5.0% or less) (Sultana et al, 1996; Shephard et al, 2012). To the extent that symptoms help identify an obvious benign cause of hematuria (e.g., infection), and the hematuria resolves after management of this (culture-documented) benign cause, a complete workup can be avoided. Nevertheless, in situations in which an obvious benign cause is not definitively identified, the hematuria does not resolve after treatment of the benign cause, or the symptoms or other risk factors could be consistent with malignancy, full evaluation is recommended. Moreover, because the presence of symptomatic hematuria has been linked to an increased risk for malignancy, current AUA guidelines include several slight modifications to the recommendations for evaluation. Specifically, **cystoscopy is recommended in such patients, regardless of age** (Davis et al, 2012). Moreover, although routine cytology is not recommended as part of the routine evaluation for the asymptomatic patient with microscopic hematuria, **cytologic examination is considered an option in the setting of irritative voiding symptoms,** although cystoscopy should not be omitted even if the cytologic findings are negative (Davis et al, 2012).

GROSS HEMATURIA

The differential diagnosis for GH remains the same as outlined earlier for MH. Of note, however, **as the degree of hematuria increases, so does the likelihood of finding clinically significant lesions during evaluation.** That is, the difference between the yield of life-threatening lesions in patients with gross versus microscopic hematuria has been found to be highly significant (Mariani, 1989). Specifically, among patients with GH, 50% have been found to have a demonstrable cause, with 20% to 25% found to have a urologic malignancy, most commonly bladder cancer and kidney cancer (Lee and Davis, 1953; Khadra et al, 2000; Alishahi et al, 2002; Edwards et al, 2006).

Given the increased frequency with which clinically significant findings are associated with GH, the recommended evaluation in this setting is relatively uniform. That is, **patients presenting with GH in the absence of antecedent trauma or culture-documented UTI should be evaluated with a urine cytologic examination, cystoscopy, and upper tract imaging, preferably CT urogram.** Meanwhile, patients with GH in the setting of a culture-documented UTI should have the infection treated and then a follow-up urinalysis obtained to ensure clearance of the hematuria. The initial assessment for patients presenting with GH should include the history, physical examination, and laboratory studies recommended for patients with MH. Further, patients with GH must be assessed for hemodynamic stability with careful attention to vital signs, anemia with a complete blood count, and, for patients on anticoagulation, coagulation parameters to ensure that levels are within the therapeutic range. After initial stabilization, diagnostic evaluation should then proceed, with cause-specific management as outlined below.

Although clear recommendations are lacking for the follow-up of patients with GH who are found to have a nondiagnostic initial evaluation, the follow-up schedule as outlined for patients with asymptomatic MH may be used as a reference, with consideration given for a full repeat evaluation if episodes of GH recur.

HEMORRHAGIC CYSTITIS

Intractable hematuria localizing to the bladder, or hemorrhagic cystitis, may range in severity from a transient condition that quickly resolves after conservative management to a life-threatening condition requiring urgent intervention. Unfortunately, patients in this situation are often elderly and infirm, with medical comorbidities that complicate plans for care.

Hemorrhagic cystitis is characterized by diffuse inflammation and bleeding from the bladder mucosa (Rastinehad et al, 2007). Numerous causes for this condition have been described (Box 9-2), a few of which merit particular mention here. Bacterial infections, for example, are a common cause of GH, with symptomatic resolution typically noted after appropriate treatment. Meanwhile, viral-induced hemorrhagic cystitis may affect children and immunosuppressed adults particularly, as following renal or bone marrow transplantation. **BK virus, a member of the polyomavirus family, is the most common virus associated with hemorrhagic cystitis** (Gorczynska et al, 2005), and adenovirus, particularly types 11 and 35, has been correlated with hemorrhagic cystitis in children and renal transplant patients (Lee et al, 1996; Hofland et al, 2004). Treatment for viral hemorrhagic cystitis is primarily supportive, with hydration, diuresis, and bladder irrigation, although case reports of antiviral therapy exist (Rastinehad et al, 2007).

Hemorrhagic cystitis also may result from exposure to the oxazaphosphorine class of chemotherapeutic agents, specifically **cyclophosphamide and ifosfamide.** Indeed, hemorrhagic cystitis has been reported to occur in 2% to 40% of patients treated with cyclophosphamide (Rastinehad et al, 2007) and is dose dependent.

BOX 9-2 Differential Diagnosis for Hemorrhagic Cystitis*

Infectious
  Bacterial
  Viral (especially BK virus, adenovirus)
  Fungal
  Parasitic
Trauma
  External
  Postsurgical (e.g., transurethral resection of the bladder)
Malignancy
  Bladder primary
  Bladder invasion from local/distant primary
Vascular malformation
Chemical exposure
  Cyclophosphamide
  Ifosfamide
  Busulfan
  Thiotepa
  Temozolomide
  Aniline dye
  Ether
  Nonoxynol-9 (accidental urethral insertion of vaginal contraceptive)
Radiation therapy history (e.g., prostate cancer, cervical cancer)
Medication induced
  Penicillin and derivatives (via immune reaction)
  Bleomycin
  Danazol
  Tiaprofenic
  Allopurinol
  Phensuximide
  Methenamine mandelate
  Acetic acid
Manifestation of systemic disease
  Amyloidosis
  Rheumatoid arthritis
  Crohn disease

*Bleeding localized to bladder after diagnostic workup for gross hematuria with cystoscopy, urine cytology, and upper tract imaging is without clear cause of alternative bleeding source

Bladder toxicity results from renal excretion of the metabolite acrolein, which is produced by the liver and which stimulates bladder mucosal sloughing and subsequent tissue edema/fibrosis (O'Reilly et al, 2002). The onset of hematuria is typically within 48 hours of treatment (Cox, 1979; Stillwell and Benson, 1988). **2-Mercaptoethane sulfonate (mesna), which binds to acrolein and renders it inert, has been suggested for prophylaxis against cyclophosphamide-induced hemorrhagic cystitis** (O'Reilly et al, 2002). Nevertheless, 10% to 40% of patients will develop the condition despite preventive treatment (Shepherd et al, 1991), and debate continues as to whether mesna is more effective at preventing hemorrhagic cystitis than hyperhydration with forced diuresis and/or continuous bladder irrigation (Shepherd et al, 1991; Vose et al, 1993).

Meanwhile, **radiation therapy for pelvic malignancy represents another predisposing factor to hemorrhagic cystitis.** Indeed, moderate-to-severe hematuria has been reported in approximately 5% of patients after pelvic radiotherapy, with onset between 6 months and 10 years after treatment (Corman et al, 2003). Mechanistically, radiation damages the vascular endothelium, thereby inducing subsequent inflammation, fibrosis, and ischemia, with tissue necrosis and mucosal sloughing occurring through progressive obliterative endarteritis (Hader et al, 1993; Bevers et al, 1995;

Chong et al, 2005). In the setting of such local vascular compromise, moreover, secondary infection frequently ensues, further compromising tissue healing (Del Pizzo et al, 1998).

Management of Hemorrhagic Cystitis

The management of hemorrhagic cystitis may occasionally be guided by the particular cause for the condition (e.g., treatment of infection), although in most cases no cause-directed therapy can be offered and instead a sequential approach, depending on the severity of the condition, should be undertaken (Fig. 9-2). Supportive management in the form of increasing urine output via hydration/diuresis, catheter placement with continuous bladder irrigation, and transfusion as needed represent the mainstay of first-line therapy and typically suffice for mild cases. If hematuria continues and/or clotting of the urine cannot be controlled with bladder irrigation, cystoscopy under anesthesia with clot evacuation and fulguration of discrete bleeding sites is then recommended.

For hematuria that persists despite such conservative measures, various agents have been investigated for bleeding control. Importantly, there is a lack of large, prospective trials reporting comparative treatment efficacy and safety. Nevertheless, an overview of these measures is warranted to facilitate a systematic approach to

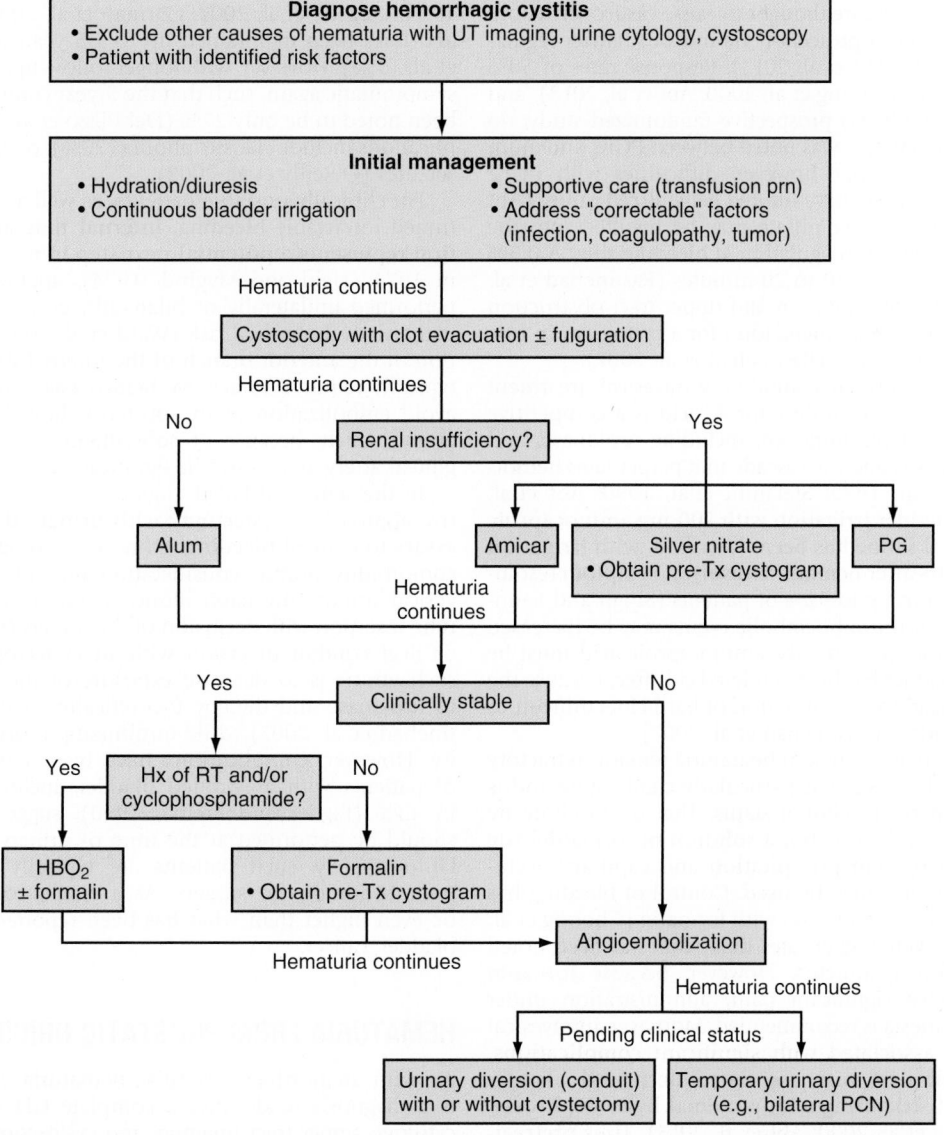

Figure 9-2. Management algorithm for patients with hemorrhagic cystitis. HBO$_2$, hyperbaric oxygen; Hx, history; PCN, percutaneous nephrostomy; PG, prostaglandin; Tx, treatment; UT, upper tract.

management. For one, alum (aluminum ammonium sulfate or aluminum potassium sulfate) may be dissolved in sterile water (50 g alum in a 5-L bag of sterile water [1% alum solution]) and then used to irrigate the bladder at a rate of 200 to 300 mL/hr. Through its action as an astringent at sites of bleeding, **alum may cause protein precipitation on the urothelial lining** (Ostroff and Chenault, 1982) **and thereby stimulate vasoconstriction and a decrease in capillary permeability** (Choong et al, 2000). **In albeit small series to date, success rates of 66% to 100% have been reported after alum instillation** (Choong et al, 2000; Abt et al, 2013). Although cell penetration and therefore overall toxicity of this agent are low (consisting mainly of suprapubic discomfort and bladder spasms), **systemic absorption may nevertheless occur and may result in aluminum toxicity, with consequent mental status changes, particularly among patients with renal insufficiency.** However, alum may be instilled without anesthesia and has an overall relatively favorable efficacy and safety profiles. Thus **this agent may be considered for first-line intravesical therapy among patients with hemorrhagic cystitis failing initial supportive measures, particularly among those who are without renal insufficiency.**

In addition, several alternative agents exist for intravesical instillation therapy. Prostaglandins (e.g., carboprost tromethamine [PGF2-α]) (Abt et al, 2013) have been used intravesically for hemorrhagic cystitis, and although the precise mechanism of activity remains unclear, these agents are thought to cause vasoconstriction, platelet aggregation, and cytoprotection via mucous barrier regulation (Choong et al, 2000; Abt et al, 2013). Response rates of 50% to 60% have been noted (Choong et al, 2000; Abt et al, 2013), and in fact in a small (19 patients) prospective randomized study, no significant difference in efficacy was noted between PGF2 and alum (Praveen et al, 1992). Notably, however, difficulties with PGF2 access, storage, and high costs have limited generalized utility (Abt et al, 2013). Alternatively, silver nitrate may be instilled into the bladder, resulting in chemical coagulation at bleeding sites. A 0.5% to 1% solution is instilled for 10 to 20 minutes (Rastinehad et al, 2007). The potential for precipitation and upper tract obstruction with this agent led to the recommendation for a cystogram to rule out reflux before administration (Rastinehad et al, 2007).

Aminocaproic acid represents another intravesical treatment alternative. A lysine analogue, aminocaproic acid is a competitive inhibitor of activators of plasminogen, including urokinase, and thus interrupts fibrinolysis and the cascade that perpetuates hemorrhage (Garber and Wein, 1989; Stefanini et al, 1990; Abt et al, 2013). **Continuous bladder irrigation with 200 mg aminocaproic acid/L of 0.9% normal saline has been described, with irrigation continued for 24 hours after hematuria resolves.** Symptom resolution has been reported in up to 92% of patients (Singh and Laungani, 1992). The risk for thromboembolic events may be increased with this treatment, and, importantly, aminocaproic acid must be given only after the bladder has been rendered clot-free, because the agent will otherwise lead to the formation of hard clots difficult to eradicate from the bladder (Rastinehad et al, 2007).

Management for patients in whom hematuria remains refractory to the aforementioned measures is particularly challenging and is often guided by the patients' clinical status. That is, for clinically stable patients, intravesical **formalin, a solution of formaldehyde that induces cellular protein precipitation and capillary occlusion** (Choong et al, 2000), **may be used.** Control of bleeding has been reported in 80% to 90% of cases with formalin (Choong et al, 2000), which are relatively higher rates than what has been noted with other intravesical treatments. However, because formalin instillation may induce significant pain, administration under general or spinal anesthesia is recommended. Moreover, intravesical **formalin therapy is associated with significant complications, including bladder fibrosis with associated decreased bladder capacity and ureteral stricturing with proximal hydronephrosis/ renal injury** (Choong et al, 2000; Abt et al, 2013). Thus **pretreatment cystogram is recommended to exclude the presence of vesicoureteral reflux and/or bladder perforation** (Donahue and Frank, 1989). If reflux is documented, placement of occlusive ureteral

catheters is recommended to limit upper tract exposure to the medication. Regardless, moreover, low concentrations of formalin (1% to 2%) should be used initially, because complication rates (albeit efficacy rates as well) have been linked to dosage (Donahue and Frank, 1989). Irrigation (with volumes up to 300 mL or to bladder capacity) (Choong et al, 2000) should be done under gravity, with the catheter no more than 15 cm above the pubic symphysis. Irrigation should be limited to 10 to 15 minutes and should be performed with the catheter on light traction to prevent urethral exposure, with care taken to protect all external areas of skin from exposure. Given the potential toxicities of formalin, together with the requirement for administration under anesthesia, this agent should be reserved for second-line therapy.

Another treatment option for patients with refractory hemorrhagic cystitis, particularly resulting from radiation therapy or cyclophosphamide-induced cystitis (Brastas et al, 2004), **is hyperbaric oxygen (HBO$_2$) therapy.** Treatment is carried out in a specially designed chamber and involves administration of 100% oxygen at a pressure of 2 to 3 atmospheres for approximately 90 minutes in 30 to 40 sessions (Bevers et al, 1995; Del Pizzo et al, 1998; O'Reilly et al, 2002). With this, local tissue oxygen tension increases and thus oxygen extraction by tissues increases, thereby diminishing edema and promoting neovascularization, critical steps in the wound healing process (Hader et al, 1993). Response rates to HBO$_2$ of 80% to 90% have been reported (Bevers et al, 1995; O'Reilly et al, 2002; Corman et al, 2003; Chong et al, 2005) and have been maintained up to 2.5 years after treatment (Weiss et al, 1994). However, with longer follow-up, most patients become symptomatic again, such that the 5-year complete response rate has been noted to be only 27% (Del Pizzo et al, 1998). Reported complications include claustrophobia (20%), otalgia (17%), and, rarely, seizures (O'Reilly et al, 2002).

For clinically unstable patients, as well as for patients with continued intractable bleeding, **internal iliac artery angioembolization represents a potential next step** in management. As reported in 1974 (Hald and Mygind, 1974), angioembolization may be performed unilaterally or bilaterally, even in debilitated patients, with relatively limited risk (Ward et al, 2003). Selective embolization of the anterior branch of the internal iliac artery bilaterally is typically required to achieve hemostasis. Care should be taken to avoid embolization of the posterior branch of the internal iliac artery, which, because of subsequent occlusion of the superior gluteal artery, may result in significant gluteal pain.

In the setting of failed angioembolization and other conservative approaches, **cystectomy with urinary diversion may be necessary to control bleeding.** Of note, pending the patients' clinical/ comorbidity profile, consideration may be been given to supravesical urinary diversion alone, including bilateral nephrostomy tube insertion with occlusion of the ureters (Gonzalez et al, 2001), or ileal conduit diversion without cystectomy. The intention of such efforts is to decrease exposure of the hemorrhagic bladder to urokinase and thereby theoretically facilitate hemostasis (Rastinehad et al, 2007) while minimizing procedure-related morbidity. However, complications have been reported in up to 80% of patients with a retained bladder, including rehospitalization in 43% (Eigner and Freiha, 1990), suggesting that cystectomy should be performed at the time of urinary diversion if feasible. Unfortunately, such patients are typically ill and therefore in poor condition for surgery. As a result, complication rates may be even higher than what has been reported after cystectomy for bladder cancer.

HEMATURIA FROM PROSTATIC ORIGIN

As with hemorrhagic cystitis, hematuria from prostatic origin is a diagnosis made after a complete GH evaluation (including cytology, upper tract imaging, and cystoscopy) to confirm that no other source of hematuria exists. Varied causes exist for prostate-related hematuria, and the severity of such bleeding likewise may range from transient self-limiting episodes to continuous bleeding resulting in the obstruction of urinary flow and in transfusion dependence. Most commonly, prostate-related bleeding is due to BPH, prostate-related infection (prostatitis), or prostate cancer (Fig. 9-3).

BPH represents the most common cause of prostate-related bleeding and has been cited as the most common cause of GH in men older than 60 (Borth and Nickel, 2006). In fact, BPH has been reported to be the only pathologic condition identified in approximately 20% of cases from hematuria studies (Hasan et al, 1994; Lynch et al, 1994). **The cause for BPH-related hematuria has been thought to be increased prostatic vascularity resulting** from higher microvessel density in hyperplastic prostate tissue (Deering et al, 1995; Foley et al, 2000; Pareek et al, 2003; Borth and Nickel, 2006). This **noted increase in microvessel density has in turn been linked to higher levels of vascular endothelial growth factor (VEGF)** (Walsh et al, 2002; Pareek et al, 2003; Borth and Nickel, 2006).

Frequently, BPH-related hematuria episodes are mild and self-limiting, such that once the diagnosis has been established, expectant management with encouraged hydration can be undertaken. Interestingly, although GH has historically been considered an indication for surgery in the setting of BPH, increased understanding of the molecular pathway contributing to the pathophysiologic process (i.e., increased VEGF) has translated into the incorporation of what may be considered targeted medical therapy in the management of patients with BPH-related hematuria.

Specifically, because the pathophysiology of BPH-related bleeding has been postulated as increased cell proliferation stimulating increased vascularity, efforts to suppress prostate growth via androgen ablation have been explored (Marshall and Narayan, 1993; Foley et al, 2000). Both estrogens and antiandrogens have, in small case reports, been associated with decreased prostate bleeding, presumably through the repression of androgen-stimulated angiogenesis and the induction of programmed cell death within the prostate (Marshall and Narayan, 1993; Rittmaster et al, 1996). In particular, finasteride, a 5α-reductase inhibitor that blocks conversion of testosterone to dihydrotestosterone and is a treatment for

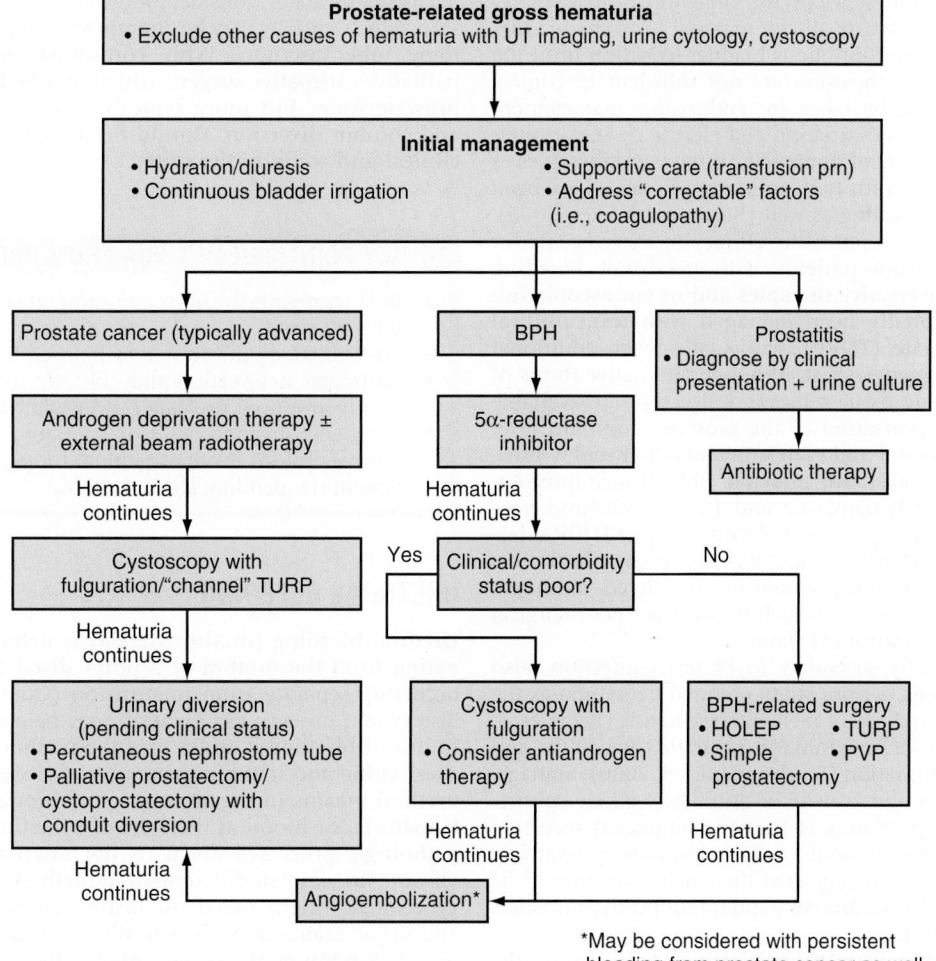

Figure 9-3. **Management algorithm for patients with persistent hematuria of prostate origin. BPH, benign prostatic hyperplasia; HOLEP, holmium laser enucleation of the prostate; PVP, photovaporization of the prostate; TURP, transurethral resection of the prostate; UT, upper tract.**

prostate-related outlet obstructive symptoms, has been investigated extensively for BPH-related bleeding. **Treatment with finasteride is associated with decreased VEGF expression** (Pareek et al, 2003), **prostate microvessel density** (Pareek et al, 2003), **and prostatic blood flow** (Frauscher et al, 2003).

Clinically, **multiple series have demonstrated efficacy of finasteride for BPH-related hematuria, including in patients being treated with anticoagulation. Symptom improvement or resolution has been consistently noted in approximately 90% of patients** (Puchner and Miller, 1995; Carlin et al, 1997; Miller and Puchner, 1998; Sieber et al, 1998; Kearney et al, 2002). A prospective randomized trial of finasteride versus expectant management in 57 patients with BPH-induced hematuria found that the rate of recurrent hematuria was significantly higher among patients in the control arm (63%) versus finasteride (14%) ($P < 0.05$), with 26% of patients in the control arm requiring surgery for bleeding versus none of the finasteride-treated patients (Foley et al, 2000). The onset of action for finasteride is variable, with improvement in bleeding noted from as short as 2 weeks to up to 9 months after initiating therapy. In addition, a randomized trial of finasteride versus cyproterone acetate versus watchful waiting demonstrated a significant decrease in recurrent hematuria in both the finasteride and in the cyproterone acetate cohorts, with no noted difference in efficacy between finasteride and cyproterone acetate in patients treated with this agent (Perimenis et al, 2002). Thus, although various forms of hormonal therapy remain options for BPH-related bleeding, the best data to date exist for 5α-reductase inhibition, which likely entails the least side-effect profile as well.

In cases of BPH-bleeding in which patients have difficulty with bladder emptying and/or presence of clot, large-bore catheter placement with irrigation to evacuate all clot material from the bladder should ensue, followed by continuous bladder irrigation until the urine has cleared. If such measures are not sufficient to control bleeding, patients should be taken for endoscopic management under anesthesia, with clot evacuation and electric or laser cauterization. Although the variety of nonspecific intravesical therapies as are used in hemorrhagic cystitis (e.g., aminocaproic acid) have been suggested for use in this setting as well (Borth and Nickel, 2006), limited evidence exists to support the efficacy of these agents for BPH-related bleeding. Thus **patients with persistent bleeding from BPH despite conservative therapies and/or endoscopic fulguration have traditionally been managed with transurethral resection of the prostate (TURP),** particularly when additional indications for BPH surgery coexist. Although alternative forms of such endoscopic prostate tissue removal/destruction are available (e.g., photoselective vaporization of the prostate, holmium laser enucleation of the prostate) and even suprapubic/retropubic prostatectomy may be undertaken, the principle with all such interventions is to remove the hyperplastic and friable transition-zone prostate tissue. In cases with persistent bleeding despite TURP, selective angioembolization (Michel et al, 2002) and even radical prostatectomy or cystoprostatectomy should be considered, although, as with hemorrhagic cystitis, often such patients are poor surgical candidates because of comorbidity status.

Prostatitis, traditionally secondary to bacterial infection, also may result in GH. Indeed, a prior study reported hematuria as the manifesting symptom in 2.5% of men with prostatitis (Rizzo et al, 2003). The mechanism of hematuria in prostatitis is unclear and may be related to inflammation (Borth and Nickel, 2006). Management in this setting should consist of antibiotics when culture-documented bacterial prostatitis is present. Significant recurrent hematuria in the setting of nonbacterial prostatitis is relatively uncommon, and it has been suggested that such cases should be treated with antibiotics in addition to standard supportive measures (Borth and Nickel, 2006).

Meanwhile, **hematuria from prostate cancer typically results in cases of significantly locally advanced tumors,** often with bladder base/trigonal invasion. Indeed, hematuria has been noted to be the most common local symptom among patients with advanced symptomatic prostate cancers (Din et al, 2009). Importantly, the hematuria in these patients, particularly in those who have previously received radiation therapy in the management of their prostate cancer, should be confirmed with endoscopic evaluation to be from a prostate source and not, for example, as a result of hemorrhagic cystitis or secondary bladder malignancy. Unfortunately, these tumors are typically invasive of the bladder and/or pelvic sidewall (T4) and the patients are often elderly and unwell. Thus treatment is primarily with palliative intent. Initial conservative measures, including catheter drainage with or without continuous bladder irrigation, suffice for most cases of mild prostatic bleeding. For patients in whom hematuria is not acutely life-threatening, palliative external beam radiotherapy with or without androgen deprivation therapy may be administered. Indeed, one series reported that hematuria from advanced prostate cancer responded to palliative radiation in 81% of patients at 6 weeks after treatment; however, durable symptom control was limited, such that the response rate 7 months after treatment in these patients was only 29% (Din et al, 2009). **Among patients who are not candidates for local therapy, as well as among patients in whom disease has recurred after previous local therapy, androgen deprivation therapy may resolve the hematuria** (Marshall and Narayan, 1993) **by decreasing prostate vascularity** (Kaya et al, 2005).

In the situation of persistent hematuria with prostate cancer, and in particular in the setting of bladder outlet obstruction, cystoscopy under anesthesia with fulguration and/or limited, or channel, transurethral resection of prostatic tissue should be undertaken. Moreover, selective internal iliac artery embolization, as has been reported for severe post-TURP bleeding (Barbieri et al, 2002; Michel et al, 2002), may be considered, although data on this approach in the setting of prostatic malignancy are scant. Ultimately, if bleeding persists or escalates, consideration should be given to urinary diversion, which initially may be attempted with percutaneous nephrostomy tube insertion. **With continued prostate hemorrhage, palliative extirpative surgery, which may be in the form of radical prostatectomy, but more typically requires cystoprostatectomy and conduit diversion, should be considered pending patients' clinical and comorbidity status.**

KEY POINTS: HEMATURIA FROM PROSTATIC ORIGIN

- BPH represents the most common cause of GH in men older than 60 years.
- 5α-Reductase inhibitors may be used for BPH-related GH.
- Androgen deprivation may be effective for patients with locally advanced prostate cancer with GH.
- Angioembolization and/or urinary diversion represent salvage options for management for patients with refractory hematuria, pending clinical status.

URETHRAL BLEEDING

Urethral bleeding (urethrorrhagia) is defined as bleeding emanating from the urethra at a point distal to the bladder neck, occurring separate from micturition (Gontero, 2013). A careful history and physical examination may help elucidate whether the source of bleeding is truly from the urethra as opposed to other sites within the lower urinary tract. For example, **blood at the urethral meatus in the absence of volitional micturition, initial hematuria, or blood at the start of urination frequently implies pathologic processes distal to the external urinary sphincter.** Of note, in women, differentiating urethral bleeding from that of gynecologic origin based on history alone may be challenging and pelvic examination is typically necessary to clarify the site of origin (Sandhu et al, 2009). Importantly, retrograde urethrogram and cystourethroscopy remain the mainstays for diagnosis in patients with suspected urethral bleeding, because direct visualization permits identification of pathologic processes in the urethra and biopsy and fulguration allow for histologic characterization and cessation of bleeding.

Causes of urethral bleeding are best classified by gender (Box 9-3). **In men, trauma to the urethral epithelium represents the most common cause of urethral bleeding.** For example, blunt trauma via straddle injury, kick to the perineum, or pelvic fracture often manifests with bleeding and concurrent urinary retention (Mundy and Andrich, 2011). Perineal or penile bruising, accompanied by a hematoma, often is a clear indication of injury related to trauma. **Retrograde urethrography is essential in instances of trauma when a urethral injury is suspected** (Avery and Scheinfeld, 2012). Meanwhile, a history of foreign body insertion in patients with hematuria may necessitate imaging to ensure no residual foreign elements remain that could perpetuate bleeding or result in subsequent calculus formation (Rahman et al, 2004). **Particular mention should be made to the evaluation of bloody urethral discharge and/or hematuria occurring in patients with a penile fracture. In this setting, prompt evaluation via retrograde urethrography or cystoscopy should be undertaken to evaluate for a urethral injury and to identify the nature and location of the injury before surgical exploration** (Avery and Scheinfeld, 2012).

Urethritis refers to infection or inflammation of the epithelial lining of the urethra and has been reported secondary to bacterial or viral infection, chemical irritants (i.e., spermicidal jelly), and, rarely, autoimmune systemic conditions (human leukocyte antigen B27 [HLA-B27] Reiter syndrome). Urethral discharge on palpation may be noted with urethritis in men. Urine microscopy and cultures, as well as urethral swabs for causative organisms, represent essential components of the evaluation.

Urethral tumors are rare, although blood per meatus may be a manifesting sign in patients with urothelial carcinoma, specifically in men who have undergone a radical cystectomy with urethra still in situ (White and Malkowicz, 2010). At the same time, urethral caruncles are benign urethral lesions typically originating from the posterior lip of the urethra, most commonly found in postmenopausal women (Conces et al, 2012). These lesions are thought to arise from prolapse of distal urethra as a consequence of estrogen deficiency. In addition to the classic presentation of dysuria, dyspareunia, and dribbling, women with a urethral diverticulum also may report intermittent episodes of bleeding, and urethral discharge may be noted on examination.

HEMATURIA ORIGINATING FROM THE UPPER URINARY TRACT

Hematuria emanating from the upper urinary tract is frequently asymptomatic, although macroscopic bleeding with clots can result in subsequent ureteral obstruction, with patients experiencing "clot colic," as well as anemia, and even rarely hemodynamic instability (Lano et al, 1979). Most often, hematuria from the upper tract manifests as total hematuria, or bleeding throughout the duration of the urinary stream (Mazhari and Kimmel, 2002), and may be characterized by wormlike clots passed per urethra. A variety of causes can result in bleeding from the upper tract (Box 9-4), with

---

BOX 9-3 Differential Diagnosis for Urethral Bleeding

MALE
Trauma
  Blunt (straddle injury, kick to perineum)
  Penetrating (foreign body insertion, failed urethral catheterization)
  Intercourse related (penile fracture, masturbation)
Urethritis
  Bacterial (gonococcal, nongonococcal)
  Viral
  Chemical
  Autoimmune (Reiter syndrome)
Malignancy
  Urothelial carcinoma
  Squamous cell carcinoma (meatus/glans)
Condyloma
Calculus disease

FEMALE
Trauma
  Blunt (pelvic fracture)
  Penetrating (foreign body)
Urethral diverticulum
Urethral caruncle
Urethritis
Malignancy
Calculus disease

BOX 9-4 Differential Diagnosis for Upper Urinary Tract Bleeding

Renal glomerular diseases
  IgA nephropathy (Berger disease)
  Thin basement membrane disease
  Acute glomerulonephritis (e.g., poststreptococcal)
  Lupus nephritis
  Hereditary nephritis (e.g., Alport syndrome)
Renal tubulointerstitial diseases
  Papillary necrosis
    Sickle cell nephropathy
    Analgesic nephropathy
  Polycystic kidney disease
  Medullary sponge kidney
Vasculitis
  Henoch-Schönlein purpura
  Wegener granulomatosis
Infection
  Pyelonephritis
  Xanthogranulomatous pyelonephritis
  Renal tuberculosis
  Fungal infection
Obstruction
  Ureteropelvic junction obstruction
  Ureteral stricture
Nephrolithiasis
Malignancy
  Renal cortical tumors (renal cell carcinoma, benign tumors)
  Upper tract urothelial carcinoma
Fibroepithelial polyp
Vascular diseases
  Renal arteriovenous malformations (congenital, acquired)
  Iliac arterio-ureteral fistula
  Renal artery aneurysm (especially ruptured)
  Renal artery pseudoaneurysm
  Renal artery and/or vein thrombosis
  Hemangioma
  Atheroembolic disease
  Nutcracker syndrome
  Loin-pain hematuria syndrome
Trauma
  Blunt
  Penetrating
Lateralizing essential hematuria

the most common causes of hematuria from the upper urinary tract including stones, trauma, and malignancy. The evaluation and management of these entities is described elsewhere. Herein, we highlight several particularly salient, albeit less frequent, causes of upper tract hematuria.

Medical Renal Disease

Glomerular diseases are a constellation of acquired or inherited conditions in which the glomeruli are damaged. Consequences include loss of RBCs and protein in the urine, with the clinical sequelae of hematuria, hypoproteinemia with associated edema, and reduced glomerular filtration rate. **Urinary findings suggestive of a glomerular cause include the presence of RBC casts in the urinary sediment, dysmorphic RBCs, and proteinuria** (Yun et al, 2004). Common acquired causes of glomerular diseases are covered in Chapter 46.

Meanwhile, tubulointerstitial diseases broadly refer to kidney diseases affecting structures in the kidney outside the glomerulus. For example, **sickle cell nephropathy is associated with sickle cell disease, whereby sickled erythrocytes decrease medullary blood flow, causing local ischemia, microinfarction, and papillary necrosis** (Pham et al, 2000). Analgesic nephropathy can likewise cause renal papillary necrosis and subsequently chronic interstitial nephritis. Percutaneous renal biopsy may be a valuable diagnostic modality when a suspicion exists for glomerular or tubulointerstitial causes of hematuria.

Vascular Conditions Affecting the Urinary Tract

A variety of vascular conditions can cause hematuria. For example, ureteroiliac artery fistula is an uncommon but potentially life-threatening cause of hematuria. **Predisposing factors include pelvic or vascular surgery, pelvic irradiation, extensive ureteral mobilization, and chronic ureteral stenting** (Muraoka et al, 2008). With regard to management, high mortality rates have been reported with surgical repair of ureteroiliac fistulas, and as such **angiographic localization with vascular stenting has become the current preferred management approach** (Keller et al, 1990). Renal arteriovenous malformations (AVMs), meanwhile, are abnormal communications between intrarenal arterial and venous systems, with congenital and acquired (iatrogenic) causes. **Acquired AVMs account for 75% of such cases and have been associated with renal biopsy, renal surgery (partial nephrectomy, nephrolithotomy), and trauma** (Muraoka et al, 2008). **Arteriography with selective angioembolization is considered the primary diagnostic and therapeutic option for suspected renal AVMs,** affording symptom resolution with maximal preservation of functional renal parenchyma. Thus **expeditious angiography should be considered for patients with a recent history of a renal procedure presenting with GH.** The goal of AVM embolization is eradication of the site where abnormal arterial and venous communication exists. Renal artery aneurysms, moreover, may be related to connective tissue disorders and are generally asymptomatic. Hypertension may be present in up to 90% of affected persons, and dissecting aneurysms may cause flank pain with GH. Renal artery aneurysms and pseudoaneurysms are generally managed via endovascular approaches in the hemodynamically stable patient, whereas surgical intervention is typically necessary in the unstable patient (Mohan and Stephens, 2013).

Additionally, "nutcracker syndrome" (i.e., renal vein entrapment syndrome) is defined as the compression of the left renal vein between the abdominal aorta posteriorly and the superior mesenteric artery anteriorly. Hematuria has been postulated to occur as a result of increase in left renal vein pressure causing small-volume rupture of thin-walled capillaries into the collecting system (Wolfish et al, 1986). Left renal vein transposition, superior mesenteric artery transposition, and nephrectomy have been described as surgical approaches for management of this condition (Hohenfellner et al, 2002). More recently, endovascular stenting to maintain a patent renal vein has been reported as well.

Lateralizing Essential Hematuria and the Evaluation of Upper Urinary Tract Bleeding

Lateralizing essential hematuria, also termed *benign essential hematuria* **or** *chronic unilateral essential hematuria,* **is defined as macroscopic hematuria cystoscopically localized to one side of the urinary system** (Nakada, 2003). Patients have typically had normal prior radiographic studies. Although rare, manifestations of lateralizing essential hematuria may range from minimally symptomatic GH to clot retention and anemia (Nakada, 2003). The differential diagnosis for this entity is as noted earlier for upper tract bleeding (see Box 9-4), although in many such cases no identifiable cause can be determined.

Cystoscopy at the time of bleeding may allow lateralization of the source of hematuria. Subsequently, in the absence of a clear cause for bleeding localized to the upper tract in a patient with lateralizing essential hematuria, direct endoscopic inspection with ureteropyeloscopy is recommended as a diagnostic and potentially therapeutic modality (Nakada, 2003). **Critical components of diagnostic ureteropyeloscopy include the judicious use of guidewires (to avoid inadvertent urothelial injury), low-pressure irrigation, and systematic evaluation of all calices from a superior-to-inferior approach** (Ankem and Nakada, 2006). Biopsy samples can be obtained for lesions suspicious for malignancy, and fulguration of such tumors or other noted sources of bleeding (i.e., hemangioma) can be accomplished as well.

KEY POINTS: URETHRAL BLEEDING AND HEMATURIA ORIGINATING FROM THE UPPER URINARY TRACT

- Urethral bleeding should be suspected with blood at the meatus and/or initial hematuria.
- A concern for traumatic urethral injury should prompt retrograde urethrogram.
- Urinary findings suggestive of a glomerular cause include the presence of RBC casts in the urinary sediment, dysmorphic RBCs, and proteinuria.
- In patients with GH after a recent renal procedure, expeditious angiography should be considered to allow for the diagnosis and management of renal AVM.

REFERENCES

The complete reference list is available online at www.expertconsult.com.

SUGGESTED READINGS

Bevers RFM, Bakker DJ, Kurth KH. Hyperbaric oxygen treatment for haemorrhagic radiation cystitis. Lancet 1995;346:803–5.

Davis R, Jones JS, Barocas DA, et al. Diagnosis, evaluation and follow-up of asymptomatic microhematuria (AMH) in adults: AUA guideline. J Urol 2012;188:2473–81.

Foley SJ, Soloman LZ, Wedderburn AW, et al. A prospective study of the natural history of hematuria associated with benign prostatic hyperplasia and the effect of finasteride. J Urol 2000;163:496–8.

Loo RK, Lieberman SF, Slezak JM, et al. Stratifying risk of urinary tract malignant tumors in patients with asymptomatic microscopic hematuria. Mayo Clin Proc 2013;88:129–38.

Muraoka N, Sakai T, Kimura H, et al. Rare causes of hematuria associated with various vascular diseases involving the upper urinary tract. Radiographics 2008;28:855–67.

10 Fundamentals of Laparoscopic and Robotic Urologic Surgery

Michael Ordon, MD, MSc, FRCSC, Louis Eichel, MD, and Jaime Landman, MD

More than 100 years ago the "father of modern medicine," Sir William Osler, challenged surgeons to perpetually refine their craft, stating, "Diseases that harm require treatments that harm less." In pursuit of this noble goal, the urologists of the 20th century brought us great achievements in our field, but it has been over the past 25 years, in particular, that the specialty of minimally invasive urology has become predominant. The earliest techniques that laid the foundation for modern laparoscopic and robotic urologic procedures were developed at academic institutions throughout the world and have continuously been validated and improved. Subsequently, an increasing number of multiinstitutional studies have emerged comparing laparoscopic and robotic procedures with their open surgical counterparts and showing equivalent efficacy and acceptable efficiency, as well as the distinct advantages of decreased postoperative pain, better cosmesis, faster recovery, a shorter hospital stay, and, in many cases, lower cost. Indeed, it has become increasingly clear that the objectives of many open urologic surgeries, be it of the adrenal gland, kidney, ureter, bladder, prostate, or lymph nodes, can now be achieved with minimally invasive surgery with less patient injury and suffering. Therefore, whereas open surgery has had a steadily diminishing role in the treatment of urologic diseases, laparoscopic and robotic surgery have moved into the mainstream of urologic surgery, and knowledge of the required principles and techniques is essential for the practicing urologist. This chapter is intended to provide a basic foundation of knowledge on which the aspiring minimally invasive urologist can build.

PREOPERATIVE PREPARATION

Patient Selection and Contraindications

Careful patient selection and identification of possible relative and absolute contraindications to laparoscopic and robotic procedures are vital to a successful outcome. To this end, a meticulous past history, focusing on prior surgeries, and physical examination, detailing the location and extent of all abdominal scars, are the initial steps in patient evaluation.

Age- and health-based laboratory studies, an electrocardiogram, and a chest radiograph should be obtained according to the same criteria established for any other significant surgical procedure that is undertaken with general anesthesia.

In patients with severe chronic obstructive pulmonary disease (COPD), further studies (i.e., arterial blood gases and pulmonary function tests) are required because of the physiologic effects of the CO_2 pneumoperitoneum. Cardiac arrhythmias should be evaluated and treated preoperatively because hypercarbia and the resulting acidosis, from the pneumoperitoneum, may have adverse effects on the myocardium, thereby exacerbating any preexisting myocardial instability.

Contraindications to laparoscopic surgery include uncorrectable coagulopathy, intestinal obstruction unless there is an intention to treat, significant abdominal wall infection, massive hemoperitoneum or hemoretroperitoneum, generalized peritonitis, and suspected malignant ascites. Select circumstances in which laparoscopy is being contemplated necessitate careful riskbenefit analysis and detailed and specific informed consent with the patient. The following conditions may portend potential difficulties with a laparoscopic approach.

Morbid Obesity

Laparoscopic procedures in morbidly obese patients are technically challenging. Difficulties may include inadequate length of instruments, decreased range of motion of trocars and instruments, need for higher pneumoperitoneum pressures to elevate the abdominal wall, and poor anatomic orientation owing to excessive amounts of adipose tissue. Traditionally, these difficulties translated into a higher rate of associated complications (Mendoza et al, 1996; Anast et al, 2004; Parker et al, 2008; Aboumarzouk et al, 2012). However, in comparison to open surgery it has been found that the laparoscopic approach to renal and adrenal procedures actually has several advantages. Studies have shown for laparoscopic adrenalectomy and nephrectomy in obese patients that the laparoscopic group had significantly superior outcomes regarding blood loss, resumption of oral intake and ambulation, narcotic analgesic requirements, median hospital stay, and convalescence compared with the open approach (Fazeli-Matin et al, 1999; Fugita et al, 2004; Kapoor et al, 2004; Shuford et al, 2004). These findings have been confirmed for complicated procedures such as laparoscopic and robotic partial nephrectomy (Colombo et al, 2007; Romero et al, 2008; Isac et al, 2012) and laparoscopic nephroureterectomy (Brown et al, 2008).

With regard to laparoscopic and robotic radical prostatectomy in obese men, it has been found that although the operation can be performed without compromising pathologic outcomes, obese patients have a greater risk of perioperative complications (26% vs. 5%) (Ahlering et al, 2005).

Extensive Prior Abdominal or Pelvic Surgery

When extensive intra-abdominal or pelvic adhesions are suspected, careful consideration must be given to the possible site of Veress needle insertion as well as to obtaining open access with a Hasson-style cannula. The Palmer point (subcostal in the midclavicular line on the left side) is the preferred site for Veress needle insertion when extensive intra-abdominal adhesions are suspected (Palmer, 1974). Alternatively, in these patients a retroperitoneal approach may be preferable to a transperitoneal approach or the procedure can be initiated retroperitoneally and the peritoneum then entered (Cadeddu et al, 1999).

Pelvic Fibrosis

Pelvic fibrosis caused by previous peritonitis, pelvic surgery, or extensive endometriosis may constitute a severe technical challenge to the laparoscopic surgeon when surgery of the lower urinary tract is indicated. Similar problems may be encountered when trying to perform pelvic lymph node dissection in patients who have a hip prosthesis; leakage of the polymethyl methacrylate cement can create a dense inflammatory reaction and fibrosis in the adjacent pelvis (Cooper et al, 1997).

Organomegaly

Known or preoperatively diagnosed organomegaly (e.g., hepatomegaly or splenomegaly) necessitates a cautious approach when obtaining the pneumoperitoneum. The site of Veress needle insertion must be chosen at a safe distance from any enlarged organs, or, preferably, open access with the Hasson cannula may be considered.

Ascites: Benign Cause

Patients with severe ascites are under increased risk of injury to the bowel owing to closer proximity of bowel loops to the anterior peritoneum. In addition, a watertight wound closure is required and a firm wound dressing should be applied to prevent prolonged postoperative leakage.

Pregnancy

Initial access to the abdomen must be obtained at a safe distance from the fundus of the gravid uterus. Therefore, trocar placement is usually performed more cephalad on the abdominal wall, depending on the fundus of the uterus. The left upper quadrant in the subcostal midclavicular line (i.e., Palmer point) is often the preferred site of access. Prolonged intra-abdominal pressures of 15 mm Hg or greater may result in hypotension owing to significantly reduced venous return because the vena cava is already mechanically compromised by the enlarged uterus. Prolonged CO_2 pneumoperitoneum, which may result in maternal hypercarbia and acidosis with subsequent adverse effects on the fetus, should be avoided. Accordingly, a working pneumoperitoneum of 10 to 12 mm Hg is recommended in the pregnant patient. **The second trimester is a preferred time for necessary surgery, given the completion of fetal organogenesis and reduced chance of inducing labor.**

As pregnancy progresses beyond the 20th week, the possibility of performing laparoscopic procedures decreases significantly, correlating with the increasing size of the gravid uterus. Of note, both laparoscopic nephrectomy and adrenalectomy have been successfully accomplished in pregnant women (Nezhat et al, 1997; O'Connor, et al, 2004; Sainsbury et al, 2004).

Hernia

A diaphragmatic hernia may result in leakage of a significant amount of CO_2 into the mediastinum, which, although rarely noted, may eventually result in clinical problems such as respiratory compromise or cardiac tamponade (e.g., pneumopericardium) (Knos et al, 1991).

Any evidence of uncorrected or surgically corrected umbilical hernia or abdominal wall hernia should rule out these sites for obtaining a pneumoperitoneum.

Iliac or Aortic Aneurysm

Significant aneurysms warrant evaluation by the vascular surgeon. If the aneurysm does not require immediate surgical correction, insertion of the Veress needle should be performed in the left upper quadrant to stay well away from the area of the aneurysm. Of course, open access with the Hasson technique can be used alternatively. Insertion of accessory trocars must be done under strict endoscopic control to avoid the area of the aneurysm.

Bowel Preparation

For extraperitoneoscopy and retroperitoneoscopy, no bowel preparation is necessary. Similarly, for transperitoneal laparoscopic or robotic procedures *not* involving the use of bowel segments for urinary tract reconstruction, a mechanical bowel preparation is not necessary. A recent large-scale propensity score-matched analysis demonstrated no benefit for mechanical bowel preparation in operative time, postoperative stay, or overall complications for patients undergoing laparoscopic nephrectomy (Sugihara et al, 2013a). Likewise, the same group found no benefit to mechanical bowel preparation in patients undergoing laparoscopic radical prostatectomy in terms of complications, operative time, and postoperative length of stay (Sugihara et al, 2013b).

More recently, emphasis has been placed on "fast-tracking" patients in an effort to streamline care and decrease length of hospital stay. Breda and associates (2007) found that a modified bowel preparation and avoidance of narcotic analgesics postoperatively (with routine administration of ketorolac) was instrumental in achieving a hospital stay of 1.1 days for patients undergoing laparoscopic donor nephrectomy. The bowel preparation consists of clear liquids for 2 days before surgery, two bottles of magnesium citrate the day before surgery, an enema the night before surgery, and nothing to eat after midnight (Breda et al, 2007).

The need for a full mechanical and antibiotic bowel preparation is subject to question and becomes an issue only if one anticipates encountering dense intra-abdominal adhesions or if the surgery involves entering the bowel. However, emerging literature suggests no benefit to a full mechanical bowel preparation for patients undergoing radical cystectomy with creation of ileal conduit or orthotopic neobladder (Hashad et al, 2012; Large et al, 2012; Raynor et al, 2013).

Preparation of Blood Products

Serum type and screen are sufficient for laparoscopic and robotic procedures with a low chance of major hemorrhage. Procedures such as laparoscopic radical nephrectomy and nephroureterectomy have a low rate of transfusion (3% to 12%), with an estimated average blood loss in the range of 106 to 255 mL (Ono et al, 1999; Dunn et al, 2000; Jeschke et al, 2000; Shalhav et al, 2000). Similarly, the transfusion rate with laparoscopic or robotic radical prostatectomy is low (2.5% at experienced centers) (Guillonneau and Vallancien 2000; Ahlering et al, 2004).

More extensive laparoscopic robotic procedures (e.g., partial nephrectomy, radical cystectomy, radical nephrectomy with inferior vena cava thrombectomy), especially early in one's experience, should be managed like any other major open surgical procedure, with packed red blood cells available before surgery. With greater experience, a type and screen may suffice for certain more extensive procedures (e.g., partial nephrectomy) because the risk for transfusion is low (6% to 7%) (Ghani et al, 2014).

IN THE OPERATING ROOM

Setup of the Operating Room

The operating room has to provide enough space to accommodate all necessary personnel and the equipment required by both the surgeon and the anesthesiologist. Positioning of equipment, surgeon, assistants, nurses, anesthesiologist, and other support staff

1. Irrigation-aspiration unit is working.
2. Electrosurgical unit is working.
3. CO_2 tank is full, with extra CO_2 tank in the room.
4. Camera is white balanced, and light source is working.
5. Insufflation is checked for flow and response to kinking of the tubing.
6. Veress needle is checked for flow and proper tip retraction.

KEY POINTS: PREOPERATIVE PREPARATION

- Careful patient selection and identification of possible relative and absolute contraindications are vital to a successful outcome of laparoscopic and robotic procedures. To this end, a meticulous past history, focusing on prior surgeries, and physical examination, detailing the location and extent of all abdominal scars, are the initial steps in patient evaluation for possible minimally invasive surgery.
- Contraindications to laparoscopic surgery include uncorrectable coagulopathy, intestinal obstruction unless treatment is intended, significant abdominal wall infection, massive hemoperitoneum or hemoretroperitoneum, generalized peritonitis, and suspected malignant ascites.

should be clearly defined and established for each laparoscopic or robotic case. All equipment must be fully functional and in operating condition before any laparoscopic procedure is started (Box 10-1). A separate tray with open laparotomy instruments must be ready for immediate use in the event of complications or problems necessitating emergent open surgery.

Patient Positioning

Positioning of the patient depends primarily on the procedure to be performed. In the supine position the arms can be tucked snugly at the sides or rest on specially designed sleds. In the Trendelenburg or lateral position, tape and security belts applied across the chest and thighs provide safe and stable positioning of the patient. In the lateral position, all bony prominences in contact with the table must be carefully padded; likewise, the point of contact between any of the positioning straps and the hip or shoulder should be padded. In the lateral position, the bottom leg is flexed approximately 45 degrees while the upper leg is kept straight; pillows are placed between the legs as a cushion and also to elevate the upper leg so that it lies level with the flank, thereby obviating any undue stretch on the sciatic nerve. Pads should be placed between the table and the knee and ankle of the lower leg because these are high-pressure areas. In the lateral decubitus position an axillary roll should be used. Application of an active warming system may prevent hypothermia, should a lengthy laparoscopic procedure be anticipated.

A host of new advances in padding and table-mounted accessories are now available, but none has been conclusively demonstrated to significantly reduce pressure on the patient's flank in the lateral position. Researchers at the University of California, Irvine, showed that women have significantly lower interface pressures than men (Deane et al, 2008). A body mass index (BMI) greater than or equal to 25, use of a kidney rest, and full-table flexion as opposed to half-table flexion were all associated with increases in interface pressures; of these, **use of the kidney rest was believed to be the most detrimental and its use beyond 20 to 30 minutes was discouraged.** Therefore, male patients with a BMI of 25 or higher

undergoing laparoscopic surgery in the lateral position with the kidney rest elevated and the table completely flexed are at highest risk of developing rhabdomyolysis from flank pressure. In this study the unaugmented operating table mattress was superior to egg crate or gel padding as an augmenting surface material; of note, egg crate padding was equal or superior to the more expensive gel padding.

Table-mounted accessories for all major commercial operating room tables now exist that aid in safely and effectively positioning patients in the lateral decubitus position and in the prone position. For laparoscopic or robotic procedures on the pelvis, the patient can be placed in Trendelenburg position with the legs on split-leg positioners (Fig. 10-1A on the Expert Consult website) or in Allen stirrups (Fig. 10-1B on the Expert Consult website). **Shoulder supports or braces should never be used in this position owing to the risk of brachial nerve injury.**

Prophylaxis and Other Preparations

Pneumatic compression stockings can be applied for antiembolic prophylaxis. In addition, the administration of 5000 units of subcutaneous heparin preoperatively is also an option. In higher-risk patients, such as the morbidly obese, both may be considered (see the discussion of early postoperative complications). Before laparoscopic or retroperitoneoscopic procedures, placement of a Foley catheter should be performed to allow for accurate measurement of urine output, to decompress the bladder to improve visibility and working space, and to reduce the risk of injury with pelvic procedures. Similarly, when needed, a nasogastric or orogastric tube can be inserted to improve the working space available in the upper abdomen.

STRATEGIC PLACEMENT OF OPERATIVE TEAM AND EQUIPMENT

Standard Laparoscopic Carts

Traditionally, the mandatory hardware for laparoscopic procedures (monitor, light source, insufflator) is located on carts or "towers" that can be rolled around the operating room and adapted to various types of surgical procedures and approaches (Fig. 10-2A on the Expert Consult website). The main laparoscopic cart should contain the insufflator, light source, camera controls, and any recording device. Ideally, the insufflator should be placed at the surgeon's eye level to allow continuous monitoring of the CO_2 pressure.

Integrated Endoscopy Systems

More recently, most major manufacturers of endoscopy equipment offer "integrated" systems that consist of flat panel displays and equipment towers that are mounted on adjustable ceiling booms (see Fig. 10-2B on the Expert Consult website). This allows the display monitors to be suspended over the patient and placed directly in front of the surgeon at any height or angle. This feature may reduce eye and body strain. Furthermore, the tower containing the light source, camera system, and insufflator can be placed in any area around the patient depending on the operation at hand.

Robotic Systems

Currently, the only robotic surgical system in widespread use for laparoscopic surgery is the da Vinci Robotic System (Intuitive Surgical, Sunnyvale, CA). The three major components of the system are the robotic tower (i.e., patient-side cart) to which are attached the instruments that are mechanically manipulated within the patient; a surgeon's console, which is the workstation at which the surgeon sits to manipulate the robotic instruments; and finally the ancillary vision cart, which supports a flat screen monitor, an insufflator, a light source, and components of the camera system (Fig. 10-3 on the Expert Consult website). Additional monitors can be linked with the robotic system and used for the assistant and support staff image viewing. The newest generation of the robotic surgical system (da Vinci Si) has the capacity for a second surgeon's console to support training and collaboration.

Placement of the Operative Team for Laparoscopic Procedures

Transperitoneal Procedures in the Upper Abdomen

Laparoscopic. For transperitoneal laparoscopic renal and adrenal surgical procedures, the patient is positioned in a modified lateral decubitus position. The surgeon and assistant usually stand in front of the abdomen with the patient in the lateral decubitus position (i.e., for a left nephrectomy the surgeon and assistant stand on the right side of the operating table). The instrument table and the scrub nurse are best located on the opposite side of the patient near the foot of the bed, such that instruments can be handed to the surgeon over the table (Fig. 10-4A). Incoming lines from insufflators, suction and irrigation, electrosurgical devices, and so on enter from the contralateral side of the table or from the ipsilateral head of the table. Additional technology (e.g., laparoscopic ultrasound probe) may be moved to the operating table depending on the surgeon's needs, as well as on the availability of space.

To provide more comfortable positioning of the surgeon's arms, a 6- × 4-foot, 6-inch lift can be used when the operating table cannot be lowered sufficiently to allow the surgeon to hold the laparoscopic instruments with his or her elbows held comfortably at the side rather than extended laterally. This is most important during suturing.

Robotic. For transperitoneal robotic-assisted laparoscopic renal and adrenal surgical procedures, the patient is again positioned in a modified lateral decubitus position. The assistant usually stands in front of the abdomen with the patient in the lateral decubitus position (i.e., for a left nephrectomy the assistant stands on the right side of the operating table). The robotic arms (i.e., patient-side cart) are brought in from the opposite side (i.e., facing the back with the patient in the lateral decubitus position), such that the robotic arms stretch over the patient and can then be docked to the preplaced ports. In general, it is best to angle the robot slightly such that the camera is pointing directly toward the site of interest. Accordingly, depending on the exact port placement, the robotic arms may be brought in at an angle toward the head of the patient, as opposed to perpendicular to the operating table, to minimize clashing of the robotic arms once docked (Fig. 10-5 on the Expert Consult website). The instrument table and the scrub nurse are best located at the foot of the bed on the same side of the patient as the surgical assistant, such that instruments can be easily handed to the surgical assistant (see Fig. 10-4B). The robotic console can be placed anywhere in the room remote from the operating table and instrument table such that it is out of the way, but in view of the patient and anesthetic monitors. All incoming lines from insufflators, suction and irrigation, and electrosurgical devices enter either from the contralateral foot side of the table or the ipsilateral head of the table.

Retroperitoneal Procedures in the Upper Abdomen

Laparoscopic. For retroperitoneal renal and adrenal procedures, the patient is placed in the true, 90-degree lateral decubitus position with the body at a right angle to the table. All of the proper steps for padding in this position should be followed (see earlier). **The table is angled at the hip to accentuate and increase the distance between the 12th rib and the iliac crest. Maximizing this distance is paramount with regard to port placement.** Both the primary surgeon and the camera assistant stand facing the patient's back (Fig. 10-6A). The scrub nurse or technician stands facing the patient's front, and instruments are handed across the patient accordingly.

Robotic. For retroperitoneal robotic-assisted renal and adrenal procedures, the patient is similarly placed in the true 90-degree lateral decubitus position. The surgical assistant can stand facing either the patient's abdomen or his or her back depending on the surgeon's preference for port placement. The instrument table and scrub nurse are best placed on the same side as the assistant near the foot of the table. The robotic arms are brought in over the head of the patient (Fig. 10-6B). Because the robotic arms are positioned over the patient's head, the anesthesiologist and the anesthetic cart and monitors should be positioned off to the side, in front of the patient, at the head of the bed.

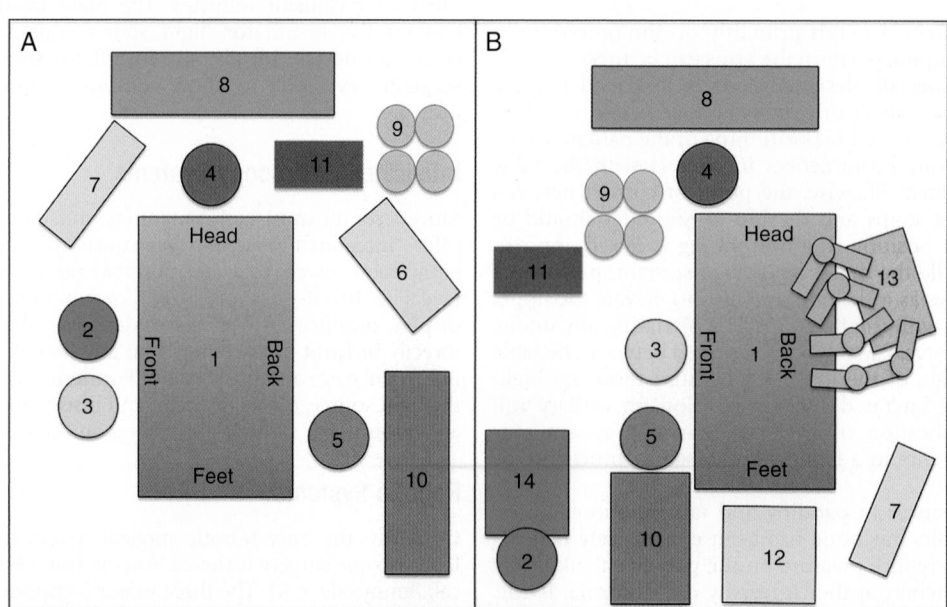

Figure 10-4. Placement of the operative team for transperitoneal procedures in the upper abdomen. A, Laparoscopic procedure. **B,** Robotic procedure. 1, Operating table; 2, surgeon; 3, assistant; 4, anesthesiologist; 5, scrub assistant; 6, laparoscopic cart or tower; 7, auxiliary video monitor; 8, anesthesia equipment; 9, suction and irrigation unit; 10, scrub assistant's instrument table; 11, electrocautery unit; 12, ancillary vision cart; 13, robotic tower; 14, surgeon's console.

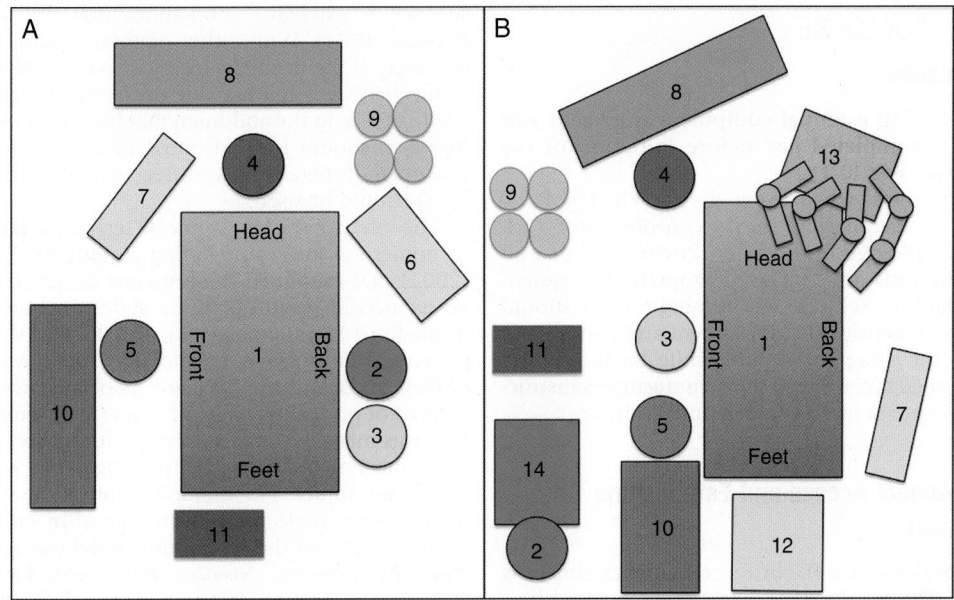

Figure 10-6. Placement of the operative team for retroperitoneal procedures in the upper abdomen. A, Laparoscopic procedure. B, Robotic procedure. 1, Operating table; 2, surgeon; 3, assistant; 4, anesthesiologist; 5, scrub assistant; 6, laparoscopic cart or tower; 7, auxiliary video monitor; 8, anesthesia equipment; 9, suction and irrigation unit; 10, scrub assistant's instrument table; 11, electrocautery unit; 12, ancillary vision cart; 13, robotic tower; 14, surgeon's console.

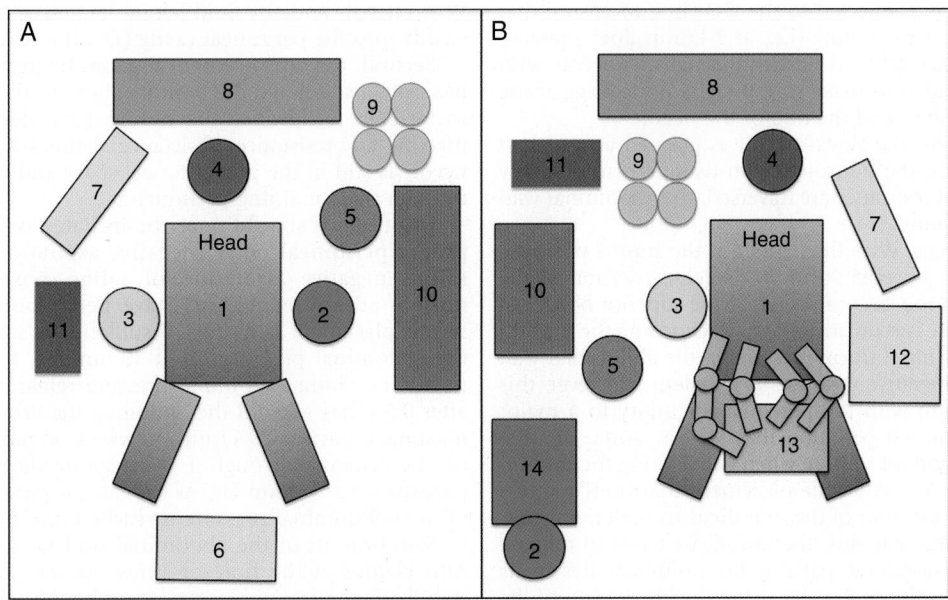

Figure 10-7. Placement of the operative team for pelvic surgery. A, Laparoscopic procedure. B, Robotic procedure. 1, Operating table; 2, surgeon; 3, assistant; 4, anesthesiologist; 5, scrub assistant; 6, laparoscopic cart or tower; 7, auxiliary video monitor; 8, anesthesia equipment; 9, suction and irrigation unit; 10, scrub assistant's instrument table; 11, electrocautery unit; 12, ancillary vision cart; 13, robotic tower; 14, surgeon's console.

Transperitoneal and Extraperitoneal Pelvic Procedures

Laparoscopic. The patient is positioned in the supine position with the legs on split-leg positioners or elevated in stirrups that have knee and leg supports to avoid perineal nerve injury. The table is angled (flexed) slightly at the hip to accentuate the pelvis. The patient's arms are tucked at the sides; plastic sleds can be used to support the arms. A slightly snug chest strap should be placed directly across the patient's chest. The table is placed in the 30-degree Trendelenburg position. The surgeon stands on the side of the table

where he or she is comfortable, and the assistant stands on the opposite side (Fig. 10-7A).

Robotic. For robotic procedures on the pelvis the patient is positioned exactly as described previously for laparoscopic pelvic procedures. After port placement the robotic arms are placed between the patient's legs, and the assistant can remain on either side of the table depending on surgeon preference (Fig. 10-7B). The scrub nurse or technician can be positioned on the same side as the assistant to facilitate passing instruments because passing instruments across the robotic arms can be cumbersome.

PERFORMING THE PROCEDURE

Before the Initial Incision

A checklist ensuring that all essential equipment is present and operational should be completed just before initiation of the pneumoperitoneum (see Box 10-1).

Additional items to check when using the da Vinci Robotic System include ensuring that all plugs for the console, vision cart, and patient-side cart are plugged into different circuits and that all cables connecting these carts are connected properly. The system should be turned on and the self-test and homing routine should be complete. The three-dimensional (3D) camera and endoscopes should be calibrated, the image black and white balanced, and target alignment performed according to the manufacturer's instructions. The patient-side cart should be draped and ready.

Achieving Transperitoneal Access and Establishing the Pneumoperitoneum

Achieving transperitoneal access is the first step before establishing a pneumoperitoneum. This can be done using either a closed (i.e., Veress needle) or open (i.e., Hasson cannula) technique.

Closed Techniques

Veress Needle. A disposable (70- or 120-mm, 14-gauge, and 2-mm outer diameter) or nondisposable Veress needle can be used. Proper needle function should be ensured before the procedure. Specifically, the blunt tip of the needle is tested to make sure it retracts easily and the needle is connected to the CO_2 line to ensure that there is no resistance to gas inflow (i.e., at 2-L/min flow, pressure remains at ≤2 mm). Last, saline is flushed through the needle with the tip manually occluded to make sure there is no leakage at the juncture between the shaft and the hub of the needle.

For proper placement the Veress needle is grasped at midshaft and is passed perpendicularly through skin using a gentle, steady pressure. Two points of resistance are traversed: the abdominal wall fascia and the peritoneum.

Sites for Needle Passage. With the patient in the supine position, the head of the bed is lowered 10 to 20 degrees; insertion of the Veress needle is commonly accomplished at the superior border of the umbilicus. There are certain advantages to choosing the umbilical area as the site for initial trocar placement: the abdominal wall is thinnest, and postoperative cosmesis is excellent. However, this point of entry is fraught with the potential for injury to a major vessel, in particular the left common iliac vessels, aorta, or vena cava. As such, it is important to note when considering the umbilical area as the site for Veress needle placement that body habitus influences the relative location of the umbilicus to underlying vascular structures. In obese patients, the umbilicus tends to migrate inferiorly, whereas in nonobese patients the umbilicus lies in its commonly described position, directly above the bifurcation of the aorta and vena cava. Thus, for umbilical access in nonobese patients the Veress needle should be passed through the abdominal wall angled toward the pelvis to avoid injury to the bowel and great vessels that lie directly beneath. In more obese patients, because the umbilicus lies more caudad, less angulation is needed and the Veress needle should be passed perpendicular to the umbilical incision (Loffer and Pent, 1976).

The right or left lower quadrant can also be used with the patient in the supine position, decreasing the likelihood of vascular injury. However, one must be cognizant of risk for colonic injury with this site. If the patient is in a lateral decubitus position, then the Veress needle can be passed two fingerbreadths medial and two fingerbreadths superior to the anterior superior iliac spine.

Other potential insertion sites when the patient is either supine or in a lateral decubitus position are at the Palmer point (i.e., subcostal in the midclavicular line on the left side) and at the corresponding site on the right side. The Palmer point is the preferred site when extensive intra-abdominal adhesions are suspected (Palmer, 1974). With either of these insertion sites care must be exercised; if the needle is inserted too deeply, there is the potential to hit the liver on either side or, rarely, the spleen on the left side. Alternatively, in the abdomen that has previously been operated on, insertion should be performed in an unscarred quadrant of the abdomen. If there is no scar-free area, then an open technique (see later) should be used.

The safety of the Veress needle technique has been demonstrated in numerous studies including a study by Chung and coworkers (2003) that examined the outcome of 622 consecutive cases with Veress needle insertion. Prior abdominal surgery had been performed in 192 patients (31%), and the BMI was 30 or greater in 98 patients. Blind Veress needle placement was successful in 579 (93%), and outcome was not associated with laterality, type of surgery, or prior surgery. In 34 cases (5%), a minor laceration to the liver was managed conservatively without sequelae; and in 21 cases (3%) the omentum or falciform ligament was traversed without significant injury. No major complications, such as vascular or hollow-organ perforation, were caused by either the Veress needle or trocar. Neither the spleen nor bowel was ever injured.

Assessing Proper Needle Placement. **First the aspiration-irrigation-aspiration test is performed.** With the use of a 10-mL syringe containing 5 mL of saline, the Veress needle is aspirated to check for blood or bowel contents. If this test result is negative, then the saline is injected into the abdominal cavity; this should occur without any resistance. Next, the plunger of the syringe is again withdrawn; no fluid should return into the barrel of the syringe. An additional injection of 2 to 3 mL of saline will help to expel any omentum that may have been sucked into the needle tip with the original aspiration technique. Last, the syringe is detached from the Veress needle and any fluid left in the hub of the needle should fall swiftly into the peritoneal cavity (i.e., **the "drop" test**).

Second, the advancement test can be performed. If the needle has truly just entered the peritoneal cavity, then the surgeon ought to be able to advance the needle 1 cm deeper without the tip meeting any resistance. Resistance at this stage usually means the needle is still in the preperitoneal space and needs to be advanced through the remaining peritoneum.

Insufflation should never be initiated unless *all* **the signs for proper peritoneal entry (negative aspiration, easy irrigation of saline, negative aspiration of saline, positive drop test, and normal advancement test) have been confirmed.** Once proper needle placement is verified, insufflation is started at 2 L/min with the abdominal pressure set at 10 mm Hg. If free flow of CO_2 is noted (i.e., intra-abdominal pressure remains <10 mm Hg), then after 0.5 L has entered the abdomen the flow can be increased to maximal capacity of 9 L/min (however, no more than 2 L/min flow can be achieved through a 14-gauge needle) and the abdominal pressure set at 15 mm Hg. As soon as the preset limit of 15 mm Hg of intra-abdominal pressure is reached, free flow stops.

Stabilization of the abdominal wall fascia with towel clips or Allis clamps at the time of Veress needle puncture may help in stabilizing the fascia; however, one should not lift up on the fascia because this will only increase the space between the fascia and the peritoneum while not changing the intra-abdominal space.

EndoTIP Entry. *See the Expert Consult website for details.*

Open Access Techniques

Hasson Technique. The pneumoperitoneum can be more easily, and in one's early experience, more safely established using the open Hasson technique; however, its use involves making a larger incision and increases the chances of port-site gas leakage during the procedure. **The open technique is recommended specifically when extensive adhesions are anticipated. Studies in general surgery have shown the open technique to be as efficient as the closed approach and slightly more or equally safe** (Bonjer et al, 1997).

In the unscarred abdomen, with the patient in the supine position, a 2-cm semicircular incision is made at the lower edge or

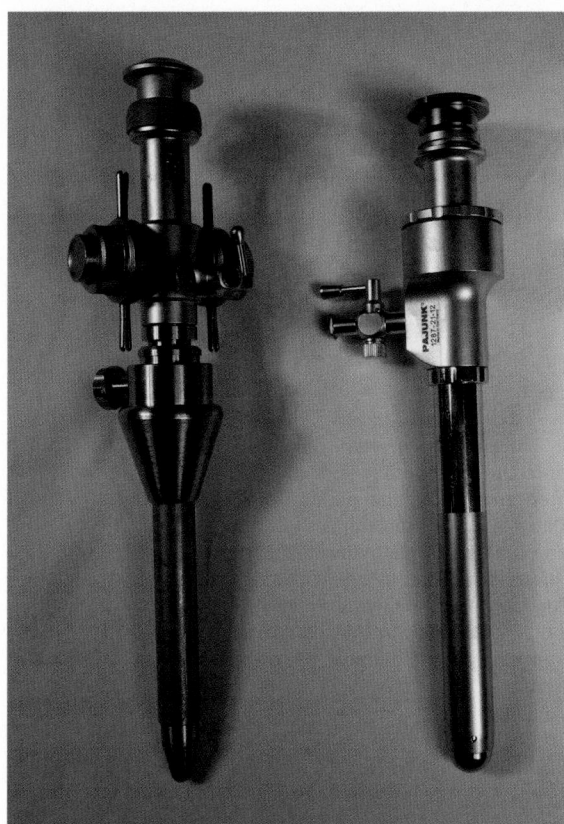

Figure 10-9. Various reusable Hasson type trocars.

slightly below the umbilicus. The fascia and peritoneum are opened individually with a transverse incision, sufficient to accommodate the surgeon's index finger. After visual and digital confirmation of entry into the peritoneal cavity, two 0 silk traction sutures are placed on either edge of the fascia. Next, the Hasson cannula is advanced through the incision with the blunt tip protruding (Fig. 10-9). The funnel-shaped adapter of the Hasson cannula is advanced until it rests firmly in the incision, and it is then tightened onto the cannula with the attached screw; fixation to the abdominal wall is provided with the fascial sutures that are wrapped around the struts on the funnel-shaped adapter of the Hasson cannula, thereby anchoring it in place. After removal of the obturator, free flow of CO_2 into the peritoneal cavity is achieved by attaching the CO_2 tubing to the cannula. The insufflator can be set at maximum inflow, thereby creating the pneumoperitoneum quickly.

A far simpler type of blunt cannula is a balloon retention device (e.g., Blunt Tip Trocar with Balloon Tip, US Surgical, Norwalk, CT or the Kii Balloon Blunt Tip System, Applied Medical Resources, Rancho Santa Margarita, CA) (Fig. 10-10 on the Expert Consult website). Once the cannula is positioned in the abdominal cavity, the balloon is inflated; the cannula is pulled upward until the balloon is snug on the underside of the abdominal wall. Next, the soft foam or rubber collar on the outside surface of the cannula is slid down until it is snug on the skin and locked in place. This process creates an excellent seal, precluding gas leakage and subcutaneous emphysema.

Hand Port Access. The pneumoperitoneum can be obtained before or after making the hand port incision. If the surgeon has little experience with achieving a pneumoperitoneum, the safest maneuver is to use an open technique and place the hand port into a 6.5- to 7.5-cm open incision and then create the pneumoperitoneum through the hand port (i.e., hand port access). For this technique, the procedure begins with making a standard midline or lower quadrant incision at the planned hand-assist site. The peritoneal cavity is entered in the standard open surgical fashion, after

which the hand-assist device is placed according to the manufacturer's instructions. Next, a blunt cannula is passed through the hand-assist device and a pneumoperitoneum is established. Additional 5-mm or 10- to 12-mm ports can be placed rapidly under manual control with the surgeon's intra-abdominal hand being used to guide the additional trocars through the abdominal wall. Alternatively, a laparoscope can be placed through the port placed in the hand-assist device for insufflation, and the rest of the trocars can then be placed under direct vision.

Technique for Laparoendoscopic Single-Site Surgery

See the Expert Consult website for details.

Achieving Retroperitoneal Access and Developing the Retroperitoneal Space

Technique for Balloon or Self-Styled Dilator Placement: Open (Hasson) Technique

The Hasson technique is the most commonly used technique because it affords the greatest precision during development of the retroperitoneal space (Gill, 1998). Initial access is obtained through a 2.0- to 2.5-cm transverse incision in the midaxillary line, just below the tip of 12th rib. The wound is opened with a pair of S-retractors. Under direct vision, the posterior layer of the lumbodorsal fascia is incised and muscle fibers are split or divided. The retroperitoneal space is entered, **under direct vision,** by making a small incision in the anterior thoracolumbar fascia with an electrocautery blade or, less commonly, by bluntly piercing the fascia digitally or with a hemostat. Care should be taken that this fascial opening is snug around the index finger and no larger, so that intraoperative air leak is minimized. Index finger palpation of the belly of the psoas muscle posteriorly and the Gerota fascia–covered inferior pole of the kidney anteriorly confirms proper entry into the retroperitoneal space (Fig. 10-11A). The index finger is used to digitally create a space in this precise location for placement of the balloon dilator; two inflations of the balloon are then done—one directed cephalad and the second directed caudad to fully dilate the retroperitoneal space (Fig. 10-11B). Thus, balloon dilation is performed anterior to the psoas muscle and fascia and outside and posterior to the Gerota fascia. In cases involving definitive ureteric mobilization (e.g., retroperitoneoscopic donor nephrectomy, nephroureterectomy), additional balloon dilation may be performed more caudad to the primary site of dilation (Gill et al, 1995). Similarly, during a retroperitoneoscopic adrenalectomy, it is helpful after the initial balloon dilation to move the balloon up higher in the retroperitoneum and perform a second, even more cephalic balloon dilation along the undersurface of the diaphragm (Sung and Gill, 2000).

Balloon Dilation. Gradual distention of a balloon dilator in the retroperitoneal space atraumatically displaces the mobile fat and moves the peritoneum forward relative to the immobile body musculature. This device thus creates a working space equivalent to the size of the balloon. Either commercially available balloon dilators (Fig. 10-12) or a self-styled dilator can be used.

See the Expert Consult website for details on commercially available balloons and self-styled dilators.
Manual Dilation. *See the Expert Consult website for details.*

Achieving Extraperitoneal Access and Developing the Extraperitoneal Space

Technique for Balloon or Self-Styled Dilator Placement: Open (Hasson) Technique

A 1.5- to 2-cm curvilinear incision is made along the inferior umbilical crease. The anterior rectus sheath is incised vertically for 1.5 cm, and the rectus muscle is separated in the midline to expose the

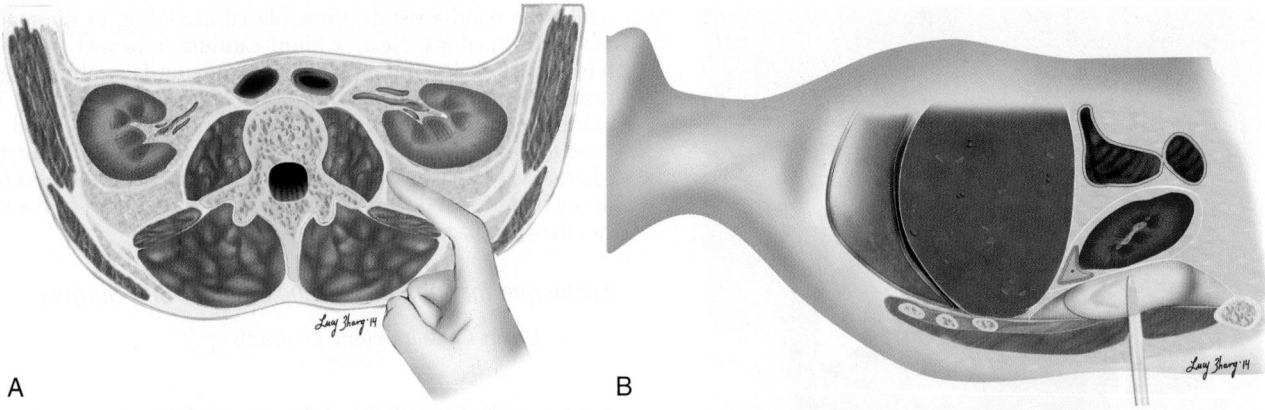

A

B

Figure 10-11. A, Access into the right retroperitoneum. Through the primary port incision at the tip of the lowest (12th) rib, open access is gained into the retroperitoneum after piercing the thoracolumbar fascia. Finger dissection is performed anterior to the psoas muscle and fascia to create a space for insertion of the balloon dilator. Confirmation that the finger dissection is indeed being performed in the proper plane is obtained by palpating the psoas and erector spinae muscles between the retroperitoneally located index finger and the fingertips of the opposite hand positioned on the patient's back. The fat-covered lower pole of the kidney can be palpated in a cephalad direction by turning the finger clockwise in the retroperitoneum on the right side. **B,** Balloon dilation in the posterior pararenal space facilitates the creation of a working space for retroperitoneal laparoscopic nephrectomy (coronal view).

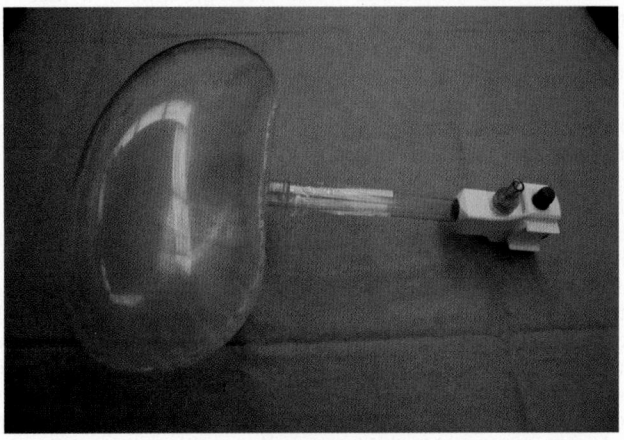

Figure 10-12. Example of a commercially available balloon dilator for creating space in the retroperitoneum: preperitoneal balloon dissector. (Courtesy Covidien Ltd., Mansfield, MA.)

posterior rectus sheath. With the surgeon's index finger positioned posterior to the rectus muscle and anterior to the posterior rectus sheath, gentle tunneling motions are made in a caudal direction until the area of the symphysis pubis is reached. At this distal location, the fascia transversalis is punctured with the fingertip, and gentle side-to-side digital dissection is performed in the prevesical space, posterior to the pubic bone. Into this predeveloped space, a balloon dilator or self-styled dilator (see earlier) is inserted and distended to create an adequate working space. Balloon dilation or self-styled dilation effectively displaces the prevesical fat and reflects the peritoneum cephalad. The balloon is initially inflated in the midline and then reinflated on either side to further expand the working area (Meraney and Gill, 2001).

Caveat: In earlier studies of retroperitoneoscopy, excessive subcutaneous emphysema and higher carbon dioxide levels were the norm owing to use of the standard Hasson cannula (Wolf et al, 1995; Ng et al, 1999); this situation was rectified with the introduction of the open access blunt balloon port, which has a balloon to secure it against the underside of the abdominal wall and a soft foam cuff to secure it to the outer abdominal wall, creating an airtight seal (Ng et al, 1999).

Limitations and Advantages of Transperitoneal versus Extraperitoneal Approach to the Flank and Pelvis

See the Expert Consult website for details.

Access Technology: Trocars, Hand Ports, and Single-Port Access

Trocars

Trocars enable the laparoscopist to introduce working instruments into the gas-filled abdomen or retroperitoneum. They also maintain the pneumoperitoneum by conveying the insufflant and may serve as pathways for delivering small amounts of dissected tissue from the surgical area. Typically a trocar consists of an outer hollow sheath (also called a *cannula* or *port*) and an inner obturator, which is removed as soon as the outer sheath has entered the peritoneal cavity.

A variety of nondisposable and disposable trocars are available (Fig. 10-13). Standard models range from 3 to 20 mm in diameter and 5 to 20 cm in length. One-way valves within the trocar allow the surgeon to exchange instruments through the port without the escape of significant amounts of gas. Some older trocar models have trapdoor or flap valves. In such trocars it is necessary to depress the valve lever to open the valve widely during retrieval of tissue or needles. More recently, **multiseal**-type valves have become available for 10- and 12-mm trocars that accommodate the passage of 5-mm and larger instruments without any air leak occurring; if large amounts of tissue are to be withdrawn, removal of the outer seal or of the entire valve is necessary for this procedure. The outer seal and valve can then be replaced before reinsertion of instruments.

Initially, only sharp-tipped or bladed trocars were available. On these trocars the sharp obturator incised the various layers of tissue as it entered the peritoneal cavity. To protect the underlying viscera from the sharp tip of these trocars, a plastic safety shield was later incorporated into the disposable trocars that would spring forward to shield the blade once the trocar entered the gas-filled abdomen. **However, bladed trocars should be only of historical interest because they have been superseded by safer noncutting dilating trocars (i.e., blunt), which no longer require a safety shield.** These trocars enter the abdomen by spreading the abdominal wall musculature, rather than cutting it. Therefore there is less chance of injuring an abdominal wall vessel, and the resulting entry site is less prone to subsequent herniation. Indeed, studies have shown the

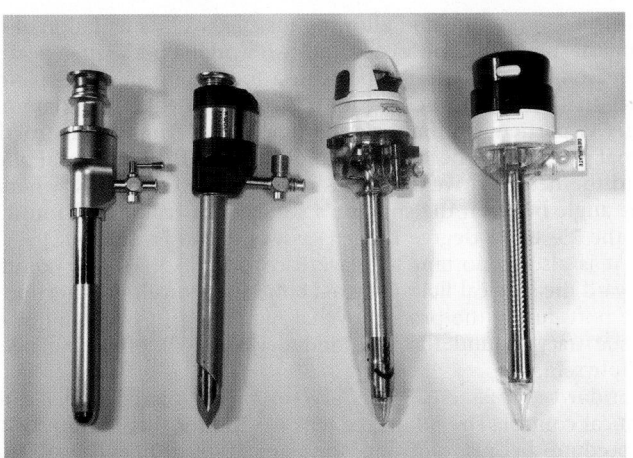

Figure 10-13. **Various trocar designs showing** *(left to right)* **reusable blunt-tipped, reusable bladed, and two disposable visual obturator fascial dilating designs.**

risk of inferior epigastric injury or port site herniation is fivefold less with blunt versus sharp trocars (Hashizume and Sugimachi, 1997; Thomas et al, 2003). In addition, a recent meta-analysis demonstrated a lower relative risk of trocar site bleeding (3% vs. 9%) and overall complications (3% vs. 10%) with blunt compared with bladed trocars (Antoniou et al, 2013).

As with the older sharp trocars, there are both disposable and nondisposable blunt trocar units. One form of blunt disposable trocar unit is the Step needle and sleeve (Covidien). This disposable system uses a needle port with an outer diameter of 2.1 mm (6.5 Fr) that incorporates a Veress needle introducer (Fig. 10-14 on the Expert Consult website). After correct and successful puncture of the abdomen and establishment of the pneumoperitoneum, the Veress needle introducer is removed and the remaining sheath is an expandable port that can then be expanded by passage of a blunt-tipped obturator to expand the collapsed sheath to 5 mm, 10 mm, or 12 mm, depending on the surgeon's needs.

Other blunt-tipped trocars are produced by all of the major trocar manufacturers. These devices have a variety of tips that enable their placement by spreading the tissues; some also have a clear plastic tip (i.e., optical trocar) such that the surgeon can pass an endoscope into the trocar to endoscopically monitor its passage through the abdominal wall and its entry into the gas-filled abdomen.

A unique reusable blunt-tipped port, the EndoTIP system (Karl Storz), is a screwlike device that has no sharp points or cutting edges (see Fig. 10-8). It comes in 5-, 10-, and 12-mm designs; however, the 10- and 12-mm trocars require use of a cumbersome reducer system because they are not a **multiseal** design (see earlier). Unlike the action of trocars with a sharp tip, the tissue is not cut but is only displaced and bluntly dilated, thereby preserving the closing mechanism of the overlying muscle and fascia. Because of its innovative design, this device reduces injury to the intra-abdominal organs, stays securely in place, and seals the point of entry against any inadvertent loss of gas.

For the da Vinci Robotic System the camera lens fits through a variety of standard 12-mm disposable trocars. The 8- and 5-mm instruments fit through proprietary reusable 8- and 5-mm trocars that couple directly with the robotic arms. These reusable metal trocars have disposable valves that must be changed with each new case and the option of a reusable blunt inner cannula or a bladeless disposable inner cannula for use during placement.

In traditional flap-valve or trap door ports, a reducer is necessary to allow downsizing of working channels in 10-mm or larger trocars to accommodate smaller, 5-mm working instruments without any leakage of CO_2. However, the development of multiseal technology and the even newer AirSeal technology (discussed later), has resulted in valves that can accommodate 5- to 12-mm instruments without the need for a reducer, which can save significant time during a long procedure.

Retention of the cannula at the port site is essential to decrease air leak and subcutaneous emphysema and facilitate the timely completion of a procedure. In the past it was necessary to affix a suture to the insufflation side port and the skin to secure the trocar. At present, myriad retention mechanisms exist to prevent dislocation of cannulae such as threaded sleeves, adjustable threaded sleeves, expandable arms, and inflatable balloons. The Blunt Tip Trocar with Balloon Tip (US Surgical) and the Kii Balloon Blunt Tip System (Applied Medical Resources) (see Fig. 10-10 on the Expert Consult website) have a retention balloon that can be inflated in the peritoneal cavity and then drawn up tightly against the peritoneal side of the abdominal wall; an outer foam or rubber sealing ring can then be advanced down the extra-abdominal shaft of the cannula, thereby sandwiching the abdominal wall between the inflated balloon and the foam or rubber seal, effectively precluding any leakage of gas during the case. **Use of this device minimizes CO_2 leakage around the primary port incision, thus reducing the incidence of subcutaneous emphysema and hypercarbia.** This is especially effective when doing retroperitoneoscopic procedures. Another self-sealing trocar, the AnchorPort (SurgiQuest, Milford, CT) has an elastic self-sealing trocar shaft that automatically forms to the patient's body wall when the inner cannula is removed, creating a tight seal.

A recent technologic advance in trocar and insufflation technology has addressed some of the limitations of existing trocar systems including air leak, need for reducers, and specimen removal. This new system, the AirSeal System (SurgiQuest), consists of a specialized Intelligent Flow System insufflator (Fig. 10-15A on the Expert Consult website) featuring a circulatory flow design, a valve-free Access Port (Fig. 10-15B and C on the Expert Consult website), and a Tri-Lumen Filtered tube set (Fig. 10-15D on the Expert Consult website). This system has the ability to provide a stable pneumoperitoneum despite continuous high-flow suction, trocar dislodgement, or excessive port-side leakage. The valve-free design of the Access Port allows smudge-free scope insertion, intact specimen removal, and easy insertion and withdrawal of instruments of varying sizes. The AirSeal System also provides continuous smoke evacuation without the fear of venting surgical smoke and plume into the operating room.

Hand-Assist Devices

A number of hand-assist devices exist, including the GelPort (Applied Medical Resources), the Omniport (Advanced Surgical Concepts, Wicklow, Ireland), and the Lap Disc (Ethicon, Cincinnati, OH).

A study of 130 urologists participating in a series of hand-assist courses evaluated these three different hand-assist devices for a variety of features. The GelPort device emerged with the highest overall score, followed by the Lap Disc and then the Omniport (Patel and Stifelman, 2004). Advantages of the GelPort included sturdiness, ease of hand exchange, maintenance of the pneumoperitoneum, and the ability to pass both a hand and a laparoscopic instrument simultaneously.

An important caveat with respect to using hand-assist devices is the impact on the surgeon. Studies have shown that compared with standard laparoscopy, pain and numbness of the surgeon's hand, wrist, and forearm and, to a lesser extent, overall fatigue are much greater with use of a hand-assist device (Monga et al, 2004; Gofrit et al, 2008).

See the Expert Consult website for details of the hand-assist devices.

Laparoendoscopic Single-Site Surgery Access Devices

See the Expert Consult website for details.

Trocar Placement

Placement of Initial Trocar

When the Veress needle technique is used, after establishment of the pneumoperitoneum an incision is made for placement of the initial trocar. Alternatively, if an incision was made for placement of the Veress needle, the edges of the wound and subcutaneous tissue are spread with blunt forceps. Next, the trocar is held in the dominant hand with the middle finger extending along the shaft and the trocar is inserted using a twisting downward motion. The nondominant hand can be placed at the level of the skin, gently holding the trocar to stabilize it and prevent a sudden advancement. If the surgical site is in the mid to upper abdomen, then the trocar is passed perpendicular to the umbilical incision; however, for pelvic procedures, the trocar is directed 70 degrees caudad. Proof of entering the gas-filled intraperitoneal cavity is the sound of CO_2 escaping from the open sidearm. After the sidearm is closed, the obturator is removed and the CO_2 insufflation line is connected to the side port of the trocar. Alternatively, if a clear blunt port (i.e., optical trocar) is used, a 0-degree laparoscopic lens is placed within the port so the entire entry of the trocar is endoscopically monitored.

Some advocate for increasing the pneumoperitoneum after achieving access with the Veress needle in preparation for initial trocar placement to decrease the risk of underlying vascular or visceral injury with trocar insertion (Vilos et al, 2007). It is recommended to increase the pressure to 20 mm Hg. However, some data exist that suggest this may not increase the volume of the pneumoperitoneum or ease of trocar insertion (McDougall et al, 1994).

When an **open technique** is performed to obtain the pneumoperitoneum, the Hasson-style cannula used to obtain access to the abdomen also serves as the initial trocar.

Hand-Assist Placement

The hand-assist device can be placed either as an initial "port," described earlier, or as a secondary port depending on the surgeon's preference. When placed as a secondary port, a Veress or Hasson pneumoperitoneum is initially established and the hand-assist device is then placed under endoscopic monitoring. Establishing the pneumoperitoneum before hand port placement can help to minimize the size of skin incision for the hand port, as the skin is on stretch. The surgeon should carefully plan out the hand port entry site as well as the additional instrument and camera port sites. Every hand port device has a "footprint" that can be drawn on the abdominal wall; that footprint varies depending on the diameter of the external appliance. **Care should be taken to plan out the additional trocar sites carefully to avoid interference between the hand port and the instrument ports;** this is most easily done once the pneumoperitoneum has been established. After the footprint has been traced, the hand port incision site is marked; the length of the incision should correspond to the surgeon's glove size (e.g., 7 glove size = 7-cm incision). The skin is incised, and the fascia is divided. The peritoneum is entered, and the insufflation is temporarily stopped. The hand port device is then placed according to the manufacturer's instructions.

Before initiating a hand-assist procedure, the surgeon is advised to wrap the arm-glove seam on the hand that is to be used through the hand port either with a 1010 drape or an Ioban (3M, St. Paul, MN) "sticky drape" to waterproof his or her arm. **Lastly, the use of a brown glove on the intra-abdominal hand is recommended because they do not reflect the light from the laparoscope and thus reduce glare** (Wolf, 2005).

Secondary Trocar Placement

After obtaining access, the first step before secondary trocar placement is to inspect the entire abdomen systematically to rule out any injury to the underlying viscera that may have occurred during access or placement of the initial trocar. After this, one can proceed with secondary port placement.

Number, size, and exact location of secondary trocars depend largely on the intended laparoscopic procedure. Their configuration should be planned so that neither the tips nor handles of the cannulas cross or come into close contact with one another (a problem termed *crossing swords* and *rollover,* respectively) such that adequate working space is provided for all instruments to be used during a

particular procedure and allowing for effective triangulation at the surgical site by the endoscope and two working ports. In general, it is reasonable to place the ports in a four-point diamond pattern such that the site of the operation is encircled within the diamond. **This is particularly important when considering reconstructive renal procedures, because the angle between the horizontal plane and the needle drivers should be less than 55 degrees, whereas the angle between the surgeon's suturing instruments should be in the 25- to 45-degree range** (Rassweiler and Frede, 2002).

It is also important to place each port so that it is pointing toward the surgical field, to avoid continued forceful redirection of the port during the procedure that may result in widening of the tissue tract around the port and development of subcutaneous emphysema.

Standard Approach. Secondary trocars are placed under direct optical control. The 30-degree lens is ideal for this portion of the procedure because turning the lens 180 degrees away from the surgical site provides the surgeon with a panoramic view of the anterior abdominal wall. The operative lights are dimmed, and the tip of the laparoscope is moved upward toward the intended site of port placement, thereby, in the thin patient, transilluminating any superficial blood vessels that need to be avoided while passing the trocar. With a blade, a skin incision is made just wide enough to accept the selected cannula. When placing secondary ports, it is of great importance to direct them toward the intended surgical field to provide tension-free maneuverability of the laparoscopic instruments. This is especially important in obese patients because the errant port will provide resistance to the surgeon throughout the rest of the procedure. Similar to placement of the initial port, all secondary ports are advanced through the abdominal wall using a slow, twisting motion and constant pressure. Each secondary port is passed into the peritoneal cavity under meticulous endoscopic monitoring. To prevent dislocation, ports that do not possess self-retaining mechanisms may be anchored to the skin using No. 2 nonabsorbable sutures. **In this regard, one should never use a metal trocar in conjunction with an outer plastic retaining ring because stray current can no longer be harmlessly dissipated through the metal cannula directly to the surrounding peritrocar abdominal wall, and hence any juxtaposed visceral structure may be damaged in an area remote to the laparoscopist's vision.**

Hand-Assist Approach. When the hand-assist device is in place, then secondary trocars can be placed with digital guidance. After inspection of the abdomen rules out any potentially interfering adhesions, the surgeon's index finger is placed on the underside of the abdominal wall at the planned site of trocar placement. A skin incision is made over the surgeon's index finger and the nonbladed trocar is passed with the other hand and guided by the surgeon's finger into the abdominal cavity. This is a very rapid and safe way to place all of the secondary nonbladed trocars.

Trocar Configuration

A number of different trocar configurations exist depending on whether one is performing transperitoneal or retroperitoneal upper abdominal laparoscopy or robotics. Details and diagrams of these configurations can be found in Chapter 61. Similarly, a number of trocar configurations exist for transperitoneal and extraperitoneal laparoscopic and robotic pelvic procedures, which are detailed in Chapter 115. Most important, regardless of the configuration chosen, is to ensure meticulous placement of the ports to minimize instrument clashing both intracorporeally and extracorporeally.

Robotic Considerations

If a robotic procedure is planned, then the camera port is a 12-mm trocar site and the two (or three if the fourth arm is used) auxiliary ports are 8 mm. **All the ports need to be placed 8 to 10 cm apart to reduce the possibility of the robotic arms clashing with each other.** In addition, if the patient is in a flank position, then the lowest port placement should not be inferior to the umbilicus or else the arm may be blocked from a full range of motion by the patient's upside leg. An assistant's port is placed on a line either caudal or inferior to the robotic arms; placement of the assistant's port between the arms of the robot makes it quite awkward for the assistant to work and limits the range of motion of the assistant's instrument owing to clashing with the arms of the robot. Of note, all 8-mm robotic ports need to be advanced to ensure that the thick black marking on the shaft of the trocar is below the abdominal wall.

Laparoscopic Instrumentation

Instruments for Visualization

To create a laparoscopic image, four components are required: the laparoscope, light source, camera, and monitor. To record the image, video recorders, digital video disc, and video printers are available.

Laparoscope and Camera
Standard Systems. The most commonly used laparoscopes have 0- or 30-degree lenses (range, 0 to 45 degrees) and are available in sizes from 2.7 to 10 mm. Typically, the 30-degree lens provides the surgeon with a more complete view of the surgical field than the 0-degree lens, allowing the surgeon to peer around vascular structures by rotating the lens. Recently, newer deflectable laparoscopes have been developed in which the tip of the endoscope can deflect in four directions up to 90 degrees (EndoEYE Deflectable-Tip Video Laparoscope [Olympus, Melville, NY]); which offers many potential angles from which to view a structure, but requires an adept assistant. Another novel endoscope design is the EndoCAMeleon (Karl Storz). This scope maintains the familiar feel of a standard rigid laparoscope but has a variable-view swing prism that enables the surgeon to change viewing angles from 0 to 30, 45, 90, or 120 degrees. An advantage of the EndoCAMeleon is that it has a standard eyepiece, allowing it to be used with most camera systems.

With standard laparoscopes, image transmission uses an objective lens, a rod-lens system with or without an eyepiece, and a fiberoptic cable. From the eyepiece, the optical image is magnified and transferred to the camera and onto the monitor. Light is transmitted from the light source through the fiberoptic cable onto the light post of the laparoscope (Fig. 10-19A on the Expert Consult website). Some newer laparoscopes have a mini charge-coupled device (CCD) camera mounted at the tip (EndoEYE [Olympus]), which improves image quality and avoids the need for an external light chord that can sometimes impede the movement of other instruments (Fig. 10-19B on the Expert Consult website).

The most vexing problem with any laparoscope is fogging of the lens. To prevent fogging of the laparoscope after insertion into the warm intraperitoneal cavity, it is advisable to initially warm the laparoscope in a container holding warm saline before it is passed into the abdomen. The most efficient way to warm the laparoscope is to use a dedicated solution warming basin that is long enough to accommodate the laparoscope; alternatively a warming thermos can be used (Applied Medical Resources). In addition, wiping the tip with a commercial defogging fluid or with povidone-iodine solution is also recommended. Should moisture buildup occur between the eyepiece and the camera, both components must be disconnected and carefully cleansed with a dry gauze pad; this is not a problem with the digital endoscopes because the only connection is from the endoscope directly into the display box.

A final important note is to ensure that the sterile scope is white balanced.

The **camera system** consists of a camera and a video monitor. All currently made cameras can be gas or liquid sterilized, thereby facilitating their use and limiting possible intraoperative contamination. For standard laparoscopes the camera is attached directly to the end of the laparoscope and transfers the view of the surgical field through a cable to the camera box unit. After reconstruction of the optical information the image is displayed on one or two video monitors.

Three-Dimensional Laparoscopic Systems. Three-dimensional laparoscopic systems offer the surgeon the distinct advantage of depth perception. Optimal 3D laparoscopy is performed with a two-lens system that duplicates the two-eye perception of 3D. In this way binocular vision is maintained. The most commonly used 3D vision system currently in use is the InSite Vision System (Intuitive Surgical), which provides vision for the da Vinci Robotic System. The laparoscope and high-definition camera are heavy (5.5 pounds for the high-definition scope and camera head) but are controlled by a robotic arm that is under direct control of the surgeon from the ergonomic console. The surgeon maintains a steady, magnified 3D view of the surgical field. Zero- and 30-degree lenses are currently available.

Handheld 3D laparoscopic systems are also available, but currently require the surgeon to wear headgear with miniature video screens to display the 3D image (EndoSite 3Di Digital Vision System [Viking Systems, La Jolla, CA]) or specialized passive polarized glasses while viewing the image on a 3D monitor (Karl Storz) (Fig. 10-20 on the Expert Consult website). A few recent studies (Honeck et al, 2012; Tanagho et al, 2012; Lusch et al, 2014) have demonstrated **superior depth perception, spatial location, and precision of surgical performance with 3D systems compared with two-dimensional (2D) systems while completing laparoscopic tasks in an ex vivo setting.**

Instrumentation for Grasping and Blunt Dissection

Most graspers and dissectors are used in their 5-mm size, but are available in a range from 3 to 12 mm, in predominantly reusable forms. Grasping instruments have either single-action (only one jaw moves during opening) or double-action (both jaws move) tip design.

Wide variations exist with regard to configuration of tip, surface characteristics of jaws, handle design, and possible electrosurgical properties. Tip designs include blunt-coarse, pointed (dolphin), straight (duck bill), curved (Maryland), and angled. The surface of the jaws may be atraumatic or traumatic. Serrated or smooth surfaces allow gentle tissue manipulation in atraumatic graspers (e.g., bowel forceps with a 3-cm long grasping jaw). Traumatic graspers have toothed or clawed surfaces on their jaws to allow them to grasp and hold tissues firmly. In addition, each of these instruments may be equipped with tip-rotation and/or articulating features. Both reusable and disposable instruments are available.

Depending on the design of the handle, grasping instruments may be locking or nonlocking. Most nonlocking forceps have a scissor-type handle. Different designs allow for locking capabilities; in particular, bar-type and spring-loaded locking handles are convenient when prolonged grasping of tissue is required. Some newer dissectors in addition to grip and rotation actually offer additional degrees of freedom by means of an articulating joint activated through wrist movements of the surgeon (RealHand [Novare Surgical Systems, Cupertino, CA]; Autonomy Laparo-Angle [Cambridge Endoscopic Devices, Framingham, MA]). **These instruments are most helpful if one is to perform a LESS procedure because the angulation of the shaft then provides the triangulation necessary for approaching the surgical field.** In addition, the shafts of these instruments may be of variable length (i.e., 34, 45, or 75 cm), again allowing for less clashing of handles during a LESS procedure.

In addition to standard dissecting instruments, both the laparoscopic suction apparatus and the "heel" of the hook electrode can be used for effective and rapid blunt dissection. Along these same lines, the development of laparoscopic "peanuts" or Kittners (i.e., 5- and 10-mm gauze-tipped disposable dissectors) has been most helpful. These dissectors can be twirled or moved side to side or up and down in an area of adipose tissue to rapidly tease away the fat surrounding vital structures such as the renal hilum or the adrenal gland. In addition, the device can be used to raise an entire "line" of tissue (e.g., pararenal fat), allowing for its rapid and safe division because neither the shaft nor tip of the Kittner will conduct electrosurgical current.

Water jet dissectors, such as the Helix Hydro-Jet (ERBE Elektromedizin, Tübingen, Germany), use an extremely thin, high-pressure laminar liquid jet to develop a cleavage plane in tissues. Pressures of 250 to 350 psi are sufficient for dissecting soft tissue while leaving vascular structures and nerves intact (Shekarriz et al, 2004). The device is activated using a foot pedal and the water jet is administered from a 5-mm wand. This device may have particular application in parenchymal transection as in partial nephrectomy or in nerve-sparing procedures such as during retroperitoneal lymph node dissection (Basting et al, 2000; Shekarriz et al, 2004). However, owing to fluid accumulation in the abdomen, changes in tissue turgor and, in particular, splash back from the fluid stream that can foul the laparoscope lens, these devices have not come into widespread use.

Instrumentation for Incising and Hemostasis

Laparoscopic scissors, scalpels, electrocautery, ultrasonic devices, and lasers (CO_2, neodymium:yttrium-aluminum-garnet [Nd:YAG], or potassium titanyl phosphate [KTP]) are used to incise or cut tissue during laparoscopic surgery. Cutting of tissue with electrocautery and lasers is achieved when the cell temperature is elevated until the concomitant gas pressure causes the cells to explode. Conversely, with ultrasonic devices the cutting mechanism is a relatively sharp blade vibrating at 25 kHz to 55 kHz over a distance of up to 100 μm.

Monopolar and bipolar electrocautery and other technologies exist for achieving hemostasis. The basic mechanism for coagulating bleeding vessels is similar among the various modalities, in that vessels are sealed and occluded with denatured protein; however, the manner in which protein is denatured is different for each modality. Electrosurgery and lasers denature protein by heating the tissues with electric current in the former and light in the latter, at a very high temperature. Conversely, ultrasonic devices denature protein by transferring mechanical energy to ultrasonic high-frequency vibration (25 kHz to 55 KHz).

Sharp Dissectors. **Laparoscopic scissors** are available in disposable and nondisposable forms. The blades of laparoscopic scissors are shorter than their open surgical counterparts. The configuration of the tip may be useful for selected situations: hooked tips for cutting sutures, microscissors for spatulating the ureter during a pyeloplasty, and curved tips for dissection. The scissors may come with either permanent blades or with replaceable tips; use of the latter ensures "sharp" scissors for each procedure. In addition, the shaft of the scissors may rotate and, in some disposable scissors, even articulate up to 90 degrees. A **laparoscopic scalpel** is also available.

Monopolar Electrosurgical Devices. For **electrosurgical incision** of tissue, a selection of different electrodes are available: needle electrodes (Corson type) produce fine cuts that are useful in making peritoneal incisions, spatula electrodes are used in blunt dissection and cutting, and hook electrodes (J and L configurations) are of particular value during dissection of vessels because tissue can be pulled away from delicate structures before the cutting current is activated. **The thinner the metal tip of the probe, the higher the density of the electrical current, and the greater the cutting power.**

As with all insulated instruments, certain precautions must be followed during monopolar electrosurgery to avoid local or distant transmitted thermal injury. Consequently, **the electrosurgical probe should not be activated unless the metal part is in complete view. The insulation of the electrosurgical instrument should be carefully checked for any damage. The probe should not be activated unless it is in direct contact with the tissue to be incised.**

To avoid the potential dangers of stray current from use of monopolar electrosurgical equipment, the surgeon can use monopolar current in conjunction with active electrode monitoring (Encision, Boulder, CO). This instrumentation is constructed such that there is ongoing feedback during activation of the electrosurgical current; therefore, any break in the insulation of the shaft results in immediate deactivation of the instrument.

For monopolar electrosurgical coagulation, the floating ball electrode (Salient Surgical Technologies, Dover, NH), which is a saline-cooled radiofrequency surface coagulator-sealer, also exists. Skimming the floating ball over a tissue surface in small circles seals

the tissue, stopping the flow of blood and other fluids by effectively shrinking the natural collagen in the tissue. The wet energy cools tissue and keeps temperatures below 100° C, preventing tissue charring and eschar formation. This device has been proven to be quite useful for coagulating the parenchymal bed after partial nephrectomy before application of a hemostatic agent and/or bolster (Stern et al, 2004; Urena et al, 2004).

Bipolar Electrosurgical Devices. The laparoscopic surgeon can also use bipolar electrosurgical devices that require less energy for performance than their monopolar counterparts. There is also a decreased likelihood of injury to surrounding tissue for a couple of important reasons. First, because the **electrical current is only passing from one jaw of the instrument to the other, it precludes the potential problem of capacitive coupling,** commonplace with monopolar electrosurgical current. Second, **with bipolar current, the extent of coagulative damage is less than with monopolar electrosurgery**: 1 to 6 mm versus 5 to 7 mm with monopolar current (Landman et al, 2003a).

One of the currently available bipolar electrosurgical devices is the LigaSure vessel-sealing system (Covidien) (Fig. 10-21 on the Expert Consult website). It consists of a 5- or 10-mm grasper-dissector connected to a bipolar radiofrequency generator. When the vascular structure is grasped by the instrument, the tissue is evaluated by a feedback-response system that subsequently delivers the optimal energy required to seal the vessel effectively. Because of the high-current and low-voltage output, the vascular structure enclosed by the jaws of the instrument degrades quickly and a protein-based seal is presumably created; this mechanism of electrical current delivery to the tissues results in less charring and less collateral thermal damage (1 to 3 mm) (Landman et al, 2003a). Indeed, use of this instrument during partial nephrectomy does not compromise the ability of the pathologist to read the surgical margin (Phillips et al, 2008). An audible signal alerts the surgeon that the sealing of the vessel is complete; the instrument has a trigger-activated blade that the surgeon can then use to cut the sealed tissue. Vessels up to and including 7 mm in diameter appear to be effectively occluded, to above normal physiologic pressures, with this device (Carbonell et al, 2003; Landman et al, 2003a). However, only one LigaSure application to the structure being sealed is recommended, because multiple applications may weaken the seal (Truong et al, 2008).

Another simultaneous vessel sealing and cutting device is the EnSeal PTC (Ethicon). This is a 5-mm instrument that can also act as a grasper-dissector. The electrode design uses a temperature-sensitive polymer that helps to limit current spread to surrounding tissues. The device has an I-beam–shaped blade that draws the jaws of the instrument together with increasing force as the blade is advanced through the tissue. Hence, the surgeon can control the rate of cutting by how quickly the instrument handle is squeezed. The device can be used to seal vessels up to 7 mm but is reported to require a longer vessel sealing time than the LigaSure V (Covidien) (Lamberton et al, 2008).

Laser Instrumentation. **Lasers** are most frequently used through the working channel of an operating laparoscope. The CO_2 laser provides excellent cutting and vaporization of surface lesions and requires a rigid hand piece and probe. In contrast, the 400- and 600-μm KTP fibers are flexible and allow for noncontact cutting and fulguration. Nd:YAG laser fibers are also flexible and allow noncontact fulguration and contact cutting. Holmium laser fibers are also flexible and are used in a contact mode for cutting. Typically, lasers are not used in urologic laparoscopy, where they have largely been supplanted by electrosurgical instruments. Only in gynecology is the CO_2 laser used extensively, in general in the treatment of endometriosis.

Ultrasound Instrumentation. Ultrasonic technology (Harmonic scalpel, Ethicon; and Sonicbeat, Olympus, Center Valley, PA) is another option for cutting and hemostasis in endoscopic surgery. It provides an especially attractive alternative to monopolar electrosurgery when one is working around particularly delicate tissues or operating on patients with an implanted pacemaker or cardioverter defibrillator (Gossot et al, 1999; Strate et al, 1999). In ultrasonic devices, electrical energy is transformed into mechanical energy by the use of a piezoelectric crystal system. Specifically, electrical energy is produced by a power-supply generator and transformed into mechanical vibration at the tip of the instrument through a piezoelectric crystal interface (Suzuki et al, 1995; Takeda et al, 1997; Gossot et al, 1999). Mechanical vibrations produced by this system in the tip of the instrument are capable of causing cavitation, coaptation and coagulation, and cutting in the targeted tissue (Strate et al, 1999). There are several important benefits to the ultrasonic system. These include the absent risk of local thermal damage and tissue charring because of a working temperature lower than 80° C. Subsequently, reduced tissue charring may result in a reduced rate of postoperative adhesions (Amaral and Chrotstek, 1997). A second benefit is that the depth of penetration is limited to the targeted tissue within a diameter of 1 mm, so there is minimal lateral thermal spread and potential for tissue damage (Landman et al, 2003a). Ultrasonic devices also minimize smoke for improved visibility in the surgical field. In addition, the ultrasonic systems eliminate other problems associated with monopolar electrosurgery, specifically, problems of remote site tissue damage caused by capacitive coupling, insulation defects in the instrumentation, and direct coupling. Lastly, as with bipolar energy, use of ultrasonic energy during partial nephrectomy does not compromise the ability of the pathologist to read the surgical margin (Phillips et al, 2008).

Potential disadvantages of ultrasonic technology include slower vessel sealing (Lamberton et al, 2008) and the fact that the metal portion of the shears becomes quite hot during activation (often over 200° C compared with the bipolar energy–based devices, which stay below 100° C) and must not come into direct contact with any bowel surrounding the area of dissection. In fact, the harmonic shears take roughly twice as long to cool to a "safe" temperature after firing (often up to 45 seconds) compared with the LigaSure device (Covidien) (Kim et al, 2008).

Combined Devices and Other Instrumentation. *See the Expert Consult website for details.*

Surgical Pharmaceuticals

Recently, a vast array of topical hemostatic agents and sealants that can be used for a variety of surgical tasks have entered the surgical realm and have become valuable additions to the surgeon's tray. A comparison of popular hemostatic agents is presented in Table 10-1.

See the Expert Consult website for further details.

Instrumentation for Suturing and Tissue Anastomosis

Needle Drivers. Suturing and knot tying are among the most difficult tasks in laparoscopic surgery. A significant amount of practice is needed to achieve a sufficient level of proficiency. **Laparoscopic needle holders** have one fixed jaw and one jaw that opens by squeezing the spring-loaded handle of the instrument. They all have a locking mechanism to secure the needle in their jaws; this is done with a ratchet, spring-loaded, or Castroviejo-type mechanism. Some needle holders also possess a feature that allows the jaws to rotate around the main axis relative to the handle. The handles may be straight or provide a pistol-type grip (Fig. 10-22 on the Expert Consult website). In addition to standard rigid needle drivers, some companies have recently developed articulating needle drivers that aid in obtaining more optimal suturing angles with the needle. The actuation of the articulation mechanism is controlled by the surgeon's wrist motion (Laparo-Angle [Cambridge Endoscopic Devices]; RealHand [Novare Surgical Systems]).

Endo Stitch. The Endo Stitch (Covidien) device is an innovative, disposable, 10-mm instrument that facilitates laparoscopic suture placement and knot tying (Adams et al, 1995). With increased experience with standard laparoscopic needle holders and especially with the advent of robotic-assisted procedures, use of the Endo Stitch has become less common.

See the Expert Consult website for further details.

Lapra-Ty clips. Lapra-Ty clips (Ethicon) are a very useful adjunct to suturing and knot tying. **The clip acts as a knot, thereby precluding time-consuming intracorporeal laparoscopic knot tying** (Fig. 10-23). These 3.5-mm clips are made of absorbable polydioxanone and are designed to provide secure anchoring of sutures for up to 14 days in low-tension to mid-tension environments (Ames et al, 2005). According to the manufacturer, these suture anchors can be secured to the end of a single strand of polyglactin 910 (Vicryl) suture as fine as 4-0. Experimental models from two different laboratories have shown that these clips are least likely to fall off polyglactin 910 sutures from size 1-0 to 3-0 (Ames et al, 2005; Weld et al, 2008). In the laboratory environment Lapra-Ty clips have been shown to be slip resistant with 2-0 Monocryl and polydioxanone suture (PDS) as well. In multiple test trials for each suture type, a percentage of monofilament sutures size 3-0 and smaller as well as 4-0 suture of any type did have slippage of the clip. Hence, it seems logical to avoid Lapra-Ty use with 4-0 suture and to avoid excessive tension when using these clips with 3-0 monofilament suture. Lapra-Ty clips can be used to secure a single suture or a running suture and for anchoring bolsters during renorrhaphy for laparoscopic or robotic partial nephrectomy (Orvieto et al, 2004).

Instrumentation for Stapling and Clipping

Stapling Devices. Various stapling devices are available for tissue occlusion and division. The Endo GIA Universal 12-mm stapler and

TABLE 10-1 Some Commonly Used Topical Tissue Sealants and Hemostatic Agents

AGENT	MANUFACTURER (TIME TO SET UP)	ACTIVE INGREDIENTS	KEY USES AND PROPERTIES
Tisseel	Baxter, Glendale, CA (20 min)	Fibrinogen CaCl Aprotinin Thrombin	Topical hemostasis Tissue glue
Crosseal	Johnson & Johnson, New Brunswick, NJ (Immediate)	Fibrinogen CaCl Aprotinin Thrombin	Topical hemostasis Tissue glue
Floseal	Baxter (2 min)	Cross-linked gelatin granules Thrombin	Topical hemostasis
EndoAvitene	Davol, Cranston, RI (Immediate)	Avitene microfibrillar collagen powder	Topical hemostasis
BioGlue	CryoLife, Kennesaw, GA (Immediate)	Bovine serum albumin and glutaraldehyde	Tissue sealant
Coseal	Baxter (Immediate)	Two polyethylene glycol polymers	Tissue sealant

CaCl, calcium chloride.

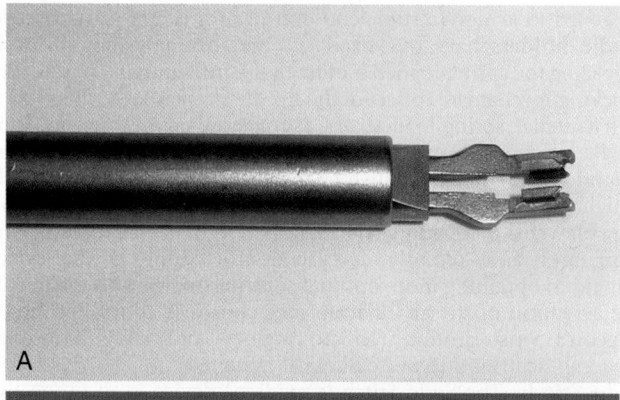

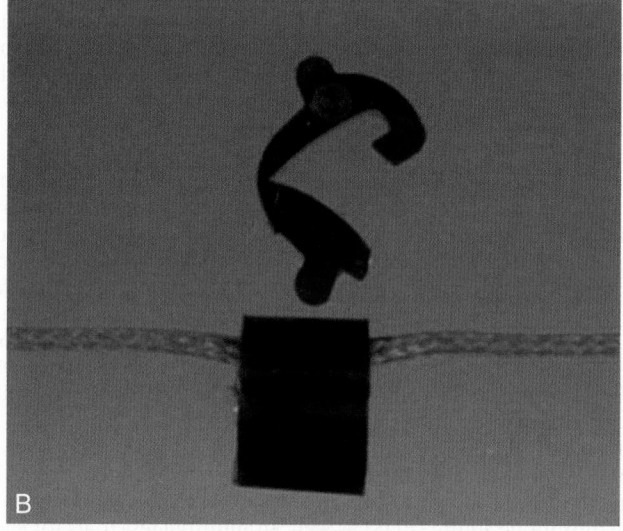

Figure 10-23. **A, Tip of laparoscopic device for applying Lapra-Ty clip (Ethicon, Somerville, NJ). B, Lapra-Ty clip affixed to a suture.**

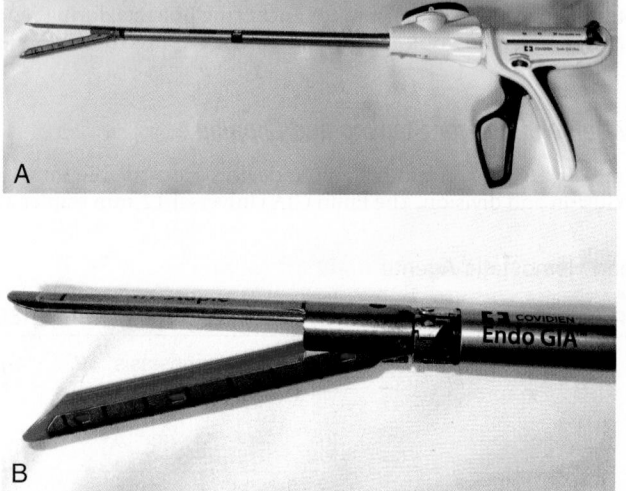

Figure 10-24. **A, Example of Endo GIA laparoscopic stapling device. B, Stapling device tip. (A, Courtesy Covidien Ltd., Mansfield, MA. All rights reserved. Used with permission of Covidien.)**

linear cutting device (Covidien) requires a 12-mm port and delivers two triple-staggered rows of staples and simultaneously cuts between the rows (Fig. 10-24). The Universal stapler can be loaded with a variety of 30-, 45-, or 60-mm loads and fired any number of times. Similarly, the ETS-Flex 45 stapler (Ethicon) also requires a 12-mm port and delivers two triple rows of staples while cutting between

rows 3 and 4. This stapler has a maximum fire limit of eight staple loads. Articulating and roticulating staplers are available from both companies, which enable the surgeon to properly align the instrument with the tissue to be occluded and divided. **Each staple load cartridge is color coded depending on the size of the staples: 2.0-mm staples (gray) or 2.5-mm staples (white) are preferred for vascular (renal vein or renal artery) stapling, whereas 3.8-mm (blue) and 4.8-mm (green) staples are used in thicker tissues (ureter, bowel, bladder).** In addition, for laparoscopic live donor nephrectomy, a single Endo-TA (linear noncutting) stapler can be used to secure the patient's side of the renal vein, thereby providing a longer donor renal vein, because there is no need to trim staples from the vessels before anastomosis in the recipient (Meng et al, 2003). Linear noncutting staplers deliver either three or four staple rows, 30 or 60 mm long. These staplers can also be used to close an enterotomy after a side-to-side bowel anastomosis. **When laparoscopic staplers are used, special attention must be paid to the markers on the cartridge to ensure that all the targeted tissue is properly situated proximal to the markers before the cartridge is fired. The stapler should not be fired across any previously placed clips because this is thought to possibly cause stapler malfunction.** Indeed, in a 9-year review of stapler use (1992 to 2001), Brown and Woo (2004) noted U.S. Food and Drug Administration–recorded reports of 112 mortalities and 2180 injuries attributed to use of the stapler; overall, malfunctions were reported 22,804 times.

Clipping Devices. Disposable and nondisposable clip appliers are available from different manufacturers and require 5-, 10-, or 12-mm laparoscopic ports. In general, they contain occlusive clips ranging in size from 6 to 11 mm. Disposable clip appliers possess a rotating shaft and multifire, self-reloading features, whereas nondisposable instruments have to be reloaded for each clip to be deployed at the site of surgery (Fig. 10-25).

Electrocoagulation must be avoided in the vicinity of clips placed for occlusion of vessels to prevent conductive tissue necrosis and subsequent clip dislocation. To ensure reliable function, the closed ends of the occlusive clips must be seen extending slightly beyond the targeted vessel and should be placed perpendicular to the longitudinal axis of the vessel.

In addition to titanium clips, polymer clips that completely encircle and lock down around a vessel are available (Weck Hem-o-lok polymer ligation clip system [Teleflex, Research Triangle Park, NC]) (see Fig. 10-25). They are available in four sizes (M, ML, L, and XL). Up to 10 mm of tissue can be ligated through a 5-mm trocar, and up to 16 mm of tissue can be ligated through a 10-mm trocar. Of note, because of results from a survey put forth by the American Society of Transplant Surgeons, in which use of these clips was associated with hemorrhage from the renal artery stump, the company producing the clips put forth a statement contraindicating their use for securing the renal artery during laparoscopic live donor nephrectomies (Friedman et al, 2006). Subsequently, a multi-institutional study of 1695 patients from nine different institutions undergoing laparoscopic donor nephrectomy with ligation of the renal artery with Hem-o-lok clips concluded that the clips were safe to use because in this review there were no adverse bleeding events (Ponsky et al, 2008a). **The authors did acknowledge, however, that proper technique of application must be strictly adhered to, including application of at least two clips on the stump of the artery, and that a 2-mm cuff of artery should be left distal to the clips** (Box 10-2). Removal of a Hem-o-lok clip is possible using the specified removal instrument, should a structure be clipped in error.

Instrumentation for Specimen Entrapment

Various organ entrapment and retrieval systems are available. Depending on the size of the tissue and on whether in situ morcellation or intact organ retrieval is planned, the laparoscopic surgeon is able to choose among different-sized sacks, materials, and designs. Studies have been conducted to test organ retrieval bags for permeability to tumor cells and bacteria before and after

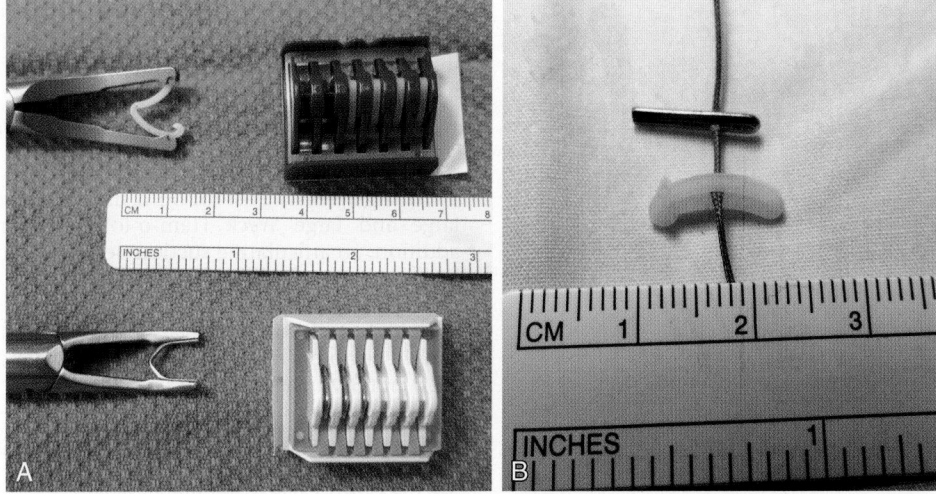

Figure 10-25. **A, Weck Hem-o-lok clip and tip of laparoscopic applier** *(top)* **(Teleflex, Research Triangle Park, NC) and metal clip and tip of laparoscopic applier** *(bottom).* **B, Metal clip** *(top)* **and Weck Hem-o-lok clip** *(bottom)* **affixed to a suture.**

BOX 10-2 Basic Principles of Hem-o-lok Clip Placement

- Complete circumferential dissection of the vessel
- Visualization of the curved tip of the clip around and beyond the vessel, often with curved end of the clip placed between artery and vein
- Confirmation of the tactile snap when the clip engages
- No cross-clipping
- Not squeezing clip handles too hard (compared with the application of metal clips)
- Careful removal of the applier after application given; the tips are sharp and can cause a laceration of nearby vessels (e.g., renal vein)
- During transaction of vessels only a partial division is performed initially to confirm hemostasis before complete transaction
- Minimum of two clips placed on the patient side of the renal hilar vessel

From Ponsky L, Cherullo E, Moinzadeh A, et al. The Hem-o-lok clip is safe for laparoscopic nephrectomy: a multi-institutional review. Urology 2008;71:593–6.

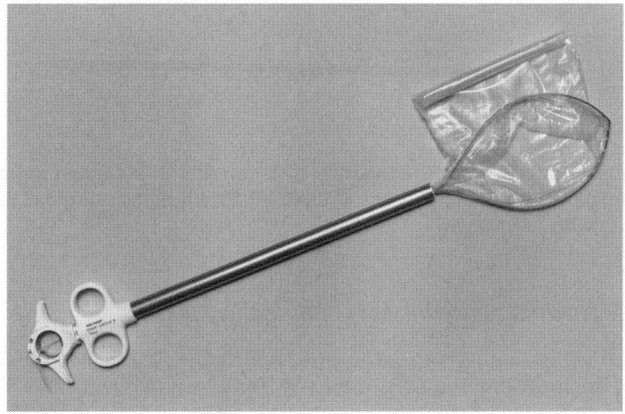

Figure 10-26. **Organ retrieval bag.**

Instrumentation for Morcellation

Various techniques of tissue morcellation have been used in laparoscopic surgery. The simplest method for fragmentation of tissue within the entrapment sack is use of the index finger, ring forceps, or Kelly clamp. Recently, however, it has been shown that ring forceps are the preferred instrument for manual morcellation because they are less likely to puncture the entrapment sack (Eichel et al, 2004).

See the Expert Consult website for further details.

Instrumentation for Retraction

Many varieties of retractors with different features are available.

See the Expert Consult website for details.

Robotic Instrumentation

For the da Vinci Robotic System (Intuitive Surgical), a wide variety of articulating instruments are available. The proprietary EndoWrist technology offers articulation at the tip of the instruments with 7 degrees of freedom and 90 degrees of articulation, mimicking the wrist movements of the surgeon at the robotic console (Fig. 10-27). A full line of 8-mm EndoWrist instruments are available, but it should be noted that all robotic instruments for the da Vinci Surgical System (except the laparoscopes) have a 10-case limit before they must be replaced. The number of "lives" left on each instrument should be recorded with each case.

morcellation, as well as for stability during morcellation and resistance to tearing forces (Urban et al, 1993; Rassweiler et al, 1998b). The originally designed (1990) LapSac (Cook Urological, Spencer, IN), which is made of nylon with a polyurethane inner coating and a polypropylene drawstring, is the least susceptible entrapment sack to tearing (Eichel et al, 2004) or leakage of cells. Up to a 2-kg specimen can be secured within the LapSac; however, deployment of the LapSac and subsequent organ entrapment remain challenging endeavors.

Other entrapment sacks offer marked advantages when the only goal is organ entrapment and intact removal, rather than morcellation. These sacks have spring wires that, when activated by the surgeon, deploy the bag after its introduction into the abdomen; this facilitates tissue entrapment because the broad wire supports stabilize the opened sack, thereby allowing the surgeon to literally scoop the specimen into the sack (Fig. 10-26). The entrapped specimen can easily be withdrawn through a hand-assist site or by enlarging a laparoscopic port site, usually to 5 to 7 cm for most specimens.

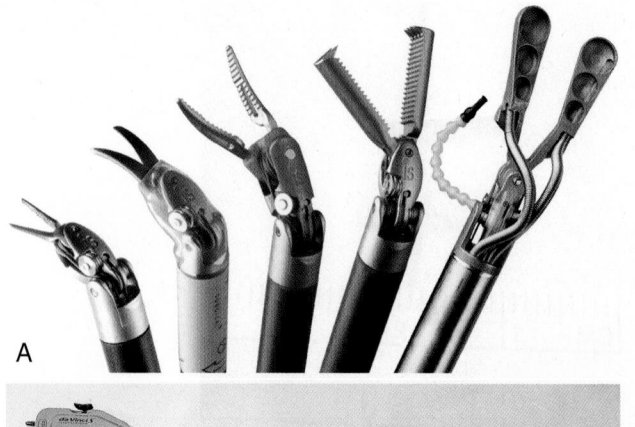

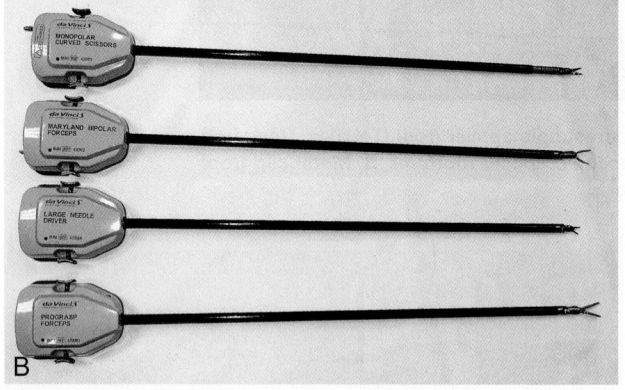

Figure 10-27. A and B, Examples of 8-mm interchangeable instruments for the da Vinci Robotic System. (© 2015 Intuitive Surgical, Inc. Used with permission.)

Instrumentation for Incising and Hemostasis

A variety of EndoWrist scissors and scalpels exist for incising tissue and include the round tip, curved and Potts scissors, and the Snap-fit scalpel instrument. EndoWrist monopolar and bipolar electrocautery instruments are available for incision, dissection, and hemostasis during procedures. Monopolar instruments include the Hot Shears curved scissors and cautery hook and spatula. Bipolar instruments include the Maryland, PK dissecting (Intuitive Surgical), fenestrated, micro, PreCise and curved bipolar forceps. An ultrasonic device (Harmonic ACE curved shears [Ethicon]) is also available for dissection and hemostasis.

Instrumentation for Grasping and Blunt Dissection

A large array of EndoWrist graspers exist that cover the range of blunt to toothed and fine to gross, for use in varying situations. The most commonly used grasper in urologic procedures is the Pro-Grasp blunt forceps.

A safety feature on all robotic grasping devices is a small Allen bolt that can manually open the jaws of the instrument in the case of a robotic arm malfunction or loss of power in which the grasper is locked onto tissue or a needle at the time of failure. Of note, robot failure is quite rare. In the series from the University of Chicago, a robot failure was recorded in less than 1% of cases, and half of these problems (e.g., failure to power up, optical malfunction) were discovered before the patient entered the operating room. In addition, in the few instances in which there was a system malfunction (e.g., loss of 3D vision, robotic arm failure) during the case (0.4%), the procedure could still be completed without converting to an open procedure (Zorn et al, 2007).

Instrumentation for Suturing and Tissue Anastomosis

Four different EndoWrist needle drivers are available for suturing. There are two sizes of needle drivers available in both the standard

and SutureCut design. The SutureCut design allows the surgeon to be able to cut the suture material using the crotch of the instrument.

Other Available 8-mm and 5-mm Instruments

A number of other robotic instruments are also available. Endo-Wrist clip appliers exist for both small titanium clips and medium-large and large Weck Hem-o-lok polymer clips (Teleflex). In addition, an articulating suction device and irrigator, a probe stabilizer, and specialty retractors exist.

A 5-mm line of instruments is also available that is slightly more limited, but still offers a relatively complete line of instruments. It should be noted, however, that the 5-mm robotic laparoscope offers a 2D not 3D image.

Instrumentation for Laparoendoscopic Single-Site Surgery

See the Expert Consult website for details.

Instrumentation for Natural Orifice Transluminal Endoscopic Surgery

See the Expert Consult website for details.

Exiting the Abdomen

Port Removal and Fascial Closure

Port removal and fascial closure are key elements of the procedure that, if not performed in a step-by-step, organized fashion, can result in major, possibly fatal, complications. Herniation, possible bowel incarceration, and postoperative hemorrhage are the results of a poorly performed or haphazard, overly rapid exiting of the abdomen.

Before port removal is initiated, the operative site and the intra-abdominal entry sites of each cannula must be carefully inspected with the intra-abdominal pressure lowered to 5 mm Hg. After achievement of perfect hemostasis, removal of all laparoscopic ports must be undertaken strictly under laparoscopic visual control, to avoid any possible acute herniation of intra-abdominal contents into the previous port sites.

Presently, with the shift away from bladed to nonbladed trocars, the need for fascial closure for even 12-mm ports has come into question. Most will recommend that **on removal of any of the blunt-tipped ports, the fascia does not need to be sutured, except for ports larger than 10 mm placed in the midline. However, a report has shown that 12-mm ports, regardless of site (i.e., midline vs. transmuscular), do not require fascial closure, provided that postoperative palpation of the entry site reveals a small defect** (Siqueira et al, 2004). **In the literature, the switch from bladed to blunt trocars has resulted in a marked decrease in abdominal wall bleeding (from 0.83% to only 0.16%) and in port site hernia formation (1.83% to 0.19%)** (Hashizume and Sugimachi, 1997; Thomas et al, 2003).

In the rare case in which bladed trocars are used, the fascia at all 10- to 12-mm port sites should be closed. After inspection at 5 mm Hg, the first 10- or 12-mm port is removed and the fascia at the entry site is secured with 0-0 Vicryl either by direct placement of a fascial suture or use of a suture-passing device (see later). **Five-millimeter ports are not closed in the adult, but are closed in the pediatric patient with a single absorbable suture.** Ideally, each fascial suture will be placed under direct endoscopic vision prior to definitive port removal. In this manner, each port is visually assessed for any bleeding at 5 mm Hg, thereby precluding the possibility of removing a port and missing an injured vessel. After removal of all ports, the CO_2 is allowed to pass out passively through the 5-mm port sites.

With regard to the hand-assist device, it should be removed before removal of the other port sites. The hand-assist device wound is then closed as one would close a typical abdominal wound. After closure, the pneumoperitoneum is reestablished and the other port sites are closed as previously described. Proceeding in this fashion precludes the chance of injuring the bowel or omentum beneath the hand-port site and ensures an airtight closure.

Instrumentation for Port Site Closure

Several possibilities for fascial closure of port sites exist. The **simplest method** is retracting the skin with retractors, grasping the fascia, and suturing it with absorbable 0-0 suture. However, in patients with a BMI above 30, securely accessing the fascia is very difficult to accomplish.

Fortunately, several devices for complete en bloc closure of fascia, muscle, and peritoneum under direct vision have been developed (Carter 1994; Monk et al, 1994; Garzotto et al, 1995; Elashry et al, 1996). These work well in patients of all sizes.

The **Carter-Thomason needle-point suture passer** (CooperSurgical, Pleasanton, CA) consists of a 5-, 10-, or 12-mm cone that has two integrated, hollow, angled, cylindric passages located 180 degrees opposite each other (Fig. 10-29). With the sharp needle-point, single-action grasper, the 0-0 Vicryl suture is inserted through one of the cylinders in the metal or plastic cone, thereby traversing muscle, fascia, and peritoneal layers in an ever-widening angle. The end of the suture is grasped with a 5-mm grasper through one of the other ports. The needle-point grasper is reintroduced through the other cylinder of the cone, and the intraperitoneal end of the suture is grasped by the needle-point grasper and pulled out of the abdomen. The cone is slid off both ends of the suture. Subsequently, closure of the fascia, muscle layer, and peritoneum is accomplished by tying the suture. **The Carter-Thomason needle-point device is not only helpful for wound closure, but also can be used as a fifth port during nephrectomy to help hold the sack open or to encircle the ureter with a vessel loop through a small stab incision.**

The **disposable Endo Close** suture carrier (Covidien) is a device with a spring-loaded suture carrier at its tip. Loaded with a suture, the device traverses fascia, muscle, and peritoneum alongside the port. After reinsertion on the opposite side of port entry, it is reloaded with the suture, aided by a 5-mm grasper, and is pulled out again so that the suture can then be tied.

A far simpler, less expensive, homemade solution is available to all surgeons for closing ports in a large patient. This **angiocatheter technique** applies the previously described principles. A 14-gauge, sheathed needle is passed alongside the port through the abdominal layers. After removal of the needle, a 0-0 Vicryl suture is inserted through the angiocatheter sheath until it is deep inside the peritoneal cavity. After the sheath is removed, the same maneuver is repeated on the opposite side, but this time a 30-inch 0-0 Prolene suture folded in half is passed into the peritoneal cavity through the sheath to act as a retrieving loop. A 5-mm grasper passed through another port is then passed through the loop of 0-0 Prolene suture and used to grasp the end of the 0-0 Vicryl suture. The 0-0

Vicryl suture is pulled through the Prolene loop and released. By pulling the Prolene loop upward through the angiocatheter sheath, the entrapped 0-0 Vicryl suture is then retrieved from the abdomen. After the angiocatheter sheath is removed, the two ends of the suture can be tied.

Closure of the Skin

The skin of all 10-mm port sites is closed with subcuticular 4-0 absorbable suture. Adhesive strips are applied to all port sites to close (for incisions <10 mm) or to further approximate (for incisions ≥10 mm) the skin. As an alternative, the skin can be closed using octylcyanoacrylate glue. This has been found to speed closure time and provide an equivalent cosmetic result compared with suturing (Sebesta and Bishoff, 2004).

KEY POINTS: PERFORMING THE PROCEDURE

- A checklist ensuring that all essential equipment is present and operational should be completed just before initiating the pneumoperitoneum. Additional items to check when using the da Vinci Robotic System include ensuring that all plugs for the console, vision cart, and patient-side cart are plugged into different circuits and that all cables connecting these carts are connected properly.
- After placement of the Veress needle, insufflation should never be initiated unless all of the signs for proper peritoneal entry (negative aspiration, easy irrigation of saline, negative aspiration of saline, positive drop test result, and normal advancement test) have been confirmed.
- The open technique is recommended specifically when extensive adhesions are anticipated.
- Noncutting dilating trocars have superseded bladed trocars because they are safer. These trocars enter the abdomen by spreading the abdominal wall musculature, rather than cutting it, and therefore there is less chance of injuring an abdominal wall vessel and the resulting entry site is less prone to subsequent herniation.

PHYSIOLOGIC CONSIDERATIONS IN THE ADULT

The rapidly expanding number of newly developed laparoscopic and robotic procedures in operative urology has resulted in an increasing need for urologists to familiarize themselves with both the physiology and the potential complications related to the pneumoperitoneum and patient positioning.

Choice of Insufflant

Carbon Dioxide

CO_2 **is the most commonly used insufflant for laparoscopic surgery and is favored by most laparoscopists thanks to its properties (colorless, noncombustible, very soluble in blood, and inexpensive).** Prolonged postoperative distention of the abdomen does not occur because CO_2 is quickly absorbed (Wolf and Stoller, 1994). It is highly soluble in water and easily diffuses in body tissues. It readily moves out of the peritoneal cavity, as a result of a high diffusion gradient caused by the difference in concentration of CO_2 between the intraperitoneal space and the surrounding components (e.g., blood). However, the characteristic of rapid absorption, which lessens the chance of a CO_2 gas embolus, may also lead to potential problems (e.g., hypercapnia, hypercarbia, associated cardiac arrhythmias). In particular, patients with COPD may not be able to compensate for the absorbed CO_2 by increased ventilation; this may result in dangerously elevated levels of CO_2 in these patients, thereby necessitating the direct testing of arterial blood gases during laparoscopy in the pulmonary compromised

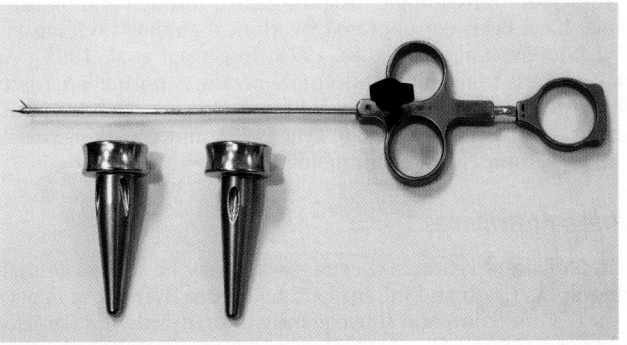

Figure 10-29. Carter-Thomason device. Cone and needle-point single-action grasper in open position.

patient. Carbon dioxide also stimulates the sympathetic nervous system, which results in an increase in heart rate, cardiac contractility, and vascular resistance. Lastly, CO_2 is also stored in various body compartments (e.g., viscera, bones, muscles). After prolonged laparoscopic procedures it may take hours before the patient has eliminated the extra CO_2 that has accumulated in these storage areas; again, this is more often the case and a problem in patients with pulmonary compromise (Lewis et al, 1972; Puri and Singh, 1992; Tolksdorf et al, 1992; Wolf and Stoller, 1994). Therefore, as previously noted, all patients, and in particular those with pulmonary disease, must be closely monitored after a lengthy laparoscopic procedure for possible signs or symptoms of hypercarbia; indeed, their greatest chance of compromise as a result of hypercarbia may occur after extubation in the postanesthesia recovery room.

Alternative Gases

Nitrous oxide is less irritating to the peritoneum and causes fewer acid-base changes and cardiovascular adverse effects (e.g., arrhythmias) than CO_2 (Scott and Julian, 1972; El-Minawi et al, 1981; Minoli et al, 1982; Sharp et al, 1982). However, some studies have shown that nitrous oxide insufflation reduces cardiac output and increases mean arterial pressure, heart rate, and central venous pressure (Marshall et al, 1972; Shulman and Aronson, 1984). Because nitrous oxide supports combustion, it can be used only during laparoscopic procedures that do not involve the use of electrosurgical instruments.

Helium is an inert and noncombustible insufflant. Initial studies performed in various animal models showed favorable effects on arterial partial pressure of CO_2 and pH with **no evidence of hypercarbia** (Fitzgerald et al, 1992; Leighton et al, 1993; Rademaker et al, 1995). These results were corroborated by clinical studies (Bongard et al, 1991; Fitzgerald et al, 1992; Leighton et al, 1993; Neuberger et al, 1994; Rademaker et al, 1995; Jacobi et al, 1997). **Therefore, helium is particularly useful for the patient with pulmonary disease in whom hypercarbia would be poorly tolerated.** In a relatively recent study from Johns Hopkins University, 10 patients at high risk for hypercarbia underwent laparoscopic renal surgery with helium insufflation. These patients were successfully managed, with only one patient developing an end-tidal CO_2 over 45 mm Hg (Makarov et al, 2007). **Likewise, if hypercarbia develops during a laparoscopic procedure with CO_2, rather than aborting the procedure or converting to an open approach the surgeon can change the insufflant to helium and usually salvage the case** (Brackman et al, 2003). There is also evidence that the use of helium may cause a decrease in tumor cell growth and inflammatory reactions within the peritoneal cavity (Jacobi et al, 1997, 1999; Dahn et al, 2005). Helium insufflation can be used for laparoscopic procedures (e.g., cholecystectomy, appendectomy, hernia repair) performed with local and regional anesthesia in high-risk patients, not only because of its favorable metabolic features, but also because of its lack of peritoneal irritation and its association with decreased postoperative pain (Crabtree and Fishman, 1999). **However, laparoscopists have to bear in mind that helium may be associated with a higher risk of gas embolism because of its lower blood solubility.** When helium is going to be used, it is advised to initially obtain the pneumoperitoneum with CO_2 and then change to helium, thereby lowering the chances of a helium gas embolus. Also, helium is significantly more expensive than CO_2. Lastly, with use of helium a separate "yoke" (i.e., line from the gas tank to the insufflator) is needed; accordingly, one needs to make sure that a "helium yoke" is available in the operating room or make arrangements to have one provided when performing laparoscopy on patients with severe pulmonary compromise. In practice, the use of helium may be quite difficult; however, argon may also be used in circumstances when hypercarbia occurs. Indeed, the gas from the argon beam coagulator can be used to maintain the pneumoperitoneum. However, with argon being an inert gas, like helium, the same precautions apply (Badger et al, 2008).

Other insufflants (e.g., room air, oxygen) have been used to establish a pneumoperitoneum in the past. However, possible serious side effects (e.g., air embolus, intra-abdominal explosion, combustion with oxygen and room air) have terminated their clinical use. Other options for insufflants include some of the other noble gases (e.g., xenon, argon, and krypton), which are inert and nonflammable; however, their widespread clinical use has not been adopted because of their high cost and poor solubility in blood.

Choice of Pneumoperitoneum Pressure

Overall, the most commonly selected pressure for performing laparoscopy is 15 mm Hg; however, recent studies support a pressure of 12 mm Hg as more optimal, because this results in no perturbations in cardiac parameters (i.e., no change in stroke volume) versus a pressure of 15 mm Hg (Mertens zur Borg et al, 2004). Working at lower pneumoperitoneum pressures has also been found to reduce postoperative pain (Sarli et al, 2000). Using an even lower working pressure of 10 mm Hg has been shown to result in a marked reduction in oliguria (McDougall et al, 1994), but this is likely at the expense of smaller working space. Conversely, a pressure of 20 mm Hg has been noted to produce a 22% increase in insufflant filling volume and possibly less venous bleeding during the procedure (Adams et al, 1999). However, the absolute benefit of increased insufflant filling is debatable; McDougall and colleagues (1994) noted that, despite the increased volume, there was only a very small increase in abdominal girth at higher pressures.

Various cardiovascular, renal, and respiratory effects seen during different intra-abdominal pressures in the supine state are summarized in Table 10-2. It is of note that these physiologic parameters may be further altered (i.e., overridden or reversed) owing to the health of the individual patient and to changes in the patient's position.

Cardiovascular Effects of the Pneumoperitoneum

Venous Flow

Animal studies have shown that the effects of the pneumoperitoneum on venous return depend on atrial pressures, which, in turn, are a reflection of the hydration state of the subject (Ivankovich et al, 1975; Diamant et al, 1978; Kashtan et al, 1981). If atrial pressures are low (normal or hypovolemic state), then, during a pneumoperitoneum of up to 20 mm Hg, venous return is reduced owing to increased compression of the vena cava from the pneumoperitoneum. If atrial pressures are high (hypervolemic state), the vena cava resists elevated intra-abdominal pressure and venous return is actually enhanced. However, these principles apply only to an intra-abdominal pressure of up to 20 mm Hg. By further increasing pneumoperitoneum pressures, especially to 40 mm Hg and above, capacitance vessels are collapsed, vascular resistance increases, blood flow decreases markedly, and venous return is significantly reduced. Lower extremity venous return is also reduced by elevated intra-abdominal pressures. Reduced venous blood flow in the lower extremities could facilitate deep vein thrombosis; however, this remains a rare clinical complication of laparoscopy (Jorgensen et al, 1993).

These pathophysiologic insights, gained through animal experiments, have been corroborated by clinical studies (Kelman et al, 1972; Motew et al, 1973; Lee, 1975; Jorgensen et al, 1993). As a result of these trials, intra-abdominal pressures during laparoscopy should not be allowed to exceed 20 mm Hg over extended periods (Arthur, 1970; Seed et al, 1970; Lee, 1975), and a working pressure of 10 to 12 mm Hg is recommended.

Cardiac Arrhythmias

Tachycardia and ventricular extrasystoles may be seen as results of hypercapnia (Scott and Julian, 1972). Peritoneal irritation may lead to vagal stimulation and subsequently to bradyarrhythmias (Doyle and Mark, 1989). Also, dysrhythmias can serve as clinical warning signs for the occurrence of pneumothorax, hypoxia, and gas embolism (Wolf and Stoller, 1994).

TABLE 10-2 Pressure Effects: 5, 10, 20, and 40 mm Hg

EFFECTS	5 mm Hg	10 mm Hg	20 mm Hg	40 mm Hg
CARDIOVASCULAR				
Heart rate	↑	↑	↑	↓
Mean arterial pressure	↑	↑	↑	↑
Systemic vascular resistance	↑	↑	↑	↑
Venous return	→/↓	↓↑	↓↑	↓
Cardiac output	→/↓	→/↑	→/↓	↓
RENAL				
Glomerular filtration rate	→	↓	↓↓	↓↓
Urine output	→	↓	↓↓	↓↓
RESPIRATORY				
End-tidal CO_2	→	→/↑	→/↑	↑
P_{CO_2}	→	↑	↑	↑
Arterial pH	→	→/↓	↓	↓

CO_2, carbon dioxide; P_{CO_2}, partial pressure of carbon dioxide.

Unreliability of Central Venous Pressure Readings

As previously noted, intravenous pressures may actually rise with low intra-abdominal pressures. In addition, increasing intra-abdominal pressures may artificially elevate central venous pressure readings owing to an increase in intrathoracic pressure. Therefore, it is important for the anesthetist *not* to rely on central venous pressure readings for any clinical decision making.

Respiratory Effects of the Pneumoperitoneum

Pressure-Mediated Effects

Owing to increased intra-abdominal pressure, diaphragmatic motion is limited. Pulmonary dead space remains unchanged, but functional reserve capacity decreases (Wolf and Stoller, 1994). The average peak airway pressure needed to keep up a constant tidal volume increases parallel to the increasing intra-abdominal pressure (Alexander et al, 1969; Motew et al, 1973; Wolf and Stoller, 1994).

Although usually not of great clinical importance in a healthy patient population, it is advisable to use positive end-expiratory pressure techniques when patients with lung disease undergo general anesthesia for a laparoscopic procedure (Ekman et al, 1988; Wolf and Stoller, 1994; Hazebroek et al, 2002).

Non–Pressure-Related Respiratory Effects

The head-down position, commonly used in laparoscopic procedures, has an adverse effect on respiration. It elevates the diaphragm and decreases vital capacity. It can also lead to a dislocation of the endotracheal tube that, in turn, may cause right main bronchus intubation. Although of little clinical significance in healthy patients, the head-down position may cause pulmonary edema in patients with increased left-sided heart pressures (Prentice and Martin, 1987). Also, during lengthy procedures performed with the patient in the head-down position, it is useful to limit fluid administration if possible because it will minimize facial swelling postoperatively.

Renal Effects of the Pneumoperitoneum

Increased intra-abdominal pressure was found to be associated with a significant decrease in urinary output. A number of investigators, with the oldest study dating back to 1923, have observed **oliguria** and anuria associated with an ongoing increase in intra-abdominal pressure (Thorington and Schmidt, 1923; Harmann

et al, 1982; Richards et al, 1983). Decreased renal vein blood flow and direct renal parenchymal compression, rather than marked hormonal changes or ureteral compression, have been shown to be the likely reasons for the oliguric state (Chiu et al, 1994; McDougall et al, 1996). Of interest, renal cortical blood flow decreases with increasing intra-abdominal pressures, whereas renal medullary blood flow increases up to pressures of 20 mm Hg; above this level, medullary blood flow also decreases (Chiu et al, 1994).

In general, if one desires to avoid an oliguric state during a laparoscopic procedure, a pressure of 10 mm Hg or less is recommended. In addition, clinically the use of furosemide (Lasix), mannitol (12.5 to 25 g), and dopamine at 2 µg/kg/min can help to overcome oliguria. With this regimen and judicious fluid administration, the patient can usually be maintained with a urine output in excess of 100 mL/hr. The key is to use these pharmaceutical modalities in lieu of excessive hydration and fluid boluses (Perez et al, 2002), which may lead to significant fluid overload and edema.

Effects of the Pneumoperitoneum on Mesenteric Blood Flow and Intestinal Motility

Decreased blood flow during laparoscopic procedures was found not only in the kidney, but also in mesenteric vessels and other organs (e.g., liver, pancreas, stomach, spleen, small and large intestines) (Caldwell and Ricotta, 1987; Ishizaki et al, 1993; Hashikura et al, 1994). This may rarely lead to mesenteric thrombosis with catastrophic results. This complication may take days to develop (Schorr, 1998).

Open, incisional abdominal surgery usually results in some postoperative impairment of gastric and intestinal emptying owing to intestinal paralysis (physiologic ileus) (Kemen et al, 1991). It is interesting to note that clinical observation and studies undertaken during laparoscopic and open surgical cholecystectomy have shown that laparoscopic surgery causes less significant disturbances of the gastrointestinal motility pattern, therefore resulting in no or less postoperative physiologic ileus than occurs with open surgery (Sezeur et al, 1993; Halevy et al, 1994). The exact mechanisms responsible for this difference have yet to be defined; however, it is postulated that perhaps it is related to the hypercarbia (Aneman et al, 2000). In addition, intestinal perfusion does not change significantly during prolonged pneumoperitoneum at a pressure of 15 mm Hg with CO_2 or helium (Goitein et al, 2005); however, at least in the rat model, there does seem to be an increase in bacterial translocation that is proportional to the pneumoperitoneum pressure (Sukhotnik et al, 2006).

Also, despite the increased intra-abdominal pressures associated with laparoscopy, there has been no increased incidence of gastroesophageal reflux and regurgitation in patients undergoing laparoscopic procedures (Schippers et al, 1992).

Acid-Base Metabolic Effects of Pneumoperitoneum

Animal and human studies have demonstrated that prolonged laparoscopic procedures may result in hypercarbia and respiratory acidosis (Motew et al, 1973). Because there is no increase in ventilatory dead space during laparoscopy, the resulting respiratory acidosis has been attributed to transperitoneal absorption of CO_2 during establishment and maintenance of the pneumoperitoneum (Motew et al, 1973; Leighton et al, 1993). Although the resulting mild respiratory acidosis does not adversely affect otherwise normal patients and can be corrected by increasing the minute ventilation, increased absorption of CO_2 can become dangerous in patients with COPD owing to their impaired ability to release pulmonary CO_2. **To ensure proper monitoring of acid-base status, intermittent arterial blood gas sampling should be performed in patients with COPD, during any laparoscopic procedure that requires more than 1 hour of CO_2 insufflation; also in patients with COPD, arterial blood gas sampling should continue in the postanesthesia recovery area because after extubation these patients may be at risk of significant hypercarbia owing to subsequent mobilization of procedurally absorbed CO_2.**

The potential for developing hypercarbia exists during both transperitoneal and preperitoneal laparoscopy. Carbon dioxide is absorbed from the peritoneal membrane during transperitoneal laparoscopy and from preperitoneal adipose and connective tissue during retroperitoneoscopy and extraperitoneoscopy (Collins, 1981). Others have also implicated the disrupted microvascular and lymphatic channels for CO_2 absorption during preperitoneal laparoscopy (Glascock et al, 1996). Several studies have demonstrated that CO_2 absorption during either transperitoneal or retroperitoneal laparoscopy increases significantly during the initial 30 to 60 minutes of the procedure and reaches a steady-state plateau thereafter (Wolf et al, 1995; Ng et al, 1999). Which one of the two approaches is associated with greater CO_2 absorption remains a debated issue. Although some studies have demonstrated greater absorption during transperitoneal laparoscopy (Giebler et al, 1997), others have demonstrated greater absorption during retroperitoneal laparoscopy using a standard Hasson cannula (Wolf et al, 1995). However, in another study, no significant clinical difference was seen (Ng et al, 1999), provided a balloon tip–type cannula was used that tightly sealed the site of entry between the balloon and soft cuff carried on the shaft of the cannula.

Although transperitoneal and retroperitoneoscopic approaches are routinely used safely at numerous centers worldwide, vigilant perioperative anesthetic management is essential to prevent the development of potential complications related to CO_2 buildup, particularly in patients with preexisting airway and cardiovascular compromise. End-tidal CO_2 and O_2 saturation should be monitored intraoperatively with a capnometer. Furthermore, arterial blood gases are obtained during prolonged laparoscopic procedures and in patients with increased risk of developing hypercarbia (owing to airway disease, renal failure, congestive heart failure, or advanced age). **A rise in end-tidal CO_2 should prompt the anesthesiologist to adjust the respiratory rate and tidal volume to enhance CO_2 elimination. Simultaneously, the surgeon should decrease the insufflation pressure of CO_2 or, if necessary, desufflate the abdomen until the hypercarbia has resolved.**

Hemodynamic Effects Related to Patient Position and Type of Approach

Several animal and human studies have examined hemodynamic changes resulting from different surgical positions during laparoscopy (Kelman et al, 1972; Joris et al, 1993; Williams and Murr,

1993). In the supine position, cardiac output remains unchanged or decreases when intra-abdominal pressures are less than 15 mm Hg, whereas mean arterial pressure (MAP) and systemic vascular resistance increase (Pearle, 1996). If pneumoperitoneum pressures are increased beyond 20 mm Hg, cardiac output is reduced because of decreasing venous return and hence MAP decreases. Alternatively, in the head-up position, heart rate increases, MAP decreases, systemic vascular resistance increases, and cardiac output decreases. In the head-down position, heart rate drops, MAP rises, systemic vascular resistance falls, and cardiac output increases (Pearle, 1996). These results have also been shown to hold true in steep Trendelenburg position used for laparoscopic and robotic radical prostatectomy (Falabella et al, 2007). The head-down position seems to be favorable for the laparoscopy patient owing to higher cardiac output caused by increased venous return.

There is some evidence that the extraperitoneal approach may be beneficial with regard to hemodynamic effects compared with transperitoneal laparoscopy. Giebler and coworkers (1997) demonstrated that transperitoneal laparoscopy was associated with more pronounced changes in cardiac output ($P = .001$), pulmonary artery pressure ($P = .007$), central venous pressure ($P = .001$), iliac venous pressure ($P = .001$), and inferior vena caval pressure gradient ($P = .00001$) as compared with retroperitoneal laparoscopy. With regard to pelvic laparoscopy, Meininger and associates (2004) compared the effects of prolonged intraperitoneal and extraperitoneal CO_2 insufflation on hemodynamics and gas exchange. With both insufflation methods, arterial CO_2 pressure increased rapidly, reaching higher levels with extraperitoneal insufflation. Therefore patients managed with extraperitoneal insufflation required significantly higher minute ventilation. Heart rate and central venous pressure increased in both groups, whereas mean arterial blood pressure and pH decreased in both groups.

Hormonal and Metabolic Effects during Laparoscopic Surgery

As in other surgical procedures, several hormones (e.g., β-endorphin, cortisol, prolactin, epinephrine, norepinephrine, dopamine) have been noted to increase during laparoscopic surgery as a response to tissue manipulation, intraoperative trauma, and postoperative pain (Cooper et al, 1982; Lehtinen et al, 1987; Lefebvre et al, 1992). The clinical significance of increased serum arginine vasopressin levels seen in open surgery and in response to intraperitoneal insufflation during laparoscopy remains unexplained (Cochrane et al, 1981; Melville et al, 1985; Solis Herruzo et al, 1989).

Several adverse metabolic changes observed during open cholecystectomy are less pronounced with laparoscopic cholecystectomy: (1) reduced postoperative plasma glucose elevation, (2) less decrease in insulin sensitivity, and (3) reduced hepatic stress response (Thorell et al, 1993; Jakeways et al, 1994; Glerup et al, 1995).

One important feature of the catabolic response is a complex intra-organ shift of nitrogen; this reaction has been best characterized in the liver (Glerup et al, 1995). The conversion of amino acids to urea by the liver is much higher after open cholecystectomy than it is after laparoscopic cholecystectomy. Hence, the catabolic reaction of the body is decreased with a laparoscopic versus an open approach (Fischer, 1995). Indeed, in the laparoscopic patient, the reduced postoperative hepatic catabolic stress associated with reduced tissue loss of amino-nitrogen may, in some way, be responsible for the more rapid convalescence that is the hallmark of laparoscopy in general. Lastly, catabolic responses, in the form of released cytokines and opioids, resulting from augmented neurohumoral stimuli caused by incisional tissue trauma may also be lessened with a laparoscopic approach (Fischer, 1995).

Immunologic Effects of Laparoscopic Surgery

A number of animal and clinical studies measuring a wide spectrum of inflammatory response mediators (e.g., C-reactive protein, interleukin-6) and other markers of cellular immune functions (pan–T cells [CD3], helper T cells [CD4], suppressor cells [CD8], and natural killer cells [CD16]); delayed-type hypersensitivity skin tests; serial phytohemagglutinin-induced T-cell proliferation) have suggested that laparoscopic procedures in general result in less immunosuppression than do their open counterparts (Kloosterman et al, 1994; Trokel et al, 1994; Cristaldi et al, 1997; Karayiannakis et al, 1997; Nguyen et al, 1999; Bolla and Tuzzato, 2003). This may also play a role in hastening convalescence after laparoscopic procedures. Some data have suggested that the CO_2 pneumoperitoneum in and of itself, as opposed to exposure of tissues to room air, results in a more favorable immunologic state (Watson et al, 1995). Also, experimental evidence shows that less tumor cell growth occurs after laparoscopic procedures than after open procedures (Bouvy et al, 1997). Although these data are intriguing, further well-designed, prospectively randomized clinical studies are needed to compare immunologic responses after laparoscopic versus open surgical procedures for urologic cancer. Indeed, in a study by Landman and colleagues (2004) there was no discernible difference in immunologic parameters between patients undergoing open or transperitoneal laparoscopic radical or total nephrectomy for renal cancer. Ultimately, whether a decrease in inflammatory response mediators and improved postlaparoscopic immune status will translate into a better long-term prognosis for patients with urologic cancers remains to be determined.

KEY POINTS: PHYSIOLOGIC CONSIDERATIONS IN THE ADULT

- Carbon dioxide is the most commonly used insufflant because it is noncombustible and rapidly absorbed in the blood.
- Helium is particularly useful for the patient with pulmonary disease in whom hypercarbia would be poorly tolerated.
- Intra-abdominal pressures during laparoscopy should not be allowed to exceed 20 mm Hg over extended periods, and a working pressure of 10 to 12 mm Hg is recommended.

COMPLICATIONS AND TROUBLESHOOTING IN LAPAROSCOPIC AND ROBOTIC SURGERY

Historically, in large series the overall incidence of laparoscopic complications in urology has been in the range of 4% and **mortality has been distinctly unusual, with a rate of 0.03% to 0.08%** (Mintz 1977; Winfield et al, 1991; Fahlenkamp et al, 1999). More contemporary series demonstrate a complication rate in the range of 13% to 22% (Table 10-3) (Vallancien et al, 2002; Parsons et al,

TABLE 10-3 Major Complications of Transperitoneal Abdominal Surgery

TOTAL PROCEDURES	894* (100% ABDOMINAL)	1311† (84% PELVIC)
Overall complications	13.2%	22.6%
Intraoperative/postoperative	5.7%/7.5%	3.6%/19%
Death	0.2%	0%
Vascular injury	2.8%	0.5%
Bowel injury	1.1%	1.2%
Adjacent organ injury	1.1%	0.8%
Conversion rate	1.7%	1.7%

*Data from Parsons JK, Varkarakis I, Rha KH, et al. Complications of abdominal urologic laparoscopy: longitudinal five-year analysis. Urology 2004;63:27–32.
†Data from Vallancien G, Cathelineau X, Baumert H, et al. Complications of transperitoneal laparoscopic surgery in urology: review of 1,311 procedures at a single center. J Urol 2002;168:23–6.

2004; Permpongkosol et al, 2007), likely representative of the introduction of new, more sophisticated laparoscopic procedures and more widespread use of laparoscopy. Vascular followed by adjacent organ injuries are the most common complications (Permpongkosol et al, 2007; Breda et al, 2009). The following section covers the myriad complications that can occur with any laparoscopic or robotic procedure. Recognition, resolution, and prevention of these various problems are discussed.

Minimizing the Incidence of Complications during the Learning Curve

Early in one's experience with laparoscopic and robotic surgery, it is wise to first apply this approach to low-risk surgical candidates of normal body habitus. In addition, it is advisable and recommended by many laparoscopic organizations, as well as by hospital credentialing boards, that the neophyte minimally invasive surgeon seek training in three arenas: (1) in-depth instructional courses, including didactic, "live-case" transmissions and "hands-on" laboratory sessions; (2) preceptor training in which the surgeon-in-training views five or more procedures being done by an already skillful laparoscopic or robotic surgeon; and (3) a mentoring experience, during which a trained laparoscopic or robotic surgeon oversees the initial procedures performed by the surgeon-in-training (Society of American Gastrointestinal and Endoscopic Surgeons, 2010). Further training can be obtained through self-teaching using videotapes, a laparoscopic box trainer, and virtual reality (VR) simulators. A laparoscopic box trainer is extremely helpful for developing one's sense of laparoscopic proprioception and for becoming facile with laparoscopic suturing and knot tying. Data have clearly shown benefits for individuals who have taken the time to practice their laparoscopic skills using a box trainer in all areas of laparoscopy (cutting, clipping, and suturing) compared with individuals who had no such training (Derossis et al, 1998). Similarly, participation in a 1-week mini-residency has been found to increase the likelihood that participants would perform more complex laparoscopic procedures (81% of participants) (Corica et al, 2006). In addition, VR simulators have been shown to improve the operative performance of surgical trainees with limited laparoscopic experience when compared with no training or with box-trainer training (Nagendran et al, 2013).

Aside from training in the basic psychomotor skills, neophyte minimally invasive surgeons must be educated with regard to prevention, recognition, and appropriate treatment of complications.

General Procedural Complications
Malfunction of Equipment

A successful outcome of any laparoscopic or robotic procedure depends not only on the psychomotor technical skills of the surgeon, but also on a proper working knowledge of all the equipment involved in performing these procedures. To ensure undisturbed functioning of all technology, the surgeon must be supported by well-trained staff who are capable not only of quickly recognizing any equipment malfunction, but also of providing an immediate, adequate response to correct problems. In this regard, the Society of American Gastrointestinal Endoscopic Surgeons has issued a troubleshooting guide for video and electronic failure. For integrated operating room systems offered by most major equipment manufacturers and the da Vinci Robotic System, the surgeon and operating room staff need to receive in-depth training on the system's operation, capabilities, and limitations. In this way, equipment failure will be minimized. In addition, the contact information for both the equipment vendor's troubleshooting experts and any in-house support should be readily available.

With regard to the da Vinci Robotic System, equipment malfunction is rare. In a review of 11 institutions with a total of 8240 cases reviewed, the overall incidence of malfunction was 0.4%. Of the 34 cases with malfunction, 24 cases were canceled before the procedure, 2 cases were converted to laparoscopic procedures, and 8 were converted to open surgery (Lavery et al, 2008).

Complications Related to Obtaining the Pneumoperitoneum

Complications Associated with Closed Access (Veress Needle Placement)

Preperitoneal Placement. Preperitoneal placement of the Veress needle may preclude successful trocar placement. If not recognized early, 1 to 2 L of CO_2 may be instilled, and once this much CO_2 has been insufflated into the preperitoneal space, many signs indicative of correct intraperitoneal insufflation may be present (e.g., distention, tympanic sound on percussion) thereby misleading the surgeon until the first trocar is placed. **The first sign of preperitoneal insufflation is that there may be a steep rise in pressure with only 500 mL of CO_2; plus, if more CO_2 is instilled, unequal distention of the abdomen occurs.** If this early sign is missed, then the laparoscope reveals only fat after trocar placement; the intraperitoneal viscera are not seen.

The next step is to evacuate the CO_2 through the sidearm of the trocar and proceed with an open insertion technique. The initial incision can be widened, and the peritoneal surface can be grasped with a pair of Allis clamps and incised. A Hasson cannula is placed and the peritoneal cavity is insufflated.

Several steps can be taken to avoid this complication. First, if the Veress needle is preperitoneal on initial insufflation, pressures are usually higher than the maximal initial allowable pressure of 10 mm. Second, if the Veress needle is preperitoneal, it cannot be easily advanced 1 cm deeper without resistance. If one has truly entered the peritoneal cavity properly, the Veress needle should be able to be moved 0.5 to 1 cm deeper without meeting any resistance.

Vascular Injuries. During initial placement of the Veress needle at the umbilicus, minor or major intra-abdominal blood vessels may be punctured by the 14-gauge needle. The first sign of intravascular entry is blood appearing in the hub of the needle. Aspiration results in additional blood filling the syringe. As long as the needle has not been manipulated, it can usually be withdrawn without excessive bleeding. An alternative site for Veress needle placement or open cannula insertion should be used at this point. On proper entry into the peritoneal cavity and establishment of a pneumoperitoneum, **it is important that the path of the initial Veress needle passage be traced. The prior site of the Veress needle passage should be carefully inspected at a pressure of 5 mm Hg. Any site of bleeding can be expeditiously treated by applying gentle pressure and the application of a surgical hemostatic agent as needed.**

To prevent this problem it is important when using an umbilical approach to direct the Veress needle toward the pelvis. One technique to help prevent this problem, when using an umbilical access, is to pass the Veress needle after making a 12-mm incision, bluntly spreading the subcutaneous fat, and grasping and stabilizing the anterior fascia with a pair of Allis clamps. These maneuvers become especially important in children, who have less space between intra-abdominal structures and the abdominal wall.

Surgeons should also be cognizant that any hemodynamic instability associated with loss of "working space" within the abdomen during the procedure might represent an expanding "unseen" retroperitoneal hematoma from unrecognized Veress needle injury.

Prevention of vascular complications can be further achieved by using a nonumbilical site for Veress needle passage (i.e., just superior and medial to the iliac crest or subcostal in the midclavicular line) where no major vessels are placed in danger.

Visceral Injuries. During Veress needle placement, intra-abdominal organs may be punctured. The initial signs of this complication consist of aspiration of blood, urine, or bowel contents through the Veress needle or, in the case of a solid organ, high pressures on initial insufflation.

Management consists of simply removing the Veress needle. The Veress needle may then be reintroduced at a different site, or an open Hasson technique can be used through a separate incision site. On entry into the abdomen, any bleeding site on the liver or spleen

can be treated with gentle pressure, an argon beam coagulator, or the application of a surgical hemostatic agent as needed. General surgical consultation should be sought in those cases in which there is difficulty achieving hemostasis.

Bowel or bladder entry by the Veress needle needs no further treatment other than needle withdrawal. Placing a nasogastric tube and a transurethral indwelling bladder catheter to decompress the stomach and bladder, respectively, before Veress needle passage can help to prevent these problems.

Complications during Open Access (Hasson Technique). Potential problems associated with open access are similar to, albeit less frequent than, problems associated with a closed Veress needle access. The principal risk with the open access is injury to underlying viscera while traversing the peritoneum. In a densely scarred abdomen, the bowel may be adherent to the underside of the abdominal wall and hence may still be injured. If a bowel injury is recognized early, it can often be repaired through the same incision that was made for insertion of the Hasson cannula. Although vascular injury with this approach is distinctly rare, the surgeon must realize that even with open access this devastating complication can occur (Hanney et al, 1999).

Complications Related to Insufflation and Pneumoperitoneum

Bowel Insufflation. If entry into the bowel is not recognized at the time of irrigation and aspiration through the Veress needle, then the surgeon may well insufflate the small or large bowel. **The first sign of this problem is asymmetrical abdominal distention followed by flatus and insufflation of only a small amount of CO_2 (<2 L) before high pressures are reached.**

If this complication is suspected, then the insufflation line should be disconnected; the outflow of gas will immediately confirm bowel entry. The needle can be withdrawn, and open access cannula placement should be done at a different abdominal site. Prevention of this problem is ensured if one properly performs the aspiration, irrigation, and aspiration tests recommended for safe Veress needle placement and if one avoids sites of prior surgery. Alternatively, initial use of open access technique should avoid this complication.

Gas Embolism. Carbon dioxide gas has favorable solubility in blood, as opposed to air, helium, or nitrous oxide; however, use of CO_2 may still result in a gas embolus. The most common cause of CO_2 embolism is puncture of a blood vessel or organ with the Veress needle, followed by insufflation; this can occur only when the surgeon has ignored the previously described tests for proper entry into the peritoneal cavity. The first sign of intravascular insufflation is acute cardiovascular collapse. Other signs include dysrhythmias, tachycardia, cyanosis, and pulmonary edema. **The diagnosis is usually made by the anesthesiologist based on an abrupt increase of end-tidal CO_2 accompanied by a sudden decline in oxygen saturation and then a marked decrease in end-tidal CO_2** (Loris, 1994). Sometimes, a "millwheel" precordial murmur can be auscultated (Keith et al, 1974). In addition, the anesthesiologist may notice foaming of a blood sample, if drawn, as a result of the presence of insufflated CO_2.

The treatment is immediate cessation of insufflation and prompt desufflation of the peritoneal cavity. The patient, if at all possible, is turned to a left lateral decubitus (i.e., right side up), head-down position in hopes of minimizing right ventricular outflow problems and forcing the air embolus to rise into the apex of the right ventricle. The patient is hyperventilated with 100% oxygen. Advancement of a central venous line into the right side of the heart with subsequent attempts to aspirate gas may rarely be helpful. The use of hyperbaric oxygen and cardiopulmonary bypass have also been reported (McGrath et al, 1989; Diakun, 1991; Abdel-Meguid and Gomella, 1996).

This devastating complication can be precluded by meticulous attention to Veress needle and initial trocar placement and performance of each of the recommended tests for intraperitoneal entry. Insufflation should never be initiated if the surgeon has even the slightest doubt about correct positioning of the Veress needle; instead, the surgeon should withdraw the Veress needle and pass it at an alternate site or should immediately proceed with open access.

Barotrauma. Prolonged elevated pressures (>15 mm Hg) may result in barotrauma (McGrath et al, 1989; Diakun, 1991; Abdel-Meguid and Gomella, 1996). Prolonged high pressures may be caused by insufficient and infrequent monitoring of CO_2 pressure, malfunction of the insufflator, or additional pressures produced by auxiliary devices (e.g., argon beam coagulator, CO_2-cooled laser). Furthermore, barotrauma may be caused by ventilation techniques using positive end-expiratory pressure resulting in rupture of a pulmonary bleb or bulla.

The initial sign of barotrauma may be hypotension caused by decreased cardiac output, secondary to an acute drop in venous return caused by compression of the vena cava. Also, a pneumothorax or pneumomediastinum may develop because of the high ventilation pressures. In addition, increased intra-abdominal pressures may exacerbate a hiatal hernia.

The anesthesiologist, who will notice an increase in ventilation pressures, usually alerts the surgeon to excessive intra-abdominal pressure. The surgeon should desufflate the abdomen and, once the hemodynamic changes have been reversed, reinitiate the pneumoperitoneum at 10 mm Hg. Any malfunctioning insufflator should be replaced. Also, if one is using an argon beam coagulator or a CO_2-cooled laser device, the sidearm on one port should be left open to allow excess high-pressure gas to escape while the device is being activated.

Barotrauma secondary to insufflator malfunction can be avoided by routinely troubleshooting the insufflator before every case.

Subcutaneous Emphysema. Subcutaneous emphysema develops owing to improper placement of the Veress needle or, more commonly, to leakage of CO_2 around ports. The latter situation occurs when a secure seal around the Hasson cannula is not obtained, port site incisions are too large, the procedure is particularly lengthy, or high intra-abdominal pressures are used. The pathognomonic sign is crepitus over the abdomen and thorax; in male patients, a pneumoscrotum may also develop.

If the problem is caused by improper placement of the Veress needle, then withdrawal of the Veress needle and use of the open technique are recommended. If the problem develops intraoperatively, the surgeon should check for gas leakage around a port site, including the Hasson cannula if the open technique was used. If leakage is found, the surgeon can either place a purse-string suture around the port or, preferably, change the trocar to a larger size or switch to a balloon trocar, which creates a tight seal between the intra-abdominal balloon and outer cuff. Also, the surgeon should consider reducing the insufflation pressure. This complication is eminently avoidable if the surgeon adheres to all the diagnostic tests for proper Veress needle placement and ensures all port site incisions are carefully tapered to the size of the port to be placed. In this regard, it is important to place each port so that it is pointing toward the surgical field, to avoid the continued forceful redirection of the port during the procedure that results in widening of the tissue tract around the port and subsequent escape of CO_2 into the surrounding subcutaneous tissues.

Several studies have demonstrated that the incidence of subcutaneous emphysema is higher during retroperitoneal laparoscopy than during transperitoneal laparoscopy, albeit without any clinically significant sequelae (Wolf et al, 1995; Zhao et al, 2008). In any event, the risk of surgical emphysema and other CO_2-related sequelae during retroperitoneoscopic and extraperitoneoscopic surgery can be effectively minimized by working at a lower pressure (i.e., 12 mm Hg vs. 15 mm Hg) (Rassweiler et al, 1998a) and using a balloon trocar to seal the initial entry site (Gill, 1998; Ng et al, 1999).

Pneumomediastinum, Pneumothorax, and Pneumopericardium. Gas leaking along major blood vessels through congenital defects or secondary enlargement of openings in the diaphragm may lead to pneumomediastinum, pneumopericardium, or

pneumothorax (Kalhan et al, 1990; Pascual et al, 1990; See et al, 1993; Abreu et al, 2004; Zhao et al, 2008). Although a pneumomediastinum is usually not associated with specific clinical symptoms, a pneumopericardium may result in impaired cardiac function. The incidence of the pneumopericardium is estimated to be 0.8% (Abreu et al, 2004). The diagnosis is usually made on a chest radiograph taken in the recovery room, except in rare instances when cardiac impairment occurs during the procedure. If there is sudden cardiac decompensation during a procedure, the same maneuvers should be undertaken as described for treatment of a suspected gas embolism, including interruption of the procedure and desufflation of the abdomen. If there is a strong suspicion of pericardial tamponade, pericardiocentesis is indicated.

A pneumothorax may be associated with pneumomediastinum, barotrauma, or direct puncture of the pleural space with a trocar (Doctor and Hussain, 1973; Kalhan et al, 1990; Pascual et al, 1990). The incidence of this complication has been found to be 1.6% to 4.0% (Abreu et al, 2004; Zhao et al, 2008). Like subcutaneous emphysema, the incidence of pneumothorax is more common in retroperitoneal procedures (Zhao et al, 2008). The earliest signs of this problem may be the development of subcutaneous emphysema, especially in the neck and chest area. More ominous signs, such as hypotension and decreased breath sounds with an increase in ventilatory pressure, are indicative of a *tension* pneumothorax. Although a chest radiograph will confirm the diagnosis, the development of pulmonary collapse with loss of breath sounds on one side mandates immediate decompression of the chest by passage of a 16-gauge needle into the second or third intercostal space in the midclavicular line followed by tube thoracostomy, if a tension pneumothorax is suspected (See et al, 1993).

Prevention of these problems is similar to the means to avoid subcutaneous emphysema: Keep the intra-abdominal pressure preferably at 12 mm Hg, make sure all port site incisions are tight around the laparoscopic cannulae, and make sure all cannulae are well seated in the peritoneal cavity. In addition, all trocars must remain below the 12th rib. While dissecting in the upper quadrants of the abdomen, especially during laparoscopic ablative renal surgery, the surgeon should be aware of the anatomic relationships of the kidneys, adrenal glands, and great vessels to the diaphragm to avoid direct injury.

Complications Related to Initial "Blind" Placement of the First Trocar after Obtaining a Veress Needle Pneumoperitoneum

With the advent of nonbladed trocars (several of which also have clear tips for direct visualization of individual abdominal wall layers during port placement), the likelihood of catastrophic injuries to vital structures has been markedly reduced (Thomas et al, 2003).

Injury to Gastrointestinal Organs. Perforation of the small or large intestine during passage of the primary port is the most common cause of trocar-induced injury of gastrointestinal organs. Other organs (e.g., stomach) are affected much less frequently. Given the lateral positioning of the spleen and liver, injury of these organs with the passage of the primary trocar is distinctly unusual. The first sign that one has entered the bowel depends on whether the injury is through one wall or both walls of the bowel. In the former instance, as soon as the laparoscope is introduced the surgeon sees the mucosal folds of the interior of the bowel. However, with a through-and-through injury the diagnosis is not made until the first secondary trocar is passed; **at that time the surgeon should routinely pass the laparoscope through the secondary port to inspect the puncture site of the initial port.** The trocar will be seen passing completely through both walls of the bowel. If the surgeon fails to perform this maneuver routinely this injury will not be noted until the end of the case when the trocars are being removed, thereby resulting in a broader injury and a prolonged time of intraperitoneal contamination. A missed bowel injury of this nature leads to peritonitis when diagnosed intraoperatively, and possible death when discovered only in the postoperative period.

In the case of a one-wall injury of the bowel, the surgeon can elect to leave the trocar in place and pass a second trocar in another location using an open access technique. On inspection of the abdomen the site of injury to the bowel will be immediately apparent because the initial trocar will still be residing in the bowel. At this time, the surgeon may elect to open and repair the bowel or, if skilled in laparoscopy, may place two more ports and proceed to close the bowel using laparoscopic suturing or stapling techniques. An intraoperative consultation with a general surgeon should be obtained regardless of whether the urologist performs the repair; from a medicolegal and quality of care standpoint, involvement of the general surgeon at the time of the acute event facilitates subsequent care should further complications arise while ensuring the best possible repair of the injury at the time of the acute event.

When the injury to the bowel is a through-and-through injury, it can similarly be repaired with an open or laparoscopic approach. In either case, the abdomen should be irrigated with 4 to 5 L of saline containing an antibiotic solution, and the patient must be placed on broad-spectrum antibiotic coverage.

Perforation of the stomach is distinctly rare; however, to best preclude this problem patients should refrain from oral intake for 12 hours before surgery. The management of this complication is the same as for injury to the bowel, with primary closure and general surgery consultation. In addition, when the stomach is noted to be distended, a nasogastric or orogastric tube should be placed to decompress the stomach and facilitate further trocar insertion.

Injury to Intra-Abdominal Vessels. Major vascular injury is a rare but serious complication, occurring in 0.11% to 2% of cases (Hanney et al, 1995; Geers and Holden, 1996; Usal et al, 1998; Lin and Grow, 1999; Vallancien et al, 2002; Parsons et al, 2004). It is far more common in procedures related to the retroperitoneum, as opposed to pelvic laparoscopy. The aorta and common iliac arteries are most frequently involved. The inferior vena cava is less affected because of its lateral location in relation to the aorta; likewise, the common iliac vein is rarely involved given its posterior position in relation to the common iliac artery. Rarely, in a patient with adhesions or prior surgery, intestinal mesenteric vessels servicing a "fixed" loop of bowel may be injured. In addition, the epigastric vessels are at risk for injury during trocar placement.

The first sign of a major vascular complication is the onset of sudden hypotension and associated tachycardia. If the trocar has not been moved, then, as the obturator is withdrawn, the diagnosis is made immediately based on whether there is a pulsatile (arterial) or nonpulsatile (venous) profuse bleeding from the trocar sheath. If the trocar has been displaced from the injured vessel, then, depending on the vessel injured, when the laparoscope is introduced the surgeon will see blood rapidly accumulating in the abdominal cavity, a mesenteric hematoma, blood dripping from the trocar entry site, or, rarely, blood that preferentially accumulates retroperitoneally, in which case the space within the peritoneal cavity will appear to be markedly reduced and actively decreasing because of the expanding retroperitoneal hematoma.

The response to injury to a major arterial or venous structure must be rapid. A vascular or trauma surgeon should be called to the room. If blood is coming through the trocar, then the trocar should be closed and left in place. An emergency laparotomy is performed, and the trocar is followed to its point of entry into the vessel. The injured vessel should be controlled proximal and distal to the site of trocar injury with vessel loops or bulldog clamps, or alternatively a Satinsky clamp can be placed to isolate the area of injury so that as the trocar is withdrawn the wound can be controlled and repaired quickly. If the injury is discovered at the time of passage of the laparoscope (i.e., the trocar is no longer residing in the vessel), then the sheath and laparoscope can be swung up to the underside of the abdominal wall and an immediate cutdown can be done on top of the laparoscope and sheath, thereby providing for a rapid and safe laparotomy. Alternatively in this situation, the procedure can be converted to a hand-assist approach and the surgeon can then use the intra-abdominal hand to control the bleeding vessel.

BOX 10-3 Contents of Hemorrhage Tray for Laparoscopic Surgery

Laparoscopic Satinsky clamp
Ten-millimeter suction-irrigation tip
Endo Stitch device with 4-0 absorbable suture
Lapra-Ty clip applier and a packet of Lapra-Ty clips
Six-inch length of 4-0 vascular suture on an SH needle with a Lapra-Ty clip preplaced on the end
Two laparoscopic needle drivers
Topical hemostatic agent of choice

The best way to handle this complication is to avoid it completely. In this regard, knowledge of the exact location and possible anatomic variations of major intra-abdominal blood vessels is mandatory. The preoperative computed tomography (CT) scan should be reviewed before operating to look for vena caval or other abnormalities of the great vessels. Because of limited intraperitoneal space, special care must be given to trocar placement in children and very thin adults. It is important to note that several maneuvers can be used to help prevent vascular injury. These include ensuring that all the safety signs of passage of a Veress needle are present before proceeding with trocar passage, obtaining an adequate pneumoperitoneum before trocar passage (intra-abdominal pressure may be raised to 25 mm Hg temporarily for placement of the primary trocar), passing the initial trocar under direct endoscopic control (i.e., optical trocar), using blunt nonbladed trocars, and avoiding initial trocar passage through an abdominal scar.

Furthermore, it is helpful to consider having a "hemorrhage" tray available in the operating room at all times (Box 10-3). This laparoscopic tray should contain a Satinsky clamp, a 10-mm suction tip for large clot evacuation, an Endo Stitch device with 4-0 Vicryl suture, a Lapra-Ty clip applier and a rack of Lapra-Ty clips (six clips per rack), two laparoscopic needle holders, and 4-0 vascular suture. With this tray available, some injuries to major venous structures can be successfully resolved laparoscopically.

Injury to the Urinary Tract. Urinary tract injuries during laparoscopy are most commonly associated with trocar passage, specifically injury to the bladder at the time of initial trocar placement. The incidence varies widely in the gynecologic literature, ranging from 0.02% to 8.3% (Ostrzenski and Ostrzenska, 1998; Lin and Grow, 1999; Soong et al, 2007). Chances of this problem occurring have been greatly reduced by the introduction of blunt trocars.

The initial sign of this problem is pneumaturia or gross hematuria. The diagnosis can be confirmed by retrograde intravesical instillation of indigo carmine diluted with saline; this allows the surgeon to rapidly identify the cystotomy site. The injury can be repaired laparoscopically with laparoscopic suturing techniques; however, extensive defects may require open surgical repair (Ostrzenski and Ostrzenska, 1998). These injuries should always be closed and not left to heal on their own with prolonged Foley catheter drainage.

Prevention of this problem is simple. Preoperative placement of a urethral catheter to drain the bladder is recommended for all major laparoscopic urologic cases. Not only does it largely preclude bladder injury, but it also provides the necessary means for monitoring urine output during major laparoscopic procedures.

Complications Related to Placement of Secondary Trocars

Bleeding at the Sheath Site. Blood dripping from the port entry site and onto the underlying abdominal viscera is the first sign of an injured abdominal wall vessel. The exact site of hemorrhage is determined by cantilevering the trocar into each of the four quadrants and noting which position of the trocar tamponades the bleeding.

Definitive therapy for this problem can be undertaken in one of three ways. The simplest method, albeit the most costly, is the insertion of curved electrosurgical scissors or forceps through another port, which can then be articulated up into the port site to coagulate the bleeding.

The least expensive method is to suture the area of hemorrhage. This can be accomplished by inserting a straight Keith needle with a 0-0 absorbable suture from the outside of the abdomen at one side of the affected quadrant and then grasping the needle with laparoscopic forceps and pushing it back out of the abdomen at the opposite side of the affected quadrant until it can be recovered on the surface of the abdomen (Fig. 10-30). This broad suture is then tied over a gauze 4- × 4-inch bolster on the abdominal surface; the port can be used throughout the procedure. Alternatively, various port closure devices, in particular the Carter-Thomason device, may be used to similarly pass a suture to control the bleeding (Ortega, 1996). Ultimately, at the end of the procedure a device of this nature should be used to definitively close the port site and occlude the injured vessel no matter which of the aforementioned techniques is used.

This problem can often be avoided by routinely transilluminating the abdominal wall, especially in the thin patient, before trocar placement so large surface vessels and overlying peritoneal vessels can be avoided and to help identify the area of the inferior epigastric vessels. In addition, the routine spreading of the subcutaneous tissues at the proposed port site with a blunt clamp (e.g., Kelly clamp) may be helpful, and the use of only **blunt trocars has been shown to reduce the chance of vascular wall injury significantly** (Bhoyrul et al, 2000). In particular, a fivefold decrease in epigastric vessel injury has been demonstrated with blunt trocars (reduced incidence from 0.83% to 0.16%) (Hashizume and Sugimachi, 1997; Thomas et al, 2003). The incidence of any abdominal wall bleeding has also be shown to be dramatically reduced (3% vs. 9%) with blunt vs. bladed trocars

(Antoniou et al, 2013). Placing trocars either in the midline or at least 6 cm lateral to the midline has also been shown to reduce the risk of epigastric vessel injury (Hashizume and Sugimachi, 1997).

Trocar Position–Related Problems. Three potential problems may occur when the secondary trocars are not properly positioned: "crossing swords," "striking handles," and "rollover." The problem of crossing swords is caused by the trocars being placed too close to one another; as a result, the intra-abdominal portions of two trocars cross each other so that the two trocars cannot be easily used to deliver instruments to the same surgical site. Similarly, the problem of striking handles is also caused by trocars being placed too close to one another. As a result, the upper portions of the trocars strike one another on the abdominal surface, again precluding delivery of instruments to a specific surgical site. Rollover is a variant of the crossing swords problem, but it occurs between the laparoscope and an instrument. Instead of running parallel to the surgical site, the primary cannula holding the laparoscope and one of the instrument-holding secondary ports are pointed toward each other. Consequently, as the instrument is advanced toward the surgical site, it strikes and is deflected by the larger laparoscope, thereby rolling over the laparoscope and hence suddenly moving out of the field of view.

By definition, these problems are more likely to occur during LESS. Because the ports are purposely placed in close proximity to one another, the surgeon must use advanced techniques or special equipment to overcome these pitfalls. This special equipment may include articulating instrumentation, instruments with different shaft lengths, and a low-profile 5-mm laparoscope.

When the da Vinci Robotic System is used, the ports should be placed at least 8 to 10 cm away from one another to avoid robotic arm collision—the robotic equivalent of striking handles. This can sometimes be challenging in thin patients with limited abdominal wall space.

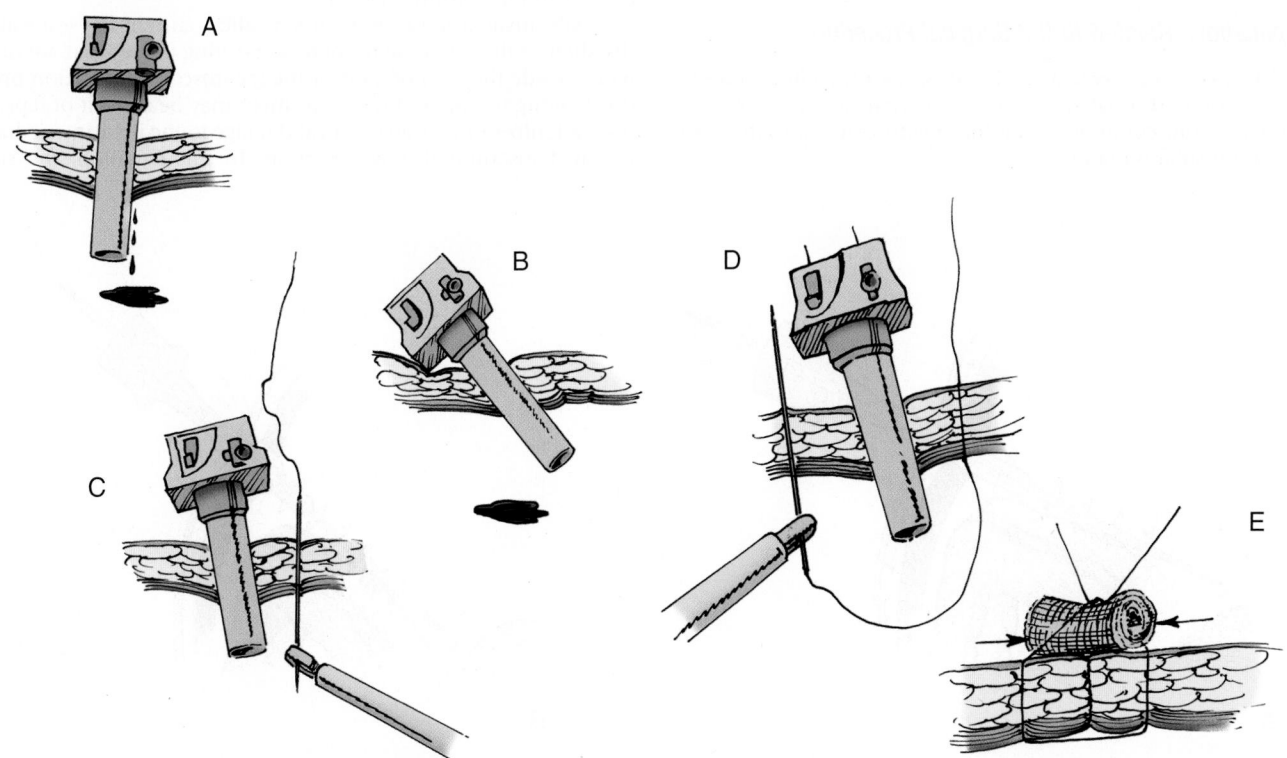

Figure 10-30. **A,** Bleeding at the cannula site. **B,** Cannula can be cantilevered into each of the four different quadrants to identify the source of bleeding. **C and D,** Straight Keith needle may be used to traverse the site of bleeding. **E,** Suture is tied down over a gauze bolster. (From Clayman RV, McDougall EM, editors. Laparoscopic urology. St. Louis: Quality Medical Publishing; 1993.)

Usually these problems are a minor annoyance, and the surgeon and assistant need to experience the problem only once to adjust for it. To compensate for the problem of striking handles, if it should occur, the sheaths can be withdrawn a bit from the abdomen, thereby increasing the space between the handles of the instruments. The problems of crossing swords and rollover can be remedied by moving the handles of the crossing trocars closer to each other, thereby moving the tips of the trocars farther apart. When this is done to correct a rollover, the surgical site may be displaced into one corner of the monitor; however, the desired delivery of the instrument to the surgical site can then be accomplished. A 30-degree laparoscopic lens can usually allow the laparoscope to be placed parallel to the instrument it is rolling over and then rotated to maintain the operative site image and eliminate the rollover.

The best way to handle these situations is to properly place and direct each trocar at the beginning of the case, to avoid encountering these problems. For some procedures, such as pyeloplasty, this may be accomplished by placing all the trocars on the same line (i.e., midline) so they are all working parallel to one another, whereas for procedures such as nephrectomy the goal is to place the trocars so that they surround the surgical site, forming a diamond pattern within which the kidney lies. Regardless, each trocar needs to be inserted such that it points to the pathology; this precludes the problem of having to redirect the trocar throughout the case, adding to surgeon fatigue and unnecessary trauma to the peritoneum and abdominal wall musculature. **Lastly, if trocar interactions become particularly vexing during a procedure, the surgeon should not hesitate to place an additional 5-mm trocar in a more conducive site to eliminate the problem.**

Complications Related to General Anesthesia Unique to Laparoscopy

See the Expert Consult website for details.

Complications Related to the Surgical Procedure

Bowel Injury: Electrosurgical. Electrosurgically induced thermal injury may occur through of one of four mechanisms: inappropriate direct activation; coupling to another instrument; capacitive coupling; and insulation failure.

Active electrode trauma by unintended activation causes direct bowel or other organ injury and may occur when the electrosurgical instrument is left unobserved within the peritoneal cavity, when it is out of the camera's view, or when someone other than the primary surgeon carries out electrode activation. Furthermore, active electrode trauma may be seen when coagulation extends beyond the intended site (thermal spread) and reaches other adjacent structures (e.g., bowel, blood vessels, ureter). This is more commonly seen when high electrocoagulation settings (i.e., >30 watts) are used.

Direct coupling may occur when the active electrosurgical instrument touches another instrument that is in direct contact with other tissue (e.g., bowel). If this happens outside the field of view of the laparoscope, it may remain unnoticed by the surgical team.

Injury caused by capacitive coupling occurs when the surrounding charge, which is intrinsic to all activated monopolar electrodes, is not allowed to conduct back to and disperse through the abdominal wall (Zucker et al, 1995; Munro, 1997). This condition may develop when a metal cannula is anchored to the skin with a nonconductive plastic grip, which, as previously noted, should never be done (Fig. 10-31). As a result, the electrical field, which builds up around the activated electrosurgical instrument and is conducted to the metal trocar through which it has been placed, cannot then be conducted to the abdominal wall because the plastic retainer acts as an insulator. This may lead to a high power density along the portion of the metal cannula that is inside the abdomen. The electrical charge built up on the cannula can then travel to other tissues in contact with the cannula. Similarly, capacitive coupling may constitute a risk when electrosurgical probes are used through operating laparoscopes, which are, in turn, inserted through plastic sheaths. The metal shaft of the laparoscope then becomes a repository for electrical current and may discharge this energy to any tissue in contact with the laparoscope. The risk of this complication is also increased when older generators with high-voltage output and/or electrodes with thicker diameters are used, especially in coagulation rather than cutting mode (Munro, 1997).

Lastly, insulation breakdown may allow current to escape along the shaft of the instrument, thereby harming tissues that are otherwise outside the field of view of the laparoscope. Insulation breakdown along the shaft of the instrument may be a result of repeated use, resterilization, or mechanical damage to the instrument during repeated insertion through a trocar. In this situation, the small

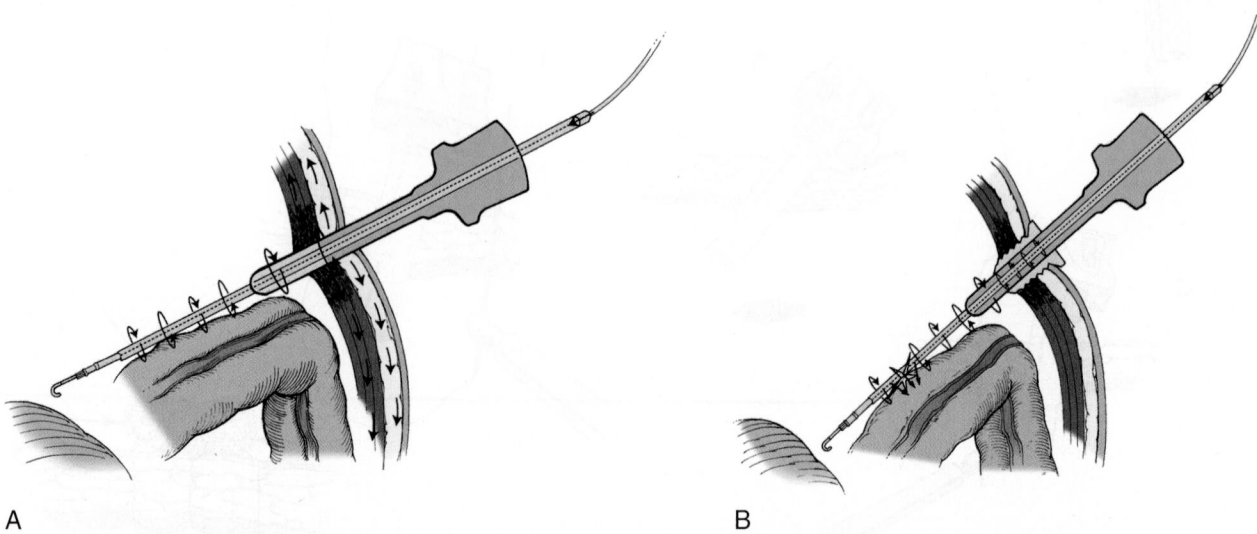

A   B

Figure 10-31. Capacitive coupling. A, Charge surrounding the activated monopolar electrode is conducted back to the all-metal cannula and dispersed by the abdominal wall. B, The electrosurgical instrument is being used through a metal cannula that has been anchored to the skin with a nonconductive plastic grip; accordingly, the electrical field cannot be conducted to the abdominal wall because the plastic retainer acts as an insulator; a stronger electrical charge is thus conducted to any other tissue in contact with the cannula.

break in insulation results in an area of very high power density that then discharges to the nearest soft tissue.

Intraoperatively, thermal injuries of the bowel may manifest as whitish spots on the serosal lining. In severe cases, the muscularis mucosae or the intestinal lumen may be seen. However, in many patients, thermal injury to the bowel is not recognized at the time of the procedure. **Postoperatively, the patient with unrecognized bowel trauma may not develop fever, nausea, or signs of peritonitis for many days, as the full extent of bowel necrosis may take up to 18 days to fully develop** (Abdel-Meguid and Gomella, 1996). Therefore, the problem may not become evident until the patient has actually been discharged from hospital.

Accordingly, bowel injury must be ruled out for any patient who develops a fever beyond postoperative day 1 or who complains of increasing abdominal discomfort. Although many patients may have the typical signs of fever, abdominal pain, ileus, and nausea and vomiting, this is not always the case. Instead many **patients may have low-grade temperature, leukopenia, and persistent and relatively extreme pain at the trocar site closest to the bowel injury** (Bishoff et al, 1999). Alternatively, laboratory values may be remarkable for leukocytosis with an associated left shift (i.e., increased percentage of neutrophils). In some patients, this occurs in the face of a normal or even low leukocyte count, making the left shift a more reliable sign than the absolute white cell count. Abdominal radiographs are notoriously inaccurate because the CO_2 from the laparoscopy may remain as free air for up to 9 days after the procedure; however, an ileus pattern is usually present. A more sensitive test is an abdominal CT scan with oral contrast accompanied by delayed films.

Minor postoperative thermal injuries of the bowel discovered late in the postoperative period (i.e., more than 5 to 7 days postoperatively) may be managed conservatively, aided by administration of antibiotics and an elemental diet. Indeed, a closed fistula may develop that will heal with this approach. However, if the patient does not respond rapidly or develops worsening peritonitis, open surgical exploration is mandatory. Thermal injury caused by monopolar cautery often results in tissue damage that extends beyond the visible area of necrosis. With this in mind, the surgeon should perform a bowel resection with a safety margin of 6 cm on either side before completing an end-to-end anastomosis (Abdel-Meguid and Gomella, 1996).

Thermal injury caused by bipolar electrosurgery is more confined to the visible area of damage. These injuries occur only as a result of direct firing of the instrument on the bowel. If the injury is small, it can be managed by simple excision of the defect and closure of the bowel wall. Bipolar injuries that involve more than half the circumference of the bowel should be treated by excision of the affected segment of the bowel followed by end-to-end anastomosis (Abdel-Meguid and Gomella, 1996).

The goal of every laparoscopic surgeon is to never experience a thermal complication. To this end there are several actions the surgeon can take to lessen the risks. First, electrosurgical instruments must be carefully inspected before use for any "breaks" in the insulation; if these are found, the instrument must be sent for recoating. Second, electrosurgical instruments should never be left untended within the abdomen; when not in use they must be removed from the abdomen. Third, *only* the primary surgeon should control electrode activation. Fourth, isolation of the area to be cauterized from the surrounding tissues (vessels, nerves, ureter), as well as use of bipolar electrocautery, reduces the risk of thermal spread and injury to other tissues. Fifth, the electrosurgical device should never be activated unless the entire extent of the metal portion of the instrument is in view. This includes not only the active tip of the instrument, but also any exposed, uncoated metal joints that may lie just behind the tip of the instrument. In this manner both inadvertent direct injury to adjacent tissue and direct coupling to another instrument can be avoided. Sixth, problems of capacitive coupling can be precluded by not creating a situation in which a mixture of conducting and nonconducting elements is used by the surgeon (e.g., metal trocars combined with plastic retainers). In addition, use of modern generators and small-diameter

electrodes can significantly decrease the risk of capacitive coupling (Munro, 1997), as can the use of blended or pure cutting current. The high voltages needed for pure coagulation current pose the greatest threat for electrosurgical injury, especially through the mechanism of capacitive coupling and insulation failure. Lastly, an active electrode monitoring system (Encision, Boulder, CO) is extremely helpful. With this system, any sudden break in the insulation of the electrosurgical instrument (e.g., with scissors or hook electrode) results in immediate shutdown of the electrosurgical current, thereby precluding an electrosurgical injury.

Bowel Injury: Mechanical. Inadvertent mechanical damage can be caused by a wide variety of sharp and blunt instruments (e.g., laparoscopic graspers, scissors, retractors). This type of injury is more visible to the surgeon and is usually discovered intraoperatively or at the end of the procedure. Direct visual identification during the procedure allows the surgeon to repair the injury laparoscopically, even though the patient has not had a formal bowel preparation. Given its localized nature, bowel resection is rarely necessary. The abdomen should be irrigated copiously at the end of the procedure with 4 to 5 L of an antibiotic-containing solution.

If mechanical bowel injury is missed during the procedure, then postoperative symptoms typically develop much earlier than with an electrosurgical injury. Fever, nausea, ileus, and peritonitis develop in the very early postoperative period, and the diagnosis is confirmed by an abdominal CT scan with oral contrast. This type of injury should be managed with immediate return to the operating room to correct the problem by local excision or resection of bowel with subsequent end-to-end anastomosis and copious irrigation of the abdomen.

Delicate handling of tissue with laparoscopic instruments by the main surgeon and the assistants is essential to avoiding this complication. Atraumatic graspers should always be used when handling bowel. Likewise, it is important that all instruments be introduced under strict visual guidance into the peritoneal cavity. Instruments should never be left unattended and should be withdrawn from the abdominal cavity when not in use. Attentiveness, economy of motion, and deftness of touch are essential characteristics of both the successful open and laparoscopic surgeon.

Vascular Injury. Fortunately, direct major vascular injury during laparoscopic dissection is a rare event. The use of only blunt trocars, the small nature of the instrumentation, the limitations on surgical speed, and the magnification of the surgical field by the laparoscope all combine to decrease this potential problem.

During right renal dissection, in particular, the chance of a vena cava, renal vein, or gonadal vein injury is heightened. When this occurs the surgeon can undertake several steps to resolve the bleeding. **First, the pneumoperitoneum pressure can be raised to 25 mm Hg, thereby slowing or stopping any venous bleeding.** With the use of the irrigator-aspirator, the blood can be cleared and the bleeding site identified. Next, through one of the 12-mm ports, a gauze sponge or pledget can be introduced into the abdomen and handled with a grasping forceps, thereby allowing the surgeon to identify and tamponade the area of bleeding. If the injury is small, then it may respond simply to direct pressure. Alternatively, surgical pharmaceuticals such as fibrin glue or gelatin matrix thrombin sealant (e.g., Floseal [Baxter, Deerfield, IL]) may be applied. If the injury is larger, then the surgeon must decide whether to convert to an open or hand-assist procedure or to attempt to secure and repair the injury laparoscopically. Depending on the severity of injury, a vascular surgery consultation may be appropriate. If a laparoscopic repair is attempted, intracorporeal suturing and possibly the use of a laparoscopic Satinsky clamp may be required. Throughout this period, it is essential for the anesthesiologist to administer sufficient fluids or blood replacement to preclude a hypovolemic state because the hypovolemic patient has a higher risk of possible air embolism at these higher intra-abdominal pressures (O'Sullivan et al, 1997).

If the surgeon is able to gain temporary control of the vessel with a grasper, then it is often helpful to place an extra 5-mm port that can be used by the assistant for suction and irrigation or to optimize the plan of approach to the injury, thereby facilitating laparoscopic suturing. Either way, the additional port allows the surgeon to repair the bleeding site using two hands and with excellent visualization of the surgical field.

Alternatively, the surgeon can convert from standard laparoscopy to a hand-assisted approach. The hand, in this case, is valuable because it can rapidly tamponade the bleeding site. In this regard it is recommended, if at all possible, to pinch the sidewalls of the vein (e.g., inferior vena cava) closed rather than just putting direct pressure on the top of the injury; the latter approach has a tendency to result in a gradual enlargement of the hole in the vein. Also, if the hole is pinched closed, a Satinsky clamp can be more easily passed beneath the surgeon's fingers to provide reliable control of the injury in preparation for a sutured repair.

Minor arterial injuries usually respond to tamponade. Larger aortic or renal artery injuries are much more difficult to resolve laparoscopically. Although the latter, if it occurs during a planned nephrectomy, can be handled by expeditiously taking the renal artery with a vascular stapler, the former may lead to immediate conversion and open repair. As mentioned earlier, addition of an additional 5-mm port can be very useful to help establish a clear field and provide the surgeon with two hands to control the injury. If conversion to an open procedure is necessary, the area of injury should be tamponaded with laparoscopic forceps and the surgeon can proceed to rapidly make a midline or subcostal incision by swinging one of the ports up to the underside of the abdominal wall and cutting down on the shaft of the port. The tamponading laparoscopic forceps are important to directing the surgeon immediately to the site of injury, which can then be properly repaired. Again, a vascular surgeon should be called into the room as necessary.

As mentioned previously in this chapter, because most bleeding episodes are unexpected, it is wise to have in the room a hemorrhage tray equipped with all instruments necessary to control bleeding and for potential open conversion (see Box 10-3).

Nerve Injury. Nerve injury is invariably a result of patient positioning in combination with the duration of the procedure. The exact incidence of this problem is not known. A survey of neuromuscular injuries associated with laparoscopic urologic surgery completed by 18 urologists from 15 institutions in the United States, published in 2000, found that of a total of 1651 procedures there were 46 neuromuscular injuries in 45 patients (2.8%). This included abdominal wall neuralgia (14), extremity sensory deficit (12), extremity motor deficit (8), clinical rhabdomyolysis (6), shoulder contusion (4), and back spasm (2) (Wolf et al, 2000).

If the patient is inadequately positioned and/or padded, nerve damage may result from abnormal nerve stretching or compression. Among position-related nerve injuries, the brachial plexus appears to be most at risk. Injury may be inflicted in several ways: (1) abduction of the arm beyond 90 degrees, (2) extreme outward rotation of the head of the humerus, and (3) compression damage when shoulder braces are used in the Trendelenburg position (Phong and Koh, 2007), which pushes the clavicle into the retroclavicular space. In particular, this has been reported as a problem with robotic radical prostatectomy when a steep Trendelenburg position is required and strapping the patient might be necessary to avoid slippage. Other nerves that can be affected by positioning include the femoral nerve, because of extreme lateral rotation and abduction of the hip joint, specifically in the lithotomy position, and the sciatic nerve, because of stretching along the superior leg when the patient is in the lateral decubitus position (Hershlag et al, 1990; Abdel-Meguid and Gomella, 1996; Liss et al, 2013). In addition, nerves may be injured during the surgery itself because of either direct mechanical injury or monopolar electrosurgical current.

Nerve palsy caused by positioning is recognized only postoperatively, often on the first postoperative day when the patient tries to ambulate. From both a medical and a legal standpoint, a neurology consultation should be obtained as soon as the patient calls the surgeon's attention to a possible nerve injury. Neurologic examination with possible nerve conduction studies to document acute damage is important. Physical therapy may facilitate recovery. However, recovery in these cases, if it does not occur within the first few postoperative days, is often slow, requiring months.

Prevention is paramount. Table-mounted accessories for all major commercial operating room tables now exist that aid in safely and effectively positioning patients in the lateral decubitus position and in the prone position. If the arms are to be at the patient's sides, they should be pronated to protect the brachial plexus. If the patient is to be in a lateral decubitus position, all bony prominences should be padded with additional gel pads (i.e., hip, knee, and ankle on the downside leg), and a pillow is always placed between the legs. Padding should also be placed beneath Velcro straps and tape, which may be used on the upside hip and shoulder. If the patient is in the lithotomy position with steep Trendelenburg, as is often required during laparoscopic or robotic radical prostatectomy, shoulder braces should not be used owing to risk of brachial plexus injury. Instead, use of well-padded wide straps directly across the upper chest and use of the surgical beanbag (Carey and Leveillee 2007) are excellent ways to secure the patient. Extreme abduction of the hip is also to be avoided; meticulous care to position the patient with attention to hip flexion should be taken when the patient is placed in lithotomy for a prolonged period. Padding must be checked each time the table position is changed, and the patient should be rechecked if he or she is suspected of sliding on the table.

Injury to the Urinary Tract, Spleen, or Pancreas. Similar to open surgery, during laparoscopic or robotic surgical procedures the urinary tract, spleen, or pancreas may be injured.

See the Expert Consult website for a discussion of the incidence, presentation, management and prevention.

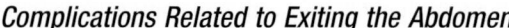

Complications Related to Exiting the Abdomen

Bowel Entrapment. During removal of laparoscopic ports and desufflation of the pneumoperitoneum, omentum or bowel may be entrapped at one of the port sites. If missed during the process of cannula removal, then in the early postoperative period, usually on the second or third postoperative day, the patient may develop an ileus and point tenderness at the port site incision.

The treatment is operative. The pneumoperitoneum is reestablished through one of the unaffected port sites, and three ports are replaced: one for the camera and two for grasping forceps. The entrapped bowel is visualized, and an atraumatic bowel clamp is placed on the bowel on either side of the area of herniation. Once this is done, the skin sutures of the affected port site are carefully cut and the wound is opened. The surgeon uses a fingertip to manually reduce the bowel into the abdominal cavity. The bowel can then be carefully inspected; if it appears viable, which is usually the case, it can be left in place and the port site closed. Rarely are formal bowel resection and reanastomosis required.

This particular problem is the result of a technical error. Indeed, most laparoscopic ports have a hole drilled into the side of the port within a few millimeters of the end of the port's shaft. This hole equalizes the pressure in the port and the abdomen as the port is pulled out of the abdomen, thereby precluding any bowel being withdrawn with the port. Furthermore, if each port site is endoscopically inspected at the time of cannula removal, bowel or omentum that may have entered the port site can be readily identified and positioned back into the abdominal cavity. When the last endoscope-bearing port is removed, the assistant should pull up on the closure sutures or on a fascial clamp, and the surgeon should back the cannula out of the wound and up onto the shaft of the endoscope so that the endoscope is the last thing to leave the abdomen.

Bleeding at the Sheath Site. Bleeding at the sheath site was previously discussed under Complications Related to Placement of Secondary Trocars. However, there are times when this problem does not become apparent until the end of the procedure owing to tamponade from the trocar itself. Again, it is essential to inspect each trocar site at 5 mm Hg to rule out this problem.

Early Postoperative Complications

Pain. Pain may be localized or diffuse. Early in the postoperative course, port site discomfort is to be expected. However, if postoperative pain is limited to a port site, it may also be secondary to herniation (immediate or late), bowel injury, or infection (late). Localized pain combined with a subcutaneous bulge may indicate a rectus sheath hematoma, bleeding and hematoma formation at a port site, or a port site hernia. Pain at a port site without swelling may be due to a particularly broad fascial suture or palpation of the knot of a port site fascial suture in a thin patient. Ultimately, if port site pain appears to be increasing on subsequent postoperative days, herniation should be suspected.

Immediate, severe, diffuse abdominal pain may be related to the release of noxious material during the procedure (e.g., cyst fluid in patients with autosomal-dominant polycystic kidney disease) or to a bowel injury. Immediate postoperative scapular discomfort may be a result of the CO_2 pneumoperitoneum itself causing some irritation of the diaphragm. Rarely, this discomfort may be sufficiently severe to mimic the symptoms of a pulmonary embolus. Of note is that this pain is invariably along the area of the right posterior shoulder region. Delayed diffuse abdominal discomfort and development of peritoneal signs or simply ongoing abdominal discomfort accompanied by low-grade fever may be results of an unsuspected bowel injury.

Incisional Hernia. In adults, the occurrence of an incisional hernia is usually confined to port sites larger than 10 mm. However, in the pediatric population, this complication can occur even with 5-mm ports. The patient usually reports localized discomfort accompanied by nausea and signs of ileus. Rarely, diffuse abdominal pain and/or signs of a complete bowel obstruction may be present. Examination reveals tenderness and, at times, swelling overlying the affected port site. A plain film of the abdomen may show an ileus pattern; however, the definitive study is abdominal CT, which can actually reveal the bowel protruding above the fascial level.

Laparoscopic repair with dissection of the hernia and subsequent intra-abdominal closure can be accomplished. The method for performing this procedure has already been described. In complicated cases in which a strangulated hernia is suspected or confirmed laparoscopically, general surgical consultation should be sought.

As discussed previously, **the risk of incisional hernia can be greatly reduced by using nonbladed as opposed to bladed trocars.** When bladed trocars are used, hernias can be avoided by performing a meticulous fascial suture closure of all trocar entry sites 10 mm or larger in all adults. In children, it is advisable to perform fascial closure of any "bladed" port site 5 mm or larger. The fascial layer is usually closed with an absorbable suture as previously described. **For patients in whom only nonbladed trocars have been used, fascial closure is indicated only of midline ports 10 mm or larger** (Kang et al, 2012) **or any port site that has been unduly stretched.** Indeed, some authors recommend no closure even of midline nonbladed trocar sites (Siqueira et al, 2004). Although there have been a few reports of a hernia developing after use of a nonbladed trocar (Lowry et al, 2003; Kouba et al 2007; Zemet et al 2012), this is distinctly rare. Indeed, the incidence of postoperative hernia formation fell from 1.8% with bladed trocars to only 0.19% for nonbladed trocars (Boike et al, 1995; Hashizume and Sugimachi, 1997; Thomas et al, 2003). Of note, with midline hand-assist approaches, a higher incidence of hernia formation has been identified than would otherwise be expected: 4.0% to 7.3% (Troxel and Das, 2005). Therefore some authors have recommended closure of this midline incision with interrupted nonabsorbable suture rather than a running closure (Troxel and Das, 2005).

In addition, transverse midline fascial incision has been shown to be superior to vertical midline fascial incision for reducing hernia risk (Brown and Goodfellow 2005; Halm et al, 2009). Specifically, for robotic radical prostatectomy the change from vertical to horizontal incisions for the camera port and subsequent prostate removal port site has resulted in a reduction in incisional hernias of 5.4% to 0.4% (Liss et al, 2013).

Deep Venous Thrombosis and Pulmonary Embolism. Although it seems reasonable to expect decreased venous return and hence increased stasis with concomitant higher risk of deep venous

thrombosis (DVT) and pulmonary embolism (PE) in patients undergoing laparoscopy, this is remarkably **not** the case. Indeed, there is no evidence that this complication occurs more often during laparoscopic or robotic procedures versus open surgery (Abdel-Meguid and Gomella, 1996; Secin et al, 2008).

Thus far there have been no randomized controlled trials addressing the issue of DVT prophylaxis in patients undergoing laparoscopic and robotic surgery. **The American Urological Association has released a Best Practice Policy Statement for the prevention of DVT in patients undergoing urologic surgery. Noting the lack of data available directly pertaining to laparoscopic and robotic surgery, the panel recommended the use of pneumatic compression stockings placed at the time of laparoscopic procedure for all patients. In addition, they acknowledged that certain high-risk groups may require the use of low-dose unfractionated heparin or low-molecular-weight heparin before, during, or after surgery.**

Pneumatic compression stockings should be placed preoperatively and continued for 48 to 72 hours postoperatively. In addition, in morbidly obese patients or in individuals at high risk for thrombosis (smoking, past history of DVT), the addition of unfractionated perioperative heparin (5000 units 2 hours preoperatively and then every 12 hours postoperatively) has also been recommended (Clagett et al, 1995; Capan and Miller, 1999, Secin et al, 2008). Of note, **with specific respect to upper retroperitoneal (renal, adrenal, ureter) laparoscopic procedures, at least one study** (Montgomery and Wolf, 2005) **indicated that sequential pneumatic compressive stockings provide equivalent DVT prophylaxis compared with subcutaneous fractionated heparin and that the use of subcutaneous heparin may increase the incidence of hemorrhagic complications.** However, it must be stressed that this was a nonrandomized study obtained from a prospective database augmented by retrospective chart review.

Wound Infections. Overall, this is a rare complication with standard laparoscopy. However, with the hand-assist approach a higher incidence of wound infections has been noted. In one report the postoperative wound infection rate at the hand-assist site was 9% (Nelson and Wolf, 2002). Prevention of this complication is similar to open surgery and includes attention to antiseptic preparation and sterile draping of the abdominal wall, irrigation of each port site at the end of the procedure, and meticulous closure of the wound.

Rhabdomyolysis. Rhabdomyolysis is a devastating complication after laparoscopic surgery. The exact incidence of this problem is not known, but one survey of neuromuscular injuries associated with laparoscopic urologic surgery found that of a total of 1651 procedures there were 6 cases (0.4%) of clinical rhabdomyolysis (Wolf et al, 2000). In a more recent study, it was estimated that the occurrence of this problem among patients undergoing retroperitoneal laparoscopic procedures (e.g., renal, ureteral, adrenal) was higher at 1% (Reisiger et al, 2005). Rhabdomyolysis is invariably associated with male patients undergoing longer laparoscopic renal procedures, especially if the kidney rest has been used for the entire case. Although extra padding applied to pressure areas can be useful in avoiding nerve compression and rhabdomyolysis, gel pads and foam egg crate padding have not been conclusively demonstrated to significantly reduce pressure on the patient's flank in the lateral position (Deane et al, 2008). As discussed previously, **male patients with a BMI of 25 or greater undergoing laparoscopic surgery in the lateral position with the kidney rest elevated and the table completely flexed are at highest risk of developing rhabdomyolysis as a result of flank pressure.**

Rhabdomyolysis manifests immediately in the postanesthesia recovery room with the patient complaining of severe pain in the downside hip area. Brown urine may also be noted. The serum creatine kinase value invariably exceeds 5000 units/dL.

Prevention of this problem is essential. This can, to some extent, be done by avoiding use of the kidney rest or using it for only the earliest part of the case (i.e., less than an hour) and avoiding prolonged periods of hypotension during the procedure (Cadeddu et al, 2001; Kuang et al, 2002; Parsons et al, 2004;

Reisiger et al, 2005). Lastly, with increasing skill and experience, few procedures should proceed beyond 5 hours.

Late Postoperative Complications

Complications beyond the 3-week postoperative period are rare. These primarily include lymphatic complications and incisional hernia. The latter is addressed in the prior discussion because it can also appear as an early postoperative complication.

See the Expert Consult website for further details.

KEY POINTS: COMPLICATIONS AND TROUBLESHOOTING IN LAPAROSCOPIC AND ROBOTIC SURGERY

- Early in one's experience with laparoscopic and robotic surgery, it is wise to apply the minimally invasive approach to low-risk surgical candidates of normal body habitus.
- The first sign of gas embolism is an abrupt increase of end-tidal CO_2 accompanied by a sudden decline in oxygen saturation and then a marked decrease in end-tidal CO_2.
- Electrosurgically induced thermal bowel injury may occur through one of four mechanisms: inappropriate direct activation; coupling to another instrument; capacitive coupling; and insulation failure.
- Careful planning of trocar placement is essential to avoid crossing swords, striking handles, rollover, and robotic arm collisions.

TRAINING AND PRACTICING LAPAROSCOPIC AND ROBOTIC SURGERY

See the Expert Consult website for details.

CONCLUSION

Laparoscopic procedures unthinkable in early 1990 are now performed routinely. Furthermore, the use of a robotic surgical platform to perform complex reconstructive procedures is improving the precision and often the outcomes of these operations and, more important, making it possible for a greater number of urologists to perform high-quality laparoscopic procedures. The widespread adoption of laparoscopy and robotic-assisted laparoscopy highlights the importance of having a detailed and robust understanding of the basics of minimally invasive surgery including the physiologic effects of the pneumoperitoneum, obtaining access, and managing complications. As robotics and flexible endoscopically guided technologies advance in the future, we may see adoption of NOTES and our patients may undergo operations that leave no visible scar. The benefit will be both more proficient laparoscopic and robotic surgeons who can handle any procedure and any complication without the massive incisions of years past, and patients treated with a truly minimally invasive technique. Such should be the next step of our surgical path of discovery and evolution. At that point Osler's 20th century admonition, "Diseases that harm require treatments that harm less," will be truly fulfilled. We are as yet still on the bridge to the future.

ACKNOWLEDGMENT

Special thanks to Dr. Robert Sowerby for his hard work and help with chapter figures.

REFERENCES

The complete reference list is available online at www.expertconsult.com.

SUGGESTED READINGS

Antoniou SA, Antoniou GA, et al. Blunt versus bladed trocars in laparoscopic surgery: a systematic review and meta-analysis of randomized trials. Surg Endosc 2013;27(7):2312–20.

Bhoyrul S, Payne J, et al. A randomized prospective study of radially expanding trocars in laparoscopic surgery. J Gastrointest Surg 2000;4(4):392–7.

Bishoff JT, Allaf ME, et al. Laparoscopic bowel injury: incidence and clinical presentation. J Urol 1999;161:887–90.

Bongard F, Planim M, et al. Using helium for insufflation during laparoscopy. JAMA 1991;266(3131).

Breda A, Bui MH, Liao JC, et al. Association of bowel rest and ketorolac analgesia with short hospital stay after laparoscopic donor nephrectomy. Urology 2007;69(5):828–31.

Breda A, Finelli A, et al. Complications of laparoscopic surgery for renal masses: prevention, management, and comparison with the open experience. Eur Urol 2009;55(4):836–50.

Brown SL, Woo EK. Surgical stapler–associated fatalities and adverse events reported to the Food and Drug Administration. J Am Coll Surg 2004;199(3):374–81.

Brown SR, Goodfellow PB. Transverse versus midline incisions for abdominal surgery. Cochrane Database Syst Rev 2005;CD005199.

Cadeddu JA, Wolfe JS Jr, et al. Complications of laparoscopic procedures after concentrated training in urological laparoscopy. J Urol 2001;166(6):2109–11.

Fahlenkamp D, Rassweiler J, et al. Complications of laparoscopic procedures in urology: experience with 2,407 procedures at 4 German centers. J Urol 1999;162:765–70.

Frede T, Stock C, et al. Geometry of laparoscopic suturing and knotting techniques. J Endourol 1999;13(3):191–8.

Ghani KR, Sukumar S, et al. Practice patterns and outcomes for open and minimally invasive partial nephrectomy since the introduction of robotic partial nephrectomy: results from the Nationwide Inpatient Sample. J Urol 2014;191(4):907–12.

Halm JA, Lip H, et al. Incisional hernia after upper abdominal surgery: a randomized controlled trial of midline versus transverse incision. Hernia 2009;13:275–80.

Landman J, Kerbl K, et al. Evaluation of a vessel sealing system, bipolar electrosurgery, harmonic scalpel, titanium clips, endoscopic gastrointestinal anastomosis vascular staples and sutures for arterial and venous ligation in a porcine model. J Urol 2003;169(2):697–700.

Liu CD, McFadden DW. Laparoscopic port sites do not require fascial closure when nonbladed trocars are used. Am Surg 2000;66(9):853–4.

Montgomery JS, Wolf JS Jr. Venous thrombosis prophylaxis for urological laparoscopy: fractionated heparin versus sequential compression devices. J Urol 2005;173(5):1623–6.

Orvieto MA, Chien GW, Laven B, et al. Eliminating knot tying during warm ischemia time for laparoscopic partial nephrectomy. J Urol 2004;172(6 Pt 1):2292–5.

Parsons JK, Varkarakis I, Rha KH, et al. Complications of abdominal urologic laparoscopy: longitudinal five-year analysis. Urology 2004;63(1):27–32.

Patel R, Stifelman MD. Hand-assisted laparoscopic devices: the second generation. J Endourol 2004;18(7):649–53.

Patel VR, Palmer KJ, Coughlin G, et al. Robot-assisted laparoscopic radical prostatectomy: perioperative outcomes of 1500 cases. J Endourol 2008;22(10):2299–305.

Pearle M. Physiologic effects of pneumoperitoneum. St. Louis: Quality Medical Publishing; 1996.

Pempongkosol S, Link RE, et al. Complications of 2,775 urological laparoscopic procedures: 1993 to 2005. J Urol 2007;177(2):580–5.

Ponsky L, Cherullo E, et al. The Hem-o-lok clip is safe for laparoscopic nephrectomy: a multi-institutional review. Urology 2008;71(4):593–6.

Recart A, Duchene D, et al. Efficacy and safety of fast-track recovery strategy for patients undergoing laparoscopic nephrectomy. J Endourol 2005;19(10):1165–9.

Secin FP, Jiborn T, et al. Multi-institutional study of symptomatic deep venous thrombosis and pulmonary embolism in prostate cancer patients undergoing laparoscopic or robot-assisted laparoscopic radical prostatectomy. Eur Urol 2008;53(1):134–45.

Vallancien G, Cathelineau X, et al. Complications of transperitoneal laparoscopic surgery in urology: review of 1,311 procedures at a single center. J Urol 2002;168(1):23–6.

Wolf JS. Tips and tricks for hand-assisted laparoscopy. AUA Update Ser 2005;24(2):10–5.

Wolf JS, Stoller M. The physiology of laparoscopy: basic principles, complications and other considerations. J Urol 1994;152:294–302.

11 Basic Energy Modalities in Urologic Surgery

Shubha De, MD, FRCPC, Manoj Monga, MD, FACS, and Bodo E. Knudsen, MD, FRCSC

Tissue Dissection and Cauterization

Intracorporeal Lithotripters

TISSUE DISSECTION AND CAUTERIZATION

Electrosurgery

Electrosurgery is the application of electrical current to tissue to achieve the effects of cutting, coagulation, desiccation, or fulguration. Monopolar and bipolar electrosurgery techniques are used in urology in numerous applications. An understanding of the basic scientific principles as well as the tissue effects is necessary for the surgeon to use the technology in a safe and efficient manner. Although the technology can be of great assistance to the surgeon, improper settings or poor application can result in patient injury (Massarweh et al, 2006).

Electrosurgical technology was first developed in the late 1800s. The technology originated from spark gap transmitters that were used to generate radio waves at that time. The waveform produced was of a steady frequency but varied in amplitude. Using a combination of inductors and capacitors, the waveform could be smoothed out, although this resulted in some power loss. French scientists in the 1890s experimented with the technology and determined that the raw output from the spark gap transmitter could coagulate tissue, and the smoothed-out current could cut tissue. Around the turn of the 20th century, the technology began to be used in clinical surgical cases in Europe (Van Way, 2000; Massarweh et al, 2006).

In the 1920s, Bovie, an electrical engineer at the Massachusetts Institute of Technology, studied the work of his predecessors and developed a cutting loop that delivered electrical energy that could be used for cutting, coagulation, and desiccation. On October 1, 1926, at the Peter Bent Brigham Hospital in Boston, Cushing used the device to remove a highly vascular myeloma from the head of a patient that previously had been deemed inoperable because of the vascularity of the mass (Van Way, 2000; Massarweh et al, 2006).

Monopolar Electrosurgery

Basic Physics. Electrosurgery uses radiofrequency current in the range of 400,000 to 600,000 Hz to pass through tissue and create the desired effects. The generators deliver more than 100 W of power to the tissue at voltages ranging from 100 to 5000 volts. As the current is delivered to the tissue, the tissue is heated, and the effect occurs. **In contrast, with electrocautery, the instrument itself is heated and then applied to the tissue. Ohm's law, Current (I) = voltage (V)/resistance (R), applies and states that the current is determined by the applied voltage and the tissue's resistance.** The higher the resistance of the tissue, the greater the voltage needed to drive the current through the tissue. Current is calculated as the flow of electrons during a specific period of time. Voltage is used to drive the current through the resistance, which in surgery is the tissue. When alternating current is used, resistance is termed *impedance*. As the resistance increases, the amount of voltage to drive the same amount of current also increases. As tissues become cauterized, their impedance increases, and a higher voltage is needed for the current to penetrate the tissue beneath (Van Way, 2000; Van Way and Hinrichs, 2000; Jones et al, 2006; Massarweh et al, 2006).

Cutting and coagulation currents can be applied and use similar frequencies. **For coagulation to occur, the current is interrupted approximately 30,000 times per second. This interruption results in short bursts of radiofrequency energy. For cutting current, the radiofrequency current is delivered continuously** (Fig. 11-1). With continuous energy delivery, the cells heat up rapidly to the point of boiling and then rupture, which results in the cutting effect. With coagulation, because the energy is interrupted, the cells are allowed to cool as the energy is cycled off, and the cells dry out instead of rupturing (Van Way, 2000; Jones et al, 2006; Massarweh et al, 2006).

Most generators also offer blended cutting, which adds some coagulation properties to the cutting current. This blended cutting is produced when the cutting current is interrupted similar to coagulation current. In contrast to coagulation current, where the generator output is concentrated into two or three cycles, blended cutting delivers more cycles to the tissue. The number of cycles delivered determines the degree of cutting versus coagulation. For example, a Blend 1 setting may allow 50% of the current through, whereas a Blend 3 setting might allow only 10% of the energy through, resulting in a greater coagulation effect (Van Way, 2000; Jones et al, 2006; Massarweh et al, 2006; Vilos and Rajakumar, 2013).

Modern electrosurgical generators are capable of high voltage and high wattage. This capability allows for either type of current to cut or coagulate. However, differences remain, and the coagulation current results in much more widespread tissue damage and charring but deeper hemostasis owing to the higher voltages used compared with a lower voltage cutting current. **Cutting current employs voltages 10 to 20 times less than coagulation but is still greater than 100 volts. Alternatively, coagulation current is delivered in short bursts at much higher voltage but with less current flow at the same amount of power.** The desiccation of the tissue results in increased impedance and lower current flow compared with cutting. Desiccation results in drying of the tissue and coagulation of blood vessels. The tissue is typically pale and dry with an eschar developing next to the electrode (Goddard et al, 1972; Van Way, 2000; Van Way and Hinrichs, 2000; Jones et al, 2006; Massarweh et al, 2006; Vilos and Rajakumar, 2013).

Fulguration results when the electrode is placed about 2 to 5 mm from the tissue. Electrical energy in the form of a spark arcs from the electrode to the tissue. A coagulation current setting on the generator usually is used, producing a darker char on the tissue with a superficial eschar. Fulguration can be effective at achieving hemostasis, but care must be taken to ensure the eschar is not too superficial, allowing for bleeding deeper in the tissue below the coagulum (Van Way, 2000; Jones et al, 2006).

Argon Beam Coagulator. Traditional monopolar devices do not work well in a liquid environment, such as when there is significant blood in the targeted field. The fluid results in dispersion of the current rendering it ineffective. To address this shortcoming, the argon beam coagulator was developed. **It works by adding a column of argon gas that passes over the electrode, and then electrosurgical energy ionizes the argon gas and helps to displace the blood in the surgical field. Because it is a noble gas, the current from the electrode is effectively transmitted to the underlying tissue. The**

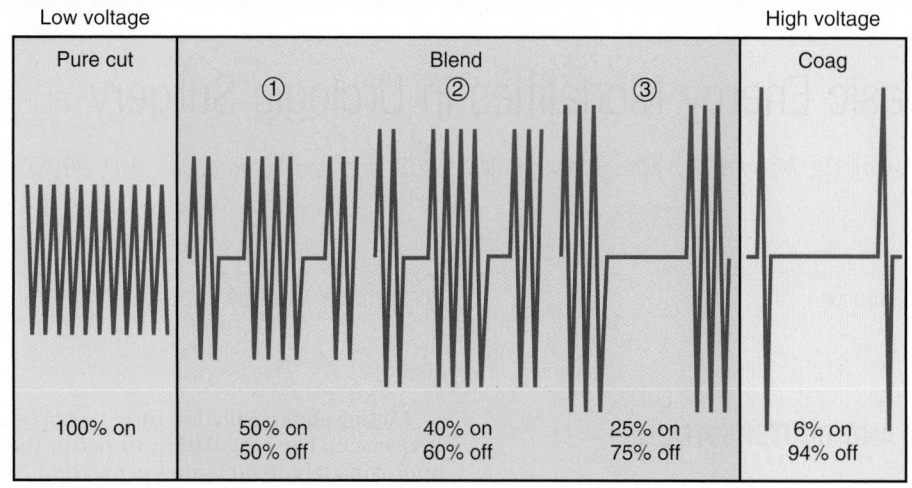

Figure 11-1. Instrument settings relating voltage and current. Pure cut uses continuous delivery, whereas coagulation uses interrupted delivery. Blended modes modify the degree of interruption to desired effect.

current follows the beam of gas and allows for diffuse superficial coagulation; this is ideal for obtaining hemostasis over a broad surface, such as during a partial nephrectomy. Typically, the argon beam coagulator is held slightly farther from the tissue at about 5 to 10 mm. It uses a standard generator and grounding pad but is operated at a higher power setting compared with traditional monopolar cautery in coagulation mode to desiccate the target tissues (Massarweh et al, 2006).

Generator Settings. When adjusting the generator settings, it is important to set the generator at a high enough power setting to achieve effective cutting and coagulation. Setting the generator too low results in an inability of the electrode to cut the tissue and poor or limited effect of the coagulation. For coagulation to occur, approximately 30 to 50 W is needed. For cutting, setting the generator at 60 W is a reasonable starting point subsequently adjusting the power as needed. Typically, fatty tissue is less conductive than muscle and may require higher settings of approximately 80 W. This information is intended as a rough guideline only; experience with individual generators varies (Van Way, 2000; Massarweh et al, 2006; Vilos and Rajakumar, 2013).

Although coagulation current may be used to "cut" tissue using lower power settings, it results in greater collateral damage compared with using a cutting setting. Although it may be reasonable to use coagulation when dividing muscle, it is better practice to use pure cut or cut on a blend setting to produce less charring and less ancillary tissue damage (Massarweh et al, 2006).

Safety

The incidence of electrosurgical injuries is estimated to be 2 to 5 per 1000 (Loffer and Pent, 1975; Nduka et al, 1994; Hulka et al, 1997). Understanding the principles of the electrosurgical devices and operating them within their safety parameters can help to decrease the risk of unintentional injuries.

During monopolar electrosurgery, the patient is part of a complete electrical circuit. Current is initially produced in the generator and is conducted over wires to the electrosurgical electrode. The electrode is used to deliver the current to the surgical site where it is focused. The current is distributed through the patient's body to the dispersive electrode (grounding pad), where it leaves the patient's body and travels over wires back to the generator to complete the circuit. **This system is designed to concentrate the energy at the tip of the electrode and then disperse it widely while traveling through the patient's body. If the current is allowed to concentrate in other locations, potential morbidity could ensue.**

Most electrosurgical injuries occur at the grounding pad site. Historically, the grounding pad was a metal plate that had contact gel applied to it before placing it in contact with the patient. Modern grounding pads are called dispersive electrodes and function in a similar but safer manner. The old-style metal grounding pads that were used with conductive gel could dry out during a case. Rather than have the current travel through a large contact patch, the dried-out pad could result in a very small contact patch that focused the current and resulted in electrical burns on the skin and underlying structures. Modern dispersive electrodes do not dry out and produce a safer, stable contact patch with the patient. Modern generators have a built-in self-test system that monitors the status of the dispersive electrode. If the generator becomes dislodged or loses contact in some way, the system shuts itself down and the ground fault warning is activated (Nduka et al, 1994; Hutchisson et al, 1998; Alkatout et al, 2012).

Injuries can ensue from inadvertent activation of the electrosurgical electrode. Injury can occur if a foot pedal is accidentally depressed and the electrode burns the drape or burns the patient at a site not intended. Handheld electrodes with a finger actuator are less likely to cause such an injury, although it is still possible. Other injuries can occur if electrosurgical energy is applied to unintended structures during surgery; this can occur when blood vessels and nerves are running close together. For example, the parasympathetic nerves that run near the prostate and are responsible for erections may be inadvertently injured when hemostasis is obtained with coagulation. During laparoscopic nephrectomy, the heel of a monopolar hook electrode may be inadvertently brought into contact with the bowel while activated, resulting in a bowel injury. Keeping the instruments in view, being aware of the surrounding structures, using low but effective power settings, and maintaining a general awareness of the instruments may help reduce such injuries.

The tissues of the body vary in their impedance (ability to conduct electrical energy). Structures such as blood vessels have lower impedance and preferentially conduct and concentrate current, whereas fat has high impedance. Tissue impedance is an important consideration when operating on structures such as the bowel, where current could get concentrated in the thin vascular pedicle that supports the structure. Current concentrated in the pedicle could damage the vascular supply to the tissue.

In patients with pacemakers or implantable cardioversion devices, the manufacturer should be consulted before surgery involving monopolar cautery to ensure that interference with the devices does not occur during surgery. The devices may need to be temporarily deactivated during the procedure.

Prosthetic joints can also affect current conduction but are not an absolute contraindication to use of monopolar cautery. Ideally, the direct path of the electrical circuit should be directed away from the prosthetic joint. For example, if the patient has a right hip prosthesis, the dispersion electrode pad should be placed on the contralateral hip (Massarweh et al, 2006).

Insulation failures can occur if there is a breakdown in the insulating material that surrounds the electrosurgical electrode. Usually only the tip of the electrode is left without surrounding insulation, but if defects occur in other locations, the current may arc out in these spots leading to unintended injuries. Such an occurrence is more likely when higher voltage coagulation modes are used. Reused instruments may be more likely to experience such failures because the defects in the insulation may occur during the reprocessing, although disposable devices could also have defects (Massarweh et al, 2006). Several clinical reports of insulation failures during robotic-assisted laparoscopic surgery have been published (Mues et al, 2011; Cormier et al, 2012). A 33% failure rate of the first-generation robotic monopolar scissors tip cover accessory after one clinical use has been described (Engebretsen et al, 2013).

The surgeon is also at risk for electrosurgical burns. Surgical gloves do not provide much insulation from electrical current. Current can penetrate gloves when they become wet, through capacitance conducting, or when mechanical breakdown of the glove occurs (Tucker and Ferguson, 1991).

Capacitive Coupling. Capacitive coupling is the transfer of energy within an electrical network by means of the capacitance between circuit nodes. Capacitive coupling occurs when two conductive elements are spaced apart by an insulator and energy is stored creating an electrostatic field. When the net charge exceeds the insulator's capacity, current is transmitted from the first conductor to the second. This occurrence is rare but can lead to complications during laparoscopic procedures using electrosurgery. When an active electrode that is surrounded by insulation is passed down a metal trocar, capacitive coupling can occur. However, it can also occur with plastic trocars. The injuries typically occur out of the surgeon's field of vision. An active electrode monitoring system and limiting the amount of time that high-voltage settings are used can decrease the risk of capacitive coupling (Tucker and Voyles, 1995; Vilos et al, 2001; Jones et al, 2006; Wang and Advincula, 2007).

General Safety Tips. Using the lowest possible energy setting that achieves the desired surgical effect is the simplest of the basic principles for the safe use of electrosurgical instruments. Rather than starting at a high setting, the surgeon should slowly ramp up the energy setting until the desired effect is reached. With higher settings, the potential for arcing and capacitive coupling increases. The settings should not exceed settings recommended by the manufacturer.

During surgical use, the electrode tip can become coated with eschar, which causes an increase in impedance and can lead to arcing, spark generation, and ignition of the eschar. A scratch pad can be used to clean the eschar, but this can cause grooves to form on the electrode, which can promote further eschar buildup. Alternatively, a sponge can be used to clean the electrode tip. A sponge effectively clears the eschar and does not cause scratches to the electrode (Massarweh et al, 2006).

A common technique during open surgical procedures is for the surgeon to grasp a bleeding vessel with a forceps or hemostat and then have the assistant touch the instrument with the activated electrode of the Bovie; this delivers current through the instrument to the bleeding vessel. During these maneuvers, the surgeon must be careful not to touch the patient with his or her free hand. Doing so would create an alternative circuit that could allow the current to travel to a different part of the patient's body. Keeping a firm grasp on the forceps can also help to reduce the possibility of current traveling in an alternate path (Hutchisson et al, 1998; Jones et al, 2006; Alkatout et al, 2012).

Basic principles that should be observed include keeping the operating field neatly organized and not tangling cords when multiple corded instruments are used. Care should be taken not to wrap cords around metal instruments because insulation defects could lead to burns. The handheld electrodes should be secured in an insulated holster when not being used rather than resting them on the patient; this reduces the possibility of burns or injury through inadvertent activation (Massarweh et al, 2006).

Types of Electrosurgical Instruments

Monopolar Devices. Electrosurgical instruments can be divided into two categories of delivery devices—monopolar and bipolar. For monopolar devices, the Bovie is the most widely used example and has broad applications in many surgical specialties including urology. The size and shape of the electrode affect its interaction with the tissue. A smaller contact area results in higher current concentration, whereas a larger contact area results in the current being more dispersed. Greater power settings would be needed with the larger electrode to achieve a similar tissue effect. Many systems allow the surgeon to select the tip appropriate to the given procedure, and the tips can be changed if needed during the procedure to fit the application (Massarweh et al, 2006; Vilos and Rajakumar, 2013).

Bipolar Devices. In contrast to monopolar systems in which a circuit is created by delivering the energy via an electrode and then removed from the patient using a dispersive electrode (grounding pad), **bipolar delivery does not require a dispersive electrode. Rather, the active and return electrodes are integrated in the delivery hand piece.** The tissue contained between the electrodes is the target tissue.

Bipolar "vessel sealing" devices have been developed that use computing technology built into the electrosurgical generators. These closed-looped feedback systems allow for vascular structures up to 7 mm in diameter to be fused and can help obviate the need for sutures, clips, or surgical staples. Several studies have confirmed the effectiveness of such devices demonstrating clinically equivalent burst pressures when compared with surgical staples, sutures, and titanium clips. Compared with the harmonic scalpel, burst pressures were higher for vessels 4 to 7 mm in diameter (Kennedy et al, 1998; Harold et al, 2003; Landman et al, 2003; Takada et al, 2005). The LigaSure vessel sealing system (Covidien, Dublin, Ireland) has been used successfully for radical prostatectomy and cystectomy with a benefit in operating time and blood loss demonstrated compared with conventional vessel ligation. However, long-term damage to neurovascular structures was not addressed in these studies (Sengupta and Webb, 2001; Daskalopoulos et al, 2004). In a study comparing the use of the LigaSure device with a harmonic scalpel during laparoscopic radical prostatectomy, a benefit in functional outcomes including return to continence and erectile function was demonstrated in favor of the LigaSure device (Pastore et al, 2013).

Ultrasonic Instrumentation (High-Frequency Vibratory Device)

Ultrasonic devices offer an alternative to electrosurgical instruments. **These devices have elements that vibrate at ultrasonic frequencies of approximately 55,000 Hz. Mechanical energy and heat are generated, and these cause the denaturation of proteins and the formation of a coagulum that can seal small vessels. Depending on the instrument, vessels 2 to 3 mm in diameter can be sealed, and vessels up to 5 mm in diameter can be sealed with some newer instruments.** Newer instruments also produce less heat and charring to the surrounding tissue, limiting thermal injury. The heat generated is usually less than 80° C. The device is best applied to the tissue in a tension-free manner; this allows the instrument to divide the tissue effectively while coagulating at the same time, limiting blood loss. Aerosolized fatty droplets may develop as the tissue is divided, and this can negatively affect visualization through the laparoscope. Examples of such devices are the Ultra Shears (Covidien), Harmonic Scalpel (Ethicon Endo-Surgery, Johnson & Johnson, New Brunswick, NJ), and Thunderbeat (Olympus, Tokyo, Japan). Devices for open and laparoscopic surgery have been developed. The Harmonic Scalpel has been shown to allow for effective tissue dissection and bleeding control during laparoscopic partial nephrectomy (Harris, 1978; Helal et al, 1997; Tremp et al, 2011).

A study comparing the vessel sealing times and thermal spread of two bipolar vessel sealing systems (LigaSure and PK [Gyrus ACMI, Southborough, MA]) and an ultrasonic device (Harmonic Scalpel) was performed. This study demonstrated that the two bipolar systems had faster vessel-sealing times with higher burst pressures compared with the ultrasonic device. However, the ultrasonic device had less thermal spread and smoke production (Lamberton et al, 2008). The smoke plume produced by ultrasonic devices may also be less toxic compared with electrosurgically generated smoke (Fitzgerald et al, 2012).

Laser Instrumentation: Soft Tissue Applications

A laser is a device that emits light through the process of optical amplification by the stimulated emission of electromagnetic radiation. The word *laser* is derived from an acronym for "*l*ight *a*mplification by *s*timulated *e*mission of electromagnetic radiation." In the 1980s, lasers first became of interest to researchers and clinicians in urology, and at the present time a wide range of lasers are employed to treat various soft-tissue and stone conditions. Although the holmium:yttrium-aluminum-garnet (Ho:YAG) laser has become the accepted gold standard for the treatment of urinary calculi at this time, various wavelengths of lasers are employed to treat soft-tissue conditions such as stricture disease, benign prostatic hyperplasia (BPH), urothelial cell cancer, and genital skin lesions (Marks and Teichman, 2007; Heinrich et al, 2010; Zarrabi and Gross, 2011).

Lasers are a source of electromagnetic radiation that emit a beam of energy that may include nonoptical wavelengths and visible light. The properties of this light create the therapeutic effects used during surgical procedures. General components exist with all lasers including an energy source, an active medium, and a resonant cavity. Light is generated with the active medium, which can be a solid, liquid, or gas. For the laser action to occur, most of the atoms or molecules within the active medium must be brought simultaneously to a higher energy state by an energy source; this is also referred to as pumping. The energy source energizes the atoms in the active medium and produces a population inversion, which is an excited state in which the atoms or molecules are primed for stimulated emission (Troup, 1963; Siegman, 1986).

Numerous types of energy sources drive lasers. Broadly, either electrical current or a different wavelength of light is used. The pump light can be generated by a flash lamp or a different wavelength laser. The specific energy source used depends on the type of laser; however, all are designed to produce laser light in a collimated beam (Siegman, 1986; Teichmann et al, 2007).

Light exists as electromagnetic waves representing spatial concentrations of energy. Each wave exists as a bundle of energy or as a particle called a photon. Photons are emitted and stimulate surrounding atoms and cause additional photons to be released. These have the same energy and travel in phase with the initial stimulating wave. The result is that the entire light is the same wavelength and travels in the same direction. The highly ordered, in-phase light arrangement is termed *coherence*. A long tube or cylinder is ideal for this process but not practical. A resonant cavity is created using mirrors to reflect light, allowing it to have many passes through the medium. A small portion of the amplified light escapes out of the resonant cavity and forms the beam of laser light (Stein and Kendall, 1984a; Stein, 1986; Welch et al, 1989).

Laser light has specific properties. It is monochromatic and of a single wavelength. The light is coherent with a uniform spatial relationship between all portions of the electromagnetic wave. It has directionality with minimal divergence, which allows it to maintain brightness over long distances. It is the high concentration of the bright laser light when focused on a small spot that gives it the properties to be a useful surgical tool but also a potential hazard (Stein and Kendall, 1984a; Welch et al, 1989).

The wavelength of laser light can vary and may be in the ultraviolet, the visible, or the infrared portions of the optical spectrum. Most lasers emit one or a couple of wavelengths; examples include the argon (488 nm—blue; 514 nm—green), the neodymium:YAG (Nd:YAG; 1064 nm and 1318 nm), and the Ho:YAG (2100 nm) lasers (Stein and Kendall, 1984a; Teichmann et al, 2007).

Pulsed and Continuous Wave Lasers

Depending on how the excitation energy is applied and how the laser cavity is configured, the output beam of laser light is either pulsed wave or continuous wave. The duration and energy of individual pulses can vary and depend on the type of laser. Pulses may be delivered individually, in groups, or continuously over a wide range of frequencies. A laser is considered continuous wave if the output emission is greater than 0.25 second. Clinically, a continuous wave laser delivers output that is continuous and of a constant amplitude; this allows for a stable, easy-to-control instrument. In contrast, a pulsed wave laser delivers bursts of energy, which works well for stone fragmentation but may be more difficult to control during soft-tissue interactions (Teichmann et al, 2007; Zarrabi and Gross, 2011).

The power of the laser is equal to the energy over time (P = energy/time or W = J/sec), and a high degree of power can be reached with even a small amount of energy if very short pulses are used. Several technique exist that can compress or shorten the pulse. Examples include Q-switching and mode locking. Q-switching involves interrupting the light beam in a controlled fashion so that the laser action is delayed until maximal population inversion has occurred in the active medium. It generates lower pulse repetition rates, higher pulse energy, and longer pulse duration compared with mode locking, another technique used to shorten the pulse. Mode locking, which can be combined with Q-switching, can create ultrashort pulses by fixing the way photons bounce back and forth in the resonant cavity. It can create very high power pulses because of their ultrashort duration (Stein and Kendall, 1984a; Teichmann et al, 2007; Zarrabi and Gross, 2011).

Delivery Systems

All medical lasers have a delivery system that allows for the laser energy to be directed to the intended target site. Delivery systems may be fixed rigid systems such as articulating arms or flexible systems such as fiberoptic glass fibers. Fiberoptic systems are generally inexpensive and quite versatile; however, fiberoptic materials are unable to transmit all laser wavelengths. For example, the carbon dioxide (CO_2) laser, with a wavelength of 10.6 µm, does not pass through quartz or glass fiber optics, and instead a more rigid system composed of an articulating arm with a series of mirrors is employed. The final tissue interface usually contains a focusing device to optimize the laser energy delivery (Stein and Kendall, 1984a, 1984b; Marks and Teichman, 2007; Teichmann et al, 2007; Zarrabi and Gross, 2011).

Light-Tissue Interaction

Laser light is absorbed by tissue in a wavelength-dependent fashion. However, some of the light, independent of the wavelength, may be reflected by the boundary layer of the tissue. This light is lost for the surgical purpose and may cause heating and collateral damage in the surrounding tissue. The optical properties of the tissue and the surrounding irrigant can affect the degree of reflection. Because this process is not dependent on the wavelength, reflection is often not considered when selecting a wavelength for surgical lasers (Teichmann et al, 2007).

Some scattering of the laser energy may also occur. By scattering, some of the intended laser energy is taken out of the surgical field. The degree of scattering varies with the wavelength of the laser. Typically, lasers with shorter wavelengths have a much greater amount of scatter compared with lasers of longer wavelengths. This

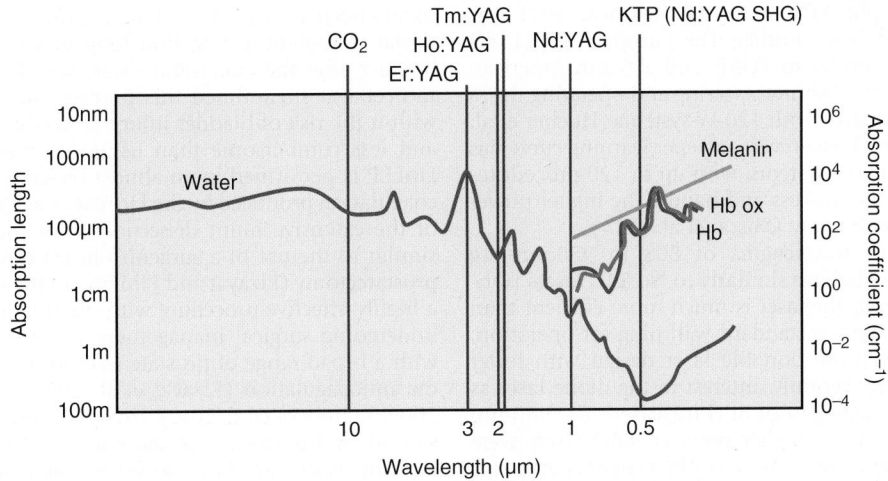

Figure 11-2. **Comparison of various laser wavelengths and absorptions in various media. CO₂, carbon dioxide; Er:YAG, erbium:YAG; Hb, hemoglobin; HbO₂, oxyhemoglobin; Ho:YAG, holmium:YAG; KTP, potassium titanyl phosphate; Nd:YAG, neodymium:YAG; SHG, second harmonic generation; Tm:YAG, thulium:YAG.**

is an important consideration in selecting an appropriate laser for surgical applications (Teichmann et al, 2007).

The most important light-tissue interaction is absorption. When the laser beam enters into a medium in which it is absorbed, the intensity of the laser energy decreases in an exponential fashion that is consistent with Beer-Lambert law. This law states that a logarithmic dependence exists between the transmission of light through a substance, the product of the absorption coefficient of the substance, and the distance the light travels through the material. Absorbed laser energy is converted to heat and increases the temperature of the target tissue. If enough heat is generated, coagulation and subsequently vaporization can occur. A chromophore is required for absorption to occur. In the body, melanin, hemoglobin, and water are available chromophores with hemoglobin and water being most important for urologic applications (Teichmann et al, 2007; Zarrabi and Gross, 2011) (Fig. 11-2).

Types of Lasers

Neodymium:Yttrium-Aluminum-Garnet. **The Nd:YAG laser has a wavelength of 1064 nm and has a tissue depth of penetration of about 1 cm.** It has hemostatic and coagulative tissue properties. Historically it has been used in urology for the treatment of BPH with visual laser ablation of the prostate (VLAP) and interstitial laser coagulation of the prostate. During VLAP, a side-firing laser fiber is used to direct the laser beam at 60- to 90-degree angles. The fiber is held off the prostatic tissue, and an area of heat-induced coagulative necrosis is produced as the tissue is targeted. The coagulated tissue is not entirely cleared at the time of surgery, but rather a sloughing process occurs in the weeks after surgery with associated edema. Prolonged postoperative catheterization may be needed in 30% of individuals (Norris et al, 1993; Cowles et al, 1995; Muschter, 2003).

Interstitial laser coagulation of the prostate involves placing laser-diffusing fibers directly into the adenoma of the prostate and can be performed either transurethrally or via a perineal approach. Similar to VLAP, the tissue undergoes coagulative necrosis and subsequently atrophies. The procedure can be safely performed in anticoagulated patients, but significant postoperative tissue edema can occur. Prolonged periods of catheterization after surgery—often 7 to 21 days—are required because of the high risk of urinary retention. Published re-treatment rates of up to 20% at 2 years and 50% at 54 months suggest poor long-term durability (Perlmutter and Muschter, 1998; Daehlin and Frugard, 2007). With the advent of newer laser technology and techniques, the use of the Nd:YAG laser for BPH has largely been abandoned.

Potassium Titanyl Phosphate. **The potassium titanyl phosphate (KTP) laser, commonly referred to as the "green light" laser, is a frequency-doubled Nd:YAG laser. The Nd:YAG laser beam is passed through a KTP crystal, which results in doubling of the frequency and halves the wavelength to 532 nm resulting in a visibly green laser beam. This wavelength is strongly absorbed by hemoglobin and in well-vascularized tissue has only 1 to 2 mm of tissue penetration compared with 10 mm for the standard Nd:YAG laser.** The KTP laser is widely used for photoselective vaporization of the prostate in which the well-vascularized prostate tissue is treated in a noncontact fashion with a side-firing laser fiber. The targeted tissue quickly increases in temperature above the boiling point and is vaporized leaving behind a rim of coagulated tissue that provides a layer of hemostasis. In contrast to VLAP, the limited depth of tissue penetration results in less tissue edema, and prolonged catheterization is usually not required (Barber and Muir, 2004; McAllister and Gilling, 2004; Teichmann et al, 2007; Zarrabi and Gross, 2011).

The early KTP laser systems were low-powered 34-W systems and were used in conjunction with a standard Nd:YAG laser. A hybrid surgical technique evolved in which the surgeon first performed a VLAP with the Nd:YAG laser and then used the KTP laser to perform bladder neck incisions. The goal was to try to reduce the prolonged catheterization and bothersome postoperative lower urinary tract symptoms after standard VLAP (Barber and Muir, 2004). Subsequently, a higher powered 60-W KTP laser was developed. This KTP laser was a pulsed wave system but allowed for rapid delivery of the pulses that simulated the effect of a continuous wave laser. This laser permitted the photoselective vaporization of the prostate procedure to be performed independently of the standard Nd:YAG laser. Further refinement resulted in the development of an 80-W KTP laser, which demonstrated favorable outcomes and complications comparable to traditional transurethral resection of the prostate (TURP) (Kuromatsu et al, 2006; Ruszat et al, 2008).

Lithium Triborate. The 120-W lithium triborate (LBO) laser was developed in an effort to increase the efficiency of the tissue vaporization compared with the 80-W KTP laser, especially for men with large prostates in whom procedures remained time-consuming (Wosnitzer and Rutman, 2009). The LBO remains a 532-nm wavelength laser. The higher power allows the distance between the fiber tip and the target prostate tissue to be increased to 3.0 mm versus 0.5 mm for the KTP laser. The greater distance may help preserve the laser fiber and make it technically easier to use. However, hemostasis with the higher-powered system appears to be less compared with the 80-W system (Heinrich et al, 2010). Most recently, a 180-W LBO laser that works in conjunction with a liquid-cooled fiber delivery system (GreenLight XPS, AMS, Minnetonka, MN) was developed to increase efficiency further. The European GOLIATH study confirmed efficacy similar to TURP, and a North American multicenter trial demonstrated shorter lasering and operating times for the 180-W system compared with 120-W systems (Hueber et al, 2013; Bachmann et al, 2014). However, a steeper learning curve has been reported with the 180-W systems, with up to 120 procedures needed to work through the process and handle the higher power of the system safely and effectively (Misrai et al, 2014).

Diode. Diode lasers with wavelengths of 808 to 980 nm are absorbed well in water and behave similarly to Nd:YAG lasers (Orihuela et al, 1996). However, the laser is much more efficient than the Nd:YAG and requires only a standard wall plug for operation; this allows for a smaller, more portable laser design with fewer cooling requirements. More recently, interest in the diode laser as a tool for the surgical management of BPH increased. The 980-nm diode laser was used when the higher powered LBO lasers were found to be not quite as effective in terms of hemostasis compared with the older 80-W KTP lasers. The diode laser appears to provide better hemostasis compared with the LBO laser but a higher complication rate; postoperative frequency and urgency and epididymitis have been associated with its use (Chiang et al, 2010).

Holmium:YAG. The Ho:YAG laser is a 2140-nm pulsed laser that is used for soft-tissue and lithotripsy applications in urology. **The 2140-nm wavelength is strongly absorbed in water, traveling only about 0.5 mm in the fluid medium, making it ideal for the urologic environment. In the prostate, the absorption depth is about 0.4 mm resulting in a high-energy density that leads to the rapid vaporization of tissue.** Heat is also generated during this process and allows for coagulation of small blood vessels up to a depth of approximately 2 mm.

It is held that the onset of vaporization occurs in the irrigant that is adjacent to the tip of the laser fiber. With each pulse of the laser, a steam bubble of a few millimeters in diameter is created. The bubble is not visible because it is present for only about 500 μsec—about the same length of time as the laser pulse duration. During holmium laser enucleation of the prostate (HoLEP), the laser pulses create the steam bubbles, which lead to the separation of the prostatic adenoma from the capsule of the prostate. Tissue vaporization occurs and leads to the white fibrous appearance of the tissue. The heat generated during the process allows for hemostasis to occur in the adjacent tissue. For persistently bleeding vessels, the laser can be "defocused" by increasing the distance between the fiber tip and the target bleeding vessel; this results in only the coagulation effect occurring with limited or no vaporization.

Before the development of the HoLEP technique, the use of the Ho:YAG laser for the treatment of BPH went through a series of steps. Similar to the KTP laser, the Ho:YAG laser was initially combined with the Nd:YAG laser to perform hybrid techniques in which the Nd:YAG was used first to perform VLAP, and then the Ho:YAG was used to make bladder neck incisions that reduced the need for prolonged postoperative catheterization (Gilling and Fraundorfer, 1998). These hybrid techniques subsequently led to holmium laser ablation of the prostate in which the laser energy was used to vaporize the prostatic tissue. This was a relatively easy procedure to learn but did require a high-powered Ho:YAG laser (80 to 100 W) and a side-firing laser fiber. However, the rate of vaporization was slow, and long procedure times were needed to treat men with large prostates adequately. The side-firing fibers would also fail if held too closely to the tissue, likely owing to thermal breakdown (Tan et al, 2003). The development of holmium laser resection of the prostate followed. This technique involved cutting pieces of the prostate off as it was resected, similar to a TURP. The sizes of the pieces could be larger than typical TURP chips but had to be small enough to be able to irrigate them out of the bladder at the completion of the resection. This technique was more challenging than holmium laser ablation of the prostate and remained time-consuming in patients with large prostates (Cresswell et al, 1997).

The next development was HoLEP, in which the median and two lateral lobes are enucleated and pushed into the bladder in a manner mimicking an open prostatectomy. Before the introduction of an effective tissue morcellator, some surgeons employed a traditional transurethral resection loop to cut up the adenoma in the bladder after the enucleation was completed. However, the tissue morcellator streamlined this process, and although it still carries with it the risk of bladder injury, it would appear to be much safer and less cumbersome than using a transurethral resection loop. HoLEP is performed in an almost bloodless field as a result of the coagulation produced by the Ho:YAG wavelength but also as a result of the extensive blunt dissection from the tip of the endoscope, similar to the use of a surgeon's finger during an open retropubic prostatectomy (Elzayat and Elhilali, 2006). HoLEP has proven to be a highly effective procedure with durable long-term results in men undergoing surgical management of BPH. It is effective for men with a broad range of prostate sizes and can be performed in men on anticoagulation (Elzayat et al, 2005, 2006; Tyson and Lerner, 2009; Krambeck et al, 2010). However, adoption of HoLEP has been slowed by the steep learning curve and the availability of other techniques that are easier to learn (Bae et al, 2010).

Thulium:YAG. The thulium:YAG (Thu:YAG) laser is a continuous wave laser operating at a wavelength of approximately 2000 nm. It differs from the Ho:YAG laser in that the thulium ions are excited by high-power laser diodes as opposed to flashlamp excitation with the Ho:YAG. As a result, there is less heat generation and increased power efficiency by a factor of five with the Thu:YAG laser, and no special electrical installation is needed to operate the laser (Teichmann et al, 2007). The slightly shorter wavelength compared with the Ho:YAG laser results in slightly less depth of tissue penetration. The continuous wave output promotes more of a direct cutting action of the laser versus tissue tearing and splattering with the pulsed output of the Ho:YAG. As the tissue is cut with the Thu:YAG, a seam of coagulated tissue is created and produces hemostasis. The coagulated tissues retain some water for efficient absorption of the laser energy during subsequent tissue passes (Teichmann et al, 2007).

Similar to other lasers, the Thu:YAG has been used in a variety of manners to treat BPH. Early reports described a tangerine technique in which the prostate was cut into slices with the laser (Xia et al, 2005). Hybrid techniques involving both vaporization and resection (vaporesection) were developed and shown to be effective (Bach et al, 2010). Thulium laser enucleation of the prostate followed and was demonstrated to have results similar to HoLEP (Lancono et al, 2012; Zang et al, 2012).

Carbon Dioxide. The CO_2 laser produces a beam of infrared light with a wavelength of 9.4 to 10.6 μm. It is strongly absorbed by water and used for numerous medical purposes including dermatologic applications. It is a continuous wave laser and highly efficient with a ratio of output power to pump power of 20%. The infrared beam is delivered with a rigid arm containing a series of mirrors (Stein and Kendall, 1984b; Malek, 1992). In urology, it is primarily used to treat skin lesions such as condyloma, but it is also used to treat penile carcinoma when an organ-preserving strategy is employed (Finkelstein, 1984; Bandieramonte et al, 2008; Colecchia et al, 2009).

INTRACORPOREAL LITHOTRIPTERS

Table 11-1 summarizes characteristics of commonly used intracorporeal lithotripters.

Electrohydraulic Lithotripsy

Electrohydraulic lithotripsy (EHL) has been implemented in biliary, pancreatic, and renal calculi. Initially employed in 1950 for bladder stones using 9-Fr probes, renal applications through flexible ureteroscopy became possible with technologic advances. First described in 1988, at a time when laser fiber technology was unable to flex in the same way, EHL became an innovative strategy to treat lower pole kidney stones endoscopically. Since then, more contemporary modalities have improved efficiency, while minimizing complication risks.

TABLE 11-1 Characteristics of Commonly Used Intracorporeal Lithotripters

MODALITY	BLADDER	URETER	KIDNEY	FLEXIBLE	CONTACT	MECHANISM OF ACTION	TISSUE EFFECTS	ADVANTAGES	DISADVANTAGES	PROBE SIZES (FR)
EHL	✓	✓	✓	✓	1 mm from stone	Electrical spark produces vapor bubble and subsequent cavitation bubble creates shockwaves that fracture stones	>1 mm distance from mucosa <500 mJ—no injury; >1000 mJ—ureteric perforation	Able to reach lower pole; Inexpensive	Significant tissue damage at higher energy; Durability of probe tip	1.6, 1.9, 3.3, 9
Ultrasonic	✓	✓	✓	✓	Direct contact	Rapidly vibrating probe tip results in fragmentation, while simultaneous aspiration removes debris	Mucosal stripping; No muscularis damage	Most efficient single modality; In-line suction for simultaneous stone removal	Reduced efficiency in hard stones	2.5, 3, 4.5, 9
Pneumatic	✓	✓	✓		Direct contact	Ballistic tip repeatedly strikes stone similar to jackhammer	Focal areas of hemorrhage and mucosal erosions; Least traumatic of all intracorporeal lithotripters	Least traumatic; Works well on harder stones; Least expensive	Least efficient; Significant retropulsion	2.4, 3, 4.8, 6, 10.5
Ho:YAG laser	✓	✓	✓	✓	Direct contact	Photothermal energy transfer rapidly heats and disintegrates stone producing fine fragments	Thermal injury to depth of 0.5-1.0 mm	Flexible enough to reach lower pole; Smallest fragments; Works on all stone compositions; Can be used for nonstone indications	Mucosal injuries with 0.5-1 mm depth of penetration; Fiber breakage can damage flexible scope; High initial cost	200-μm, 365-μm, 550-μm, 1000-μm
Combination ultrasonic/pneumatic	✓		✓		Direct contact	Simultaneous pneumatic and ultrasonic lithotripsy	Subepithelial denudation, muscularis rupture	More efficient than pneumatic or ultrasonic alone; Works on all stone compositions	Only rigid probes available; Requires large-diameter working channel	9.9 (Swiss LithoClast Ultra); 11.25 (CyberWand)

EHL, electrohydraulic lithotripsy; Ho:YAG, holmium:YAG.

Physics and Mechanism of Action

Two electrodes are positioned at the tip of the probe, creating a spark when triggered. **Immersed in a liquid, the electrical spark creates an immediate transition from fluid to gas, creating a rapidly expanding plasma shockwave radiating from the spark outward 360 degrees. The collapse of this shockwave creates a cavitation bubble, which creates a secondary shockwave and high-pressure microjets** (Vorreuther et al, 1995).

By adjusting spark discharge, the electrical and subsequent acoustic fragmentation potential can be optimized. Vorreuther and Engelking (1992b) identified that higher voltage shocks produce linearly increasing peak pressures and steeper shockwave fronts. Lower capacity probes produced shorter currents and shorter sparks with more narrow pulse widths. Because fluid vaporization provides the force required for fragmentation, a small space between the probe and stone is recommended during fragmentation. Typically, 1 mm is required because increasing the probe-to-stone distance leads to exponential decreases in shockwave power.

Probes between 1.9 and 3.3 Fr are available. Thinner probes are considered more versatile because of their application in flexible and semirigid ureteroscopy. Reducing probe diameter does not clearly lessen fragmentation potential; however, durability is decreased (Elashry et al, 1996). Pressure generated by EHL probes is estimated using the formula: Maximum pressure = energy/(pulse duration × fiber cross-sectional diameter).

Tissue Effect

Vorreuther and colleagues (1995) attempted to quantify tissue damage resulting from the use of a 3.3-Fr Wolf EHL probe. Using freshly harvested human ureters, histologic changes were measured after direct contact with the EHL probe. At 100 mJ, only punctate mucosal injuries were noted, whereas increasing to 400 to 600 mJ caused superficial mechanical defects in the muscularis. Increasing the energy to 1000 mJ caused transmural perforations. Microscopically, no thermal injuries were noted, and defects appeared to be due to mechanical disruptions, although limited to the cross-sectional diameter of the probe. When maintaining constant energy levels, altering voltage and/or capacity did not affect the resulting histologic findings. No damage was encountered at a distance of 1 mm between the probe tip and mucosa, even at maximal energy and pulse rates (Vorreuther et al, 1995). In a porcine model, bladder exposure to varying energy and total pulse numbers was performed using a 3-Fr probe. Scanning electron microscopy identified that the depth of mechanical mucosal denudation correlated independently with the energy setting and number of delivered pulses (Wu et al, 1994).

When tested in an intact ureter, the probe tip was centered in the lumen, and no histologic damage was encountered at energy settings less than 500 mJ/pulse. When energy levels reached 1000 mJ, a single pulse could produce a 1-cm longitudinal ureteric perforation. Thought to be secondary to cavitation bubbles, which can reach 1.5 cm in diameter at greater than 1300 mJ, the rapid expansion effectively burst the ureter (Vorreuther et al, 1995). The safe use of this (and any other) lithotripter requires a working knowledge of the physics behind stone fragmentation and the collateral effects on surrounding fluid and tissues (Fig. 11-3).

See the Expert Consult website for further details.

Chemical stone composition has been shown to affect fragmentation efficiency during EHL ureteroscopy. A review of operating room times for 193 patients was compared with the chemical composition of ureteric stones. Uric acid stones required the most time, followed by calcium oxalate monohydrate, and in multivariate analysis, stone size was negatively associated with successful fragmentation (Song et al, 2012). This association may be due to the smooth outer surface and lamination of uric acid stones being more difficult for shockwave-generated fragmentation.

See the Expert Consult website for further details.

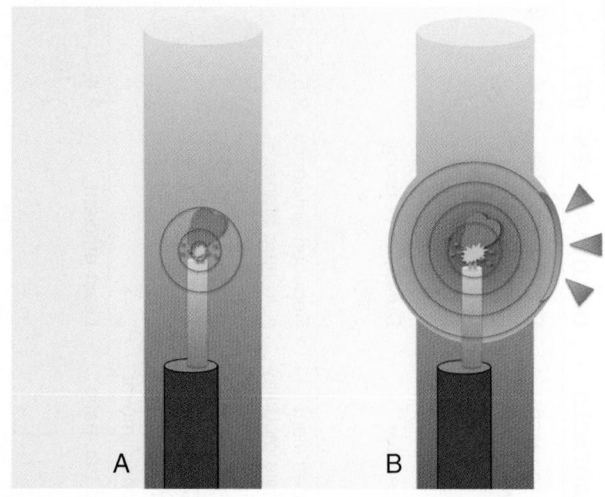

Figure 11-3. **A,** Electrohydraulic lithotripter probe spark producing a concentric shockwave within the ureter. **B,** Higher energy settings create cavitation bubbles up to 1.5 cm, increasing the risk of ureteric injury and/or perforation.

KEY POINTS: ELECTROHYDRAULIC LITHOTRIPSY

- EHL probes create a spark, which produces a rapidly expanding plasma shockwave and cavitation bubble with high-pressure microjets.
- Increasing the distance from the target reduces its peak pressure exponentially.
- At less than 500 mJ, mucosal injuries are rare; at greater than 1000 mJ, the risk of tissue damage is increased.
- A 1.9-Fr probe can be used with flexible ureteroscopy and allows active deflection for acceptable rates of stone fragmentation in all calyces.
- Chemical stone composition and surface characteristics affect the efficiency of EHL fragmentation.

Pneumatic Lithotripsy

Pneumatic lithotripsy provides a versatile and dependable approach to urolithiasis throughout the genitourinary tract. Early clinical reports confirmed the efficacy of pneumatic lithotripsy, and success rates of 95% (Teh et al, 1998) have been reported. **With good fragmentation effect in hard stone compositions and attractive safety ratings, it continues to be popular globally in upper and lower tract stone disease.**

Basic Physics

Pneumatic lithotripsy uses ballistic forces to transfer kinetic energy from a handheld probe to the stone surface (Michel et al, 2008). Either compressed gas (medical air or CO_2 cartridges) or electromagnetic oscillations are used to drive a projectile forcefully against the probe tip, thrusting it forward like a piston. **Repetitive strikes (LithoClast [Boston Scientific, Marlborough, MA/Electro Medical Systems, Dallas, TX]), 12 Hz; electrokinetic lithotripter, 15 to 30 Hz) from the probe tip act as a jackhammer, fragmenting stones at the point of contact. When applied to compliant surfaces such as soft tissue, the impact energy is absorbed and dispersed, whereas rigid objects are not compliant resulting in fracture.** Pneumatic lithotripters are safe for use in close proximity to the mucosa because soft tissue injuries from probe contact are relatively mild (see later). Other advantages of pneumatic lithotripters are their durability, simplicity of use, and completely reusable components (Hofbauer et al, 1995). Adding to dependability are the successful fragmentation of all chemical stone composition

(Teh et al, 1998) and the ability to use interchangeable probes to facilitate stone breakage anywhere in the genitourinary tract.

Probes are available in diameters of 0.8 mm (2.4 Fr), 1 mm (3 Fr), 1.6 mm (4.8 Fr), 2 mm (6 Fr), and 3.5 mm (10.5 Fr). In a head-to-head bench comparison of pneumatic (4.8-Fr probe, 2.5 bar), EHL (3-Fr probe, 80% power), laser (0.32-mm fiber, 100 mJ), and ultrasonic (4.5-Fr probe, power setting 3) lithotripters by Teh and colleagues (1998), fragmentation efficacy index (minutes/gram of fragmented stone) was compared. Pneumatic lithotripsy (5.00 ± 0.94 min/g) was the least efficient, whereas ultrasonic was the most efficient (8.49 ± 1.15 min/g), followed by laser (7.62 ± 0.78 min/g) and EHL lithotripters (6.60 ± 1.58 min/g). When increasing probe sizes at constant pressures (2 bar), incremental improvements in fragmentation were noted (3 Fr = 14 min/g, 6 Fr = 6 min/g). Pneumatic lithotripsy is effective in fragmenting harder stones and is less efficient in very soft stones; this is likely because the jackhammer effect produces numerous tiny fragments or because, in the case of extremely soft stones (i.e., matrix stones), the probe punches holes into stones without fragmentation.

Tissue Effects

A survival porcine model was used to test the short-term and long-term effects of 5- to 7-second bursts of LithoClast mucosal exposure to bladder and ureteric urothelium. A short duration was selected to simulate inadvertent contact experienced during stone fragmentation. Histologic changes in immediately sacrificed animals included focal areas of hemorrhage with mucosal erosions and transmural edema. At 3 and 6 weeks, the treated areas were unidentifiable, and histology failed to identify any significant changes. All animals experienced 24 to 48 hours of hematuria but failed to show any other systemic or diagnostic differences (Denstedt et al, 1995).

In a four-way comparison of intracorporeal lithotripters on iatrogenic urothelial trauma, **Piergiovanni and associates (1994) found perpendicular exposure to pneumatic probes to be the least traumatic (compared with laser, ultrasonic lithotripsy, and EHL).** Assessing perforation thresholds for each modality, at 250 pulses, the 0.8-mm probe perforated ureteric walls, whereas larger probes (1- and 2-mm probes) were unable to perforate the ureter or bladder, regardless of total number of pulses.

See the Expert Consult website for further details.

The hand piece houses the piezoelectric interface, and waves propagate as mechanical vibrational energy longitudinally down a solid or metal probe to where contact is made with the stone (Segura and LeRoy, 1984). **As the metal probe vibrates, when contact is made with the stone, this reverberation transmitted to the stone causes fracturing** (Teh et al, 1998) **along with the mechanical trauma of the oscillating metal tip against the surface** (LeRoy and Segura, 1984). Solid metal probes disintegrate stones by transmitting mechanical energy in a transverse plane, rather than longitudinally as with hollow probes. Local fracture can produce fine debris, which is aspirated by the probe; or if the probe is applied to fault lines, regional breakage can be created leading to larger fragments.

Tissue Effects

Using an amplitude of 50 μm, no perforations could be created in rabbit bladders. Edema and submucosal hemorrhages were caused when only suction was applied, and irrigation (20 mL/min) kept frictional heating to a minimum. Metal splinters were observed embedding into the bladder wall, but after 9 weeks, minimal inflammation was noted on histology (Stackl and Marberger, 1985).

Piergiovanni and coworkers (1994) compared the Olympus ultrasonic lithotripter with EHL, pneumatic, and Ho:YAG laser lithotripters to assess tissue effects on a porcine bladder. **Ureteral and bladder perforations were impossible with perpendicular application of the ultrasonic and pneumatic probes.** Histologic analysis immediately after application displayed denuded epithelial layers and edema.

When applied to immediately removed human renal pelvis samples (postnephrectomy), perpendicular application of suction alone caused 50% to 80% mucosal denudation, whereas the ultrasonic probe (21,000 Hz) caused 100% mucosal stripping, with no evidence of muscularis injury, regardless of application time (Khemees et al, 2013a). A case report from 1988 described symptomatic hyponatremia during cystolithotripsy using an ultrasonic lithotrite and distilled water with a resulting intraperitoneal perforation. Although this treatment is not common practice today, it highlights that clinical conditions may not always reflect animal or in vitro models, and caution should still be exercised (Batra et al, 1988).

See the Expert Consult website for further details.

KEY POINTS: PNEUMATIC LITHOTRIPSY

- Pneumatic lithotripsy uses compressed air to drive a projectile forcefully against the probe tip, transmitting repetitive ballistic forces to the stone surface similar to a jackhammer.
- Causing limited mucosal erosions and transmural edema, pneumatic lithotrites cause the least amount of trauma compared with other intracorporeal lithotripters.
- The efficiency of stone fragmentation is improved by increasing probe diameter and pulse frequency independently.
- Stone migration is a significant disadvantage when treating ureteric stones with pneumatic lithotripsy.

KEY POINTS: ULTRASONIC LITHOTRIPSY

- Piezoceramic crystals produce directional sound waves of 23,000 to 27,000 Hz. Vibrational energy is transmitted from the probe tip to the stone surface, and fragment debris are aspirated through the central lumen of the tip.
- In vitro testing shows that direct contact with the urothelium causes mucosal stripping, although deeper perforations are difficult to achieve.
- Ultrasonic lithotripsy is useful in large soft stones; however, for harder stones, ultrasonic lithotripsy is most efficacious when paired with pneumatic lithotripsy in dual modality lithotrites.

Ultrasonic Lithotripsy

Ultrasonic lithotripsy affords a straightforward method of stone fragmentation, while simplifying extraction. **Instead of manually extracting fragments after treatment, a central channel for suction provides simultaneous stone debris aspiration during lithotripsy.** The most common applications at the present time are percutaneous nephrolithotomy and cystolithotripsy, although applications in ureteroscopy exist.

Basic Physics

Ultrasonic lithotrites pass electrical current through piezoceramic crystals, producing directional sound waves of 23,000 to 27,000 Hz.

Holmium:YAG and Erbium:YAG Laser Lithotripsy

See the Expert Consult website for details.

Basic Physics

Laser physics for tissue-based applications are discussed in detail in Laser Instrumentation: Soft Tissue Applications.

Early on, questions existed surrounding the mechanism of lithotripsy of holmium lasers. Preceding technologies, such as the ruby and Nd:YAG lasers, used photoacoustic or photomechanical processes, where light energy created shockwaves that fragmented stones. In contrast, photothermal stone breakage during holmium laser use was hypothesized based on early observations of "glowing hot stones." Photothermal processes involve direct light energy absorption ("photo") by stone surfaces causing rapid temperature ("thermal") increases, before significant heat diffusion can occur.

Using a combination of techniques, Chan and colleagues (1999) identified the predominant mode of Ho:YAG lithotripsy to be photothermal. Mass loss experiments showed less fragmentation when stones −80° C were treated. As expected with a thermal mechanism, more energy was required to increase temperatures to ejection thresholds when starting below physiologic temperatures. After treatment, chemical analysis of all stone types showed thermal breakdown components. Finally, synchronized photography failed to identify fragmentation during bubble expansion or collapse, and measured pressures were too low (2 to 20 bar) to induce fracture.

Ablation crater volumes are associated with the irradiated surface photon density (fluence) and pulse energy. A "Moses effect" occurs by the rapid vaporization of fluid creating a vapor channel between the fiber tip and stone surface, allowing for more direct energy transfer. Although photoacoustic forces are not thought to contribute to fracture, interstitial water vaporization is likely involved with fragment ejection. Tensile and compressive forces, which dictate Nd:YAG lithotripsy, ESWL, and EHL, are not important (Chan et al, 1999).

Ho:YAG lasers produce fine fragments in large part owing to photothermal energy absorption by urolithiasis; this results in the breakdown and disintegration of the heated area, causing craters and fragmentation (Qiu et al, 2010). As a result of the relatively long pulse rate (250 to 350 μsec), the Ho:YAG laser is considerably less efficient than other shorter pulse lasers. Because Er:YAG lasers have a shorter pulse duration and longer wavelength (2940 μm), they can still produce small fragments, but with improved efficiency over Ho:YAG lithotripsy.

The Er:YAG laser uses optical energy, and similar to Ho:YAG, irradiation of the stone's surface leads to increasing temperatures. Er:YAG lasers produce a 2940-nm wavelength, which has a fivefold increase in photothermal absorption by urolithiasis. Although shockwave production is insufficient for stone breakage in Ho:YAG lasers, Er:YAG lasers also show improved photoacoustic vapor bubble force transmission. With higher acoustic transients, the Er:YAG laser forms a torpedo-shaped vapor bubble in the interfacing fluid between probe and stone. The vapor bubble of the Ho:YAG laser is pear-shaped, leading to increased energy loss laterally, producing weak shockwaves with minimal effect on stone fracture.

The radiant threshold for Er:YAG to initiate lithotripsy is 0.47 J/cm² at 2940 nm for calcium oxalate monohydrate compared with a Ho:YAG threshold of 7.36 J/cm². Deeper craters and larger ablation volumes are produced at this wavelength (Lee et al, 2006). **The combination of effective photothermal and photoacoustic lithotripsy of Er:YAG leads to faster fragmentation, with larger subsequent pieces.** In vitro studies showed larger fragments are created by Er:YAG; however, calcium oxalate monohydrate and cystine stone lithotripsy resulted in fragments less than 1 mm for both lasers, which clinically would be considered equivalent. Soft tissue depth of penetration is 0.79 μm, which is a significant improvement in safety compared with Ho:YAG (0.5 to 1 mm).

A problem with Er:YAG laser technology is that the hydroxy silica quartz fibers used in Ho:YAG machines are not compatible. Although sapphire fibers used with Er:YAG are too brittle and thick to be used in routine endourologic procedures, salivary stones were treated in wet-field applications using semirigid instrumentation (Raif et al, 2006). ZBLAN fluoride glass fibers have favorable properties in regard to reflection losses and light attenuation. However, because of a much lower melting point, durability is inadequate for clinical use. Before this technology can be applied to kidney stones, improved mechanical, thermal, and chemical fiber reliability is required. Hybrid fibers using fluoride cores with sapphire protection tips and circumferential cladding may help provide the transmission and flexibility required for endourology (Qiu et al, 2010).

See the Expert Consult website for further details.

A technique dubbed "popcorning" uses both the photoacoustic and the photothermal mechanisms of laser lithotripsy. **Photoacoustic and photothermal properties of a laser are functions of pulse duration and energy. Longer pulse duration produces greater photothermal functionality.** Although most Ho:YAG lasers have fixed durations of 250 to 350 μm, adjustable units are becoming more common. Shorter pulses yield higher peak power in resulting shockwaves. In a ureteric model, increasing pulse duration from 300 to 700 μm reduced stone retropulsion by 50% (Finley et al, 2005). Pulse duration is inversely related to power and can manipulate stone motion depending on the circumstance; this can be helpful in difficult-to-reach anatomy (i.e., lower pole stones) or when numerous fragments exist in a confined area (i.e., minor calyx). The fiber tip is placed several millimeters away from the stones (and mucosa), and shockwaves produced by vapor bubbles collapsing cause stones to bounce like popcorn. As stones are agitated, intermittent contact with the laser fiber causes photothermal disintegration. As time passes, the "popcorning" effect continues to produce smaller and smaller fragments, resulting in a fine stone dust, which is passed without consequence. An in vitro experiment identified settings of 1.0 J and 20 Hz as giving the most efficient fragmentation when using this technique (Chawla et al, 2008).

See the Expert Consult website for further details.

KEY POINTS: HOLMIUM:YAG LASER LITHOTRIPSY

- Laser lithotripsy has brought versatility to intracorporeal lithotripsy by allowing safe fragmentation in virtually all areas of the genitourinary tract.
- Ho:YAG laser fragmentation is predominantly due to photothermal decomposition and possibly photoacoustic propulsion of fragments.
- Laser output can be adjusted based on rate (Hz), energy (J), pulse duration (μsec), and fiber size (μm).
- Maximal deflection is achieved with 200-μm fibers during flexible ureteroscopy; however, maximal efficiency is seen with 360-μm fibers.
- Proper laser fiber handling can help reduce scope damage and prolong the life of reusable fibers.
- Techniques used during stone fragmentation include painting and "popcorning," which create fine stone dust (precluding removal), or crude fragmentation for basket extraction.
- Laser lithotripsy can produce the smallest fragments and is efficacious in all stone compositions.

Dual Modality Lithotripters

Newer modalities have been developed by combining ultrasonic and pneumatic lithotripters into a single hand piece. The Swiss LithoClast Ultra and CyberWand (Olympus, Southborough, MA) use different strategies to capitalize on the advantages of each modality. Pneumatic lithotripsy is effective at fragmenting harder stones, whereas ultrasonic action produces smaller fragments, while simultaneously removing them from the field. These hybrid systems are available only as rigid probes and can be used only in transurethral or percutaneous procedures (Fig. 11-5).

LithoClast Ultra

The LithoClast Ultra was the first dual modality lithotripter, combining two independently functioning hand pieces that are fixed together. **The front piece houses the ultrasonic lithotripter, with a central channel allowing throughway for the slender pneumatic probe.** The 1-mm solid pneumatic probe sits within the suction channel of the 3.3-mm hollow ultrasonic probe. Fine-tuning of positioning of the pneumatic probe tip (relative to the ultrasonic tip) can be achieved using the depth wheel built into the hand piece. Pneumatic activity can be triggered as needed or continuously

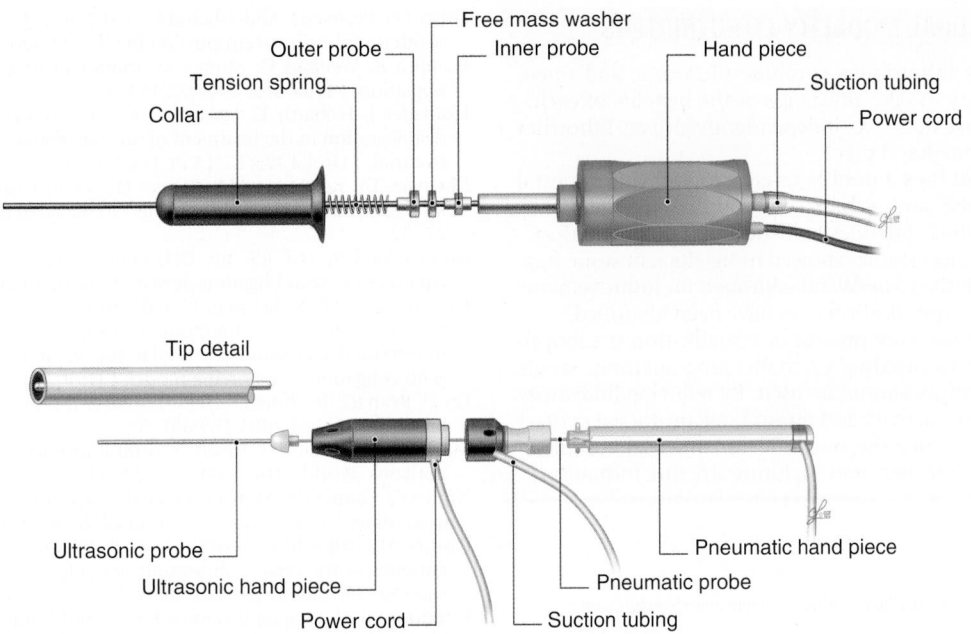

Figure 11-5. **Dual modality lithotripter configurations.**

from 2 to 12 cycles per second. The ultrasonic probe can be adjusted based on power and duty cycle. A composite pedal allows selective or combined use of each modality. Three cords attach to the hand piece for medical air, ultrasonic power, and suction. In-line suction allows continuous fragment removal and collection (using a stone trap) and hand piece cooling.

For maximal control, the tip of the pneumatic probe should be slightly recessed from the outer ultrasonic probe. In this way, the ultrasonic probe can make maximal contact with the stone surface, and pneumatic retropulsion is limited. When activated, the pneumatic tip advances and strikes the stone beyond the ultrasonic probe tip. If large immobile stones are being treated (i.e., staghorn calculi), better fragmentation can be achieved by adjusting the pneumatic probe 2.5 mm past the ultrasonic sheath; however, simultaneous treatment of smaller fragments may become more challenging (VonDerHaar et al, 2010).

CyberWand

The CyberWand uses an ultrasonic hand piece producing vibrational energy by means of a piezoceramic crystal. Disposable probes are made of an inner 2.77-mm and outer 3.75-mm cylindrical metal tube. The inner probe screws onto the handset extending 1 mm past the tip of the outer sheath. The fixed inner probe vibrates at a frequency of 21,000 Hz. Owing to a free mass washer and dampening spring, the free-floating outer probe vibrates at approximately 1000 Hz, oscillating longitudinally 1 mm. Selecting "large stone" on the foot pedal couples both sheaths. **Ultrasonic energy from the inner sheath is transmitted to the outer, which moves in a ballistic manner, similar to pneumatic lithotripters** (Auge et al, 2002). The "small stone" pedal allows for finer control and activates only the ultrasonic action of the inner probe. The hollow lumen of the inner sheath of the probe incorporates irrigation suction, which simultaneously clears stone debris during fragmentation, while cooling the hand piece.

Noise levels related to CyberWand fragmentation (93 dB) were determined to be the loudest (at ear level) compared with the Storz Ultrasonic lithotrite (Storz, El Segundo, CA; 77 dB), Olympus LUS-2 single modality ultrasonic lithotripter (Olympus, Southborough, MA; 68 dB), and Ho:YAG laser (60 dB). If used for more than 90 minutes per day, only the CyberWand is above the threshold set by the U.S. Department of Labor and Occupational Health and Safety Administration for risk of noise-related occupational hearing loss (Soucy et al, 2008).

Tissue Effects

Using fresh human urothelium from nephrectomy specimens, perpendicular application of the CyberWand and LithoClast was done for 2 to 8 seconds. Tissue effects were compared with untreated areas and control specimens (suction-only probe contact). Suction alone showed 50% to 80% denudation of urothelium, with no changes identified in the subepithelial or muscular layer. The CyberWand "small stone" setting showed 100% urothelial denudation, with separation of the subepithelial connective tissue layer and no muscular damage. During use with the "large stone" setting, a greater amount of subepithelial edema and muscular rupture was noted with increasing contact time to the mucosa.

For ultrasonography-only settings, the Swiss LithoClast Ultra and CyberWand ("small stone" setting) showed 100% urothelial denudation, with separation of the subepithelial connective tissue layer and no muscular damage. With 2 seconds of exposure, minimal tissue damage was noted. **Increasing contact time led to increased mucosal denudation and submucosal vacuolation. Muscle rupture worsened with increasing exposure times except for the single modality "small stone" setting on the CyberWand, which was unable to cause muscle rupture.** Based on these findings, the authors concluded that both modalities were safe, although contact time when using dual modality settings should be minimized when possible (Khemees et al, 2013a).

Clinical Use

Several studies showed the combination of pneumatic and ultrasonic lithotripters is more efficient compared with pneumatic or ultrasonic lithotripsy alone. Each modality separately cleared phantom stones 3.8 times (pneumatic) and 1.7 times (ultrasonic) slower than combination lithotripsy with the Swiss LithoClast Ultra (Soucy et al, 2008). An in vitro experiment using gypsum stones was performed to compare penetration times of the CyberWand and Swiss LithoClast Ultra. Penetration times were 41% shorter with the CyberWand with no significant differences in overheating, blockages, or malfunctioning (Kim et al, 2007).

See the Expert Consult website for further details.

KEY POINTS: DUAL MODALITY LITHOTRIPTERS

- Dual modality lithotripters combine ultrasonic and pneumatic lithotripsy to take advantage of the benefits of each.
- Swiss LithoClast uses two independently driven lithotrites combined in one hand piece.
- The CyberWand uses a double-layered probe with a central ultrasonic probe and a passively coupled low-frequency outer probe, which provides ballistic stone fragmentation.
- In vitro and clinical studies showed more efficient stone fragmentation with the CyberWand, although no improvements in stone-free or complication rates have been identified.
- When friable tissues are present or visualization is suboptimal secondary to bleeding or challenging anatomy, single modality lithotripsy should be used. By reducing lithotripsy to ultrasonic only activity and minimizing urothelial contact time, one can reduce the potential for mucosal complications (i.e., bleeding, perforation, future stricture formation).

REFERENCES

 The complete reference list is available online at www.expertconsult.com.

SUGGESTED READINGS

Anastasiadis A, Onal B, Modi P, et al. Impact of stone density on outcomes in percutaneous nephrolithotomy (PCNL): an analysis of the Clinical Research Office of the Endourological Society (CROES) PCNL global study database. Scand J Urol 2013;47:509–14.

Bachmann A, Tubaro A, Barber N, et al. 180-W XPS GreenLight laser vaporisation versus transurethral resection of the prostate for the treatment of benign prostatic obstruction: 6-month safety and efficacy results of a European multicentre randomised trial—the GOLIATH study. Eur Urol 2014;65:931–42.

Chawla SN, Chang MF, Chang A, et al. Effectiveness of high-frequency holmium:YAG laser stone fragmentation: the "popcorn effect." J Endourol 2008;22:645–50.

Cone EB, Eisner BH, Ursiny M, et al. Cost effectiveness comparison of renal calculi treated with ureteroscopic laser lithotripsy versus shock wave lithotripsy. J Endourol 2014;28:639–43.

Finley DS, Petersen J, Abdelshehid C, et al. Effect of holmium:YAG laser pulse width on lithotripsy retropulsion in vitro. J Endourol 2005;19:1041–4.

Hendlin K, Weiland D, Monga M. Impact of irrigation systems on stone migration. J Endourol 2008;22:453–8.

Hofbauer J, Höbarth K, Marberger M. Electrohydraulic versus pneumatic disintegration in the treatment of ureteral stones: a randomized, prospective trial. J Urol 1995;153(3 Pt 1):623–5.

Khemees TA, Kenneson MA, Zynger DL, et al. Histologic impact of dual-modality intracorporeal lithotripters to the renal pelvis. Urology 2013;82:27–32.

Lamberton GR, Hsi RS, Jin DH, et al. Prospective comparison of four laparoscopic vessel ligation devices. J Endourol 2008;22:2307–12.

Landman J, Kerbl K, Rehman J, et al. Evaluation of a vessel sealing system, bipolar electrosurgery, harmonic scalpel, titanium clips, endoscopic gastrointestinal anastomosis vascular staples and sutures for arterial and venous ligation in a porcine model. J Urol 2003;169:697–700.

Lee H, Ryan RT, Teichman JM, et al. Stone retropulsion during holmium:YAG lithotripsy. J Urol 2003;169:881–5.

Marks AJ, Teichman JM. Lasers in clinical urology: state of the art and new horizons. World J Urol 2007;25:227–33.

Nduka CC, Super PA, Monson JR, et al. Cause and prevention of electrosurgical injuries in laparoscopy. J Am Coll Surg 1994;179:161–70.

Pastore AL, Palleschi G, Silvestri L, et al. Prospective randomized study of radiofrequency versus ultrasound scalpels on functional outcomes of laparoscopic radical prostatectomy. J Endourol 2013;27:989–93.

Piergiovanni M, Desgrandchamps F, Cochand-Priollet B, et al. Ureteral and bladder lesions after ballistic, ultrasonic, electrohydraulic, or laser lithotripsy. J Endourol 1994;8:293–9.

Ruszat R, Seitz M, Wyler SF, et al. GreenLight laser vaporization of the prostate: single-center experience and long-term results after 500 procedures. Eur Urol 2008;54:893–901.

Seitz C, Tanovic E, Kikic Z, et al. Impact of stone size, location, composition, impaction, and hydronephrosis on the efficacy of holmium:YAG-laser ureterolithotripsy. Eur Urol 2007;52:1751–7.

Teichman JM, Vassar GJ, Glickman RD. Holmium:yttrium-aluminum-garnet lithotripsy efficiency varies with stone composition. Urology 1998;52:392–7.

Van Way CW, Hinrichs CS. Electrosurgery 201: basic electrical principles. Curr Surg 2000;57:261–4.

VonDerHaar JN, McAteer JA, Williams JC Jr, et al. In vitro evaluation of the Lithoclast Ultra Vario combination lithotrite. Urol Res 2010;38:485–9.

Vorreuther R, Corleis R, Klotz T, et al. Impact of shock wave pattern and cavitation bubble size on tissue damage during ureteroscopic electrohydraulic lithotripsy. J Urol 1995;153(3 Pt 1):849–53.

12 Infections of the Urinary Tract

Anthony J. Schaeffer, MD, Richard S. Matulewicz, MS, MD, and David James Klumpp, PhD

Urinary tract infections (UTIs) are common, affect men and women of all ages, and vary dramatically in their presentation and sequelae. They are a common cause of morbidity and can lead to significant mortality. Although the urinary tract is normally free of bacterial growth, bacteria that generally ascend from the rectal reservoir may cause UTIs. When bacterial virulence increases or host defense mechanisms decrease, bacterial inoculation, colonization, and infection of the urinary tract occur. Careful diagnosis and treatment result in successful resolution of infections in most instances. A better understanding of the pathogenesis of UTIs and the role of host and bacterial factors has improved the ability to identify patients at risk and prevent or minimize sequelae. Clinical manifestations can vary from asymptomatic bacterial colonization of the bladder to irritative symptoms such as frequency and urgency associated with bacterial infection; upper tract infections associated with fever, chills, and flank pain; and bacteremia associated with severe morbidity, including sepsis and death. New antimicrobial agents that achieve high urinary and tissue levels, can be administered orally, and are not nephrotoxic have significantly reduced the need for hospitalization for severe infection. Shorter-course therapy and prophylactic antimicrobial agents have reduced the morbidity and cost associated with recurrent cystitis in women. Although the vast majority of patients respond promptly and are cured by therapy, early identification and treatment of patients with complicated infections that place them at significant risk remains a clinical challenge to urologists.

DEFINITIONS

UTI is an inflammatory response of the urothelium to bacterial invasion that is usually associated with bacteriuria and pyuria.

Bacteriuria **is the presence of bacteria in the urine, which is normally free of bacteria.** It has been assumed to be a valid indicator of either bacterial colonization or infection of the urinary tract. Although this is usually true, studies in animals (Hultgren et al, 1985; Mulvey et al, 1998) and humans (Elliott et al, 1985) have indicated that bacteria may be in the urothelium in the absence of bacteriuria. Alternatively, bacteriuria may represent bacterial contamination of an abacteriuric specimen during collection.

The possibility of contamination increases as the reliability of the collection technique decreases from suprapubic aspiration to catheterization to voided specimens. The term *significant bacteriuria* has a clinical connotation and is used to describe the number of bacteria in a suprapubically aspirated, catheterized, or voided specimen that exceeds the number usually caused by bacterial contamination of the skin, the urethra, or the prepuce or introitus, respectively. Hence it represents a UTI.

Bacteriuria can be *symptomatic* **or** *asymptomatic*. When it is detected by population studies (screening surveys), *screening bacteriuria* is a more precise and descriptive term than *asymptomatic bacteriuria*, especially because the latter term is clinically useful for describing the presence or absence of symptoms in an individual patient.

Pyuria, **the presence of white blood cells (WBCs) in the urine, is generally indicative of infection and/or an inflammatory response of the urothelium to the bacterium, stones, or other indwelling foreign body. Bacteriuria without pyuria is generally indicative of bacterial colonization without infection of the urinary tract. Pyuria without bacteriuria warrants evaluation for tuberculosis, stones, or cancer.**

Infections are often defined clinically by their presumed site of origin. *Cystitis* describes a clinical syndrome of dysuria, frequency, urgency, and occasionally suprapubic pain. These symptoms, although generally indicative of bacterial cystitis, may also be associated with infection of the urethra or vagina or noninfectious conditions such as interstitial cystitis, bladder carcinoma, or calculi. Conversely, patients may be asymptomatic and have infection of the bladder and possibly the upper urinary tract.

Acute pyelonephritis is a clinical syndrome of chills, fever, and flank pain that is accompanied by bacteriuria and pyuria, a combination that is reasonably specific for an acute bacterial infection of the kidney. The term should not be used if flank pain is absent. It may have no morphologic or functional components detectable by routine clinical modalities. There may be serious difficulties in diagnosing spinal cord–injured and elderly patients who may be unable to localize the site of their discomfort.

Chronic pyelonephritis describes a shrunken, scarred kidney, diagnosed by morphologic, radiologic, or functional evidence of renal disease that may be postinfectious but is frequently not associated with UTI. Bacterial infection of the kidney may cause a *focal, coarse scar* in the renal cortex overlying a calyx, almost always accompanied by some calyceal distortion (Fig. 12-1), which can be detected radiographically or by gross examination of the kidney. Less commonly, renal scarring from infection can result in atrophic pyelonephritis or generalized thinning of the renal cortex, with a small kidney appearing radiographically similar to one with postobstructive atrophy (Fig. 12-2).

UTIs may also be described in terms of the anatomic or functional status of the urinary tract and the health of the host.

Uncomplicated describes an infection in a healthy patient with a structurally and functionally normal urinary tract. The majority of these patients are women with isolated or recurrent bacterial cystitis or acute pyelonephritis, and the infecting pathogens are usually susceptible to and eradicated by a short course of inexpensive oral antimicrobial therapy.

A *complicated* infection is associated with factors that increase the chance of acquiring bacteria and decrease the efficacy of therapy (Box 12-1). The urinary tract is structurally or functionally abnormal, the host is compromised, and/or the bacteria have increased virulence or antimicrobial resistance. The majority of these patients are men.

Renal diseases that reduce the concentrating ability of the kidney or neurologic conditions that alter bladder-emptying capabilities are commonly encountered functional abnormalities.

Examples of anatomic abnormalities include obstruction associated with calculi or enlargement of the prostate or congenital or acquired sites of residual urine, such as calyceal or bladder diverticula. A complicated infection is frequently caused by bacteria that have exposure to many antimicrobial agents.

Chronic is a poor term that should be avoided in the context of UTIs, except for chronic pyelonephritis or bacterial prostatitis, because the duration of the infection is not defined.

UTIs may also be defined by their relationship to other UTIs:

A *first* or *isolated* infection is one that occurs in an individual who has never had a UTI or has one remote infection from a previous UTI.

An *unresolved* infection is one that has not responded to antimicrobial therapy and is documented to be the same organism with a similar resistance profile.

A *recurrent* infection is one that occurs after documented, successful resolution of an antecedent infection. Consider these two different types of recurrent infection:

1. *Reinfection* describes a new event associated with reintroduction of bacteria into the urinary tract from outside.
2. *Bacterial persistence* refers to a recurrent UTI caused by the same bacteria reemerging from a focus within the urinary tract, such as an infectious stone or the prostate. *Relapse* is frequently used interchangeably. These definitions require careful clinical and bacteriologic assessment and are important because they influence the type and extent of the patient's evaluation and treatment.

Antimicrobial prophylaxis is the prevention of reinfections of the urinary tract by the administration of antimicrobial drugs. If the term is used correctly in reference to the urinary tract, it can be assumed that bacteria have been eliminated before prophylaxis is begun. **Surgical antimicrobial prophylaxis entails administration of an antimicrobial agent before and for a *limited* time after a procedure to prevent local or systemic postprocedural infections.**

Antimicrobial suppression is the prevention of growth of a focus of bacterial persistence that cannot be eradicated. A low, nightly dosage of an antimicrobial agent usually results in the urine showing no growth, as in the case of a stone colonized with bacteria (i.e., infection stone) or in bacterial prostatitis caused by *Escherichia coli*. *Suppressive* is also a useful term when recurrent acute symptoms are prevented in a poor-risk patient, such as one with a large staghorn calculus in whom the antimicrobial agent reduces but does not eliminate the bacteria in the urine.

Domiciliary or *outpatient* *UTIs* occur in patients who are not hospitalized or institutionalized at the time they become infected. **The infections are generally caused by common bowel bacteria** (e.g., Enterobacteriaceae or *Enterococcus faecalis*) which are susceptible to most antimicrobial agents.

Nosocomial or *health care–associated* *UTIs* occur in patients **who are hospitalized or institutionalized,** and these are typically caused by *Pseudomonas* and other more antimicrobial-resistant strains.

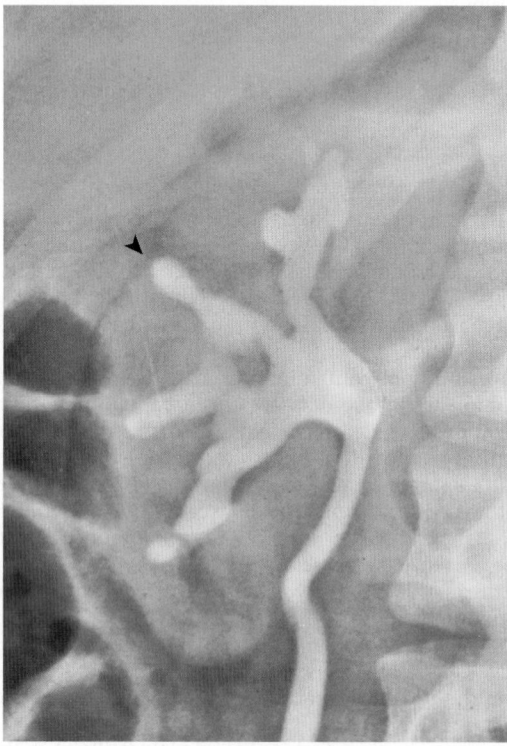

Figure 12-1. Excretory urogram demonstrates focal, coarse scarring in the right kidney of an 18-year-old girl with a history of many recurrent fevers between 2 months and 2 years of age. A cystogram when the patient was 2 years old established an atrophic left kidney with marked reflux up to the left kidney and slight reflux up to the right kidney. Excretory urography at the age of 6 years established severe atrophy of the left kidney. She had no infections between the ages of 6 and 15 years. Several reinfections occurred at the age of 15 years, and they ceased with prophylactic therapy. Her blood pressure has remained normal, and her serum creatinine level was 0.9 mg/dL at the age of 18 years. At 21 years of age she stopped antimicrobial prophylaxis for 18 months without infections or introital colonization with Enterobacteriaceae. Note that all calyces are blunted and that one extends to the capsule *(arrowhead)* because of atrophy of the overlying cortex.

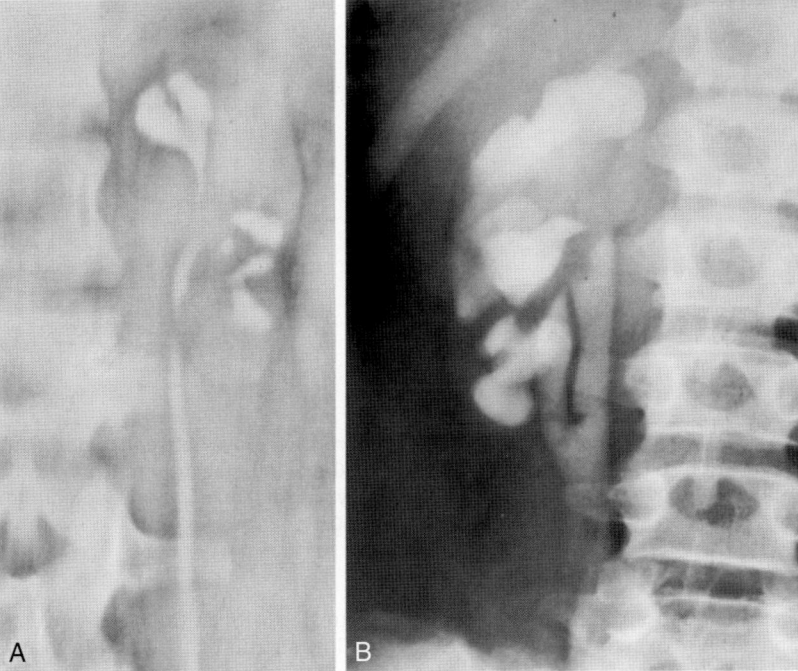

Figure 12-2. **A,** Excretory urogram of the contralateral left kidney from the same patient as in Figure 12-1. The severe pyelonephritic atrophy, undoubtedly caused by febrile urinary infections during early infancy with reflux into different segments of the kidney, produced irregular cortical scarring. Note how all the calyces extend to the capsule with irregular, intervening areas of cortex. **B,** Pyelonephritic atrophy, suggestive of postobstructive atrophy, in a 20-year-old woman with spina bifida, neurogenic bladder, and many episodes of fever and bacteriuria in early childhood. Observe the uniform, regular atrophy of the renal cortex that suggests reflux of bacteria simultaneously into virtually all nephrons. This type of pyelonephritic atrophy is uncommon compared with that shown in A and is characteristic of obstruction with superimposed infection.

BOX 12-1 Factors That Suggest a Complicated Urinary Tract Infection

Functional or anatomic abnormality of urinary tract
Male gender
Pregnancy
Elderly patient
Diabetes
Immunosuppression
Childhood urinary tract infection
Recent antimicrobial agent use
Indwelling urinary catheter
Urinary tract instrumentation
Hospital-acquired infection
Symptoms for more than 7 days at presentation

From Schaeffer AJ. Urinary tract infections. In: Gillenwater JY, Grayhack JT, Howards SS, et al, editors. Adult and pediatric urology. Philadelphia: Lippincott Williams & Wilkins; 2002. p. 212.

KEY POINTS: DEFINITIONS

- Infection of the urinary tract occurs when bacterial virulence increases and/or host defense mechanisms decrease.
- The majority of patients respond promptly to short courses of antimicrobial therapy.
- Early identification and treatment of complicated UTIs is essential to prevent major sequelae or death.

INCIDENCE AND EPIDEMIOLOGY

UTIs are considered to be the most common bacterial infection. They account for more than 7 million visits to physicians' offices and necessitate or complicate over 1 million office visits and 1 million emergency department visits, resulting in 100,000 hospitalizations annually (Patton et al, 1991; Hooton and Stamm, 1997; Foxman 2002). **They account for 1.2% of all office visits by women and 0.6% of all office visits by men** (Schappert, 1997).

The overall **prevalence of bacteriuria in women** has been estimated at 3.5%, with prevalence generally increasing with age in a linear trend (Evans et al, 1978). Surveys screening for bacteriuria have shown that about 1% of schoolgirls (aged 5 to 14 years) (Kunin et al, 1962) have bacteriuria and that this figure increases to about 4% by young adulthood and then by an additional 1% to 2% per decade of age (Fig. 12-3). **Nearly 30% of women will have had a symptomatic UTI requiring antimicrobial therapy by age 24, and almost half of all women will experience a UTI during their lifetime.** The prevalence of bacteriuria in young women is 30 times more than in men. However, **with increasing age, the ratio of women to men with bacteriuria progressively decreases. At least 20% of women and 10% of men older than 65 years have bacteriuria** (Boscia and Kaye, 1987; Juthani-Mehta, 2007).

The incidence of bacteriuria also increases with institutionalization or hospitalization and concurrent disease (Sourander, 1966). In a study of women and men older than 68 years, Boscia and Kaye (1987) found that 24% of functionally impaired nursing home residents had bacteriuria, compared with 12% of healthy domiciliary subjects (Boscia et al, 1986). UTIs account for approximately 38% of the 2 million nosocomial infections each year (Sedor and Mulholland, 1999; Lo et al, 2008); **catheter-associated UTIs (CAUTIs) are the most common nosocomial infection.** More than

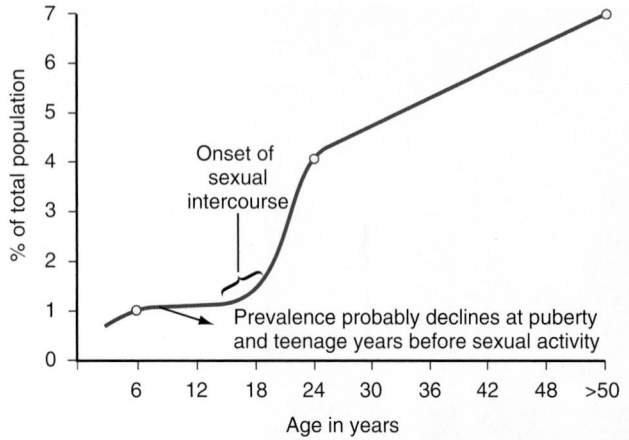

Figure 12-3. Prevalence of bacteriuria in females as a function of age. (From Stamey TA. The prevention of recurrent urinary infections. New York: Science and Medicine; 1973.)

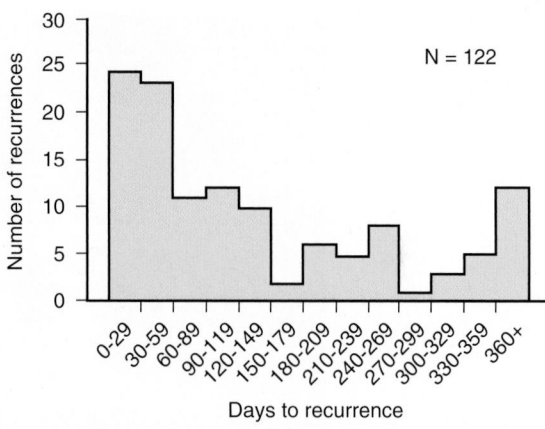

Figure 12-4. Days between recurrent urinary tract infections grouped by 30-day intervals. (From Kraft JK, Stamey TA. The natural history of symptomatic recurrent bacteriuria in women. Medicine 1977;56: 55–60.)

80% of nosocomial UTIs are secondary to an indwelling urethral catheter (Sedor and Mulholland, 1999; Foxman, 2002). **The incidence of UTIs is also increased during pregnancy and in patients with spinal cord injuries, diabetes, multiple sclerosis, and human immunodeficiency virus (HIV) infection/acquired immunodeficiency syndrome (AIDS).**

The **financial impact** of community-acquired UTIs is nearly $1.6 billion in the United States alone (Foxman, 2002); the annual cost of nosocomial UTIs has been estimated to range from between $515 million and $548 million (Jarvis, 1996). Each CAUTI is estimated to cost between $589 and $758 (Tambyah et al, 2002; Anderson et al, 2007). In patients requiring intensive care, the cost is roughly $2,000 per nosocomial UTI (Chen et al, 2009).

Little is known about the natural history of untreated bacteriuria in women because most women are treated when they are diagnosed, but a few studies in which treatment with antimicrobial agents is compared with placebo have been done. These show that 57% to 80% of bacteriuric women who are untreated or treated with placebo clear their infections spontaneously (Mabeck, 1972; Guttmann, 1973). Mabeck (1972) found that 8 of 53 bacteriuric women placed on placebo needed treatment with an antimicrobial agent because of symptoms, but 32 of the remaining 45 women cleared without treatment within a month, and 43 of the 45 had spontaneously cleared of bacteriuria within 5 months; only 2 women remained persistently bacteriuric.

Once a patient has an infection, he or she is likely to develop subsequent infections. Many adults had UTIs as children, underscoring the importance of genotypic factors in UTIs (Gillenwater et al, 1979). Of 45 women with untreated UTIs whose infection cleared, 20 (46%) had recurrences within a year (Mabeck, 1972). When women with recurrent bacteriuria were observed after treatment, about one sixth (37 of 219) had a very high recurrence rate (2.6 infections per year), whereas the remaining women had a recurrence rate of only 0.32 per year (Mabeck, 1972). Similar separation was seen in a prospective study, in which only 28.6% of 60 women who experienced their first symptomatic UTI had recurrent infections over the first 18 months of observation, as opposed to recurrences in 82.5% of 106 women who had had previous UTIs (Harrison et al, 1974). **Other investigators also have found that the probability of recurrent UTIs increases with the number of previous infections and decreases in inverse proportion to the elapsed time between the first and the second infections** (Mabeck, 1972). Of these recurrent infections, 71% to 73% are caused by reinfection with different organisms, rather than recurrence with the same organism (Mabeck, 1972; Guttmann, 1973).

Women with frequent reinfections have a rate of 0.13 to 0.25 UTIs per month (1.6 to 3.1 infections per year) when the infections are treated with antimicrobial agents (Mabeck, 1972; Guttmann, 1973; Kraft and Stamey, 1977; Vosti, 2002).

In a prospective long-term study of 235 women with more than 1000 confirmed infections studied over a period ranging from 1 to nearly 20 years, about half of the patients had clusters of infections, which ranged in frequency from 2 to 12 infections per cluster. Infections were followed by remission-free intervals that averaged approximately 1 year. **Most reinfections occurred after 2 weeks** (Harrison et al, 1974) and within 5 months (Mabeck, 1972), and most occurred early in this interval (Kraft and Stamey, 1977; Vosti, 2002) (Fig. 12-4). Rates of reinfection were independent of bladder dysfunction, radiologic changes of chronic pyelonephritis, and vesicoureteral reflux (Guttmann, 1973). The reinfections did not occur evenly over time. In the Stanford series (Kraft and Stamey, 1977), 23 women with frequent recurrent infections were studied with monthly urine cultures when asymptomatic and with immediate cultures when symptomatic for cystitis, for a mean of 3 years. Thirty-four percent of infections were followed by infection-free intervals of at least 6 months (average, 12.8 months), and 22 of the 23 women had such intervals. However, even these long intervals were followed by further infections (Kraft and Stamey, 1977), thus underscoring the importance of genotypic factors in the pathogenesis of UTIs in women (Schaeffer et al, 1981).

When the Stanford data (Kraft and Stamey, 1977) on recurrent UTIs in highly susceptible females is analyzed by examining sets of infections separated by remissions of at least 6 months, 69% of the sets contain only one infection. After this first set, the remaining sets show a 33% remission rate in infections, which means a patient who has two or more infections within 6 months has only a 33% probability of remaining free of infection for the next 6 months. Therefore, **if antimicrobial prophylaxis is started after the second or any succeeding infection within a set, about two thirds of the women will benefit.**

Whether a patient receives no treatment at all or short-term, long-term, or prophylactic antimicrobial treatment, the risk of recurrent bacteriuria remains the same; prophylactic antimicrobial therapy reduces reinfections but does not alter the underlying predisposition to recurring infection. Asscher and associates (1973) found that reinfections occurred in 17 patients (34%) treated with a 7-day course of nitrofurantoin and in 13 patients (29%) receiving placebo during a 3- to 5-year follow-up. Mabeck (1972) found that 46% (20 of 43) of untreated patients had recurrent infections by 12 months compared with about 40% of treated patients who had recurrences. Both studies suggest that it makes little difference whether a UTI is cured with an antimicrobial agent or is allowed to clear spontaneously—the susceptibility to recurrent UTI remains the same. Moreover, patients with frequent UTI who take prophylactic antimicrobial agents for extended periods (≥6 months) may decrease their infections during the time of prophylaxis, but the rate of infection returns to the pretreatment rate after prophylaxis is stopped (Stamm et al, 1980a; Vosti, 1975). Even long interruptions in the pattern of recurrence, therefore, do not appear to alter the patient's basic susceptibility to infections.

The sequelae of complicated UTIs are substantial. It is well established in the presence of obstruction, infection stones, diabetes mellitus, and other risk factors that UTIs in adults can lead to progressive renal damage (Freedman, 1975). **The long-term effects of uncomplicated recurrent UTIs are not completely known, but, so far, no association between recurrent infections and renal scarring, hypertension, or progressive renal azotemia has been established** (Asscher et al, 1973; Freedman, 1975). Indeed, one investigator was unable to find a single case of unequivocal nonobstructive chronic pyelonephritis in 22 patients in whom chronic pyelonephritis was the cause of end-stage renal failure (Schechter et al, 1971). Similar data were reported by Huland and Busch (1982).

In pregnant women, the prevalence and rate of recurrent infection are the same, but their bacteriuria progresses to acute clinical pyelonephritis more frequently than in nonpregnant women. This variation in the natural history of recurrent infections in females is discussed in a later section on UTIs in pregnancy.

KEY POINTS: INCIDENCE AND EPIDEMIOLOGY

- UTIs are the most common bacterial infection.
- They cause significant morbidity but do not cause renal damage unless comorbidities are present.
- Prophylactic antimicrobial therapy reduces morbidity and the time to recurrent bacteriuria, but the risk of recurrence remains the same.

PATHOGENESIS

UTIs are a result of interactions between the uropathogen and the host. Successful infection of the urinary tract is determined in part by the virulence factors of the bacteria, the inoculum size, and the inadequacy of host defense mechanisms. These factors also play a role in determining the ultimate level of colonization and damage to the urinary tract. Whereas increased bacterial virulence appears to be necessary to overcome strong host resistance, bacteria with minimal virulence factors are able to infect patients who are significantly compromised.

Routes of Infection

Ascending Route

Most bacteria enter the urinary tract from the bowel reservoir via ascent through the urethra into the bladder. Adherence of pathogens to the introital and urothelial mucosa plays a significant role in ascending infections. This route is further enhanced in individuals with significant soilage of the perineum with feces, women who use spermicidal agents (Hooton et al, 1996; Foxman, 2002; Handley et al, 2002), and patients with intermittent or indwelling catheters.

Although cystitis is often restricted to the bladder, approximately 50% of infections can extend into the upper urinary tract (Busch and Huland, 1984). The weight of clinical and experimental evidence strongly suggests that **most episodes of pyelonephritis are caused by retrograde ascent of bacteria from the bladder through the ureter to the renal pelvis and parenchyma. Although reflux of urine is probably not required for ascending infections, edema associated with cystitis may cause sufficient changes in the ureterovesical junction to permit reflux.** Once the bacteria are introduced into the ureter, they may ascend to the kidney unaided.

However, this ascent would be greatly increased by any process that interferes with the normal ureteral peristaltic function. Gram-negative bacteria and their endotoxins, as well as pregnancy and ureteral obstruction, have a significant antiperistaltic effect.

Bacteria that reach the renal pelvis can enter the renal parenchyma by means of the collecting ducts at the papillary tips and then ascend upward within the collecting tubules. This process is hastened and exacerbated by increased intrapelvic pressure from ureteral obstruction or vesicoureteral reflux, particularly when it is associated with intrarenal reflux.

Hematogenous Route

Infection of the kidney by the hematogenous route is uncommon in normal individuals. However, the kidney is occasionally secondarily infected in patients with *Staphylococcus aureus* bacteremia originating from oral sites or with *Candida fungemia*. Experimental data indicate that infection is enhanced when the kidney is obstructed (Smellie et al, 1975).

Lymphatic Route

Direct extension of bacteria from the adjacent organs via lymphatics may occur in unusual circumstances, such as a severe bowel infection or retroperitoneal abscesses. There is little evidence that lymphatic routes play a significant role in the vast majority of UTIs.

Urinary Pathogens

Most UTIs are caused by facultative anaerobes usually originating from the bowel flora. Uropathogens such as *Staphylococcus epidermidis* and *Candida albicans* originate from the flora of the vagina or perineal skin.

***E. coli* is by far the most common cause of UTIs, accounting for 85% of community-acquired and 50% of hospital-acquired infections.** Other gram-negative Enterobacteriaceae, including *Proteus* and *Klebsiella*, and gram-positive *E. faecalis* and *Staphylococcus saprophyticus* are responsible for the remainder of most community-acquired infections. **Nosocomial infections** are caused by *E. coli, Klebsiella, Enterobacter, Citrobacter, Serratia, Pseudomonas aeruginosa, Providencia, E. faecalis,* and *S. epidermidis* (Kennedy et al, 1965). Less common organisms such as *Gardnerella vaginalis, Mycoplasma* species, and *Ureaplasma urealyticum* may infect patients with intermittent or indwelling catheters (Josephson et al, 1988; Fairley and Birch, 1989).

E. coli strains mediating extraintestinal infections are typically grouped into broad phylogenetic classes by multiplex polymerase chain reaction (Clermont et al, 2000), where 70% of uropathogenic *E. coli* (UPEC) isolates fall into the B2 group (Johnson et al, 2001). More recent studies have used multilocus sequence typing to further define and characterize *E. coli* strains mediating UTI and other infections at the level of "sequence type." *E. coli* **sequence type ST131 (serotype O25b:H4) merits special attention as a rapidly emerging cause of multidrug-resistant infections, including UTI** (Johnson et al, 2010; Kudinha et al, 2013). Although first noted for extended-spectrum β-lactamases, fluoroquinolone resistance is a hallmark phenotype among ST131 isolates. Recent work with geographically diverse ST131 isolates revealed that a single ST131 subclonal lineage, *H30*, has emerged within approximately a decade as the major cause of multidrug-resistant *E. coli* infections and is highly associated with recurrent UTI and sepsis (Johnson et al, 2013; Tchesnokova et al, 2013). However, because ST131 isolates were not more virulent in a murine sepsis model, it is likely that the epidemiologic success of ST131 is due to enhanced fitness in early infection events or transmission (Johnson et al, 2012).

The prevalence of infecting organisms is influenced by the patient's age. For example, *S. saprophyticus* is now recognized as causing approximately 10% of symptomatic lower UTIs in young, sexually active females (Latham et al, 1983), whereas it rarely causes infection in males and elderly individuals. A seasonal variation with a late summer to fall peak has been reported (Hovelius and Mardh, 1984).

Fastidious Organisms

Anaerobes in the Urinary Tract

Although symptomatic anaerobic infections of the urinary tract are documented, they are uncommon. However, the distal urethra, perineum, and vagina are normally colonized by anaerobes. Whereas 1% to 10% of voided urine specimens are positive for anaerobic organisms (Finegold, 1977), anaerobic organisms found in suprapubic aspirates are much more unusual (Gorbach and Bartlett, 1974). Clinically symptomatic UTIs in which only anaerobic organisms are cultured are rare, but **these organisms must be suspected when a patient with bladder irritative symptoms has cocci or gram-negative rods seen on microscopic examination of the centrifuged urine** (catheterized, suprapubic aspirated, or voided midstream urine) **and routine quantitative aerobic cultures fail to grow organisms** (Ribot et al, 1981).

Anaerobic organisms are frequently found in **suppurative infections** of the genitourinary tract. In one study of suppurative genitourinary infections in males, 88% of scrotal, prostatic, and perinephric abscesses included anaerobes among the infecting organisms (Bartlett and Gorbach, 1981). The organisms found are usually *Bacteroides* species, including *B. fragilis*, *Fusobacterium* species, anaerobic cocci, and *Clostridium perfringens* (Finegold, 1977). The growth of clostridia may be associated with cystitis emphysematosa (Bromberg et al, 1982).

Mycobacterium tuberculosis *and Other* Nontuberculous Mycobacteria

Mycobacterium tuberculosis and other nontuberculous mycobacteria may be found when cultures for acid-fast bacteria are requested; **they do not grow under routine aerobic conditions and may be found during evaluation for sterile pyuria.** It has been emphasized that the mere presence of mycobacteria may not indicate tissue invasion. Therefore factors such as symptoms, endoscopic or radiologic evidence of infection, abnormal urine sediment, the absence of other pathogens, repeated demonstration of the organism, and the presence of granulomas should be considered before therapy is instituted (Brooker and Aufderheide, 1980; Thomas et al, 1980). (*M. tuberculosis* is discussed in Chapter 17.)

Chlamydia

Chlamydiae are not routinely grown in aerobic culture but have been implicated in genitourinary infections. (Their role in the urinary tract is discussed in Chapter 15.)

Bacterial Virulence Factors

Virulence characteristics play a role in determining both if an organism will invade the urinary tract and the subsequent level of infection within the urinary tract. It is generally believed that uropathogenic strains resident in the bowel flora, such as UPEC, can infect the urinary tract not only by chance but also by the expression of virulence factors that enable them to adhere to and colonize the perineum and urethra and migrate to the urinary tract where they establish an inflammatory response in the urothelium (Schaeffer et al, 1981; Yamamoto et al, 1997; Schlager et al, 2002; Moreno et al, 2008). The same virulence factors can be found on bacterial strains that cause recurrent UTI in patients (Foxman et al, 1995). Some of these virulence determinants are located on one of approximately 20 UPEC-specific pathogenicity-associated islands ranging in size from 30 to 170 kb (Hacker et al, 1999; Oelschlaeger et al, 2002). These pathogenicity islands collectively increase the size of the pathogen genome by about 20% over a commensal strain. A recent genomic analysis of a UPEC strain revealed the presence of genes for putative chaperone-usher systems, as well as autotransporter proteins that may function as adhesins, toxins, proteases, invasins, serum resistance factors, or motility mediators (Henderson and Nataro, 2001). One UPEC-specific autotransporter, Sat, seems toxic to urinary tract cells in vitro (Guyer et al, 2000) and can cause cytoplasmic vacuolation and severe histologic damage in mouse kidneys (Guyer et al, 2002). Another toxin, hemolysin (HlyA), forms pores in a variety of host cell membranes (Uhlen et al, 2000). In addition to proteases and toxins, UPEC produces several iron acquisition systems, including aerobactin (Johnson et al, 1988; Johnson, 2003) and the more recently described IroN system (Russo et al, 1999; Sorsa et al, 2003). Lastly, most UPEC strains produce an acid polysaccharide capsule that protects the bacteria from phagocytosis by human polymorphonuclear leukocytes and inhibits activation of complement (Johnson, 2003).

Early Events in UPEC Pathogenesis

Bacterial Adherence

Bacterial adherence to vaginal and urothelial epithelial cells is an essential step in the initiation of UTIs. This interaction is influenced by the adhesive characteristics of the bacteria, the receptive characteristics of the epithelial surface, and the fluid bathing both surfaces. Bacterial adherence is a specific interaction that plays a role in determining the organism, the host, and the site of infection. Portions of this section on bacterial adherence have been published (Schaeffer et al, 1981).

Bacterial Adhesins. UPEC expresses a number of adhesins that allow it to attach to urinary tract tissues (Mulvey, 2002). These adhesins are classified as either **fimbrial** or **afimbrial**, depending on whether the adhesin is displayed as part of a rigid fimbria or pilus (Fig. 12-5). Bacteria may produce a number of antigenically and functionally different pili on the same cell; others produce a single type; in some, no pili are seen (Klemm, 1985). A typical piliated cell may contain 100 to 400 pili. The pilus is usually 5 to 10 nm in diameter, is up to 2 μm long, and appears to be composed primarily of subunits known as *pilin* (Klemm, 1985). Pili are defined functionally by their ability to mediate hemagglutination of specific types of erythrocytes. The most well-described pili are types 1, P, and S.

Type 1 (Mannose-Sensitive) Pili. Type 1 pili are commonly expressed on both nonpathogenic and pathogenic *E. coli*. Type 1 pili consist of a helical rod composed of repeating FimA subunits joined to a 3-nm wide distal tip structure containing the adhesin FimH (Jones et al, 1995). These pili mediate hemagglutination of guinea pig erythrocytes (Duguid et al, 1979). The reaction is inhibited by the addition of mannose; thus type 1 pili are termed *mannose-sensitive hemagglutination* (MSHA) (Svenson et al, 1984; Reid and Sobel, 1987).

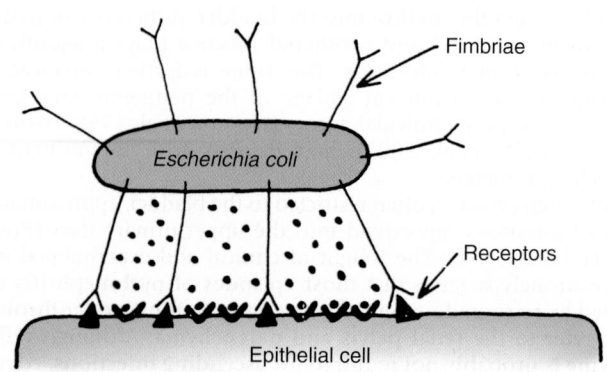

Figure 12-5. Bacterial adherence. Adhesins on pili (fimbriae) mediate attachment to specific epithelial cell receptors.

The role of type 1 pili as a virulence factor in UTIs has been established. This evidence has been obtained (1) from the analysis of bacteria isolated from the urine of patients with UTIs, which were found to express mannose-sensitive (MS) adhesins (Ljungh and Wadstrom, 1983); (2) from studies with animal models (Fader and Davis, 1982; Hagberg et al, 1983a, 1983b; Iwahi et al, 1983; Hultgren et al, 1985) in which inoculation of type 1 piliated organisms into the bladder resulted in significantly more colonization of the urinary tract than inoculation of nonpiliated organisms; and (3) from the observation that anti–type 1 pili antibodies and competitive inhibitors such as methyl-α-D-mannopyranoside protected mice from contracting UTIs (Aronson et al, 1979; Hultgren et al, 1985). **Recent studies have demonstrated that interactions between FimH and receptors expressed on the luminal surface of the bladder epithelium are critical for the ability of many UPEC strains to colonize the bladder and cause disease** (Connell et al, 1996; Langermann et al, 1997; Thankavel et al, 1997; Mulvey et al, 1998).

P (Mannose-Resistant) Pili. P pili confer tropism to the kidney, the designation "P" standing for pyelonephritis (Mulvey, 2002). P pili, which are found in most pyelonephritogenic strains of UPEC, mediate hemagglutination of human erythrocytes that is not altered by mannose and is thus termed *mannose-resistant hemagglutination* (MRHA) (Kallenius et al, 1979). The adhesin PapG, at the tip of the pilus, recognizes the α-D-galactopyranosyl-(1-4)-β-D-galactopyranoside moiety present in the globoseries of glycolipids (Kallenius et al, 1980; Leffler and Svanborg-Eden, 1980), which are found on P blood group antigens and on uroepithelium (Svenson et al, 1983).

The MRHA adhesins of UPEC that do not show the digalactoside-binding specificity have been provisionally named *X adhesins* (Vaisanen et al, 1981). In some strains of UPEC, hemagglutination is mediated by nonpiliated adhesins or hemagglutinins (Duguid et al, 1979).

Svanborg-Eden and coworkers (1978) were the first to report a correlation between bacterial adherence and severity of UTIs. They showed that UPEC strains from girls with acute pyelonephritis had high adhesive ability, whereas strains causing asymptomatic bacteriuria or from the feces of healthy girls had low bacterial adherence. Between 70% and 80% of the pyelonephritic strains, but only 10% of the bowel isolates, had adhesive capacity. Furthermore, P pili were present in 91% of urinary strains causing pyelonephritis, 19% of strains causing cystitis, and 14% of strains causing asymptomatic bacteriuria but only 7% of bowel isolates from healthy children, highlighting the correlation between bacterial adherence and UTIs (Kallenius et al, 1981).

Whereas MRHA and P pili are strongly associated with pyelonephritis, these virulence factors are not associated with renal scarring and reflux caused by bacterial infection (Vaisanen et al, 1981). Studies suggest minimal correlation between P-piliated *E. coli* strains and recurrent pyelonephritis with gross reflux in girls (Lomberg et al, 1983). Thus it would appear that P pili in acute pyelonephritis are important mainly in nonrefluxing or minimally refluxing children.

Other Adhesins. S pili, which bind to sialic acid residues via the SfaS adhesin, have been associated with both bladder and kidney infection (Mulvey, 2002). F1C pili bind to glycosphingolipids in renal epithelial cells and induce an interleukin-8 inflammatory response (Backhed et al, 2002).

UPEC also expresses a group of afimbrial adhesins (AFA), which have been clustered with the Dr adhesin family for their recognition of decay-accelerating factor and for their similar genetic structure. Decay-accelerating factor is found on numerous different epithelial sites, and Dr adhesins are known to bind to many locations throughout the urinary tract (Anderson et al, 2004b).

Catch Bonds. Not surprisingly, UPEC adhesins have evolved to meet the physical dynamics of the urinary tract, and this is best understood for FimH. Using hemagglutination assays and flow cell approaches, **the affinity of *E. coli* expressing specific FimH alleles for erythrocytes was found to be enhanced by shear stress**, and mutations that abolished FimH-erythrocyte interactions in static conditions did not impact dynamic affinities (Thomas et al, 2002). Conversely, static conditions reduced FimH-erythrocyte interactions. Known as *catch bonds*, this fingertrap-like mechanism is mediated by shear-altered interactions between the FimH pilin and mannose-binding domains that result in force-induced tightening of the mannose-binding pocket (Le Trong et al, 2010). Similar shear-enhanced binding now appears widespread in biology and includes *E. coli* P-fimbriae (reviewed in Sokurenko et al, 2008). The implications of catch bonds for UPEC adherence and UTI pathogenesis are obvious. **Enhanced adherence in the presence of shear would promote UPEC retention in the urethra and bladder during voiding and in the ureters against peristalsis. In the absence of shear, reduced FimH affinity would facilitate diffusion and thereby promote ascending infection.**

Phase Variation of Bacterial Pili in Vivo

Early evidence for the role of type 1 and P pili in adherence in UTIs in humans was contradictory. Pili were visible by electron microscopy on *E. coli* in the urine of 31 of 37 patients (Ljungh and Wadstrom, 1983). Conversely, no MS adhesins were found in 22 of 24 urine isolates from patients with indwelling catheters (Ofek et al, 1981), and 19 of 20 samples from patients with acute UTIs were devoid of pili and nonadherent until subcultured in broth (Harber et al, 1982). Assessment of pili production by clinical *E. coli* isolates demonstrates that environmental growth conditions can produce rapid changes in pilus expression (Duguid et al, 1966; Goransson and Uhlin, 1984; Hultgren et al, 1986), wherein cells switch back and forth between piliated and nonpiliated phases (Eisenstein, 1981). For example, some bacteria grown in a broth medium express pili, whereas the same strain grown on the same medium in a solid state will cease production of pili. **This process, called *phase variation*, can also occur in vivo and has obvious biologic and clinical implications.** For example, the presence of type 1 pili may be advantageous to the bacteria for adhering to and colonizing the bladder mucosa but disadvantageous because the pili enhance phagocytosis and killing by neutrophils (Silverblatt et al, 1979).

An animal model of ascending UTIs and studies of bacterial isolates from different sites in patients with UTI provide evidence that phase variation can occur during *E. coli* UTI in vivo. Type 1 piliated *E. coli* organisms that were capable of phase variation were introduced into the mouse bladder in the piliated phase, and the bacteria recovered from the bladder and urine 24 or more hours after inoculation were tested for piliation. All of the animals had bladder colonization, and 78% of the bacteria recovered showed type 1 piliation. The bacteriologic state of the urine often differed from that of the bladder. The urine was sterile in 59% of the animals with bladder colonization, and the organisms recovered from the urine were often nonpiliated.

When bladder and kidney cultures were examined 1, 3, and 5 days after intravesical inoculation of piliated bacteria, organisms recovered from the bladder remained piliated, whereas organisms recovered from the kidney showed significantly less piliation (Schaeffer et al, 1987) (Fig. 12-6).

Studies in humans using indirect immunofluorescence of fresh urine bacteria have confirmed in vivo expression and phase variation of pili. Analysis of the urine of adults with lower UTI detected type 1 pili in 31 of 41 specimens and P pili in 6 of 18 specimens (Kisielius et al, 1989). The piliation status of the bacterial population in the urine was heterogeneous, varying from predominantly piliated to a mixture of piliated and nonpiliated cells (Fig. 12-7). Strains isolated from different sites in the urogenital tract showed variation in the state of piliation. These results demonstrate that type 1 and P pili are expressed and subject to phase variation in vivo during acute UTIs.

This process of phase variation has obvious biologic and clinical implications. For example, the presence of type 1 pili may be advantageous to the bacteria for initially adhering to and colonizing the bladder mucosa. Subsequently, type 1 pili may be unnecessary for strains in suspension in urine and in fact detrimental because they enhance apoptosis, phagocytosis, and killing by neutrophils

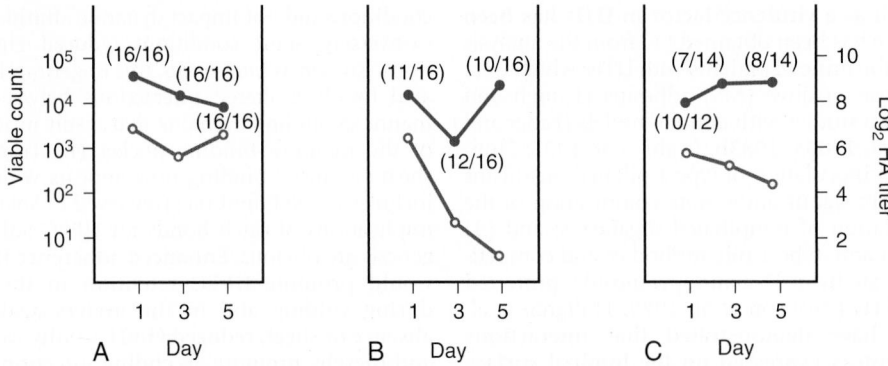

Figure 12-6. Time study after intravesical inoculation with *Escherichia coli* strain I-I49 that compared the mean viable bacteria count *(solid circles)* and hemagglutination (HA) titer *(open circles)* for bladders (A), kidneys (B), and urine specimens (C) from the same animals. Each point is the mean of all the animals tested. The numbers in parentheses show the proportion of animals inoculated that gave positive cultures. The HA titers were tested after 18 hours of growth on agar. The HA titer of bacteria recovered from the kidney decreased significantly by day 5 ($P < 0.001$). (From Schaeffer AJ, Schwan WR, Hultgren SJ, et al. Relationship of type 1 pilus expression in *Escherichia coli* to ascending urinary tract infections in mice. Infect Immun 1987;55:373–80.)

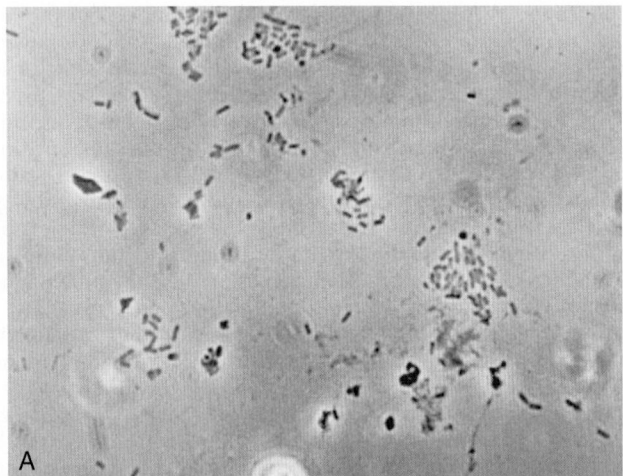

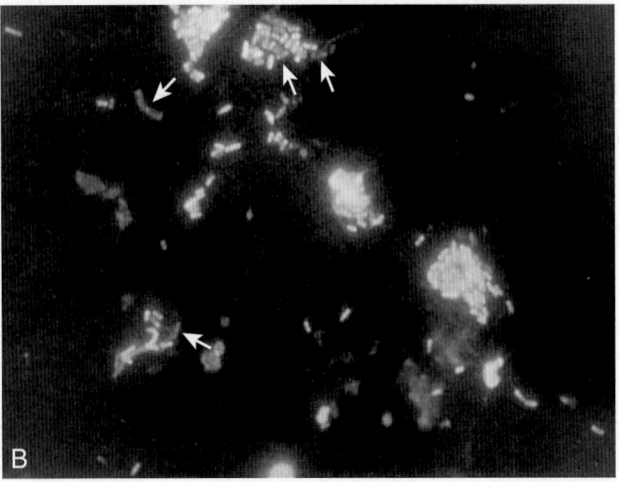

Figure 12-7. Phase-contrast micrograph (A) and immunofluorescence micrograph (B) of a sample stained with antiserum to type 1 pili of strain I-49 and with fluorescein isothiocyanate–conjugated second antibody against nonadherent *Escherichia coli* in the urine of a patient with acute urinary tract infection show a mixture of piliated and nonpiliated *(arrows in B)* cells. (From Kisielius PV, Schwan WR, Amundsen SK, et al. In vivo expression and variation of *Escherichia coli* type 1 and P pili in the urine of adults with acute urinary tract infections. Infect Immun 1989;57:1656–62.)

(Silverblatt et al, 1979; Mulvey et al, 1998). In the kidney, P pili may then take over as the primary mediator of bacterial attachment via their binding to the glycolipid receptors (Stapleton et al, 1995).

Epithelial Cell Receptivity

Vaginal Cells

The significance of epithelial cell receptivity in the pathogenesis of ascending UTI has been studied initially by examining adherence of *E. coli* to vaginal epithelial cells and uroepithelial cells collected from voided urine specimens. Fowler and Stamey (1977) established that certain indigenous microorganisms (e.g., lactobacilli, *S. epidermidis*) avidly attached themselves to washed epithelial cells in large numbers. When vaginal epithelial cells were collected from patients susceptible to reinfection and compared with such cells obtained from controls resistant to UTI, the *E. coli* strains that cause cystitis adhered much more avidly to the epithelial cells from the susceptible women. **These studies established increased adherence of pathogenic bacteria to vaginal epithelial cells as the first demonstrable biologic difference that could be shown in women susceptible to UTI.**

Subsequently, **Schaeffer and colleagues (1981) confirmed these vaginal differences in women, but in addition they observed that the increased bacterial adherence was also characteristic of buccal epithelial cells.** As can be seen in Figure 12-8, there is a striking similarity in the ability of both cell types to bind to the same *E. coli* strain. In addition, there was a significant relationship between vaginal cell and buccal cell receptivity. Seventy-seven different *E. coli* strains were tested for their ability to bind to vaginal and buccal epithelial cells. A direct nonlinear relationship between buccal and vaginal adherence in controls and patients was confirmed for urinary, vaginal, and anal isolates. Thus high vaginal cell receptivity was associated with high buccal cell receptivity.

These observations emphasize that the increase in receptor sites for UPEC on epithelial cells from women with recurrent UTIs is not limited to the vagina and thus suggest that a genotypic trait for epithelial cell receptivity may be a major susceptibility factor in UTIs. This concept was extended by examining the human leukocyte antigens (HLAs), which are the major histocompatibility complex in humans and have been associated statistically with many diseases (Schaeffer et al, 1983). The A3 antigen was identified in 12 (34%) of the patients, which is significantly higher than the 8% frequency observed in healthy controls. Thus, HLA-A3 may be associated with increased risk of recurrent UTIs.

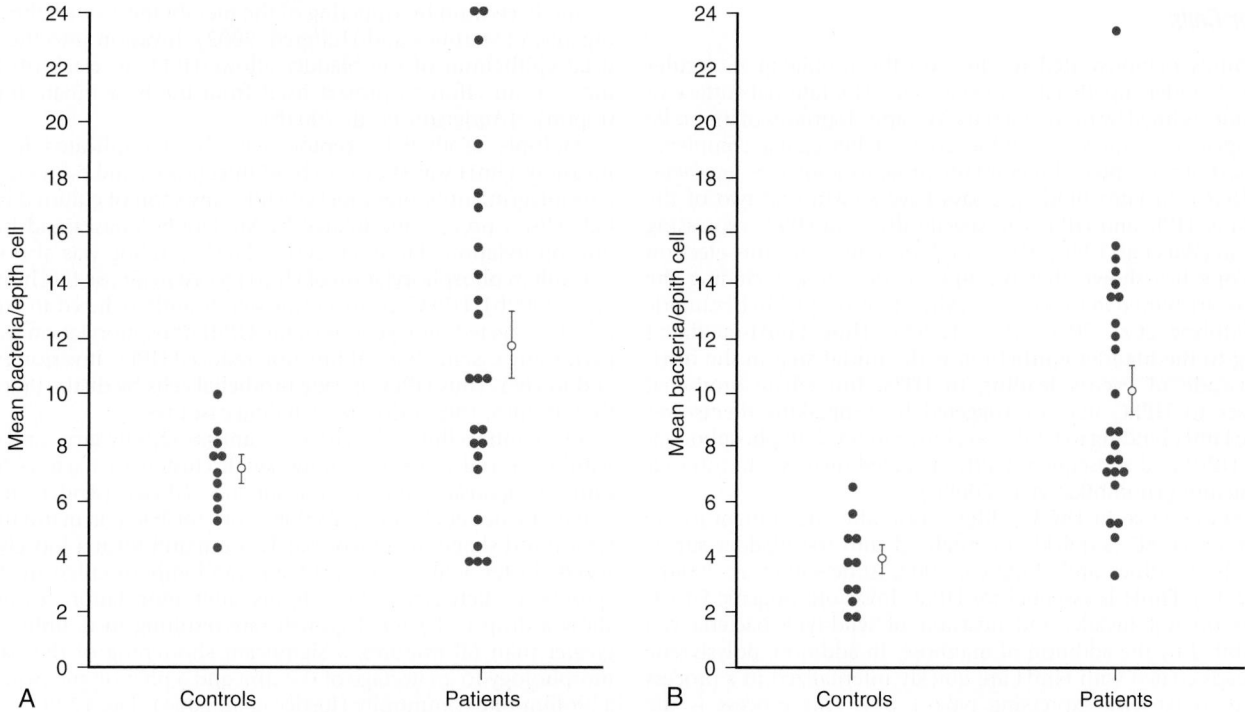

Figure 12-8. In vitro adherence of *Escherichia coli* to vaginal (A) and buccal (B) cells from healthy controls and patients with recurrent urinary tract infections. Values represent an average of 14 (A) and 11 (B) determinations in each individual. The *open circles* and *bars* represent the means + standard error of the mean. (From Schaeffer AJ, Jones JM, Dunn JK. Association of in vitro *Escherichia coli* adherence to vaginal and buccal epithelial cells with susceptibility of women to recurrent urinary tract infections. N Engl J Med 1981;304:1062–6.)

Variation in Receptivity. A small variation in both vaginal cell and buccal cell receptivity may be observed from day to day in healthy controls. Adherence ranges from 1 to 17 bacteria per cell and appears to be both cyclic and repetitive. When adherence was correlated with the days of a woman's menstrual cycle, higher values were noted in the early phase, diminishing shortly after the time of expected ovulation (day 14). The number of bacteria per epithelial cell often correlated with the value obtained on the same day of the menstrual cycle 1 or 2 months previously. Premenopausal women are particularly susceptible to attachment of uropathogenic *E. coli* and nonpathogenic lactobacilli at certain times during the menstrual cycle and to *E. coli* during the early stages of pregnancy. **The importance of such hormones as estrogens in the pathogenesis of UTI is therefore a matter of great interest, especially because the clinical urologist may see women who have recurrent cystitis at regular intervals, possibly in response to these hormonal changes.**

Reid and Sobel (1987) found that uropathogens attached in larger numbers to uroepithelial cells from women older than 65 years of age than to cells from premenopausal women 18 to 40 years of age. Raz and Stamm (1993) noted that **susceptibility to recurrent UTI was increased by the lowered estrogen levels found in the postmenopausal women and that estrogen replacement decreased uropathogenic bacterial colonization and the incidence of UTI.**

Blood group antigens and carbohydrate structures bound to membrane lipids or proteins also constitute an important part of the uroepithelial cell membrane. The **presence or absence of blood group determinants on the surface of uroepithelial cells may influence an individual's susceptibility to a UTI.** Sheinfeld and associates (1989) determined the blood group phenotypes in women with recurrent UTI and compared them with those of age-matched women controls. There is a higher frequency of Lewis nonsecretor Le(a+b-) and recessive Le(a-b-) phenotypes among women with recurrent UTIs. There was no significant difference in the distribution of ABO or P blood group phenotypes. The Lewis antigen controls fucosylation. The protective effect in women with the secretor Le(a-b+) phenotype may be due to fucosylated structures at the vaginal cell surface or in the overlying mucus, which decreases availability of putative receptors for *E. coli* (Navas et al, 1993). The nonsecretor status has also been associated with female acute uncomplicated pyelonephritis, especially in premenopausal women (Ishitoya et al, 2002). Stapleton and coworkers (1995) have shown that unique *E. coli*–binding glycerides are found in vaginal epithelial cells from nonsecretors but not from secretors. **These studies individually and collectively support the concept that there is an increased epithelial receptivity for *E. coli* on the introital, urethral, and buccal mucosa that is characteristic of women susceptible to recurrent UTIs and may be a genotypic trait.**

The possibility that vaginal mucus might influence bacterial receptivity was investigated by Schaeffer and colleagues (1994). Type 1 piliated *E. coli* bound to all of the vaginal fluid specimens (Venegas et al, 1995). The binding capacity of vaginal fluid from women colonized with *E. coli* in vivo was greater than that from noncolonized women (Schaeffer et al, 1999). The importance of vaginal fluid in bacteria/epithelial cell interactions was investigated in an in vitro model that measured the effect of vaginal fluid on the binding of bacteria to an epithelial cell line (Gaffney et al, 1995). Vaginal fluid from colonized women enhanced binding of bacteria to epithelial cells. Conversely, vaginal fluid from noncolonized women inhibited adherence. Thus the **vaginal fluid appears to influence adherence to cells** and, presumably, vaginal mucosal colonization. Subsequent studies demonstrated that secretory IgA is the primary glycoprotein responsible for vaginal fluid receptivity (Rajan et al, 1999).

Bladder Cells

FimH binds mannosylated residues on the uroplakin molecules covering bladder superficial epithelial cells. The luminal surface of the bladder is lined by umbrella cells. The apical surfaces of umbrella cells appear as a quasi-crystalline array of hexagonal complexes composed of four integral membrane proteins known as *uroplakins* (Sun, 1996). In vitro binding assays have shown that two of the uroplakins, UPIa and UPIb, can specifically bind UPEC expressing type 1 pili (Wu et al, 1996). High-resolution freeze-fracture electron microscopy has shown that the tips of these pili, including the adhesins, are buried in the central cavity of the uroplakin hexameric rings (Mulvey et al, 2000) (Fig. 12-9A). **Thus FimH-mediated binding to the bladder epithelium is the initial step in the intricate cascade of events leading to UTIs.** Immediate urothelial responses to UPEC may be triggered by uroplakins themselves because FimH binding to UPIb was shown to result in phosphorylation of UPIII and subsequent UPIII-mediated increases in intracellular calcium (Thumbikat et al, 2009b).

UPEC Persistence in the Bladder. Soon after attachment to the epithelium, UPEC is quickly internalized into the bladder superficial cells (Martinez and Hultgren, 2002; Anderson et al, 2004b) (Fig. 12-9B). FimH is essential for UPEC invasion; isogenic FimH-mutants do not invade, and invasion of wild-type bacteria can be inhibited by the addition of mannose. In addition, polystyrene latex beads coated with FimH are quickly internalized in a process identical to bacteria expressing type 1 pili. This process is the result of localized actin rearrangement and engulfment of the bound bacterium by zippering of the membrane around the microorganism (Martinez and Hultgren, 2002). Invasion into the superficial epithelium of the bladder allows UPEC to establish a new niche in an effort to protect itself from the host innate immune response (Anderson et al, 2004b).

Multiple urothelial receptors have been implicated in UPEC invasion. FimH was shown to bind integrins α_3 and β_1 in vitro, and anti-integrin antibodies blocked UPEC invasion of cultured urothelial cells, a process modulated by Src family kinases and integrin phosphorylation (Eto et al, 2007). FimH binding was also shown to result in phosphorylation of UPIII by casein kinase II (Thumbikat et al, 2009b). UPEC invasion was significantly reduced in cultured cells by targeted mutagenesis of the UPIII phosphorylation site, and perturbing casein kinase II function reduced UPEC invasion in vitro and in vivo. Thus UPEC invade urothelial cells by distinct receptors that, in turn, trigger diverse signaling cascades.

Once intracellular, the UPEC organisms rapidly grow and divide within the cell cytosol, forming small clusters of bacteria termed *early intracellular bacterial communities* (IBCs) (Anderson et al, 2004b; Justice et al, 2004). As they grow, the bacteria maintain their typical rod shape of approximately 3 μm and form a loosely organized cluster, with microorganisms randomly oriented in the cell cytoplasm. Between 6 to 8 hours after inoculation, early IBCs show a drop in bacterial growth rate resulting in doubling times greater than 60 minutes, a significant shortening of the bacterial morphology to an average of 0.7 μm, and a phenotypic switch into a biofilm-like community (Justice et al, 2004) (Fig. 12-9C). Similar bacteria-engorged urothelial cells have been identified in 22% of

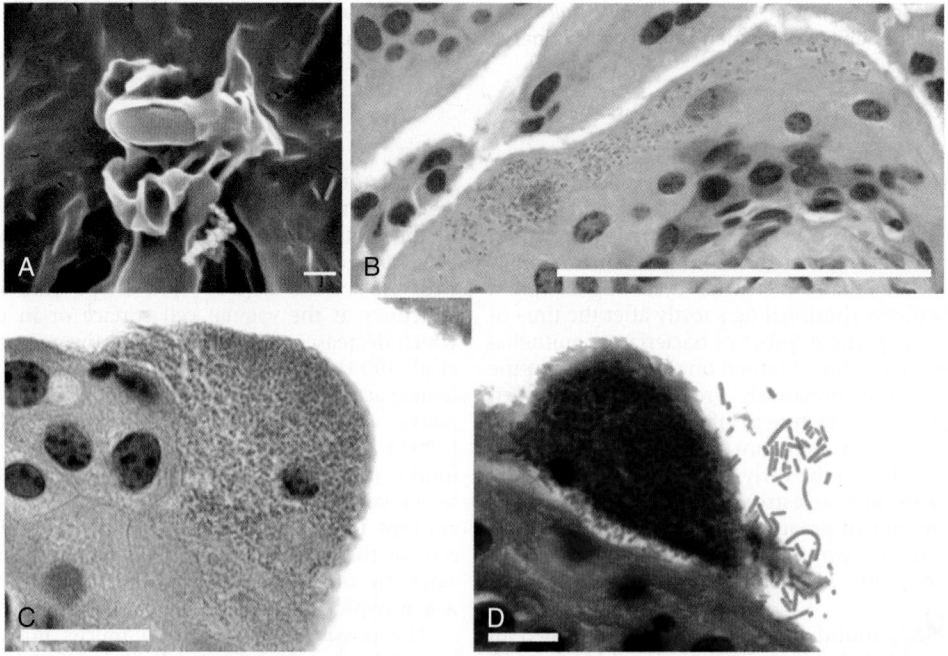

Figure 12-9. Uropathogenic *Escherichia coli* (UPEC) binds, invades, and multiplies inside the superficial cells of the bladder epithelium. A, Scanning electron microscopy shows a single UPEC bound to the surface of a bladder cell. Type 1 pilus–mediated contact between bacterium and host cell initiates signaling cascades in the bladder cell, leading to localized actin rearrangements and membrane protrusions around the bacterium. Scale bar, 0.5 μm. **B,** Once inside the bladder superficial cells, UPEC rapidly multiplies to form disordered bacterial clusters in the host cell cytoplasm, called an early intracellular bacterial community (IBC). Bacteria are visible as dark-staining rods inside the cell in this hematoxylin and eosin (H&E)-stained thin bladder section. Scale bar, 100 μm. **C,** H&E-stained thin bladder section reveals a middle IBC, wherein the constituent bacteria have organized themselves into a biofilm-like state within the bladder cell. Scale bar, 20 μm. **D,** A late IBC, visible by H&E staining, is typified by detachment of peripheral bacteria and fluxing of these organisms into the bladder lumen. Scale bar, 10 μm. **(From Anderson GG, Martin SM, Hultgren SJ. Host subversion by formation of intracellular bacterial communities in the urinary tract. Microbes Infect 2004;6:1094–101.)**

voided urine specimens from patients with UTI with *E. coli* (Rosen et al, 2007). Importantly, **UPEC isolated from the human IBC-like cells were capable of infecting mice and recapitulating IBCs** (Garofalo et al, 2007).

Biofilms shield bacteria from environmental challenges such as antimicrobial agents and the host immune response (Donlan and Costerton, 2002). **Characteristics of the biofilm that increase protection include the slower growth rate of the bacteria with associated physiologic changes, expression of factors that inhibit antimicrobial activity, and the inability of the antimicrobial agent to penetrate the biofilm matrix** (Anderson et al, 2004b). The biofilm also protects the bacteria from neutrophils because they are unable to effectively penetrate the IBC and engulf the bacteria. In animal models, bacteria on the edge of IBCs eventually detach, differentiate to typical rod morphology, become motile, and then escape the host cell into the bladder lumen in a process called *fluxing* (Mulvey et al, 2001) (Fig. 12-9D). These bacteria may become highly filamentous, reaching up to 70 μm or greater in length. This process occurs by approximately 24 hours after inoculation (Justice et al, 2004). It is possible that the filaments may help the bacteria evade the immunologic response.

The escaped bacteria re-adhere and reinvade superficial cells to lead to second IBC formation. In subsequent rounds, further IBC formation occurs. After a few days, the invasive bacteria become more quiescent. In animal models, the bacteria can persist in this dormant reservoir state for some time before reemerging to cause recurrent UTIs (Anderson et al, 2004a). Indeed, in murine UTI, individuals with sterile urine nonetheless may contain thousands of viable UPEC within bladder tissue (Mulvey et al, 2001), suggesting that IBCs may be a transient intermediate in the establishment of stable UPEC reservoirs within the bladder. Exfoliation of superficial urothelial cells (see later) exposes underlying transitional cells. In contrast to the cytosolic UPEC aggregates characteristic of IBCs, UPEC invasion of transitional cells results in membrane-bound bacteria limited to two to four bacteria per cell (Justice et al, 2004). These intracellular UPEC remain quiescent, and thus such transitional cells are referred to as *quiescent intracellular reservoirs* (QIR) (Mysorekar and Hultgren, 2006). However, chemically perturbing the urothelium to evoke urothelial differentiation caused reemergence of UPEC from QIR marked by significant bacterial proliferation. Together, these findings suggest that bladder reservoirs of intracellular UPEC may contribute to recurrent UTI in susceptible individuals as the transitional cells undergo differentiation.

Natural Defenses of the Urinary Tract

Periurethral and Urethral Region

The normal flora of the vaginal introitus, the periurethral area, and the urethra usually contain microorganisms such as lactobacilli, coagulase-negative staphylococci, corynebacteria, and streptococci that form a barrier against uropathogenic colonization (Fair et al, 1970; Pfau and Sacks, 1977; Marrie et al, 1978). Changes in the vaginal environment related to estrogen, cervical IgA (Stamey et al, 1978), and low vaginal pH (Stamey and Timothy, 1975) may alter the ability of these bacteria to colonize. More commonly, however, acute changes in colonization have been associated with use of antimicrobial agents and spermicidal agents that alter the normal flora and increase the receptivity of the epithelium for uropathogens.

Little is known about the factors that predispose patients to urethral colonization with uropathogens. The proximity of the urethral meatus to the vulvar and perianal areas suggests that contamination occurs frequently. The nature of urethral defense mechanisms other than flow of urine is largely unknown. Bacterial multiplication in the normal urethra may be inhibited by the indigenous flora (Chan et al, 1984). Although colonization of the periurethral and urethral regions is prerequisite to most infections, the ability of the organisms to overcome the normal defense mechanisms of the urine and the bladder is clearly pivotal.

Urine

In general, fastidious organisms that normally colonize the urethra will not multiply in urine and rarely cause UTIs (Cattell et al, 1974). In contrast, urine will usually support the growth of nonfastidious bacteria (Asscher et al, 1968). **Urine from normal individuals may be inhibitory, especially when the inoculum is small** (Kaye, 1968). The **most inhibitory factors are the osmolality, urea concentration, organic acid concentration, and pH. Bacterial growth is inhibited by either very dilute urine or a high osmolality when associated with a low pH.** Much of the antimicrobial activity of urine is related to a high urea and organic acid content (Solomon et al, 1983). From a clinical perspective, however, these conditions do not appear to significantly distinguish between patients who are susceptible or resistant to infection.

Uromodulin (Tamm-Horsfall protein), a kidney-derived mannosylated protein that is present in an extraordinarily high concentration in the urine (>100 mg/mL), **may play a defensive role by saturating all the mannose-binding sites of the type 1 pili, thus potentially blocking bacterial binding to the uroplakin receptors of the urothelium** (Duncan, 1988; Kumar and Muchmore, 1990).

Recent studies have exploited next-generation DNA-sequencing technology to quantify any bacteria in normal urine and thus characterize the normal female urinary microbiome. Flora were identified in urine obtained by suprapubic aspiration from healthy participants that differed from voided urine and contained species that were uncultivatable under either aerobic or anaerobic conditions (Wolfe et al, 2012). Aspirated urine (or urine obtained by catheter) that was culture-negative revealed diverse genera in a majority of participants. And while urine culture remains the gold standard for assessing UTI, this work also suggests a more complex bladder ecology: a single participant whose urine culture was positive for *E. coli* had relative DNA abundance of approximately 45% *Aerococcus*, 21% *Actinobaculum*, and only 2% *E. coli*. The authors then ask whether clinical symptoms reflect the low-abundance uropathogen, the more abundant fastidious bacteria, or both. Because most healthy participants exhibited urinary flora, future studies should define the role of the urinary microbiome in resistance and susceptibility to UTI.

Bladder

Bacteria presumably make their way into the bladder fairly often. Whether small inocula of bacteria persist, multiply, and infect the host depends in part on the ability of the bladder to empty (Cox and Hinman, 1961). Additional factors responsible for defense involve both innate and adaptive immunity and exfoliation of epithelial cells.

Immune Response

Pathogen Recognition. The host recognition of the pathogen is mediated by a series of pathogen-associated molecular pattern receptors (PAMPs), such as Toll-like receptors (TLRs) (Anderson et al, 2004b), which provide the link between recognition of invading organisms and development of the innate immune response. TLRs recognize molecular patterns that are conserved among many species of pathogens, such as lipopolysaccharide (LPS) and peptidoglycan (PG), and activate signaling pathways that initiate immune and inflammatory responses to kill pathogens. Superficial bladder epithelial cells express TLR4 on their membranes, which along with CD14 recognize LPS from the bacteria and activate the innate immune response (Anderson et al, 2004a). The newly identified TLR11, which recognizes UPEC and protects the kidneys from ascending infection, is also expressed on uroepithelial cells, as well as renal cells (Zhang et al, 2004).

The innate system response to an infection in the bladder or kidneys is primarily local inflammation.

The innate immune response occurs more rapidly than the adaptive response and involves a variety of cell types, including

polymorphonuclear leukocytes, neutrophils, macrophages, eosinophils, natural killer cells, mast cells, and dendritic cells. In addition, increased transcription of inducible nitric oxide synthase by polymorphonuclear leukocytes results in high levels of nitric oxide and related breakdown products that also have toxic effects on the bacteria (Poljakovic et al, 2001; Poljakovic and Persson, 2003). The innate response aids in establishing adaptive immunity because of interactions of macrophages, dendritic cells, and natural killer cells with T and B lymphocytes. Adaptive immunity involves the specific recognition of pathogens by T and B lymphocytes and production of high-affinity antibodies, a process that occurs 7 to 10 days after infection.

For additional data regarding the immunologic response to UTI, the idea of immunization, and the roles of lipopolysaccharide, see the Expert Consult website.

Multiple Roles for Lipopolysaccharide. Because TLR signaling triggers innate immune responses and mediates innate-adaptive interactions, diverse pathogens target TLR signaling. Consistent with this, TLR modulation has been identified in UPEC. UPEC was found to modulate urothelial inflammatory responses at the levels of nuclear factor-κB (NF-κB) activation and cytokine suppression, and this inflammatory suppression is widespread among clinical *E. coli* strains (Klumpp et al, 2001; Hunstad et al, 2005; Billips et al, 2007). In contrast to bacteria that modulate inflammatory responses through the action of secreted virulence factors, UPEC genetic screens identified genes associated with modification of TLR ligands (Hunstad et al, 2005; Billips et al, 2008). One such screen revealed that UPEC genes inhibiting urothelial cytokine responses were *waaL*, *ampG*, and *alr*, genes encoding LPS O-antigen ligase, muropeptide permease, and alanine racemase, respectively (Billips et al, 2008). WaaL is involved in LPS biosynthesis, whereas both *ampG* and *alr* contribute to peptidoglycan metabolism, ligands for TLR4 and TLR2, respectively. UPEC strains with targeted deletions of *waaL* or *ampG* were attenuated in a murine UTI model (Billips et al, 2008), indicating that modulation of TLR-mediated responses is important to UTI pathogenesis by UPEC. In a similar genetic screen, LPS biosynthesis operons *rfa* and *rfb* and the membrane protein isomerase *surA* were found to mediate cytokine suppression (Hunstad et al, 2005). Some UPEC strains even encode direct inhibitors of TLR signaling (Cirl et al, 2008). Together, these findings suggest that **UPEC enhances virulence by modulating inflammatory responses at the level of TLR recognition, thereby extending a "window of opportunity"** to establish infection by evading innate surveillance mechanisms.

Studies in murine UTI also suggest that these observations can be exploited for the development of novel vaccines against UPEC because immunizing with the *waaL* mutant of UPEC strain NU14 conferred protection against challenge with wild-type NU14 (Billips et al, 2009). Immunization with the *waaL* mutant of NU14, a phylogenetic group B2 strain, also conferred protection against other B2 strains, as well as A and D strains, and prevented kidney infection. Consistent with TLR-mediated skewing of immune responses (Schnare et al, 2001), *waaL* mutant also promoted bladder sterilization of stable UPEC reservoirs, indicating enhanced cell-mediated immunity. These findings suggest that **UPEC mutants represent live-attenuated vaccine candidates for recurrent UTI.**

LPS has also emerged as a key determinant of the symptomatic response to *E. coli* in the urinary tract in recent studies using tactile allodynia as a measure of pelvic pain in murine UTI. The cystitis isolate NU14 evoked an acute pelvic pain response, whereas the asymptomatic bacteriuria *E. coli* strain 83972 did not, thus recapitulating the spectrum of human symptomatic response to bladder colonization (Rudick et al, 2010). Surprisingly, purified LPS preparations from NU14 and 83972 yielded the same pain/no pain responses as intact bacteria, yet the level of neutrophil influx and cytokines induced by each LPS was similar. Pain responses were also mediated by the LPS receptor TLR4. The O-antigen moiety that defines *E. coli* serotypes is an important determinant of the bacterial pain phenotype because, depending

upon O-antigen status, it was shown that a single *E. coli* strain could be shifted from an acute pain phenotype to a chronic pain phenotype, to a null pain phenotype (Rudick et al, 2012). Again, although pain responses were dependent upon TLR4, bacteria that elicited distinct pain responses induced similar pathology and neutrophil influx. These findings indicate that **LPS defines the pain phenotype of *E. coli* and that bacterial pain is not correlated with inflammation.** Moreover, because some strains lacking O antigen caused pain that persisted long after bacterial clearance, these findings demonstrate that *E. coli* can cause post-UTI chronic pain.

Induced Exfoliation. Mulvey and colleagues (1998) demonstrated that exfoliation and excretion of infected and damaged superficial cells is mediated by type 1 piliated bacteria that induce programmed cell death. By utilizing an in vivo mouse model, it has been demonstrated that mice exhibiting a strong exfoliation response to UPEC infiltration are unlikely to form IBCs (Anderson et al, 2004b). However, mice with a much milder exfoliation response tend to form biofilms, which become sequestered in the bladder and presumably could lead to recurrent UTIs. It has also been shown that many uropathogenic bacteria can suppress NF-κB, increase apoptosis, and decrease the inflammatory responses (Klumpp et al, 2001), a process that could lead to subsequent bacterial invasion into deeper tissues. Thus in some instances apoptosis may be a bacterial offense maneuver rather than a host defense.

The same UPIII–casein kinase II signaling cascade mediating UPEC invasion also drives FimH-induced urothelial apoptosis (Thumbikat et al, 2009b). Consistent with this, increased UPIII expression during urothelial differentiation sensitizes urothelial cells to UPEC and FimH-induced apoptosis (Thumbikat et al, 2009a). However, because FimH-induced urothelial apoptosis and successful establishment of the UPEC intracellular life cycle are mutually exclusive, UPEC and/or host factors must define individual urothelial cell fates and thus the bifurcation between invasion and apoptosis.

Alterations in Host Defense Mechanisms

Obstruction

Obstruction to urine flow at all anatomic levels is a key factor in increasing host susceptibility to UTI. Obstruction inhibits the normal flow of urine, and the resulting stasis compromises bladder and renal defense mechanisms. **Stasis also contributes to the growth of bacteria in the urine and their ability to adhere to the urothelial cells.** In the animal model of experimental hematogenous pyelonephritis, the kidney is relatively resistant to infection unless a ureter is ligated. Under these circumstances, only the obstructed kidney becomes infected (Beeson and Guze, 1956). Clinical observations support the role of obstruction in pathogenesis of UTI and in increasing severity of infection. **Mild episodes of cystitis or pyelonephritis can become life threatening when obstruction to urine flow becomes present.** Although obstruction clearly increases the severity of infection, it need not be a predisposing factor. For example, men with large residual urine may remain uninfected for years. However, if they are catheterized, even small inocula may lead to severe infections that are difficult to eradicate.

Vesicoureteral Reflux

Hodson and Edwards (1960) first described the association of vesicoureteral reflux, UTI, and renal clubbing and scarring. **Children with gross reflux and UTIs usually develop progressive renal damage manifested by renal scarring, proteinuria, and renal failure. Those with a lesser degree of reflux usually improve or completely recover spontaneously or after treatment of the UTI. In adults, the presence of reflux does not appear to decrease renal function unless there are stasis and concurrent UTIs.**

Underlying Disease

There is a high incidence of renal scarring in patients with underlying conditions that cause chronic interstitial nephritis, virtually all of which produce primary renal papillary damage. These conditions include diabetes mellitus, sickle cell disorders, adult nephrocalcinosis, hyperphosphatemia, hypokalemia, analgesic abuse, sulfonamide nephropathy, gout, heavy-metal poisoning, and aging (Freedman, 1979).

Diabetes Mellitus

An increased incidence of clinical asymptomatic and symptomatic UTIs appears to occur in women with diabetes mellitus, but there is no substantial increase among diabetic men (Vejlsgaard, 1973; Ooi et al, 1974; Forland et al, 1977; Meiland et al, 2002). Diabetes also results in three times more hospitalizations for acute pyelonephritis among women (10.86/10,000) than for men (3.32/10,000) (Nicolle et al, 1996). Autopsy studies have shown the incidence of pyelonephritis to be fourfold to fivefold higher in diabetic than in nondiabetic individuals (Robbins and Tucker, 1944). However, such studies may be misleading because it is difficult to distinguish renal parenchymal changes resulting from pyelonephritis from the interstitial inflammatory changes of diabetic nephropathy.

Although most UTIs in diabetic patients are asymptomatic, diabetes appears to predispose the patient to more severe infections. There is no evidence that increased frequency of infection is due to glycosuria (Geerlings et al, 2000). One study using antibody-coated bacteria techniques to localize the site of infection showed the upper urinary tract to be involved in nearly 80% of diabetic patients with UTIs (Forland et al, 1977). This evidence of increasing immunologic response in diabetic patients who acquire bacteriuria suggests renal parenchymal involvement and a potential increase in morbidity.

Infections are frequently caused by atypical organisms such as yeast and result in upper tract infections and significant sequelae such as emphysematous pyelonephritis, papillary necrosis, perinephric abscess, or metastatic infection (Wheat, 1980; Stapleton, 2002).

Renal Papillary Necrosis

The role of infection in the development and progression of renal papillary necrosis (RPN) is controversial. **Multiple predisposing conditions have been associated with the development of RPN, particularly diabetes, analgesic abuse, sickle cell hemoglobinopathy, and obstruction** (Box 12-2).

BOX 12-2 Conditions Associated with Renal Papillary Necrosis

Diabetes mellitus
Pyelonephritis
Urinary tract obstruction
Analgesic abuse
Sickle cell hemoglobinopathies
Renal transplant rejection
Cirrhosis of the liver
Dehydration, hypoxia, and jaundice of infants
Miscellaneous: renal vein thrombosis, cryoglobulinemia, renal candidiasis, contrast media injection, amyloidosis, calyceal arteritis, necrotizing angiitis, rapidly progressive glomerulonephritis, hypotensive shock, acute pancreatitis

From Eknoyan G, Qunibi WY, Grissom RT, et al. Renal papillary necrosis: an update. Medicine 1982;61:55.

Clinically, RPN is a spectrum of disease. Patients may have an acute fulminating illness with rapid progression or may have a chronic disease that is incidentally discovered. Some patients may chronically pass necrotic tissue in their urine (Hernandez et al, 1975), and some may never pass papillae (Lindvall, 1978). Retained necrotic papillae may calcify, especially in association with infection. Furthermore, this necrotic tissue may form the nidus for chronic infection. Opportunistic fungal infections have been reported (Madge and Lombardias, 1973; Juhasz et al, 1980; Vordermark et al, 1980; Tomashefski and Abramowsky, 1981). Renal sonography may be useful to diagnose RPN (Buonocore et al, 1980; Hoffman et al, 1982).

The early diagnosis of RPN is important to improve prognosis and reduce morbidity. In addition to chronic infection, patients with analgesic abuse–associated papillary necrosis may have an increased incidence of urothelial tumors; routine urinary cytologic examinations may be helpful to diagnose these tumors early (Jackson et al, 1978). In patients who have analgesic abuse–induced RPN, the disease stabilizes if the analgesic intake is stopped (Gower, 1976). Furthermore, adequate antimicrobial therapy to control infection and early recognition and treatment of ureteral obstruction caused by sloughed necrotic tissue can minimize a decline in renal function. **A patient who suffers from an acute ureteral obstruction caused by a sloughed papilla and who has a concomitant UTI has a urologic emergency.** In this case, immediate removal of the obstructing papilla by stone basket (Jameson and Heal, 1973) or acute drainage of the kidney by ureteral catheter or percutaneous nephrostomy is necessary.

Other conditions that may increase the susceptibility of the kidney to infection include hypertension and vascular obstruction (Freedman, 1979). The association of renal infection with several other renal diseases, including glomerulonephritis, atherosclerosis, and tubular necrosis, which are not associated with papillary necrosis, does not lead to pyelonephritis and scarring.

Human Immunodeficiency Virus

UTIs are fivefold more prevalent in HIV-positive individuals than in control subjects (Schonwald et al, 1999). Furthermore, the pathologic flora is typically more reminiscent of complicated UTIs. It also appears that HIV-positive patients with UTIs have a tendency for recurrence and require longer treatment.

Pregnancy

The prevalence of bacteriuria in pregnant women varies from 4% to 7%, and the incidence of acute clinical pyelonephritis ranges from 25% to 35% in untreated bacteriuric women (Stamey, 1980). This is probably the result of dilation of the ureters and pelvis of the kidney secondary to pregnancy-related hormonal alterations. In addition, urine obtained from pregnant women exhibits a more suitable pH for growth of *E. coli* in all stages of gestation (Asscher et al, 1973). **It is not surprising that untreated bacteriuria in the first trimester is accompanied by a substantial increase in the incidence of acute pyelonephritis because half of these women have upper tract bacteriuria** (Fairley et al, 1966).

For further details, see the Expert Consult website.

Spinal Cord Injury with High-Pressure Bladders

Of all patients with bacteriuria, no group compares in severity and morbidity with those who have spinal cord injury. Nearly all these patients require catheterization early after their injuries because of bladder overactivity or flaccidity, and significant numbers develop ureterectasis, hydronephrosis, reflux, and renal calculi. Bacteriologic and urodynamic advances in the management of these patients have vastly reduced their morbidity and mortality. Special problems associated with spinal cord injury are presented in a later section.

CLINICAL MANIFESTATIONS

Symptoms and Signs

Cystitis is usually associated with dysuria, frequency, and/or urgency. Suprapubic pain and hematuria are less common. Lower tract symptoms are commonly present and usually predate the appearance of upper tract symptoms by several days. Pyelonephritis is classically associated with fever, chills, and flank pain. Nausea and vomiting may be present. Renal or perirenal abscess may cause indolent fever and flank mass and tenderness. In the elderly, the symptoms may be much more subtle (e.g., epigastric or abdominal discomfort) or the patient may be asymptomatic (Romano and Kaye, 1981). Patients with indwelling catheters often have asymptomatic bacteriuria, but fever associated with bacteremia may occur rapidly and become life threatening.

Diagnosis

Presumptive diagnosis of UTI is made by direct or indirect analysis of the urine and is confirmed by urine culture. The urine and the urinary tract are normally free of bacteria and inflammation. False-negative urinalysis and culture can occur in the presence of UTI, particularly early in an infection when the numbers of bacteria and WBCs are low or diluted by increased fluid intake and subsequent diuresis. Occasionally, the urine may be free of bacteria and WBCs despite bacterial colonization and inflammation of the uroepithelium (Elliott et al, 1985; Hultgren et al, 1985). False-positive urinalysis and culture are caused by contamination of the urine specimen with bacteria and WBCs during collection. This is most likely to occur in voided specimens but can also occur during urethral catheterization. Suprapubic aspiration of bladder urine is least likely to cause contamination of the specimen; therefore it provides the most accurate assessment of the status of bladder urine.

Urine Collection

Voided and Catheterized Specimens. Diagnostic accuracy can be improved by reducing bacterial contamination when the urine is collected. In circumcised men, voided specimens require no preparation. For men who are not circumcised, the foreskin should be retracted and the glans penis washed with soap and then rinsed with water before specimen collection. The first 10 mL of urine (representative of the urethra) and a midstream specimen (representative of the bladder) should be obtained. Prostatic fluid is obtained by performing digital prostatic massage and collecting the expressed prostatic fluid on a glass slide. In addition, collection of the first 10 mL of voided urine after massage will reflect the prostatic fluid added to the urethral specimen. Catheterization of a male patient for urine culture is not indicated unless the patient cannot urinate.

In women, contamination of a midstream urine specimen with introital bacteria and WBCs is common, particularly when the woman has difficulty spreading and maintaining separation of the labia. Therefore the female should be instructed to spread the labia, wash and cleanse the periurethral area with moist gauze, and then collect a midstream urine specimen. Cleansing with antiseptics is not recommended because they may contaminate the voided specimen and provide a false-negative urine culture. The voided specimen is contaminated if it shows evidence of vaginal epithelial cells and lactobacilli on urinalysis, and a midcatheterized specimen should be collected.

Catheterization and collection of a midcathterized specimen is more accurate than a voided specimen, but carries a risk of iatrogenic infection. Although a single dose of an oral antimicrobial agent such as trimethoprim-sulfamethoxazole (TMP-SMX) may be effective for prophylaxis because antimicrobial usage encourages development of bacterial resistance, prophylaxis should be limited to high-risk patients.

Suprapubic Aspiration. Suprapubic aspiration is highly accurate, but because it carries some morbidity there is limited clinical usefulness except for a patient who cannot urinate on command, such as patients with spinal cord injuries. It is highly useful in newborns (Newman et al, 1967) and in patients with paraplegia. A single aspirated specimen reveals the bacteriologic status of the bladder urine without introducing urethral bacteria, which can start a new infection.

Before a suprapubic aspiration is performed, the patient should force fluids until the bladder is full. The site of the needle puncture is in the midline, between the symphysis pubis and the umbilicus and directly over the palpable bladder. The full bladder in the male is usually palpable because of its greater muscle tone; unfortunately, the full bladder in the female is frequently not palpable. In such patients, the physician performing the aspiration must rely on the observation that suprapubic pressure directly over the bladder produces an unmistakable desire to urinate. After determining the approximate site for needle puncture, the local area is shaved and the skin is cleansed with an alcohol sponge; a cutaneous wheal is raised with a 25-gauge needle and any local anesthetic. A 3.5-inch spinal, 22-gauge needle is introduced through the anesthetized skin. The progress of the needle is arrested just below the skin within the anesthetized area, and with a quick plunging action, similar to that of any intramuscular injection, the needle is advanced into the bladder. Most patients experience more discomfort from the initial anesthetization of the skin than during the second stage when the needle is advanced into the bladder. After the needle has been introduced, a 20-mL syringe is used to aspirate 5 mL of urine for culture and 15 mL of urine for centrifugation and urinalysis. The obturator is reintroduced into the needle, and both needle and obturator are withdrawn. A small dressing is placed over the needle site in the skin. If urine is not obtained with complete introduction of the needle, the patient's bladder is not full and is usually deep within the retropubic area. When no urine is obtained on the first attempt, it is probably wise to wait until the bladder is full.

Urinalysis

For patients with urinary symptoms, microscopic urinalysis for bacteriuria, pyuria, and hematuria should be performed. Urinalysis provides rapid identification of bacteria and WBCs and presumptive diagnosis of UTI. Usually, the sediment from an approximately 5- to 10-mL specimen obtained by centrifugation for 5 minutes at 2000 rpm is analyzed. Microscopic bacteriuria is found in more than 90% of infections with counts of 10^5 colony-forming units (cfu) per milliliter of urine or greater and is a highly specific finding (Stamm, 1982; Jenkins et al, 1986). However, bacteria are usually not detectable microscopically with lower colony count infections (10^2 to 10^4/mL). This important error (i.e., a false-negative result) occurs because of the limitation imposed by the microscope on the volume of urine that can be observed. If the volume of urine that can easily rest beneath a standard 22-mm cover glass is carefully measured (0.01 mL) and the number of high dry fields (×570 magnification) present beneath the cover glass is estimated, it is disturbing to find that one high dry field represents a volume of approximately 1/30,000 mL. There are excellent studies showing that the bacterial count must be approximately 30,000/mL before bacteria can be found in the sediment, stained or unstained, spun or unspun (Sanford et al, 1956; Kunin, 1961). **For these** reasons, a negative urinalysis for bacteria never excludes the presence of bacteria in numbers of 30,000/mL and less.

The second error of urinalysis (i.e., a false-positive result) is the reverse of the first error: bacteria are seen in the microscopic sediment, but the urine culture shows no growth. The voided urine from a female patient can contain many thousands of lactobacilli and corynebacteria. These bacteria are readily seen under the microscope; and although they are gram-positive, they often appear gram-negative (gram-variable) if stained. Strict anaerobes, usually gram-negative bacilli, also make up a significant mass of the normal vaginal flora (Marrie et al, 1978).

In practice, these problems can be minimized by using other information provided by urinalysis that can help the clinician to decide whether a patient has a UTI such as pyuria (Stamm et al, 1982b). The validation of the midstream urine specimen can be questioned if numerous squamous epithelial cells (indicative of preputial, vaginal, or urethral contaminants) are present.

Pyuria and hematuria are good indicators of an inflammatory response. Although the number of WBCs per high-power field in a centrifuged urine sample is useful, it is important to remember that other factors can influence the number of cells seen. These include the state of hydration; the intensity of tissue reaction; the method of urine collection; the volume, speed, and time of centrifugation; and the volume in which the sediment is resuspended.

The presence of bacteriuria has a sensitivity for UTI of 40% to 70%, and a specificity of 85% to 95%, depending on the number of bacteria observed (Fihn, 2003).

Significant pyuria can be determined simply and reliably with a microscope by accurately examining the centrifuged sediment or by using a hemocytometer to count the number of WBCs in the unspun urine. One to 2 WBCs per high-power field (HPF) in sediment from a centrifuged specimen represents about 10 WBCs/mm^3 in an unspun specimen. More than 2 WBCs per HPF in a centrifuged specimen or 10 WBCs/mm^3 of urine correlates well with the presence of bacteriuria and is rarely seen in nonbacteriuric patients (Stamm et al, 1981). In clinical studies, determination of pyuria in voided urine specimens has a reported sensitivity of 80% to 95% and a specificity of 50% to 76% for UTI (depending on the definition of infection, the patient population, and the method used to evaluate for pyuria) (Stamm, 1982; Schultz et al, 1984; Wong et al, 1984; Wigton et al, 1985).

The absence of pyuria should cause the diagnosis of UTI to be questioned until urine culture data are available. Conversely, many diseases of the urinary tract produce significant pyuria in the absence of bacteriuria. Whereas tuberculosis is the well-recognized example of abacterial pyuria, staghorn calculi and stones of smaller size can produce intense pyuria with clumps of WBCs in the absence of UTI. Almost any injury to the urinary tract, from chlamydial urethritis to glomerulonephritis and interstitial cystitis, can elicit large numbers of fresh polymorphonuclear leukocytes (glitter cells). Depending on the stage of hydration, the intensity of the tissue reaction producing the cells, and the method of urine collection, any number of WBCs can be seen in the microscopic sediment in the presence of an uninfected urinary tract.

Microscopic hematuria is found in 40% to 60% of cases of cystitis and is uncommon in other dysuric syndromes (Stamm et al, 1980b; Wigton et al, 1985).

Rapid Screen Methods. Biochemical and enzymatic tests have been devised to detect bacteriuria and pyuria (Pezzlo, 1988). The Griess test detects the presence of **nitrite** in urine that is formed when bacteria reduce the nitrate normally present in urine. Tests for detecting pyuria by determining **leukocyte esterase activity** have also been developed (Chernow et al, 1984). In a study comparing traditional urine culture with these indirect tests, the combination of nitrite and leukocyte esterase tests (either test positive) had a sensitivity of 71% and a specificity of 83% when compared with 10^3 cfu/mL or greater of urine cultures (Pfaller and Koontz, 1985). However, several investigators (Pels et al, 1989; Hurlbut and Littenberg, 1991) noted substantial variability in the sensitivity and specificity results, which could be markedly influenced by the types of patients and infections chosen to evaluate the tests. This concept

of spectrum bias was illustrated by a study that reported differences in the sensitivity of reagent strip testing, ranging from 56% to 92%, by changing only the groups of patients included in the analysis. Although false-positive results are relatively uncommon, the borderline sensitivity of these tests, especially among patients with less characteristic symptoms of UTIs, does not allow these inexpensive tests to replace careful microscopic urinalysis in symptomatic patients (Semeniuk and Church, 1999). **Their main role is in screening asymptomatic patients** (Pezzlo, 1988).

Urine Culture

Two techniques for urine culture are available. **Direct surface plating** of a known amount of urine on split-agar disposable plates is the traditional quantitative culture technique used by most microbiology laboratories. One half of the plate is blood agar, which grows both gram-positive and gram-negative bacteria, and the other is desoxycholate or eosin-methylene blue (EMB), which grows gram-negative bacteria (some of them, such as *E. coli*, in a very characteristic manner). Simple curved-tip eye droppers are sufficient to deliver about 0.1 mL of urine onto each half of the plate. After overnight incubation, the number of colonies is estimated, often identified (after some experience), and multiplied by 10 to report the number of cfu per milliliter of urine. The technique has been presented elsewhere in detail (Stamey, 1980).

A simpler but somewhat less accurate technique is the use of **dip slides** (Fig. 12-10). These inexpensive plastic slides are attached to screw-top caps; they have soy agar (a general nutrient agar to grow all bacteria) on one side and EMB or MacConkey agar for gram-negative bacteria on the opposite side. A slide is dipped into urine, the excess is allowed to drain off, and the slide is replaced in its plastic bottle and incubated. The volume of urine that attaches to the slide is between 1/100 mL and 1/200 mL. Hence, the colony count is 100 to 200 times the number of colonies that become visible with incubation. In actual practice, the growth is compared with a visual standard and reported as such. The species of bacteria is more difficult to recognize when this technique is used, but the technique is completely adequate.

The urine must be refrigerated immediately on collection and should be cultured within 24 hours of refrigeration. One advantage to the dip slide is the ease with which the urine can be immediately cultured without the necessity of refrigeration. Patients can culture their own urine at home, keep the slide at room temperature, and bring it to the office within 48 hours.

Although most bacteria allowed to incubate for several hours in bladder urine reach cfu counts of 10^5/mL, this statistical

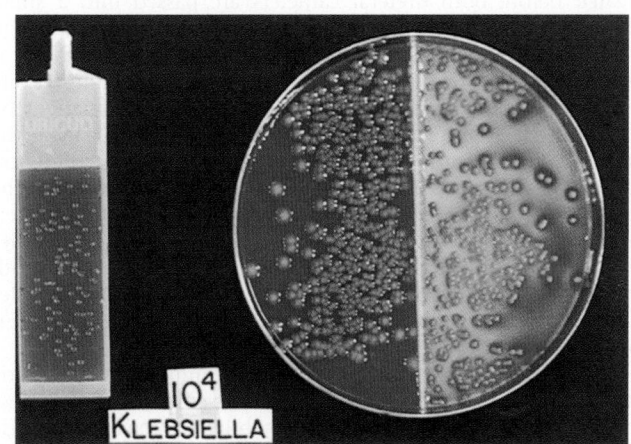

Figure 12-10. The dip slide on the left is compared with a split-agar surface plate on the right. The urine contained 10,000 colonies of *Klebsiella* per milliliter (about 200 times the number of colonies on the dip slide and 10 times the number on either side of the split-agar plate).

number is fraught with two limitations. The first is that 20% to 40% of women with symptomatic UTIs present with bacteria counts of 10^2 to 10^4 cfu/mL of urine (Stamey et al, 1965; Mabeck, 1969; Kunz et al, 1975; Kraft and Stamey, 1977), probably because of the slow doubling time of bacteria in urine (every 30 to 45 minutes) combined with frequent bladder emptying (every 15 to 30 minutes) from irritation. **Thus, in dysuric patients, an appropriate threshold value for defining significant bacteriuria is 10^2 cfu/mL of a known pathogen** (Stamm and Hooton, 1993). Fortunately, most of these patients have symptoms of UTI and pyuria on urinalysis.

The **second limitation of the 10^5 cutoff is overdiagnosis.** Women susceptible to infection often carry large numbers of pathogenic bacteria on the perineum that contaminate otherwise sterile bladder urine. Uncircumcised men may harbor uropathogenic bacteria on their foreskins. In the original studies by Kass (1960), a single culture of 10^5 cfu/mL or more had a 20% chance of representing contamination. There is no statistical way to avoid these two major limitations on the interpretation of the midstream voided culture in women and in uncircumcised men without careful preparation.

Localization

Kidney

Fever and Flank Pain. Fever and flank pain are thought to indicate pyelonephritis, but few studies have tested the hypothesis. Aggressive localization studies in children and adults (Huland and Busch, 1982; Busch and Huland, 1984), as well as in patients with end-stage renal disease (Huland et al, 1983), have shown substantial incidences of fever and even flank pain in bacteriuric patients in whom infection was localized to the bladder (see the later section on Acute Pyelonephritis).

Ureteral Catheterization. Ureteral catheterization allows not only separation of bacterial persistence into upper and lower urinary tracts but also separation of the infection between one kidney and the other, and even localization of infection to ectopic ureters or to nonrefluxing ureteral stumps (by using saline solution irrigation) (Stamey, 1980).

Stamey began in 1959 to localize the site of bacteriuria by ureteral catheterization studies; the technique was published in 1963 (Stamey and Pfau, 1963) and the results in 1965 (Stamey et al, 1965). The technique is simple but exacting; the urologist should consult a more detailed description (Stamey, 1980) before actually performing this localization technique. The validity depends on controlling the number of bacteria from the bladder that contaminate the ureteral catheters as they pass through the bladder into the ureteral orifices. The bladder must be thoroughly irrigated before both ureteral catheters are passed into a small volume of residual irrigating fluid. A sample is obtained through both ureteral catheters simultaneously, and then each catheter is passed into the ureter or renal pelvis. Four serial cultures are obtained from each kidney. It is mandatory that the patient be started on the appropriate antimicrobial agent before leaving the cystoscopy room. In addition to quantitative bacterial counts on each specimen, determination of either specific gravity or urine creatinine levels on the renal samples can be very helpful in interpreting a change in diuresis in relation to bacterial counts. Examples of infections localized to the bladder, to one kidney, and to both kidneys have been published (Stamey, 1980). Clinical examples of results from each site are shown in Table 12-1 on the Expert Consult website.

When this technique was applied to large numbers of bacteriuric patients, 45% were found to have bladder infection only; 27%, unilateral renal bacteriuria; and 28%, bilateral renal bacteriuria (Table 12-2 on the Expert Consult website) (Stamey et al, 1965). These figures have been confirmed by at least five investigators in three countries (the United States, England, and Australia) and can be taken as a good approximation for any general bacteriuric adult population. Although renal stones and other kidney abnormalities in the presence of bacteriuria can increase the proportion of

renal infections, the urologist should never assume the kidney is involved if an important decision is to be made.

Tissue and Stone Cultures. It is clinically useful to culture stones removed from the urinary tract to document that bacteria reside within their interstices. Tissue cultures are primarily useful for research information.

Using sterile technique at the operating table, the surgeon places the stone or fragment of tissue into a sterile culture tube containing 5 mL of saline solution; the culture is packed in ice and sent to the bacteriologic laboratory, where, after agitation of the stone or tissue in the 5 mL of saline solution, 0.1 mL is surface-streaked on both blood agar and EMB agar. The saline solution is then poured off the specimen, and, with sterile forceps, the stone or tissue is transferred to a second 5 mL of sterile saline solution. After agitation to ensure a reasonable washing action, the saline solution is again decanted and the specimen is transferred to a third 5 mL of saline solution and finally to a fourth 5 mL of saline solution. This last saline solution wash is cultured quantitatively in the same manner as the first. The remainder of this fourth 5 mL of saline solution is poured with the stone into a sterile mortar and pestle dish.

After the stone is crushed (or the tissue is ground in a tissue blender) in the fourth saline solution wash, 0.1 mL is again cultured on both blood agar and EMB agar. The difference in colony counts between the first and the fourth saline solution washes represents the washing effect of the saline solution transfers on the surface bacteria of the stone or tissue. The difference between the fourth saline wash before and after crushing (or grinding, for tissue) represents the difference between surface bacteria and bacteria within the specimen.

Prostate and Urethral Localization Studies. The technique for localizing infections to the urethra or prostate is covered in detail in Chapter 13.

KEY POINTS: CLINICAL MANIFESTATIONS

- The urine and the urinary tract are normally sterile.
- Bacteriuria and WBCs provide a presumptive diagnosis of UTI.
- In diagnosing patients, 10^2 cfu/mL confirms a symptomatic UTI.

IMAGING TECHNIQUES

Imaging studies are not required in most cases of UTI because clinical and laboratory findings alone are sufficient for correct diagnosis and adequate management of most patients. However, infection in most men or a compromised host, febrile infections, signs or symptoms of urinary tract obstruction, failure to respond to appropriate therapy, and a pattern of recurrent infections suggesting bacterial persistence within the urinary tract warrant imaging for identification of underlying abnormalities that require modification of medical management or percutaneous or surgical intervention.

Indications

Radiologic studies are unnecessary for evaluation of most women with genitourinary infections. Several reports of women patients with recurrent UTIs show that excretory urograms are unnecessary for routine evaluation if women who have special risk factors are excluded (Fair et al, 1979; Engel et al, 1980; Fowler and Pulaski, 1981; Fairchild et al, 1982). In none of these studies did excretory urograms yield information that was useful in the management of these patients. Furthermore, excluding excretory urograms in the routine evaluation of such patients represents a substantial financial saving.

However, in high-risk patients, including women with febrile infections and most men, radiologic studies may determine acute

BOX 12-3 Indications for Radiologic Investigation in Acute Clinical Pyelonephritis

Potential ureteral obstruction (e.g., caused by stone, ureteral stricture, tumor)

History of calculi, especially infection (struvite) stones

Potential papillary necrosis (e.g., patients with sickle cell anemia, severe diabetes mellitus, analgesic abuse)

History of genitourinary surgery that predisposes to obstruction, such as ureteral reimplantation or ureteral diversion

Poor response to appropriate antimicrobial agents after 5 to 6 days of treatment

Diabetes mellitus

Polycystic kidneys in patients in dialysis or with severe renal insufficiency

Neuropathic bladder

Unusual infecting organisms, such as tuberculosis, fungus, or urea-splitting organisms (e.g., *Proteus*)

BOX 12-4 Correctable Urologic Abnormalities That Cause Bacterial Persistence

Infection stones

Chronic bacterial prostatitis

Unilateral infected atrophic kidneys

Ureteral duplication and ectopic ureters

Foreign bodies

Urethral diverticula and infected periurethral glands

Unilateral medullary sponge kidneys

Nonrefluxing, normal-appearing, infected ureteral stumps after nephrectomy

Infected urachal cysts

Infected communicating cysts of the renal calyces

Papillary necrosis

Perivesical abscess with fistula to bladder

infectious processes that require further intervention or may find the cause of complicated infections.

First, radiologic procedures are needed in patients with risk factors that may require intervention in addition to antimicrobial treatment (Box 12-3).

A UTI associated with possible urinary tract obstruction must be evaluated. These are patients with calculi, especially infection (struvite) stones; ureteral tumors; ureteral strictures; congenital obstructions; or previous genitourinary surgery, such as ureteral reimplantation or urinary diversion procedures that may have caused obstruction. Patients with **diabetes mellitus** can develop special complications from UTIs; they may acquire emphysematous pyelonephritis or papillary necrosis. **Impacted necrotic papillae** may cause acute ureteral obstruction. Patients with **polycystic kidney disease who are on dialysis** are particularly prone to developing perinephric abscesses.

Urologic imaging is indicated in patients whose symptoms of acute clinical pyelonephritis persist after 5 to 6 days of appropriate antimicrobial therapy; they often have perinephric or renal abscesses. In addition, **patients with unusual organisms,** including urea-splitting organisms (e.g., *Proteus* species), should be examined for abnormalities within the urinary tract, such as obstructing stones, strictures, or fungus balls.

The second reason for radiologic evaluation is to diagnose a focus of bacterial persistence. **In patients whose bacteriuria fails to resolve after appropriate antimicrobial therapy or who have rapid recurrence of infection, abnormalities that cause bacterial persistence should be sought.** Although these patients are uncommon, it is important to identify them because they may have correctable urologic abnormalities that represent the only surgically curable causes of recurrent UTIs. Acquired or congenital urologic abnormalities that can cause unresolved or recurrent UTIs are listed in Box 12-4.

Ultrasonography

The renal ultrasound study is an important renal imaging technique because it is noninvasive, easy to perform, and rapid and offers no radiation or contrast agent risk to the patient. It is particularly useful in identifying calculi and hydronephrosis, pyonephrosis, and perirenal abscesses. A single radiograph for calculi should accompany ultrasonography. Ultrasonography is also useful for diagnosing postvoid residual urine. A disadvantage is that the study is dependent on the interpretative and performance skills of the examiner. Furthermore, the study may be technically poor in patients who are obese or who have dressings, drainage tubes, or open wounds overlying the area of interest.

Computed Tomography and Magnetic Resonance Imaging

The radiologic modalities that offer the best anatomic detail are CT and MRI. They are more sensitive than excretory urography or ultrasonography in the diagnosis of acute focal bacterial nephritis, renal and perirenal abscesses, and radiolucent calculi (Kuhn and Berger, 1981; Mauro et al, 1982; Wadsworth et al, 1982; Soulen et al, 1989; Soler et al, 1997). When used to localize renal and perirenal abscesses, CT improves the approach to surgical drainage and permits percutaneous approaches. MRI has not superseded CT in the evaluation of renal inflammation, but it has provided some advantages in delineating extrarenal extension of inflammation.

Voiding Cystourethrogram

The voiding cystourethrogram is an important examination in assessing vesicoureteral reflux. It may be used to evaluate patients with neuropathic bladders and the rare female patient who has a urethral diverticulum causing her persistent infections.

Radionuclide Studies

Hippuran I-131 and technetium-99m (^{99m}Tc) glucoheptonate scans are used to detect focal parenchymal damage, renal function impairment, and decreased renal perfusion in acute renal infections (McAfee, 1979). Although gallium-67 scanning has been reported to be useful in the diagnosis of pyelonephritis and renal abscess, it is uncommonly required and may be positive in noninfectious entities. Indium-111–labeled WBC studies have limited efficacy in establishing the presence of an inflammatory focus, particularly when the patient's clinical presentation does not suggest an infectious process.

KEY POINTS: IMAGING TECHNIQUES

- Imaging studies are not required in most women with UTIs.
- Men and compromised patients or those who do not respond to therapy require imaging to identify abnormalities.
- CT and MRI provide the best anatomic data on the site, cause, and extent of infection.

PRINCIPLES OF ANTIMICROBIAL THERAPY

Therapy for UTIs must ultimately eliminate bacterial growth in the urinary tract. This can occur within hours if the proper antimicrobial agent is used (Stamey, 1980). **Efficacy of the antimicrobial therapy is critically dependent on the antimicrobial levels in the**

TABLE 12-3 Serum and Urinary Antimicrobial Levels in Adults*

ANTIMICROBIAL AGENT	DOSE (mg)	PEAK SERUM LEVEL (mg/L)	PERCENTAGE BOUND TO PROTEIN	HALF-LIFE SERUM PEAK (hr)	MEAN (ACTIVE) URINE LEVELS* (g/mL)	DOSE EXCRETED IN URINE (%)	DOSE ACTIVE IN URINE (IF DIFFERENT) (%)
Ampicillin	250 PO qid	3 at 2 hr	15	1	350	42	–
Carbenicillin	764 PO qid	11-17 at 1.5 hr	60	1.2	1000	40	–
Cephalexin	250 PO qid	9 at 2 hr	12	0.9	800	98	–
Ciprofloxacin	500 PO bid	2.3 at 1.2 hr	35	3.9	200	50	–
Colistin	75 IM bid	1.8 at 4 hr	10	2	34	75	50
Gentamicin	1 mg/kg IM tid (200 mg/day)	4 at 1 hr	Negligible	2	125	80	–
Kanamycin	500 IM bid	18 at 1 hr	Negligible	2	750	94	–
Levofloxacin	500 mg PO qd	6.0 mg/L	30-50	6	N/A	95	95
Nalidixic acid	1000 PO qid	34 at 2-23 hr	85	1.5	75	79	5
Nitrofurantoin	100 PO qid	<2		0.3	150	42	–
Penicillin G	500 PO qid	1 at 1 hr	60	0.5	300	60-85	–
Sulfamethizole	250 PO qid		98	10	700	95	85
Tetracycline hydrochloride	250 PO qid	2-3 at 4 hr	31	6	500	60	–
Trimethoprim-sulfamethoxazole	160/800 PO bid	1.7/32 at 2 hr	45/66	10/9	150/400	55/50	–/37
Trimethoprim	100 PO bid	1.0 at 2-4 hr	45	10	92	55	–

*These average urinary concentrations are based on the amount of biologically active drug excreted by normal kidneys at a urine flow rate of 1200 mL/24 hr.

Modified from Stamey TA. The pathogenesis and treatment of urinary infections. Baltimore: Williams & Wilkins; 1980. p. 59.

urine and the duration that this level remains above the minimal inhibitory concentration of the infecting organism (Hooton and Stamm, 1991). Hence, resolution of infection is closely associated with the susceptibility of the bacteria to the concentration of the antimicrobial agent achieved in the urine (McCabe and Jackson, 1965; Stamey et al, 1965, 1974). The concentration of useful antimicrobial agents in the serum and urine of healthy adults is shown in Table 12-3, which demonstrates that the urinary levels are often several hundred times greater than the serum levels. Inhibitory concentrations in urine are achieved after oral administration of all commonly used antimicrobial agents, except for the macrolides (erythromycin). The question of serum levels versus urinary levels is a practical one because the policy of testing antimicrobial susceptibility agents at concentrations obtainable only in the serum discourages the physician from using drugs that are effective at the urinary level; for example, oral penicillin G for *E. coli* and *Proteus mirabilis* and tetracycline for *P. aeruginosa*.

The concentration of the antimicrobial agent achieved in blood is not important in treatment of uncomplicated UTIs. However, blood levels are critical in patients with bacteremia and febrile urinary infections consistent with parenchymal involvement of the kidney and prostate.

In patients with renal insufficiency, dosage modifications are necessary for agents that are cleared primarily by the kidneys and cannot be cleared by another mechanism. In renal failure, the kidneys may not be able to concentrate an antimicrobial agent in the urine; hence, difficulty in eradicating bacteria may occur. Urinary tract obstruction may also reduce concentration of antimicrobial agents within the urine.

A decision regarding the antimicrobial selection and the duration of therapy must consider the spectrum of activity of the drug against the known pathogen or the most probable pathogen based on the presumed source of acquisition of infection, whether the infection is judged to be uncomplicated or complicated, potential adverse effects, and cost. An often underemphasized but important characteristic is the drug's impact on the bowel and vaginal flora and the hospital bacterial environment. Bacterial susceptibility will vary dramatically in patients exposed to antimicrobial agents and in individuals in inpatient and outpatient settings. It is imperative that each clinician keep abreast of changes that affect antimicrobial use and susceptibility patterns.

Bacterial Resistance

In the past several years, the frequency and spectrum of antimicrobial-resistant UTIs have increased in both the hospital and community. The increasing frequency of drug resistance has been attributed to combinations of microbial characteristics, bacterial selection pressure caused by antimicrobial use, and societal and technologic changes that enhance the transmission of drug resistance (Shepherd and Pottinger, 2013). Resistance patterns have been shown to vary by geographical location (Manges et al, 2001).

Bacterial resistance may occur because of inherited chromosomal-mediated resistance or by acquired chromosomal- or extrachromosomal (plasmid)-mediated resistance caused by exposure of an organism to antimicrobial agents.

Inherited chromosomal resistance exists in a bacterial species because of the absence of the proper mechanism on which the antimicrobial agent can act. For example, *Proteus* and *Pseudomonas* species are always resistant to nitrofurantoin.

Acquired chromosomal resistance occurs during therapy for UTIs. Before antimicrobial therapy, relatively resistant bacteria called *mutators* may be present in the urine at very low concentrations. Frequencies in mutations for high-level antimicrobial resistance are 1000-fold higher in mutators than in normal strains, indicating the increased adaptability of these strains (Miller et al, 2004). The remainder of the bacteria, which are susceptible to the administered antimicrobial agent, will be eradicated by therapy, but within 24 to 48 hours a repeat urine culture will show high bacterial counts of the resistant mutant. In essence, the antimicrobial therapy has selected out the resistant mutant. This phenomenon is most likely to occur when the antimicrobial level in the urine is close to or below the minimal inhibitory concentration of the drug. **Selection of resistant clones in the course of therapy for a previously sensitive bacteriuric population occurs between 5% and 10% of the time, clearly not an insignificant factor and one that must be considered in resolving bacteriuria.** Underdosing and noncompliance, as well as diuresis induced by increased fluid intake, can contribute to this process. Therefore the clinician should select an antimicrobial agent with a urinary concentration that exceeds the minimal inhibitory concentration by the widest margin possible, avoid underdosing, and emphasize patient compliance.

Extrachromosomal-mediated resistance may be acquired and transferable via plasmids, which contain the genetic material for the resistance. **This so-called R-factor resistance occurs in the bowel flora and is much more common than selection of preexisting mutants in the urinary tract. All antimicrobial classes are capable of causing plasmid-mediated resistance. However, for the fluoroquinolones, resistance is rarely transmitted by plasmids, and nitrofurantoin plasmid-mediated resistance has not been reported.** Therefore patients previously exposed to β-lactams, aminoglycosides, sulfonamides, TMP, and tetracycline will often have R-factor resistance to both the antimicrobial agent to which the bacteria were exposed and also to other antimicrobial agents. In addition, the plasmids carrying the resistant genetic material are transferable both within species and across genera. Thus, for example, a patient receiving tetracycline may harbor several bowel strains that are resistant to tetracycline, ampicillin, sulfonamides, and TMP. **Because the bowel flora is the major reservoir for bacteria that ultimately colonize the urinary tract, infections that occur after antimicrobial therapy and that can cause plasmid-mediated resistance are commonly caused by organisms with multidrug resistance. However, resistant *E. coli* in the bowel flora that infect the urinary tract almost always show susceptibility to nitrofurantoin or to the quinolones.**

Antimicrobial resistance is also influenced by the duration and amount of antimicrobial agent used. For example, documented increased use of fluoroquinolones in the hospital setting has been directly associated with increased resistance of bacteria (particularly *Pseudomonas*) to the fluoroquinolones. Resistance tends to increase the longer the agent is used. Conversely, reduction in duration of therapy and in the amount of the drug used may lead to reemergence of more susceptible strains.

Most studies reporting antimicrobial resistance have been based on surveys of laboratory isolates, generally without correlation with clinical or epidemiologic factors (e.g., the presence and nature of symptoms, age, sex, and whether the infection was complicated). Gupta and colleagues (2011) determined the prevalence of and trends in antimicrobial resistance among uropathogens isolated from a large, well-defined population of women with acute uncomplicated cystitis. The prevalence of resistance to TMP-SMX and ampicillin is greater than 20% in many countries worldwide (Gupta et al, 2011) and resistance to cephalothin has increased significantly, whereas resistance to nitrofurantoin and ciprofloxacin has remained uncommon. **However, fluoroquinolone resistance of *E. coli* is still less than 10% in most parts of North America and Europe** (Gupta et al, 2011). **Fluoroquinolone resistance was also associated with more frequent multidrug resistance** (Karlowsky et al, 2006). More recent single-center hospital studies have found resistance patterns to be even higher, roughly 26% (Siddiqui, 2008). In a transplant unit, where fluoroquinolones are commonly administered prophylactically, *E. coli* resistance can be 80%. **Previous use of fluoroquinolones and the presence of underlying urologic diseases were the strongest determinants for UTIs caused by resistant strains** (Ena et al, 1995). Fluoroquinolone resistance is an increasing problem in some European countries. A multiple-resistant phenotype involving fluoroquinolone resistance is now present in most countries in Europe, and this phenotype is selected for not only by the use of quinolones but also by the use of ampicillin, sulfamethoxazole, and TMP-MX (Kahlmeter and Menday, 2003). This is a concern because fluoroquinolones, which are associated with chromosomal-mediated but not plasmid-mediated resistance, are the current drug of choice for patients who have been exposed to agents causing plasmid-mediated resistance.

The clinical significance of these in vitro trends in resistance has been addressed in studies that correlated in vitro resistance to TMP-SMX with clinical outcome in uncomplicated cystitis and pyelonephritis (Gupta and Stamm, 2002). Clinical failures occurred in 40% to 50% of women if the bacteria were resistant and the bacteriologic failure approached 60%. (For further information on the role of TMP-SMX in prophylaxis, see Bladder Infections later in this chapter.)

Antimicrobial Formulary

The mechanism of action, reliable coverage, and common adverse reactions, precautions, and contraindications for antimicrobial agents used in the treatment of UTIs are indicated in Tables 12-4, 12-5, and 12-6, respectively.

TABLE 12-4 Mechanism of Action of Common Antimicrobials Used in the Treatment of Urinary Tract Infections

DRUG OR DRUG CLASS	MECHANISM OF ACTION	MECHANISMS OF DRUG RESISTANCE
β-Lactams (penicillins, cephalosporins, aztreonam)	Inhibition of bacterial cell wall synthesis	Production of β-lactamase Alteration in binding site of penicillin-binding protein Changes in cell wall porin size (decreased penetration)
Aminoglycosides	Inhibition of ribosomal protein synthesis	Downregulation of drug uptake into bacteria Bacterial production of aminoglycoside-modifying enzymes
Quinolones	Inhibition of bacterial DNA gyrase	Mutation in DNA gyrase-binding site Changes in cell wall porin size (decreased penetration) Active efflux
Fosfomycin	Inhibition of bacterial cell wall synthesis	Novel amino acid substitutions or the loss of function of transporters
Nitrofurantoin	Inhibition of several bacterial enzyme systems	Not fully elucidated—develops slowly With prolonged exposure
Trimethoprim-sulfamethoxazole	Antagonism of bacterial folate metabolism	Draws folate from environment (enterococci)
Vancomycin	Inhibition of bacterial cell wall synthesis (at β-lactams)	Enzymatic alteration of peptidoglycan at different point than target

TABLE 12-5 Reliable Coverage of Antimicrobials Used in the Treatment of Urinary Tract Infections of Commonly Encountered Pathogens*

ANTIMICROBIAL AGENT OR CLASS	GRAM-POSITIVE PATHOGENS	GRAM-NEGATIVE PATHOGENS
Amoxicillin or ampicillin	*Streptococcus* Enterococci	*Proteus mirabilis*
Amoxicillin with clavulanate	*Streptococcus* Enterococci	*P. mirabilis* *Klebsiella* species
Ampicillin with sulbactam	*Staphylococcus* (not MRSA) Enterococci	*P. mirabilis* *Haemophilus influenzae, Klebsiella* species
Antistaphylococcal penicillins	*Streptococcus* *Staphylococcus* (not MRSA)	None
Antipseudomonal penicillins	*Streptococcus* Enterococci	Most, including *Pseudomonas aeruginosa*
First-generation cephalosporins	*Streptococcus* *Staphylococcus* (not MRSA)	*Escherichia coli* *P. mirabilis* *Klebsiella* species
Second-generation cephalosporins (cefamandole, cefuroxime, cefaclor)	*Streptococcus* *Staphylococcus* (not MRSA)	*E. coli, P. mirabilis* *H. influenzae, Klebsiella* species
Second-generation cephalosporins (cefoxitin, cefotetan)	*Streptococcus*	*E. coli, Proteus* species (including indole-positive) *H. influenzae, Klebsiella* species
Third-generation cephalosporins (ceftriaxone)	*Streptococcus* *Staphylococcus* (not MRSA)	Most, excluding *P. aeruginosa*
Third-generation cephalosporins (ceftazidime)	*Streptococcus*	Most, including *P. aeruginosa*
Aztreonam	None	Most, including *P. aeruginosa*
Aminoglycosides	*Staphylococcus* (urine)	Most, including *P. aeruginosa*
Fluoroquinolones	*Streptococcus**	Most, including *P. aeruginosa*
Nitrofurantoin	*Staphylococcus* (not MRSA) Enterococci	Many Enterobacteriaceae (not *Providencia, Serratia, Acinetobacter*) *Klebsiella* species
Fosfomycin	Enterococci	Most Enterobacteriaceae (not *P. aeruginosa*)
Pivmecillinam	None	Most, excluding *P. aeruginosa*
Trimethoprim-sulfamethoxazole	*Streptococcus* *Staphylococcus*	Most Enterobacteriaceae (not *P. aeruginosa*)
Vancomycin	All, including MRSA	None

MRSA, methicillin-resistant *Staphylococcus aureus*.
*Depends on the antimicrobial agent.

TABLE 12-6 Common Adverse Reactions, Precautions, and Contraindications for Antimicrobial Agents Used in Treatment of Urinary Tract Infection

DRUG OR DRUG CLASS	COMMON ADVERSE REACTIONS	PRECAUTIONS AND CONTRAINDICATIONS
Amoxicillin or ampicillin	Hypersensitivity (immediate or delayed) Diarrhea (especially with ampicillin), GI upset AAPMC Maculopapular rash (not hypersensitivity) Decreased platelet aggregation	Increased risk of rash with concomitant viral disease, allopurinol therapy
Amoxicillin with clavulanic acid	Increased diarrhea, GI upset with amoxicillin/clavulanic acid	
Ampicillin with sulbactam	Same as with amoxicillin/ampicillin	
Antistaphylococcal penicillins	Same as with amoxicillin/ampicillin GI upset (with oral agents) Acute interstitial nephritis (especially with methicillin)	

TABLE 12-6 Common Adverse Reactions, Precautions, and Contraindications for Antimicrobial Agents Used in Treatment of Urinary Tract Infection—cont'd

DRUG OR DRUG CLASS	COMMON ADVERSE REACTIONS	PRECAUTIONS AND CONTRAINDICATIONS
Antipseudomonal penicillins	Same as with amoxicillin/ampicillin Hypernatremia (these drugs are given as sodium salt; especially carbenicillin, ticarcillin) Local injection site reactions	Use with caution in patients very sensitive to sodium loading.
Cephalosporins	Hypersensitivity (less than with penicillins) GI upset (with oral agents) Local injection site reactions AAPMC Positive Coombs test Decreased platelet aggregation (especially with cefotetan, cefamandole, cefoperazone)	Should not be used in patients with immediate hypersensitivity to penicillins; may use with caution in patients with delayed hypersensitivity reactions
Aztreonam	Hypersensitivity (less than with penicillins)	Less than 1% incidence of cross-reactivity in penicillin- or cephalosporin-allergic patients; may be used with caution in these patients
Aminoglycosides	Ototoxicity: vestibular and auditory components Nephrotoxicity: nonoliguric azotemia Neuromuscular blockade with high levels	Avoid in pregnant patients, except in pyelonephritis. Avoid if possible in patients with severely impaired renal function, diabetes, or hepatic failure. Use with caution in myasthenia gravis patients (owing to potential for neuromuscular blockade). Use with caution with other potentially ototoxic and nephrotoxic drugs.
Fluoroquinolones	Mild GI effects; dizziness, lightheadedness; photosensitivity Central nervous system effects, including dizziness, tremors, confusion, mood disorder, hallucinations Tendon rupture	Avoid in children or pregnant patients due to arthropathic effects. Concomitant antacid, iron, zinc, or sucralfate use dramatically decreases oral absorption; use another antimicrobial agent or discontinue sucralfate use while on quinolones. Space administration of quinolones from antacids, iron, or zinc products by at least 2 hr to ensure adequate absorption. Ensure adequate patient hydration. These agents can significantly increase theophylline plasma levels (ciprofloxacin and enoxacin seem to have a greater effect than norfloxacin or ofloxacin); avoid quinolones or monitor theophylline levels closely. These agents can lower seizure threshold; avoid in patients with epilepsy and in patients with other risk factors (medications or illness) that may lower the seizure threshold. Monitor glucose levels in patients on antidiabetic agents because hypoglycemia and hyperglycemia have been reported in patients treated concurrently with fluoroquinolones and antidiabetic agents. These agents can enhance warfarin effects; closely monitor coagulation tests.
Fosfomycin	Headache GI upset Vaginitis	Hypersensitivity to fosfomycin or any component of the formulation
Pivmecillinam	Rash GI upset	Use with caution in patients with penicillin hypersensitivity.

Continued

TABLE 12-6 Common Adverse Reactions, Precautions, and Contraindications for Antimicrobial Agents Used in Treatment of Urinary Tract Infection—cont'd

DRUG OR DRUG CLASS	COMMON ADVERSE REACTIONS	PRECAUTIONS AND CONTRAINDICATIONS
Nitrofurantoin	GI upset Peripheral polyneuropathy (especially in patients with impaired renal function, anemia, diabetes, electrolyte imbalance, vitamin B deficiency, and debilitated) Hemolysis in patients with G6PD deficiency Pulmonary hypersensitivity reactions can range from acute to chronic and include cough, dyspnea, fever, and interstitial changes.	Do not use in patients with low creatinine clearance (<50 mL/min) because adequate urine concentrations will not be achieved. Monitor long-term patients closely. Avoid concomitant probenecid use, which blocks renal excretion of nitrofurantoin. Avoid concomitant magnesium or quinolones, which are antagonistic to nitrofurantoin.
Trimethoprim-sulfamethoxazole	Hypersensitivity, rash GI upset Photosensitivity Hematologic toxicity (AIDS patients)	Higher incidence of all adverse reactions occurs in AIDS patients and the elderly. Avoid in pregnant patients. Avoid in patients receiving warfarin; concomitant use can significantly elevate prothrombin time.
Vancomycin	"Red-man syndrome": flushing, fever, chills, rash, hypotension (histaminic effect) Nephrotoxicity and/or ototoxicity when combined with other nephrotoxic and/or ototoxic drugs Local injection site reactions	Use with caution with other potentially ototoxic and nephrotoxic drugs.

AAPMC, antimicrobial-associated pseudomembranous colitis; AIDS, acquired immunodeficiency syndrome; GI, gastrointestinal; G6PD, glucose-6-phosphate dehydrogenase.
Modified from McEvoy GK, editor. American Hospital Formulary Service drug information. Bethesda (MD): American Society of Health-System Pharmacists; 1995.

Nitrofurantoin

Nitrofurantoin is effective against common uropathogens, but it is not effective against *Pseudomonas* and *Proteus* species (Iravani, 1991). It is rapidly excreted from the urine but does not obtain therapeutic levels in most body tissues, including the gastrointestinal (GI) tract. Therefore it is not useful for upper tract and complicated infections (Wilhelm and Edson, 1987). It has minimal effects on the resident bowel and vaginal flora and has been used effectively in prophylactic regimens for more than 40 years. Acquired bacterial resistance to this drug is exceedingly low. Nitrofurantoin should be used only during the first two trimesters of pregnancy. Nitrofurantoin can cause GI upset and rare pulmonary issues when used chronically. Nitrofurantoin should also be avoided in patients with suspicion of or known glucose-6-phosphate dehydrogenase (G6PD) deficiency because it can lead to hemolytic anemia.

Trimethoprim/Sulfamethoxazole

The combination of TMP-SMX has been the most widely used antimicrobial agent for the treatment of acute UTIs. TMP alone is as effective as the combination for most uncomplicated infections and may be associated with fewer side effects (Johnson and Stamm, 1989); however, the addition of SMX contributes to efficacy in the treatment of upper tract infection via a synergistic bactericidal effect and may diminish the emergence of resistance (Burman, 1986) and attains therapeutic levels in most tissues. TMP alone or in combination with SMX is effective against most common uropathogens, with the notable exception of *Enterococcus* and *Pseudomonas* species. TMP and TMP-SMX are inexpensive and have minimal adverse effects on the bowel flora. Disadvantages are relatively common adverse effects, consisting primarily of rashes and gastrointestinal complaints (Cockerill and Edson, 1991). TMP-SMX should be avoided during pregnancy.

Fosfomycin

Fosfomycin, an oral bactericidal antimicrobial agent similar to phosphonic acid in chemical structure, is active against most uropathogens. Its major benefit is its limited cross-resistance between most other common antibacterial agents, as well as its efficacy against the majority of gram-negative organisms and vancomycin-resistant *Enterococcus* (VRE). Further, it has been shown to be effective as a single-dose agent when used as an empirical treatment for uncomplicated cystitis. It is generally well tolerated with low incidences of GI upset and headache and very rare adverse events seen in multiple trials (Patel et al, 1997).

Fluoroquinolones

Fluoroquinolones share a common predecessor in nalidixic acid and inhibit DNA gyrase, a bacterial enzyme integral to replication. The fluoroquinolones have a broad spectrum of activity that makes them ideal for the empirical treatment of UTIs. They are highly effective against Enterobacteriaceae, as well as *P. aeruginosa*. Activity is also high against *S. aureus* and *S. saprophyticus*, but, in general, antistreptococcal coverage is marginal. Most anaerobic bacteria are resistant to these drugs; therefore the normal vaginal and bowel flora are not altered (Wright et al, 1993). Bacterial resistance initially appeared to be uncommon, but it is being reported at an increasing rate because of indiscriminate use of these agents (Wright et al, 1993; Vromen et al, 1999).

These drugs are not nephrotoxic, but renal insufficiency prolongs the serum half-life, requiring adjusted dosing in patients with creatinine clearances of less than 30 mL/min. Adverse reactions are uncommon; gastrointestinal disturbances are more common. Hypersensitivity, skin reactions, mild central and peripheral nervous system reactions, and even acute renal failure have been reported (Hootkins et al, 1989). Achilles tendon disorders, including rupture, have been estimated to occur in 20 cases per 100,000 and therefore fluoroquinolone use should be discontinued at the first sign of tendon pain (Greene, 2002). The mechanism of tendon rupture is unclear, but ciprofloxacin stimulates matrix-degrading protease activity from fibroblasts and exerts an inhibitory effect on fibroblast metabolism and synthesis of matrix ground substance, factors that may contribute to tendinopathy (Williams et al, 2000). Administration of the fluoroquinolones to immature animals has caused damage to the developing cartilage; therefore they are currently contraindicated in children, adolescents, and pregnant or nursing women (Christ et al, 1988). There are important drug interactions associated with the fluoroquinolones. The World Health Organization (WHO) warns of rare increases in the anticoagulant effects of Coumadin when taken with fluoroquinolones. Antacids containing magnesium or aluminum interfere with absorption of fluoroquinolones (Davies and Maesen, 1989). Certain fluoroquinolones (enoxacin and ciprofloxacin) elevate plasma levels of theophylline and prolong its half-life (Wright et al, 1993). For most uncomplicated UTIs, the fluoroquinolones have been only slightly more effective than TMP-SMX. However, as resistance to TMP-SMX increases, the fluoroquinolones have distinct advantages in empirical treatment of patients recently exposed to antimicrobial agents and in the outpatient treatment of complicated UTIs (Dalkin and Schaeffer, 1988; Gupta et al, 1999). **They may be considered as first-line agents in areas where a significant level of resistance (>20%) exists (in common bacteria) to agents such as ampicillin and TMP-SMX.**

Cephalosporins

All three generations of cephalosporins have been used for the treatment of acute UTIs (Wilhelm and Edson, 1987). In general, as a group, activity is high against Enterobacteriaceae and poor against enterococci. First-generation cephalosporins have greater activity against gram-positive organisms, as well as common uropathogens such as *E. coli* and *Klebsiella pneumoniae*, whereas second-generation cephalosporins have activity against anaerobes. Third-generation cephalosporins are more reliably active against community-acquired and nosocomial gram-negative organisms than other β-lactam antimicrobials. **Selective pressure engendered by these broad-spectrum agents should limit their use to complicated infections and situations in which parenteral therapy is required and resistance to standard antimicrobial agents is likely. They are also safe for use during pregnancy.**

Aminopenicillins

Ampicillin and amoxicillin have been used often in the past for the treatment of UTIs, but the emergence of resistance in 40% to 60% of common urinary isolates has lessened the usefulness of these drugs (Hooton and Stamm, 1991; Gupta et al, 2011). The effects of these agents on the normal bowel and vaginal flora can predispose patients to reinfection with resistant strains and often lead to candidal vaginitis (Iravani, 1991). The addition of the β-lactamase inhibitor clavulanate to amoxicillin greatly improves activity against β-lactamase–producing bacteria resistant to amoxicillin alone. However, its high cost and frequent gastrointestinal side effects limit its usefulness. The extended-spectrum penicillin derivatives (e.g., pivmecillinam, piperacillin, mezlocillin, azlocillin) retain ampicillin's activity against enterococci and offer activity against many ampicillin-resistant gram-negative bacilli. **This makes them attractive agents for use in patients with nosocomially acquired UTIs and as the initial parenteral treatment of acute uncomplicated pyelonephritis acquired outside of the hospital, although less expensive agents are equally effective.**

Aminoglycosides

When combined with TMP-SMX or ampicillin, aminoglycosides are the first drugs of choice for febrile UTIs. Their nephrotoxicity and ototoxicity are well recognized; hence, careful monitoring of

patients for renal and auditory impairment associated with infection is indicated. Once-daily aminoglycoside regimens have been instituted to maximize bacterial killing by optimizing the peak concentration-to-minimal inhibitory concentration ratio and reduce the potential for toxicity (Fig. 12-11) (Nicolau et al, 1995). Administering an aminoglycoside as a single daily dose can take advantage not only of its concentration-dependent killing ability but also of two other important characteristics: time-dependent toxicity and a more prolonged postantimicrobial effect (Gilbert, 1991; Zhanel et al, 1991). The regimen consists of a fixed 7 mg/kg dose of gentamicin or 5 to 7 mg/kg tobramycin. Subsequent interval adjustments are made by using a single concentration in serum and a nomogram designed for monitoring of once-daily therapy (Fig. 12-12). Antimicrobial doses are given at the interval determined by the drug concentration of a sample obtained after the start of the initial infusion. For example, if the serum concentration was 7 mg/mL 10 hours after the start of the infusion, subsequent 7-mg/kg doses would be given every 36 hours. This regimen is

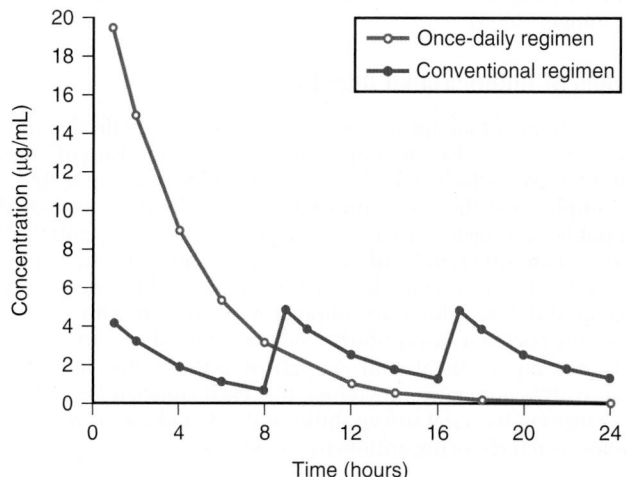

Figure 12-11. Simulated concentration-versus-time profile of once-daily (7 mg/kg/24 hr) and conventional (1.5 mg/kg/8 hr) regimens for patients with normal renal function. (From Nicolau DP, Freeman CD, Belliveau PP, et al. Experience with a once-daily aminoglycoside program administered to 2,184 adult patients. Antimicrob Agents Chemother 1995;39:650–5.)

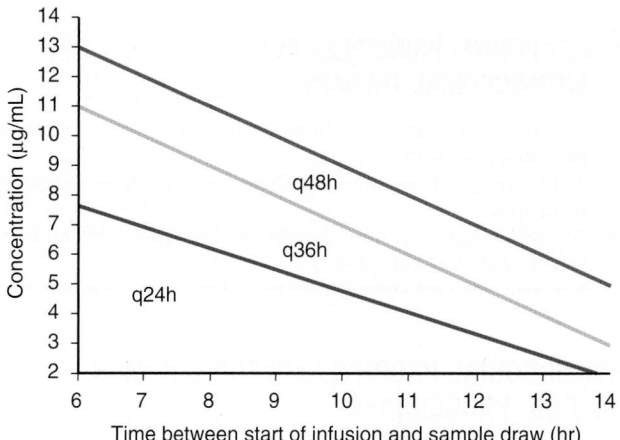

Figure 12-12. Once-daily aminoglycoside nomogram for gentamicin and tobramycin at 7 mg/kg. (From Nicolau DP, Freeman CD, Belliveau PP, et al. Experience with a once-daily aminoglycoside program administered to 2,184 adult patients. Antimicrob Agents Chemother 1995;39:650–5.)

clinically effective, reduces the incidence of nephrotoxicity, and provides a cost-effective method for administering aminoglycosides by reducing ancillary service times and serum aminoglycoside determinations.

Aztreonam

Aztreonam has a similar spectrum of activity as the aminoglycosides, and as with all β-lactams, it is not nephrotoxic. However, its spectrum of activity is less broad than the third-generation cephalosporins. **It should be used primarily in patients who have penicillin allergies.**

Pivmecillinam

Pivmecillinam is a penicillin-like β-lactam antibiotic which is the prodrug of mecillinam. It has high activity against gram-negative organisms and is primarily used in Nordic countries for empirical treatment of uncomplicated cystitis. **It is not currently available in the United States,** but it has been shown to have low resistance patterns (roughly 2% of *E. coli*) as well as being safe and effective (Graninger, 2003).

Choice of Antimicrobial Agents

Many antimicrobial agents have been shown to be effective in the treatment of UTIs. **Factors important in aiding selection of empirical therapy include whether the infection is complicated or uncomplicated; the spectrum of activity of the drug against the probable pathogen; a history of hypersensitivity; potential side effects, including renal and hepatic toxicity; and cost.** In addition, favorable or unfavorable effects of the antimicrobial agent on the vaginal and bowel flora are important in women with recurrent UTIs. The bacterial susceptibility and cost of the drug vary dramatically among inpatient and outpatient settings throughout the country. It is imperative, therefore, that each clinician keep abreast of changes in bacterial susceptibility and cost and use current information when choosing antimicrobial agents.

Duration of Therapy

The duration of therapy needed to cure a UTI appears to be related to a number of variables, including the extent and duration of tissue invasion, the bacterial concentration in urine, the achievable urine concentration of the antimicrobial agent, and risk factors (see later) that impair the host and natural defense mechanisms.

minutes and 120 minutes before the procedure (Bratzler and Houck, 2004). **Efficacious levels should be maintained for the duration of the procedure and, in special circumstances, a limited time (24 hours, at most) after the procedure** (Bratzler and Houck, 2004). Although prospective studies addressing prophylaxis for urologic procedures exist, most focus on only a narrow spectrum of procedures. However, application of the principles of these studies with additional consideration of both the patient and the type of procedure provides a framework for determining when and what type of antimicrobial prophylaxis may be indicated. An additional, nontraditional type of prophylaxis in urology entails periprocedural treatment of the urinary tract with an antimicrobial agent to prevent local or systemic sequelae from the manipulation of colonized hardware such as a stent or urethral catheter.

A wide array of patients undergo invasive procedures in urology. The ability of a host to respond to bacteriuria or bacteremia and the sequelae of a possible infection are two important considerations when assessing the need for antimicrobial prophylaxis. Factors that affect the host's ability to respond to infection include advanced age, anatomic anomalies, poor nutritional status, smoking, chronic corticosteroid use, other concurrent medication use, and immunodeficiencies such as untreated HIV infection (Box 12-5). Additionally, chronic indwelling hardware, infected endogenous material such as stones, distant infectious sites, and prolonged hospitalizations also increase the risk of infectious complications by increasing the local bacterial concentration and/or altering the spectrum of bacterial flora. The potential seeding of artificial heart valves or prosthetic joints increases the sequelae of a systemic infection in hosts who otherwise may not be at an increased risk of infection. Thus a thorough history and examination of the patient is crucial in directing antimicrobial prophylaxis before a urologic procedure.

The type of procedure will also help direct the timing, duration, and spectrum of antimicrobial prophylaxis needed (see Table 12-7 for a summary of antimicrobial prophylaxis recommendations). Consideration should be given to the extent of the local tissue injury incurred and the anticipated type of flora at the site.

Antimicrobial prophylaxis is not without morbidity because allergic complications, although rare, may result in minor reactions such as rash or gastric disturbances or significant sequelae such as early withdrawal of therapy, allergic nephritis, or anaphylaxis.

Urethral Catheterization and Removal

The indications for the routine use of prophylactic antimicrobial agents before urethral catheterization vary and depend on the health, sex, and specific living circumstances of the individual

---

KEY POINTS: PRINCIPLES OF ANTIMICROBIAL THERAPY

- Effective antimicrobial therapy must eliminate bacterial growth in the urinary tract.
- Antimicrobial resistance is increasing because of excessive utilization.
- Antimicrobial selection should be influenced by efficacy, safety, cost, and compliance.

ANTIMICROBIAL PROPHYLAXIS FOR COMMON UROLOGIC PROCEDURES

Principles

Surgical antimicrobial prophylaxis entails treatment with an antimicrobial agent before and for a *limited* time after a procedure to prevent local or systemic postprocedural infections. For most procedures, prophylaxis should be initiated between 30

BOX 12-5 Host Factors That Increase the Risk of Infection

Advanced age
Anatomic anomalies
Poor nutritional status
Smoking
Chronic corticosteroid use
Immunodeficiency
Chronic indwelling hardware
Infected endogenous/exogenous material
Distant coexistent infection
Prolonged hospitalization

Data from Cruse PJ. Surgical wound infection. In: Wonsiewicz MJ, editor. Infectious disease. Philadelphia: WB Saunders; 1992. p. 758–64; and Mangram AJ, Horan TC, Pearson ML, et al. Guideline for prevention of surgical site infection, 1999. Hospital Infection Control Practices Advisory Committee. Infect Control Hosp Epidemiol 1999;20:250–78; quiz 279–80.

patient, as well as the indication for catheterization (Schaeffer 2006). The risk of infection after one-time urethral catheterization is 1% to 2% in healthy domiciliary women; however, this risk rises significantly in hospitalized patients (Turck et al, 1962; Thiel and Spuhler, 1965). Thus, for patients with risk factors for infection (see Box 12-5), antimicrobial prophylaxis with an oral agent such as TMP-SMX or a fluoroquinolone should decrease the risk of postprocedural infection (see Table 12-7).

Prolonged use of an indwelling urethral catheter is common in hospitalized patients and is associated with an increased risk of bacterial colonization, with a 3% to 10% incidence of bacteriuria per catheter day in one study and 100% incidence of bacteriuria with long-term catheterization (>30 days) (Kass, 1956; Nickel et al, 1985; Liedl, 2001). **Prophylactic administration of antimicrobial agents during catheterization is not generally recommended** because bacterial resistance can develop rapidly and complicate subsequent antimicrobial treatment (Clarke et al, 2005). This is supported by the Cochrane Database of Systematic Reviews that concluded that antimicrobials given postprocedurally until removal or for the first three postoperative days did not reduce rates of bacteriuria or infection (Niël-weise and van den Broek, 2005).

The natural history of bacteriuria after catheter removal has not been comprehensively studied. Harding and associates (1991) reported that in asymptomatic bacteriuric women who had been

TABLE 12-7 Guide for Antimicrobial Prophylaxis for Uncomplicated Urologic Procedures

PROCEDURE	ORGANISMS	PROPHYLAXIS INDICATED	ANTIMICROBIAL(S) OF CHOICE	ALTERNATIVE ANTIMICROBIAL(S)	DURATION OF THERAPY[a]
LOWER TRACT INSTRUMENTATION					
Removal of external urinary catheter	GU tract[b]	If risk factors[c]	Fluoroquinolone TMP-SMX[d]	Aminoglycoside ± ampicillin 1st/2nd gen. cephalosporin[d]	≤24 hr[d]
Cystography, urodynamic study, or simple cystourethroscopy	GU tract	If risk factors[c]	Fluoroquinolone TMP-SMX	Amoxicillin/clavulanate Aminoglycoside ± ampicillin 1st/2nd gen. cephalosporin	≤24 hr
Cystourethroscopy with manipulation[e]	GU tract	All	Fluoroquinolone TMP-SMX	Amoxicillin/clavulanate	≤24 hr
Prostate brachytherapy or cryotherapy	Skin	Uncertain	1st gen. cephalosporin	Aminoglycoside ± ampicillin 1st/2nd gen. cephalosporin Amoxicillin/clavulanate Clindamycin[f]	≤24 hr
Transrectal prostate biopsy	Intestine[g]	All	Fluoroquinolone Targeted prophylaxis[h]	TMP-SMX Aminoglycoside ± metronidazole or clindamycin[f]	≤24 hr
UPPER TRACT INSTRUMENTATION					
Shockwave lithotripsy	GU tract	All	Fluoroquinolone TMP-SMX	Aminoglycoside ± ampicillin 1st/2nd gen. cephalosporin	≤24 hr
Percutaneous renal surgery	GU tract and skin[i]	All	1st/2nd gen. cephalosporin Aminoglycoside + metronidazole or clindamycin	Amoxicillin/clavulanate Ampicillin/sulbactam Fluoroquinolone	≤24 hr
Ureteroscopy	GU tract	All	Fluoroquinolone TMP-SMX	Aminoglycoside ± ampicillin 1st/2nd gen. cephalosporin Amoxicillin/clavulanate	≤24 hr
OPEN OR LAPAROSCOPIC SURGERY					
Vaginal surgery	GU tract, skin, and group B *Streptococcus*	All	1st/2nd gen. cephalosporin Aminoglycoside + metronidazole or clindamycin	Ampicillin/sulbactam	≤24 hr
Without entering urinary tract	Skin	If risk factors	1st gen. cephalosporin	Fluoroquinolone	Single dose
Involving entry into urinary tract	GU tract and skin	All	1st/2nd gen. cephalosporin Aminoglycoside + metronidazole or clindamycin	Clindamycin	≤24 hr

Continued

TABLE 12-7   Guide for Antimicrobial Prophylaxis for Uncomplicated Urologic Procedures—cont'd

PROCEDURE	ORGANISMS	PROPHYLAXIS INDICATED	ANTIMICROBIAL(S) OF CHOICE	ALTERNATIVE ANTIMICROBIAL(S)	DURATION OF THERAPY[a]
Involving intestine[j]	GU tract, skin, and intestine	All	2nd/3rd gen. cephalosporin Aminoglycoside + metronidazole or clindamycin	Ampicillin/sulbactam Fluoroquinolone	≤24 hr
Involving implanted prosthesis	GU tract and skin	All	Aminoglycoside + 1st/2nd gen. cephalosporin or vancomycin	Ampicillin/sulbactam Ticarcillin/clavulanate Piperacillin/tazobactam Fluoroquinolone Ampicillin/sulbactam Ticarcillin/clavulanate Piperacillin/tazobactam	≤24 hr

Order of agents in each column is not indicative of preference. The absence of an agent does not preclude its appropriate use depending on specific situations.

[a]Additional antimicrobial therapy may be recommended at the time of removal of an externalized urinary catheter.

[b]GU tract: common urinary tract organisms are *E. coli, Proteus* species, *Klebsiella* species, *Enterococcus.*

[c]If urine culture shows no growth before the procedure, antimicrobial prophylaxis is not necessary.

[d]Or full course of culture-directed antimicrobial agents for documented infection (which is treatment, not prophylaxis).

[e]Includes transurethral resection of bladder tumor and prostate, and any biopsy, resection, fulguration, foreign body removal, urethral dilation or urethrotomy, or ureteral instrumentation, including catheterization or stent placement/removal.

[f]Clindamycin or an aminoglycoside + metronidazole or clindamycin is an alternative to penicillins and cephalosporins in patients with penicillin allergy, even when not specifically listed.

[g]Intestine: common intestinal organisms are *E. coli, Klebsiella* species, *Enterobacter, Serratia* species, *Proteus* species, *Enterococcus,* and anaerobes.

[h]Perform prebiopsy rectal swab culture and bacterial susceptibility; select appropriate antimicrobial prophylaxis.

[i]Skin: common skin organisms are *S. aureus,* coagulase-negative *Staphylococcus* species, group A *Streptococcus* species.

[j]For surgery involving the colon, bowel preparation with oral neomycin + either erythromycin base or metronidazole can be added to or substituted for systemic agents.

gen., generation; GU, genitourinary; TMP-SMX, trimethoprim-sulfamethoxazole.

Drug doses: ampicillin, 25 mg/kg/dose; gentamicin, 1.5 mg/kg/dose; cefazolin, 25 mg/kg/dose.

Modified from Wolf JS Jr, Bennett CJ, Dmochowski RR, et al. Best practice policy statement on urologic surgery antimicrobial prophylaxis. J Urol 2008;179:1379-90.

catheterized for 4 to 6 days, 25% developed a UTI within 14 days of catheter removal. In this study, 1-day treatment with TMP-SMX was as effective as a 10-day course at resolving infections. Similar studies on the natural history of postcatheterization bacteriuria have not been performed in male patients. Note that antimicrobial treatment before removal of an indwelling catheter in a patient suspected of having bacteriuria is not considered prophylaxis but rather is treatment for a presumptive UTI; duration of treatment generally should follow previously outlined guidelines for uncomplicated or complicated UTIs.

Data from Polastri and colleagues (1990) suggest that antimicrobial prophylaxis for chronic indwelling catheter changes is not indicated. In their study of 46 catheter changes, bacteremia occurred 4% of the time and, when noted, was associated with very low concentrations of bacteria in the cultures. Systemic sequelae were not noted.

Urodynamics

Urodynamics, like cystoscopy, is a minimally traumatic procedure with limited urothelial injury that poses a small risk of local infection in hosts with normal anatomy and immune response. Several recent studies support this notion. In a series of women with urinary incontinence randomized to receive 1 day of nitrofurantoin or placebo, Cundiff and coworkers (1999) noted no difference in postprocedural UTI (5% vs. 7%) 1 week after evaluation. Similarly, Peschers and associates (2001) reported infections 1 week after multichannel urodynamics in 5% and 6% in nondiabetic women

treated with placebo or co-trimoxazole. Conversely, Kartal and colleagues (2006) demonstrated a reduction in UTIs from 14% to 1% with administration of a single dose of ciprofloxacin in a blinded 192-patient trial. Most series examining the use of antimicrobial prophylaxis exclude patients with altered anatomy such as large prostates or comorbidities, including neurogenic bladder, spinal cord injury, or diabetes, all factors that increase the risk of infection. This is illustrated in work performed by Payne and colleagues in which frequencies of bacteriuria after urodynamics were much higher in men (36%) compared with the women studied (15%) (Payne et al, 1988). **In sum, antimicrobial prophylaxis should be considered for patients with a more complex clinical history or anatomy such as men with large postvoid residuals or spinal cord–injured patients.**

Transrectal Ultrasound-Guided Prostate Biopsy

The use of prophylactic antimicrobials for transrectal ultrasound-guided prostate (TRUSP) biopsy reduces postprocedural fever and UTI in most studies. The class and duration of antimicrobial treatment are more varied and controversial. Antimicrobial prophylaxis with fluoroquinolones has been shown to significantly reduce the rates of infectious complications compared to placebo (8% vs. 25%) (Sieber et al, 1997; Taylor and Bingham, 1997a, 1997b; Kapoor et al, 1998; Shandera et al, 1998; Tal et al, 2003; Zani et al, 2011).

However, **several recent studies have highlighted an increasing trend of infectious complications caused by fluoroquinolone-resistant organisms** among men undergoing TRUSP (Binsaleh et al, 2004; Han et al, 2005; Feliciano et al, 2008; Ng and Chan, 2008; Lange et al, 2009; Young et al, 2009; Zaytoun et al, 2011). Prevalence rates for colonization with fluoroquinolone-resistant organisms in this patient population have been reported to be as high as 22% (Liss et al, 2011). Nevertheless more than 90% of urologists continue to use fluoroquinolones empirically for antimicrobial prophylaxis before TRUSP (Shandera et al, 1998). The increasing prevalence of infectious complications with fluoroquinolone-resistant bacteria in men undergoing TRUSP suggests that this approach may be injudicious for some patients (Taylor et al, 2012). Indeed, of fluoroquinolone-resistant strains obtained by rectal swabs of men prior to prostate biopsy, 70% were ST131 isolates (Liss et al, 2013). See Urinary Pathogens earlier in chapter for more in-depth information on ST131 and resistance.

Empiric prophylaxis with a combination of aminoglycosides and fluoroquinolones has been effective in recent studies (Kehinde et al, 2013; Ho et al, 2009), but it is inevitable that this approach will also eventually fail because of antimicrobial resistance. **Rectal swab culture obtained before TRUSP allows for the isolation and identification of fluoroquinolone-resistant organisms from a patient's native intestinal flora.** In a study using targeted prophylaxis based on bacterial sensitivities of rectal swabs prior to TRUSP, 19.6% of men had fluoroquinolone-resistant organisms. There were no infectious complications in the men who received targeted prophylaxis, while there were infectious complications, including sepsis, in 2.6% on empiric prophylaxis (Taylor et al, 2012). Cost-effectiveness analysis revealed that targeted prophylaxis yielded a cost savings of $4,499 per post TRUSP infectious complication averted. Per estimation, 38 men would need to undergo rectal swab before TRUSP to prevent one infectious complication. Thus a benefit to screening before TRUSP and targeted prophylaxis should be considered as a thoughtful, predictable alternative to empiric prophylaxis.

Recent studies suggest a single-dose/day of fluoroquinolones is as effective as 3 days of treatment (Sabbagh et al, 2004). Together these data suggest that a minimum of 1 day of an antimicrobial agent is indicated for transrectal ultrasound-guided prostate biopsies.

Shockwave Lithotripsy

The incidence of UTIs after shockwave lithotripsy is reported to range from 0% to 28% without antimicrobial prophylaxis. A recent meta-analysis of contemporary randomized controlled trials examined the utility and cost-effectiveness of antimicrobial prophylaxis for shockwave lithotripsy and demonstrated, in individuals with sterile preprocedure urine cultures, a reduction in the rate of UTIs after shockwave lithotripsy from 5.7% to 2.1% (Pearle and Roehrborn, 1997). This analysis also demonstrated cost-effectiveness of prophylaxis when consideration was given for the treatment of the rare but more morbid complications of urosepsis and pyelonephritis. A history of a recent UTI or of infection stones should warrant a full treatment course of antimicrobial agents before shockwave lithotripsy.

Endoscopic Procedures: Lower Urinary Tract

Cystoscopy

Cystoscopy is a minimally traumatic procedure with limited urothelial injury performed on a diverse spectrum of patients, including young healthy women and older men. Several prospective trials (Manson, 1988; Clark and Higgs, 1990; Burke et al, 2002) of patients with preprocedure sterile urine report culture-proven rates of UTI between 2.2% and 7.8% after cystoscopy without antimicrobial prophylaxis. In Clark's report the risk of infection was higher in patients with a previous history of UTI. In a similarly designed study, Rane and colleagues (2001) reported a significantly higher postprocedure culture-proven infection rate of 21% without antimicrobial prophylaxis. More recently, Johnson and colleagues (2007) reported a randomized controlled trial of over 2000 patients that demonstrated reductions in bacteriuria with administration of

single-dose trimethoprim or ciprofloxacin. In all the studies, single doses of antimicrobial agents reduced infections to between 1% and 5%. In none of these studies were significant systemic infections reported after the cystoscopic procedures.

Together these studies illustrate two key concepts: (1) despite appropriate periprocedural preparation, a small inoculum of bacteria is likely introduced into the bladder during cystoscopy, and (2) the significance of the bacteriuria is dependent on host factors, including the ability to mount an appropriate immune response to bacterial inoculation and the ability to clear the bacterial inoculation. For example, in a man with urinary retention, a small inoculum of bacteria could persist and divide in the retained fraction of urine and result in a symptomatic infection. In a host with a reduced ability to respond to infection, this bacteriuria could become significant. In contrast, a middle-aged woman undergoing cystoscopy for microscopic hematuria is more likely to efficiently empty her bladder and clear the inoculum but may be exposed to an increased inoculum of bacteria if inappropriately prepared for the examination. **Thus we recommend prophylaxis when aberrant host factors could increase the probability or significance of an infection** (see Table 12-7). A single dose of a fluoroquinolone is commonly used but other agents such as trimethoprim have also been utilized.

Transurethral Resection of the Prostate and Bladder

Therapeutic transurethral lower urinary tract procedures increase the risk of localized infections compared with simple diagnostic cystoscopy. Although not delineated in any prospective studies, several risk factors likely increase infectious complications, including trauma to the mucosa, increased duration and/or degree of difficulty of the procedure, pressurized irrigants, and manipulation or resection of infected material. The most well-studied lower urinary tract procedure is **transurethral resection of the prostate**. In a meta-analysis of 32 studies (Berry and Barratt, 2002), a risk reduction was noted in bacteriuria from 26% to 9% on postoperative urine cultures obtained 2 to 5 days after the procedure for patients treated with prophylactic antimicrobial agents. Similarly, septicemia (defined as rigors, persistently elevated temperature [>38.5° C], and an elevated C-reactive protein level) decreased from 4.4% to 0.9% with antimicrobial prophylaxis. The most effective antimicrobial classes included fluoroquinolones, aminoglycosides, cephalosporins, and TMP-SMX. **Single doses of antimicrobial agents did lower the relative risk of bacteriuria but not as significantly as antimicrobial agents administered for short courses (2 to 5 days) while the urethral catheter remained in place.** Although continuation of antimicrobial therapy while the catheter is in place is not truly prophylaxis, continuation of the initial prophylactic antimicrobial agent for an anticipated short period of time (with catheter in place) does not increase the risk of developing antimicrobial-resistant organisms. No recent trials have investigated prophylaxis for **transurethral resection of bladder tumors; however, evidence from transurethral resection of the prostate procedures would suggest that prophylaxis would reduce bacteriuria in these procedures.**

Patients who are known preoperatively to have UTIs should have the infections eradicated before the procedure is started; hence, in these patients, preoperative antimicrobial agents are therapeutic and not prophylactic. Failure to eradicate bacteriuria results in bacteremia in 50% of patients (Morris et al, 1976).

Diagnostic and therapeutic upper tract studies that are performed with pressurized irrigants may induce urothelial injury. Prophylaxis with antimicrobial agents that cover uropathogens is indicated.

Endoscopic Procedures: Upper Urinary Tract

Ureteroscopy

Diagnostic and therapeutic upper tract endoscopic procedures have an increased risk of localized infections compared with simple diagnostic cystoscopy because of several factors, including increased trauma to the mucosa, increased duration and/or degree of difficulty of most ureteroscopic procedures, increased pressure of irrigants, and (when applicable) manipulation or resection of infected material. **The use of antimicrobial prophylaxis is supported** by a randomized trial by Knopf and colleagues (2003) in which prophylactic fluoroquinolone administration significantly reduced postprocedure UTIs in a healthy population of individuals with ureteral stones and uninfected preoperative urine. If an infection or infectious material is suspected, culture and a full treatment course of an appropriate antimicrobial are recommended before the procedure. Some urologists advocate for medical diuresis during the procedure with furosemide.

Percutaneous Procedures

Percutaneous renal surgery is commonly performed for large renal stones, ureteropelvic junction obstruction, and transitional cell carcinoma surveillance. Pyrexia and bacteremia occur frequently and likely stem from a combination of renal parenchymal injury, pressurized irrigation, and, in some cases, manipulation of infectious stones. Several studies demonstrated a relationship between the risk of postoperative infectious complications (including bacteriuria and sepsis) and the duration of the procedure and amount of irrigant used (Dogan et al, 2002). **If preoperative urine cultures are positive, treatment of the infection should occur before surgery. Conversely, if preoperative cultures are negative, antimicrobial prophylaxis covering common urinary pathogens should be instituted** (Wolf et al, 2008) (see Table 12-7).

Open and Laparoscopic Surgery

Open surgical procedures can be classified as clean, clean contaminated, contaminated, and dirty (Table 12-8). **Antimicrobial prophylaxis is indicated for clean contaminated and contaminated wounds, whereas antimicrobial treatment with an appropriate agent should be instituted for dirty-infected wounds.** To date, no large studies have evaluated the risk of surgical site infections for different laparoscopic urologic procedures. However, data in the general surgery literature suggest that the laparoscopic approach lowers the risk of surgical site infections (Kluytmans, 1997). Clean surgeries in urology include radical nephrectomy if the urinary tract is not entered. **All urologic procedures in which the urinary tract**

is opened electively are considered clean contaminated procedures, whereas entry into an infected urinary tract is considered a contaminated procedure and carries a higher rate of surgical site infection (Cruse, 1992). **Antimicrobial agents should be active against the most likely infecting organism and should be administered within 1 hour of the procedure and discontinued 24 hours after** because several studies have failed to demonstrate beneficial effects of long courses of prophylaxis (Conte et al, 1972; Goldmann et al, 1977). In the United States, first-generation cephalosporins are commonly used for prophylaxis of clean contaminated procedures because they have low incidences of allergic reactions, long half-lives, and low cost. For patients with a β-lactam allergy, the 2004 National Surgical Infection Prevention Project (NSIPP) guidelines recommend either vancomycin or clindamycin. Prophylaxis for urinary reconstruction with intestine requires increased anaerobic coverage, and thus use of second-generation cephalosporins is recommended (Bratzler and Houck, 2004). When use of the colon or appendix is anticipated for urologic reconstruction, the 2004 NSIPP recommendations include orally administered antimicrobial bowel preparation (neomycin plus erythromycin or neomycin plus metronidazole) 18 to 24 hours before surgery and parenteral cefotetan or cefoxitin 30 to 60 minutes before incision (Bratzler and Houck, 2004). Recommendations for patients with a β-lactam allergy include clindamycin plus gentamicin, aztreonam, or ciprofloxacin. Dirty wounds in urology include all abscesses and traumatic perforation of the genitourinary tract. Treatment of a dirty wound should begin with broad coverage of anticipated organisms and intraoperative wound cultures. Subsequent therapy and treatment duration depends on the sensitivities of the cultured organism.

Special Considerations
Patients with Risk of Endocarditis

The risk of infectious endocarditis (IE) after urologic procedures is low. Previous guidelines from the American Heart Association (AHA) had recommended routine prophylaxis, but the current recommendation is that the use of prophylactic antibiotics solely to prevent IE is **not recommended** (Wilson et al, 2007). However, these guidelines do acknowledge that instrumentation of the GU tract may result in transient enterococcal bacteremia. The evidence supporting this claim is anecdotal, and no data exist to demonstrate either a conclusive link between this bacteremia and IE or that administration of antimicrobial prophylaxis prevents IE. Regardless, the guidelines do state that for patients with certain concomitant conditions (prosthetic cardiac valve, previous IE, congenital heart disease, cardiac transplantation) and an active infection or colonization who are to undergo GU tract manipulation, including elective cystoscopy, antibiotic therapy to sterilize the urine may be reasonable (Class IIb evidence). Amoxicillin or ampicillin is suggested as a first-line agent for enterococci, vancomycin for those who cannot tolerate ampicillin, or culture-directed agents as possible (Wilson et al, 2007).

Patients with Indwelling Orthopedic Hardware

Bacterial seeding of implanted orthopedic hardware is a rare but morbid event. A joint commission of the American Urological Association (AUA), the American Academy of Orthopaedic Surgeons (AAOS), and infectious disease specialists convened in 2003 and released an advisory statement on antimicrobial prophylaxis for urologic patients with total joint replacement (American Urological Association and American Academy of Orthopaedic Surgeons, 2003) (Table 12-9). **In general, antimicrobial prophylaxis for urologic patients with total joint replacements, pins, plates, or screws is not indicated. Prophylaxis is advised for individuals at higher risk of seeding a prosthetic joint, including those with recently inserted implants (within 2 years) and/or host risk factors as delineated earlier.** Prophylaxis on the basis of potential seeding of a prosthetic joint should be instituted for procedures

TABLE 12-8 Surgical Wound Classification

TERM	DESCRIPTION
Clean	Uninfected wound without inflammation or entry into the genital, urinary, or alimentary tract Primary wound closure ± closed drainage
Clean contaminated	Uninfected wound with controlled entry into the genital, urinary, or alimentary tract Primary wound closure ± closed drainage
Contaminated	Uninfected wound with major break in sterile technique (gross spillage from gastrointestinal tract or nonpurulent inflammation) Open fresh accidental wounds
Dirty infected	Wound with preexisting clinical infection or perforated viscera Old traumatic wounds with devitalized tissue

Modified from Mangram AJ, Horan TC, Pearson ML, et al. Guideline for prevention of surgical site infection, 1999. Hospital Infection Control Practices Advisory Committee. Infect Control Hosp Epidemiol 1999;20:250–78; quiz 279–80.

TABLE 12-9 Antimicrobial Regimens for Patients with Indwelling Orthopedic Hardware

PATIENT TYPE	ANTIMICROBIAL RECOMMENDATION
Total joint inserted >2 yr ago, pins, plates, screws + no host risk factors	Not recommended empirically
Total joint inserted <2 yr ago or aberrant host factor(s)	Oral quinolone or ampicillin, 2 g IV + gentamicin, 1.5 mg/kg IV, 30-60 min before procedure Substitute vancomycin, 1 g IV, over 1-2 hr before procedure if ampicillin allergy

From American Urological Association and American Academy of Orthopaedic Surgeons. Antibiotic prophylaxis for urological patients with total joint replacements. J Urol 2003;169:1796–7.

BOX 12-6 Risk Factors for Urinary Tract Infections

REDUCED URINE FLOW
Outflow obstruction, prostatic hyperplasia, prostatic carcinoma, urethral stricture, foreign body (calculus)
Neurogenic bladder
Inadequate fluid uptake (dehydration)

PROMOTE COLONIZATION
Sexual activity—increased inoculation
Spermicide—increased binding
Estrogen depletion—increased binding
Antimicrobial agents—decreased indigenous flora

FACILITATE ASCENT
Catheterization
Urinary incontinence
Fecal incontinence
Residual urine with ischemia of bladder wall

---

including stone manipulation, transmural incision of the urinary tract, upper tract endoscopic procedures, procedures involving bowel segments, and transrectal prostate biopsy. Additionally, patients with recent prosthetic joints or compromised host factors and urinary diversions, indwelling stents or catheters, a recent history of urinary retention, or UTIs should receive antimicrobial prophylaxis before urinary tract procedures. The AUA Advisory Statement recommends for these patients either an oral quinolone or ampicillin, 2 g intravenous (IV) (vancomycin, 1 g IV over 1 to 2 hours for ampicillin-allergic patients), and gentamicin, 1.5 mg/kg IV, 30 to 60 minutes before the procedure.

KEY POINTS: ANTIMICROBIAL PROPHYLAXIS FOR COMMON UROLOGIC PROCEDURES

- Antimicrobial prophylaxis entails treatment with an antimicrobial agent before and for a limited time after a procedure to prevent local or systemic postprocedural infections.
- The type of procedure and competency of the host defenses determine the need for antimicrobial prophylaxis.
- Special considerations for antimicrobial prophylaxis include patients undergoing TRUSP, those with a risk of endocarditis, and patients with indwelling orthopedic hardware.

BLADDER INFECTIONS

Uncomplicated Cystitis

Most cases of uncomplicated cystitis occur in women. Each year, approximately 10% of women report having had a UTI and more than 50% of all women have at least one such infection in their lifetime (Foxman et al, 2000). Uncomplicated cystitis occasionally occurs in prepubertal girls, but it increases greatly in incidence in late adolescence and during the second and fourth decades of life. Twenty-five to 30 percent of women 20 to 40 years of age have a history of UTIs (Kunin, 1987). **Although it is much less common, young men may also experience acute cystitis without underlying structural or functional abnormalities of the urinary tract** (Krieger et al, 1993). Risk factors (Box 12-6) include sexual intercourse and use of spermicides (Hooton et al, 1996; Foxman, 2002; Handley et al, 2002). Sexual transmission of uropathogens has been suggested by demonstrating identical *E. coli* in the bowel and urinary flora of sex partners (Johnson and Stamm, 1989).

Clinical Presentation

The presenting symptoms of cystitis are variable but usually include dysuria, frequency, and/or urgency (Fig. 12-13). **Suprapubic pain, hematuria, or foul-smelling urine may develop. The probability of cystitis in a woman with these symptoms alone or in combination is 50% to 90%, respectively** (Bent et al, 2002). When a woman who previously has had cystitis has symptoms suggesting a recurrence, the probability that an infection is present is about 90% (Gupta et al, 2001). By definition, acute cystitis is a superficial infection of the bladder mucosa, so fever, chills, and other signs of dissemination are not present. Some patients may experience suprapubic tenderness, but most have no diagnostic physical findings. In women, physical examination should include the possibility of vaginitis, herpes, and urethral pathology, such as a diverticulum.

A remarkably narrow spectrum of etiologic agents with highly predictable profiles of antimicrobial susceptibility causes infections in young women with acute uncomplicated cystitis. *E. coli* **is the causative organism in 75% to 90% of cases of acute cystitis in young women** (Latham et al, 1983; Ronald, 2002). *S. saprophyticus,* **a commensal organism of the skin, is the second most common cause of acute cystitis in young women, accounting for 10% to 20% of these infections** (Jordan et al, 1980). **Other organisms less commonly involved include** *Klebsiella* **and** *Proteus* **species and** *Enterococcus.* **In men,** *E. coli* **and other Enterobacteriaceae are the most commonly identified organisms.**

Laboratory Diagnosis

The presumptive laboratory diagnosis of acute cystitis is based on microscopic urinalysis, which indicates microscopic pyuria, bacteriuria, and occasionally hematuria. Indirect dipstick tests for bacteria (nitrite) or pyuria (leukocyte esterase) may also be informative and more convenient but are less sensitive than microscopic examination of the urine. Dipsticks are most accurate when the presence of either nitrite or leukocyte esterase is considered a positive result. Urine culture remains the definitive test; and in symptomatic patients, the presence of 10^2 cfu/mL or more of urine usually indicates infection (Stamm et al, 1982b). However, as previously discussed, different thresholds are needed based on different clinical situations.

However, routine urine cultures are often not necessary. It is generally more cost-effective to manage many patients who have symptoms and urinalysis findings characteristic of uncomplicated cystitis without an initial urine culture because treatment decisions

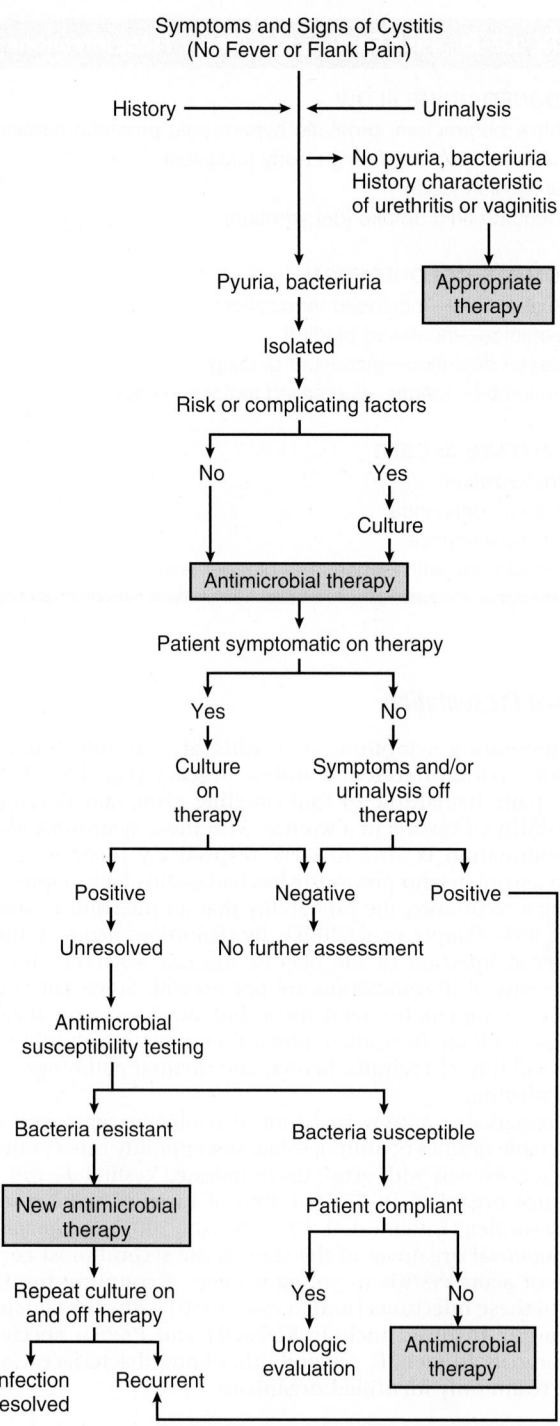

Figure 12-13. Management of acute cystitis.

are usually made and therapy is often completed before culture results are known (Komaroff, 1986). This position was supported by a cost-effectiveness study (Carlson and Mulley, 1985) in which it was estimated that the routine use of pretherapeutic urine cultures for lower UTI increases costs by 40% but decreases the overall duration of symptoms by only 10%.

Thus, in women with recent onset of symptoms and signs suggesting acute cystitis and in whom factors associated with upper tract or complicated infection are absent, a urinalysis that is positive for pyuria, bacteriuria, or hematuria, or a combination should provide sufficient documentation of UTI, and a urine culture may be omitted (McIsaac et al, 2002). **A urine culture should be obtained for patients in whom symptoms and urine examination findings leave the diagnosis of cystitis in doubt.** Pretherapeutic cultures and susceptibility tests are also essential

in the management of patients with recent antimicrobial therapy or UTI. In these situations, various pathogens may be present and antimicrobial therapy is less predictable and must be tailored to the individual organism (Stamm, 1986).

Differential Diagnosis

Cystitis must be differentiated from other inflammatory infectious conditions in which dysuria may be the most prominent symptom, including vaginitis, urethral infections caused by sexually transmitted pathogens, and miscellaneous noninflammatory causes of urethral discomfort (Komaroff, 1984). Characteristic features of the history, physical examination, and voided urine or other specimens allow patients with dysuria to be assigned to one of these diagnostic categories. **Vaginitis** is characterized by irritative voiding associated with vaginal irritation and is subacute in onset. A history of vaginal discharge or odor and multiple or new sexual partners is common. Frequency, urgency, hematuria, and suprapubic pain are not present. Physical examination reveals a vaginal discharge, and examination of vaginal fluid demonstrates inflammatory cells. Differential diagnosis includes herpes simplex virus, gonorrhea, *Chlamydia*, trichomoniasis, yeast, and bacterial vaginosis. **Urethritis** causes dysuria that is usually subacute in onset and is associated with a history of discharge and new or multiple sexual partners. Frequency and urgency of urination may be present but are less pronounced than in patients with cystitis, and fever and chills are absent. Urethral discharge with inflammatory cells or initial pyuria in the male is characteristic. The common causes of urethritis include *Neisseria gonorrhoeae*, *Chlamydia*, herpes simplex virus, and trichomoniasis. Appropriate cultures and immunologic tests are indicated. **Urethral injury** associated with sexual intercourse, chemical irritants, or allergy may also cause dysuria. A history of trauma or exposure to irritants and a lack of discharge or pyuria are characteristic.

Management

Antimicrobial Selection. Oral antimicrobial agents for treatment of acute uncomplicated cystitis are listed in Table 12-10.

Nitrofurantoin has maintained an excellent level of activity over 4 decades and is well tolerated, but it is more expensive than TMP-SMX and is considerably less active against aerobic gram-negative rods other than *E. coli*. Furthermore, it is usually prescribed for 5 days and may cause gastrointestinal upset. It is not associated with plasmid-mediated resistance, however, so it is an excellent choice for patients with recent exposure to most other antimicrobial agents. The high in vitro resistance to ampicillin and sulfonamide and the high cost of amoxicillin/clavulanate and the cephalosporins limit their usefulness.

TMP and TMP-SMX are effective and inexpensive agents for empirical therapy, resulting in bacteriologic cure (i.e., eradication of the pathogen from the urine) within 7 days after the start of treatment in approximately 94% of women (Warren et al, 1999). **They are recommended in areas where the prevalence of resistance to these drugs among *E. coli* strains causing cystitis is less than 20%** (Gupta et al, 2011). The probability of resistant strains can be predicted in part from the history of recent antimicrobial usage. Women who have taken TMP-SMX recently are approximately 16 times as likely to be infected with an isolate resistant to this agent compared with women who have not taken the antimicrobial agent recently. In addition, those who have taken any other antimicrobial agent are more than twice as likely to be infected with a resistant isolate (Brown et al, 2002). With a 30% rate of resistance to TMP-SMX, the bacteriologic eradication rate is predicted to be 80% and the clinical cure rate is predicted to be 85% (Gupta et al, 2001). When used alone, TMP is as efficacious as TMP-SMX and is associated with fewer side effects, presumably because of the absence of the sulfa component (Harbord and Gruneberg, 1981). It can be prescribed to patients who are allergic to sulfa. However, TMP can cause hypersensitivity and rashes that may be erroneously attributed to sulfa (Alonso et al, 1992).

TABLE 12-10 Treatment Regimens for Acute Cystitis

CIRCUMSTANCES	ROUTE	DRUG	DOSAGE (mg)	FREQUENCY PER DOSE	DURATION (DAYS)	COST PER DAY
WOMEN						
Healthy	Oral	Nitrofurantoin macrocrystals	100 mg	bid	5	$3.24
		TMP-SMX	1 double-strength tablet (160-800 mg)	bid	3	$0.26
		Trimethoprim	100 mg	bid	3	$1.32
		Fosfomycin trometamol	3 g	Single dose	—	$47.99
		Pivmecillinam	400 mg	bid	3-7	Not available in the U.S.
		Ciprofloxacin	250 mg†	bid	3	$0.50
		Levofloxacin	250 mg†	qd	3	$5.07
Symptoms for >7 days, recent urinary tract infection, age >65 yr, diabetes, diaphragm use		TMP-SMX or fluoroquinolone	As above	As above	7	As above
Pregnancy	Oral	Amoxicillin	As above	As above	3-7	$0.68
		Cephalexin	As above	As above		$1.76
		Nitrofurantoin macrocrystals	As above	As above		As above
		TMP-SMX*	As above	As above		As above
MEN						
Healthy and age <50 yr	Oral	TMP-SMX	As above	As above	7	As above
		Ciprofloxacin	500 mg	bid	7	As above
		Levofloxacin	500 mg	qd	7	As above

*Use of TMP-SMX during the first trimester of pregnancy is cautioned because there is early potential for teratogenicity and late potential for kernicterus after delivery.
†Fluoroquinolones should be reserved for important infections other than acute cystitis except in select situations.
Modified from Schaeffer AJ. Urinary tract infections. In: Gillenwater JY, Grayhack JT, Howards SS, et al, editors. Adult and pediatric urology. Philadelphia: Lippincott Williams & Wilkins; 2002. p. 211–72; and Gupta K, Hooton TN, Naber KG, et al: International clinical practice guidelines for the treatment of acute uncomplicated cystitis and pyelonephritis in women: a 2010 update by the Infectious Diseases Society of America and the European Society for Microbiology and Infectious Diseases. Clin Infect Dis 2011;52:e103–20.

Fosfomycin trometamol (3 g in a single dose) is an appropriate choice for therapy where it is available because of minimal resistance and propensity for collateral damage, but it may have inferior efficacy compared with standard short-course regimens according to data submitted to the U.S. Food and Drug Administration (FDA) and summarized in the Medical Letter (A-I) (Fosfomycin for urinary tract infections, 1997; Gupta et al, 2011).

Pivmecillinam (400 mg twice daily for 3 to 7 days) is an appropriate choice for therapy in regions where it is available (availability limited to some European countries; not licensed and/or available for use in North America) because of minimal resistance and propensity for collateral damage, but it may have inferior efficacy compared with other available therapies (A-I) (Gupta et al, 2011).

The fluoroquinolones offer excellent activity, and are well tolerated. Resistance to the fluoroquinolones remains below 5% in most places (Fihn et al, 1988); however, it is increasing in certain areas. Twice-daily and once-daily extended-release fluoroquinolones are equally effective (Henry et al, 2002). They have a high propensity for collateral damage (i.e., ecological adverse effects, such as drug resistance) and should be reserved for important infections other than acute cystitis and thus should be considered alternative antimicrobials for acute cystitis (Gupta et al, 2011). Their use for uncomplicated cystitis should be limited to patients who are allergic to TMP-SMX, to patients with previous exposure to antimicrobial agents causing bacterial resistance, and to areas where the prevalence of resistance to TMP or TMP-SMX is 20% or greater (Warren et al, 1999; Hooton et al, 2004).

The effects of an antimicrobial agent on the vaginal flora are also important in recurrence of bacteriuria (Fihn et al, 1988). The concentrations of TMP and the fluoroquinolones that have been studied in vaginal secretions are high, eradicating E. coli but minimally altering normal anaerobic and microaerophilic vaginal flora (Hooton and Stamm, 1991). Single-dose regimens using these drugs are less effective than multiple-day regimens in this regard (Fihn et al, 1988), which probably explains why there are more early recurrent infections after single-dose therapy with these drugs. Nitrofurantoin and β-lactam drugs are generally not effective in eliminating E. coli from the vagina.

Duration of Therapy. Three-day therapy is the preferred regimen for uncomplicated cystitis in women (Norrby, 1990; Warren et al, 1999). In an excellent review of more than 300 separate clinical trials of single-dose, 3-day, or 7-day treatment with TMP, TMP-SMX, fluoroquinolones, and β-lactam antimicrobial therapies, it was concluded that, irrespective of the antimicrobial used, 3-day therapy is more effective than single-dose therapy. Three-day therapy with TMP-SMX, TMP, amoxicillin, or cloxacillin has been associated with cure rates similar to longer courses of therapy and an incidence of adverse effects about as low as that seen with single-dose therapy and lower than seen with longer courses of therapy (Charlton et al, 1976; Kunin, 1985; McCue, 1986; Warren et al, 1999). Because 7-day therapy often causes more adverse effects, it is recommended only for women with symptoms of 1 week or more, men, and individuals with possible complicating factors. Other options include nitrofurantoin, perhaps as 7-day therapy, and fosfomycin single-dose therapy; each of these requires further study. β-Lactams as a group are less effective in treatment of cystitis than TMP, TMP-SMX, and the fluoroquinolones.

Seven-day therapy is the preferred regimen in uncomplicated cystitis in men.

Cost of Therapy. The cost of treating a UTI involves not only the initial evaluation and cost of the drug but also what occurs subsequently. The most important prediction of high cost-effectiveness is high efficacy against the most common urinary pathogen, *E. coli*. The lower the effectiveness against this bacterium, the greater the number of revisits, cases of progression to pyelonephritis, and follow-up costs. Antimicrobial cost is a poor prediction of cost-effectiveness, as illustrated by the finding that the most expensive and least expensive drugs, the fluoroquinolones and TMP-SMX, are approximately equally cost-effective (Rosenberg, 1999). Both of these drugs are more cost-effective than nitrofurantoin and amoxicillin.

Follow-Up

Approximately 90% of women are asymptomatic within 72 hours after initiating antimicrobial therapy (Fihn et al, 1988). A follow-up visit or culture is not required in young women who are asymptomatic after therapy. A follow-up visit, urinalysis, and urine culture are recommended in older women or those with potential risk factors and in men. Urologic evaluation is unnecessary in women and is usually unnecessary in young men who respond to therapy (Lipsky, 1989; Abarbanel et al, 2003). However, UTIs in most men should be considered complicated until proven otherwise. Andrews and associates (2002) showed that approximately 50% of men with UTIs have a significant abnormality. Furthermore, if a patient does not respond to therapy, appropriate microbiologic urologic evaluations should be undertaken for the causes of unresolved and complicated UTIs.

Asymptomatic Bacteriuria

Asymptomatic bacteriuria is a microbiologic diagnosis based on the isolation of a specified quantitative count of bacteria in a properly collected specimen of urine from a patient who is without symptoms or signs referable to UTI. In healthy individuals, the absence of symptoms is clear cut, but, for example, in catheterized or neurologically compromised patients, it may be difficult to discern whether the UTI is truly asymptomatic. Kass (1962) originally proposed that for asymptomatic women two consecutive voided urine specimens with isolation of the same bacterial strain in quantitative counts of 10^5 cfu/mL is consistent with asymptomatic bacteriuria. In men, a single clean-catch voided specimen with similar counts is adequate. A single catheterized urine specimen with a solitary isolate with a quantitative count of 10^2 cfu/mL identifies bacteriuria in women or men (Nicolle et al, 2005). The prevalence of pyuria in women with asymptomatic bacteriuria ranges from approximately 30% in young women (Hooton et al, 2000) to 100% in catheterized patients. In addition, many coexisting factors, such as stones, can incite inflammation in these patients, and therefore the presence or absence of pyuria is not sufficient to diagnose bacteriuria nor does it differentiate symptomatic from asymptomatic patients or provide indication for antimicrobial treatment (Nicolle et al, 2005).

The prevalence of asymptomatic bacteriuria varies widely and depends on the age, sex, and the presence of other genitourinary abnormalities (Table 12-11). *E. coli* is the most common isolate among patients with bacteriuria, and it contains fewer virulence characteristics than isolates from patients with symptomatic infections (Svanborg and Godaly, 1997). Other Enterobacteriaceae (e.g., *P. mirabilis*) and gram-positive uropathogens, including group B streptococci and coagulase-negative staphylococci, become more prevalent in concert with increased underlying abnormalities. For patients who are institutionalized and/or with indwelling urologic devices, *P. aeruginosa*, *Proteus*, and other highly resistant organisms are more prevalent.

TABLE 12-11 Prevalence of Asymptomatic Bacteriuria in Selected Populations

POPULATION	PREVALENCE (%)	REFERENCE
Healthy, premenopausal women	1.0-5.0	Nicolle, 2003
Pregnant women	1.9-9.5	Nicolle, 2003
Postmenopausal women aged 50-70 years	2.8-8.6	Nicolle, 2003
Diabetic patients		
Women	9.0-27	Zhanel, 1991
Men	0.7-11	Zhanel, 1991
Elderly persons in the community		
Women	10.8-16	Nicolle, 2003
Men	3.6-19	Nicolle, 2003
Elderly persons in a long-term care facility		
Women	25-50	Nicolle, 1997
Men	14-50	Nicolle, 1997
Patients with spinal cord injuries		
Intermittent catheter use	23-89	Bakke and Digranes, 1991
Sphincterotomy and condom catheter in place	57	Waites et al, 1993b
Patients undergoing hemodialysis	28	Chaudhry, 1993
Patients with indwelling catheter use		
Short-term	9-23	Stamm, 1991
Long-term	100	Warren, 1982

From Nicolle LE, Bradley S, Colgan R, et al. Infectious Diseases Society of America guidelines for the diagnosis and treatment of asymptomatic bacteriuria in adults. Clin Infect Dis 2005;40:643–54.

Management of asymptomatic bacteriuria is determined by the population and their risk for adverse outcome, which can be prevented with antimicrobial treatment of asymptomatic bacteriuria (Nicolle et al, 2005) (Table 12-12). These recommendations are based on the observation that in adult populations asymptomatic bacteriuria has not been shown to be harmful. Furthermore, although persons with bacteriuria are at increased risk of symptomatic urinary tract infections, treatment of asymptomatic bacteriuria does not decrease the frequency of symptomatic infections or improve other outcomes. Thus, in populations other than those for whom treatment has been documented to be beneficial (e.g., pregnant women and patients undergoing urologic interventions), screening for or treatment of asymptomatic bacteriuria is not appropriate and should be discouraged (Nicolle et al, 2005).

Complicated Cystitis

Complicated UTIs are those that occur in a patient with a compromised urinary tract or that are caused by a very resistant pathogen (Box 12-7). These complicating factors may be readily apparent from the severity of the presenting illness or the past medical history. However, they may not be obvious at first and may only become evident from subsequent failure of the patient to respond to appropriate therapy (see later discussion on unresolved or recurrent UTIs).

The clinical spectrum ranges from mild cystitis to life-threatening kidney infections and urosepsis (kidney infections and urosepsis are discussed subsequently). These infections can be caused by a broad range of bacteria with resistance to multiple antimicrobial agents. Therefore urine cultures are mandatory to identify the bacteria and its antimicrobial susceptibility.

Because of the wide range of host conditions and pathogens and a lack of adequate controlled trials, guidelines for empirical therapy are limited. For patients with mild to moderate illness who can be treated as an outpatient with oral therapy, the fluoroquinolones provide a broad spectrum of activity with excellent urine and tissue levels and safety. If the susceptibility pattern of the pathogen is known, TMP-SMX may be effective (Table 12-13).

For patients requiring hospitalization, IV antimicrobials should be administered based on the susceptibility patterns of the known uropathogens at that institution.

Because therapy will be compromised without addressing complicating factors, every effort should be made to correct any underlying urinary tract abnormalities and treat host factors that exacerbate the infection.

Therapy is usually continued for 10 to 14 days and switched from parenteral to oral therapy when the patient is afebrile and clinically stable. Repeat urine cultures should be performed if the patient fails to respond to therapy.

Unresolved UTIs

Clinical Presentation

Unresolved infection indicates that initial therapy has been inadequate in eliminating symptoms and/or bacterial growth in the urinary tract. If the symptoms of UTI do not resolve by the end of treatment or if symptoms recur shortly after therapy, urinalysis and urine culture with susceptibility testing should be obtained. If the patient's symptoms are significant, empirical therapy with a fluoroquinolone is appropriate, pending results of the culture and susceptibility testing.

The causes of unresolved bacteriuria during antimicrobial therapy are shown in Box 12-8. **Most commonly, the bacteria are resistant to the antimicrobial agent selected to treat the infection.** Typically, the patient has received the antimicrobial therapy in the recent past and developed bowel colonization with resistant bacteria. β-lactams, tetracycline, and sulfonamides are notorious for causing plasmid-mediated R factors that simultaneously carry resistance to multiple antimicrobial agents. **The second most common cause is development of resistance in a previously susceptible population of bacteria during the course of treatment of UTIs.** This problem occurs in approximately 5% of the patients receiving antimicrobial therapy. It is easy to recognize clinically because the culture on therapy shows that the previous susceptible population has been replaced by resistant bacteria of the same species. It can be shown that resistant organisms were actually present

TABLE 12-12 Screening for and Treatment of Asymptomatic Bacteriuria

Premenopausal nonpregnant women	Not recommended
Pregnant women	Recommended
Diabetic women	Not recommended
Older persons residing in the community	Not recommended
Elderly institutionalized subjects	Not recommended
Subjects with spinal cord injuries	Not recommended
Patients with indwelling urethral catheters	Not recommended
Note: Antimicrobial treatment of asymptomatic women with catheter-associated bacteriuria that persists 48 hours after catheter removal may be considered.	
Urologic interventions	Recommended
Immunocompromised patients and transplant patients	Not recommended

From Nicolle LE, Bradley S, Colgan R, et al. Infectious Diseases Society of America guidelines for the diagnosis and treatment of asymptomatic bacteriuria in adults. Clin Infect Dis 2005;40:643–54.

BOX 12-7 Complicating Host Factors

Functional/structural abnormalities of urinary tract
Recent urinary tract instrumentation
Recent antimicrobial agent use
Diabetes mellitus
Immunosuppression
Pregnancy
Hospital-acquired infection

TABLE 12-13 Treatment of Complicated Urinary Tract Infections

COMMON PATHOGENS	MITIGATING CIRCUMSTANCES	RECOMMENDED EMPIRICAL TREATMENT
E. coli, Proteus species, *Klebsiella* species, *Pseudomonas* species,	Mild-to-moderate illness, no nausea or vomiting—outpatient therapy	Oral* ciprofloxacin or ofloxacin for 10-14 days
Serratia species, enterococci, staphylococci	Severe illness or possible urosepsis—hospitalization required	Parenteral† ampicillin and gentamicin, ciprofloxacin, levofloxacin, ceftriaxone, aztreonam, ticarcillin-clavulanate or imipenem-cilastatin until fever gone; then oral* trimethoprim-sulfamethoxazole, norfloxacin, ciprofloxacin, or levofloxacin for 14-21 days

*Oral regimens for pyelonephritis and complicated urinary tract infection: trimethoprim-sulfamethoxazole, 160 and 800 mg q12h; ciprofloxacin, 500 mg q12h; levofloxacin, 500 mg/day.

†Parenteral regimens: ciprofloxacin, 400 mg q12h; levofloxacin, 250 mg/day; gentamicin, 1 mg/kg q8h; ceftriaxone, 1 to 2 g/day; ampicillin, 1 g q6h; imipenem-cilastatin, 250 to 500 mg q6-8h; ticarcillin-clavulanate, 3.1 g q6h; and aztreonam, 1 g q8-12h.

Modified from Stamm WE, Hooton TM. Management of urinary tract infections in adults. N Engl J Med 1993;329:1328–34. Copyright 1993, Massachusetts Medical Society. All rights reserved.

BOX 12-8 Causes of Unresolved Bacteriuria, in Descending Order of Importance

Bacterial resistance to the drug selected for treatment
Development of resistance from initially susceptible bacteria
Bacteriuria caused by two different bacterial species with mutually exclusive susceptibilities
Rapid reinfection with a new, resistant species during initial therapy for the original susceptible organism
Azotemia
Papillary necrosis from analgesic abuse
Giant staghorn calculi in which the "critical mass" of susceptible bacteria is too great for antimicrobial inhibition
Self-inflicted infections or deception in taking antimicrobial drugs (a variant of Munchausen syndrome)

before contact with the initial antimicrobial agent, but they were present in such low numbers that it was impossible to detect by in vitro susceptibility studies before therapy. When the antimicrobial concentration in the urine is insufficient to kill all the bacteria present, the more resistant forms will emerge. This characteristically is seen in patients who are underdosed or who are poorly compliant and hence have inadequate dose regimens. **The third cause is the presence of an unsuspected, second pathogen that was present initially and is resistant to the antimicrobial therapy chosen.** Treatment of the dominant organism unmasks the presence of the second strain. **The fourth cause is rapid reintroduction of a new resistant species while the patient is undergoing initial therapy.** Rapid reinfection that mimics unresolved bacteriuria should alert the clinician to the possibility of an enterovesical fistula.

If the culture obtained on therapy shows that the initial species is still present and susceptible to the antimicrobial chosen to treat the infection, the unresolved infection must be caused by either inability to deliver an adequate concentration of antimicrobial agents into the urinary tract or an excessive number of bacteria that "override" the antimicrobial activity. In patients with azotemia, a determination of urinary antimicrobial concentrations usually shows that the level of the drug is below the minimal inhibitory concentration of the infecting organism.

In patients with papillary necrosis, severe defects in the medullary concentrating ability dilute the antimicrobial agent. A large mass of bacteria within the urinary tract is most commonly associated with a giant staghorn calculus. Even though adequate urinary levels of bactericidal drugs are present, the concentration is inadequate to sterilize the urine. This occurs because even susceptible bacteria cannot be inhibited once they reach a certain critical density, particularly if attached to a foreign body.

The last cause of unresolved bacteriuria occurs in those patients who have variants of Munchausen syndrome. These patients secretly inoculate their bladders with uropathogens or omit their oral antimicrobial agents while steadfastly asserting that they never miss a dose. The patient with Munchausen syndrome presents with an inconsistent clinical history and invariably a normal urinary tract on urologic imaging. Careful bacteriologic observations usually indicate the implausibility of the clinical picture.

Laboratory Diagnosis

Urinalysis and urine culture are mandatory to determine the cause of unresolved bacteriuria. The first four causes that are associated with resistant bacteria require no further evaluation. However, if reculture shows that the bacteria are sensitive to the antimicrobial agent the patient is taking, renal function and radiologic evaluation should be performed to identify renal or urinary tract abnormalities.

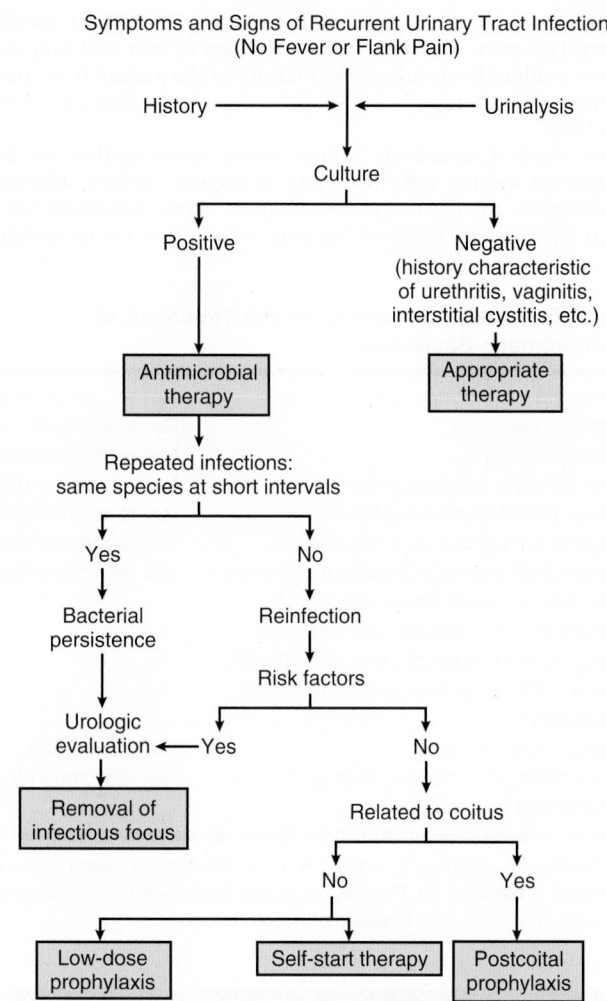

Figure 12-14. **Management of recurrent urinary tract infection.**

Management

Initial empirical antimicrobial selection should be based on the assumption that the bacteria are resistant. Therefore an antimicrobial agent different from the original agent should be selected. Fluoroquinolones offer excellent coverage in most cases and should be given for 7 days. When the bacterial susceptibilities are available, adjustments can be made if necessary. Urine cultures should be performed during and 7 days after therapy to ensure microbiologic efficacy.

Recurrent UTIs

Recurrent UTIs are caused by either reemergence of bacteria from a site within the urinary tract (bacterial persistence) or new infections from bacteria outside the urinary tract (reinfection). Clinical identification of these two types of recurrence is based on the pattern of recurrent infections (Fig. 12-14). Bacterial persistence must be caused by the same organism in each instance, and infections that occur at close intervals are characteristic. Conversely, reinfections usually occur at varying and sometimes long intervals and often are caused by different species. The distinction between bacterial persistence and reinfection is important in management because patients with bacterial persistence can usually be cured of the recurrent infections by identification and surgical removal or correction of the focus of infection. Conversely, women with reinfection usually do not have an alterable urologic abnormality and require long-term medical management. Reinfections in men are uncommon and may be associated with an underlying abnormality, such as urethral stricture; therefore, at a minimum, endoscopic evaluation is indicated.

Bacterial Persistence

Once the bacteriuria has resolved (i.e., the urine shows no growth for several days after the antimicrobial agent has been stopped), recurrence with the same organism can arise from a site *within* the urinary tract that was excluded from the high urine concentrations of the antimicrobial agent. The 12 correctable urologic abnormalities that cause bacteria to persist within the urinary tract between episodes of recurrent bacteriuria are listed in Box 12-4. The relationship of these abnormalities to bacterial persistence, as well as the documentation that surgical excision removes the infection as a source of recurrent bacteriuria, is presented elsewhere in detail (Stamey, 1980). Once the urologist recognizes that the cause of the patient's recurrent bacteriuria is bacterial persistence, Box 12-4 should serve as a checklist for known, correctable causes. Some of the causes are subtle, and many require cystoscopic localization of the infection with ureteral catheters to accurately define the focus of bacterial persistence.

Although patients with bacterial persistence are relatively uncommon, their identification is important because they represent the only surgically curable cause of recurrent UTIs. A systematic radiologic and endoscopic evaluation of the urinary tract is mandatory. CT and cystoscopy provide the initial screening. Retrograde urography may be required in selected patients to delineate abnormalities, such as diverticulum or nonrefluxing ureteral stump.

Urea-Splitting Bacteria That Cause Struvite Renal Stones. The infection that ultimately leads to an infection stone commonly begins inconspicuously as inadequately treated cystitis. Most patients with *P. mirabilis* cystitis do not form struvite stones. But **struvite stones form in those patients who have a protracted infection with *P. mirabilis*,** an infection that is often asymptomatic or minimally symptomatic. *P. mirabilis* causes intense alkalinization of the urine with precipitation of calcium, magnesium, ammonium, and phosphate salts and the subsequent formation of branched struvite renal stones. Bacteriuria in most of these patients with struvite stones recurs almost immediately on stopping antimicrobial therapy, usually within 5 to 7 days. The bacteriologic consequences are substantial because the **bacteria persist inside these struvite stones even when the urine shows no growth**. Indeed, struvite infection stones, together with the occasional oxalate or apatite stone that becomes secondarily colonized, constitute the major cause of bacterial persistence in women in the absence of azotemia.

Underlying urinary tract abnormalities are not a prerequisite for this type of infection. However, patients with indwelling catheters, urinary diversions, or other urinary tract abnormalities are particularly susceptible to these infections. Urea-splitting organisms, such as *P. mirabilis*, cause infection stones that are relatively radiolucent. If such a stone is suspected, plain film tomograms or CT scans without contrast medium enhancement should be obtained (Greenberg et al, 1982). Medical management with continued suppressive antimicrobial therapy and acidification temporarily relieves symptoms and retards deterioration of renal function in some patients. **Complete removal of the calculus is generally required for bacteriologic cure and to prevent renal damage caused by obstruction** (Silverman and Stamey, 1983). Percutaneous nephrolithotomy and extracorporeal shockwave lithotripsy are now the preferred treatment for most renal and upper ureteral calculi.

When extracorporeal shockwave lithotripsy is used to fragment infection stones, the patient should be maintained on appropriate antimicrobial therapy until the fragments pass. Occasionally, long-term antimicrobial therapy can result in eradication of bacteriuria even if some fragments persist after lithotripsy, presumably because the shockwaves have rendered the entrapped bacteria more susceptible to antimicrobial therapy (Michaels et al, 1988). **If percutaneous or open surgery is used, all the residual particles of struvite stones must be removed at surgery to prevent recurrent bacteriuria from bacterial persistence in the calculus.**

Rocha and Santos (1969) have shown that soaking these stones in iodine and alcohol for 6 hours will not kill the bacteria within the interior of the stone. **The importance of recognizing this fact is twofold: (1) The bacteria cannot be killed by antimicrobial therapy, even though the urine may show no growth for months or even years** (Shortliffe et al, 1984), **and (2) any fragments left behind at the time of surgical removal leave residual bacteria within the interstices of the stone; these bacteria ensure recurrence of the staghorn calculus with its attendant morbidity.**

If fragments remain after surgery, a small, multihole polyethylene catheter should be left for postoperative irrigation with Renacidin or Suby G solution (Silverman and Stamey, 1983). Follow-up radiographs are essential to ensure that all the stone fragments are removed, and cultures must demonstrate that the urease-splitting bacteria are eradicated.

Most of the other congenital or acquired abnormalities listed in Box 12-4 require surgical removal for eradication of the source of bacterial persistence. Chronic bacterial prostatitis is treated initially with long-term antimicrobial therapy and, in select cases, by radical transurethral resection (Meares, 1978).

In patients in whom the focus of infection cannot be eradicated, long-term, low-dose antimicrobial suppression is necessary to prevent symptoms of infection. The antimicrobial drugs used for low-dose prophylaxis will also be effective for bacterial suppression if the persistent strain is susceptible. These include nitrofurantoin, TMP-SMX, cephalexin, and the fluoroquinolones.

Reinfections

Patients with recurrent infections caused by different species or occurring at long intervals almost invariably have reinfections. These reinfections most often occur in women and girls and are associated with ascending colonization from the bowel flora. Reinfections in men are often associated with a urinary tract abnormality. The possibility of a vesicoenteric or vesicovaginal fistula should be considered when the patient has any history of pneumaturia, fecaluria, diverticulitis, obstipation, previous pelvic surgery, or radiation therapy. **Evaluation of the patient with presumed reinfections must be individualized.**

Failure to recognize and correct abnormalities that reduce formation, transmission, and elimination of urine by the urinary tract increases the incidence of reinfection in susceptible patients and reduces the effectiveness of antimicrobial therapy. Abnormalities should be corrected and urinary tract function restored by medical, pharmacologic, or surgical management. A thorough urologic evaluation is essential in all men and in women with evidence of upper tract infections (fevers, chills, flank pain, hemorrhagic cystitis, or other risk factors, such as history of unexplained hematuria, obstructive symptoms, neurogenic bladder dysfunction, renal calculi, fistula, analgesic abuse, or severe disease such as diabetes mellitus). In women, diaphragm-spermicide use has been associated with an increased risk of UTI and vaginal colonization with *E. coli* (Hooton et al, 1991b). Spermicides containing the active ingredient nonoxynol-9 may provide a selective advantage in colonizing the vagina, perhaps by a reduction in vaginal lactobacilli and through enhancement of adherence of *E. coli* to epithelial cells (Hooton et al, 1991a; Gupta et al, 2000). Thus spermicides should be discontinued in women with recurrent UTI, and other forms of contraception should be used.

Postmenopausal women have frequent reinfections (Hooton and Stamm, 1991; Raz and Stamm, 1993). These infections are **sometimes attributable to residual urine** after voiding, which is often associated with bladder or uterine prolapse. **In addition, the lack of estrogen causes marked changes in the vaginal microflora,** including a loss of lactobacilli and increased colonization by *E. coli* (Raz and Stamm, 1993). Estrogen replacement frequently restores the normal vaginal environment, allows recolonization with lactobacilli, and thus eliminates bacterial uropathogenic colonization. A reduced incidence of UTIs has been documented with this approach (Raz and Stamm, 1993).

Urinary tract imaging will demonstrate the anatomy of the urinary tract and provide reasonable assessment of its functional status. In healthy women, upper tract abnormalities associated with reinfections are very rare; therefore routine urologic imaging is not indicated. Cystoscopy should be performed in men or women who have frequent reinfections and symptoms suggestive of obstruction, bladder dysfunction, and fistula. If the patient has residual urine that is judged to be significant (e.g., 100 mL) and due to a narrowing of the urethra, a single dilation of the urethra to improve bladder emptying would appear appropriate. There is little evidence, however, that repeated urethral dilation is indicated in the routine management of most women.

Antimicrobial management in women who have had two or more symptomatic UTIs over a 6-month period or three or more episodes within a 12-month period involves one of three regimens: low-dose continuous prophylaxis, self-start intermittent therapy, or postintercourse prophylaxis.

Low-Dose Continuous Prophylaxis

Biologic Basis of Successful Prophylaxis: Antimicrobial Effect on Bowel and Vaginal Bacterial Flora. The success of prophylaxis depends, in large part, on the effect an antimicrobial agent has on the introital and bowel reservoirs of pathogenic bacteria. Antimicrobial agents that eliminate pathogenic bacteria from these sites and/or do not cause bacterial resistance at the sites can be effective for antimicrobial prophylaxis of UTIs (Table 12-14).

Winberg and his colleagues were among the first to emphasize that oral antimicrobial therapy causes resistant strains in the bowel flora and subsequent resistant UTIs (Lincoln et al. 1970; Winberg et al, 1973). The increase in resistant strains of *E. coli* is well documented, as is the proliferation of other Enterobacteriaceae species, *Candida albicans*, enterococci, and other pathogenic bacteria in the bowel and vaginal flora that accompanies even short-term, full-dose oral administration of tetracyclines, ampicillin, sulfonamides, amoxicillin, and cephalexin (Sharp, 1954; Daikos et al, 1968; Hinton, 1970; Lincoln et al, 1970; Datta et al, 1971; Gruneberg et al, 1973; Winberg et al, 1973; Toivanen et al, 1976; Ronald et al, 1977; Preiksaitis et al, 1981). These ecologic changes may interfere with antimicrobial prophylaxis in the urinary tract and must be considered in the choice of prophylactic agents.

Effective Drugs. The oral antimicrobial agents with minimal adverse effects on the bowel and vaginal flora are TMP-SMX or TMP alone, nitrofurantoin, cephalexin (in minimal dosage), and the fluoroquinolones.

TMP-SMX eradicates gram-negative aerobic flora from the bowel and vaginal fluid. Vaginal fluid measurements of TMP and

TABLE 12-14   Low-Dose Prophylaxis for Recurrent Urinary Tract Infections in Women

INVESTIGATORS	REGIMEN	INFECTIONS PER PATIENT-YEAR
Bailey et al (1971)	Nitrofurantoin, 50 or 100 mg daily	0.09
	Nitrofurantoin, 50 mg daily	0.19
	Placebo	2.1
Harding and Ronald (1974)	Sulfamethoxazole, 500 mg daily	2.5
	TMP-SMX, 40 and 200 mg daily	0.1
	Methenamine mandelate, 2 g daily, plus ascorbic acid, 2 g	1.6
Kasanen et al (1974)	Nitrofurantoin, 50 mg daily	0.32
	Methenamine hippurate, 1 g daily	0.39
	Trimethoprim, 100 mg daily	0.13
	TMP-SMX, 80 and 400 mg daily	0.19
Gower (1975)	Cephalexin, 125 mg daily	0.10
Stamey et al (1977)	TMP-SMX, 40 and 200 mg daily	0.00
	Nitrofurantoin macrocrystals, 100 mg daily	0.74
Harding et al (1979)	TMP-SMX, 40 and 200 mg three times weekly	0.1
Stamm et al (1980)	TMP-SMX, 40 and 200 mg daily	0.15
	Trimethoprim, 100 mg daily	0.00
	Nitrofurantoin macrocrystals, 100 mg daily	0.14
	Placebo	2.8
Brumfitt et al (1981)	Nitrofurantoin, 50 mg twice daily	0.19
	Methenamine hippurate, 1 g twice daily	0.57
Harding et al (1982)	TMP-SMX, 40 and 200 mg three times weekly	0.14
Brumfitt et al (1983)	Trimethoprim, 100 mg daily	1.53
	Methenamine hippurate, 1 g daily	1.38
	Povidone-iodine wash, twice daily	1.79
Wong et al (1985)	TMP-SMX, 40 and 200 mg daily	0.2
	Self-administered cotrimoxazole, 4 × 80 and 400 mg	2.2
Martinez et al (1985)	Cephalexin, 250 mg daily	0.18
Brumfitt et al (1985)	Trimethoprim, 100 mg daily	1.00
	Nitrofurantoin macrocrystals, 100 mg daily	0.16
Nicolle et al (1989)	Nitrofurantoin, 200 mg daily	0.00

TMP-SMX, trimethoprim-sulfamethoxazole.
Modified from Nicolle LE, Ronald AR. Recurrent urinary tract infection in adult women: diagnosis and treatment. Infect Dis Clin North Am 1987;1:793–806.

SMX in patients showed that TMP infused across the noninflamed vaginal wall and produced concentrations that exceeded serum levels (Stamey and Condy, 1975); SMX was undetectable in vaginal fluid. These observations on diffusion and concentration of TMP and vaginal fluid and on the effects of TMP-SMX in clearing Enterobacteriaceae from the rectal and vaginal flora clearly indicate why TMP-SMX is such a powerful prophylactic agent for the prevention of reinfections in the female. These important biologic effects occur in addition to the bactericidal levels of TMP-SMX that are present in the urine during nightly prophylaxis.

Kasanen and his colleagues (1978) in Finland studied the bowel flora in volunteers and patients who took 100 mg of TMP per day for periods of 3 weeks to 36 months; 4 of 20 patients treated for long periods developed coliforms resistant to TMP (>8 µg/mL). Svensson and his associates (1982) gave 100 mg of TMP once daily for 6 months to 26 patients with recurrent UTIs. The infection recurrence rate before prophylaxis was 26 per 100 months compared with 3.3 recurrences per 100 months during prophylaxis ($P = .001$). The postprophylactic infection rate returned to 23 recurrences per 100 months. It is important to note that all E. coli UTIs after prophylaxis were sensitive to TMP, the number of rectal Enterobacteriaceae was markedly reduced during prophylaxis, and, although a 10% incidence of TMP-resistant organisms from rectal swabs was observed less than 1 month into prophylaxis, there was no significant further accumulation of resistant bacteria.

These studies on TMP alone suggest that it should be as effective as TMP-SMX for prophylactic prevention of recurrent UTIs. Stamm and coworkers (1980a) noted only one resistant strain of E. coli in 316 rectal, urethral, and vaginal isolates from 15 patients receiving 100 mg of TMP and 15 others receiving 40 mg of TMP with 200 mg of SMX nightly for 6 months; their unbelievably low recovery of TMP-resistant E. coli was due to their method of sampling, which did not include streaking cultures from these colonization sites directly onto media containing TMP.

These studies on TMP-SMX and TMP prophylactic therapy usually have been limited to 6 months to test continuing susceptibility in patients with reinfections. Two studies (Pearson et al, 1979; Harding et al, 1982), however, continued TMP-SMX prophylaxis from 2 to 5 years without showing any increase in "breakthrough" infections or any increase in TMP-resistant recurrent infections. Indeed, in the 15 patients treated for 2 years with one-half tablet of TMP-SMX thrice weekly (Harding et al, 1982), 100 of 116 cultures from the periurethral area (91%) and 60 of 97 cultures from the anal canal (68%) showed no aerobic gram-negative bacilli at these colonization sites.

Nitrofurantoin, which does not alter the bowel flora, is present for brief periods at high concentrations in the urine and leads to repeated elimination of bacteria from the urine, presumably interfering with bacterial initiation of infection. Because of either its complete absorption in the upper intestinal tract or its degradation and inactivation in the intestinal tract, it produces minimal effects on bowel flora (Stamey et al, 1977). Unlike the situation in prophylaxis with TMP-SMX that eliminates colonization, in prophylaxis with nitrofurantoin colonization of the vaginal introitus with Enterobacteriaceae continues throughout therapy. The bacteria colonizing the vagina nearly always remain susceptible because of the lack of bacterial resistance in the bowel flora. Patients on long-term therapy should be monitored for adverse reactions, (e.g., pulmonary fibrosis). **The risk of an adverse reaction increases with age, with the greatest number occurring in patients older than 50 years. If a patient develops a chronic cough, the drug should be discontinued and a chest radiograph obtained.**

Fairley and his associates (1974) first reported on the prophylactic efficacy of 500 mg of **cephalexin** per day in preventing recurrent infections during a 6-month period of observation. Of the 22 patients, 17 remained free of infection, an impressive record because several patients had papillary necrosis, chronic pyelonephritis, and even renal calculi. Gower (1975) treated 25 women with 125 mg of cephalexin nightly for 6 to 12 months and found only 1 infection, whereas 13 of 25 women receiving a placebo had infection.

Martinez and coworkers (1985) studied the effect on the vaginal and rectal flora of 250 mg of cephalexin nightly for 6 months in 23 patients with reinfections of the urinary tract. Throughout prophylaxis, 22 of the 23 patients maintained a sterile urine; a single patient developed two enterococcal UTIs, both of which responded to nitrofurantoin. No change was detected in the rectal or vaginal carriage of Enterobacteriaceae. More importantly, not a single resistant strain of E. coli was detected in 154 cultures obtained at monthly intervals during cephalexin therapy. These results are in contrast to those of Preiksaitis and colleagues (1981), who found rectal Enterobacteriaceae resistance in 38% of patients when cephalexin was administered at a dose of 500 mg four times daily for 14 days. **Cephalexin at 250 mg or less nightly is an excellent prophylactic agent because bowel flora resistance does not develop at this low dosage.**

With short-course fluoroquinolone therapy (Hooton et al, 1989), eradication of Enterobacteriaceae from the bowel and vaginal (Nord, 1988; Tartaglione et al, 1988) flora has been documented—observations that have been exploited in the use of these agents for prophylaxis. More recently, Nicolle and coworkers (1989) documented the prophylactic efficacy of norfloxacin for the prevention of recurrent UTIs in women. Of 11 women who completed 1 year of prophylaxis (200 mg orally), all remained free of infection. By comparison, the majority of individuals receiving placebos developed UTIs. The drug was well tolerated. In addition to preventing symptomatic UTIs, norfloxacin virtually eradicated periurethral and bowel colonization with aerobic gram-negative organisms. A larger study by Raz and Boger (1991) confirmed these results.

Because the fluoroquinolones are expensive and can be used only in nonpregnant women, we favor their use only when antimicrobial resistance or patient intolerance to TMP-SMX, TMP, nitrofurantoin, or cephalexin occurs. Further studies are required to determine the minimal effective regimen and efficacy of the fluoroquinolones for prophylaxis of recurrent UTIs in women.

Efficacy of Prophylaxis. Low-dose continuous prophylaxis is indicated when the urine culture shows no growth (usually when a patient has completed antimicrobial therapy). Nightly therapy is then begun with one of the following drugs: (1) nitrofurantoin, 50 to 100 mg half-strength (HS) (Stamey et al, 1977); (2) TMP-SMX, 40 to 200 mg (Stamm et al, 1982a); (3) TMP, 50 mg (Stamm et al, 1982a); or (4) cephalexin (Keflex), 250 mg (Martinez et al, 1985). **Prophylactic therapy has been repeatedly documented as being effective in the management of women with recurrent UTIs, with recurrences decreased by 95% when compared with placebo or with the patients' prior experiences as controls.** These reported results of prophylaxis, together with agents and doses, have been summarized by Nicolle and Ronald (1987) (see Table 12-14). These studies consistently show a remarkable reduction in the reinfection rate from 2.0 to 3.0 per patient-year to 0.1 to 0.4 per patient-year with the use of prophylaxis. Urinary antiseptics, such as methenamine mandelate or hippurate, have resulted in some decrease in recurrences, but they are not as effective as antimicrobial agents.

Every-other-night therapy is also effective and is probably practiced by most patients. **When breakthrough infections occur, they are not necessarily accompanied by symptoms; therefore we advocate monitoring for infections every 1 to 3 months, even in asymptomatic patients. Breakthrough infections usually respond to full-dose therapy with the drug used for prophylaxis. However, cultures and susceptibility tests may indicate that another drug is indicated. After the infection is cured, prophylaxis may be reinstituted. Low-dose prophylaxis is usually discontinued after about 6 months, and the patient is monitored for reinfection.** Approximately 30% of women will have spontaneous remissions that last up to 6 months (Kraft and Stamey, 1977). Unfortunately, many of the remissions are followed by reinfections, and low-dose prophylaxis must be reinstituted. At this point, many patients prefer an alternative form of management.

Self-Start Intermittent Therapy. With self-start intermittent therapy, the patient is given a dip slide device to culture the urine and is instructed to perform a urine culture when symptoms of UTI occur (Schaeffer and Stuppy, 1999; Blom et al, 2002). The patient is also provided a 3-day course of empirical, full-dose antimicrobial therapy to be started immediately after performing the culture. It is important that the antimicrobial agent selected for self-start therapy have a broad spectrum of activity and achieve high urinary levels to minimize development of resistant mutants. In addition, there should be minimal or no side effects on the bowel flora. Fluoroquinolones are ideal for self-start therapy because they have a spectrum of activity broader than any of the other oral agents and are superior to many parenteral antimicrobials, including aminoglycosides. Nitrofurantoin and TMP-SMX are acceptable alternatives, although they are somewhat less effective. Antimicrobial agents such as tetracycline, ampicillin, SMX, and cephalexin in full doses should be avoided because they can give rise to resistant bacteria (Wong et al, 1985).

The culture is brought to the office as soon as possible. If the culture is positive and the patient is asymptomatic, a culture is performed 7 to 10 days after therapy to determine efficacy. In most cases, the therapy is limited to two inexpensive dip slide cultures and a short course of antimicrobial therapy. If the patient has symptoms that do not respond to initial antimicrobial therapy, a repeat culture and susceptibility testing of the initial culture specimen are performed and therapy adjusted accordingly. If symptoms of infection are not associated with positive cultures, urologic evaluation should be performed to rule out other causes of irritative bladder symptoms, including carcinoma in situ, interstitial cystitis, and neurogenic bladder dysfunction. Our experience with this technique has been very favorable and is particularly attractive to patients who have less frequent infections and are willing to play an active role in their diagnosis and management.

Postintercourse Prophylaxis. Antimicrobial management through postintercourse prophylaxis is based on research establishing that sexual intercourse can be an important risk factor for acute cystitis in women (Nicolle et al, 1982). Diaphragm users have a significantly greater risk of UTI than do women who use other contraceptive methods (Fihn et al, 1985). Postintercourse therapy with antimicrobial agents, such as nitrofurantoin, cephalexin, TMP-SMX, or a fluoroquinolone taken as a single dose, will effectively reduce the incidence of reinfection (Pfau et al, 1983; Melekos et al, 1997).

Other Strategies. Cranberry juice contains proanthocyanidins that block adherence of pathogens to uroepithelial cells in vitro (Foo et al, 2000). Randomized trials in low-risk patients show that 200 to 750 mL daily of cranberry or lingonberry juice or cranberry-concentrate tablets reduce the risk of symptomatic, recurrent infection by 12% to 20% (Avorn et al, 1994; Kontiokari et al, 2001; Stothers, 2002; McMurdo et al, 2009). However, the actual cranberry content of juices and tablets varies substantially; therefore their efficacy is not predictable (Consumer Reports, 2001; Klein, 2002). Furthermore, other trials of cranberry products show no benefit and there is no evidence that they are effective for treatment of UTIs (Jepson et al, 2001; Raz et al, 2004).

Other factors, such as hygiene, frequency and timing of voiding, wiping patterns, use of hot tubs, and type of undergarments, have not been shown to predispose women to recurrent infection, and there is no rationale for giving women specific instructions regarding them.

KEY POINTS: BLADDER INFECTIONS

- Uncomplicated cystitis should be treated for 3 days.
- Asymptomatic bacteriuria should be treated only in pregnant women and prior to urologic intervention.
- Recurrent UTIs caused by bacterial persistence require urologic management; reinfections can be managed medically.

KIDNEY INFECTIONS

Renal Infection (Bacterial Nephritis)

Although renal infection is less prevalent than bladder infection, it often is a more difficult problem for the patient and his or her physician because of its often varied and morbid presentation and course, the difficulty in establishing a firm microbiologic and pathologic diagnosis, and its potential for significantly impairing renal function. **Although the classic symptoms of acute onset of fever, chills, and flank pain are usually indicative of renal infection, some patients with these symptoms do not have renal infection. Conversely, significant renal infection may be associated with an insidious onset of nonspecific local or systemic symptoms, or it may be entirely asymptomatic.** Therefore a high clinical index of suspicion and appropriate radiologic and laboratory studies are required to establish the diagnosis of renal infection.

Unfortunately, **the relationship between laboratory findings and the presence of renal infection often is poor. Bacteriuria and pyuria, the hallmarks of UTI, are not predictive of renal infection. Conversely, patients with significant renal infection may have sterile urine if the ureter draining the kidney is obstructed or the infection is outside of the collecting system.**

The pathologic and radiologic criteria for diagnosing renal infection may also be misleading. Interstitial renal inflammation, once thought to be caused predominantly by bacterial infection, is now recognized as a nonspecific histopathologic change associated with a variety of immunologic, congenital, or chemical lesions that usually develop in the absence of bacterial infection. Infectious granulomatous diseases of the kidney often have either radiologic or pathologic characteristics that mimic renal cystic disease, neoplasia, or other renal inflammatory disease.

The effect of renal infection on renal function is varied. Acute or chronic pyelonephritis may transiently or permanently alter renal function, but nonobstructive pyelonephritis is no longer recognized as a major cause of renal failure (Baldassarre and Kaye, 1991; Fraser et al, 1995). However, pyelonephritis, when associated with urinary tract obstruction or granulomatous renal infection, may lead rapidly to significant inflammatory complications, renal failure, or even death.

Pathology

The opportunity for pathologic confirmation of **acute bacterial nephritis** is rare. The kidney may be edematous. Focal acute suppurative bacterial nephritis caused by hematogenous dissemination of bacteria to the renal cortex is characterized by multiple focal areas of suppuration on the surface of the kidney (Fig. 12-15). Histologic examination of the renal cortex shows focal suppurative destruction of glomeruli and tubules. Adjacent cortical structures and the medulla are not involved in the inflammatory reaction. **Acute ascending pyelonephritis** is characterized by linear bands of inflammation extending from the medulla to the renal capsule (Fig. 12-16). Histologic examination usually reveals a focal wedge-shaped area of acute interstitial inflammation with the apex of the wedge in the renal medulla. Polymorphonuclear leukocytes or a predominantly lymphocytic and plasma cell response are seen. Bacteria also may be present.

The changes that appear to be most specific for **chronic pyelonephritis** are evident on careful gross examination of the kidney and consist of a cortical scar associated with retraction of the corresponding renal papilla (Hodson, 1965; Hodson and Wilson, 1965; Heptinstall, 1974; Freedman, 1979). The kidney shows evidence of patchy involvement with numerous chronic inflammatory foci mainly confined to the cortex but also involving the medulla (Fig. 12-17).

The scars may be separated by intervening zones of normal parenchyma, causing a grossly irregular renal outline. The microscopic appearance, as with most chronic interstitial disease, includes the presence of lymphocytes and plasma cells. Although glomeruli within scars may be surrounded by a cuff of fibrosis or be partially

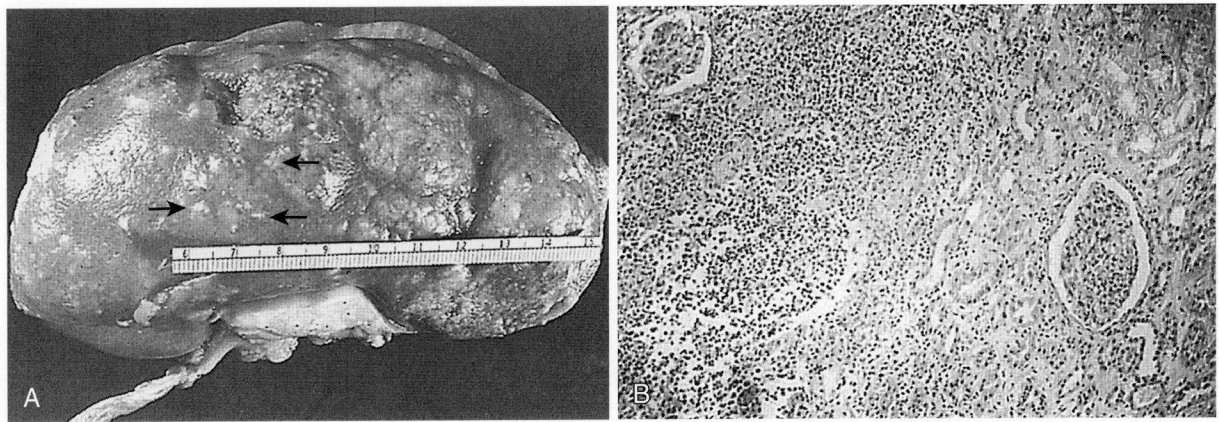

Figure 12-15. Acute focal suppurative bacterial nephritis. A, Surface of kidney. *Arrows* indicate focal areas of suppuration. B, Renal cortex showing focal suppuration destruction of glomeruli and tubules. (From Schaeffer AJ. Urinary tract infections. In: Gillenwater JY, Grayhack JT, Howards SS, et al, editors. Adult and pediatric urology. Philadelphia: Lippincott Williams & Wilkins; 2002. p. 211–72.)

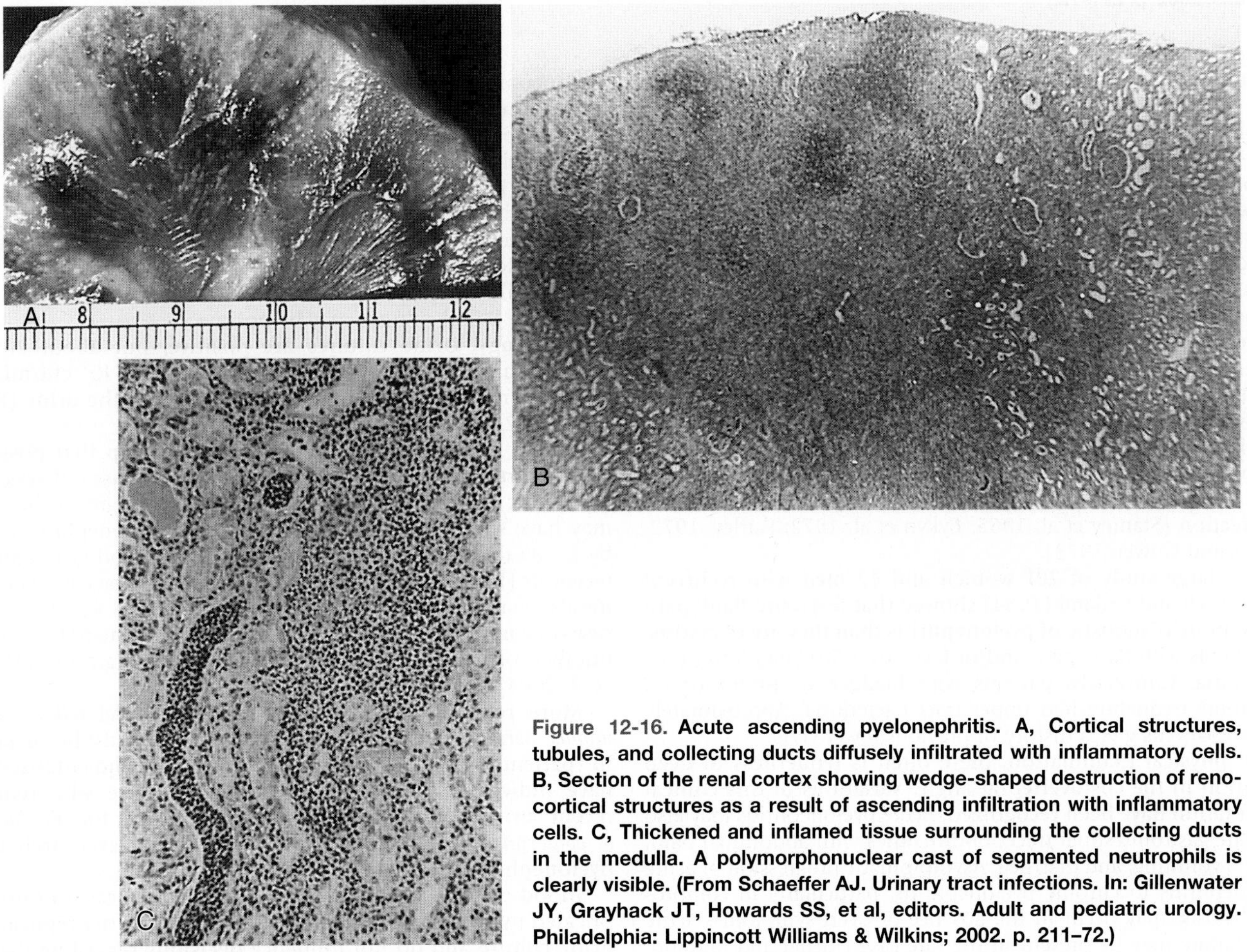

Figure 12-16. Acute ascending pyelonephritis. A, Cortical structures, tubules, and collecting ducts diffusely infiltrated with inflammatory cells. B, Section of the renal cortex showing wedge-shaped destruction of renocortical structures as a result of ascending infiltration with inflammatory cells. C, Thickened and inflamed tissue surrounding the collecting ducts in the medulla. A polymorphonuclear cast of segmented neutrophils is clearly visible. (From Schaeffer AJ. Urinary tract infections. In: Gillenwater JY, Grayhack JT, Howards SS, et al, editors. Adult and pediatric urology. Philadelphia: Lippincott Williams & Wilkins; 2002. p. 211–72.)

or completely hyalinized, glomeruli outside these severely scarred zones are relatively normal. Vascular involvement is variable, but in patients with hypertension, nephrosclerosis may be found. Papillary abnormalities include deformity, sclerosis, and sometimes necrosis. Studies in animals have clearly indicated the critical role of the papilla in the initiation of pyelonephritis (Freedman and Beeson, 1958). However, these changes are not necessarily specific for bacterial infection and may occur in the absence of infection as

a result of other disorders such as analgesic abuse, diabetes, and sickle cell disease.

Acute Pyelonephritis

Although pyelonephritis is defined as inflammation of the kidney and renal pelvis, the diagnosis is clinical. True infection of the "upper urinary tract" can be proved by catheterization tests (ureteral

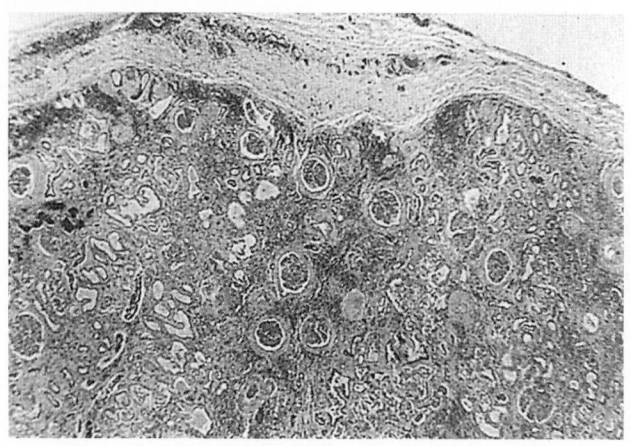

Figure 12-17. Chronic pyelonephritis. The renal cortex shows thickened fibrous capsule and focal retracted scar on surface of kidney. Focal destruction of tubules in center of picture is accompanied by periglomerular fibrosis and scarring. (From Schaeffer AJ. Urinary tract infections. In: Gillenwater JY, Grayhack JT, Howards SS, et al, editors, Adult and pediatric urology. Philadelphia: Lippincott Williams & Wilkins; 2002. p. 211–72.)

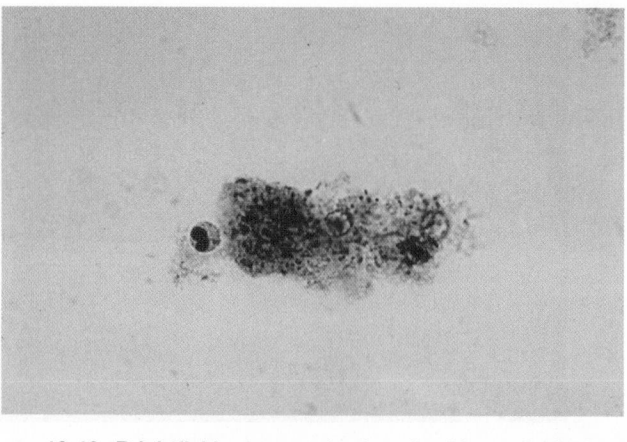

Figure 12-18. Brightfield micrograph of a mixed bacterial leukocyte cast from patient with acute pyelonephritis. Only the bacteria and the nucleus of a leukocyte stain strongly. Many bacteria are clearly demonstrated by through-focusing (toluidine blue O stain, magnification ×640). (From Lindner LE, Jones RN, Haber MH. A specific urinary cast in acute pyelonephritis. Am J Clin Pathol 1980;73:809–11.)

catheterization or bladder washout) as described in this chapter, but these are impractical and unnecessary in most patients with acute pyelonephritis. None of the noninvasive tests that have been developed to determine infection in the kidney or bladder are totally reliable.

Clinical Presentation. The clinical spectrum ranges from gram-negative sepsis to cystitis with mild flank pain (Stamm and Hooton, 1993). The classic presentation is an abrupt onset of chills, fever (100.3° F or greater), and unilateral or bilateral flank or costovertebral angle pain and/or tenderness. These so-called upper tract signs are often accompanied by dysuria, increased urinary frequency, and urgency.

Although some authors regard loin pain and fever in combination with significant bacteriuria as diagnostic of acute pyelonephritis, it is clear from localization studies using ureteral catheterization (Stamey and Pfau, 1963) or the bladder washout technique (Fairley et al, 1967) that **clinical symptoms correlate poorly with the site of infection** (Stamey et al, 1965; Eykyn et al, 1972; Fairley, 1972; Smeets and Gower, 1973).

In a large study of 201 women and 12 men with recurrent UTIs, Busch and Huland (1984) showed that fever and flank pain are no more diagnostic of pyelonephritis than they are of cystitis. Of patients with flank pain and/or fever, over 50% had lower tract bacteriuria. Conversely, patients with bladder symptoms or no symptoms frequently had upper tract bacteriuria. Approximately 75% of patients give a history of previous lower UTIs.

On physical examination, there often is tenderness to deep palpation in the costovertebral angle. Variations of this clinical presentation have been recognized. Acute pyelonephritis may also simulate gastrointestinal tract abnormalities with abdominal pain, nausea, vomiting, and diarrhea. Asymptomatic progression of acute pyelonephritis to chronic pyelonephritis, particularly in compromised hosts, may occur in the absence of overt symptoms. Acute renal failure may be present in the rare case (Richet and Mayaud, 1978; Olsson et al, 1980).

Laboratory Diagnosis. The patient may have leukocytosis with a predominance of neutrophils. **Urinalysis usually reveals numerous WBCs, often in clumps, and bacterial rods or chains of cocci.** Leukocytes exhibiting brownian motion in the cytoplasm (glitter cells) may be present if the urine is hypotonic, but they are not in themselves diagnostic of pyelonephritis. **The presence of large amounts of granular or leukocyte casts in the urinary sediment is suggestive of acute pyelonephritis.** A specific type of urinary cast characterized by the presence of bacteria in its matrix has been demonstrated in the urine of patients who have had acute

pyelonephritis (Fig. 12-18) (Lindner et al, 1980). Bacteria in the casts were not easily distinguished by simple brightfield microscopy without special staining of the sediment. Staining of the sediment with a basic dye such as dilute toluidine blue or KOVA stain (I.C.L. Scientific, Fountain Valley, CA) demonstrated the bacteria in casts without difficulty. Blood tests may show leukocytosis with a predominance of neutrophils, increased erythrocyte sedimentation rate, elevated C-reactive protein levels, and elevated creatinine levels if renal failure is present. In addition, creatinine clearance may be decreased. Blood cultures may be positive.

Bacteriology. Urine cultures are positive, but about 20% of patients have urine cultures with fewer than 10^5 cfu/mL and therefore negative results on Gram staining of the urine (Rubin et al, 1992).

E. coli, which constitutes a unique subgroup that possesses special virulence factors, accounts for 80% of cases. If vesicoureteral reflux is absent, a patient bearing the P blood group phenotype may have special susceptibility to recurrent pyelonephritis caused by *E. coli* that have P pili and bind to the P blood group antigen receptors (Lomberg et al, 1983). Bacterial K antigens and endotoxins also may contribute to pathogenicity (Kaijser et al, 1977). Many cases of community-acquired pyelonephritis are caused by a limited number of multiantimicrobial-resistant clonal groups (Manges et al, 2004).

More resistant species, such as *Proteus, Klebsiella, Pseudomonas, Serratia, Enterobacter,* or *Citrobacter,* should be suspected in patients who have recurrent UTIs, are hospitalized, or have indwelling catheters, as well as in those who required recent urinary tract instrumentation. Except for *E. faecalis, S. epidermidis,* and *S. aureus,* gram-positive bacteria rarely cause pyelonephritis.

Blood cultures are positive in about 25% of cases of uncomplicated pyelonephritis in women, and the majority replicate the urine culture and do not influence decisions regarding therapy. Therefore blood cultures should not be routinely obtained for the evaluation of uncomplicated pyelonephritis in women. **However, they should be performed in men and women with systemic toxicity or in those requiring hospitalization or with risk factors such as pregnancy** (Velasco et al, 2003).

Renal Ultrasonography and Computed Tomography. These studies are commonly used to evaluate patients initially for complicated UTIs or factors or to reevaluate patients who do not respond after 72 hours of therapy (see later). Ultrasonography (Fig. 12-19) and CT show renal enlargement, hypoechoic or attenuated parenchyma, and a compressed collecting system. They also may delineate focal bacterial nephritis and obstruction. When parenchymal destruction becomes pronounced, a more disorganized parenchyma and abscess formation associated with complicated renal and perirenal infections may be identified (Soulen et al, 1989).

Differential Diagnosis. Acute appendicitis, diverticulitis, and pancreatitis can cause a similar degree of pain, but the location of the pain often is different. Results of the urine examination are usually normal. Herpes zoster can cause superficial pain in the region of the kidney but is not associated with symptoms of UTI; the diagnosis will be apparent when shingles appear.

Management

Initial Management. Infection in patients with acute pyelonephritis can be subdivided into (1) uncomplicated infection that does not warrant hospitalization, (2) uncomplicated infection in patients

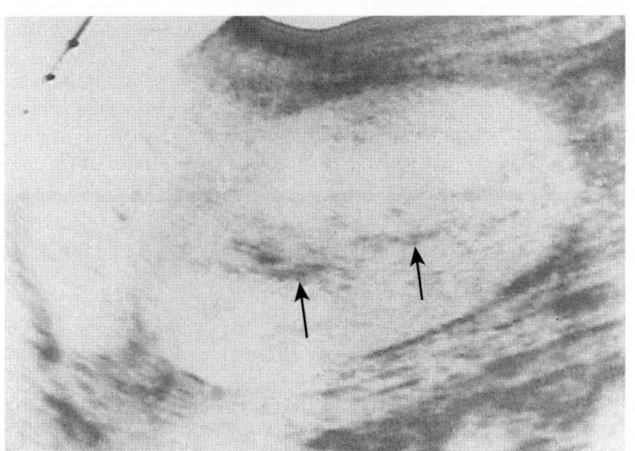

Figure 12-19. Acute pyelonephritis. Ultrasound image of the right kidney demonstrates renal enlargement, hypoechoic parenchyma, and compressed central collecting complex *(arrows).* **(From Schaeffer AJ. Urinary tract infections. In: Gillenwater JT, Grayhack JT, Howards SS, et al, editors. Adult and pediatric urology. Philadelphia: Lippincott William & Wilkins; 2002. p. 211–72.)**

with normal urinary tracts who are ill enough to warrant hospitalization for parenteral therapy, and (3) complicated infection associated with hospitalization, catheterization, urologic surgery, or urinary tract abnormalities (Fig. 12-20).

It is critical to determine whether the patient has an uncomplicated or complicated UTI because significant abnormalities have been found in 16% of patients with acute pyelonephritis (Shen and Brown, 2004). In patients with presumed uncomplicated pyelonephritis who will be managed as outpatients, initial radiologic evaluation can usually be deferred. **However, if there is any reason to suspect a problem or if the patient will not have reasonable access to imaging if there should be no change in condition, we prefer renal ultrasonography to rule out stones or obstruction.** In patients with known or suspected complicated pyelonephritis, CT provides excellent assessment of the status of the urinary tract and the severity and extent of the infection.

For patients who will be managed as outpatients, single-drug oral therapy with a fluoroquinolone is more effective than TMP-SMX for patients with domiciliary infections (Talan et al, 2000). Many physicians administer a single parenteral dose of an antimicrobial agent (ceftriaxone, gentamicin, or a fluoroquinolone) before initiating oral therapy (Israel et al, 1991; Pinson et al, 1994). If a gram-positive organism is suspected, amoxicillin or amoxicillin/clavulanic acid is recommended (Warren et al, 1999).

If a patient has an uncomplicated infection but is sufficiently ill to require hospitalization (high fever, high WBC count, vomiting, dehydration, evidence of sepsis), has complicated pyelonephritis, or fails to improve during the initial outpatient treatment period, a parenteral fluoroquinolone, an aminoglycoside with or without ampicillin, or an extended-spectrum cephalosporin with or without an aminoglycoside is recommended (Warren et al, 1999) (Table 12-15). If gram-positive cocci are causative, ampicillin/sulbactam with or without an aminoglycoside is recommended.

Hospitalization, IV fluids, and antipyretics are required.

An obstructed kidney has difficulty concentrating and excreting antimicrobial agents. Any substantial obstruction must be relieved expediently by the safest and simplest means.

A Gram stain of the urine sediment is helpful to guide the selection of the initial empirical antimicrobial therapy. In all cases,

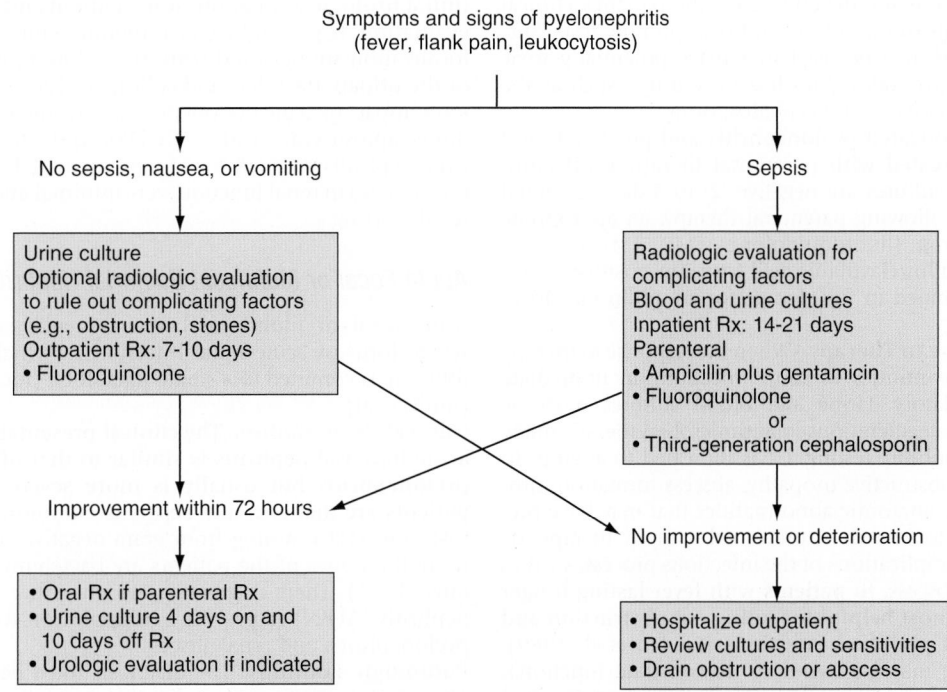

Figure 12-20. Management of acute pyelonephritis.

TABLE 12-15 Treatment Regimens for Acute Complicated and Uncomplicated Pyelonephritis in Women

CIRCUMSTANCES	ROUTE	DRUG	DOSAGE	FREQUENCY PER DOSE	DURATION (DAYS)
Outpatient—moderately ill, no nausea or vomiting	Oral	TMP-SMX DS	160-800 mg	bid	10-14
		Ciprofloxacin	500 mg	bid	
		Levofloxacin	500 mg	qd	3-7
Inpatient—severely ill, possible sepsis	Parenteral	Ampicillin and gentamicin	1 g 1.5 mg/kg	qid tid	14
		Ciprofloxacin	400 mg	bid	
		Levofloxacin	500 mg	qd	10
		Ceftriaxone	1 to 2g	qd	Take until afebrile, then take oral
		TMP-SMX or fluoroquinolone			
		Ceftriaxone	1-2 g	qd	14
Pregnant	Parenteral	Ampicillin and gentamicin	1 g 1 mg/kg	qid tid	
		Aztreonam	1 g	tid-qid	Take until afebrile, then take oral
	Oral	Cephalexin	500 mg	bid	

DS, double strength; TMP-SMX, trimethoprim-sulfamethoxazole.
Modified from Stamm WE, Hooton TM. Management of urinary tract infections in adults. N Engl J Med 1993;329:1328–34. Copyright 1993, Massachusetts Medical Society. All rights reserved.

antimicrobial therapy should be active against potential uropathogens and achieve antimicrobial levels in renal tissue and urine.
Subsequent Management. Even though the urine usually becomes sterile within a few hours of starting antimicrobial therapy, patients with acute uncomplicated pyelonephritis may continue to have fever, chills, and flank pain for several more days after initiation of successful antimicrobial therapy (Behr et al, 1996). They should be observed.

Ambulatory patients should be treated with a fluoroquinolone for 7 days (Talan et al, 2000). Fluoroquinolone therapy is associated with greater bacteriologic and clinical cure rates than 14-day TMP-SMX therapy (Talan et al, 2000). Alterations in antimicrobial therapy may be made depending on the patient's clinical response and the results of the culture and susceptibility tests. Susceptibility tests should also be used to replace potentially toxic drugs, such as aminoglycosides, with less toxic drugs, such as the fluoroquinolones, aztreonam, and cephalosporins.

Patients with complicated pyelonephritis and positive blood cultures should be treated with parenteral therapy until clinically stable. If blood cultures are negative, 2- to 3-day parenteral therapy is sufficient. Following parenteral therapy, an appropriate oral antimicrobial drug (fluoroquinolone, TMP, TMP-SMX, or amoxicillin or amoxicillin/clavulanic acid for gram-positive organisms) should be continued in full dosage for an additional 10 to 14 days.
Unfavorable Response to Therapy. When the response to therapy is slow or the urine continues to show infection, an immediate reevaluation is mandatory. Urine and blood cultures must be repeated and appropriate alterations in antimicrobial therapy made on the basis of susceptibility testing. CT is indicated to attempt to identify unsuspected obstructive uropathy, abscess formation, urolithiasis, or underlying anatomic abnormalities that may have predisposed the patient to infection, prevented a rapid therapeutic response, or caused complications of the infectious process, such as renal or perinephric abscess. **In patients with fever lasting longer than 72 hours, CT is most helpful for ruling out obstruction and identifying renal and perirenal infections** (Soulen et al, 1989). Radionuclide imaging may be useful to demonstrate functional changes associated with acute pyelonephritis (decrease in renal blood flow, delay in peak function, and delay in excretion of the

radionuclide) (Fischman and Roberts, 1982) and cortical defects associated with vesicoureteral reflux.
Follow-Up. Repeat urine cultures should be performed on the fifth to the seventh day of therapy and 10 to 14 days after discontinuing antimicrobial therapy to ensure that the urinary tract remains free of infections. Between 10% and 30% of individuals with acute pyelonephritis relapse after a 14-day course of therapy. Patients who relapse usually are cured by a second 14-day course of therapy, but occasionally a 6-week course is necessary (Tolkoff-Rubin et al, 1984; Johnson and Stamm, 1987).

Depending on the clinical presentation and response and initial urologic evaluation, some patients may require additional evaluation (e.g., voiding cystourethrogram, cystoscopy, bacterial localization studies) and correction of an underlying abnormality of the urinary tract. Raz and colleagues (2003) evaluated the long-term impact of acute pyelonephritis in women. Scanning with ^{99m}Tc-dimercaptosuccinic acid (^{99m}Tc-DMSA) 10 to 20 years after acute pyelonephritis revealed scars in approximately 50% of the patients, but changes in renal function were minimal and not associated with renal scarring.

Acute Focal or Multifocal Bacterial Nephritis

Acute focal or multifocal bacterial nephritis is an uncommon, severe form of acute renal infection in which a heavy leukocyte infiltrate is confined to a single renal lobe (focal) or multiple lobes (multifocal).
Clinical Presentation. The clinical presentation of patients with acute bacterial nephritis is similar to that of patients with acute pyelonephritis but usually is more severe. About half of the patients are diabetic, and sepsis is common. Generally, leukocytosis and UTI resulting from gram-negative organisms are found; more than 50% of the patients are bacteremic (Wicks and Thornbury, 1979). There is growing evidence that acute focal bacterial nephritis (AFBN) represents a midpoint on the spectrum between pyelonephritis and renal abscess.
Radiologic Findings. The diagnosis must be made by radiologic examination. The mass has slightly less nephrographic density than the surrounding normal renal parenchyma.

Ultrasonography and CT establish the diagnosis. On ultrasonography, the lesion is typically poorly marginated and relatively sonolucent with occasional low-amplitude echoes that disrupt the cortical medullary junction (Corriere and Sandler, 1982) (Fig. 12-21A). **Enhancement with a contrast agent is necessary with CT studies because the lesion is difficult to visualize on the unenhanced study** (Fig. 12-21B). **Wedge-shaped areas of decreased enhancement are seen.** No definite wall is evident, and frank liquefaction is absent. Conversely, abscesses tend to have liquid centers, are usually round, and are present both before and after contrast medium enhancement. More chronic abscesses may also show a ring-shaped area of increased enhancement surrounding the lesion (Corriere and Sandler, 1982). Gallium scanning reveals uptake that is in the region of and larger than the previously demonstrated mass (Rosenfield et al, 1979). In patients with multifocal disease, the findings are similar but multiple lobes are involved.

Management. Acute bacterial nephritis probably represents a relatively early phase of frank abscess formation. In a series of cases reported by Lee and coworkers (1980), a patient with acute focal bacterial nephritis progressed to abscess formation. McCoy and associates reported radiographically proven progression from acute nephritis to an abscess despite appropriate medical management (McCoy et al, 1985). Shimizu and colleagues presented a case of a 16-year-old female with CT imaging consistent with AFBN and no evidence of drainable fluid collection, which progressed by hospital day 13 to a hypodense large abscess in the area previously seen to be nephritis while being treated (Shimizu et al, 2005). **Treatment includes hydration and IV antimicrobial agents for at least 7 days, followed by 7 days of oral antimicrobial therapy.** Patients with bacterial nephritis typically respond to medical therapy, and follow-up studies will show resolution of the wedge-shaped zones of diminished attenuation. **Failure to respond to antimicrobial therapy is an indication for appropriate studies to rule out obstructive uropathy, renal or perirenal abscess, renal carcinoma, or acute renal vein thrombosis.** Long-term follow-up studies performed in a few patients with multifocal disease have demonstrated a decrease in renal size and focal calyceal deformities suggestive of papillary necrosis (Davidson and Talner, 1978).

Emphysematous Pyelonephritis

Emphysematous pyelonephritis is a urologic emergency characterized by an acute necrotizing parenchymal and perirenal infection caused by gas-forming uropathogens. The pathogenesis is poorly understood. **Because the condition usually occurs in diabetic patients, it has been postulated that the high tissue glucose levels provide the substrate for microorganisms such as** *E. coli,* **which are able to produce carbon dioxide by the fermentation of sugar** (Schainuck et al, 1968). Although glucose fermentation may be a factor, the explanation does not account for the rarity of emphysematous pyelonephritis despite the high frequency of gram-negative UTI in diabetic patients, nor does it explain the rare occurrence of the condition in nondiabetic patients.

In addition to diabetes, many patients have urinary tract obstruction associated with urinary calculi or papillary necrosis and significant renal functional impairment. The overall mortality rate has been reported to be between 19% (Huang and Tseng, 2000) and 43% (Freiha et al, 1979).

Clinical Presentation. Nearly all of the documented cases of emphysematous pyelonephritis have occurred in adults (Hawes et al, 1983). Juvenile diabetic patients do not appear to be at risk. Women are affected more often than men.

The usual clinical presentation is severe, acute pyelonephritis, although in some instances a chronic infection precedes the acute attack. **Almost all patients display the classic triad of fever, vomiting, and flank pain** (Schainuck et al, 1968). Pneumaturia is absent unless the infection involves the collecting system. Results of urine cultures are invariably positive. *E. coli* is most commonly identified. *Klebsiella* and *Proteus* are less common.

Radiologic Findings. The diagnosis is established radiographically. **Tissue gas that is distributed in the parenchyma may appear on abdominal radiographs as mottled gas shadows over the involved kidney** (Fig. 12-22). This finding is often mistaken for bowel gas. A crescentic collection of gas over the upper pole of the kidney is more distinctive. As the infection progresses, gas extends to the perinephric space and retroperitoneum. This distribution of gas should not be confused with cases of emphysematous pyelitis in which air is in the collecting system of the kidney. Emphysematous pyelitis is secondary to a gas-forming bacterial UTI, often occurs in nondiabetic patients, is less serious, and usually responds to antimicrobial therapy.

Ultrasonography usually demonstrates strong focal echoes suggesting the presence of intraparenchymal gas (Brenbridge et al, 1979; Conrad et al, 1979). **CT is the imaging procedure of choice in defining the extent of the emphysematous process and guiding management** (Figs. 12-23 and 12-24). **An absence of fluid in CT**

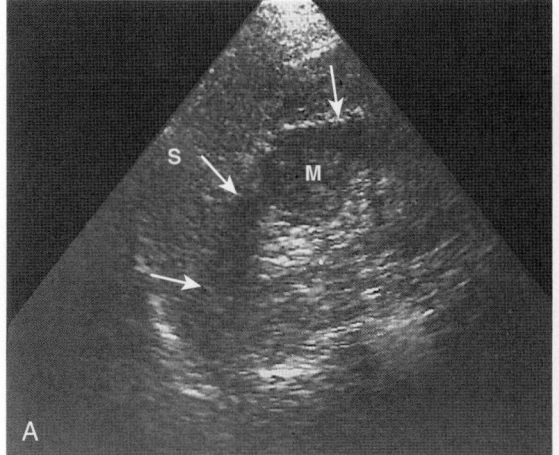
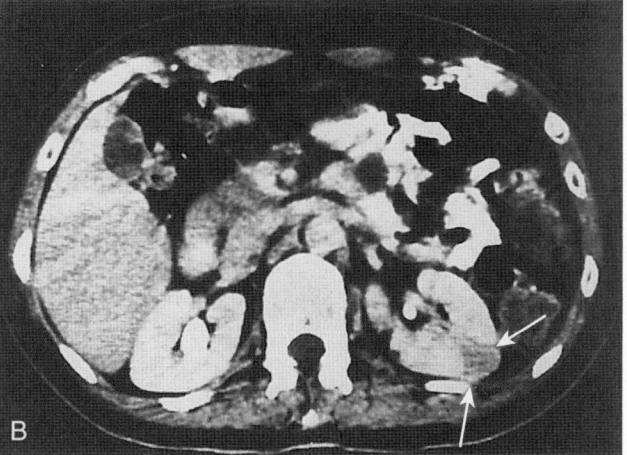

Figure 12-21. Acute focal bacterial nephritis. A, Ultrasound image; longitudinal view of the left kidney demonstrates spleen (S) and left kidney *(arrows).* Note irregular midpole mass (M) of slightly higher echo texture than surrounding normal renal parenchyma. **B,** Contrast medium–enhanced computed tomography scan demonstrates a wedge-shaped area of low density *(arrows)* in the middle portion of the left kidney. The findings resolved after antimicrobial therapy. (From Schaeffer AJ. Urinary tract infections. In: Gillenwater JY, Grayhack JT, Howards SS, et al, editors. Adult and pediatric urology. Philadelphia: Lippincott Williams & Wilkins; 2002. p. 211–72.)

images or the presence of streaky or mottled gas with or without bubbly and loculated gas appears to be associated with rapid destruction of renal parenchyma and a 50% to 60% mortality rate (Wan et al, 1996; Best et al, 1999). The presence of renal or perirenal fluid, the presence of bubbly or loculated gas or gas in the collecting system, and the absence of streaky or mottled gas patterns are associated with a less than 20% mortality rate. Obstruction is demonstrated in approximately 25% of the cases. A nuclear renal scan should be performed to assess the degree of renal function impairment in the involved kidney and the status of the contralateral kidney.

Management. Emphysematous pyelonephritis is a surgical emergency. Most patients are septic, and fluid resuscitation and broad-spectrum antimicrobial therapy are essential. If the kidney is functioning, medical therapy can be considered (Wan et al, 1996; Best et al, 1999). Nephrectomy is recommended for patients who do not improve after a few days of therapy (Malek and Elder, 1978). If the affected kidney is nonfunctioning and not obstructed, nephrectomy should be performed because medical treatment alone is usually lethal. If a kidney is obstructed, catheter drainage must be instituted. If the patient's condition improves, nephrectomy may be deferred pending a complete urologic evaluation. Although there are isolated case reports of retention of renal function after medical therapy combined with relief of obstruction, most patients require nephrectomy (Hudson et al, 1986).

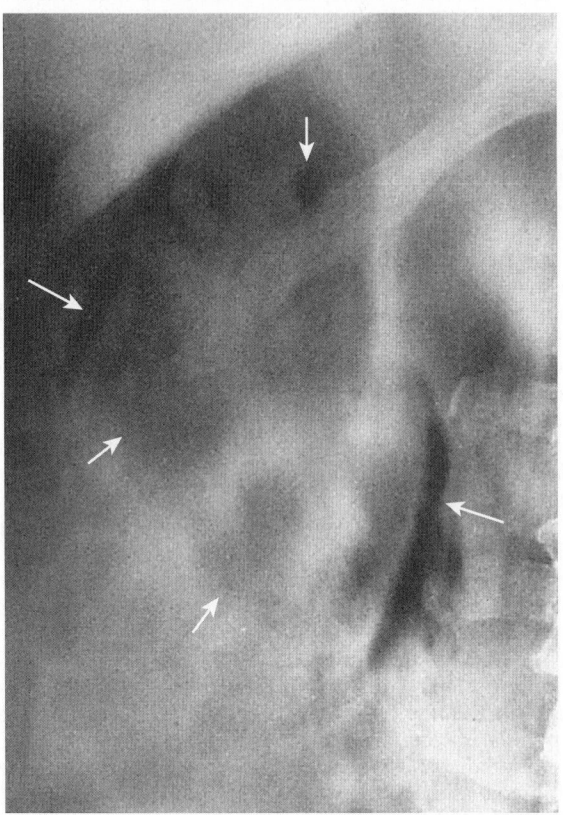

Figure 12-22. Emphysematous pyelonephritis; plain film. Extensive perinephric *(long arrows)* **and intraparenchymal** *(short arrows)* **gas secondary to acute bacterial pyelonephritis. (From Schaeffer AJ. Urinary tract infections. In: Gillenwater JY, Grayhack JT, Howards SS, et al, editors. Adult and pediatric urology. Philadelphia: Lippincott William & Wilkins; 2002. p. 211–72.)**

Renal Abscess

Renal abscess or carbuncle is a collection of purulent material confined to the renal parenchyma. Before the antimicrobial era, 80% of renal abscesses were attributed to hematogenous seeding by staphylococci (Campbell, 1930). Additionally, patients historically presenting with abscesses were young men with no prior renal disease. Although experimental and clinical data document the facility for abscess formation in normal kidneys after hematogenous inoculation with staphylococci, widespread use of antimicrobial agents since about 1950 appears to have diminished the propensity for gram-positive abscess formation (DeNavasquez, 1950; Cotran, 1969). The current index patient typically has a history of renal disease or obstruction, has no gender predominance and no laterality, and the infection is typically with a gram-negative organism.

Since about 1970, gram-negative organisms have been implicated in the majority of adults with renal abscesses. Hematogenous renal seeding by gram-negative organisms may occur, but this is not likely to be the primary pathway for gram-negative abscess formation. Clinically, there is no evidence that gram-negative septicemia antedates most lesions. Further, gram-negative hematogenous pyelonephritis is virtually impossible to produce in animals unless the kidney is traumatized or completely obstructed (Cotran, 1969; Timmons and Perlmutter, 1976). Like the normal kidney, the

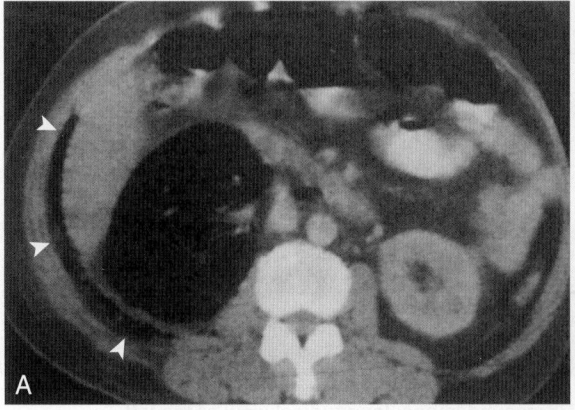
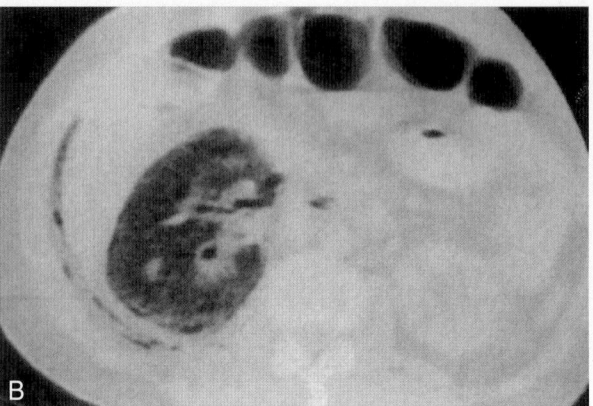

Figure 12-23. Type I emphysematous pyelonephritis with complete renal destruction in a 49-year-old woman. A, Computed tomography (CT) scan of the right kidney shows complete destruction with gas *(arrowheads)* **extending beyond the renal fascia. B, CT scan with a modified lung window display shows the characteristic streaky gas in the completely destroyed kidney. The patient died on arrival in the emergency department. (From Wan YL, Lee TY, Bullard MJ, et al. Acute gas-producing bacterial renal infection: correlation between imaging findings and clinical outcome. Radiology 1996;198:433–8.)**

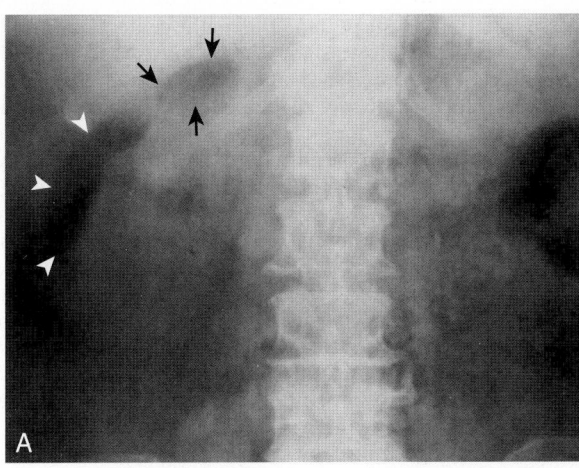
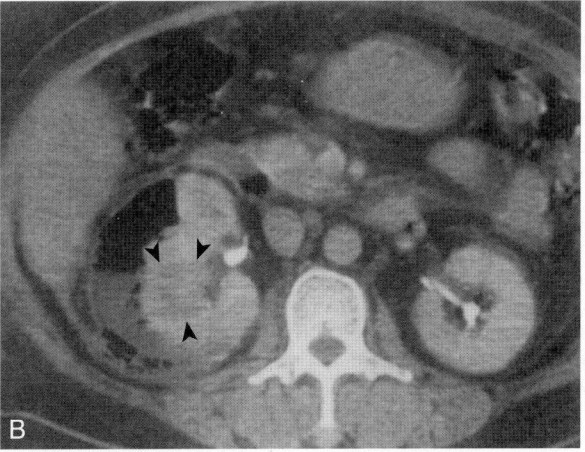

Figure 12-24. Type II emphysematous pyelonephritis in a 57-year-old woman. A, Radiograph shows crescent-shaped (white arrowheads) and loculated (black arrows) gas in the right renal area. B, Computed tomography scan obtained after administration of contrast material shows a low-attenuation area (arrowheads) in the right kidney due to acute pyelonephritis, as well as a subcapsular abscess with fluid and bubbly and loculated gas. The patient survived after percutaneous drainage was performed. (From Wan YL, Lee TY, Bullard MJ, et al. Acute gas-producing bacterial renal infection: correlation between imaging findings and clinical outcome. Radiology 1996;198:433–8.)

partially obstructed kidney rejects blood-borne gram-negative inocula. Thus ascending infection associated with tubular obstruction from prior infections or calculi appears to be the primary pathway for the establishment of gram-negative abscesses. Two-thirds of gram-negative abscesses in adults are associated with renal calculi or damaged kidneys (Salvatierra et al, 1967; Siegel et al, 1996). Although the association of pyelonephritis with vesicoureteral reflux is well established, the association of renal abscess with vesicoureteral reflux has been infrequently noted (Segura and Kelalis, 1973). Case reports in the pediatric literature exist, but literature within the adult population is sparse. More recent observations, however, indicate that reflux is frequently associated with renal abscesses and persists long after sterilization of the urinary tract (Timmons and Perlmutter, 1976; Anderson and McAninch 1980).

Clinical Presentation. The patient may present with fever, chills, abdominal or flank pain, and occasionally weight loss and malaise. Symptoms of cystitis may occur. Occasionally, these symptoms may be vague and delay diagnosis until surgical exploration or, in more severe cases, autopsy (Anderson and McAninch, 1980). **A thorough history may reveal a gram-positive source of infection 1 to 8 weeks before the onset of urinary tract symptoms or symptoms consistent with UTI or pyelonephritis in the weeks prior** (Hung et al, 2007). **The infection may have occurred in any area of the body.** Multiple skin carbuncles and IV drug abuse introduce gram-positive organisms into the bloodstream. Other common sites are the mouth, lungs, and bladder (Lyons et al, 1972). Complicated UTIs associated with stasis, calculi, pregnancy, neurogenic bladder, and diabetes mellitus also appear to predispose the patient to abscess formation (Anderson and McAninch, 1980).

Laboratory Diagnosis. The patient typically has marked leukocytosis. In Siegel and associates' (1996) series of 52 patients, blood cultures were positive 28% of the time, while Yen and colleagues (1999) published a series of 78 patients, 25 of which (32%) had positive blood cultures. When comparing positive cultures in all three types of fluids (abscess, blood, urine) only 1 patient of the 78 had identical isolates in all three. Urine and abscess culture had a 15% identical culture rate, whereas blood and abscess had a 13% identical culture rate (Yen et al, 1999). Pyuria and bacteriuria may not be evident unless the abscess communicates with the collecting system. **Because gram-positive organisms are most commonly blood-borne, urine cultures in these cases typically show no**

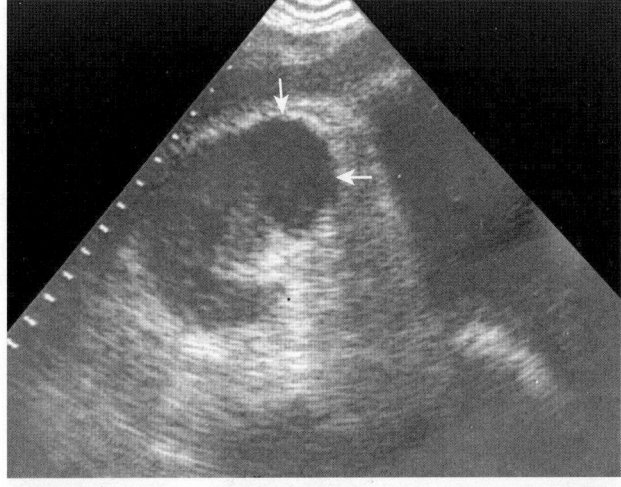

Figure 12-25. Acute renal abscess. Transverse ultrasound image of the right kidney demonstrates a poorly marginated rounded focal hypoechoic mass (arrows) in the anterior portion of the kidney.

growth or a microorganism different from that isolated from the abscess. Another study showed not only a bacteremia rate of 26% but also that positive urine cultures were only present in roughly 30% of patients (Shu et al, 2004).

Ultrasonography and CT distinguish abscess from other inflammatory renal diseases. **Ultrasonography is the quickest and least expensive method to demonstrate a renal abscess. An echo-free or low-echodensity space-occupying lesion with increased transmission is found on the ultrasound image** (Fig. 12-25). The margins of an abscess are indistinguishable in the acute phase, but the structure contains a few echoes and the surrounding renal parenchyma is edematous (Fiegler, 1983). Subsequently, the appearance tends to be that of a well-defined mass. The internal appearance, however, may vary from a virtually solid lucent mass to one with large numbers of low-level internal echoes (Schneider et al, 1976). The number of echoes depends on the amount of cellular debris within the abscess. The presence of air results in a strong echo with a shadow. Differentiation between an abscess and a tumor is impossible in many cases. Arteriography is used infrequently to demonstrate abscesses. The center of the mass tends to be hypervascular or avascular, with increased vascularity at the cortical margins and lack of vascular displacement and neovascularity.

CT appears to be the diagnostic procedure of choice for renal abscesses because it provides excellent delineation of the tissue. On CT, abscesses are characteristically well defined both before and after contrast agent enhancement. The findings depend in part on the age and severity of the abscess (Baumgarten and Baumgartner, 1997). Initially, CT shows renal enlargement and focal, rounded areas of decreased attenuation (Fig. 12-26). After several days of the onset of the infection, a thick fibrotic wall begins to form around the abscess. An echo-free or slightly echogenic mass caused by the presence of necrotic debris is seen. CT of a chronic abscess shows obliteration of adjacent tissue planes, thickening of the Gerota fascia, a round or oval parenchymal mass of low attenuation, and a surrounding inflammatory wall of slightly higher attenuation that forms a ring when the scan is enhanced with contrast material (Fig. 12-27). The ring sign is caused by the increased vascularity of the abscess wall (Callen, 1979; Gerzof and Gale, 1982).

Radionuclide imaging with gallium or indium is sometimes useful in evaluating patients with renal abscesses (see prior sections in this chapter and Chapter 2).

Management. Although the classic treatment for an abscess has been percutaneous or open incision and drainage, there is good evidence that use of IV antimicrobial agents and careful observation of a small abscess less than 3 cm or even 5 cm in a clinically stable patient is appropriate. Antibiotics, if begun early enough in the course of the process, may obviate surgical procedures (Hoverman et al, 1980; Levin et al, 1984; Shu et al, 2004). CT- or ultrasound-guided needle aspiration may be necessary to differentiate an abscess from a hypervascular tumor. Aspirated material should be cultured and appropriate antimicrobial therapy instituted on the basis of the findings.

All patients should be immediately started on IV antibiotic therapy. The selection of empirical antimicrobial therapy is dependent on the presumed source of the infection and the resistance patterns within the hospital. When hematogenous dissemination is suspected, the pathogenic organism most frequently is penicillin-resistant *Staphylococcus,* and the antimicrobial of choice therefore is a penicillinase-resistant penicillin (Schiff et al, 1977). If a history of penicillin hypersensitivity is present, the recommended drug is vancomycin. Cortical abscesses that occur in the abnormal urinary tract are associated with more typical gram-negative pathogens secondary to ascending infection and should be treated empirically with IV third-generation cephalosporins, antipseudomonal penicillins, or aminoglycosides until specific therapy can be instituted. Patients should have serial examinations with ultrasonography or CT until the abscess resolves. The radiographic evolution or resolution of the abscesses will typically further dictate clinical management. The suspicion of misdiagnosis or an uncontrolled infection with the development of perinephric abscess or infection with an organism resistant to the antimicrobial agents used in therapy should be suspected with worsening clinical picture.

After patients are started on IV antibiotic therapy and there is radiographic confirmation of abscess, the size of the abscess typically dictates management. Abscesses 3 cm or less can be managed with antibiotics alone (Shu et al, 2004; Lee et al, 2010; Siegel et al, 1996). In a series from South Korea of 49 patients with normal urinary tracts and abscesses less than 5 cm, there was 100% resolution of abscesses confirmed with CT scan with antibiotics alone (Lee et al, 2010).

Though less data exist for patients with obstruction or anomalous urinary tracts, **abscesses 3 to 5 cm in diameter should be**

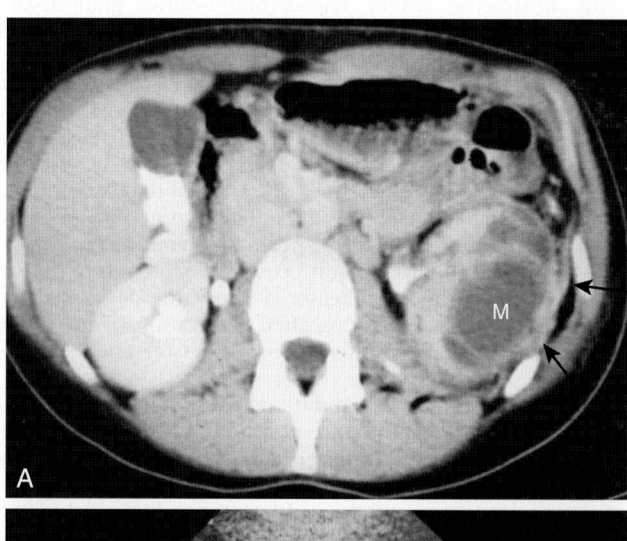

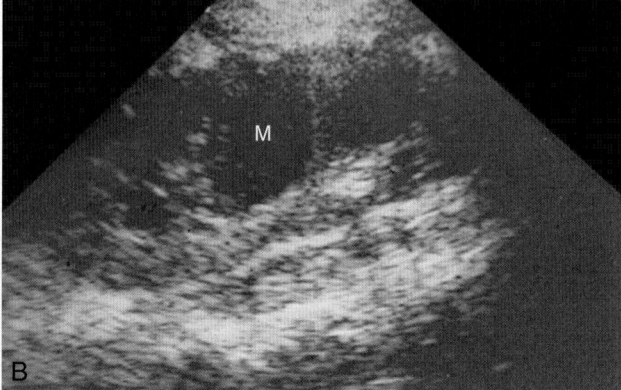

Figure 12-27. Chronic renal abscess. A, Enhanced computed tomography scan shows an irregular septated low-density mass **(M)** extensively involving the left kidney. Note thickening of perinephric fascia **(arrows)** and extensive compression of the renal collecting system. Findings are typical of renal abscess. **B,** Ultrasound longitudinal image demonstrates a septated hypoechoic mass **(M)** occupying much of the renal parenchymal volume.

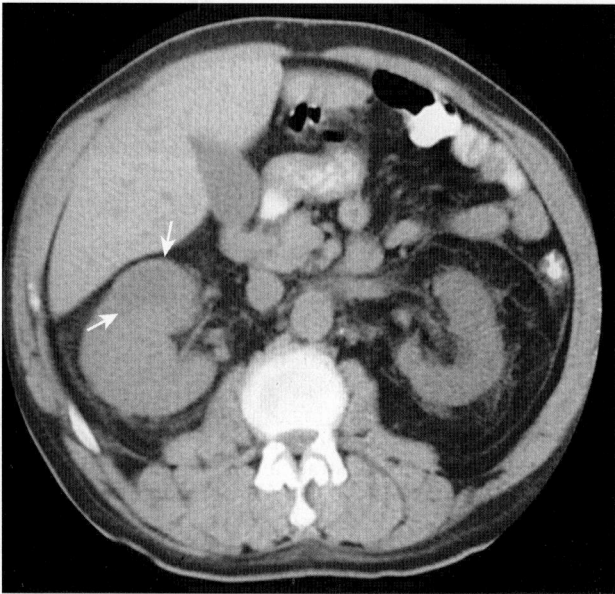

Figure 12-26. Acute renal abscess. Nonenhanced computed tomography scan through the mid pole of the right kidney demonstrates right renal enlargement and an area of decreased attenuation **(arrows).** After antimicrobial therapy, a follow-up scan showed complete regression of these findings.

conservatively managed initially in the setting of stable clinical parameters. We suggest following the clinical course and size of the abscess radiographically to assess for improvement. Should the patient progress, percutaneous drainage should be considered. Abscesses of all sizes in immunocompromised hosts or those that do not respond to antimicrobial therapy should be drained percutaneously (Fernandez et al, 1985; Fowler and Perkins, 1994; Siegel et al, 1996). **Percutaneous drainage, however, remains the first-line procedure of choice for most renal abscesses greater than 5 cm in diameter.** Typically, abscesses of this size require multiple drains, multiple drain manipulations, or eventual surgical washout and potential nephrectomy (Siegel et al, 1996).

Infected Hydronephrosis and Pyonephrosis

Infected hydronephrosis is bacterial infection in a hydronephrotic kidney. The term *pyonephrosis* refers to infected hydronephrosis associated with suppurative destruction of the parenchyma of the kidney, in which there is total or nearly total loss of renal function (Fig. 12-28). Where infected hydronephrosis ends and pyonephrosis begins is difficult to determine clinically. Rapid diagnosis and treatment of pyonephrosis are essential to avoid permanent loss of renal function and to prevent sepsis.

Clinical Presentation. The patient is usually very ill, with high fever, chills, flank pain, and tenderness. Occasionally, however, a patient may have only an elevated temperature and a complaint of vague gastrointestinal discomfort. A previous history of urinary tract calculi, infection, or surgery is common. **Bacteriuria may not be present if the ureter is completely obstructed.**

Radiologic Findings. The ultrasonographic diagnosis of infected hydronephrosis depends on demonstration of internal echoes within the dependent portion of a dilated pyelocalyceal system. CT is nonspecific but may show thickening of the renal pelvis, stranding of the perirenal fat, and a striated nephrogram. Ultrasonography demonstrates hydronephrosis and fluid debris levels within the dilated collecting system (Corriere and Sandler, 1982) (Fig. 12-29A). The diagnosis of pyonephrosis is suggested if focal areas of decreased echogenicity are seen within the hydronephrotic parenchyma.

Management. Once the diagnosis of pyonephrosis is made, the treatment is initiated with appropriate antimicrobial drugs and

drainage of the infected pelvis. A ureteral catheter can be passed to drain the kidney, but if the obstruction prevents this, a percutaneous nephrostomy tube should be placed (Camunez et al, 1989) (Fig. 12-29B). When the patient becomes hemodynamically stable, other procedures are usually needed to identify and treat the source of the obstruction.

Perinephric Abscess

Perinephric abscess **usually results from rupture of an acute cortical abscess into the perinephric space or from hematogenous seeding from sites of infection.** Patients with pyonephrosis,

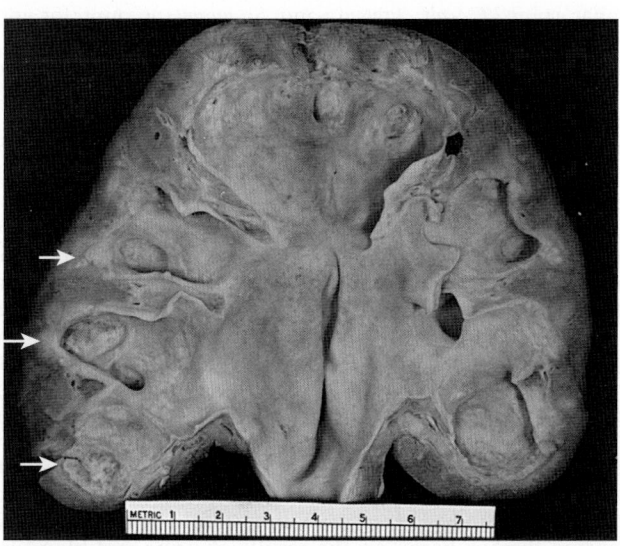

Figure 12-28. Pyonephrosis: gross specimen. The kidney shows marked thinning of the renal cortex and medulla, suppurative destruction of the parenchyma *(arrows)*, and distention of the pelvis and calyces. Previous incision released a large quantity of purulent material. The ureter showed obstruction distal to the point of section.

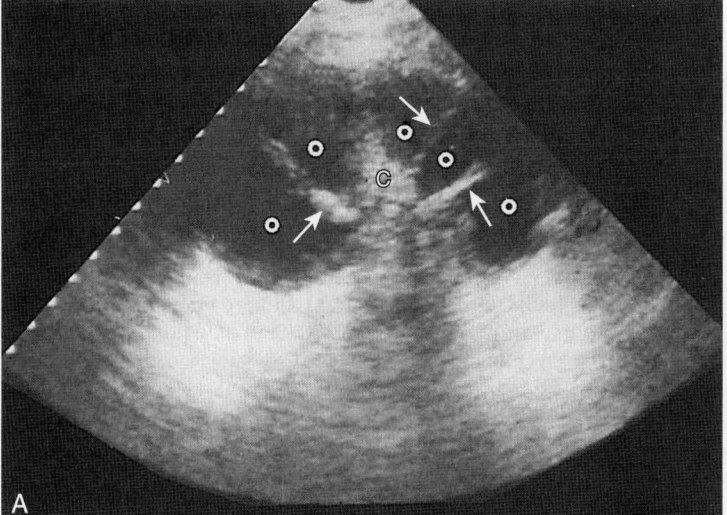

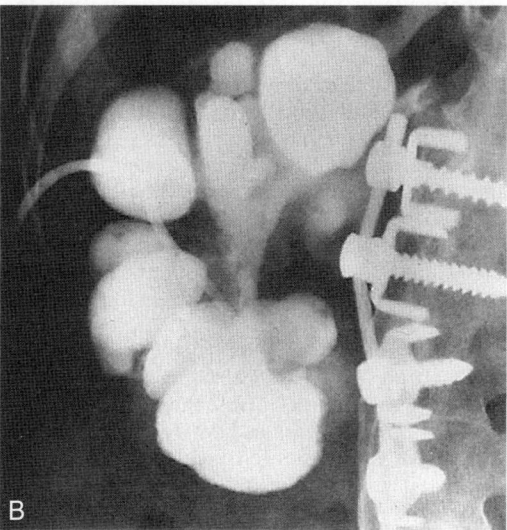

Figure 12-29. Pyonephrosis. A, Longitudinal ultrasound image of the right kidney demonstrates echogenic central collecting complex (C) with radiating echogenic septa *(arrows)* and thinned hypoechoic parenchyma. Multiple dilated calyces (o) with diffuse low-level echoes are seen. **B,** Antegrade pyelogram performed through a percutaneous nephrostomy catheter correlates well with the ultrasound image. Dilated pus-filled calyces are demonstrated. The renal pelvis is obliterated by chronic scarring and stone disease. The kidney did not regain function. (From Schaeffer AJ. Urinary tract infections. In: Gillenwater JY, et al, editors. Adult and pediatric urology. Philadelphia: Lippincott Williams & Wilkins; 2002. p. 211–72.)

particularly when a calculus is present in the kidney, are susceptible to perinephric abscess formation. **Diabetes mellitus is present in approximately one third of patients with perinephric abscess** (Edelstein and McCabe, 1988; Meng et al, 2002). **In about one third of the cases, perinephric abscess is caused by hematogenous spread, usually from sites of skin infection** (Gardiner et al, 2011). A perirenal hematoma can become secondarily infected by the hematogenous route or by direct extension of a primary renal infection. When a perinephric infection ruptures through the Gerota fascia into the pararenal space, the abscess becomes paranephric. Paranephric abscesses may also result from infectious disorders of the bowel, pancreas, or pleural cavity. Conversely, perinephric or psoas abscess may be the result of bowel perforation, Crohn disease, or spread of osteomyelitis from the thoracolumbar spine. *E. coli, Proteus,* and *S. aureus* account for most infections.

Clinical Presentation. The onset of symptoms is typically insidious. Symptoms are present for more than 5 days in most patients with perinephric abscess compared with only about 10% of patients with pyelonephritis. The clinical presentation may be similar to that of pyelonephritis; however, more than one third of patients may be afebrile. An abdominal or flank mass can be felt in about half of the cases; costovertebral angle tenderness is typically present. Psoas abscess should be suspected if the patient has a limp and flexion and external rotation of the ipsilateral hip. Laboratory features include leukocytosis, elevated levels of serum creatinine, and pyuria in more than 75% of cases. Edelstein and McCabe (1988) showed that results of urine cultures predicted perinephric abscess isolates in only 37% of cases; a blood culture, particularly with multiple organisms, was often indicative of perinephric abscess but identified all organisms in only 42% of cases. Meng et al (2002) showed that roughly 75% of patients had a positive culture. Urine was statistically significantly more sensitive than blood and abscess fluid collection in their study. **Therefore caution should be exercised when choosing therapy based on the results of urine and blood cultures because data may sometimes be inadequate. Pyelonephritis usually responds within 4 to 5 days of appropriate antimicrobial therapy; perinephric abscess does not. Thus perinephric abscess should be suspected in a patient with UTI and abdominal or flank mass or persistent fever after 4 days of antimicrobial therapy.** Perinephric abscesses are commonly seen concomitantly with renal abscesses.

CT is particularly valuable for demonstrating the primary abscess. In some cases, the abscess is confined to the perinephric space; however, extension to the flank or psoas muscle may occur (Fig. 12-30). CT is able to show with exquisite anatomic detail the route of spread of infection into the surrounding tissues (Fig. 12-31). This information may be helpful in planning the approach for surgical drainage. Ultrasonography demonstrates a diverse appearance ranging from a nearly anechoic mass displacing the kidney to an echogenic collection that tends to blend with normally echogenic fat within the Gerota fascia (Corriere and Sandler, 1982). Occasionally, a retroperitoneal or subdiaphragmatic infection may spread to the paranephric fat that is outside this fascia. The clinical symptoms of insidious onset of fever, flank mass, and tenderness are indistinguishable from those associated with perinephric abscess. UTI, however, is absent. Ultrasonography and CT can usually delineate the abscess outside the Gerota fascia.

Improved imaging techniques have decreased the mortality rate of 40% to 50% in early series to roughly 12%, but there is still an average of 3.4 days' lag time before appropriate diagnosis in a current series (Meng et al, 2002). Only 35% of patients were correctly diagnosed on presentation in the Meng series, and this lag time contributed to mortality in nearly all patients in that series. Having an appropriate threshold for imaging will continue to improve the rate of correct diagnoses.

Management. Antimicrobial agents should be immediately started upon diagnosis of perinephric abscess. Gram stain identifies the pathogenesis and guides antimicrobial therapy. An aminoglycoside together with an antistaphylococcal agent, such as methicillin or oxacillin, should be started immediately. If the

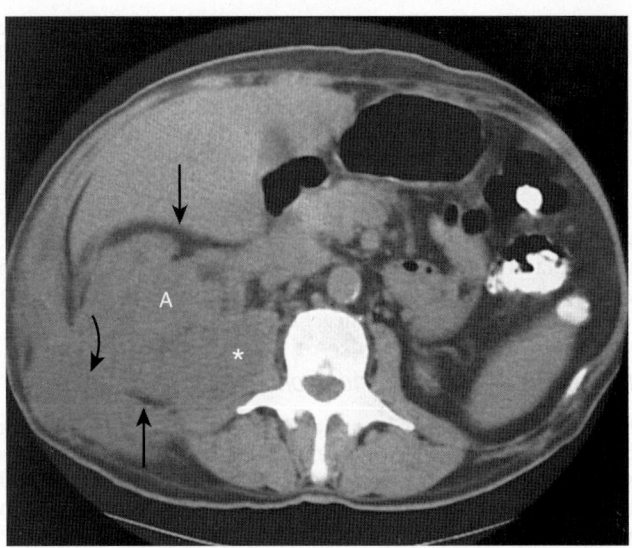

Figure 12-30. Nonenhanced computed tomography scan through the lower pole of the right kidney (previous left nephrectomy) shows extensive perinephric abscess. Extensive abscess (A) distorts and enlarges the renal contour, infiltrates perinephric fat *(straight arrows),* and also extends into the psoas muscle *(asterisk)* and the soft tissues of the flank *(curved arrow).* Also note that normal renal collecting system fat has been obliterated by the process.

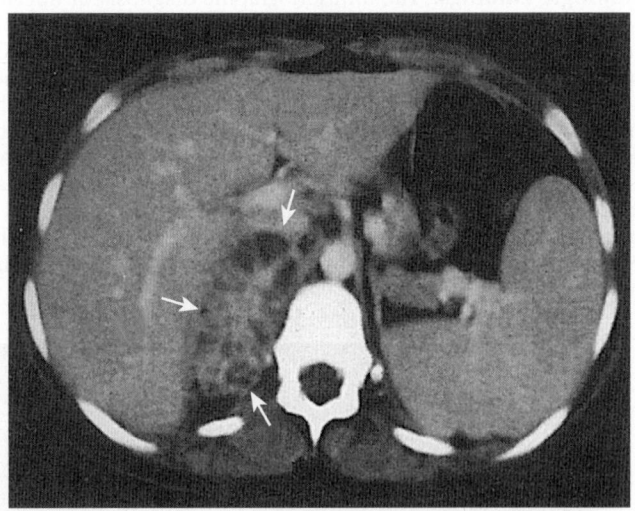

Figure 12-31. Perinephric abscess involving the right adrenal gland. Computed tomography scan shows large right pararenal mass *(arrows)* with multiple low-density areas within. At surgery, a large pararenal abscess with extensive involvement of the right adrenal was found. (From Schaeffer AJ. Urinary tract infections. In: Gillenwater JY, Grayhack JT, Howards SS, et al, editors. Adult and pediatric urology. Philadelphia: Lippincott Williams & Wilkins; 2002. p. 211–72.)

patient has a penicillin hypersensitivity, cephalothin or vancomycin may be used.

In addition to controlling sepsis and preventing further spread of infection, Meng and colleagues' series of 25 patients suggests that, for small perinephric abscesses (<3 cm), antibiotics alone can appropriately treat immune-competent patients (Meng et al, 2002). **Eight out of the 10 patients treated with antibiotics alone had full resolution after a mean of 10 days in the hospital. The average size of abscess treated was 1.8 cm.** Siegel and coworkers (1996) also showed good resolution of perinephric abscesses less than 3 cm, with cure seen in all five patients in their series.

For larger collections or those not responsive to initial antibiotic therapy, intervention is the next step in treatment. **Surgical drainage, or nephrectomy if the kidney is nonfunctioning or severely infected, was the classic treatment for perinephric abscesses. However, with the advent of the field of interventional radiology and improvements in percutaneous drainage techniques, renal ultrasonography and CT- or ultrasound-guided percutaneous aspiration and drainage of perirenal collections is now a good option for therapy.** In Meng's study, 11 of the 25 patients had percutaneous drainage in addition to antibiotics (Meng et al, 2002). The mean abscess size was 11 cm and the mean time to resolution was 25 days. Four of these patients eventually required open surgical exploration and drainage. All removed kidneys demonstrated hallmarks of minimal function. **Unlike in renal abscesses, early drainage of abscesses greater than 3 cm in diameter is recommended.**

Once the perinephric abscess has been drained, the underlying problem must be dealt with. Some conditions such as renal cortical abscess or enteric communication require prompt attention. Nephrectomy for pyonephrosis may be performed concurrent with drainage of the perinephric abscess if the patient's condition is good. In other instances it is best to drain the perinephric abscess first and correct the underlying problem or perform a nephrectomy when the patient's condition has improved. Meng's series of 11 patients with abscesses greater than 11 cm had a roughly 33% need for nephrectomy (Meng et al, 2002). Although this is a high number in patients who are likely diabetic where the nephron-sparing approach is ideal, it is decidedly lower than the historical nephrectomy rate, likely secondary to more successful percutaneous drainage rates. In three of their patients with small perinephric abscesses and hydronephrosis, antibiotics and drainage of the obstructed urinary system led to cure.

Perinephric Abscess versus Acute Pyelonephritis. It has already been emphasized that the greatest obstacle to the treatment of perinephric abscess is the delay in diagnosis. **In the series of Thorley and colleagues (1974), a common misdiagnosis was acute pyelonephritis; Meng's study showed a similar delay of roughly 3 to 4 days in appropriate diagnosis in a modern study** (Meng et al, 2002). **Thorley's study found that two factors differentiated perinephric abscess and acute pyelonephritis: (1) most patients with uncomplicated pyelonephritis were symptomatic for less than 5 days before hospitalization, whereas most with perinephric abscesses were symptomatic for longer than 5 days; and (2) no patient with acute pyelonephritis remained febrile for longer than 4 days once appropriate antimicrobial agents were started. All patients with perinephric abscesses had a fever for at least 5 days, with a median of 7 days.** Similar results were noted by Fowler and Perkins (1994).

Patients with polycystic renal disease who undergo hemodialysis may be particularly susceptible to the progression from acute UTIs to perinephric abscess. Of 445 patients undergoing chronic hemodialysis at the Regional Kidney Disease Program in Minneapolis, 5.4% had polycystic kidney disease and 33.3% of these patients developed symptomatic UTIs (Sweet and Keane, 1979). Eight (62.5%) developed perinephric abscesses, and three of these patients died. According to the investigators, all UTIs, even those that progressed to perinephric abscesses, were promptly treated with appropriate antimicrobial agents, and all patients in this group became afebrile and asymptomatic when the agents were stopped. Yet later, after various times, symptoms attributable to perinephric abscess developed in eight of the patients. The mechanism of this process is not clear, but the limited bioavailability of some antimicrobial agents in cysts is variable and could contribute to the progression of renal infection.

Chronic Pyelonephritis

In patients without underlying renal or urinary tract disease, chronic pyelonephritis secondary to UTI is a rare disease and an even more rare cause of chronic renal failure. In patients with underlying functional or structural urinary tract abnormalities, however, chronic renal infection can cause significant renal impairment. Thus it is essential that appropriate studies be used to diagnose, localize, and treat chronic renal infection.

The prevalence of chronic pyelonephritis has also been assessed in patients undergoing dialysis for end-stage renal disease. Despite a 2% to 5% prevalence of bacteriuria in women, pyelonephritis uncomplicated by obstruction or urinary tract malformation does not cause end-stage renal disease. Schechter and colleagues (1971) analyzed the cause for renal failure in 170 patients referred to them for dialysis. Chronic pyelonephritis was the primary cause of end-stage renal disease in 22 (13%) but was usually associated with an underlying structural defect. Unequivocal nonobstructive chronic pyelonephritis was not found. Symptomatic infections tended to occur before the onset of azotemia in most patients with chronic pyelonephritis. Similarly, Huland and Busch (1982) evaluated 161 patients with end-stage renal disease and found that 42 had chronic pyelonephritis. However, in addition to a history of UTIs, these 42 patients had complicating defects, such as vesicoureteral reflux, analgesic abuse, nephrolithiasis, or obstruction. Nonobstructive uncomplicated UTI alone was never found to be the cause of renal insufficiency. Thus, using end-stage renal disease seen at autopsy or at the dialysis clinic as an indicator, the prevalence of uncomplicated chronic bacterial pyelonephritis is rare.

In addition, the role of bacterial infection in development of chronic renal disease can be assessed in patients with renal interstitial and tubular damage similar to that which has classically been called chronic pyelonephritis. The frequency with which various potential causes of interstitial damage are operative in patients with interstitial nephritis was assessed by Murray and Goldberg (1975). These investigators not only concluded that UTI is rarely the sole cause of chronic renal disease in the adult but also observed that 89% of their azotemic patients had a readily identifiable primary cause of their interstitial nephritis. Thus, when patients with a clinical diagnosis of chronic interstitial nephritis are selected as the starting point, it is easy to associate many factors with this disease, but UTI does not seem to be one of them.

Clinical Presentation. There are no symptoms of chronic pyelonephritis until it produces renal insufficiency, and then the symptoms are similar to those of any other form of chronic renal failure. If a patient's chronic pyelonephritis is thought to be an end result of many episodes of acute pyelonephritis, a history of intermittent symptoms of fever, flank pain, and dysuria may be elicited. Similarly, urinary findings and the presence of renal infection correlate poorly. Bacteriuria and pyuria, the hallmarks of UTI, are not predictive of renal infection. Conversely, patients with significant renal infection may have sterile urine if the ureter draining the kidney is obstructed or the infection is outside of the collecting system.

The pathologic and radiologic criteria for diagnosing renal infection may also be misleading. Asscher (1980) has tabulated eight long-term follow-up studies from the literature on kidneys of adults with UTIs. The data from these reports on 901 patients show that bacteriuria present in otherwise healthy adults for long periods may be associated with nonexistent or extremely minimal evidence of kidney damage. Conversely, patients who have chronic pyelonephritis may have negative urine cultures.

Radiologic Findings. The diagnosis of chronic pyelonephritis can be made with the greatest confidence on the basis of pyelographic findings. The essential features are asymmetry and irregularity of the kidney outlines, blunting and dilation of one or more calyces, and cortical scars at the corresponding site (Fig. 12-32). In the absence of stones, obstruction, and tuberculosis, and with the single exception of analgesic nephritis with papillary necrosis (which can be readily excluded by history), chronic pyelonephritis is virtually the only disease that produces a localized scar over a deformed calyx (Stamey, 1980). In advanced pyelonephritis, calyceal distortion and irregularity together with cortical scars complete the picture. Regardless of the etiology of chronic pyelonephritis, CT findings will be consistent with atrophy, cortical/parenchymal thinning, calyceal clubbing, and possible hypertrophy of residual normal tissue and asymmetry (Craig et al, 2008). D'Souza and colleagues (1995) showed a linear relationship between renal

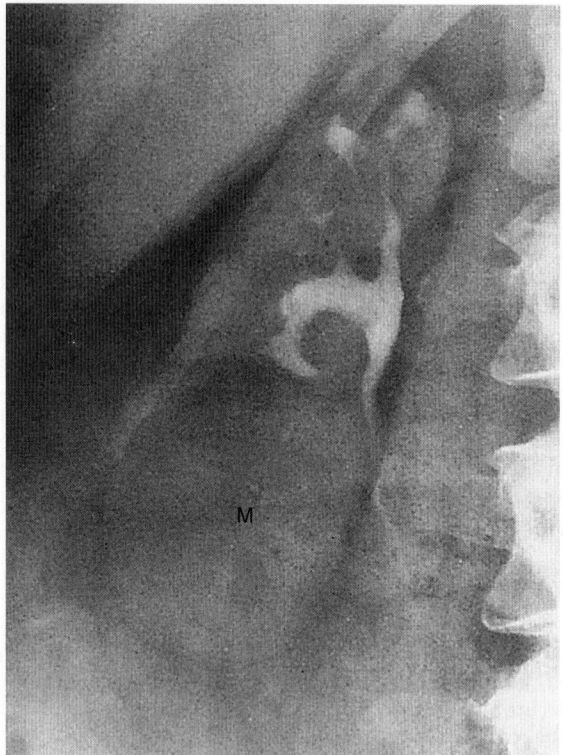

Figure 12-32. Chronic pyelonephritis. Ten-minute excretory urogram demonstrates irregular renal outline with upper pole parenchymal atrophy. Note significant loss of renal cortical thickness over blunted and dilated calyces. Lower pole mass (M) is a simple cyst. (From Schaeffer AJ. Urinary tract infections. In: Gillenwater JY, Grayhack JT, Howards SS, et al, editors. Adult and pediatric urology. Philadelphia: Lippincott Williams & Wilkins; 2002. p. 211–72.)

parenchymal volume loss and function decline as assessed by DMSA scan. Hodson and Wilson (1965) pointed out that renal infarction, an extremely rare condition, may closely resemble pyelonephritic scars but that the renal pyramid remains with renal infarction in contradistinction to pyelonephritis.

Pathology. In chronic pyelonephritis, the gross kidney is often diffusely contracted, scarred, and pitted. The scars are Y-shaped, flat, broad-based depressions with red-brown granular bases. The scarring is often polar with underlying calyceal blunting. The parenchyma is thin, and the corticomedullary demarcation is lost. **Histologic changes are patchy.** There is usually an interstitial infiltrate of lymphocytes, plasma cells, and occasional polymorphonuclear cells. Portions of the parenchyma may be replaced by fibrosis, and, although glomeruli may be preserved, periglomerular fibrosis is often seen. In some affected areas, glomeruli may be completely fibrosed and tubules atrophied. Leukocyte and hyaline casts are sometimes present in the tubules; the latter may cause resemblance to the thyroid colloid, hence the description *renal thyroidization* (Braude, 1973). In general, the changes are nonspecific; they also may be seen in toxic exposures, postobstructive atrophy, hematologic disorders, postirradiation nephritis, ischemic renal disease, and nephrosclerosis.

Management. Management of radiographic evidence of pyelonephritis should be directed at treating infection if present, preventing future infections, and monitoring and preserving renal function. The treatment of existing infection must be based on careful antimicrobial susceptibility tests and selection of drugs that can achieve bactericidal concentrations in the urine and yet are not nephrotoxic. Achievement of acceptable bactericidal levels of a drug in the urine of a patient with chronic pyelonephritis may be difficult because the diminished concentrating ability of pyelonephritis may impair excretion and concentration of the antimicrobial agent. The

duration of antimicrobial therapy is often prolonged to maximize the chance of cure. With patients in whom renal damage develops or progresses in the presence of UTI, the working hypothesis should be that there is an underlying renal, usually papillary, lesion or underlying urologic condition, such as obstruction or calculus, which has increased susceptibility to renal damage. Appropriate nephrologic and urologic evaluation should be undertaken to identify and, if possible, correct these abnormalities.

Bacterial "Relapse" from a Normal Kidney

The concept that bacteria persist in the renal parenchyma between bacteriuric episodes and cause "relapsing" UTIs was based on a study by Turck and colleagues (1968) that suggested that bacterial persistence could be recognized by simply identifying two consecutive recurrent infections with the same organism. Unfortunately, this study did not indicate whether the urine was cultured during therapy to ensure that the original infection had actually been eradicated. It is possible that some of these so-called relapses were in fact unresolved initial infections and that ureteral edema associated with catheterization may have impeded clearance of the initial infecting strain.

Subsequent studies summarized by Stamey (1980) and Forland and associates (1977) have shown that in a normal urinary tract recurrent infections are not caused by relapse from bacterial persistence in the kidney. With ureteral catheterization techniques, Cattell and colleagues (1973) localized the site of bacteriuria in 42 patients who had follow-up for 6 months after therapy. He analyzed the response to antimicrobial therapy of 2 weeks' duration. Of the 26 patients who were cured of their initial infection, 16 had recurrence with the same organism, 8 had upper tract infections, and 8 had bladder bacteriuria.

Most of the changes of chronic pyelonephritis seem to occur in infancy, probably because the growing kidney is most susceptible to scarring. A review that examined the long-term effect of UTIs in adults concluded that renal damage is rare in nonobstructive UTIs (Stamey, 1980), but it does occur (Bailey et al, 1969; Davies et al, 1972; Davidson and Talner, 1973; Feldberg, 1982).

The association between hypertension and the pyelonephritic kidney has been addressed by Pfau and Rosenmann (1978), who concluded that the association of chronic pyelonephritis and hypertension is usually coincidental. Their conclusion agrees with that of a study by Parker and Kunin (1973) that examined 74 women who had been admitted to the hospital 10 to 20 years previously for pyelonephritis. Only 14.5% of these women had hypertension, a rate similar to that found in a random female population of the same age.

Infectious Granulomatous Nephritis

Xanthogranulomatous Pyelonephritis

Xanthogranulomatous pyelonephritis (XGP) is a rare, severe, chronic renal infection typically resulting in diffuse renal destruction. Most cases are unilateral and result in a nonfunctioning, enlarged kidney associated with obstructive uropathy secondary to nephrolithiasis. XGP is characterized by accumulation of lipid-laden foamy macrophages. It begins within the pelvis and calyces and subsequently extends into and destroys renal parenchymal and adjacent tissues. It has been known to imitate virtually every other inflammatory disease of the kidney, as well as renal cell carcinoma, on radiographic examination (Malek and Elder, 1978; Tolia et al, 1980). In addition, the microscopic appearance of XGP has been confused with clear cell adenocarcinoma of the kidney on frozen section and has led to radical nephrectomy (Anhalt et al, 1971; Malek and Elder, 1978; Flynn et al, 1979; Lorentzen and Nielsen, 1980; Tolia et al, 1980). The entity is uncommon and is found in only about 0.6% (Malek et al, 1972) to 1.4% (Ghosh, 1955) of patients with renal inflammation who are evaluated pathologically.

Pathogenesis. The primary factors involved in the pathogenesis of XGP are nephrolithiasis, obstruction, and infection (Gregg et al, 1999). Nephrolithiasis has been noted in as many as 83% of the patients in various series; approximately half of the renal stones have been of the staghorn type (Parsons et al, 1983; Chuang et al, 1992; Nataluk et al, 1995). It has been proposed clinically and demonstrated experimentally that primary obstruction followed by infection with *E. coli* can lead to tissue destruction and collections of lipid material by macrophages (Povysil and Konickova, 1972). These macrophages (xanthoma cells) are distributed in sheets around parenchymal abscesses and calyces and are intermixed with lymphocytes, giant cells, and plasma cells. The bacteria appear to be of low virulence because spontaneous bacteremia has rarely been described. Other possible interrelated factors include venous occlusion and hemorrhage, abnormal lipid metabolism, lymphatic blockage, failure of antimicrobial therapy in UTI, altered immunologic competence, and renal ischemia (Friedenberg and Spjut, 1963; Mering et al, 1973; Goodman et al, 1979; McDonald, 1981; Tolia et al, 1981). The concept that XGP is related to incomplete bacterial degradation and altered host response has received mixed support (Nielsen and Lorentzen, 1981; Khalyl-Mawad et al, 1982). Thus it appears that there is probably no single factor that is instrumental in the pathogenesis of this disease. Rather, there is an inadequate host acute inflammatory response within an obstructed, ischemic, or necrotic kidney.

Pathology. The kidney is usually massively enlarged and has a normal contour. XGP may be diffuse, as in approximately 80% of the patients, or segmental. In the diffuse form of the disease, the entire kidney is involved, whereas in segmental XGP, only the parenchyma surrounding one or more calyces or one pole of a duplicated collecting system is involved. On sectioning, the kidney usually demonstrates nephrolithiasis and peripelvic fibrosis. The calyces are dilated and filled with purulent material, but fibrosis surrounding the pelvis usually prevents dilation. The papillae are often destroyed by papillary necrosis (Goodman et al, 1979). In advanced stages of the disease, multiple parenchymal abscesses are filled with viscous pus and lined by yellowish tissue (Fig. 12-33A). The cortex is often thin and replaced by xanthogranulomatous tissue. The capsule is often thickened, and extension of the inflammatory process into the perinephric or paranephric space is common (Goodman et al, 1979; McDonald, 1981; Gregg et al, 1999).

On microscopic examination, the yellowish nodules that line the calyces and surround the parenchymal abscesses contain dark sheets of lipid-laden macrophages (foamy histiocytes with small, dark nuclei and clear cytoplasm) intermixed with lymphocytes, giant cells, and plasma cells (Fig. 12-33B). Xanthogranulomatous cells are not specific to XGP but may be present anywhere inflammation or obstruction coexists. The origin of the fatty substance is disputed. Cholesterol esters that make up a part of the lipid might be derived from lysis of erythrocytes after hemorrhage (Saeed and Fine, 1963).

Clinical Presentation. XGP should be suspected in patients with UTIs and a **unilateral enlarged nonfunctioning or poorly functioning kidney with a stone or a mass lesion indistinguishable from malignant tumor. Most patients present with flank pain (69%), fever and chills (69%), and persistent bacteriuria (46%)** (Malek and Elder, 1978). **Additional vague symptoms, such as malaise, may be present. On physical examination, 62% of the patients had a flank mass and 35% had previous calculi** (Malek and Elder, 1978). Less commonly, hypertension, hematuria, or hepatomegaly is the presenting complaint. The medical history is often positive for UTIs and urologic instrumentation (Malek and Elder, 1978; Flynn et al, 1979; Goodman et al, 1979; Grainger et al, 1982; Yazaki et al, 1982; Petronic et al, 1989; Eastham et al, 1994; Nataluk et al, 1995). Diabetics also appear to be at greater risk of

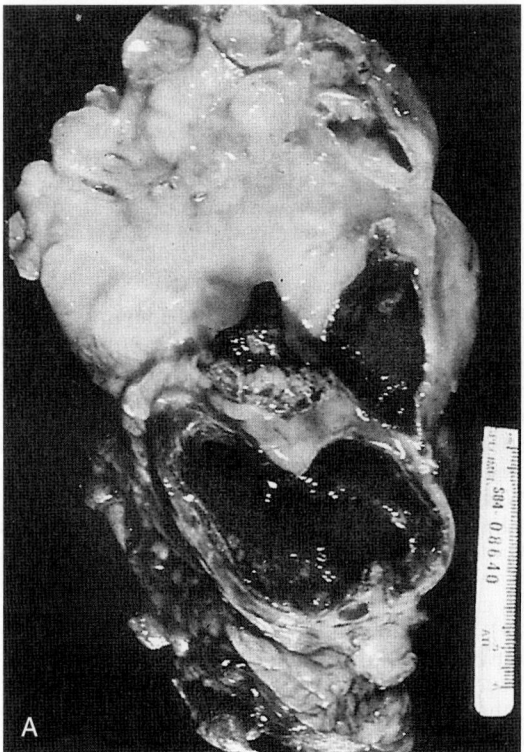
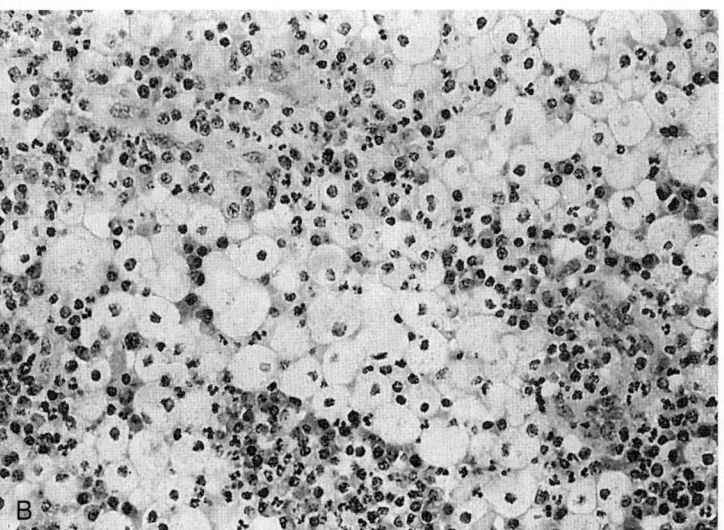

Figure 12-33. Xanthogranulomatous pyelonephritis. A, Gross specimen. Kidney is massively enlarged, measuring 23 × 12 cm; the normal architecture is replaced by a shaggy yellow upper pole mass corresponding to xanthogranulomatous inflammation and numerous distorted and dilated calyces. **B,** Microscopically, the shaggy yellow tissue is composed primarily of lipid-laden histiocytes mixed with other inflammatory cells. (From Schaeffer AJ. Urinary tract infections. In: Gillenwater JY, Grayhack JT, Howards SS, et al, editors. Adult and pediatric urology. Philadelphia: Lippincott Williams & Wilkins; 2002. p. 211–72.)

developing the disease (Eastham et al, 1994). Although it may occur at any age, the peak incidence of XGP is in the fifth to the seventh decade. Women are more commonly affected than men. There is no predilection for either kidney.

Bacteriology and Laboratory Diagnosis. Although review of the literature shows *Proteus* to be the most common organism involved with XGP (Anhalt et al, 1971; Tolia et al, 1981), *E. coli* is also common. The prevalence of *Proteus* organisms may reflect their association with stone formation and subsequent chronic obstruction and irritation. Malek and Elder (1978), in their analysis of 26 cases, found that renal tissue cultures grew bacteria in 22 of 23 cases. Anaerobes also have been cultured (Malek and Elder, 1978).

Approximately 10% of patients have mixed cultures. About one third of patients have no growth in their urine, probably because many patients have recently taken or are taking antimicrobial agents when cultures are obtained. The infecting organism may be revealed only by tissue cultures obtained during surgery. Urinalysis usually shows pus and protein. In addition, blood tests often reveal anemia and may show hepatic dysfunction in up to 50% of the patients (Malek and Elder, 1978).

XGP is almost always unilateral; therefore azotemia or frank renal failure is uncommon (Goodman et al, 1979; Gregg et al, 1999).

CT is probably the most useful radiologic technique in evaluating patients with XGP (Fig. 12-34). **Fifty to eighty percent of patients show the classic triad of unilateral renal enlargement with little or no function and a large calculus in the renal pelvis** (Elder, 1984). **CT usually demonstrates a large, reniform mass with the renal pelvis tightly surrounding a central calcification but without pelvic dilatation** (Solomon et al, 1983; Goldman et al, 1984; Hartman, 1985). Renal parenchyma is replaced by multiple water-density masses representing dilated calyces and abscess cavities filled with varied amounts of pus and debris. On enhanced scans, the walls of these cavities demonstrate a prominent blush owing to the abundant vascularity within the granulation tissue. The cavities themselves, however, fail to enhance, whereas tumors and other inflammatory lesions usually do. The CT scan is particularly helpful in demonstrating the extent of renal involvement and may indicate whether adjacent organs or the abdominal wall are involved by XGP (Eastham et al, 1994; Kaplan et al, 1997).

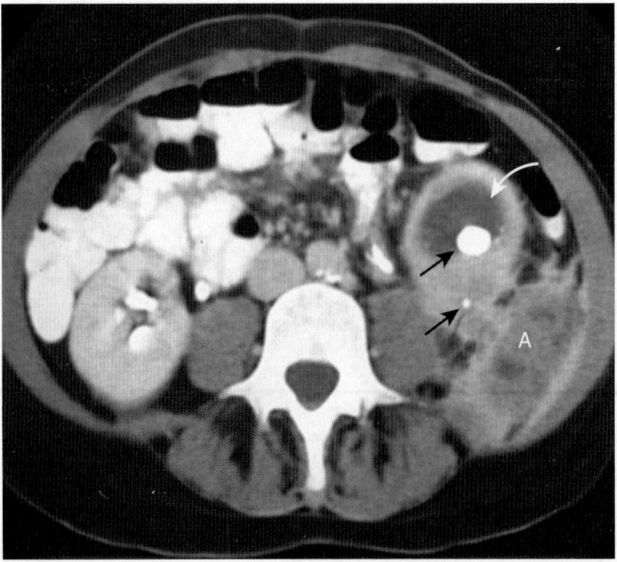

Figure 12-34. Xanthogranulomatous pyelonephritis. Enhanced computed tomography scan shows collecting system and parenchymal calculi *(straight black arrows)* with lower pole pyonephrosis *(curved white arrow)* and an irregular, predominantly low-density perinephric abscess (A) extending into the soft tissues of the flank.

Ultrasonography usually demonstrates global enlargement of the kidney (Merenich and Popky, 1991). The normal renal architecture is replaced by multiple hypoechoic fluid-filled masses that correspond to debris-filled, dilated calyces or foci of parenchymal destruction (Fagerholm, 1983; Hartman et al, 1984). With focal involvement, a solid mass involving a segment of the kidney is demonstrated with an associated calculus in the collecting system or ureter. Renal cell carcinoma and other solid renal lesions must be considered in the differential diagnosis (Elder, 1984).

Radionuclide renal scanning using ^{99m}Tc-DMSA is used to confirm and quantify the differential lack of function in the involved kidney (Gregg et al, 1999). MRI has not yet superseded CT in the evaluation of renal inflammation, but it provides some advantages in delineating extrarenal extension of inflammation (Soler et al, 1997). Lesions of XGP may appear as cystic foci of intermediate intensity signal on T1-weighted images and hyperintensity on T2-weighted images. Arteriography shows hypervascular areas, but there may be some hypovascular areas (Malek and Elder, 1978; Van Kirk et al, 1980; Tolia et al, 1981). Therefore radiologic studies, although distinctive, often cannot be used to differentiate between XGP and renal cell carcinoma.

Differential Diagnosis. Diagnosis of segmental XGP without calculi may be difficult. XGP in association with massive pelvic dilation cannot be distinguished from pyonephrosis. When XGP occurs within a small contracted kidney, the radiographic findings are nonspecific and nondiagnostic. Renal parenchymal malacoplakia may show renal enlargement and multiple inflammatory masses replacing the normal renal parenchyma, but calculi are usually not present. Renal lymphoma may be associated with multiple hypoechoic masses surrounding the contracted, nondilated pelvis, but lymphoma is usually clinically obvious, and renal involvement is usually bilateral and not associated with calculi (Hartman, 1985).

Management. **The primary obstacle to the correct treatment of XGP is incorrect diagnosis.** Today with CT technology, the diagnosis of XGP is made preoperatively nearly 90% of the time (Eastham et al, 1994; Nataluk et al, 1995). Antimicrobial therapy may be necessary to stabilize the patient preoperatively, and, **occasionally, long-term antimicrobial therapy will eradicate the infection and restore renal function** (Mollier et al, 1995). Because the renal abnormality may be diagnosed preoperatively as a renal tumor and/or is diffuse, **nephrectomy is usually performed.** If localized XGP is diagnosed preoperatively or at exploration, it is amenable to partial nephrectomy (Malek and Elder, 1978; Tolia et al, 1980; Osca et al, 1997).

The lipid-laden macrophages associated with XGP, however, closely resemble clear cell adenocarcinoma and may be difficult to distinguish solely on the basis of frozen section. Furthermore, XGP has been associated with renal cell carcinoma, papillary transitional cell carcinoma of the pelvis or bladder, and infiltrating squamous cell carcinoma of the pelvis (Schoborg et al, 1980; Pitts et al, 1981; Tolia et al, 1981); thus, if malignant renal tumor cannot be excluded, nephrectomy should be performed. When diffuse and extensive disease into the retroperitoneum exists, removal of the kidney and perinephric fat may be needed. Under these circumstances, the surgery may be difficult and may involve dissection of granulomatous tissue from the diaphragm, great vessels, and bowel (Malek and Elder, 1978; Flynn et al, 1979). It is important to remove the entire inflammatory mass because in nearly three fourths of patients, xanthogranulomatous tissue is infected. If incision and drainage alone are performed rather than nephrectomy, the patient may continue to suffer from protracted debilitating illness and may develop a renal cutaneous fistula; an even more difficult nephrectomy will then be necessary. One early case-matched series of laparoscopic nephrectomies performed for XGP concluded that the benefits of laparoscopic surgery do not extend to the treatment of this disease (Bercowsky et al, 1999); however, a larger review of a modern XGP experience suggests that laparoscopic nephrectomy is a reasonable treatment approach. Some studies suggest a retroperitoneal approach laparoscopically and, if transperitoneal, the use of a hand-assist port (Tobias-Machado et al, 2005). High conversion rates were seen across multiple studies (Korkes et al, 2008)

Malacoplakia

Malacoplakia, from the Greek word meaning "soft plaque," is an unusual inflammatory disease that was originally described to affect the bladder but has been found to affect the genitourinary and gastrointestinal tracts, skin, lungs, bones, and mesenteric lymph nodes. It is an inflammatory lesion described originally by Michaelis and Gutmann (1902). It was characterized by von Hansemann (1903) as soft, yellow-brown plaques with granulomatous lesions in which the histiocytes contain distinct basophilic lysosomal inclusion bodies or Michaelis-Gutmann bodies. Although its exact pathogenesis is unknown, malacoplakia probably results from abnormal macrophage function in response to a bacterial infection, which is most often *E. coli.*

Pathogenesis. The pathogenesis is unknown, but several theories are popular. In 93 patients who had cultures of urine, diseased tissue, or blood, 89.4% had coliform infections (Stanton and Maxted, 1981). Moreover, 40% of the patients in this review had an immunodeficiency syndrome, autoimmune disease, carcinoma, or another systemic disorder. **This association of coliform infections and compromised health status in patients with malacoplakia is well recognized.**

It is hypothesized that bacteria or bacterial fragments form the nidus for the calcium phosphate crystals that laminate the Michaelis-Gutmann bodies. Most investigations into the pathogenesis of this disease support theories that a defect in intraphagosomal bacterial digestion accounts for the unusual immunologic response that causes malacoplakia.

Pathology. The diagnosis is made by biopsy. The lesion is characterized by large histiocytes, known as *von Hansemann cells,* and small basophilic, extracytoplasmic, or intracytoplasmic calculospherules called *Michaelis-Gutmann bodies,* which are pathognomonic (Fig. 12-35). Electron microscopy has revealed intact coliform bacteria and bacterial fragments within phagolysosomes of the foamy-appearing malacoplakic histiocytes (Lewin et al, 1976; Stanton and Maxted, 1981). In their review of the subject, Stanton and Maxted (1981) and Esparza and associates (1989) emphasized that, although pathognomonic for the disease, Michaelis-Gutmann bodies may be absent in early malacoplakia and are not necessary for the diagnosis.

It has been shown that macrophages in malacoplakia involving the kidney and bladder contain large amounts of immunoreactive α_1-antitrypsin (Callea et al, 1982). The amount of α_1-antitrypsin remains unchanged during the morphogenetic stages of the pathologic process. Macrophages from other pathologic processes, closely resembling malacoplakia but without Michaelis-Gutmann bodies, do not contain α_1-antitrypsin except for a few macrophages in

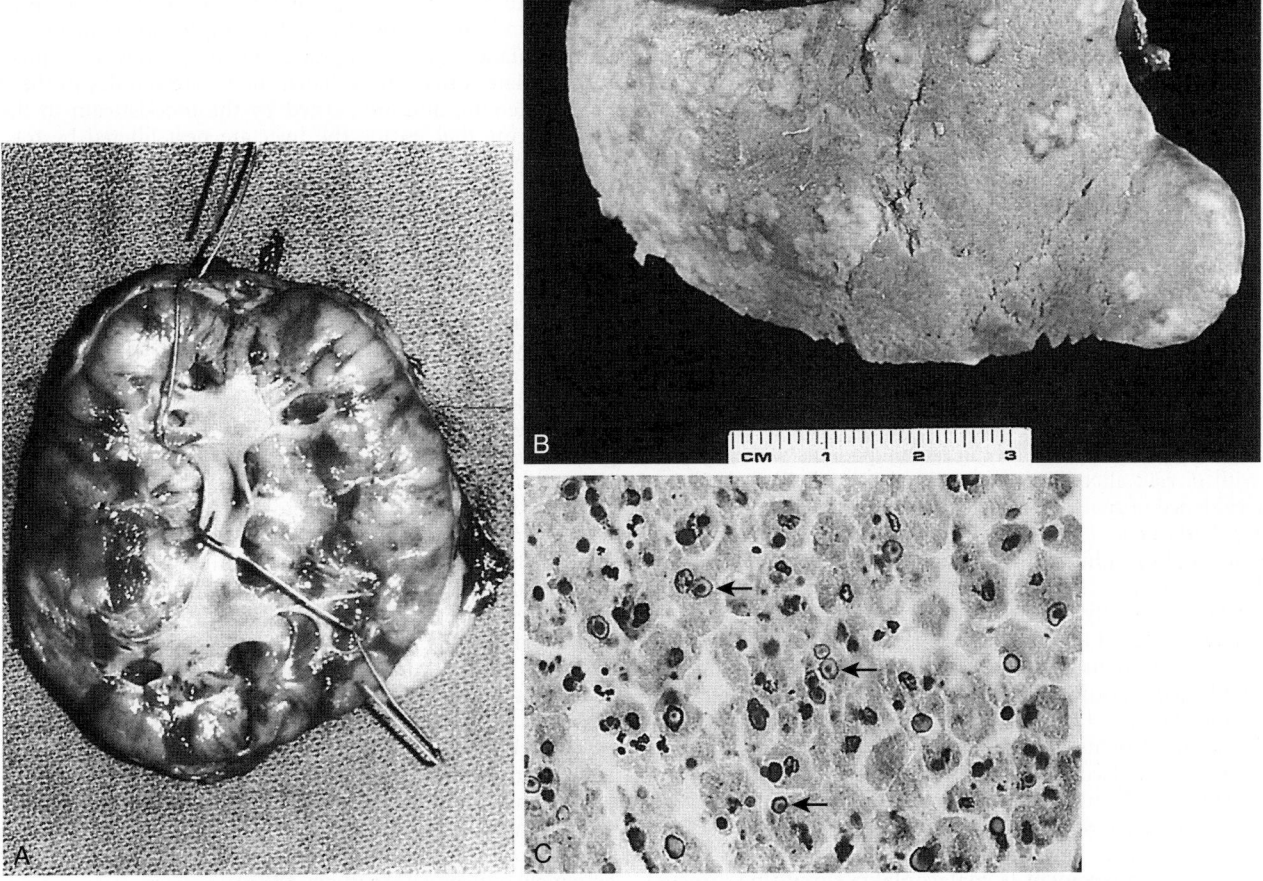

Figure 12-35. Renal parenchymal malacoplakia. **A,** Cut surface demonstrates extensive cortical and upper medullary replacement by multifocal, confluent, tumorlike masses. **B,** Cortical surface exhibits multiple, firm, plaquelike lesions. **C,** Hallmark of malacoplakia is demonstration of the Michaelis-Gutmann body *(arrows),* which represents incompletely destroyed bacteria surrounded by lipoprotein membrane (hematoxylin and eosin stain). (From Hartman DS. Radiologic pathologic correlation of the infectious granulomatous diseases of the kidney: I and II. Monogr Urol 1985;6:3.)

tuberculosis and XGP. **Therefore immunohistochemical staining for α₁-antitrypsin may be a useful test for an early and accurate differential diagnosis of malacoplakia.**

Clinical Presentation. Most patients are older than 50 years. The ratio of females to males with malacoplakia within the urinary tract is 4:1, but this disparity does not occur in other body tissues (Stanton and Maxted, 1981). The patients often are debilitated and immunosuppressed and have other chronic diseases. The symptoms of bladder malacoplakia are bladder irritability and hematuria. Cystoscopy reveals mucosal plaques or nodules. As these lesions progress, they may become fungating, firm, sessile masses that cause filling defects of the bladder, ureter, or pelvis on excretory urograms. The distal ureter may become strictured or stenotic and cause subsequent renal obstruction or nonfunction (Sexton et al, 1982). A typical patient with renal parenchymal disease may have one or more radiographic masses and chronic *E. coli* infections. Renal parenchymal malacoplakia may be complicated by renal vein thrombosis and inferior vena cava thrombosis (McClure, 1983). When malacoplakia involves the testis, epididymo-orchitis is present. Malacoplakia of the prostate is rare, but, when it occurs, it may be confused with carcinoma clinically (Shimizu et al, 1981). Mortality can exceed 50%, and the morbidity can be substantial (Stanton and Maxted, 1981).

Radiologic Findings. Multifocal malacoplakia on excretory urography typically presents as enlarged kidneys with multiple filling defects. Renal calcification, lithiasis, and hydronephrosis are absent. The multifocal nature is best appreciated by using ultrasonography, CT, or arteriography. Ultrasound examination may demonstrate renal enlargement and distortion of the central echo complex. The masses are often confluent, resulting in an overall increase in the echogenicity of the renal parenchyma (Hartman et al, 1980). On CT, the foci of malacoplakia are less dense than the surrounding enhanced parenchyma (Hartman, 1985). Arteriography typically reveals a hypovascular mass without peripheral neovascularity (Cavins and Goldstein, 1977; Trillo et al, 1977).

Unifocal malacoplakia on excretory urography appears as a noncalcified mass that is indistinguishable from other inflammatory or neoplastic lesions. Ultrasonography and CT may demonstrate a solid or cystic structure, depending on the degree of internal necrosis. Angiography may demonstrate neovascularity (Trillo et al, 1977). Extension beyond the kidney, which can occur with either multifocal or uniform malacoplakia, is best demonstrated by CT.

Differential Diagnosis. The differential diagnosis includes renal cystic disease, neoplasia, and renal inflammatory disease (Hartman, 1985). Malacoplakia should be considered when one or more renal masses are observed, particularly in female patients with recurrent UTIs with *E. coli*, altered immune response syndromes, or cystoscopic evidence of malacoplakia or filling defects in the collecting system (Charboneau, 1980). Malacoplakia should also be suspected when these radiographic findings occur in a renal transplant patient who has persistent UTI despite appropriate antimicrobial therapy. Cystic disease generally can be excluded by careful sonographic and CT evaluations. Renal involvement with metastatic disease or lymphomas usually occurs late in the course of the disease, which is well established. Multifocal renal cell carcinoma is most often seen in the context of von Hippel-Lindau disease with its other clinical manifestations. Patients with XGP usually have signs and symptoms of UTI. As with malacoplakia, the involved kidney is enlarged but renal calculi and obstruction are common. Multiple renal abscesses are often associated with hematogenous dissemination resulting from cardiac disease.

Management. Management of malacoplakia should be directed at control of the UTIs, which should stabilize the disease process. This subject is well reviewed by Stanton and Maxted (1981). Although multiple long-term antimicrobial agents, including many antituberculosis agents, have been used, the sulfonamides, rifampin, doxycycline, and TMP are thought to be especially useful because of their intracellular bactericidal activity (Maderazo et al, 1979). Fluoroquinolones are taken up by macrophages directly and have

also proven effective in the management of malacoplakia (Vallorosi et al, 1999). Other investigators have used ascorbic acid and cholinergic agents such as bethanechol in conjunction with antimicrobial therapy and have reported good results (Abdou et al, 1977; Zornow et al, 1979; Stanton et al, 1983). Both agents are thought to increase intracellular cyclic guanosine monophosphate levels, which have been postulated as the biologic defect causing macrophage dysfunction. Surgical intervention, however, may be necessary if the disease progresses in spite of antimicrobial treatment. Nephrectomy is usually performed for the treatment of symptomatic unilateral renal lesions.

The long-term prognosis appears to be related to the extent of the disease. When parenchymal renal malacoplakia is bilateral or occurs in the transplanted kidney, death usually occurs within 6 months (Bowers and Cathey, 1971; Deridder et al, 1977). Patients with unilateral disease usually have a long-term survival after nephrectomy.

Renal Echinococcosis

Echinococcosis is a parasitic infection caused by the larval stage of the tapeworm *Echinococcus granulosus.* The disease is prevalent in dogs, sheep, cattle, and humans in South Africa, Australia, New Zealand, Mediterranean countries (especially Greece), and some parts of the former Soviet Union. In the United States, the disease is rare, but it is found in immigrants from Eastern Europe or other foreign endemic areas or as an indigenous infection among American Indians in the Southwest and in Eskimos (Plorde, 1977).

Pathogenesis and Pathology. Echinococcosis is produced by the larval form of the tapeworm, which in its adult form resides in the intestine of the dog, the definitive host. The adult worm is 3 to 9 mm long. The ova in the feces of the dog contaminate grass and farmlands and are ingested by sheep, pigs, or humans, the intermediate hosts. Larvae hatch, penetrate venules in the wall of the duodenum, and are carried by the bloodstream to the liver. Those larvae that escape the liver are next filtered by the lungs. Approximately 3% of the organisms that escape entrapment in the liver and lungs may then enter the systemic circulation and infect the kidneys. The larvae undergo vesiculation, and the resultant hydatid cyst gradually develops at a rate of about 1 cm/yr. Thus the cyst may take 5 to 10 years to reach pathologic size.

Echinococcosis cysts of the kidney are usually single and located in the cortex (Nabizadeh et al, 1983). The wall of the hydatid cyst has three zones: a peripheral zone of fibroblasts derived from tissues of the host becomes the adventitia and may calcify; an intermediate laminated layer becomes hyalinized; and a single inner layer is composed of nucleated epithelium and is called the *germinal layer*. The germinal layer gives rise to brood capsules that increase in number, become vacuolated, and remain attached to the germinal membrane by a pedicle. New larvae (scoleces) develop in large numbers from the germinal layer within the brood capsule (Fig. 12-36). The hydatid cyst is also filled with fluid. When brood capsules detach, they enlarge and move freely in the fluid and are then called daughter cysts. Hydatid sand is composed of free larvae and daughter cysts.

Clinical Presentation. The symptoms of echinococcosis are those of a slowly growing tumor. Most patients are asymptomatic or have a flank mass, dull pain, or hematuria (Gilsanz et al, 1980; Nabizadeh et al, 1983). Because the cyst is focal, it rarely affects renal function. Rarely, the cyst ruptures into the collecting system, and the patient may experience severe colic and passage of debris resembling grape skins in the urine (hydatiduria). The cyst may also rupture into an adjacent viscus or the peritoneal cavity. The fluid is extremely antigenic (Hartman, 1985).

Laboratory Diagnosis. If cyst rupture occurs, the definitive diagnosis can be established by identifying daughter cysts in the urine or by identifying the laminated wall of the cyst (Sparks et al, 1976). Fewer than half of the patients have eosinophilia. The most reliable diagnostic test uses partially purified hydatid arc 5 antigens in a double-diffusion test (Coltorti and Varela-Diaz, 1978). Complement fixation, hemagglutination (HA), and the Casoni

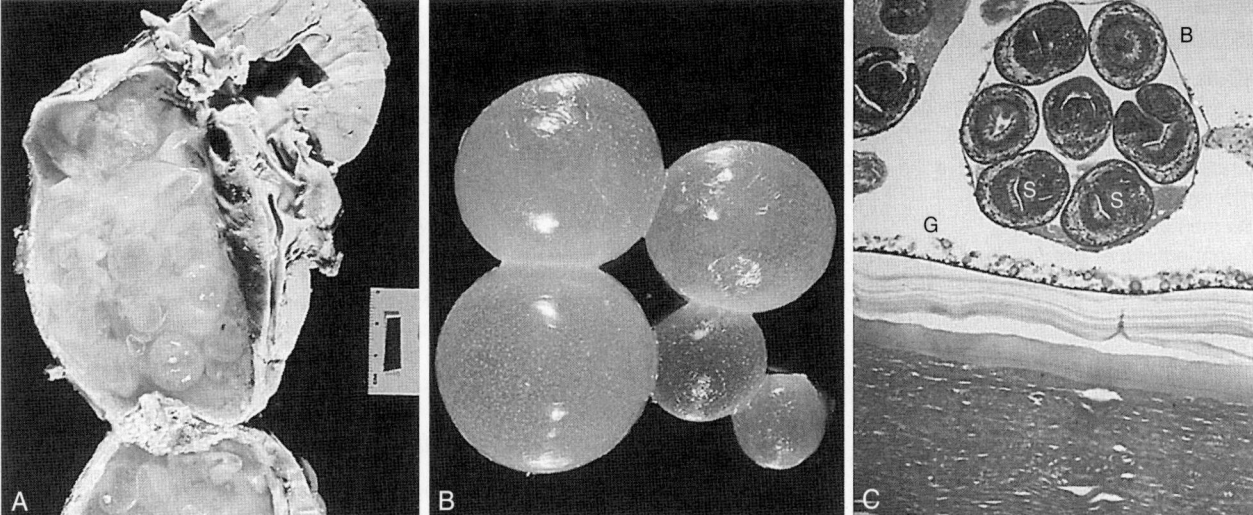

Figure 12-36. **Echinococcosis. A,** Gross specimen. A cystic mass measuring 7 × 11 cm in lower pole. Smaller daughter cysts are identified within the larger cystic mass. **B,** Gross specimen. Daughter cysts represent brood capsules that have detached and move freely. **C,** Photomicrograph. Brood capsules (B) arising from the germinal layer (G) contain viable and degenerating scoleces (S). (From Hartman DS. Radiologic pathologic correlation of the infectious granulomatous diseases of the kidney: III and IV. Monogr Urol 1985;6:26.)

intradermal skin tests are less reliable but, when combined, are positive in about 90% of patients (Sparks et al, 1976).

Radiologic Findings. **Excretory urography typically shows a thick-walled cystic mass, occasionally calcified** (Buckley et al, 1985). If the cyst ruptures into the collecting system, daughter cysts may be outlined in the pelvis as an irregular mass or as multiple solitary lesions (Gilsanz et al, 1980). Occasionally, direct filling of the cyst with contrast medium occurs.

Ultrasonography and CT are useful in characterizing the mass. Ultrasonography usually demonstrates a multicystic or multiloculated mass. A sudden change in position may demonstrate bright falling echoes corresponding to hydatid sand, which can be observed during real-time evaluation of hydatid cysts (Saint Martin and Chiesa, 1984).

On CT, several patterns of renal echinococcosis may be recognized. The most specific is a cystic mass with discrete, round daughter cysts and a well-defined enhancing membrane (Martorana et al, 1981). The less specific pattern is that of a thick-walled multiloculated cystic mass (Gilsanz et al, 1980). The presence of daughter cysts within the mother cyst differentiates the lesion from a simple renal cyst and from renal abscesses, infected cysts, and necrotic neoplasm.

Both CT and ultrasonography are useful in evaluating the liver. Angiography is seldom required. **Diagnostic aspiration should not be performed because of the danger of rupture and spillage of the highly antigenic cyst contents and risk of fatal anaphylaxis.** Nevertheless, Baijal and coworkers (1995) described a percutaneous management of renal hydatidosis as a minimally invasive diagnostic and therapeutic option.

Management. **The prognosis of echinococcosis is good but depends on the site and size of the cysts.** Medical treatment with benzimidazole compounds such as mebendazole or albendazole has shown limited success with significant side effects (Nabizadeh et al, 1983).

Surgery remains the mainstay of treatment of renal echinococcosis (Poulios, 1991). **The cyst should be removed without rupture to reduce the chance of seeding, antigen reaction, and recurrence.** If the cyst wall is calcified, the larvae are probably dead and the risk of seeding is low, although a daughter cyst may be viable. If the cyst ruptures or cannot be removed and marsupialization is required, the contents of the cyst initially should be aspirated and filled

with a scolicidal agent such as 30% sodium chloride, 0.5% silver nitrate, 2% formalin, or 1% iodine for approximately 5 minutes to kill the germinal portion (Sparks et al, 1976; Nabizadeh et al, 1983; Shetty et al, 1992).

KEY POINTS: KIDNEY INFECTIONS

- Acute pyelonephritis classically presents as the abrupt onset of chills, fever, and flank or costovertebral angle tenderness but can present as symptoms as mild as cystitis or as severe as sepsis.
- Emphysematous pyelonephritis is a life-threatening infection diagnosed radiographically by the presence of gas in the parenchyma or collecting system and managed surgically.
- Renal abscesses are well delineated by CT and are classically managed with IV antimicrobial agents and drainage. Smaller abscesses may be amenable to conservative treatment with medical management.
- Pyonephrosis is a bacterial infection in a hydronephrotic kidney. Prompt diagnosis is critical; treatment entails intravenous antimicrobial agents and drainage of the obstructed renal unit.
- XGP is a chronic renal infection that is often found in poorly functioning renal units obstructed secondary to nephrolithiasis. XGP can be mistaken for renal tumors.
- Malacoplakia is an unusual inflammatory disease thought to result from abnormal macrophage function. Michaelis-Gutmann bodies are lysosomal inclusion bodies that characterize this disease microscopically.

BACTEREMIA, SEPSIS, AND SEPTIC SHOCK

Sepsis is a clinical syndrome characterized by extremes of body temperature, heart rate, respiratory rate, and WBC count that occurs in response to an infection. A detailed list of potential characteristics can be found in Box 12-9. Severe sepsis and septic shock are extensions of the sepsis spectrum and involve acute organ dysfunction and life-threatening hypotension not

BOX 12-9 Potential Characteristics of Sepsis Spectrum

GENERAL
Fever (core temperature >38.3°C)
Hypothermia (core temperature <36°C)
Heart rate >90 min, 1 or 2 SD above the normal value for age
Tachypnea
Altered mental status
Significant edema or positive fluid balance (20 mL/kg/24 hr)
Hyperglycemia (plasma glucose >120 mg/dL or 7.7 mmol/L) in the absence of diabetes

INFLAMMATORY
Leukocytosis (WBC count >12,000/μL)
Leukopenia (WBC count <4000/μL)
Normal WBC count with >10% immature forms

ORGAN DYSFUNCTION
Arterial hypoxemia (PaO$_2$/FIO$_2$ >300)
Acute oliguria (urine output 0.5 mL/kg in 1 hr for at least 2 hr)
Creatinine increase of 0.5 mg/dL
Coagulation abnormalities (INR 1.5 or aPTT >60 sec)
Ileus (absent bowel sounds)
Thrombocytopenia (platelet count <100,000/μL)
Hyperbilirubinemia (plasma total bilirubin >4 mg/dL or 70 mmol/L)

TISSUE PERFUSION
Hyperlactatemia (>1 mmol/L)
Decreased capillary refill or mottling

INR, international normalized ratio; aPTT, activated partial thromboplastin time.
From Levy MM, Fink MP, Marshall JC, et al. 2001 SCCM/ESICM/ACCP/ATS/SIS International Sepsis Definitions Conference. Crit Care Med 2003;31:1250–6.

responsive to fluid resuscitation (Dellinger et al, 2008). A typical host response to infection involves localized containment and elimination of bacteria and repair of damaged tissue. This process is facilitated by macrophages and dendritic cells and orchestrated by CD4$^+$ T helper cells via the release of both proinflammatory and anti-inflammatory molecules (cytokines, chemokines, interferons). Sepsis occurs when a local infectious process becomes an uncontrolled systemic blood-borne inflammatory response resulting in damage to tissues or organs remote from the initial site of infection or injury. The extremes of the spectrum are lethal in one in four patients, and there are an estimated 750,000 cases (3 cases per 1000 population) of sepsis or septic shock in the United States each year (Rivers et al, 2001; Dellinger et al, 2008). Much like other medical emergencies, including polytrauma, acute myocardial infarction, and stroke, early recognition and appropriate treatment significantly influence outcome; these are commonly known as "the golden hours."

Definitions

- **Bacteremia:** the presence of viable bacteria in the blood
- **Systemic inflammatory response syndrome (SIRS):** a clinical syndrome characterized by the 2001 International Sepsis Definitions Conference (Levy et al, 2003) as extremes of body temperature, heart rate, ventilation, and immune response. **SIRS can occur in response to multiple insults, including systemic infection, trauma, thermal injury, or a sterile inflammation.**
- **Sepsis:** SIRS and infection either documented or strongly suspected
- **Severe sepsis:** sepsis plus sepsis-induced organ dysfunction or tissue hypoperfusion, typically systolic blood pressure (SBP)

less than 90 mm Hg or mean arterial pressure (MAP) less than 70 mm Hg
- **Septic shock:** an extreme form of sepsis with sepsis-induced hypotension persisting despite adequate fluid resuscitation; findings may include elevated lactic acid or oliguria

Pathophysiology

Initial studies of pathophysiologic features of septic shock concentrated on the interactions of lipopolysaccharides (LPS) from the gram-negative bacterial cell wall with various innate immune system pathways. More recent investigations now focus on understanding the activation and regulation of both the innate and acquired immune systems and the array of cytokines that are released during localized and systemic inflammatory responses.

Bacterial Cell Wall Components in Septic Shock

The exotoxins produced by some bacteria (e.g., exotoxin A produced by *P. aeruginosa*) can initiate septic shock. **However, the bacteria themselves, and in particular their cell wall components, are primarily responsible for the development of septic shock. These components activate numerous innate immunologic pathways, including macrophages, neutrophils, and dendritic cells and the complement system. The prime initiator of gram-negative bacterial septic shock is endotoxin, an LPS component of the bacterial outer membrane.** Endotoxin can directly activate the coagulation, complement, and fibrinolytic systems, leading to the release of small molecules that cause vasodilation and increased endothelial permeability (Tapper and Herwald, 2000).

Cytokine Network

Monocytic cells appear to have a pivotal role in mediation of the biologic effects of SIRS and septic shock. Monocytes can remove and detoxify LPS and be beneficial to the host. However, LPS-stimulated monocytes produce cytokines such as tumor necrosis factor (TNF) and interleukin (IL)-1. The intravascular activation of inflammatory systems involved in septic shock is mainly the consequence of an overproduction of these and other cytokines. Production of these cytokines is modulated by CD4$^+$ T helper cells. Type I CD4$^+$ T helper cells release proinflammatory cytokines including TNF-α, interferon-γ, and IL-2. These cytokines are also produced by macrophages, endothelial cells, and other cells stimulated by microbial products. The systemic release of large amounts of the cytokine TNF is associated with death from septic shock in humans (Waage et al, 1987; Calandra et al, 1988; Girardin et al, 1988). However, despite the fact that TNF is classically regarded as a central mediator of pathophysiologic changes associated with sepsis, the role of attenuation of this and other proinflammatory cytokines remains unclear. For example, in one animal model of peritonitis, survival was worsened by the administration of antibodies blocking TNF (Eskandari et al, 1992). Also, patients suffering from rheumatoid arthritis treated with TNF-α agents remain susceptible to the development of septic shock. Lastly, a meta-analysis of clinical trials utilizing anti-inflammatory agents in sepsis suggested these agents were generally harmful in all but a small subset of patients (Hotchkiss and Karl, 2003). More recently, anti-inflammatory cytokines, including IL-4 and IL-10, released by type II CD4$^+$ T helper cells, have also been noted to be elevated in sepsis, further illustrating the complex regulation of both proinflammatory and anti-inflammatory cytokines in a septic patient. In summary, both proinflammatory and anti-inflammatory cytokines are elements of early sepsis; however, the role of cytokine modulation in the treatment of sepsis remains unclear.

Clinical Presentation and Diagnosis

Early signs of systemic inflammatory response syndrome include temperature extremes (>38°C [100.4°F] or <36°C [96.8°F]), tachycardia (heart rate >90 beats/min), tachypnea, and altered

mental status. The classic bedside findings differentiating septic shock from other types of shock include a warm patient, brisk capillary refill, and a bounding pulse reflecting pyrexia, peripheral vasodilation, and decreased systemic vascular resistance. Other diagnostic criteria include evidence of organ dysfunction such as hypotension, oliguria, or ileus and laboratory abnormalities including leukocytosis or leukopenia, hyperbilirubinemia, hyperlactatemia, hyperglycemia, coagulation abnormalities, and elevated C-reactive protein and procalcitonin (see Box 12-9). The classic clinical presentation of fever and chills followed by hypotension is manifest only in about 30% of patients with gram-negative bacteremia (McClure, 1983). Even before temperature extremes and the onset of chills, bacteremic patients often begin to hyperventilate. Thus the **earliest metabolic change in septicemia is a resultant respiratory alkalosis.** In critically ill patients, the sudden onset of hyperventilation should lead to blood drawing for culture and careful evaluation of the patient. **Changes in mental status can also be important clinical clues.** Although the most common pattern is lethargy or obtundation, an occasional patient may become excited, agitated, or combative. Cutaneous manifestations such as the bull's-eye lesion associated with *P. aeruginosa* may be identified.

Metastatic infections secondary to genitourinary tract bacteremia have been described (Siroky et al, 1976). In this review of 137 patients who developed metastatic infections from bacteremia with a genitourinary source, 79% had undergone prior urologic instrumentation, 59% developed skeletal infections, mainly of the spine, and 29% developed endocarditis, most commonly caused by *E. faecalis.*

Bacteriology

In classic studies of sepsis syndrome and septic shock, gram-negative bacteria were predominant organisms isolated in 30% to 80% of cases and gram-positive bacteria in 5% to 24% (Ispahani et al, 1987; Calandra et al, 1988; Bone, 1991). Although *E. coli* is the most common organism causing gram-negative bacteremia, many nosocomial catheter-associated infections are caused by highly resistant gram-negative organisms: *P. aeruginosa, Proteus, Providencia,* and *Serratia. Acinetobacter* and *Enterobacter* are also emerging as important nosocomial pathogens. In a large series, *E. coli* caused about one third of the cases; the *Klebsiella-Enterobacter-Serratia* family, approximately 20%; and *Pseudomonas, Proteus, Providencia,* and anaerobic species, approximately 10% each (Kreger et al, 1980). Anaerobic organisms may cause bacteremia when the source is a postsurgical intra-abdominal abscess or transrectal prostatic biopsy. **More recent studies suggest the incidence of sepsis caused by both gram-positive bacterial and fungal organisms is increasing** (Martin et al, 2003) **and reinforce the need for initial broad-spectrum antimicrobial coverage.**

Management

The principles of management of sepsis include resuscitation, supportive care, monitoring, administration of broad-spectrum antimicrobial agents, and drainage or elimination of infection (Sessler et al, 2004; Dellinger et al, 2008). Although the identification and early intervention of sepsis by the urologist is important, the use of expert consultants is also recommended because management of sepsis and the critically ill patient is complex and always evolving. Early goal-directed therapy remains the standard approach since it was shown to be significantly beneficial in a 263-patient study by Rivers and colleagues in 2001.

Principles of resuscitation include support of the airway and breathing and optimization of perfusion with the use of invasive pressure monitoring with central access (Rivers et al, 2001). Intubation and mechanical ventilation may be required in patients who are obtunded and unable to protect their airway. Supplemental oxygen may be instituted, but supranormal oxygen delivery is no longer considered a goal of therapy (Dellinger et al, 2008). **Tissue perfusion should first be optimized** with fluid resuscitation to restore mean circulating filling pressures; this may include both crystalloid and or colloid/blood products. If additional blood pressure support is needed, vasoactive agents including phenylephrine, norepinephrine, vasopressin, and dopamine can be instituted; however, low-dose dopamine administration for renal protection is no longer recommended by critical care experts. Other principles of resuscitation and supportive care include optimization of oxygen delivery, correction of coagulopathies if clinically significant, maintenance of blood glucose levels below 110 mg/dL with intensive insulin therapy (Van den Berghe et al, 2001), and implementation of hemofiltration as needed (Schiffl et al, 2002). The use of hydrocortisone therapy in septic shock patients did not show a survival or disease-specific benefit in patients in a large study (Sprung et al, 2008).

Identification of the presumptive source of infection and cultures from corresponding fluids and blood should be obtained before the initiation of antimicrobial therapy. Multiple blood cultures for aerobic and anaerobic organisms should be obtained. In addition, all potential sources of bacteremia must be cultured (i.e., urine, sputum, and wounds). Careful attempts to identify the source of infection should be made because the choice of appropriate antimicrobial coverage depends on the organisms that are thought most likely to cause the infection. The severity of the underlying disease and the possibility of synergistic interactions are also important considerations. **If the urinary tract is the most likely portal of entry, a broad spectrum antimicrobial either alone or in combination with an aminoglycoside should be administered. Three clinical factors have been predictive of the subsequent isolation of a resistant pathogen: (1) the use of an antimicrobial drug in the last month, (2) advanced age, and (3) male sex** (Leibovici et al, 1992). If the infection is hospital acquired, or if the patient has had multiple infections or is immunocompromised or severely ill, an aminoglycoside and anti-*Pseudomonas* β-lactam or a third-generation cephalosporin should be used. When identification and drug susceptibilities of the offending organism are known, antimicrobial therapy should be changed to use the lowest cost, least toxic antimicrobial with the narrowest antimicrobial coverage. Antimicrobial treatment should be continued until the patient has been afebrile for 3 to 4 days and is clinically stable. Local infections that may have provided the focus for the bacteremia should be treated individually as appropriate. The surviving sepsis campaign suggests the initiation of broad-spectrum antibiotics within 1 hour of diagnosis of septic shock (Dellinger et al, 2008).

KEY POINTS: BACTEREMIA, SEPSIS, AND SEPTIC SHOCK

- Sepsis is a clinical syndrome characterized by extremes of body temperature, heart rate, respiratory rate, and WBC count that occurs in response to an infection.
- The principles of management of sepsis include resuscitation, supportive care, monitoring, administration of broad-spectrum antimicrobial agents, and drainage or elimination of infection.
- The surviving sepsis campaign and early goal-directed therapy has been shown to improve outcomes in critically ill patients.

BACTERIURIA IN PREGNANCY

Asymptomatic bacteriuria is one of the most common infectious issues encountered during pregnancy. The prevalence of asymptomatic bacteriuria does not change with the occurrence of pregnancy and ranges from 2% to 7% (Hooton et al, 2000). The risk of acquiring bacteriuria during pregnancy increases with lower socioeconomic class, multiparity, and sickle cell traits (Patterson and Andriole, 1987; Stenqvist et al, 1989).

The site of bacteriuria in pregnant female patients probably also reflects the situation before conception. In two studies that localized the origin of the bacteriuria, one using the Stamey ureteral catheterization technique and the other the Fairley bladder washout, upper tract infections were found in 44% and 24.5% of pregnant female patients, respectively (Fairley et al, 1966; Heineman and Lee, 1973). In nonpregnant females with recurrent bacteriuria, Stamey (1980) has reported about a 50% probability that the origin is in the upper tract. With other techniques, which may reflect the severity of tissue infection rather than the location of infection, the results are similar; approximately 50% of women with screening bacteriuria of pregnancy are fluorescent antibody-positive (Fa+) and thus have evidence of upper tract infection (Harris et al, 1976). Fairley and his group (1973) found that the site of infection is unrelated to the likelihood that pyelonephritis will develop during pregnancy.

Spontaneous resolution of bacteriuria in pregnant women is unlikely unless treated. Nonpregnant patients often clear their asymptomatic bacteriuria (Hooton et al, 2000), but pregnant women become symptomatic more frequently and tend to remain bacteriuric (Elder et al, 1971).

Pyelonephritis develops in 1% to 4% of all pregnant women (Sweet, 1977) and in 20% to 40% of pregnant women with untreated bacteriuria (Pedler and Bint, 1987; Wright et al, 1993). Of the women who develop pyelonephritis during pregnancy, 60% to 75% acquire it during the third trimester (Cunningham et al, 1973), when hydronephrosis and stasis in the urinary tract are most pronounced. From 10% to 20% of pregnant women who get pyelonephritis develop it again before or just after the delivery (Cunningham et al, 1973; Gilstrap et al, 1981). Moreover, a third of pregnant women who develop pyelonephritis have a documented prior history of pyelonephritis (Gilstrap et al, 1981).

The increased likelihood that bacteriuria may progress to acute pyelonephritis during pregnancy alters the morbidity of bacteriuria for this group. Treatment of screening bacteriuria of pregnancy decreases the incidence of acute pyelonephritis during pregnancy from a range of 13.5% to 65% to a range of 0% to 5.3% (Sweet, 1977).

Pathogenesis

The anatomic and physiologic changes induced by the gravid state significantly alter the natural history of bacteriuria (Patterson and Andriole, 1987). These changes may cause pregnant women to be more susceptible to pyelonephritis and may require alteration of therapy. These changes have been well summarized in several reviews (Davidson and Talner, 1978; Waltzer, 1981).

Anatomic and Physiologic Changes during Pregnancy
Increase in Renal Size

Renal length increases approximately 1 cm during normal pregnancy. It is thought that this does not represent true hypertrophy but is the result of increased renal vascular and interstitial volume. No histologic changes have been identified in renal biopsies (Waltzer, 1981).

Smooth Muscle Atony of the Collecting System and Bladder

The collecting system, especially the ureters, undergoes decreased peristalsis during pregnancy, and most women in their third trimester show significant ureteral dilatation (Davison and Lindheimer, 1978; Kincaid-Smith, 1978; Waltzer, 1981) (Fig. 12-37).

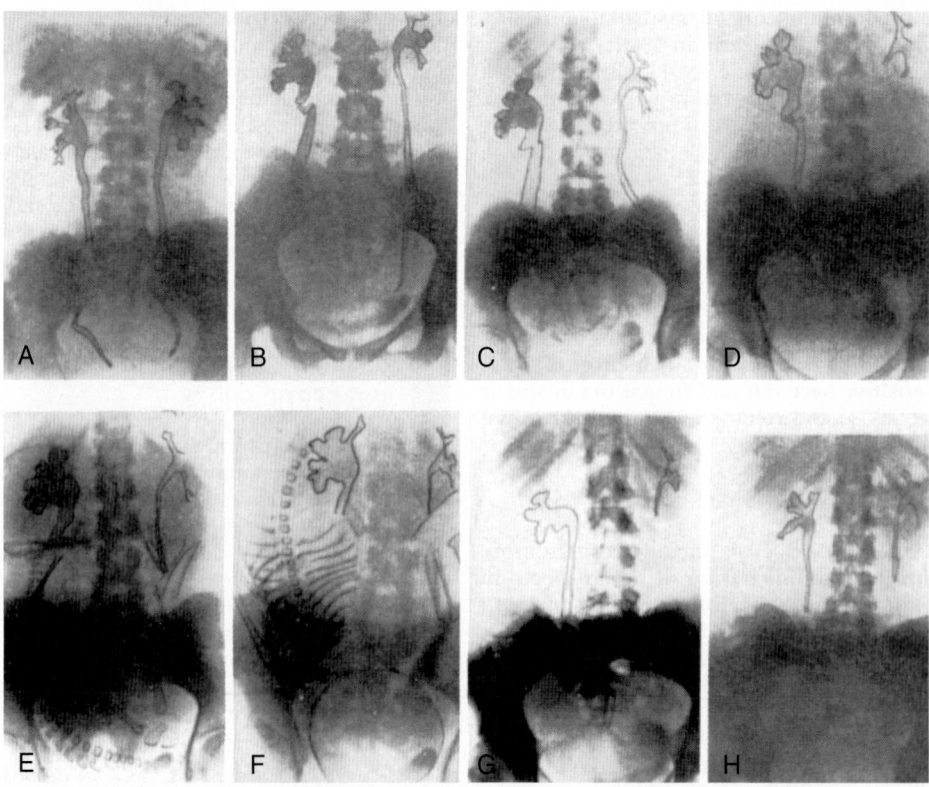

Figure 12-37. Progressive hydroureter and hydronephrosis observed on intravenous pyelogram during a normal pregnancy. A, 15 weeks; B, 18 weeks; C, 22 weeks; D, 26 weeks; E, 34 weeks; F, 39 weeks; G, 1 week postpartum; H, 6 weeks postpartum. Bilateral hydroureter and hydronephrosis are shown as early as 15 weeks (A). B to H, Successive urograms are from one patient during a normal pregnancy. Dilation occurs mainly on the right side, and both urinary tracts are normal by 6 weeks after delivery. (From Hundley JM, Walton HJ, Hibbits JT, et al. Physiologic changes occurring in the urinary tract during pregnancy. Am J Obstet Gynecol 1935;30:625–49.)

This hydroureter has been attributed both to the muscle-relaxing effects of increased progesterone during pregnancy and to mechanical obstruction of the ureters by the enlarging uterus at the pelvic brim. Progesterone-induced smooth muscle relaxation also may cause an increased bladder capacity (Waltzer, 1981). Later in pregnancy, the dilation may be the result of the obstructive effect of the enlarging uterus (Poole and Thorsen, 1999).

Bladder Changes

The enlarging uterus displaces the bladder superiorly and anteriorly. The bladder becomes hyperemic and may appear congested endoscopically (Waltzer, 1981). Estrogen stimulation probably causes bladder hypertrophy, as well as squamous changes of the urethra (Waltzer, 1981).

Augmented Renal Function

The transient increases in glomerular filtration rate and renal plasma flow during pregnancy have been well summarized by several authors and are probably secondary to the increase in cardiac output (Zacur and Mitch, 1977; Davison and Lindheimer, 1978; Kincaid-Smith, 1978; Waltzer, 1981). **Glomerular filtration increases by 30% to 50%, and urinary protein excretion increases. The significance of these physiologic changes is apparent when the normal serum creatinine and urea nitrogen values for pregnant women are surveyed** (Table 12-16). **Values considered normal in nonpregnant women may represent renal insufficiency during pregnancy.**

Davison and Lindheimer (1978) recommend that pregnant patients with serum creatinine levels greater than 0.8 mg/dL or urea nitrogen levels greater than 13 mg/dL undergo further evaluation of renal function. Similarly, **urinary protein in pregnancy is not considered abnormal until greater than 300 mg of protein in 24 hours is excreted.**

These significant physiologic changes in pregnancy, which may develop as early as the first trimester, lead to urinary stasis and mild hydroureteronephrosis and contribute to development of pyelonephritis.

Recent studies of *E. coli* adhesins and their respective specific tissue receptors have established an adhesin-based mechanism of pyelonephritis-induced preterm births and low birth weights in mice (Kaul et al, 1999). There is a higher incidence of *E. coli*–bearing Dr adhesins during the third trimester of pregnancy in women with gestational pyelonephritis (Nowicki et al, 1994) and an upregulation of Dr adhesin in the kidney, endometrium, and placenta during the third trimester of pregnancy (Martens et al, 1993). When infected intravesically with *E. coli*–bearing Dr adhesin, nearly 90% of mice that were hyporesponsive to bacterial lipopolysaccharide and had a deficient immune response delivered preterm, compared with 10% of mice infected with *E. coli* without Dr adhesin. Also, there was a significant reduction in fetal birth weight in the Dr adhesin–infected group. Bacterial tissue culture showed systemic spread of the *E. coli*–bearing Dr adhesins to the placentae and fetuses.

TABLE 12-16 Average Values for Serum Creatinine and Urea Nitrogen

	NONPREGNANT FEMALES (mg/dL)	PREGNANT FEMALES (mg/dL)
Serum creatinine	0.7	0.5
Urea nitrogen	13.0	9.0

Data from Davison JM, Lindheimer MD. Renal disease in pregnant women. Clin Obstet Gynecol 1978;21:411.

Complications Associated with Bacteriuria during Pregnancy

Prematurity and Prenatal Mortality

In the preantimicrobial era, pregnant women with symptomatic UTIs and bacterial pyelonephritis were reported to have a high incidence of prematurity, low birth weight, and death (Gilstrap et al, 1981). The relationship between asymptomatic bacteriuria and prematurity is less clear. Gilstrap and colleagues (1981) found no difference in pregnancy among patients treated for asymptomatic bacteriuria as compared with nonbacteriuric controls. However, Cunnington's review suggests that ascending GU tract infections may contribute to up to 50% of premature deliveries, especially before 30 weeks' gestation (Cunnington et al, 2013). **Because women with asymptomatic bacteriuria are at higher risk for developing a symptomatic UTI that results in adverse fetal sequelae, complications associated with bacteriuria during pregnancy and pyelonephritis and its possible sequelae such as sepsis in the mother, all women with asymptomatic bacteriuria should be treated** (Smaill, 2001).

Maternal Anemia

Although several studies suggest that bacteriuria untreated during pregnancy is associated with maternal anemia, not all studies support this. Some difficulties in interpreting the results of these surveys have been caused by inadequate documentation of bacteriuria. In one survey in which urine cultures were obtained by suprapubic aspiration, the data suggest that pregnant patients requiring three or more treatments for bacteriuria have lower levels of serum hemoglobin and folate than controls (McFadyen et al, 1973). In another study from England, investigators showed a statistically significant difference in the incidence of anemia between 410 bacteriuric pregnant women and 409 control pregnant women (Williams et al, 1973). In this survey, 14.6% of bacteriuric women and 10% of control women were anemic at the first prenatal visit. This separation increased during the third trimester (32 weeks), when 25% of women treated with placebo alone had anemia, but only 16.8% of those women treated with antimicrobial agents had anemia. Furthermore, in the 31 untreated (placebo-treated) bacteriuric women who subsequently developed pyelonephritis, the incidence of anemia was 45.2%. These investigators concluded that "untreated bacteriuria increases the likelihood of developing anemia during pregnancy and that this risk is enhanced by the development of acute pyelonephritis, even if it is treated promptly."

Laboratory Diagnosis

Significant false-negative rates occur if screening is conducted by urinalysis or reagent strip testing (McNair et al, 2000; Preston et al, 1999). **Therefore an initial screening culture should be performed in all pregnant women during the first trimester** (Stenqvist et al, 1989). If the culture shows no growth, repeat cultures are generally unnecessary because **patients who have no growth in their urine early in their pregnancy are unlikely to develop bacteriuria later** (Norden and Kass, 1968; McFadyen et al, 1973). Pregnant women with a history of recurrent UTI or vesicoureteral reflux may benefit from antimicrobial prophylaxis (Bukowski et al, 1998).

Management

Selection of an antimicrobial agent to treat the bacteriuria must be made, however, with special considerations given to maternal and fetal toxicity. The physiologic changes of pregnancy may decrease tissue and serum drug concentrations. Maternal expanded fluid volume, the distribution of the drug in the fetus, increased renal blood flow, and increased glomerular filtration decrease the serum drug concentration. **If the culture is positive, special consideration must be given to the selection of antimicrobial agents**

TABLE 12-17 Oral Antimicrobial Agents Used in Pregnancy

DRUG	DOSAGE	COMMENTS
AGENTS CONSIDERED SAFE		
Penicillins		
Ampicillin	500 mg qid	Extensively used
Amoxicillin	250 mg tid	Safe and effective
Penicillin V	500 mg qid	Used less frequently but achieves excellent urinary levels
Cephalosporins		
Cephalexin	500 mg qid	Extensively used
Cefaclor	500 mg qid	Somewhat more effective against gram-negative organisms
Nitrofurantoin	100 mg qid	May be used during the first two trimesters; may result in hemolytic anemia in patients with G6PD deficiency
AGENTS THAT SHOULD BE AVOIDED		
Fluoroquinolones		Possible damage to immature cartilage
Chloramphenicol		Associated with "gray baby" syndrome
Trimethoprim		May cause megaloblastic anemia because of anti–folic acid action
Erythromycin		Associated with maternal cholestatic jaundice
Tetracyclines		May cause acute liver decompensation in the mother and inhibition of new bone growth in the fetus

G6PD, glucose-6-phosphate dehydrogenase.
Modified from Schaeffer AJ. Urinary tract infections. In: Gillenwater JY, Grayhack JT, Howards SS, et al, editors. Adult and pediatric urology. Philadelphia: Lippincott Williams & Wilkins; 2002. p. 211–72.

chosen to treat infection to prevent fetal toxicity. **The pathogens are similar to those seen in nonpregnant women** (MacDonald et al, 1983). Table 12-17 lists the antimicrobial agents and dosing for use in pregnancy. The **aminopenicillins and cephalosporins are considered safe and generally effective throughout pregnancy. In patients with penicillin allergy, nitrofurantoin is a reasonable alternative. It may be used safely during the first two trimesters in patients without glucose-6-phosphate dehydrogenase deficiency.** Given the low efficacy of short-course β-lactam therapy in nonpregnant women, it is prudent to prescribe a full 3- to 7-day course of therapy in pregnant women. A recent Cochrane Review completed by Widmer and colleagues suggests that there is not adequate evidence at this time to suggest a single dose treatment to be noninferior to standard 7-day treatment (Widmer et al, 2011). Follow-up cultures should be obtained to document absence of infection. If the culture is positive, the cause of bacteriuria must be determined to be lack of resolution, bacterial persistence, or reinfection. If the infection is unresolved, proper selection and administration of another drug probably will solve the problem. If the problem is bacterial persistence or rapid reinfection, antimicrobial suppression of infection or prophylaxis (Pfau and Sacks, 1992) throughout the remainder of the pregnancy should be considered.

Pregnant women with acute pyelonephritis should be hospitalized and treated initially with parenteral antimicrobial agents. More than 95% of these patients respond within 24 hours using ampicillin and an aminoglycoside (Cunningham et al, 1973) or cephalosporins (Sanchez-Ramos et al, 1995). Appropriate oral agents should then be given for at least 14 days (Faro et al, 1984). After the treatment course is completed, low-dose prophylaxis with nitrofurantoin, amoxicillin, or cephalexin has been shown to be effective in preventing reinfection (Van Dorsten et al, 1987; Sandberg and Brorson, 1991). The efficacy of postcoital prophylaxis with either cephalexin (250 mg) or nitrofurantoin (50 mg) has been reported (Pfau and Sacks, 1992).

Drugs that are relatively contraindicated during pregnancy include the fluoroquinolones, TMP, chloramphenicol, erythromycin, tetracycline, sulfonamides, and sometimes nitrofurantoin (Nicolle, 1987). Fluoroquinolones are contraindicated because of their effects on immature cartilage. TMP may have teratogenic effects and should be avoided, especially in the first trimester. The "gray baby" syndrome is a toxic effect of chloramphenicol

on neonates resulting from the inability of the infant to metabolize or excrete the drug. Erythromycin may cause cholestatic jaundice in the mother. Tetracycline may cause fetal malformations and maternal liver decompensation. Sulfonamides may cause kernicterus and neonatal hyperbilirubinemia and should be avoided in the third trimester. As mentioned above, nitrofurantoin can cause hemolytic anemia in both mother and child when glucose-6-phosphate dehydrogenase deficiency is present (Nicolle, 1987).

Pregnancy in Women with Renal Insufficiency

With current management of recurrent UTIs, infections alone are no contraindication to pregnancy. In patients who have renal insufficiency with or without UTIs, Davison and Lindheimer (1978) emphasize that renal function should be carefully evaluated by both serum creatinine levels and creatinine clearance before a woman is counseled about conceiving or continuing a pregnancy. Although little is known about the outcome of pregnancies with differing degrees of renal insufficiency, it is known that **normal pregnancy is rare if the preconception serum creatinine level exceeds 3 mg/dL (about 30 mL/min clearance).**

The degree of renal function impairment is the major determinant for pregnancy outcome. **The fetal survivors of pregnant women with mild or moderate renal disease (serum creatinine <1.4 mg/dL and from 1.4 mg/dL to 2.4 to 2.8 mg/dL, respectively) is only slightly diminished, and irreversible deterioration of maternal renal function is uncommon.** However, the perinatal mortality is approximately four times higher with severe disease. The rate of perinatal morbidity caused by low birth weight or prematurity doubles from mild to moderate renal disease and again from moderate to severe disease (Vidaeff et al, 2008).

BACTERIURIA IN THE ELDERLY

UTIs in the elderly are a common and expanding health problem (Kaye, 1980). In 2003, there were almost 34 million Americans older than 65 years (U.S. Census Bureau, 2003). As the life expectancy increases, the diagnosis, treatment, morbidity, and mortality of UTIs in the elderly will assume increasing importance.

KEY POINTS: BACTERIURIA IN PREGNANCY

- Screening for bacteriuria with a culture should be performed in all pregnant women during the first trimester.
- The prevalence of bacteriuria does not change with the occurrence of pregnancy; however, unlike in nonpregnant women, spontaneous resolution of bacteriuria in pregnant women is unlikely.
- All pregnant women with bacteriuria should be treated.
- Bacteriuria more commonly progresses to acute pyelonephritis during pregnancy.
- Pyelonephritis develops in 1% to 4% of all pregnant women (Sweet, 1977) and in 20% to 40% of pregnant women with untreated bacteriuria.
- Pregnant women with acute pyelonephritis should be hospitalized and treated initially with parenteral antimicrobial agents.

Epidemiology

At least 20% of women and 10% of men older than 65 years have bacteriuria (Boscia and Kaye, 1987). In contrast to young adults, in whom bacteriuria is 30 times more prevalent in women than in men, the ratio in women to men with bacteriuria progressively decreases to 2 : 1. Most elderly patients with bacteriuria are asymptomatic; estimates among women living in nursing homes range from 17% to 55%, as compared with 15% to 31% for their male cohorts (Nicolle, 1994). The prevalence of bacteriuria in the elderly increases with age (Table 12-18) (Sourander, 1966; Brocklehurst et al, 1968) and concurrent disease (Fig. 12-38) and may exceed 50% in selective groups (Boscia and Kaye, 1987; Schaeffer, 1991). Risk factors can be compounded. In a study of 373 women and 150 men older than 68 years, 24% of functionally impaired nursing home residents had bacteriuria compared with 12% of healthy domiciliary subjects (Boscia et al, 1986). Longitudinal studies have clarified the dynamic aspect of bacteriuria in the elderly with frequent, spontaneous alteration between positive and negative urine cultures (Monane et al, 1995) (Fig. 12-39). There is only a small pool of elderly patients with persistent bacteriuria (Kaye, 1980). The incidence of asymptomatic bacteriuria is much more common than is apparent from a single survey, implying that most elderly will eventually have episodes of bacteriuria (Boscia et al, 1986).

Pathogenesis

The pathophysiology of increased susceptibility is multifactorial and poorly understood. **Age-related changes include decline** in cell-mediated immunity, neurogenic bladder dysfunction, increased perineal soiling as a result of fecal and urinary incontinence, increased incidence of urethral catheter placement, and, in women, changes in the vaginal environment associated with estrogen depletion (Schaeffer, 1991; Raz and Stamm, 1993). Increased receptivity of uroepithelial cells (Reid et al, 1984) and a decrease in prostatic and vaginal antimicrobial factors associated with changes in pH and levels of zinc and hormones have been observed (Boscia et al, 1986). Bacteriologic characteristics of infection in the elderly differ from those in younger patients (Baldassarre and Kaye, 1991). *E. coli* **remains the most common uropathogen, causing 75% of these infections.** There is a **significant increase in the incidence of** *Proteus, Klebsiella, Enterobacter, Serratia,* **and** *Pseudomonas* **species, as well as enterococci.** Bacteriuria caused by gram-positive bacteria is much more common in elderly men than in elderly women (Jackson et al, 1962). *S. saprophyticus* is not seen in this population. Polymicrobial bacteriuria is more common among the elderly (Nicolle et al, 1987). The shift in the pattern of uropathogens, the high frequency of polymicrobial infections, and antimicrobial resistance in UTIs in the elderly are due in large part to the high frequency of institutionalization and hospitalization, catheterization, and antimicrobial usage in this population (Fig. 12-40).

Laboratory Diagnosis

Diagnosis of bacteriuria and UTIs in the elderly can be difficult. **Urinary tract symptoms are often absent, and concomitant disease can mask or mimic UTI. Even severe upper tract infections may not be associated with fever or leukocytosis** (Baldassarre and Kaye, 1991). Therefore a high index of suspicion is warranted, and diagnosis should rely on the results of a carefully obtained urinalysis and culture. **The presence of greater than 10^5 cfu/mL of urine remains the standard for diagnosis** in these patients. However, **counts of 10^2 or more bacteria are clinically**

TABLE 12-18 Bacteriuria in Two Population Surveys

AGE (yr)	MEN (%)	WOMEN (%)
65-70	2-3	20-21
>80	21-22	23-50

Data from Brocklehurst JC, Dillane JB, Griffiths L, et al. Prevalence and symptomatology of urinary infection in an aged population. Gerontol Clin 1968;10:242–53; and Sourander LB. Urinary tract infections in the aged: an epidemiological study. Ann Med Intern Fenn 1966;55:7–55.

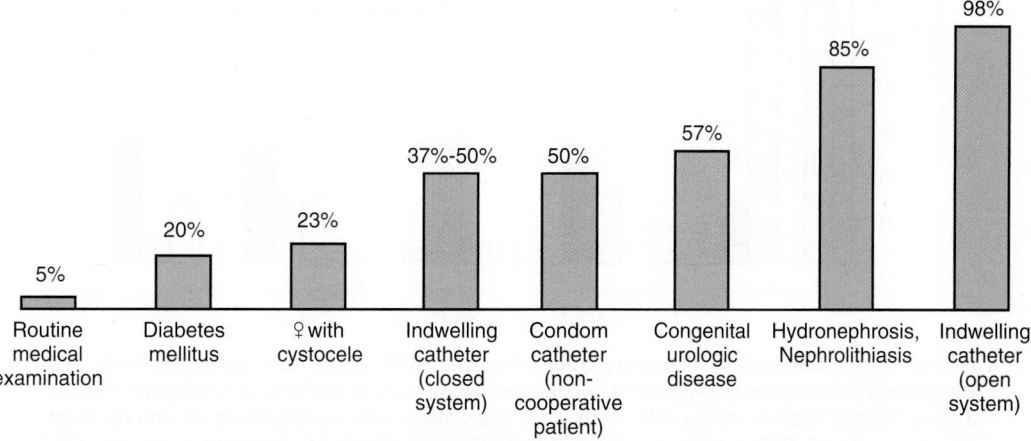

Figure 12-38. Frequency of significant bacteriuria related to underlying disease. (Modified from Jackson GG, Arana-Sialer JA, Andersen BR, et al. Profiles of pyelonephritis. Arch Intern Med 1962;110:63–75.)

significant in catheterized specimens (Kunin, 1987; Nicolle et al, 2005).

Pyuria alone is not a good predictor or an indication for antimicrobial treatment of bacteriuria in this population (Ouslander et al, 1996; Nicolle et al, 2005). Boscia and associates (1989) reported that more than 60% of women with pyuria of 10 WBCs/mm³ or greater (noted in midstream specimens) did not have a concurrent bacteriuria. However, **the absence of pyuria was a good predictor of the absence of bacteriuria.**

Because urinary tract abnormalities can often predispose and complicate bacteriuria in the elderly, a thorough urologic evaluation is warranted. Renal dysfunction, calculi, hydronephrosis, urinary retention, neurogenic bladder dysfunction, and other abnormalities should be identified by serum creatinine measurement, excretory urography, CT, ultrasonography, urodynamics, and/or cystoscopy. The timing and sequence of these tests should be dictated by the clinical setting.

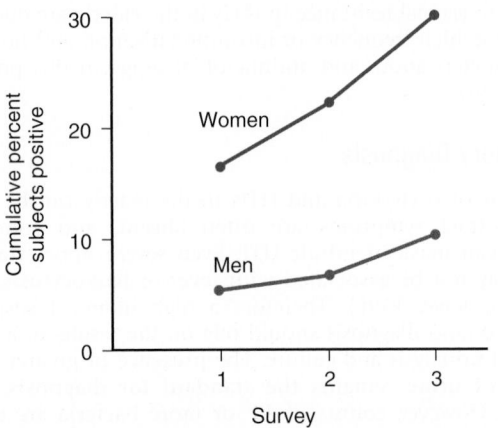

Figure 12-39. **Cumulative percentage of subjects (age = 65 years) with at least one positive urine culture survey result over three surveys performed at 6-month intervals. (From Boscia JA, Kobasa WD, Knight RA, et al. Epidemiology of bacteriuria in an elderly ambulatory population. Am J Med 1986;80:208–14.)**

Significance of Screening Bacteriuria

Screening for asymptomatic bacteriuria in elderly residents in the community or long-term care facilities is not recommended (Nicolle et al, 1983; Nordenstam et al, 1986; Boscia et al, 1987; Abrutyn et al, 1994). **There is no documented relationship between asymptomatic bacteriuria and uncomplicated UTIs and worsening renal function in this population. The treatment of asymptomatic bacteriuria to improve incontinence has not been justified** (Baldassarre and Kaye, 1991; Ouslander et al, 1995). Although studies have demonstrated decreased survival in bacteriuric patients compared with nonbacteriuric control subjects, it is unclear whether increased mortality rates and bacteriuria are causally related (Baldassarre and Kaye, 1991; Abrutyn et al, 1994).

Studies that have found a significantly increased mortality among persons with bacteriuria have looked at populations that were heterogeneous in terms of age and underlying disease (Dontas et al, 1981; Latham et al, 1985). An age difference of only 2 years increases mortality by 20% (Dontas et al, 1968). Therefore, in the studies mentioned previously (Dontas et al, 1968) and others (Abrutyn et al, 1994), it is not clear how much of the observed association between bacteriuria and mortality was due to differences in age between the bacteriuric and the abacteriuric groups. In a study of bacteriuria and mortality in a homogeneous 70-year-old population, the association between bacteriuria and mortality was weaker and linked to fatal diseases not attributable to bacteriuria (Dontas et al, 1968). Nicolle and associates (1987) randomized institutionalized women with bacteriuria to treatment or observation and followed these patients for more than 1 year. Treatment did not result in improved survival and was associated with a number of adverse effects.

Bacteriuria that leads to UTIs in elderly subjects in the presence of underlying structural urinary tract abnormalities (e.g., obstruction with hydronephrosis) or systemic conditions (e.g., severe diabetes mellitus) are clinically significant, can lead to renal failure, and require prompt therapy. In addition, UTIs caused by urea-splitting bacteria, such as *Proteus* or *Klebsiella* species that cause formation of infection stones, may also lead to severe renal damage.

Sepsis and its sequelae (sepsis syndrome and septic shock) are increasingly common in the elderly. This is in part due to the

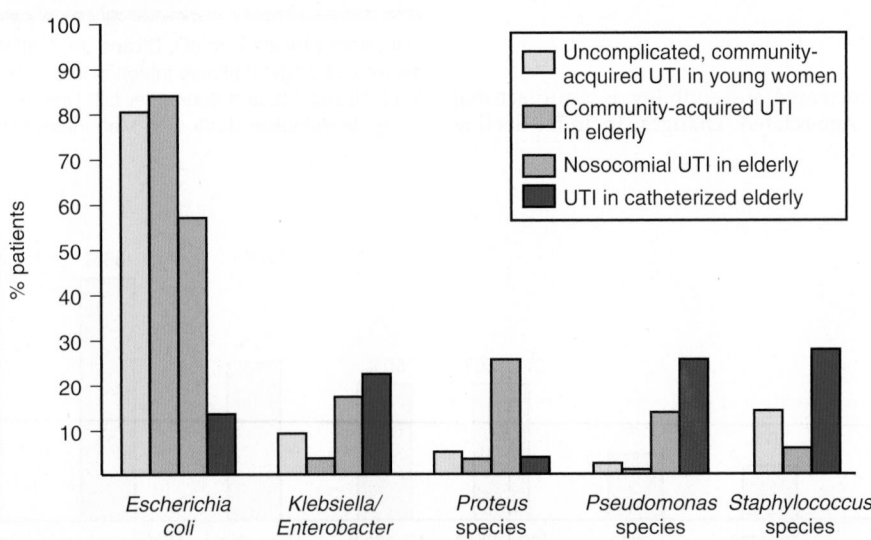

Figure 12-40. **Microbiology of urinary tract infections (UTI). (Data from Stark RP, Maki DG. Bacteriuria in the catheterized patient: what quantitative level of bacteriuria is relevant? N Engl J Med 1984;311:560–4; Kunin CM. Detection, prevention, and management of urinary tract infections. 4th ed. Philadelphia: Lea & Febiger, 1978, p xiii; Nicolle LE, Bjornson J, Harding GK, et al. Bacteriuria in elderly institutionalized men. N Engl J Med 1983;309:1420–5; and Krieger JN, Kaiser DL, Wenzel RP. Urinary tract etiology of bloodstream infections in hospitalized patients. J Infect Dis 1983;148:57–62.)**

aggressive use of catheters (Kunin et al, 1992) and other invasive equipment, implantation of prosthetic devices, and the administration of chemotherapy to cancer patients or corticosteroids in other immunosuppressed patients with organ transplants or inflammatory diseases. In addition, modern medical care has given longer life spans to the elderly and patients with metabolic, neoplastic, or immunodeficiency disorders, who remain at increased risk for infection.

Management

Prospective randomized comparative trials of antimicrobial or no therapy in elderly male and female nursing home residents with asymptomatic bacteriuria consistently document no benefit of antimicrobial therapy. There was no decrease in symptomatic episodes and no improvement in survival. In fact, treatment with antimicrobial therapy increases the occurrence of adverse drug effects and reinfection with resistant organisms and increases the cost of treatment. **Therefore asymptomatic bacteriuria in elderly residents of long-term care facilities should not be treated with antimicrobial agents.**

If patients present with lower tract symptoms, 7 days of therapy is recommended. For individuals presenting with fever or more severe systemic infection 10 to 14 days of therapy is recommended. The goal in this population is to eliminate symptoms but not sterilize the urine (McMurdo and Gillespie, 2000).

The 10% to 15% decrease in susceptibility of uropathogens to β-lactams, TMP-SMX, and fluoroquinolones in isolates from nursing home residents is disturbing and most likely due to a pattern of empirical prescribing in the nursing homes. In contrast, the susceptibility of isolates from patients with acute uncomplicated UTI in an outpatient setting has not changed appreciably in 10 years. The difference in susceptibility between the isolates from the outpatient and nursing home settings can be attributed to the presence of additional risk factors for antimicrobial resistance in the latter group. These risk factors include frequent antimicrobial usage, overcrowding, underlying pathology, and the presence of catheters and other invasive devices. Antimicrobial use needs to be guided by current surveillance studies of targeted uropathogenic bacteria and implemented (Vromen et al, 1999).

The elderly population is more susceptible than young patients to the toxic and adverse effects of antimicrobial agents (Grieco, 1980; Carty et al, 1981; Boscia et al, 1986) because the metabolism and excretion of antimicrobial agents may be impaired, and the resulting increased serum levels can further damage renal function. Interactions with other medications can occur (Stahlmann and Lode, 2003). The safety margin between therapeutic and toxic doses is significantly narrowed. Therefore antimicrobial agents must be used judiciously, and dosing and drug levels should be carefully monitored.

The fluoroquinolones are effective in this population, and the side effects are not more apparent than in a younger population. However, fluoroquinolones can cause QT interval prolongation, and therefore they should be avoided in patients with known prolongation of the QT interval, patients with uncorrected hypokalemia or hypomagnesemia, and patients receiving some antiarrhythmic agents (Stahlmann and Lode, 2003).

Chondrotoxicity of fluoroquinolones has led to restricted use in pediatric patients, but there is no indication that similar effects could occur in joint cartilage of adults. Tendinitis and tendon ruptures have occurred in rare cases. Chronic renal diseases, concomitant use of corticosteroids, and age older than 60 years have been recognized as risk factors for fluoroquinolone-induced tendon disorders (Stahlmann and Lode, 2003).

CATHETER-ASSOCIATED BACTERIURIA

Catheter-associated bacteriuria is the most common hospital-acquired infection, accounting for up to 40% of such infections and more than 1 million per year (Haley et al, 1985; Stamm,

---

KEY POINTS: BACTERIURIA IN THE ELDERLY

- Bacteriuria is very common in both elderly women and men.
- Screening for bacteriuria is not recommended in elderly patients because there is no relationship between asymptomatic bacteriuria and uncomplicated UTIs and deteriorating renal function; asymptomatic bacteriuria should not be treated.
- Infections of the urinary tract may present as subtle signs, and a high index of suspicion is often required for diagnosis.
- Treatment of symptomatic UTI requires modifications for physiologic and pathophysiologic conditions of the elderly.

1991). **The development of bacteriuria in the presence of an indwelling catheter is inevitable and occurs at an incidence of approximately 10% per day of catheterization. Sterile and clean intermittent catheterization has been associated with rates of bacteriuria ranging from 1% to 3% per catheterization** (Warren, 1997). **The most important risk factors associated with increased likelihood of developing catheter-associated bacteriuria are duration of catheterization, female gender, absence of systemic antimicrobial agents, and catheter-care violations** (Stamm, 1991). **Most catheter-associated UTIs are asymptomatic.** In patients with short-term catheter placement, only 10% to 30% of bacteriuric episodes produce typical symptoms of acute infection (Haley et al, 1981; Hartstein et al, 1981). Similarly, although patients with long-term catheters are bacteriuric, the incidence of febrile episodes occurs at a rate of only 1 per 100 days of catheterization (Warren, 1991). The **financial impact** of community-acquired UTIs is nearly $1.6 billion in the United States alone (Foxman, 2002); the annual cost of nosocomial UTIs has been estimated to range from between $515 million and $548 million (Jarvis, 1996). Each catheter-associated urinary tract infection (CAUTI) is estimated to cost between $589 and $758 (Tambyah et al 2002; Anderson et al 2007). In patients requiring intensive care, the cost is roughly $2,000 per nosocomial UTI (Chen et al, 2009). The nosocomial costs for *E. coli* infections with relatively susceptible strains are considerably lower than for those caused by resistant gram-negative bacteria, which often require expensive parenteral antimicrobial therapy (Tambyah et al, 2002). Recently, the Center for Medicare and Medicaid Services (CMS) announced that it will no longer reimburse hospitals for the extra costs resulting from catheter-associated UTIs.

Pathogenesis

Bacteria enter the urinary tract of a catheterized patient by several routes. **Bacteria can be introduced at the time of initial catheter placement** by either mechanical inoculation of urethral bacteria or contamination from poor technique. **Subsequently, the bacteria most commonly gain access via a periurethral or intraluminal route** (Stamm, 1991). In women, periurethral entry is the most prevalent. Daifuku and Stamm (1984) found that among 18 women who developed catheter-associated bacteriuria, 12 had antecedent urethral colonization with the infecting strain. **Bacteria may also enter the drainage bag and follow the intraluminal route to the bladder.** This route is particularly common in patients who are clustered among other patients with indwelling catheters (Maizels and Schaeffer, 1980; Tambyah et al, 1999).

The urinary catheter system provides a unique environment that allows for two distinct populations of bacteria: those that grow within the urine and another population that grows on the catheter surface. A biofilm represents a microbial environment of bacteria embedded in an extracellular matrix of bacterial products and host proteins that often lead to catheter encrustation (Stamm, 1991; Bonadio et al, 2001). Certain bacteria, particularly of the *Pseudomonas* and *Proteus* species, are adept at biofilm growth, which may explain their higher incidence in this clinical setting (Mobley and Warren, 1987). The uropathogens isolated from the catheterized urinary tract often differ from those found in noncatheterized ambulatory patients. *E. coli* is still the most common organism isolated, but *Pseudomonas*, *Proteus*, and *Enterococcus* species are very prevalent (Warren, 1991). In patients with long-term catheterization of more than 30 days, the bacteriuria is usually polymicrobial and the presence of four or five pathogens is not uncommon (Warren et al, 1982). Although certain species may persist for long periods, the bacterial populations in these patients tend to be dynamic.

Clinical Presentation

Most patients are asymptomatic. Suprapubic discomfort and development of fever, chills, or flank pain may indicate a symptomatic UTI.

Laboratory Diagnosis

Significant bacteriuria in patients with catheters is present when greater than 100 cfu/mL is present because even this low level progresses to greater than 10^5 cfu/mL in almost all patients (Maizels and Schaeffer, 1980; Stark and Maki, 1984). Pyuria is not a discriminate indicator of infection in this population.

Management

Careful aseptic insertion of the catheter and maintenance of a closed dependent drainage system are essential to minimize development of bacteriuria. The catheter-meatal junction should be cleaned daily with water, but antimicrobial agents should be avoided because they lead to colonization with resistant pathogens, such as *Pseudomonas*.

Incorporation of silver oxide (Schaeffer et al, 1988) or silver alloy (Saint et al, 1998) into the catheter and hydrogen peroxide into the drainage bag has been reported to decrease the incidence of bacteriuria in some studies (Schaeffer et al, 1988) but not in other populations (Stamm, 1991). **The major benefit of silver alloy is in decreasing the likelihood of bacteriuria in hospitalized adults catheterized for the short-term** (Saint et al, 2000; Newton et al, 2002; Brosnahan et al, 2004). If an asymptomatic catheterized patient has had an indwelling catheter for 3 or more days and will have the catheter removed, a dipstick test can be used to rule out bacteriuria (Tissot et al, 2001). **Concurrent administration of systemic antimicrobial agents transiently decreases the incidence of bacteriuria associated with short-term catheterization, but after 3 to 4 days the incidence of bacteriuria is similar to the rate in catheterized patients not taking systemic antimicrobials agents, and the prevalence of resistant bacteria and side effects is substantial.** The concept of instilling nonvirulent bacteria into the bladder to completely block colonization and infection by pathogens has been tested in patients with spinal cord injuries (Hull et al, 2000). Patients successfully colonized with the nonvirulent strain had reduced symptomatic UTI and a subjective improvement in quality of life.

Patients with indwelling catheters should be treated only if they become symptomatic (e.g., febrile). Urine cultures should be performed before initiating antimicrobial therapy. The antimicrobial agent should be discontinued within 48 hours of resolution of the infection. If the catheter has been indwelling for several weeks, encrustation may shelter bacteria from the antimicrobial agent; therefore the catheter should be changed.

When a catheter is to be removed and there is a high probability of bacteriuria or the dipstick test is positive, a culture should be obtained 24 hours before removal (Tissot et al, 2001). **If the probability is low or the dipstick is negative, a culture may not be necessary. The patient should be started on empirical antimicrobial therapy such as TMP-SMX or a fluoroquinolone just before decatheterization and maintained on therapy for 2 days. A post-therapy culture should be obtained 7 to 10 days later to confirm the eradication of the bacteriuria.**

KEY POINTS: CATHETER-ASSOCIATED BACTERIURIA

- Careful aseptic insertion of the catheter and maintenance of a closed, dependent drainage system are essential to minimize development of bacteriuria.
- The development of catheter-associated bacteriuria is inevitable.
- If an infection is suspected in a catheterized patient, a culture should be obtained and antimicrobial therapy initiated before decatheterization.
- Only symptomatic catheter-associated UTIs require treatment.
- Antimicrobial therapy should be continued for 2 to 3 days and a post-therapy culture obtained 7 to 10 days later.

MANAGEMENT OF URINARY TRACT INFECTIONS IN PATIENTS WITH SPINAL CORD INJURY

Patients with spinal cord injury have unique concerns that affect the risk, diagnosis, and management of UTIs, which are all considered complicated.

Epidemiology

UTIs are among the most common urologic complications of spinal cord injury. It has been estimated that approximately 33% of spinal cord–injured patients have bacteriuria at any time (Stover et al, 1989) and that eventually almost all spinal cord–injured patients will become bacteriuric and many will suffer significant morbidity and mortality. One prospective study of patients on intermittent catheterization or condom catheterization reported an incidence of significant bacteriuria of 18 episodes per person per year and an annual incidence of febrile UTIs of 1.8 per person per year (Waites et al, 1993a). In addition, **UTI is the most common cause of fever in the spinal cord–injured patient** (Beraldo et al, 1993). **The 1992 National Institute on Disability and Rehabilitation Research Consensus Conference examined the problems associated with UTIs in spinal cord–injured patients** (National Institute on Disability and Rehabilitation Research, 1993). **Among the risk factors identified were impaired voiding, overdistention of the bladder, elevated intravesical pressure, increased risk of urinary obstruction, vesicoureteral reflux, instrumentation, and increased incidence of stones.** Other factors that have been implicated are decreased fluid intake, poor hygiene, perineal colonization, decubiti, and other evidence of local tissue trauma, and reduced host defense associated with chronic illness (Gilmore et al, 1992; Waites et al, 1993a).

Pathogenesis

The method of bladder management has profound impact on UTI. The National Institute on Disability and Rehabilitation Research Consensus Conference noted that indwelling catheters were most likely to lead to UTI and that the vast majority of patients with an indwelling catheter for 30 days are bacteriuric (National Institute on Disability and Rehabilitation Research, 1993). Suprapubic catheters and indwelling urethral catheters eventually have an equivalent infection rate (Kunin et al, 1987; Tambyah and Maki, 2000; Biering-Sorensen, 2002). However, the onset of bacteriuria may be delayed using a suprapubic catheter compared with a urethral catheter. During a 2-year period, 170 patients with spinal cord injury were evaluated regarding type of urinary drainage and infection (Warren et al, 1982). In patients using indwelling urethral catheters, all urine cultures were positive. The corresponding values for the suprapubic catheter group were 44%. Condom drainage systems are also associated with an incidence of bacteriuria from 63% (Dukes, 1928) to almost 100% (Pyrah et al, 1955).

Since its introduction by Lapides and colleagues (1972), clean (but not sterile) intermittent catheterization (CIC) has earned general recognition in the management of spinal cord injury patients (National Institute on Disability and Rehabilitation Research, 1993). **Although never rigorously compared with indwelling urethral catheterization, CIC has been shown to decrease lower tract complications by maintaining low intravesical pressure and reducing the incidence of stones** (Stover et al, 1989). CIC also appears to reduce complications associated with an indwelling catheter, such as UTI, fever, bacteremia, and local infections such as epididymitis and prostatitis. Weld and Dmochowski (2000) followed 316 patients with spinal cord injury with different bladder management for a mean of 18.3 years and recorded all complications. The CIC group had statistically significantly lower complication rates compared with the urethral catheterization group and no significantly higher complication rates relative to all other management methods for each type of complication studied. Thus it is generally agreed that **CIC places patients with spinal cord injury at the lowest risk for significant long-term urinary tract complications** (Stamm, 1975).

There is conflicting evidence over the value of sterile versus nonsterile or "no touch" methods of CIC. Some studies have reported a lower incidence of infection in patients treated with sterile techniques (Foley, 1929), whereas others have not (Pyrah et al, 1955; Nyren et al, 1981). Bennett and coworkers (1997) reported on a sterile method of CIC that uses an introducer tip to bypass the distal 1.5 cm of the urethra and showed a significant decrease in UTI with the use of the urethral introducer tip. Different types of catheters have been used for CIC. The low-friction catheters might be less traumatic for the urethra (Casewell and Phillips, 1977; Garibaldi et al, 1980), but their impact on bacteriuria and UTI has to be studied.

Clinical Presentation

The majority of patients with spinal cord injury with bacteriuria are asymptomatic. Because of a loss of sensation, patients usually do not experience frequency, urgency, or dysuria. More often, they complain of flank, back, or abdominal discomfort, leakage between catheterizations, increased spasticity, malaise, lethargy, and/or cloudy, malodorous urine. UTI is the most common cause of fever in spinal cord–injured patients (Beraldo et al, 1993).

Bacteriology and Laboratory Diagnosis

Urinalysis will show bacteriuria and pyuria. Pyuria is not diagnostic of infections because it may occur from the irritative effects of the catheter. The National Institute on Disability and Rehabilitation Research Consensus Statement recommended the following criteria for the diagnosis of significant bacteriuria in spinal cord–injured patients (National Institute on Disability and Rehabilitation Research, 1993). Any detectable bacteria from indwelling or suprapubic catheter aspirates was considered significant because the vast majority of patients with an indwelling catheter and low-level bacteriuria showed an increase to greater than 10^5 cfu/mL within a short period of time (Cardenas and Hooton, 1995). For patients on CIC, greater than or equal to 10^2 cfu/mL was considered significant. For catheter-free males, a clean voided specimen showing greater than or equal to 10^4 cfu/mL was considered significant.

Bacteriuria in patients with spinal cord injury differs from that in patients with intact spinal cords in its etiology, complexity, and antimicrobial susceptibility and is influenced by the type and duration of catheterization. E. coli is isolated in approximately 20% of patients. Enterococci, P. mirabilis, and Pseudomonas are more common among spinal cord–injured patients than patients with intact spinal cords. Other common organisms are Klebsiella species, Serratia species, Staphylococcus, and Candida species. Most bacteriuria in short-term catheterization is of a single organism, whereas patients catheterized for longer than a month will usually demonstrate a polymicrobial flora caused by a wide range of gram-negative and gram-positive bacterial species (Edwards et al, 1983). Such specimens commonly have two to four bacterial species, each at concentrations of 10^5 cfu/mL or more (Monson and Kunin, 1974; Nickel et al, 1987). Some may have up to six to eight species at that concentration (Monson and Kunin, 1974). This phenomenon is due to an incidence of new episodes of bacteriuria approximately every 2 weeks and the ability of these strains to persist for weeks and months in the catheterized urinary tract (Edwards et al, 1983; Gabriel et al, 1996). Two of the most persistent species are E. coli and Providencia stuartii. P. stuartii is rarely found outside the long-term catheterized urinary tract and may use the catheter itself as a niche (Lindberg et al, 1975; Hockstra, 1999).

Management

Because of the diverse flora and high probability of bacterial resistance, a urine culture must be obtained before initiating empirical therapy. For afebrile patients, an oral fluoroquinolone is the agent of choice (Cardenas and Hooton, 1995). β-Lactams, TMP-SMX, and nitrofurantoin are not recommended because of the high prevalence of bacterial resistance to these drugs. An indwelling catheter should be changed to ensure maximal drainage and eliminate bacterial foci in catheter encrustations. **Spinal cord–injured patients with fever or chills are usually admitted and treated with a parenteral aminoglycoside and a penicillin or a third-generation cephalosporin** (Cardenas and Hooton, 1995). In this patient population consultation with a physician with expertise in antimicrobial management may be necessary, especially in a patient with recurrent infections.

If clinical improvement does not occur within 24 to 48 hours, reculture and adjustment of antimicrobial therapy based on the initial culture and susceptibility should be performed. Imaging studies should be obtained to rule out obstruction, stones, and abscess. The duration of therapy is not established, but 4 to 5 days is recommended for the mildly symptomatic patient and 10 to 14 days for sicker patients (Cardenas and Hooton, 1995). Post-therapy cultures are usually not necessary because asymptomatic recolonization is common and not clinically significant. However, if a urea-splitting bacterium is identified, a follow-up culture should be obtained to ensure its eradication. Spinal cord–injured patients with recurrent symptomatic UTIs should undergo urinary tract imaging and urodynamic testing and a review of their bladder management program with particular attention to catheter drainage, intermittent catheterization techniques, and frequency of intermittent catheterization or voiding schedule (Cardenas and Hooton, 1995).

Antimicrobial prophylaxis is not supported for most patients who have neurogenic bladder caused by spinal cord injury (Morton et al, 2002). Antimicrobial prophylaxis did not significantly decrease symptomatic UTIs and resulted in an approximately twofold increase in antimicrobial-resistant bacteria.

Recurrent UTIs may be associated with high storage pressures, and intervention to decrease storage pressure may decrease the incidence of symptomatic UTI. Evidence from studies in spinal cord–injured patients suggests that bladder catheterization for longer than 10 years is associated with an increased risk of carcinoma of the bladder. West and colleagues (1999) examined two databases with more than 33,000 spinal cord–injured patients and identified 130 patients with bladder cancer (0.4%) during a 5-year period. Several risk factors for bladder cancer have been proposed. Vereczky and associates (cited in Weyrauch and Bassett, 1951) tested different risk factors based on the outcome of 153 spinal cord–injured patients in which 7 were diagnosed with bladder cancer. Of a total of 31 possible predictors, only duration of catheterization was significant. **Chronic infection and inflammation of the bladder mucosa could be the carcinogenic stimulus in these patients** (Pyrah et al, 1955). **Nitrosamines produced in infected urine have also been implicated** (Najenson et al, 1969).

For further discussion of spinal cord injury and urinary infection, see Chapter 75.

OTHER INFECTIONS

Fournier Gangrene

Fournier gangrene is a potentially life-threatening form of necrotizing fasciitis involving the male genitalia. It is also known as idiopathic gangrene of the scrotum, streptococcal scrotal gangrene, perineal phlegmon, and spontaneous fulminant gangrene of the scrotum (Fournier, 1883, 1884). As originally reported by Baurienne in 1764, and by Fournier in 1883, it was characterized by an abrupt onset of a rapidly fulminating genital gangrene of idiopathic origin in previously healthy young patients that resulted in gangrenous destruction of the genitalia. The disease now differs from these descriptions in that it involves a broader age range, including older patients (Bejanga, 1979; Wolach et al, 1989), follows a more indolent course, and has a less abrupt onset; and, in approximately 95% of the cases, a source can now be identified (Macrea, 1945; Burpee and Edwards, 1972; Kearney and Carling, 1983; Jamieson et al, 1984; Spirnak et al, 1984).

Infection most commonly arises from the skin, urethra, or rectal regions. An association between urethral obstruction associated with strictures and extravasation and instrumentation has been well documented. **Predisposing factors include diabetes mellitus, local trauma, paraphimosis, periurethral extravasation or urine, perirectal or perianal infections, and surgery such as circumcision or herniorrhaphy. In cases originating in the genitalia, specifically as a result of urethral obstruction, the infecting bacteria probably pass through Buck fascia of the penis and spread along the dartos fascia of the scrotum and penis, Colles fascia of the perineum, and Scarpa fascia of the anterior abdominal wall.** In view of the typical foul odor associated with this condition, a major role for anaerobic bacteria is likely. **Wound cultures generally yield multiple organisms, implicating anaerobic-aerobic synergy** (Meleney, 1933; Miller, 1983; Cohen, 1986). Mixed cultures containing facultative organisms (*E. coli*, *Klebsiella*, enterococci) along with anaerobes (*Bacteroides*, *Fusobacterium*, *Clostridium*, microaerophilic streptococci) have been obtained from the lesions.

Clinical Presentation

Patients frequently have a history of recent perineal trauma, instrumentation, urethral stricture associated with sexually transmitted disease, or urethral cutaneous fistula. Pain, rectal bleeding, and a history of anal fissures suggest a rectal source of infection. Dermal sources are suggested by history of acute and chronic infections of the scrotum and spreading recurrent hidradenitis suppurativa or balanitis.

The infection commonly starts as cellulitis adjacent to the portal of entry. Early on, the involved area is swollen, erythematous, and tender as the infection begins to involve the deep fascia. **Pain is prominent, and fever and systemic toxicity are marked** (Paty and Smith, 1992). The swelling and crepitus of the scrotum quickly increase, and dark purple areas develop and progress to extensive gangrene. If the abdominal wall becomes involved in an obese patient with diabetes, the process can spread very rapidly. Specific genitourinary symptoms associated with the condition include dysuria, urethral discharge, and obstructed voiding. Alterations in mental status, tachypnea, tachycardia, and temperature greater than 38.3°C (101°F) or less than 35.6°C (96°F) suggest gram-negative sepsis.

Laboratory Diagnosis and Radiologic Findings

Anemia occurs secondary to a decreased functioning erythrocyte mass caused by thrombosis and ecchymosis coupled with decreased production secondary to sepsis (Miller, 1983). Elevated serum creatinine levels, hyponatremia, and hypocalcemia are common. Hypocalcemia is believed to be secondary to bacterial lipases that destroy triglycerides and release free fatty acids that chelate calcium in its ionized form.

Because crepitus is often an early finding, a plain film of the abdomen may be helpful in identifying air. Scrotal ultrasonography is also useful in this regard. Biopsy of the base of an ulcer is characterized by superficially intact epidermis, dermal necrosis, and vascular thrombosis and polymorphonuclear leukocyte invasion with subcutaneous tissue necrosis. Stamenkovic and Lew (1984) noted that the use of frozen sections within 21 hours after the onset of symptoms could confirm a diagnosis earlier and lead to early institution of appropriate treatment.

Management

Prompt diagnosis is critical because of the rapidity with which the process can progress. The clinical differentiation of necrotizing fasciitis from cellulitis may be difficult because the initial signs including pain, edema, and erythema are not distinctive. However, **the presence of marked systemic toxicity out of proportion to the local finding should alert the clinician.** Intravenous hydration and antimicrobial therapy are indicated in preparation for surgical debridement. Antimicrobial regimens include broad-spectrum antibiotics (β-lactam plus β-lactamase inhibitor) such as piperacillin-tazobactam, especially if *Pseudomonas* is suspected, ampicillin plus sulbactam, or vancomycin or carbapenems plus clindamycin or metronidazole (Morpurgo and Galandiuk, 2002).

Immediate debridement is essential. In the patient in whom diagnosis is clearly suspected on clinical grounds (deep pain with patchy areas of surface hypoesthesia or crepitation, or bullae and skin necrosis), direct operative intervention is indicated. **Extensive incision should be made through the skin and subcutaneous tissues, going beyond the areas of involvement until normal fascia is found. Necrotic fat and fascia should be excised, and the wound should be left open. A second procedure 24 to 48 hours later is indicated if there is any question about the adequacy of initial debridement. Orchiectomy is almost never required,** because the testes have their own blood supply independent of the compromised fascial and cutaneous circulation to the scrotum. **Suprapubic diversion should be performed in cases in which urethral trauma or extravasation is suspected. Colostomy should be performed if there is colonic or rectal perforation.** Hyperbaric oxygen therapy has shown some promise in shortening hospital stays, increasing wound healing, and decreasing the gangrenous spread when used in conjunction with debridement and antimicrobials (Paty and Smith, 1992). Once wound healing is complete, reconstruction (e.g., using myocutaneous flaps) improves cosmetic results.

Outcome

The mortality rate averages approximately 20% (Cohen, 1986; Baskin et al, 1990; Clayton et al, 1990) but ranges from 7% to 75%.

Higher mortality rates are found in diabetics, alcoholics, and those with colorectal sources of infection who often have a less typical presentation, greater delay in diagnosis, and more widespread extension. Regardless of the presentation, **Fournier gangrene is a true urologic emergency that demands early recognition, aggressive treatment with antimicrobial agents, and surgical debridement to reduce morbidity and mortality.**

Periurethral Abscess

Periurethral abscess is a life-threatening infection of the male urethra and periurethral tissues. Initially, the area of involvement can be small and localized by Buck fascia. However, when Buck fascia is penetrated, there can be extensive necrosis of the subcutaneous tissue and fascia. Fasciitis can spread as far as the buttocks posteriorly and the clavicle superiorly. Rapid diagnosis and treatment are essential to reduce the morbidity and high mortality historically associated with this disease.

Pathogenesis

Periurethral abscess is frequently a sequela of gonorrhea, urethral stricture disease, or urethral catheterization. Frequent instrumentation is also associated with periurethral abscess formation. The source of the infecting organism is the urine. Gram-negative rods, enterococci, and anaerobes are most frequently identified. The presence of multiple organisms is common. Anaerobes, normal residents of the male urethra, are also frequently found in wound cultures.

Clinical Presentation

Presenting signs and symptoms include scrotal swelling in 94% of patients, fever (70%), acute urinary retention (19%), spontaneously drained abscess (11%), and dysuria or urethral discharge (5% to 8%). The average interval between initial symptoms and presentation is 21 days. Urinalysis of the first glass specimen reveals pyuria and bacteriuria.

Management

Treatment consists of immediate suprapubic urinary drainage and wide debridement. Antimicrobial therapy with an aminoglycoside and a cephalosporin is usually adequate for empirical coverage. More selective antimicrobial therapy can be instituted when the antimicrobial susceptibility of the organisms is available. Perineal urethrostomy or chronic suprapubic diversion occasionally has been helpful to prevent recurrences, and it should be considered in patients with diffuse stricture disease. The presence of a malignancy is unusual, but biopsy is important.

KEY POINTS: OTHER INFECTIONS

- Fournier gangrene is necrotizing fasciitis arising from the perineal skin, scrotum, urethra, or rectum.
- Emergent surgical debridement and broad-spectrum antimicrobial agents are the essentials of treatment of Fournier gangrene.
- Periurethral abscess can occur secondarily to urethral stricture or catheterization; treatment entails surgical debridement, suprapubic urinary drainage, and antimicrobial agents.

REFERENCES

The complete reference list is available online at www.expertconsult.com.

SUGGESTED READINGS

Anderson GG, Dodson KW, Hooton TM, et al. Intracellular bacterial communities of uropathogenic *Escherichia coli* in urinary tract pathogenesis. Trends Microbiol 2004;12:424–30.

Asscher AW, Chick S, Radford N, et al. Natural history of asymptomatic bacteriuria in nonpregnant women. In: Brumfitt W, Asscher AW, editors. Urinary tract infection. London: University Press; 1973. p. 51.

Dajani AS, Taubert KA, Wilson W, et al. Prevention of bacterial endocarditis: recommendations by the American Heart Association. JAMA 1997;277:1794–801.

Eknoyan G, Qunibi WY, Grissom RT, et al. Renal papillary necrosis: an update. Medicine (Baltimore) 1982;61:55–73.

Elliott TS, Reed L, Slack RC, et al. Bacteriology and ultrastructure of the bladder in patients with urinary tract infections. J Infect 1985;11:191–9.

Foxman B. Epidemiology of urinary tract infections: incidence, morbidity, and economic costs. Am J Med 2002;113(Suppl. 1A):5S–13S.

Gupta K, Scholes D, Stamm WE. Increasing prevalence of antimicrobial resistance among uropathogens causing acute uncomplicated cystitis in women. JAMA 1999;281:736–8.

Hooton TM, Stamm WE. Management of acute uncomplicated urinary tract infection in adults. Med Clin North Am 1991;75:339–57.

Hultgren SJ, Porter TN, Schaeffer AJ, et al. Role of type 1 pili and effects of phase variation on lower urinary tract infections produced by *Escherichia coli*. Infect Immun 1985;50:370–7.

Hultgren SJ, Schwan WR, Schaeffer AJ, et al. Regulation of production of type 1 pili among urinary tract isolates of *Escherichia coli*. Infect Immun 1986;54:613–20.

Mabeck CE. Treatment of uncomplicated urinary tract infection in nonpregnant women. Postgrad Med J 1972;48:69–75.

Martinez JJ, Hultgren SJ. Requirement of Rho-family GTPases in the invasion of type 1-piliated uropathogenic *Escherichia coli*. Cell Microbiol 2002;4:19–28.

Mulvey MA. Adhesion and entry of uropathogenic *Escherichia coli*. Cell Microbiol 2002;4:257–71.

Mulvey MA, Lopez-Boado YS, Wilson CL, et al. Induction and evasion of host defenses by type 1-piliated uropathogenic *Escherichia coli*. Science 1998;282:1494–7.

Mulvey MA, Schilling JD, Martinez JJ, et al. Bad bugs and beleaguered bladders: interplay between uropathogenic *Escherichia coli* and innate host defenses. Proc Natl Acad Sci U S A 2000;97:8829–35.

National Institute on Disability and Rehabilitation Research. The prevention and management of urinary tract infections among people with spinal cord injuries. National Institute on Disability and Rehabilitation Research consensus statement. January 27-29, 1992. SCI Nurs 1993;10:49–61.

Nicolle LE, Bradley S, Colgan R, et al. Infectious Diseases Society of America guidelines for the diagnosis and treatment of asymptomatic bacteriuria in adults. Clin Infect Dis 2005;40:643–54.

Schaeffer AJ, Jones JM, Dunn JK. Association of in vitro *Escherichia coli* adherence to vaginal and buccal epithelial cells with susceptibility of women to recurrent urinary-tract infections. N Engl J Med 1981;304:1062–6.

Stamey TA. Pathogenesis and treatment of urinary tract infections. Baltimore: Williams & Wilkins; 1980.

Stamey TA, Govan DE, Palmer JM. The localization and treatment of urinary tract infections: the role of bactericidal urine levels as opposed to serum levels. Medicine (Baltimore) 1965;44:1–36.

Stamm WE. Recent developments in the diagnosis and treatment of urinary tract infections. West J Med 1982;137:213–20.

Stamm WE. Catheter-associated urinary tract infections: epidemiology, pathogenesis, and prevention. Am J Med 1991;91:65S–71S.

Turck M, Goffe B, Petersdorf RG. The urethral catheter and urinary tract infection. J Urol 1962;88:834–7.

Vromen M, van der Ven AJ, Knols A, et al. Antimicrobial resistance patterns in urinary isolates from nursing home residents: fifteen years of data reviewed. J Antimicrob Chemother 1999;44:113–6.

Warren JW, Abrutyn E, Hebel JR, et al. Guidelines for antimicrobial treatment of uncomplicated acute bacterial cystitis and acute pyelonephritis in women. Infectious Diseases Society of America (IDSA). Clin Infect Dis 1999;29:745–58.

13 Inflammatory and Pain Conditions of the Male Genitourinary Tract: Prostatitis and Related Pain Conditions, Orchitis, and Epididymitis

J. Curtis Nickel, MD, FRCSC

Prostatitis and Chronic Pelvic Pain Syndrome

Other Inflammatory and Pain Conditions of the Lower Urinary Tract

PROSTATITIS AND CHRONIC PELVIC PAIN SYNDROME

Historical Perspective

The clinical presentation, pathology, and microscopic evaluation of prostate-specific specimens of prostatitis patients were firmly established (Young et al, 1906) by the turn of the 20th century. Bacterial and cytologic localization studies of the lower urinary tract were described shortly thereafter (Hitchens and Brown, 1913) and standardized by 1930 (Von Lackum, 1927, 1928; Nickel, 1930, 1999c). **The primary form of therapy for prostatitis during most of the 20th century was repetitive prostate massage** (Farman, 1930; O'Conor, 1936; Henline, 1943; Campbell, 1957). Antimicrobial therapy became the mainstay of therapy with the introduction of sulfanilamide in the 1930s (Ritter and Lippow, 1938). However, even in the 1950s and 1960s, the significance of inflammatory cells and bacteria in the expressed prostatic secretion (EPS) was questioned (O'Shaughnessy et al, 1956; Bowers and Thomas, 1958; Bourne and Frishette, 1967), and it was even recognized that, in many cases, antibiotics were performing little better than placebo in the treatment of prostatitis (Gonder, 1963).

The next era of prostatitis management began in the 1960s with Meares and Stamey's (1968) description of the four-glass lower urinary tract segmented localization study. Prostatic massage as the mainstay of prostatitis therapy was abandoned, and antimicrobial therapy was rationalized for the very small percentage of patients with bacteria localized to prostate-specific specimens. Unfortunately, the vast majority of patients who were diagnosed with a nonbacterial cause continued to suffer the indignities of dismal urologic management (Nickel, 1998b). The establishment of new definitions and a classification system, better understanding of the etiopathogenesis, completion of randomized placebo-controlled trials with validated outcome indices, and the evolving insight that patients with prostatitis have variable clinical phenotypes have radically changed the way this condition is managed.

Epidemiology

Prostatitis is the most common urologic diagnosis in men younger than 50 years and the third most common urologic diagnosis in men older than 50 years after benign prostatic hyperplasia (BPH) and prostate cancer (Collins et al, 1998). As part of the International Consultation on Urologic Disease (ICUD) preparation for the male lower urinary tract symptoms (LUTS) guideline, the prevalence and incidence of prostatitis and/or chronic pelvic pain syndrome were estimated (Nickel et al, 2013b). Of 24 studies identified, 13 were from North America (Moon et al, 1997; Roberts et al, 1998; Collins et al, 1998, 2002; Nickel et al, 2001a;

Roberts et al, 2002; Clemens et al, 2006, 2007; Daniels et al, 2007; Walz et al, 2007; Tripp et al, 2008; Wallner et al, 2009; Cheng et al, 2010); six from Asia (Ku et al, 2001; Tan et al, 2002; Cheah et al, 2003a; Kunishima et al, 2006; Liang et al, 2009; Lan et al, 2011); two from Europe (Mehik et al, 2000; Marszalek et al, 2007); two from Africa (Ejike et al, 2008; Tripp et al, 2012); and one from Australia (Ferris et al, 2010). Compiling the results of all studies, which included a total of 336,846 patients, a prevalence of 7.1% was estimated (range was from 2.2% to 16% with a median prevalence rate of 6.7%). Thirteen of these studies were population based and examined 48,824 patients. The prevalence overall was 7.7% with a range of 2.2% to 14.2% with a median prevalence rate of 8.4%. Five studies depended on physician diagnoses of prostatitis-like symptoms, including those using large databases to extract codes made by physicians for diagnosis. The reported prevalence ranged from 2.7% to 8.8%. The overall prevalence for these studies was 10,592 patients diagnosed out of 186,533 examined (mean 5.7%; median 8%). Five studies used patient recollection of a diagnosis of prostatitis. Of 101,489 patients, 9388 self-reported a diagnosis of prostatitis for a prevalence of 9.3%, ranging from 4.3% to 16%. The mean prevalence in studies according to continent of origin was 6.9% in North America, 7.5% in Asia, 7.6% in Australia, 8.6% in Europe, and 12.1% in Africa. A detailed discussion of this epidemiologic review can be found in the 2012 International Consultation report (Nickel et al, 2013b).

One study evaluated the incidence of male chronic pelvic pain syndrome (CPPS) in a managed care population (Clemens et al, 2005). The incidence was 3.30 cases per 1000 men per year, representing an incidence of 267,000 cases per year if these data can be extrapolated to the overall U.S. population. Prostatitis results in a substantial number of physician visits. The Urologic Diseases in America study reported an annualized visit rate of 1798 per 100,000 population for prostatitis (Pontari et al, 2007). Patients with symptoms of prostatitis appear to be at increased risk for persistent symptoms and for recurrent episodes. Participants with a previous diagnosis of prostatitis had a much higher cumulative probability of subsequent episodes of prostatitis (Roberts et al, 1998; Turner et al, 2004b).

In summary, the prevalence of prostatitis-like symptoms ranges from 2.2% to 16%, with a median prevalence rate approximating 7% for chronic prostatitis and CPPS.

Chronic prostatitis is associated with substantial costs and significant predicted resource consumption (Calhoun et al, 2004; Turner et al, 2004a; Duloy et al, 2007; Clemens et al, 2009). Overall spending in the United States for the diagnosis and management of prostatitis, exclusive of pharmaceutical spending, totaled 84 million dollars in 2000 and appears to be increasing (Pontari et al, 2007). This economic factor needs increased attention when evaluating the incidence and treatment of this prevalent condition.

Histopathology

For the pathologist, prostatitis is defined as an increased number of inflammatory cells within the prostatic parenchyma (Cotran et al, 1999). Prostatic inflammation may or may not be noted in patients with a diagnosis of prostatitis (True et al, 1999), BPH (Nickel et al, 1999c), or prostate cancer (Zhang et al, 2000) and is noted in autopsy series in as many as 44% of prostate tissue samples from men without any definitive prostate disease (McNeal, 1968).

Consistently, fairly distinct although often coexisting patterns of chronic inflammation can be found in the prostate glands of patients with or without prostate disease. The most common pattern of inflammation is a lymphocytic infiltrate in the stroma immediately adjacent to the prostatic acini (Kohnen and Drach, 1979; Nickel et al, 1999c). The intensity of the inflammatory process varies considerably from only scattered lymphocytes to dense lymphoid nodules. Stromal lymphocytic infiltrates frequently coexist with periglandular inflammation. Sheets, clusters, and occasional nodules of lymphocytes and scattered plasma cells are seen within the fibromuscular stroma with no apparent relationship to the ducts and acini. Infiltrates of inflammatory cells restricted to the glandular epithelium and lumen are found in association with prostatitis and BPH but can be found in asymptomatic patients. The intraepithelial inflammatory cells may be neutrophils, lymphocytes, macrophages, or all of these, whereas neutrophils and macrophages are typically found in the lumen. A more detailed description of histologic inflammatory patterns in the prostate is available (Nickel et al, 2001d). Figure 13-1 illustrates the various inflammatory patterns seen in a prostate specimen from a patient with chronic prostatitis (CP).

Corpora amylacea, which may develop from the deposition of prostatic secretions around a sloughed epithelial cell or other irritant, are not usually associated with inflammation unless they become large enough to distend or obstruct the prostatic gland (Attah, 1975). Prostatic calculi may contribute to prostatic inflammation by obstructing central prostate ducts and thus preventing drainage or providing a nidus in which bacteria can survive host defenses and antibiotics (Meares, 1974; Roberts et al, 1997).

Granulomatous prostatitis presents a nonspecific and variable histologic pattern typified by heavy lobular, mixed, inflammatory infiltrates that include abundant histiocytes, lymphocytes, and plasma cells. Small, discrete granulomas may be present, or the pattern may be typified by well-defined granulomas. Granulomatous prostatic inflammation is a common consequence of surgery (Eyre et al, 1986) or bacille Calmette-Guérin (BCG) therapy (Lafontaine et al, 1997) and a rare event in patients with systemic tuberculosis (Saw et al, 1993).

Etiology

Microbiology

Gram-Negative Uropathogens. Acute bacterial prostatitis is a generalized infection of the prostate gland and is associated with both lower urinary tract infection (UTI) and generalized sepsis. Chronic bacterial prostatitis is associated with recurrent lower UTIs (i.e., cystitis) secondary to areas of focal uropathogenic bacteria residing in the prostate gland. The most common cause

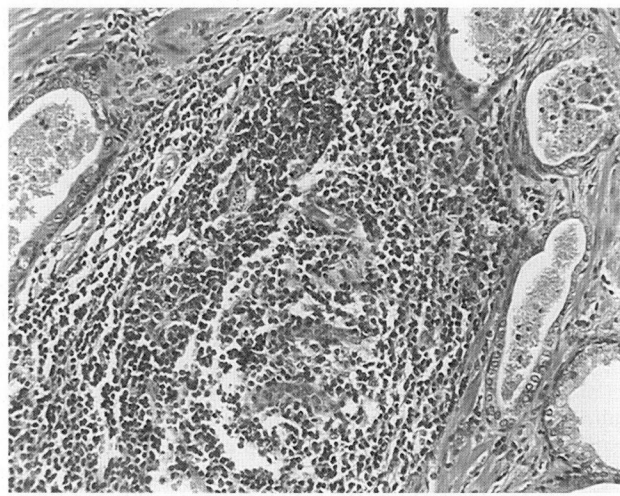

Figure 13-1. Histologic preparation of a prostate specimen demonstrating areas of glandular, periglandular, and stromal inflammation (×400). **(Courtesy Dr. Alexander Boag.)**

of bacterial prostatitis is the Enterobacteriaceae family of gram-negative bacteria, which originate in the gastrointestinal flora. The most common organisms are strains of *Escherichia coli*, which are identified in 65% to 80% of infections (Stamey, 1980; Lopez-Plaza and Bostwick, 1990; Weidner et al, 1991b; Schneider et al, 2003). *Pseudomonas aeruginosa, Serratia* species, *Klebsiella* species, and *Enterobacter aerogenes* are identified in a further 10% to 15% (Meares, 1987; Weidner et al, 1991b). However, in acute bacterial prostatitis, the organisms that result from previous manipulation of the lower urinary tract (including prostate biopsy) show different patterns of virulence and resistance (e.g., to quinolones and cephalosporins) compared with the organisms associated with spontaneous acute prostatitis (Millán-Rodríguez et al, 2006; Ha et al, 2008). Positive culture for extended-spectrum β-lactamase (ESBL) *E. coli* after prostate biopsy appears to be a risk factor for progression to CP (Oh et al, 2013).

Urovirulence factors play a significant role in the pathogenesis of bacterial prostatitis (Ruiz et al, 2002; Johnson et al, 2005). For instance, bacterial P fimbriae (or pili) bind to the urothelial receptors, and this subsequently facilitates ascent into the urinary tract as well as establishing deep infections in the prostate gland itself (Dilworth et al, 1990; Neal et al, 1990; Andreu et al, 1997). Colonization of the lower urinary tract by *E. coli* is also facilitated by the presence of type 1 fimbria, also known as *mannose-sensitive fimbria.* The receptor is a common moiety of the uroepithelial uromucoid; this association has been shown to be important in the development of cystitis in humans, and its presence in prostatitis has also been documented (Correll et al, 1996). Phase variation of type 1 pili during the establishment of acute bacterial prostatitis may occur in the setting of prostatitis (Schaeffer, 1991). Multiple virulence factors appear to be necessary to produce prostatitis (Mitsumori et al, 1999; Ruiz et al, 2002). Bacteria reside deep in the ducts of the prostate gland and when threatened with host defense and antimicrobial therapy tend to form aggregates (also called *biofilms*), which appears to be a protective mechanism allowing bacteria to persist in the prostate gland even when the cystitis is treated with antibiotics (Nickel and Costerton, 1993; Nickel et al, 1994). Hemolysin appears to be a virulence factor associated with *E. coli* acute prostatitis, but hemolysin may also be associated with increased ability of certain strains of *E. coli* to persist in the prostate as biofilms in patients with chronic bacterial prostatitis (Soto et al, 2007).

Gram-Positive Bacteria. Enterococci are believed to account for 5% to 10% of documented prostate infections (Drach, 1974a; Meares, 1987; Bergman, 1994). The role of other gram-positive organisms, which are also commensal organisms in the anterior urethra, is controversial (Fowler and Mariano, 1984a; Jimenez-Cruz et al, 1984; Krieger et al, 2002). An etiologic role for gram-positive organisms such as *Staphylococcus saprophyticus*, hemolytic streptococci, *Staphylococcus aureus*, and other coagulase-negative staphylococci has been suggested by a number of authors (Drach, 1974a, 1986; Bergman, 1994). Nickel and Costerton (1992) have shown coagulase-negative *Staphylococcus* to be present in the EPS as well as transperineal prostate biopsy tissue of men with CP (microscopy and culture). Although this and other studies (Carson et al, 1982; Pfau, 1983; Bergman et al, 1989; Wedren, 1989) suggested that coagulase-negative staphylococci are involved in the pathogenesis of CP, these studies did not conclusively demonstrate that these bacteria were actually causing the inflammation and symptom complex rather than simply colonizing the prostate (Krieger et al, 2002). However, eradication of gram-positive bacteria in the prostate of men experiencing recent onset of prostatitis symptoms resulted in similar clinical results compared with men with gram-negative uropathogens localizing to the prostate (Magri et al, 2007a; Nickel and Xiang, 2008). In both cases, eradication of the bacteria localized to the prostate was strongly correlated with a good clinical outcome. However, the inconsistent localization of gram-positive bacteria in prostate-specific specimens from patients with CP suggests that this relationship may not be as strong as suggested (e.g., Krieger et al, 2005).

Anaerobic Bacteria. In studies in which the prostate-specific specimens were cultured anaerobically, anaerobic bacteria could be identified in a small number of patients (Nielsen and Justesen, 1974; Mardh and Colleen, 1975; Szoke et al, 1998). This has not been a consistent finding, and the role of anaerobic bacteria is essentially unknown.

Corynebacterium **Infection.** *Corynebacterium* species have usually been acknowledged as prostate nonpathogens but have been suggested as potential etiologic agents in this disease (Riegel et al, 1995; Domingue, 1998). Domingue and colleagues (1997) suggested that these difficult-to-culture coryneforms could be missed by routine culturing of EPS. Direct Gram staining of the EPS showed gram-variable pleomorphic coccobacillary rods that do not usually grow on routine media. The presence of these pleomorphic swollen rods was also shown by fluorescent acridine orange staining. Tanner and associates (1999), using polymerase chain reaction (PCR) techniques, were able to identify a bacterial signal (phylogenetically gram-positive organisms with predominance of *Corynebacterium* species) in 65% of 17 patients with CP. Approximately half these patients tended to respond to antimicrobial therapy, whereas patients in whom molecular signals for these bacteria could not be identified did not.

Chlamydial Infection. The evidence supporting the role of *Chlamydia trachomatis* as an etiologic agent in chronic prostatic inflammation is both confusing and conflicting. Mardh and Colleen (1972) found that one third of men with CP had antibodies to *C. trachomatis* compared with 3% of controls. Shortliffe and coworkers (1992) found that 20% of patients with nonbacterial prostatitis had antichlamydial antibody titers in the prostatic fluid. Koroku and associates (1995) detected *C. trachomatis*–specific immunoglobulin A (IgA) in 29% of men with chronic nonbacterial prostatitis. Bruce and colleagues (1981), on examination of early morning urine, prostatic fluid, or semen, found that 56% of patients with "subacute or chronic prostatitis" were infected with *C. trachomatis*. In a follow-up study, Bruce and Reid (1989) found that 6 of 55 men with abacterial prostatitis, including 31 believed to have chlamydial prostatitis, met strict criteria for positive diagnosis for chlamydial prostatitis based on identification of the organisms by culturing or immunofluorescence. Kuroda and colleagues (1989) identified *C. trachomatis* in the urethras of 20% of men with prostatitis. Other investigators have come to similar conclusions (Nilsson et al, 1981; Weidner et al, 1983). *Chlamydia* has also been isolated in prostate tissue specimens. Poletti and coworkers (1985) isolated *C. trachomatis* from prostate samples obtained by transrectal aspiration biopsy of men with "nonacute abacterial prostatitis." Abdelatif and colleagues (1991) identified intracellular *Chlamydia* through use of "in situ hybridization techniques" in transurethral prostate chips from 30% of men with histologic evidence of "chronic

abacterial prostatitis." Shurbaji and associates (1998) identified *C. trachomatis* in paraffin-embedded secretions in 31% of men with histologic evidence of prostatitis compared with none in patients with BPH without inflammation.

Although Mardh and Colleen (1972) suggested that *C. trachomatis* may be implicated in as many as one third of men with CP, their follow-up studies employing culturing and serologic tests could not confirm *C. trachomatis* as an etiologic agent in idiopathic prostatitis (Mardh and Colleen, 1975; Mardh et al, 1978). Shortliffe and Wehner (1986) came to a similar conclusion when their group evaluated antichlamydial antibody titers in prostatic fluid. Twelve percent of controls (compared with 20% of patients with nonbacterial prostatitis) had detectable antibodies. Berger and coworkers (1989) could not culture *C. trachomatis* from the urethras in men with CP, nor did they find a serologic or local immune response to *C. trachomatis* in such patients. Doble and associates (1989b) were not able to culture or detect by immunofluorescence *Chlamydia* in transperineal biopsy specimens of abnormal areas of the prostate in men with chronic abacterial prostatitis. Krieger and colleagues (1996b) were able to find *Chlamydia* in only 1% of prostate tissue biopsy specimens from men with CP. A further localization and culture series by Krieger and associates (2000) also failed to culture *Chlamydia* from either urethral or prostate specimens. Further elucidation of the role of chlamydial etiology of prostate infection is required before any definitive statement can be made regarding the association between isolation of this organism and its prostatic origin and effect (Weidner et al, 2002). That being said, antimicrobial therapy for presumed chlamydial prostate infection does result in amelioration of symptoms in many cases (Skerk et al, 2002b, 2003; Perletti et al, 2013).

Ureaplasma **Infection.** *Ureaplasma urealyticum* is a common organism isolated from the urethra of both asymptomatic men and men with nonspecific urethritis. Weidner and colleagues (1980) found high *U. urealyticum* concentrations in prostate-specific specimens in patients with signs and symptoms of abacterial prostatitis. Isaacs (1993) and associates cultured *U. urealyticum* from prostate secretions in 8% of patients with chronic nonbacterial prostatitis. Fish and Danziger (1993) found significant *U. urealyticum* concentrations in 13% of patients with prostatitis. Treatment with specific antimicrobial therapy cleared the organisms in all cases. Ohkawa and associates (1993a) isolated *U. urealyticum* cells from the prostates of 18 of 143 patients with CP. Antibiotics eradicated the organism in all, improved the symptoms in 10, and cleared the leukocytes in the EPS in 4 (Ohkawa et al, 1993b).

Other investigators (Mardh and Colleen, 1975), employing similar techniques, were unable to implicate *U. urealyticum* in patients with nonbacterial prostatitis. The problems encountered in all these studies include the absence of controls and the fact that it was difficult to account for possible urethral contamination in collecting specific prostate specimens. However, macrolides do appear to successfully improve CP symptoms when *Ureaplasma* or *Mycoplasma* organisms are identified in prostate specimens (Perletti et al, 2013).

Other Microorganisms. *Candida* (Golz and Mendling, 1991; Indudhara et al, 1992) and other mycotic infections such as aspergillosis and coccidioidomycosis (Schwarz, 1982; Chen and Schijj, 1985; Campbell et al, 1992; Truett and Crum, 2004) have been implicated in prostatic inflammation. However, in most cases it was usually an isolated finding in immunosuppressed patients or those with systemic fungal infection. Viruses (Doble et al, 1991; Benson and Smith, 1992) have also been implicated in prostatic inflammation, but no systematic evaluation of the role of these agents in prostatitis has been undertaken. *Trichomonas* has been described in the prostate glands of patients complaining of prostatitis-like symptoms (Kuberski, 1980; Gardner et al, 1996; Skerk et al, 2002a). *Helicobacter pylori* antibodies were positive in serum in 76% of men with CP compared with 62% in controls ($P < .05$). Although this is significantly greater, a large number of the patients without symptoms were seropositive (Karatas et al, 2010).

A newer concept is that it may not be the specific type of bacteria, but that the virulence of bacteria in men with CPPS may

be greater, resulting in symptoms or even causing symptoms that persist after eradication of the bacterial organism (Ivanov et al, 2009; Ivanov et al, 2010; Rudick et al, 2011; Galeone et al, 2013; Quick et al, 2013). It is interesting to note that the symptom patterns for patients who develop CPPS associated with previous bacterial infection may be different from those in patients who develop the syndrome not related to previous infection (Magri et al, 2013). **Nonculturable Microorganisms.** There are significant limitations to the culture techniques used to attempt to identify causative microorganisms associated with prostatitis (Lowentritt et al, 1995; Domingue et al, 1997; Domingue, 1998). Bacteria may exist in aggregated biofilms adherent to the prostatic ductal walls or within the obstructed ducts in the prostate (Nickel and MacLean, 1998). Nickel and Costerton (1993) observed that 60% of patients with previously diagnosed chronic bacterial prostatitis who progressed to sterile EPS cultures but continued to have symptoms despite antimicrobial therapy had positive cultures in prostate biopsy specimens showing an organism similar to the initial organism. As discussed earlier, such organisms appear to persist in small aggregates or biofilms in the ducts and acini of the prostate gland.

Berger and associates (1997) cultured urine specimens and transperineal prostate biopsies specifically for commensal and fastidious organisms. These investigators demonstrated that in prostate biopsy cultures men with evidence of inflammation in EPS are more likely to have bacteria isolated, positive cultures for anaerobic bacteria, higher total bacterial counts, and more bacterial species isolated than men without EPS inflammation. Krieger and colleagues (1996b), Riley and coworkers (1998) and Tanner and associates (1999), used a combination of clinical, culture, and molecular biologic methods (PCR) and found a strong correlation between inflammation and EPS and the detection of bacteria-specific 16S rRNA (gram-negative and gram-positive organisms) in the prostate tissue. But other researchers did not find any association between culture and PCR findings in men with nonbacterial prostatitis compared with men with prostatitis symptoms (Keay et al, 1999; Lee et al, 2003; Leskinen et al, 2003b). Nanobacteria are intriguing organisms that are difficult to isolate and culture, but may be implicated in some chronic urologic conditions including CP (Wood and Shoskes, 2006). A number of investigators (Shoskes et al, 2005; Zhou et al, 2008) have demonstrated the possibility that nanobacteria associated with and without prostatic calculi may be implicated in some cases of CP.

It has been estimated that less than 10% of all environmental bacteria have been identified (Domingue, 1998), so it is possible that fastidious and nonculturable microorganisms might be present in the prostate gland and that such organisms might be involved in the inflammatory process and subsequent development of symptoms.

Altered Prostate Host Defense

Risk factors that allow bacterial colonization or infection of the prostate with potentially pathogenic bacteria include intraprostatic ductal reflux (Kirby et al, 1982); **phimosis** (VanHowe, 1998); **specific blood groups** (Lomberg et al, 1986); **unprotected penetrative anal rectal intercourse; UTI; acute epididymitis** (Berger et al, 1987); **indwelling urethral catheters and condom catheter drainage** (Meares, 1998); **and transurethral surgery, especially in men who have untreated, infected urine** (Meares, 1989). Secretory dysfunction of the prostate characterized by an alteration in the composition of prostatic secretions can be diagnostic of patients with prostatitis—that is, a decrease in the levels of fructose; citric acid; acid phosphatase; the cations zinc, magnesium, and calcium; and the zinc-containing prostatic antibacterial factor—whereas pH, the ratio of isoenzymes lactate dehydrogenase-5 to lactate dehydrogenase-1, and inflammatory proteins such as ceruloplasmin and complement C3 are increased (Meares, 1989). These defined alterations in the prostate secretory function have also been blamed for adversely affecting the normal antibacterial nature of prostatic secretions. A decrease in prostatic antibacterial factor may reduce the intrinsic antibacterial activity of the prostatic fluid (Fair

et al, 1976), whereas the alkaline pH may hamper diffusion of certain basic antimicrobial drugs into the prostatic tissue and fluid (Fair and Cordonnier, 1978). However, caution is warranted because it is not known whether these compositional changes are a cause or a consequence of inflammation. It has further been suggested that the metabolic syndrome (Wang et al, 2013) and endothelial dysfunction with arterial stiffness (Shoskes et al, 2011) may be risk, mechanistic, or associated factors, likely through alteration of inflammatory pathways.

Dysfunctional Voiding

Anatomic or neurophysiologic obstruction resulting in high-pressure dysfunctional flow patterns has been implicated in the pathogenesis of prostatitis syndrome. Blacklock (1974, 1991) demonstrated that bladder neck, prostatic, and urethral anatomic abnormalities predisposed some men to developing prostatitis. Urodynamic studies confirm that many patients, particularly those with prostatodynia, have decreased maximal urinary flow rates and obstructive-appearing flow patterns (Barbalias et al, 1983; Ghobish, 2002). On video-urodynamic studies, many patients with prostatitis syndromes show incomplete funneling of the bladder neck as well as vesicourethral dyssynergic patterns (Kaplan et al, 1994, 1997; Hruz et al, 2003). Investigators (Dellabella et al, 2006) have described ultrasound alterations of the preprostatic sphincter in men with CP. In a study of 48 treatment-refractory CP patients with no associated infection, Hruz et al (2003) determined that 29 (60%) had bladder neck hypertrophy diagnosed by endoscopic and urodynamic criteria. This dyssynergic voiding may lead to an autonomic overstimulation of the perineal-pelvic neural system with subsequent development of a chronic neuropathic pain or neuromuscular state. Alternatively, this high-pressure, dysfunctional voiding may result in intraprostatic ductal reflux in susceptible individuals (see the next section).

Intraprostatic Ductal Reflux

Reflux of urine and possibly bacteria into the prostatic ducts has been postulated as one of the causative mechanisms involved in the pathogenesis of chronic bacterial and nonbacterial prostatic inflammation in some individuals. Anatomically, the ductal drainage of the peripheral zone is more susceptible than other prostatic zones to intraprostatic ductal reflux (Blacklock, 1974, 1991). Kirby and associates (1982) instilled a carbon particle solution into the bladders of men diagnosed with nonbacterial prostatitis. Carbon particles were found in the EPS macrophages and prostatic acini and ductal system after surgery in men with nonbacterial prostatitis. Persson and Ronquist (1996) noted high levels of urate and creatinine in EPS, which they postulated was caused by urine reflux into the prostatic ducts. Terai and colleagues (2000) provided molecular epidemiologic evidence for ascending infection in acute bacterial prostatitis.

Prostatic calculi are composed of substances found only in urine, not in prostatic secretions (Sutor and Wooley, 1974; Ramiraz et al, 1980), **further evidence that urinary intraprostatic reflux occurs and likely contributes to the formation of prostatic calculi. If pathogenic bacteria reflux into the prostate gland, they may exist in protected aggregates within prostatic calculi themselves** (Mazzoli, 2010). High culture counts of pathogens encrusted in prostatic calculi were demonstrated by Eykyn and colleagues (1974). This type of bacterial colonization in protective bacterial aggregates or biofilms associated with prostatic calculi may lead to recalcitrant CP and subsequent recurrent UTIs despite what seems to be adequate antibiotic therapy. Ludwig and coworkers (1994), employing transrectal ultrasonography, showed that men with chronic inflammatory prostatitis had a significantly increased frequency of prostatic calculi compared with men without prostate inflammation. It appears that prostatic calcification is common in patients with nonbacterial CP and is associated with greater inflammation, bacterial colonization, pelvic floor spasm, and symptom duration (Shoskes et al, 2007). The inflammation resulting from chemical, bacterial, or immunologic stimulation has been shown to possibly cause an increase in intraprostatic pressures, measurable with transperineally inserted pressure transducers (Mehik et al, 2002).

Immunologic Alterations

The local prostatic immune system is activated by infection in bacterial prostatitis. In acute bacterial prostatitis, serum and prostatic fluid antigen-specific (i.e., bacterial antigen) IgG and IgA can be detected immediately after the onset of infection, and, after successful antibiotic therapy the levels decline to normal over the next 6 to 12 months (Meares, 1977; Fowler and Mariano, 1984b; Kumon, 1992; Meares, 1998). **Prostate-specific antigen (PSA) levels can be markedly elevated during an acute episode of bacterial prostatitis (Dalton, 1989; Moon et al, 1992; Neal et al, 1992) and slowly resolve to normal levels over the course of 6 weeks to many months, provided there is no recrudescence of the infection.** In chronic bacterial prostatitis, no serum Ig elevation is detected, whereas prostatic fluid IgA and IgG levels are both increased (Shortliffe and Wehner, 1986; Kumon, 1992). After successful antibiotic therapy, IgG levels return to normal after several months, but the IgA (particularly secretory IgA) levels remain elevated for almost 2 years (Shortliffe et al, 1981a, 1981b; Fowler and Mariano, 1984b). The presence of antibody-coated bacteria detected in urine, EPS, and semen is another prominent feature of chronic bacterial prostatitis (Riedasch et al, 1984, 1991).

Noninfectious inflammation (nonbacterial prostatitis or CPPS) might also be secondary to immunologically mediated inflammation caused by some unknown antigen or perhaps even related to an autoimmune process. IgA and IgM antibody levels (not microorganism specific) are elevated (Shortliffe and Wehner, 1986; Shortliffe et al, 1989, 1992), and similar antibodies as well as fibrinogen and complement C3 (Vinje et al, 1983; Doble et al, 1990) have been identified in prostatic biopsy samples from patients with CP. Both animal model studies (Donadio et al, 1998; Ceri et al, 1999; Lang et al, 2000; Breser et al, 2013; Chen et al, 2013; Quick et al, 2013) and human studies (Alexander et al, 1997; Batstone et al, 2002; Maake et al, 2003; Motrich et al, 2007) have suggested that prostatitis may be an autoimmune process. A number of candidates have been suggested for the self-antigen, including PSA (Ponniah et al, 2000). Other specific immunologic and neuroendocrine alterations such as cytokine production (Alexander et al, 1998; Jang et al, 2003), nerve growth factor (Miller et al, 2002), and mast cell activation (Done et al, 2012) have a subsequent role to play in the process of inflammation. Specifically, interleukin-10 (IL-10) has been implicated in the cause and clinical manifestations of CP (Miller et al, 2002; Shoskes et al, 2002), but other cytokines such as IL-1β and tumor necrosis factor–α (TNF-α) have also been implicated (Nadler et al, 2000). IL-8 is the most common cytokine localized to the semen in men with CP (Khadra et al, 2006; Penna et al, 2007). There may be a genetic phenotype that promotes specific immunologic parameters that predispose to immunologically induced prostatic inflammation (Shoskes et al, 2002; Riley et al, 2002). These immunophenotypic patterns have even been observed in noninflammatory category IIIB CP/CPPS (Barghorn et al, 2001). **One of the newest concepts emerging in the literature is that CPPS can exist through persistent immunologic mechanisms long after the bacteria have been eradicated** (Ivanov et al, 2009, 2010; Rudick et al, 2011; Galeone et al, 2013; Quick et al, 2013). **Whatever the initiating event, the immunologic cascade appears to have an important role in the development of prostatitis or CPPS in patients who develop prostatic inflammation** (Moon, 1998; Kumon, 1999).

Chemically Induced Inflammation

Investigators have demonstrated that urine and its metabolites (e.g., urate) are present in the prostatic secretion of patients with CP (Persson and Ronquist, 1996). These investigators have hypothesized that the prostatic inflammation and subsequent symptoms

may be simply the result of a chemically induced inflammation secondary to the noxious substances in the urine that have refluxed into the prostatic duct.

Pelvic Floor Muscle Abnormalities

Investigators (Zermann et al, 1999) **have proposed that the sensory or motor disturbances or both consistent with neural dysregulation of the lower urinary tract may be a consequence of acquired abnormalities in the central nervous system (CNS).** Certainly, extraprostatic tenderness is identified in many patients with CP (Berger et al, 2007; Shoskes et al, 2008). Zermann and Schmidt (1999) described 103 patients with chronic pelvic pain whom they evaluated at a specialized neurourologic unit. They showed that a majority of the men had insufficient conscious control of their somatically innervated striated pelvic floor muscles. The patients showed various levels of identity with their pelvic floor muscles, but none were able to demonstrate the full range of pelvic floor contraction and relaxation repetitively and effortlessly. This was true whether or not there was evidence of inflammation. The researchers concluded that their findings reflect a functional disassociation between the CNS and the peripheral target, the pelvic floor muscles.

Other clinicians (Anderson, 1999; Potts, 2003; Hetrick et al, 2003; Shoskes et al, 2008; Anderson et al, 2009b) have proposed that the source of the pain is specifically at the pelvic musculature attachment area at the sacrum, coccyx, ischial tuberosity, pubic rami, and endopelvic fascia. These areas are immediately adjacent to the prostate and bladder and can be recognized by the demonstration of a hyperirritable spot or myofascial trigger point that is painful on compression. It is hypothesized that the formation of myofascial trigger points in this area results from mechanical abnormalities in the hip and lower extremities, chronic holding patterns such as those that occur during toilet training, sexual abuse, repetitive minor trauma and constipation, sports that create chronic pelvic stimulation, traumatic or unusual sexual activity, recurrent infections, and surgery (Anderson, 1999). More recently, it has been hypothesized that the pain experienced in some men with CPPS may be explained by pudendal nerve entrapment, which causes subsequent neuropathic pain (Antolak et al, 2002).

Neural Sensitization

The pain associated with the CP syndromes is similar in many respects to neuropathic pain. Objective autonomic nervous system changes can be observed in men with CP, suggesting that altered autonomic nervous system responses may be responsible for the pain associated with CPPS (Miller et al, 2002; Yang et al, 2003; Yilmaz et al, 2007, 2010). Pain that may have originated in the prostate or pelvic floor muscles, through mechanisms of cross-sensitization may have spread to adjacent organs and/or structures. Only recently have researchers begun to understand the complexity of overlapping neuropathways and possible mechanisms underlying pelvic organ crosstalk (Malykhina, 2007) including that from bowel (Takahashi et al, 2013). It now appears that actual measurable changes (functional and anatomic) in brain function can be observed in men with long-standing CPPS (Farmer et al, 2011; Mordasini et al, 2012).

It has recently been shown that **men with CP showed evidence of dysfunctional hypothalamic-pituitary-adrenal axis function** reflected in augmented awakening cortisol responses (Anderson et al, 2008), which can be further induced by stress (Anderson et al, 2009a). Another study evaluating adrenocortical hormone abnormalities in men with CP suggested that some men with this condition may even meet the diagnostic criteria for nonclassic congenital hyperplasia (Dimitrakov et al, 2008).

Psychosocial Associations

Psychological factors have always been considered to play an important role in the development or exacerbation of CP syndromes. Some researchers who have investigated the psychopathology of these patients concluded that this syndrome should be viewed as a psychosomatic disorder (Mendlewich et al, 1971; Mellan et al, 1973; Keltikangas-Jarvinen et al, 1982). De la Rosette and associates (1993b) compared a group of 50 CP patients with a group of 50 patients seen for vasectomy and showed that although there were significant statistical differences between the groups (with CP patients demonstrating consistently higher personality disorder scores), these differences in scores were quite small compared with those between prostatitis and psychiatric patients. Berghuis and coworkers (1996) compared 51 prostatitis patients with a group of 34 men without any chronic pain condition and concluded that depression and psychological disturbances are common among prostatitis patients. Egan and Krieger (1994) compared prostatitis patients with those seeking treatment for chronic low back pain. Major depression was more common in prostatitis patients, but back pain caused more somatically focused depression and anxiety. Ku et al (2002) suggested that depression and weak masculine identity may be associated with an early stage of CP. A large case-control study confirmed that depression and panic disorders are significantly more common in men with chronic pelvic pain conditions than in controls (Clemens et al, 2008). **These more recent studies demonstrate that psychological factors are involved in the disease, but it seems unjustified to label this group of patients as "neurotic" or as having a psychopathologic condition.** However, recent analyses of the large prostatitis cohorts showed that **psychological variables, such as depression, maladaptive coping techniques (e.g., pain catastrophizing, pain-contingent resting), poor social support, anxiety, and stress are important in CP outcomes** (Tripp et al 2005; Ulrich et al, 2005; Tripp et al, 2006; Nickel et al, 2008c; Chung and Lin, 2013; Kwon and Chang, 2013). Factors such as catastrophizing are particularly important because they have been found to be stronger predictors of patient pain reports than depression (Tripp et al, 2006), indicating that negative cognitive appraisals of pain experience may be a primary target for psychosocial interventions. This may be especially important given the strong association that pain catastrophizing has been shown to have with elevations in depression, disability, and lower quality of life in patients with CP (Tripp et al, 2005, 2006; Nickel et al, 2008c; Hedelin, 2012; Tripp et al, 2013).

Association with Interstitial Cystitis or Bladder Pain Syndrome

Interstitial cystitis, now referred to by many as *bladder pain syndrome*, is an ill-defined CPPS occurring primarily in females, and a number of investigators have hypothesized that CPPS in men may have a similar cause (Pontari, 2006; Forrest et al, 2007). Unfortunately, the cause of interstitial cystitis remains unknown, but the pathogenic mechanisms are theorized to be very similar to those that cause CP and/or chronic pelvic pain in men (Sant and Nickel, 1999; Eisenberg and Moldwin, 2003; Parsons 2003). Some researchers have proposed that in some patients diagnosed with prostatitis, a bladder-orientated interstitial cystitis mechanism actually accounts for the symptoms, and the prostate is only indirectly involved (Sant and Kominski, 1997). Certainly, the pain and voiding symptoms of interstitial cystitis and CP overlap to some extent (Miller et al, 1995; Novicki et al, 1998; Sant and Nickel, 1999; Forrest and Schmidt, 2004), and men with prostatitis diagnoses have cystoscopic (Berger et al, 1998), urodynamic (Siroky et al, 1981), and potassium sensitivity testing (Parsons and Albo, 2002; Parsons et al, 2005) findings very similar to those of patients with interstitial cystitis. However Yilmaz and coworkers (2004) did not confirm positive potassium sensitivity testing results in prostatitis patients, and Keay and colleagues (2004) showed that men diagnosed with CP (pain only) have normal antiproliferative factor (APF) activity whereas men diagnosed with interstitial cystitis (pain and irritative voiding symptoms) have detectable levels of urine APF.

Summary: Pathophysiology of Prostatitis and Related Syndromes

It is likely that nonbacterial prostatitis syndromes have a multifactorial cause—either a spectrum of causative mechanisms or, more likely, a progression or cascade of events that occur after one or more of the initiating factors described in the previous section. In a review on mechanisms involved in the pathogenesis of CP, Pontari and Ruggieri (2004) concluded that "the symptoms of chronic prostatitis/chronic pelvic pain syndrome appear to result from an interplay between psychological factors and dysfunction in the immune, neurological and endocrine systems." Figure 13-2 describes a suggested pathophysiologic scenario that could potentially involve most of the proposed and interrelated causes described in this section.

KEY POINTS: ETIOLOGY

- Gram-negative Enterobacteriaceae and *Enterococcus* species are responsible for most cases of bacterial prostatitis.
- Other microorganisms might be implicated.
- Nonbacterial prostatitis and chronic pelvic pain syndromes are caused by an interrelated cascade of inflammatory, immunologic, endocrine, muscular, neuropathic, and psychologic mechanisms that begin with an initiator in a genetically or anatomically susceptible man.

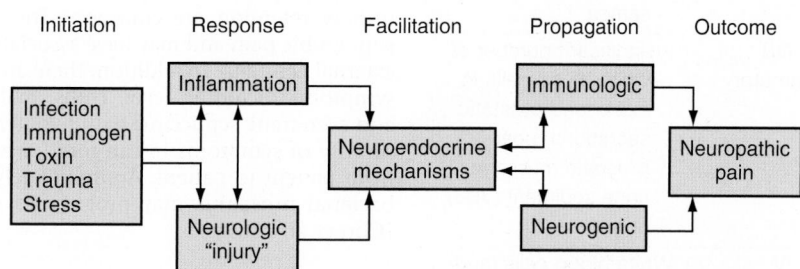

Figure 13-2. The cause and pathogenesis of chronic prostatitis/chronic pelvic pain syndrome (category III CPPS) appear to involve a pluricausal, multifactorial mechanism. An initiating stimulus, such as infection, reflux of some toxic or immunogenic urine substance, or perineal or pelvic trauma, starts a cascade of events in an anatomically or genetically susceptible man, resulting in a local response of inflammation or neurogenic injury or both. Further interrelated immunologic, neuropathic, endocrinologic, and psychologic mechanisms propagate or sustain the chronicity of the initial (or ongoing) event. The final outcome is the clinical manifestation of chronic perineal or pelvic pain and associated symptoms with local and central neuropathic mechanisms involving areas outside the prostate or pelvic area.

Definition and Classification

The traditional classification system is based on the landmark paper by Meares and Stamey (1968) describing the differential diagnosis of the prostatitis syndromes. This classic paper describes in great detail the serial cultures (and treatment) in four patients with CP and introduced the so-called *Meares-Stamey four-glass test*. This localization test, which segmentally assesses inflammation and cultures of the male lower urinary tract, is described in detail in the section on lower urinary tract evaluation. **Based on 10 years of clinical experience with this test, a classification system describing four categories of prostatitis was described by Drach and colleagues in 1978. Differentiation of the four categories depended on an analysis of prostatic fluid, which included microscopy (examination for white blood cells (WBCs), inflammatory cell clumps, mucous debris, oval fat bodies, and macrophages) and culturing (identifying traditional uropathogens).** This traditional classification system, which categorizes patients into those with acute bacterial prostatitis, chronic bacterial prostatitis, nonbacterial prostatitis, or prostatodynia, is described in Table 13-1.

The limitations of the traditional diagnostic algorithm and traditional classification system led to the development of the National Institutes of Health (NIH) classification system (see Table 13-1) (Krieger et al, 1999). The new definition recognized that pain is the main symptom in "abacterial chronic prostatitis" (with variable voiding and sexual dysfunction), and it was the optimal criterion to differentiate CP patients from control patients or patients experiencing other genitourinary problems (e.g., BPH). **The NIH classification differed from the traditional system in two main areas: the descriptions of category III CP/CPPS, and category IV asymptomatic inflammatory prostatitis.**

Category I is identical to the acute bacterial prostatitis category of the traditional classification system. **Category II** is identical to the traditional chronic bacterial prostatitis classification, except that it now usually refers to patients with recurrent lower UTIs (with a prostate nidus of infection) (Schaeffer, 2006). **Category III** is defined as the "presence of genitourinary pain in the absence of uropathogenic bacteria detected by standard microbiological methodology." This syndrome is further categorized into **category IIIA**, or inflammatory CP/CPPS (based on the presence of excessive leukocytes in EPSs or post–prostatic massage urine or semen), and **category IIIB** or noninflammatory CP/CPPS (no significant leukocytes in similar specimens). The inclusion of **category IV**, or asymptomatic inflammatory prostatitis, addressed one of the major problems and omissions of the traditional classification system. Patients are classified as having category IV prostatitis by the presence of significant leukocytes (or bacteria or both) in prostate-specific specimens (EPS, semen, and tissue biopsy specimens) in the absence of typical chronic pelvic pain.

The value of this classification system, not only in clinical research studies but also in clinical practice, has been generally accepted (Nickel et al, 1999d).

TABLE 13-1 Classification System for the Prostatitis Syndromes

TRADITIONAL	NATIONAL INSTITUTES OF HEALTH	DESCRIPTION
Acute bacterial prostatitis	Category I	Acute infection of the prostate gland
Chronic bacterial prostatitis	Category II	Chronic infection of the prostate gland
N/A	Category III Chronic pelvic pain syndrome (CPPS)	Chronic genitourinary pain in the absence of uropathogenic bacteria localized to the prostate gland employing standard methodology
Nonbacterial prostatitis	Category IIIA Inflammatory CPPS	Significant number of white blood cells in expressed prostatic secretions, post–prostatic massage urine sediment (VB3), or semen
Prostatodynia	Category IIIB Noninflammatory CPPS	Insignificant number of white blood cells in expressed prostatic secretions, post–prostatic massage urine sediment (VB3), or semen
N/A	Category IV Asymptomatic inflammatory prostatitis (AIP)	White blood cells (and/or bacteria) in expressed prostatic secretions, post–prostatic massage urine sediment (VB3), semen or histologic specimens of prostate gland

> **KEY POINT: CLASSIFICATION**
>
> - The National Institutes of Health classification of the prostatitis syndromes has now become recognized as the best system for research and clinical practice.

Clinical Presentation

Category I: Acute Bacterial Prostatitis

Acute bacterial prostatitis, category I, is a rare but important lower urinary tract infectious disease. It is characterized by an acute onset of pain combined with storage (irritative) and voiding (obstructive) urinary symptoms in a patient with manifestations of a systemic febrile illness. The patient typically reports urinary frequency, urgency, and dysuria. Obstructive voiding complaints including hesitancy, poor interrupted stream, strangury, and even acute urinary retention are common. The patient notes perineal and suprapubic pain and may have associated pain or discomfort of the external genitalia. In addition, there are usually significant systemic symptoms including fever, chills, malaise, nausea and vomiting, and even frank septicemia with hypotension. The combination and severity of symptoms in category I, acute bacterial prostatitis, vary from patient to patient. Approximately 5% of patients with acute bacterial prostatitis may progress to chronic bacterial prostatitis (Cho et al, 2005).

Category II: Chronic Bacterial Prostatitis

The most important clue in the diagnosis of category II, chronic bacterial prostatitis, is a history of documented recurrent UTIs. From 25% to 43% of patients diagnosed with chronic bacterial prostatitis through use of a four-glass test had a history of recurrent UTIs (Weidner and Ludwig, 1994; Wright et al, 1994). Patients may be relatively asymptomatic between acute episodes, or they may present with a long history of a CPPS, which is described extensively in the next section. The prevalence of bacterial prostatitis ranges from 5% to 15% of prostatitis cases (Schaeffer et al, 1981; Krieger and Egan, 1991; Weidner and Ludwig, 1994). In one of the largest and most comprehensive clinical series, Weidner and associates (1991b) found significant bacteriuria (with uropathogenic organisms) in 4.4% of patients with symptoms of CP.

Category III: Chronic Prostatitis/Chronic Pelvic Pain Syndrome

The presenting symptoms of patients with inflammatory category IIIA CP/CPPS are indistinguishable from those of patients with noninflammatory category IIIB disease. The symptoms experienced by patients with CP/CPPS have been studied extensively by Krieger and colleagues (1996a). They evaluated 50 patients with CP/CPPS seen in a prostatitis clinic (compared with 75 control patients). Alexander and Trissel (1996) surveyed a cohort of 163 prostatitis patients on the Internet. These symptoms were best defined in the development of prostatitis symptom scores by Neal and Moon (1994), Krieger and colleagues (1996a), Nickel and Sorensen (1996), and Brahler and coworkers (1997). **The predominant symptom in all these studies was pain, which was most commonly localized to the perineum, suprapubic area, and penis but can also occur in the testes, groin, or low back. Pain during or after ejaculation is one of the most prominent, important, and bothersome features in many patients** (Shoskes et al, 2004). Storage and voiding urinary symptoms including urgency, frequency, hesitancy, and poor interrupted flow are associated with this syndrome in many patients. Erectile dysfunction and sexual disturbances have been reported in patients with CPPS (Mehik et al, 2001; Liang et al, 2004; Zaslau et al, 2005; Muller and Mulhall, 2006; Smith et al, 2007a, 2007b; Lee et al, 2008b; Magri et al, 2008; Chung et al, 2012) but are not pathognomonic features of this syndrome. The best description of the CP/CPPS patient was provided by the NIH Chronic Prostatitis Cohort Study (Schaeffer et al, 2002). A detailed description of 488 men with CP/CPPS noted that the most frequently reported pain or discomfort was in the perineum, followed by pain or discomfort in the suprapubic area. Over half of the men had pain or discomfort during or after sexual climax (ejaculatory pain may be the most discriminatory symptom). A recent analysis of an international cohort of 1563 CP/CPPS patients was undertaken by Wagenlehner and colleagues (2013) to determine the prevalence and impact of pain locations and types to improve the strategy of individualized phenotypically guided treatment. This assessment confirmed that perineal pain or discomfort was the most prevalent pain symptom (63%), followed by testicular pain (58%), pain in the pubic area (42%), and pain in the penis (32%); reports of pain during ejaculation and voiding were 45% and 43%, respectively. Further study of this cohort showed that pain has more impact on quality of life than urinary symptoms; pain severity and frequency are more important than pain localization or type.

By definition, the syndrome becomes chronic after 3 months' duration. The symptoms tend to wax and wane over time; approximately one third of patients improve over 1 year (usually patients with a shorter duration of illness and fewer symptoms) (Nickel et al, 2002; Turner et al, 2004b; Propert et al, 2006b). An age-matched case-control study of risk factors in men with CP/CPPS (Pontari et al, 2005) showed that compared with asymptomatic controls, men with CP/CPPS reported a significantly greater lifetime prevalence of nonspecific urethritis (12% vs. 4%), cardiovascular disease (11% vs. 2%), neurologic disease (41% vs. 14%), psychiatric conditions (29% vs. 11%), and blood or infectious disease (41% vs. 20%).

The impact of this condition on health status is significant. The quality of life of many patients diagnosed with CP/CPPS is greatly diminished. Wenninger and associates (1996), employing a generic health status measure, the Sickness Impact Profile, showed that the mean scores were within the range of scores reported in the literature for patients with a history of myocardial infarction, angina, or Crohn disease. McNaughton Collins and coworkers

(2001b) employed similar quality-of-life assessment instruments in the NIH Chronic Prostatitis Cohort Study of almost 300 patients and confirmed this finding. These investigators noted that the mental health component was affected more than the physical component of the quality-of-life assessment. CP/CPPS patients' quality of life was lower than that observed in the most severely ill subgroups of men with congestive heart failure and diabetes mellitus. This significant impact on quality of life has also been reported in a cohort of CP/CPPS patients evaluated in a primary care setting (Turner et al, 2002). Patients with a diagnosis of CP/CPPS may have depression (Tripp et al, 2005, 2006), stress (Ulrich et al, 2005), or a history of abuse (sexual, physical, or emotional) (Hu et al, 2007). Depression, maladaptive coping techniques (e.g., catastrophizing and pain-contingent resting) and poor social support are associated with a poorer quality of life (Nickel et al, 2008c).

Category IV: Asymptomatic Inflammatory Prostatitis

Category IV, asymptomatic inflammatory prostatitis, by definition does not cause symptoms. The patients have BPH, an elevated PSA level, prostate cancer, or infertility. Subsequent microscopy of EPS or semen and/or histologic examination of BPH tissue, prostate cancer specimens, or prostate biopsy specimens disclose evidence of prostatic inflammation.

Evaluation
Symptom Assessment

For CP/CPPS, which is defined primarily by its symptom complex, analysis of specific prostatitis-like symptoms, the quality of life, the patient's functional status, and the patient's satisfaction with medical care will result in not only better evaluation of the prostatitis patient but also improved therapeutic follow-up. Scientifically validated symptom indices not only improve the care of patients but also optimize clinical decision making in terms of comparing clinical trial outcomes. Since the early 1990s, several different symptom indices have been described in clinical research (Neal and Moon, 1994; Krieger et al, 1996a; Nickel and Sorensen, 1996; Brahler et al, 1997; Chiang et al, 1997) and have been sporadically employed in clinical practice (McNaughton Collins and O'Leary, 1999). Although each of these symptom indices was successful at the time it was developed for the specific purpose or study, none was believed to be ideal for use in general research or clinical practice because they were not validated according to the rigorous standards that now must be met for an accepted urologic disease-specific index (O'Leary et al, 1992).

The NIH Chronic Prostatitis Collaborative Research Network (CPCRN) developed a reproducible and valid instrument to measure the symptoms and quality of life of patients with CP for use in research protocols as well as clinical practice (Litwin et al, 1999). The steps followed in the development of the NIH–Chronic Prostatitis Symptom Index (NIH-CPSI) included a systematic literature review, focus groups, cognitive testing, an expert panel review, a validation test, and psychometric analyses. **The final CPSI consists of nine questions that address the three most important domains of the CP experience. Pain (which is the primary symptom of CP/CPPS) was captured in four questions that focused on its location, severity, and frequency. Urinary function, the second most important component of patients' symptoms, was captured in two questions, one concerning storage (irritative) and the other voiding (obstructive) function. The quality of life or impact was captured in three additional questions that asked about the effect of symptoms on daily activities. The NIH-CPSI** (Fig. 13-3) **has now been accepted by the international prostatitis research community as an accepted outcome measure** (Nickel et al, 1999d) **and has shown validity and responsiveness in primary care samples** (Turner et al, 2003) **and clinical trials** (Propert et al, 2006a). It has been translated and validated in many languages other than English (Collins et al, 2001; Kunishima et al, 2002; Leskinen et al, 2003a; Schneider et al, 2004; Karakiewicz

NIH-Chronic Prostatitis Symptom Index (NIH-CPSI)

Pain or Discomfort

1. In the last week, have you experienced any pain or discomfort in the following areas?

	Yes	No
a. Area between rectum and testicles (perineum)	❏ 1	❏ 0
b. Testicles	❏ 1	❏ 0
c. Tip of the penis (not related to urination)	❏ 1	❏ 0
d. Below your waist, in your pubic or bladder area	❏ 1	❏ 0

2. In the last week, have you experienced:

	Yes	No
a. Pain or burning during urination?	❏ 1	❏ 0
b. Pain or discomfort during or after sexual climax (ejaculation)?	❏ 1	❏ 0

3. How often have you had pain or discomfort in any of these areas over the last week?

❏ 0 Never
❏ 1 Rarely
❏ 2 Sometimes
❏ 3 Often
❏ 4 Usually
❏ 5 Always

4. Which number best describes your AVERAGE pain or discomfort on the days that you had it, over the last week?

❏	❏	❏	❏	❏	❏	❏	❏	❏	❏	❏
0	1	2	3	4	5	6	7	8	9	10

NO PAIN · · · PAIN AS BAD AS YOU CAN IMAGINE

Urination

5. How often have you had a sensation of not emptying your bladder completely after you finished urinating, over the last week?

❏ 0 Not at all
❏ 1 Less than 1 time in 5
❏ 2 Less than half the time
❏ 3 About half the time
❏ 4 More than half the time
❏ 5 Almost always

6. How often have you had to urinate again less than two hours after you finished urinating, over the last week?

❏ 0 Not at all
❏ 1 Less than 1 time in 5
❏ 2 Less than half the time
❏ 3 About half the time
❏ 4 More than half the time
❏ 5 Almost always

Impact of Symptoms

7. How much have your symptoms kept you from doing the kinds of things you would usually do, over the last week?

❏ 0 None
❏ 1 Only a little
❏ 2 Some
❏ 3 A lot

8. How much did you think about your symptoms, over the last week?

❏ 0 None
❏ 1 Only a little
❏ 2 Some
❏ 3 A lot

Quality of Life

9. If you were to spend the rest of your life with your symptoms just the way they have been during the last week, how would you feel about that?

❏ 0 Delighted
❏ 1 Pleased
❏ 2 Mostly satisfied
❏ 3 Mixed (about equally satisfied and dissatisfied)
❏ 4 Mostly dissatisfied
❏ 5 Unhappy
❏ 6 Terrible

Scoring the NIH-Chronic Prostatitis Symptom Index Domains

Pain: Total of items 1a, 1b, 1c, 1d, 2a, 2b, 3, and 4 = ____

Urinary Symptoms: Total of items 5 and 6 = ____

Quality of Life Impact: Total of items 7, 8, and 9 = ____

Figure 13-3. The National Institutes of Health Chronic Prostatitis Symptom Index (NIH-CPSI) captures the three most important domains of the prostatitis experience: pain (location, frequency, and severity), voiding (irritative and obstructive symptoms), and quality of life (including impact). This index is useful in research studies and clinical practice. (From Litwin MS, McNaughton Collins M, Fowler FJ, et al. The NIH Chronic Prostatitis Symptom Index [NIH-CPSI]: development and validation of a new outcome measure. J Urol 1999;162:369–75.)

et al, 2005). The symptom index has also proved its usefulness in the evaluation and follow-up of patients in general clinical urologic practice (Nickel, 1999d; Nickel et al, 2001c). Cut-off levels for pain severity categories were mild, 0 to 3; moderate, 4 to 6; and severe, 7 to 10 for CPSI item 4 (0 to 10); CPSI pain domain (0 to 21) scores were mild, 0 to 7; moderate, 8 to 13; and severe, 14 to 21 (Wagenlehner et al, 2013).

KEY POINT: SYMPTOM ASSESSMENT

- The validated National Institutes of Health Chronic Prostatitis Symptom Index (NIH-CPSI) is a useful research and clinical tool for evaluating chronic prostatitis and chronic pelvic pain syndrome patients.

Physical Examination

Physical examination is an important part of the evaluation of a patient with prostatitis, and although not confirmatory in making a definitive diagnosis, it is very helpful in further classifying the disorder and even directing therapy. It assists in ruling out other perineal, anal, neurologic, pelvic, or prostate abnormalities and is an integral part of the lower urinary tract evaluation by providing prostate-specific specimens (Nickel, 2002a).

In **category I**, acute bacterial prostatitis, the patient may be systemically toxic—that is, flushed, febrile, tachycardic, tachypneic, and even hypotensive. The patient usually has suprapubic discomfort and perhaps has clinically detectable acute urinary retention. Perineal pain and anal sphincter spasm may complicate the digital rectal examination. The prostate itself is usually described as hot, boggy, and exquisitely tender. The expression of prostatic fluid is believed to be totally unnecessary and perhaps even harmful.

The physical examination of a patient with **category II**, chronic bacterial prostatitis, and **category III** CPPS is usually unremarkable (except for pain). Careful examination and palpation of external genitalia, groin, perineum, coccyx, external anal sphincter (tone), and internal pelvic floor and side walls may pinpoint prominent areas of pain or discomfort (Shoskes et al, 2008; Anderson et al, 2009b). The findings of pelvic floor dysfunction and spastic pain, myofascial pain, or painful trigger points has significant implications for developing treatment plans. **The digital rectal examination should be performed after the patient has produced preprostatic massage urine specimens (see later) and after the perineal and pelvic examination. The prostate may be normal in size and consistency, and it has also been described as enlarged and boggy (loosely defined by me as softer than normal). The degree of elicited pain during prostatic palpation is variable and is unhelpful in differentiating a prostatitis syndrome.** The prostate should be carefully checked for prostatic nodules before a vigorous prostatic massage is performed to produce prostate-specific specimens (EPS and post–prostatic massage urine sample).

Lower Urinary Tract Cytologic Examination and Culture Techniques. In patients with category I, acute bacterial prostatitis, a urine culture is the only laboratory evaluation of the lower urinary tract required. It has been suggested that the vigorous prostatic massage necessary to produce EPS can exacerbate the clinical situation, although such fears have never been substantiated in the literature. A midstream urine specimen will show significant leukocytosis and bacteriuria microscopically, and culturing usually discloses typical uropathogens. Blood cultures may show the same organism.

In 1968, Meares and Stamey described the classic four-glass urine collection technique to distinguish urethral, bladder, and prostate infections in men with CP, and for three decades this has remained the gold standard for the evaluation of this lower urinary tract syndrome. The voided bladder–1 (VB1) specimen includes the first 10 mL of urine and represents the urethral specimen. The voided bladder–2 (VB2) specimen is similar to a midstream urine collection and represents the bladder urine. EPS should be collected directly into a sterile container during prostatic massage. The voided bladder–3 (VB3) specimen, the first 10 mL of urine voided after prostatic massage, includes any EPS trapped in the prostatic urethra. All four specimens are to be sent to the clinical microbiology laboratory for quantitative culture. Aliquots of the three urine specimens are centrifuged for 5 minutes and the sediment examined under high power for leukocytes (including aggregates of leukocytes), macrophages, oval fat bodies, erythrocytes, bacteria, and fungal hyphae. A wet mount of a drop of EPS can be examined under a coverslip in a similar manner. Some researchers (Muller et al, 2001; Krieger et al, 2003) point out that quantitative determination of the EPS WBC concentration by a counting chamber method is superior to the standard wet mount method but probably only indicated in research studies. In fact, the NIH Chronic Prostatitis Cohort Study (Schaeffer et al, 2002; Nickel et al, 2003a) suggested that leukocyte determination did not appear to add significant clinical information to the assessment of a patient with CP/CPPS.

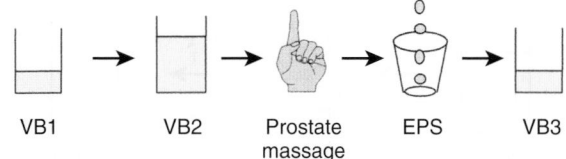

4-Glass Test (Meares-Stamey Test)

Classification	Specimen	VB1	VB2	EPS	VB3
CAT II	WBC	–	+/–*	+	+
	Culture	–	+/–*	+	+
CAT IIIA	WBC	–	–	+	+
	Culture	–	–	–	–
CAT IIIB	WBC	–	–	–	–
	Culture	–	–	–	–

Figure 13-4. Technique and interpretation of the Meares-Stamey four-glass lower urinary tract localization test for chronic prostatitis and chronic pelvic pain syndrome. CAT, category; EPS, expressed prostatic secretion; VB, voided bladder; WBC, white blood cell.

Figure 13-4 illustrates the technique and interpretation of the four-glass test.

Category II, chronic bacterial prostatitis, is diagnosed if there is a 10-fold increase in bacteria in the EPS or VB3 specimen compared with the VB1 and VB2 specimens. In a patient who has acute cystitis this localization is impossible, and in this case the patient can be treated with a short course (1 to 3 days) of therapy with an antibiotic such as nitrofurantoin, which penetrates the prostate poorly but eradicates the bladder bacteriuria. Subsequent localization of bacteria in the post–prostatic massage urine or EPS is then diagnostic of category II prostatitis. Category IIIA CP/CPPS is diagnosed when no uropathogenic bacteria are cultured, but excessive leukocytosis (usually defined as more than 5 to 10 WBCs per high-power field [HPF]) is noted in the prostate-specific specimens (EPS or VB3 or both). Category IIIB CP/CPPS is diagnosed when no uropathogenic bacteria are cultured and there is no significant leukocytosis noted on microscopic examination of EPS or the sediment of VB3.

Although the four-glass test remains the gold standard diagnostic evaluation of prostatitis patients, numerous surveys (Moon, 1997; Nickel et al, 1998a; McNaughton Collins and O'Leary, 1999; McNaughton Collins et al, 2000a) have confirmed that clinicians have more or less abandoned this time-consuming and expensive rigorous evaluation. **The pre-massage and post-massage test (or two-glass test), originally suggested by Weidner and Ebner** (1985) **and popularized by Nickel** (1995, 1996, 1997a), **is a simple, cost-effective screen to categorize patients with CP.** The patient provides a midstream pre-massage urine specimen and a urine specimen (initial 10 mL) after prostatic massage. Microscopy (sediment) and culturing of these two screening urine specimens allows categorization of the majority of patients with a CP syndrome. Figure 13-5 illustrates the technique and interpretation of the two-glass pre-massage and post-massage test.

In a retrospective personal series and a review of series in the literature, Nickel (1997a) noted that this test had 91% sensitivity and specificity compared with the gold standard Meares-Stamey test. Its limitations were thought to be the result of the exclusion of the urethral and EPS specimen. However, in patients without clinical urethritis, Krieger and associates (2000) demonstrated that urethral swabs are more efficient in picking up urethral inflammation than the VB1 specimen. But in this series of 235 patients, only 3% had more than 1 WBC/HPF. Therefore the urethral specimens rarely resulted in detection of significant urethral inflammation, and in this series rarely did cultured organisms change the direction of clinical therapy in patients with prostatitis (without clinical urethritis). In the same study (Krieger et al, 2000) comparing EPS with post–prostatic massage urine, the investigators demonstrated that EPS examination detected 76%, whereas post-massage urine

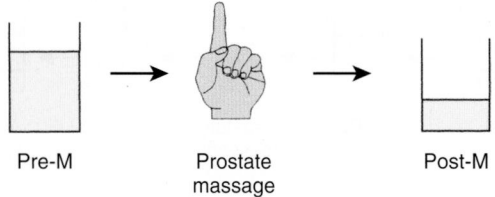

Pre-M → Prostate massage → Post-M

2-Glass Test (PPMT)

Classification	Specimen	Pre-M	Post-M
CAT II	WBC	+/–*	+
	Culture	+/–*	+
CAT IIIA	WBC	–	+
	Culture	–	–
CAT IIIB	WBC	–	–
	Culture	–	–

Figure 13-5. Technique and interpretation of the pre- and post-massage two-glass lower urinary tract localization test for chronic prostatitis and chronic pelvic pain syndrome. CAT, category; PPMT, pre- and post-massage test; WBC, white blood cell.

examination detected 82% of the patients who had inflammation on one or both tests. Ludwig and associates (2000), in a series of 328 patients in whom both EPS and a VB3 specimen were obtained, demonstrated that VB3 is almost as accurate as EPS (92% sensitivity; 99% specificity) in detecting prostate-specific inflammation. Seiler and associates (2003) came to the same conclusion in their study of 143 CP patients. Nickel and colleagues from the NIH CPCRN examined a cohort of 353 CP/CPPS men with complete four-glass data and noted that the two-glass test predicted a positive four-glass result with clinically acceptable accuracy (over 95% of men would have had the same diagnosis if the four-glass test were performed) (Nickel et al, 2006). This test, however, is only a screening test, and in patients in whom it is important to localize bacteria to the prostate versus the urethra (e.g., patients with recurrent UTIs, suspicion of urethral abnormality), a follow-up VB1 specimen or urethral swab may be very helpful. If typical urethral organisms are localized to the prostate when the pre-massage and post-massage test is used and the clinician is inclined to consider them pathogenic and subsequently treat the patients, urethral and EPS specimens to definitively localize the specific bacteria to the prostate are appropriate. As a general rule, it is always best to examine the EPS (if obtainable) microscopically.

The significance and diagnostic value of semen analysis in chronic bacterial prostatitis have been extensively debated and remain controversial. In a small study of 70 men with CP and 17 asymptomatic controls, Zegarra Montes and colleagues (2008) concluded that although a positive semen culture in a symptomatic patient may be useful to make a decision to start antibiotic treatment, a negative culture does not rule out the condition. Segmented lower urinary tract urine specimens are required for a definitive diagnosis. Data analyzed by Magri and associates (2009), in which 696 symptomatic patients were subjected to a four-glass test followed by semen culture and analysis, support the usefulness of semen analysis in the diagnostic workup of prostatitis patients but only when this test is used to complement the four-glass Meares and Stamey test.

> **KEY POINT: LOWER URINARY TRACT CULTURE TECHNIQUE**
>
> - The two-glass pre- and post-massage test is a simple, useful screen for inflammation and infection of the lower urinary tract in patients with chronic prostatitis.

Microbiologic Considerations

The Prostatitis Syndrome classification system depends on culturing for standard uropathogens. The Enterobacteriaceae (e.g., *E. coli, Serratia, Klebsiella, Proteus, Pseudomonas*) represent the most common uropathogens, followed by gram-positive enterococci. However, as discussed earlier in the section on etiology, other gram-positive organisms that typically colonize the urethra (*Staphylococcus epidermidis, S. saprophyticus, Streptococcus* species, *Corynebacterium*, and *Bacteroides*) can be localized to prostate specimens, including semen (>10-fold colony-forming unit count in prostate-specific specimens compared with pre–prostatic massage specimens), and their association with the prostatic inflammation symptom complex remains unclear. At this time, these patients are still considered to have category III CP/CPPS, but this may change as more research results become available and the current understanding of bacterial pathogenicity in the prostate gland evolves (Nickel and Moon, 2005; Nickel and Xiang, 2008). In patients with acute prostatitis, a blood culture should be considered, particularly if the patient has signs and symptoms of systemic infection (Etienne et al, 2010).

Cytologic Considerations

The differentiation of the two subtypes of category III CP/CPPS depends on cytologic examination of the urine or EPS or both. The urine specimens are centrifuged for 5 minutes; the sediment is resuspended under a coverslip and examined at high power (×300 to ×400), and the wet mount of a drop of EPS is examined under a coverslip at the same power. WBCs have traditionally been reported as numbers of leukocytes per high-power field (Fig. 13-6). **There is no validated cutoff point for the level of WBCs per high-power field that is required to differentiate an inflammatory from a noninflammatory CP/CPPS. Although the suggested limits have ranged from as low as 2 (Anderson and Weller, 1979) to as high as 20 (Blacklock and Beavis, 1978), the consensus appears to favor 5 to 10 WBCs/HPF in EPS as the upper level of normal** (Meares and Stamey, 1968; Pfau et al, 1978; Schaeffer et al, 1981). But inflammatory cells in the EPS fluctuate over time (Anderson and Weller, 1979; Schaeffer et al, 1981) and with the frequency of ejaculation (Jameson, 1967; Yavascaoglu et al, 1999). A disadvantage of looking at a drop of prostatic fluid or urine sediment is that the cells may clump or aggregate, which renders quantifying them virtually impossible. Also, an unstained specimen does not allow differentiation of the types of WBCs present (e.g., polymorphonuclear leukocytes, lymphocytes, monocytes, macrophages). If accuracy is required (e.g., for research), then the WBCs can be counted in a glass hemacytometer (so they may be quantified as cells per square millimeter) and subsequently stained to differentiate the inflammatory cell subtype (Anderson and Weller, 1979).

The clinical relevance of adding cytologic examination of semen specimens (which is difficult without special staining techniques) is unknown. Certainly, semen examination increases the percentage of patients identified as having inflammatory category IIIA CP/CPPS (Krieger et al, 2000).

Nickel and colleagues (2003a) compared the number of WBCs in the EPS in patients with CP/CPPS with the number in EPS specimens from normal asymptomatic control men and noted that although there was a statistically significant difference in WBC counts in the CP/CPPS men, the clinical significance was not apparent (i.e., 50% of CPPS men had >5 WBCs/HPF compared with 40% of control men). The relevance of examining urine and EPS for white cells in routine clinical practice has been challenged (Nickel et al, 2003a). In fact, **my colleagues and I have not been able to confirm the association between histologically proven prostate inflammation and prostatitis symptoms** (Nickel et al, 2007), **further confusing the issue of whether it is necessary to determine prostate-specific specimen inflammation,** which is really just a surrogate for prostate inflammation. However, some investigators (Nickel, 2002b) have recommended that a separate aliquot of urine be examined cytologically for malignant cells, particularly

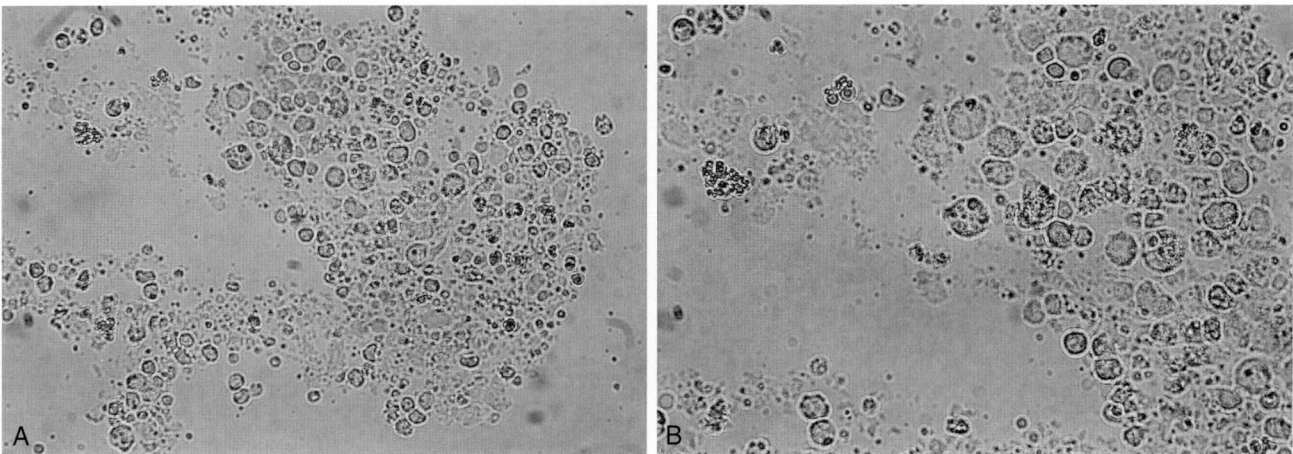

Figure 13-6. A and B, Unstained photomicrographs showing individual white blood cells, clumps of white blood cells, and lipid-laden macrophages in the expressed prostatic secretion of a patient with category IIIA chronic pelvic pain syndrome (**A**, ×250; **B**, ×400).

if the symptom complex includes storage urinary symptoms, dysuria, and/or suprapubic or bladder pain.

Urodynamics

Pain is the dominant symptom in patients with CP/CPPS, but a wide constellation of storage and voiding symptoms is associated with this syndrome. Proposed causes to account for the persistent urinary symptoms include detrusor vesical neck or external sphincter dyssynergia, proximal or distal urethral obstruction, and fibrosis or hypertrophy of the vesical neck (Blacklock, 1974; Bates et al, 1975; Orland et al, 1985; Blacklock, 1986; Theodorou et al, 1999). These abnormalities can often be clarified and diagnosed by urodynamics, particularly video-urodynamics. Others have suggested that men with defined primary voiding dysfunction have been misdiagnosed with CP (Webster et al, 1980; Siroky et al, 1981; Murnaghan and Millard, 1984). Siroky and associates (1981) noted that urodynamics revealed that 50% of 47 men with recurrent urinary symptoms, perigenital pain, or both who had previously been diagnosed as having CP had bladder acontractility during a study with nonrelaxing perineal floor (striated muscle spasm) and that another 36% had detrusor overactivity with appropriate striated sphincter relaxation. Barbalias (1990) and Barbalias and colleagues (1983) noted decreased peak and mean urinary flow rates, a significantly elevated maximal urethral closing pressure, and incomplete funneling of the bladder neck accompanied by urethral narrowing at the level of the external urinary sphincter during voiding with urodynamic evaluation of men diagnosed with CP. Hellstrom and colleagues (1987) also noted elevated urethral pressures, "hyperreflexia" of the external urethral sphincter, and intraprostatic reflux in three patients with unremitting symptoms of chronic nonbacterial prostatitis.

Kaplan and associates (1994, 1996, 1997) postulated that chronic lower urinary tract symptoms in young men are often misdiagnosed as chronic nonbacterial prostatitis when in fact they indicate a cohort of men with undiagnosed chronic voiding dysfunction. This conclusion is based on the video-urodynamic studies of 137 consecutive men 50 years of age or younger diagnosed with CP that did not respond to standard therapy (Kaplan et al, 1996). These researchers demonstrated a variety of urodynamic abnormalities in this selected population, including 54% of patients with primary vesical neck obstruction, 24% with functional obstruction localized to the membranous urethra (pseudodyssynergia), 17% with impaired bladder contractility, and 5% with an acontractile bladder. They noted detrusor overactivity in 49% of the men. Simple documentation of uroflowmetry and residual urine bladder scan abnormalities may suggest proceeding to more sophisticated urodynamics (Ghobish, 2000). Other groups dispute the benefits

of urodynamics and have noted very few urodynamic abnormalities in the typical patients with classic CP symptoms (Mayo et al, 1998).

Endoscopy

Clinical experience (rather than controlled clinical studies) suggests that lower urinary tract endoscopy (i.e., cystoscopy) is not indicated in the majority of men with CP/CPPS. However, cystoscopy is indicated in patients in whom the history (e.g., hematuria), lower urinary tract evaluation (e.g., VB1 urinalysis), or ancillary studies (e.g., urodynamics) indicate the possibility of a diagnosis other than CP/CPPS. In these patients, lower urinary tract malignancy, stones, urethral strictures, bladder neck abnormalities, and other lower urinary tract abnormalities that can be surgically corrected occasionally are discovered. Cystoscopy can probably be justified in men whose condition is refractory to standard therapy.

Ultrasonography

Transrectal ultrasonography has become one of the best radiologic methods to evaluate prostate disease and has become an especially helpful clinical tool for the assessment of prostate volume and ultrasound guidance of biopsy needles. **The diagnostic value of ultrasonography in differentiating benign from malignant prostate disease is controversial, and the further differentiation of the various benign conditions of the prostate is even more so.** Di Trapani and colleagues (1988) described inhomogeneous echo structures, constant dilatation of periprostatic venous plexus, elongated seminal vesicles, and thickening of the inner septa in patients with prostatitis. Doble and Carter (1989) described seven ultrasound signs associated with the presence of symptoms of CP compared with controls, and although the sensitivity increased with higher leukocyte counts, the signs were not sufficiently specific to differentiate clinical groups.

Peeling and Griffiths (1984) described the heterogeneity of the echo pattern and prostatic calculi as ultrasound features related to prostatitis. Ludwig and coworkers (1994) described the ultrasound features such as prostatic calcifications and seminal vesicle abnormalities that appear to be indicative of signs of inflammation but not proof of the presence of CP. Harada and associates (1980) concluded that the presence of stones is not related to a specific prostate disease process. De la Rosette and colleagues (1992b) performed ultrasonography in 22 patients with nonbacterial prostatitis and compared the results with those of a control group of 22 patients without lower urinary tract symptoms. This study indicated that there were no significant differences in ultrasound patterns of patients with nonbacterial prostatitis and the control group.

Others have employed color Doppler ultrasonography (Veneziano et al, 1995) and automated computer analysis (de la Rosette et al, 1995) in an attempt to improve the value of transrectal ultrasonography in the evaluation of prostatitis patients; however, the results are not conclusive enough to indicate that this is a clinically useful tool.

Transrectal ultrasonography can be valuable in diagnosing medial prostatic cysts in patients with prostatitis-like symptoms (Dik et al, 1996), **diagnosing and draining prostatic abscesses** (Granados et al, 1992), **or diagnosing and draining obstructed seminal vesicles** (Littrup et al, 1988). It is not required in all cases of acute bacterial prostatitis but rather only in those patients in whom appropriate antimicrobial therapy is failing (Horcajada et al, 2003).

Transabdominal (Khorasani et al, 2012) and pelvic floor (Davis et al, 2011) ultrasound have been suggested as modalities that could be used in assessing pelvic floor mobility; however, their use has not been standardized to a point at which it could be recommended in clinical practice.

Prostate Biopsy

Occasionally, because of an elevated PSA level or abnormal digital rectal examination findings, prostate biopsy is indicated (Kawakami et al, 2004). Some clinicians will consider starting patients with elevated screening PSA levels and a history of prostatitis or symptoms of CPPS on antibiotics, but this practice is reasonable only in patients with acute or chronic bacterial prostatitis (Nickel, 2002e), conditions that invariably lead to elevated PSA levels. The diagnosis of CP/CPPS should be used only as a reason against a prostate biopsy if the clinician is looking for an excuse not to perform a biopsy (Nickel, 2002e). Antimicrobial or anti-inflammatory treatment of category IV asymptomatic prostatitis detected on biopsy in men with elevated PSA is controversial, and no evidence-based recommendations can be made. Reviews on PSA and prostatitis are available (Kawakami et al, 2004, Hochreiter, 2008, Sandhu, 2009).

Out of desperation, urologists sometimes resort to prostate biopsy in an attempt either to demonstrate histologic evidence of prostatic inflammation or to culture an organism that cannot be cultured with the standard approach. The importance and interpretation of prostate biopsies in prostatitis performed for reasons other than prostate cancer screening are unclear. Doble and associates (1990) demonstrated immune complexes in the prostates of patients with prostatitis but found culture of the prostatic tissue unhelpful (Doble et al, 1989a). Nickel and Costerton (1993) were able to confirm the presence of potentially uropathogenic bacteria in patients with a documented history of chronic bacterial prostatitis in which EPS cultures became sterile after antibiotic therapy. Berger and associates (1997) also confirmed the presence of potential uropathogenic bacteria in prostate biopsy specimens (which correlated to some extent with prostatic inflammation in EPS) in patients in whom the same bacteria did not grow in standard prostatic specimens (e.g., EPS). Krieger and colleagues (1996b) demonstrated the possible presence of microorganisms in the prostate glands of a majority of men with CP syndrome through use of the molecular biologic technique of PCR. **At this time, histologic, culture, and molecular biologic evaluations of prostate biopsy specimens in patients with CP/CPPS remain research tools only.**

Evaluation of Suspected Seminal Vesiculitis

Occasionally, seminal vesiculitis can occur as a consequence of local bacterial infection in acute and chronic bacterial prostatitis (Zeitlin, 1999), and patients can develop seminal vesicle abscesses (Stearns, 1963; Kennelly and Oesterling, 1989). Seminal vesicle abscesses were traditionally diagnosed clinically by a positive ejaculate culture and seminal vesiculography (Dunnick et al, 1982; Baert et al, 1986) but are now imaged with computed tomography (Patel and Wilbur, 1987), transrectal ultrasonography (Littrup et al, 1988), magnetic resonance imaging (MRI) (Sue et al, 1989), or recently with

technetium-99m ciprofloxacin radioisotope scan (Choe et al, 2003).

Other Potential Markers

Wishnow and associates (1982) found that control patients (10 patients) and men with chronic abacterial prostatitis (4 patients) had no antibodies to gram-negative bacterial antigens, in contrast to men with bacterial prostatitis (6 patients). They hypothesized that immunologic analysis may provide a better diagnostic tool than culturing and microscopy. Shortliffe and coworkers (1981a, 1981b, 1986, 1989, 1992) found that the total IgA and IgG levels in the prostatic fluid in men with chronic abacterial prostatitis were higher than those in controls. They also discovered that prostatic fluid from control or abacterial prostatitis patients did not contain specific antibodies to gram-negative urinary pathogens (in contrast to men with bacterial prostatitis). Nickel and colleagues (2001b) used a similar antibody screening procedure in evaluation of 102 men with CP/CPPS who were subsequently treated with quinolone antibiotics. However, "antibody-positive" patients did not have a better response to antibiotic therapy than "antibody-negative" patients after 12 weeks of therapy. Li and associates (2001) demonstrated increased endotoxin concentrations in EPS and VB3 of men with bacterial prostatitis and inflammatory category IIIA CPPS and suggested that endotoxin levels might be used to identify these categories of patients with CP.

Alexander and colleagues (1998) discovered that men with chronic abacterial prostatitis had higher mean levels of the pro-inflammatory cytokines IL-1α and TNF-α in seminal plasma compared with controls. Ruggieri and coworkers (2000) noted that levels of both IL-1α and IL-8 were significantly higher in semen in category IIIA patients (leukocytes) than in category IIIB patients, but there was no statistically significant difference in levels of TNF-α, IL-1α, or IL-6. This group found no correlation between cytokine levels and the number of leukocytes in EPS. The increased IL-8 levels in the semen of patients with prostatitis symptoms was confirmed by Khadra and coworkers (2006) and Penna and associates (2007), suggesting that this could be a surrogate marker for CP/CPPS. Nadler and colleagues (2000) found that mean levels of IL-1α in EPS were higher in men with inflammatory chronic abacterial prostatitis and noninflammatory chronic bacterial prostatitis compared with controls. Hochreiter and associates (2000a) did find a direct significant correlation between the number of leukocytes in EPS and IL-1α levels in EPS. **One of the most intriguing possible biomarkers includes monocyte chemoattractant protein–1 and macrophage inflammatory protein–1α detected in EPS. Both of these chemokines are elevated in category IIIA and IIIB CP/CPPS, and macrophage inflammatory protein–1α may be a further marker for clinical pain in these patients** (Desireddi et al, 2008). The sensitivity, specificity, and, more important, the clinical applicability of all these immunologic tests is really unknown, and none of them is yet indicated in clinical practice.

Marmar and associates (1980) hypothesized that zinc levels in EPS would be a useful marker for prostatitis and found that, indeed, zinc levels in men with chronic abacterial prostatitis and bacterial prostatitis were significantly lower than zinc levels in control patients and men with prostatodynia. However, Zaichick and colleagues (1996) found no differences in zinc levels between patients with chronic abacterial prostatitis, those with BPH, and controls. At this time the measurement of zinc levels in prostatic or semen specimens is clinically unhelpful.

Tanner and associates (1999) detected positive signals (rRNA-based molecular technique with prostatic fluid) in 65% of patients with CP. The condition of 7 of 11 patients with bacterial signals but none of 6 patients without bacterial signals was improved on antibiotic therapy. The same group (Shoskes and Shahed, 2000) subsequently confirmed this finding with a larger cohort of patients. These results are intriguing, and controlled studies evaluating the potential clinical significance of differentiating patients based on molecular biologic techniques are required.

An Approach to Diagnosis and Classification

A diagnostic algorithm that provides a practical approach to the workup of the majority of men with CP/CPPS is shown in Figure 13-7. Box 13-1 shows the tests recently recommended by the ICUD Guidelines for Male LUTS (Nickel et al, 2013b).

Phenotype Assessment in Chronic Prostatitis and Chronic Pelvic Pain Syndrome

Researchers and clinicians have become aware that patients with urologic CPPS, such as CP/CPPS, are not a homogeneous group of patients with identical causative mechanisms, genitourinary pain, urinary symptoms, and/or psychosexual problems but rather a heterogeneous group of individual patients with widely differing clinical phenotypes. This realization led the NIH to fund the Multidisciplinary Approach to the Study of Chronic Pelvic Pain (MAPP) study group (www.mappnetwork.org) to explore basic science (particularly biomarker and causative studies) and epidemiology to

---

KEY POINTS: LOWER URINARY TRACT EVALUATION

- Mandatory evaluation includes history-taking, physical examination, urinalysis, and urine culture.
- Recommended evaluation includes lower urinary tract localization test, National Institutes of Health Chronic Prostatitis Symptom Index (NIH-CPSI), sexual functioning assessment, flow rate, residual urine determination, and urine cytology.

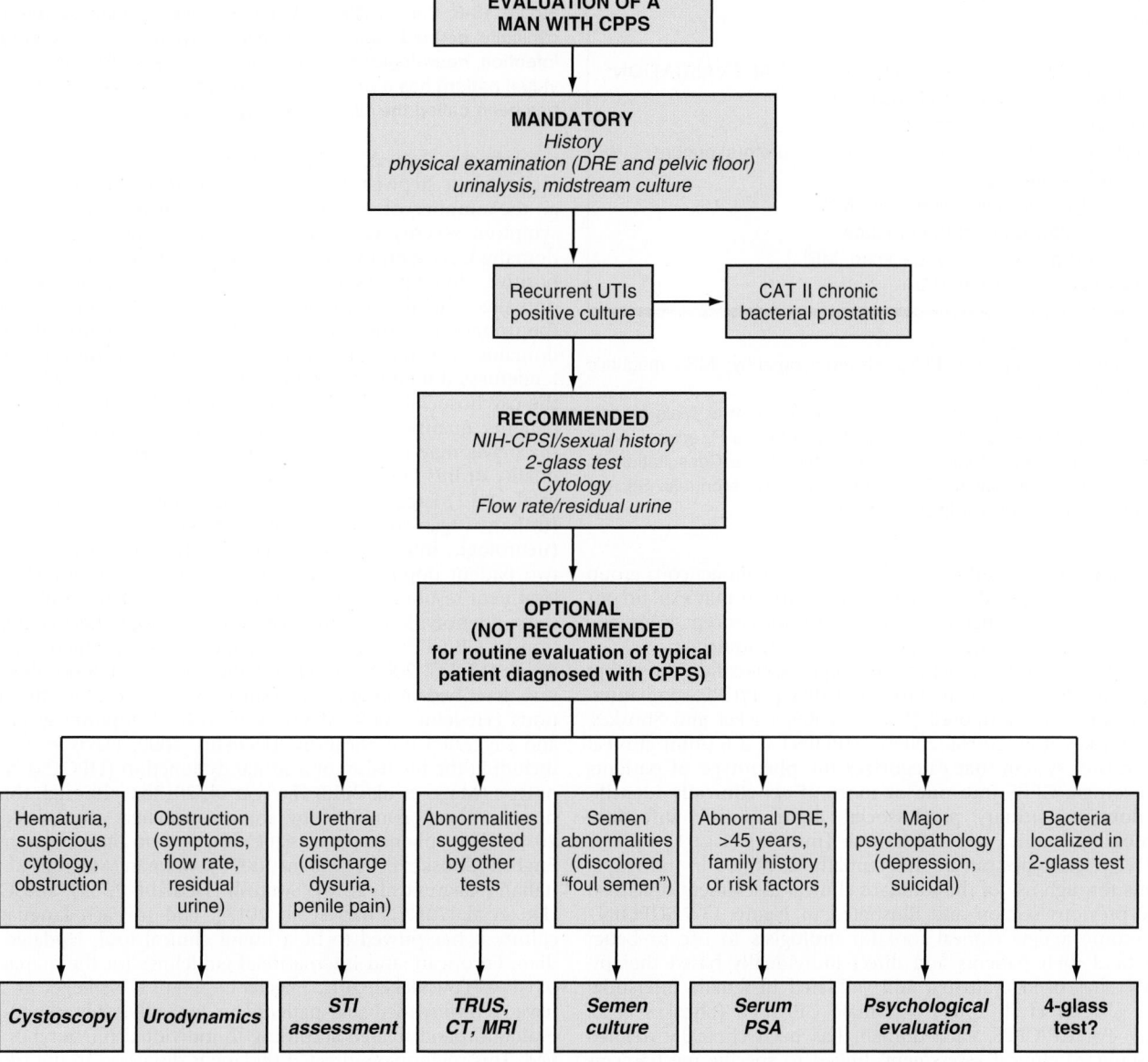

Figure 13-7. A suggested diagnostic algorithm from the 2012 International Consultation on Urological Diseases (ICUD) recommendations for the evaluation of patients with chronic prostatitis and chronic pelvic pain syndrome (CPPS). CAT, category; CT, computed tomography; DRE, digital rectal examination; MRI, magnetic resonance imaging; NIH-CPSI, National Institutes of Health Chronic Prostatitis Symptom Index; PSA, prostate-specific antigen; STI, sexually transmitted infection; TRUS, transrectal ultrasonography; UTIs, urinary tract infections. (Modified from Nickel JC, Wagenlehner F, Pontari M, et al. Male chronic pelvic pain syndrome (CPPS). In: Chapple C, Abrams P, editors. Male lower urinary tract symptoms (LUTS). An International Consultation on Male LUTS, Fukuoka, Japan, Sept 30-Oct 4, 2012. Montreal: Société Internationale d'Urologie (SIU); 2013. p. 331–72.)

BOX 13-1 Evaluation of the Typical Man with Chronic Pelvic Pain Syndrome

MANDATORY

History

Physical examination, including digital rectal examination and pelvic floor assessment

Urinalysis and culture

RECOMMENDED

Two-glass lower urinary tract evaluation

Symptom inventory or index (National Institutes of Health Chronic Prostatitis Symptom Index [NIH-CPSI])

Sexual functioning assessment (questionnaire)

Flow rate

Residual urine determination

Urine cytology

NOT RECOMMENDED FOR ROUTINE INITIAL EVALUATION*

Four-glass lower urinary tract evaluation

Semen analysis and culture

Sexually transmitted infection evaluation or urethral culture

Pressure-flow studies

Video-urodynamics (including flow-EMG)

Transrectal ultrasound of the prostate

Pelvic imaging—ultrasound, CT scan, MRI

Prostate-specific antigen (PSA)

*Optional in selected patients.

CT, computed tomography; EMG, electromyography; MRI, magnetic resonance imaging.

Modified from Nickel JC, Wagenlehner F, Pontari M, et al. Male chronic pelvic pain syndrome (CPPS). In: Chapple C, Abrams P, editors. Male lower urinary tract symptoms (LUTS). An International Consultation on Male LUTS, Fukuoka, Japan, Sept 30-Oct 4, 2012. Montreal: Société Internationale d'Urologie (SIU); 2013. p. 331–72.

UPOINT: THE "SNOWFLAKE HYPOTHESIS"

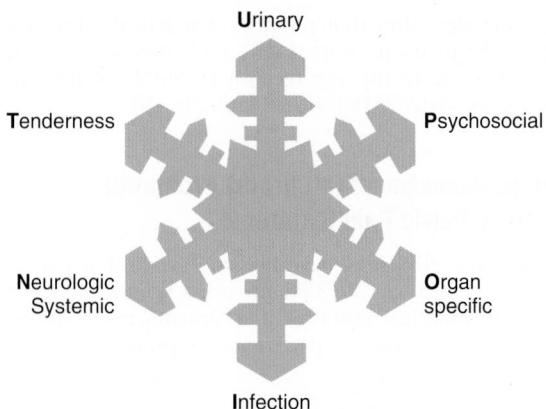

Figure 13-8. The UPOINT phenotypic classification system has six clinically defined domains (*u*rinary, *p*sychosocial, *o*rgan-specific, *i*nfection, *n*eurologic/systemic, and *t*enderness). Because each individual patient has a unique phenotype, the six-point UPOINT system has been called the "snowflake hypothesis."

better understand the differences in this very heterogeneous group of patients. It is hoped that "phenotyping" patients may explain our very inconsistent therapeutic results and that the concept eventually may be applicable to direct better management strategies.

In 2009, a clinically practical phenotyping classification system for patients diagnosed with urologic CPPS (CP/CPPS and interstitial cystitis) was proposed (Nickel, 2009; Nickel and Shoskes, 2009; Shoskes et al, 2009a, 2009b). **UPOINT is a 6-point clinical classification system that categorizes the phenotype of patients with urologic CPPS into one or more of six clinically identifiable domains: *u*rinary, *p*sychosocial, *o*rgan-specific, *i*nfection, *n*eurologic/systemic, and *t*enderness (muscle)** (Fig. 13-8). The UPOINT phenotypes can be differentially identified in individual patients through use of the standard clinical assessment described in the previous section and illustrated in Figure 13-7. UPOINT has become a new clinical tool for urologists to use to better understand their patients and direct individually based therapy. UPOINT has been evaluated and validated in female interstitial cystitis (Nickel et al, 2009) and male CP/CPPS (Shoskes et al, 2009a). For CP/CPPS, each domain has been clinically defined with standard clinical assessment, linked to specific mechanisms of symptom production or propagation, and associated with specific therapy (details described in the section on treatment).

In one study researchers determined the phenotype of a cohort of men with documented CP/CPPS through use of the UPOINT system and assessed the frequency of individual domains and their effect on symptom severity (Shoskes et al, 2009a). The percentages of patients positive for each domain were 52%, 34%, 61%, 16%, 37%, and 53% for the urinary, psychosocial, organ-specific, infection, neurologic/systemic, and tenderness domains,

respectively. Only 22% were positive for only one domain, and a significant stepwise increase was found in the total CPSI score as the number of positive domains increased (in other words, symptom severity was associated with the number of identified domains). As symptom duration increased, so did the number of positive domains (suggesting a phenotype progression). The domains with the most significant effect on symptoms included the urinary, psychosocial, organ-specific, and neurologic/systemic domains. For pain, the psychosocial, neurologic/systemic, and tenderness domains had significantly greater scores, whereas only the psychosocial and neurologic/systemic domains influenced the patients' quality of life. This suggests that domains active outside the pelvis may have the most profound effect on symptoms and quality of life. Further evaluation of CP/CPPS patients (Samplaski et al, 2012) suggests clustering of domains specific to the pelvis (urinary, organ-specific, and tenderness) versus systemic domains (neurologic, infection, and psychosocial). This perspective implies two patient populations that may differ in pathophysiology and treatment response. It is postulated that identifying and managing these phenotypic domains may result in more effective amelioration of CP/CPPS symptoms and greater improvement in quality of life (Nickel, 2009; Nickel and Shoskes, 2009). Since this system was described, numerous investigators have assessed its implications (Hedelin, 2009; Magri et al, 2010; Samplaski et al, 2012) and suggested modifications (Hedelin, 2009; Davis et al 2013a), including the inclusion of a sexual dysfunction (UPOINT"s") phenotype (Magri et al, 2010; Davis et al, 2013b), although this addition has been contested by some researchers (Samplaski et al, 2011). This phenotype classification system has been used in English (Shoskes et al, 2009a, 2009b), German (Magri et al, 2010), Italian (Magri et al, 2010), Swedish (Hedelin, 2009), and Chinese (Liu et al, 2012; Zhao et al, 2013), and in each language and culture it has proved to be a useful clinical tool. Updated Canadian, European, and International guidelines for the management of CP/CPPS (Nickel, 2011; Engeler et al, 2013; Nickel et al, 2013b) have recommended that patients be clinically phenotyped during evaluation and treated according to individual phenotypes identified. This phenotype-directed therapy is discussed in the treatment section. My colleagues and I are currently testing specific questionnaires that will provide urologists with a clinical instrument to identify the six major phenotypes and also the further subclassifications that will likely be relevant within each specific domain. A better understanding of cause, mechanisms of disease, and disease progression and the discovery of specific biomarkers (e.g., from the NIH MAPP study) that will allow better phenotype identification will further improve our understanding and management of CP/CPPS.

Treatment

This section presents the rationale for each of the various treatments advocated for the prostatitis syndromes and reviews the clinical trial data that support (or not) the use of those specific therapeutic modalities in clinical practice. Recent rigorous prospective studies in chronic bacterial prostatitis and randomized placebo-controlled trials employing standardized definitions and validated outcomes in CP/CPPS have allowed us to develop best-evidence–based treatment strategies in a therapeutic field that used to be based on poor clinical data, dogma, and anecdotal experience (McNaughton Collins et al, 2000b, 2001a; Nickel, 2002c, 2002d, 2004; Schaeffer, 2006; Nickel, 2008b; Anothaisintawe et al, 2011; Nickel, 2011; Cohen et al, 2012; Thakkinstian et al, 2012; Engeler et al, 2013; Nickel et al, 2013b) (Tables 13-2 and 13-3).

Antimicrobials

Rationale. It is generally accepted that acute and chronic bacterial prostatitis are directly related to bacterial infection of the prostate gland. Many urologists further believe that, although bacteria are cultured in only 5% to 10% of cases of prostatitis, bacteria may be the cause of CP symptoms in a significant percentage of patients with this syndrome. **Antimicrobial therapy is the most commonly prescribed treatment for the CP syndromes** (Moon, 1997; Nickel et al, 1998a; McNaughton Collins et al, 2000b, 2001a; Taylor et al, 2008), independent of culture status.

Pharmacology and Pharmacokinetics. Most antimicrobial pharmacokinetic studies were performed in animal models (dogs and rats) (Madsen et al, 1978; Nickel, 1997b). Stamey (1980) and Stamey and associates (1970) found that acid antibiotic drugs can be detected in prostatic secretions only in very low concentrations, even when plasma concentrations of the drug are very high. Alkaline antibiotic drugs are found in concentrations greater than the simultaneous plasma levels. This phenomenon of ion trapping, and the fact that drug penetration was believed to be a passive transport mechanism based on diffusion and concentration, suggested that drug penetration is dependent on the lipid solubility, degree of ionization, degree of protein binding, and size and shape of the antimicrobial molecule. In dogs, the pH of plasma was found to be 7.4, whereas that of prostatic secretion is 6.4. Therefore, in this model, weak acids (low pKa) concentrate on the plasma side, whereas antibiotics with a higher pKa (weak bases) concentrate in the prostatic secretion.

Because infection may alter the local prostatic environment, thus changing the pharmacokinetic parameters, animal models were developed that introduced infection into the process (Baumueller and Madsen, 1977; Madsen et al, 1994; Nickel et al, 1995). All these animal studies (with and without infection) showed that trimethoprim concentrates in prostatic secretion and prostatic interstitial fluid (exceeding plasma levels), whereas sulfamethoxazole and ampicillin do not. The fluoroquinolones, which are neither pure acids nor bases but have characteristics of both, being zwitterionic drugs (i.e., those that have two pKa values) (Gasser et al, 1986), should allow drug concentration in the prostate at various pH ranges. Carbenicillin and the aminoglycosides did not concentrate in prostatic fluid in dog models.

It is difficult to extrapolate the animal pharmacokinetic studies to humans (Sharer and Fair, 1982). **Fair and Cordonnier (1978) found that the prostatic secretion of normal men is** slightly alkaline (pH of approximately 7.3) but also that the pH of prostatic secretion in men with prostatic infection is markedly increased (pH of approximately 8.3). This has been confirmed in other studies (Anderson and Fair, 1976; Blacklock and Beavis, 1978; Pfau et al, 1978), **and because the pH gradation is crucial to ion trapping, the results from animal studies should not be applied directly to humans. Unfortunately, drug diffusion studies are difficult to perform in humans, and most studies determine antibiotic concentrations in transurethrally resected BPH adenomas. These studies are further complicated because the high drug concentrations in urine can substantially alter the results.** Employing a method to reduce urine contamination, Naber and Madsen (1999) demonstrated that for most fluoroquinolones the ratio of concentrations in prostatic fluid to concentrations in plasma is less than 1 (norfloxacin ratio 0.12, ciprofloxacin ratio 0.18 to 0.26, lomefloxacin ratio 0.48). Concentrations in seminal fluid usually exceed corresponding plasma concentrations of ciprofloxacin and ofloxacin, with ciprofloxacin demonstrating the highest ratio of seminal fluid to plasma (Naber, 1999). The numerous studies evaluating fluoroquinolone concentrations in prostatic tissue demonstrated that the fluoroquinolone concentration in the adenoma tissue is usually higher than that in plasma.

Clinical Trial Data. Unless the patient has a significant anatomic abnormality of the lower urinary tract or develops a prostate abscess, antimicrobial therapy is universally successful in eradicating the bacteria and curing the patient with acute bacterial prostatitis (Nickel and Moon, 2005). **In the acutely inflamed prostate gland the pharmacokinetic considerations described in the previous section probably do not play a significant role in antibiotic penetration,** and it is believed that most antibiotics achieve reasonable intraprostatic concentrations in the acute phase of the disease. Although prospective clinical trial data are unavailable, **most experts suggest therapy initially with parenteral antibiotics (depending on the seriousness of the infection) followed by oral antibiotics with wide-spectrum antimicrobial activity** (Becopoulos et al, 1990). The most common drugs suggested for initial therapy (Neal, 1999; Benway and Moon, 2008; Ludwig, 2008) are a combination of penicillin (i.e., ampicillin) and an aminoglycoside (i.e., gentamicin), second- or third-generation cephalosporins, or one of the fluoroquinolones. This traditional approach has changed recently because of the increasing risk of post–prostate biopsy prostate infection with ESBL microorganisms (Ozden et al, 2009; Oh et al, 2013). There are now identified risk factors for this shift, one of which is previous exposure to fluoroquinolones (Mosharafa et al, 2011; Ekici et al, 2012). Both the microorganisms (Bang et al, 2013) and the longer, more difficult clinical treatment course of the prostatitis after urologic intervention (Kim et al, 2012) illustrate the differences with spontaneous acute prostatitis. In patients with acute prostatitis with ESBL or suspected ESBL organisms (usually associated with transrectal prostate biopsies), treatment with a carbapenem (ertapenem, imipenem, or meropenem), amikacin, or colistin for at least 10 to 14 days is recommended (Paterson and Bonomo, 2005; Pallett and Hand, 2010; Fournier et al, 2013). **Once the acute infection has settled down, therapy should be continued with one of the oral antimicrobial agents appropriate for the treatment of chronic bacterial prostatitis (e.g., trimethoprim or fluoroquinolones or ESBL-effective antimicrobial therapy based on sensitivity analysis). The duration of optimal therapy is unknown; between 2 and 4 weeks has been suggested** (Bjerklund Johansen et al, 1998; Nickel, 1998a; Wagenlehner et al, 2007; Ludwig, 2008). It has been suggested that ineffective treatment of acute bacterial prostatitis may lead to the emergence of a CP category (Rudick et al, 2011; Galeone et al, 2013), particularly if the organism was post–prostate biopsy ESBL *E. coli* (Oh et al, 2013).

In the 1970s to 1990s the most commonly used antimicrobial agents in the treatment of CP were trimethoprim-sulfamethoxazole (co-trimoxazole) (Moon, 1997; Nickel et al, 1998a) **and, to a lesser extent, trimethoprim alone.** In patients with chronic bacterial prostatitis, eradication of pathogens (the only objective

TABLE 13-2 Randomized Placebo-Controlled Clinical Trials Evaluating Therapy for Chronic Prostatitis and Chronic Pelvic Pain Syndrome (CP/CPPS)*

ACTIVE AGENT	REFERENCE	DURATION	PATIENTS (N)		RESPONDERS (%)		CHANGE IN NIH-CPSI		TREATMENT EFFECT
			ACTIVE	PLACEBO	ACTIVE	PLACEBO	ACTIVE	PLACEBO	
Levofloxacin	Nickel et al, 2003b	6 wk	35	45	42	37	−5.4	−2.9	2.5
Tetracycline	Zhou et al, 2008	12 wk	24	24	NK	NK	−18.5†	−1.0	17.5†
Ciprofloxacin	Alexander et al, 2004	6 wk	49	49	22	22	−6.2	−3.4	2.8
Tamsulosin			49		24		−4.4		1.0
Ciprofloxacin and tamsulosin			49		10		−4.1		0.7
Terazosin	Cheah et al, 2003b	14 wk	43	43	NK	NK	−14.3†	−10.2	4.1†
Alfuzosin	Mehik et al, 2003	24 wk	17	20	65†	24	−9.9†	−3.8	6.1†
Tamsulosin	Nickel et al, 2004a	6 wk	27	30	52	33	−9.1†	−5.5	3.6†
Alfuzosin	Nickel et al, 2008c	12 wk	138	134	49.3‡ 34.8§	49.3‡ 33.6§	−7.1	−6.5	0.6
Doxazosin	Tugcu et al, 2007	24 wk	30	30	66†	33	−12.4†	−1.0	11.4
Tamsulosin (0.2 mg)	Chen et al, 2011	24 wk	50	50	50	50	−7.5†	−4.0	3.5†
Silodosin 4 mg	Nickel et al, 2011a	12 wk	45	54	63	35	−12.1†	−8.5	3.6†
Silodosin 8 mg			52		51		−10.2		1.7
Rofecoxib 25 mg	Nickel et al, 2003c	6 wk	53	59	46	40	−4.9	−4.2	0.7
Rofecoxib 50 mg	Nickel et al, 2003c	6 wk	49	59	63†	40	−6.2	−4.2	2.0
Prednisone	Bates et al, 2007	4 wk	6	12	50	50	NK	NK	No significant difference
Celecoxib	Zhao et al, 2009	6 wk	32	32	78†	32	−8.0†	−4.0	4.0†
Tanezumab	Nickel et al, 2012	Single IV dose	30	32	24	23.1	−4.3	−2.8	1.5
Pentosan polysulfate	Nickel et al, 2005a	16 wk	51	49	37	18	−5.9	−3.2	2.7
Finasteride	Nickel et al, 2004b	24 wk	33	31	33	16	−3.0	−0.8	2.2
Mepartricin	De Rose et al, 2004	8 wk	13	13	NK	NK	−15.0†	−5.0	10.0†
Quercetin	Shoskes et al, 1999	4 wk	15	13	67†	20	−7.9†	−1.4	6.5†
Pollen extract (Cernilton)	Wagenlehner et al, 2009	12 wk	70	69	62.9†	41.8	−7.5†	−5.4	2.1†
Pregabalin	Pontari et al, 2010	6 wk	103	106	47.2‡ (31†)§	35.8‡ (19)§	−6.6†	−4.2	2.4†

*These studies met the evidence-based criteria updated by the 2012 International Consultation on Urologic Disease (ICUD) committee (Nickel et al, 2013b), which included randomized, placebo-controlled design with National Institutes of Health Chronic Prostatitis Symptom Index (NIH-CPSI) as one of the outcomes.
†Significant difference between active and placebo (P < .05).
‡Primary end point (CPSI responders—see text).
§Global Response Assessment responders.
NK, not known.

measurement in most CP studies) with trimethoprim-sulfamethoxazole or trimethoprim alone ranged from a low of 0% (Smith et al, 1979) to a high of 67% (Paulson and White, 1978), with most studies demonstrating an efficacy rate between 30% and 50% (Meares, 1973; Drach, 1974b; Meares, 1975; McGuire and Lytton, 1976; Meares, 1978). It appears that longer-duration therapy (90 days) provides the best clinical results. **Trimethoprim-sulfamethoxazole is less effective both in bacterial eradication and cost-effectiveness when compared with the newer fluoroquinolones (Kurzer and Kaplan, 2002).**

TABLE 13-3 Sham Controlled Trials Evaluating Nonmedical Therapies Using the National Institutes of Health Chronic Prostatitis Symptom Index (NIH-CPSI) as an Outcome Parameter

THERAPY	REFERENCE	DURATION OF THERAPY AND FOLLOW-UP (WEEKS)	PATIENTS (N)		CHANGE IN NIH-CPSI		TREATMENT EFFECT
			ACTIVE	SHAM	ACTIVE	SHAM	
Directed physiotherapy*	FitzGerald et al, 2009	12	10	11	−14.4	−6.8	7.6
Posterior tibial nerve stimulation	Kabay et al, 2009	12	45	44	−13.4	−1.4	12.0†
Acupuncture	Lee et al, 2008a	10	44	45	−10	−6	4.0†
Electroacupuncture	Lee and Lee, 2009	6	12	12	−9.5	−3.5	6.0†
Extracorporeal shock wave therapy	Zimmermann et al, 2009	4	30	30	−3.7	−0.1	3.6†
Extracorporeal shock wave therapy	Vahdatpour et al, 2013	4 (assessed at 12 weeks)	20	20	−7.1	−0.2	6.9†
Botulinum toxin A	Gottsch et al, 2011	4	13	16	+0.4	−2.2	2.6

*The randomized therapy was not sham but rather relaxation massage therapy.
†Statistically significant difference between groups.

Except for the well-studied fluoroquinolones, most antibiotics (including minocycline, cephalexin, and carbenicillin) do not demonstrate significant clinical efficacy in clinical studies in which patients were observed for sufficient time (Paulson and White, 1978; Oliveri et al, 1979; Mobley, 1981). One notable exception has been the macrolides erythromycin (Mobley, 1974), azithromycin (Skerk et al, 2003), and clarithromycin (Skerk et al, 2002b), particularly when *C. trachomatis* is implicated. A recent Cochrane review (Perletti et al, 2013) concluded that although the microbiologic and clinical cure rates were higher for the macrolides compared with fluoroquinolones for the treatment of intracellular pathogens (*Chlamydia* or *Mycoplasma*), there was no significant difference between azithromycin and clarithromycin.

The fluoroquinolones have demonstrated improved therapeutic results, especially in prostatitis caused by *E. coli* and other members of the Enterobacteriaceae but not necessarily in prostatitis caused by *P. aeruginosa* or enterococci. Naber (1999) analyzed the many studies available in the literature evaluating fluoroquinolones in the treatment of CP and found eight comparable studies in which the diagnosis was obtained by localization studies and in which the patients were observed for a sufficient time after completion of therapy (Weidner et al, 1987; Pust et al, 1989; Heidler, 1990; Schaeffer and Darras, 1990; Pfau, 1991; Weidner et al, 1991a; Ramirez et al, 1994; Koff, 1996); in these studies the researchers evaluated norfloxacin, ciprofloxacin, ofloxacin, and lomefloxacin. In 2005, Naber, reporting at the Sixth International Consultation on New Developments in Prostate Cancer and Prostate Disease, Paris, June, 2005 (Schaeffer et al, 2006), added three more recent studies that met these strict criteria (Naber et al, 2000, Naber and European Lomefloxacin Prostatitis Study Group, 2002; Bundrick et al, 2003) with a further addition from 2008 (Naber et al, 2008). The overall conclusion was that fluoroquinolones were the optimal antimicrobial agent for the treatment of chronic bacterial prostatitis. In a 2013 Cochrane review, Perletti and colleagues (2013) undertook an ambitious comprehensive review of antimicrobial therapy for chronic bacterial prostatitis by evaluating and comparing 18 clinical trials (Smith et al, 1979; Paulson et al, 1986; Cox, 1989; Ohkawa et al, 1993b; Koff 1996; Bustillo et al, 1997; Naber and European Lomefloxacin Prostatitis Study Group, 2002; Skerk et al, 2002a, 2002b; Bundrick et al, 2003; Skerk et el, 2003, 2004a, 2004b, 2006; Giannarini et al, 2007; Aliaev et al, 2008; Cai et al, 2009, 2010; Zhang et al, 2012) that met strict inclusion criteria including standardized microbiologic diagnoses and outcomes (microbiologic and clinical) in randomized controlled studies in which the comparison was with placebo, different administration schedules, or another antibiotic or combinations of antibiotics plus other agents. The authors concluded that there are no significant differences in microbiologic and clinical efficacy or in adverse effect rates among the oral fluoroquinolones ciprofloxacin, levofloxacin, lomefloxacin, ofloxacin, and prulifloxacin. As mentioned previously, the macrolides appear to be superior to the fluoroquinolones for the treatment of proven chlamydial infection. The authors further concluded that there is inconclusive randomized controlled evidence regarding the role of combination treatments of chronic bacterial prostatitis with antimicrobial and nonantimicrobial substances, such as phosphodiesterase-5 inhibitors or herbal preparations.

For CP caused by *E. coli*, treatment duration of 1 month for the fluoroquinolones seems to be superior to the usual 3-month treatment with trimethoprim-sulfamethoxazole. It has been suggested that antibiotics should be continued only for 4 to 6 weeks if pretreatment cultures are positive and/or the patient has reported positive effects from treatment (Wagenlehner et al, 2007); however, the duration of therapy cannot be confirmed from analysis of available studies (Perletti et al, 2013). Some clinicians have observed that as many as 20% of patients in whom an initial treatment period fails could be rescued with a second cycle of treatment with another antibiotic (Magri et al, 2007b). In microbiologically diagnosed chronic bacterial prostatitis, eradication of bacteria is associated with both short-term and long-term clinical success (Nickel and Xiang, 2008). This appears to be true in men with recent onset of prostatitis associated with bacterial localization with the traditional uropathogens (gram-negative uropathogens and *Enterococcus* species) as well as nontraditional bacteria (gram-positive bacteria such as coagulase-negative staphylococcal and streptococcal species) (Magri et al, 2007a; Nickel and Xiang, 2008). A number of investigators (Baert and Leonard, 1988; Jimenez-Cruz et al, 1988; Yamamoto et al, 1996; Guercini et al, 2005b) have advocated direct injection of antibiotics into the prostate gland, but this method has never been rigorously evaluated or become popular among urologists. It appears that men with chronic bacterial prostatitis and prostatic calculi are more difficult to cure (Zhao et al, 2012). Many physicians have resorted to prolonged therapy with low-dose prophylactic or suppressive antimicrobials for recurrent or refractory prostatitis, respectively, although this practice has not been confirmed with clinical studies.

Many studies evaluating physicians' practice patterns in prostatitis syndromes (de la Rosette et al, 1992a; Moon, 1997; Collins et al, 1998; Nickel et al, 1998a; McNaughton Collins et al, 2000a; Taylor et al, 2008) have confirmed that most patients diagnosed with CP, irrespective of culture results, are treated with antimicrobial therapy. Older studies have generally indicated that approximately 40% of patients with nonbacterial CP have some symptomatic improvement with antimicrobial therapy (Berger et al, 1989; Weidner, 1992; de la Rosette et al, 1993a; Ohkawa et al, 1993b; Bergman, 1994; Bjerklund Johansen et al, 1998; Tanner et al, 1999; Nickel et al, 2001b). Antibiotic therapy may benefit CP/CPPS patients by three different mechanisms: a strong placebo effect, the eradication or suppression of noncultured microorganisms (Nickel et al, 2001b), or the independent anti-inflammatory effect of some antibiotics (Yoshimura et al, 1996; Galley et al, 1997). It has been suggested by a European consensus group evaluating the role of antibiotics in the treatment of CP (Bjerklund Johansen et al, 1998; Engeler et al, 2013) that antibiotics could be considered empirical treatment for category IIIA CP/CPPS, but the benefits should be appraised after a minimum of 2 to 4 weeks of therapy. The antibiotics could be continued for 4 to 6 weeks if the patient reports positive effects from treatment (Wagenlehner et al, 2007). These recommendations remain controversial (Taylor et al, 2008), particularly because new data appear to provide conflicting interpretations. Two multicenter randomized placebo-controlled studies have assessed the efficacy of 6 weeks of levofloxacin (Nickel et al, 2003b) and ciprofloxacin (Alexander et al, 2004) in men with CP/CPPS. In these trials the participants had chronic symptoms for a long duration (many years) and had been heavily treated (including treatment with antibiotics). In the study by Nickel and associates (2003b) 80 patients were randomized to levofloxacin or placebo, whereas in the NIH-sponsored study reported by Alexander and colleagues (2004) 196 men with CP/CPPS were randomized in a 2 × 2 factorial design to ciprofloxacin, tamsulosin, the combination of ciprofloxacin and tamsulosin, or placebo. In both of these prospective-designed controlled multicenter trials, no significant difference was reported between the fluoroquinolone and placebo in terms of symptom amelioration. **Antibiotics should not be prescribed for previously treated men with CP/CPPS of long duration.** However, two prospective trials comparing the effect of 4 to 6 weeks of antibiotics (Magri et al, 2007a; Nickel and Xiang, 2008) in men with localization of both traditional uropathogens and organisms not usually believed to be uropathogenic (and therefore classified as category III CP/CPPS) showed similar eradication and clinical success rates (75% to 80%). Furthermore, in the study by Nickel and Xiang (2008), the eradication of those organisms, whether or not they were considered to be uropathogens, correlated with both short- and long-term clinical success. Because the majority of patients in Nickel and Xiang's study (2008) had a short history of prostatitis and were antibiotic naive for that episode, it was concluded that **antibiotic treatment may be considered for antibiotic-naive patients with a recent diagnosis of prostatitis, regardless of culture status.**

α-Adrenergic Blocker Therapy

Rationale. Patients with CP/CPPS have significant lower urinary tract symptoms, which appear to be related to poor relaxation of the bladder neck during voiding (Barbalias et al, 1983; Murnaghan and Millard, 1984; Blacklock, 1986; Hellstrom et al, 1987; Barbalias, 1990; Kaplan et al, 1997). The subsequent turbulent "dysfunctional" voiding may predispose the patient to reflux of urine into the prostatic ducts, causing intraprostatic inflammation and subsequently pain (Kirby et al, 1982). **The bladder neck and prostate are rich in α receptors, and it is hypothesized that α-adrenergic blockade may improve outflow obstruction, improving urinary flow and perhaps diminishing intraprostatic ductal reflux.**

Clinical Trial Data. A number of older clinical trials suggested that the α-adrenergic blockers diphenoxybenzamine (Dunzendorfer, 1983), phenoxybenzamine (Osborn et al, 1981), alfuzosin (de la Rosette et al, 1992c; Barbalias et al, 1998), terazosin (Neal and Moon, 1994; Barbalias et al, 1998; Lacquaniti et al, 1999; Gül et al, 2001), doxazosin (Evliyaoglu and Burgut, 2002), and tamsulosin (Lacquaniti et al, 1999) resulted in significant symptomatic improvement of prostatitis-related symptoms; however, these trials were small, most were uncontrolled, and outcome measures were not validated. Studies by Barbalias and associates (1998) and Youn et al (2008) further seemed to indicate that the combination of

antibiotics and α-adrenergic blockers improved the clinical result in patients with chronic bacterial prostatitis.

At least six randomized placebo-controlled trials with clearly defined CP/CPPS patients (NIH classification) and employing the NIH-CPSI as the outcome parameter appear to have confirmed the efficacy of α-adrenergic blockers but only in men who have recent-onset disease and have not been heavily pretreated and who are on therapy for longer than 6 weeks. Cheah and colleagues (2003b) randomized 86 patients with CP to either terazosin or placebo for 14 weeks. Patients on terazosin had a 50% reduction in mean symptom score compared with 37% in the placebo-treated group. Terazosin resulted in modest but significant improvement in all domains of the NIH-CPSI. Mehik and colleagues (2003) followed 19 patients randomized to 6 months of alfuzosin treatment and 20 patients on 6 months of placebo therapy, and both groups were followed for a further 6 months after discontinuing the active or placebo medication. Patients in the alfuzosin group had a significant amelioration of symptoms compared with the placebo therapy group that was evident at 4 months and became even more clinically significant by 6 months. At 6 months, 65% of alfuzosin patients were rated as responders compared with 24% of the placebo group. The beneficial effect appeared to wear off over the next 6 months after the alfuzosin was discontinued. Nickel and colleagues (2004c) randomized 57 men with CP/CPPS to tamsulosin, 0.4 mg, or placebo after a 2-week placebo run-in and observed the two groups for 6 weeks. Patients treated with tamsulosin had a statistically significant (but only modest clinically significant) treatment effect compared with patients taking a placebo. A significant treatment effect was not observed in patients who had mild symptoms, but patients with severe symptoms (75th percentile) had a statistically and clinically significant response compared with placebo. It appears that the response to α-adrenergic blockers is durable, for at least up to 24 to 38 weeks as long as the patient stays on the medication (Mehik et al, 2003; Cheah et al, 2004). Another study (Tugcu et al, 2007) included 90 treatment-naive patients with CP/CPPS randomized to receive doxazosin, 4 mg/day, alone or a triple therapy (doxazosin, 4 mg/day, plus an anti-inflammatory agent—ibuprofen, 400 mg/day—and a myorelaxant—thiocolchicoside, 12 mg/day) or placebo. Over 6 months, the total NIH-CPSI score significantly improved in the doxazosin group (from 23.1 to 10.5 points) and triple-therapy groups (from 21.9 to 9.2), and it remained stable in the placebo group (from 22.9 to 21.9). Chen and colleagues (2011) examined a total of 100 men diagnosed with CP/CPPS randomly allocated to receive either 0.2 mg of tamsulosin daily or placebo for 6 months. The tamsulosin patients had modest satisfactory improvements compared with the placebo group during treatment. Six months after initiation of treatment, the mean decrements of total NIH-CPSI score in the tamsulosin and placebo groups were 7.5 ± 1.9 and 4.0 ± 2.3, respectively ($P < .01$). After cessation of therapy, the significant difference waned gradually. Two years after cessation of therapy, the mean decrements in total NIH-CPSI score in the two groups were 3.0 ± 1.3 and 1.9 ± 0.9, respectively ($P > .05$). This suggests that in patients who respond to α blockers, the therapy must be continued long term. Finally, Nickel and coworkers (2011a) evaluated the efficacy and safety of two doses of silodosin versus placebo in 151 men with CP/CPPS who had not been treated previously with α blockers. Patients randomized to silodosin 4 mg experienced a significant decrease in total NIH-CPSI of −12.1 versus placebo (−8.5). At this dose, men also had a significant decrease in the urinary and quality of life subscore as well as the physical component of the Medical Outcomes Study Short Form 12 quality-of-life assessment. During global response assessment 56% of patients receiving 4 mg of silodosin versus 29% receiving placebo reported moderate or marked improvement (also significant). Increasing the dose of silodosin to 8 mg resulted in no incremental treatment effects.

In contrast, the results from the NIH CPCRN randomized controlled trial (Alexander et al, 2004) comparing 6 weeks of ciprofloxacin, tamsulosin, and the combination of ciprofloxacin and tamsulosin with placebo in very chronic and heavily pretreated patients failed to show any improvement in patients

treated with tamsulosin (with or without ciprofloxacin) compared with patients treated with placebo. A number of meta-analyses and comprehensive reviews of these data have suggested that α-adrenergic blockers provide significant symptom amelioration only after more than 6 weeks of therapy in less heavily treated patients with recent onset of moderate to severe symptoms (Yang et al, 2006; Mishra et al, 2007; Nickel, 2008a). **To test this hypothesis, an NIH multicenter, randomized, double-blind, placebo-controlled trial was conducted to evaluate the efficacy of 12 weeks of alfuzosin or placebo to reduce symptoms in 272 randomized men with CP/CPPS diagnosed within 2 years previously and who had not been previously treated with an α-adrenergic blocker** (Nickel et al, 2008a). The rate of the primary outcome (reduction of at least 4 points in NIH-CPSI total score from baseline) was 49% in both treatment groups. The response rates at 12 weeks measured with a global response assessment were also similar: 34% and 35% for the placebo and alfuzosin groups, respectively ($P = .90$). **These important findings did not support the use of α-adrenergic blockers in recently diagnosed α-adrenergic blocker–naive men with CP/CPPS.**

Anti-Inflammatory Agents and Immune Modulators

Rationale. Prostatic inflammation is associated with category IIIA CP/CPPS, and elevated cytokine levels are noted in the semen (Alexander et al, 1998; Ruggieri et al, 2000) and EPS (Hochreiter et al, 2000b; Nadler et al, 2000) of patients with inflammatory CPPS. **Nonsteroidal anti-inflammatory drugs, corticosteroids, and immunosuppressive drugs theoretically should improve the inflammatory parameters within the prostate and possibly result in a reduction of symptoms** (Pontari, 2002).

Clinical Trial Data. Canale and associates (1993a) found that nimesulide (a nonsteroidal anti-inflammatory drug) quickly reduced inflammatory-type symptoms such as dysuria, strangury, and painful ejaculation. A second study by Canale and colleagues (1993b) found that, by the rectal route, ketoprofen was inferior to nimesulide (both drugs were used as suppositories). Prednisolone has been suggested as a potent anti-inflammatory for CP (Bates and Talbot, 2000), and a randomized study presented by Dimitrakov and associates (2004) indicates that high-dose methylprednisolone (followed by rapid tapering of dose) may have more efficacy than placebo, even after 12 months, but the side effect profile makes this type of therapy less attractive. A small randomized trial evaluating oral corticosteroids did not show superiority of the active therapy over placebo (Bates et al, 2007).

The new class of cyclooxygenase-2 inhibitors has proved successful for long-term treatment of other chronic inflammatory conditions such as rheumatoid arthritis and chronic osteoarthritis; many urologists have employed these medications for prostatitis patients, with some anecdotal successes reported. The results of a North American randomized controlled trial comparing the cyclooxygenase-2 inhibitor rofecoxib with placebo indicated that many men with CPPS benefited (in terms of pain and quality of life) from rofecoxib therapy compared with placebo. In this study, in which 161 patients were randomized to rofecoxib 25 mg, rofecoxib 50 mg, or placebo, only patients on the high dose showed any clinical improvement compared with the placebo. Very few patients, however, had complete resolution of their symptoms (Nickel et al, 2003c). Another study from China (Zeng et al, 2004) assessing the effectiveness of two doses of the cyclooxygenase-2 inhibitor celecoxib also demonstrated a dose-dependent response (200 mg twice a day for 6 weeks was more effective than 200 mg once a day). Zhao et al (2009) randomized 64 patients with category IIIA CPPS to celecoxib (200 mg daily) and placebo for 6 weeks with 8 weeks of follow-up. These researchers showed that celecoxib provides significant symptomatic improvement, but the benefit was limited to the duration of the therapy. At this time, high-dose, long-duration monotherapy with cyclooxygenase-2 inhibitors is not recommended.

Because the clinical and pathologic characteristics are similar to those of interstitial cystitis and there is evidence that pentosan polysulfate, a glycosaminoglycan drug that has been used in the treatment of interstitial cystitis and provides significant anti-inflammatory effects (Sunaga et al, 2012), Wedren (1987) compared the efficacy of pentosan polysulfate with placebo. In this small study the treated group was noted to have a statistically significant improvement in symptoms, but the major symptom that improved was nonspecific myalgias and arthralgias. An uncontrolled pilot study evaluating oral pentosan polysulfate in 32 men with CPPS demonstrated amelioration of symptoms and improvement in the quality of life in over 40% after treatment for 6 months (Nickel et al, 2000). The results of a multicenter, randomized, placebo-controlled trial that randomized 100 men to pentosan polysulfate, 900 mg/day (three times the usual dose), or placebo indicated this medication provided modest benefit for some men with CPPS (Nickel et al, 2005a).

Thalidomide, a cytokine modulating drug, was assessed in 30 men with chronic abacterial prostatitis and abnormal semen cytokine levels (IL-2, IL-6, IL-8, IL-10, and TNF-α) in a randomized placebo-controlled trial (Guercini et al, 2005a). Despite a significant reduction in cytokine levels in semen, no difference in symptom relief was noted. A similar lack of efficacy was noted in a small placebo-controlled trial evaluating the leukotriene antagonist zafirlukast (Goldmeier et al, 2005).

The potential of various anti-inflammatory agents, immune modulators, and cytokine inhibitors makes these classes of drugs potentially useful as adjunctive therapy for the CP syndromes, but clinical trials suggest that they are not a useful monotherapy.

Muscle Relaxants

Rationale. Many investigators believe that CPPS is the ultimate reflection of a smooth and skeletal neuromuscular dysregulatory phenomenon in the perineum or pelvic floor (Osborn et al, 1981; Egan and Krieger, 1997; Anderson, 1999; Zermann and Schmidt, 1999). **The use of α blockers to relax smooth muscle** (see earlier discussion of α-adrenergic blockers) **and skeletal muscle relaxants combined with adjuvant medical and physical therapies has been advocated and promoted** (Anderson, 1999; Zermann and Schmidt, 1999).

Clinical Trial Data. In one of the few studies to compare muscle relaxants with placebo, Osborn and associates (1981) conducted a prospective double-blind study comparing phenoxybenzamine, baclofen (a striated muscle relaxant), and placebo in 27 patients with prostatodynia (category IIIB). Patients were treated with each agent for 1 month in a crossover trial. Symptomatic improvement was seen in 37% of the patients treated with baclofen compared with 8% treated with placebo. Simmons and Thin (1985) compared diazepam with an antibiotic in patients with chronic abacterial prostatitis and found no difference in symptom improvement between the diazepam group (8 of 11 men improved) and the antibiotic group (7 of 12 men improved). Unfortunately **these studies were hindered by a lack of controlled and defined entry criteria and no quantified measurement of patients' responses and therefore the role of muscle relaxants has yet to be determined.**

Hormone Therapy

Rationale. Prostate growth and function are influenced by the local hormonal milieu, especially by androgens. **Theoretically, anti-androgens (including 5α-reductase inhibitors) could result in regression of prostatic glandular tissue (inflammation is believed to begin at the level of the ductal epithelium), decreased intra-prostatic pressure** (Mehik et al, 2002), **improved voiding parameters (especially in older patients with BPH and prostatitis), and reduced intraprostatic ductal reflux** (Nickel, 1999a).

Clinical Trial Data. Holm and Meyhoff (1996) were the first to note that the 5α-reductase inhibitor finasteride had potential in alleviating symptoms by observing the effect of finasteride therapy in four patients with CP or prostatodynia. Leskinen and colleagues

(1999) randomized 41 patients with chronic idiopathic prostatitis (i.e., nonbacterial prostatitis and prostatodynia) to treatment with placebo (25%, or 10 patients) or finasteride (75%, or 31 patients) for 1 year. Compared with placebo, finasteride reduced prostatitis and BPH symptom scores; however, there was no statistically significant difference in pain between the two groups. The baseline characteristics of the two groups were not comparable, and the enrolled patients consisted of an unknown mixed population with inflammatory and noninflammatory prostatitis syndromes. A randomized open-label comparative trial in CP/CPPS men showed significantly more improvement in men treated for a year with finasteride compared with saw palmetto, an herbal therapy (Kaplan et al, 2004). A randomized controlled trial compared the reduction of NIH-CPSI in 64 men with CP/CPPS randomized to finasteride or placebo (Nickel et al, 2004b). Six months of finasteride resulted in a numerical but not statistically significant reduction in symptoms compared with the symptom reduction noted in the placebo group. In the 4-year Reduction by Dutasteride of Prostate Cancer Events (REDUCE) prostate cancer reduction trial, dutasteride therapy produced statistically and possibly clinically significant benefits compared with placebo in the men with preexisting prostatitis or prostatitis symptoms (Nickel et al, 2011b). **Finasteride and dutasteride cannot be recommended as a monotherapy except in men with associated BPH.**

Testosterone and dihydrotestosterone are not the only hormones with a possible effect on prostate inflammation; estrogens may also play a role. A number of small, poorly controlled studies (Cavallini, 2001; Saita et al, 2001) suggested that mepartricin (a drug that lowers estrogen levels in the prostate) may be useful in the treatment of CP/CPPS. A small prospectively designed trial randomized 26 men with CP/CPPS to 60 days of therapy with mepartricin or placebo (De Rose et al, 2004). The study showed a statistical and perhaps clinically significant benefit (60% vs. 20% improvement, respectively) that should stimulate further research in the role of hormonal manipulation (in this case estrogens) in the treatment of CP/CPPS.

Phytotherapeutic Agents

Rationale. A number of plant extracts have been shown in many in vitro experiments to have 5α-reductase activity, α-adrenergic blockade activity, effects on bladder contractility, and antiinflammatory properties (Lowe and Fagelman, 1999; Shoskes, 2002).

Clinical Trial Data. Three specific phytotherapeutic agents have been tested in well-controlled clinical trials: Cernilton, a pollen extract (Buck et al, 1989; Rugendorff et al, 1993; Wagenlehner et al, 2009); Quercetin, a natural bioflavonoid (Shoskes et al, 1999); and *Serenoa repens* (saw palmetto berry) extract (Kaplan et al, 2004; Reissigl et al, 2004). Rugendorff and coworkers (1993) noted that over half of 72 patients with CP without other lower urinary tract abnormalities had favorable improvements in pain and irritative voiding symptoms when treated with Cernilton, but no control group was included in this study. A randomized study of pollen extract (Cernilton) in 122 men with category IIIA CP/CPPS showed that men receiving the active treatment had statistically significant improvements in the pain and quality-of-life components of the CPSI (Wagenlehner et al, 2009). A controlled, randomized study of a similar preparation, Prostat/Poltit (grass pollen extract, including rye pollen), in 60 patients showed greater improvement in patients receiving active therapy compared with placebo, but no validated outcome index was incorporated into the study design (Elist, 2006). Shoskes and associates (1999) randomized 15 patients to the bioflavonoid Quercetin and 13 patients to placebo for 1 month. Sixty-seven percent of the patients in the treatment group were considered responders compared with only 20% of the patients in the placebo arm. Kaplan and associates (2004) noted possible benefits with the use of saw palmetto but did not note any appreciable long-term improvement in any CP/CPPS parameters when compared with 12 months of finasteride in a randomized open-label comparative study. However, Reissigl and colleagues (2004) reported that there

was moderate to marked improvement in more than 60% of 72 CP/CPPS patients after 12 months of therapy with *S. repens* extract compared with less than 25% in the 70 men in the placebo-treated group. However, further follow-up did not support the durability of this therapy (Reissigl et al, 2005). **Phytotherapy for CP/CPPS may look promising, but further multicenter randomized controlled trials with well-characterized, standardized, and stable herbal components should be considered to assess their role in therapy.**

Neuromodulator Therapy

Rationale. One proposed mechanism is that CP/CPPS, particularly chronic, long-standing cases, represents a neurogenic pain syndrome and that the subsequent pain is actually a neuropathic pain (Pontari and Ruggieri, 2004). Patients with CP/CPPS have a history of neurologic disease that is almost five times more likely among cases than control subjects (Pontari et al, 2005), and men with CP/CPPS have been found to have abnormalities of both the afferent and efferent autonomic nervous systems (Yang et al, 2003; Yilmaz et al, 2007; Yang, 2013). This type of neuropathic pain related to CNS sensitization responds to gabapentinoids in other chronic pain conditions (Rosenstock et al, 2004; Crofford et al, 2005).

Clinical Trial Data. A recent NIH CPCRN randomized placebo-controlled trial evaluated the effect of the gabapentinoid pregabalin on symptoms of men with long-standing, treatment-refractory CP/CPPS (Pontari et al, 2010). Among the 103 men assigned to pregabalin, 47% reported at least a 6-point decrease in total NIH-CPSI score at 6 weeks (primary end point) compared with 35.8% of 106 men assigned to placebo ($P = .072$). The NIH-CPSI total score decreased by a mean of 6.6 and 4.2 points (of 43) in the pregabalin and placebo groups, respectively ($P = .008$), whereas significantly more men in the pregabalin arm reported they were markedly or moderately improved compared with placebo (31% and 19%, respectively; $P = .023$). Although 6 weeks of pregabalin therapy was not superior to placebo for treating symptoms of CP/CPPS based on the primary end point, the impressive differences in secondary end points suggest that pregabalin may prove effective in some men with long-standing CP/CPPS. A recent well-powered study evaluating tanezumab (Nickel et al, 2012), a humanized monoclonal antibody directed against nerve growth factor, was not able to show significant benefit in a generally unselected population of men with CP/CPPS; however, a signal suggested that it might be beneficial in selected men (perhaps those with expression of nerve growth factor), a concept that should further explored (Watanabe et al, 2011). **It appears that for neuromodulatory therapy to be effective, it will need to be targeted toward a specific patient phenotype; however, biomarkers, either clinically or laboratory derived, have yet to be confirmed.**

Allopurinol

Rationale. Persson and Ronquist (1996) theorized that the intraprostatic ductal reflux of urine increases the concentration of metabolites containing purine and pyrimidine bases in the prostatic ducts, causing inflammation.

Clinical Trial Data. Persson and associates (1996) compared allopurinol therapy with placebo in a double-blind controlled study in 54 men. The allopurinol groups had lower levels of serum urate, urine urate, and EPS urate and xanthine. With variations in accepted statistical methodology, the investigators were able to show a difference in the mean patient-reported discomfort score between the study and the control groups at certain times in this trial with 330 days of follow-up. However, a re-examination of the data with use of more standardized statistical analyses did not convince other groups that changes in the urine and prostatic secretion of purine and pyrimidine bases resulted in significant amelioration of symptoms in this particular trial (Nickel et al, 1996). A follow-up randomized clinical trial further showed no advantage of allopurinol compared with placebo (Ziaee et al, 2006).

Prostatic Massage

Prostatic massage has been the principal therapy for prostatitis since the turn of the 20th century (O'Conor, 1936; Campbell, 1957). With the introduction of the scientific approach advocated by Meares and Stamey in 1968, prostatic massage became important only as a diagnostic tool, but as a therapy it was abandoned by urologists. It eventually regained some popularity, primarily because of the failure of standard medical therapy in patients with refractory symptoms of CP. Its benefits are believed to arise from draining theoretically occluded prostatic ducts and improving circulation and antibiotic penetration (Hennenfent and Feliciano, 1998). Independent but uncontrolled studies (Nickel et al, 1999b; Shoskes and Zeitlin, 1999) found clinical benefits in one third to two thirds of patients treated with repetitive prostatic massage (two to three times per week) for 4 to 6 weeks along with antibiotic therapy. However, another trial indicated that prostatic massage does not significantly improve the response of men with CP/CPPS treated with antibiotics (Ateya et al, 2006). It appears that some patients may improve with prostatic massage, but a panel of North American prostatitis experts (Nickel et al, 1999a) could not come to a consensus on the potential overall benefit or even the mechanism of achievement of that benefit if it does occur. **A subsequent systematic review of the literature concluded that evidence for a role of repetitive prostatic massage as an adjunct in the management of CP is at most "soft" but that the practice could be considered as part of multimodal therapy in selected patients** (Mishra et al, 2008). It has been suggested that frequent ejaculation may achieve the same function as prostatic massage (Yavascaoglu et al, 1999).

Pelvic Floor Physiotherapy (Including Directed Perineal and/or Pelvic Floor Massage and Myofascial Trigger Point Release)

Most clinicians recognize that men with prostatitis syndromes, especially category III CPPS, have specific anatomic areas that cause discomfort. Anderson (1999) believes that prolonged or chronic tension, distention, or distortion in the muscle bands (e.g., in the perineum) leads to a painful trigger point that is responsible for the pain. Predisposing factors leading to the formation of myofascial trigger points in the perineum or pelvis may include mechanical abnormalities in the hip and lower extremities, chronic urinary holding patterns (dysfunctional toilet training), sexual abuse, repetitive minor trauma, constipation, trauma, unusual sexual activity, recurrent infections or surgery, and perhaps stress and anxiety (Anderson et al, 2009a). Treatment of these trigger points includes heat therapy, physiotherapy massage, ischemic compression, stretching, anesthetic injections, acupuncture, electroneural modulation, and mind-body interactions such as progressive relaxation exercises, yoga, and hypnosis (Potts, 2003). Anderson and associates (2005) report that employing these techniques with a team consisting of a urologist, physiotherapist, and psychologist results in more than half of patients having or demonstrating a clinically detectable improvement. A case study analysis indicates that this may be an effective therapeutic approach in some patients (Anderson et al, 2005) and may result in improvement not just in pain but also in sexual function (Anderson et al, 2006). This technique has been further refined and modified by employing relaxation training (Anderson et al, 2011b) This technique has even been described as self-treatment using a "myofascial trigger point wand" (Anderson et al, 2011a). Certainly, many physicians managing CP/CPPS have found that directed physiotherapy results in significant benefits for selected patients with pelvic floor pathology diagnosed on physical examination (Van Alstyne et al, 2010). An NIH pilot study of men and women with chronic pelvic pain randomized to treatment with either relaxation massage or specific pelvic massage therapy demonstrated improvement; however, the beneficial effects were mainly found in women at 6 months, and the investigators could not corroborate these findings in the 23 randomized men (FitzGerald et al, 2009). In contrast, Marx and coworkers (2009), who randomized 35 men to osteopathic therapy, noted statistically significant

differences in favor of the osteopathy group ($P < .0005$). Long-term follow-up of 19 of the 20 men randomized to the treatment arm continued to show benefits for 5 years (Marx et al, 2013). **Most clinicians with experience in the field believe that variations of pelvic floor physiotherapy can be extremely helpful in patients with demonstrable pelvic floor pathology that was found to be refractory to other therapies** (Fitzgerald et al, 2013).

Pudendal Nerve Entrapment Therapy

It has been hypothesized that the symptoms of CPPS could be caused by entrapment of the pudendal nerve, perhaps between the sacrotuberous and sacrospinous ligaments, in the canal of Alcock or by the falciform process of the sacrotuberous ligament (Robert et al, 1998). Pudendal nerve blocks (Thoumas et al, 1999; McDonald and Spigos, 2000; Peng and Tumber, 2008) and neurolysis surgery (Robert et al, 1993; Mauillon et al, 1999) have been suggested for treatment. The role of the pudendal nerve in chronic perineal pain deserves more scientific scrutiny.

Biofeedback

It is possible that the voiding and pain symptoms associated with CP/CPPS may be secondary to some form of pseudodyssynergia during voiding or repetitive perineal muscle spasm; biofeedback has the potential to improve this process. Kaplan and associates (1997), Nadler (2002), Ye and colleagues (2003), and Cornel and coworkers (2005) have demonstrated in small uncontrolled studies that biofeedback does ameliorate specific prostatitis-like symptoms in some men. Controlled clinical trials will be necessary to evaluate this mode of therapy.

Acupuncture

Acupuncture is an accepted traditional Chinese therapy for chronic pain, including pain from prostatitis (Ge et al, 1988; Katai, 1992; Ikeuchi and Iguchi, 1994). Chen and Nickel (2003) determined in a pilot study of 12 treatment-refractory men that acupuncture was safe and provided effective and durable symptom improvement. A subsequent study comparing 10 weeks of acupuncture versus sham acupuncture treatment indicated that the active acupuncture proved to be almost twice as likely as sham treatment to improve CP/CPPS symptoms (Lee et al, 2008a). A subsequent trial evaluating electroacupuncture versus sham therapy (Lee and Lee, 2009) also confirmed the efficacy of this approach. A 2011 analysis by Lee and associates further confirmed that sham therapy comparison in acupuncture trials was feasible (Lee et al, 2011). A subsequent systemic review (Posadzki et al, 2012) concluded that acupuncture is a reasonable choice of therapy for selected men with CP/CPPS.

Psychological Support

Data from the NIH Prostatitis Cohort (Tripp et al, 2004, 2005, 2006; Nickel et al, 2008c) support a biopsychosocial model that associates the chronic pain and poor quality of life of CP/CPPS with depression and suggest that physicians may be able to advise patients to avoid certain pain coping strategies that can be associated with greater depression. Nickel and colleagues (2008b) have developed an evidence-based cognitive behavioral treatment program for men with CP/CPPS (described in Tripp et al, 2011). This program specifically targets empirically supported biopsychosocial variables (e.g., pain catastrophizing, depressive thinking, social support) and encourages patients to critically evaluate their patterns of thinking and to entertain novel thinking and behavioral responses to their troublesome symptoms, with an end objective to improve overall quality of life. A pilot evaluation of the program demonstrated significant merit in this approach (Tripp et al, 2011).

Studies also show that the maladaptive pain coping technique of employing "pain-contingent resting" (using rest rather than more active behaviors to control pain) is reported by CP/CPPS patients in response to their pain (Tripp et al, 2006; Nickel et al, 2008c). It was suggested by Tripp and coworkers (2006) that such sedentary behaviors in the presence of pain may be associated with elevated disability in men with CP/CPPS. A double-blind randomized study showed that men participating in aerobic exercise were significantly better than those who were randomized to stretching and motion exercise, suggesting that increased physical activity is a valid option in men with CP/CPPS (Giubilei et al, 2007). The results of a study examining perceived helpfulness of medical and self-management strategies suggested that clinicians may find it useful to support patients' use of safe, inexpensive self-management approaches, such as warm baths, increased water intake, exercise, and avoidance of prolonged sitting (Turner et al, 2006). It further appears that the support of a patient's partner can have a negative or positive impact on pain, disability, and sexual functioning (Smith et al, 2007b; Ginting et al, 2011).

Lifestyle Modification and Other Conservative Therapies

Conservative therapy should always be considered the primary therapy for CP/CPPS, despite the lack of evidence. Expert opinion and experience attest to the fact that conservative nonmedical and/or invasive therapies may provide the most benefit (Turner et al, 2006; Herati and Moldwin, 2013). My experience suggests that education (sometimes the only therapy required); avoidance of food, drink, and/or activities that exacerbate the symptoms; low-impact exercise (walking, elliptical machine, swimming, yoga, stretching); local heat therapy (hot water bottle, heating pad, hot tub or bath); and positive attitude and development of personal coping skills provide the basis on which all the other therapies rest. **Most of these interventions, even diet modification** (Herati et al, 2013), **have not been proven in randomized clinical trials in CP/CPPS specifically; however, they have proven their worth in clinical practice** (Turner et al, 2006) **and in use with other pain syndromes** (Giubilei et al, 2007).

Minimally Invasive Therapies

Balloon Dilatation. Lapatin and coworkers (1990) employed balloon dilatation in an uncontrolled trial of seven patients with nonbacterial prostatitis and prostatodynia and showed improvement in voiding symptoms during a 1- to 5-month follow-up. Pain and discomfort were not assessed. This treatment effect has never been substantiated, and balloon dilatation has not been routinely employed in clinical practice. Suzuki and coworkers (1995) combined the potential beneficial effects of balloon dilatation with prostatic hyperthermia in five men with CP/CPPS and demonstrated significant improvement in symptoms in one patient and partial improvement in three. Nickel and associates (1998b) were not able to duplicate this beneficial effect in a small pilot trial evaluating the "hot balloon" (heating by radiofrequency energy rather than laser energy).

Transurethral Needle Ablation. Chiang and associates (1997) employed transurethral needle ablation (TUNA) of the prostate in seven patients with chronic nonbacterial prostatitis, assessed the patients before and after therapy (6 months of follow-up) with a modification of the Symptom Severity Index (Nickel and Sorensen, 1996), and reported favorable results in four. A follow-up study by Chiang and Chiang (2004) showed significant improvement in symptoms in the majority of 32 patients treated with TUNA. However, Leskinen and colleagues (2002) investigated the effectiveness and durability of TUNA in 25 patients randomized to TUNA and eight patients randomized to sham treatment, and they reported that the efficacy of TUNA in CP/CPPS is comparable to that of sham treatment and so could not recommend TUNA as therapy for CP/CPPS.

Extracorporeal Shockwave Therapy. Extracorporeal shockwave lithotripsy has been suggested for the symptomatic relief of local perineal symptoms associated with CP/CPPS (Zimmerman et al, 2008). Zimmerman and colleagues (2009) randomized 60 men to perineal extracorporeal shockwave therapy (ESWT) or placebo and showed statistically significant beneficial effects in comparison with placebo. Another study randomized 40 patients to ESWT or placebo (Vahdatpour et al, 2013), and this study again showed significant improvement in the treated group. This modality of therapy certainly should be further considered for a larger confirmatory clinical trial, especially because there seem to be few complications.

Minimally Invasive Neuromodulation Therapies. Neuromodulation techniques used for chronic pelvic pain conditions include sacral nerve stimulation (SNS), percutaneous tibial nerve stimulation (PTNS), and pudendal nerve stimulation (Yang, 2013). Ruedi and associates (2003) suggested that high-frequency electrostimulation may be harnessed to treat CP. Others (Schneider et al, 2013) have evaluated electrostimulation therapies and suggest that they might be beneficial. In a study published in the non-English literature, Yang and colleagues (2011) randomly divided a total of 140 patients with diagnosed CP/CPPS into a control group (n = 20), a biofeedback group (n = 40), an electrical stimulation group (n = 40), and a biofeedback plus electrical stimulation group (n = 40). Each treatment appeared to be better than the control group, with combination therapy being the most effective. In a study to evaluate posterior tibial nerve stimulation (Kabay et al, 2009), a total of 89 patients with therapy-resistant pelvic pain were randomized to receive either nerve stimulation (n = 45) or sham treatment (n = 44). The authors demonstrated that percutaneous PTNS may relieve pain in patients with category IIIB CP/CPPS. SNS has been studied in interstitial cystitis (bladder pain syndrome) (Yang, 2013), but the typical pain and lack of voiding symptoms in male CPPS make it much more difficult to treat and assess using this strategy (Yang et al, 2003). Yang (2013) reviewed the invasive neuromodulation literature and concluded that these modalities of therapy may eventually be proven to provide benefits for patients with CPPS. However, because of the paucity of data and the limitations of small studies, the conclusions of the existing literature must be carefully considered.

Microwave Hyperthermia and Thermotherapy. It is believed that the heat applied to the prostate gland by the microwave process could shorten the natural resolution of the inflammatory process, perhaps by accelerating the process of fibrosis or scar formation in the area of chronic inflammation. In addition, heat therapy, particularly with the higher temperatures achieved with transurethral microwave thermotherapy, could alter the afferent nerve fibers that convey the objective symptom of pain from the inflamed prostate gland (intraprostatic sympathectomy) (Perachino et al, 1993). It may even be possible that the microwave energy kills nonculturable or cryptic bacteria within the prostate gland (Sahin et al, 1998).

Although many uncontrolled trials employing heat therapy have shown benefit (Nickel, 1999b; Zeitlin, 2002), only three published studies have used sham controls, and unfortunately the NIH-CPSI was not available as an outcome parameter for these studies. Vassily and associates (1999) noted symptom improvement in 75% of men in a transrectal microwave hyperthermia–treated group compared with 52% of men in the sham-treated group. Shaw and colleagues (1993) documented treatment success (defined as a greater than 50% improvement in symptoms) in 55% of the men in a transrectal microwave hyperthermia group (15 patients) compared with 10% of patients treated with sham therapy (13 patients) at 3 months. Nickel and Sorensen (1996) examined the safety and efficacy of transurethral microwave thermotherapy in 20 men randomized to therapy or sham. At 3 months' follow-up, the transurethral microwave thermotherapy–treated patients had significantly improved symptom scores compared with sham-treated patients (7 of 10 men treated with transurethral microwave thermotherapy had a favorable result compared with 1 of 10 men treated with a sham therapy). A recently reported study in men with CP/CPPS treated with cooled transurethral microwave thermotherapy using the NIH-CPSI as an outcome (Kastner et al, 2004) again suggested that thermotherapy remains a promising treatment for intractable CP, particularly when it is associated with concomitant BPH. Although this prospective study showed a significant reduction in NIH-CPSI score compared with baseline in 35 men followed for 12 months, it was not a randomized sham controlled trial. Heat therapy appears to be a promising therapeutic approach but, until larger-scale studies have been performed, should be restricted to patients with refractory or end-stage symptoms. In 2012, Gao and colleagues attempted to relate improvement they observed with transrectal hyperthermia with physiologic changes in the prostate.

Other Minimally Invasive Surgical Procedures. Serel and colleagues (1997) reported significantly meaningful beneficial effects of use of the neodymium:yttrium-aluminum-garnet laser in 30 patients with chronic abacterial prostatitis and prostatodynia. A number of other minimally invasive treatments have been examined in small pilot studies. These include pelvic and sacral electromagnetic therapy (Leippold et al, 2005; Rowe et al, 2005; Kim et al, 2013). It has been suggested that injection of botulinum toxin directly into the prostate may benefit some patients (Chuang and Chancellor, 2006). Botulinum toxin A (BTX-A) injection was evaluated in a small pilot study in which 29 patients were randomized to receive either BTX-A 100 U or normal saline injected into the perineal body and bulbospongiosus muscle (Gottsch et al, 2011). Total CPSI score did not reach significance in the BTX-A-treated group compared with controls; however, the CPSI pain subdomain score reached statistical significance in the BTX-A patients compared with controls ($P = .05$), with 30% of treated patients compared with 13% of placebo patients achieving at least minimal responder status ($P = .0002$).

Some minimally invasive surgical procedures (electrical neuromodulation, extracorporeal shock wave therapy, electroacupuncture, and perhaps transurethral microwave thermotherapy (TUMT) and botulinum toxin injection may be beneficial for treatment for CP/CPPS in selected patients (see Table 13-3); however, large, well-designed sham-controlled trials are required before these therapies can be considered recommended.

Traditional Surgery

In acute bacterial prostatitis (category I), urinary obstruction is a very common symptom. Traditionally it has been suggested that the insertion of a suprapubic cystotomy tube is the optimal therapy because an indwelling Foley catheter may further obstruct urethral ducts, resulting in the potential for development of prostate abscesses (Dajani and O'Flynn, 1968; Pai and Baht, 1972; Weinberger et al, 1988). **In most patients, however, an in-and-out catheterization to relieve the initial obstruction or short-term (12 hours) indwelling catheterization with a small-caliber Foley catheter is appropriate. A developing prostate abscess, best detected with transrectal ultrasonography or computed tomography** (Rovik and Doehlin, 1989), **that fails to respond quickly to antibiotics is optimally drained by the transurethral incision route** (Pai and Baht, 1972). **However, transperineal incision and drainage** (Granados et al, 1992) **must be considered when the abscess has penetrated beyond the prostatic capsule or penetrated through the levator ani muscle. More recently it has been suggested that percutaneous drainage of the abscess is the most effective and less morbid procedure** (Varkarakis et al, 2004).

Surgery does not have an important role in the treatment of most CP syndromes unless a specific indication is discovered during the evaluation of the patient (Kirby, 1999). These indications are usually noted during specific and ancillary investigations such as cystoscopy, transrectal ultrasonography, urodynamics, computed tomography, or MRI. Certainly, patients with urethral strictures benefit from surgical correction. Kaplan and associates (1994) have suggested that men with chronic nonbacterial prostatitis-like symptoms and urodynamic evidence of vesical neck obstruction benefit from endoscopic incision of the bladder neck.

Seminal vesicle abscesses can be managed with antibiotic therapy, transrectal aspiration, and, if necessary, an operation to remove the seminal vesicles. Traditionally, seminal vesiculectomy was performed as a difficult open procedure, but laparoscopic excision of the seminal vesicles was reported to be the least morbid procedure (Nadler and Rubenstein, 2001).

Radical transurethral resection of the prostate (Barnes et al, 1982; Sant et al, 1984) has been advocated in patients who have

either relapsing or refractory chronic bacterial prostatitis (category II) secondary to bacterial persistence within the prostate gland. Although prostatic calculi are not pathognomonic of prostatitis (Harada et al, 1980), it has been clearly shown that bacteria can persist in protective biofilms or aggregates within the interstices or on the surface of the calculus material (Meares, 1974; Nickel et al, 1994). Theoretically, removal of all the infected material, including potentially infected calculi, can be achieved (with appropriate intraoperative radiographs or ultrasound studies), but except for small anecdotal case series (Barnes et al, 1982; Sant et al, 1984) there is no substantial proof in the literature as to the efficacy of major prostate surgery in category II CP. Radical transurethral resection of the prostate has not been advocated for category III CP/CPPS, but open radical prostatectomy has been shown anecdotally to benefit a few patients with symptoms of nonbacterial prostatitis or prostatodynia or both (Davis and Weigel, 1990; Frazier et al, 1992). **No definitive clinical series or long-term follow-up has ever been presented, and this type of surgery should not be encouraged or recommended at this time.**

Phenotype Directed Multimodal Treatment Strategy

There are a number of reasons why the majority of randomized placebo- or sham-controlled trials reported in the literature and this chapter have been "negative" or only modestly "positive," making it difficult to develop evidence-based management guidelines. The first reason is that treatments based on a single causative mechanism may be doomed to fail when tested in the whole CP/CPPS population. As discussed earlier in the section on etiology, most of the mechanisms examined are based on sound scientific theory, and all are associated with at least some confirmatory clinical data. But it appears that patients have differing mechanisms and pathogenic progressions. We must accept that there is no one all-encompassing causative mechanism responsible for all cases of CP/CPPS. As further discussed in the section on evaluation, it is now evident that patients also have quite heterogeneous clinical phenotypes. In addition, one cannot be sure that the patients routinely managed in clinical practice are the same patients who have been enrolled in clinical trials. In fact, the most rigorously designed NIH-sponsored randomized controlled trials (Alexander et al, 2004; Nickel et al, 2008b; Pontari et al, 2010) did not enroll over 90% of the CP/CPPS patients who were screened. Finally, were the negative trials reported in the literature and this chapter really negative? A reappraisal of the study results would suggest otherwise. Antibiotics tended to work better in less chronic heavily pretreated patients (marginally significant improvement in levofloxacin trial [Nickel et al, 2003b] compared with ciprofloxacin trial [Alexander et al, 2004]), further substantiated by the 75% improvement seen with use of ciprofloxacin or levofloxacin treatment in patients with very early presentation (within 4 to 8 weeks of symptoms associated with that particular episode) (Nickel and Xiang, 2008). Whereas large NIH-sponsored multicenter studies failed to confirm the benefits of α-adrenergic blockers in both chronic heavily pretreated (Alexander et al, 2004) and recently diagnosed α-adrenergic blocker–naive (Nickel et al, 2008b) CP/CPPS patients, at least six other randomized controlled trials (Cheah et al, 2003b; Mehik et al, 2003; Nickel et al, 2004b; Tugcu et al, 2007; Chen et al, 2011; Nickel et al, 2011a) with less rigorous selection criteria did show significant efficacy with α-adrenergic blockers. Although the results of trials examining anti-inflammatory agents (Nickel et al, 2003b), pentosan polysulfate (Nickel et al, 2005a), finasteride (Nickel et al, 2004b), celecoxib (Zhao et al, 2009), tanezumab (Nickel et al, 2012), and the neuromodulator pregabalin (Pontari et al, 2010) were considered only marginally positive or even negative based on the primary end point analysis, these trials showed efficacy for many of the validated outcomes (including responder analyses using the validated subjective global or global response assessment scale) of statistical or marginal significance. In fact, when examined using a network meta-analysis approach, Anothaisintawee and colleagues (2011) evaluated all randomized controlled data for medical therapies and concluded that there was a statistically significant improvement compared with placebo for almost all of these therapies. However, **the clinical significance of this benefit and the disconnect between symptom score improvement and responder data indicate that these treatments are not very effective when used indiscriminately in the entire CP/CPPS population.** It is very likely that we will never discover a single overall cure for all patients diagnosed with this condition. This reevaluation of trial results, however, strongly suggests that some patients do, in fact, respond to these various therapies. **Multimodal therapy using multiple concurrent treatment strategies appears to offer the best results** (Shoskes et al, 2003; Shoskes and Katz, 2005), **at least compared with a sequential monotherapy approach** (Nickel et al, 2004a; Nickel, 2008b). However, a number of well-controlled prospective studies did not demonstrate increased efficacy of combining α-adrenergic blockers and antibiotics (Alexander et al, 2004) or α-adrenergic blockers and anti-inflammatory agents (Batstone et al, 2005). The explanation for this difficulty in treating CP may be that the patients become peripherally and centrally sensitized and that treatment targeted to the local initiators of the early process may not work as well when the condition becomes chronic and outside the pelvis (Yang et al, 2003; Pontari and Ruggieri, 2004; Pontari, 2007). We must be able to identify patients who may respond to specific therapies, and at this time the UPOINT clinical phenotyping system comprehensively described in the evaluation section may be the best approach.

It has been suggested that **UPOINT will be a new clinical tool for urologists to use to direct individually based therapy.**

Each domain has been clinically defined using standard clinical assessment and linked to specific mechanisms of symptom production or propagation (see evaluation section for details). Each of these domains has been associated with specific therapy based on best evidence and expert experience (Fig. 13-9). One clinical trial assessing this approach in CP/CPPS showed what appeared to be a superior clinical benefit. In this study by Shoskes and associates (2010) almost 100 consecutive men referred to a tertiary CP clinic were categorized according to the UPOINT system and then treated according to an algorithm similar to that described in this chapter (see Fig. 13-9) and followed for 6 months. A 6-point decrease in NIH-CPSI total score is believed to be a clinically significant achievement in these chronic heavily pretreated patients, and 84% of men reported this level of improvement at 6 months. The overall NIH-CPSI mean score in the group decreased from 25.2 (±6.1) to 13.2 (±7.2) a clinically and statistically significant ($P < .0001$) result. Based on previous clinical trial data, poor clinical experience with providing treatment benefits to CP/CPPS patients, initial studies, and ongoing experience in the clinic, the European (Engeler et al, 2013), Canadian (Nickel, 2011), and International Consultation on Urinary Disease (Nickel et al, 2013b) guidelines suggest that a phenotypic approach to therapy as described by the UPOINT system be considered for clinical practice. (Criteria for inclusion in the specific CP/CPPS domains and suggested directed therapies are shown in Fig. 13-9.)

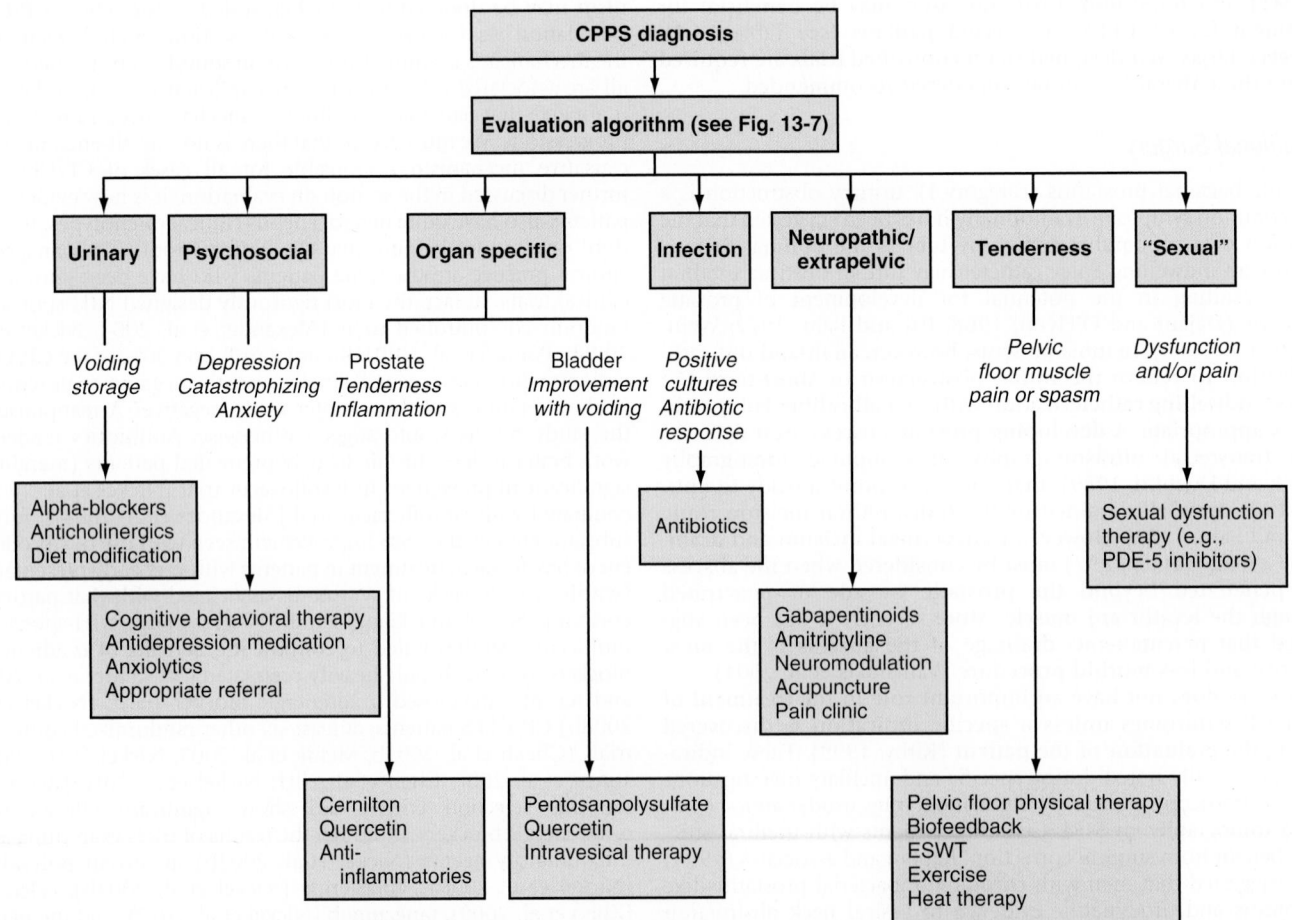

Figure 13-9. A suggested diagnostic and therapeutic algorithm for the treatment of patients with chronic prostatitis and chronic pelvic pain syndrome (CPPS) based on the UPOINT clinical phenotyping strategy. ESWT, extracorporeal shockwave therapy; PDE-5, phosphodiesterase type 5. (Modified from Nickel JC. Prostatitis. CUA Guideline. Can Urol Assoc J 2011;5:306–15; and Nickel JC, Wagenlehner F, Pontari M, et al. Male chronic pelvic pain syndrome (CPPS). In: Chapple C, Abrams P, editors. Male lower urinary tract symptoms (LUTS). An International Consultation on Male LUTS, Fukuoka, Japan, Sept 30-Oct 4, 2012. Montreal: Société Internationale d'Urologie (SIU); 2013. p. 331–72.)

Treatment Summary

Acute bacterial prostatitis is relatively simple to treat; the bacteria are eradicated with appropriate antibiotic therapy. However, ESBL infection related to prostate biopsy is becoming a worldwide problem. The objective for chronic bacterial prostatitis is similar—eradication of bacteria—but long-term symptom amelioration sometimes eludes us. Our standard therapies for CP/CPPS, when used as monotherapy, offer only modest improvement in symptoms (Nickel et al, 2004a, 2008b). Box 13-2 outlines a list of the various standard therapies that are currently recommended. Table 13-4 describes the standard doses of the various medical therapies.

To evaluate and compare the many clinical trials assessing the various therapies advocated for CP/CPPS it is important to clearly define and classify the patient population (NIH classification system), determine results by using a standardized outcome index (NIH-CPSI), prospectively compare a treated group with a similar group randomized to placebo, and fulfill the requirements of peer review for publication in a reputable journal (Nickel et al, 1999b; Propert et al, 2002). In the past several years the results of a significant number of such trials have been published (Nickel, 2004; Schaeffer, 2006; Nickel, 2008a; Anothaisintawe et al, 2011; Nickel, 2011; Cohen et al, 2012; Thakkinstian et al, 2012; Engeler et al, 2013; Nickel et al, 2013a), allowing the reader to assess and compare the efficacy of antibiotics, α-adrenergic blockers, anti-inflammatory agents, phytotherapies, hormonal agents, and minimally invasive approaches in CP/CPPS (see Tables 13-2 and 13-3). A patient-directed phenotypic strategy (such as the UPOINT approach), developing a unique best-evidence multimodal treatment plan for each individual, may be the optimal way to use the available clinical trial data to ultimately improve patient management in CP/CPPS (see Fig. 13-9).

BOX 13-2 Suggested Therapies for Chronic Prostatitis and Chronic Pelvic Pain Syndrome (National Institutes of Health Category III)

RECOMMENDED

1. α-Blocker therapy as part of a multimodal treatment strategy for newly diagnosed, α blocker–naive patients who have voiding symptoms.
2. Antimicrobial therapy trial for selected newly diagnosed, antimicrobial-naive patients.
3. Selected phytotherapies: Cernilton and Quercetin.
4. Multimodal therapy directed by clinical phenotype.
5. Directed physiotherapy. Although level 1 evidence is not available, evidence from multiple weak trials and vast clinical experience strongly suggests benefit for selected patients.

NOT RECOMMENDED

1. α-Blocker monotherapy, particularly in patients previously treated with α-blockers.
2. Anti-inflammatory monotherapy.
3. Antimicrobial therapy as primary therapy, particularly for patients in whom treatment with antibiotics has previously failed.
4. 5α-Reductase inhibitor monotherapy; can be considered in older patients with coexisting benign prostatic hyperplasia.
5. Most minimally invasive therapies such as transurethral needle ablation (TUNA), laser therapies.
6. Invasive surgical therapies such as transurethral resection of the prostate (TURP) and radical prostatectomy.

REQUIRING FURTHER EVALUATION

1. Low-intensity shock wave treatment.
2. Acupuncture.
3. Biofeedback.
4. Invasive neuromodulation (e.g., pudendal nerve modulation).
5. Electromagnetic stimulation.
6. Botulinum toxin A injection.
7. Medical therapies including mepartricin, muscle relaxants, neuromodulators, immunomodulators.

Modified from Nickel JC, Wagenlehner F, Pontari M, et al. Male chronic pelvic pain syndrome (CPPS). In: Chapple C, Abrams P, editors. Male lower urinary tract symptoms (LUTS). An International Consultation on Male LUTS, Fukuoka, Japan, Sept 30-Oct 4, 2012. Montreal: Société Internationale d'Urologie; 2013. p. 331–72.

KEY POINTS: THERAPY

- The following medical therapies have been evaluated in standardized randomized placebo-controlled trials in chronic pelvic pain syndrome (CPPS): antibiotics, α-adrenergic blockers, anti-inflammatory agents, hormonal therapies, phytotherapies, and pregabalin. The following minimally invasive therapies have been evaluated in randomized placebo- or sham-controlled trials in CPPS: extracorporeal shockwave therapy (ESWT), transurethral microwave therapy (TUMT), and neuromodulation (electrostimulation, botulinum toxin).
- The following therapies have shown benefits in placebo- or sham-controlled studies in CPPS: marked benefit—none; moderate benefit in some selected trials—α-adrenergic blockers and pregabalin; and modest benefit—anti-inflammatory agents, phytotherapies, ESWT, TUMT, selected neurostimulation.
- Specific multimodal therapy directed at individual UPOINT phenotypes may result in better management outcomes.

OTHER INFLAMMATORY AND PAIN CONDITIONS OF THE LOWER URINARY TRACT

Orchitis

Definition and Classification

By definition, orchitis is inflammation of the testis, but the term has been used to describe testicular pain localized to the testis without objective evidence of inflammation. **Acute orchitis** represents sudden occurrence of pain and swelling of the testis associated with acute inflammation of that testis. **Chronic orchitis** involves inflammation and pain in the testis, usually without swelling, persisting for more than 6 weeks. A classification (Nickel and Beiko, 2001) based on cause is presented in Box 13-3.

Pathogenesis and Etiology

Isolated orchitis is a relatively rare condition and is usually viral in origin. It spreads to the testis by a hematogenous route. Most cases of orchitis, particularly bacterial, occur secondary to local spread of an ipsilateral epididymitis and are referred to as *epididymo-orchitis.* UTIs are usually the underlying source in boys and elderly men. In young sexually active men, sexually transmitted diseases are often responsible (Berger, 1998). Truly noninfectious orchitis is often idiopathic or related to trauma, although autoimmune disease has rarely been implicated (Pannek and Haupt, 1997). It may be impossible to clinically distinguish chronic orchitis from chronic orchialgia.

Bacterial orchitis is usually associated with epididymitis and is therefore often caused by urinary pathogens, including *E. coli* and *Pseudomonas.* Less commonly, *Staphylococcus* species or *Streptococcus* species are responsible. The most common sexually transmitted

TABLE 13-4   Suggested Medical Therapy for Chronic Prostatitis and Chronic Pelvic Pain Syndrome

DRUG CLASS	SPECIFIC THERAPY	DOSE	DURATION OF THERAPY (WK)	EVIDENCE
Antibiotics	TMP-SMX	160/800 mg bid	12	See text for summary of clinical trial data.
	Norfloxacin	400 mg bid	4-12	
	Ciprofloxacin	500 mg bid	4-12	
	Ofloxacin	300 mg bid	4-12	
	Lomefloxacin	400 mg qd	4-12	
	Levofloxacin	500 mg qd	4-12	
α-Adrenergic blockers	Terazosin	5 mg qd	>14	Cheah et al, 2003b
	Alfuzosin	10 mg qd	>12	Mehik et al, 2003
				Nickel et al, 2008b
	Tamsulosin	0.4 mg qd	>6	Nickel et al, 2004c
				Alexander et al, 2004
	Silodosin	4 mg qd	>12	Nickel et al, 2011a
Phytotherapy	Pollen extract	1 tab tid	24	Buck et al, 1989
				Rugendorff et al, 1993
				Wagenlehner et al, 2009
	Quercetin	500 mg bid	4	Shoskes et al, 1999
	Saw palmetto	150 mg qd	24	Reissigl et al, 2004
Anti-inflammatory agents	Nimesulide	100 mg bid	2-4	Canale et al, 1993a
	Rofecoxib	25-50 mg qd	>6	Nickel et al, 2003c
	Other NSAIDs	Various	2-4	Evans, 1999
	Indomethacin			
	Diclofenac			
	Ibuprofen			
	Pentosan polysulfate	100 mg tid	24	Wedren, 1987
				Nickel et al, 2000
				Nickel et al, 2005a
Hormonal agents	Finasteride	5 mg qd	24	Leskinen et al, 1999
				Nickel et al, 2004b
	Mepartricin	40 mg qd	8	De Rose et al, 2004
Gabapentinoids	Pregabalin	50-100 mg tid	6	Pontari et al, 2010

NSAIDs, nonsteroidal anti-inflammatory drugs; TMP-SMX, trimethoprim-sulfamethoxazole.

BOX 13-3   Classification of Orchitis

Acute bacterial orchitis
    Secondary to urinary tract infection
    Secondary to sexually transmitted disease
Nonbacterial infectious orchitis
    Viral
    Fungal
    Parasitic
    Rickettsial
Noninfectious orchitis
    Idiopathic
    Traumatic
    Autoimmune
Chronic orchitis
Chronic orchialgia

---

microorganisms responsible are *Neisseria gonorrhoeae, C. trachomatis,* and *Treponema pallidum.* Xanthogranulomatous orchitis, usually associated with *Proteus* and *E. coli,* is an extremely rare inflammatory destructive lesion of the testes that is treated with orchiectomy (Al-Said et al, 2007; Kang et al, 2007).

Mycobacterial infections, tuberculosis (Chen et al, 2004; Park et al, 2008; Gomez-Garcia et al, 2010), and BCG therapy (Hill et al,

2008) can also cause orchitis. The most common cause of **viral orchitis** is mumps (Jalal et al, 2004; Masarani et al, 2006; Emerson et al, 2007; Davis et al, 2010), but infectious mononucleosis has also been implicated (Weiner, 1997). **Fungal infections** occasionally involve the testis, with candidiasis, aspergillosis, histoplasmosis, coccidioidomycosis, blastomycosis, and actinomycosis all having been reported as causes of orchitis (Wise, 1998). **Parasitic infections** rarely cause orchitis in the Western Hemisphere, but filariasis (Hazen Smith and von Lichtenberg, 1998) and trypanosomiasis (Ehrhardt et al, 2006) have been described in some endemic areas of Africa, Asia, and South America.

Autoimmune orchitis can be a relevant cause of decreased fecundity in males with the concomitant presence of anti-sperm antibodies. Causes of this variant of orchitis and/or testicular vasculitis are associated with autoimmune diseases, mainly those with primary vasculitis such as polyarteritis nodosa, Behçet disease, and Henoch-Schönlein purpura (Hedger, 2011; Silva et al, 2012).

Diagnosis

In patients with **acute infectious orchitis,** history discloses a recent onset of testicular pain, often associated with abdominal discomfort, nausea, and vomiting. These symptoms may be preceded by symptoms of parotitis in boys or young men, by UTIs in boys or elderly men, or alternatively by symptoms of a sexually transmitted disease in sexually active men. Although the process is usually unilateral, it is sometimes bilateral, especially if viral. Physical examination may reveal a toxic and febrile patient. The skin of the involved hemiscrotum is erythematous and edematous, and the testis is quite tender to palpation or can be associated with a transilluminating hydrocele. The patient should be clinically assessed for prostatitis and urethritis. For acute noninfectious orchitis the clinical picture resembles the just-presented description except that these patients lack the toxic appearance and fever.

For **chronic orchitis and orchialgia** there may have been a history of previous episodes of testicular pain, usually secondary to acute bacterial orchitis, trauma, or other causes. The patient has chronic testicular (and possibly epididymal) pain to a degree that could seriously affect his day-to-day functioning and quality of life. Patients with this diagnosis usually become very frustrated with this problem. On examination the patient does not appear toxic and does not have a fever. The scrotum is not usually erythematous, but the testis may be somewhat indurated and is almost always tender to palpation.

Laboratory tests employed to assist in the diagnosis include urinalysis, urine microscopy, and urine culture. For a patient in whom a sexually transmitted disease is suspected, a urethral swab should also be taken for culture. If the diagnosis is not evident from the history, physical examination, and these simple tests, scrotal ultrasonography should be performed (to rule out malignancy in patients with chronic orchitis or orchialgia). Color Doppler ultrasonography is a reasonably reliable method for evaluating patients with scrotal diseases, including swelling and pain (Rizvi et al, 2011), and MRI has been suggested as a second-line investigation (Parenti et al, 2009; Makela et al, 2011). The most important differential diagnosis in young men and boys is testicular torsion. Testicular torsion is often difficult to differentiate from an acute inflammatory condition. Scrotal ultrasound evaluations (with use of Doppler imaging to determine testicular blood flow) are especially helpful in differential diagnosis (Mernagh et al, 2004; Gunther et al, 2006), but occasionally the diagnosis will be missed (particularly with intermittent or partial torsion) and the clinician should err in favor of the surgically correctable diagnosis of torsion.

Treatment

General principles of therapy include bed rest, scrotal support, hydration, antipyretics, anti-inflammatory agents, and analgesics. **Antibiotic therapy** (specific for UTIs, prostatitis, or sexually transmitted diseases) should be employed for infectious orchitis and is ideally based on culture and sensitivity testing but may be based on microscopic or Gram stain results. Orchitis resulting from *Mycobacterium tuberculosis* infection requires treatment with antituberculous drugs (rifampin, isoniazid, and pyrazinamide or ethambutol) and rarely surgery (Gomez-Garcia et al, 2010). There are no specific antiviral agents available to treat orchitis caused by mumps, and the previously mentioned supportive measures are important. If early testing findings are negative or results are unavailable, empirical treatment should be initiated, directed at the most likely pathogens based on the available clinical information; a fluoroquinolone would be the best agent in this scenario. Most patients can be readily managed on an outpatient basis. Surgical intervention is rarely indicated, unless testicular torsion (or rarely xanthogranulomatous orchitis) is suspected (as discussed previously). Spermatic cord blocks with injection of a local anesthetic may sometimes be needed to relieve severe pain. Abscess formation is rare; if it does occur, then percutaneous or open drainage is necessary. Glucocorticoids and immunosuppressive drugs may be indicated in autoimmune orchitis-associated active systemic autoimmune diseases (Silva et al, 2012).

Treatment of chronic orchitis or orchialgia is supportive. Anti-inflammatory agents, analgesics, support, heat therapies, and nerve blocks all have a role in ameliorating symptoms. Neuromodulation, usually medical (tricyclic antidepressants or gabapentinoids), can be helpful, and SNS has been suggested as a potential treatment modality (McJunkin et al, 2009), but the evidence is not really available to justify this invasive procedure at this time. It is generally believed that the condition is self-limited but could take years (and sometimes decades) to resolve. **Orchidectomy is indicated only in**

cases in which pain control is refractory to all other measures (and even this might not be successful in alleviating the chronic pain) (Nariculam et al, 2007).

Epididymitis

Definitions and Classification

Epididymitis by definition is inflammation of the epididymis. Acute epididymitis represents sudden occurrence of pain and swelling of the epididymis associated with acute inflammation of the epididymis (Nickel et al, 2002). **Chronic epididymitis** refers to inflammation and pain in the epididymis, usually without swelling (but with induration in long-standing cases), persisting for over 6 weeks (Nickel et al, 2002). Inflammation is not always clinically evident in many cases of localized epididymal pain. Approximately 1 man in 100 attending a North American urology clinic has a diagnosis of epididymitis (Nickel et al, 2005b). In the late 1990s the average cost per episode of epididymitis managed in the United States was $368 (Gift and Owens, 2006), a cost considerably less than that reported for men with a diagnosis of CP. A classification for epididymitis is presented in Box 13-4 (Nickel et al, 2002).

Pathogenesis and Etiology

Acute epididymitis usually results from the spread of infection from the bladder, urethra, or prostate via the ejaculatory ducts and vas deferens into the epididymis. The process starts in the tail of the epididymis and then spreads through the body of the structure to the head of the epididymis. In infants and boys, epididymitis is often related to a UTI and/or an underlying genitourinary congenital anomaly (Merlini et al, 1998) or even to the presence of a foreskin (Bennett et al, 1998). In elderly men, BPH and associated stasis, UTI, and catheterization are the most common causes of epididymitis. Bacterial prostatitis and/or seminal vesiculitis are associated with epididymal infection in postpubertal males of all ages (Furuya et al, 2004). In sexually active men younger than 35 years of age, epididymitis is commonly the result of a sexually transmitted infection (Berger, 1998). In most cases of acute epididymitis, the testis is also involved in the process and thus the condition is referred to as *epididymo-orchitis*.

Chronic epididymitis may result from inadequately treated acute epididymitis, recurrent epididymitis, or some other cause including associations with other disease processes such as Behçet disease (Cho et al, 2003; Arromdee and Tanakitivirul, 2006; Pektas et al, 2008) or treatment with amiodarone (Nikolaou et al, 2007). The cause of chronic epididymalgia is usually unclear. Certainly one of the best known and studied is the chronic epididymitis

---

BOX 13-4 Classification of Epididymitis

Acute bacterial epididymitis
    Secondary to urinary tract infection
    Secondary to sexually transmitted disease
Nonbacterial infectious epididymitis
    Viral
    Fungal
    Parasitic
Noninfectious epididymitis
    Idiopathic
    Traumatic
    Autoimmune
    Amiodarone-induced
    Associated with a known syndrome (e.g., Behçet disease)
Chronic epididymitis
Chronic epididymalgia

or epididymalgia that occurs in some men after a vasectomy. About 1 in 100 men describe severe pain 6 months after a vasectomy that noticeably affects their quality of life (up to 15% of men report some discomfort 6 months after the procedure) (Leslie et al, 2007).

The most common causative microorganisms in the pediatric and elderly age groups are the coliform organisms that cause bacteriuria (Berger et al, 1979). In men younger than age 35 who are sexually active with women, the most common offending organisms causing epididymitis are the usual bacteria that cause urethritis, namely *N. gonorrhoeae* and *C. trachomatis* (Ito et al, 2012). In homosexual men who practice anal intercourse, *E. coli* and *Haemophilus influenzae* are most commonly responsible. Both tuberculosis (Liu et al, 2005; Tsili et al, 2008) and mycobacteria, such as BCG (Harada et al, 2006), can be associated with epididymitis. As with orchitis, viral, fungal, mycoplasmal, and parasitic microorganisms have all been implicated in epididymitis (Berger, 1998; Hazen Smith and von Lichtenberg, 1998; Wise, 1998; Scagni et al, 2008). Rarely, epididymitis as a complication of brucellosis has been described (Akinci et al, 2006; Queipo-Ortuno et al, 2006; Colmenero et al, 2007).

Diagnosis

Both acute infectious and acute noninfectious epididymitis manifest in much the same way as do acute infectious and acute noninfectious orchitis, respectively. Physical examination localizes the tenderness to the epididymis. However, in many cases the testis is also involved in the inflammatory process and subsequent pain; this is referred to as *epididymo-orchitis*. The spermatic cord is usually tender and swollen. Early in the process only the tail of the epididymis is tender, but the inflammation quickly spreads to the rest of the epididymis, and if it continues to the testis then the swollen epididymis becomes indistinguishable from the testis.

There may be no clinical or etiologic differentiation between chronic epididymitis and epididymalgia. The patient usually has a long-standing history of pain (waxing and waning or constant) localized to the epididymis, and, as with chronic orchitis and orchialgia, these symptoms may have a significant impact on the patient's quality of life (Nickel et al, 2002).

Laboratory tests should include Gram staining of a urethral smear and a midstream urine specimen. Gram-negative bacilli can usually be identified in patients with underlying cystitis. If the urethral smear reveals the presence of intracellular gram-negative diplococci, a diagnosis of infection with *N. gonorrhoeae* is established. If only WBCs are seen on the urethral smear, a diagnosis of *C. trachomatis* will be established two thirds of the time. A urethral swab and midstream urine specimen should be sent for culture and sensitivity testing. When an infant or young boy is diagnosed with epididymitis, he should be further evaluated with abdominopelvic ultrasonography, voiding cystourethrography, and possibly cystoscopy (Shortliffe and Dairiki, 1998; Al-Taheini et al, 2008). If the diagnosis is uncertain, duplex Doppler scrotal ultrasonography to look for increased blood flow to the affected epididymis may be performed (also to rule out torsion as described in the section on orchitis) (Mernagh et al, 2004; Rizvi et al, 2011). Ultrasonography can sometimes be helpful to rule out other epididymal and scrotal pathology (Lee et al, 2008). MRI can be considered a second-line investigation (Parenti et al, 2009; Makela et al, 2011).

Treatment

Management of acute infectious epididymitis depends on the likely cause and organism (Tracy et al, 2008). **The Centers for Disease Control and Prevention's 2006 guidelines for the treatment of infectious epididymitis included ceftriaxone or doxycycline for men younger than age 35 years and levofloxacin or ofloxacin for men older than age 35 years** (Centers for Disease Control and Prevention et al, 2006). The guidelines updated in 2010 (Centers for Disease Control and Prevention, 2010) have not changed the ceftriaxone recommendation but suggest that azithromycin could

be used instead of doxycycline. The recent U.K. guidelines (Street et al, 2011) are very similar.

For chronic epididymitis, a 4- to 6-week trial of antibiotics that would potentially be effective against possible bacterial pathogens and particularly *C. trachomatis* may be appropriate (Nickel, 2005). Anti-inflammatory agents, analgesics, scrotal support, and nerve blocks have all been recommended as empirical treatment (Nickel, 2005). It is generally believed that chronic epididymitis is a self-limited condition that will eventually "burn out," but this could take years (or even decades). **Surgical removal of the epididymis (epididymectomy) should be considered only when all conservative measures have been exhausted and the patient accepts that the operation will have at best a 50% chance of curing his pain** (Padmore et al, 1996; Tracy et al, 2008; Calleary and Masood, 2009). Successful spermatic cord block (temporary pain relief) does seem to predict a better result with surgery (Benson et al, 2013). Better surgical results (up to 70%) have also been reported for epididymectomy for postvasectomy pain (Siu et al, 2007; Lee et al, 2011). It has recently been reported that inhibition of adhesion and fibrosis after epididymectomy with local application of hyaluronic acid and carboxymethylcellulose improves pain relief and patient satisfaction (Chung et al, 2013). Many clinicians have shown that microsurgical denervation of the spermatic cord may achieve the same results as a complete epididymectomy (Choa et al, 1992; Heidenreich et al, 2002; Strom and Levine, 2008; Parekattil et al, 2013).

KEY POINTS: ORCHITIS AND EPIDIDYMITIS

- Orchitis usually occurs with epididymitis (except for viral causation).
- The cause of epididymitis and orchitis is usually related to the age of the patient.
- Acute presentation is usually related to infection or ischemia.
- In the young patient the most important differential diagnosis is torsion of the testis.
- Treatment of chronic epididymitis or epididymo-orchitis is difficult.

REFERENCES

The complete reference list is available online at www.expertconsult.com.

SUGGESTED READINGS

Anothaisintawee T, Attia J, Nickel JC, et al. The management of chronic prostatitis/chronic pelvic pain syndrome: a systematic review and network meta-analysis. JAMA 2011;305:78–86.

Drach GW, Fair WR, Meares EM, et al. Classification of benign diseases associated with prostatic pain: prostatitis or prostatodynia? J Urol 1978;120(2):266.

Kavoussi PK, Costabile RA. Orchialgia and the chronic pelvic pain syndrome. World J Urol 2012;31:773–8.

Krieger JN, Nyberg LJ, Nickel JC. NIH consensus definition and classification of prostatitis. JAMA 1999;282:236–7.

Litwin MS, McNaughton Collins M, Fowler FJ Jr, et al. The National Institutes of Health Chronic Prostatitis Symptom Index: development and validation of a new outcome measure. J Urol 1999;162(2):369–75.

Nickel JC, Alexander RB, Schaeffer AJ, et al. Leukocytes and bacteria in men with chronic prostatitis/chronic pelvic pain syndrome compared to asymptomatic controls. J Urol 2003;170(3):818–22.

Nickel JC, Shoskes D. Phenotypic approach to the management of chronic prostatitis/chronic pelvic pain syndrome. Curr Urol Rep 2009;10(4):307–12.

Nickel JC, Shoskes DA, Wagenlehner FM. Management of chronic prostatitis/chronic pelvic pain syndrome (CP/CPPS): the studies, the evidence and the impact. World J Urol 2013;31:747–53.

Nickel JC, Wagenlehner F, Pontari M, et al. Male chronic pelvic pain syndrome (CPPS). In: Chapple C, Abrams P, editors. Male lower urinary tract symptoms (LUTS). An International Consultation on Male LUTS,

Fukuoka, Japan, Sept 30-Oct 4, 2012. Montreal: Societe Internationale d'Urologie (SIU); 2013. p. 331–72.

Pontari MA, Ruggieri MR. Mechanisms in prostatitis/chronic pelvic pain syndrome. J Urol 2004;172(3):839–45.

Schaeffer AJ. Chronic prostatitis and chronic pelvic pain syndrome. N Engl J Med 2006;355:1690–8.

Schaeffer AJ, Landis JR, Knauss JS, et al. Chronic Prostatitis Collaborative Research Network Group. Demographic and clinical characteristics of men with chronic prostatitis: the National Institutes of Health chronic prostatitis cohort study. J Urol 2002;168(2):593–8.

Tracy CR, Steers WD, Costabile R. Diagnosis and management of epididymitis. Urol Clin North Am 2008;35(1):101–8.

Wagenlehner FME, VanTill JW, Magri V, et al. National Institutes of Health Chronic Prostatitis Symptom Index (NIH-CPSI) symptom evaluation in multinational cohorts of patients with chronic prostatitis/chronic pelvic pain syndrome. Eur Urol 2013;63(5):953–9.

Weidner W, Schiefer HG, Krauss H, et al. Chronic prostatitis: a thorough search for etiologically involved microorganisms in 1461 patients. Infection 1991;19:119–25.

14 Bladder Pain Syndrome (Interstitial Cystitis) and Related Disorders

Philip M. Hanno, MD, MPH

Definition	Diagnosis
Historical Perspective	Classification
Epidemiology	Treatment
Etiology	Principles of Management
Pathology	

Bladder pain syndrome or interstitial cystitis (BPS/IC) is a condition **diagnosed on a clinical basis** and requiring a high index of suspicion on the part of the clinician. It is a deceptively intricate disorder that **should be considered in the differential diagnosis of the patient with chronic pelvic pain, pressure, or discomfort often exacerbated by bladder filling, and associated with at least one other urinary symptom, often urinary frequency.** One can argue that it is a *symptom complex* because it has a differential diagnosis that should be explored in a timely fashion before or at the time of initiation of empirical therapy (Blaivas, 2007). It is a diagnosis of exclusion in a patient who has experienced the symptoms for at least 6 weeks. Once other conditions have been ruled out, it can be considered a syndrome that typically responds to one of a variety of therapeutic approaches in the majority of cases. **Symptoms compatible with the diagnosis are now thought to affect up to 3% of the female population** (Berry et al, 2011). **Although the female-to-male ratio has historically been about 5 : 1, newer epidemiologic data suggest that male symptom prevalence may approach that of female symptom prevalence in the United States** (Suskind et al, 2013a).

The perception that the original term, *interstitial cystitis*, was not at all descriptive of the clinical syndrome, or even the pathologic findings in many patients, led to the current effort to reconsider the name of the disorder and even the way it is positioned in the medical spectrum (Hanno, 2008a). **What was originally considered a bladder disease is now considered a chronic pain syndrome** (Janicki, 2003) **that may begin as a pathologic process in the bladder in most but not all patients and eventually can develop into a condition that, in a small subset of those affected, even cystectomy may not benefit** (Baskin and Tanagho, 1992). Its relationship to type 3 chronic pelvic pain syndrome (CPPS) or nonbacterial prostatitis is unclear (Chai, 2002; Hakenberg and Wirth, 2002). Its association with other chronic pain syndromes has taken on more importance recently as a promising clue in unlocking the challenging etiologic and therapeutic puzzle of this condition (Rodriguez et al, 2009).

BPS/IC encompasses a major portion of the "painful bladder" disease complex. **Painful bladder disorders involve a large group of patients with bladder, urethral, and/or pelvic pain; irritative voiding symptoms (urgency, frequency, nocturia, dysuria); and sterile urine cultures.** Painful bladder conditions with well-established causes include radiation cystitis, cystitis caused by microorganisms that are not detected by routine culture methodologies, ketamine cystitis (Winstock et al, 2012), and systemic disorders that affect the bladder. In addition, many gynecologic disorders can mimic BPS/IC (Kohli et al, 1997; Howard 2003a, 2003b). BPS/IC has no easily discernible cause.

The symptoms are allodynic, an exaggeration of normal sensations. There are no pathognomonic findings on pathologic examination, and even the finding of petechial hemorrhages on the bladder mucosa during cystoscopy after bladder hydrodistention under anesthesia is no longer considered the sine qua non of BPS/IC (Erickson, 1995; Waxman et al, 1998; Erickson et al, 2005). **BPS/IC is truly a diagnosis of exclusion.** It may have multiple causes and represent a final common reaction of the bladder to different types of insult. Misdiagnosis as a psychological problem, an overactive bladder, or chronic urinary infection has plagued patients with the syndrome. **A distinct subgroup of patients with discrete inflammatory lesions in the bladder lining (Hunner lesions) involves specific characteristics, and successful treatment of this subgroup is available** (Nordling et al, 2012).

DEFINITION

"It resembles a constellation of stars; its components are real enough but the pattern is in the eye of the beholder" (Mäkelä and Heliövaara, 1991). This evocative description of fibromyalgia could equally apply to BPS/IC. Indeed, it has been argued, not necessarily convincingly, that each medical specialty has at least one somatic syndrome (irritable bowel syndrome, chronic pelvic pain, fibromyalgia, tension headache, noncardiac chest pain, hyperventilation syndrome) that might be better conceptualized as a part of a general functional somatic syndrome than with the symptom-based classification that we have now, which may be more reflective of professional specialization and access to care (Wessely and White, 2004).

BPS/IC is a clinical diagnosis based primarily on chronic symptoms of pain perceived by the patient to emanate from the bladder and/or pelvis associated with urinary urgency or frequency in the absence of another identified cause for the symptoms. It has been defined and redefined over the last century, and as the problem of definition has become more prominent lately, so have the number of definitions and attempts to crystallize just what the diagnosis means (Box 14-1). **The International Continence Society (ICS) prefers the term *painful bladder syndrome*, defined as "the complaint of suprapubic pain related to bladder filling, accompanied by other symptoms such as increased daytime and night-time frequency, in the absence of proven urinary infection**

BOX 14-1 History of Definitions of Bladder Pain Syndrome, Painful Bladder Syndrome, and Interstitial Cystitis Syndrome

- *1887, Skene (Skene, 1887):* An inflammation that has destroyed the mucous membrane partly or wholly and extended to the muscular parietes.
- *1915, Hunner (Hunner, 1915):* A peculiar form of bladder ulceration whose diagnosis depends ultimately on its resistance to all ordinary forms of treatment in patients with frequency and bladder symptoms (spasms).
- *1951, Bourque (Bourque, 1951):* Patients who suffer chronically from their bladder—the ones who are distressed, not only periodically but constantly, having to urinate at all hours of the day and of the night and suffering pains every time they void.
- *1978, Messing and Stamey (Messing and Stamey, 1978):* Nonspecific and highly subjective symptoms of around-the-clock frequency, urgency, and pain somewhat relieved by voiding when associated with glomerulations on bladder distention under anesthesia.
- *1990, Revised National Institute of Diabetes and Digestive and Kidney Diseases (NIDDK) criteria (Wein et al, 1990):* Pain associated with the bladder or urinary urgency, and glomerulations or Hunner ulcer on cystoscopy under anesthesia, in patients with symptoms for 9 months or longer—at least eight voids per day, one void per night, and cystometric bladder capacity less than 350 mL.
- *1997, NIDDK Interstitial Cystitis Data Base study entry criteria (Simon et al, 1997):* Unexplained urgency or frequency (seven or more voids per day) or pelvic pain, of at least 6 months' duration in the absence of other definable causes.

- *2008, European Society for the Study of Interstitial Cystitis (ESSIC) (van de Merwe et al, 2008):* Chronic (longer than 6 months) pelvic pain, pressure, or discomfort perceived to be related to the urinary bladder accompanied by at least one other urinary symptom such as persistent urge to void or frequency. Confusable diseases as the cause of the symptoms must be excluded.
- *2009, Japanese Urological Association (Homma et al, 2009):* A disease of the urinary bladder diagnosed by three conditions: (1) lower urinary tract symptoms such as urinary frequency, bladder hypersensitivity, and/or bladder pain; (2) bladder pathology proven endoscopically by Hunner ulcer and/or mucosal bleeding after overdistention; and (3) exclusion of confusable diseases such as infection, malignancy, or calculi of the urinary tract.
- *2009, Society for Urodynamics and Female Urology (SUFU) informal international dialogue consensus meeting (Hanno and Dmochowski, 2009):* An unpleasant sensation (pain, pressure, discomfort) perceived to be related to the urinary bladder, associated with lower urinary tract symptoms of longer than 6 weeks' duration, in the absence of infection or other identifiable causes.
- *2011, American Urological Association:* An unpleasant sensation (pain, pressure, discomfort) perceived to be related to the urinary bladder, associated with lower urinary tract symptoms of longer than 6 weeks' duration, in the absence of infection or other identifiable causes.

---

or other obvious pathology" (Abrams et al, 2002). **The ICS reserves the diagnosis of *interstitial cystitis* for patients with "typical cystoscopic and histological features," without further specifying these. This definition may miss 36% of patients, primarily because it confines the pain to a suprapubic location and mandates a relationship of pain to bladder filling** (Warren et al, 2006).

In the absence of clear criteria for IC, this chapter will refer to BPS/IC and IC interchangeably, because all but recent literature terms the syndrome *interstitial cystitis*. The definition of the European Society for the Study of Interstitial Cystitis (ESSIC) is a clinically useful one, and changes made since its original iteration have likely made it more sensitive and inclusive (Mouracade et al, 2008). Minor modifications made at a meeting under the auspices of the Society for Urodynamics and Female Urology (SUFU) may be preferred by some clinicians. The SUFU definition was adopted in the guidelines of the American Urological Association (AUA) along with the nomenclature *interstitial cystitis/bladder pain syndrome* (Hanno et al, 2011). Perhaps more than for most diseases, how we arrived at this point is instructive and critical to an overall understanding of BPS/IC. The paradigm change that has resulted in morphing what was originally considered a bladder disease (aptly named *interstitial cystitis*) to a chronic pain syndrome *(bladder pain syndrome)* also merits discussion.

HISTORICAL PERSPECTIVE

Recent historical reviews confirm that IC was recognized as a pathologic entity during the 19th century (Christmas and Sant, 1997; Parsons and Parsons, 2004). Joseph Parrish, a Philadelphia surgeon, described three patients with severe lower urinary tract symptoms in the absence of a bladder stone in an 1836 text (Parrish, 1836), and termed the disorder *tic douloureux of the bladder*. Teichman argued that this may represent the first description of IC (Teichman

et al, 2000). Fifty years later Skene used the term *interstitial cystitis* to describe an inflammation that had "destroyed the mucous membrane partly or wholly and extended to the muscular parietes" (Skene, 1887).

Early in the 20th century, at a New England Section meeting of the AUA, Guy Hunner reported on eight women with a history of suprapubic pain, frequency, nocturia, and urgency lasting an average of 17 years (Hunner, 1915, 1918). He drew attention to the disease, and the red, bleeding areas he described on the bladder wall came to be called *Hunner ulcers*. As Walsh (1978) observed, this has proved to be unfortunate. In the early part of the 20th century, the very best cystoscopes available gave a poorly defined and ill-lit view of the fundus of the bladder. It is not surprising that when Hunner saw red and bleeding areas high on the bladder wall, he thought they were ulcers. For the next 60 years, urologists would look for ulcers and fail to make the diagnosis in their absence. The disease was thought to be focal, rather than a pancystitis.

Hand (1949) authored the first comprehensive review about the disease, reporting on 223 patients. In looking back, his paper was truly a seminal one, years ahead of its time. Many of his epidemiologic findings have held up to this day. His description of the clinical findings bears repeating. "I have frequently observed that what appeared to be a normal mucosa before and during the first bladder distention showed typical interstitial cystitis on subsequent distention." He noted "small, discrete, submucosal hemorrhages, showing variations in form ... dot-like bleeding points ... little or no restriction to bladder capacity." He portrayed three grades of disease, with grade 3 matching the small-capacity, scarred bladder described by Hunner. Sixty-nine percent of patients had grade 1 disease, and only 13% had grade 3.

Walsh (1978) later coined the term *glomerulations* to describe the petechial hemorrhages that Hand had described. But it was not until Messing and Stamey (1978) discussed the "early diagnosis" of IC that attention turned from looking for an ulcer to make the diagnosis to the concepts that (1) symptoms and glomerulations at the time of bladder distention under anesthesia were the disease hallmarks, and (2) the diagnosis was primarily one of exclusion.

Bourque's "Aunt Minnie description" of IC (i.e., it is hard to define, but one knows it when one sees it) is more than 60 years old and is worth recalling. "We have all met, at one time or another, patients who suffer chronically from their bladder; and we mean the ones who are distressed, not only periodically but constantly, having to urinate often, at all moments of the day and of the night, and suffering pains every time they void. We all know how these miserable patients are unhappy, and how those distressing bladder symptoms get finally to influence their general state of health physically at first, and mentally after a while" (Bourque, 1951).

Although memorable, this description and others like it were not suitable for defining this disease in a manner that would help physicians make the diagnosis and design research studies to learn more about the problem. Physician interest and government participation in research were sparked through the efforts of a group of frustrated patients led by Dr. Vicki Ratner, an orthopedic surgery resident in New York City, who founded the first patient advocacy group, the Interstitial Cystitis Association, in the living room of her small New York City apartment in 1984 (Ratner et al, 1992, 1997). The first step was to develop a working definition of the disease. The modern history of BPS/IC is best viewed through the development of the modern definition.

Evolution of the Definition

There are data to suggest that true urinary frequency in women can be defined as regularly having to void at intervals of less than 3 hours, and that of women older than 40 years, 25% have nocturia at least once (Glenning, 1985; Fitzgerald and Brubaker, 2003). Whereas bladder capacity tends to fall in women by the eighth and ninth decades of life, bladder volume at first desire to void tends to rise as women age (Collas and Malone-Lee, 1996). Based on a 90th percentile cutoff to determine the ranges of normality, the highest "normal" frequency ranges in the fourth decade range from six for men to nine for women (Burgio et al, 1991). **Large variation in the degree of bothersomeness with varying rates of frequency** (Fitzgerald et al, 2002) **makes a symptomatic diagnosis of BPS/IC based on an absolute number of voids subject to question,** and frequency per volume of intake or even the concept of "perception of frequency" as a problem may be more accurate than an absolute number.

In an effort to define IC so that patients in different geographic areas and under the care of different physicians could be compared, the National Institute of Diabetes and Digestive and Kidney Diseases (NIDDK) held a workshop in August 1987 at which consensus criteria were established for the diagnosis of IC (Gillenwater and Wein, 1988). These criteria were not meant to define the disease, but rather to ensure that groups of patients included in basic and clinical research studies would be relatively comparable. After pilot studies were carried out to test the criteria, they were revised at another NIDDK workshop a year later (Wein et al, 1990). These criteria are presented in Box 14-2.

Although meant initially to serve only as a research tool, the NIDDK "research definition" became a de facto definition of this disease, diagnosed by exclusion and colorfully termed a "hole in the air" by Hald (George et al, 1986). Certain of the exclusion criteria serve mainly to make one wary of a diagnosis of IC, but should by no means be used for categoric exclusion of such a diagnosis. However, because of the ambiguity involved, these patients should probably be eliminated from research studies or categorized separately. In particular, exclusion criteria 4, 5, 6, 8, 9, 11, 12, 17, and 18 are only relative. The percentage of patients with idiopathic "sensory urgency" (hypersensitivity without decreased compliance or detrusor overactivity [DO]) who have BPS is unclear (Frazer et al, 1990). **The specificity of the finding of bladder glomerulations before or after distention has come into question** (Erickson 1995; Waxman et al, 1998; Tomaszewski et al, 2001). Similarly, **the sensitivity of glomerulations is also unknown, but clearly patients with IC symptoms can demonstrate an absence**

> **BOX 14-2** National Institute of Diabetes and Digestive and Kidney Diseases (NIDDK) Diagnostic Criteria for Interstitial Cystitis
>
> To be diagnosed with interstitial cystitis, patients must have either glomerulations on cystoscopic examination or a classic Hunner ulcer, and they must have either pain associated with the bladder or urinary urgency. An examination for glomerulations should be undertaken after distention of the bladder under anesthesia to 80 to 100 cm H_2O for 1 to 2 minutes. The bladder may be distended up to two times before evaluation. The glomerulations must be diffuse—present in at least three quadrants of the bladder—and there must be at least 10 glomerulations per quadrant. The glomerulations must not be along the path of the cystoscope (to eliminate artifact from contact instrumentation). The presence of any one of the following excludes a diagnosis of interstitial cystitis:
>
> 1. Bladder capacity of greater than 350 mL on awake cystometry using either a gas or liquid filling medium
> 2. Absence of an intense urge to void with the bladder filled to 100 mL of gas or 150 mL of liquid filling medium
> 3. The demonstration of phasic involuntary bladder contractions on cystometry using the fill rate just described
> 4. Duration of symptoms less than 9 months
> 5. Absence of nocturia
> 6. Symptoms relieved by antimicrobial agents, urinary antiseptic agents, anticholinergic agents, or antispasmodic agents
> 7. A frequency of urination while awake of fewer than eight times per day
> 8. A diagnosis of bacterial cystitis or prostatitis within a 3-month period
> 9. Bladder or ureteral calculi
> 10. Active genital herpes
> 11. Uterine, cervical, vaginal, or urethral cancer
> 12. Urethral diverticulum
> 13. Cyclophosphamide or any type of chemical cystitis
> 14. Tuberculous cystitis
> 15. Radiation cystitis
> 16. Benign or malignant bladder tumors
> 17. Vaginitis
> 18. Age younger than 18 years

From Wein AJ, Hanno PM, Gillenwater JY. Interstitial cystitis: an introduction to the problem. In: Hanno PM, Staskin DR, Krane RJ, et al, editors. Interstitial cystitis. London: Springer-Verlag; 1990. p. 13–5.

---

of glomerulations under anesthesia (Awad et al, 1992; Al Hadithi et al, 2002). **Bladder ulceration has been considered rare** (Sant, 1991). A California series found 20% of patients to have ulceration (Koziol, 1994). Hunner lesions have been recognized more commonly as more urologists and gynecologists have become aware of the sometimes subtle findings suggesting a lesion and are present in up to 50% of patients in Scandinavia (Logadottir et al, 2012). Specific pathologic findings represent a glaring omission from the criteria because **there is a lack of consensus as to which pathologic findings, if any, are required for, or even suggestive of, a tissue diagnosis** (Hanno et al, 1990, 2005a; Tomaszewski et al, 1999, 2001).

The unexpected use of the NIDDK research criteria by the medical community as a definition of IC led to concerns that many patients with this syndrome might be misdiagnosed. The multicenter Interstitial Cystitis Data Base (ICDB) study through NIDDK accumulated data on 424 patients with IC, enrolling patients from May 1993 through December 1995. Entry criteria were much more

BOX 14-3 Interstitial Cystitis Data Base (ICDB) Study Eligibility Criteria

1. Informed consent to participate in the study
2. Willing to undergo a cystoscopy under general or regional anesthesia when indicated, during the course of the study
3. At least 18 years of age
4. Symptoms of urinary urgency, frequency, or pain for more than 6 months
5. Urinating at least seven times per day, or having some urgency or pain (measured on linear analog scales)
6. No history of current genitourinary tuberculosis
7. No history of urethral cancer
8. No history of bladder malignancy, high-grade dysplasia, or carcinoma in situ
9. Males: no history of prostate cancer
10. Females: no occurrence of ovarian, vaginal, or cervical cancer in the previous 3 years
11. Females: no current vaginitis, clue cells, or *Trichomonas* or yeast infection
12. No bacterial cystitis in the previous 3 months
13. No active herpes in the previous 3 months
14. No antimicrobials for urinary tract infections in previous 3 months
15. Never treated with cyclophosphamide
16. No radiation cystitis
17. No neurogenic bladder dysfunction (e.g., from spinal cord injury, stroke, Parkinson disease, multiple sclerosis, spina bifida, or diabetic cystopathy)
18. No bladder outlet obstruction (determined by urodynamic investigation)
19. Males: no bacterial prostatitis for previous 6 months
20. Absence of bladder, ureteral, or urethral calculi for previous 3 months
21. No urethritis for previous 3 months
22. No urethral dilation, cystometrogram, bladder cystoscopy under full anesthesia, or a bladder biopsy in previous 3 months
23. Never having had an augmentation cystoplasty, cystectomy, cystolysis, or neurectomy
24. No urethral stricture of less than 12 Fr

From Simon LJ, Landis JR, Erickson DR, et al. The Interstitial Cystitis Data Base study: concepts and preliminary baseline descriptive statistics. Urology 1997;49:64–75.

symptom driven than those promulgated for research studies (Simon et al, 1997) and are noted in Box 14-3. In an analysis of the defining criteria (Hanno et al, 1999a, 1999b), it appeared the NIDDK research criteria fulfilled their mission. Fully 90% of expert clinicians agreed that patients diagnosed with IC by those criteria in the ICDB indeed had the disorder. However, 60% of patients deemed to have IC by these experienced clinicians would not have met NIDDK research criteria. The ESSIC definition (pelvic pain for longer than 6 months; pressure or discomfort perceived to be related to the urinary bladder accompanied by at least one other urinary symptom such as persistent urge to void or frequency; exclusion of confusable diseases as the cause of the symptoms) (van de Merwe et al, 2008) allows the inclusion of more patients in the IC/BPS syndrome, facilitating diagnosis and treatment in many patients who would otherwise remain undiagnosed (Proaño et al, 2013). **Whereas IC symptom and problem indices have been developed and validated** (O'Leary et al, 1997; Goin et al, 1998), **these are not intended to diagnose or define IC but rather to measure the** severity of symptomatology and monitor disease progression or regression (Moldwin and Kushner, 2004).

IC/BPS is now viewed not only through the paradigm of a chronic pain syndrome that manifests through bladder-related symptoms, but as a syndrome that may not be a true disease of the bladder alone in many patients (Hanno, 2008b). This paradigm is reflected in the current Multidisciplinary Approach to the Study of Chronic Pelvic Pain (MAPP) Research Network (mappnetwork.org), a 10-year ongoing research project of the National Institutes of Health. The subgroup of patients with Hunner lesions do seem to have a primary bladder disease, but their symptom complex is indistinguishable from that of the general IC/BPS population without the aid of endoscopic examination (Nordling et al, 2012). On average, these patients are two decades older than non-Hunner patients and have a smaller bladder capacity when under anesthesia (Logadottir et al, 2012).

Nomenclature and Taxonomy

In accordance with the guidelines of the AUA, this chapter uses the terminology of the International Consultation on Incontinence—*bladder pain syndrome*—but keeps the term *interstitial cystitis* to facilitate recognition and understanding. This change implies that it is the symptoms that drive treatment, and **whether *interstitial cystitis* should refer to a distinct subgroup of the bladder pain syndrome (i.e., those with a Hunner lesion) is, as yet, unclear** (Hanno et al, 2011; Fall and Peeker, 2013; Hanno et al, 2013).

The literature over the last 170 years has seen numerous changes in description and nomenclature of the disease. The syndrome has variously been referred to as *tic douloureux of the bladder, interstitial cystitis, cystitis parenchymatosa, Hunner ulcer, panmural ulcerative cystitis, urethral syndrome,* and *painful bladder syndrome* (Skene, 1887; Hunner, 1918; Powell and Powell, 1949; Bourque, 1951; Christmas and Sant, 1997; Teichman et al, 2000; Dell and Parsons, 2004). The term *interstitial cystitis,* which Skene is credited with coining and Hunner brought into common usage, is a misnomer; in many patients not only is there no interstitial inflammation, but histopathologically there may be no inflammation at all (Lynes et al, 1990a; Denson et al, 2000; Tomaszewski et al, 2001; Rosamilia et al, 2003). Focusing exclusively on the urinary bladder, the term *interstitial cystitis* furthermore does not do justice to the condition from both the physician's and the patient's perspectives. The textual exclusiveness ignores the high comorbidity with various pelvic, extrapelvic, and nonurologic symptoms and associated disorders (Clauw et al, 1997) that frequently precede or develop after the onset of the bladder condition (Wu et al, 2006).

With the formal definition of the term *painful bladder syndrome* by the ICS in 2002, the terminology discussion became an intense international focal point (Abrams et al, 2002).

- In Kyoto at the International Consultation on Interstitial Cystitis, Japan (ICICJ) in March 2003, it was agreed that the term *interstitial cystitis* should be expanded to *interstitial cystitis/chronic pelvic pain syndrome* when pelvic pain is at least of 3 months' duration and associated with no obvious treatable condition or pathology (Ueda et al, 2003).
- ESSIC held its first meeting in Copenhagen soon after Kyoto. Nomenclature was discussed but no decision was reached; the meeting concentrated on how to evaluate patients for diagnosis (Nordling et al, 2004).
- At the 2003 meeting of the NIDDK entitled "Research Insights into Interstitial Cystitis," it was concluded that "interstitial cystitis" would ultimately be replaced as a sole name for this syndrome. This was to be a gradual process over several years. At the meeting the condition was referred to as *interstitial cystitis/painful bladder syndrome* in keeping with ICS nomenclature (Hanno et al, 2005b).
- At the 2004 inaugural meeting of the Multinational Interstitial Cystitis Association in Rome, it was concluded that the syndrome should be referred to as *painful bladder syndrome/interstitial cystitis* or *PBS/IC* to indicate an intellectual and taxonomic hierarchy within the acronym (Hanno et al, 2005b).

TABLE 14-1   European Society for the Study of Interstitial Cystitis Classification System

BIOPSY	CYSTOSCOPY WITH HYDRODISTENTION			
	NOT DONE	NORMAL	GLOMERULATIONS*	HUNNER LESION†
Not done	XX	1X	2X	3X
Normal	XA	1A	2A	2A
Inconclusive	XB	1B	2B	3B
Positive‡	XC	1C	2C	3C

*Cystoscopy granulations grade II to III.
†With or without glomerulations.
‡Histology showing inflammatory infiltrates and/or detrusor mastocytosis and/or tissue granulation and/or interfascicular fibrosis.
From van de Merwe JP, Nordling J, Bouchelouche P, et al. Diagnostic criteria, classification, and nomenclature for painful bladder syndrome/interstitial cystitis: an ESSIC proposal. Eur Urol 2008;53:60.

- The International Consultation on Incontinence in 2004, cosponsored by the ICS and the Société Internationale d'Urologie in association with the World Health Organization, included the syndrome as a part of its consultation. The chapter in the report was entitled "Painful Bladder Syndrome (Including Interstitial Cystitis)," suggesting that the IC formed an identifiable subset within the broader syndrome. Because such a distinction is difficult to define, within the body of the chapter, coauthored by nine committee members and five consultants from four continents, the syndrome was referred to as *PBS/IC* (one inclusive entity) (Hanno et al, 2005a). **IC may be a subgroup that encompasses patients with typical histologic and cystoscopic features** (Peeker and Fall, 2002a), **but what these features are is still controversial and somewhat vague.**
- In June 2006 Abrams and colleagues published an editorial focusing on the nomenclature problem (Abrams et al, 2006). They noted, "It is an advantage if the medical term has clear diagnostic features that translate to a known pathophysiologic process so that effective treatment may be given. Unfortunately, the latter is not the case for many of the pain syndromes suffered by patients seen at most pain, gynecologic, and urologic clinics. For the most part these "diagnoses" describe syndromes that do not have recognized standard definitions, yet imply knowledge of a pathophysiologic cause for the symptoms. Unfortunately the terminology used to describe the condition may promote erroneous thinking about treatment on the part of physicians, surgeons and patients. These organ based diagnoses are mysterious, misleading and unhelpful, and can lead to therapies that are misguided or even dangerous." The editorial went on to note that use of a single pathologic descriptive term (*interstitial cystitis*) for a spectrum of symptom combinations ill serves patients. The umbrella term *painful bladder syndrome* was proposed, with a goal to define and investigate subsets of patients who could be clearly identified within the spectrum of PBS. It would fall within the rubric of CPPS. Affected patients would be identified according to the primary organ that appeared to be affected on clinical grounds. Pain not associated with an individual organ would be described in terms of the symptoms.

One can see in this the beginnings of a new paradigm that might be expected to change the emphasis of both clinical and basic science research and that removes the automatic presumption that the end organ in the name of the disease should necessarily be the sole or primary target of such research.

- At the major biannual IC research conference in the fall of 2006, held by the NIDDK ("Frontiers in Painful Bladder Syndrome/Interstitial Cystitis"), the ESSIC group was given a block of time in which to present thoughts and conclusions. Because the term *painful bladder syndrome* (1) did not fit into the taxonomy of other pelvic pain syndromes such as urethral or vulvar pain syndromes, (2) as defined by the ICS missed more than a third of affected patients, and (3) is a term open to different interpretations, ESSIC suggested that *painful bladder*

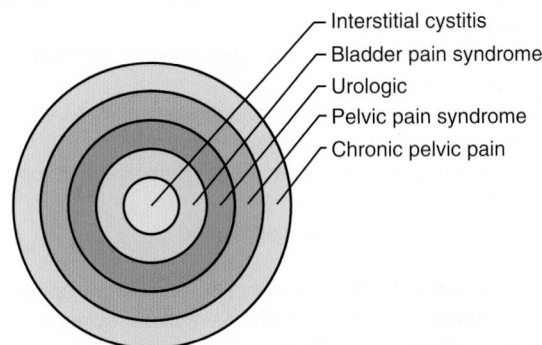

Figure 14-1. Conceptualization of pelvic pain syndrome classification. (From Hanno PM. Interstitial cystitis/painful bladder syndrome/bladder pain syndrome: the evolution of a new paradigm, Proceedings of the International Consultation on Interstitial Cystitis, Japan: Comfortable Urology Network; 2008. p. 2–9.)

syndrome be redesignated as *bladder pain syndrome* followed by a type designation. BPS is indicated by two symbols: The first corresponds to cystoscopy with hydrodistention (CHD) findings (1, 2, or 3, indicating increasing grade of severity), and the second to biopsy findings (A, B, and C, indicating increasing grade of pathologic severity) (Table 14-1). Although neither CHD nor bladder biopsy was prescribed as an essential part of the evaluation, categorizing patients in terms of whether either procedure was performed, and, if so, the results, made it possible to follow patients with similar findings and study each identified cohort to compare natural history, prognosis, and response to therapy (van de Merwe et al, 2008).

- As Baranowski and colleagues conceived it in early 2008, **BPS is thus defined as a pain syndrome with a collection of symptoms, the most important of which is pain perceived to be in the bladder** (Baranowski et al, 2008). **IC is distinguished as an end-organ, visceral-neural pain syndrome, whereas BPS can be considered a pain syndrome that involves the end-organ (bladder) and neurovisceral (myopathic) mechanisms. In IC, one expects end-organ primary pathology. This is not necessarily the case in the broader BPS.**

A didactically very demonstrative way to conceptualize the dawning shift in conception of the condition is with the drawing of a target (Fig. 14-1). There may be many causes of chronic pelvic pain. When a cause cannot be determined, the condition is characterized as pelvic pain syndrome. To the extent that it can be distinguished as urologic, gynecologic, dermatologic, and the like, it is further categorized by organ system. A urologic pain syndrome can sometimes be further differentiated based on the site of perceived pain. Bladder, prostate, testicular, and epididymal pain syndromes follow. Finally, types of BPS can be further defined as IC or simply categorized by ESSIC criteria. Patient groups have expressed their concerns with regard to any nomenclature change that potentially drops the term *interstitial cystitis* because the U.S. Social Security Administration and private insurers recognize IC but not the term *bladder pain syndrome*, and benefits potentially could be adversely affected. Whether the term *interstitial cystitis*, as difficult as it is to define and as potentially misleading as it is with regard to cause and end-organ involvement, should be maintained is a subject of ongoing controversy (Hanno and Dmochowski, 2009).

> ### KEY POINTS: DEFINITION
>
> - The *painful bladder disease complex* includes a large group of patients with bladder and/or urethral and/or pelvic pain, irritative voiding symptoms, and sterile urine cultures, many with specific identifiable causes.
> - *Bladder pain syndrome* comprises a part of this complex and is a clinical diagnosis based primarily on chronic symptoms of pain perceived by the patient to emanate from the bladder and/or pelvis associated with urinary urgency or frequency *in the absence* of other identified causes for the symptoms.
> - Whether the older term *interstitial cystitis* should refer to a distinct subgroup of BPS (i.e., those with Hunner lesions) is, as yet, unclear.

Urgency is a common complaint of this group of patients. **The ICS definition of urgency** (Abrams et al, 2002), "the complaint of a sudden compelling desire to pass urine, which is difficult to defer," **could be interpreted as compatible with either DO or BPS/IC depending on the weight one attaches to the word** *sudden*. There are those who see hypersensitivity or sensory urgency as bridging both overactive bladder and BPS/IC (Haylen et al, 2007; Yamaguchi et al, 2007), and the issue has been nicely addressed by Homma (2008). **Pain and pressure are more involved in the frequency of BPS/IC, and fear of incontinence seems the reason for the urgency of overactive bladder** (Abrams, 2005). Although BPS patients may have significantly higher voiding frequencies, smaller voided volumes, and narrower ranges of voided volume compared with overactive bladder patients (Kim et al, 2014), one cannot distinguish between the two syndromes based on a voiding diary. Urgency is not required to define BPS/IC, as it would tend to obfuscate the borders of overactive bladder and BPS/IC, and is unnecessary for definition purposes. The term *urgency* as it is comprehended by patients is not a well-defined and commonly understood symptom that can be used to clearly discriminate between BPS/IC and overactive bladder (Clemens et al, 2011). Figure 14-2 (Abrams et al, 2005)

is a graphic depiction of one view of the relationship between these two sometimes confused conditions. The 14% incidence of urodynamic DO in the BPS/IC patients (Nigro et al, 1997a) is probably close to what one might expect in the general population if studied urodynamically (Salavatore et al, 2003).

Still, there remains some ambiguity, and further research is necessary with regard to urgency (Hanno et al, 2009). Studies are hampered by the fact that patients tend to use words to describe lower urinary tract symptoms, but attribute different meanings to the words than do physicians and researchers (Digesu et al, 2008). An analysis of urgency by the University of Maryland group reported that 65% of patients with BPS experienced an urge to urinate to relieve pain, with 46% agreeing that they had an urge to relieve pain and not to prevent incontinence. Still, 21% reported that urgency arose from fear of impending incontinence and that this sensation was not present before the onset of BPS symptoms (Diggs et al, 2007). In some patients the term connotes an intensification of the normal urge to void, and in others it is a different sensation (Blaivas et al, 2009).

New efforts to phenotype the chronic urologic pain syndromes (BPS and chronic nonbacterial prostatitis and CPPS in men) are currently being explored (Shoskes et al, 2009). One of these is the MAPP Research Network, a 10-year ongoing research project of the National Institutes of Health (mappnetwork.org). Patients with Hunner lesions would seem to have a more bladder-centric disorder and are less likely to have comorbid conditions (Peters et al, 2011). The hope is that looking at psychological, physical, and organ-specific parameters of affected patients, and specifically focusing on associated disorders, will aid in proper selection of therapeutic agents that may have selective specificity for different symptom constellations, and also may improve productivity and results of research on etiology, prognosis, and new therapeutic agents.

> ### KEY POINTS: URGENCY
>
> - Urgency has been defined as the complaint of a sudden compelling desire to pass urine, which is difficult to defer.
> - What the patient believes precipitates the sensation is not a part of the definition, and this has resulted in some ambiguity. Fear of incontinence is more consistent with overactive bladder, whereas pressure, pain, or discomfort suggests BPS.

EPIDEMIOLOGY

Prevalence

Epidemiology studies of BPS/IC have been hampered by many problems (Bernardini et al, 1999). The lack of an accepted definition, the absence of a validated diagnostic marker, and questions regarding etiology and pathophysiology make much of the literature difficult to interpret. This is most apparent when one looks at the variation in **prevalence reports** in the United States and around the world. These **range from 1.2 to 4.5 per 100,00 females in Japan** (Ito et al, 2000) **to a figure in American women of 20,000 per 100,000 according to a questionnaire-based study** (Parsons and Tatsis, 2004). **Tea consumption and smoking were purported to be risk factors in a large Swedish twin study** (Tettamanti et al, 2011); **however the per capita consumption of tea in the United Kingdom is more than double that of the vast majority of the world's population, and no study reports a higher prevalence of BPS in that country.**

It has been estimated that the prevalence in the population of chronic pain from benign causes is at least 10% (Verhaak et al, 1998). Numerous case series have, until recently, formed the basis of epidemiologic information regarding BPS/IC. Farkas and associates discussed IC in adolescent girls (Farkas et al, 1977). Hanash and Pool reviewed their experience with IC in men (Hanash and Pool, 1969). Geist and Antolak reviewed and added to reports of

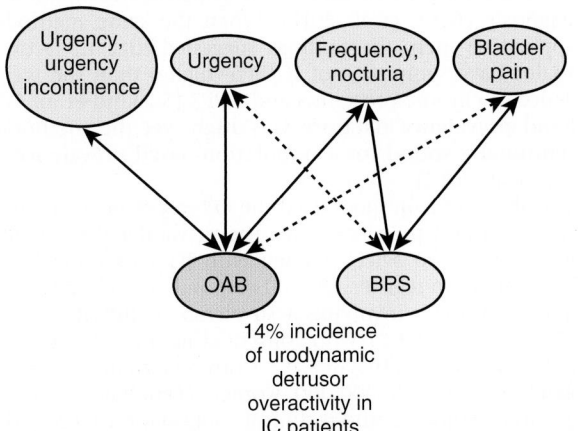

Figure 14-2. Overactive bladder (OAB) and its relationship to bladder pain syndrome (BPS). IC, interstitial cystitis. (From Abrams P, Hanno P, Wein A. Overactive bladder and painful bladder syndrome: there need not be confusion. Neurourol Urodyn 2005;24:149–50.)

disease occurring in childhood (Geist and Antolak, 1970). **A childhood presentation is extremely rare and must be differentiated from the much more common and benign-behaving** *extraordinary urinary frequency syndrome of childhood,* a self-limited condition of unknown cause (Koff and Byard, 1988; Robson and Leung, 1993). Nevertheless, there is a small cohort of children with chronic symptoms of bladder pain, urinary frequency, and sensory urgency in the absence of infection who have been evaluated with urodynamics, cystoscopy, and bladder distention and have findings consistent with the diagnosis of BPS/IC. In a review of 20 such children by Close and colleagues, the median age of **onset was younger than 5 years, and the vast majority of patients had long-term remissions with bladder distention** (Close et al, 1996).

A study conducted at the Scripps Research Institute (Koziol et al, 1993) included 374 patients at Scripps as well as some members of the Interstitial Cystitis Association, the large patient support organization. The findings of a more recent but similar study in England (Tincello and Walker, 2005) concurred with the Scripps findings of urgency, frequency, and pain in the vast majority of these patients, devastating effects on quality of life, and often unsuccessful attempts at therapy with a variety of treatments. Although such reviews provide some information, they would seem to be necessarily biased by virtue of their design.

Several population-based studies have been reported in the literature (Fig. 14-3), and these studies tend to support the reviews of selected patients or from individual clinics and the comprehensive follow-up case-control study by Koziol (1994). The first population-based study (Oravisto, 1975) included "almost all the patients with interstitial cystitis in the city of Helsinki." This superb, brief report from Finland surveyed all diagnosed cases in a population approaching 1 million. The prevalence of the disease in women was 18.1 per 100,000. The joint prevalence in both sexes was 10.6 cases per 100,000. The annual incidence of new cases in women was 1.2 per 100,000. Severe cases accounted for about 10% of the total. Ten percent of cases were in men. The disease onset was typically subacute rather than insidious, and full development of the classic symptom complex occurred over a relatively short time. IC does not progress continuously, but usually reaches its final stage rapidly (within 5 years in the Koziol study (Koziol et al, 1993) and then continues without significant change in symptomatology. Subsequent major deterioration was found by Oravisto to be unusual. The duration of symptoms before diagnosis was 3 to 5 years in the Finnish study. Analogous figures in a classic U.S. paper a quarter of a century earlier were 7 to 12 years (Hand, 1949).

Another early population study, this in the United States, first demonstrated the potential extent of what had been considered a very rare disease (Held et al, 1990). The following population groups were surveyed: (1) 127 board-certified urologists who completed a random survey; (2) 64 IC patients selected by the surveyed urologists and divided among the last patient with IC seen and the last patient with IC diagnosed; (3) 904 female patients belonging to the Interstitial Cystitis Association; and (4) 119 persons from the

U.S. population who completed a random phone survey. This 1987 study found the following:

1. 43,500 to 90,000 diagnosed cases of IC in the United States (twice the Finnish prevalence)
2. Up to a fivefold increase in IC prevalence if all patients with painful bladder and sterile urine had been given the diagnosis, yielding up to half a million possible cases in the United States
3. Median age of onset 40 years
4. Late deterioration in symptoms unusual
5. 50% temporary spontaneous remission rate, mean duration 8 months
6. 10 times higher incidence of childhood bladder problems in IC patients versus controls
7. Double the incidence of a history of urinary tract infection versus controls
8. 14% of IC patients were Jewish (15% in Koziol sample [Koziol, 1994]) versus 3% Jewish individuals in the general population sample
9. Lower quality of life than in dialysis patients
10. Costs including lost economic production in 1987 of $427 million

Other population studies followed. Jones and colleagues obtained their data from self-report of a previous diagnosis of IC in the 1989 National Household Interview Survey (Jones and Nyberg, 1997). The survey estimated that 0.5% of the population, or more than 1,000,000 people in the United States, reported having had a diagnosis of IC. There was no verification of this self-report by medical records. Bade and colleagues performed a physician questionnaire–based survey in the Netherlands that yielded an overall prevalence of 8 to 16 per 100,000 females, with diagnosis heavily dependent on pathology and presence of mast cells (Bade et al, 1995). This prevalence in females compares with 4.5 per 100,00 in Japan (Ito et al, 2000). The Nurses' Health Study I and II (Curhan et al, 1999) showed a prevalence of IC of 52 to 67 per 100,000 in the United States, twice the prevalence in the Held study (Held et al, 1990) and threefold higher than in the Netherlands (Bade et al, 1995). It improved on previous studies by using a large sample derived from a general population and careful ascertainment of the diagnosis. If the 6.4% confirmation rate of these studies were applied to the Jones and colleagues National Health Interview Survey data, the prevalence estimates of the two studies would be nearly identical.

The most sophisticated population-based prevalence study was conducted by the Rand Corporation. With use of a case definition with an 83% specificity, a random sample of 146,231 households was contacted by telephone and 12,752 women completed the questionnaire; 2.7% met the high-specificity definition of BPS. Less than 10% of these women had a clinical diagnosis of BPS/IC. The figures correspond to 3.3 million women in the United States aged 18 or older with symptoms compatible with the diagnosis (Berry et al, 2011). When the same methodology was applied to men, the findings suggested that 1.9% of adult U.S. males have symptoms of IC/BPS, higher than the weighted prevalence of chronic prostatitis and CPPS (Suskind et al, 2013a). **The Rand prevalence data are very high, yet the methodology is exceptionally sound for a population-based prevalence study** (Konkle et al, 2012).

Leppilahti and colleagues used the O'Leary-Sant interstitial cystitis symptom and problem index (never validated for making a diagnosis per se) to select women with IC symptoms from the Finnish population register. Of 1331 respondents, 32 had moderate or severe symptoms involving a suspicion of BPS/IC (symptom score 7 or higher). Of 21 who consented to clinical evaluation, 7 had probable or possible BPS/IC. Corrected estimates yielded a prevalence of 300 per 100,000 women (Leppilahti et al, 2002, 2005). Similar studies without clinical confirmation suggested prevalence in Austrian women of 306 per 100,000 (Temml et al, 2007) and in Japanese women of 265 per 100,000 (Inoue et al, 2009). With use of the Bristol Female Lower Urinary Tract Symptoms questionnaire, prevalence of BPS symptoms of 100 per 100,000 Fuzhou Chinese women was reported (Song et al, 2009).

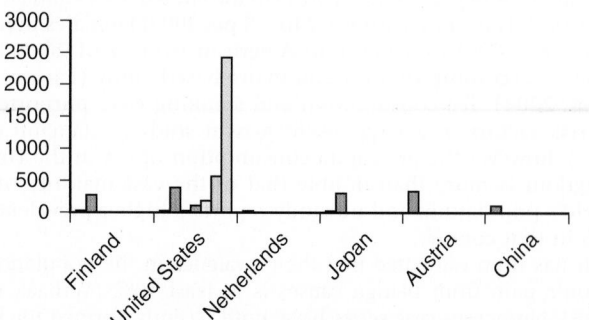

Figure 14-3. Prevalence of bladder pain syndrome per 100,000 females in reported studies from around the world. See text for details.

Roberts and colleagues, using a physician diagnosis as the arbiter of IC, found annual incidence in Olmsted County, Minnesota of 1.6 per 100,000 in women and 0.6 per 100,000 in men, a figure remarkably similar to that of Oravisto in Helsinki (Roberts et al, 2003). The cumulative prevalence by age older than 80 years in the Minnesota study was 114 per 100,000, a figure comparable to that in the Nurses' Health Study if one takes into account the younger age group in the Curhan data. Clemens calculated a prevalence of diagnosed disease in a managed care population of 197 per 100,000 women and 41 per 100,000 men, but when the diagnosis was tested by eliminating those who had not been evaluated with endoscopy or in whom exclusionary conditions existed, the numbers dropped considerably (Clemens et al, 2005). The Boston Area Community Health (BACH) Survey estimated a prevalence of BPS symptoms of 1% to 2% of the population depending on the definition used (Clemens et al, 2007). A population-based study in Korea found a prevalence in women of 0.26% (Choe et al, 2011). A Japanese study estimated the incidence of hospital admissions related to IC/BPS at 1.35 per 100,000 person-years (Sugihara et al, 2012).

With regard to office visits to practices with an interest in urologic problems, 2.8% of patients in Canadian urologist offices had BPS/IC (Nickel et al, 2005b), and probable BPS/IC was found in 0.57% of patients in a primary care office in Michigan (Rosenberg and Hazzard, 2005).

Until the Rand study, a reasonable prevalence estimate (recognizing that a consistent definition of the condition had not been used in epidemiologic studies) appeared to be about 300 per 100,000 in females, and in males 10% to 20% of the estimate in females. It now appears the problem may be 10 times greater.

Whether the considerable variability in prevalence in studies within the United States and around the world is related to methodology or true differences in incidence is an important question yet to be answered. One reason may be that pain that the patient perceives to be related to the bladder is a problematic concept, because most patients have different reasons for reaching that conclusion (Warren et al, 2011b). It is clear that the prevalence of BPS/IC symptoms is much greater than the prevalence of a physician diagnosis of the disease (Clemens et al, 2007). Familial occurrence of BPS/IC has been reported (Dimitrakov, 2001). **A hereditary aspect to incidence has been suggested** by Warren in a pioneering study. He found that adult female first-degree relatives of patients with IC may have a prevalence of IC 17 times that found in the general population. This, together with previously reported evidence showing a greater concordance of IC among monozygotic than dizygotic twins, suggests but does not prove a genetic susceptibility to IC that could partially explain the discord in prevalence rates in different populations (Warren et al, 2001b, 2004).

KEY POINT: PREVALENCE

- Prevalence studies show wide variation; however, more modern studies of the prevalence of BPS/IC per 100,000 women tend to show higher values.

Prevalence of BPS/IC per 100,000 Women

Oravisto, 1975 (Finland)	18
Jones and Nyberg, 1997 (United States)	500
Held et al, 1990 (United States)	30
Bade et al, 1995 (Netherlands)	12
Curhan et al, 1999 (United States)	60
Ito et al, 2000 (Japan)	4.5
Roberts et al, 2003 (United States)	1.6
Leppilahti et al, 2005 (Finland)	300
Clemens et al, 2007 (United States)	197
Temml et al, 2007 (Austria)	306
Song et al, 2009 (China)	100
Berry et al, 2011 (United States)	2700

Characteristics and Natural History

Before the Rand study (Suskind et al, 2013a), **most studies had shown a female-to-male preponderance of 5 : 1 or greater** (Clemens et al, 2005; Hanno et al, 2005a). In the absence of a validated marker, it is often difficult to distinguish BPS/IC from CPPS (nonbacterial prostatitis, prostatodynia) that affects males (Forrest and Schmidt, 2004), and the percentage of men with BPS/IC may actually be higher (Miller et al, 1995, 1997; Novicki et al, 1998). **Men tend to be diagnosed at an older age and have a higher percentage of Hunner lesions in the case series reported** (Novicki et al, 1998; Roberts et al, 2003). **Costs of the disorder are not insignificant and can range from $4000 to $7000 dollars per year, not including lost wages, costs preceding diagnosis, costs of alternative therapies, and costs attributable to misdiagnosis** (Clemens et al, 2008c, 2009b).

Patients with BPS/IC analyzed across a wide spectrum of ages at time of diagnosis show different symptom profiles. Those diagnosed at the youngest ages experienced significantly more urinary urgency, frequency, dysuria, dyspareunia, and pain in their external genitalia. Older patients had a higher incidence of nocturia, urinary incontinence, and Hunner lesions (Rais-Bahrami et al, 2012). Patients with mild disease symptoms at onset appear to show symptom stability at 3 years, whereas those with concomitant chronic fatigue syndrome at symptom onset tend to show symptom progression of BPS/IC over time (Warren et al, 2013a).

The ICDB cohort of patients has been carefully studied, and the findings seem to bear out those of other epidemiologic surveys (Propert et al, 2000). Patterns of change in symptoms with time suggest regression to the mean and an intervention effect associated with the increased follow-up and care of cohort participants. **Although all symptoms fluctuated, there was no evidence of significant long-term change in overall disease severity. The data suggest that BPS/IC is a chronic disease, and no current treatments have a significant impact on symptoms over time in the majority of patients.** Quality-of-life studies suggest that BPS/IC patients are six times more likely than individuals in the general population to cut down on work time because of health problems, but only half as likely to do so as patients with arthritis (Shea-O'Malley and Sant, 1999). There is an associated high incidence of comorbidity including depression, chronic pain, and anxiety and overall mental health issues (Michael et al, 2000; Rothrock et al, 2002; Hanno et al, 2005a). Disability may be partially explained by the impact of negative affect and catastrophizing (Katz et al, 2013). **There seems to be no effect on pregnancy outcomes** (Onwude and Selo-Ojeme, 2003).

Female patients with BPS/IC seem to report significant dyspareunia and other manifestations of sexual dysfunction. **All domains of female sexual function including sexually related distress, desire, and orgasm frequency can be affected** (Ottem et al, 2007; Peters et al, 2007b). Sexual function is an important predictor of physical quality of life and was the only strong predictor of mental quality of life in one study of patients with severe BPS/IC (Nickel et al, 2007).

The BACH Survey (Link et al, 2008) **showed an overall prevalence of symptoms suggestive of BPS of 2%, with twice as many women as men affected.** It was most common among middle-aged respondents, with an earlier peak in women. It was most common among minorities and those of lower socioeconomic status (SES), and SES seemed to overcome any effect of race or ethnicity. **Emotional, sexual, and physical abuse was shown to be a risk factor** in the BACH Survey (Link and Lutfey, 2007), and this has been borne out in other studies. A Michigan study compared a control group of 464 women with 215 BPS/IC patients and found that 22% of the control group had experienced abuse versus 37% of the patient group (Peters et al, 2007b). Those with a history of sexual abuse may have more pain and fewer voiding symptoms (Seth and Teichman, 2008). How reliable these data are is not clear, and it would be wrong to jump to any conclusions about abuse in an individual patient. However, practitioners need to have sensitivity to the possibility of an abusive relationship history in all pain patients, and BPS patients in particular. When patients are found to have multiple diagnoses, the rate of previous abuse also increases, and these patients may need referral for further counseling at a traumatic stress center (Fenton et al, 2008).

> **KEY POINTS: NATURAL HISTORY**
>
> - The female-to-male preponderance had been estimated at 5 : 1. Newer data suggest the prevalence may be similar in males and females.
> - Symptoms tend to fluctuate, with the majority of patients showing no long-term deterioration.
> - There is no deleterious effect on pregnancy outcomes.
> - Men are diagnosed at an older age and have a higher prevalence of Hunner lesions.
> - Quality of life in almost all domains is significantly affected.

Associated Disorders

Knowledge of associated diseases is relevant for the clues it engenders with regard to cause and possible treatment of this enigmatic pain syndrome. It is well known that patients with chronic pain syndromes including chronic fatigue syndrome, fibromyalgia, and temporomandibular disorder share key symptoms and can often develop overlapping conditions including chronic pelvic pain (Aaron and Buchwald 2001; Aaron et al, 2001). Female patients with BPS/IC report significantly more nonpain symptoms and pain outside the pelvis than control female urology patients. In contrast to males with CPPS and nonbacterial prostatitis, females with BPS/IC are more likely to endorse multiple bothersome, medically unexplained symptoms across multiple organ systems (Lai et al, 2012). Bladder symptoms do not uniformly predate the nonbladder symptoms (Clemens et al, 2012). The number of functional somatic syndromes is perhaps the strongest risk factor for development of other non–bladder pain syndromes in the BPS/IC population. This is especially true for irritable bowel syndrome, fibromyalgia, and chronic fatigue syndrome (Warren et al, 2013a). These associated syndromes have an equivalent negative impact to BPS/IC in terms of quality of life (Suskind et al, 2013b).

In a case-control study Erickson found that patients with IC had higher scores than controls for pelvic discomfort, backache, dizziness, chest pain, aches in joints, abdominal cramps, nausea, palpitations, and headache (Erickson et al, 2001). Buffington theorizes that a common stress-response pattern of increased sympathetic nervous system function in the absence of comparable activation of the hypothalamic-pituitary-adrenal axis may account for some of these related symptoms (Buffington, 2004). Both depression and panic attacks have a high prevalence in patients with BPS/IC symptoms (Watkins et al, 2011). It has been suggested that panic disorder, a diagnosis associated with some BPS/IC patients (Clemens et al, 2008a), may sometimes be a part of a familial syndrome that includes IC, thyroid disorders, and other disorders of possible autonomic or neuromuscular control (Weissman et al, 2004; Subaran et al, 2012). Depression has been associated with BPS/IC in both men and women (Clemens et al, 2008a; Hall et al, 2008), but whether this is an association or effect of the disorder is uncertain (FitzGerald et al, 2007).

Newly diagnosed patients are most concerned with the possibility that BPS/IC could be a forerunner of bladder carcinoma. Until recently, no reports have ever documented a relationship to suggest that IC is a premalignant lesion. Utz and Zincke discovered bladder cancer in 12 of 53 men treated for IC at the Mayo Clinic (Utz and Zincke, 1974). Initial misdiagnosis was likely. Three of 224 women were eventually diagnosed with bladder cancer. Four years later, additional cases were reported (Lamm and Gittes, 1977). Tissot and colleagues reported that 1% of 600 patients previously diagnosed as having IC were found to have transitional cell carcinoma as the cause of symptoms (Tissot et al, 2004). Somewhat ominously, 2 of these patients had no hematuria. In all patients, irritative symptoms resolved after treatment of the malignancy. From this experience has come the dictum that all patients with presumed IC should undergo cystoscopy, urine cytology, and bladder biopsy of any suspicious lesion to be sure that a bladder carcinoma is not masquerading as BPS/IC. It would seem that **in the absence of microhematuria, and with negative cytology, the risk of missing a cancer is negligible, but not zero. A study from Taiwan reports a 2.95 relative risk of developing bladder cancer in BPS/IC patients compared with controls based on data analyzed from the Taiwan National Health Insurance Program** (Keller et al, 2013b). **This leaves the question still unresolved.**

A large-scale survey of 6783 individuals diagnosed by their physicians as having BPS/IC studied the incidence of associated disease in this population (Alagiri et al, 1997). Data from the 2405 responders were validated by comparison with 277 nonresponders (Fig. 14-4). **Allergies** were the most common association, with over 40% affected. Allergy was also the primary association in Hand's study (Hand, 1949). Thirty percent of patients had a diagnosis of **irritable bowel syndrome**, a finding confirming that of Koziol (1994). Altered visceral sensation has been implicated in irritable bowel syndrome in that these patients experience intestinal pain at intestinal gas volumes that are lower than those that cause pain in healthy persons (Lynn and Friedman, 1993), strikingly similar to the pain on bladder distention in IC.

Fibromyalgia, another disorder frequently considered functional because no specific structural or biochemical cause has been found, is also overrepresented in the BPS/IC population. This is a painful nonarticular condition predominantly involving muscles; it is the commonest cause of chronic, widespread musculoskeletal pain. It is typically associated with persistent fatigue, nonrefreshing sleep, and generalized stiffness. Women are affected at least 10 times more often than men (Consensus document on fibromyalgia, 1993). The association is intriguing because both conditions have similar demographic features, modulating factors, associated symptoms, and response to tricyclic compounds (Clauw et al, 1997; Chelimsky et al, 2012).

Diagnosed **vulvodynia, migraine headaches, endometriosis, chronic fatigue syndrome, incontinence, and asthma had similar prevalence as in the general population.** Several publications have noted an association between BPS/IC and systemic lupus erythematosus (SLE) (Fister, 1938; Boye et al, 1979; de la Serna and Alarcon-Segovia, 1981; Weisman et al, 1981; Meulders et al, 1992). The question has always been whether the bladder symptoms represent an association of these two disease processes or rather are a manifestation of lupus involvement of the bladder (Yukawa et al, 2008) or even a myelopathy with involvement of the sacral cord in a small group of these patients (Sakakibara et al, 2003). The beneficial response of the cystitis of SLE to steroids (Meulders et al, 1992) tends to support the latter view. No association with discoid lupus has been demonstrated (Jokinen et al, 1972b). Overall, the incidence of collagen-vascular disease in the IC population is low. Parsons found only 2 of 225 consecutive IC patients to have a history of autoimmune disorder (Parsons, 1990).

The National Health Insurance Research Database of the Taiwan National Health Insurance Programme has yielded data on many associations with BPS, some of which await confirmation from further population-based research. These include depression, anxiety, urinary calculus, erectile dysfunction, reflux esophagitis, coronary heart disease, obstructive sleep apnea, rheumatoid arthritis, and ischemic stroke (Chung et al, 2013, 2014a, 2014b, 2015; Kang et al, 2013; Keller et al, 2013a, 2013c, 2013d; Chen et al, 2014b). A study using this database has looked at a multitude of other illnesses using a logistic regression analysis, and only metastatic cancer did not show a statistically higher prevalence rate in BPS patients, making the data somewhat difficult to interpret (Keller et al, 2012).

Inflammatory bowel disease was found in over 7% of the IC population Alagiri studied, a figure 100 times higher than in the general population and never corroborated by other epidemiologic studies (Alagiri et al, 1997). Although unexplained at this time, abnormal leukocyte activity has been implicated in both conditions (Bhone et al, 1962; Kontras et al, 1971).

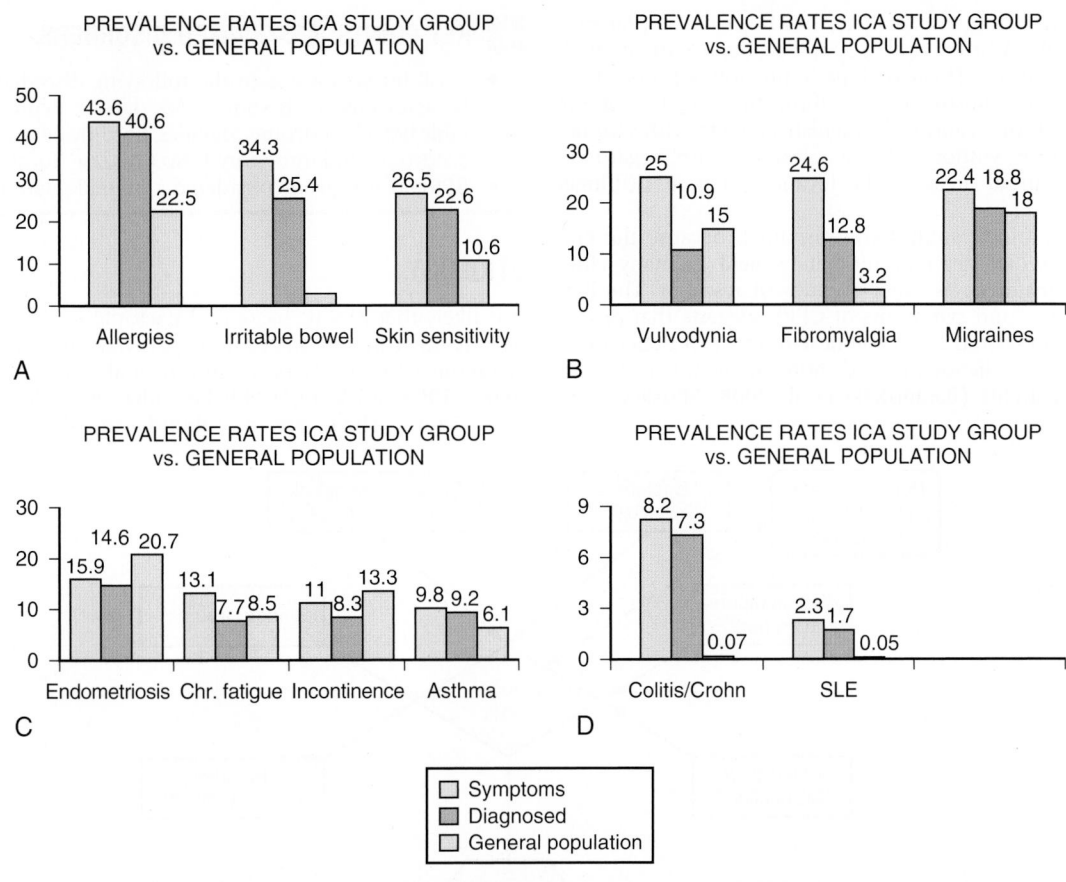

Figure 14-4. A through D, Comparison of disease prevalence rates among the Interstitial Cystitis Association (ICA) study group patients who report symptoms of a disorder, who have been diagnosed with a disorder, and the general population. Chr., chronic; SLE, systemic lupus erythematosus. (From Alagiri M, Chottiner S, Ratner V, et al. Interstitial cystitis: unexplained associates with other chronic pain syndromes. Urology 1997;49[Suppl. 5A]:52–7.)

The University of Maryland group sought antecedent nonbladder syndromes in 313 patients with incident BPS/IC and compared them with 313 matched controls (Warren et al, 2009). They found 11 antecedent syndromes were more often diagnosed in those with BPS/IC, and most syndromes appeared in clusters. The **most prominent cluster (45%) comprised fibromyalgia–chronic widespread pain, chronic fatigue syndrome, sicca syndrome, and/or irritable bowel syndrome**. Most of the other syndromes and identified clusters were associated with it. These researchers found probable chronic fatigue syndrome in 20% of BPS/IC patients, probable fibromyalgia in 22%, and probable irritable bowel in 27% of the BPS patients. Far fewer had physician-reported diagnoses of these syndromes, and odds ratios (ORs) for BPS/IC versus controls were 2.5 to 2.9. BPS/IC was significantly associated with previous female hormone use, a history of fewer pregnancies (in premenopausal women), and antecedent nonbladder syndromes (Warren et al, 2011a). Perhaps not surprisingly, in the month before the onset of BPS/IC, the approximated annual incidence of nonbladder pelvic surgeries was 15 times higher and of hysterectomy 25 times higher than the incidences in previous years and similarly higher than controls. The rate declined to preindex levels over the first 2 years of BPS/IC (Warren et al, 2013b). Although one could postulate that the surgery was an initiating factor, it may be more likely that the pelvic pain from undiagnosed BPS was what prompted the pelvic surgery in the first place.

Study of a managed care database in Portland, Oregon revealed that patients coded for gastritis (OR = 12.2), child abuse (OR = 9.3), fibromyalgia (OR = 3.0), anxiety disorder (OR = 2.8), headache (OR = 2.5), or depression (OR = 2.0) were commonly diagnosed with BPS/IC (Clemens et al, 2008b).

Women with BPS experience very high levels of sexual dysfunction (Bogart et al, 2011). **An unexplained disorder that has been associated with IC is vulvodynia with focal vulvitis** (Gardella et al, 2011; Reed et al, 2012). Vulvar vestibulitis syndrome is a constellation of symptoms and findings involving and limited to the vulvar vestibule and consisting of (1) severe pain on vestibular touch to attempted vaginal entry, (2) tenderness to pressure localized within the vulvar vestibule, and (3) physical findings confined to vulvar erythema of various degrees (Marinoff and Turner, 1991). McCormack reported on 36 patients with focal vulvitis, 11 of whom also had IC (McCormack, 1990). Fitzpatrick added 3 more patients (Fitzpatrick et al, 1993). Vulvodynia is associated not only with BPS/IC but also with irritable bowel syndrome and fibromyalgia (Nguyen et al, 2013). The concordance of these noninfectious inflammatory syndromes involving the tissues derived from the embryonic urogenital sinus and the similarity of the demographics argue for a common cause.

An association has been reported between IC and **Sjögren syndrome** (SS), an autoimmune exocrinopathy with a female preponderance manifested by dry eyes, dry mouth, and arthritis, but which can also include fever, dryness, and gastrointestinal and lung problems. Van de Merwe and colleagues (1993) investigated 10 IC patients for the presence of SS. Two patients had both keratoconjunctivitis sicca and focal lymphocytic sialoadenitis, allowing a primary diagnosis of SS. Only 2 patients had neither finding. He later reported an incidence of 28% of SS in patients with IC (van de Merwe et al, 2003). The incidence of symptoms of BPS/IC in patients with SS has been estimated to be up to 5% (Leppilahti et al, 2003). Patients with SS may have bladder symptoms from DO, and each patient requires careful individual evaluation before a diagnosis of BPS/IC is made (Lee et al, 2011a).

A negative correlation with diabetes has been noted (Parsons, 1990; Koziol, 1994; Warren et al, 2009). Although patients with multiple pain locations (increased pain phenotype) may have poorer psychosocial adjustment and diminished quality of life (Tripp et al, 2012), one cannot distinguish patients with Hunner lesions from those without Hunner lesions with regard to the number of painful areas or the location of pain (Killinger et al, 2013).

Further epidemiologic studies are warranted, because the epidemiology of this disorder may ultimately yield as many clues into cause and treatment as other avenues of research. The heterogeneity of causes and symptoms of CPPS suggests that proper clinical phenotyping could foster the development of better treatments for individual phenotypes and more successful treatments for all affected patients (Baranowski et al, 2008; Shoskes et al, 2009).

KEY POINTS: ASSOCIATED DISORDERS

- Look for symptoms of the following disorders, which may be associated with some cases of BPS: depression, SS, irritable bowel syndrome, allergies, fibromyalgia, chronic fatigue syndrome, inflammatory bowel disease, focal vulvitis.
- BPS has not been considered a premalignant condition.

ETIOLOGY

It is likely that BPS/IC has a multifactorial cause that may act predominantly through one or more pathways, resulting in the typical symptom complex (Holm-Bentzen et al, 1990; Mulholland and Byrne, 1994; Erickson, 1999; Levander, 2003; Keay et al, 2004b) (Fig. 14-5). There are an abundance of theories regarding

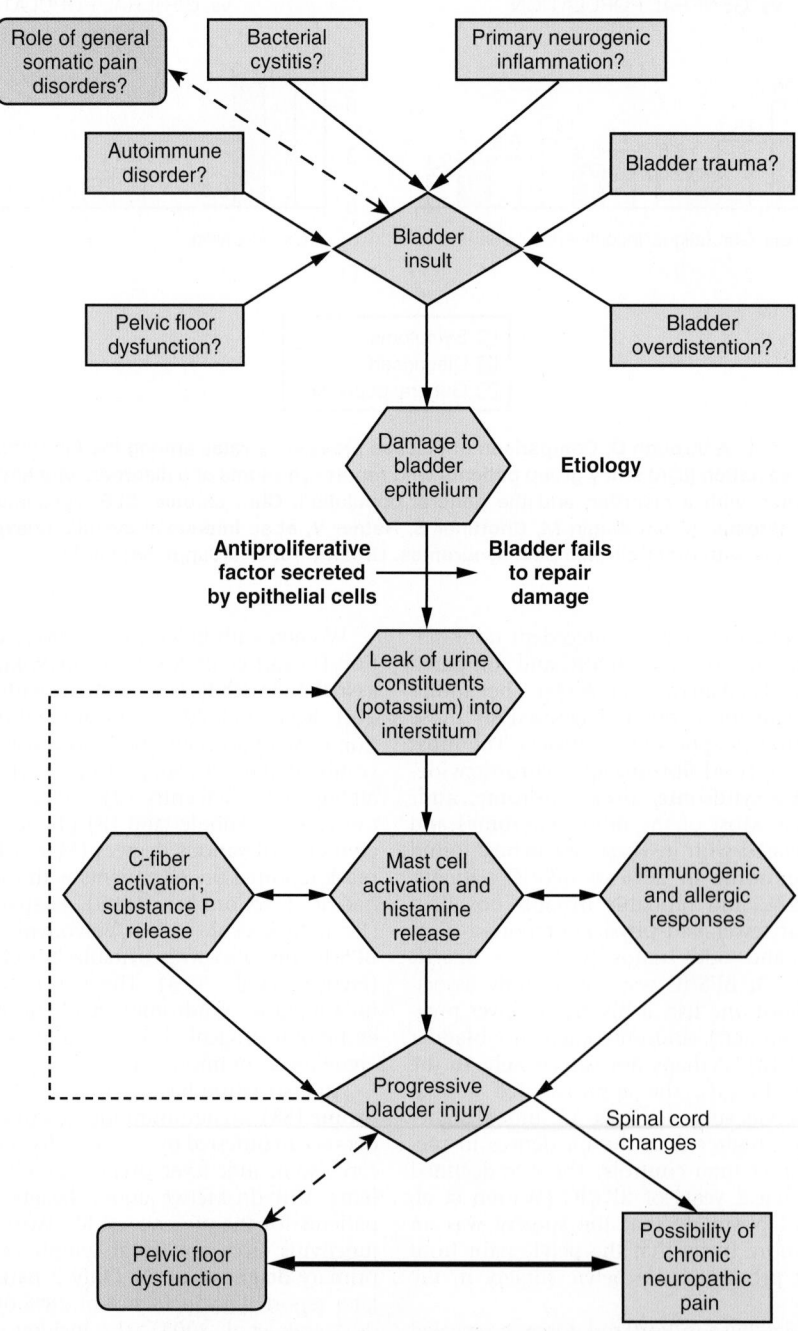

Figure 14-5. Hypothesis of causative cascade of bladder pain syndrome. (From Hanno P, Dinis P, Lin A, et al. Bladder pain syndrome. In: Abrams P, Cardozo L, Khoury S, et al, editors. Incontinence. Paris: International Consultation on Urological Diseases/European Association of Urology; 2013. p. 1583–649.)

its pathogenesis, but confirmatory evidence gleaned from clinical practice has proven sparse. Among numerous **proposals** that are further explored in this section are **"leaky epithelium," mast cell activation,** and **neurogenic inflammation,** or **some combination** of these and other **factors leading to a self-perpetuating process resulting in chronic bladder pain and voiding dysfunction** (Elbadawi, 1997). Irritable bowel syndrome, fibromyalgia, chronic fatigue syndrome, and various other chronic pain disorders may precede or follow the development of BPS/IC in some patients (Kim and Chang, 2012), but development of associated syndromes is not inevitable by any means, and their relationship to the cause is currently unknown (Warren et al, 2009). It has been postulated that neural cross-talk in the dorsal root ganglia, in the spinal cord, and at the level of the brain might play a role in the development of chronic pain disorders and their clinical associations through central sensitization (Furuta et al, 2012a). In rats, injection of hydrochloric acid into the gluteus can induce plantar hypersensitivity and urinary frequency for up to 2 weeks after the injection (Furuta et al, 2012b).

A discussion of animal models and the possible role of infection, autoimmunity, inflammation, mast cells, histamine, epithelial permeability, antiproliferative factor (APF), neurogenic factors, cross-sensitization, urine abnormalities, genetic factors, stress, and pelvic floor dysfunction can be found on the Expert Consult website.

PATHOLOGY

Pathology can be consistent with the diagnosis of BPS, but **there is no histology pathognomonic of this syndrome. The role of histopathology in the diagnosis of BPS is primarily one of excluding other possible diagnoses. One must rule out carcinoma and carcinoma in situ, eosinophilic cystitis, and tuberculous cystitis, as well as any other entities with a specific tissue diagnosis** (Hellstrom et al, 1979; Johansson and Fall, 1990; Tsiriopoulos et al, 2006).

Although earlier reports described a chronic, edematous pancystitis with mast cell infiltration, submucosal ulcerations, and involvement of the bladder wall and chronic lymphocytic infiltrate (Smith and Dehner, 1972; Jacobo et al, 1974), these were cases culled from patients with severe disease and not representative of the majority of cases currently diagnosed. **The pathologic findings in BPS are not consistent.** There has been a great variation in the reported histologic appearance of biopsy specimens from BPS patients, and even variation among samples taken from the same patients over time (Gillenwater and Wein, 1988).

Lépinard and colleagues (1984) reported a pancystitis affecting the three layers of bladder wall. In nonulcerative disease the vesical wall was never normal, epithelium being thinned and muscle being affected. Johansson and Fall looked at 64 patients with ulcerative disease and 44 with nonulcerative IC (Johansson and Fall, 1990). The former group had mucosal ulceration and hemorrhage, granulation tissue, intense inflammatory infiltrate, elevated mast cell counts, and perineural infiltrates. The nonulcerative group, despite having the same severe symptoms, had a relatively unaltered mucosa with a sparse inflammatory response, the main feature being multiple, small mucosal ruptures and suburothelial hemorrhages that were noted in a high proportion of patients. As these specimens were almost all taken immediately after hydrodistention, how much of the admittedly minimal findings in the nonulcerative group was purely iatrogenic is a matter of speculation.

Completely normal biopsy specimens are not uncommon in the nonulcerative BPS group (Johansson and Fall, 1994). **Transition from nonulcerative to ulcerative BPS is a rare event** (Fall et al, 1987), and **pathologically the two types of IC may be completely separate entities.** Although mast cells are more commonly seen in the detrusor in ulcerative BPS (Holm-Bentzen et al, 1987a), they are also common in patients with idiopathic bladder instability (Moore et al, 1992). Mastocytosis in BPS is best documented by tryptase immunocytochemical staining (Theoharides et al, 2001). Larsen and colleagues recommend taking biopsy specimens from

the detrusor of patients with suspected BPS and examining them with tryptase-stained 3-micron-thick sections, with every seventh section used for quantification. They consider 27 mast cells/mm^2 indicative of mastocytosis (Larsen et al, 2008). Despite attempts to develop a diagnostic algorithm based on the detrusor-to-mucosa mast cell ratio and nerve fiber proliferation (Hofmeister et al, 1997), **mast cell counts per se have no place in the differential diagnosis of this clinical syndrome.**

Mast cells could be valuable in clinical phenotyping, but as yet that is unproven. Mast cells trigger inflammation that is associated with local pain, but the mechanisms mediating pain are unclear. In a murine model of neurogenic cystitis, Rudick and colleagues demonstrated that mast cells promote cystitis pain and bladder pathophysiology through the separable actions of histamine and TNF, respectively (Rudick et al, 2008). Therefore, pain is independent of pathology and inflammation, and histamine receptors may represent direct therapeutic targets for the pain of BPS and other chronic pain conditions.

Lynes and coworkers concluded that biopsy specimens are often not helpful in confirming the diagnosis (Lynes et al, 1990a). Although BPS patients in their study had a higher incidence and degree of denuded epithelium, ulceration, and submucosal inflammation, none of these findings was pathognomonic. In addition, these "typical" findings occurred only in BPS patients with pyuria or small bladder capacity. Epithelial and basement membrane thickness, submucosal edema, vascular ectasia, fibrosis, and detrusor muscle inflammation and fibrosis were not significantly different in the BPS and control patients.

Attempts to definitively diagnose BPS by electron microscopy have also been unsuccessful. Collan's group, in the first such study (Collan et al, 1976), wrote that the similarity of the ultrastructure of epithelial cells in controls and IC patients makes it improbable that the disease process originates in the epithelium. Other investigators found no differences in the morphologic appearances of the glycocalyx and of urothelial cells in patients with IC when compared with controls (Dixon et al, 1986). Anderstrom and colleagues saw no surface characteristics specific for IC (Anderstrom et al, 1989), but believed that the mucin layer covering the urothelial cells seemed reduced in IC compared with controls, a fact disputed by Nickel in a very elegant paper (Nickel et al, 1993). Elbadawi and Light observed ultrastructural changes sufficiently distinctive to be diagnostic in specimens submitted for pathologic confirmation of nonulcerative IC (Elbadawi and Light, 1996). Marked edema of various tissue elements and cells appeared to be a common denominator of many observed changes. The wide-ranging discussion of the etiology of IC in his paper is fascinating, but the pathologic findings are potentially marred by the methodology, in that specimens were obtained after diagnostic hydrodistention (Elbadawi, 1997).

So what is the place of pathologic examination of tissue in BPS? Attempts to classify the painful bladder by the pathoanatomic criteria described by Holm-Bentzen (1989) are of questionable value. There is a group of patients with what she describes as *nonobstructive detrusor myopathy* (Holm-Bentzen et al, 1985). In her series, these patients with degenerative changes in the detrusor muscle often had residual urine, a history of urinary retention, and an absence of sensory urgency on cystometry with bladder capacities over 400 mL. Most of these signs would not be clinically confused with BPS. A similar English series (Christmas et al, 1996b), however, included patients who met NIDDK research criteria and associated detrusor myopathy with diminished detrusor compliance and ultimate bladder contracture.

The ICDB study worked backward from symptoms to pathology and concluded that certain symptoms are predictive of specific pathologic findings (Tomaszewski et al, 1999, 2001). Denson and colleagues analyzed forceps biopsy specimens from 65 females and 4 males with BPS (Denson et al, 2000). Ten percent of specimens showed vasodilatation or submucosal edema. Inflammation was absent in 30% of patients, and mild in another 41%. Cystoscopic changes did not correlate with degree of inflammation. Hanus and colleagues studied 84 biopsy specimens from 112 BPS patients and reported a linear relationship between the mean bladder capacity under anesthesia and severity of glomerulations (Hanus et al, 2001). They did not find a correlation between severity of symptoms and histopathologic changes observed with light or electron microscopy.

Rosamilia reviewed the pathology literature pertaining to BPS and presented her own data (Rosamilia et al, 2003; Hanno et al, 2005a). She compared forceps biopsy specimens from 35 control and 34 BPS/IC patients, 6 with bladder capacities less than 400 mL under anesthesia. Epithelial denudation, submucosal edema, congestion and ectasia, and inflammatory infiltrate were increased in the BPS group. Submucosal hemorrhage did not differentiate the groups, but denuded epithelium was unique to the BPS group and more common in those with severe disease. The most remarkable finding in her study was that histologic parameters were normal and indistinguishable from control subjects in 55% of BPS subjects. Method of biopsy can be important in interpreting findings, because transurethral resection biopsy specimens tend to show mucosal ruptures, submucosal hemorrhage, and mild inflammation (Johansson and Fall, 1990), whereas histology is normal approximately half the time with cold-cup forceps biopsy specimens (Mattila, 1982; Lynes et al, 1990a; Rosamilia et al, 2003).

Histopathology plays a supportive diagnostic role at best (Johansson et al, 1997). **Major reconstructive procedures appear to have better outcomes in patients with pathology consistent with Hunner lesions** (Rössberger et al, 2007). **Inflammatory features can be seen in 24% to 76% of patients without a visible Hunner lesion** (Erickson et al, 2008b). Although studies have suggested that a severely abnormal pathology may be associated with poor prognosis (McDougald and Landon, 2003; Nordling et al, 2004), this is not necessarily the case (MacDermott et al, 1991a). At this point in time, excluding other diseases that are pathologically identifiable is the primary clinical use of bladder biopsy in this group of patients.

> ### KEY POINTS: PATHOLOGY
>
> - The role of histopathology is primarily to exclude other possible diagnoses that might be responsible for the symptoms.
> - There is no histology pathognomonic of BPS, and one cannot make the diagnosis on pathology alone in the absence of the cardinal symptoms.
> - Completely normal-appearing bladder biopsy specimens in symptomatic patients are not uncommon.

DIAGNOSIS

BPS/IC can be considered a functional pain disorder (Mayer and Bushnell, 2009) and one of the chronic visceral pain syndromes affecting the urogenital and rectal area, many of which are well described but poorly understood (Wesselmann et al, 1997; Wesselmann, 2001). These include vulvodynia, orchalgia, penile pain, perineal pain, and rectal pain. In men, many of the entities have now been included in the rubric of CPPS and can be difficult to distinguish from BPS/IC (Hakenberg and Wirth, 2002; Forrest and Schmidt, 2004). The diagnosis of BPS/IC is by its very nature based on the definition. In the past this was, by default, the symptom criteria enumerated by the NIDDK (Hanno et al, 1999a, 1999b) (see Box 14-2). **It has now morphed largely into a diagnosis of chronic pain, pressure, or discomfort associated with the bladder, usually accompanied by urinary frequency in the absence of any identifiable cause** (Hanno et al, 2005a, 2005b). Diagnostic approaches vary widely, and **general agreement on a diagnostic algorithm remains a future goal** (Chai, 2002; Nordling, 2004; Nordling et al, 2004). The disorder can be very difficult to diagnose until symptoms become well established, unless one has a high level of suspicion (Porru et al, 2004). **Frequency and pelvic pain of long duration perceived to be related to the bladder unrelated**

to other known causes establishes a working diagnosis. It is often difficult for patients to distinguish between sensations of pain, pressure, discomfort, and urgency. **Ask a patient why he or she voids hourly, and the patient usually will state that it is because of discomfort rather than convenience.** Heavy reliance on other aspects of the NIDDK research criteria will result in underdiagnosing more than half of patients (Hanno et al, 1999b). **IC symptom scales** (O'Leary et al, 1997; Goin et al, 1998; Moldwin and Kushner, 2004), **such as the AUA symptom score for BPH, are designed to evaluate the severity of symptomatology and monitor disease progression or regression with or without treatment. They have not been validated as diagnostic criteria.**

One must rule out infection and less common conditions including but not limited to carcinoma (Utz and Zincke, 1974; Tissot et al, 2004), eosinophilic cystitis (Hellstrom et al, 1979; Sidh et al, 1980; Littleton et al, 1982; Aubert et al, 1983; Abramov et al, 2004), **malakoplakia, schistosomiasis, scleroderma** (Batra and Hanno, 1997), **and detrusor endometriosis** (Sircus et al, 1988; Price et al, 1996). In men under the age of 50, video-urodynamics are useful to rule out voiding dysfunction resulting from vesical neck obstruction, "pseudo" dyssynergia, or impaired contractility (Kaplan et al, 1996). Musculoskeletal dysfunction may also play a role in causation or increasing symptom severity and should be looked for in the diagnostic phase of evaluation (Prendergast and Weiss, 2003). Reports of successful treatment of IC symptoms by laparoscopic adhesiolysis (Chen et al, 1997) or urethral diverticulum excision (Daneshgari et al, 1999) give credence to the fact that IC is a diagnosis of exclusion. Many drugs including cyclophosphamide, aspirin, nonsteroidal anti-inflammatory agents, and allopurinol have caused a nonbacterial cystitis that resolves with drug withdrawal (Bramble and Morley, 1997; Gheyi et al, 1999).

Ketamine hydrochloride, commonly used as an anesthetic agent, is an NMDA receptor antagonist. It has a rapid onset and short duration of action and produces a cataleptic-like state wherein the patient is dissociated from the surrounding environment by direct action on the cortex and limbic system. In some parts of the world such as Taiwan, it is an increasingly popular choice among young drug users, especially within dance club venues. It can cause dysuria, lower urinary tract symptoms, pelvic pain, and impaired bladder functional capacity. At endoscopy, ulceration with severe diffuse bladder hemorrhage and low capacity has been described (Chen et al, 2011; Middela and Pearce, 2011). **Decreased E-cadherin and increased apoptosis are more severe in ketamine cystitis than BPS** (Lee et al, 2013). **Treatment is cessation of abuse of the drug.**

Tarlov cysts are present in 4.6% of the population. When present at lumbosacral levels, symptoms may include perineal pressure and pain and voiding hallmarks of BPS. Successful treatment with epidural steroids has been reported (Freidenstein et al, 2012).

Various gynecologic problems can mimic the pain of IC (Kohli et al, 1997). The **pelvic congestion syndrome,** a condition of the reproductive years and equally prevalent among parous and nulliparous women, manifests with shifting location of pain, deep dyspareunia and postcoital pain, and exacerbation of pain after prolonged standing (Stones, 2003). Similar symptoms can be seen in BPS/IC. Other gynecologic disorders can include **pelvic tumors, vaginal atrophy, vulvodynia, vestibulitis, pelvic relaxation, pelvic adhesive disease, levator ani myalgia, and undiagnosed chronic pelvic pain** (Myers and Aguilar, 2002). **Pelvic surgery is more common in women with a diagnosis of BPS/IC than in a control population** (Ingber et al, 2008). **In Ingber's series, the diagnosis of BPS/IC occurred 1 to 5 years after hysterectomy in most patients, suggesting that pelvic surgery may be performed for pain related to undiagnosed BPS.**

Endometriosis can be a cause of pelvic pain (Evans et al, 2007), an idea largely based on findings of two randomized, placebo controlled studies of laser laparoscopy (Sutton et al, 1995, 1997; Abbott et al, 2004). Nevertheless, it is disconcerting that **any claim linking endometriosis with pain fails to account for the common experience that identical lesions can be found in symptomatic and asymptomatic women** (Vercellini, 1997). From 2% to 43% of asymptomatic women are found to have endometriosis (Moen and Stokstad, 2002). Furthermore, there does not appear to be any risk for patients with asymptomatic mild endometriosis to develop symptoms even after more than 10 years (Moen and Stokstad, 2002). Although 70% to 90% of women with chronic pelvic pain have endometriosis, this does not definitively establish causation (Gambone et al, 2002). **For these reasons, laparoscopy, which is not considered essential before initiation of hormonal treatment of endometriosis (Ling, 1999; Howard, 2003b), should not be considered a part of any routine evaluation of BPS/IC unless an experienced practitioner believes it is likely to benefit the patient.**

A presumptive diagnosis can be made merely by ruling out known causes of frequency, pain, and urgency in a patient with compatible chronic symptoms (Box 14-5). This holds true for adolescents as well as adults (Yoost et al, 2012). Often this will involve a complete history, physical examination, appropriate cultures, and local cystoscopy. A finding of tenderness on examination

of the anterior vaginal wall with an empty bladder at the initial examination can lead one to suspect BPS (Paulson and Paulson, 2011). **In the absence of microhematuria the value of cytology is questionable** (Duldulao et al, 1997), **but it is something we still consider important, especially if bladder carcinoma in situ is a serious possibility, as in patients older than 40 and those with a smoking history.** The report of a large series of BPS/IC patients indicating that 1% actually had transitional cell carcinoma and that four of the six cancer patients did not have microhematuria provides evidence for the justification of local cystoscopic examination (Tissot et al, 2004).

It must be recognized that one may sacrifice a certain level of confidence in the diagnosis without the supporting evidence that can be furnished by additional studies. In a long-term illness such as BPS/IC, many patients and physicians ultimately want to base a diagnosis and treatment plan on the most complete data set possible (Rovner and Wein, 1999). **A more thorough evaluation would also include a urodynamic evaluation and cystoscopy under anesthesia with hydrodistention of the bladder** (Hanno et al, 1990; Hanno, 1994b). **Bladder biopsy is indicated only if necessary to rule out other disorders that might be suggested by the cystoscopic appearance. Cystoscopy under anesthesia with bladder distention has been important in the identification of a Hunner lesion.** Experimental data suggest that measurement of increased nitric oxide levels in the bladder can also accurately identify those with ulcerative disease (Logadottir et al, 2004). In general, the diagnosis is subject to more rigorous testing in Europe (Fall et al, 2008) than in North America, where symptoms in the absence of other obvious causes seems to be the gold standard (Nordling, 2004; Nordling et al, 2004; Hanno et al, 2005a). Japanese guidelines are listed in Box 14-6.

Although sensations reported during cystometric bladder filling are subjective, they have a normal pattern and may be helpful in distinguishing bladder pathology (Wyndaele, 1998). Many dispute the need for urodynamic study (Cameron and Gajewski, 2009), but Siroky and Kim argue that not only can it help to assess

---

BOX 14-5 International Consultation on Incontinence 2009: Diagnosis of Bladder Pain Syndrome

HISTORY
General thorough medical history emphasizing the following:
1. Previous pelvic surgery
2. Previous urinary tract infection
3. Bladder history and urologic diseases
4. Location of pelvic pain and relationship to bladder filling and emptying
5. Characteristics, onset, correlation of pain with other events
6. Previous pelvic irradiation
7. Autoimmune diseases
8. Associated syndromes (irritable bowel, fibromyalgia, chronic fatigue)

PHYSICAL EXAMINATION
Physical examination emphasizing the following:
1. Standing: kyphosis, scars, hernia
2. Supine: abduction and adduction of hips, hyperesthetic areas
3. Females: vaginal examination with pain mapping of vulvar region, vaginal palpation for tenderness of the bladder, urethra, levator and adductor muscles of the pelvic floor
4. Males: digital rectal examination with pain mapping of the scrotal-anal region and palpation of tenderness of the bladder, prostate, levator and adductor muscles of the pelvic floor and scrotal contents

LABORATORY TESTING
1. Urinalysis
2. Urine culture
3. Urine cytology in risk groups

SYMPTOM EVALUATION
1. Voiding diary
2. O'Leary-Sant symptom and problem index
3. Visual analog scale for pain in the last 24 hours

OTHER EVALUATIONS
Urodynamics (optional)
Cystoscopy with or without hydrodistention under anesthesia (optional)
Bladder biopsy (optional)

From Hanno P, Lin AT, Nordling J, et al. Bladder pain syndrome. In: Abrams P, Cardozo L, Khoury S, et al, editors. Incontinence. Paris: Health Publication; 2009. p. 1459–518.

BOX 14-6 Recommended Tests for Diagnosis of Interstitial Cystitis from the Japanese Urological Association

MANDATORY
Clinical history
Physical examination
Urinalysis

RECOMMENDED
Urine culture
Urine cytology
Symptom scores
Quality-of-life scores
Frequency-volume chart
Residual urine measurement
Prostate-specific antigen
Cystoscopy
Hydrodistention

OPTIONAL
Ultrasonography
Urodynamic study
X-ray examination
Potassium test
Biopsy

From Homma Y, Ueda T, Ito T, et al. Japanese guideline for diagnosis and treatment of interstitial cystitis. Int J Urol 2009;16:4–16. Copyright © Japanese Urological Association.

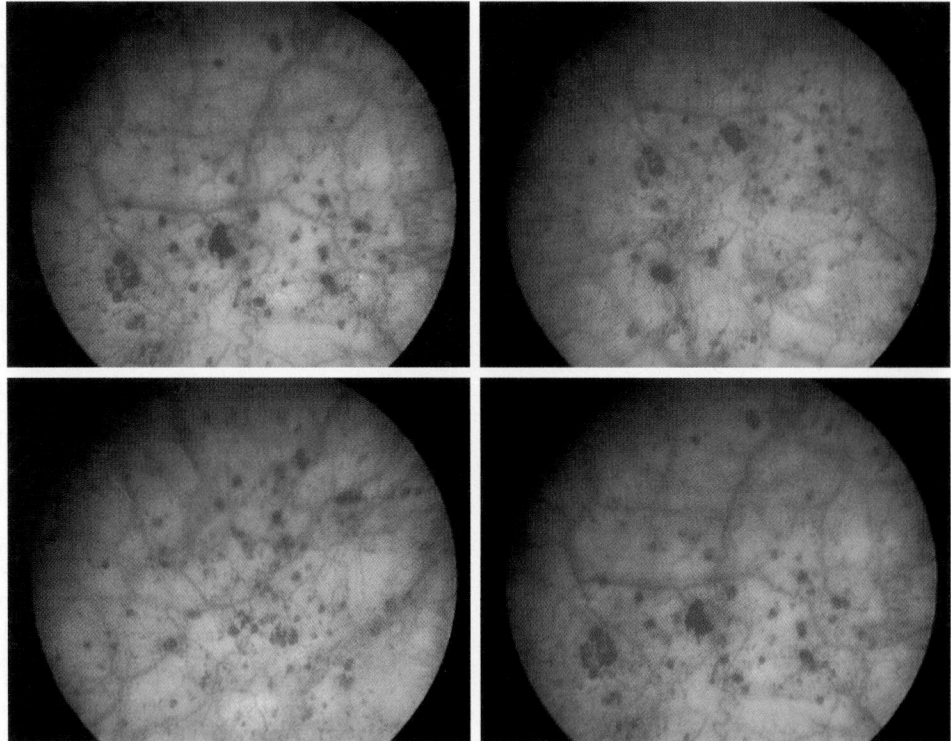

Figure 14-9. Typical appearance of glomerulations after bladder distention in a patient with nonulcerative bladder pain syndrome.

bladder compliance and sensation and reproduce the patient's symptoms during bladder filling, but it can help to rule out DO (Siroky, 1994; Kim et al, 2009b). Women with pain on filling can be indistinguishable from those with DO in their perception of bladder fullness (Creighton et al, 1991). **One should be wary of diagnosing BPS/IC in patients with discrete, involuntary bladder contractions whose symptoms respond to antimuscarinic therapy. The two problems may coexist in 15% to 19% of patients** (Gajewski et al, 1997, Kirkemo et al, 1997), **but the pathophysiology is possibly very different.** Patients who respond to anticholinergic medication tend not to respond to standard therapy for BPS (Perez-Marrero et al, 1987). If involuntary contractions are noted and the patient's symptoms of frequency and pain continue despite treatment for overactive bladder, one is on firmer ground in considering a diagnosis of BPS/IC. Complex cases may benefit from full video-urodynamic studies (Carlson et al, 2001).

Cystometry in conscious BPS patients typically demonstrates normal function, the exception being decreased bladder capacity and hypersensitivity. Pain on bladder filling that reproduces the patient's symptoms is very suggestive of the diagnosis. Volume at strong desire to void has been purported to be a predictor of treatment outcome (Kuo and Kuo, 2013). **Bladder compliance in patients with BPS/IC is normal, as hypersensitivity would prevent the bladder from filling to the point of noncompliance** (Siroky, 1994; Rovner and Wein, 1999). The possible addition of a second cystometrogram after instillation of intravesical lidocaine to help determine if pain is bladder related is a provocative issue worth further study (Teichman et al, 1997). It is not uncommon to find evidence of outlet obstruction in BPS/IC, presumably related to associated pelvic floor dysfunction (Cameron and Gajewski, 2009).

Long before it was considered a diagnostic tool, CHD was used as a therapeutic modality for BPS (Bumpus, 1930). **CHD under anesthesia allows for sufficient distention of the bladder to afford visualization of either glomerulations** (Fig. 14-9) **or Hunner lesions** (Fig. 14-10). **After filling to 80 cm water pressure for 1 to 2 minutes, the bladder is drained and refilled. The terminal portion of the effluent is often blood tinged. Reinspection will reveal the pinpoint petechial hemorrhages that develop

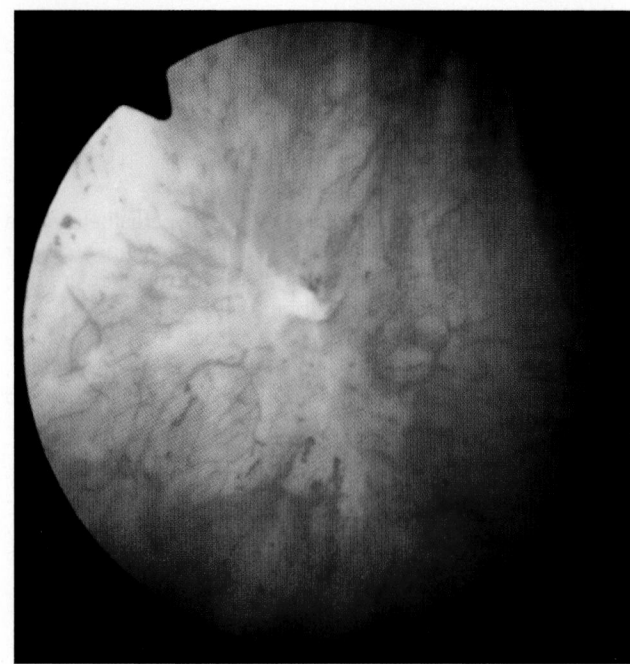

Figure 14-10. Typical appearance of Hunner lesion in a patient with bladder pain syndrome before bladder distention.

throughout the bladder after distention and are not usually seen during examination without anesthesia (Nigro et al, 1997b).

Glomerulations are not specific for BPS/IC (Erickson, 1995; Waxman et al, 1998), and only when seen in conjunction with the clinical criteria of pain and frequency can the finding of glomerulations be viewed as potentially significant. **Glomerulations can be seen after radiation therapy, in patients with carcinoma, after exposure to toxic chemicals or chemotherapeutic agents, and often in patients on dialysis or after urinary diversion when the bladder has not filled for prolonged periods. They have been reported in the majority of men with prostate pain syndromes, begging the question as to whether CPPS in men is closely linked with IC (Berger et al, 1998). They are observed in up to 20% of men undergoing transurethral prostatectomy for lower urinary tract symptoms (Furuya et al, 2007). We have speculated that they may simply reflect the response of the bladder to distention after a prolonged period of chronic underfilling because of sensory urgency, rather than resulting from a primary pathologic process. Although the presence of a Hunner ulcer has been associated with pain and urinary urgency, neither the finding of bloody irrigating fluid nor of glomerulations is strongly associated with any particular symptom in patients in the ICDB (Messing et al, 1997).

Further confusion arises when the patient demonstrates the symptoms of IC but the cystoscopic findings under anesthesia are completely normal. This occurred in 8.7% of patients undergoing CHD entered into the IC database (Messing et al, 1997). Awad and colleagues recognized this entity soon after the NIDDK research criteria had been described. They reported on a series of patients in whom the symptomatology, urodynamic evaluation findings, histology, and response to therapy were identical to IC but in whom findings on CHD were normal. It was termed *idiopathic reduced bladder storage* (Awad et al, 1992). Clinical, urodynamic, and cystoscopic data strongly suggest that the presence of glomerulations is not selecting out a meaningful difference in patients with symptoms of BPS/IC (Al Hadithi et al, 2002). **The presence of cystoscopic abnormalities such as glomerulations on cystoscopy under anesthesia meeting the NIDDK criteria may identify a group of patients with worse daytime frequency and nocturia, lower mean voiding volumes, and lower bladder capacity under anesthesia, but does not have any relationship to biopsy findings, bladder pain, or urgency** (Erickson et al, 2005; Boudry et al, 2013).

The Search for a Marker

What is the value of a "diagnostic test" in what is essentially a clinical syndrome defined by a symptom complex? If a patient has chronic pain associated with the bladder usually accompanied by urinary frequency with no discernible cause, we diagnose BPS/IC. In essence, once we have ruled out well-characterized pathologic entities, the patient makes the diagnosis by relating symptoms, much as a patient with impotence makes that diagnosis. Testing for impotence may give clues as to the cause, but we cannot rule out impotence by doing a test in a patient who cannot function sexually!

This is not to say that establishment of a valid diagnostic marker would not be a major advance in our understanding of IC. Just as with phenotyping, it will be important largely to the extent that it can predict prognosis in a given group of patients, predict response to therapy in a given group of patients, and/or distinguish between BPS/IC and another possible cause of the symptom complex that has been diagnosed. Ultimately, marker identification may enable us to stratify patients with the symptom complex in such a way that treatments will be specific to the specific cause (i.e., disease) the patient has. As various causes are identifiable, the diagnosis of BPS may itself become a rarity, much like what has happened to "acute urethral syndrome" (Stamm et al, 1980).

In just such an effort, numerous investigators have looked at the mast cell as a possible diagnostic marker for IC. The current standard involves detrusor muscle biopsy specimens examined with tryptase staining of 3-μm thick sections, with every seventh section used for quantification (Larsen et al, 2008). Twenty-seven mast cells per cubic millimeter is considered indicative of mastocytosis. The results in the past have been very contradictory, **and at this time, in terms of the use of mast cell criteria in diagnosis, the issue remains moot** (Kastrup et al, 1983; Feltis et al, 1987; Holm-Bentzen et al, 1987a; Lynes et al, 1987; Hanno et al, 1990; Christmas and Rode, 1991; Moore et al, 1992; Dundore et al, 1996; Hofmeister et al, 1997). Methylhistamine, a histamine metabolite found in the urine and thought to reflect mast cell activation, was not associated

with symptom scores, response to bladder distention, cystoscopic findings, or bladder biopsy features including mast cell determination by tryptase staining (Erickson et al, 2004).

Attempts have been made to look at other markers (Erickson, 2001), including eosinophil cationic protein (Lose et al, 1987), GAG excretion (Hurst et al, 1993), and urinary histamine and methylhistamine (El Mansoury et al, 1994). Proposals for measuring smooth muscle isoactin expression (Rivas et al, 1997) and urinary levels of neurotrophin-3, nerve growth factor, glial cell line–derived neurotrophic factor, and tryptase (Okragly et al, 1999) have been suggested. Low levels of GP51, a urinary glycoprotein with a molecular weight of 5 kDa, have been documented in IC patients compared with normal controls and patients with other urinary tract disease (Byrne et al, 1999). Cell cultures (Elgavish et al, 1997) have been proposed as a screening technique.

The measurement of elevated nitric oxide levels in air instilled and incubated in the bladder has been proposed for office screening (Lundberg et al, 1996; Ehrén et al, 1999). Increased levels of endogenously formed nitric oxide in patients with IC correspond to increased iNOS mRNA expression and protein levels in these patients. Furthermore, iNOS was found to be localized to the urothelium, but it was also found in macrophages in the bladder mucosa (Koskela et al, 2008). The simple technique allows for discrimination of ulcer from nonulcer disease (Logadottir et al, 2004) and may provide an objective measure of treatment response (Hosseini et al, 2004).

The urine APF identified by Keay (see earlier) may prove to be an accurate marker of BPS/IC if it can be confirmed by other centers and become a biochemical rather than biologic assay. **It appears to have the highest sensitivity and specificity of the variety of possible markers tested** and fits nicely into an etiologic schema (Keay et al, 2001a, 2001b; Erickson et al, 2002). It has also been shown to differentiate men with BPS/IC symptoms from controls and to differentiate men with bladder-associated pain and irritative voiding symptoms from those with pelvic or perineal pain alone and other nonspecific findings compatible with CPPS in men (CPPS III), previously referred to as *nonbacterial prostatitis* (Keay et al, 2004a). This question—whether CPPS and BPS/IC are two different disorders—will doubtless be the subject of future research and is an integral question that the NIDDK is hoping to answer with current research (www.mappnetwork.org). Data regarding the reproducibility of APF and any practical clinical uses are lacking.

Much work in markers is ongoing. Uroplakin III-delta 4 is a potential marker for identifying nonulcerative IC (Zeng et al, 2007). The feasibility of diagnosing IC in humans and domestic cats from the spectra of dried serum films (DSFs) using infrared microspectroscopy has been reported (Rubio-Diaz et al, 2009).

Potassium Chloride Test

Parsons has championed an intravesical KCl challenge, comparing the sensory nerve provocative ability of sodium versus potassium using a 0.4-M KCl solution. Pain and provocation of symptoms constitutes a positive test result. **Whether the results indicate abnormal epithelial permeability in the subgroup of positive patients or hypersensitivity of the sensory nerves is unclear.** Normal bladder epithelium can never be absolutely tight, and there is always some leak, however small (Hohlbrugger and Sant, 1997). The concentration of potassium used is 400 mEq/L, far exceeding the physiologic urinary concentrations of 20 to 80 mEq/L depending on dietary intake (Vander, 1995). Healthy controls can distinguish KCl from sodium chloride, although they don't experience severe pain (Roberto et al, 1997). **The hope is that this test may stratify patients into those who will respond to certain treatments (perhaps those designed to fortify the GAG layer), but to date this information is lacking** (Teichman and Nielsen-Omeis, 1999).

Used as a diagnostic test for IC, the KCl test is not valid (Chambers et al, 1999). The gold standard in defining BPS/IC for research purposes has been the NIDDK criteria. These criteria are recognized to constitute a set of patients that virtually all researchers can agree have BPS/IC, though they are far too restrictive to be used in clinical practice (Hanno et al, 1999b). Thus, this group of patients should virtually all be positive if the KCl test is to have the sensitivity needed to aid in diagnosis. **Up to 25% of patients meeting the NIDDK criteria will have a negative KCl test result** (Parsons et al, 1998). **In the group of patients in whom it should perform best, it is lacking in sensitivity.**

When we look at the specificity side of the equation, in the universe of unselected persons, studies reported a 36% false-positive rate in asymptomatic men (Yilmaz et al, 2004) and a 33% positive rate in a fixed population of Turkish textile workers (Sahinkanat et al, 2008). In the patient population with confounding conditions for which we would want help in sorting out BPS/IC from other disorders, 25% of patients with overactive bladder test positive and virtually all patients with irritative symptoms from radiation cystitis and urinary tract infection test positive (Parsons et al, 1994b, 1998). The results with chronic prostatitis and CPPS in men are variable, but 50% to 84% of men have been reported to test positive (Parsons and Albo, 2002; Yilmaz et al, 2004; Parsons et al, 2005). In women with pelvic pain the results are similar (Parsons et al, 2002b), and based on these findings Parsons has expressed the view that BPS/IC may affect over 20% of the female population of the United States (Parsons et al, 2002a). Another way to interpret the findings would be that the KCl test is very nonspecific, missing a significant number of BPS/IC patients and overdiagnosing much of the population.

Prospective and retrospective studies looking at the KCl test for diagnosis in patients with symptoms of BPS/IC have found no benefit of the test in comparison with standard techniques of diagnosis (Chambers et al, 1999; Gregoire et al, 2002; Kuo, 2003), and it is not useful for monitoring results of treatment (Sairanen et al, 2007). The development of a painless modification of the KCl test (Daha et al, 2003) using cystometric capacity and a 0.2-M solution may improve acceptability among patients, but further research is needed to determine what place, if any, this test will have in the diagnostic or treatment algorithm.

Confusable Diseases (Differential Diagnosis)

The diagnosis of BPS can be made on the basis of exclusion of confusable diseases and confirmed by the recognition of the presence of the specific combination of symptoms and signs of BPS. If the main urinary symptoms are not explained by a single diagnosis, the presence of a second diagnosis is possible. One must remember that BPS may occur together with confusable diseases such as chronic or remitting urinary infections or endometriosis. Table 14-3 summarizes confusable diseases related to BPS and their mode of exclusion based on aforementioned diagnostic

TABLE 14-3 Diseases That May Be Mistaken for Bladder Pain Syndrome

CONFUSABLE DISEASE	EXCLUDED OR DIAGNOSED BY
Carcinoma and carcinoma in situ	Cystoscopy and biopsy
Infection with:	
Common intestinal bacteria	Routine bacterial culture
Chlamydia trachomatis, Ureaplasma urealyticum, Mycoplasma hominis, Mycoplasma genitalium, Corynebacterium urealyticum, Candida species, *Mycobacterium tuberculosis*	Special cultures Dipstick; if "sterile" pyuria, culture for *M. tuberculosis*
Herpes simplex and human papillomavirus	Physical examination
Radiation	Medical history
Chemotherapy, including immunotherapy with cyclophosphamide	Medical history
Anti-inflammatory therapy with tiaprofenic acid	Medical history
Bladder neck obstruction and neurogenic outlet obstruction	Uroflowmetry and ultrasonography
Bladder stone	Imaging or cystoscopy
Lower ureteral stone	Medical history and/or hematuria; upper urinary tract imaging (CT or IVP)
Urethral diverticulum	Medical history and physical examination
Urogenital prolapse	Medical history and physical examination
Endometriosis	Medical history and physical examination
Vaginal candidiasis	Medical history and physical examination
Cervical, uterine, and ovarian cancer	Physical examination
Incomplete bladder emptying (retention)	Postvoid residual urine volume measured by ultrasound evaluation
Overactive bladder	Medical history and urodynamics
Prostate cancer	Physical examination and PSA test
Benign prostatic obstruction	Uroflowmetry and pressure-flow studies
Chronic bacterial prostatitis	Medical history, physical examination, culture
Chronic nonbacterial prostatitis	Medical history, physical examination, culture
Pudendal nerve entrapment	Medical history, physical examination; nerve block may prove diagnosis
Pelvic floor muscle–related pain	Medical history, physical examination

CT, computed tomography; IVP, intravenous pyelogram; PSA, prostate-specific antigen.
From van de Merwe JP, Nordling J, Bouchelouche P, et al. Diagnostic criteria, classification, and nomenclature for painful bladder syndrome/interstitial cystitis: an ESSIC proposal. Eur Urol 2008;53:60–7.

proposals and procedures as outlined by the ESSIC group (van de Merwe et al, 2008).

KEY POINTS: DIAGNOSIS

- BPS remains a diagnosis of exclusion in patients who meet the symptomatic criteria for diagnosis after confusable disorders have been ruled out.
- Cystoscopy with bladder distention under anesthesia aids in the diagnosis of a Hunner lesion but is not considered a prerequisite for beginning treatment.
- Cystoscopy and upper tract imaging are mandatory in patients with hematuria who have not been previously evaluated for this finding.
- Urodynamics are optional and usually reserved for complex cases. There are no commonly available laboratory markers that substantially contribute to diagnosis.

CLASSIFICATION

IC was originally described as a bladder disease with severe inflammation of the bladder wall described by Hunner as an ulcer (Hunner, 1915). The lesion is, however, not an ulcer, but a vulnus (weakness, vulnerability) that can ulcerate on distention, and the name of the bladder lesion has consequently been changed to *Hunner lesion* (van de Merwe et al, 2008). The finding of a Hunner lesion could therefore originally be regarded as a diagnostic criterion for IC. Messing and Stamey introduced glomerulations alone as another typical finding for IC, and this was included in the NIDDK criteria (Wein et al, 1990).

Magnus Fall proposed that patients with Hunner lesions (classic IC) and patients with glomerulations (non-Hunner type) represented two different subtypes (Fall et al, 1987). They may have different clinical pictures, different outcomes, and different responses to treatment (Peeker and Fall, 2002b). Patients with Hunner lesions were found to have a 5-fold to 20-fold increase in the chemokines CXCL-10 and CXCL-1, interleukin-6, and nerve growth factor when compared with BPS patients without Hunner lesions (Tyagi et al, 2012). Different expression patterns of the genes involved in pronociceptive inflammatory reactions suggest distinct pathophysiologies for Hunner lesion patients compared with patients with BPS without Hunner lesions (Homma et al, 2013).

Thus, patients fulfilling the NIDDK criteria represent at least two (and possibly more) different patient populations. Moreover, up to 60% of patients clinically believed to have BPS by experienced clinicians do not fulfill the NIDDK criteria (Hanno et al, 1999b) and whether or not these patients are comparable to the patients fulfilling the NIDDK criteria is unknown. Finally, Japanese urologists consider that *interstitial cystitis* should be preserved as a disease name reserved for patients with urinary symptoms and cystoscopic findings of glomerulations or Hunner lesion as outlined in the NIDDK criteria (Homma, 2008).

In an attempt to unite these different philosophies into a coherent schema, ESSIC proposed a classification of BPS based on findings during CHD and morphologic findings in bladder biopsy specimens (van de Merwe et al, 2008) (see Table 14-1). The classification includes groups not having had CHD (group X) as well as groups not having had morphologic investigation of bladder biopsy specimens (group XX). By using this classification, future researchers will be able to identify whether findings of glomerulations and/or Hunner lesion as well as morphologic changes in bladder biopsy specimens do have significant importance for disease prognosis and/or treatment outcome (Geurts et al, 2011).

TREATMENT
Conservative Therapies

Once the diagnosis has been made, one must decide whether to institute therapy or employ a policy of conservative watchful

waiting. **If the patient has not had an empirical course of antibiotics for their symptoms by the time the BPS/IC diagnosis is made, such a trial is reasonable.** Doxycycline has been reported efficacious in a Swiss study (Burkhard et al, 2004). Further attempts to alleviate symptoms with antibiotics are unlikely to be worthwhile and are not recommended in the absence of positive cultures. **Stress reduction, exercise, warm tub baths, and efforts by the patient to maintain a normal lifestyle all contribute to overall quality of life** (Whitmore, 1994). In a large patient survey, dietary changes, application of heat or cold, and stress reduction all had positive response rates in over 80% of responders (O'Hare et al, 2013). In a controlled study of 45 PBS/IC patients and 31 healthy controls, higher levels of stress were related to greater pain and urgency in patients with IC but not in the control group (Rothrock et al, 2001). Maladaptive strategies for coping with stress may adversely affect symptoms (Rothrock et al, 2003).

Biofeedback, soft-tissue massage, and other physical therapies may aid in muscle relaxation of the pelvic floor (Mendelowitz et al, 1997; Meadows, 1999; Holzberg et al, 2001; Lukban, et al, 2001; Markwell, 2001). This is a reasonable intervention, given the strong association of pelvic floor dysfunction and BPS/IC (Peters et al, 2007a; Bassaly et al, 2011). A preliminary NIDDK trial demonstrated the feasibility of such a study and strongly suggested the efficacy of physical therapy when compared with global therapeutic massage (FitzGerald et al, 2009). This was confirmed in a randomized controlled trial comparing 10 scheduled treatments of myofascial physical therapy versus global therapeutic massage at 11 North American clinical centers. The Global Response Assessment (GRA) response rate was 26% in the global therapeutic massage group and 59% in the myofascial physical therapy group ($P = .0012$) (FitzGerald et al, 2012).

Mendelowitz and Moldwin had a 69% success rate in 16 patients treated with electromyographic biofeedback (Mendelowitz et al, 1997), but treatment response did not correlate to changes in muscle identification, and the placebo effect may have been considerable. **Acupuncture** has been used for BPS/IC and many other chronic pain syndromes. There is **limited evidence that it is more effective than nontreatment for chronic pain** and inconclusive evidence that acupuncture is more effective than placebo, sham acupuncture, or standard care (Ezzo et al, 2000). **BPS/IC results with acupuncture have been disappointing** (Geirsson et al, 1993).

Diet

Elaborate dietary restrictions are unsupported by any literature, but many patients do find their symptoms are adversely affected by specific foods and would do well to avoid them (Koziol et al, 1993; Koziol, 1994). **Often these include caffeine, alcohol, artificial sweeteners, hot peppers, and beverages that might acidify the urine, such as cranberry juice** (Shorter et al, 2007). Several acid-sensing ion channel subunits are expressed in human bladder, and the upregulation of some of these channels in BPS/IC patients suggests involvement in increased pain and hyperalgesia (Sanchez-Freire et al, 2011). **Anecdotal association of IC with many foods has spawned the recommendation of various "interstitial cystitis diets" with little in the way of objective, scientific basis** (Box 14-7). The only placebo-controlled dietary study, although small, failed to demonstrate a relationship between diet and symptoms (Fisher et al, 1993). Bade and colleagues found that IC patients tend to have a healthier diet than the general population but could discern no rationale for dietary or fluid intake change other than decreasing caffeine intake (Bade et al, 1997b). Nguan and coworkers performed a prospective, double-blind, crossover study consisting of crossover instillations of urine at physiologic pH (5.0) and neutral buffered pH (7.5) (Nguan et al, 2005). There was no statistically significant difference in subjective pain scores, suggesting that adjusting urine pH with diet or dietary supplements may have little influence on symptomatology. Orange and grapefruit juices, rich in potassium and citrate, tend to increase urinary pH (Wabner and Pak, 1993) but are avoided by many IC patients based on "IC diet" recommendations and their personal experience with food-related

---

BOX 14-7   Interstitial Cystitis Association Recommendations of Foods to Avoid

Milk and dairy products
- Aged cheeses
- Sour cream
- Yogurt
- Chocolate

Vegetables
- Fava beans
- Lima beans
- Onions
- Tofu
- Soybeans
- Tomatoes

Fruits
- Apples
- Apricots
- Avocados
- Bananas
- Cantaloupes
- Citrus fruits
- Cranberries
- Grapes
- Nectarines
- Peaches
- Pineapples
- Plums

Fruits—cont'd
- Pomegranates
- Rhubarb
- Strawberries
- Juices from above fruits

Carbohydrates and grains
- Rye bread
- Sourdough bread

Meats and fish
- Aged, canned, cured processed, smoked meats and fish

Nuts

Beverages
- Alcoholic beverages including beer and wine
- Carbonated drinks
- Coffee
- Tea
- Fruit juices

Seasonings
- Mayonnaise
- Ketchup
- Mustard
- Salsa

Seasonings—cont'd
- Spicy foods (Chinese, Mexican, Indian, Thai)
- Soy sauce
- Miso
- Salad dressing
- Vinegar

Preservatives and additives
- Benzyl alcohol
- Citric acid
- Monosodium glutamate
- Artificial sweeteners
- Preservatives
- Artificial ingredients
- Food coloring

Miscellaneous
- Tobacco
- Caffeine
- Diet pills
- Junk foods
- Recreational drugs
- Allergy medications with ephedrine or pseudoephedrine
- Certain vitamins

Modified from Interstitial Cystitis Association. Understanding the interstitial cystitis/painful bladder syndrome diet, <http://www.ichelp.org/document.doc?id=7>; 2009 [accessed 29.10.14].

---

flares. Alkalinizing the urine may be worth trying, but supporting studies are lacking. Some patients have had benefit with calcium glycerophosphate, an over-the-counter food acid–reducing agent (Hill et al, 2008; O'Hare et al, 2013), but supporting controlled trials are lacking. A controlled method to determine dietary sensitivities, such as an elimination diet, may play an important role in patient management (Friedlander et al, 2012).

In a large National Institutes of Health study, patients with newly diagnosed BPS/IC were treated with a focus on four targeted areas: (1) controlling or managing symptoms, (2) controlling fluid intake, (3) changing the diet to one that might improve symptoms, and (4) bladder training and urge suppression. A behavioral approach to stress and pain management was also used to help patients learn skills to reduce stress in their lives. Of 135 patients randomized to this approach without additional medication, 45% were moderately or markedly improved at the 12-week end point (Foster et al, 2010). In another trial, hydrodistention followed by bladder training produced a statistically significant better response at 24 weeks post-procedure than hydrodistention alone (Hsieh et al, 2012).

Unfortunately, education and self-help are often not sufficient, and most patients will require one or more of a variety of therapies.

Oral Therapies (Table 14-4)

Amitriptyline

Amitriptyline, a tricyclic antidepressant, has become a staple of oral treatment for BPS/IC. The tricyclics possess varying degrees of at **least three major pharmacologic actions:** (1) They have central and peripheral anticholinergic actions at some but not all sites, (2) they block the active transport system in the presynaptic nerve ending that is responsible for the reuptake of the released amine neurotransmitters serotonin and noradrenaline, and (3) they are sedatives, an action that occurs presumably on a central basis but perhaps is related to their antihistaminic properties. Amitriptyline, in fact, is one of the most potent tricyclic antidepressants in terms of blocking H_1-histaminergic receptors (Baldessarini et al, 1985).

There is also evidence that they desensitize α_2 receptors on central noradrenergic neurons. Paradoxically, they also have been shown to block α-adrenergic receptors and serotonin receptors. Theoretically, tricyclic agents have actions that might tend to stimulate predominantly β-adrenergic receptors in bladder body smooth musculature, an action that would further facilitate urine storage by decreasing the excitability of smooth muscle in that area (Barrett et al, 1987).

Hanno and Wein first reported a therapeutic response in IC after noting a "serendipitous" response to amitriptyline in one of their patients concurrently being treated for depression (Hanno and Wein, 1987). The following year, a similar report appeared relating a response to desipramine hydrochloride (Renshaw, 1988). Reasoning that a drug used successfully at relatively low doses for many types of chronic pain syndromes, that would also have anticholinergic properties, β-adrenergic bladder effects, sedative characteristics, and strong H_1-antihistaminic activity, would seem to be ideal for IC, the first clinical trial was carried out with promising results (Hanno et al, 1989). A subsequent follow-up study (Hanno, 1994a) reported that in 28 of 43 patients who could tolerate therapy for at least a 3-week trial at a dose of 25 mg at bedtime gradually increasing to 75 mg at bedtime over 2 weeks, 18 had total remission of symptoms with a mean follow-up of 14.4 months, 5 dropped out because of side effects, and 5 derived no clinical benefit. Benefits were apparent within 4 weeks. In all patients, hydrodistention and intravesical DMSO therapy had failed. **Sedation was the main side effect.** Kirkemo and colleagues treated 30 patients and had a 90% subjective improvement rate at 8 weeks (Kirkemo et al, 1990). Both studies noted that patients with bladder capacities over 450 to 600 mL under anesthesia seemed to have the best results. Another uncontrolled study of 11 patients with urinary frequency and pelvic pain (Pranikoff and Constantino, 1998) related success in 9 of the patients, with 5 reporting complete resolution of symptoms and 4 significant relief. Two patients could not tolerate the medication. In a 4-month intent-to-treat placebo-controlled double-blind trial of 50 patients, 63% on amitriptyline at doses of 25 to 75 mg (dose as tolerated) before bed reported good or excellent satisfaction versus

TABLE 14-4 Grade and Level of Evidence According to Oxford System for Oral and Intravesical Therapies

TREATMENT	ICI*	EAU†	GIANNANTONI‡
ORAL THERAPIES			
Amitriptyline	B: 2	A: 1	A: 1
Analgesics	C: 4	C: 2	
Hydroxyzine	D: 1	A: 1	
PPS	D: 1	A: 1	C: 1
Cyclosporine	C: 3	A: 1	A: 1
L-Arginine	–A: 1		A: 1
Antibiotics regimens	D: 4		
Azathioprine	D: 4		
Benzydamine	D: 3		
Chloroquine derivatives	D: 4		
Cimetidine	C: 3		
Doxycycline	D: 4		
Duloxetine	–C: 4		
Gabapentin	C: 4		
Methotrexate	D: 4		
Misoprostol	D: 4		
Montelukast	D: 4		
Nalmefene	–A: 1		
Nifedipine	D: 4		
Quercetin	D: 4		
Tanezumab	D: 1		
Suplatast tosilate	D: 3		
Vitamin E	D: 4		
INTRAVESICAL THERAPIES			
Lidocaine	C: 2		
DMSO	B: 2	A: 1	
Heparin	C: 3		
Hyaluronic acid	D: 1	B: 2	
Chondroitin sulfate	D: 4	B: 2	A: 1
PPS	D: 4	A: 1	
Capsaicin/RTX	–A: 1		
BCG	–A: 1		A: 1
Oxybutynin	D: 4		
BTX (intramural)	A: 1		A: 1

BCG, bacille Calmette-Guérin; BTX, botulinum toxin; DMSO, dimethyl sulfoxide; EAU: European Association of Urology; ICI, International Consultation on Incontinence, 2012; PPS, pentosan polysulfate; RTX, resiniferatoxin.

*Hanno P, Dinis P, Lin A, et al. Bladder pain syndrome. In: Abrams P, Cardozo L, Khoury S, et al, editors. Incontinence. Paris: International Consultation on Urological Diseases/European Association of Urology; 2013. p. 1583–649.
†Fall M, Baranowski AP, Elneil S, et al. EAU guidelines on chronic pelvic pain. Eur Urol 2010;57:35–48.
‡Giannantoni A, Bini V, Dmochowski R, et al. Contemporary management of the painful bladder: a systematic review. Eur Urol 2012;61:29–53.
From Committee on Bladder Pain Syndrome. Fifth International Consultation on Incontinence; 2012 Feb; Paris, France.

4% on placebo (van Ophoven et al, 2004a). At 19-month follow-up there was little tachyphylaxis, and good response rates were observed in the entire spectrum of BPS/IC symptoms (van Ophoven and Hertle, 2005).

The large, double-blind, randomized controlled trial by the NIDDK comparing education and behavioral modification with and without oral amitriptyline showed a 55% response in the arm that included both medication and conservative therapy compared with a 45% response to education and behavioral

therapy alone (Foster et al, 2010). The difference was not statistically significant. However, if only patients who could tolerate 25 mg or more of medication or placebo are included, the success compared with conservative therapy alone was 73% compared with 53% at 12 weeks. Frequency and O'Leary-Sant symptom and problem scores also showed significant improvement. Thus, on an intent-to-treat basis, there was not significant benefit from amitriptyline, but in the 62% of patients who could tolerate these relatively low doses of drug, the benefits appear substantial (Yang et al, 2014). Patients should be cautioned about fatigue, constipation, dry mouth, increased appetite, and dizziness. Slowly titrating the dose on a weekly basis, beginning at 10 mg before bed and increasing by 10 mg weekly to a maximum tolerated dose of 50 mg before bed seems to minimize side effects. Amitriptyline appears to have efficacy that is unrelated to the presence or absence of a Hunner lesion, and cystoscopy shows no predictive value for treatment outcome (Sun et al, 2014). It may also be beneficial in treating the vulvar pain syndrome that sometimes accompanies BPS (Ventolini, 2013).

Amitriptyline has proven analgesic efficacy with a median preferred dose of 50 mg in a range of 25 to 150 mg daily. This range is lower than traditional doses for depression of 150 to 300 mg. The speed of onset of effect is much faster (1 to 7 days) than reported in depression, and the analgesic effect is distinct from any effect on mood (McQuay and Moore, 1997). Tricyclic antidepressants are contraindicated in patients with long QT syndrome or significant conduction system disease (bifascicular or trifascicular block) after recent myocardial infarction (within 6 months), unstable angina, congestive heart failure, frequent premature ventricular contractions, or a history of sustained ventricular arrhythmias. They should be used with caution in patients with orthostatic hypotension (Low and Dotson, 1998). Doses greater than 100 mg are associated with increased relative risk of sudden cardiac death (Ray et al, 2004).

Other Antidepressants

Other tricyclic antidepressants have been used for BPS. One trial employed the combination of doxepin and piroxicam, a cyclooxygenase-2 (COX-2) inhibitor. Twenty-six of 32 patients (81%) experienced remission of symptoms (Wammack et al, 2002). Another study reported satisfactory outcome with desipramine (Renshaw, 1988). The safety and efficacy of duloxetine, a serotonin and norepinephrine reuptake inhibitor, for BPS/IC was assessed in an observational study of 48 women (van Ophoven and Hertle, 2007). Patients were prospectively treated for 2 months after an uptitration protocol to the target dose of 40 mg duloxetine twice daily. Five patients were identified as responders and 17 patients dropped out because of side effects including nausea in all 17 patients. No severe adverse events were reported. In the 5 responders, the 40-mg twice daily dose was required for efficacy to be seen. Overall, duloxetine did not result in clinically meaningful improvement of symptoms.

Antihistamines

The use of antihistamines goes back to the late 1950s and stems from work by Simmons, who postulated that the local release of histamine may be responsible for or may accompany the development of IC (Simmons, 1961). He reported on 6 patients treated with pyribenzamine. The results were far from dramatic, with only half the patients showing some response. The therapy is notable for this disease in that it was very logically conceived. It has been Theoharides who has spearheaded mast cell research in this field and been a major modern proponent of antihistamine therapy (Theoharides, 1994). He has used the unique piperazine H_1-receptor antagonist hydroxyzine, a first-generation antihistamine (Simons, 2004), which can block neuronal activation of mast cells (Minogiannis et al, 1998). In 40 patients treated with 25 mg before bed increasing over 2 weeks (if sedation was not a problem) to 50 mg at night and 25 mg in the morning, virtually every symptom evaluated improved by 30%. Only 3 patients had absolutely no response. As with many IC drug reports, these responses were evaluated subjectively and without blinding or placebo control. A subsequent study suggested improved efficacy in patients with documented allergies and/or evidence of bladder mast cell activation (Theoharides et al, 1997; Theoharides and Sant, 1997). **No significant response to hydroxyzine was found in an NIDDK placebo-controlled trial** (Sant et al, 2003).

Why an H_2-antagonist would be effective is unclear, but uncontrolled studies show improvement of symptoms in two thirds of patients taking cimetidine in divided doses totaling 600 mg (Seshadri et al, 1994; Lewi, 1996). It proved effective in a double-blind, placebo-controlled trial (Thilagarajah et al, 2001), but histologic studies show the bladder mucosa to be unchanged before and after treatment, and the mechanism of any efficacy remains unexplained (Dasgupta et al, 2001). Cimetidine is a common treatment in the United Kingdom, where over a third of patients reported having used it (Tincello and Walker, 2005).

Sodium Pentosan Polysulfate

Parson's suggestion that a defect in the epithelial permeability barrier, the GAG layer, contributes to the pathogenesis of IC has led to an attempt to correct such a defect with the synthetic sulfated polysaccharide sodium pentosan polysulfate (PPS), a heparin analogue available in an oral formulation, 3% to 6% of which is excreted into the urine (Barrington and Stephenson, 1997). It is sold under the trade name Elmiron. **Study findings have been contradictory.**

Fritjofsson treated 87 patients in an open multicenter trial in Sweden and Finland (Fritjofsson et al, 1987). Bladder volume with and without anesthesia was unchanged. Relief of pain was complete in 35% and partial in 23% of patients. Daytime frequency decreased from 16.5 to 13 and nocturia decreased from 4.5 to 3.5. Mean voided volumes increased by almost a tablespoon in the nonulcer group. Holm-Bentzen studied 115 patients in a double-blind, placebo-controlled trial (Holm-Bentzen et al, 1987b). Symptoms, urodynamic parameters, cystoscopic appearance, and mast cell counts were unchanged after 4 months. Bladder capacity under anesthesia increased significantly in the group with mastocytosis, but this had no bearing on symptoms or awake capacity.

Parsons had a more encouraging initial experience (Parsons et al, 1983), and subsequently the results of two placebo-controlled multicenter trials in the United States were published (Mulholland et al, 1990; Parsons et al, 1993). In the initial study, overall improvement of more than 25% was reported by 28% of the PPS-treated group versus 13% of the placebo group. In the latter study the respective figures were 32% on drug versus 16% on placebo. Average voided volume on PPS increased by 20 mL. No other objective improvements were documented. An NIDDK 2 × 2 factorial study to evaluate PPS and hydroxyzine looked at each drug used alone and in combination and compared results with a placebo group (Sant et al, 2003). Patients were treated for 6 months. No statistically significant response to either medication was documented. No significant trend was seen in the PPS treatment groups (34%) compared with non-PPS groups (18%). Of the 29 patients on PPS alone, 28% had a global response (the primary end point) of moderate or marked improvement versus 13% on placebo, a number remarkably similar to the results in the 3-month pivotal trials, although not reaching statistical significance in the 6-month study. A subsequent industry-sponsored trial showed no dose-related efficacy response in the range of 300 to 900 mg daily; however, adverse events *were* dose related (Nickel et al, 2005a). Another 6-month trial that compared PPS with cyclosporine A yielded a 19% response rate for PPS compared with a 75% global response to cyclosporine A (Sairanen et al, 2005).

Long-term experience with PPS in uncontrolled studies is consistent with efficacy in a subset of patients (Al-Zahrani and Gajewski 2011) **that may drop below 30% of those initially treated** (Jepsen et al, 1998). **Tachyphylaxis seems to be uncommon in responders. A phase 4 study mandated by the U.S. Food and**

Drug Administration (FDA) and initiated in July 2004 was terminated in January 2011. **It evaluated the safety and efficacy of PPS, comparing 100 mg once a day, 100 mg three times a day, and placebo for 24 weeks in 66 study locations in 369 patients. The study was terminated when interim analysis showed that study continuation was futile and the drug was ineffective** (http://clinicaltrials.gov/ct2/show/results/NCT00086684?term=elmiron&rank=1).

Adverse events with PPS occurred in less than 4% of patients at the dose of 100 mg three times daily (Hanno, 1997) **and included reversible alopecia, diarrhea, nausea, and rash. Rare bleeding problems have been reported** (Rice et al, 1998). It promotes cellular proliferation in vitro in the MCF-7 breast cancer cell line, and caution has been suggested in prescribing it in groups at high risk for breast cancer and premenopausal females (Zaslau et al, 2004). **A 3- to 6-month treatment trial is usually required to see symptom improvement.** In a small trial, PPS has shown efficacy when administered intravesically (Bade et al, 1997a). It may be of value in the management of radiation cystitis (Parsons, 1986; Hampson and Woodhouse, 1994) and cyclophosphamide cystitis (Toren and Norman, 2005), but **its value in the treatment of BPS/IC seems marginal.**

Immunomodulator Drugs

Cyclosporine. Cyclosporine, a widely used immunosuppressive drug in organ transplantation, was the subject of a novel BPS trial (Forsell et al, 1996). Eleven patients received cyclosporine for 3 to 6 months at an initial dose of 2.5 to 5 mg/kg daily and a maintenance dose of 1.5 to 3 mg/kg daily. Micturition frequency decreased, and mean and maximum voided volumes increased significantly. Bladder pain decreased or disappeared in 10 patients. After cessation of treatment, symptoms recurred in the majority of patients.

In a longer-term follow-up study, 20 of 23 refractory IC patients on cyclosporine therapy followed for a mean of 60.8 months became free of bladder pain. Bladder capacity more than doubled. Eleven patients subsequently stopped therapy, and in 9, symptoms recurred within months but responded to reinitiating cyclosporine (Sairanen et al, 2004). Sairanen and colleagues further found that cyclosporine A was far superior to sodium PPS in all clinical outcome parameters measured at 6 months (Sairanen et al, 2005). Patients who responded to cyclosporine A had a significant reduction of urinary levels of EGF (Sairanen et al, 2008). Data from three centers in the United States reported success in 23 of 34 patients with Hunner lesions and 3 of 10 patients without Hunner lesions (Forrest et al, 2012). A 3- to 4-month trial was suggested to gauge treatment success. Measurement of luminal nitric oxide has correlated lower levels with treatment response to cyclosporine (Ehrén et al, 2013). A case report highlighted success in a patient with primary SS and BPS (Emmungil et al, 2012).

Suplatast Tosilate. Suplatast tosilate (IPD-1151T) is an immunoregulator that selectively suppresses IgE production and eosinophilia via suppression of helper T cells that produce IL-4 and IL-5. It is used in Japan to treat allergic disorders including asthma, atopic dermatitis, and rhinitis. Ueda and colleagues reported a small study in 14 women with IC (Ueda, 2000). Treatment for 1 year resulted in a significantly increased bladder capacity and decreased urinary urgency, frequency, and lower abdominal pain in 10 women. Concomitant changes occurred in blood and urine markers, suggesting an immune system response. Larger, multicenter, randomized controlled trials in the United States and Japan have not led to the governmental approval of the BPS/IC indication or the introduction of the drug into the United States.

Azathioprine and Chloroquine Derivatives. In a single report in 1976, Oravisto and colleagues used azathioprine or chloroquine derivatives for BPS patients not responding to other treatments (Oravisto and Alfthan, 1976). About 50% of patients responded.

Mycophenolate Mofetil. In an aborted multicenter randomized placebo-controlled NIDDK trial, mycophenolate mofetil (CellCept) 1 to 2 g daily in divided doses failed to show efficacy in the treatment of symptoms of refractory BPS/IC. The trial, which included

59 patients randomized 2 : 1 to the active arm, was halted when the FDA issued a new black box warning for the drug (*miscarriage and congenital malformations have been associated with its use*), and **an interim analysis showed no benefit** (Yang et al, 2011).

Adalimumab. A randomized double-blind placebo-controlled trial of this TNF-inhibiting anti-inflammatory agent failed to demonstrate positive proof of concept for this drug, which is approved for use in the treatment of rheumatoid, psoriatic, and other types of arthritis; plaque psoriasis; Crohn disease; and ulcerative colitis (Bosch, 2014).

Miscellaneous Agents

L-Arginine. Foster and Weiss were the original proponents of L-arginine in the therapy of IC (Foster et al, 1997). Eight patients with IC were given 500 mg of L-arginine three times daily. After 1 month, urinary NOS activity increased 8-fold and 7 of the 8 patients noticed improvement in symptoms. An open-label study of 11 patients showed improvement in all 10 of the patients who remained on L-arginine for 6 months (Smith et al, 1997).

An open-label study of 9 women in Sweden failed to find any change in symptom scores or in nitric oxide production in the bladder (Ehrén et al, 1998). A placebo-controlled randomized trial of 53 BPS/IC patients could find no difference on an intention-to-treat analysis between drug- and placebo-treated patients (Korting et al, 1999). A smaller randomized placebo-controlled crossover trial of 16 BPS patients found no clinically significant improvement with L-arginine and concluded that it could not be recommended for IC treatment (Cartledge et al, 2000).

The body of evidence does not support the use of L-arginine for the relief of symptoms of IC.

Quercetin. Quercetin, a bioflavonoid available in many over-the-counter products, may have the anti-inflammatory effects of other members of this class of compounds found in fruits, vegetables, and some spices. Katske and colleagues administered 500 mg twice daily to 22 BPS patients for 4 weeks (Katske et al, 2001). All but 1 patient had some improvement in the O'Leary-Sant symptom and problem scores as well as in a global assessment score. Further larger studies with placebo controls are necessary to determine efficacy.

Antibiotics. Warren and colleagues (2000) randomized 50 patients to receive 18 weeks of placebo or antibiotics including rifampin plus a sequence of doxycycline, erythromycin, metronidazole, clindamycin, amoxicillin, and ciprofloxacin for 3 weeks each. Intent-to-treat analysis demonstrated that 12 of 25 patients in the antibiotic and 6 of 25 patients in the placebo group reported overall improvement, whereas 10 and 5, respectively, noticed improvement in pain and urgency. The study was complicated by the fact that 16 of the patients in the antibiotic group underwent new BPS therapy during the study, as did 13 of the placebo patients. There was no statistical significance reached. What was statistically significant was the occurrence of adverse events in 80% of participants who received antibiotics compared with 40% in the placebo group. Nausea and/or vomiting and diarrhea were the predominant side effects. Most patients on antibiotics correctly guessed what treatment arm they were in, and those who guessed correctly were significantly more likely to note improvement after the study. No duration in improvement after completion of the trial of antibiotics was reported.

Burkhard and colleagues recorded a 71% success rate in 103 women with a history of urinary urgency and frequency and chronic urethral and/or pelvic pain often associated with dyspareunia and/or a history of recurrent urinary tract infection (Burkhard et al, 2004). This was a large, inclusive group and one that is probably broader than the BPS on which we are focusing. Nevertheless, Burkhard recommended empirical doxycycline in this group. The overwhelming majority of BPS patients have been treated with empirical antibiotics before diagnosis.

At this time there is no evidence to suggest that antibiotics have a place in the therapy of BPS in the absence of a culture-documented infection (Maskell, 1995). **Nevertheless, it would not be unreasonable to treat patients with *one* empirical course of antibiotic, if they have never been on an antibiotic for their urinary symptoms.**

Methotrexate. Low-dose oral methotrexate significantly improved bladder pain in four of nine women with BPS but did not change urinary frequency, maximum voided volume, or mean voided volume (Moran et al, 1999). No placebo-controlled RCT has been done with this agent.

Montelukast. Mast cell triggering releases two types of proinflammatory mediators, including granule stored preformed types such as heparin and histamine and newly synthesized prostaglandins and leukotrienes B_4 and C_4. Classic antagonists, such as montelukast, zafirlukast, and pranlukast, block cysteinyl leukotriene-1 receptors. In a pilot study (Bouchelouche et al, 2001b), 10 women with IC and detrusor mastocytosis received 10 mg of montelukast daily for 3 months. Frequency, nocturia, and pain improved dramatically in 8 of the patients. Further study would seem to be warranted, especially in patients with detrusor mastocytosis, defined as more than $28/mm^2$ (Traut et al, 2011).

Nifedipine. The calcium channel antagonist nifedipine inhibits smooth muscle contraction and cell-mediated immunity. In a pilot study (Fleischmann, 1994), 30 mg of an extended-release preparation was administered to 10 female patients and titrated to 60 mg daily in 4 of the patients who did not get symptom relief. Within 4 months, 5 patients showed at least a 50% decrease in symptom scores, and 3 of the 5 were asymptomatic. No further studies have been reported.

Misoprostol. The oral prostaglandin analogue misoprostol was studied in 25 patients at a dose of 600 μg daily (Kelly et al, 1998). At 3 months 14 patients were significantly improved, and at 6 months 12 patients still had a response. A cytoprotective action in the urinary bladder was postulated.

Dextroamphetamine. A single anecdotal series of six patients reported benefit from use of 30 mg of dextroamphetamine sulfate daily, with return of symptoms on discontinuation of medication (Check et al, 2013).

Phosphodiesterase Inhibitors. The use of phosphodiesterase (PDE) inhibitors for BPS has long been considered. PDE type 5 (PDE5) inhibitors are hypothesized to relax smooth muscle or structures involved in afferent signaling and suppress smooth muscle spontaneous activity (Truss et al, 2001; Hanna-Mitchell and Birder, 2011; Chen et al, 2014a). Trials using them for BPS are underway.

Analgesics

The long-term, appropriate use of pain medications forms an integral part of the treatment of a chronic pain condition such as IC. Most patients can be helped markedly with medical pain management using pain medications commonly used for chronic neuropathic pain syndromes including antidepressants, anticonvulsants, and opioids (Wesselmann et al, 1997). Many nonopioid analgesics including acetaminophen and the nonsteroidal anti-inflammatory drugs (NSAIDs) and even antispasmodic agents (Rummans, 1994) have a place in therapy along with agents designed to specifically treat the disorder itself.

Studies on the use of analgesics for BPS are sparse, and most data have been inferred from non-BPS types of pain and expert opinion. Health professionals should ask about pain, and the patient's self-report should be the primary source of assessment. Clinicians should assess pain with easily administered rating scales and should document the efficacy of pain relief at regular intervals after starting or changing treatment.

Unlike opioids, with increasing doses acetaminophen, aspirin, and the other NSAIDs all reach a ceiling for their maximum analgesic effect (Drugs for pain, 1998). Gabapentin, introduced in 1994 as an anticonvulsant, has found efficacy in neuropathic pain disorders including diabetic neuropathy (Backonja et al, 1998) and postherpetic neuralgia (Rowbotham et al, 1998). It demonstrates synergism with morphine in neuropathic pain (Gilron et al, 2005). It may give some benefit in CPPS and BPS/IC (Sasaki et al, 2001). Pregabalin is also reported to be effective for neuropathic pain and the pain of fibromyalgia (Freynhagen et al, 2005; Arnold et al, 2008).

With the results of major surgery anything but certain, the use of long-term opioid therapy in the patient in whom more conservative therapies have failed may also be considered (Box 14-8). Opiates are seldom the first choice of analgesics in chronic pain states, but they should not be withheld if less powerful analgesics have failed (Portenoy et al, 1997; Bennett, 1999). This is a difficult decision that requires much thought and discussion between patient and urologist, and involvement of a pain specialist is indicated. A single practitioner has to take responsibility for pain treatment and write all prescriptions for pain medications (Brookoff and Sant, 1997). Opioids are effective for most forms of moderate and severe pain and have no ceiling effect other than that imposed by adverse effects. The common side effects include sedation, nausea, mild confusion, and pruritus. In general, these are transient and easily managed. Respiratory depression is extremely rare if they are used as prescribed. Constipation is common and a mild laxative is typically necessary. The major impediment to the proper use of these drugs when they are prescribed for long-term nonmalignant pain is the fear of addiction. Studies suggest the risk is low (Gourlay, 1994). The long-acting narcotic formulations that result in steady levels of drug over many hours are preferable.

Chronic pain patients often receive inadequate doses of short-acting pain medications, which put them on cycles of short-term relief, anxiety, and pain. It leads to doctor-shopping and drug-seeking behavior confused by physicians with drug addiction. Although physical dependence on opioids will be unavoidable, physical addiction, a chronic disorder characterized by the compulsive use of a substance resulting in physical, psychological, or social harm to the user and the continued use despite that harm, is rare. Chronic opioid therapy can be considered in carefully selected patients. It is best administered in a pain clinic setting and necessitates frequent reassessment by both patient and physician (Portenoy and Foley, 1986).

BOX 14-8 General Guidelines for the Use of Opioids in Chronic or Nonacute Urogenital Pain

1. All other reasonable treatments must have been tried and failed.
2. The decision to instigate long-term opioid therapy should be made by an appropriately trained specialist in consultation with another physician (preferably the patient's family doctor).
3. When there is a history or suspicion of drug abuse, a psychiatrist or psychologist with an interest in pain management and drug addiction should be involved.
4. The dose required needs to be calculated by careful titration.
5. The patient should be made aware of (and possibly give written consent regarding) the following:
   a. Opioids are strong drugs and associated with addiction and dependency.
   b. Opioids will normally be prescribed from only one source.
   c. The drugs will be prescribed for fixed periods of time and a new prescription will not be available until the end of that period.
   d. The patient will be subjected to spot urine and possibly blood checks to ensure that the drug is being taken as prescribed and that nonprescribed drugs are not being taken.
   e. Inappropriate aggressive behavior associated with demanding the drug will not be accepted.
   f. Hospital specialist review will normally occur at least once a year.
   g. The patient may be requested to attend a psychiatric or psychological review.
   Failure to comply with the above may result in the patient being referred to a drug dependency agency and the use of therapeutic, analgesic opioids being stopped.
6. Morphine is the first-line drug, unless there are contraindications to morphine or special indications for another drug. The drug should be prescribed in a slow-release or modified-release form. Short-acting preparations are undesirable and should be avoided where possible. Parenteral administration is undesirable and should be avoided when possible.

From Fall M, Baranowski A, Elneil S, et al. Guidelines on chronic pelvic pain. European Association of Urology; 2008. p. 1–99. www.uroweb.org/professional-resources/guidelines/.

KEY POINTS: ORAL THERAPIES

- Few of the oral therapies commonly used for the treatment of BPS have unequivocal evidence of efficacy in large, multicenter, randomized controlled clinical trials.
- There is little evidence that any of these therapies change the natural history of the disease, although many seem effective in individual patients.

Intravesical Therapies (see Table 14-4)

The use of silver nitrate and Clorpactin is described on the Expert Consult website.

Dimethyl Sulfoxide

A mainstay of the treatment of BPS is the intravesical instillation of 50% DMSO (Sant, 1987). It is sometimes administered in a solution with sodium bicarbonate, heparin, and/or steroid, but its only FDA-approved use is as a stand-alone treatment (Stav et al, 2012; Gafni-Kane et al, 2013). DMSO is a byproduct of the wood pulp industry and a derivative of lignin. It has exceptional solvent properties and is freely miscible with water, lipids, and organic agents. One must be cognizant of systemic absorption of coadministered agents. Pharmacologic properties include membrane penetration, enhanced drug absorption, anti-inflammatory action (Kim et al, 2011), analgesic effects, collagen dissolution, muscle relaxation, and mast cell histamine release. In vitro effects on bladder function belie its positive effects in vivo (Freedman et al, 1989), where histamine release has not been demonstrated after treatment (Stout et al, 1995). It has been suggested that DMSO actually desensitizes nociceptive pathways in the lower urinary tract (Birder et al, 1997). Tests for DMSO for treatment of human illness began in the 1960s in the areas of musculoskeletal inflammation and the cutaneous manifestations of scleroderma.

Stewart and colleagues are credited for popularizing intravesical DMSO for BPS/IC (Stewart et al, 1967). In the mid 1960s he applied it to the skin over the suprapubic area in a group of patients refractory to conventional forms of therapy. Results were poor, but intravesical delivery of 50 mL of a 50% solution instilled for 15 minutes by catheter and repeated at intervals of 2 to 4 weeks showed positive effects lasting 2 to 12 months in six of eight patients. The absence of side effects, other than a garlic-like odor on the breath, and the lack of a need for inpatient administration were significant breakthroughs over previous treatments. Further reports by this group confirmed safety and efficacy (Stewart et al, 1971, 1972; Stewart and Shirley, 1976; Shirley et al, 1978) with symptom-free intervals of 1 to 3 months in 73% of patients. Ek reported a 70% success rate but found that most patients ultimately required retreatment or further therapy with other modalities (Ek et al, 1978). Prospective series of Fowler (Fowler, 1981) and Barker and colleagues (Barker et al,

1987) revealed symptomatic success rates higher than 80%, although relapse was not uncommon. Fowler noted only minimal improvements in functional bladder capacity and attributed the beneficial effects of DMSO to a direct effect on the sensory nerves of the bladder. Perez-Marrero compared DMSO with saline and showed a 93% objective improvement and 53% subjective improvement compared with 35% and 18%, respectively, for saline (Perez-Marrero et al, 1988). Patients with bladder instability do not respond (Emerson and Feltis, 1986). Stav and Hung reported 60% success rates and recommended it be considered a first-line therapy (Stav et al, 2012; Hung et al, 2012).

With its ease of administration (Biggers, 1986), **low morbidity, and reasonable symptomatic results, DMSO certainly merits its place as a useful treatment for BPS/IC.** In vivo studies on rat bladder strips exposed to various concentrations of DMSO for 7 minutes showed absence of electrical field stimulation contraction at a 40% concentration and diminished compliance at 30% concentration (Melchior et al, 2003). Concentrations of 25% or less had negligible effects in this model. How it relates to use of DMSO in humans is unknown. A rare case of eosinophilic cystitis has been reported after DMSO instillation (Abramov et al, 2004).

DMSO is often administered as part of an "intravesical cocktail" (50 mL Rimso-50 + 10 mg Kenalog + 44 mEq sodium bicarbonate + 20,000 to 40,000 units intravesical heparin) weekly for 6 weeks. If there is a good clinical response, maintenance therapy consisting of administration of the cocktail monthly for 6 months has been employed. There are no controlled studies as to the efficacy of this combined therapy, nor are there long-term safety studies reported. There is an inherent problem in doing placebo-controlled trials with DMSO because the strong garlic odor resulting from instillation quickly unblinds any trial.

Glycosaminoglycans

Exogenous GAGs have been shown to be effective in providing an epithelial permeability barrier in bladders in which the epithelium has been injured with protamine (Nickel et al, 1998). **Heparin,** which can mimic the activity of the bladder's own mucopolysaccharide lining (Hanno et al, 1978b), has anti-inflammatory effects as well as actions that inhibit fibroblast proliferation, angiogenesis, and smooth muscle cell proliferation. Because of its numerous effects, the possibility that heparin could be used for therapeutic reasons other than the control of coagulation has been the subject of much inquiry and speculation (Lane and Adams, 1993). Weaver first reported on the use of intravesical heparin for IC treatment (Weaver et al, 1963). Given intravesically, there is virtually no systemic absorption, even in an inflamed bladder (Caulfield et al, 1995). Although uncontrolled studies suggested some beneficial effect for subcutaneous administration (Lose et al, 1983, 1985), the obvious risks of anticoagulation and osteoporosis have prevented this form of administration from undergoing further trials and general usage. Ten thousand units can be administered intravesically in sterile water either alone or with DMSO at varying intervals with good results reported (Perez-Marrero et al, 1993; Parsons et al, 1994a). Kuo reported 50% or greater improvement in the International Prostate Symptom Score in 29 of 40 women with IC treated with 25,000 units intravesically twice weekly for 3 months (Kuo, 2001).

Parsons has used daily intravesical doses of 40,000 units of heparin in 20 mL of sterile water administered by the patient daily and held for 30 to 60 minutes. "Reasonable improvement of symptoms" can be expected between 6 months and 2 years after initiation of therapy (Parsons, 2000). Adding alkalinized lidocaine to the heparin instillation provides better pain relief (Parsons, 2005). The addition of 8 mL of 2% lidocaine and 4 mL of 8.4% sodium bicarbonate may improve results (Welk and Teichman, 2008). In fact, a combination of 200 mg of lidocaine with 8.4% sodium bicarbonate (10 mL total solution) *without* heparin showed a 30% response rate 3 days after completion of daily intravesical administration for 5 days and was statistically superior to a placebo cocktail (Nickel et al, 2009b). A Japanese study reported high success rates with weekly intravesical instillation of 20,000 units of heparin with 5 mL of 4% lidocaine and 25 mL of 7% sodium bicarbonate for 12 weeks (Nomiya et al, 2013). Intravesical administration of a solution of lidocaine and heparin has been proposed as a treatment for symptom flare (Parsons et al, 2012).

Another GAG analogue, **PPS,** administered intravesically (300 mg twice weekly in 50 mL of normal saline) showed some modest benefit in a small trial (Bade et al, 1997a). A 41-patient trial comparing oral PPS with oral and intravesical administration showed that the 24% reduction in O'Leary-Sant scores with oral therapy alone rose to a 46% reduction in the group that also received intravesical PPS (Davis et al, 2008).

The nonsulfated GAG **hyaluronic acid** has also been used intravesically. Trials using 40 mg dissolved in 40 mL of normal saline weekly for 4 to 6 weeks and then monthly treatments thereafter have had response rates varying from 71% (Morales et al, 1996) to 30% (Porru et al, 1997). In the summer of 2003 Bioniche Life Sciences and in the spring of 2004 Seikagaku Corporation reported double-blind, placebo-controlled, multicenter clinical studies of their hyaluronic acid preparations (40 mg or 200 mg per milliliter, respectively), and neither showed significant efficacy of sodium hyaluronate compared with placebo. These negative studies have not been published in peer-reviewed literature. Neither preparation has been approved for use for BPS/IC in the United States. An Austrian open-label study showed that 13 of 27 patients with BPS and a positive potassium test result responded to intravesical hyaluronic acid 40 mg weekly for 10 weeks, though initial nonresponders at 5 weeks also were treated with intravesical PPS 200 mg three times weekly for the remaining 5 weeks (Daha et al, 2008). The best results for hyaluronic acid come from Riedl, who studied 126 patients with a positive modified potassium test result who could hold the solution for 2 hours, using 40 mg weekly for a minimum 10 weeks; 84% had significant improvement (Riedl et al, 2008). Treatment-resistant cases have been managed with a combination of sequential bladder distention under anesthesia accompanied by a hyaluronic acid instillation every 1 to 3 months depending on response with a 74% success rate in 23 patients (Ahmad et al, 2008). Although hyaluronic acid has been seemingly efficacious in uncontrolled trials (Van Agt et al, 2011; Engelhardt et al, 2011; Figueiredo et al, 2011; Lv et al, 2012; Lai et al, 2013), **the efficacy of hyaluronic acid for BPS/IC remains unproven in controlled and blinded trials** (Iavazzo et al, 2007). It remains unapproved for BPS in the United States.

Chondroitin sulfate plays an important role for bladder barrier function (Janssen et al, 2013). Hurst has shown by immunohistochemistry a deficit of chondroitin sulfate from the luminal bladder surface in IC patients (Hurst, 2003). Intravesical chondroitin sulfate inhibited recruitment of inflammatory cells in an experimental "leaky bladder" model of cystitis (Engles et al, 2012). Small uncontrolled studies using intravesical **chondroitin sulfate** have shown success rates of 33% to 75% (Steinhoff et al, 2002; Sorensen, 2003; Tornero et al, 2013). A multicenter, open-label study using a 2% solution of sodium chondroitin sulfate weekly for 6 weeks and then monthly for 4 months had a 60% response rate with no safety issues (Nickel et al, 2009a). A larger follow-up study failed to demonstrate significant efficacy (Nickel et al, 2012; Thakkinstian and Nickel, 2013). A large open-label experience using the device for all forms of "chronic cystitis" concluded that it was effective in improving urgency, voided volumes, and nocturia, and well tolerated when administered weekly for a maximum of eight instillations (Nordling and van Ophoven, 2008).

The GAGs have been combined for instillation with good results reported in uncontrolled studies (Cervigni et al, 2008; Cervigni et al, 2012; Porru et al, 2012; Giberti et al, 2013).

A large analysis of GAG layer replenishment therapy with intravesical GAGs concluded that despite the fact that GAG intravesical therapy has been in use for over two decades, most of the studies have been uncontrolled, have been poorly done, and have had a small number of patients. Large-scale randomized controlled trials are urgently needed to underline the benefit of this type of therapy. Distinct patient groups (well phenotyped) need to be confirmed by definite diagnostic findings (Madersbacher et al, 2013). Another review sadly concludes that "randomized controlled trials have suggested the GAG analogues are at best as good as placebo" (Chintea and Belal, 2013).

Other Intravesical Therapies

 The use of doxorubicin, BCG, capsaicin, and resiniferatoxin (RTX) is described on the Expert Consult website.

KEY POINTS: INTRAVESICAL THERAPIES

- The potential for high efficacy combined with safety and a low side effect profile that is gained by applying a treatment directly to the bladder lining has made research into new methods of intravesical therapy a high priority of researchers and pharmaceutical companies.
- Patients in whom pain and other symptoms are not related directly to bladder pathology would not be expected to respond well to this type of organ-directed therapy.

Intradetrusor Therapies

The therapeutic value of **botulinum toxin type A (BTX-A)** stems partially from its ability to temporarily inhibit the release of acetylcholine and other neurotransmitters and to cause flaccid paralysis in a dose-related manner in skeletal muscle. It can correct focal dystonia when injected into a muscle. Intradetrusor BTX-A has now been approved for use in the United States in the management of refractory neurogenic and idiopathic DO. BTX-A also has analgesic properties (Rajkumar and Conn, 2004). Initially this effect was thought to be a result of relief of muscle spasm. However, botulinum has been shown to reduce peripheral sensitization by inhibiting the release of several neuronal signaling markers, including glutamate and substance P, and reducing *c-Fos* gene expression. It may affect the sensory feedback loop to the central nervous system by decreased input from the muscle tissue, possibly by inhibiting acetylcholine release from gamma motor neurons innervating intrafusal fibers of the muscle spindle (Rosales et al, 1996). It inhibits the release of sensory neurotransmitters from isolated bladder preparations in rat bladder models of both acute injury and chronic inflammation (Lucioni et al, 2008). Chronic inflammation and apoptosis is significantly reduced after repeated BTX-A injections in patients with BPS (Shie et al, 2013). BTX-A has been used effectively for years in different conditions with muscular hypercontractions. Intravesical BTX administration blocks the acetic acid–induced calcitonin gene–related peptide (CGRP) release from afferent nerve terminals in the bladder mucosal layer in rats (Chuang et al, 2004). In an animal model of bladder permeability barrier disruption, intravesical BTX-A minimized bladder irritability and restored afferent neural responses to baseline levels (Vemulakonda et al, 2005). These results support clinical trials of BTX-A for the treatment of BPS/IC and other types of visceral pain (Chancellor and Yoshimura, 2004).

A multi-institutional case series using Botox or Dysport intravesical injections in 13 patients with refractory BPS/IC reported improvement in 9 patients. Improvements in symptoms lasted a mean of 3.72 months (range 1 to 8 months). No systemic complications were observed, although 2 patients had a diminished flow with some need to strain to void (Smith and Chancellor, 2004). Rackley and colleagues at the Cleveland Clinic reported no change in objective or subjective outcome measures in a series of 10 BPS/IC patients in whom the trigone was spared in the injection technique (Rackley et al, 2005). A 1-year follow-up in 15 patients treated with 200 units of BTX-A in 20 mL of normal saline showed that the success rate fell from 86.6% at 3 months to 26.6% at 5 months and was 0 at 12 months (Giannantoni et al, 2008). Bladder biopsy 2 weeks after BTX-A intradetrusor injection showed that

nerve growth factor production levels fell to those of controls in patients who responded (Liu et al, 2009). It is hypothesized that treatment-refractory patients may have developed antibodies after initial BTX injection (Schulte-Baukloh et al, 2008).

The Portuguese group from Oporto has championed limiting injections to 100 units divided into 10 injection sites, all in the trigone. More than 50% of patients experienced efficacy with a duration of 9 months, and no voiding dysfunction was noted (Pinto et al, 2010). There appears to be little tachyphylaxis associated with the treatment, and repeated injections at regular intervals or when symptoms recur remain effective (Kuo, 2013; Pinto et al, 2013). **Onabotulinum toxin A appears to be a reasonable treatment for BPS that is refractory to standard conservative, oral, and intravesical treatment** (Mangera et al, 2011; Yokoyama et al, 2012). When injected into the trigone in 10-unit aliquots (100 units total), the risk of impaired bladder emptying seems to be minimized.

Submucosal injection of 10 mL of 40 mg/mL **triamcinolone acetonide** injected in 0.5-mL aliquots was used for the treatment of Hunner lesions in 30 patients (Cox et al, 2009). Seventy percent of patients were very much improved, and duration of improvement was estimated to be 7 to 12 months.

Neuromodulation

Because PBS/IC is a chronic pain syndrome, it is reasonable to consider therapeutic options that directly interface with the nervous system. This approach is further supported by the association of pelvic floor dysfunction with pelvic pain syndromes (Zermann et al, 1999).

Pain diversion by **transcutaneous electrical nerve stimulation (TENS)** is routine in a variety of painful conditions (Fall, 1987). Fall and colleagues were the first to use electrical stimulation in IC, reporting on 14 women treated successfully with long-term intravaginal nerve stimulation or TENS (Fall et al, 1980). Subsequently McGuire noted improvement in 5 of 6 patients treated with electrical stimulation (McGuire et al, 1983).

The primary intention in applying peripheral electrical nerve stimulation in IC is to relieve pain by stimulating myelinated afferents to activate segmental inhibitory circuits. As a secondary effect, urinary frequency may also be reduced. In the most complete review of the subject (Fall and Lindstrom, 1994), 33 patients with ulcerative IC and 27 patients with nonulcerative IC were treated by means of suprapubic TENS. Electrodes were positioned 10 to 15 cm apart immediately above the pubic symphysis. High- or low-frequency (2 to 50 Hz) TENS was employed. If there was no effect with high-frequency TENS after 1 month, low-frequency TENS was used. Application of 30 to 120 minutes of TENS was prescribed daily. Pain improved more than frequency. Good results or remission was described in 26% of nonulcerative IC patients and a surprising 54% of patients with ulcerative disease. Fall and Lindstrom (1994) caution that the experience is based on open studies, relatively few patients, and the knowledge of a significant placebo effect with peripheral pain stimulation.

Acupuncture has been used to treat frequency, urgency, and dysuria (Chang, 1988). Twenty-two of 26 patients treated at the SP 6 point had clinically symptomatic improvement. A study looking at both acupuncture and TENS in IC showed limited effects of both modalities (Geirsson et al, 1993). Lumbar epidural blockade was the subject of a positive case report (Pelaez et al, 2004), but in an earlier series resulted in only short-term (mean 15 days) pain relief in IC (Irwin et al, 1993). Posterior tibial nerve stimulation was successful in 60% of 37 patients with symptoms of bladder overactivity in an uncontrolled Dutch study (van Balken et al, 2001). An Australian double-blind placebo-controlled study of transdermal posterior tibial nerve laser therapy showed no benefit in 56 patients when comparing active with placebo arms, but the placebo effect was remarkably strong, indicating the importance of such trials in evaluation of invasive therapies (O'Reilly et al, 2004). A Chinese study of posterior tibial nerve stimulation twice weekly for 5 weeks in BPS/IC patients failed to show improvement in pain scores, and none of the 18 patients thought the treatment had a significant effect (Zhao et al, 2008).

Direct sacral nerve stimulation has been explored in the treatment of BPS and urgency and frequency and is referred to as **neuromodulation,** a technique whose urologic potential was developed through the basic and clinical research of Tanagho and Schmidt (Schmidt, 1993; Fandel and Tanagho, 2005). They and others have observed that patients who do best with this treatment modality are those who have identifiable pain *and* dysfunction in the pelvic muscles (Everaert et al, 2001; Siegel et al, 2001; Aboseif et al, 2002). Patients reporting pelvic pain in the absence of demonstrable pelvic floor dysfunction and levator tenderness did poorly (Schmidt, 2001). As initially practiced, trial stimulation was performed with a percutaneous temporary electrode for a 3- to 4-day temporary stimulation period to access efficacy. The S3 nerve was most frequently used. A wire electrode was inserted into the foramen and connected to an external pulse generator (Medtronic, Minneapolis, MN). If the trial was successful, the patient was considered for implantation of a permanent neural prosthesis. More recently, a staged procedure has supplanted the traditional percutaneous approach, as the response to stimulation can be better assessed with more accurate lead placement and stability than through the more hit-or-miss percutaneous lead placement (Peters et al, 2003). Peters's test-to-implant rate increased from 52% to 94%. Other reports have noted a test-to-implant rate with the percutaneous technique of 76% in 33 PBS/IC patients (Whitmore et al, 2003) to 40% in 211 patients with refractory urge incontinence, urgency-frequency syndrome, and urinary retention (Scheepens et al, 2002b).

Neuromodulation has been shown to be effective in treating refractory urinary urge incontinence (Schmidt et al, 1999; Spinelli et al, 2001). Studies on therapeutic potential in BPS/IC followed (van Kerrebroeck, 1999). The University of Maryland group described a decrease in antiproliferative activity and normalization of HB-EGF levels in patients with successful test stimulation (Chai et al, 2000a). Peters and coworkers reported success in two thirds of BPS/IC patients with sacral nerve stimulation (Peters et al, 2003). GRA score as determined by the patients correlated with objective findings (Peters et al, 2008). Another study (Comiter, 2003) noted that 17 of 25 patients were successful with test stimulation and went on to permanent implantation of the InterStim device (Medtronics, St. Paul, MN). Devices in 13 of 15 who underwent staged implantation were permanently implanted versus in 4 of 10 undergoing percutaneous test stimulation. With a mean follow-up of 14 months, 16 of 17 patients were judged to have a successful outcome, yielding an intent-to-treat success rate of 64%. Although sacral neuromodulation can decrease narcotic requirements significantly in refractory BPS/IC, the majority of patients taking chronic narcotics for pain will likely continue to use them for pain relief even after implantation (Peters and Konstandt, 2004). One center reported a long-term improvement rate of 45% for the urgency and frequency indication (Elhilali et al, 2005). Treatment results do not appear to be age dependent (Peters et al, 2013b). Sexual functioning in women may improve as well (Yih et al, 2013). **Several studies now attest to the benefits of sacral neuromodulation for BPS** (Ghazwani et al, 2011; Marinkovic et al, 2011; Vaarala et al, 2011; Tirlapur et al, 2013b).

Unilateral stimulation should be performed before bilateral sacral stimulation is considered (Oerlemans and van Kerrebroeck, 2008). A bilateral test stimulation could be indicated when a unilateral test fails (Steinberg et al, 2007). The only prospective randomized crossover trial to compare the unilateral with bilateral sacral nerve stimulation found no significant differences comparing the results (Scheepens et al, 2002a). The presence of pain is a predictor of adverse events (White et al, 2009), and although sacral neuromodulation is effective in 56% of patients with urgency and frequency, when pain is the major complaint, caution is indicated. Nevertheless, **reviews of multiple, largely uncontrolled anecdotal studies show success rates of 60% to 80% for chronic pelvic pain** (Marcelissen et al, 2011; Srivastava, 2012). **Surgical revision rates are 7% to 0%** (van Kerrebroeck et al, 2007; Gajewski and Al-Zahrani, 2011). When used for BPS symptoms, frequent reprogramming is

often required (Maxwell et al, 2008). The presence of urgency may be a positive predictor of long-term success (Gajewski and Al-Zahrani, 2011).

> ### KEY POINTS: NEUROMODULATION
>
> - The association of pelvic floor dysfunction with pelvic pain syndromes makes neuromodulation a rational therapeutic alternative.
> - Patients with pelvic pain in the absence of demonstrable pelvic floor dysfunction and levator tenderness may not respond as well as those with urgency and frequency associated with pelvic floor dysfunction. Controlled trials of sacral nerve stimulation for BPS are needed.

Surgical Therapy

Hydrodistention

Hydrodistention of the bladder under anesthesia, while technically a surgical treatment, is often the first therapeutic modality employed, often as a part of the diagnostic evaluation. **Because there have been no standard methods of distention** (Turner and Stewart, 2005), **results vary markedly.** Frontz first suggested hydraulic overdistention of the bladder for IC in 1922 (Frontz, 1922), and Bumpus reported the first series 8 years later (Bumpus, 1930). Simple bladder filling at cystoscopy will give relief to some patients (Hald et al, 1986); other researchers have reported use of an office-based procedure with intravesical lidocaine anesthesia and electromotive drug administration (Rose et al, 2005); and Dunn reported on 25 patients undergoing distention under anesthesia to the level of the systolic blood pressure for up to 3 hours (Dunn et al, 1977). Sixteen of the patients were symptom free with a mean follow-up of 14 months; 2 patients experienced bladder rupture. **The bladder in IC patients can be very thin, and the possibility of perforation or rupture must always be kept in mind and discussed with the patient** (Badenoch, 1971; Hamer et al, 1992). **Prolonged distention probably has little or no benefit over a short-term distention measured in minutes** (Taub and Stein, 1994; McCahy and Styles, 1995). Using epidural anesthesia and a balloon distention technique to the mean arterial pressure for 3 hours continuously, Glemain and colleagues reported good but transient efficacy in patients with a bladder capacity greater than 150 mL on predistention cystometry (Glemain et al, 2002). In their prospective series of 30 patients, 18 had maintained a therapeutic response at 6 months and 13 at 1 year of follow-up. Moderate hematuria was almost universal, worsening of symptoms occurred in 5% of patients, and low back and hypogastric pain were common sequelae. One bladder rupture, one episode of sepsis, and one episode of prolonged retention occurred.

Our method is to perform an initial cystoscopic examination (the findings of which are usually unremarkable), obtain urine for cytology, and distend the bladder for 1 to 2 minutes at a pressure of 80 cm H_2O. The bladder is emptied and then refilled to allow observation for glomerulations or ulceration. A therapeutic hydraulic distention follows for another 8 minutes. Biopsy, if indicated, is performed after the second distention. Therapeutic responses in patients with a bladder capacity under anesthesia of less than 600 mL showed 26% with an excellent and 29% with a fair result compared with 12% excellent and 43% fair in patients with larger bladder capacities (Hanno and Wein, 1991). Most favorable responses were extremely brief, however, with the exceptional patient noting improvement for 6 months, thus being a candidate for repeat therapeutic distention.

Acute hydrodistention does not seem to result in any long-term bladder dysfunction (Kang et al, 1992; Lasanen et al, 1992). **Any efficacy is probably related to damage to mucosal afferent nerve endings** (Dunn et al, 1977). It has no benefits in patients with DO

(Taub and Stein, 1994; McCahy and Styles, 1995). Over half of men with prostate pain and without bacteriuria may have glomerulations. Symptoms in this group have been reported to improve with hydrodistention (Berger et al, 1998). **Although many patients with IC have sensory urgency at awake capacities of less than 100 mL, hydrodistention under anesthesia seems to allow for "staging" of the disease, giving the clinician some idea of the capacity he or she has to work with conservative therapies.** A capacity under anesthesia of under 200 mL would not bode well for the likelihood of success of medical therapy. Fortunately, these cases are relatively rare.

Surgical Considerations

Major extirpative and/or reconstructive surgical therapy for BPS is an option after all trials of conservative treatment have failed— a point that cannot be overemphasized. BPS/IC, although a cause of significant morbidity, is a nonmalignant process with a temporary spontaneous remission rate of up to 50% (Held et al, 1990) that does not directly result in mortality. Deaths are either self-inflicted or the result of complications of therapy. **Nowhere does the caveat** *primum non nocere* **bear more relevance; the treatment must be no worse than the disease process** (Siegel et al, 1990). Surgery should be reserved for the motivated and well-informed patient who falls into the category of having extremely severe, unresponsive disease, a group that comprises less than 10% of patients (Irwin and Galloway, 1994; Parsons, 2000).

Historical Procedures

Many surgical approaches have been employed for IC, and it is worth mentioning a few for historical perspective alone. Sympathectomy and intraspinal alcohol injections have been used to treat pelvic pain (Greenhill, 1947). Differential sacral neurotomy was reported in 3 patients with good results (Meirowsky, 1969), but like most deinnervation procedures never gained popularity because of subsequent poor results. Transvesical infiltration of the pelvic plexuses with phenol failed in 5 of 5 patients with IC (Blackford et al, 1984). With a significant complication rate of 17% (McInerney et al, 1991), it is rarely if ever currently used for sensory urgency disorders or detrusor hyperreflexia. There are several reports on cystolysis going back to Richer in 1929 (Bourque, 1951). Worth and Turner-Warwick reported some short-term benefit, but unpredictable long-term results (Worth and Turner-Warwick, 1973; Worth, 1980). Freiha and Stamey used cystolysis in 6 IC patients with good results in 4 (Freiha and Stamey, 1979). Albers reported long-term follow-up in 11 IC patients and only 1 success (Albers and Geyer, 1988). Denervation procedures have a notoriously high late-failure rate, and the procedure is not justified for BPS/IC (Walsh, 1985; Stone, 1991). In fact, Rogers has concluded that there exist no convincing clinical studies to recommend surgical procedures to interrupt visceral nerve pathways in women with any type of chronic pelvic pain (Rogers, 2003).

Surgery for Hunner Lesion

Transurethral resection of a Hunner lesion as initially reported by Kerr can provide symptomatic relief (Kerr, 1971). Fall resected ulcerated lesions in 30 patients, resulting in initial disappearance of pain in all and a decrease in urinary frequency in 21 (Fall, 1985). Similar results have been attained with the neodymium-yttrium-aluminum-garnet (YAG) laser (Shanberg et al, 1985, 1989; Rofeim et al, 2001). The majority of patients require repeat fulguration as recurrence of the lesions and symptoms is to be expected over ensuing months to years (Hillelsohn et al, 2012). Extreme caution is critical with use of a laser in a BPS/IC bladder, because forward scatter through these thin bladders with resulting bowel injury is an ever-present danger. There would seem to be no justification in the literature for using the laser to treat areas of glomerulation or in the nonulcerative form of the disease (Shanberg et al, 1997).

Major Surgical Procedures

Supratrigonal cystectomy and the formation of an enterovesical anastomosis with bowel segments (substitution cystoplasty) has been a popular surgical procedure for intractable IC. The diseased bladder is resected in its entirety, sparing only a 1-cm cuff around the trigone to which the bowel segment is anastomosed (Worth et al, 1972; Irwin and Galloway, 1994). Although it is not always clear in the literature how much bladder has been resected, the results reported using these procedures for IC have been mixed at best. Badenoch operated on 9 patients, with 4 becoming much worse and 3 ultimately undergoing urinary diversion (Badenoch, 1971). Flood and colleagues reviewed 122 augmentation procedures, 21 of which were done for IC. Patients with IC had the poorest results of any group, with only 10 having an "excellent" outcome (Flood et al, 1995). Wallack reported 2 successes (Wallack et al, 1975); Seddon had success in 7 of 9 patients (Seddon et al, 1977); and Freiha ended up performing formal urinary diversion in 2 of 6 patients treated with augmentation cecocystoplasty (Freiha et al, 1980). Weiss had success in 3 of 7 patient treated with sigmoidocystoplasty (Weiss et al, 1984), and Lunghi had no excellent results in 2 patients with IC (Lungi et al, 1984). Webster reviewed his data in 19 patients and concluded that only patients with bladder capacities under anesthesia less than 350 mL should undergo substitution cystoplasty (Webster and Maggio, 1989). Hughes lowered the threshold to less than 250 mL (Hughes et al, 1995).

More recent series on subtotal cystectomy plus augmentation have been somewhat more positive (Costello et al, 2000; Chesa et al, 2001). Peeker had good results in all 10 patients with ulcerative IC but poor results in the 3 patients operated on with nonulcerative disease (Peeker et al, 1998). He no longer performs the procedure in the latter group. Linn had success in 20 of 23 patients (only 2 with ulcerative IC) treated with subtotal cystectomy and orthotopic bladder substitution with an ileocecal pouch (Linn et al, 1998). He recommends a supratrigonal cystectomy. A Spanish series reported success in 13 of 17 procedures with a mean follow-up of 94 months (Rodriguez Villamil et al, 1999). The University of Alabama group reported long-term success in 1 of 4 patients with orthotopic neobladders and 1 of 3 with augmentation cystoplasty (Lloyd, 1999). A German report on substitution cystoplasty sparing the trigone was quite enthusiastic, detailing a 78% pain-free rate in 18 patients treated with ileocecal augmentation (10) or ileal substitution (8) at a mean follow-up of 57 months (van Ophoven et al, 2002). Two patients failed to get any pain relief, and 4 required either long-term intermittent catheterization or suprapubic drainage to empty the neobladder.

Not all patients empty the bladder spontaneously after substitution cystoplasty. Although the need for clean intermittent catheterization would not obviate a successful outcome in the patient treated for bladder contraction from tuberculous cystitis, it can be a painful disaster in the IC patient. Nurse and colleagues have gone one step further, recommending trigone biopsy before substitution cystoplasty (Nurse et al, 1991). Diversion and/or total cystourethrectomy is recommended if the trigone is affected by IC. It is not clear how this is determined histologically, as IC has no pathognomonic findings by histology and in general is not a localized process. Nielsen and coworkers described eight women treated with substitution cystoplasty (Nielsen et al, 1990). Treatment in six patients failed, and the results of postoperative biopsies from the trigone showed no difference in the amount of fibrosis, degree of degenerative changes in the muscle, and mast cell density between the two cured patients and the others.

There has been a controversy over whether the IC process can occur in a transposed bowel patch (McGuire et al, 1973; Kisman et al, 1991; Singh and Thomas, 1996) or even in the ureter (Smith and Christmas, 1996). If so, not only would this be a relative contraindication to bladder augmentation, but it would also provide support for the view that a substance in the urine might be involved in pathogenesis. There is, however, evidence that inflammation and fibrosis are the usual reactions of bowel to exposure to urine;

therefore, pathologic findings alone would not be conclusive of spread of IC in such patients (MacDermott et al, 1990).

Augmentation cystoplasty has many potential complications, from the rare incidence of bladder neoplasm (Golomb et al, 1989) to the more common complication of upper tract obstruction (Cheng and Whitfield, 1990). In the best of hands, complications can involve almost 50% of patients, necessitating surgical intervention in 25% (Khoury et al, 1992; Bunyaratavej et al, 1993). Although problems are more common in patients operated on for disorders other than IC, **the risk-benefit ratio of substitution cystoplasty seems to have discouraged its use in the last several years.**

Urinary diversion with or without cystourethrectomy is the ultimate surgical answer to the dilemma of IC, akin to cutting the "Gordian knot." If diversion alone is chosen, one must keep in mind potential problems that can befall the remaining bladder, including pyocystis, hemorrhage, severe pain, and unremitting feelings of incomplete emptying and spasm (Eigner and Freiha 1990; Adeyoju et al, 1996). Bladder carcinoma has also been reported after urinary diversion but is not specifically associated with BPS (Hanno and Tomaszewski, 1982). Consideration of cystourethrectomy is **indicated only in patients who are miserable, in whom all other therapies have failed, and who have demonstrated chronicity such that remission is considered extremely unlikely.** Fortunately, few patients fall into this category. **Theoretically, conduit diversion seems to be reasonable if one is concerned about disease occurring in any continent storage type of reconstruction.** The extended simple cystectomy performed for intractable IC may lend itself to anterior enterocele formation from weakening of the anterior vaginal wall, and prevention of this entity is warranted at the time of cystectomy (Anderson et al, 1998).

Bejany and Politano reported excellent results in 5 patients treated with total bladder replacement and recommended neobladder reconstruction (Bejany and Politano, 1995). Keselman and colleagues had 2 failures in 11 patients treated with continent diversion and attributed this to surgical complications (Keselman et al, 1995). A Finnish group noted failure in 2 of 4 patients treated with cystectomy and conduit diversion because of persistent pain (Lilius et al, 1973). Baskin and Tanagho also cautioned about persistence of pelvic pain after cystectomy and continent diversion, discussing 3 such patients (Baskin and Tanagho, 1992). A similar report followed (Irwin and Galloway, 1992). Webster and coworkers had 10 failures in 14 patients treated with urinary diversion and cystourethrectomy (Webster et al, 1992). Ten patients had persistent pelvic pain, and 4 of them also complained of pouch pain. Only 2 patients had symptom resolution. An English study of 27 patients who underwent cystectomy and bladder replacement with a Kock pouch noted successful treatment of pain in all patients, but follow-up was limited (Christmas et al, 1996a). Parsons suggests that pouch pain will occur in 40% to 50% of patients within 6 to 36 months of surgery (Parsons, 2000).

Attempts have been made to improve results by limiting the operation to those without detrusor mastocytosis (Trinka et al, 1993) and those without "neuropathic pelvic pain" (Lotenfoe et al, 1995). Based on the experience of the past decades, it is unclear if these efforts will prove any more successful. It would seem that risks of failure peculiar to IC include both the development of pain over time in any continent storage mechanism that is constructed, and the risk of phantom pain in the pelvis that persists despite the fact that the stimulus that initially activated the nociceptive neurons (diseased bladder) has been removed (Cross, 1994). Brookoff has proposed trying a differential spinal anesthetic block before considering cystectomy (Brookoff and Sant, 1997). If the patient continues to perceive bladder pain after a spinal anesthetic at the T10 level, it can be taken as an indicator that the pain signal is being generated at a higher level in the spinal cord and that surgery on the bladder will not result in pain relief. Some patients with intractable urinary frequency will opt for simple conduit urinary diversion alone, feeling that their quality of life will be improved independent of the pain piece of the puzzle. Despite all of the problems, many patients will do well after major surgery, and quality of life can measurably improve (Rupp et al, 2000). In the

event of neobladder pain after subtotal cystectomy and enterocystoplasty or continent diversion, it appears safe to retubularize a previously used bowel segment to form a urinary conduit for a straightforward urinary diversion without significant risk of conduit pain (Elzawahri et al, 2004).

The Gothenburg experience was recently reviewed, looking at results in 47 patients subjected to reconstructive or extirpative surgery (Rössberger et al, 2007). This included 23 substitution cystoplasties, 12 conduit diversions, and 10 Kock pouches. Twenty-eight of 34 patients with classic Hunner lesions had complete symptom resolution from the initial surgical procedure. Four of the remaining 6 required urinary diversion, cystectomy, or ulcer resection in a trigonal remnant, but ultimately did well. Only 3 of 13 patients with non-Hunner disease had successful symptom resolution after reconstructive surgery, 2 of whom required conduit diversion. Peeker's group concluded that only patients with Hunner lesions refractory to standard therapy could be expected to do well after major surgery.

A Thai experience using cystectomy and ileal neobladder in women in whom conservative therapy failed reported good results in all 35 patients treated (Kochakarn et al, 2007). Spontaneous voiding with minimal residual urine was found in 33 patients, and the remaining 2 patients had spontaneous voiding with residual urine requiring clean intermittent catheterization.

Forty years ago, Pool recognized that "surgical treatment has not been the boon many had hoped it would be" (Pool, 1967). "Diversion of the urine is not the entire answer to the situation. Removal of the lesion in the bladder has been of no benefit. Likewise, removal of almost the entire mobile portion of the bladder proved to be a failure." Blaivas and colleagues (2005) described results of augmentation enterocystoplasty and continent diversion in 76 consecutive patients with benign disease with a mean 9-year follow-up. The procedures in all 7 patients with the diagnosis of IC were classified as failures, whereas 67 of the remaining 69 patients were cured or improved. When one of the deans of major urologic reconstruction writes, "I find it very difficult to justify such extensive surgery (continent diversion, cystourethrectomy) with such limited results and for these reasons have not been involved in surgery for IC over the past 3 years" (Webster, 1993), it is obvious that one should think carefully and proceed with surgery only after a complete discussion with a very motivated and well-informed patient. Recent reports seem to be more sanguine with regard to these procedures.

KEY POINTS: SURGICAL THERAPY

- Major surgery for BPS is a reasonable alternative for patients with severe symptoms in whom standard attempts at treatment have failed and when the disease course suggests that spontaneous remission of symptoms is unlikely.
- Patients with a small bladder capacity under anesthesia are less likely to respond to conservative attempts at therapy.
- Patients with a Hunner lesion may have the best results with major surgery.
- If one conceptualizes BPS as two disorders, one of pain and the other of frequency, it becomes easier for the patient and physician to rationalize the decision.
- Conduit urinary diversion can be relied on to resolve the frequency symptoms, and if the patient would consider this alone to make for a successful procedure, there is reason to seriously consider this option.
- Diversion, and even cystectomy with diversion, cannot guarantee a pain-free result, and it is critical for the patient to factor this into the decision about this often irrevocable step.

A simple ileal conduit without cystectomy or attempt at continent diversion can be an acceptable treatment choice with good clinical results and resulting quality-of-life improvement (Norus et al, 2014). Cystectomy may add complications and need for reoperation (Peters et al, 2013a). Subtotal cystectomy with bladder augmentation may fail to give pain relief in more than one third of patients (Andersen et al, 2012).

Assessing Treatment Results

The diversity of BPS/IC therapies underscores the lack of understanding about the treatment of this syndrome (Rovner et al, 2000). It has been not only a difficult condition to diagnose, but also a difficult condition for which to assess therapeutic impact. **There is a 50% incidence of temporary remission unrelated to therapy, with a mean duration of 8 months** (Held et al, 1990). **A recent meta-analysis of articles published from 1990 to 2010 on management of BPS/IC concluded that there is limited evidence proving efficacy of treatment and attributed the lack of definitive conclusions to the great heterogeneity in methodology, symptom assessment, duration of treatment, and follow-up in both randomized controlled trials and nonrandomized reports** (Giannantoni et al, 2012). This should not be interpreted to conclude that all treatments for the affected individual are ineffective, but rather that demonstrating treatment effects in populations of patients has been problematic for the reasons noted. The lack of knowledge about how the syndrome should be best phenotyped stands out as an important missing piece.

A somewhat surprising finding from the ICDB was that although there was initial improvement in symptoms partially because of regression to the mean (Sech et al, 1998) and the intervention effect, there was no evidence of a long-term change in average symptom severity over the 4-year course of follow-up (Propert et al, 2000). In a chronic, devastating condition with primarily subjective symptomatology, no known cause, and no cure, patients are desperate and often seem to respond to any new therapy (Fig. 14-11). They are often victims of unorthodox health care providers with untested forms of therapy—some medical, some homeopathic, and some even surgical.

The Placebo Conundrum

Where possible, the results of randomized controlled studies should be used for decision making. Placebo-controlled, double-blind studies are optimal in this disorder for which there is no generally effective standard therapy.

Placebo effects influence patient outcomes after any treatment that the clinician and patients believe is effective, including surgery. Placebo effects plus disease natural history and regression to the mean can result in high rates of good outcomes, which may be misattributed to specific treatment effects (Gillespie et al, 1991; Gillespie, 1994; Turner et al, 1994; Propert et al, 2000). Unfortunately, **too few BPS treatments have been subjected to a placebo-controlled trial.** This is not to say that what seems effective is not, but rather that a high index of skepticism is healthy, even in treatments tested in controlled trials (Schulz et al, 1995).

Whereas in many diseases an argument can be made against using a true placebo control as opposed to an orthodox treatment of approved or accepted value (Rothman and Michels, 1994), a good case for true placebo comparison can readily be made for BPS. The vagaries of the natural history, the general lack of progression of symptom severity over time, and the fact that the condition is not life-threatening mean that there is little to lose and much to gain by subjecting new treatments to the rigorous scrutiny of placebo control. Many patients who volunteer for such trials have already run the gamut of accepted (although, in general, unproved) therapies. It has long been recognized in protocols that use subjective criteria for assessment that "improvement" may be expected in up to 35% of placebo-treated patients (Benson and Epstein, 1976). The spontaneous remission rate (although temporary) for BPS is 11% (Oravisto and Alfthan, 1976) to 50% (Held et al, 1990), and this in combination with the placebo improvement make efficacy difficult to prove.

Even in placebo-controlled trials, it is reasonable to surmise that some degree of unblinding may occur as a result of somatic or

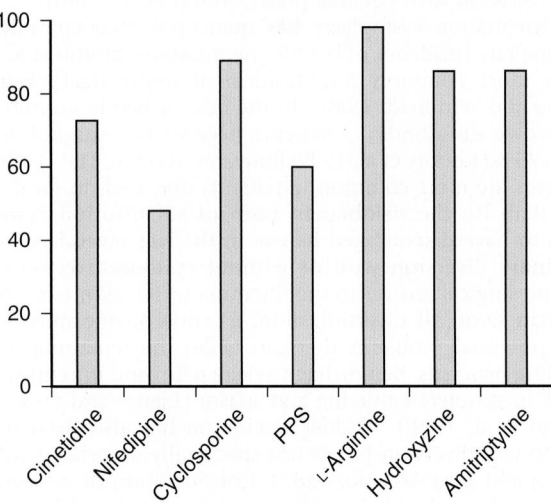

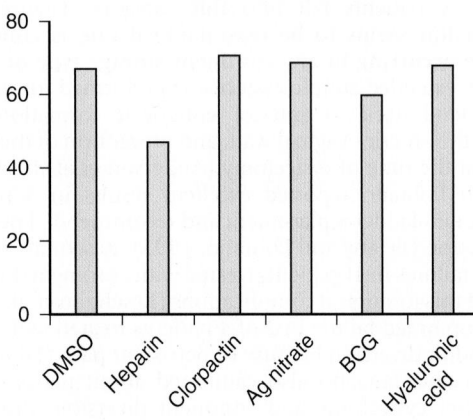

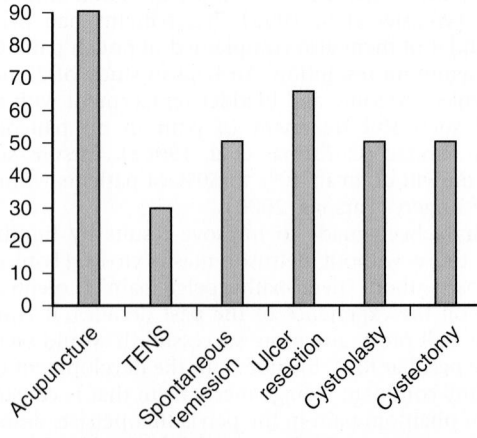

Figure 14-11. Selected reported treatment outcomes in uncontrolled studies in the bladder pain syndrome and interstitial cystitis literature: Percentage of patients initially improved. Ag nitrate, silver nitrate; BCG, bacillus Calmette-Guérin; DMSO, dimethyl sulfoxide; PPS, sodium pentosan polysulfate; TENS, transcutaneous electrical nerve stimulation.

psychological side effects of the active arm, impairing the validity of the trial results and giving the active arm a slight edge over placebo (DuBeau et al, 2005; Rees et al, 2005). Failure to recognize unblinding can easily bias results of a study and has not been routinely measured in clinical trials (Desbiens, 2002). When occurring late in a study after one would expect onset of a therapeutic effect, unblinding could be the result of side effect profile or drug efficacy. Early in the trial it reflects poor placebo or study design. The degree of blinding needs to be ascertained throughout the trial. This is of specific concern in BPS and any disorder in which primary outcomes may be subject to patient-specific psychological and physiologic factors.

The ethics and necessity of placebo-controlled trials have been questioned, especially in situations in which an effective treatment exists and also in which delay in treatment has been shown to result in disease progression (Streiner, 1999; Anderson, 2006; Polman et al, 2008). However, there are methodologic concerns with equivalence and noninferiority active agent comparison trials (Streiner, 2007). These include an inability to determine if the treatments are equally good or equally bad and the possibility that successive noninferiority trials can lead to a gradual decrease in treatment efficacy. Although the use of placebo-controlled trials raises ethical concerns when proven effective treatment exists for the condition under investigation, they are ethically justified, provided that stringent criteria for protecting research subjects are satisfied (Miller et al, 2004).

The value of placebo-controlled trials is aptly illustrated by the recent decisions by pharmaceutical manufacturers not to pursue FDA approval in the United States for seemingly promising intravesical therapies for BPS/IC (Morales et al, 1996; Chancellor and de Groat, 1999) after placebo-controlled trials failed to establish efficacy. These include low-concentration hyaluronic acid (Bioniche, Canada), high-concentration hyaluronic acid (Seikagaku, Tokyo), and RTX (ICOS, Bothell, WA). Nalmefene, an initially promising oral therapy in the 1990s (Stone, 1994), also failed phase 3 trials (IVAX, Miami, FL). Placebo trials are impractical in surgery, and it can be difficult to evaluate surgical reports. The many older medications currently used off-label might not meet success if tested in the stringent manner in which new molecular entities are tested. The expense of testing therapies currently used off-label often requires dependence on the largesse of government agencies such as the National Institutes of Health (Propert et al, 2002; Sant et al, 2003; Mayer et al, 2005).

Finally, in considering objective changes, the concept of statistical versus clinical significance is paramount. Investigators should, but rarely do, point out differences between statistical improvement and what they consider to be clinically significant improvement (Wein and Broderick, 1994). As Gertrude Stein reportedly stated, "A difference, to be a difference, must make a difference." An increase in bladder capacity of 30 mL may be statistically significant but clinically irrelevant. Number-needed-to-treat and number-needed-to-harm data (McQuay, 2003) may be particularly important in BPS/IC and have not typically been included in efficacy analysis.

Clinical Symptom Scales

BPS/IC symptom questionnaires include the University of Wisconsin Interstitial Cystitis Inventory, the O'Leary-Sant IC symptom index and IC problem index, and the Pelvic Pain and Urgency/Frequency (PUF) scale.

The **University of Wisconsin IC scale** includes seven PBS/IC symptom items (Table 14-5). **It has not been validated for identification or diagnosis of BPS/IC. It captures severity of symptom expression** (Keller et al, 1994; Goin et al, 1998). BPS/IC patients do not appear to indiscriminately report higher scores than controls for different somatic and general complaints (Porru et al, 2005). Unlike the other two instruments, it addresses some quality-of-life issues, and this is an advantage when such issues are subject of investigation. Its most attractive aspects are its clinically apparent face validity and its ease of implementation.

The O'Leary-Sant indices (Table 14-6) are a **validated** questionnaire that was originally developed by focus groups, subjected to test-retest reliability analysis, and validated by administration to IC patients and asymptomatic controls (O'Leary et al, 1997; Lubeck

TABLE 14-5 University of Wisconsin Symptom Instrument

SYMPTOM	SCORE 1-6 (0 = NOT AT ALL, 6 = A LOT)
1. Bladder discomfort	___
2. Bladder pain	___
3. Other pelvic discomfort	___
4. Headache	___
5. Backache	___
6. Dizziness	___
7. Feelings of suffocation	___
8. Chest pain	___
9. Ringing in ears	___
10. Getting up at night to go to the bathroom	___
11. Aches in joints	___
12. Swollen ankles	___
13. Nasal congestion	___
14. Flu	___
15. Abdominal cramps	___
16. Numbness or tingling in fingers or toes	___
17. Nausea	___
18. Going to the bathroom frequently during the day	___
19. Blind spots or blurred vision	___
20. Heart pounding	___
21. Difficulty sleeping because of bladder symptoms	___
22. Sore throat	___
23. Urgency to urinate	___
24. Coughing	___
25. Burning sensation in bladder	___

From Sirinian E, Azevedo K, Payne CK. Correlation between 2 interstitial cystitis symptom instruments. J Urol 2005;173:835–40.

et al, 2001). The questionnaire centers on three questions related to urgency and frequency and one on bladder-associated pain. It does not address generalized pelvic pain or symptomatology associated with sexual activity. This is not because these questions were not considered in the formulation of the questionnaire. Of 73 questions in the preliminary instrument covering domains of urinary symptoms, pain, sexual function, menstrual variability, and general health, only the four questions now in the instrument were needed to reliably and validly describe the illness experience of those with IC and distinguish these patients from those without the disorder (O'Leary and Sant, 1997).

Another instrument is the **PUF questionnaire** (Parsons et al, 2002a) (Table 14-7). It was specifically designed to include questions that directly reflect a wide variety of the symptoms experienced by patients who are affected by this disorder. One third of the questions address pelvic pain, including pain anywhere in the pelvis: the vagina, labia, lower abdomen, urethra, perineum, testes, penis, or scrotum. A large study using the PUF questionnaire has concluded that up to 23% of female Americans have BPS/IC (Parsons et al, 2002a). This makes one wary as to the usefulness and face-validity of the PUF (Ito et al, 2003). A total score of 10 to 14 indicates a 74% likelihood of a positive potassium test (PST); 15 to 19 indicates 76%; 20+ indicates 91%. To the extent that the PST is suspect, the reliability of PUF data comes into question. Question 4 of the PUF is problematic. Patients who are sexually active can gain up to 6 more points than those who are not, and

TABLE 14-6 O'Leary-Sant Indices

INTERSTITIAL CYSTITIS SYMPTOM INDEX	INTERSTITIAL CYSTITIS PROBLEM INDEX
During the past month:	During the past month, how much has each of the following been a problem for you?
Q1. How often have you felt the strong need to urinate with little or no warning? 0. ____ Not at all 1. ____ Less than 1 time in 5 2. ____ Less than half the time 3. ____ About half the time 4. ____ More than half the time 5. ____ Almost always	Q1. Frequent urination during the day 0. ____ No problem 1. ____ Very small problem 2. ____ Small problem 3. ____ Medium problem 4. ____ Big problem
Q2. How often have you had to urinate less than 2 hours after you finished urinating? 0. ____ Not at all 1. ____ Less than 1 time in 5 2. ____ Less than half the time 3. ____ About half the time 4. ____ More than half the time 5. ____ Almost always	Q2. Getting up at night to urinate 0. ____ No problem 1. ____ Very small problem 2. ____ Small problem 3. ____ Medium problem 4. ____ Big problem
Q3. How often did you most typically get up at night to urinate? 0. ____ None 1. ____ Once 2. ____ 2 times 3. ____ 3 times 4. ____ 4 times 5. ____ 5 times	Q3. Need to urinate with little warning 0. ____ No problem 1. ____ Very small problem 2. ____ Small problem 3. ____ Medium problem 4. ____ Big problem
Q4. Have you experienced pain or burning in your bladder? 0. ____ Not at all 2. ____ A few times 3. ____ Fairly often 4. ____ Usually 5. ____ Almost always	Q4. Burning, pain, discomfort, or pressure in your bladder 0. ____ No problem 1. ____ Very small problem 2. ____ Small problem 3. ____ Medium problem 4. ____ Big problem
Add the numerical values of the checked entries.	**Add the numerical values of the checked entries.**
Total score: _____	**Total score:** _____

From O'Leary MP, Sant GR, Fowler FJ, et al. The interstitial cystitis symptom index and problem index. Urology 1997;49:58–63.

patients who over time begin sexual activity because they are feeling better can actually accumulate a falsely elevated PUF score because of this anomaly.

None of the questionnaires has been shown to be of value in diagnosis (Moldwin and Kushner, 2004), **although they may suggest who should be screened further for the syndrome** (Kushner and Moldwin, 2006). **The O'Leary-Sant scales and University of Wisconsin instrument correlate strongly in a large population of patients with BPS/IC** (Sirinian and Payne, 2001). **Both the O'Leary-Sant and University of Wisconsin questionnaires are responsive to change over time and thus good for following the natural history of the disorder and the results of treatment.**

Treatment outcome studies have also used the **Global Response Assessment (GRA)**, a balanced patient self-report on overall response to therapy, developed for NIDDK-sponsored multicenter therapeutic trials (Sant et al, 2003) (Box 14-9). A one-category change in GRA correlates with a 1.2-point change in the O'Leary-Sant and a 3.1-point change in the University of Wisconsin instruments (Propert et al, 2006). More recently, the validated Genitourinary Pain Index (GUPI) has been used to assess the degree of symptoms in men and women with genitourinary complaints (Clemens et al, 2009a) (Figs. 14-12 and 14-13).

PRINCIPLES OF MANAGEMENT

The information currently available in the literature does not lend itself to easily formulating a diagnostic or treatment guideline that would be universally accepted. Different groups of experts would undoubtedly create different best practices. The algorithms for diagnosis and management constructed by the AUA (Hanno et al, 2011) and the International Consultation on Incontinence are presented in Figures 14-14 and 14-15. The compromise approach constructed by an experienced cross section of urologists and gynecologists from around the world at the International Consultation on Incontinence 2012 meeting in Paris seems reasonable and allows for significant latitude in individual practice and patient preference (Hanno et al, 2013). It is outlined in the following sections.

Definition of Bladder Pain Syndrome

(In the absence of a universally agreed-on definition, the ESSIC definition is given along with the definition of the AUA.)

ESSIC: Chronic pelvic pain, pressure, or discomfort of longer than 6 months' duration perceived to be related to the urinary

TABLE 14-7 Pelvic Pain and Urgency/Frequency Patient Symptom Scale

Patient's Name: _____ Today's Date: _____
Please circle the answer that best describes how you feel for each question.

	0	1	2	3	4	SYMPTOM SCORE	BOTHER SCORE
1. How many times do you go to the bathroom during the day?	3-6	7-10	11-14	15-19	20+		
2. a. How many times do you go to the bathroom at night?	0	1	2	3	4+		
b. If you get up at night to go to the bathroom, does it bother you?	Never bothers	Occasionally	Usually	Always			
3. Are you currently sexually active? YES ____ NO ____							
4. a. If you are sexually active, do you now or have you ever had pain or symptoms during or after sexual activity?	Never	Occasionally	Usually	Always			
b. If you have pain, does it make you avoid sexual activity?	Never	Occasionally	Usually	Always			
5. Do you have pain associated with your bladder or in your pelvis (vagina, labia, lower abdomen, urethra, perineum, penis, testes, or scrotum)?	Never	Occasionally	Usually	Always			
6. a. If you have pain, is it usually		Mild	Moderate	Severe			
b. Does your pain bother you?	Never	Occasionally	Usually	Always			
7. Do you still have urgency after you go to the bathroom?	Never	Occasionally	Usually	Always			
8. a. If you have urgency, is it usually		Mild	Moderate	Severe			
b. Does your urgency bother you?	Never	Occasionally	Usually	Always			

Total Score (Symptom Score + Bother Score)
Symptom Score (1, 2a, 4a, 5, 6a, 7, 8a)
Bother Score (2b, 4b, 6b, 8b)
Total score ranges are from 1 to 35.

From Parsons CL, Dell J, Stanford EL, et al. Increased prevalence of interstitial cystitis: previously unrecognized urologic and gynecologic cases identified using a new symptom questionnaire and intravesical potassium sensitivity. Urology 2000;60:573–8.

BOX 14-9 Global Response Assessment

−3: Markedly worse
−2: Moderately worse
−1: Slightly worse
0: No change
+1: Slightly improved
+2: Moderately improved
+3: Markedly improved

Data from Sant GR, Propert KJ, Hanno PM, et al. A pilot clinical trial of oral pentosan polysulfate and oral hydroxyzine in patients with interstitial cystitis. J Urol 2003;170(3):810–5.

bladder and accompanied by at least one other urinary symptom such as a persistent urge to void or urinary frequency. Confusable diseases as the cause of the symptoms must be excluded.

AUA guideline definition: An unpleasant sensation (pain, pressure, discomfort) perceived to be related to the urinary bladder, associated with lower urinary tract symptoms of more than 6 weeks' duration, in the absence of infection or other identifiable causes.

Nomenclature

The scientific committee of the International Consultation voted to use the term *bladder pain syndrome* for the disorder that has been commonly referred to as *interstitial cystitis.* The term *painful bladder syndrome* was dropped from the lexicon. The term *interstitial cystitis* implies an inflammation within the wall of the urinary bladder, involving gaps or spaces in the bladder tissue. This does not accurately describe the majority of patients with this syndrome. *Painful bladder syndrome* as defined by the ICS is too restrictive for the clinical syndrome.

Properly defined, the term *bladder pain syndrome* appears to fit in well with the taxonomy of the International Association for the Study of Pain (IASP) (see later) and focuses on the actual symptom complex rather than on what appears to be a long-held misconception of the underlying pathology.

Bladder Pain Syndrome (XXIII-2) (per IASP)

BPS is the occurrence of persistent or recurrent pain perceived in the urinary bladder region and accompanied by at least one other symptom, such as pain worsening with bladder filling and daytime and/or nighttime urinary frequency. There is no proven infection or other obvious local pathology. BPS is often associated with negative cognitive, behavioral, sexual, or emotional consequences as well

Female Genitourinary Pain Index

1. In the last week, have you experienced any pain or discomfort in the following areas?

a. Entrance to vagina $\square_1$ Yes $\square_0$ No
b. Vagina $\square_1$ Yes $\square_0$ No
c. Urethra $\square_1$ Yes $\square_0$ No
d. Below your waist, in your pubic or bladder area $\square_1$ Yes $\square_0$ No

2. In the last week, have you experienced:

a. Pain or burning during urination? $\square_1$ Yes $\square_0$ No
b. Pain or discomfort during or after sexual intercourse? $\square_1$ Yes $\square_0$ No
c. Pain or discomfort as your bladder fills? $\square_1$ Yes $\square_0$ No
d. Pain or discomfort relieved by voiding? $\square_1$ Yes $\square_0$ No

3. How often have you had pain or discomfort in any of these areas over the last week?

$\square_0$ Never $\square_1$ Rarely $\square_2$ Sometimes $\square_3$ Often $\square_4$ Usually $\square_5$ Always

4. Which number best describes your AVERAGE pain or discomfort on the days you had it, over the last week?

$\square$ $\square$ $\square$ $\square$ $\square$ $\square$ $\square$ $\square$ $\square$ $\square$ $\square$
0   1   2   3   4   5   6   7   8   9   10
No pain   Pain as bad as you can imagine

5. How often have you had a sensation of not emptying your bladder completely after you finished urinating, over the last week?

$\square_0$ Not at all $\square_1$ Less than 1 time in 5 $\square_2$ Less than half the time $\square_3$ About half the time $\square_4$ More than half the time $\square_5$ Almost always

6. How often have you had to urinate again less than two hours after you finished urinating, over the last week?

$\square_0$ Not at all $\square_1$ Less than 1 time in 5 $\square_2$ Less than half the time $\square_3$ About half the time $\square_4$ More than half the time $\square_5$ Almost always

7. How much have your symptoms kept you from doing the kinds of things you would usually do, over the last week?

$\square_0$ None $\square_1$ Only a little $\square_2$ Some $\square_3$ A lot

8. How much did you think about your symptoms, over the last week?

$\square_0$ None $\square_1$ Only a little $\square_2$ Some $\square_3$ A lot

9. If you were to spend the rest of your life with your symptoms just the way they have been during the last week, how would you feel about that?

$\square_0$ Delighted
$\square_1$ Pleased
$\square_2$ Mostly satisfied
$\square_3$ Mixed (about equally satisfied and dissatisfied)
$\square_4$ Mostly dissatisfied
$\square_5$ Unhappy
$\square_6$ Terrible

Figure 14-12. Female Genitourinary Pain Index.

Male Genitourinary Pain Index

1. In the last week, have you experienced any pain or discomfort in the following areas?

a. Area between rectum and testicles (perineum) $\square_1$ Yes $\square_0$ No
b. Testicles $\square_1$ Yes $\square_0$ No
c. Tip of penis (not related to urination) $\square_1$ Yes $\square_0$ No
d. Below your waist, in your pubic or bladder area $\square_1$ Yes $\square_0$ No

2. In the last week, have you experienced:

a. Pain or burning during urination? $\square_1$ Yes $\square_0$ No
b. Pain or discomfort during or after sexual climax (ejaculation)? $\square_1$ Yes $\square_0$ No
c. Pain or discomfort as your bladder fills? $\square_1$ Yes $\square_0$ No
d. Pain or discomfort relieved by voiding? $\square_1$ Yes $\square_0$ No

3. How often have you had pain or discomfort in any of these areas over the last week?

$\square_0$ Never $\square_1$ Rarely $\square_2$ Sometimes $\square_3$ Often $\square_4$ Usually $\square_5$ Always

4. Which number best describes your AVERAGE pain or discomfort on the days you had it, over the last week?

$\square$ $\square$ $\square$ $\square$ $\square$ $\square$ $\square$ $\square$ $\square$ $\square$ $\square$
0   1   2   3   4   5   6   7   8   9   10

No   Pain as bad as you
pain   can imagine

5. How often have you had a sensation of not emptying your bladder completely after you finished urinating, over the last week?

$\square_0$ Not at all $\square_1$ Less than 1 $\square_2$ Less than half the $\square_3$ About half $\square_4$ More than $\square_5$ Almost
                time in 5   time   the time   half the time   always

6. How often have you had to urinate again less than two hours after you finished urinating, over the last week?

$\square_0$ Not at all $\square_1$ Less than 1 $\square_2$ Less than half the $\square_3$ About half $\square_4$ More than $\square_5$ Almost
                time in 5   time   the time   half the time   always

7. How much have your symptoms kept you from doing the kinds of things you would usually do, over the last week?

$\square_0$ None $\square_1$ Only a little $\square_2$ Some $\square_3$ A lot

8. How much did you think about your symptoms, over the last week?

$\square_0$ None $\square_1$ Only a little $\square_2$ Some $\square_3$ A lot

9. If you were to spend the rest of your life with your symptoms just the way they have been during the last week, how would you feel about that?

$\square_0$ Delighted
$\square_1$ Pleased
$\square_2$ Mostly satisfied
$\square_3$ Mixed (about equally satisfied and dissatisfied)
$\square_4$ Mostly dissatisfied
$\square_5$ Unhappy
$\square_6$ Terrible

Figure 14-13. Male Genitourinary Pain Index.

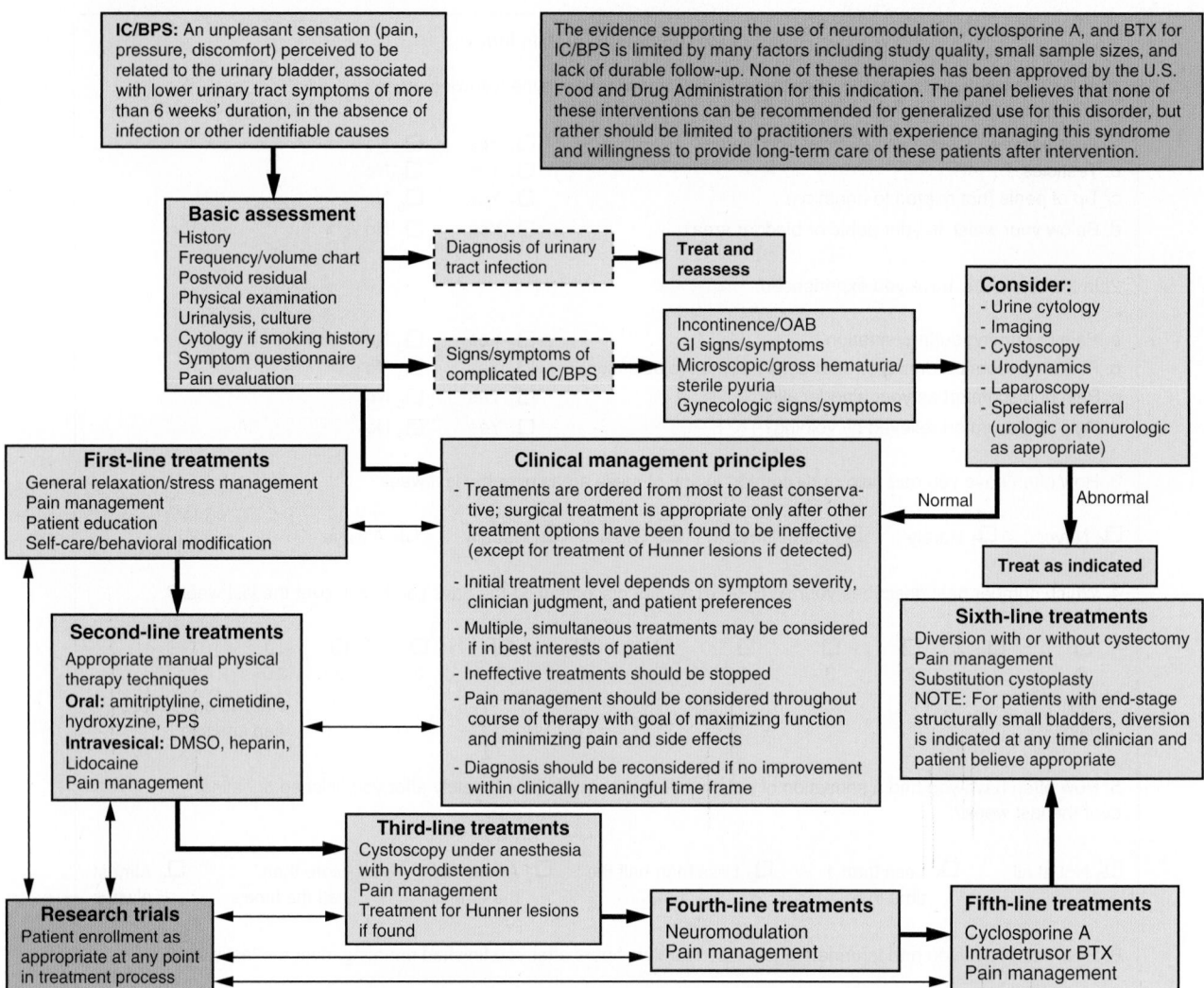

Figure 14-14. Diagnosis and treatment algorithm for interstitial cystitis/bladder pain syndrome (IC/BPS) of the American Urological Association. BTX, botulinum toxin; DMSO, dimethyl sulfoxide; GI, gastrointestinal; OAB, overactive bladder; PPS, pentosan polysulfate. (From Hanno PM, Burks DA, Clemens JQ, et al; Interstitial Cystitis Guidelines Panel of the American Urological Association Education and Research, Inc. AUA guideline for the diagnosis and treatment of interstitial cystitis/bladder pain syndrome. J Urol 2011;185[6]:2162–70. Copyright © 2010 American Urological Association Education and Research, Inc.)

as with symptoms suggestive of lower urinary tract and sexual dysfunction.

History and Initial Assessment

Patients whose symptoms meet the requirements of the definition of BPS should be evaluated. The presence of commonly associated disorders including irritable bowel syndrome, chronic fatigue syndrome, and fibromyalgia in the presence of the cardinal symptoms of BPS also suggests the diagnosis. Abnormal gynecologic findings in women and well-characterized confusable diseases that may explain the symptoms must be ruled out.

The initial assessment consists of a frequency and volume chart, focused physical examination, urinalysis, and urine culture. Urine cytology, cystoscopy, and urodynamic evaluation are recommended if clinically indicated and/or the diagnosis is in doubt. Patients with urinary infection should be treated and reassessed. Those with recurrent urinary infection, abnormal urinary cytology, and microscopic or gross hematuria are evaluated with appropriate imaging and endoscopic procedures, and only if findings are unable to explain the symptoms are they diagnosed with BPS.

Initial Treatment

The initial treatment of BPS consists of the following:
- Patient education
- Dietary manipulation
- Nonprescription analgesics
- Stress reduction
- Pelvic floor relaxation techniques

In the patient with findings suggesting pelvic floor dysfunction, pelvic floor physical therapy with myofascial trigger point release and intravaginal Thiele massage is often an effective therapeutic intervention. The **treatment of pain** needs to be addressed directly, and in some instances referral to an anesthesia or pain center can be an appropriate early step in conjunction with ongoing treatment of the syndrome.

When conservative therapy fails or symptoms are severe and conservative management is unlikely to succeed, the following can be prescribed:
- Oral medication
- Intravesical treatment

It is recommended to initiate a single form of therapy and observe results, adding other modalities or substituting other

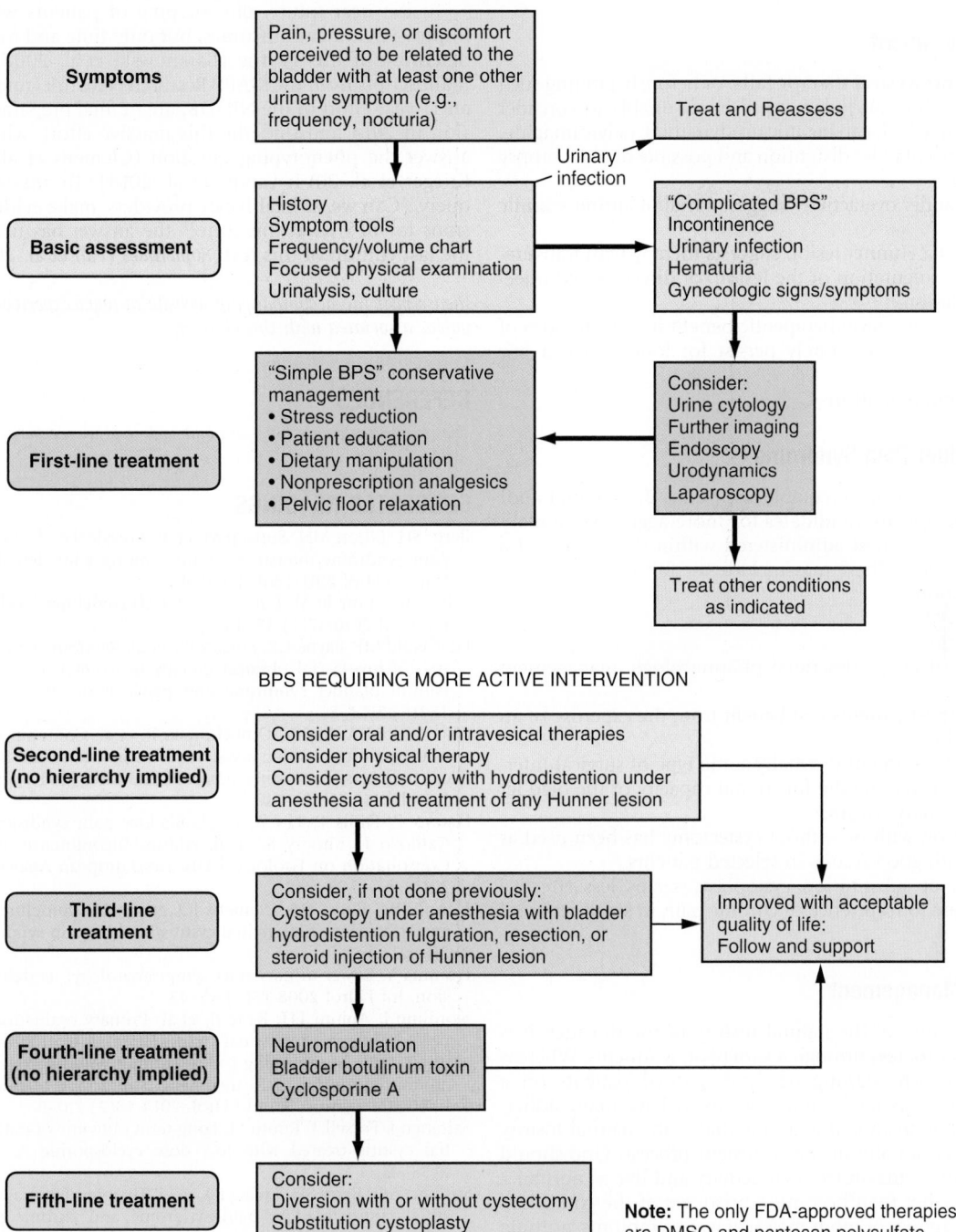

Figure 14-15. Algorithm for diagnosis and treatment of bladder pain syndrome (BPS) according to the Committee on Bladder Pain Syndrome of the Fifth International Consultation on Incontinence, held in Paris in February 2012, under the auspices of the International Consultation on Urological Diseases and enabled by the generous support of the European Association of Urology. Pain management is a primary consideration at every step of algorithm. Patient enrollment in an appropriate research trial is a reasonable option at any point. Evidence supporting neuromodulation, cyclosporine A, and botulinum toxin for BPS indication is limited. These interventions are appropriate only for practitioners with experience treating BPS and willingness to provide long-term care postintervention. DMSO, dimethyl sulfoxide; FDA, U.S. Food and Drug Administration. (From Hanno P, Dinis P, Lin A, et al. Bladder pain syndrome. In: Abrams P, Cardozo L, Khoury S, et al, editors. Incontinence. Paris: International Consultation on Urological Diseases/European Association of Urology; 2013. p. 1583–649.)

modalities as indicated by degree of response or lack of response to treatment.

Secondary Assessment

If initial oral or intravesical therapy fails, or before beginning such therapy based on clinician judgment, it is reasonable to consider **further evaluation**, which can include urodynamics, pelvic imaging, and cystoscopy with bladder distention and possible bladder biopsy under anesthesia.

- Findings of bladder overactivity suggest a trial of antimuscarinic therapy.
- The presence of a Hunner lesion suggests therapy with transurethral resection, fulguration of the lesion, or direct steroid injection into the lesion.
- Distention itself can have therapeutic benefit in 30% to 50% of patients, though benefits rarely persist for longer than a few months.
- **Grade of recommendation: C**

Refractory Bladder Pain Syndrome

Patients with persistent, unacceptable symptoms despite oral and/or intravesical therapy are candidates for more aggressive modalities. Many of these are best administered within the context of a clinical trial if possible. These may include the following:

1. Neuromodulation
2. Intradetrusor BTX
3. Oral cyclosporine A
4. Clinical trials of newly described pharmacologic management techniques

At this point, most patients will benefit from the expertise of an anesthesia pain clinic.

The last step in treatment is usually some type of surgical intervention aimed at increasing the functional capacity of the bladder or diverting the urinary stream.

- Urinary diversion with or without cystectomy has been used as a last resort with good results in selected patients.
- Augmentation or substitution cystoplasty seems less effective and more prone to recurrence of chronic pain in small reported series.

Philosophy of Management

I believe that, because of the natural history of the disorder, it is best to cautiously progress through a variety of treatments. Whereas the shotgun approach, starting newly diagnosed patients on a variety of simultaneous medications, seems to have many adherents, employing one treatment at a time makes the natural history of the disease itself an ally in the treatment process. One should encourage patients to maximize their activity and live as normal a life as possible, rather than becoming prisoners of the condition. Although some activities or foods may aggravate symptoms, nothing has been shown to negatively affect the disease process itself. Therefore patients should feel free to experiment and judge for themselves how to modify their lifestyle without the guilt that comes from feeling they have harmed themselves if symptoms flare.

Dogmatic restriction and diet are to be avoided unless they are shown to improve symptoms in a particular patient.

In the near future, phenotyping of patients with BPS/IC may improve treatment outcomes, but only time and future studies will determine if this is true (Baranowski et al, 2008). Foundational manuscripts from the MAPP Research Network (mappnetwork.org), an 11-year effort of the NIDDK, are in final preparation for submission in 2014 and underlie this massive effort, which will help to answer the phenotyping question (Clemens et al, 2014a, 2014b; Krieger et al, 2014; Landis et al, 2014). To answer the perennial query, "Can we, as health care providers, make evidence-based decisions for BPS/IC at this time?" the answer has not changed since the last edition of this text: *Sometimes* (Fall et al, 2008).

Please visit the accompanying website at www.expertconsult.com to view videos associated with this chapter.

REFERENCES

The complete reference list is available online at www.expertconsult.com.

SUGGESTED READINGS

Berry SH, Elliott MN, Suttorp M, et al. Prevalence of symptoms of bladder pain syndrome/interstitial cystitis among adult females in the United States. J Urol 2011;186(2):540–4.

Fall M, Baranowski AP, Elneil S, et al. EAU guidelines on chronic pelvic pain. Eur Urol 2010;57(1):35–48.

FitzGerald MP, Payne CK, Lukacz ES, et al. Randomized multicenter clinical trial of myofascial physical therapy in women with interstitial cystitis/painful bladder syndrome and pelvic floor tenderness. J Urol 2012; 187(6):2113–8.

Giannantoni A, Bini V, Dmochowski R, et al. Contemporary management of the painful bladder: a systematic review. Eur Urol 2012;61(1):29–53.

Hand JR. Interstitial cystitis: report of 223 cases (204 women and 19 men). J Urol 1949;61:291–310.

Hanno P, Dinis P, Lin A, et al. Bladder pain syndrome. In: Abrams P, Cardozo L, Khoury S, et al, editors. Incontinence. Paris: nternational Consultation on Urological Diseases/European Association of Urology; 2013. p. 1583–649.

Hanno PM, Burks DA, Clemens JQ, et al. AUA guideline for the diagnosis and treatment of interstitial cystitis/bladder pain syndrome. J Urol 2011; 185(6):2162–70.

Homma Y. Lower urinary tract symptomatology: its definition and confusion. Int J Urol 2008;15(1):35–43.

Nordling J, Anjum FH, Bade JJ, et al. Primary evaluation of patients suspected of having interstitial cystitis (IC). Eur Urol 2004;45(5):662–9.

Norus T, Fode M, Nordling J. Ileal conduit without cystectomy may be an appropriate option in the treatment of intractable bladder pain syndrome/interstitial cystitis. Scand J Urol. 2014;48(2):210–5.

Sairanen J, Forsell T, Ruutu M. Long-term outcome of patients with interstitial cystitis treated with low dose cyclosporine A. J Urol 2004;171: 2138–41.

Suskind AM, Berry SH, Ewing BA, et al. The prevalence and overlap of interstitial cystitis/bladder pain syndrome and chronic prostatitis/chronic pelvic pain syndrome in men: results of the RAND Interstitial Cystitis Epidemiology male study. J Urol 2013;189(1):141–5.

van de Merwe JP, Nordling J, Bouchelouche P, et al. Diagnostic criteria, classification, and nomenclature for painful bladder syndrome/interstitial cystitis: an ESSIC proposal. Eur Urol 2008;53(1):60–7.

15 Sexually Transmitted Diseases*

Michel Arthur Pontari, MD

EPIDEMIOLOGY OF SEXUALLY TRANSMITTED DISEASES

The Centers for Disease Control and Prevention (CDC) publishes annual reports on the number of cases of sexually transmitted diseases (STDs) in the United States (CDC, 2013). Data from 2012 are summarized in Tables 15-1 and 15-2. Overall, the estimate is that nearly 20 million new STDs occur every year in the United States, half among people aged 15 to 24 years. This group accounted for 58% of gonorrhea and 69% of chlamydia cases in 2012. Another group with disproportionate risk is men who have sex with men (MSM). This group now accounts for 75% of all primary and secondary syphilis cases. Factors that increase the risk of acquiring an STD include a higher number of lifetime sex partners, unprotected sex without use of a condom, risky sex partners, and the effect of alcohol or drugs on sexual decision making (Pollack et al, 2013).

Centers for Disease Control and Prevention Screening Recommendations

1. Annual chlamydia screening for all sexually active women age 25 and younger, as well as for women with risk factors such as new or multiple sex partners.
2. Annual gonorrhea screening for at-risk sexually active women, including women with new or multiple sex partners, or women who are living in areas with high rates of disease.
3. Syphilis, human immunodeficiency virus (HIV), and chlamydia screening for all pregnant women, and gonorrhea screening for at-risk pregnant women starting early in pregnancy, with repeat testing as needed.
4. At least once-per-year screening for syphilis, chlamydia, gonorrhea, and HIV for all sexually active gay, bisexual, and other MSM. Men who have multiple or anonymous partners should be screened more frequently for STDs, at 3- to 6-month intervals. More frequent screening is also recommended for MSM who use illicit drugs, particularly methamphetamine, or whose sex partners use them.

---

*The Centers for Disease Control and Prevention (CDC) provides national guidelines on the diagnosis and treatment of sexually transmitted diseases. The 2010 guidelines were used at the time this chapter was written (CDC, 2010c). These guidelines are periodically updated based on review of the most recent literature, and the reader is encouraged to check for updates from the CDC before treating patients with sexually transmitted diseases. Guidelines also include instructions for partner treatment and recommendations on follow-up.

Diseases That Must Be Reported to Local Health Authorities

Syphilis, gonorrhea, chlamydia, chancroid, HIV infection, and acquired immunodeficiency syndrome (AIDS) are reportable diseases in every state. Check requirements for reporting other STDs by state.

URETHRITIS

Urethritis, or urethral inflammation, can be the result of STDs. Symptoms include urethral discharge, pruritus, and dysuria. Several organisms can cause urethritis. Two broad classes are gonococcal urethritis (GU), caused by *Neisseria gonorrhoeae*, and nongonococcal urethritis (NGU), caused by all other organisms.

Diagnosis

Traditionally, urethritis is documented based on examination of the purulent discharge with Gram stain showing more than 5 white blood cells (WBCs) per high-power field (HPF), and documenting the presence or absence of white cells with intracellular gram-negative diplococci indicating GU. Looking at the urethral fluid can yield false-negative results, with reported sensitivity for more than 5 WBCs/HPF as low as 29% for chlamydial infection (Janier et al, 1995). Another criterion is a positive leukocyte esterase test result on first void urine or microscopic examination of first void urine sediment demonstrating more than 10 WBCs/HPF (CDC, 2010c). Nucleic acid amplification tests (NAATs) performed on urine can be used to look for *N. gonorrhoeae* and *Chlamydia trachomatis* (Geisler et al, 2005). **Culture and hybridization tests that require urethral swab specimens are available. However, NAATs are preferred because of their higher sensitivity** (Geisler, 2011), **and urethral swabs are no longer recommended for evaluation of urethritis.** All patients should be tested for both gonorrhea and chlamydia, given the high association of coinfection.

Gonococcal Infections

Neisseria gonorrhoeae is a gram-negative diplococcus. It is the second most common bacterial cause of STDs in the United States (CDC, 2013). The incubation period ranges from 3 to 14 days. Men will usually have symptoms that cause them to seek treatment soon enough to prevent transmission to others. This could include urethritis, epididymitis, proctitis or prostatitis. Women are frequently asymptomatic. Complications in women include pelvic inflammatory disease (PID), tubal scarring, infertility, ectopic pregnancy, and chronic pelvic pain (Short et al, 2009). Disseminated gonorrhea is rare today but can produce arthritis, dermatitis, meningitis, and

TABLE 15-1 Sexually Transmitted Disease Cases, 2012, Reported per 100,000 Population

	CASES REPORTED, 2012	RATE PER 100,000 PEOPLE	NOTES ON CHANGES
Chlamydia	1,422,976	456.7	Stable since 2011
Gonorrhea	334, 826	107.5	4.1% increase since 2011
Syphilis, primary and secondary	15, 667	5.0	11.1% increase since 2011
Chancroid	15		Decline 1987-2001, steady fluctuation since then

TABLE 15-2 Sexually Transmitted Disease Cases, 2012, Reported by Initial Visits to Physicians' Offices

SEXUALLY TRANSMITTED DISEASE	NUMBER OF CASES REPORTED DURING INITIAL VISITS TO PHYSICIANS' OFFICES
Genital herpes	228,000
Genital warts	353,000
Vaginal trichomoniasis	219,000
Other vaginitis	3,452,000

endocarditis. Gonorrheal infection can also increase the risk of contracting and transmitting HIV (Cohen et al, 1997).

Treatment

Dual therapy is required for both *N. gonorrhoeae* and chlamydia because of the high rate of coinfection. Gonorrhea treatment is hindered by the ability of gonorrhea to develop antimicrobial resistance. As of 2007, quinolones are no longer recommended in the United States for treatment of gonorrhea and associated conditions such as PID (CDC, 2007). As of August 2012, because of high resistance, cefixime is no longer recommended as first-line therapy to treat gonorrhea (CDC, 2012; Kirkcaldy et al, 2013). Current treatment of uncomplicated gonococcal infections of the cervix, urethra, and rectum involves ceftriaxone 250 mg IM single dose *plus* azithromycin 1 gm orally in a single dose or doxycycline 100 mg orally twice per day for 7 days. Because NAATs cannot provide susceptibility results, in cases of treatment failure a culture test should be performed along with antimicrobial susceptibility testing. All persons with gonorrhea should be tested for other STDs including chlamydia, syphilis, and HIV. Treatment is no different in persons with HIV. In persons with a history of penicillin allergy, third-generation cephalosporins have a low incidence of cross-reactivity, lower than the 5% to 10% in first-generation cephalosporins.

Nongonococcal Urethritis

Chlamydia trachomatis accounts for 15% to 40% of cases of NGU, with less common causes including *Mycoplasma genitalium* (15% to 25%), *Trichomonas vaginalis,* adenoviruses, and herpes simplex virus type 1 (HSV-1); a pathogen is not identified in 20% to 50% of cases (Deguchi and Maeda, 2002; Bradshaw et al, 2006; Tabrizi et al,

2007). HSV-1 urethritis may be associated with oral sex (Bradshaw et al, 2006).

Chlamydia

Chlamydia is the most common bacterial sexually transmitted STD in the United States. The 1,422,976 cases of *C. trachomatis* infection reported to the CDC in 2012 comprised the largest number of cases ever reported to the CDC for any condition (CDC, 2013). The incubation period ranges from 3 to 14 days. The prevalence of chlamydia is highest in persons 25 years of age or older (Geisler, 2011). Other sequelae of chlamydial infection in males include epididymitis and Reiter syndrome (Geisler et al, 2008). One of the main concerns with untreated chlamydial infections in men is transmission to their female partners (Geisler, 2011). Up to 75% of women with chlamydial infection can be asymptomatic. Ascending chlamydial infection can result in scarring of the fallopian tubes, PID, risk for ectopic pregnancy, pelvic pain, and infertility. The risk of untreated chlamydial infection producing PID is estimated to be between 9.5% and 27% (Gottlieb et al, 2013).

Mycoplasma genitalium *and* Ureaplasma

Mycoplasmas are the smallest prokaryotes capable of autonomous replication. The genus *Mycoplasma* belongs to the class Mollicutes, along with *Ureaplasma.* Mycoplasmas lack a cell wall and cannot be Gram stained. They contain a terminal adhesion structure that helps them attach to epithelial cells (Cazanave et al, 2012). *M. genitalium* was first described as a pathogen in urethritis in 1980, and considerable evidence since has established this organism as a cause of acute NGU (Manhart et al, 2011). Most infected patients are symptomatic, but approximately 25% may have asymptomatic urethral infection (Taylor-Robinson and Jensen, 2011). *M. genitalium* can become intracellular, which can establish a chronic infection and aid in avoidance of both immune response and antibiotics (McGowin et al, 2009). The prevalence of *M. genitalium* in chronic urethritis is estimated at 12% to 41% (Manhart et al, 2011). Risk factors for infection with *M. genitalium* in men are young age, sexual intercourse in the past month, and a sex partner with a recent history of STD diagnosis or treatment (Mena et al, 2002). Culture is very difficult, and the diagnosis is made by nuclear amplification or polymerase chain reaction (PCR), but no commercially available test is available (Cazanave et al, 2012; Sena et al, 2012).

Other species of Mollicutes include *Ureaplasma urealyticum* and *Ureaplasma parvum* (Cazanave et al, 2012). The evidence for *Ureaplasma* as a causative agent in NGU is conflicting (Taylor-Robinson et al, 1979). In a case control study of 329 men with symptoms of urethritis and controls without symptoms, both *U. urealyticum* and *U. parvum* were found more often in controls than in cases and therefore were not considered to be associated with NGU in this population (Bradshaw et al, 2006). A more recent series reported *U. urealyticum* in 24% of cases of NGU (Wetmore et al, 2011a). An explanation for the difference among numerous studies has been proposed by Wetmore and colleagues (2011b). In a case control series of men with clinical signs and symptoms of NGU and controls from an STD clinic or emergency room, the overall association of *U. urealyticum* and NGU was marginal, and *U. parvum* was not associated with NGU. However, in men with fewer than 10 lifetime vaginal sex partners, *U. urealyticum* was significantly associated with NGU. The hypothesis proposed is that adaptive immunity by repeated or prolonged exposure to *U. urealyticum* through multiple sex partners may result in asymptomatic infection without signs of urethral inflammation.

Trichomonas

Trichomonas vaginalis is a flagellated parasite that exclusively infects the urinary tract (Muzny and Schwebke, 2013). *T. vaginalis* is a common vaginal pathogen but also can cause urethritis in men. Among men attending an STD clinic, the prevalence is reported at

3% to 17% (Schwebke and Hook, 2003; Bachmann et al, 2011). Wet mounts examined for *T. vaginalis* have been traditionally used for diagnosis, with a sensitivity of only 60%; culture has also been used as the gold standard of diagnosis. Both are being supplanted by NAATs (Schwebke et al, 2011).

Treatment of Nongonococcal Urethritis

Patients are treated initially for both *N. gonorrhoeae* and chlamydia. Treatment is azithromycin 1 g orally as a single dose or doxycycline 100 mg orally twice per day for 7 days.

Recurrent and Persistent Urethritis

Persons who were noncompliant with the initial regimen or reexposed to an untreated sex partner can be treated again with the initial medications. Persistent symptoms after doxycycline treatment could be caused by doxycycline-resistant *M. genitalium*, or by *T. vaginalis*. A urine specimen can be sent for testing (Schwebke and Hook, 2003). Alternative regimens include metronidazole 2 g orally in a single dose or tinidazole 2 g orally in a single dose plus azithromycin 1 g orally in single dose (if not used in initial episode). Another choice for second-line therapy is moxifloxacin 400 mg orally for 7 days, which is effective against *M. genitalium* (Bradshaw et al, 2008). The resistance rate for *M. genitalium* to azithromycin has been reported at 16% to 24% (Bradshaw et al, 2008; Twin et al, 2012). In men with persistent symptoms, urologic evaluation does not usually identify a specific cause for the urethritis. One consideration is to make sure there is not pain elsewhere in the pelvis, which could indicate chronic pelvic pain syndrome as opposed to localized urethritis (Nickel et al, 2003).

EPIDIDYMITIS

Acute epididymitis is characterized by pain, swelling, and inflammation of the epididymis that lasts less than 6 weeks (Tracy et al, 2008). The testis is usually involved (epididymo-orchitis). Among sexually active men younger than 35 years, acute epididymitis is frequently caused by *C. trachomatis* or *N. gonorrhoeae*. Among MSM, acute epididymitis can be caused by enteric organisms such as *Escherichia coli* and *Pseudomonas* as a result of anal intercourse. Sexually transmitted acute epididymitis is usually also accompanied by urethritis, although this can be asymptomatic. In men older than 35 years, a sexually transmitted cause is uncommon, and the infecting organism is usually associated with bacteriuria from obstruction or benign prostatic hyperplasia (BPH), with *E. coli* the most common organism (Berger et al, 1979). There can be atypical organisms in men with HIV, including cytomegalovirus (CMV), *Salmonella*, *Ureaplasma*, *Corynebacterium*, *Mycoplasma*, and fungi (Parr et al, 1993; Hohmann, 2001). Chronic epididymitis is characterized by more than 6 weeks of pain in the scrotum, testicle, and epididymis. Chronic infectious epididymitis is most commonly seen with tuberculosis (TB), as a consequence of hematogenous spread rather than seeding of the urinary tract from the kidneys (Heaton et al, 1989).

The diagnosis of acute epididymitis includes ruling out testicular torsion, especially in younger patients. Scrotal ultrasonography can be helpful but is not always diagnostic (Pontari, 2013). The evaluation of acute epididymitis should include either a Gram stain of urethral secretions as noted earlier for urethritis, a urine dip for leukocyte esterase on first-void urine, or microscopic examination of the first-void urine demonstrating more than 10 WBCs/HPF. Urine can be sent for NAAT (CDC, 2010c). Empirical therapy is indicated before laboratory test results are available. First-line therapy in men younger than 35 years is ceftriaxone 250 mg IM plus doxycycline 100 mg orally twice per day for 10 days. For patients with suspected enteric organisms, treatment is ceftriaxone plus levofloxacin 500 mg orally twice per day for 10 days (CDC, 2010c).

GENITAL ULCERS

In the United States, most young sexually active patients who have ulcers (Table 15-3) have either genital herpes or syphilis, with genital herpes being more common. Less common causes are chancroid and donovanosis. Ulcers may also be associated with noninfectious causes such as yeast, trauma, malignancy, aphthae, fixed drug eruption, and psoriasis (CDC, 2010c). In addition to a history and physical examination, all patients with ulcers need serologic testing for syphilis and a darkfield examination if possible, culture or PCR testing for HSV, and diagnostic serology for determining the specific type of HSV. In environments where chancroid is prevalent, a test for *Haemophilus ducreyi* should be performed. Patients who are not known to be HIV positive should be tested for HIV. Even after complete diagnostic evaluation, 25% of patients with genital ulcers will have no laboratory-confirmed diagnosis. Biopsy of ulcers is indicated if they are unusual or do not respond to initial therapy.

Syphilis

Syphilis is caused by *Treponema pallidum*, a coiled spirochete bacterium. *Treponema pallidum* cannot be easily cultured. Transmission is usually by sexual contact, through microabrasions in skin and mucosal membranes in patients with primary and secondary syphilis (Ho and Lukehart, 2011). The risk increases with increasing numbers of sexual partners (French, 2007). Syphilis replicates at the site of the infection and divides every 30 to 33 hours (Fieldsteel et al, 1981). It is estimated that 50% to 60% of sexual contacts of individuals with early syphilis will acquire syphilis (Schober et al, 1983).

Primary Syphilis

The lesions occur at the initial site of infection. The incubation is typically 2 to 3 weeks but can range from 9 to 90 days for the appearance of lesions after infection (French, 2007). The lesions are usually single and painless but can be multiple, and up to one quarter of chancres can be painful (Read and Donovan, 2012). Local nontender lymphadenopathy is common. Untreated lesions heal spontaneously in 3 to 8 weeks (Ho and Lukehart, 2011). In men,

TABLE 15-3 Genital Ulcer Disease

DISEASE	LESIONS	LYMPHADENOPATHY	SYSTEMIC SYMPTOMS
Primary syphilis	**Painless,** indurated, with a clean base, usually singular	Nontender, rubbery, nonsuppurative bilateral lymphadenopathy	None
Genital herpes	**Painful** vesicles, shallow, usually multiple	Tender, bilateral inguinal adenopathy	Present during primary infection
Chancroid	Tender papule, then **painful,** undermined purulent ulcer, single or multiple	Tender, regional, painful, suppurative nodes	None
Lymphogranuloma	Small, **painless** vesicle or papule progresses to an ulcer	Painful, matted, large nodes with fistulous tracts	Present after genital lesion heals

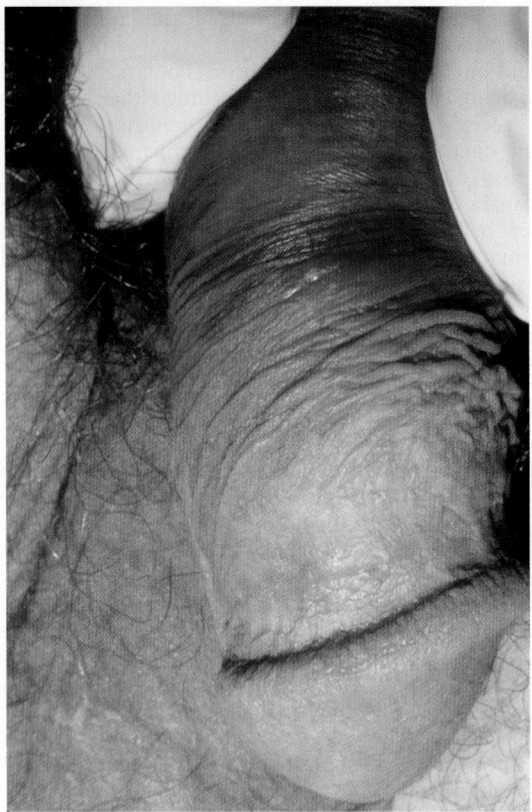

Figure 15-1. **Syphilis with penile chancre.**

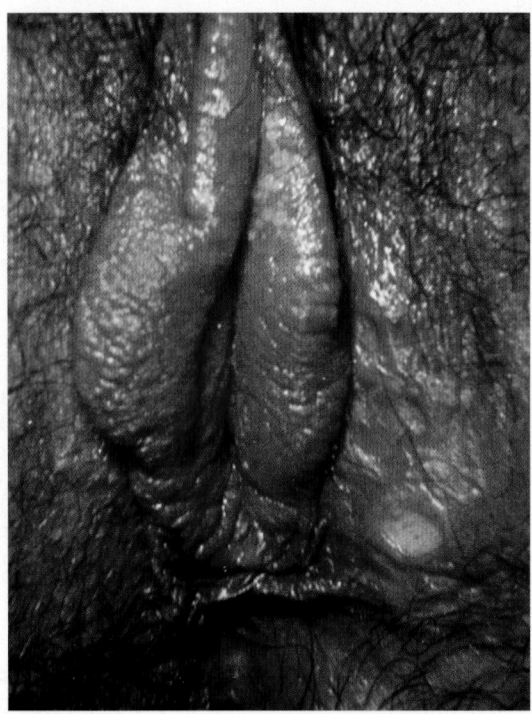

Figure 15-2. **Syphilis with vulvar chancre.**

lesions are typically on the glans or the coronal or perineal area (Fig. 15-1), and on the labia or perianal area in women (Fig. 15-2).

Secondary Syphilis

Treponema pallidum eventually becomes a systemic infection with bacteremia. Secondary syphilis appears 3 to 5 months after the

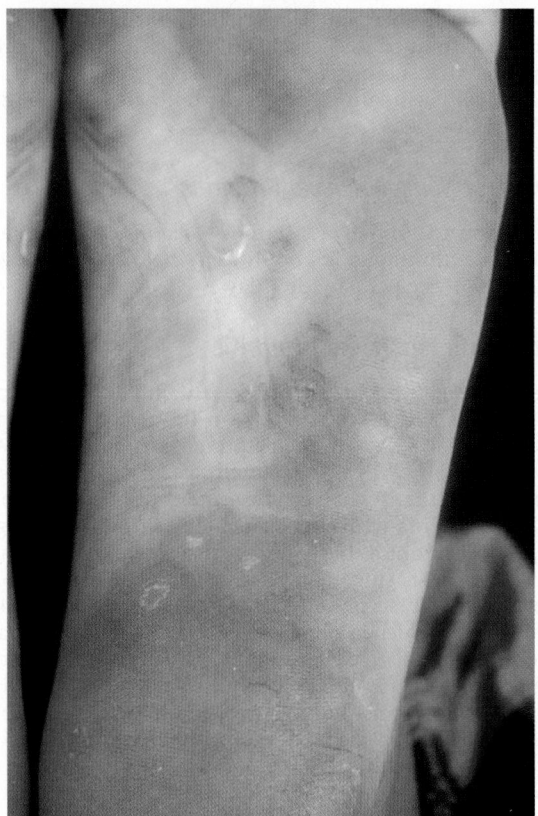

Figure 15-3. **Secondary syphilis affecting the soles of the feet.**

initial infection and is characterized by a maculopapular rash, which is often widespread and involves the scalp, palms, and soles of the feet in 75% of patients (Fig. 15-3) (Read and Donovan, 2012). The rash can ulcerate and lead to condyloma lata, which are wartlike lesions. Additional symptoms include fever, malaise, weight loss, patchy alopecia, and ocular inflammation (Mindel et al, 1989). There is also a broad vasculitis that in approximately 10% of patients may to manifestations such as hepatitis, iritis, nephritis, and neurologic problems including headache and cranial nerve involvement, especially VIII (auditory). Relapses usually occur in the first year after infection and rarely after the second year. The infection then becomes latent and asymptomatic.

Latent Syphilis

Latent syphilis is defined as seroreactivity with no clinical evidence of disease and is arbitrarily divided into early and late latent infection. To be diagnosed with early latent syphilis, the patient must have no signs of primary or secondary disease and have positive syphilis serology, preceded by negative serology in the past year, or recent contact with an infectious patient (CDC, 2010c). Asymptomatic patients with no evidence of recent negative serology or previous treatment are classified as having syphilis of unknown duration and are considered to have late latent syphilis (Read and Donovan, 2012).

Tertiary or Late Syphilis

About 35% of individuals with late latent syphilis will develop the late manifestations of syphilis, which include neurosyphilis, cardiovascular syphilis, and gummatous syphilis. These are rare outside of developing countries. Neurosyphilis can be seen in secondary syphilis, and meningovascular syphilis also occurs in tertiary syphilis. The incubation period is usually 5 to 12 years. After 10 to 20 years, the spinal column and brain can also be involved. The spinal cord syndrome is called *tabes dorsalis,* and the brain syndrome is also called *general paralysis of the insane* (Danielsen et al, 2004;

French, 2007). Cardiovascular syphilis occurs 15 to 30 years after infection and may occur in any large vessel (French, 2007).

Tests for Syphilis

Darkfield Examination. Cultures of *T. pallidum* are not possible in vitro. Direct tests include identification of *T. pallidum* under a dark-ground microscope from samples taken from a lesion, with a sensitivity rate of up to 97% (Wheeler et al, 2004). This, however, requires trained personnel.

Serology

Nontreponemal Tests. Measurement of antibodies is important for the screening and diagnosis of syphilis. There are two categories of tests: nontreponemal, which are directed against phospholipids, and treponemal, which are directed against *T. pallidum* polypeptides. Nontreponemal antibodies bind lipids that have bound to the treponeme and become antigenic (Lafond and Lukehart, 2006). Nontreponemal antibodies are detected with the rapid plasma reagin (RPR) test, the Venereal Disease Research Laboratory (VDRL) test, and the toluidine red unheated serum test (TRUST). Results are positive within 21 days but sometimes as long as 6 weeks after infection. They are universally positive in secondary syphilis (Read and Donovan, 2012). **Nontreponemal test results need confirmation with a treponemal test because they can be positive in other conditions such as viral infections, pregnancy, malignancies, autoimmune disease, and advanced age** (Larsen et al, 1995). False-negative reactions occur if there is an excess of antibodies that overwhelm the assay, called the *prozone effect* (CDC, 2010c). **Nontreponemal tests are used to monitor disease activity. A fourfold change in titer equivalent to a change of two dilutions (e.g., from 1:16 to 1:4) is considered necessary to demonstrate a clinically significant difference. The same test should be used in a given person because the tests are not directly comparable** (CDC, 2010c). Nontreponemal tests usually become nonreactive with time after treatment, but in some patients levels of the antibodies can persist for a long time, including for the lifetime, a response referred to as the *serofast reaction* (CDC, 2010c).

Treponemal Tests. Treponemal antibodies are detected by immunofluorescence in the fluorescent treponemal antibody absorption (FTA-ABS) test or by agglutination in the microhemagglutination assay for *T. pallidum* (MHA-TP), the *T. pallidum* hemagglutination assay (TPHA), or the *T. pallidum* particle agglutination (TP-PA) test. False-positive results are uncommon but can occur in patients with collagen disease, systemic lupus erythematosus, and other infections (Hart, 1986). **Treponemal test results remain positive for life except in 15% to 25% of patients treated early for primary syphilis** (Young et al, 2009). **Treponemal tests are not used to determine disease activity or treatment response.**

Other Tests. Polymerase chain reaction to identify *T. pallidum* may prove to be useful, with a sensitivity of 94.7% and specificity of 98.6% reported (Palmer et al, 2003). Rapid syphilis tests including enzyme-linked immunosorbent assays (ELISAs) are also available and are U.S. Food and Drug Administration (FDA) approved and cheaper than the nontreponemal tests usually used for initial diagnosis. They can give results in 5 to 20 minutes but cannot distinguish between active and treated syphilis (Ho and Lukehart, 2011). A newer paradigm of testing is to use the rapid test first, and if the result is positive, to perform a nontreponemal test with titers to guide management. If the nontreponemal test result is negative, a different treponemal test should be performed.

Coinfection with Human Immunodeficiency Virus

Of patients becoming infected with syphilis, up to 25% are HIV infected, and the incidence rate for syphilis in HIV patients has been reported as 77 times that of the general population (Chesson et al, 2005). The clinical course of syphilis in a person with HIV is similar to that in immunocompetent persons. However, HIV-positive patients may have larger ulcers in the primary phase and may be at risk for a more rapid progression to neurosyphilis with a CD4 count

of 350 or lower and/or a nontreponemal serologic test result of 1:32 or higher (French, 2007). Occasionally an unusual serologic response may occur with a false-negative result. If the clinical course strongly suggests syphilis and serologic test results are negative, consider other tests such as biopsy of lesion or rash (CDC, 2010c). **All patients with syphilis should be tested for HIV.**

Treatment of Syphilis

The standard treatment for all stages of syphilis is penicillin G. The stage and clinical manifestations of syphilis determine the preparation, dosage, and length of treatment. Treatment guidelines from the CDC are presented in Table 15-4 (CDC, 2010c). Not considered appropriate treatment are combinations of benzathine and procaine penicillin (Bicillin C-R), nor is oral penicillin. Patients with HIV receive the same treatment regimen as non–HIV-infected persons. **A reaction consisting of fever, malaise, nausea, and vomiting, called the Jarisch-Herxheimer reaction, can occur. This is not an allergic reaction to penicillin but occurs with treatment of the treponemes, and more commonly with treatment with penicillin and in early syphilis. It may also be associated with chills and exacerbation of secondary rash. Treatment is with bed rest and nonsteroidal anti-inflammatory medications.** Signs of treatment failure include persistent or recurring signs and symptoms of syphilis, and sustained fourfold increase in

TABLE 15-4 Treatment of Syphilis (Centers for Disease Control and Prevention 2010 Guidelines for Treatment of Sexually Transmitted Diseases)

STAGE OF SYPHILIS	PENICILLIN TREATMENT	PENICILLIN-ALLERGIC PATIENTS
Primary, secondary, and early latent syphilis, no neurologic involvement	Benzathine penicillin G 2.4 million units IM, single dose	Doxycycline 100 mg PO bid for 2 wk Tetracycline 500 mg PO qid for 2 wk
Late latent or latent syphilis of unknown duration, no neurologic involvement	Benzathine penicillin G 2.4 million units IM once per week for 3 wk	Doxycycline 100 mg PO bid for 28 days Tetracycline 500 mg PO qid for 28 days
Tertiary (late) syphilis without neurologic involvement	Benzathine penicillin G 2.4 million units IM once per week for 3 wk	Consult infectious disease specialist
Neurosyphilis Alternative regimen	Aqueous crystalline penicillin G 3-4 million units IV q4h, or continuous IV infusion for total 18-24 million units per day, for 10-14 days Procaine penicillin 2.4 million units IM daily plus probenecid 500 mg PO qid, both for 10-14 days	

nontreponemal test result or failure to decrease fourfold within 6 months of therapy. Patients should be (1) retested for HIV, (2) evaluated for neurosyphilis with cerebrospinal fluid (CSF) examination, and (3) re-treated with weekly injections of benzathine penicillin G, 2.4 million units IM for 3 weeks, unless neurosyphilis is diagnosed.

Herpes

Herpes simplex virus type 1 and HSV-2 are double-stranded DNA viruses. They share 83% sequence homology of their protein coding regions and share similar structure of their genomes (Gupta et al, 2007). They can be distinguished serologically. HSV-1 causes mainly oral infections but now accounts also for at least half of first episodes of genital HSV infections (Roberts et al, 2003). This is thought to be a combination of later acquisition of oral HSV-1, which would confer immunity to the genital infection, and increase in oral sex in young adults (Halpern-Felsher et al, 2005). HSV-2 causes genital herpes and is transmitted by sexual contact. Women are more susceptible to HSV-2 infection than men and are more likely to have symptomatic infections (Langenberg et al, 1999). Most HSV-2 transmission thus occurs from individuals who do not know they are infected (Mertz, 2008). In a study of 5452 adults attending primary care offices in the United States, the seroprevalence of HSV-2 was 25.5%, but only 12% of these patients reported a history of prior infection (Leone et al, 2004). HSV-2 infection seems to protect against HSV-1 infection, but HSV-1 gives only a small amount of protection from infection with HSV-2 (Looker and Garnett, 2005).

Pathophysiology

Herpes simplex virus initiates replication in epithelial cells at the site of entry, damages the cells, and enters the ends of peripheral sensory nerves. It is then transported in a retrograde manner to the cell body in the sensory root ganglia. In the initial infection, herpes also spreads to the local and regional lymph nodes. Once in the nerve cell body, HSV enters a latent state (Jerome et al, 1998). Recurrence and reactivation of virus occur with transportation in the peripheral nerves back to the mucosal or skin surface. Events that trigger reactivation of HSV include local trauma such as surgery or ultraviolet light, immunosuppression, or fever (Gupta et al, 2007). Recurrence can lead to recurrence of lesions from mucosal or skin disruption or may occur in the absence of recognizable lesions. This is termed *asymptomatic* or *subclinical shedding* (Wald et al, 1995; Wald et al, 2000).

Natural History and Diagnosis

The classic first presentation of primary herpes is clusters of erythematous papules and vesicles on the external genitalia that do not follow a neural distribution (Figs. 15-4 and 15-5). This usually occurs 4 to 7 days after sexual intercourse (Looker and Garnett, 2005). Many herpetic lesions do not have the classic appearance and may look like fissures or furuncles, and in women may manifest as vulvar erythema (Koutsky et al, 1992). Patients have pain, burning, or itching, and 80% of women report dysuria. Other associated symptoms include fever, headache, malaise, and myalgias (Corey et al, 1983). Tender inguinal and femoral lymph nodes may be present. Primary genital HSV-1 infection cannot be distinguished from HSV-2 infection on clinical examination alone, but requires laboratory testing. Over the next 2 to 3 weeks, 75% of patients have new lesions, which can progress to vesicles and pustules and can coalesce into ulcers before crusting and healing (Corey et al, 1983). Possible complications include aseptic meningitis and autonomic dysfunction that can lead to urinary retention (Corey et al, 1983).

Recurrent Episodes

A primary genital herpes infection with either HSV-1 or HSV-2 is more severe in the absence of preexisting HSV-1 immunity (Corey

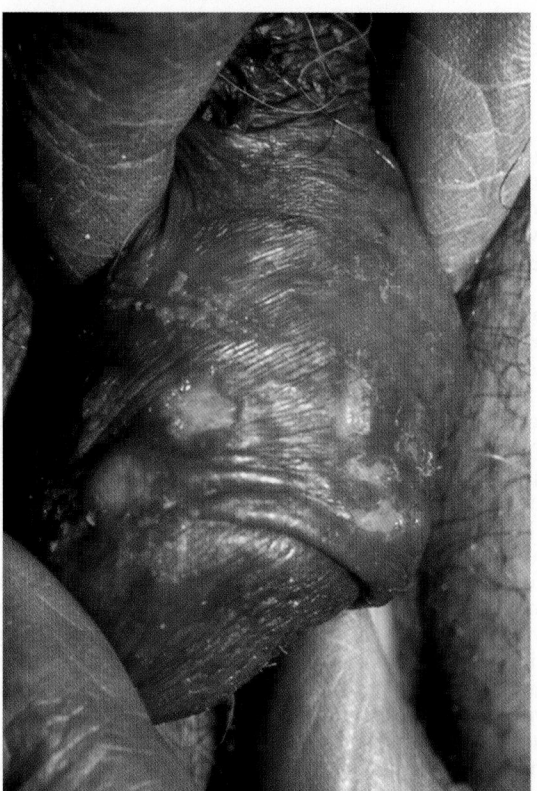

Figure 15-4. Herpes simplex virus infection on the penis.

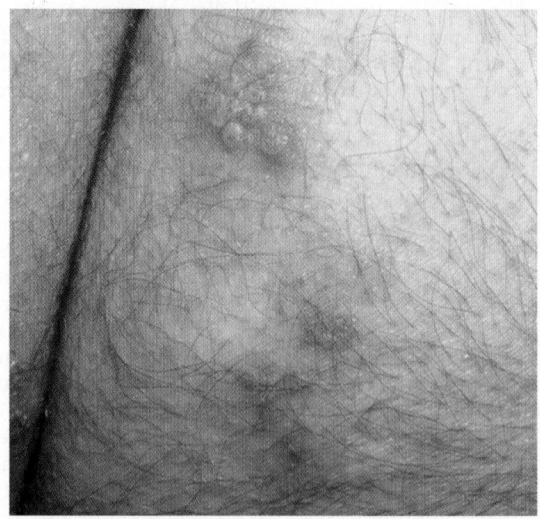

Figure 15-5. Typical vesicular eruption of herpes simplex virus.

et al, 1983). Subsequent recurrent episodes with established immunity are milder than the initial infection. **Genital HSV-1 recurs much less frequently (0.02 recurrences per month) than genital HSV-2 infections (0.23 recurrences per month), on the order of 10-fold less** (Lafferty et al, 1987a). Although shedding is greatest in the first 6 to 12 months, it can continue for years (Schacker et al, 1998; Benedetti et al, 1999). Lesions heal in 5 to 10 days in the absence of antiviral treatment. HSV recurrences decrease after the first year, although some spike in recurrences in HSV-2 even after 4 years of follow-up have been noted (Benedetti et al, 1999).

Diagnosis and Testing for Herpes Simplex Virus

A definitive diagnosis of HSV subtype should be made both to confirm the diagnosis and to obtain important prognostic

TABLE 15-5 Recommended Oral Treatment for Genital Herpes Simplex Virus Infection

AGENT	FIRST CLINICAL EPISODE	EPISODIC THERAPY	SUPPRESSIVE THERAPY
Acyclovir	400 mg tid for 7-10 days *or* 200 mg 5 times/day for 7-10 days	400 mg tid for 5 days *or* 800 mg tid for 2 days *or* 800 mg bid for 5 days	400 mg bid
Famciclovir	250 mg bid for 7-10 days	125 mg bid for 5 days *or* 1000 mg bid for 1 day *or* 500 mg once, followed by 250 mg bid for 2 days	250 mg bid
Valacyclovir	1 g bid for 7-10 days	500 mg bid for 3 days *or* 1 g sid for 5 days	500 mg sid *or* 1 g sid

Modified from Workowski KA, Berman S; Centers for Disease Control and Prevention (CDC). Sexually transmitted diseases treatment guidelines, 2010. MMWR Recomm Rep 2010;59(RR-12):1–110.

information, given the clinical disparity between genital HSV-1 and HSV-2. In patients with lesions, fluid can be obtained from the base of the genital lesion and sent for viral culture, HSV antigen detection, or PCR of HSV DNA (Rose et al, 2008; Nguyen et al, 2010). The detection rate for HSV from lesions is 80% for primary infections but only 25% to 50% for recurrent lesions, and even less if the lesion has begun to heal (Lafferty et al, 1987b). In patients with no active lesions, serology must be used—that is, testing for antibodies. Specific immunoglobulin G (IgG) testing for glycoprotein G of HSV-1 or HSV-2 can distinguish the two types of HSV (Ashley, 2001). Serology is recommended for confirmation of a clinical diagnosis of genital herpes in patients with recurrent genital symptoms, atypical lesions, or healing ulcers and negative viral cultures. Type-specific antibodies to herpesvirus can take from 2 weeks to 3 months to develop; thus in a person with newly acquired herpes, an initial negative serology followed by a positive test after 12 weeks confirms a new infection (CDC, 2010c).

Treatment *(Table 15-5)*

Currently available medications to treat herpes do not eradicate the virus, but aim to reduce the signs and symptoms of infection and to prevent new lesions. Available drugs include acyclovir (intravenous only), valacyclovir, and famciclovir (CDC, 2010c). Treatment for a first clinical episode should be started on clinical grounds before laboratory confirmation of diagnosis. Treatment is usually 7 to 10 days but should be extended if lesions are not adequately healed (CDC, 2010c). Intravenous acyclovir (5 to 10 mg/kg every 8 hours) may be needed for those with neurologic complications, those unable to take oral medications, or those with widespread disease (e.g., immunocompromised patients) (Gupta et al, 2007). **Treatment of recurrent episodes reduces their severity and duration. Oral therapy within 24 hours of the first signs or symptoms of recurrence increases the chance of resolving a recurrence without lesions** (Leone et al, 2002; Wald et al, 2002; Aoki et al, 2006). In patients with frequent recurrences, daily suppressive therapy can be used to reduce recurrences by 70% to 80% (Wald et al, 2006). Patients with HIV can have prolonged or severe episodes of HSV infection, and HSV shedding is increased in HIV-infected persons. Doses and durations of medications are increased for suppression and treatment of episodic HSV infections in persons with HIV (CDC, 2010c).

Chancroid

Chancroid is caused by the gram-negative bacterium *H. ducreyi* (Lewis, 2003). Infection leads to anogenital ulceration and lymphadenitis with progression to bubo formation (Lewis and Ison, 2006). The incubation period is 3 to 10 days, with the initial

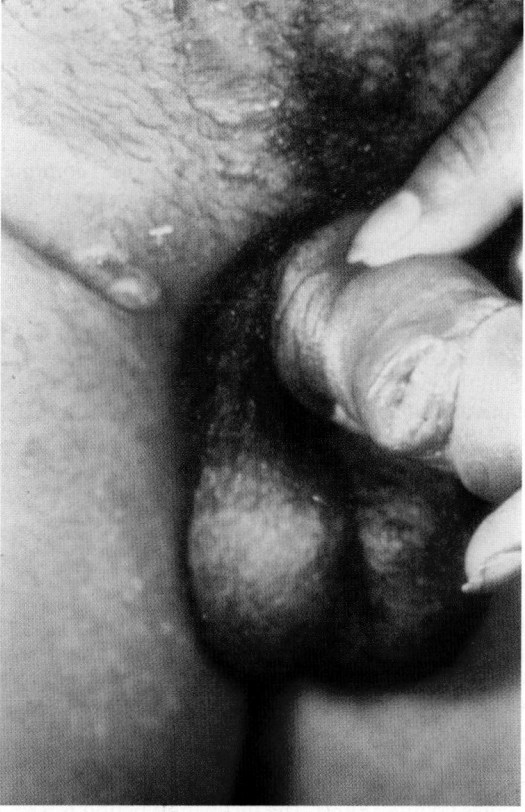

Figure 15-6. Chancroid with regional adenopathy.

presentation of a papule that may progress to form an ulcer (Fig. 15-6) (Lewis and Ison, 2006). Circumcised men are at lower risk of being infected with chancroid (Weiss et al, 2006). The prevalence of chancroid has declined in the United States (CDC, 2013), but chancroid is still endemic in other parts of the world such as Africa, Asia, Latin America, and parts of the Caribbean; a genital ulcer in a person with a history of travel to these areas should raise suspicion for chancroid (Lewis and Ison, 2006). Chancroid, like genital herpes and syphilis, is a risk factor for transmission of HIV (Magro et al, 1996).

A definitive diagnosis of chancroid requires culture on media not routinely available (Lockett et al, 1991). There are no FDA-approved tests. **The CDC suggests that a probable diagnosis of chancroid can be made if (1) the patient has one or more painful ulcers;**

(2) no evidence of *T. pallidum* is present on darkfield examination of ulcers or by serologic testing for syphilis performed at least 7 days after onset of the ulcers; (3) ulcers and lymphadenopathy, if present, are typical for chancroid; and (4) results of tests for HSV on the ulcer exudate are negative (CDC, 2010c). Treatment is with azithromycin 1 g in a single dose or ceftriaxone 250 mg IM in single dose or ciprofloxacin 500 mg orally twice per day for 3 days or erythromycin base 500 mg orally three times per day for 7 days. Patients should be tested for HIV at the time of diagnosis of chancroid. If initial test results were negative, repeat testing at 3 months for syphilis and HIV should be performed. Patients with HIV are less likely to respond to treatment, have slower healing of ulcers, and may require longer courses of therapy (CDC, 2010c).

Granuloma Inguinale

Granuloma inguinale is an infection by the intracellular gram-negative bacterium *Klebsiella granulomatis* (formerly called *Calymmatobacterium granulomatis*) that produces genital ulcers. Granuloma inguinale does not usually occur in the United States. The most common locations in the world for granuloma inguinale are Papua New Guinea, South Africa, parts of India and Brazil, and the aboriginal community in Australia (Lagergard et al, 2011). The incubation period averages 50 days (O'Farrell, 2002). The disease manifests as painless, slowly progressive ulcers on the genitals and perineum. Despite the name, inguinal involvement is uncommon (10%) (Velho et al, 2008). The lesions are described as beefy red because of high vascularity, and they bleed easily. The most common site of extragenital spread is the mouth, producing loss of teeth from bone destruction, but it can also occur in the pelvis, intra-abdominal organs, and other bones (especially the tibia) (Velho et al, 2008).

The bacterium is a strict human pathogen, which makes culture difficult. Diagnosis requires visualization of dark-staining Donovan bodies on crush preparation or biopsy, described by Donovan in 1905 (Richens, 2006). These are intracellular inclusions of the bacteria within the cytoplasm of macrophages and appear deep purple when stained with Wright, Giemsa, or Leishman stain (Lagergard et al, 2011). There are no FDA-cleared molecular tests for detection of *K. granulomatis*. Treatment is with doxycycline 100 mg orally twice per day for at least 3 weeks and until all lesions have healed (CDC, 2010c).

Lymphogranuloma Venereum

Lymphogranuloma venereum (LGV) is an infection by *Chlamydia*, specifically serovars L1, L2 or L3 (Mabey and Peeling, 2002). Traditionally, LGV is rare in developed countries but is endemic in parts of Africa, Asia, South America and the Caribbean (Mabey and Peeling, 2002). However, the incidence of LGV, especially in MSM, has been rising since the infection was first described in Western Europe in 2003, and LGV is occurring worldwide including in the United States (White, 2009). The incubation period is 3 to 30 days. A self-limited genital ulcer or papule sometimes is present at the site of infection but usually has disappeared by the time of presentation. The secondary stage is the most common presentation in heterosexuals and is marked by tender inguinal and/or femoral lymphadenopathy, typically unilateral (Fig. 15-7). Inguinal lymph nodes are more common in men because the lymph drainage of the cervix and vagina are to the retroperitoneal rather than the inguinal lymph nodes (Mabey and Peeling, 2002). Inguinal lymph nodes above and below the inguinal ligament can give rise to the "groove sign" in 10% to 20% of patients (Schachter and Osoba, 1983). Rectal exposure in women or MSM can result in proctitis with hemorrhoids, rectal or anal pain, rectal discharge, constipation, and fever (Arnold et al, 2013). A third stage can develop. If left untreated, LGV proctocolitis can develop into chronic colorectal fistulas and strictures. Chronic infection can also lead to lymphatic obstruction with elephantiasis of the genitalia in either sex. LGV does not appear to occur more frequently or with any more virulence in HIV-positive individuals (Jebbari et al, 2007).

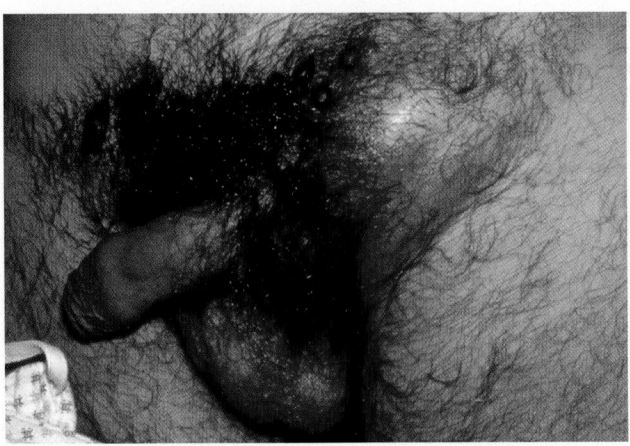

Figure 15-7. Lymphogranuloma venereum with inguinal adenopathy.

Diagnosis is made by swab of lesions or aspiration of buboes from genitals or lymph nodes, sent for culture, direct immunofluorescence, or nucleic acid detection. NAATs are used for urethral specimens but are not FDA approved for rectal specimens. *Chlamydia* serology with complement fixation titers exceeding 1 : 64 can support the diagnosis of LGV (CDC, 2010c). When specific diagnostic testing is not available, the patient should be presumptively treated for LGV. Treatment is with doxycycline 100 mg orally twice per day for 21 days (CDC, 2010c).

Human Papillomavirus

Human papillomavirus (HPV) is a double-stranded DNA virus belonging to the Papillomaviridae family. More than 100 types of HPV exist, of which more than 40 types of HPV can infect the genital area and be sexually transmitted (Dunne et al, 2011). Types 6 and 11 are nononcogenic and are responsible for about 90% of anogenital warts (Gissmann et al, 1983; Garland et al, 2009). Other subtypes including 16 and 18 account for cervical cancer and other types of anogenital cancer including vulvar, vaginal, anal, and penile cancers (De Vuyst et al, 2009; Li et al, 2011). Although certain HPV types are associated with certain morphologic characteristics, the association is not absolute. The usual keratinizing squamous cell penile cancer is associated with HPV in only 11% of patients, with much higher rates of HPV DNA positivity strongly associated with either basaloid or warty changes (47%) or purely basaloid changes (75%) (Giuliano et al, 2008).

More than 50% of sexually active persons will become infected at least once in their lifetime (Myers et al, 2000). Approximately 70% of HPV infections resolve spontaneously in 1 year and 90% in 2 years, and HPV persistence develops in the remaining persons (Veldhuijzen et al, 2010). Transmission can occur from asymptomatic and subclinical patients. Among asymptomatic women in the general population, the prevalence of HPV infection ranges from 2% to 44%, and among men from 2.3% to 34.8% (Burchell et al, 2006). HPV infection starts at the basal cell layer of stratified squamous epithelial cells, which then stimulates cell proliferation in the epithelium. HPV warts can also occur in the urethra and can cause hematuria, dysuria, or difficulty voiding. Bowenoid papulosis involves reddish brown verrucous papules on the penis that are a low-grade carcinoma in situ with a chance of malignant transformation of 2% to 3% (Cubie, 2013). Buschke-Lowenstein tumors, or giant condyloma acuminatum, are large verrucous exophytic lesions on the penis or perineum, associated with HPV-6 or HPV-11. These tumors are considered a low-grade verrucous carcinoma, and in general only local invasion is present (Armstrong et al, 2009; Cubie, 2013).

Lesions such as warts can be seen clinically (Figs. 15-8 and 15-9), but HPV virus can also be present and subclinical. Latent viruses are detectable only through demonstration of HPV DNA in skin or

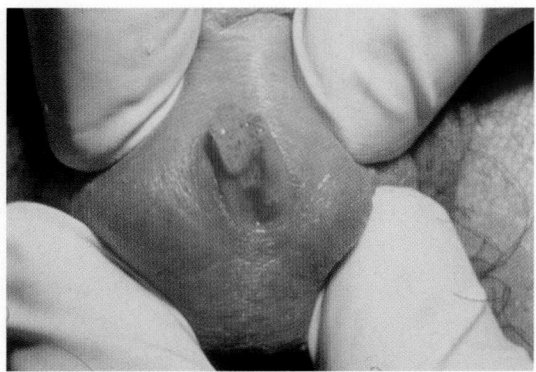

Figure 15-8. Meatal wart caused by human papillomavirus.

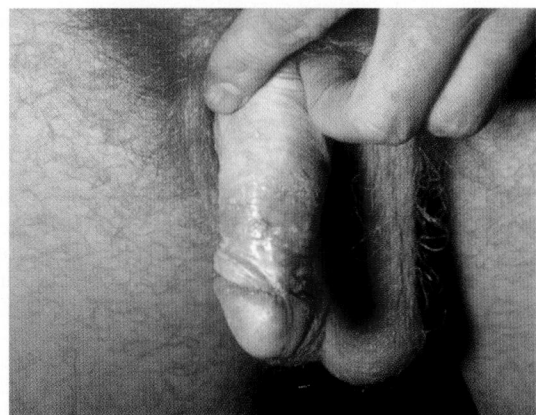

Figure 15-9. Penile warts.

mucosa (Cubie, 2013). The use of acetic acid to detect nonvisible skin lesions is not recommended because of the large number of false-positive results. HPV tests that detect viral nucleic acid (i.e., DNA or RNA) or capsid protein are available for women older than 30 years undergoing cervical cancer screening. These tests should not be used for men, for women younger than 20 years, or as a general test for STDs (CDC, 2010c). In the following situations, biopsy may be warranted to rule out a malignant lesion: (1) the diagnosis is uncertain; (2) the patient is immunocompromised; (3) the warts are pigmented, indurated, or fixed; (4) the lesions do not respond to or they worsen with standard treatment; (5) there is persistent ulceration or bleeding.

Treatment

The goal of treatment is removal of the warts; treatment will not eradicate the infection. Treatment is guided by wart size, number, and location, and patient preference. Treatment regimens are divided into patient-applied and provider-applied modalities (CDC, 2010c).

Patient-applied treatments for HPV (note: these are not approved for use during pregnancy):

1. Podofilox 0.5% solution or gel up to 0.5 mL/day, applied twice per day for 3 days, then no therapy for 4 days, up to four cycles. Total wart area should not exceed 10 cm^2.
2. Imiquimod cream 5% once daily at bedtime, three times per week up to 16 weeks; should be washed off 6 to 10 hours after application.
3. Sinecatechins 15% ointment (sinecatechins are major poly-phenols found in green tea leaves) (Dunne et al, 2011), three times per day for up to 16 weeks. This should not be washed off after application. Avoid sexual contact with the ointment on the skin. Not recommended in patients with HIV, those

who are otherwise immunocompromised, or those with herpes.

Provider-administered treatments:

4. Podophyllin resin 10% to 25% in tincture of benzoin, applied to wart and allowed to dry. This can be repeated weekly. To avoid complications from systemic absorption and toxicity, ensure that (1) application is limited to an area less than 10 cm^2 or less than 0.5 mL of podophyllin is used and (2) the treatment area does not contain any open lesions or wounds.
5. Cryotherapy such as liquid nitrogen, which induces cytolysis. Application can be repeated every 1 to 2 weeks. Providers should be trained in the use of this method. Large warts may need local anesthesia because of possible pain with application.
6. Trichloroacetic acid (TCA) or bichloroacetic acid (BCA) 80% to 90%; these acids destroy warts by chemical coagulation of wart proteins. Apply to wart and allow to dry before patient stands up; if intense pain ensues after administration, neutralize the acid with soap and water or sodium bicarbonate. Can be repeated weekly.
7. Surgical therapy including direct excision with scissors, tangential shave excision, curettage, or laser therapy using a CO$_2$ laser (Aynaud et al, 2008). Consider collaboration with a plastic surgeon for large lesions that require large areas of excision, especially on the penis or in the groin creases.

Urethral warts are usually caused by HPV subtypes at low risk for malignancy (Beutner et al, 1999). Treatments for urethral meatal warts include cryotherapy with liquid nitrogen and podophyllin 10% to 25% compounded in tincture of benzoin. The adjacent skin must be dry before treatment. Men with external urethral warts should undergo urethroscopy to rule out intraurethral warts (Fralick et al, 1994). Bladder warts may also be present. 5-Fluorouracil has been used intraurethrally, but its use is limited by the significant inflammation produced. Holmium laser can be used for lesions in the urethra and bladder. A biopsy is recommended to rule out any malignant or precancerous lesions.

Human Papillomavirus Vaccine

In June 2006, a quadrivalent HPV vaccine (Gardasil) was licensed for use in the United States in girls and women aged 9 to 26 years (Markowitz et al, 2007) In October 2009, this vaccine also was licensed for use in boys and men aged 9 to 26 years (CDC, 2010b). This vaccine provides protection against HPV types 6, 11, 16, and 18. In October 2009, a bivalent HPV vaccine (Cervarix) that provides protection against types 16 and 18 was licensed for use in girls and women aged 10 to 25 years (CDC, 2010a). Overall the bivalent vaccine prevents HPV types that cause 70% of cervical cancer and the quadrivalent vaccine prevents HPV types that cause 70% of cervical cancers and 90% of genital warts. Either vaccine is recommended for girls starting at age 11 to 12 and can be given to girls as young as age 9. Girls and women aged 13 to 26 who have not started or completed the vaccine series should also receive the vaccine. It is most effective if started before the onset of sexual activity. The vaccine is given as a three-dose series of intramuscular shots over a 6-month period. Women should still undergo regular cervical cancer screening because 30% of cervical cancer is caused by other HPV subtypes. The vaccines are not licensed for use in women older than 26 years in the United States (Dunne et al, 2011).

The quadrivalent vaccine is used in males to prevent genital warts and in both genders to prevent anal cancer (Dunne et al, 2011). MSM are particularly at risk for developing anal intraepithelial neoplasia and anal cancer (Burchell et al, 2006). As in women and girls, it is best started before the onset of sexual activity. The vaccines are designed to prevent infection and are not effective in clearing an infection once established (Markowitz, 2007). The use of the vaccine is still relatively low, with 49% of girls and women aged 13 to 19 having received at least one dose and 32% having received three doses in a 2010 survey. Despite

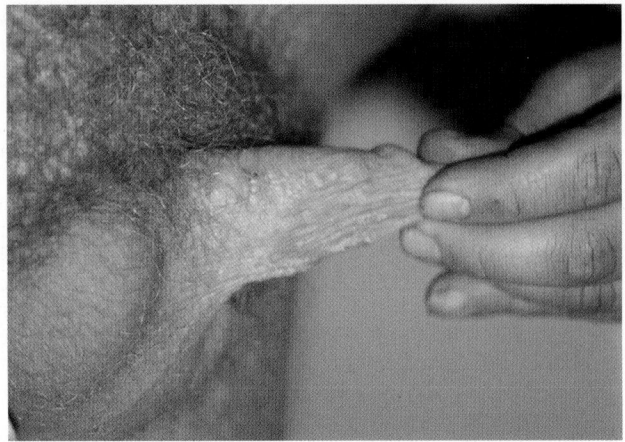

Figure 15-10. **Scabies affecting the penis.**

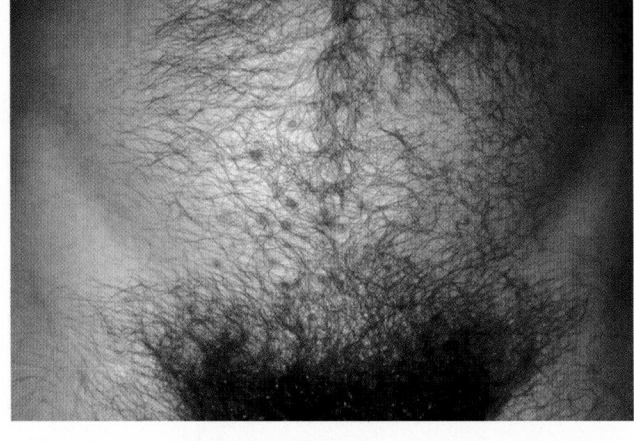

Figure 15-11. **Molluscum contagiosum on the abdomen.**

low rates of use, the prevalence of vaccine HPV subtypes in girls and women declined from 11.5% during the years 2003-2006 to 5.1% during the period 2007-2010 after initiation of the vaccine (Markowitz et al, 2013).

Scabies

Scabies is a skin infection caused by the mite *Sarcoptes scabiei* var. *hominis* and has been known for over 2500 years (Chosidow, 2000). The female lays eggs in the skin, and transmission is by person-to-person skin-to-skin contact with passage of pregnant female mites. This can occur during sexual contact (Fig. 15-10). Scabies also commonly passes from person to person in crowded conditions (Hay et al, 2013) and by contact with infected bedding or clothing. Symptoms usually do not appear for 2 to 6 weeks after infestation, and infected persons can pass the mites in the absence of symptoms (Chosidow, 2000). The most common symptoms are skin rash and itching, especially at night, from an allergic reaction to the mite proteins. Female scabies mites can tunnel under the skin, producing tiny raised and crooked or serpiginous lines on the skin. Scratching at a sore can lead to infection with *Staphylococcus aureus* or β-hemolytic streptococci. These secondary infections have been associated with poststreptococcal glomerulonephritis (Svartman et al, 1972).

A more concentrated area of mites can form a crust and is called *crusted* or *Norwegian scabies*. This may occur in persons who have difficulty scratching or are prevented from scratching, such as those with spinal cord injury or mental disability, and also occurs in elderly and immunocompromised persons, including those with HIV infection. These individuals are very contagious (Chosidow, 2000). Diagnosis is made by demonstration of mites, mite eggs, or fecal matter (scybala) on microscopic examination of a skin scraping. Treatment is with permethrin cream (5%) applied to all areas of the body from the neck down and washed off after 8 to 14 hours or ivermectin 200 μg/kg orally, repeated in 2 weeks. An alternative is lindane (1%) lotion or cream, but this is used only if the patient cannot tolerate other therapies or if other therapies have failed, because lindane toxicity causes central nervous system (CNS) effects, seizures, and aplastic anemia (Chosidow, 2006). Bedding and clothing should be decontaminated by washing and drying on the hot cycles, or by removal and placement in a decontamination bag for longer than 72 hours. Scabies do not generally survive more than 2 or 3 days away from human skin.

Pediculosis Pubis *(Phthirus pubis):* Pubic or Crab Louse

Pediculosis (lice) has been known for 10,000 years (Orion et al, 2004). Lice are obligate bloodsucking parasites of humans. The pubic lice are much shorter than those that occur on the scalp or body. Transmission requires close contact. The female's life cycle

lasts for 1 to 3 months. Females lay eggs (nits) at the skin-hair junction; they mature into lice in 20 days. Pubic lice infestation is common in sexually active persons and tends to recur in gay men. Transmission is not prevented with use of condoms. Pubic lice specifically have a serrated surface on their claws to facilitate clinging to flat, hairless surfaces (Orion et al, 2006). In children, the presence of pubic lice does not imply a definite sexual contact, as they can be acquired by contact with an infected parent (Chosidow, 2000).

The typical presentation is pruritus, which is caused by a delayed hypersensitivity reaction to the lice. First exposure can result in symptoms in 2 to 6 weeks (Orion et al, 2004). Symptoms develop more quickly with subsequent exposures, on the order of 1 to 2 days. Eggs remain in situ after releasing their larvae (nymphs), and empty shells can remain on the hair for many months after the infection has been eradicated; therefore the diagnosis is only by identifying live lice or viable eggs (Chosidow, 2000). Treatment is permethrin 1% cream rinse applied to affected areas and washed off after 10 minutes or pyrethrins with piperonyl butoxide applied to affected areas and washed off after 10 minutes (CDC, 2010c). Bedding and clothing should be decontaminated by dry cleaning; washing and drying at high temperature; or removal from body contact for 72 hours. Patients with pediculosis pubis should be evaluated for other STDs.

Molluscum Contagiosum

Molluscum contagiosum is a superficial skin disease caused by the pox virus. The virus contains double-stranded DNA and replicates entirely in the cytoplasm of infected cells, independent of the host nucleus (Myskowski, 1997). It can be sexually transmitted. Characteristic lesions are small, discrete waxy papules 3 to 5 mm in diameter, with a central depression (Fig. 15-11). The central core can be expressed, producing a white material. Localized eczematous dermatitis is commonly seen around the lesions (Chen et al, 2013). The infection is usually self-limited and spontaneously disappears in 6 to 12 months, but may take up to 4 years to resolve. However, infection in immunocompromised individuals, such as those with HIV, is typically more severe and extensive. Patients with HIV may develop widespread and large lesions including "giant" lesions larger than 15 mm in diameter (Cronin et al, 1996). Increase in the number of lesions can be seen in HIV patients as a manifestation of the immune reconstitution syndrome, which occurs shortly after the initiation of antiretroviral therapy (ART) in severely immunocompromised patients (Pereira et al, 2007). Diagnosis is generally on the basis of the characteristic appearance of skin lesions. Biopsy is indicated in cases of unclear diagnosis, especially in immunocompromised patients with unusual presentations in which malignancy must be excluded (Trope and Lenzi, 2005). Skin biopsy will show typical "molluscum bodies" or Henderson-Patterson bodies, which are eosinophilic inclusions in the epidermis (Eleftheriou et al, 2011).

One option for treatment is waiting, because the infection is generally self-limited. Rapid treatment options include cryotherapy (freezing the lesions), curettage with piercing of the lesion and removal of the contents, and laser therapy. Oral therapy with cimetidine has been used (Dohil and Prendiville, 1996). Topical therapies include podophyllotoxin cream 0.5% in men (this cannot be used in pregnant women because of fetal toxicity), iodine and salicylic acid, potassium hydroxide (KOH), cantharidin (a blistering agent), and imiquimod (Gottlieb and Myskowski, 1994). A first treatment in HIV patients is to use ART. The number of molluscum contagiosum lesions is inversely proportional to the CD4 cell count (Myskowski, 1997). Regression of recalcitrant molluscum contagiosum lesions after initiation of ART has been reported (Cattelan et al, 1999). Systemic and topical cidofovir may be beneficial in treating large molluscum contagiosum lesions associated with immunosuppression (Davies et al, 1999).

Vaginitis

Vaginal infections are characterized by discharge, itching, or odor. Three diseases most frequently associated with vaginal discharge are bacterial vaginosis (BV), trichomoniasis, and candidiasis. BV and trichomoniasis are sexually transmitted. The diagnosis can be made via Amsel's criteria: pH, a KOH test, and microscopic examination of fresh samples of the discharge (Table 15-6).

Bacterial Vaginosis

Bacterial vaginosis is caused by replacement of the normal hydrogen peroxide–producing *Lactobacillus* species in the vagina with high concentrations of anaerobic bacteria including *Prevotella*, *Mobiluncus*, *Gardnerella vaginalis*, *Ureaplasma*, *Mycoplasma*, and other fastidious anaerobes. Although BV is the most common diagnosis in women seeking care for vaginal symptoms, most women with BV are asymptomatic. Women with BV are at risk for acquisition of some STDs including HIV, *N. gonorrhoeae*, *C. trachomatis*, and HSV-2. Diagnosis can be made by Gram stain, evaluating for relative amounts of *Lactobacillus* and other bacteria characteristic of BV. Characteristic findings for BV on microscopic examination are clue cells, which are vaginal epithelial cells covered with bacteria. Recommended treatment regimens include metronidazole 500 mg orally twice per day for 7 days or metronidazole 0.75%, one full applicator (5 g) intravaginally once per day for 5 days or clindamycin cream 2%, one full applicator (5 g) intravaginally at bedtime for 7 days (CDC, 2010c). Note that clindamycin is oil based and may weaken condoms and diaphragms for 5 days after use.

Trichomoniasis

Trichomoniasis is caused by the protozoan *T. vaginalis*. The discharge from trichomoniasis is diffuse, malodorous, and yellow green with vulvar irritation; however, not all women infected are symptomatic. Diagnosis is usually by microscopy of vaginal secretions showing the *Trichomonas* organisms. The sensitivity of microscopy is only 60% to 70%. There are two FDA-approved rapid tests for *Trichomonas*: the OSOM Trichomonas Rapid Test (Sekisui Diagnostics, Lexington, MA), which uses immunochromatographic capillary flow dipstick technology, and the Affirm VPIII (Becton, Dickinson and Company, Sparks, MD), which is a nucleic acid probe test. Culture is also available for *T. vaginalis*. Treatment is metronidazole 2 g orally in a single dose or tinidazole 2 g orally in single dose (CDC, 2010c). **Patients are advised to abstain from alcohol consumption for 24 hours after taking metronidazole and 72 hours after tinidazole.** Evidence suggests interaction between HIV and *T. vaginalis* such that *T. vaginalis* infection in HIV-infected women might enhance HIV transmission by increasing genital shedding of the virus (Wang et al, 2001). In women with HIV, a multidose treatment regimen of metronidazole, 500 mg orally given twice per day for 7 days, is recommended instead of one 2-g dose (Kissinger et al, 2008; Kissinger et al, 2010).

Candidiasis

Vulvovaginal candidiasis is usually caused by *Candida albicans* but occasionally by other species of *Candida* or yeasts. Vaginal candidiasis is classified as complicated or uncomplicated based on clinical criteria (CDC, 2010c). Uncomplicated cases involve infections that are sporadic or infrequent, produce mild to moderate symptoms, are likely to be caused by *C. albicans*, and occur in immunocompetent women. Complicated cases involve recurrent candidiasis (four or more episodes of symptomatic vulvovaginal candidiasis in 1 year), severe infection, non–*C. albicans* cause, and women with uncontrolled diabetes, debilitation, or immunocompromise. Approximately 10% to 20% of cases of vulvovaginal candidiasis will be complicated. Vaginal cultures should be obtained in patients with recurrent vulvovaginal candidiasis because conventional antimycotic treatments are not as effective against atypical species such as *Candida glabrata*. The diagnosis is made via wet prep with saline or KOH; a Gram stain of vaginal discharge that demonstrates yeast, hyphae, or pseudohyphae; or a culture that shows *Candida* or other yeast species. Wet mounts should first be done for all patients, and culture used for those with symptoms with negative wet mounts.

Treatment for uncomplicated vulvovaginal candidiasis includes numerous over-the-counter intravaginal agents including butoconazole or clotrimazole creams, miconazole as a cream or intravaginal suppository, or tioconazole ointment. Prescription treatment formulations include butoconazole cream, terconazole cream or vaginal suppository, nystatin vaginal suppository, or one oral dose of fluconazole 150 mg (CDC, 2010c). A woman who has persistent symptoms or a recurrence 2 months after having used an over-the-counter treatment should be evaluated. In cases of recurrence, a longer duration of therapy such as 7 to 14 days of topical therapy or a dose of fluconazole every third day for a total of three doses is

TABLE 15-6 Differential Diagnosis of Vaginitis in Women

	VAGINAL DISCHARGE	pH	WHITE BLOOD CELLS	MICROSCOPY	SYMPTOMS
Normal	White, thick, smooth	≤4.5	Absent	Lactobacilli	None
Candidiasis	White, thick, curdlike	≤4.5	Absent	Mycelia	Vulvar pruritus, external or superficial dysuria
Trichomoniasis	Frothy or purulent	≥4.5	Present	Mobile trichomonads present Amine odor	Vulvar erythema and edema, punctate strawberry lesions on cervix
Bacterial vaginosis	Thin, white homogeneous	≥4.5	Absent	Paucity of lactobacilli (75% of patients) Amine odor Clue cells	Fishy odor and increased vaginal discharge

recommended (CDC, 2010c) Treatment for non–*C. albicans* vulvovaginal candidiasis is not standardized.

HUMAN IMMUNODEFICIENCY VIRUS/ACQUIRED IMMUNODEFICIENCY SYNDROME AND THE UROLOGIST

HIV is a retrovirus that infects T cells and dendritic cells (Klasse, 2012). HIV spreads through blood, semen, vaginal fluid, or breast milk. The resultant immunosuppression leads to AIDS. The diagnosis of AIDS is made if the CD4 count is less than 200 cells/mm³ or if there is a serious opportunistic infection, neoplasm, or other life-threatening condition. A total of 26 conditions are AIDS defining, including cervical cancer, lymphomas, and infections with *Candida* and CMV (National Institutes of Health, 2013).

Estimates of the national HIV incidence in the United States are calculated by the CDC. At the end of 2010, approximately 1.1 million Americans were living with HIV, and it was estimated that 16% did not know they were infected (Lansky et al, 2010). Approximately 50,000 new infections occur each year, a number that has remained stable since the mid-1990s (Hall et al, 2008). HIV occurs more often in some populations. Of new infections, two thirds occur in MSM, with over half occurring in young black men. Heterosexuals accounted for one quarter of all new infections in 2010, two thirds of those being women. Injections drug users made up 8% to 10% of new cases (Lansky et al, 2010). The most affected age group was 25 to 34 years (31%), followed by 13 to 24 years (26%) and 35 to 44 years (24%) (CDC, 2014).

See Expert Consult website for details.

Diagnosis of Human Immunodeficiency Virus Infection

The CDC recommends HIV screening for all patients aged 13 to 64 in health care settings (Branson et al, 2006). Patients should be counseled and notified that testing will be performed and given the option to decline or defer testing. Written consent is not usually required. Diagnosis of HIV includes using serologic tests that detect antibodies against HIV-1 (and HIV-2) and virologic tests that detect HIV antigens or RNA. The initial test is a screening test for antibodies, the conventional or rapid enzyme immunoassay (EIA). The initial result can be obtained in 30 minutes. Positive or reactive screening tests must be confirmed by a supplemental antibody test, Western blot and indirect immunofluorescence assay (IFA), or virologic test, the HIV-1 RNA assay (CDC, 2004). A positive confirmation test result establishes the diagnosis. HIV is detectable in 95% of patients within 3 months after infection. During this initial 3-month period, the "window" period, the screening test result may be negative but the person may still be infected. Virologic tests for HIV-1 RNA can be used to detect an acute infection in persons negative for HIV antibodies. This should be used with the initial antibody test in the setting of suspicion of acute retroviral syndrome (see the discussion of acute infection). A positive RNA test result should be confirmed by a subsequent antibody test. The majority of infections in the United States are HIV-1. HIV-2 infection should be suspected in persons with an unusual clinical presentation or with risk factors including having lived or having a sex partner from an endemic area (West Africa, Portugal), having a sex partner known to be HIV-2 positive, or having had a blood transfusion or nonsterile injection in an endemic area (CDC, 2004, 2010c).

See Expert Consult website for details.

Urologic Manifestations of Human Immunodeficiency Virus Infection

Interaction with other Sexually Transmitted Diseases

Testing for HIV is recommended in anyone with a diagnosed STD or who is at risk for an STD (CDC, 2010c). In many populations, the pattern of HIV acquisition parallels that of other STDs (Quinn et al, 1988; Clottey and Dallabetta, 1993); the presence of an STD increases the risk for both transmitting and acquiring HIV infection. STDs that produce ulcers are particularly associated with HIV; the adjusted OR for the effect of genital ulcer disease on increase in the risk of acquiring HIV is 2.2 to 11.3 (Quinn et al, 1990; Hook et al, 1992; Fleming and Wasserheit, 1999).

Several factors likely contribute to this association (Fleming and Wasserheit, 1999). Genital ulcers bleed frequently during intercourse, potentially leading to increased infectiousness. HIV has been detected in genital ulcer exudates (Kreiss et al, 1989). In HIV-seronegative individuals, ulcers may increase susceptibility to infection by disrupting mucosal integrity and by recruiting HIV-susceptible immune cells to the site of the ulcer, as in *H. ducreyi* infection (Magro et al, 1996). HSV infection may make keratinocytes also vulnerable to HIV, expanding the targets for infection (Heng et al, 1994). HSV also increases HIV replication in persons infected with both viruses (Van de Perre et al, 2008). Non–ulcer-producing STDs such as chlamydia and gonorrhea increase HIV shedding by recruiting HIV inflammatory cells in infected individuals (Moss et al, 1995). HIV shedding is associated with gonorrhea, cervicitis, and vaginitis in women (Mostad et al, 1997); higher levels are associated with concomitant infection with *M. genitalium* (Manhart et al, 2008). HIV-infected patients can also have larger lesions as in the case of HPV with giant condyloma (Fig. 15-16).

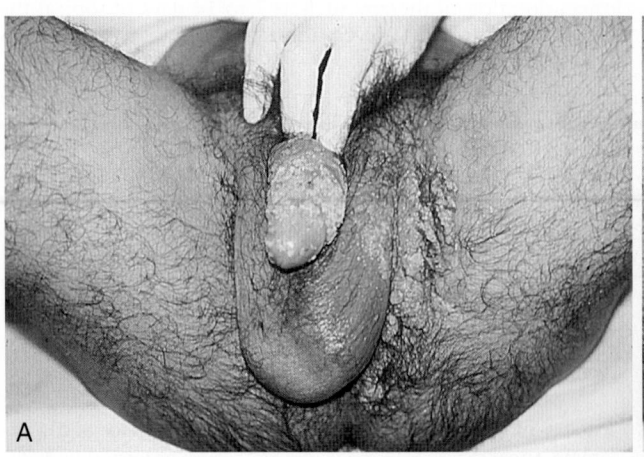
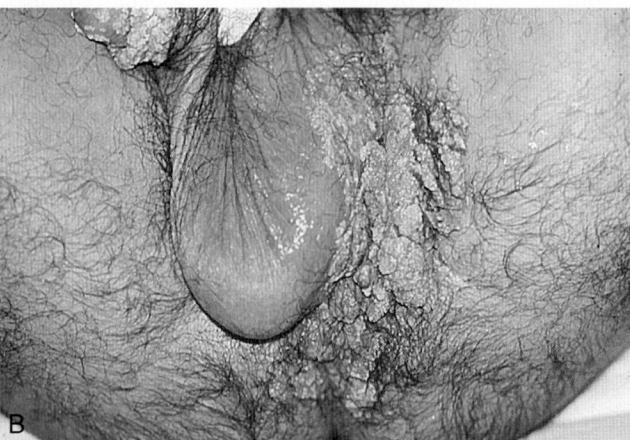

Figure 15-16. A and **B,** Acquired immunodeficiency syndrome patient with extensive genital condyloma.

Renal Infections

Mycobacterial infection of the kidney is detected at autopsy in 6% to 23% of AIDS patients, and a significant number had no symptoms before death (Shindel et al, 2011a). Persons with HIV infection are more likely to develop clinical TB if infected, including renal and other extrapulmonary disease (Weiss et al, 1998). Treatment for TB may include rifampin, which induces cytochrome P450 and lowers concentrations of protease inhibitors and NNRTIs. HIV patients being treated for TB should be monitored carefully, and drug levels may have to be monitored and adjusted (Sterling et al, 2010). Other renal infections that occur in AIDS include CMV (van der Reijden et al, 1989) and *Aspergillus* and *Toxoplasma* infections. Abscesses may develop that require drainage, percutaneous or open, or nephrectomy.

Prostatitis

Prostate infection may be more common in men with HIV. One study of 209 hospitalized men with HIV reported bacterial prostatitis in 8%, with the incidence increasing from 3% in men with asymptomatic HIV infection to 14% in patients with AIDS (Leport et al, 1989). Most of the men were symptomatic with fever and urinary symptoms; prostate tenderness was not universal but was found on examination in 41%. Prostatitis is usually caused by *E. coli*, but in HIV-infected men many other organisms can cause prostate infection, including *S. aureus, Klebsiella pneumoniae, Pseudomonas aeruginosa, Serratia marcescens, Salmonella* Typhi, *Mycobacterium tuberculosis* and *Mycobacterium avium intracellulare*, and CMV (Weinberger et al, 1988; Benson and Smith, 1992). Fungal infections also can cause prostatitis, particularly in immunocompromised patients with T-cell counts below 200 cells/μL. Organisms include *C. albicans, Aspergillus fumigatus, Cryptococcus neoformans*, and *Histoplasma capsulatum* (Santillo and Lowe, 2006).

In men with HIV, cultures should be performed not only for the usual bacteria, but also for more atypical organisms including aerobes, anaerobes, fungi, and *M. tuberculosis* (Heyns and Fisher, 2005). The usual treatment in these men is a 4- to 6-week course of antimicrobials; in men with HIV, consideration should be given to low antimicrobial suppression for some time to reduce the risk of recurrence (Santillo and Lowe, 2006). In patients who are already being treated with ART and still persistently immunocompromised, lifetime suppressive antimicrobials have been recommended to reduce risk of progression to prostatic abscess (Lee et al, 2001). Prostate abscess can develop from relapsing or untreated infection and usually occurs in more severely immunocompromised patients. The incidence of prostate abscess in men with HIV has been reduced by use of ART, which has decreased the incidence of opportunistic infections (Murphy et al, 2001), and also by the use of long-term antibiotics in HIV men with bacterial or atypical urinary tract infections (UTIs). Diagnosis is made by transrectal ultrasound or computed tomography (CT) scan. It is important to prevent progression to sepsis by using broad-spectrum antimicrobials and performing surgical drainage.

Urinary Tract Infection

In a prospective study of urine cultures in a group of HIV-positive men, 30% of the group with CD4 counts below 200 had an episode of bacteriuria, which was significantly greater than in the group with CD4 counts of 200 to 500 (11%) and above 500 (0%) (Hoepelman et al, 1992). There was no association with age or practice of anal intercourse. Of the episodes of bacteriuria, 42% were asymptomatic. The incidence of bacteriuria also increases with progression to AIDS (De Pinho et al, 1994). The bacteria found in UTI in HIV-infected individuals may be different as well. Data from a single site showed that over a 9-year period, the most common organism causing UTI in HIV-infected patients, men and women, was *Enterococcus* (26%), whereas in uninfected controls it was *E. coli* (64.8%). *Proteus* was also found five times more often in the HIV-infected group (Schonwald et al, 1999). In severely immunocompromised patients, unusual organisms may cause UTIs, including CMV (Benson et al, 1988). The mucosa may appear normal with a CMV infection, and deep biopsies may be needed to diagnose CMV interstitial cystitis (Whitaker et al, 2008). Other urinary infections include fungi such as *Cryptococcus, Candida*, or *Aspergillus* (Kiertiburanakul et al, 2004); other viruses including erythrovirus B19 (parvovirus B19) (Christensen et al, 2001) and adenovirus; and parasites such as *Toxoplasma gondii* and *Mycobacterium* (Heyns et al, 2009).

Overall, the incidence of bacteriuria does not appear to be greater in women with HIV but can be associated with the amount of viral load (Park et al, 2002). The management of UTI may be complicated by the concomitant use of other antibiotics for prophylaxis for other infections in HIV-infected patients. The use of co-trimoxazole as prophylaxis against pulmonary infection did not reduce the risks of UTI in a series of HIV-positive patients (Evans et al, 1995). However, the use of the other antibiotics may select out for antibiotic resistance. Among the bacterial isolates found in 350 episodes of symptomatic UTI in HIV-infected subjects, 29 of 36 *E. coli* isolates were multidrug resistant. Overall, 83% of bacterial isolates were resistant to trimethoprim-sulfamethoxazole (Vignesh et al, 2008). These findings should help inform empirical therapy for symptomatic UTI in these patients.

Testis, Epididymis and Seminal Vesicles

HIV in semen is the main vector for transmission and can persist despite high loads of ART (Roulet et al, 2006). The interstitium of the testis contains cells that have the receptors and coreceptors CXCR4, CCR5, CD4, and DC-SIGN, and is permissive to HIV infection. These cells appear to be macrophages (Roulet et al, 2006). The seminal vesicles also appear to be a reservoir for HIV, again with infection located in macrophages (Deleage et al, 2011).

The most common intrascrotal pathology in men with HIV/AIDS is testicular atrophy. This can arise from endocrine imbalances, febrile episodes, malnutrition, testicular infections, and toxic effects of therapy (Leibovitch and Goldwasser, 1994). A correlation has also been shown with body mass index (BMI); underweight HIV patients were 3.5 times more likely to have testicular atrophy on autopsy (Mhawech et al, 2001). The histology in men with HIV is peritubular interstitial inflammation, interstitial fibrosis, and thickening of the basement membrane (De Paepe et al, 1989). Spermatogenesis is decreased and maturation arrest is observed (Leibovitch and Goldwasser, 1994). HIV itself is thought to be cytotoxic to germ and Sertoli cells; on average, 30% of germ cells are infected (Shevchuk et al, 1998).

The testes may also be directly infected by opportunistic infections. Up to 39% of examined testes in autopsy series may have an opportunistic infection (Leibovitch and Goldwasser, 1994). The most common pathogens are CMV, *T. gondii*, and *M. avium intracellulare* (Lo and Schambelan, 2001). Treatment requires initial antibiotic therapy followed by a period of maintenance suppression, particularly if *Salmonella* is identified as the causative organism (Shindel et al, 2011a). Patients with AIDS are also prone to develop tuberculous epididymitis (Heyns et al, 2009). As a result of atrophy, infection, or other insult, testicular failure can occur. **In combination with extratesticular causes, testosterone levels fall with progressive HIV disease** (Lo and Schambelan, 2001; Moreno-Perez et al, 2010a).

Renal Function

Many factors affect renal function in patients with HIV/AIDS (Miro et al, 2012). HIVAN has received considerable attention because of the rapid clinical decline in these patients, the progression to irreversible renal failure, and the predilection for African Americans (Pardo et al, 1984; Rao et al, 1984). The classic clinical presentation is that of rapidly progressive azotemia with severe proteinuria, often nephrotic range, and little or no peripheral edema. The initial pathologic lesions described were global or focal segmental glomerulosclerosis (FSGS). Other features added to the description include collapse of glomerular capillary loops, called "collapsing glomerulopathy" (Weiss et al, 1986). A recent review of a large case series of kidneys with HIVAN also described a new variant, termed the "fetal variant" because histologically it resembles a fetal glomerulus (Wearne et al, 2012). There appears to be a spectrum of histologic findings now associated with HIVAN, making the consensus definition in flux (Wearne et al, 2012).

The pathogenesis of HIVAN involves infection of renal epithelial cells by HIV virus, including podocytes, glomerular parietal epithelial cells, and tubular cells (Leventhal and Ross, 2008). Infection can be by cell free virus or by transfer of virus from infected T cells to renal tubular epithelial cells (Chen et al, 2011). The *vpr* and *nef* gens of HIV-1 are the most responsible for inducing HIVAN (Leventhal and Ross, 2008). Recently the genetic predisposition to HIVAN has been characterized. African-Americans carrying two variants of the *APOL-1* gene are at very high risk to develop HIVAN. These genes encode a secreted lipid binding protein called *apolipoprotein-1 (apoL1)*. The variants G1 and G2 are common in African chromosomes but absent in European chromosomes; these variants lyse trypanosomes, including *Trypanosoma brucei rhodesiense,* which causes African sleeping sickness (Genovese et al, 2010). Thus, these loci are thought to be selected out in this population. The presence of these two genes together increases the risk by 29-fold, resulting in a 50% risk of development of HIVAN in untreated individuals (Kopp et al, 2011) as compared with a 12% baseline risk (Shahinian et al, 2000). FSGS found in individuals with the two risk genes also occurs at an earlier age and progresses much more rapidly (Kopp et al, 2011). There also may be a contribution from the myosin heavy chain gene 9 *(MYH9)*, which is a locus adjacent to the *APOL-1* gene on chromosome 22 and has been implicated in rare kidney disease producing glomerulosclerosis and podocyte effacement (Hays and Wyatt, 2012). Podocyte specific deletion of *Myh9* predisposes mice to renal injury (Johnstone et al, 2011). *APOL-1* and *MYH9* are likely contributors to HIVAN, but not the only contributors (Kopp et al, 2008).

The incidence of HIVAN can be decreased by treatment to reduce the viral load (Lucas et al, 2004). The study by Wearne and colleagues from South Africa (Wearne et al, 2012) included findings from a time when ART had not yet been endorsed or provided by the South African government. Therefore data are available on the untreated natural history of HIVAN. The 50% survival of those patients with HIVAN without ART was 4.47 months. The use of ART, no matter when started, reduced the mortality by 57%. Patients with better estimated glomerular filtration rate (eGFR) at presentation had better outcomes (adjusted hazard ratio [AHR] 0.72).

Voiding Dysfunction

Early series on voiding dysfunction in HIV-positive patients reported on neurogenic bladder in patients largely with AIDS and neurologic complications (Gyrtrup et al, 1995; Menéndez et al, 1995). Detrusor areflexia was commonly seen in patients with AIDS (Khan et al, 1992), but more patients with non-AIDS HIV had detrusor hyperreflexia (overactivity) (Kane et al, 1996). With the use of ART, patients are living longer and having less severe complications, and therefore it is expected that there will be an increase in incidence of voiding dysfunction as a result of aging in this group. In an Internet survey of MSM, HIV status was an independent risk factor for bothersome lower urinary tract symptoms (LUTS), and a history of AIDS was a risk factor for severe disease. Other risk factors for moderate but not severe LUTS were UTI, prostatitis, and gonorrhea. Although the cause of the association is not known, this study raised the question as to whether a direct toxic effect of the virus or ART leads to LUTS (Breyer et al, 2011).

Hematuria

A study from 1995 reviewed the records of 1326 patients with HIV in the U.S. Air Force. Urinalysis was performed and found a high rate of hematuria at 25%. Of the 67 patients with hematuria who underwent evaluation, management was affected in three patients (4%). The recommendation at that time was that in young asymptomatic HIV-positive patients with microscopic hematuria, a urologic evaluation could be omitted (Cespedes et al, 1995). Of note in this study is that grade 1 hematuria was defined as 1 to 4 red blood cells (RBCs) per HPF; given the current definition of microhematuria as 3 or more RBCs per HPF, some of these patients who were diagnosed with microhematuria might not be diagnosed according to current criteria. Of the men with renal cell cancer in a recent series of patients with HIV, 44% had hematuria on presentation (Gaughan et al, 2008). Given the greater life expectancy of patients infected with HIV on ART, hematuria in the setting of HIV infection should be evaluated as in other individuals.

Erectile Dysfunction

The prevalence of mild, moderate, and severe erectile dysfunction (ED) is reported as being higher in HIV-infected than uninfected men for all decades of age. On multivariate analysis, HIV infection is the strongest predictor of ED, with an OR of 42.26 ($P < .001$) (Crum et al, 2005; Ende et al, 2006; Crum-Cianflone et al, 2007; Zona et al, 2012). Other studies have shown that progression to AIDS also leads to greater ED (Shindel et al, 2011b). ED is common in HIV-infected men under age 50, reported as 50% of infected men younger than age 30 years, 48% of those aged 31 to 40 years, and 53% of those aged 41 to 50 years (Zona et al, 2012). HIV also leads to an increased risk and earlier onset by 10 to 15 years of other comorbidities including coronary disease, diabetes, and bone fractures (Guaraldi et al, 2011). Thus, ED is thought to be one of the manifestations of an early aging phenomenon that is being seen in HIV-infected individuals. Other factors also influence the development of ED in this population, including depression (Crum-Cianflone et al, 2007), psychological distress associated with changes in body composition (lipodystrophy) (Guaraldi et al, 2012), hypogonadism (Crum et al, 2005; Zona et al, 2012), and diabetes (Shindel et al, 2011b). Endothelial dysfunction as measured by brachial artery flow-mediated dilation was not associated with ED in men with HIV (Guaraldi et al, 2012).

The role of ART in the development of ED in men with HIV is uncertain. Several studies have shown an association with ART, including duration of ART (Moreno-Perez et al, 2010b), and particularly protease inhibitors (Martinez et al, 1999; Lamba et al, 2004; Asboe et al, 2007). Other studies have not confirmed these associations (Ende et al, 2006; Zona et al, 2012). One consideration in treating ED in men with HIV is the possible interaction of phosphodiesterase type 5 (PDE5) inhibitors and antiretroviral medications. PDE5 inhibitors depend on CYP3A for clearance, and all protease inhibitors and NNRTIs are inhibitors of CYP3A to some extent (Rosen et al, 2006). This can lead to a significant increase in the serum dose of PDE5 inhibitors, and therefore they should be started at the lowest dose possible in patients taking these ART medications (Merry et al, 1999).

Stones and Human Immunodeficiency Virus

One of the complications of some medications for treatment of HIV is stone formation. The protease inhibitors specifically may cause stone formation. Indinavir can form crystals in the urine (Kopp et al, 1997). The incidence of indinavir stones is reported to be as high as 22% (Brodie et al, 1998). The risk has been reported to be greater in patients with hepatitis (Malavaud et al, 2000) or hemophilia (Brodie et al, 1998). Indinavir stones are typically radiolucent on both plain film and CT scan but can also be mixed with calcium and appear radiopaque (Sundaram and Saltzman, 1999). Newer inhibitors including lopinavir, atazanavir, amprenavir, and nelfinavir have also been associated with the development of stones, but with less frequency than reported for indinavir (Shindel et al, 2011a). The incidence of stones with atazanavir was 0.97% in one series (Couzigou et al, 2007). One possible risk factor for atazanavir stones is the discontinuation of tenofovir. Concomitant administration of tenofovir lowers circulating levels of atazanavir, so discontinuation increases plasma levels;

this was thought to play in a role in several cases of atazanavir stones (Fabbiani et al, 2011).

Hydration after taking protease inhibitors is suggested as means to reduce the risk of stone formation (Daudon et al, 1997). In patients with protease stones and in whom conservative management is possible as a first-line step, discontinuation of the drug and hydration should be tried. Success with these measures approaching 70% has been reported (Kohan et al, 1999). Patients with HIV can have other conditions that contribute to stone formation including dehydration with high specific gravity, low pH, hyperoxaluria, hypercalciuria, and hypocitraturia (Gagnon et al, 2000; Nadler et al, 2003). One other type of stone reported to be more common in HIV patients is ammonium acid urate stones, possibly reflecting chronic diarrhea and malnutrition of chronic disease (Nadler et al, 2003).

Human Immunodeficiency Virus and Neoplasms

In the earlier history of HIV infection, the predominant oncologic problems were AIDS-defining cancers, Kaposi sarcoma (KS), non-Hodgkin lymphoma, and, in women, invasive cervical cancer. With the advent of more effective therapies, ART has markedly improved life expectancy, turning HIV into a chronic disease. The emphasis has shifted to non–AIDS-defining cancers (Bonnet et al, 2009). Overall, patients with HIV compared with the general population still have a greater risk to develop not only non–AIDS-defining cancers with a viral pathogenesis but also non–virus-related cancers, estimated at a twofold risk in a recent study (Albini et al, 2013). Several factors have been suggested to explain this increased risk, including high-risk behaviors such as tobacco smoking, which is two to three times more prevalent in HIV-infected patients (Rahmanian et al, 2011); immunodeficiency (Grulich et al, 2007); inflammation (Borges et al, 2013); and age itself, because people are living longer with HIV infection (Albini et al, 2013). For the urologist, KS has the greatest relevance of the AIDS-defining cancers, given the possibility of KS lesions on the penis. There are increasing data regarding the rates and clinical course of non–AIDS-defining urologic malignancies.

Kaposi Sarcoma

Kaposi sarcoma was described in 1872 by Moritz Kaposi, who described three cases of fatal pigmented hemangiosarcomas in elderly men (Ruocco et al, 2013). Four forms are described: classic as described by Kaposi; an African endemic form occurring in young black men aged 25 to 40; an iatrogenic form first seen in the 1970s in patients on immunosuppressive therapy; and first reported in 1981 the form of KS in young homosexual men called the "epidemic form" (Hymes et al, 1981; Ruocco et al, 2013). KS is the second most common tumor in HIV-infected patients worldwide (Martellotta et al, 2009). However, the incidence of KS has decreased dramatically since the advent of the use of ART. In one recent prospective study, no new cases were noted in the period 1997 to 2000 (Speeckaert et al, 2011). Patients with KS typically have a CD4 cell count below 150 cells/mm^3 and a viral load higher than 10,000 copies/mL (Gallafent et al, 2005). A cluster of patients having KS despite being on ART, and with CD4 cell counts above 300 cells/mm^3 and viral loads below 300 copies/mL for at least 2 years, has been reported (Maurer et al, 2007).

The causative agent found in more than 90% of KS patients of all four types is human herpesvirus 8 (KSHV/HHV-8), a double-stranded DNA virus (Chang et al, 1994; Buonaguro et al, 1996). HHV-8 is now considered a necessary condition for the development of KS, but not all persons with HHV-8 get KS, and genetic, immunologic, and environmental factors are thought to be required as cofactors for KS to develop (Ruocco et al, 2013). KSHV infection leads to proliferation of both endothelial and spindle cells, the predominant cell type in KS, and angiogenesis (Martellotta et al, 2009; Ma et al, 2013). KS typically manifests with disseminated pigmented skin lesions, a few millimeters to several centimeters, from pink to purple or brown, often associated with edema and

lymph node and visceral involvement in up to 50% of patients. Other common sites of involvement are the oral cavity, gastrointestinal (GI) tract, and lungs (Mitsuyasu, 1993). The prognosis depends on the extent of the tumor, status of the immune system by CD4 count, and presence of systemic illness. The 3-year survival for patients with good risk is 80% to 88%, and for those with poor risk factors it is 53% (Nasti et al, 2003). Treatment depends on the type and is either local or systemic (Curatolo et al, 2012; Ruocco et al, 2013). For systemic therapy, one mainstay for epidemic KS is ART, which can produce a remission rate of 35% to 50% (Nguyen et al, 2008; Ruocco et al, 2013). Lesions typically start to decrease in size a few weeks to months after the initiation of treatment (Spano et al, 2008). KS may flare dramatically initially after the initiation of ART in what is called the *immune reconstitution inflammatory syndrome* (IRIS), seen in HIV-positive patients with initial low CD4 counts and high viral load (Leidner and Aboulafia, 2005). Onset of IRIS is as early as 3 weeks, with a mean onset of 5 weeks, and the syndrome can be fatal (Leidner and Aboulafia, 2005). First-line chemotherapy for advanced disease is liposomal anthracyclines (pegylated liposomal doxorubicin, daunorubicin citrate liposome DNX). Pegylated liposomes accumulate preferentially in highly vascularized KS lesions and are more effective than conventional chemotherapy regimens and with fewer side effects (Krown et al, 2004). Second-line therapy is paclitaxel or docetaxel (Lim et al, 2005; Cianfrocca et al, 2010).

Non–AIDS-Defining Urologic Malignancies

Testicular Tumors. The risk of testis tumors in early studies was reported to be 20 to more than 50 times greater in men with HIV than in uninfected men, and in general for seminoma. Later studies looking at men with HIV infection but after the development of ART have put the relative risk at a still significant level but much lower. Powles and colleagues found a relative risk for nonseminomatous germ cell tumors (NSGCTs) and seminoma of 4.36 (95% CI 2.71 to 6.55) and 5.45 (95% CI 3.35 to 8.10) (Powles et al, 2003). In a review of more than 260,000 men in the United States from 1980 to 2003, the risk for seminoma was 1.9 (95% CI 1.6 to 2.2) and there was no increased for NSGCTs (Goedert et al, 2007). An increased risk of 3.11 (95% CI 1.48 to 6.52) was recently reported from an Italian cohort, with no distinction between seminoma and nonseminoma tumors (Albini et al, 2013). The treatment for HIV-positive men with testes germ cell tumors is the same as for uninfected individuals (Powles et al, 2003). HIV-infected men are also at risk for testicular non-Hodgkin lymphoma, which may be disseminated at time of presentation, but tend to have the same response to therapy as uninfected individuals (Heyns et al, 2009).

Prostate Cancer. The relative risk of prostate cancer in men with HIV compared with uninfected individuals has been reported as either being no different or being even less, at 0.70 (Grulich et al, 2007; Bedimo et al, 2009; Albini et al, 2013). It has been postulated that ART may have a protective effect on prostate cancer independent of effect on increasing the CD4+ count (Chao et al, 2012). Radiotherapy in HIV-positive men is not associated with an increase in complications or effect on CD4 count (Ng et al, 2008). An increase in infectious complications with radical prostatectomy may be seen in patients with lower CD4 counts and higher viral loads, but no other adverse perioperative complications or differences in response to therapy (Huang et al, 2006). In a series of patients undergoing robot-assisted laparoscopic radical prostatectomy for prostate cancer, patients infected with HIV had a higher rate of transfusion and ileus compared with men without HIV; no other complications were different in the two groups, and prostate-specific antigen (PSA) was undetectable at 8 months in all HIV-positive men (Silberstein et al, 2010). PSA levels do not appear to be different in men based on their HIV status (Vianna et al, 2006; Pantanowitz et al, 2008). HIV-positive patients are reported to have a greater likelihood of a positive prostate biopsy compared with uninfected men (OR 3.9, 95% CI 1.3 to 11.5) (Hsiao et al, 2009), but the Gleason score on biopsies is not different (Pantanowitz et al, 2008). Overall, the evaluation and treatment of prostate cancer in patients with HIV do not appear to be significantly different from those in uninfected men (Levinson et al, 2005). Given that the median survival after starting ART is estimated to be over 13 years (Walensky et al, 2006), patients with HIV should be screened and treated as uninfected men.

Kidney Cancer. An increased risk of renal cell carcinoma and HIV infection has been reported. In a study of more than 300,000 adults aged 15 to 69 years with HIV/AIDS in multiple geographic locations in the United States, compared with the expected population-based incidence rates, kidney cancer was 1.5 times more likely in the HIV population, similar to another large study of more than 444,000 patients (Frisch et al, 2001; Grulich et al, 2007). There was no increase in risk with progression to AIDS, arguing against immunosuppression as a contributing factor (Frisch et al, 2001). Much higher risks of developing renal cell cancer in HIV infection were reported in a single-site series from Cleveland (United States)—an increased risk of 8.5 times, as well as presentation 15 years younger than expected (Baynham et al, 1997)—and from Uganda (Africa), reporting a relative risk of up to 16 times (Mbulaiteye et al, 2006). A case series of nine men with renal cell carcinoma found diagnosis at a median age of 48, no association with immunosuppression, and a clinical presentation or response to treatment that appeared similar to that of uninfected individuals (Gaughan et al, 2008). The differential diagnosis of renal mass in an HIV-infected person should also include lymphoma.

Penile Cancer. The relative risk of penile cancer is reported to be approximately four times higher than in men without infection (Frisch et al, 2001; Grulich et al, 2007). Men with HIV have a high prevalence of high-risk HPV types, 16 and 18, in the anus, penis, and mouth, without evidence of any lesions in these areas (Sirera et al, 2006). This occurs in both MSM and heterosexual men (Videla et al, 2013). The risk of penile cancer increases the closer a man is to having AIDS or the longer he has had AIDS (Chaturvedi et al, 2009). Although squamous cell cancers can be more aggressive in HIV-positive individuals (Nguyen et al, 2002), early lesions such as penile intraepithelial carcinoma can still respond to treatment with local therapy (Ramoni et al, 2009).

Bladder Cancer. In large series reporting the incidence of cancer in HIV-positive patients compared with those without infection, bladder cancer is not more frequent than in uninfected persons (Frisch et al, 2001; Grulich et al, 2007; Mbulaiteye et al, 2006). A suggestion of a reduced risk has been reported (Layman and Engels, 2008). A case series of patients with bladder cancer and HIV indicated no difference in clinical course or response to treatment (Gaughan et al, 2009). One possible difference in treatment of HIV-positive patients is to use caution in deciding to use intravesical bacille Calmette-Guérin (BCG). The effectiveness of BCG is dependent on a functioning immune system, and therefore the agent is not typically used in immunocompromised patients. There is the theoretic risk of disseminated infection. One case report has documented bilateral interstitial pneumonitis in an HIV-infected patient after intravesical therapy with BCG (Kristjansson et al, 1993). However, in the case series by Gaughn and colleagues, one of their HIV patients received BCG without complications (Gaughan et al, 2009).

KEY POINTS

- Patients with urethritis need to be treated for both gonorrhea and chlamydia. In addition to microscopic examination of urethral discharge, urine should be sent for nucleic acid amplification testing for both gonorrhea and chlamydia. Urethral swab is no longer indicted.
- Most genital ulcers in the United States are either herpes or syphilis, with most being herpes. Chancroid occurs in some parts of the United States, but donovanosis usually does not. LGV is increasing in incidence in MSM, including in the United States.
- Vaccines to prevent HPV-associated disease such as genital warts and anal cancer in both genders and cervical cancer in females are now available and recommended for men and women younger than age 26, preferably to start before onset of sexual activity.
- Testing for HIV is recommended in anyone with an STD or at risk of acquiring an STD.
- Treatment of HIV with ART is indicated in all infected persons regardless of CD4 count.
- HIV is becoming a chronic disease, and many of the associated problems are from aging and chronic disease instead of immunosuppression.

REFERENCES

The complete reference list is available online at www.expertconsult.com.

SUGGESTED READINGS

Beutner KR, Wiley DJ, Douglas JM, et al. Genital warts and their treatment. Clin Infect Dis 1999;28:S37–56.

Deeks SG, Lewin SR, Havlir DV. The end of AIDS: HIV infection as a chronic disease. Lancet 2013;382:1525–33.

Dunne EF, Friedman A, Datta SD, et al. Updates on human papillomavirus and genital warts and counseling messages from the 2010 sexually transmitted diseases treatment guidelines. Clin Infect Dis 2011;53:S143–52.

Ho EL, Lukehart SA. Syphilis: using modern approaches to understand an old disease. J Clin Invest 2011;121:4584–92.

Lewis DA, Ison CA. Chancroid. Sex Transm Infect 2006;82:19–20.

Patel R, Rompalo A. Managing patients with genital herpes and their sexual partners. Infect Dis Clin North Am 2005;19:427–38.

Steinbrook R. Preexposure prophylaxis for HIV infection. JAMA 2012;308:865–6.

Taylor-Robinson D, Jensen JS. *Mycoplasma genitalium:* from chrysalis to multicolored butterfly. Clin Microbiol Rev 2011;24:498–514.

Thompson MA, Aberg JA, Hoy JF, et al. Antiretroviral treatment of adult HIV infection: 2012 recommendations of the International Antiviral Society—USA Panel. JAMA 2012;308:387–402.

Wetmore CM, Manhart LE, Lowens MS, et al. Demographic, behavioral, and clinical characteristics of men with nongonococcal urethritis differ by etiology: a case-comparison study. Sex Transm Dis 2011a;38:180–6.

16 Cutaneous Diseases of the External Genitalia

Richard Edward Link, MD, PhD, and Theodore Rosen, MD

The diagnosis and treatment of cutaneous diseases of the external genitalia remain important elements of urologic practice. Often overlooked during formal urology residency training, this topic lies at the interface of multiple specialties, including urology, diagnosis of infectious diseases, rheumatology, allergy-immunology, and dermatology.

INTRODUCTION TO BASIC DERMATOLOGY

Dermatology is the clinical discipline focused on the normal biology and pathogenesis of diseases and disorders of the skin. The diagnosis of skin disease depends critically on the history and physical examination, with laboratory testing often relegated to a peripheral and confirmatory role. In many cases, visual inspection alone will suffice to narrow the diagnosis significantly. On the other hand, the skin has a limited repertoire of morphologic expression. Therefore one should not hesitate to perform a skin biopsy, when indicated, or to order a variety of laboratory investigations when needed to distinguish between two or more clinical mimics.

The skin is divided into three layers: the epidermis, dermis, and subcutaneous tissue. The epidermis, composed of stratified squamous epithelia, can vary in thickness from 0.05 to 1.5 mm depending on location. Melanocytes (pigment-producing cells) populate the lower layers of the epidermis. The dermis, composed of collagen, elastin, and reticular fibers, can be divided into two layers: the thin superficial layer (papillary dermis) and the thicker deeper layer (reticular dermis). Located within the dermis are mesenchymal structures, such as blood vessels and nerves. The bottom layer of the skin, known as subcutaneous tissue, is largely composed of fat.

Literally hundreds of cutaneous diseases exist that may involve the external genitalia. In addition, within each disease there may be significant variation in appearance and symptoms as the process for each condition evolves. For this reason, a methodical and systematic approach is essential to reach a rational diagnosis. The dermatologic history should focus on the duration, rate of onset, location, associated symptoms, family history, allergies, occupation, and previous treatment of the condition (Habif, 2004). Common symptoms include pruritus (itching), burning, stinging, and pain. The *lack* of symptoms, such as pain, can be important in arriving at the correct diagnosis and should therefore be noted.

The physical examination should address the distribution of primary and secondary skin lesions. **It is important to perform a thorough skin survey and not to focus solely on the area of affected genital skin.** Most skin conditions begin with a characteristic primary lesion that is an important key to diagnosis. A precise description of this lesion includes documenting its color (red, brown, black, yellow, white, blue, or green) and morphology (macule, papule, plaque, nodule, pustule, vesicle, bulla, or wheal; Table 16-1) (Habif, 2004). Because of the mucosal nature of genital skin, papular and macular lesions may present as erosions in this area (Margolis, 2002). Secondary skin lesions develop as the skin condition evolves or are caused by scratching, rubbing, or superinfection. A secondary lesion should also be classified morphologically as a scale, crust, erosion, ulcer, atrophy, thickening, or scar (Table 16-2).

After gross morphology is determined, laboratory testing may serve to confirm the diagnosis. To identify cutaneous fungi such as dermatophytes and *Candida* species, potassium hydroxide (KOH) or periodic acid–Schiff staining may be applied to scraped or touched skin specimens. KOH dissolves keratin, leaving fungal hyphal walls prominently visible under the microscope. Likewise, Tzanck preparations may aid in identifying viral agents such as herpes simplex, varicella zoster, and molluscum contagiosum.

For difficult cases or those in which malignancy is suspected, skin biopsy may be indicated. A variety of techniques exist for this purpose, including curettage, punch, shave, and incisional and complete excisional biopsies. For small scrotal or phallic shaft lesions, these techniques can usually be performed in the office setting under local anesthesia. For larger lesions or those involving the urethral meatus, biopsy in the operating room is recommended. It is often possible to determine the correct diagnosis with a very small (2 to 3 mm) punch biopsy. The resultant defect can easily be closed with one or two 6-0 or 7-0 nylon sutures, thereby avoiding any substantial scar.

Additional diagnostic maneuvers that may prove invaluable in select situations include serologic testing (e.g., serologic tests for syphilis), culture (e.g., culture for *Pseudomonas aeruginosa*), and immunohistochemistry stains of biopsy specimens (e.g., examination for specific types of cytokeratins associated with different variants of lichen sclerosus).

DERMATOLOGIC THERAPY

Medical therapy for dermatologic conditions consists of a broad range of topical and systemic compounds.

For systemic therapy, useful drug classes include antibiotics, antifungals, antivirals, anti-inflammatories, and antipruritics. Less commonly used agents, including chemotherapeutic and biologic drugs (e.g., methotrexate, cyclophosphamide, adalimumab, etanercept, infliximab, and ustekinumab), immunosuppressants (e.g., azathioprine, cyclosporine, tacrolimus), and hydroxyurea, will be discussed within the specific disease entities.

TABLE 16-1   Primary Cutaneous Lesions

PRIMARY LESION	DESCRIPTION
FLAT	
Macule	A circumscribed, **flat** discoloration that may be brown, blue, red, or hypopigmented
ELEVATED, SOLID	
Papule	An **elevated, solid** lesion up to 0.5 cm in diameter of variable color. Papules may become confluent to become plaques
Nodule	A circumscribed, **elevated solid** lesion >0.5 cm in diameter
Plaque	A circumscribed, **elevated**, superficial, **solid** lesion >0.5 cm in diameter
FLUID-FILLED	
Vesicle	A circumscribed **collection of free fluid** ≤0.5 cm in diameter
Bulla	A circumscribed **collection of free fluid** >0.5 cm in diameter
Pustule	A circumscribed collection of leukocytes and free fluid **(pus)**
Wheal (hive)	A firm **erythematous plaque** resulting from **infiltration** of the dermis with fluid (may be transient)

From Habif TP. Clinical dermatology: a color guide to diagnosis and therapy. Edinburgh: Mosby; 2004.

TABLE 16-2   Secondary Cutaneous Lesions

SECONDARY LESION	DESCRIPTION
Scale	Excess dead epidermal cells that are produced by abnormal keratinization and shedding
Crust	A collection of dried serum and cellular debris (a scab)
Erosion	A focal loss of epidermis. Erosions do not penetrate below the dermoepidermal junction and they heal without scarring
Ulcer	A focal loss of epidermis and dermis, which heals with scarring
Fissure	A linear loss of epidermis and dermis with sharply defined, vertical walls
Atrophy	A depression in the skin resulting from thinning of the epidermis or dermis
Scar	An abnormal formation of connective tissue implying dermal damage

From Habif TP. Clinical dermatology: a color guide to diagnosis and therapy. Edinburgh: Mosby; 2004.

A lack of familiarity with cutaneous diseases affecting the genitalia may lower the threshold of urologists in prescribing systemic antibiotics for these conditions. Unfortunately, these agents carry significantly greater risks than topical preparations, including promotion of resistant organisms, interaction with other medications, and disruption of the normal bowel and vaginal flora. It is worth noting that alterations in bacterial flora or in their antimicrobial susceptibility patterns may persist for protracted periods, thus emphasizing the need for truly appropriate antibiotic use (Jernberg et al, 2010). Similar caveats apply to systemic antifungal agents such as fluconazole, ketoconazole, and terbinafine. Superficial dermatophytes, such as those causing tinea cruris, generally respond well to diligent application of topical antifungal preparations. **Systemic antifungals are only indicated for very extensive cutaneous dermatophytosis, endemic mycoses with skin involvement, deep infection involving the hair follicles (Majocchi granuloma), or fungal infections in severely immunocompromised individuals** (Lesher and McConnell, 2003). In some cases, even in immunocompetent individuals, systemic antifungals are necessary to treat infections resistant to local therapy (Lesher, 1999). On the other hand, warnings have emphasized the need to avoid the routine use of some systemic antifungal medications (such as ketoconazole) for superficial cutaneous infections because of the unpredictable risk of life-threatening hepatotoxicity and adrenal insufficiency (U.S. Food and Drug Administration, 2013). Systemic anti-inflammatory agents, in particular the glucocorticosteroids (GCS), deserve additional attention. Oral GCS are absorbed in the jejunum with peak plasma concentrations occurring in 30 to 90 minutes (Lester, 1989). Despite short plasma half-lives of 1 to 5 hours, the duration of effect of GCS lasts between 8 and 48 hours, depending on the agent (Nesbitt, 2003). These drugs have **widespread** anti-inflammatory effects. They release neutrophils from bone marrow but they inhibit their movement to sites of inflammation in tissue. They also impair both T-cell activation and antigen presentation by dendritic cells (Nesbitt, 2003). **For short-term (≤3 weeks) treatment of dermatologic conditions such as allergic contact dermatitis** (Feldman, 1992), **a single morning dose of GCS is administered to minimize suppression of the hypothalamic-pituitary-adrenal axis** (Myles, 1971). Prednisone is generally the GCS of choice because of its low cost, intermediate duration of action, and variety of dosage forms, although methylprednisolone may be substituted to reduce the mineralocorticoid effects (Wolverton, 2001). **Longer-term treatment with systemic GCS may lead to a wide variety of adverse effects including osteoporosis, cataract formation, hypertension, obesity, hyperglycemia, aseptic necrosis of the femoral head, immunosuppression, and psychiatric changes** (Nesbitt, 2003). For this reason, the use of topical steroids (see later) is preferable to reliance on systemic GCS, whenever clinically feasible.

Topical preparations are the mainstay of therapy for a wide range of cutaneous diseases affecting the genitalia. Urologists tend to be less familiar with the use of these medications than are dermatologists. **Topical medications can be broken down into five general classes: emollients, anti-inflammatories, antibiotics, antifungals, and chemotherapeutic agents.**

Topical preparations include active ingredients and they also include a vehicle that determines the rate at which the active ingredients are absorbed by the skin. Emollients restore water and lipids to the epidermis and are useful for dry-skin diseases. Emollients should be applied to moist skin for maximal effect, such as after bathing. Preparations containing urea (e.g., Carmol, vanadine) or lactic acid (Lac-Hydrin, AmLactin) may be particularly potent hydrating agents (Habif, 2004). It has been noted that ceramides (combinations of a fatty acid and a sphingoid base), the main natural intercellular lipids in the outermost layer of skin, are critical for maintaining normal cutaneous hydration and barrier function (Weber et al, 2012). For this reason, new formulations containing ceramides (CeraVe) may also be particularly useful for skin conditions characterized by xerosis (dryness). Topical corticosteroids are potent anti-inflammatory agents available in a myriad of preparations and strengths. A detailed review of the use and dosing of topical corticosteroids is beyond the scope of this chapter, and the reader is directed to several excellent dermatology textbooks for more detail (Habif, 2004). **It is important to recognize that even topical corticosteroids can include significant adverse effects, both from systemic absorption and also from the results of local application. Local effects include epidermal atrophy and the development of striae on the upper portion of the inner thigh,**

dermal changes (telangiectasias, hypopigmentation), allergic reactions, and negative alterations in the usual course of skin infections and infestations (Burry, 1973). In most cases, atrophy is a reversible process that can be expected to resolve during the course of several months (Sneddon, 1976). Atrophy is particularly troublesome if corticosteroids are applied under the foreskin, which can serve as an occlusive "dressing" and can enhance penetration of the drug (Fig. 16-1) (Goldman and Kitzmiller, 1973).

A variety of physical modalities have also been applied to treat dermatologic problems, including ultraviolet light therapy, photodynamic therapy, laser therapy, and cryosurgery. Ultraviolet light therapy, with both broadband and narrow-band ultraviolet B (UVB), has been used to treat atopic dermatitis, psoriasis, seborrheic dermatitis, and vitiligo (Honigsmann and Schwarz, 2003). There are now several convenient single-wavelength UVB (308 nm) laser units with small spot sizes, which are particularly useful for treating vexing localized areas of genital psoriasis or vitiligo; such narrow spectrum machines are believed not to carry the risk of inducing the nonmelanoma skin cancer that is associated with broadband full-body light boxes. Psoralens, when combined with long-wave ultraviolet A radiation (psoralen ultraviolet A [PUVA] therapy), generate a phototoxic effect that is beneficial for treating psoriasis (Honigsmann, 2001; Stern, 2007), vitiligo (Honigsmann and Schwarz, 2003), atopic dermatitis (Morison, 1992), and lichen planus (Honigsmann and Schwarz, 2003). In general, the narrow-band UVB boxes and lasers have supplanted PUVA therapy, as the latter carries a substantial risk of squamous cell carcinoma (SCC) when performed throughout a prolonged period (Stern and PUVA Follow-Up Study, 2012). Photodynamic therapy involves the use of cytotoxic oxygen radicals generated from photoactivated molecules to achieve a therapeutic response (Tope and Shaffer, 2003; Braathen et al, 2007). Photodynamic therapy is a new arena of dermatologic therapy and holds promise for treating a variety of inflammatory, malignant, and infectious skin conditions. For example, photodynamic therapy is effective, both as monotherapy and in combination with cryosurgery, CO_2 laser ablation, and curettage, in the management of large or resistant condyloma acuminata or in genital warts occurring during pregnancy (Scheinfeld, 2013b). The downside to this promising modality is that there is not yet an established optimum regimen for off-label use, including for genital warts. Laser and cryosurgery play a relatively small role in the management of genital lesions, although the CO_2 laser has been used effectively to manage genital condyloma acuminata, and cryosurgery may be useful for genital and suprapubic molluscum contagiosum.

ALLERGIC DERMATITIS

Allergic or "eczematous" dermatitis consists of a group of allergy-mediated processes leading to pruritic skin lesions (Box 16-1).

Atopic Dermatitis (Eczema)

Atopic dermatitis (AD) is a chronic relapsing dermatitis with a predilection for skin flexures that is associated with intense pruritus and damage to the epidermis (Williams, 2005). **The characteristic lesions are erythematous papules and thin plaques with secondary excoriations** (Fig. 16-2) (Kang et al, 2003). In

---

BOX 16-1 Differential Diagnosis of Allergic Dermatitis

Eczema
Allergic dermatitis
Seborrheic dermatitis
Intertrigo
Contact dermatitis
Irritant dermatitis
Balanoposthitis
Zoon balanitis
Candidal-related illness
Impetigo
Herpes simplex
Herpes zoster
Drug reaction

From Margolis DJ. Cutaneous disease of the male external genitalia. In: Walsh PC, editor. Campbell's urology. Philadelphia: Saunders; 2002.

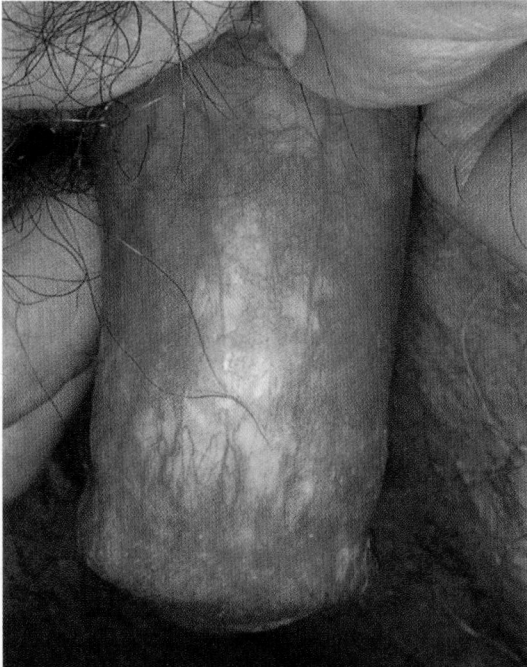

Figure 16-1. Steroid atrophy of penile shaft skin after application of corticosteroid under the foreskin for 8 weeks. (From Habif TP. Clinical dermatology. Edinburgh: Mosby; 2004. p. 36.)

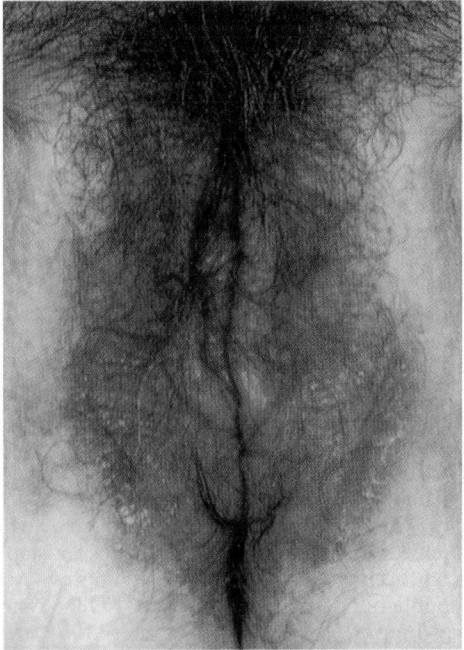

Figure 16-2. Eczema involving the vulva. (From du Vivier A. Atlas of clinical dermatology. London: Churchill Livingstone; 2002. p. 687.)

general, the lesions do not have a precise border as is common for papulosquamous disorders (Margolis, 2002). Although any age can be affected, 90% of AD patients manifest their condition before the age of 5 years (Rajka, 1989). AD is associated with susceptibility to a wide variety of substances that act as irritants (e.g., fragrances, preservatives, and various proteins). Patients suffering from AD also have a propensity to develop asthma and allergic rhinitis.

The genetic susceptibility to AD has been extensively explored. In a study of 372 AD patients, 73% had a positive family history for atopy. Likewise, twin concordance studies have demonstrated an AD risk of 0.86 for monozygotic twins compared to only 0.21 for dizygotic twins. These findings have spurred an intense search for genes involved in atopy and AD (Wollenberg and Bieber, 2000). Although no single gene has been found to be a unique marker for the disease, at least 11 genetic foci seem to be closely associated with AD (Kang et al, 2003; Ellinghaus et al, 2013). The single most important genetic defects confer an inability to synthesize functional filaggrin properly. This structural abnormality results in both a "leaky" epithelial barrier and chronic immune activation, which contribute to the pathophysiology of this common skin disease (Heimall and Spergel, 2012).

Intense pruritus is the hallmark of AD, and controlling the patient's urge to scratch is critical for successful treatment (Przybilla et al, 1994). Itching is often worse during evening hours and can be exacerbated by sweating, occlusive undergarments, or wool clothing (Kang et al, 2003). Scratching of lesions may contribute to the clinical complications of AD, including superinfection with *Staphylococcus aureus* species (Ogawa et al, 1994). There is growing evidence that bacterial toxins may serve as superantigens that drive an inflammatory cascade that sustains AD (Skov and Baadsgaard, 2000; Skov et al, 2000).

Clinically, there is no pathognomonic laboratory test, biopsy result, or single clinical feature that allows the definitive diagnosis of AD. The association with a personal or family history of atopy is a critical clue to the diagnosis (Kang et al, 2003). For patients presenting with genital findings, extragenital involvement is commonplace.

A variety of "trigger factors" have been implicated in the exacerbation of AD, including chemicals, detergents, and household dust mites. Removal of these factors from the environment may be beneficial on an individualized basis. Dust mite exposure, in particular, has received significant attention in the literature. Although several studies have demonstrated modest improvement in AD with mite reduction (Kubota et al, 1992; Tan et al, 1996), others report that reduction is associated with no significant clinical benefit (Colloff et al, 1989; Gutgesell et al, 2001).

Treatments for AD include gentle cleaning with nonalkali soaps or soap substitutes (e.g., Cetaphil, Aquanil) and the frequent use of emollients. Evaporation of liquid from the skin may trigger AD (Kang et al, 2003), so frequent bathing is not encouraged. Soaking may help during episodes of bacterial superinfection but should be discontinued after the infection has resolved (Margolis, 2002). Topical corticosteroids may be needed to control pruritus but should only be used for short courses with a rapid taper to avoid local complications of skin atrophy and dyschromia. Topical macrolide immunomodulatory agents such as tacrolimus and pimecrolimus have shown efficacy in the treatment of AD (Meagher et al, 2002; Nghiem et al, 2002; Luger and Paul, 2007; Leung et al, 2009), and these agents may decrease the need for corticosteroids during long-term therapy (Zuberbier et al, 2007). Antihistamines such as diphenhydramine or a variety of nonsedating agents, such as cetirizine, loratadine, and analogues of these, may be helpful in breaking the "itch-scratch cycle" in AD, particularly when administered before bedtime (Kang et al, 2003). Oral antistaphylococcal drugs have not been shown to significantly improve AD in a randomized, double-blind trial (Ewing et al, 1998). Systemic treatment with azathioprine, corticosteroids, cyclosporine, methotrexate, or mycophenolate mofetil may rarely be indicated for severe, widely disseminated cases (Cooper, 1993; Salek et al, 1993; Denby and Beck, 2012).

Contact Dermatitis

Contact dermatitis can be broken down into two distinct entities: irritant contact dermatitis (ICD) and allergic contact dermatitis (ACD). Although the mechanisms differ significantly, the clinical presentation of ICD and ACD may be similar. Most notably, the affected area is usually sharply limited to an area of skin exposure to true allergen or irritating chemical. The primary mode of treatment is to identify and reduce exposure to the offending agent.

ICD results from a direct cytotoxic effect of an irritant chemical touching the skin and is responsible for approximately 80% of contact dermatitis cases (Marks et al, 2002). Examples of offending agents include soaps, solvents, metal salts, and acid- or alkali-containing compounds. Occupational ICD is a serious public health problem and contributes to costs on the scale of $1 billion annually in the United States (Cohen, 2000). The clinical manifestations of ICD depend on the identity of the irritating substance as well as the duration of contact, concentration, temperature, pH, and location of exposure. Acute ICD, such as might result from an occupational accident, generally peaks within minutes to hours after exposure and then begins to heal. Symptoms of burning, stinging, and soreness may be accompanied by erythema, edema, bullae, or frank necrosis in a sharply defined area corresponding to the exposed skin (Cohen and Bassiri-Tehrani, 2003). There are also a variety of subacute forms of ICD that result from repeated subthreshold skin insults. Pruritus is much more common in these more chronic conditions, and the skin lesions are not as well demarcated. The mainstay of treatment for ICD lies in avoiding skin contact with the causative irritants through the use of protective clothing, safe occupational practices, and the use of skin barrier preparations such as ointments, emollient creams, or protective foams. Some commercially available barrier products include Atopiclair, Biafine, EpiCeram, MimyX, Neosalus Foam, and PruMyx (Berndt et al, 2000; Draelos, 2012).

In contrast, ACD represents a local type IV hypersensitivity reaction to a skin allergen to which an individual has been previously exposed and sensitized. The typical appearance is a well-demarcated pruritic eruption, which may manifest blistering or weeping in the acute phase or the development of scaly plaques more chronically (Mowad and Marks, 2003). In 2003 and 2009, the North American Contact Dermatitis Group (NACDG) reported a long list of common allergens implicated in ACD based on patch testing results (Zug et al, 2009). Similar lists that were produced subsequently contain the same set of allergens, with only a few exceptions. Patch testing is a simple technique of exposing an area of skin to a variety of potential allergens at a known concentration in a grid template (Fig. 16-3). Generally performed by dermatologists, patch testing can help to confirm both the diagnosis of ACD and the allergen involved. The most common sensitizing allergen identified by the NACDG was nickel sulfate (Zug et al, 2009), which is a common component of costume jewelry and belt buckles (Fig. 16-4). Although traditionally a cause of earlobe dermatitis from pierced earrings, nickel sensitivity may be a potential cause of genital ACD resulting from the increasing prevalence of genital piercing. Other important allergens include textile dyes, topical antibiotics, perfumes and other fragrance materials, formaldehyde-releasing preservatives, the latex in condoms, and topical corticosteroids. When ACD is suspected, one should always inquire about the use of over-the-counter products such as genital moisturizers, antiyeast and anti-itch preparations, and lubricants used during sexual intercourse. Oral antihistamines may be helpful for the symptomatic control of ACD in combination with the removal of the inciting allergen. Severe ACD should *not* be treated with a short course of systemic steroids, but rather with a 3-week tapering dose of prednisone.

Erythema Multiforme and Stevens-Johnson Syndrome

Erythema multiforme (EM) is a generalized skin disease that may involve the genitalia. **EM can be subdivided into minor and major forms.**

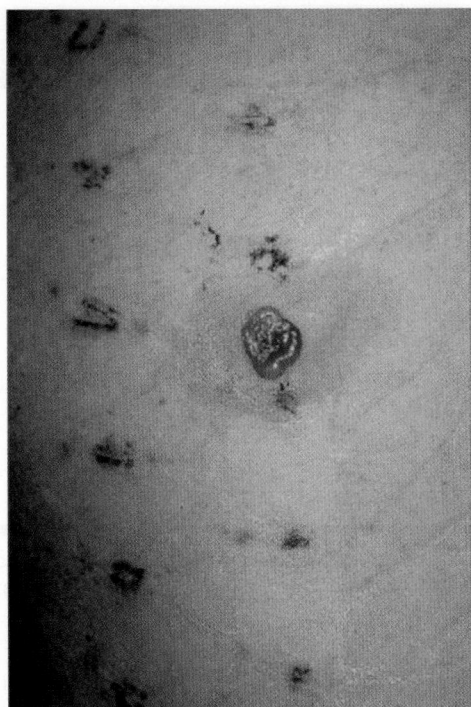

Figure 16-3. An example of patch testing with a positive response to nickel. (From Bolognia JL, Jorizzo JL, Rapini RP. Dermatology. Edinburgh: Mosby; 2003. p. 233.)

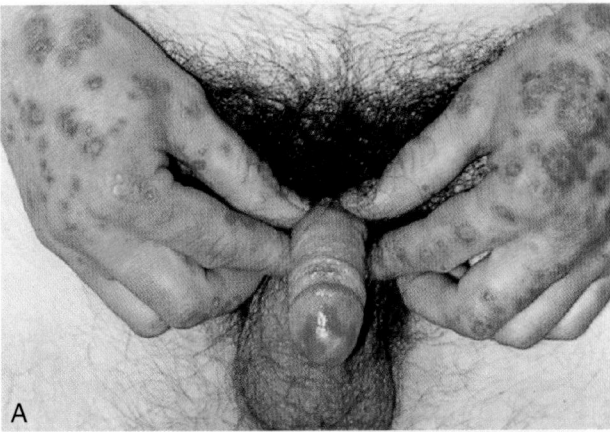

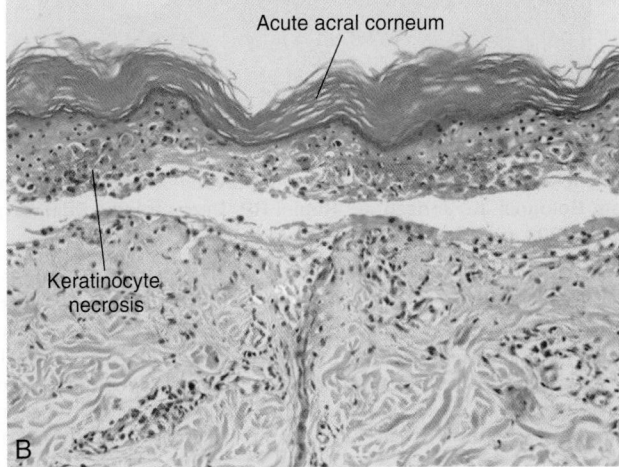

Acute acral corneum

Keratinocyte necrosis

Figure 16-5. Erythema multiforme (EM). A, Targetoid lesions of the hands and penis. B, Typical microscopic picture of EM with a normal stratum corneum, necrotic keratinocytes in the epidermis and a lymphoid infiltrate. (A, From Korting GW. Practical dermatology of the genital region. Philadelphia: Saunders; 1981. p. 16; B, from Elston DM, Ferringer T. Dermatopathology. Edinburgh: Saunders; 2009. p. 147.)

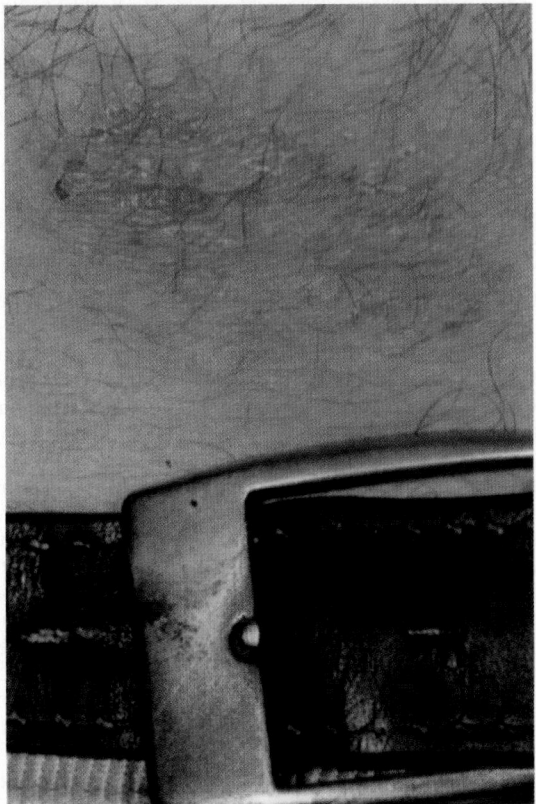

Figure 16-4. Contact dermatitis caused by a nickel allergy from a belt buckle. (From Habif TP. Clinical dermatology. Edinburgh: Mosby; 2004. p. 94.)

EM minor was first described in 1860 by an Austrian dermatologist, Ferdinand von Hebra (von Hebra, 1860). **This condition is an acute, self-limited skin disease characterized by the abrupt onset of symmetrical fixed red papules that may evolve into target lesions** (Weston, 1996). EM is a clinical rather than a histologic

diagnosis. Papules and target lesions are usually grouped and can be present anywhere on the body, including the genitalia (Fig. 16-5A). There is also a predilection for involvement of the oral mucous membranes, as well as the palms and soles.

The majority of cases of recurrent EM minor are precipitated by human herpesvirus 1 and 2 (Schofield et al, 1993; Nikkels and Pierard, 2002), **with herpetic lesions usually preceding the development of target lesions by 10 to 14 days** (Lemak et al, 1986). Although continuous suppressive acyclovir may prevent EM episodes in patients with herpes infection (Tatnall et al, 1995), administration of the drug after development of target lesions is of no benefit (Huff, 1988). The natural history of EM minor is spontaneous resolution after several weeks without sequelae (Schofield et al, 1993), although recurrences are common (Huff and Weston, 1989). Oral antihistamines may provide symptomatic relief. For immunosuppressed patients, the time course of EM minor outbreaks may be longer and the frequency of recurrence may be greater (Schofield et al, 1993).

The major form of EM has been called Stevens-Johnson syndrome (SJS) in the past, although there remains some controversy as to whether EM major and SJS are distinct entities or are part of a spectrum of disease (Bachot and Roujeau, 2003; Williams and Conklin, 2005). SJS is a much more serious illness than EM minor and it includes features similar to extensive skin burns (Parrillo, 2007). In its more severe forms, SJS may mimic life-threatening toxic epidermal necrolysis. Admission to the intensive care unit or burn unit may significantly reduce the morbidity and mortality of

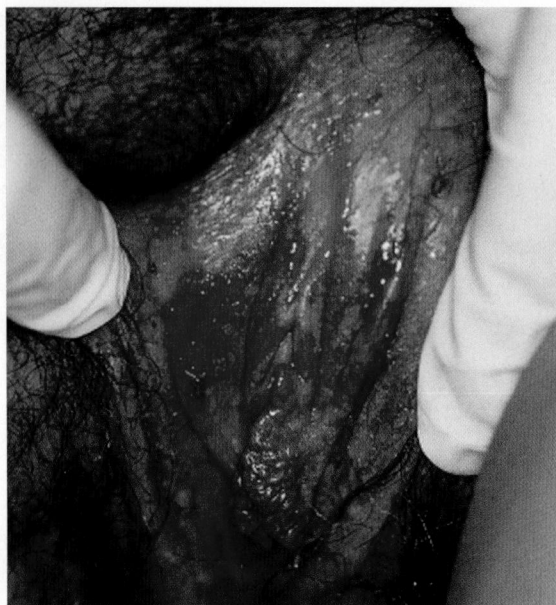

Figure 16-6. Labial erosions in a case of Stevens-Johnson syndrome. (From Bolognia JL, Jorizzo JL, Rapini RP. Dermatology. Edinburgh: Mosby; 2003. p. 319.)

BOX 16-2   Differential Diagnosis of Papulosquamous Lesions

Psoriasis
Seborrheic dermatitis
Dermatophyte infection
Erythrasma
Secondary syphilis
Pityriasis rosea
Discoid lupus
Mycosis fungoides
Lichen planus
Fixed drug eruption
Reactive arthritis
Pityriasis versicolor
Bowen disease
Extramammary Paget disease

From Margolis DJ. Cutaneous disease of the male external genitalia. In: Walsh PC, editor. Campbell's urology. Philadelphia: Saunders; 2002.

this condition (Wolf et al, 2005). **Most patients with SJS exhibit a prodromal upper respiratory illness (fever, cough, rhinitis, sore throat, and headache), which progresses after 1 to 14 days to the abrupt development of red macules with blister formation and areas of epidermal necrosis. Genital involvement includes erythema and erosions of the labia** (Fig. 16-6), **penis, and perianal region.**

A vast array of inciting factors has been implicated in the development of SJS, with drug exposures being the most commonly identified. Among the most common offending agents are nonsteroidal anti-inflammatory agents, sulfonamides (particularly cotrimoxazole), tetracycline and doxycycline, penicillin and cephalosporins, and a wide range of anticonvulsants (Chan et al, 1990). In contrast to EM minor, there is rarely an association with an infectious agent (Weston, 2003). **SJS generally presents a protracted course of 4 to 6 weeks and may include a mortality rate approaching 30%. Severe scarring of denuded skin may result in a range of complications including joint contractures, labial synechia, vaginal stenosis, urethral meatal stenosis, and anal strictures** (Brice et al, 1990; Weston, 2003). Treatment involves immediate removal of the offending drug and supportive care similar to the management of severe burns. There is currently no strong evidence for any specific medical therapy for SJS (Weston, 2003), and the role of systemic corticosteroids in treating SJS remains controversial (Rasmussen, 1976; Tripathi et al, 2000; Weston, 2003). Newer modalities anecdotally reported to act as effective interventions include cyclosporine (3 to 5 mg/kg/day), tumor necrosis factor (TNF)-α inhibitors, plasmapheresis, and, especially noted, intravenous immunoglobulin (Mockenhaupt, 2011; Worswick and Cotliar, 2011). Care of the SJS patient is best accomplished via a multispecialty team approach.

PAPULOSQUAMOUS DISORDERS

Papulosquamous disorders are a disparate group of diseases that share a common primary lesion: scaly papules and plaques (Box 16-2).

Psoriasis

Psoriasis is a common disease affecting up to 2% of the population (Christophers, 2001; Nestle et al, 2009). For patients with a predisposition, which is likely polygenic in nature, triggering factors such as trauma, infection, psychological stress, or new medications can elicit a flare in the psoriatic phenotype. One third of affected patients have a family history of psoriasis (Melski and Stern, 1981; Hensler and Christophers, 1985; Margolis, 2002).

The characteristic lesion is a sharply demarcated erythematous plaque with silvery-white scales (van de Kerkhof, 2003). Its pattern can be limited to the elbows or knees or can be distributed on the entire surface of the skin. Although psoriasis can appear at any age, two peaks of onset have been identified: 20 to 30 and 50 to 60 years of age. Patients complain of a significant impairment in their quality of life as a result of pruritus and bleeding, as well as the cosmetic and psychosocial impact of these visible plaques.

Psoriatic involvement of the genitalia is relatively common although it is usually within the context of a generalized cutaneous disorder. **Patients may present with concerns for malignancy or sexually transmitted disease (STD) when psoriatic lesions are present on the genitalia.** Genital psoriasis leads to impaired self-esteem and reduced sexual self-image, thereby interfering with normal intimate relationships, particularly in women (Magin et al, 2010; Meeuwis et al, 2011). The presence of characteristic lesions on the elbows, knees, buttocks, nails, scalp, and umbilicus may help direct the diagnosis (Fig. 16-7A) (Margolis, 2002). When lesions are present in the inguinal folds and intergluteal cleft, scaling may be absent (so-called inverse psoriasis) (Goldman, 2000). When evaluating nonscaling erythematous plaques in the inguinal folds, the diagnosis of fungal involvement (i.e., tinea or Candida) should be considered and ruled out by KOH preparation or fungal culture. In circumcised men, psoriatic plaques are often present on the glans and corona whereas in uncircumcised men, lesions are commonly hidden under the preputial skin (Buechner, 2002). In some cases, however, psoriasis involves the entire penis and scrotum (Fig. 16-8).

Psoriasis is a chronic disease with a relapsing and remitting course. A variety of topical and systemic therapies have been developed and are applied to this difficult problem. Despite the variety of therapy, however, as many as 40% of psoriasis sufferers express frustration at the ineffectiveness of current treatments (Krueger et al, 2001). **For genital psoriasis, the mainstay of therapy is the use of low-potency topical corticosteroid creams for short courses** (Kalb et al, 2009). Examples include a preparation of 3% liquor carbonis detergens (a tar derivative) in 1% hydrocortisone cream or hydrocortisone butyrate 0.1% (Fisher and Margesson, 1998). These preparations should not be used for more than 2 weeks continuously on thin genital skin or in areas occluded by skin folds (Margolis, 2002). Other topical therapies for psoriasis include vitamin D₃ analogues (calcitriol, calcipotriene), topical calcineurin inhibitors (pimecrolimus cream and tacrolimus ointment), and low-potency retinoids, although these agents are sometimes too irritating or not sufficiently effective. Photochemotherapy combining an ingested psoralen with ultraviolet radiation (PUVA) has been used extensively to treat psoriasis (Stern, 2007). However, a dose-dependent increase in the risk of genital SCC has been associated with high-dose PUVA therapy for psoriasis elsewhere on the body (Stern, 1990; Stern et al, 2002). Genital shielding during PUVA therapy is strongly recommended; therefore this modality is contraindicated for treating psoriatic lesions localized to genital skin. For patients with extensive psoriasis, systemic therapy with methotrexate, cyclosporine, retinoids, or one of the approved TNF-α inhibitors (adalimumab, etanercept) or IL12/23 inhibitors (ustekinumab) may be appropriate. The 308-nm excimer laser (Gerber et al, 2003) is now approved for psoriasis treatment. Experimental therapies that have shown promise in treating psoriasis include vitamin D receptor ligands (Bos and Spuls, 2008) and antibodies or antisense oligonucleotides against T-lymphocyte surface molecules (Gottlieb et al, 2000b), TNF (Chaudhari et al, 2001; Bos and Spuls, 2008), or intracellular adhesion molecules (Gottlieb et al, 2000a).

Reactive Arthritis (Formerly Reiter Syndrome)

Reactive arthritis (formerly Reiter syndrome) is composed of urethritis, arthritis, ocular findings, oral ulcers, and skin lesions. Only about one third of all patients with this disorder demonstrate all of the manifestations. The skin findings, particularly when present on the genitalia, may be mistaken for psoriatic lesions (Fig. 16-9). Reactive arthritis is more common in men than in women and is rarely diagnosed in children. **Reactive arthritis is generally preceded by an episode of either urethritis *(Chlamydia, Gonococcus)* or gastrointestinal infection *(Yersinia, Salmonella, Shigella, Campylobacter, Neisseria* or *Ureaplasma* species) and is more common in human immunodeficiency virus (HIV)-positive patients** (Rahman et al, 1992; Margolis, 2002; Wu and Schwartz,

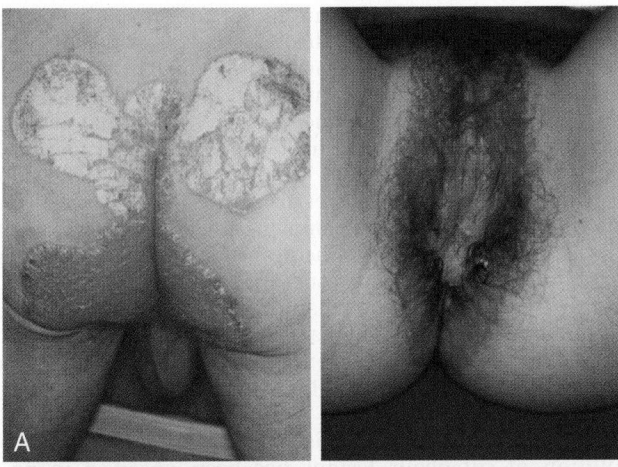

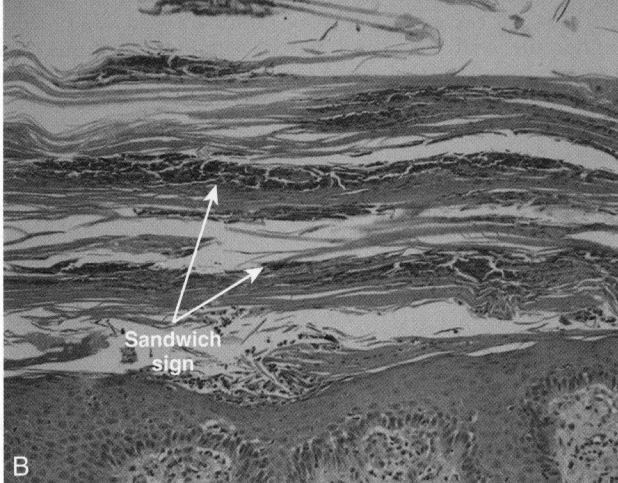

Figure 16-7. Psoriasis. A, Silver scales on an erythematous base. B, Alternating neutrophils and parakeratosis in the stratum corneum of plaque psoriasis (sandwich sign). (A, From Callen JP, Greer DE, Hood AF, et al. Color atlas of dermatology. Philadelphia: Saunders; 1993. p. 320; B, from Elston DM, Ferringer T. Dermatopathology. Edinburgh: Saunders; 2009. p. 152.)

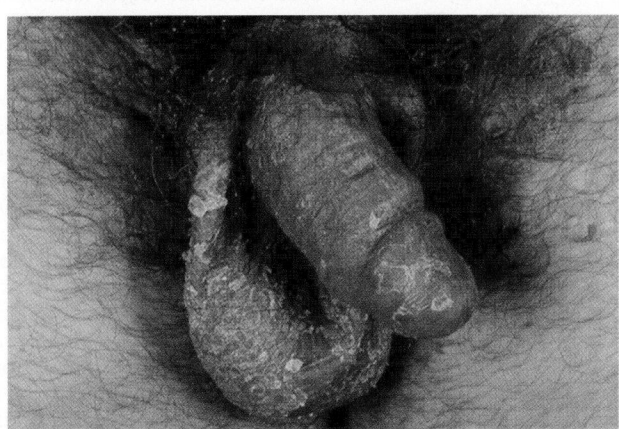

Figure 16-8. Psoriasis involving the entire penis and scrotum. (From Bolognia JL, Jorizzo JL, Rapini RP. Dermatology. Edinburgh: Mosby; 2003. p. 130.)

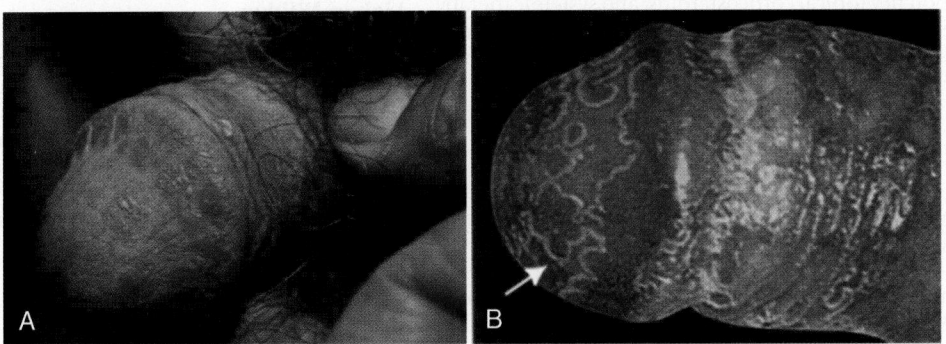

Figure 16-9. Comparison of psoriasis (A) and reactive arthritis (B) (balanitis circinata) involving the glans penis. Note the highly characteristic coalescence of lesions in this case of reactive arthritis forming a wavy pattern *(arrow).* (From Habif TP. Clinical dermatology. Edinburgh: Mosby; 2004. p. 217.)

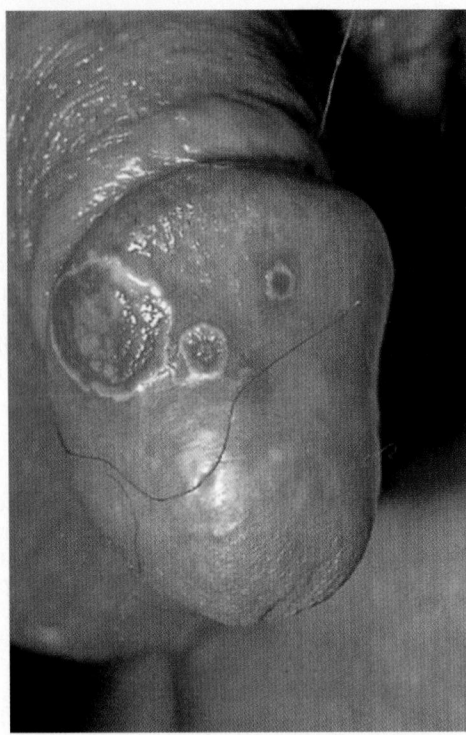

Figure 16-10. Erosive psoriaform lesions of the glans penis (reactive arthritis; balanitis circinata) may also lack the wavy pattern, making them difficult to differentiate from genital psoriasis. (From Callen JP, Greer DE, Hood AF, et al. Color atlas of dermatology. Philadelphia: Saunders; 1993. p. 160.)

2008). **There is a strong genetic association with the human leukocyte antigen (HLA)-B27 haplotype.** Whether or not cross-reactivity between bacterial antigens and HLA-B27 leads to autoimmunity in reactive arthritis remains controversial (Ringrose, 1999; Yu and Kuipers, 2003).

Conjunctivitis is the most common ocular manifestation, although iritis, uveitis, glaucoma, and keratitis may occur. Polyarthritis and sacroiliitis are the most common orthopedic complaints and may lead to chronic disability in a small minority of cases (van de Kerkhof, 2003). Scaly, erythematous psoriaform skin lesions appearing on the penis are referred to as *balanitis circinata* (Fig. 16-10), and similar lesions on the soles are referred to as *keratoderma blennorrhagicum*. **These lesions may be difficult to distinguish from psoriasis, and histologic analysis of biopsy specimens cannot consistently differentiate the two conditions** (Margolis, 2002). The course of reactive arthritis involving the genitalia is usually self-limited, lasting a few weeks to months. Lesions may respond to low-potency topical corticosteroids, and systemic therapy is rarely required. Lesions on soles, however, are more persistent; these respond well to the application of potent topical retinoids such as tazarotene (Lewis et al, 2000).

Lichen Planus

Lichen planus (LP), the prototype of the lichenoid dermatoses, is an idiopathic inflammatory disease of the skin and mucous membranes. The characteristic "lichenoid tissue reaction" is characterized by epidermal basal cell damage that is associated with a massive infiltration of mononuclear cells in the papillary dermis (Shiohara and Kano, 2003). Cutaneous LP may affect up to 1% of the adult population (Boyd and Neldner, 1991) and oral lesions may be present in as many as 4% (Scully et al, 1998). The pathogenesis of LP appears related to an autoimmune reaction against basal keratinocytes, which express altered self-antigens on their surfaces (Morhenn, 1986).

The primary lesion of LP is a small, polygonal-shaped, violaceous, flat-topped papule. These lesions may be widely separated or may coalesce into larger plaques that may ulcerate, particularly on mucosal surfaces. LP commonly involves the flexor surfaces of the extremities, the trunk, the lumbosacral area, the oral mucosa, and the glans penis (Margolis, 2002). **On the male genitalia, the clinical presentation of LP can be quite variable and includes isolated or grouped papules, a white reticular pattern, or an annular (ringlike) arrangement with or without ulceration** (Fig. 16-11). In some cases, the lesions appear to form linear patterns related to skin trauma (the so-called Koebner phenomenon, which is also seen with psoriasis). On the female genitalia, painful erosion of erythematous plaques is common; in long-standing LP of the vulva, some areas of hyperhydrated hyperkeratosis (manifesting as white plaques) may surround shallow erosions. In women, more than in men, concomitant oral LP may be found on the buccal mucosa or tongue (Santegoets et al, 2010). The differential diagnosis of LP includes invasive and in situ SCC, Zoon balanitis, psoriasis, secondary syphilis, herpes and extramammary Paget disease, and lupus erythematosus. Biopsy may be necessary to establish the diagnosis, particularly when the lesions are small, multiple, and ulcerated (Shiohara and Kano, 2003). Lichenoid reactions can also occur in response to ingested drugs and contact allergens, and a careful search for potential offending agents is appropriate.

The natural history of LP is benign and the spontaneous resolution of cutaneous lesions has been observed in up to two thirds of cases after 1 year (Shiohara and Kano, 2003), although the oral form may persist significantly longer, and isolated cases of SCC arising within chronic genital LP have been reported (Mignogna et al, 2000). Although bothersome pruritus (more often in men) or pain/burning (more often in women) is common with LP, asymptomatic lesions on the genitalia do not require treatment. The primary modality of treatment for symptomatic genital LP is the application of an ultrapotent topical corticosteroid (such as clobetasol 0.05% or halobetasol 0.05%). There is also a role for topical calcineurin inhibitors (pimecrolimus cream, tacrolimus ointment) in the management of genital LP (Luger and Paul, 2007). For severe cases, systemic corticosteroids (15 to 20 mg/day; 2- to 6-week course) (Boyd and Neldner, 1991) have been shown to shorten the time course to clearance of LP lesions from 29 weeks to 18 weeks (Cribier et al, 1998). Other systemic therapies for severe LP include cyclosporine, tacrolimus, griseofulvin, metronidazole, and acitretin (Ho et al, 1990; Boyd and Neldner, 1991; Cribier et al, 1998; Buyuk and Kavala, 2000; Madan and Griffiths, 2007), although randomized trials demonstrating efficacy are generally lacking. In fact, as pointed out in an exhaustive meta-analysis, there is no overwhelmingly reliable evidence for the efficacy of *any* single treatment for erosive mucosal LP, including application of an ultrapotent topical steroid, which is the widely accepted first-line therapy (Cheng et al, 2012).

Lichen Nitidus

Lichen nitidus (LN) is an unusual inflammatory eruption characterized by tiny, discrete, flesh-colored papules arranged in large clusters. Although there is some debate as to whether LN may represent a variant of LP (Aram, 1988), the two entities are histologically distinct. LN has a dense, well-circumscribed, lymphohistiocytic infiltrate that is closely apposed to the epidermis (Shiohara and Kano, 2003). Commonly involved sites include the flexor aspects of the upper extremities, the genitalia, the trunk, and the dorsal aspects of the hands. Nail involvement is common. Similar to LP, the natural history of LN is one of spontaneous resolution, with the majority of patients (69%) manifesting the disease for less than 1 year (Lapins et al, 1978). Patients should be reassured that these genital lesions are not infectious and should resolve with time. For symptomatic pruritus, genital lesions usually respond to mid- to low-potency topical corticosteroids and oral antihistamines (Shiohara and Kano, 2003).

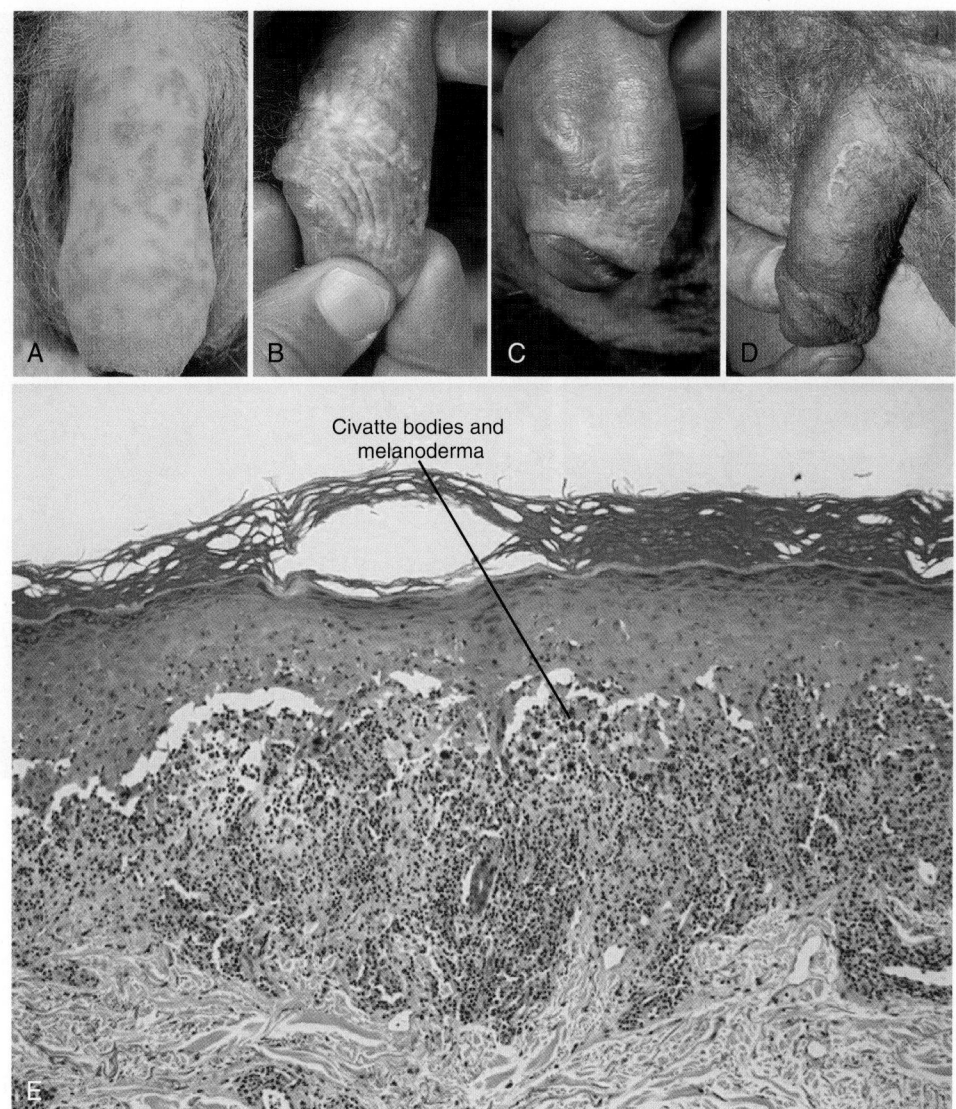

Figure 16-11. **Lichen planus (LP). Various presentations of LP on the male genitalia. A and B, Both individual and grouped purple papules on the penile shaft, some oriented in a linear pattern. C, A white reticular pattern sometimes seen in LP. D, An annular (ringlike) arrangement with a shiny surface. E, Histologically, LP is characterized by destruction of the basal layer, a sawtooth rete ridge pattern, the presence of Civatte bodies and dermal melanocytes, and the absence of parakeratosis or eosinophils. (A, From Korting GW. Practical dermatology of the genital region. Philadelphia: Saunders; 1981. p. 29; B, C, and D, from du Vivier A. Atlas of clinical dermatology. London: Churchill Livingstone; 2002. p. 100; E, from Elston DM, Ferringer T. Dermatopathology. Edinburgh: Saunders; 2009. p. 137.)**

Lichen Sclerosus

Lichen sclerosus et atrophicus (LS) is a chronic inflammatory disease of unknown etiology with a predilection for the external genitalia. LS is 6 to 10 times more prevalent in women than in men, generally presenting either around the time of menopause or in the prepubertal years (Wojnarowska and Cooper, 2003). It tends to affect older men (>60 years of age) (Ledwig and Weigand, 1989) and can be associated with pain during voiding or erection (Margolis, 2002). There is a strong familial predisposition for this disorder, suggesting a genetic contribution (Sherman et al, 2010). For patients with genital LS, 15% to 20% experience extragenital disease (Powell and Wojnarowska, 1999). LS is ultimately a scarring disorder characterized by tissue pallor, loss of architecture resulting from fibrosis, and hyperkeratosis (Fig. 16-12). Some cases of LS may demonstrate prominent purpura and fissuring; the former may be so severe as to obscure the typical "white" color of the disease. The

glans penis and foreskin are usually affected, and the perianal involvement common in women is usually absent. Preputial scarring from LS can lead to phimosis, and circumcision is usually curative, although recurrence in the circumcision scar may occur. The late stage of this disease is called *balanitis xerotica obliterans*, which can involve the penile urethra and result in troublesome urethral strictures. In women, the disease can eventually lead to vulvar adhesions, labial fusion, clitoral phimosis, and vaginal obstruction. LS can also be the cause of considerable genital itching, burning, pain, and dyspareunia in women.

Despite the similarities in name, LS shares little in common with LP and LN other than pruritus and a predilection for the genital region. **Another critical distinction is that LS has been associated with SCC of the penis and vulva, particularly those variants not associated with human papillomavirus (HPV), and LS may represent a premalignant condition** (Velazquez and Cubilla, 2003; Bleeker et al, 2009; van de Nieuwenhof et al, 2011).

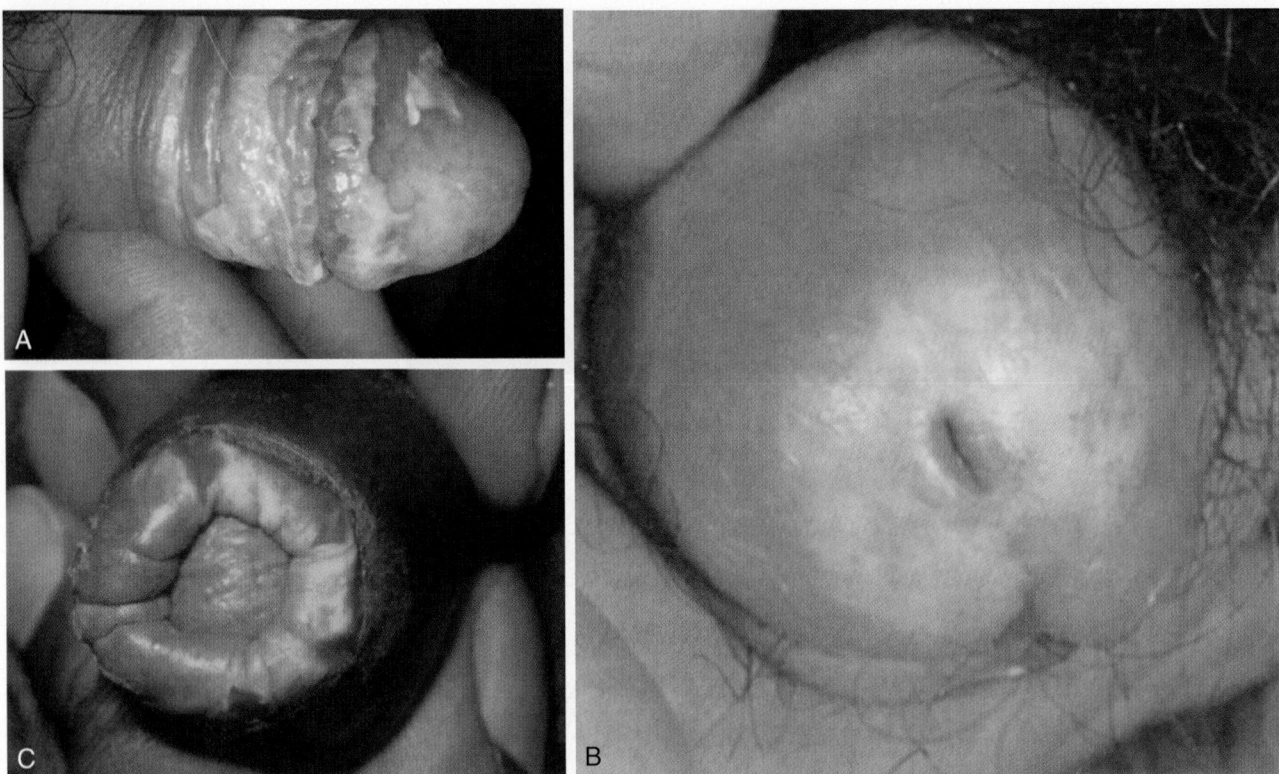

Figure 16-12. A to C, Lichen sclerosus et atrophicus (balanitis xerotica obliterans) of the penis. Note the erythematous and white plaques involving the penile shaft, preputial skin, and glans. (A, From Callen JP, Greer DE, Hood AF, et al. Color atlas of dermatology. Philadelphia: Saunders; 1993. p. 327; B, from du Vivier A. Atlas of clinical dermatology. London: Churchill Livingstone; 2002. p. 716; C, from Bolognia JL, Jorizzo JL, Rapini RP. Dermatology. Edinburgh: Mosby; 2003. p. 1101.)

LS includes specific histologic features, including basal cell vacuolation, epidermal atrophy, marked dermal edema, collagen homogenization, focal perivascular infiltrate of the papillary dermis, and plugging of the ostia of follicular and eccrine structures (Margolis, 2002). Biopsy is worthwhile both to confirm the diagnosis and to exclude malignant change (Powell and Wojnarowska, 1999). It has been suggested that the expression of selected cellular markers (such as p53, survivin, telomerase, Ki-67, and cyclin D1) can help distinguish between indolent LS and LS with true malignant potential (Carlson et al, 2013). In the future, biopsy specimens may routinely be investigated for these (and other) protein markers to determine prognosis.

From a management standpoint, long-term follow-up of patients with LS is important because of the association with SCC. The application of potent topical steroids (such as clobetasol propionate 0.05% or halobetasol 0.05%) for long courses (3 months) is well established as a treatment for LS in women, and may both improve symptoms and reverse the disease process (Dalziel et al, 1991). This regimen is contrary to the usual policy of avoiding long courses of steroid application to genital skin. The efficacy of similar approaches has not been definitively confirmed in adult men, although benefits have been demonstrated in the pediatric age group (Kiss et al, 2001). A European, multicenter, phase II trial also supported the safety and efficacy of topical tacrolimus in the treatment of long-standing LS (Hengge et al, 2006). The application of topical and administration of systemic retinoids, as well as photodynamic therapy, may be therapeutic options in rare cases refractory to standard therapeutic interventions. Because of a high rate of recurrence (40% to 50%) after seemingly successful initial therapy, some experts suggest the routine use of proactive (prophylactic) maintenance therapy with either midpotency topical steroids (such as mometasone furoate 0.1%) or topical calcineurin inhibitors (Virgili et al, 2013).

Fixed Drug Eruption

A fixed drug eruption occurs in response to oral medications, usually 1 to 2 weeks after the first exposure, and commonly involves the lips, face, hands, feet, and genitalia, particularly the glans penis (Fig. 16-13). After subsequent re-exposure to the drug, the reaction presents in the exact same location, usually within 24 hours (hence the term "fixed"). The most common medications causing this reaction are sulfonamides, nonsteroidal anti-inflammatory agents, barbiturates, tetracyclines, carbamazepine, phenolphthalein, oral contraceptives, and salicylates (Kauppinen and Stubb, 1985; Stubb et al, 1989; Thankappan and Zachariah, 1991). There have been isolated reports of fixed drug eruption associated with urologic drugs, such as finasteride, tadalafil, and fluconazole (administered for vulvovaginal candidiasis).

When present on the penile shaft or glans, these lesions are usually solitary, violaceous-colored, inflammatory plaques, which may become erosive and painful (Margolis, 2002). On the genitalia, the differential diagnosis includes herpes simplex infection or an insect bite. Removing the offending agent usually results in resolution of the lesion, although a postinflammatory brown pigmentation may remain. There should be no long-lasting residual functional defect from this process.

Seborrheic Dermatitis

Seborrheic dermatitis (SD) is a common skin disease characterized by the presence of sharply demarcated pink-yellow to red-brown plaques covered with an adherent flaky scale. It shares a variety of features in common with eczematous dermatitis and could easily be grouped in that category. Common dandruff is a mild form of SD localized to the scalp. It has a predilection for areas rich in sebaceous glands and is generally present only during the

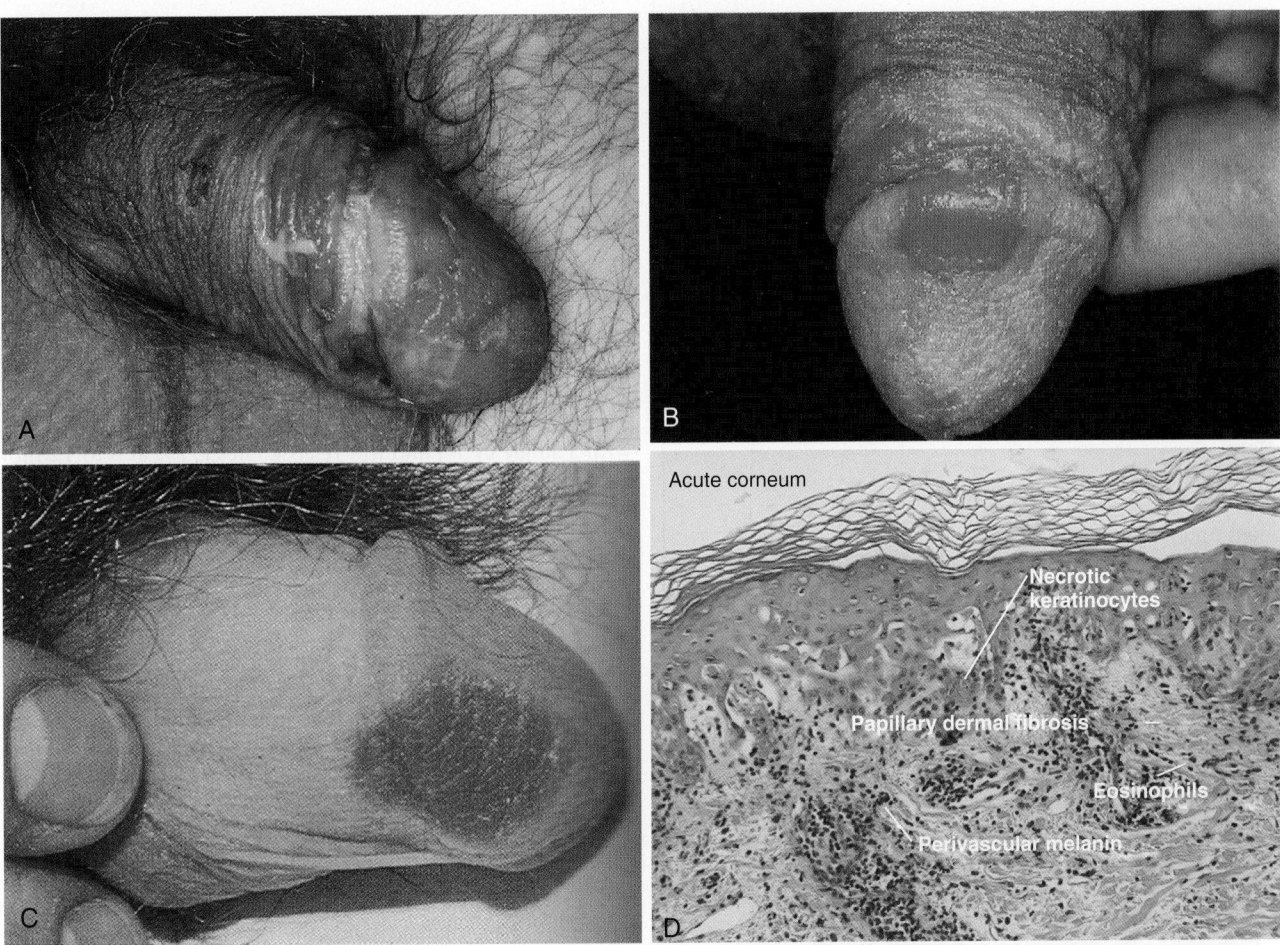

Figure 16-13. Fixed drug eruptions. A to C, Involvement of the penis. D, Histologic features include a normal stratum corneum with chronic changes in the superficial dermis including an eosinophilic infiltrate. (A, From Callen JP, Greer DE, Hood AF, et al. Color atlas of dermatology. Philadelphia: Saunders; 1993. p. 160; B, from Bolognia JL, Jorizzo JL, Rapini RP. Dermatology. Edinburgh: Mosby; 2003. p. 345; C, from Habif TP. Clinical dermatology. Edinburgh: Mosby; 2004. p. 492; D, from Elston DM, Ferringer T. Dermatopathology. Edinburgh: Saunders; 2009. p. 149.)

first few months of life or postpuberty, when sebaceous glands are active. Commonly affected areas include the scalp, eyebrows, nasolabial folds, ears, and chest, although the anus, glans penis, and pubic areas may also be involved (Margolis, 2002). Circumcision may be somewhat protective against the development of SD. In one study of 357 patients, the risk of developing penile SD was 2.5 times greater in the uncircumcised state (Mallon et al, 2000).

Adult SD includes a chronic relapsing course (Webster, 1991). **This condition is particularly common in patients with Parkinson disease, and up to 83% of acquired immunodeficiency syndrome (AIDS) patients may manifest SD (**Froschl et al, 1990; Gupta and Bluhm, 2004). Particularly in immunosuppressed individuals, SD may involve a significant proportion of the body surface area. **Extensive and/or severe SD should raise concerns for possible underlying HIV infection (**Fritsch and Reider, 2003). SD may be pruritic, and differentiation from psoriasis may occasionally be problematic. Unlike psoriasis, however, SD rarely involves the nails and tends to have a thinner associated scale.

Controversy concerning the etiology of SD revolves around a possible autoimmune response to a component of normal skin flora, the yeast *Malassezia furfur (Pityrosporum ovale)*. Although *M. furfur* can be isolated from the lesions of SD, the number of organisms is only about twice that observed in normal control skin (Nenoff et al, 2001). Likewise, severely SD-affected HIV patients do not harbor more organisms than HIV patients who do not manifest

SD (Pechere et al, 1999). Another factor potentially linked to SD is an elevated level of triglycerides and cholesterol at the skin surface (Fritsch and Reider, 2003).

Creams or foams containing topical antifungals (i.e., ketoconazole) are the mainstay of SD treatment on the body and include a 75% to 90% response rate (Faergemann, 2000; Fritsch and Reider, 2003; Elewski et al, 2007). For hair-bearing areas, "antidandruff" shampoos containing zinc, salicylic acid, selenium sulfide, tar, ciclopirox olamine, or 1% to 2% ketoconazole are effective (Margolis, 2002; Squire and Goode, 2002). Because of the chronic and relapsing nature of SD, treatment often must be repetitive and prolonged. Low-potency topical corticosteroids may play a role during the initial treatment of severe cases, but they should not be the primary mode of treatment for this condition because of the potential for local steroid side effects.

VESICOBULLOUS DISORDERS

Vesicobullous disorders are uncommon conditions often characterized by autoimmune damage to the epidermis or basement membrane (Box 16-3). Although intact blisters may be found on the groin and suprapubic skin per se, the rupture of vesicles and bullae on the genitalia may only leave behind residual erosions (Margolis, 2002).

From Margolis DJ. Cutaneous disease of the male external genitalia. In: Walsh PC, editor. Campbell's urology. Philadelphia: Saunders; 2002.

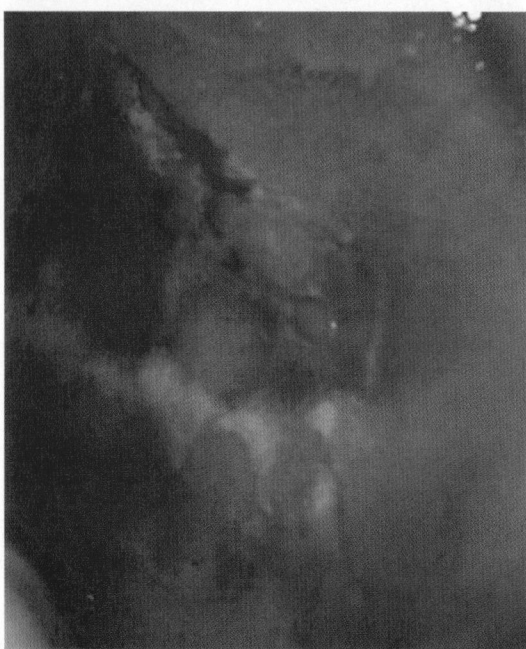

Figure 16-14. Characteristic painful oral mucosal erosions in pemphigus vulgaris. (From Bolognia JL, Jorizzo JL, Rapini RP. Dermatology. Edinburgh: Mosby; 2003. p. 455.)

Pemphigus Vulgaris

Pemphigus is a family of autoimmune blistering diseases characterized by intraepidermal blisters resulting from the loss of keratinocyte cell-cell adhesion (Martel and Joly, 2001). These blisters are located in the deep epidermis close to the basal cell layer. The proposed immunopathology includes the development of autoantibodies directed against keratinocyte cell surface markers and desmosomes (Amagai et al, 1996; Zhou et al, 1997; Joly et al, 2000).

Almost all pemphigus patients will exhibit painful oral mucosal erosions and more than half will experience cutaneous blisters that may involve the genitalia. Characteristic oral lesions are therefore an important clue to the diagnosis (Fig. 16-14). The cutaneous blisters are thin-walled and easily broken to leave behind a painful erosion. The loss of epidermal cohesion seen in pemphigus leads to the characteristic Asboe-Hansen sign: spreading of fluid under the adjacent normal-appearing skin away from the direction of pressure on the blister (Amagai, 2003). **In severe cases without appropriate treatment, pemphigus may lead to fatal septicemia as a result of the loss of the epidermal barrier function of large areas of affected skin.** Treatment for pemphigus traditionally depends on systemic corticosteroids, although minimization of steroid dose is an important goal to limit side effects. The addition of immunosuppressive agents such as azathioprine, cyclophosphamide, and mycophenolate mofetil may be beneficial because of their corticosteroid-sparing effect (Amagai, 2003). In recent years, the use of rituximab as monotherapy (1000 mg administered intravenously on days 1 and 15; repeated in 1 month if necessary) has gained considerable support because of high efficacy rates (>70% with a single cycle) and low relapse rates (22% at 8 to 12 months) (Leshem et al, 2013). The infusion of intravenous immunoglobulin may also prove effective and presents an inherent advantage of lowering infectious complication rates (Ruocco et al, 2013). The management of pemphigus is difficult and should always be performed in concert with a dermatologist or a rheumatologist who has experience with this disease.

Bullous Pemphigoid

Bullous pemphigoid (BP) is a subepidermal blistering disease that is more common in men and generally afflicts patients older than 60 years of age (Rzany and Weller, 2001). There is enrichment for specific HLA class II alleles in BP patients as compared to normal controls (Delgado et al, 1996), supporting an autoimmune mechanism of pathogenesis. In BP, autoantibodies against specific proteins involved in cell-cell adhesion (BP180, BP230) are present. These proteins are components of hemidesmosomes, which are structures that mediate epidermal-stromal adhesion. Binding of autoantibodies to these structures leads to complement activation and a cascade of events resulting in tissue damage, epidermal-dermal separation, and blister formation (Kitajima et al, 1994; Lin et al, 1997).

The clinical presentation of BP can be highly variable. It generally begins with a nonbullous phase characterized by severe itching and nonspecific skin findings. As the disease moves into the bullous phase, vesicles and blisters appear on normal skin or, most characteristically, on areas containing confluent erythematous plaques. The blisters are tense, tend to form on flexor surfaces, and may involve the inner thighs and genitalia (Fig. 16-15A). Mucous membranes may also be involved, although this is less common than in pemphigus. **The diagnosis is made by a combination of clinical, histologic, and, often most importantly, immunohistochemical features such as the deposition of IgG antibodies along the basement membrane** (Fig. 16-15B) (De Jong et al, 1996). Treatment of BP in the United States is traditionally similar to that described for pemphigus, with systemic corticosteroids and various immunosuppressives playing primary roles (Kirtschig and Khumalo, 2004). However, based on the results of several randomized comparative studies, the Europeans favor the use of superpotent topical steroids for the management even of extensive pemphigoid (Joly et al, 2002, 2009). Certainly, treatment of limited-extent pemphigoid should rely heavily on topical, rather than systemic, corticosteroids. For treatment-resistant cases, oral methotrexate, intravenous immunoglobulin, plasmapheresis, or intravenous rituximab may be beneficial (Hatano et al, 2003; Lee et al, 2003; Ruetter and Luger, 2004; Wetter et al, 2005; Shetty and Ahmed, 2013).

Dermatitis Herpetiformis and Linear IgA Bullous Dermatosis

Both of these entities are blistering autoimmune skin diseases associated with the deposition of IgA antibodies at the basement membrane.

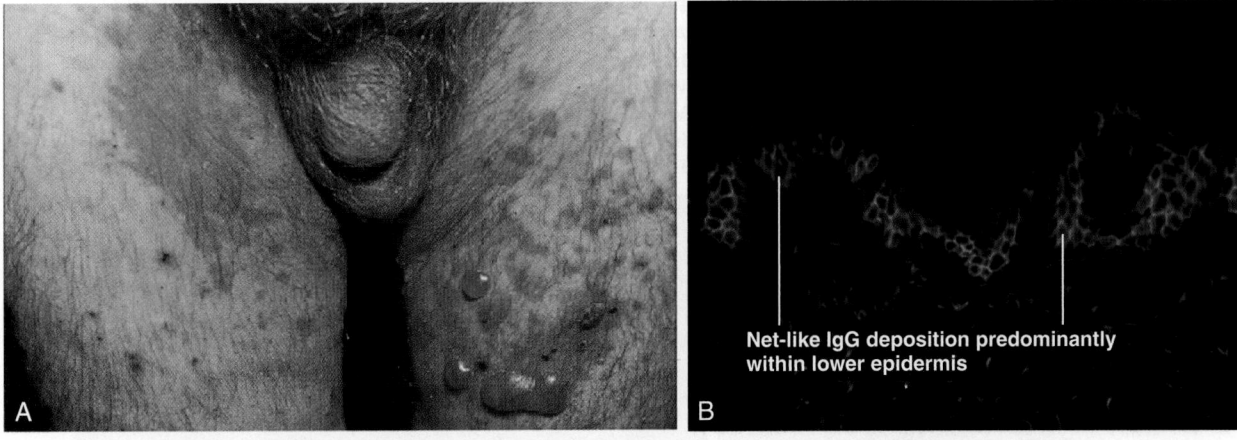

Figure 16-15. Bullous pemphigoid (BP). A, Involvement of the inner thighs. Note the confluent plaques and tense blisters in the inguinal area. **B,** Direct immunofluorescence of BP showing deposition of autoantibodies (IgG) at the dermoepidermal junction. (A, From Bolognia JL, Jorizzo JL, Rapini RP. Dermatology. Edinburgh: Mosby; 2003. p. 465); B, from Elston DM, Ferringer T. Dermatopathology. Edinburgh: Saunders; 2009. p. 169.)

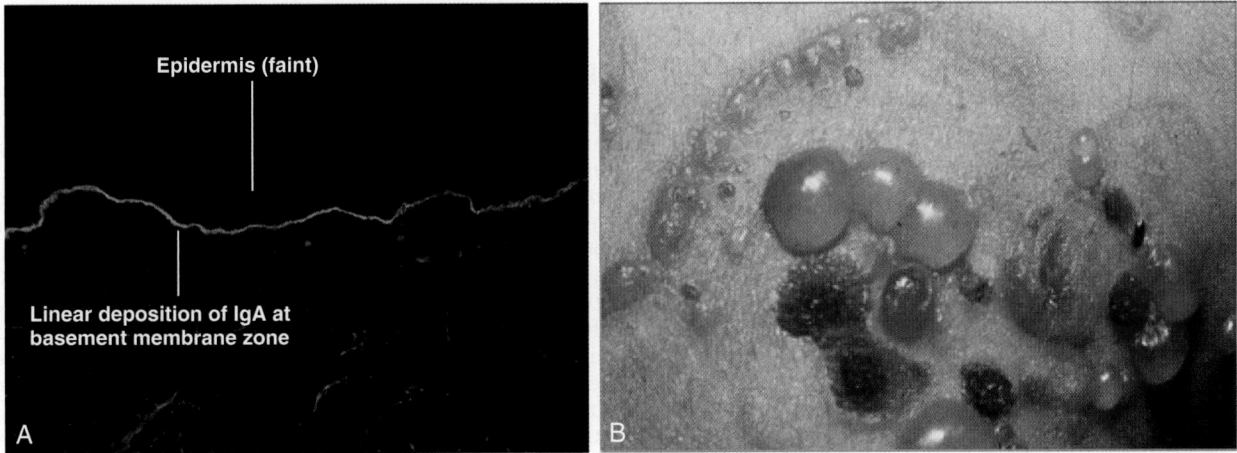

Figure 16-16. Linear IgA bullous dermatosis. A, Direct immunofluorescence showing linear deposition of IgA along the dermoepidermal junction. **B,** Typical circumferential and linear patterns of vesicles. (A, From Elston DM, Ferringer T. Dermatopathology. Edinburgh: Saunders; 2009. p. 170; B, from Bolognia JL, Jorizzo JL, Rapini RP. Dermatology. Edinburgh: Mosby; 2003. p. 485.)

Dermatitis herpetiformis is a cutaneous manifestation of celiac disease and is generally associated with gluten sensitivity (Karpati, 2004). It is most common in people of northern European origin. There is a close association of dermatitis herpetiformis with certain HLA class II DQ2 alleles (DQA1*0501, DQB1*02) (Reunala, 1998). Pruritic plaques, papules, and vesicles in a symmetrical distribution characterize dermatitis herpetiformis. These vesicles may form "herpetiform" groups on an erythematous base. Patients may also complain of pain and burning over the lesions. Diagnosis can be confirmed by biopsy and direct immunofluorescence, which shows a granular pattern of IgA deposition at the basement membrane. Treatment includes the use of dapsone and a strict gluten-restricted diet (Frodin et al, 1981; Andersson and Mobacken, 1992).

Linear IgA bullous dermatosis (LABD), in contrast, is not associated with celiac disease. As the name implies, a linear pattern of antibody deposition at the basement membrane is found on immunohistochemistry in LABD (Fig. 16-16). Characteristic clinical features include vesicles and bullae arranged in a combination of circumferential and linear orientations. Treatment with either sulfapyridine or dapsone is usually effective in controlling LABD, and long-term spontaneous remission rates of 30% to 60% have been described (Wojnarowska et al, 1988). In contrast to both pemphigus and BP, neither dermatitis herpetiformis nor LABD commonly affects genital or perigenital skin.

Hailey-Hailey Disease

Hailey-Hailey disease is an autosomal dominant blistering dermatosis related to various mutations in the ATP2C1 gene. The ATP2C1 gene encodes the protein product hSPCA1, which is a Ca^{2+}/Mn^{2+} transporter. This protein is responsible for calcium homeostasis in the Golgi apparatus required for the post-translational processing of junctional proteins involved in proper epidermal cell-cell adhesion. Hailey-Hailey disease usually develops within the second or third decade of life (Burge, 1992). It has a characteristic predilection for the intertriginous areas including the neck, axillae, groin, and perianal region (Fig. 16-17). In women, disease in the inframammary folds is common although vulvar disease is unusual (Wieselthier and Pincus, 1993). Symptoms include an unfortunate combination of pruritus, pain, and a foul odor. As heat and sweating exacerbate the condition, Hailey-Hailey disease tends to worsen dramatically during the summer months (Burge, 1992). Skin findings include confluent areas of fragile vesicles and blisters, which form as a result of the

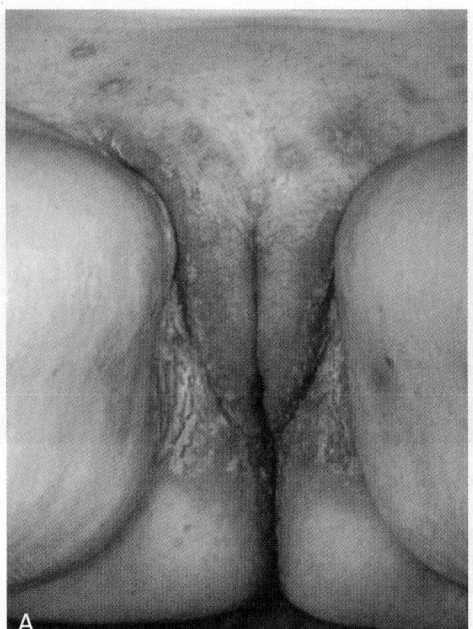

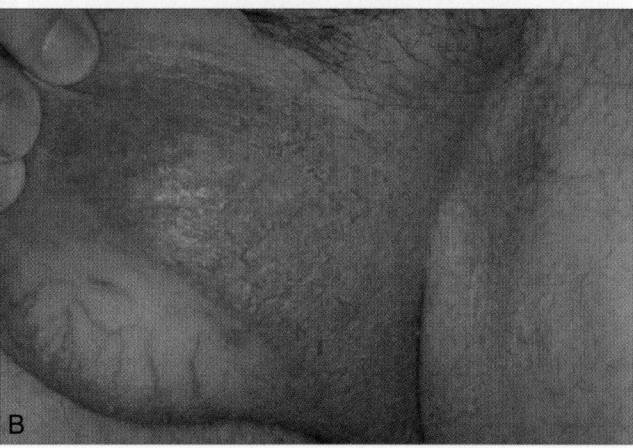

Figure 16-17. Genital presentations of Hailey-Hailey disease. A, The vulva and groin are covered in a vesicular eruption that has become confluent and macerated. **B,** Erythematous plaque with maceration of the inguinal canal and scrotum. (A, From du Vivier A. Atlas of clinical dermatology. London: Churchill Livingstone; 2002. p. 688; B, from Bolognia JL, Jorizzo JL, Rapini RP. Dermatology. Edinburgh: Mosby; 2003. p. 830.)

BOX 16-4 Differential Diagnosis of Ulcers

Syphilis
Chancroid
Herpes simplex
Crohn disease
Aphthous ulcer
Behçet disease
Granuloma inguinale
Genital bite wound
Lymphogranuloma venereum
Factitial dermatitis
Wegener granulomatosis
Leukocytoclastic vasculitis
Pyoderma gangrenosum

From Margolis DJ. Cutaneous disease of the male external genitalia. In: Walsh PC, editor. Campbell's urology. Philadelphia: Saunders; 2002.

---

aberrant keratinocyte cell adhesion. Lesions may be confined to the axilla or groin, and superinfection with yeast, bacteria or herpes simplex virus may compound the problem. Histologic examination may be helpful in differentiating Hailey-Hailey disease from impetigo, pemphigus, intertrigo, and Darier disease (Margolis, 2002). **Treatment includes wearing lightweight, breathable clothing to avoid friction and sweating. Lesions may respond to topical or intralesional corticosteroids, with the caveats mentioned previously about the use of these agents on intertriginous skin. For disease that is resistant to medical therapy, wide excision and skin grafting have been effective, as have local ablative techniques such as dermabrasion, photodynamic therapy, and CO_2 or erbium-YAG laser vaporization** (Hamm et al, 1994; Christian and Moy, 1999; Hohl et al, 2003). An innovative approach to this disorder is to inject infected areas with botulinum toxin type A; this therapy greatly reduces sweating and thereby reduces disease severity (Bessa et al, 2010).

NONINFECTIOUS ULCERS

Genital ulcers can be a result of both infectious and noninfectious causes (Box 16-4).

Aphthous Ulcers and Behçet Disease

Aphthous ulcers are small, painful erosions that commonly involve the oral cavity (so-called canker sores) but they can occasionally be present on the genitalia. **When oral and genital aphthous ulcers coexist, the clinician should seriously consider the diagnosis of Behçet disease (BD).** BD is a generalized relapsing and remitting ulcerative mucocutaneous disease that likely involves a genetic predisposition and an autoimmune mode of pathogenesis (Sakane, 1997; Mendes et al, 2009). Although many genetic loci have been implicated, perhaps the strongest association is with HLA B51. Oxidative stress related to the overproduction of superoxide radicals by neutrophils has also been implicated in the development of this condition (Freitas et al, 1998; Najim et al, 2007). However, a large number of other etiopathogenetic mechanisms have been proposed and supported by experimental findings (such as IL-10 gene mutations) (Remmers et al, 2010). The notable variability in efficacy for any of the therapeutic interventions enumerated later suggests that pathways of inflammation in BD are unlikely to be uniform. BD has a high prevalence in Turkey (80 per 100,000), Israel (15 per 100,000), and Japan (10 to 12 per 100,000), but it is quite rare in the United States (0.12 to 5.0 per 100,000) (Arbesfeld and Kurban, 1988; Calamia et al, 2009). Affected individuals may also suffer from epididymitis, thrombophlebitis, aneurysms (particularly of the pulmonary artery), and gastrointestinal, neurologic, and arthritic problems (Koc et al, 1992; Tuzun et al, 1997; Cetinel et al, 1998; Krause et al, 1999; Aykutlu et al, 2002; Margolis, 2002). BD occurs with roughly similar frequency among males and females, although men typically experience a more severe course.

Mucocutaneous lesions of the oral cavity and genitalia (Fig. 16-18) and ocular involvement (uveitis) form a triad of clinical features in BD. The genital lesions are larger and generally more painful than the oral lesions. Optic involvement occurs in 90% of cases and may lead to blindness (Moschella, 2003). The Behçet International Study Group has defined the diagnosis as recurrent oral ulceration plus any two of the following: recurrent genital ulceration, eye lesions, cutaneous lesions, and skin sensitivity to needle puncture (pathergy test) (Criteria for diagnosis of Behçet's disease. International Study Group for Behçet's Disease, 1990). Other causes for genital ulceration, however, including simple aphthous ulcers, primary syphilis, herpes simplex, and chancroid, must be considered before a diagnosis of BD is made (Margolis, 2002). While using these accepted criteria, it should be noted that oral ulceration is the most sensitive lesion and genital ulceration is the most specific lesion. The latter therefore is the most clinically useful

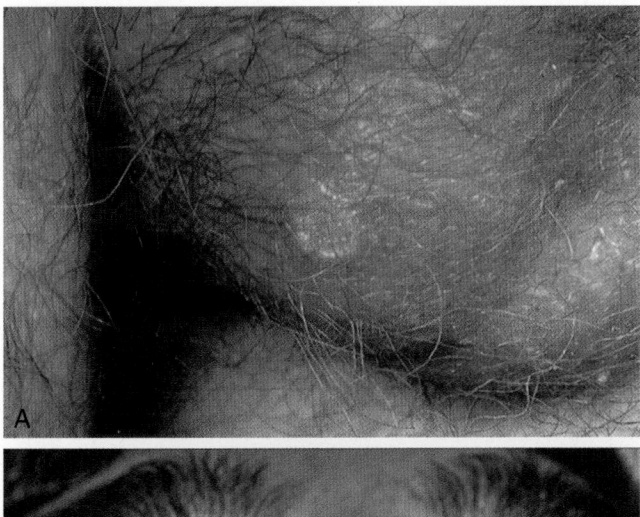

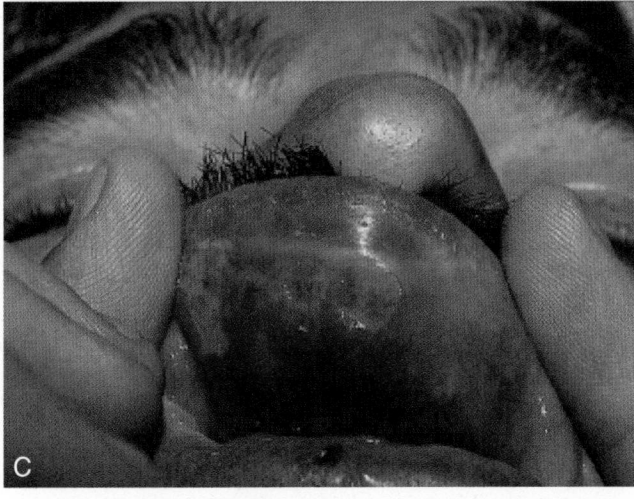

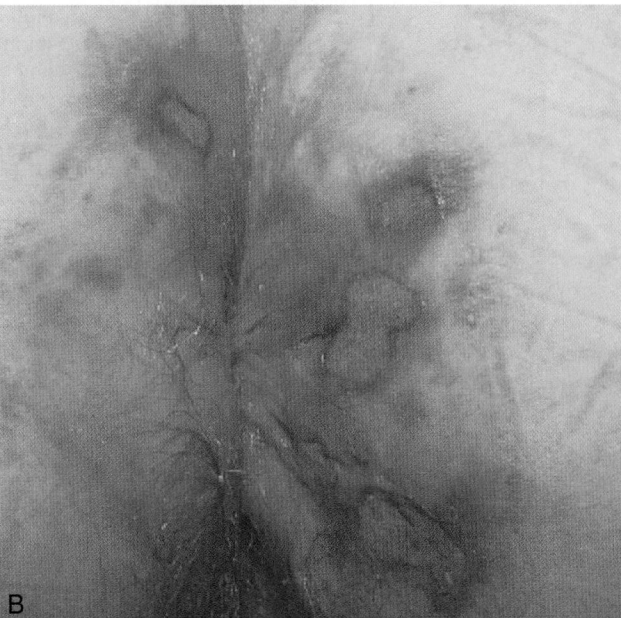

Figure 16-18. Scrotal (A), perianal (B), and oral (C) ulcers seen in Behçet disease. (A, From du Vivier A. Atlas of clinical dermatology. London: Churchill Livingstone; 2002. p. 713; B and C, from Bolognia JL, Jorizzo JL, Rapini RP. Dermatology. Edinburgh: Mosby; 2003. p. 419.)

lesion in diagnosing BD according to this schema. Nonetheless the diagnosis of BD depends exclusively on the aggregate clinical findings, as there are no specific laboratory, radiologic, genetic, or histologic findings that conclusively confirm this diagnosis (Hatemi et al, 2013).

The clinical course of BD is protean, and randomized controlled trials in support of specific therapy are currently limited (Kaklamani and Kaklamanis, 2001). A wide range of topical and systemic agents has been applied to treat BD with variable success, including corticosteroids, dapsone, colchicine, immunosuppressants, 5-aminosalicylic acid (5-ASA) derivatives, cyclosporine A, and TNF-α inhibitors (especially infliximab and adalimumab) (Moschella, 2003; Kose et al, 2009). It has become clear that earlier and more aggressive treatment of BD-associated significant organ involvement with immunosuppressives and biologics has improved the overall outcome. Rheumatologic consultation is advised when this diagnosis is suspected.

Pyoderma Gangrenosum

Pyoderma gangrenosum (PG) is a rare ulcerative skin disease associated with systemic illnesses including inflammatory bowel disease, arthritis, collagen vascular disease, chronic active hepatitis, HIV infection, and myeloproliferative disorders (Moschella, 2003). It most commonly affects women between the second and fifth decade of life and likely has an autoimmune pathogenesis given its association with other autoimmune diseases. Between 20% and 50% of cases, however, are idiopathic. The annual incidence of PG in the United States is about 1 case per 100,000 individuals.

The classic morphologic presentation of PG is painful cutaneous and mucous membrane ulceration, often with extensive loss of tissue and a purulent base (Fig. 16-19). Although unusual, PG can

involve the penis, scrotum, vulva, and peristomal sites (Cairns et al, 1994). As was the case in BD, no specific diagnostic laboratory test or histopathologic feature is pathognomonic for PG, although a history of an underlying systemic disease may raise suspicion. Aside from ulcerative STDs, the differential diagnosis of penile PG includes calciphylaxis, BD, necrotizing fasciitis, cutaneous metastatic Crohn disease, deep fungal infection, pemphigus vegetans, Fournier gangrene, neoplastic conditions, erosive LP, trauma, and factitious damage (Badgwell and Rosen, 2006). Treatment includes a combination of local and systemic corticosteroid therapy with or without adjunctive immunosuppressants (i.e., cyclosporine) (Chow and Ho, 1996). Minocycline, sulfasalazine, and thalidomide have been used in combination with corticosteroids in a small number of cases. Genital PG may also be amenable to topical treatment with calcineurin inhibitors (Lally et al, 2005).

Traumatic Causes

Cutaneous lesions of the genitalia, including ulceration, can be caused by local trauma, which should be included in the differential diagnosis. **This can be either accidental ("innocent trauma") or self-inflicted ("factitial dermatitis" or "dermatitis artefacta").** Accidental injuries may be a result of trauma during sexual practices (including genital bite wounds), ornamentation (i.e., piercing), or unusual hygiene practices (i.e., cleaning) (Margolis, 2002). **Factitial dermatitis is a psychocutaneous disorder in which the individual self-inflicts cutaneous lesions usually for an unconscious motive or because of an underlying mental illness (Fig. 16-20). Factitial lesions are occasionally produced deliberately with the hope of some secondary gain (such as product liability litigation).** An association between factitial dermatitis and borderline personality disorder appears to exist (Koblenzer, 2000). Other disorders to be considered include Munchausen syndrome by proxy, body

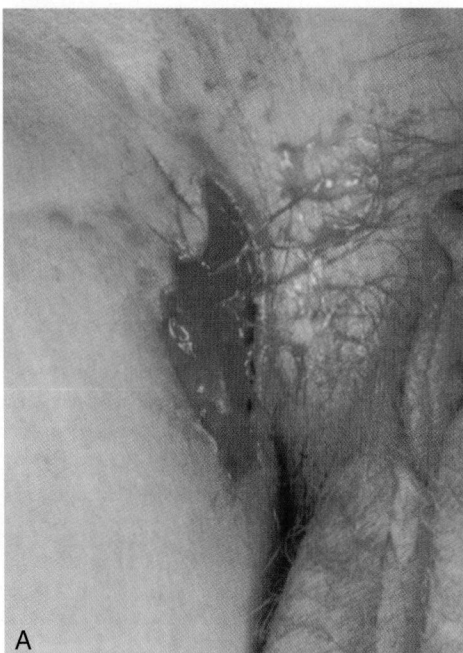

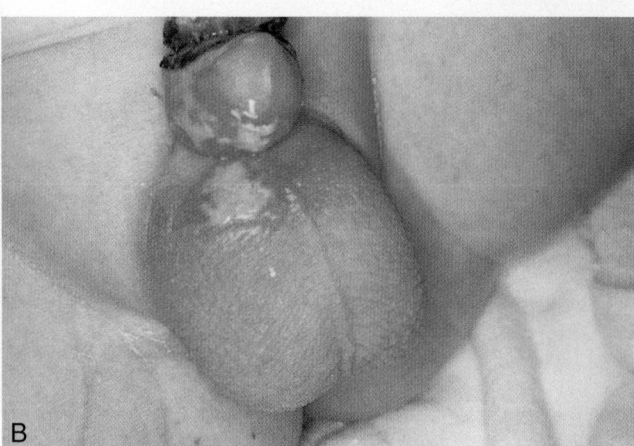

Figure 16-19. Pyoderma gangrenosum involving the inner thigh of a woman with rheumatoid arthritis (A) and the penis and scrotum (B). (A, From du Vivier A. Atlas of clinical dermatology. London: Churchill Livingstone; 2002. p. 387; B, from Callen JP, Greer DE, Hood AF, et al. Color atlas of dermatology. Philadelphia: Saunders; 1993. p. 330.)

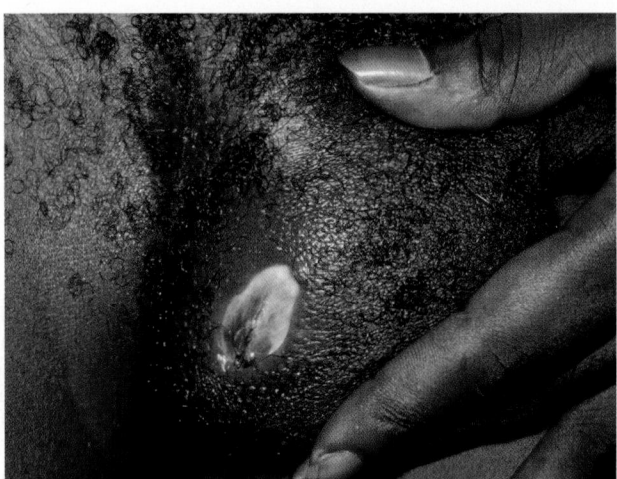

Figure 16-20. Factitial ulcer of the scrotum caused by repeated picking at the scrotal skin.

dysmorphic disorder, and malingering, if secondary-gain issues exist. Although rare, factitial dermatitis should always be considered in the differential diagnosis of unusual genital lesions, including oddly configured erosions and ulcerations (Verma et al, 2012).

INFECTIONS AND INFESTATIONS

Sexually Transmitted Diseases

STDs with genital cutaneous manifestations include lymphogranuloma venereum, granuloma inguinale, herpes simplex, chancroid, molluscum contagiosum, HPV, and syphilis (Fig. 16-21). These conditions are discussed in detail in Chapter 15.

Balanitis and Balanoposthitis

Balanitis is an inflammatory disorder of the glans penis. When the process involves the preputial skin in uncircumcised men, it is termed balanoposthitis. In children, bacterial infections are the predominant cause. In adult men, the cause may be intertrigo, ICD,

local trauma, or candidal and bacterial infections (Fig. 16-22). Treatment includes removal of irritating agents, improved hygiene, topical antibiotics and antifungals, and occasionally short courses of low-potency topical corticosteroids (Margolis, 2002). When treatment fails, the differential should include neoplastic diseases, Zoon balanitis, psoriasis, and alternative infectious agents such as HPV (Wikstrom et al, 1994). Balanoposthitis tends to occur in patients with phimosis and circumcision may be curative in select recurrent cases. Balanoposthitis may also result from bacterial superinfection in the setting of poor hygiene and neutropenia (Manian and Alford, 1987).

Cellulitis and Erysipelas

Cellulitis is an infection of the deep dermis and subcutaneous tissues most commonly caused by gram-positive organisms (*S. pyogenes* and *S. aureus*) (Lewis, 1998). In immunocompetent individuals, organisms usually gain entry to the site of infection through a break in the skin barrier. In immunocompromised patients, a blood-borne route of infection is more common. Systemic signs of illness include fever, chills, and general malaise. Local signs include erythema (rubor), warmth (calor), pain (dolor), and swelling (tumor) at the site with indistinct borders (Fig. 16-23). Treatment includes systemic antibiotics with activity against *S. pyogenes* and *S. aureus* species. The clinician may be forced to rely on known local antimicrobial sensitivity patterns, because obtaining satisfactory material for culture may be difficult. In cases associated with diabetes, mixed flora may be present and antibiotic coverage should be broadened. Marking the zone of cellulitis at the onset of therapy is an important step to allow progression and resolution of cellulites to be monitored during therapy.

Erysipelas is a superficial bacterial skin infection limited to the dermis with lymphatic involvement. This disease commonly occurs at the extremes of age and often involves the face. In contrast to the cutaneous lesion of cellulitis, erysipelas generally exhibits a raised and distinct border at the interface with normal skin. The causative organism is usually *S. pyogenes*.

Fournier Gangrene (Necrotizing Fasciitis of the Perineum)

Fournier gangrene (FG) is a potentially life-threatening progressive infection of the perineum and genitalia (Morpurgo and Galandiuk, 2002). In the genital region, most cases of FG are caused by mixed

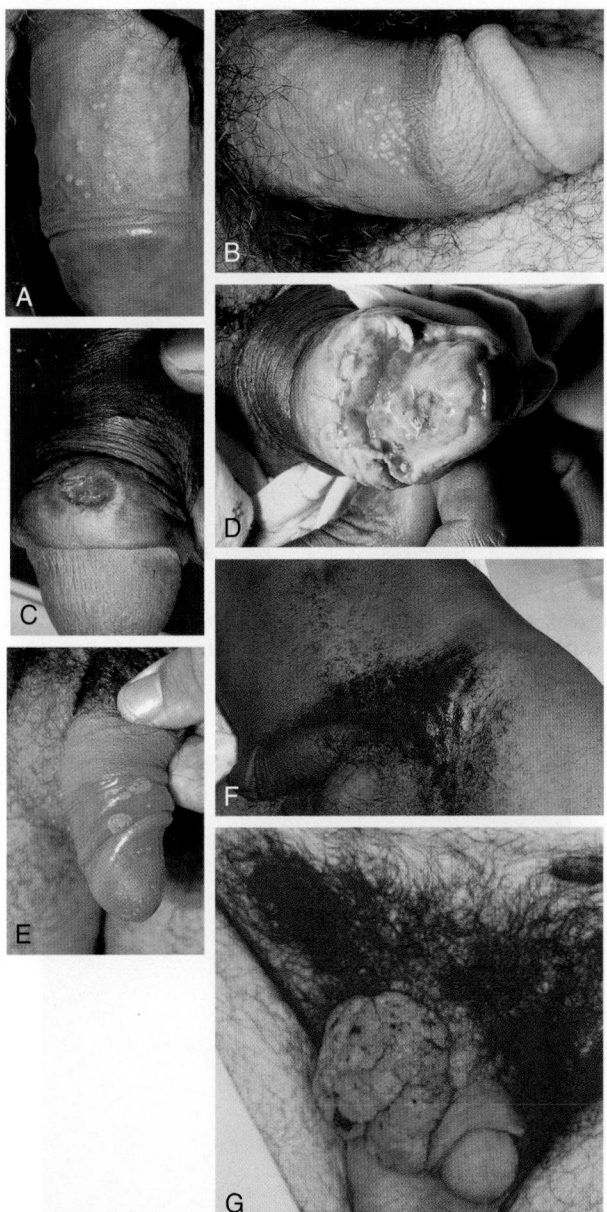

Figure 16-21. Genital lesions associated with sexually transmitted diseases. A, Herpes simplex virus. B, Molluscum contagiosum. C, Syphilitic chancre. D, Granuloma inguinale. E, Chancroid. F, Lymphogranuloma venereum. G, Condyloma accuminata. (From Callen JP, Greer DE, Hood AF, et al. Color atlas of dermatology. Philadelphia: Saunders; 1993.)

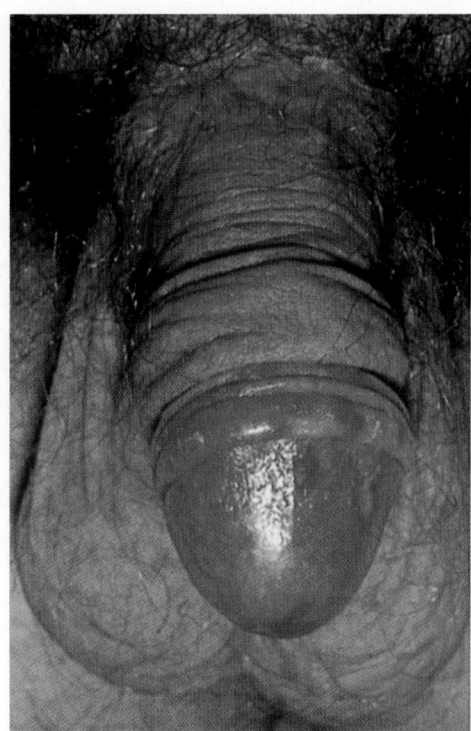

Figure 16-22. Candidal balanoposthitis. (From Korting GW. Practical dermatology of the genital region. Philadelphia: Saunders; 1981. p. 159.)

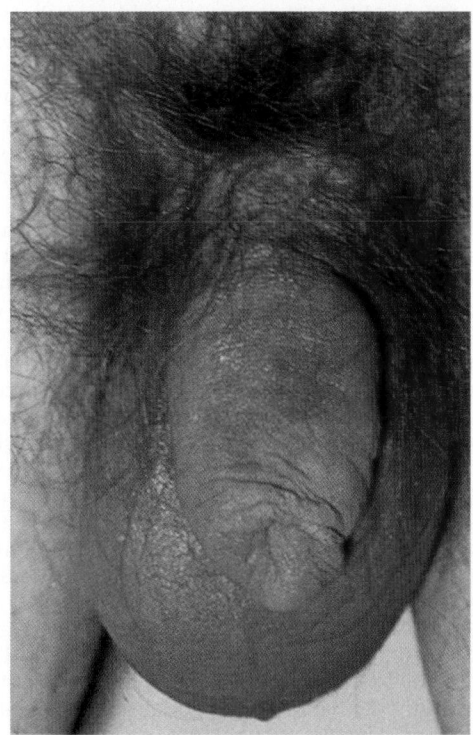

Figure 16-23. Penoscrotal cellulitis. (From Korting GW. Practical dermatology of the genital region. Philadelphia: Saunders; 1981. p. 37.)

bacterial flora, which include gram-positive, gram-negative, and anaerobic bacteria. *Escherichia coli*, *Bacteroides* spp., *S. pyogenes*, and *S. aureus* are common etiologic pathogens. Risk factors for developing FG include underlying alcoholism, diabetes, cancer and malnutrition, advanced age, recent urogenital or colorectal instrumentation or trauma, and preexisting peripheral vascular disease. However, group A streptococcal necrotizing fasciitis can occur in healthy immunocompetent individuals.

The hallmark of FG is a rapid progression from the signs and symptoms of cellulitis (erythema, swelling, and pain) to blister formation, to clinically visible ischemia, and ultimately to foul-smelling necrotic lesions (Fig. 16-24). **Infection may spread along fascial planes and hence the exterior skin findings may represent only a small proportion of the underlying infected and necrotic tissue. The diagnosis of FG is a surgical emergency, as progression from genitalia to perineum to abdominal wall may occur**

extremely rapidly (often within hours). Spread of tissue infection is accompanied by an ever-increasing risk of bacterial septicemia, usually the eventual cause of death. The exclusion of FG therefore should be a priority during every consultation for soft tissue infection of the genitalia. Pain out of proportion to

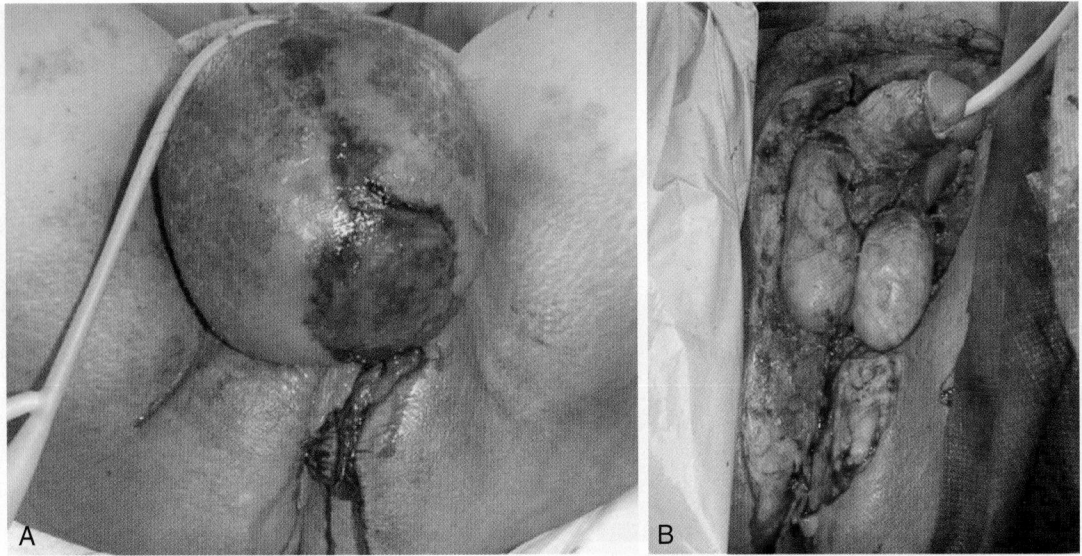

Figure 16-24. Fournier gangrene of the scrotum. A, Surface appearance of scrotum and perineum showing area of frank necrosis. B, Extent of soft tissue debridement required to achieve margins of viable tissue. Note that the testes within their tunica vaginalis compartment are spared.

the visible extent of infection should raise suspicion for FG. The skin may also exhibit a grayish cast or fetid odor uncharacteristic of uncomplicated genital cellulitis. Imaging of the genitalia with plain radiographs, computed tomography, and/or bedside ultrasonography (Amendola et al, 1994; Avery and Scheinfeld, 2013) may demonstrate gas bubbles within the tissue, although the delay associated with imaging should not postpone surgical intervention in obvious cases.

Treatment involves a combination of broad-spectrum antibiotics and extensive surgical debridement to margins of healthy bleeding tissue. These patients will often require a second-look operation after 24 to 48 hours to exclude further disease progression (Gurdal et al, 2003). During surgical debridement for scrotal FG, the testicles and other structures within the tunica vaginalis can almost always be spared, although loss of tissue in the abdominal wall may be extensive because of bacterial spread along fascial planes. The indications for adjunctive hyperbaric oxygen therapy in FG remain controversial, although several groups have reported favorable results (Dahm et al, 2000; Eke, 2000; Jallali et al, 2005). There may also be potential benefit to the use of vacuum-assisted closure devices in FG (Czymek et al, 2009). However, despite aggressive modern management, the mortality of FG may be as high as 16% to 40% (Dahm et al, 2000; Eke, 2000; Blume et al, 2003; Yeniyol et al, 2004; Sorensen et al, 2009). A number of different numeric scoring scales have been applied to FG in an attempt to predict proactively the patients who are at the highest risk for mortality and who should receive the most aggressive intervention. These include the FG Severity Index and the Uludag FG Severity Index, as well as the more general Age-Adjusted Charlson Comorbidity Index (ACCI) and the recently introduced surgical Apgar Score (sAPGAR). A study verified that *all* of these scoring systems are valid methods for assessing patients in the setting of FG, and adoption of one may assist the clinician in making therapeutic decisions (Vyas et al, 2013).

Among patients who survive an episode of FG, there most likely will be ongoing disability and reduced functionality for months to years. Sexual dysfunction is quite common (~65%) (Czymek et al, 2013). Therefore FG survivors should expect to receive long-term care from a variety of specialists.

Folliculitis

Folliculitis is a common disorder characterized by perifollicular pustules on an erythematous base (Kelly, 2003). It occurs most

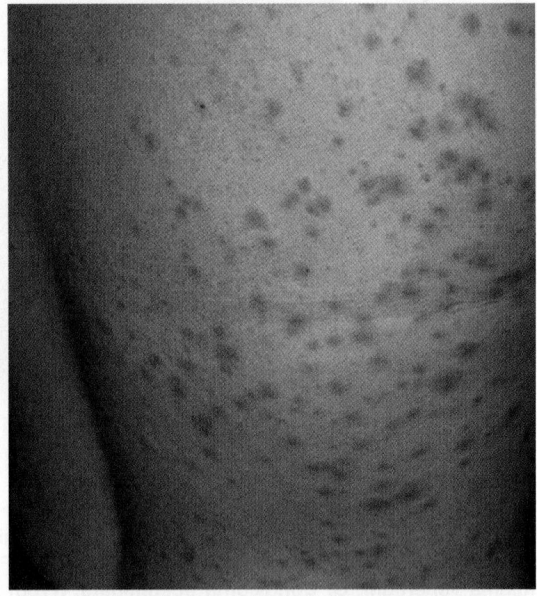

Figure 16-25. Pseudomonal folliculitis caused by the use of a hot tub. (From Bolognia JL, Jorizzo JL, Rapini RP. Dermatology. Edinburgh: Mosby; 2003. p. 554.)

frequently in heavily hair-bearing areas such as the scalp, beard, axilla, groin, and buttocks and can be exacerbated by local trauma from prolonged occlusion (e.g., truck drivers), shaving, rubbing, or clothing irritation (Margolis, 2002). Patients may complain of pruritus or pain over the area; conversely, symptoms may be entirely absent. Cultures are generally negative, although a variety of infectious organisms have been associated with folliculitis including *S. aureus*, *Pseudomonas* spp., fungi, and herpes simplex virus. Folliculitis has also been associated with the use of contaminated hot tubs and swimming pools, with the offending organism usually *Pseudomonas aeruginosa* (Fig. 16-25) (Gregory and Schaffner, 1987; Rolston and Bodey, 1992). Treatment for folliculitis includes good hygiene, removal of offending irritants, and appropriate topical or systemic antiviral, antibiotic, or antifungal agents. The results of a surveillance study indicate that 96% of *P. aeruginosa* isolates tested from swimming pools and hot tubs were multidrug resistant (Lutz and Lee, 2011). These results may have important implications for immune-suppressed individuals, where infection with multidrug-resistant *P. aeruginosa* has a greater potential impact. Failure to respond to conservative measures should lead to lesion culture with concomitant antimicrobial susceptibility testing.

Furunculosis

Both furuncles and abscesses are walled-off collections of pus. **Although abscesses can occur anywhere on the body, a furuncle is by definition associated with a hair follicle.** Furuncles tend to occur in areas prone to minor trauma including the groin and buttocks (Fig. 16-26). *S. aureus* is the most common causative organism although anaerobes may be present. Risk factors include diabetes mellitus, obesity, poor hygiene, and immunosuppression (Brook and Finegold, 1981). Warm compresses may be beneficial, and larger lesions may require incision and drainage, as for any abscess. When there is associated cellulitis, a systemic antibiotic with activity against staphylococci should be administered. In today's environment of methicillin-resistant staphylococci, coverage for such organisms is advisable if they are prevalent within the clinician's community.

Hidradenitis Suppurativa (Acne Inversa)

Hidradenitis suppurativa (HS) is a chronic disease of apocrine gland-bearing skin with a predilection for the axillae and anogenital regions (Kelly, 2003; Alikhan et al, 2009). **The condition generally begins after puberty and a familial form with an autosomal dominant pattern of inheritance has been described** (Von Der Werth et al, 2000). Originally believed to be a disease of apocrine glands, HS is now thought to be an epithelial disorder of hair follicles (Jansen et al, 2001). Although superinfection of HS lesions may occur, bacterial infection does not appear to be the primary initiator. During the pathogenesis of HS, hair follicles become plugged and swollen. **Rupture of follicular contents (including bacteria and keratin) into the surrounding dermis initiates a marked inflammatory response with the formation of abscesses and sinus tracts** (Slade et al, 2003).

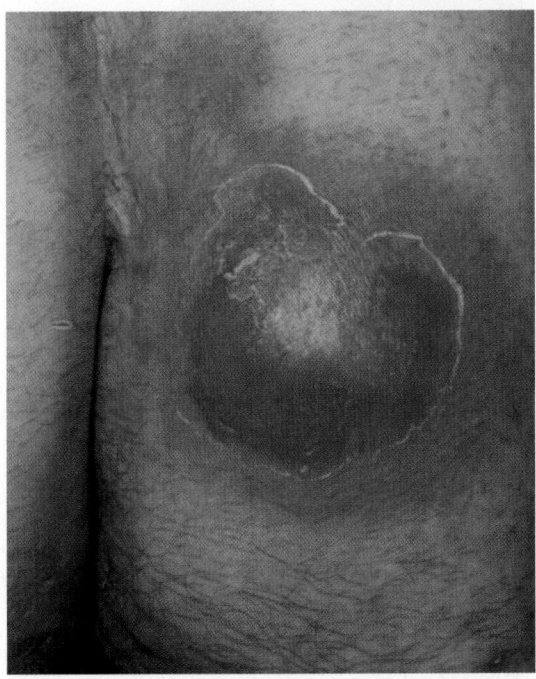

Figure 16-26. A large furuncle located on the buttocks. (From Habif TP. Clinical dermatology: Edinburgh: Mosby; 2004. p. 284.)

The clinical features of HS include painful inflammatory nodules and sterile abscesses developing in the axillae, groin, perianal, and inframammary areas (Fig. 16-27) (Kelly, 2003). With time, draining sinus tracts and hypertrophic scars develop. Serious complications of HS can occur, including hypoproteinemia, secondary amyloidosis, the development of fistulae to the urethra (Gronau and Pannek, 2002), bladder, peritoneum and rectum (Nadgir et al, 2001), and SCC in areas of heavy scarring (Altunay et al, 2002; Rosenzweig et al, 2005).

Treatment of HS includes improvement in hygiene, weight reduction, and efforts to minimize friction and moisture in affected areas (i.e., loose undergarments, absorbent powder) (Kelly, 2003). No single therapeutic intervention is universally effective. Topical clindamycin or the combination of oral clindamycin or minocycline with oral rifampicin may be beneficial for some patients (Gener et al, 2009). In a double-blind randomized trial, systemic therapy with tetracycline was no more effective than topical clindamycin in HS (Jemec and Wendelboe, 1998). Other oral agents that sometimes prove beneficial include dapsone (50 to 200 mg/day), zinc (40 to 80 mg/day elemental zinc), retinoids (acitretin 25 to 50 mg/day or isotretinoin 1 mg/kg/day), cyclosporine (4 mg/kg/day), and hormone blockers (spironolactone and oral contraceptives in women and finasteride and dutasteride in men) (Scheinfeld, 2013a). Systemic corticosteroids may improve HS, but relapse is the rule after cessation of therapy (Slade et al, 2003). Lithium may exacerbate HS or limit its response to conventional medical therapy (Gupta et al, 1995). Although recurrent incision and drainage of HS lesions are discouraged, wide and deep excision with skin grafting has been effective (Rompel and Petres, 2000; Bocchini et al, 2003). A variety of new approaches, including the use of the CO_2 and Nd:YAG lasers to treat HS, are under investigation (Lapins et al, 1994; Madan et al, 2008; Tierney et al, 2009). Off-label administration of TNF-α blockers (particularly subcutaneous adalimumab: 40 mg/wk) has proven variably effective in the management of HS in select patients when surgery is simply not feasible (Shuja et al, 2010).

Corynebacterial Infection (Trichomycosis Axillaris and Erythrasma)

Trichomycosis axillaris is a superficial bacterial infection of axillary and pubic hair caused by corynebacteria. Yellow, red, or black nodules are visible on the hair shafts (Fig. 16-28) and there is frequently a characteristic odor (Blume et al, 2003). There is an association with hyperhidrosis (Margolis, 2002). The differential diagnosis includes infestation with pediculosis pubis or fungal infection (piedra) (Avram et al, 1987), although examination with magnification can generally distinguish trichomycosis axillaris from these conditions. Shaving can provide immediate improvement, and antibacterial soaps may prevent further infection (Blume et al, 2003). For pubic trichomycosis axillaris, clindamycin gel, bacitracin, and oral erythromycin have also proven effective (Bargman, 1984; Blume et al, 2003).

Erythrasma is a *Corynebacterium minutissimum* infection of the skin that results in sharply bordered, light red to dark brown, scaling patches in moist areas, particularly the groin and axilla. These lesions may be pruritic or asymptomatic and may be confused with dermatophyte infection (tinea cruris) (Sindhuphak et al, 1985). Under a Wood light, the lesions show a characteristic bright coral-red fluorescence (see Fig. 16-28) (Halprin, 1967). Effective treatments include antibacterial soaps, topical aluminum chloride, topical clindamycin 1% solution or gel, miconazole 1% cream, and oral erythromycin (500 to 1000 mg/day) (Cochran et al, 1981; Holdiness, 2002).

Ecthyma Gangrenosum

Ecthyma gangrenosum is a rare cutaneous manifestation of pseudomonal septicemia that presents most commonly on the

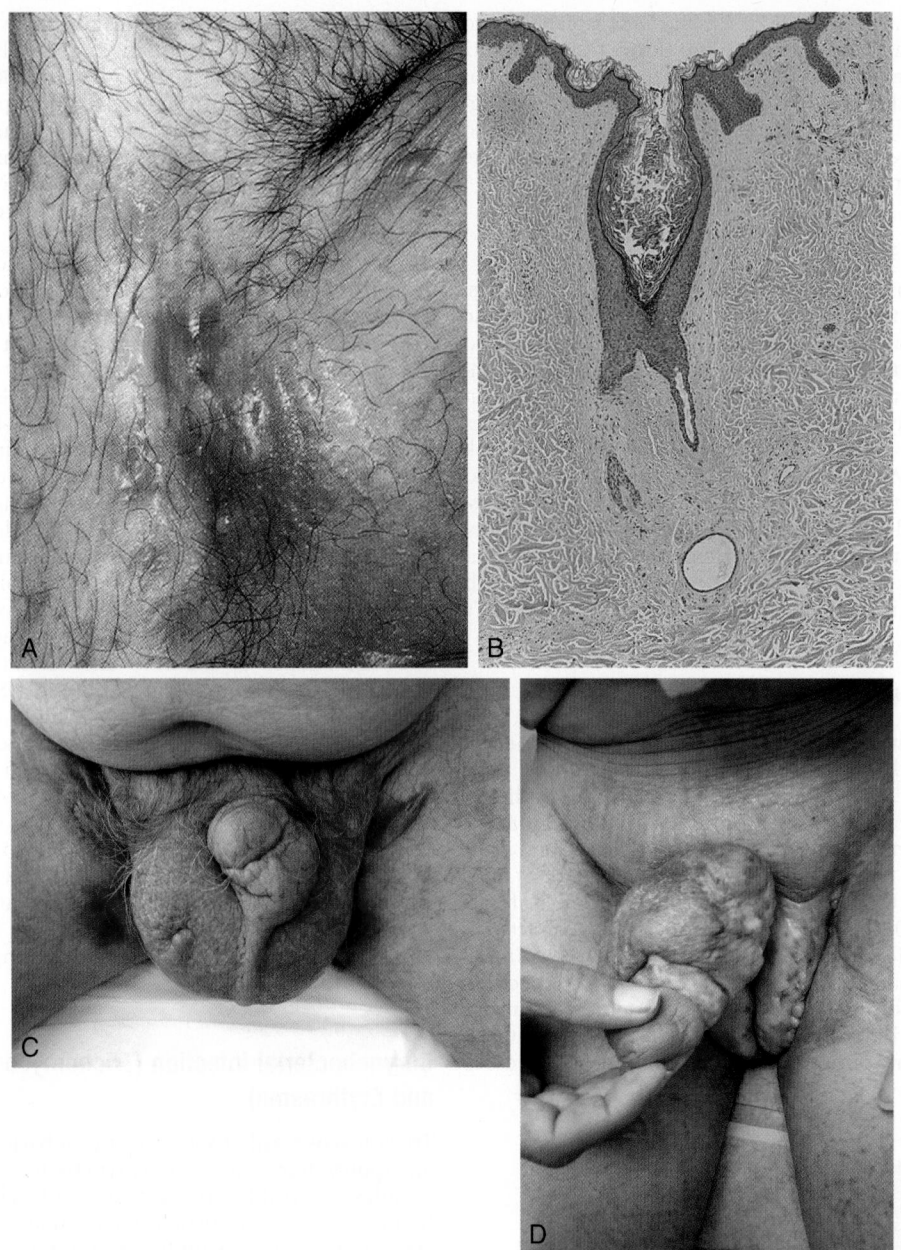

Figure 16-27. Hidradenitis suppurativa. A, Characteristic painful papules and draining sinus tracts. B, Histology shows follicular plugging and connection to a dilated apocrine duct. C and D, Examples of severe genital involvement of hidradenitis, which would make surgical management difficult. (A, From du Vivier A. Atlas of clinical dermatology. London: Churchill Livingstone; 2002. p. 712; B, from Bolognia JL, Jorizzo JL, Rapini RP. Dermatology. Edinburgh: Saunders; 2008. Fig. 39.13.)

anogenital area in debilitated, immunosuppressed, or neutropenic patients. The lesions of ecthyma gangrenosum are tender grouped erythematous macules that may progress to form bullae or rupture to produce a gangrenous ulcer covered by a thick, black eschar (Fig. 16-29) (Blume et al, 2003). On histologic examination, necrotizing vasculitis and gram-negative organisms are present. The differential diagnosis includes PG, necrotizing vasculitis, cryoglobulinemia, and septic emboli containing other organisms including *Candida, Aspergillus, Citrobacter, E. coli, Aeromonas hydrophila,* and *Fusarium* (Altwegg and Geiss, 1989; Martino et al, 1994; Gucluer et al, 1999; Reich et al, 2004). Consistent with the underlying sepsis, ecthyma gangrenosum carries a poor prognosis and immediate treatment with intravenous antipseudomonal antibiotics is

indicated. Wound debridement may also be necessary (Collini et al, 1986).

Genital Bite Wounds

Following deliberate or accidental bite wounds to the genitalia, a normal component of the human oral flora, *Eikenella corrodens,* may be implanted into genital skin. This results in the rapid development of extremely painful, necrotic ulcerations at the bite site(s) (Fig. 16-30) (Rosen and Conrad, 1999; Rosen, 2005). The rapidity of ulceration, extraordinary degree of discomfort, and a history of traumatic orogenital contact help distinguish this type of infection from the more common STDs and other genital ulcers. The

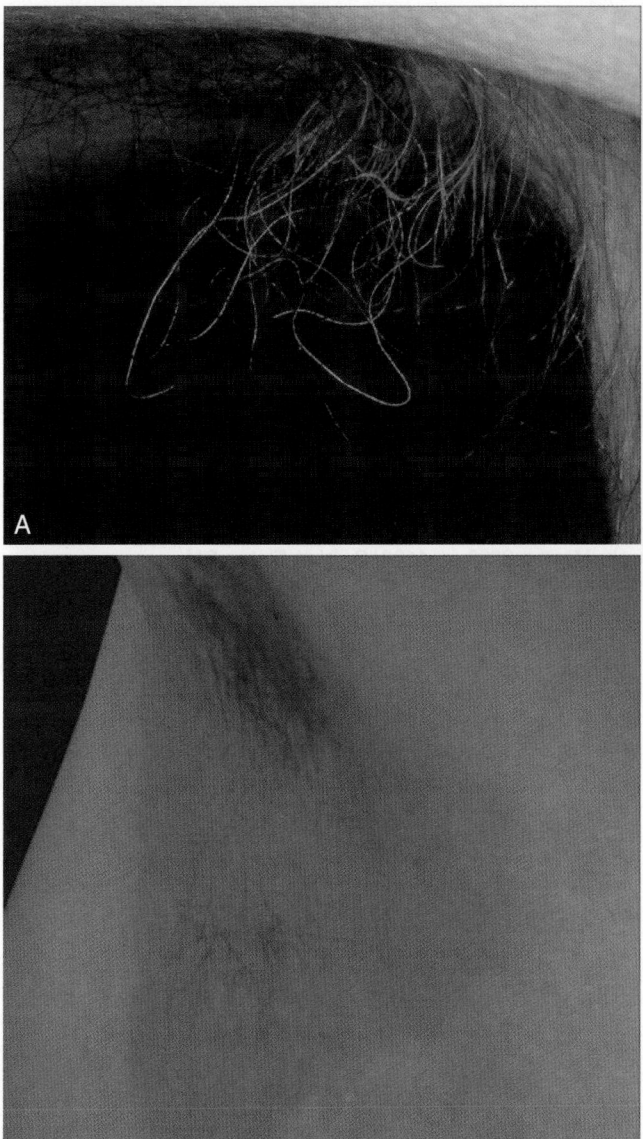

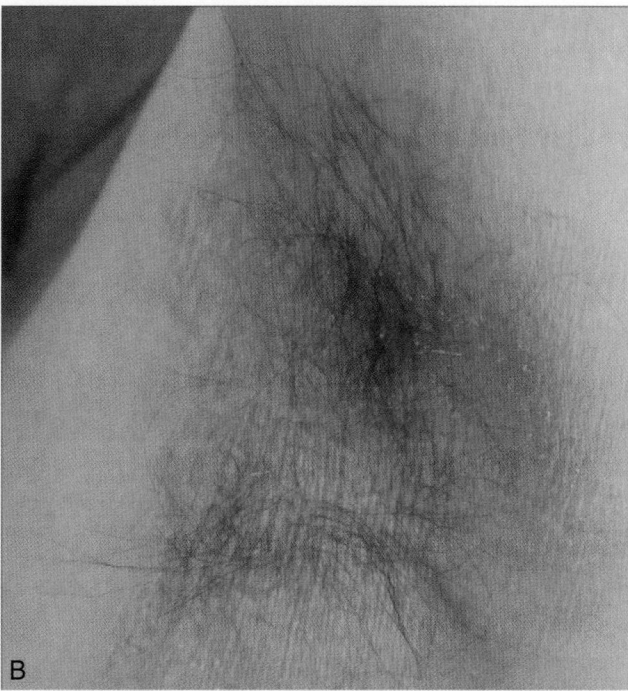

Figure 16-28. Corynebacterial infections of the skin. A, Tricho-mycosis axillaris. B and C, Erythrasma under white light (B) and Wood lamp (C) showing coral-red fluorescence. (From Bolognia JL, Jorizzo JL, Rapini RP. Dermatology. Edinburgh: Mosby; 2003.)

treatment is high-dose oral amoxicillin-clavulanate (1500 mg/day) until healing occurs.

Candidal Intertrigo

Fungal infection of macerated skin folds can occur with candidal species and involve the finger webs and intertriginous areas. Affected pruritic skin is reddened and characteristic satellite lesions may be present (Fig. 16-31). The differential diagnosis includes dermatophyte infection (tinea cruris), pemphigoid, psoriasis, SD, and contact dermatitis (Margolis, 2002). Fungal forms (round yeast cells as well as elongate pseudohyphae) can be seen in scraped skin preparations after treatment with KOH, and culture is usually unnecessary. Daily topical treatment with any imidazole antifungal agent for at least 2 weeks is usually necessary for intertrigo, and oral antifungals (such as fluconazole 150 mg/day) are occasionally required (Cullin, 1977). Maneuvers to decrease moisture and skin maceration, such as the use of drying powders and loose clothing, may also help prevent relapse. Candida intertrigo may be a presenting sign of diabetes, and appropriate laboratory testing should be performed to rule this out as a predisposing condition.

Dermatophyte Infection

Dermatophytes are fungi of three genera *(Trichophyton, Microsporum, Epidermophyton)* that have the propensity to invade and grow within keratinized tissues such as the skin, hair, and nails. These fungi produce keratinases, which break down keratin and facilitate invasion (Viani et al, 2001). In addition, mannans in the cell wall of some dermatophytes produce immunoinhibitory effects (Dahl, 1994).

Tinea cruris is the term applied to dermatophyte infection of the groin and genital area and is commonly known as "jock itch." More common in males than females, this condition is favored by hot, humid environments and concomitant dermatophyte infection of the feet *(tinea pedis)*. Obesity may also be a significant risk factor (Scheinfeld, 2004). The inner thighs and inguinal region are the most commonly affected areas and the scrotum and penis are usually spared in men. However, isolated penile dermatophytosis has been well described (Pielop and Rosen, 2001). **Conversely, significant scrotal involvement should raise suspicion for cutaneous candidiasis as an alternative diagnosis** (Sobera and Elewski, 2003). Characteristic lesions in tinea cruris are sharply demarcated with a raised erythematous border

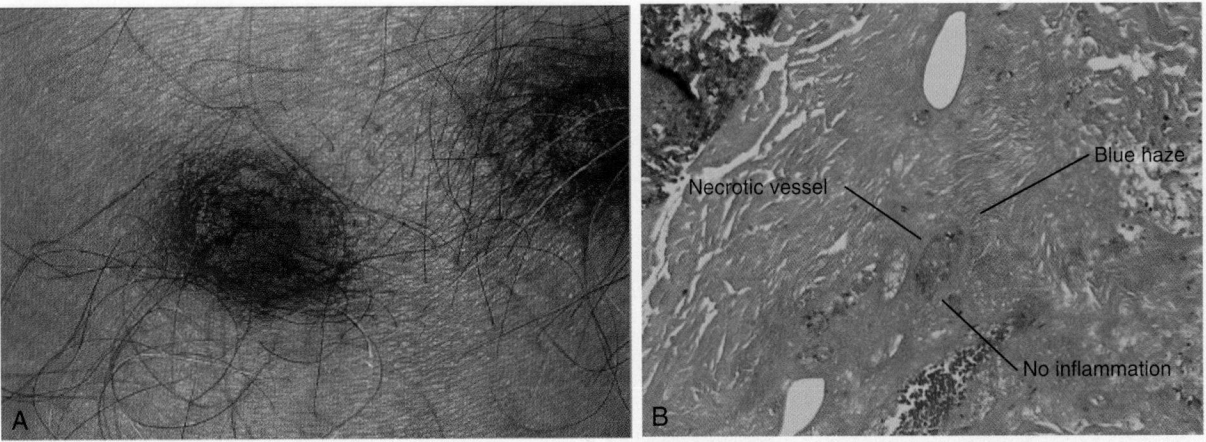

Figure 16-29. Ecthyma gangrenosum. A, Involvement on the chest wall. Note the necrotic center and erythematous border around the lesion. B, Histologically, necrotic vessels surrounded by a "blue haze" of organisms characterize ecthyma gangrenosum. (A, From Bolognia JL, Jorizzo JL, Rapini RP. Dermatology. Edinburgh: Mosby; 2003. p. 1132; B, from Elston DM, Ferringer T. Dermatopathology. Edinburgh: Saunders; 2009. p. 263.)

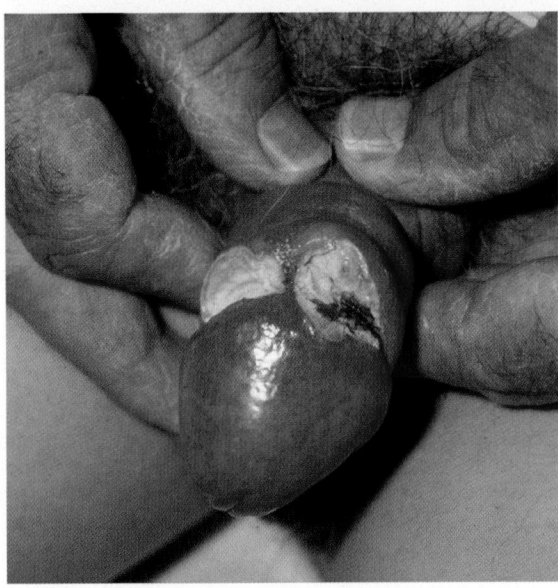

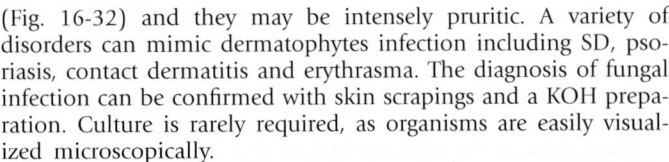

Figure 16-30. Ulceration following a human bite wound to the penile shaft.

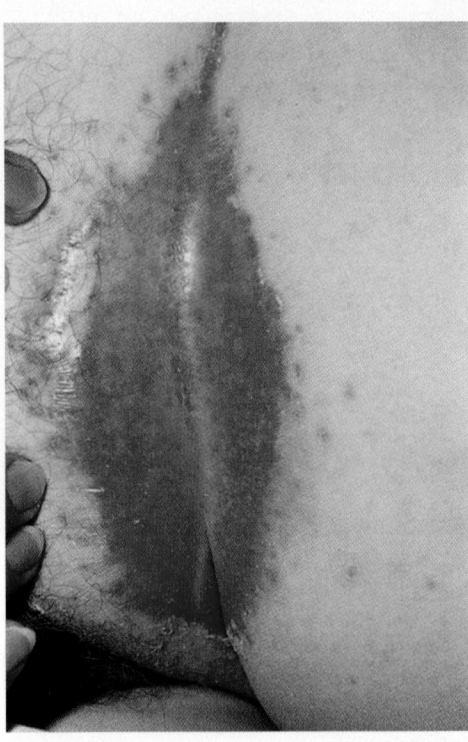

Figure 16-31. Candidal intertrigo with erythema, areas of tissue maceration, and satellite lesions. (From Callen JP, Greer DE, Hood AF, et al. Color atlas of dermatology. Philadelphia: Saunders; 1993. p. 318.)

(Fig. 16-32) and they may be intensely pruritic. A variety of disorders can mimic dermatophytes infection including SD, psoriasis, contact dermatitis and erythrasma. The diagnosis of fungal infection can be confirmed with skin scrapings and a KOH preparation. Culture is rarely required, as organisms are easily visualized microscopically.

Good hygienic practices can be beneficial in preventing recurrent disease, including wearing loose clothing, cleaning of contaminated garments, weight reduction, and the use of topical powders to keep the intertriginous areas dry (Sobera and Elewski, 2003). Topical antifungal preparations are the primary agents for treatment, with the powdered forms having the added benefit of drying moist areas. Care should be taken to treat only active disease and not the postinflammatory hyperpigmentation that can occur with recurrent chronic dermatophyte infection (Margolis, 2002). Systemic antifungals are rarely necessary to treat groin infection with dermatophytes. However, should this prove necessary, the current drug of choice is terbinafine in a dose of 250 mg/day for 1 week (Farag et al, 1994).

Infestation

Pediculosis pubis and scabies *(Sarcoptes scabiei)* are the most common infestations involving the genital region.

Infestation with the crab louse *(Phthirus pubis)* causes pediculosis pubis, a pruritic disorder of the genitalia, which may coexist with other STDs (Opaneye et al, 1993; Varela et al, 2003). In one study of adolescent males, patients with pediculosis pubis showed a risk of concomitant gonorrhea or chlamydial infection more than twofold higher than normal controls (Pierzchalski et al, 2002). Louse infestation is not limited to the genitals and may involve other hair-bearing areas such as the eyelashes, beard, and axillae (Meinking, 1999). The diagnosis is confirmed by

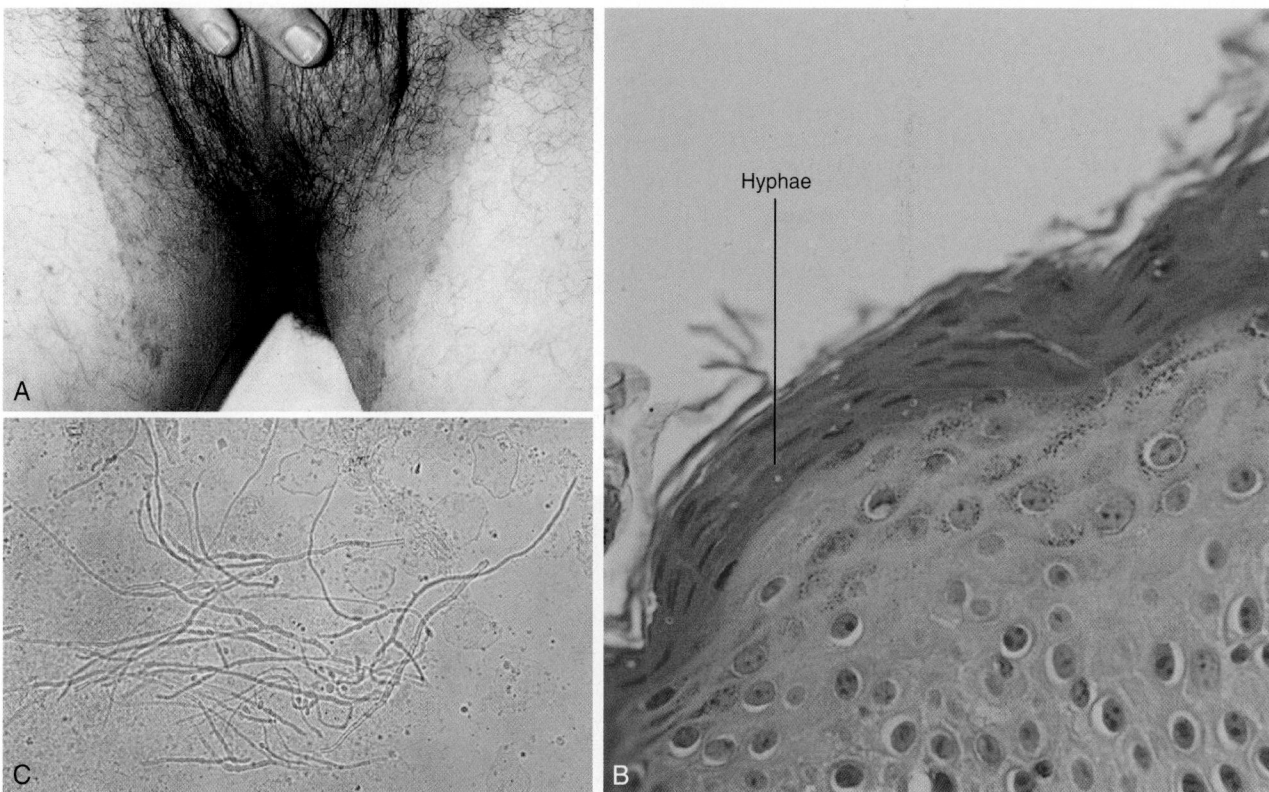

Figure 16-32. Dermatophyte infection. A, *Tinea cruris* showing areas of postinflammatory hyperpigmentation and active infection at the border of the lesions. B, Histologically, fungal hyphae are localized within a compact stratum corneum layer. C, Potassium hydroxide preparation from a scraping showing fungal forms. (A, From Callen JP, Greer DE, Hood AF, et al. Color atlas of dermatology. Philadelphia: Saunders; 1993. p. 318; B and C, from Elston DM, Ferringer T. Dermatopathology. Edinburgh: Saunders; 2009. p. 275.)

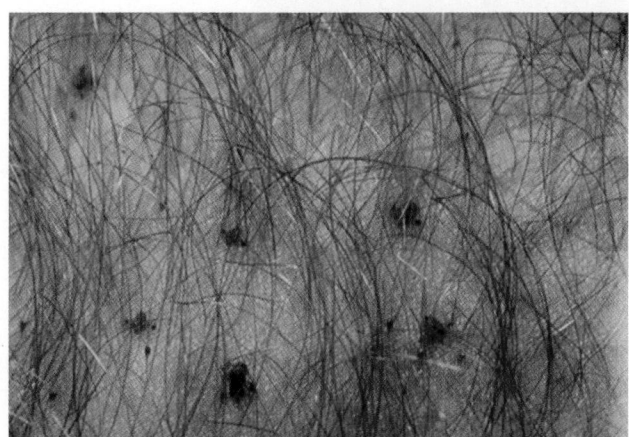

Figure 16-33. Pediculosis pubis. Several crab lice are visible. (From du Vivier A. Atlas of clinical dermatology. London: Churchill Livingstone; 2002. p. 338.)

identification of crab lice attached to hairs (Fig. 16-33), often with associated perifollicular erythema. **Transmission of pediculosis pubis is usually though sexual contact, although contaminated clothing, bedding, and towels have also been implicated in some cases** (Meinking, 1999). **The standard treatment is the application of 5% permethrin cream overnight to all affected hair-bearing areas with a repeat application 1 week later** (Meinking et al, 2003). Note that the second application of permethrin is important, as the rate of treatment success with

a single application may be as low as 57% (Kalter et al, 1987). For rare cases refractory to topical therapy or those involving the eyelashes *(tinea palpebrarum)*, the addition of oral ivermectin may be curative (Burkhart and Burkhart, 2000). Interestingly, because of the adoption of the widespread removal of pubic hair among young adults of both genders ("Brazilian waxing"), the incidence of pubic louse infestation in industrialized countries has fallen dramatically in recent years.

Another important infestation involving the genitalia is scabies, caused by the female itch mite *Sarcoptes scabiei*. **Scabies is a worldwide problem and factors such as overcrowding, delayed treatment of primary cases, and poor public awareness encourage spread** (Meinking et al, 2003). Transmission is common between close contacts and family members (Burkhart et al, 2000). The number of mites living on an immunocompetent host is usually small (<100) (Arlian et al, 1988), although far greater numbers may be recovered in cases of immunosuppression (so-called crusted or Norwegian scabies). The incubation period before symptoms develop after infestation can vary from days to months in duration, but is most typically about 6 weeks.

Severe pruritus is the hallmark of scabies, often accentuated at night or after bathing (Meinking et al, 2003). In both genders, the genital areas are commonly affected. Small erythematous and pruritic papules are present, and excoriations with secondary bacterial infection may occur (Fig. 16-34). **Thin, gray or white burrows may be visible and are pathognomonic for scabies infestation. Crusted scabies affecting genital skin presents as it does in other anatomic sites: with thickly crusted plaque(s)** (Perna et al, 2004). In the absence of visible burrows, a broad differential must be considered including AD, pyoderma, psoriasis, and other insect bites. As in the case of pediculosis pubis, the

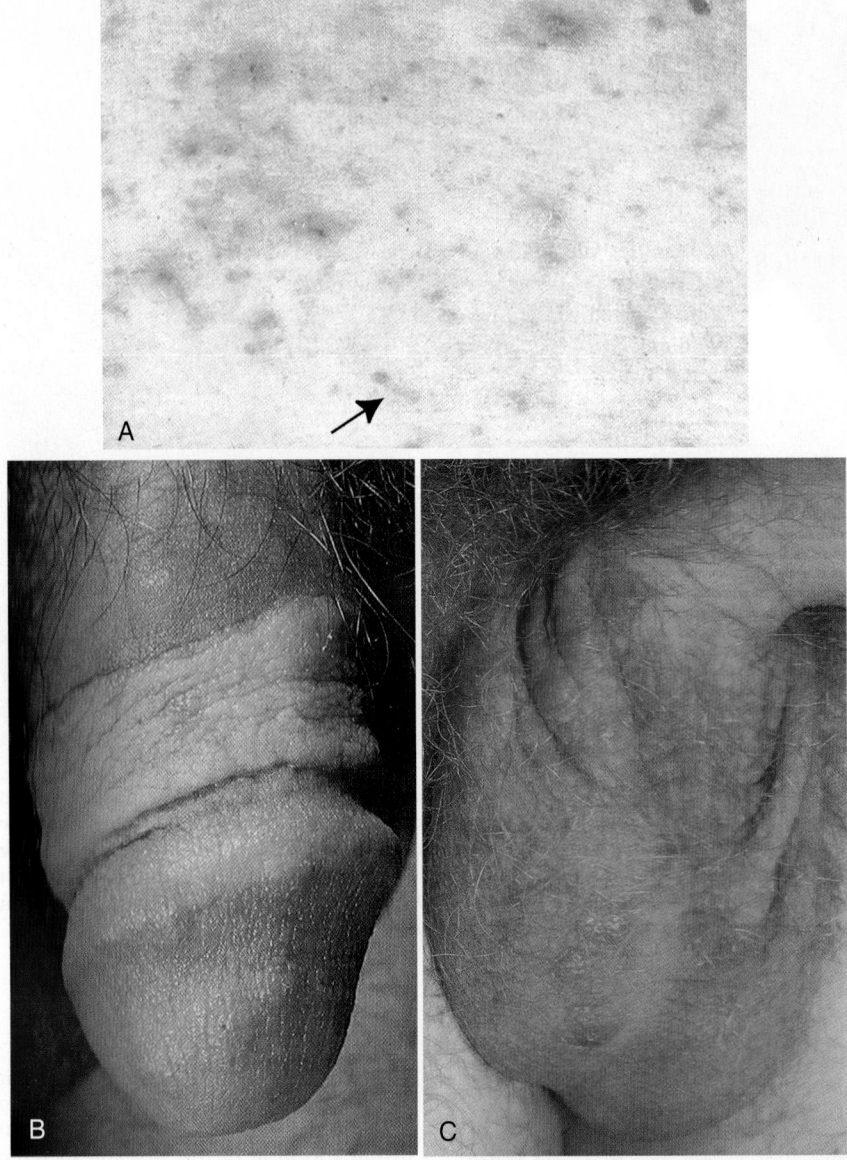

Figure 16-34. Scabies. A, A papular eruption with visible characteristic burrows *(arrow)*. **B** and **C,** Classic established genital scabies with eroded papules on the glans penis and scrotum. **(A,** From du Vivier A. Atlas of clinical dermatology. London: Churchill Livingstone; 2002. p. 332; **B** and **C,** from Habif TP. Clinical dermatology. Edinburgh: Mosby; 2004. p. 501.)

treatment of choice for scabies is 5% permethrin cream applied to the entire body overnight with a second application 1 week later. An alternative topical scabicide, lindane, is not favored because of both central nervous system toxicity in children and a rising rate of resistance among mites (Purvis and Tyring, 1991; Elgart, 1996; Boix et al, 1997). Oral ivermectin (200 μg/kg/dose, 2 doses administered 2 weeks apart) is an alternate regimen that has been successfully used to treat scabies (Chouela et al, 2002; Heukelbach et al, 2004; Karthikeyan, 2005). A randomized comparative trial showed that permethrin was slightly more effective than ivermectin when the latter is only provided as a single dose (Goldust et al, 2012). **Note that pruritus may persist for several weeks despite successful treatment and that all intimate contacts should also be treated to prevent reinfestation.** Even with effective treatment, itchy nodules may remain on the glans penis; intralesional injections of minute amounts of dilute triamcinolone acetonide (2 to 3 mg/mL) may facilitate resolution of these post-scabies nodules.

NEOPLASTIC CONDITIONS

Squamous Cell Carcinoma in Situ

Squamous cell carcinoma in situ (SCCis) is a full thickness intraepidermal carcinoma (Miller and Moresi, 2003). Bowen originally described this condition in 1912, hence the term "Bowen disease" (Bowen, 1912). On extragenital sites, there is a strong association between SCCis and ultraviolet light exposure (Reizner et al, 1994). **Commonly presenting in the seventh decade of life with a slight female predominance (Hemminki and Dong, 2000; Arlette, 2003), SCCis usually has an indolent clinical course and rarely progresses to invasive disease. When it occurs on mucosal surfaces of the male genitalia, most notably the glans penis of uncircumcised men, this entity is referred to as erythroplasia of Queyrat** (Fig. 16-35). Yet another name for this entity is penile intraepithelial neoplasia. In the female, the comparable SCCis on the vulva would be called vulvar intraepithelial neoplasia. In these locations, coinfection with HPV types 8, 16 (70%), and other serotypes (30%) has been identified (Wieland et al, 2000). Other risk factors for SCCis include ionizing radiation, immunosuppression, thermal injury, arsenic exposure, chronic dermatoses (such as long-standing LP), and LS of the glans penis (Euvrard et al, 1995; Nasca et al, 1999; Powell et al, 2001; Centeno et al, 2002; Arlette, 2003).

SCCis lesions are sharply demarcated, solitary, pink to red scaly plaques, which may be confused with basal cell carcinoma, eczema, seborrhea, or psoriasis. SCCis on or near the vulva may be heavily pigmented and resemble both melanoma and external genital warts. When localized to the penile shaft, SCCis may have a more thickened, verrucoid appearance. Although usually asymptomatic, these lesions may also be pruritic or painful. The diagnosis is confirmed by histologic evaluation and several areas should be sampled to exclude the presence of dermal invasion (Margolis, 2002).

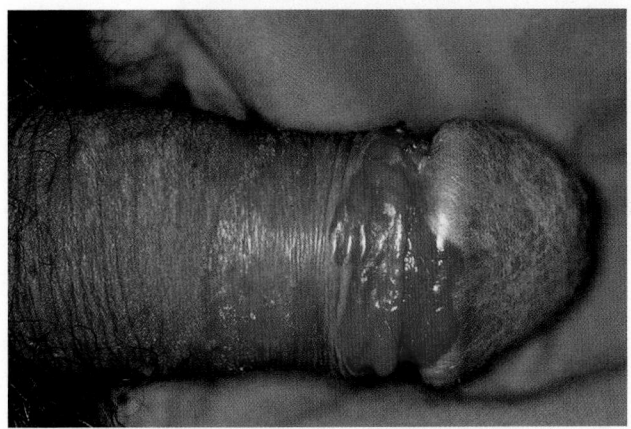

Figure 16-35. Erythroplasia of Queyrat. Squamous cell carcinoma involving the glans penis. (From Callen JP, Greer DE, Hood AF, et al. Color atlas of dermatology. Philadelphia: Saunders; 1993. p. 330.)

Primary treatment of SCCis involves either surgical excision or tissue ablation. For accessible areas, such as the scrotum, simple excision with a 5-mm margin is favored (Bissada, 1992; Margolis, 2002). For areas where tissue preservation is more critical, Mohs microsurgery, laser therapy, and cryoablation may play a role (Sonnex et al, 1982b; van Bezooijen et al, 2001; Leibovitch et al, 2005). Topical treatment with either 5-fluorouracil or imiquimod 5% has also proven effective for management of selected cases of SCCis involving the genitalia (Gerber, 1994; Orengo et al, 2002; Arlette, 2003; Micali et al, 2003).

Bowenoid Papulosis

Bowenoid papulosis is an uncommon condition found on the penis and vulva of sexually active adults, with a peak incidence in the third decade of life (Schwartz and Janniger, 1991). **It histologically resembles Bowen disease except that the abnormal keratinocytes are spread discontinuously throughout the epidermis** (Margolis, 2002). Typical lesions are multiple small erythematous papules that may coalesce to form plaques with a verrucous surface similar to a genital wart (Fig. 16-36). There is a clear association with HPV type 16. **Female partners of men with bowenoid papulosis have an increased risk of cervical neoplasia and should receive close cervical follow-up** (Rosemberg et al, 1991). In men, however, bowenoid papulosis generally has a benign course and spontaneous regression may occur (Eisen et al, 1983; Giam and Ong, 1986; Feng et al, 2013). Therefore, in a young and reliable patient, observation alone may be justified. If treatment is desired, conservative local therapy with topical agents (0.5% 5-fluorouracil, 0.5% tazarotene cream, or imiquimod 5%) or ablative measures (electrodessication, liquid nitrogen cryotherapy, laser ablation) is usually appropriate (Margolis, 2002).

Squamous Cell Carcinoma

Invasive SCC involving the genitalia (Fig. 16-37) is covered in detail in Chapter 37.

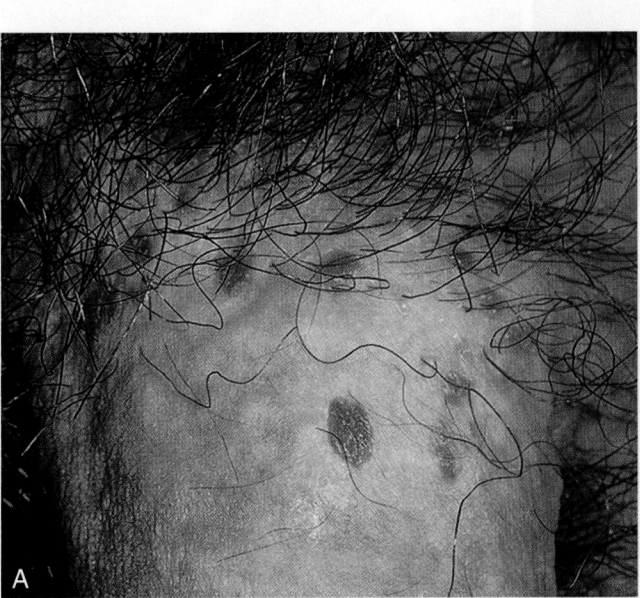

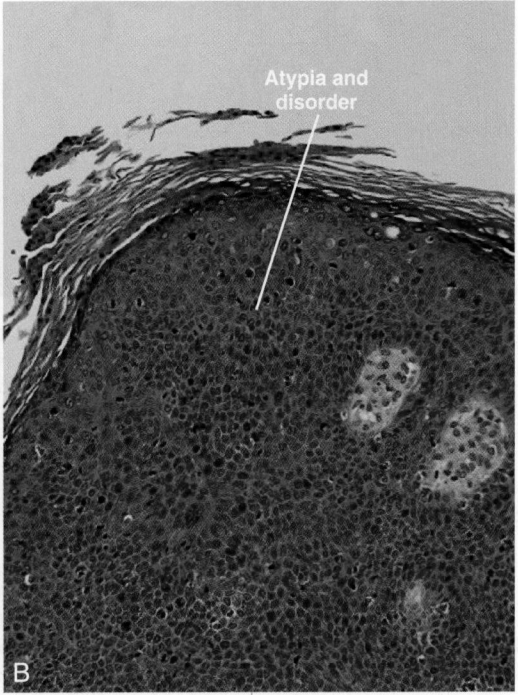

Figure 16-36. Bowenoid papulosis. A, Involvement of the penile shaft. Note multiple brown verrucous papules on the penile shaft. B, Characteristic full thickness atypia, which may be mistaken for Bowen disease. (A, From Habif TP. Clinical dermatology. Edinburgh: Mosby; 2004. p. 343; B, from Elston DM, Ferringer T. Dermatopathology. Edinburgh: Saunders; 2009. p. 293.)

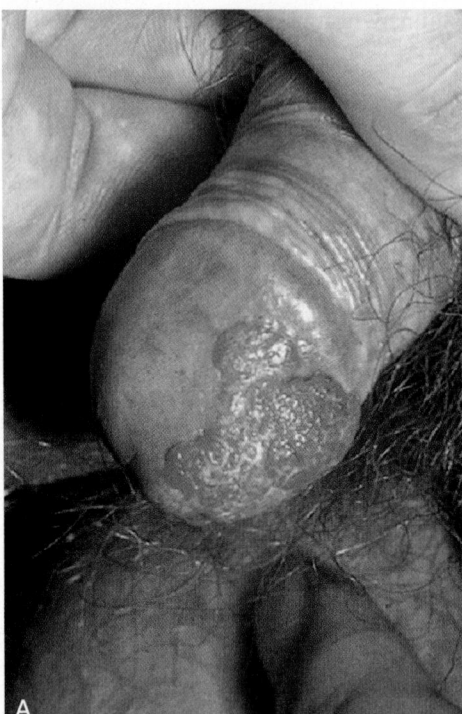

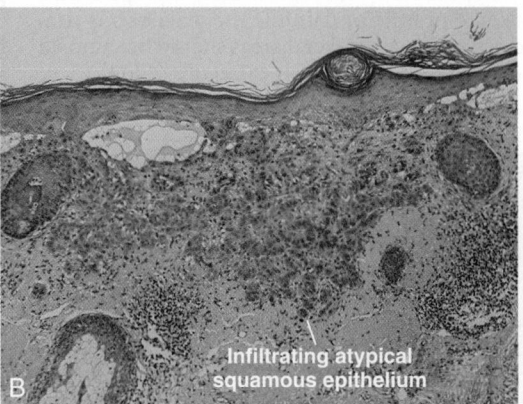

Figure 16-37. Squamous cell carcinoma (SCC). A, Exophytic erosive lesion on the glans with evident keratinization. B, Atypical keratinocytes invading the dermis in SCC. (A, From Callen JP, Greer DE, Hood AF, et al. Color atlas of dermatology. Philadelphia: Saunders; 1993. p. 129; B, from Elston DM, Ferringer T. Dermatopathology. Edinburgh: Saunders; 2009. p. 57.)

Infiltrating atypical squamous epithelium

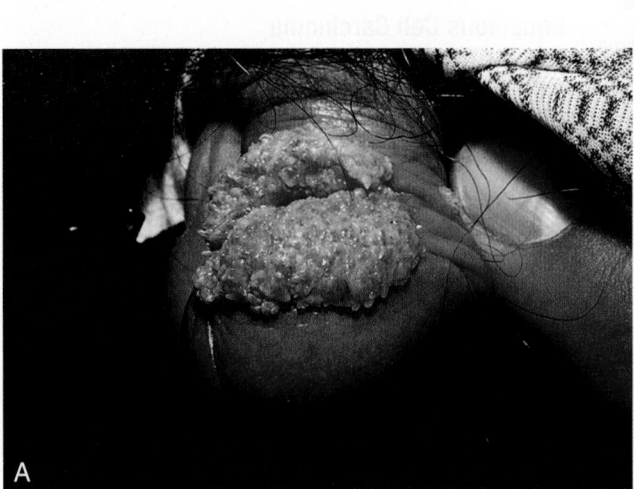

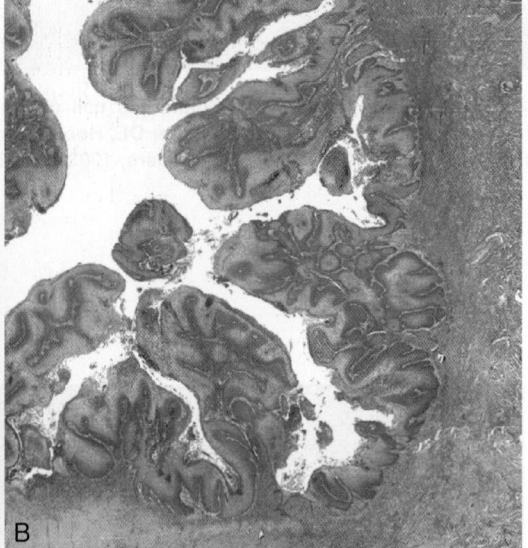

Figure 16-38. Verrucous carcinoma of the penis (Buschke-Lowenstein tumor). A, Note the exophytic and wartlike appearance. B, Histologic features of verrucous carcinoma. (A, From Callen JP, Greer DE, Hood AF, et al. Color atlas of dermatology. Philadelphia: Saunders; 1993. p. 330; B, from Elston DM, Ferringer T. Dermatopathology. Edinburgh: Saunders; 2009. p. 58.)

Verrucous Carcinoma (Buschke-Lowenstein Tumor)

Verrucous carcinoma is a locally aggressive, exophytic, low-grade variant of SCC that has little metastatic potential (Habif, 2004). The Buschke-Lowenstein tumor is a verrucous carcinoma of the anogenital mucosal surface and may represent up to 24% of all penile tumors (Schwartz, 1995). It most commonly occurs in uncircumcised men on the glans or prepuce, although similar lesions can be found on the vulva, vagina cervix, or anus. Verrucous carcinoma has been associated with HPV type 6 and 11 infection but not with the more classically oncogenic types 16 and 18 (Yasunaga et al, 1993; Chan et al, 1994; Margolis, 2002; Ahmed et al, 2006).

Verrucous carcinoma lesions have a warty appearance and are often large and fungating when presenting on the genitalia (Fig. 16-38). Aside from genital sites, these lesions can also present within the oral and nasal cavities and plantar surfaces of the feet. They are slow growing and locally destructive, often extending deeply into underlying tissue. Preferred treatment is by local excision. Mohs micrographic surgery may be helpful in tracing out the tumor and minimizing tissue loss. **Primary radiotherapy is relatively contraindicated because of the potential for anaplastic transformation with a subsequent increase in metastatic potential** (Stehman et al, 1980; Andersen and Sorensen, 1988; Fukunaga et al, 1994; Vandeweyer et al, 2001).

Basal Cell Carcinoma

Basal cell carcinoma (BCC) is the most common cutaneous neoplasm overall, arising most often on areas of chronically sun-exposed skin such as the head and neck. Genital BCC has also been described as a very rare entity, most commonly involving the scrotal skin in the male and the vulva in the female (Nahass et al, 1992; Benedet et al, 1997; Esquivias Gomez et al, 1999; Kinoshita et al, 2005). In the world medical literature, to date fewer than 100 total cases of BCC have been described involving all the potential genital sites (penis, scrotum, vulva). Several subtypes of BCC have been defined including nodular, superficial, micronodular morphea-form, and infiltrating. The nodular variant accounts for 60% of extragenital BCCs and virtually all genital BCCs, and this variant presents as a pearly, skin-toned papule or plaque often with telangiectasias overlying the tumor (Fig. 16-39) (Miller and Moresi,

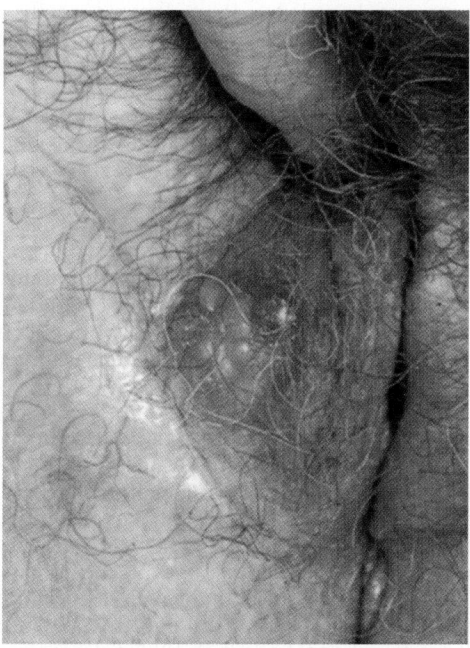

Figure 16-39. Basal cell carcinoma involving the vulva. (From du Vivier A. Atlas of clinical dermatology. London: Churchill Livingstone; 2002. p. 688.)

2003). These lesions may ulcerate centrally and manifest a very low metastatic potential. Treatment is by local excision. Because preservation of genital skin is important, both for form and function, the use of Mohs micrographic surgery may be advisable for the rare genital BCC.

Kaposi Sarcoma

Kaposi sarcoma (KS) is a disease of endothelial cell origin. Whether KS is a neoplastic or hyperplastic process remains controversial, and evidence exists both for and against clonal expansion (Rabkin et al, 1997; Gill et al, 1998). Before the onset of the AIDS epidemic, KS was considered a chronic disease afflicting elderly men of Jewish, Mediterranean, or Eastern European descent ("classic KS") (Safai, 1987). However, infection with HIV-1 has increased the incidence of KS by more than 7000-fold (Miles, 1994; Margolis, 2002). KS generally affects HIV-infected patients with advanced immune impairment (CD4+ T-cell counts of <500 cells/mm) (Tappero et al, 1993). Approximately 40% of homosexual men with AIDS have developed KS as compared to less than 5% in other risk groups (Rogers et al, 1987; North et al, 2003). There is also a clear association between infection with human herpesvirus 8 and the development of KS (Boshoff and Weiss, 1997; Weiss et al, 1998). In this regard, the other group at risk for development of KS associated with human herpesvirus 8 infection includes recipients of solid organ transplants (Riva et al, 2012).

Classic KS in immunocompetent individuals presents as slowly growing, blue-red to overtly violaceous pigmented macules on the lower extremities. Although oral and gastrointestinal lesions may occur, the genitalia are seldom involved. This is in contrast to the case with AIDS ("epidemic KS") in which a solitary genital lesion may be the first manifestation of KS (Lowe et al, 1989). **The clinical features of KS in both AIDS patients and solid organ transplant recipients are diverse, ranging from a single lesion to disseminated cutaneous and visceral disease** (Fig. 16-40). Lesions may coalesce to cover large areas of skin and may result in lymphatic or venous blockage leading to local edema (Margolis, 2002). When these lesions involve the glans penis, they can cause obstruction at the urethral meatus or fossa navicularis (Swierzewski et al, 1993). It should be noted, however, that penile KS is still rare, even among those infected with HIV-1; only about 3% of AIDS patients will ever develop KS of the genitalia (Rosen et al, 1999).

Treatment must be tailored to the individual clinical case and complete cure may be an unrealistic goal. For solitary lesions, local

Figure 16-40. Kaposi sarcoma. Classic macular lesions seen on the back (A) and glans penis (B). (A, From Callen JP, Greer DE, Hood AF, et al. Color atlas of dermatology. Philadelphia: Saunders; 1993. p. 220; B, from du Vivier A. Atlas of clinical dermatology. London: Churchill Livingstone; 2002. p. 716.)

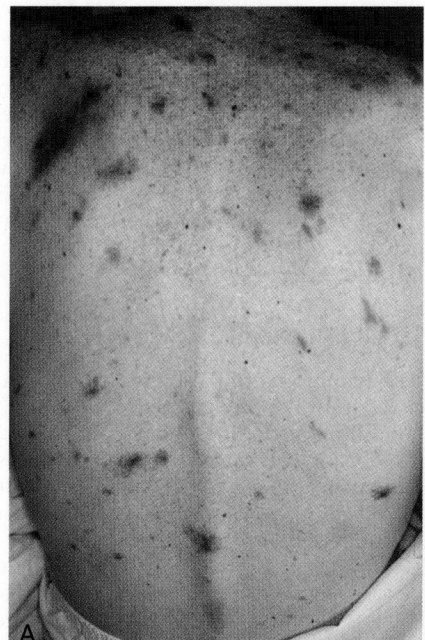

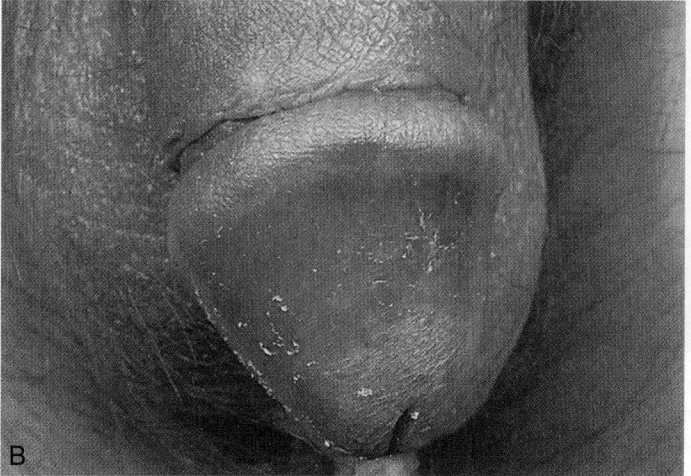

therapy such as surgical excision, laser ablation, cryotherapy, topical imiquimod 5%, or intralesional injection of chemotherapeutic agents (i.e., vinblastine) may be beneficial (Chun et al, 1999; Schwartz, 2004; Heyns and Fisher, 2005; Rosen, 2006). For extensive locoregional disease, radiotherapy (15 to 30 Gy) has an objective response rate of greater than 90% (Kirova et al, 1998; Cattelan et al, 2002). For widely disseminated KS, systemic chemotherapy with vincristine, doxorubicin, and bleomycin is the treatment of choice (Aversa et al, 1999). For KS associated with organ transplantation, reduction in the degree of postoperative immunosuppression or switching from a calcineurin inhibitor to an mTOR inhibitor may lead to KS resolution without any additional intervention (Riva et al, 2012).

Pseudoepitheliomatous, Keratotic, and Micaceous Balanitis

Pseudoepitheliomatous, keratotic, and micaceous balanitis (PEKMB) is a rare entity characterized by the development of a thick, hyperkeratotic plaque on the glans penis of older men (Fig. 16-41). The term *micaceous* refers to the white, scaly appearance of the lesions (Child et al, 2000). PEKMB was originally thought to be a purely benign process, although several case reports have documented the presence of concurrent verrucous carcinomas associated with this lesion (Child et al, 2000). Controversy remains as to whether PEKMB is a premalignant condition (Read and Abell, 1981; Beljaards et al, 1987; Jenkins and Jakubovic, 1988). Histologic examination is essential to exclude the presence of SCC and verrucous carcinoma (Margolis, 2002). PEKMB is characterized on histology by a hyperplastic epidermis with ridges extending deeply into the dermis (Jenkins and Jakubovic, 1988). These lesions should be treated locally either by surgical excision or ablative techniques, and close follow-up is essential (Read and Abell, 1981; Bargman, 1985). There are also anecdotal reports of successful treatment using topical 5-fluorouracil cream (Bargman, 1985; Krunic et al, 1996).

Melanoma

Malignant melanoma is a neoplasm arising from melanocytes. The incidence of melanoma has risen 3% to 7% during the past several decades (Nestle and Kerl, 2003). Risk factors for development of the disease include family history, certain genetic markers, fair skin, light eye color, and a history of excessive ultraviolet radiation exposure (especially multiple blistering sunburns as a child or adolescent). Primary melanoma of the male genitalia is an uncommon entity with only approximately 100 cases reported in the literature (Sanchez-Ortiz et al, 2005) and melanoma of the male urethra is even more rare (Oliva et al, 2000). The same cannot be said for

females, as melanoma comprises about 7% to 10% of all vulvar malignancies and remains the second most common such lesion after SCC (Suwandinata et al, 2007). Although vulvar melanoma is more common among Caucasian women, the prognosis is worse among African-American women (Mert et al, 2013).

Genital melanoma usually presents as a pigmented macule or papule with an irregular border, although unpigmented lesions and ulceration may also be present (Margolis, 2002). **Early diagnosis is critical because local treatment of superficial lesions with wide local excision or partial penectomy can provide excellent disease control** (Stillwell et al, 1988; Sanchez-Ortiz et al, 2005). **The same caveats are true in female patients.** In contrast, patients with biopsy-proven metastatic disease have traditionally had a universally poor prognosis despite aggressive surgical management and multiagent cytotoxic chemotherapy. In the last several years, however, several drugs have gained regulatory approval for the treatment of metastatic and unresectable melanoma as a result of an increase of knowledge in melanoma-specific molecular biology and immunology. The efficacy of small-molecule BRAF (e.g., vemurafenib, dabrafenib, trametinib) and MAP-ERK kinase (MEK) inhibitors, as well as the immune checkpoint inhibitors (e.g., ipilimumab and the anti-PD1/PDL1 antibodies lambrolizumab and nivolumab), have transformed the treatment of advanced melanoma.

Extramammary Paget Disease

Extramammary Paget disease (EPD) is an uncommon intraepithelial adenocarcinoma of sites bearing apocrine glands (Zollo and Zeitouni, 2000). The majority of patients with EPD are elderly Caucasian females, and involvement of the male penis and scrotum is exceedingly rare (Park et al, 2001; van Randenborgh et al, 2002; Yang et al, 2005). The vulva is the most commonly involved genital site in women followed by the perianal region in men (Wojnarowska and Cooper, 2003). **There is an important association between EPD and another underlying malignancy in at least 10% to 30% of cases** (Payne and Wells, 1994; Ng et al, 2001; Margolis, 2002). An investigation in a cancer specialty hospital suggested that this association might be even stronger in men than previously appreciated (Hegarty et al, 2011). In the male, associations between urethral, prostate, bladder, rectal, and apocrine malignancies with EPD have been described (Hayes et al, 1997; Salamanca et al, 2004; Hegarty et al, 2011). **It is critical therefore to perform a systematic evaluation for underlying carcinoma in all cases of EPD.**

The lesion in EPD is usually an erythematous plaque with a sharp border between normal and involved skin (Fig. 16-42). It may be asymptomatic, pruritic, or associated with burning pain. The diagnosis is confirmed histologically by the presence of vacuolated Paget cells in the epidermis that stain for glandular cytokeratins, epithelial membrane antigen, and carcinoembryonic antigen (Wojnarowska and Cooper, 2003). Treatment generally involves surgical excision or Mohs micrographic surgery, although radiotherapy, photodynamic therapy, and topical imiquimod 5% or 5-fluorouracil have also been used successfully (Sillman et al, 1985; Bewley et al, 1994; Brown et al, 2000; Brown et al, 2002; Guerrieri and Back, 2002; Moreno-Arias et al, 2003; Qian et al, 2003; Lee et al, 2009).

Cutaneous T-Cell Lymphoma

Cutaneous T-cell lymphoma (CTCL) represents a group of related neoplasms derived from T cells that home to the skin. CTCL includes a variety of conditions including mycosis fungoides, Sézary syndrome, lymphoid papulosis, and pagetoid reticulosis (Willemze, 2003). There is an increased risk of CTCL associated with HIV infection (Biggar et al, 2001). Although these disorders may involve the genitalia of both genders, extragenital disease is usually also present. CTCL accounts for the majority of primary cutaneous lymphomas with B-cell–derived lymphomas accounting for only 20% to 25% (Willemze et al, 1997, 2005). Definitive diagnosis depends on biopsy histopathology.

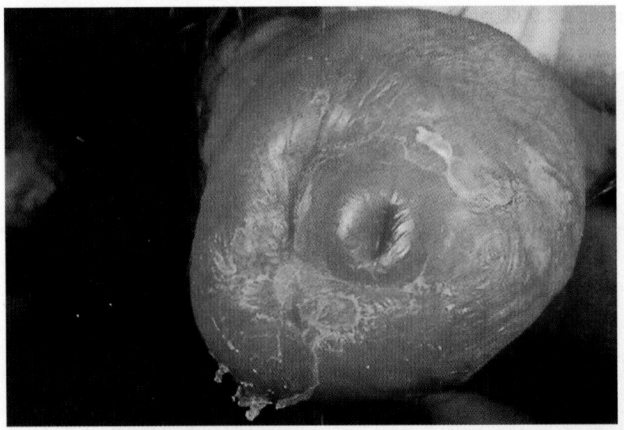

Figure 16-41. Pseudoepitheliomatous, keratotic, and micaceous balanitis. The glans becomes covered with mica (asbestos-like) scales and horny crusts. (From du Vivier A. Atlas of clinical dermatology. London: Churchill Livingstone; 2002. p. 717.)

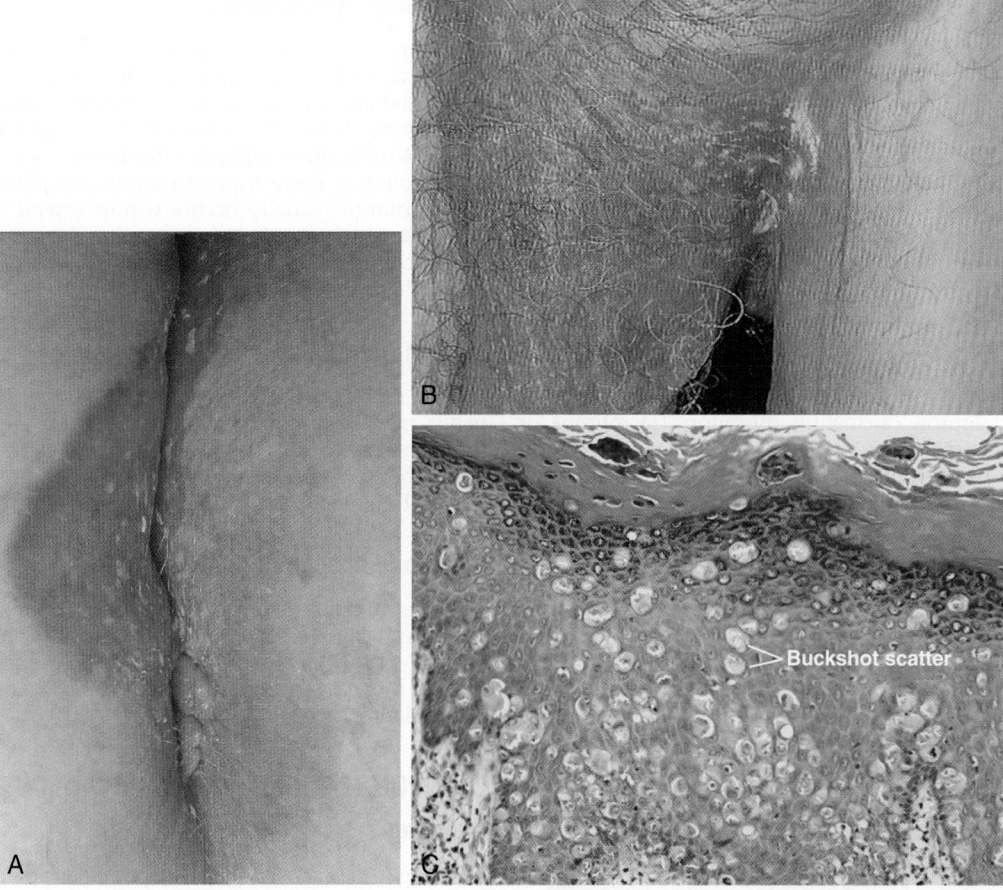

Figure 16-42. **Extramammary Paget disease involving the vulva (A) and base of scrotum (B). Note the well-demarcated border between the lesion and normal adjacent skin. C, Tumor cells distributed throughout the epidermis ("buckshot scatter"). (A, From Habif TP. Clinical dermatology. Edinburgh: Mosby; 2004. p. 764; B, from Bolognia JL, Jorizzo JL, Rapini RP. Dermatology. Edinburgh: Mosby; 2003. p. 1108; C, from Elston DM, Ferringer T. Dermatopathology. Edinburgh: Saunders; 2009. p. 66.)**

CTCL generally presents initially as pruritic patches that must be differentiated from a variety of benign dermatoses including psoriasis, eczema, superficial fungal infections, and drug reactions. **The initial lesions of CTCL have a strong predilection in both sexes to occur on suprapubic and/or buttock skin.** Patients may subsequently develop hematologic involvement (Sézary syndrome) and cutaneous plaques, erosions, ulcers, or frank skin tumors (Fig. 16-43) (Margolis, 2002). CTCL is a chronic condition that may progress throughout many years. Topical treatments include application of ultrapotent corticosteroids, nitrogen mustard, and carmustine with complete remission rates of approximately 60% (Vonderheid et al, 1989; Zackheim et al, 1998). Other treatments include radiotherapy (including total body electron beam treatment), phototherapy (PUVA), and systemic treatment with chemotherapy, interferons, or retinoids (Hoppe et al, 1990; Olsen and Bunn, 1995; Diederen et al, 2003; Querfeld et al, 2005).

BENIGN CUTANEOUS DISORDERS SPECIFIC TO THE MALE GENITALIA

Angiokeratoma of Fordyce

Angiokeratomas of Fordyce are vascular ectasias of dermal blood vessels that may be visible on the penis and scrotum of adult men (Bechara et al, 2002). These lesions appear as 1- to 2-mm red or purple papules (Fig. 16-44A) and associated generalized scrotal redness may exist (Miller and James, 2002). This is usually a benign condition without systemic manifestations, although it may rarely be a source of troublesome scrotal bleeding (Taniguchi et al, 1994; Hoekx and Wyndaele, 1998). Similar lesions can be observed in Fabry disease (Fig. 16-44B), which is a rare glycogen storage deficiency. Although treatment is usually unnecessary for angiokeratoma of Fordyce, several authors have reported success using erbium:YAG, Nd:YAG, KTP, and Argon laser photocoagulation in select cases (Occella et al, 1995; Bechara et al, 2004; Ozdemir et al, 2009).

Pearly Penile Papules

Pearly penile papules are white, dome-shaped or filiform, closely spaced small papules located on the glans penis (Fig. 16-44C). They are often arranged circumferentially at the corona. Pearly penile papules are common lesions found in up to 14% to 48% of young postpubertal adults, particularly if the penis is not circumcised (Rehbein, 1977; Khoo and Cheong, 1995; Sonnex and Dockerty, 1999). **Although pearly penile papules may occasionally be misdiagnosed as condyloma, the available evidence does not support a role for HPV in causing pearly penile papules and no association with cervical intraepithelial neoplasia in female partners has been demonstrated** (Hogewoning et al, 2003). Patients should be reassured that this is a benign condition that does not usually require treatment. If treatment is desired because of cosmetic concerns, local destruction with either the CO_2 laser or cryotherapy has been applied successfully (Ocampo-Candiani and Cueva-Rodriguez, 1996; Lane et al, 2002). **Histologically,** these lesions are angiofibromas similar to the lesions seen on the face in tuberous sclerosis.

Zoon Balanitis

Zoon balanitis, also called plasma cell balanitis and balanitis plasmacellularis, occurs in uncircumcised men from the third decade onward (Pastar et al, 2004). Smooth, moist, erythematous, well-circumscribed plaques on the glans penis characterize the disease (Fig. 16-44D). Shallow erosions are often present (Yoganathan et al, 1994) and the lesions can be quite large (up to 2 cm in diameter) (Margolis, 2002). SCC and EPD must be excluded, typically by biopsy. Circumcision appears to be proof against development of the disease and can be performed to cure the majority of cases (Sonnex et al, 1982a; Ferrandiz and Ribera, 1984). For patients averse to circumcision, topical corticosteroids may provide symptomatic relief, and topical calcineurin inhibitors (tacrolimus or pimecrolimus) and laser therapy may also play a role in alleviation (Baldwin and Geronemus, 1989; Tang et al, 2001; Albertini et al, 2002; Retamar et al, 2003; Wojnarowska and Cooper, 2003; Rallis et al, 2007).

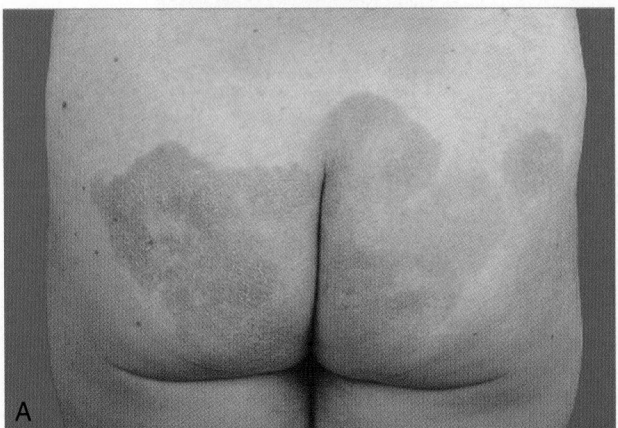

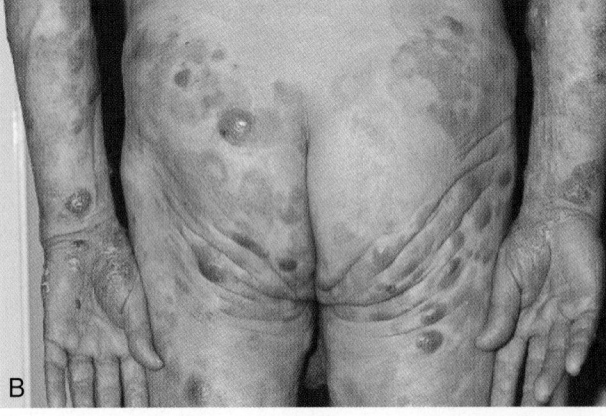

Figure 16-43. Mycosis fungoides (a cutaneous T-cell lymphoma) involving the buttocks. A shows the limited plaque stage, and B shows a more advanced case with plaques, patches, and tumors present. (From Bolognia JL, Jorizzo JL, Rapini RP. Dermatology. Edinburgh: Mosby; 2003.)

Sclerosing Lymphangitis

Nonvenereal sclerosing lymphangitis is a rare penile lesion consisting of an indurated, slightly tender cord involving the coronal sulcus and adjacent penile skin (Gharpuray and Tolat, 1991; Rosen and Hwong, 2003). It is usually flesh colored but may occasionally be red. A mechanism related to thrombosis of lymphatic vessels has been proposed. There is an association with vigorous sexual activity, and resolution usually occurs within several weeks (Sieunarine, 1987; Margolis, 2002). Although somewhat controversial, a search for concomitant gonococcal and nongonococcal urethritis may be advisable in these cases.

Median Raphe Cysts

Median raphe cysts occur in young men on the ventral aspect of the penis, most commonly near the glans (Stone, 2003). Although these cysts are believed to develop from aberrant urethral epithelium, they do not communicate with the urethra (Asarch et al, 1979). Treatment is accomplished by surgical removal.

Ectopic Sebaceous Glands

Ectopic sebaceous glands on the penile shaft may be visible as pin-sized, flesh-colored papular lesions that may be mistaken for verruca (Fig. 16-44E) (Margolis and Wein, 2002). There is no indication for treating these asymptomatic benign lesions and patient reassurance is sufficient.

COMMON MISCELLANEOUS CUTANEOUS DISORDERS
Skin Tag

Skin tags (acrochordons, fibroepithelial polyps) are soft, skin-colored, pedunculated lesions that can be present anywhere on the body but have a clear predilection for the neck, axillae, and inguinal folds. Although usually asymptomatic, these lesions may become painful secondary to local trauma or as a result of torsion and infarction in rare cases. These are common lesions, and up to 50% of all individuals may have at least one skin tag (Banik and Lubach, 1987). **It is important to distinguish these lesions from the hamartomatous skin lesions (multiple fibrofolliculomas) associated with Birt-Hogg-Dube syndrome, which are histologically distinct from common skin tags** (De la Torre et al, 1999). When skin tags cause either discomfort or cosmetic distress, they can easily be removed by snip excision and light electrocautery to the base to achieve hemostasis. When a large number of skin tags appear at a relatively young age (<40), there may be an association with both benign and malignant lower gastrointestinal tract polyposis, and gastroenterological referral for endoscopy should be considered (Piette et al, 1988).

Epidermoid Cysts

Epidermoid or epidermal-inclusion cysts are the most common cutaneous cysts, and these lesions can be found anywhere on the body including the genitalia. They are particularly common on the scrotum (Fig. 16-45E). **The term "sebaceous cyst" should be avoided because the contents of these cysts are not sebaceous in origin** (Stone, 2003). Although not painful at baseline,

Figure 16-44. Benign cutaneous disorders specific to the male genitalia. **A,** Angiokeratoma of Fordyce showing purple scrotal vascular malformations. **B,** Fabry disease: a glycogen storage deficiency with associated purple vascular malformations on the penile shaft. **C,** Pearly penile papules located on the corona of the glans penis. **D,** Zoon balanitis of the glans penis. **E,** Ectopic sebaceous glands on the penile shaft. (A, B, and E, From Callen JP, Greer DE, Hood AF, et al. Color atlas of dermatology. Philadelphia: Saunders; 1993; C and D, from Korting GW. Practical dermatology of the genital region. Philadelphia: Saunders; 1981.)

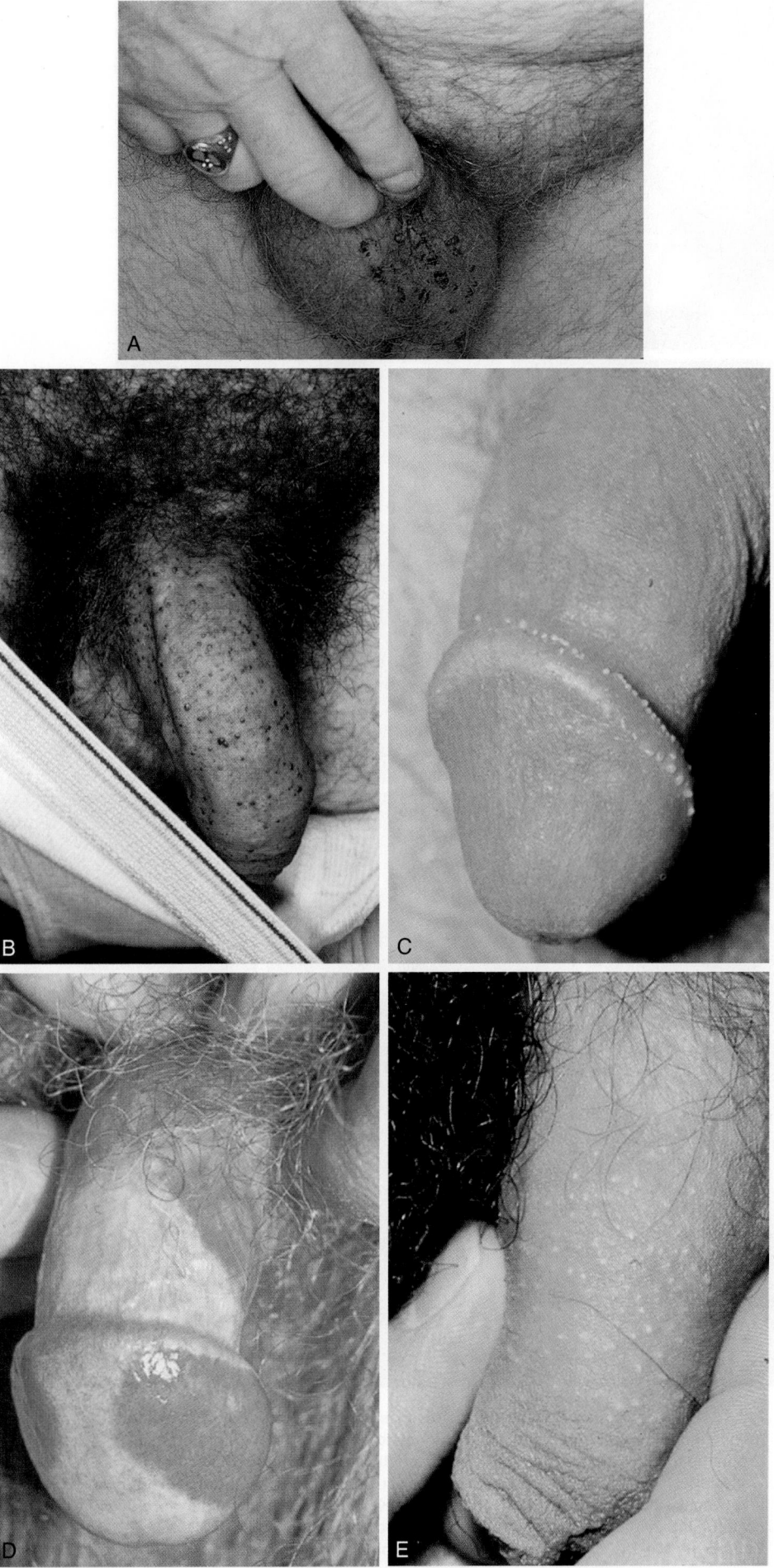

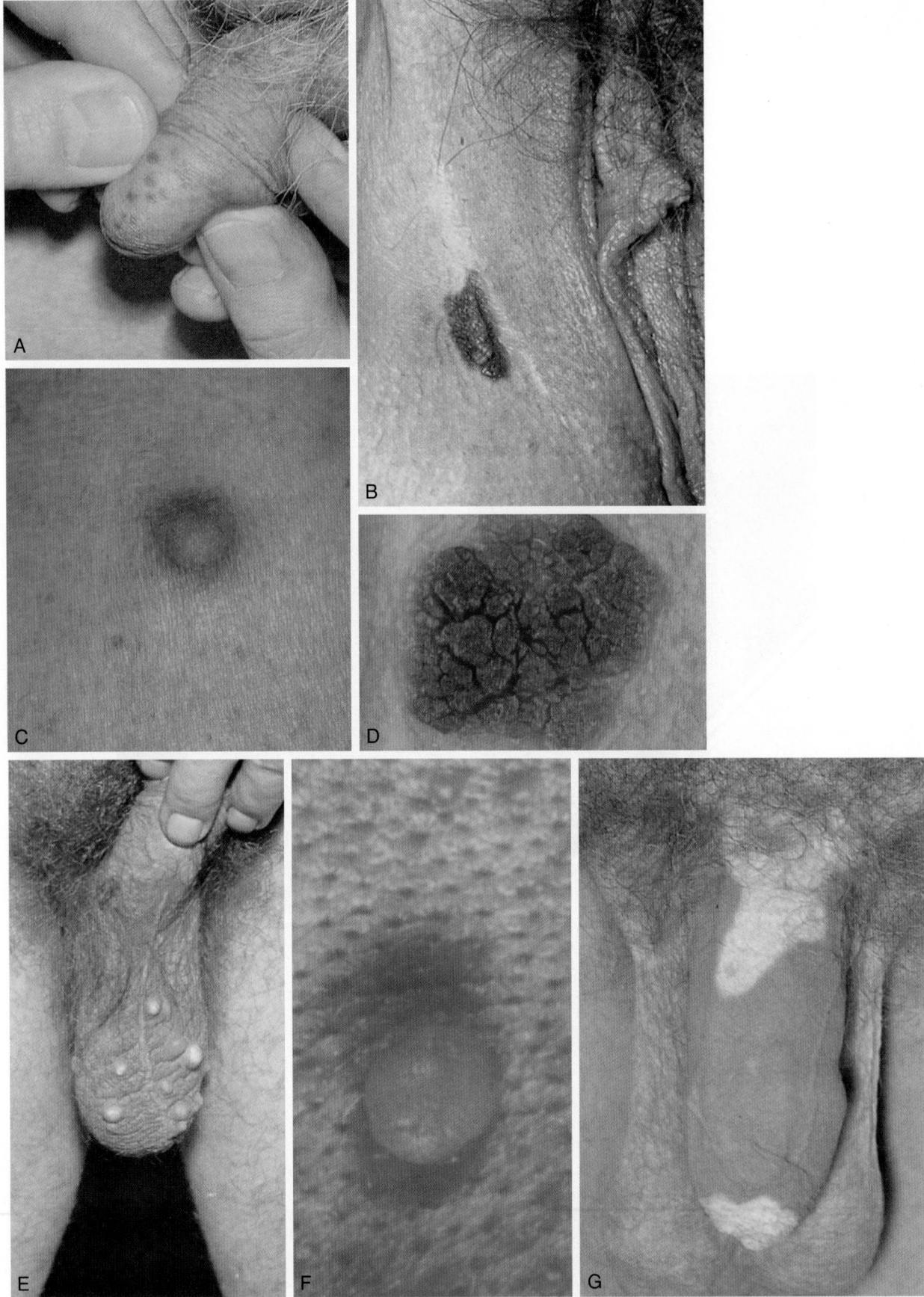

Figure 16-45. Miscellaneous cutaneous disorders. A, Lentigo simplex involving the glans penis (penile melanosis). B, A compound melanocytic nevus in the inguinal crease. C, A dermatofibroma on the lower extremity. D, A characteristic seborrheic keratosis showing the "stuck-on" waxy appearance. E, Epidermoid cysts of the scrotum. F, Pedunculated neurofibroma. G, Vitiligo involving the penile shaft. (A, B, E, and G, From Korting GW. Practical dermatology of the genital region. Philadelphia: Saunders; 1981; C, from Bolognia JL, Jorizzo JL, Rapini RP. Dermatology. Edinburgh: Mosby; 2003; D, from Habif TP. Clinical dermatology. Edinburgh: Mosby; 2004.)

rupture of the cyst wall can lead to a severe inflammatory reaction that is extremely painful. Definitive treatment requires surgical excision of the entire cyst wall to prevent cyst recurrence. Inflamed or superinfected epidermoid cysts may require incision and drainage and antibiotic therapy if there is adjacent cellulitis. Dystrophic calcification of scrotal epidermoid cysts may be a cause of scrotal calcinosis (Dare and Axelsen, 1988; Michl et al, 1994).

Seborrheic Keratosis

Seborrheic keratoses are very common beige to dark brown macules, plaques, and papules affecting individuals older than 30 years, and the incidence increases in frequency with advancing age. They are most common on the face, neck, and trunk although any body site except the palms, soles, and mucous membranes may be affected. The degree of pigmentation can vary significantly, and darker lesions may be confused with melanoma or warts (Pierson et al, 2003). **These lesions have a waxy, "stuck-on" appearance** (Fig. 16-45D) **and patients may note that they drop off spontaneously and then regrow** (Margolis, 2002). Treatment by shave excision or destruction with liquid nitrogen is usually performed for cosmetic reasons. **An abrupt increase in the size and number of multiple seborrheic keratoses has been termed the Sign of Leser-Trélat and has been implicated as a cutaneous marker of occult internal malignancy** (Chiba et al, 1996; Heaphy et al, 2000; Vielhauer et al, 2000; Ginarte et al, 2001).

Lentigo Simplex

Lentigo simplex is a condition characterized by the presence of brown-pigmented macules unrelated to sunlight exposure (Fig. 16-45A). These lesions can be found anywhere on the body including the mucous membranes and nail beds. In the genital area (benign genital lentiginosis), these lesions present commonly on the labia, vaginal introitus, perineum, and glans penis (penile melanosis). The lesions of lentigo simplex are usually smaller than those seen in melanocytic nevi. Although usually benign, the lesions of lentigo simplex may deserve biopsy evaluation in cases demonstrating atypical shape or coloration. When present in a discontinuous manner at multiple sites, the diagnosis of genital melanoma becomes less likely compared to the probability of benign genital lentiginosis. **Finally, the combination of multiple pigmented lesions associated with intestinal polyposis should raise suspicion for Peutz-Jeghers syndrome.**

Mole (Nevus)

A mole or nevus of the skin is composed of slightly altered melanocytes called "nevus cells" arranged in a cluster. The location of the cluster determines the type of nevus. Junctional nevi are located between the epidermis and dermis and are usually flat, tan to black in coloration, small (<5 mm), and sharply bordered (Margolis, 2002). Intradermal nevi have clusters within the dermis and are usually small (<5 mm), lighter in coloration, with sharp borders. Compound nevi have clusters in both locations and are usually darker and raised as a papule (Fig. 16-45B). As is the case for any pigmented lesion, marked irregularity in coloration or border, and rapid morphologic change with time, are indications for excisional biopsy.

Dermatofibroma

Dermatofibromas are small hyperpigmented nodules that occur most commonly on the lower extremities and occasionally on the genitalia (Fig. 16-45C). Pinching of these lesions causes a downward movement of the tumor (the so-called dimple sign) (Kamino and Pui, 2003). These are benign lesions with a characteristic histologic pattern of spindle-shaped fibroblasts and myofibroblasts arranged in fascicles. Treatment by surgical excision is usually unnecessary and may leave a scar that is cosmetically inferior to the original lesion (Kamino and Pui, 2003).

Neurofibroma

Neurofibromas are common tumors composed of neuromesenchymal tissue with residual nerve axons. They can be present anywhere on the body including the labia and scrotum (Yoshimura et al, 1990; Singh et al, 1992; Mishra et al, 2002; Kantarci et al, 2005). They are usually skin-colored, soft or rubbery nodular lesions, which may be pedunculated (Fig. 16-45F). **Digital pressure on the lesion causes invagination or so-called button-holing** (Habif, 2004). These can be solitary lesions or multiple, which should raise suspicion for neurofibromatosis or von Recklinghausen disease.

Capillary Hemangioma

Capillary hemangiomas are proliferations of blood vessels that are either present at birth or develop rapidly during the neonatal period. These lesions can involve the anogenital region, can lead to bleeding, or can cause obstruction of the urethra, vagina, or anus (Sharma et al, 1981; Roberts and Devine, 1983). The majority will involute during childhood or early adolescence (Margolis, 2002). An innovation in the treatment of very large, persistent, and/or obstructive hemangiomas is the systemic administration of propranolol; because this treatment is not without some risk, it should be initiated and supervised by a clinician experienced with this modality (Izadpanah et al, 2013).

Vitiligo

Vitiligo is an acquired autoimmune disorder of the skin, leading to depigmentation, affecting 0.5% to 2% of the global population (Ortonne, 2003). It might present at any age and the precise pathogenesis of vitiligo remains a topic of intense research effort. Large patches of skin become completely amelanotic. Although the skin appears white, it is otherwise completely normal. The borders with unaffected skin are usually sharp and well defined (Fig. 16-45G). This condition is particularly noticeable in darker skinned individuals and on body sites that are normally hyperpigmented. Vitiligo limited to the genitalia has been observed in less than 0.3% of the male population (Moss and Stevenson, 1981). Lesions have a tendency to enlarge circumferentially with time and might develop at sites of local trauma (Koebner phenomenon). Genital vitiligo must be differentiated from LS and postinflammatory hypopigmentation (Margolis, 2002). Treatments include temporary

---

KEY POINTS

- The diagnosis of cutaneous diseases of the external genitalia depends critically on a thorough history and physical examination. Extragenital findings may provide the key to diagnosis. The urologist should perform a thorough skin survey and should not focus solely on the area of affected genital skin.
- The side effects of topical corticosteroids are significant, both from systemic absorption and locally. Adverse effects may be worsened if these agents are applied under the foreskin, which may serve as an occlusive dressing. In general, when applied to genital skin, only low-potency topical corticosteroids should be used for short treatment courses.
- Cutaneous disorders of the external genitalia can be broken down into the general categories of allergic, papulosquamous, vesicobullous, ulcerative, infectious, neoplastic, and miscellaneous diseases.
- Histopathologic analysis of biopsy specimens plays an important role in differentiating cutaneous diseases with similar clinical features and in excluding malignancy.
- Local treatment modalities including the use of laser energy, photodynamic therapy, ultraviolet radiation, and cryotherapy are being applied successfully to a variety of genital cutaneous disorders and offer an alternative to surgical excision in some cases.

repigmentation with topical cosmetics, ultraviolet light exposure, PUVA therapy, and skin grafting. Use of the excimer laser to induce melanin production is particularly suited to the genitalia. **The diagnosis of vitiligo should prompt a screening for autoimmune thyroid disease.**

REFERENCES

 The complete reference list is available online at www.expertconsult.com.

SUGGESTED READINGS

Bhattacharya M, Kaur I, Kumar B. Lichen planus: a clinical and epidemiological study. J Dermatol 2000;27:576–82.

Bolognia JL, Jorizzo JL, Schaffer JV. Dermatology. 3rd ed. Edinburgh: Saunders; 2012.

Criteria for diagnosis of Behçet's disease. International Study Group for Behçet's Disease. Lancet 1990;335:1078–80.

Czymek R, Kujath P, Bruch HP, et al. Treatment, outcome and quality of life after Fournier's gangrene: a multicentre study. Colorectal Dis 2013;15:1529–36.

Denby KS, Beck LA. Update on systemic therapies for atopic dermatitis. Curr Opin Allergy Clin Immunol 2012;12:421–6.

Eke N. Fournier's gangrene: a review of 1726 cases. Br J Surg 2000;87:718–28.

Ellinghaus D, Baurecht H, Esparza-Gordillo J, et al. High-density genotyping study identifies four new susceptibility loci for atopic dermatitis. Nat Genet 2013;45:808–12.

Hatemi G, Yazici Y, Yazici H. Behçet's syndrome. Rheum Dis Clin North Am 2013;39:245–61.

Krueger G, Koo J, Lebwohl M, et al. The impact of psoriasis on quality of life: results of a 1998 National Psoriasis Foundation patient-membership survey. Arch Dermatol 2001;137:280–4.

Leibovitch I, Huilgol SC, Selva D, et al. Cutaneous squamous carcinoma in situ (Bowen's disease): treatment with Mohs micrographic surgery. J Am Acad Dermatol 2005;52:997–1002.

Mallon E, Hawkins D, Dinneen M, et al. Circumcision and genital dermatoses. Arch Dermatol 2000;136:350–4.

Morpurgo E, Galandiuk S. Fournier's gangrene. Surg Clin North Am 2002;82:1213–24.

Rompel R, Petres J. Long-term results of wide surgical excision in 106 patients with hidradenitis suppurativa. Dermatol Surg 2000;26:638–43.

Ruocco E, Wolf R, Ruocco V, et al. Pemphigus: associations and management guidelines: facts and controversies. Clin Dermatol 2013;31:382–90.

Sanchez-Ortiz R, Huang SF, Tamboli P, et al. Melanoma of the penis, scrotum and male urethra: a 40-year single institution experience. J Urol 2005;173:1958–65.

Scheinfeld N. Hidradenitis suppurativa: a practical review of possible medical treatments based on over 350 hidradenitis patients. Dermatol Online J 2013;19:1.

Stern RS, PUVA Follow-Up Study. The risk of squamous cell and basal cell cancer associated with psoralen and ultraviolet A therapy: a 30-year prospective study. J Am Acad Dermatol 2012;66:553–62.

Wolf R, Orion E, Marcos B, et al. Life-threatening acute adverse cutaneous drug reactions. Clin Dermatol 2005;23:171–81.

Wollenberg A, Bieber T. Atopic dermatitis: from the genes to skin lesions. Allergy 2000;55:205–13.

Worswick S, Cotliar J. Stevens-Johnson syndrome and toxic epidermal necrolysis: a review of treatment options. Dermatol Ther 2011;24:207–18.

17 Tuberculosis and Parasitic Infections of the Genitourinary Tract

Alicia H. Chang, MD, MS, Brian G. Blackburn, MD, and Michael H. Hsieh, MD, PhD

Genitourinary Tuberculosis

Parasitic Infections of the Urogenital Tract

GENITOURINARY TUBERCULOSIS

Tuberculosis (TB) can affect any organ system of the body, including the genitourinary (GU) tract. Untreated, GU TB can lead to irreparable tissue damage with serious consequences such as renal failure and infertility, making it critical for clinicians to consider TB in the differential diagnosis of GU disorders. Described as the second "great imitator" (after syphilis) (Sievers, 1961), TB can mimic many other diseases and complicate the correct diagnosis and treatment of infected patients. As TB becomes less common in industrialized nations, the diagnosis of GU TB increasingly relies on clinical recognition and a high index of suspicion.

History

Genomic analyses suggest that *Mycobacterium tuberculosis* co-evolved with humans. Its early progenitor, *Mycobacterium prototuberculosis*, possibly infected early hominids more than 3 million years ago (Gutierrez et al, 2005). Bony lesions consistent with TB have been detected in a 500,000-year-old *Homo erectus* skeleton (Kappelman et al, 2008). The oldest microbiologic confirmation of *M. tuberculosis* infection in humans dates back to the Neolithic Period with use of DNA isolated from 9000-year-old skeletons of a woman and child found in a prehistoric site in the Eastern Mediterranean (Hershkovitz et al, 2008). Microscopic and molecular findings of tubercle bacilli have been documented in Egyptian mummies from circa 3000 BC (Zimmerman 1979; Nerlich et al, 1997). Descriptions of TB can be found in written records of civilizations from ancient East Asia, to New World cultures in the Americas, to Western Hemisphere societies such as the Greeks and Romans, and continuing into modern history (Daniel, 2006). It was not until the 18th and 19th centuries, however, that TB reached epidemic proportions and ravaged Europe and North America. "Consumption," as it was known, was responsible for as many as 25% of deaths during the Industrial Age (Chalke, 1959). The turning point in the history of TB came on March 24, 1882, when Robert Koch famously presented to the scientific community the first successful isolation and identification of the tubercle bacillus (Sakula, 1982). In honor of Dr. Koch, March 24 has become World Tuberculosis Day.

Microbiology

Tuberculosis is caused by a group of closely related acid-fast bacteria referred to as the *Mycobacterium tuberculosis* complex (MTBC). The species that comprise the complex are *M. tuberculosis*, *Mycobacterium africanum*, *Mycobacterium bovis*, *Mycobacterium canettii*, *Mycobacterium microti*, *Mycobacterium caprae*, *Mycobacterium mungi*, *Mycobacterium orygis*, and *Mycobacterium pinnipedii* (Alexander et al, 2010; Coscolla et al, 2013). *M. tuberculosis* and *M. africanum* infect only humans, whereas the others infect humans and additional mammals. By far, the most frequently isolated species in human TB is *M. tuberculosis*. This species has become synonymous with TB and is often used to represent the entire complex. Although the mycobacterial species in the complex are clinically indistinguishable, drug susceptibility among them may differ. *M. bovis*, for example, has innate resistance to pyrazinamide, which is one of the first-line agents against *M. tuberculosis*.

Epidemiology

The World Health Organization (WHO) estimates that one third of the world's population is infected with MTBC in its latent form. In 2012 there were 8.6 million new cases of active TB and 1.3 million deaths from TB worldwide, a decline that has continued since the year 2000. TB mortality has fallen by 45% since 1990 (WHO, 2013). However, new obstacles in TB control have also surfaced. These include medical conditions that promote resurgence of TB such as the human immunodeficiency virus (HIV) epidemic in sub-Saharan Africa and the rapid increase in obesity and diabetes worldwide. The appearance of multidrug and extensive drug resistance also compromises TB control.

In the United States, 9945 cases of active TB were reported in 2012 (3.2 per 100,000 persons). TB incidence in the United States has been steadily declining since its resurgence in the 1980s and its peak in 1992. In the United States, TB disproportionately affects the foreign-born. In 2012, the incidence among foreign-born individuals was 11 times higher than among U.S.-born persons (Centers for Disease Control and Prevention [CDC], 2013d).

The frequency of GU involvement among patients who develop TB varies significantly depending on the population studied. In developed countries, GU TB has been found in 2% to 10% of patients with pulmonary TB. In contrast, the frequency in developing countries approaches 15% to 20% (Figueiredo and Lucon, 2008). In the developing world, the GU tract is the second most common extrapulmonary site after lymph nodes (Wong et al, 2013). In the United States, GU TB is the third most common form after pleural and lymphatic TB and is found in 27% of extrapulmonary cases (Daher Ede et al, 2013). Approximately two thirds of those affected are men. GU TB is generally a disease of adults, although it has been reported in children as young as 2 years of age (Merchant et al, 2013a).

Transmission and Host Immune Response

The initial mode of entry of MTBC into the host is via inhalation of cough-generated infectious aerosols, although there are reported cases of direct inoculation of MTBC into soft tissues (Angus et al, 2001). When the bacilli reach the alveoli, they are phagocytosed by alveolar macrophages. In some persons, MTBC organisms are killed by the macrophages at this point and effectively cleared from the body. These persons do not develop infection nor an adaptive immune response (Walzl et al, 2011). In others, MTBC bacilli escape killing, begin to replicate within macrophages, and establish infection. Up to 12 weeks may pass before a cellular immune response is detectable (Dannenberg, 1994), and before this development the tubercle bacilli can spread through the lymphatics to the hilar lymph nodes and ultimately through the bloodstream to seed distant organs.

The host attempts to contain MTBC infection by forming granulomas. Infected macrophages secrete inflammatory cytokines such as interleukin-6 (IL-6), IL-12, IL-1β, and tumor necrosis factor–α (TNF-α) and recruit a variety of immune cells to surround them. Foamy macrophages, epithelioid cells, and multinucleated giant cells (Langhans cells) cluster to the center of the granuloma and are surrounded by a cuff of lymphocytes (Silva Miranda et al, 2012). Antigen processing and presentation lead to T-cell activation and the mounting of an adaptive cellular response against MTBC (Schluger and Rom, 1998). T cells secrete cytokines such as IL-2, TNF-α, and, most important, interferon-γ (IFN-γ) to maintain the granuloma and to induce killing of the infected macrophages and the infectious bacilli. When killing is not achieved, the granuloma can still successfully sequester viable tubercle bacilli, which stop replicating and become dormant. In 90% to 95% of persons, TB is controlled at this point and enters latency (Boom et al, 2003). Latent TB is marked by cicatrization and granuloma calcification. In fewer than 5% of infected persons the initial infection fails to be controlled and progresses within the year to active TB (primary progression). After latency is established, MTBC can resurface years later to cause reactivation TB. The process of reactivation is not well understood. The development of some conditions such as old age, renal failure, diabetes mellitus, malnutrition, HIV infection, and other causes of immune suppression shifts the balance between host and pathogen in favor of the pathogen. A series of events then occur that lead to renewed bacillary replication and release, granuloma caseation (the pathognomonic lesion of TB), and reactivation. The lifetime risk of reactivation TB is estimated at 5% to 10%, although the risk is higher in patients with the medical comorbidities mentioned previously. Treatment of patients with latent TB with isoniazid (INH) for 9 months can decrease the risk of reactivation by up to 90%.

Development of Genitourinary Disease

There are four means by which GU TB develops. The principal route is via hematogenous spread of MTBC. Clinical disease may occur soon after bacilli reach the GU system, or they may enter a period of latency before becoming clinically active (Figueiredo and Lucon, 2008; Patterson et al, 2012). Typically, GU TB becomes evident after a prolonged latency, ranging up to 46 years (Christensen, 1974; Narayana, 1982). Hematogenous seeding may localize to only the GU tract or may widely disseminate to multiple organ systems. The typical sites for GU seeding are the kidneys and epididymis. Other organs of the GU tract become infected via contiguous spread from these initial landing sites.

Ascending or retrograde infection through the urinary system is the second route of infection, albeit significantly less common than hematogenous spread. This is the case in GU TB after bladder irrigation with bacille Calmette-Guérin (BCG) for the treatment of bladder cancer. BCG is a live, attenuated vaccine derived from *M. bovis*, a member of the MTBC. Although rare, GU TB complicates 0.9% of patients receiving BCG irrigation (Lamm et al, 1992). Cases described include pyelonephritis, renal abscesses, ureteric obstruction, cystitis, prostatitis, and epididymo-orchitis (Squires et al, 1999; Demers and Pelsser, 2012; Parker and Kommu, 2013).

Rarely, TB can also reach the GU system via contiguous spread from other organ systems or direct inoculation. TB is one of the few infectious diseases that do not respect anatomic boundaries. Extension of TB from the spine and psoas to the kidneys has been described (Kothari et al, 2001). Similarly, gastrointestinal (GI) TB can extend into the GU tract to form enterorenal and enterovesical fistulae (Ney and Friedenberg, 1981; Merchant et al, 2013a). Direct inoculation is exceedingly rare. Cases include autoinoculation of external genitalia from infected stool or urine, and person-to-person

genital inoculation after contact with infected genital or oral lesions (Angus et al, 2001).

Clinical Manifestations and Pathologic Features

Symptoms and signs of GU TB are often nonspecific. Patients are often treated for other bacterial infections (sometimes repeatedly) or are evaluated for possible malignancy before GU TB is entertained. Symptoms correlate with the severity and location of disease. Renal TB, for example, can be progressive and destructive but symptomatically silent until it extends into the bladder. In developed countries, where patients with TB tend to seek medical attention earlier in the disease process, 8.4% of GU TB patients are asymptomatic (Figueiredo and Lucon, 2008). The typical TB constitutional symptoms of fever, weight loss, night sweats, and malaise are present in fewer than 20% of patients (Simon et al, 1977). Up to 50% of patients with GU TB have only dysuria on presentation, 50% have storage symptoms, and 33% have hematuria and flank pain (Figueiredo and Lucon, 2008). Renal colic occurs in fewer than 10% of patients and corresponds to the passage of necrotic papillary tissue, clots, stones, and caseous phlegmon in patients with severe pyelonephritis (Simon et al, 1977; Eastwood et al, 2001). Typical laboratory findings include sterile pyuria and/or hematuria. This combination is found in more than 90% of GU TB patients in developing countries.

Kidney

The kidney is the most common site of GU TB (Wong et al, 2013). Renal infection is progressive and highly destructive over time. The pathologic findings in the kidney vary greatly depending on disease severity.

The most insidious lesions are found in patients with pulmonary TB and renal failure, with or without pyuria, who have no changes visible on imaging of the GU tract. In these patients, kidney biopsies reveal TB-induced granulomatous interstitial nephritis (Ram et al, 2011). Renal histology shows granulomas, which are sometimes caseating. In some patients, treatment reverses the associated renal insufficiency (Eastwood et al, 2001). Other microscopic changes in the kidney include glomerulonephritis from immune complex deposition or amyloidosis secondary to TB (Sun et al, 2012). In these patients, the kidneys are collateral damage of pulmonary or systemic disease.

When renal infection is the outcome of widely disseminated TB in multiple organ systems, hematogenous spread of high numbers of bacilli leads to innumerable small (3-mm), pale clumps of granulomas that look like scattered millet seeds on gross pathologic examination of the kidney. This form of disseminated TB is known as *miliary TB* and carries a high mortality. In the kidney, the "milia" can be found studding the renal cortex and medulla and do not usually affect renal function (Eastwood et al, 2001).

In more localized infection of the kidney, tubercle bacilli become lodged first in the periglomerular capillaries. Granulomas form in the renal parenchyma and coalesce. When they caseate, cavities with necrotic material form. These can result in frank abscesses, chronic pyelonephritis, and parenchymal and papillary necrosis. Sinus tracts may emerge along the flanks (Bhatt and Lodha, 2012; Patterson et al, 2012). Examination findings at this stage can include costovertebral angle tenderness (Gokce et al, 2002). As infection advances, the calyces become inflamed and eventually calcify, resulting in calyceal distortion, dilatation, and stenosis (Merchant et al, 2013a).

With enough disease progression, the kidney becomes nonfunctional, a process called *autonephrectomy* (Teo and Wee, 2011). This complication is present in up to 33% of patients with GU TB. There are two types of autonephrectomy. The first is the caseo-cavernous type, in which viable tissue is replaced with granulomas and cavities filled with inflammatory exudate. This type of autonephrectomy occurs both with and without calcification. The second type is fibrotic, with severe scarring and calcification resulting in a shrunken kidney (Fischmann, 1951).

End-stage renal failure develops in approximately 7% of patients (Figueiredo and Lucon, 2008). Chronic inflammation may lead to squamous metaplasia in the renal pelvis that persists after treatment, posing a risk for squamous cell carcinoma (Byrd et al, 1976).

Ureter

TB in the ureters occurs via descent of infection from the kidneys. As bacilli pass in the urine through the ureter, granulomas can form along the walls. Infected calculi can also descend and lodge in the ureters. The ensuing inflammation leads to scarring and strictures, commonly in the distal end of the ureter at the vesicoureteral junction (Patterson et al, 2012). Strictures can also occur throughout the ureter in a "pan-ureteral" fashion leading to a "beaded corkscrew" appearance (Wong et al, 2013). When ureters are distorted from scarring, both obstruction and urinary reflux can develop (Eastwood et al, 2001). Urinary obstruction resulting from strictures is an important cause of renal failure in GU TB (Carl and Stark, 1997).

Bladder

Descending infection to the bladder usually begins near the ureteral orifices and spreads along the lymphatics to other areas. Similar to TB in the ureters, bacilli implant in the urothelium and cause a patchy cystitis. Ulcerations may develop in areas where large granulomas coalesce. The dome of the bladder is the most affected, whereas the trigone and neck usually remain normal. Mucosal inflammation, friability, and hematuria all follow (Wong et al, 2013). After approximately a year of chronic inflammation and mucosal scarring, bladder contracture develops (Singh et al, 2013). Urinary frequency, urgency, pain, and dysuria become prominent when bladder capacity shrinks to less than 100 mL. The severely contracted "thimble" bladder typically has a capacity of less than 20 mL. Bladder contraction is a late complication of GU TB and is more common in the developing world (12% vs. 4% of GU cases in developed countries), where diagnosis occurs after disease is more advanced (Figueiredo and Lucon, 2008).

Epididymis, Vas Deferens, Testes, and Scrotum

The epididymis, the second most common GU site of hematogenous seeding after the kidney, is involved in 10% to 55% of GU TB patients. Infection is bilateral in 34%. The disease initially affects the more vascular globus minor. Granulomas in the epididymal epithelium elicit chronic inflammation leading to fibrous narrowing and obliteration of the lumen. With disease progression, large caseous granulomas result in a nodular epididymis. On examination, the epididymis may appear swollen or hardened (Fraietta et al, 2003). Granulomas may adhere to the overlying skin and ulcerate, and in up to 50% of patients a tuberculous sinus tract develops on the posterior surface of the scrotum (Ferreira et al, 2011). After the infection spreads to the vas deferens, it becomes thickened and beaded on examination as a result of nodular scarring (Kulchavenya et al, 2012).

Isolated epididymis or testicular infections are rare but have been described (Kho and Chan, 2012; Shenoy et al, 2012). More commonly, epididymal TB extends into the testes. Granulomas form within the seminiferous tubular epithelium as well as in the connective tissue of the testis. Eventually, normal tissue becomes replaced with granulomatous tissue and fibrosis. The hardened masses that develop mimic testicular tumors. Approximately 5% of patients develop hydrocele.

Prostate and Seminal Vesicles

The prostate is infected via either hematogenous spread or urinary contamination. With hematogenous spread, prostatic lesions can be found in the periphery with sparing of the urethra. Disease then remains asymptomatic and progresses to calcification and gland hardening. Infection via the urinary route often involves the urethra and manifests more like bacterial prostatitis. Prostatic nodules or

fluctuation might be palpated on examination. TB should be suspected in patients with chronic prostatitis that persists despite antibiotics. Quinolones used to treat routine bacterial prostatitis are also active against MTBC. However, the shorter courses used for bacterial prostatitis are not sufficient for TB prostatitis, and the symptoms will not resolve or will quickly recur. Prostatic abscesses are rare but do occur, particularly in acquired immunodeficiency syndrome (AIDS) patients (Figueiredo and Lucon, 2008).

TB of the seminal vesicles may cause infertility, which can be the first symptom of GU TB (Lübbe et al, 1996). The bacilli reach the seminal vesicles through the vas deferens in patients with TB of the testis or epididymis, or through the urethra and ejaculatory ducts in patients with TB of the kidneys, bladder, or prostate. Granulomas develop in the walls of the seminal vesicles, and the lumen may be filled by caseation. Eventually calcification ensues. Patients may have low-volume ejaculate, oligospermia, azoospermia, or hemospermia. TB can rarely cause seminal vesicle abscesses (Eastham et al, 1999). Physical examination might reveal enlarged seminal vesicles with earlier detection, or hardened nodules with advanced disease.

Penis and Urethra

The urethra appears somewhat resistant to TB infection and is involved in only 1.9% to 4.5% of GU TB patients. It is typically associated with prostate infection and can manifest with urethroscrotal fistulae. Isolated urethral TB is very rare but has been reported (Bouchikhi et al, 2013). Similarly, primary TB in the penis is exceedingly rare. Penile lesions begin on the skin as an inflamed papule or a keratotic plaque (also known as *lupus vulgaris*). The lesions then ulcerate and spread to the cavernous tissue. Pea-sized nodules can be felt in the cavernous bodies and urethra corresponding to coalescing granulomas. These can be painless and hard, similar to malignancy. When fibrosis develops, the penis can become distorted (Angus et al, 2001; Gupta et al, 2008b; Kar and Kar, 2012).

Orificial TB, a rapidly necrotic form of penile TB, has also been reported (Ramesh and Vasanthi, 1989). It has been described in immunocompromised or severely debilitated patients. It arises from autoinoculation of the penile skin with infected stool or urine from the patient, or rarely from hematogenous or lymphatic spread (Wilkinson et al, 2010). Painful ulcers coated with pseudomembrane appear and can erode into deeper structures (Chen et al, 2000). Orificial TB is a presentation of very advanced and severe TB elsewhere in the GU or GI tract and carries a poor prognosis.

An exceedingly rare form of penile TB is papulonecrotic tuberculid (PNT) (Dandale et al, 2013). This is a cutaneous manifestation of TB on the glans penis and can occur in other skin areas as well. PNT of the penis has been described in Japan, South Africa, and India. The tuberculids are red papules that erupt on the skin, ulcerate, and undergo varioliform scarring. Unlike primary TB of the penis, these ulcers can be painless and do not contain tubercle bacilli. The tuberculids are hypersensitivity reactions to MTBC antigens that were disseminated to the skin from other infectious foci, and as such they are culture negative and typically polymerase chain reaction (PCR) negative. Histology is often inconclusive, as mature granulomas are not always seen. The recurrent lesions are easily confused with syphilis, Behçet disease, recurrent herpes simplex, balanitis, and squamous cell carcinoma. Recognizing this entity is the first step in diagnosis, and response to empirical TB treatment despite negative cultures confirms it.

Diagnosis

In developed countries, the primary goal of the diagnostic workup is isolation of MTBC in culture for drug susceptibility testing. In the right clinical context, tissue samples demonstrating caseating granulomas can support a diagnosis of TB when cultures or DNA test results are negative. Absent those, diagnosis of patients with GU TB relies on the constellation of consistent clinical findings in a patient with probable exposure and response to empirical medical treatment. Because up to 20% of GU TB occurs concurrently with pulmonary TB (Figueiredo and Lucon, 2008), it is useful to also assess for the presence of pulmonary disease.

Culture

The current gold standard for the diagnosis of GU TB is urine acid-fast bacilli (AFB) culture. First-void urine is the best sample because urine is the most concentrated at that time. Three to five urine samples on consecutive days should be collected for maximum yield. These should be cultured immediately after collection because prolonged exposure to urine acidity can retard mycobacterial growth (American Thoracic Society, 2000a). The sensitivity of urine AFB cultures is as high as 80% when done in this manner. In real-world practice, however, sensitivity can be as low as 10% (Abbara and Davidson, 2011). Ziehl-Neelsen stains can be done on the urine as well, but the sensitivity is less than 50%. In addition, any tissue obtained from biopsy or surgery should also be cultured.

Mycobacterium tuberculosis complex has traditionally been cultured on solid, egg-based, Löwenstein-Jensen (LJ) medium. This method is laborious and time-consuming; usually 4 to 6 weeks are required before growth of MTBC can be detected. LJ remains the medium of choice in developing countries because it is the least expensive and requires no specialized equipment. In developed countries, urine is cultured on more expensive, agar-based, transparent, solid media, such as Middlebrook 7H10. With this medium, colonies can be visualized approximately 1 week earlier than with LJ media. Liquid-based detection systems such as the BACTEC Mycobacteria Growth Indicator Tube (MGIT) are also used in the developed world. The MGIT is a fully automated system that uses fluorescence quenching to detect mycobacterial growth in liquid media in as little as 10 days. Current guidelines recommend culturing on at least one solid medium concurrently with the liquid system to maximize yield (American Thoracic Society, 2000a). Other available detection methods include semiautomated systems that use radiometric liquid culture. Antibiotic susceptibility can be tested using any of the culture methods described earlier. Typically, susceptibility to first-line TB drugs is tested "in house" with use of the MGIT instrument. Susceptibility testing for second-line TB drugs is generally performed only at reference laboratories.

Nucleic Acid Amplification Tests

Several amplification tests have been developed to speed the detection of MTBC, providing results within 1 to 2 days. This can also aid detection in cases with low bacillary load, in which culture might fail to isolate the organisms. The tests have reported sensitivities ranging from 87% to 96% when compared with culture. However, nonsputum specimens such as urine contain natural inhibitors that interfere with the DNA or RNA amplification process, potentially resulting in false-negative test results (Moussa et al, 2000; Chawla et al, 2012; Mehta et al, 2012). The sensitivity of PCR tests for GU TB also depends on the type of sequence amplification used. Assays using the MTBC repetitive IS6110 insertion sequence perform better than those amplifying 16S-rRNA (Moussa et al, 2000).

In general, nucleic acid amplification tests (NAATs) are frequently underused in developed countries because culture is necessary for drug susceptibility testing. In developing countries, the cost and the need for expensive equipment have been the obstacles. Unlike cultures, NAATs cannot be used to monitor response to treatment because nucleic acids are shed from dead organisms and test results can remain positive despite adequate treatment (American Thoracic Society, 2000a).

In 2010, WHO enthusiastically endorsed the newest TB PCR assay on the market, the GeneXpert MTB/RIF. The system provides a self-contained platform that automates sputum processing, DNA extraction, and amplification in less than 2 hours. It simultaneously detects the presence of MTBC and rifampin resistance. Because more than 90% of rifampin-resistant strains are also INH-resistant, rifampin resistance serves as a surrogate marker for multidrug-resistant tuberculosis (MDR-TB) (Ioannidis et al, 2011). The assay

has been most studied with sputum samples and appears to have sensitivity similar to culture. Its use for GU TB is still being evaluated. In a small study of extrapulmonary TB that included 91 urine samples (only five of which were culture positive), the GeneXpert was 100% sensitive and 98.6% specific (Hillemann et al, 2011).

Histopathology

Histopathology shows findings consistent with TB in 38.3% of GU TB cases in developed countries and 21.9% of cases globally. Because urine cultures are sometimes negative, tissue biopsy can aid the diagnosis of GU TB (Kulchavenya et al, 2013). Although mycobacteria are often not seen, the finding of caseating granulomas in the appropriate clinical context can help establish a diagnosis of GU TB.

Screening Tests

The tuberculin skin test (TST) and interferon-gamma release assays (IGRAs) do not differentiate between latent and active TB. They have limited usefulness in the diagnosis of active disease, although they are widely used and are approved by the U.S. Food and Drug Administration (FDA) for this purpose. A positive test result cannot rule in active TB, and a negative test result cannot rule it out. The ideal use for these tests is in the screening of individuals for the presence of latent TB infection. However, in the absence of other positive test results, the use of these screening tests can sometimes help sway the physician toward making a diagnosis of active TB disease.

Tuberculin Skin Test, Purified Protein Derivative, Mantoux Test. The TST evaluates the presence of an existing cellular immune response to MTBC antigens, which should be present in persons who have been infected. Tuberculin is a sterile suspension of protein extracted from cultures of *M. tuberculosis* and is injected intradermally into the volar aspect of the forearm. After 48 to 72 hours, delayed-type hypersensitivity will cause induration at the site of injection in those with prior immune priming. The CDC guidelines for interpretation of a positive test result depend on the risk factors of the patient. Three distinct cut-points for positivity have been defined according to risk. For persons with recent contact with a patient with TB, with fibrotic changes on chest radiographs that are consistent with prior TB, or who are immunosuppressed, 5 mm of induration or more is positive. For recent immigrants from high-prevalence countries, residents of or workers in high-risk institutions, injection drug users, and persons with medical comorbidities that increase risk of active TB, 10 mm of induration or more is positive. For the general public, 15 mm or more is positive (Box 17-1) (American Thoracic Society, 2000b).

Although initial training of personnel both in test placement and interpretation is necessary, the TST has many advantages. It is cheap, does not require a laboratory, and is easy to perform. The main disadvantage is that the TST is not specific for MTBC. Vaccination with BCG and infection with nontuberculous mycobacteria may elicit a positive reaction. In addition, the TST requires a second visit from the patient for test reading, which can be difficult to ensure. False-negative results can occur in 10% to 25% of persons with active TB (Huebner et al, 1993). In one study, the TST result was positive in 85% to 95% of patients with GU TB (Figueiredo and Lucon, 2008).

Interferon-Gamma Release Assays. IGRAs are blood tests that measure the level of IFN-γ (a surrogate of cellular immune reactivity) produced in response to MTBC-specific antigens, akin to an in vitro MTBC-specific TST. Persons infected with MTBC have circulating T cells that quickly recognize MTBC antigens and secrete IFN-γ on re-exposure. The antigens used in IGRAs are absent from all BCG strains and most nontuberculous mycobacteria, and thus exposure to these organisms does not result in a positive IGRA result. Results are available after 24 hours.

There are two IGRAs available in the United States: the QuantiFERON-TB Gold In-Tube test (QFT-GIT) and the T-SPOT.TB test. The QFT-GIT is simpler to run, whereas the T-SPOT.TB

IGRA requires more steps. In the QFT-GIT, whole blood is collected in three specialized test tubes, one containing the MTBC antigens ESAT-6, CFP-10, and TB7.7, and two controls (negative and positive). The blood is incubated directly in the collection tubes for 16 to 24 hours. Plasma is then separated and IFN-γ is measured using enzyme-linked immunosorbent assay (ELISA). Test results are read as positive, negative, or indeterminate, based on the level of IFN-γ produced in relation to the negative and positive controls. In the T-SPOT.TB assay, peripheral blood mononuclear cells are separated from whole blood and then incubated with ESAT-6 and CFP-10 in wells coated with antibodies that capture IFN-γ. Enzyme-linked immunospot (ELISPOT) assay is used to detect an increase in the number of cells (appearing as spots in each test well) that secrete IFN-γ in relation to a negative control. Spots are manually counted, and the test result is read as positive, negative, or borderline. Despite the increased difficulty of performing T-SPOT.TB over QFT-GIT, it is the more sensitive test. Pooled studies estimate a sensitivity of 83% for QFT-GIT and 91% for T-SPOT, versus 89% for TST in cases of culture-confirmed TB (Mazurek et al, 2010).

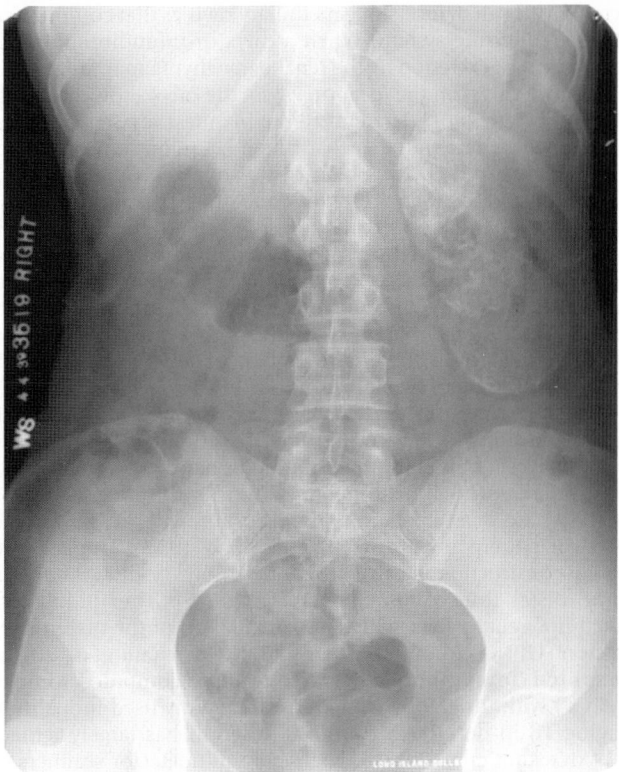

Figure 17-1. Kidney-ureter-bladder radiographic view in a patient with left renal tuberculosis with associated calcifications.

Radiography

GU TB generates a wide spectrum of imaging findings. The test of choice depends on disease location and should be driven by symptoms and other clinical data. Imaging is often the first test that indicates TB is the cause of a GU disorder.

Plain Radiography. The kidney-ureter-bladder (KUB) radiograph will frequently demonstrate calcifications caused by TB, which are present in more than 50% of patients (Merchant et al, 2013a). Initial renal lesions may appear as faint punctate calcifications within the parenchyma. As TB progresses, the KUB film may show globular calcifications that correspond to a tubercular mass (Fig. 17-1). Papillary necrosis appears as triangular ringlike calcifications in the collecting system. With fibrotic autonephrectomy, the KUB radiograph shows a small, shrunken, calcified "cement" or "putty" kidney, in which calcific rims outline the individual renal lobes; this lobar pattern is pathognomonic for end-stage renal TB.

A plain radiograph can also demonstrate renal and ureteral TB-infected calculi. Stones may take strange shapes as they form in a deformed and fibrosed renal pelvis. A stone in the shape of an upward arrowhead may indicate a renal pelvis that has been "hiked up" by contraction from scarring.

The KUB film can also show ureteral calcifications, which are characteristically intraluminal as opposed to the mural calcifications of schistosomiasis. Bladder wall calcifications are not very common except in late cases of bladder contraction. Calcifications of the prostate and seminal vesicles are seen in 10% of patients. Plain film findings suggestive of TB may be seen in surrounding tissues as well, appearing as erosions of the vertebral bodies or calcifications in cold abscesses of the psoas muscle (Teo and Wee, 2011; Merchant et al, 2013a).

Intravenous Urography. Intravenous urography (IVU) is the gold standard for imaging early renal TB. Initial erosive changes of the urothelium appear as loss of sharpness and edge irregularities (Figueiredo and Lucon, 2008). Calyceal erosions have a moth-eaten appearance (Patterson et al, 2012). Filling defects may be seen, caused by tuberculomas rupturing into the calyx or by papillary necrosis. IVU can demonstrate medullary cavities that communicate with the collecting system. When a calyx or infundibulum is stenosed, contrast excretion by the renal parenchyma may fail, creating a "phantom calyx" in the location where the calyx should be visible (Eastwood et al, 2001). Ureteral TB can manifest as a rigid, calcified, straightened, pipestem ureter that is tubular and lacks normal peristaltic activity on IVU. The ureter may also take on the appearance of a beaded corkscrew as a result of nodular fibrosis along the entire ureter. The pipestem and corkscrew findings are highly suggestive of TB, particularly when seen concurrently with either kidney or bladder abnormalities. IVU can also detect nonfunctional kidneys resulting from autonephrectomy, as well as a fibrosed, contracted bladder (Fig. 17-2). On occasion, perinephric abscess might be suggested, particularly if there is restriction of renal movement with breathing, or ureteral displacement on IVU.

The most common findings on IVU, however, are obstructive changes resulting from scarring and distortion of the collecting system: calyceal obliteration, infundibular narrowing, hydrocalycosis, segmental or total hydronephrosis, and hydroureter (Figs. 17-3 and 17-4). Calyceal dilatation and distortion will present a typical cloverleaf pattern on film (Carl and Stark, 1997). Ureterovesical junction obstruction is caused by tuberculous cystitis or strictures of the distal third of the ureter (Fig. 17-5). The finding of a "hiked-up" renal pelvis, with sharp angulation of the ureteropelvic junction (UPJ), is known as "Kerr's kink" (Merchant et al, 2013a).

Computed Tomography with Urography. Computed tomography (CT) with urography is the most frequently used modality for imaging TB in developed countries, where it has largely replaced IVU (Merchant et al, 2013b). High-end multidetector scanners can detect lesions as small as 3 to 4 mm. With the administration of intravenous contrast, CT can assess kidney function during different phases of excretion. Similar to KUB and IVU, CT reveals calcifications, scarring, and signs of obstruction (Fig. 17-6). CT is more sensitive than KUB in detecting calcifications and thickening of the collecting ducts. It is particularly useful in evaluating patients with complicated and extensive TB. Perinephric and psoas abscesses can be seen, as well as any pathology in lymph nodes, vertebrae, spleen, or liver. Pathology in the prostate and seminal vesicles can also be visualized, including enlargement, necrosis, cavitations and abscesses, and calcifications.

CT does have disadvantages. CT is less sensitive for detecting the minimal urothelial thickening, subtle papillary necrosis, and other changes of early renal TB, for which IVU is still the preferred study. In addition, CT imparts a higher radiation dose than IVU.

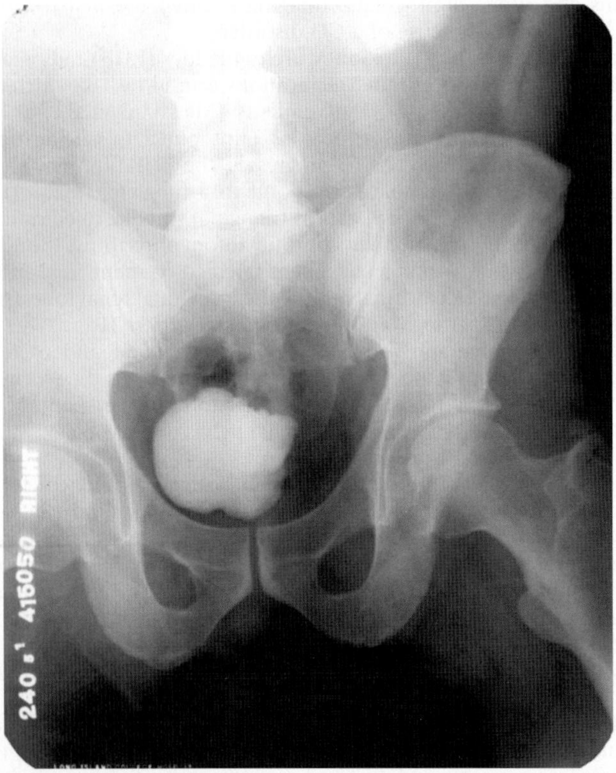

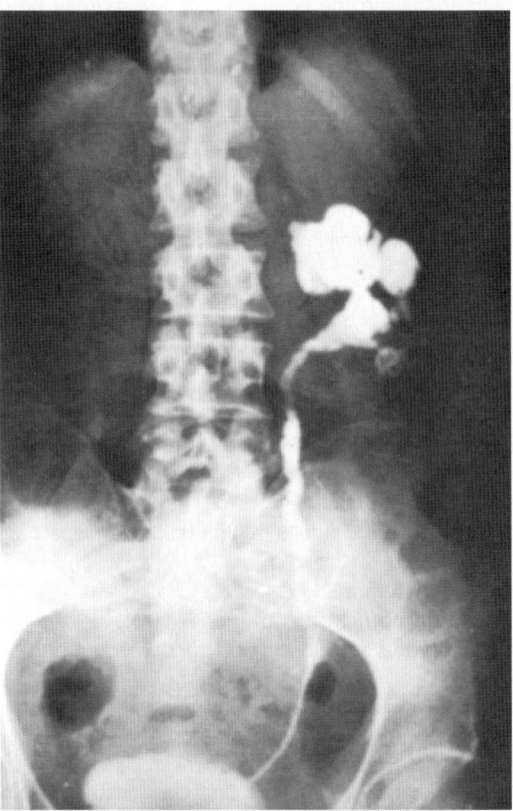

Figure 17-3. **Occluded calyx.**

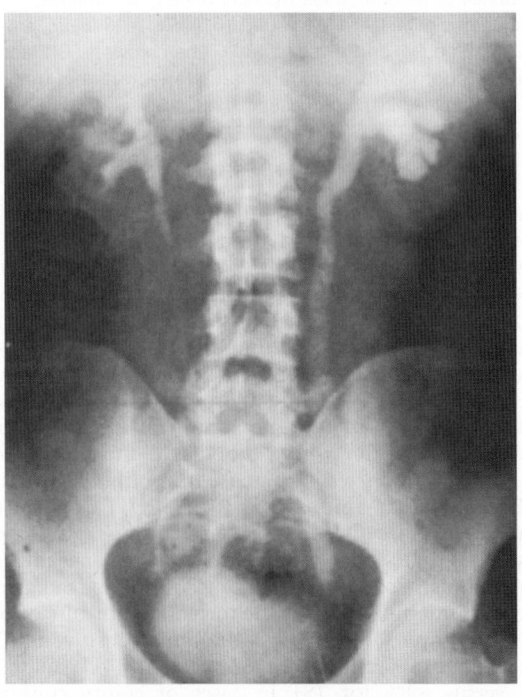

Figure 17-4. **Severe calyceal and parenchymal destruction.**

Figure 17-2. **The cystogram portion of an intravenous pyelogram in a patient with left renal tuberculosis. Note the contracted left side of the bladder that is secondary to fibrosis from the tuberculosis.**

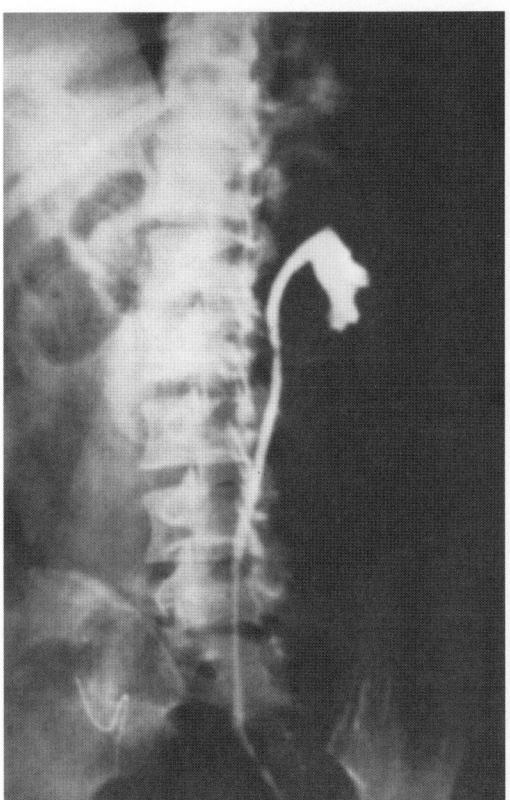

Figure 17-5. Stricture at the distal left ureter.

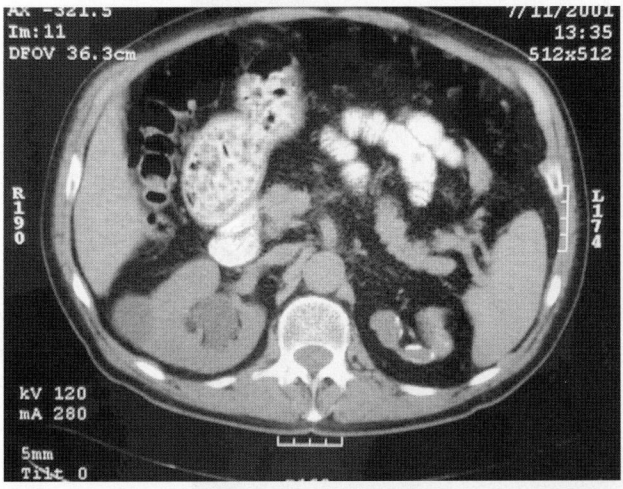

Figure 17-6. Computed tomography scan after oral contrast medium in a patient with bilateral renal tuberculosis. The right kidney is hydronephrotic secondary to infundibular stenosis but has retained good function. The left kidney is an end-stage nonfunctioning atrophic kidney with calcification.

Retrograde Pyelography and Antegrade Pyelography. Both retrograde and antegrade pyelography, with either percutaneously or endoscopically administered contrast, have been replaced by CT urography. However, when IVU or CT cannot be done because of renal insufficiency or contrast allergy, these modalities can be helpful in delineating the distortions in GU anatomy. In addition, these tests can be used in conjunction with IVU to determine whether cavitations are obstructive or nonobstructive, and whether they are in communication with the urinary collecting system or not (Merchant et al, 2013b).

Ultrasonography

Ultrasonography (US) has a limited role in the diagnosis of GU TB because findings are generally nonspecific and visualization is not as clear as with CT. It is useful in pediatric or pregnant patients because of the lack of radiation exposure. US is also less expensive than CT. US can be used to evaluate the testes, epididymis, and, with transrectal US, the prostate and seminal vesicles, which will appear thickened. US can also locate abscesses or cavities in the kidney. Cystic lesions with septations suggest chronic infection (Wong et al, 2013). Focal calcifications appear as highly echogenic areas with distal shadowing. Restriction of renal movement during breathing suggests a perinephric or psoas abscess. Like CT, US can provide concurrent information about the abdomen, such as the presence of ascites, lymphadenopathy, or omental caking. A primary use of US in GU TB is to follow hydronephrosis in patients who are receiving medical treatment because fibrosis during healing can worsen urinary obstruction.

Magnetic Resonance Imaging

Magnetic resonance imaging (MRI) is not commonly used in the workup of GU TB because of the many other imaging modalities available (Merchant et al, 2013b). Similar to US, it can be useful in pediatric or pregnant patients to avoid exposure to radiation. MRI can detect a single granuloma. Small lesions are hypointense on both T1 and T2 images. Larger lesions have central hyperintensity on T2 images because of the increased cellularity at the center of the granuloma. Larger TB lesions can mimic malignancy, and it is not always possible to differentiate the two.

A magnetic resonance urogram (MRU) can be more sensitive than IVU in showing urothelial thickening and caliectasis. The addition of diffusion-weighted imaging (DWI) can help distinguish hydronephrosis from pyonephrosis. Various techniques have been explored with MRI to study TB, including cine MRU and dynamic MRU, which can evaluate ureteral peristalsis. MRI with DWI can be used to monitor renal fibrosis. Apparent diffusion coefficients (ADCs) decrease with fibrosis and can be used to gauge the stage of TB, including the effect of treatment. Caution should be exercised with use of gadolinium in renal failure patients because of the risk of development of nephrogenic systemic fibrosis.

Cystoscopy and Ureteroscopy

Endoscopy plays a limited role in the diagnosis of TB. Although it allows direct visualization of lesions, findings can be nonspecific. They include local hyperemia, mucosal erosion, ulceration, granulomatous masses, and irregularity of the ureteral orifices. Ulcerative lesions may mimic malignancy. A "golf-hole" ureteric orifice is suggestive of TB, and, when found, upper tract imaging or endoscopy should be performed (Fig. 17-7). Biopsies should be performed when possible, especially if malignancy is a possibility. Although a positive urine culture for MTBC is sufficient for diagnosis, results may not be available quickly enough. Furthermore, in those with negative urine cultures, bladder biopsy can be 19% to 52% sensitive for TB (Figueiredo and Lucon, 2008).

Treatment

Before the development of antimicrobials, treatment of TB relied primarily on rest and nourishment in sanatoria; and in those with severe GU disease, extirpative surgery was the best hope for cure. With the development of streptomycin in 1944, followed by INH in 1952 and the rifamycins in 1957, medical treatment with antituberculous drugs replaced sanatoria and surgical procedures (Daniel, 2006). Today, most TB patients can be treated medically and in the ambulatory setting, even those with MDR-TB. Surgery now serves primarily to establish a diagnosis or as an adjunct to antibiotics in advanced cases (Abbara and Davidson, 2011).

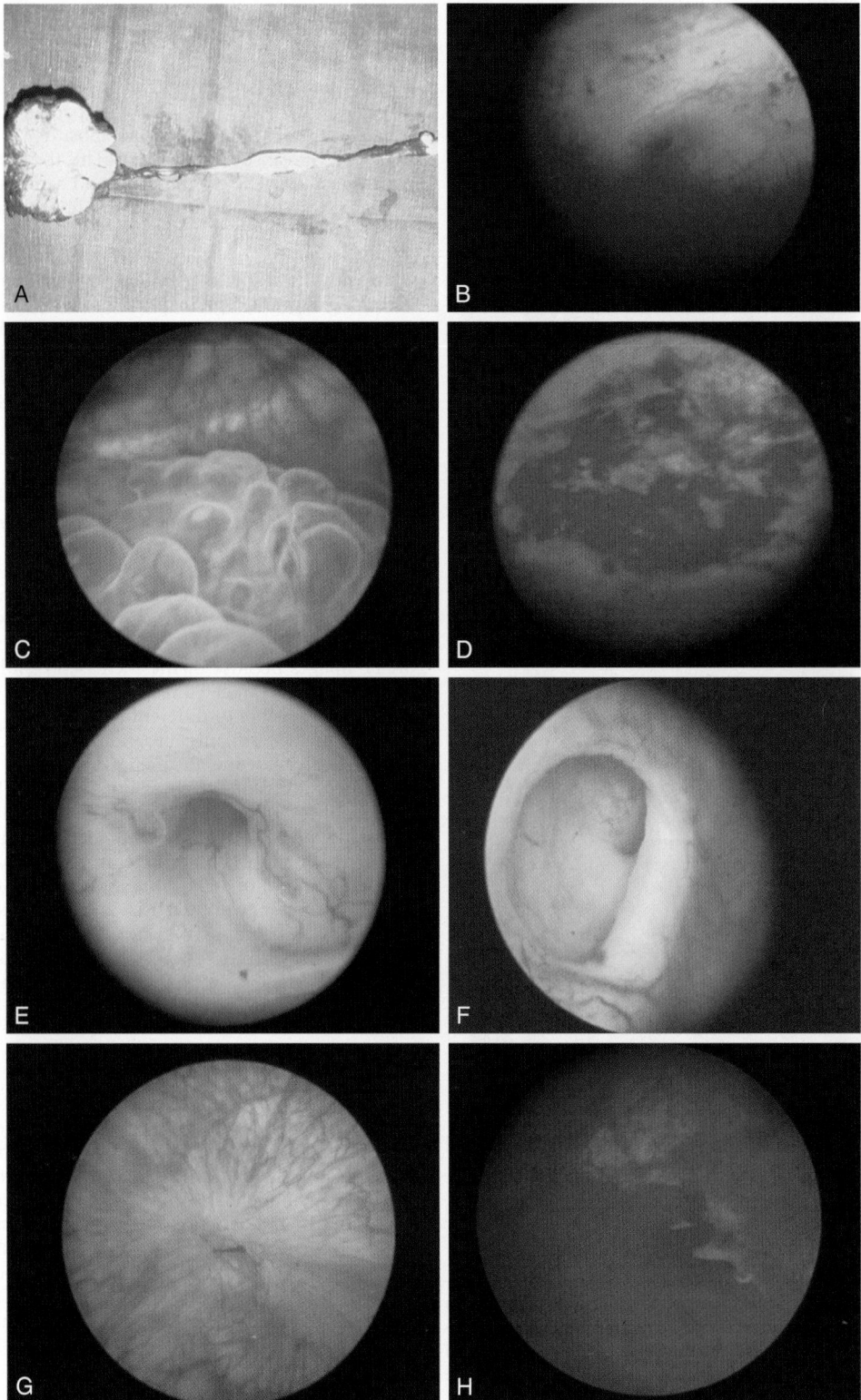

Figure 17-7. A, Extensive tuberculosis of the kidney and ureter with calcification and stricture formation. **B,** Acutely inflamed ureteric orifice. **C,** Tuberculous bullous granulations. **D,** Acute tuberculous ulcer. **E,** Tuberculous golf-hole ureter. **F,** Tuberculous golf-hole ureter, severely withdrawn. **G,** Healed tuberculous lesion. **H,** Acute tuberculous cystitis with ulceration.

Medical Therapy

Successful medical treatment of TB requires multiple drugs for several reasons (CDC, 2003). First, the tubercle bacilli exist in different microenvironments within the host. These apply different pressures on the organism and cause it to exhibit

different metabolic needs and replication speeds. The drugs vary in their activity against MTBC; some are bactericidal, whereas others are only bacteriostatic. Some drugs work best on rapidly replicating bacteria, whereas others are more effective against dormant bacilli. The drugs also penetrate differently into various tissues and perform optimally at different pHs. In addition,

TABLE 17-1 First-Line Antituberculous Drugs

DRUG/FORMULATION	ADULT DOSAGE (DAILY)[1]	ADULT DOSAGE (INTERMITTENT)[2]	MAIN ADVERSE EFFECTS
Isoniazid (INH)[3] 100-mg, 300-mg tabs 50-mg/5-mL syrup 100-mg/mL injection	5 mg/kg (max 300 mg)	15 mg/kg (max 900 mg) 3 times/wk	Hepatic toxicity, peripheral neuropathy
Rifampin (Rifadin, Rimactane)[4] 150-mg, 300-mg caps 600-mg injection powder	10 mg/kg (max 600 mg)	10 mg/kg (max 600 mg) 3 times/wk	Hepatic toxicity, flulike syndrome, pruritus, drug interactions
Rifabutin (Mycobutin)[5] 150-mg caps	5 mg/kg (max 300 mg)	5 mg/kg (max 300 mg) 3 times/wk	Hepatic toxicity, flulike syndrome, uveitis, neutropenia, drug interactions
Rifapentine (Priftin)[6] 150-mg tabs		10 mg/kg/wk PO (max 600 mg) **Continuation phase only in very select patients**	Similar to rifampin
Pyrazinamide 500-mg tabs	40-55 kg: 1000 mg 56-75 kg: 1500 mg 76-90 kg: 2000 mg	3 times/wk: 40-55 kg: 1500 mg 56-75 kg: 2500 mg 76-90 kg: 3000 mg	Arthralgias, hepatic toxicity, pruritus, rash, hyperuricemia, gastrointestinal upset
Ethambutol (Myambutol) 100-mg, 400-mg tabs	40-55 kg: 800 mg 56-75 kg: 1200 mg 76-90 kg: 1600 mg	3 times/wk: 40-55 kg: 1200 mg 56-75 kg: 2000 mg 76-90 kg: 2400 mg	Decreased red-green color discrimination, decreased visual acuity, optic neuritis

1. Or 5 times/wk directly observed therapy (DOT).
2. Intermittent therapy (administered by DOT) only during the continuation phase of therapy. The World Health Organization (WHO) no longer recommends dosage intervals less frequent than 3 times/wk.
3. Pyridoxine 25 to 50 mg should be given to prevent neuropathy in malnourished or pregnant patients and those with human immunodeficiency (HIV) infection, renal failure, thyroid disease, alcoholism, or diabetes.
4. In general, cannot be taken by HIV-infected persons taking protease inhibitors or certain non-nucleoside reverse-transcriptase inhibitors (NNRTIs).
5. When taken with efavirenz, the rifabutin dose is increased to 450 mg/day or 600 mg 3 times/wk. When taken with fosamprenavir, nelfinavir or indinavir, the rifabutin dose is 150 mg/day or 300 mg 3 times/wk. With ritonavir, atazanavir, or ritonavir combined with other protease inhibitors, the rifabutin dose is 150 mg every other day or 3 times/wk; some experts believe this dose to be subtherapeutic and recommend 150 mg daily or 300 mg 3 times/wk with close monitoring for rifabutin toxicity, particularly uveitis.
6. *Rifapentine is contraindicated in HIV-positive persons, in persons with cavitary pulmonary disease, and in persons with extrapulmonary tuberculosis.* Use of once-weekly rifapentine is not advocated by WHO.

From Drugs for tuberculosis. Treat Guidel Med Lett 2012;10(116):29–36; and modified by Centers for Disease Control and Prevention (CDC). Treatment of tuberculosis, American Thoracic Society, CDC, and Infectious Diseases Society of America. MMWR Recomm Rep 2003;52(RR-11):1–77.

multiple drug therapy prevents the emergence of drug-resistant strains.

Combination therapy with first-line antituberculous drugs achieves the best cure rates in the shortest time frame (Table 17-1). Treatment should start with these—namely, INH, rifampin, pyrazinamide, and ethambutol. Before the start of treatment, baseline measurements should include blood counts and liver and kidney function tests. Patients should also be tested for HIV and, when appropriate, hepatitis B and C. Medical therapy should be tailored according to drug susceptibility data when available. Directly observed therapy (DOT) should be employed to ensure medication adherence and minimize the likelihood of development of drug-resistant strains.

Second-line agents are reserved for patients in whom first-line agents fail or who experience side effects from first-line agents, and for cases of drug resistance. Second-line agents vary in tolerability and ease of administration (Table 17-2). Recent drugs added to the second-line agents are the fluoroquinolones and linezolid (Lee et al, 2012), both of which were developed to treat other bacterial infections, and bedaquiline—the first new drug in 40 years specifically developed for TB. It was fast-tracked by the FDA and approved for use on December 28, 2012 after completion of only phase 2b

studies. Currently, it is approved only as part of combination therapy for drug-resistant pulmonary TB (CDC, 2013b).

Genitourinary TB can be successfully treated with the standard short-course regimen of 6 months of first-line antituberculous drugs (CDC, 2003). Treatment begins with an intensive phase of 2 months of daily INH, rifampin, and pyrazinamide, followed by a continuation phase of 4 months of INH and rifampin given daily, or alternatively thrice weekly. Twice-weekly administration during the continuation phase is no longer recommended (WHO, 2010). Pyridoxine (vitamin B_6) administration minimizes the risk of INH-induced peripheral neuropathy. Ethambutol is added at the beginning of treatment pending drug susceptibilities and is discontinued if the strain is found to be susceptible to the other first-line drugs. First-line drugs reach high concentrations in the urine and work well in acidic environments. The intensive phase of treatment targets rapidly multiplying bacteria, whereas the continuation phase attempts to eradicate slow, sporadic multipliers and persistent bacteria.

Although 6 months is the duration of standard short-course therapy, clinical scenarios regularly arise that require prolongation of treatment. Both the type of clinical disease present and the antituberculous drugs used affect duration of treatment (CDC, 2003).

TABLE 17-2 Second-Line Antituberculous Drugs

DRUG/FORMULATION	ADULT DOSAGE (DAILY)[1]	MAIN ADVERSE EFFECTS
Streptomycin[2]	15 mg/kg IM, IV (max 1 g)	Vestibular and auditory toxicity, renal damage
Capreomycin (Capastat)[2]	15 mg/kg IM, IV (max 1 g)	Auditory and vestibular toxicity, renal damage, electrolyte imbalance
Kanamycin (Kantrex and others)[2]	15 mg/kg IM, IV (max 1 g)	Ototoxicity, renal damage
Amikacin (Amikin and others)[2]	15 mg/kg IM, IV (max 1 g)	Ototoxicity, renal damage
Cycloserine (Seromycin)[3]	10-15 mg/kg in 2 doses (max 500 mg bid) PO	Psychiatric symptoms, seizures
Ethionamide (Trecator-SC)	15-20 mg/kg in 1 or 2 doses (max 500 mg bid) PO	Gastrointestinal and hepatic toxicity, hypothyroidism, optic neuritis, neurotoxicity
Levofloxacin (Levaquin)	500-1000 mg PO, IV	Gastrointestinal toxicity, central nervous system effects, rash, dysglycemia, QT prolongation, tendinitis or tendon rupture
Moxifloxacin (Avelox)	400 mg PO, IV	Gastrointestinal toxicity, central nervous system effects, rash, dysglycemia, QT prolongation, tendinitis or tendon rupture
Aminosalicylic acid (PAS; Paser)	8-12 g in 2 or 3 doses PO	Gastrointestinal disturbance, hepatitis, hypothyroidism
Linezolid (Zyvox)	600 mg PO bid	Bone marrow suppression, peripheral and optic neuropathy, hepatic toxicity
Bedaquiline (Sirturo)[4]	400 mg PO	Headache, nausea, arthralgias, QT prolongation, hepatic toxicity

1. Dosage may need to be adjusted for patients with renal impairment.
2. In general, given 5 to 7 times/wk (15 mg/kg, or a maximum of 1 g per dose) for an initial 2 to 4 months, and then (if needed) 3 times/wk (20 to 30 mg/kg, or a maximum of 1.5 g per dose). Administration less frequently than 3 times/wk is no longer recommended. For patients older than 59 years, dose is reduced to 10 mg/kg (max 750 mg per dose). Dose should be decreased if renal function is diminished.
3. Some authorities recommend pyridoxine 50 mg for every 250 mg of cycloserine to decrease the incidence of adverse neurologic effects.
4. Bedaquiline is given at 400 mg orally with food, daily for 2 weeks, then 200 mg orally 3 times/wk.

From Drugs for tuberculosis. Treat Guidel Med Lett 2012;10(116):29–36; and modified by Centers for Disease Control and Prevention (CDC). Treatment of tuberculosis, American Thoracic Society, CDC, and Infectious Diseases Society of America. MMWR Recomm Rep 2003;52(RR-11):1–77; Lee M, Lee J, Carroll MW, et al. Linezolid for treatment of chronic extensively drug-resistant tuberculosis. N Engl J Med 2012;367(16):1508–18; and CDC. Provisional CDC guidelines for the use and safety monitoring of bedaquiline fumarate (Sirturo) for the treatment of multidrug-resistant tuberculosis. MMWR Recomm Rep 2013;62(RR-09):1–12.

For example, treatment for at least 9 months is recommended for extensive pockets of infection, concurrent smear-positive cavitary pulmonary disease, central nervous system involvement, or a delay in positive cultures converting to negative. If the patient is unable to take pyrazinamide for at least 2 months, because of either side effects or drug resistance, the duration of therapy should also be 9 months or longer. Some clinicians recommend 12 months of therapy for GU TB because of high relapse rates of up to 22% when therapy is given for only 6 months (Gokalp et al, 1990). Because of the complexities that often arise with regimen choice, drug interactions, and side effects, any deviation from standard short-course therapy should be discussed with specialists experienced in treating TB.

During therapy, liver enzymes should be monitored monthly in those with preexisting liver disease because all first-line agents except ethambutol can cause hepatic toxicity that can be reversed with drug discontinuation (CDC, 2003). Patients should be advised to abstain from alcohol and other hepatotoxic drugs. Although treatment is, in general, well tolerated, severe hepatic injury has occurred. Visual acuity and red-green color perception also should be monitored in patients taking ethambutol. Close follow-up of patients is necessary, not only to monitor for side effects, but also because renal lesions may worsen with drug treatment. The healing process is sometimes accompanied by new fibrosis, which can worsen urinary obstruction and bladder contraction (Psihramis and Donahoe, 1986). Steroids may help in the management of these patients (see later). Surgical intervention to relieve worsening or newly developed obstruction might be necessary.

Corticosteroids. The role of adjunctive corticosteroids for the treatment of active TB still needs to be fully elucidated. The anti-inflammatory effects of corticosteroids are thought to prevent an unchecked host immune response from causing excessive tissue destruction and scarring. They are strongly recommended for TB meningitis and TB pericarditis, and they are sometimes used in patients with severe pulmonary TB, when antibiotic treatment leads to a paradoxic worsening of symptoms (Breen et al, 2004). Steroids have also been used in a few patients with GU TB to prevent ureteral strictures and bladder contraction, but these situations are anecdotal and no clinical trials have been conducted. A recent review and meta-analysis of published clinical trials of corticosteroid use in pulmonary, meningeal, pleural, pericardial, and peritoneal TB showed that regardless of which organ system was affected, steroids reduced mortality by 17% (Critchley et al, 2013).

Surgical Therapy

About 55% of patients with GU TB will require surgical management during the course of their disease (Wong et al, 2013). Intervention is more frequent as disease advances. Surgical procedures are performed to relieve urinary obstruction and drain infected material, to remove nonworking infected kidneys in cases resisting cure, to improve medically resistant hypertension secondary to a functionally excluded kidney, or to reconstruct the urinary tract. Currently, more than half of operations performed for TB are reconstructive (Gupta et al, 2008b). The optimal timing of surgery is 4 to 6 weeks after the initiation of medical therapy. This delay allows active inflammation to subside, the bacillary load to decrease, and lesions to stabilize.

Procedures to Relieve Obstruction. Prompt relief of obstruction is emergently required in cases of uremia or sepsis. Bilateral obstruction or unilateral obstruction of a functionally solitary kidney is often the cause of renal failure. Early ureteral stenting or percutaneous nephrostomy (PCN) for tuberculous ureteral strictures limits the loss of renal function and increases the opportunity for later reconstructive surgery (Shin et al, 2002). Temporary and immediate drainage of obstruction is recommended, preferably by retrograde ureteric stenting. An indwelling double-J stent can be placed until the patient's condition has been optimized. Retrograde placement is successful in 41% of cases (Ramanathan et al, 1998). When this is not technically feasible, an antegrade, internalized or externalized ureteral stent is placed via percutaneous puncture of the obstructed kidney. If that also fails, a PCN is left in place until definitive management. Because strictures and fibrous scars may be present, more than one PCN may be necessary (Carl and Stark, 1997). PCN must be followed by correction of the cause of obstruction. A tuberculous cutaneous fistula can develop if the PCN is simply removed, although this is less likely to develop with effective concurrent medical therapy. If the kidney is unsalvageable, a nephrectomy may become necessary. High-contrast injection pressures during stent and PCN placement should be avoided to prevent possible dissemination of infection (Salem, 2008).

Nephrectomy. Organ preservation is the fundamental goal in surgical management of GU TB. However, total nephrectomy is considered in two settings. The first is the patient with a nonfunctional kidney and recalcitrant or recurrent TB despite optimal medical therapy. After nephrectomy of the infected kidney, relapse rates of less than 1% have been reported following short-course medical treatment (Figueiredo and Lucon, 2008). The second setting in which nephrectomy is considered is the patient with a nonfunctional kidney and medically resistant hypertension. Nephrectomy improves hypertension in 65% of patients (Flechner and Gow, 1980). Overall, nephrectomy is performed in 27% of GU TB patients, and the frequency is similar between developed and developing countries (Figueiredo and Lucon, 2008).

Because of the extensive fibrosis often present, the traditional approach to the kidney is through an oblique retroperitoneal incision that can be extended dorsally or ventrally as needed. In rare patients the perinephric fat may appear to have granulomatous masses or caseous cavities. These should be removed with the specimen. Individual ligation of the renal artery and vein is preferred to limit risk of late arteriovenous fistula. The ureters are usually not taken out concurrently. Care must be taken to minimize disruption of the surrounding lymphatics and to avoid entering the pleural or peritoneal space during the procedure.

More recently, laparoscopic nephrectomy has gained popularity (Lee et al, 2002; Hemal, 2011) despite concerns that extensive fibrosis associated with TB would render a laparoscopic approach suboptimal. Several investigators have reported good outcomes and suggest that it should be the preferred approach because of decreased blood loss and more rapid patient recovery (Chibber et al, 2005; Zhang et al, 2005; Gupta et al, 2008a). In experienced hands, laparoscopic nephrectomy for renal TB is a somewhat longer procedure than when it is done for other reasons, but in one study the procedure took only half an hour longer on average (Lee et al, 2002).

Ureteropelvic and Ureteral Surgery. Strictures of the UPJ and ureter may be temporarily stented to allow improvement of renal function before definitive management. Upper ureteric and mid-ureteric strictures are rare and may be amenable to endourologic treatment. Lower ureteric strictures are more common and often require open surgical intervention. The length and degree of the stricture, whether it can be passed by a guidewire or not, vascular supply to the lesion, and renal function are important factors to be considered in the management of patients (Kim et al, 1993).

Endoscopic Management. Tuberculous ureteric strictures are characterized by mucosal ischemia and dense fibrosis. Hence, success rates for endoscopic management of strictures from other causes may not necessarily apply to TB strictures. In general, short strictures with residual lumens in patients with good renal function yield the best outcome. Strictures forming during medical treatment and managed by early stenting (double-J placement) can stabilize and require no further treatment (Shin et al, 2002). Balloon dilatation

by retrograde or antegrade access has been described for TB strictures of the ureter, UPJ, ureterovesical junction, and calyceal infundibula (Murphy et al, 1982; Kim et al, 1993). A stent is often placed after dilatation. Because of high failure rates, repeated procedures are often needed.

Follow-up imaging (US or IVU) of all patients with ureteric strictures is needed, especially those managed endoscopically, because some strictures will worsen during the healing process as a result of fibrosis and cicatrization. Corticosteroids may be added if deterioration is detected. Failure to improve or progression after 6 weeks of medical treatment is an indication for open surgical management.

Open Surgical Options. Long, complex strictures require open surgical repair. Because of fibrosis, loss of elasticity, and reduced vascularity, mobilization of structures may be difficult. Repair of UPJ scarring is more challenging in patients with TB than in those with congenital stenosis. Dismembered pyeloplasty is feasible for extrarenal pelves with short-segment scarring. Nondismembered (flap) pyeloplasty is preferred for longer strictures but may not be feasible because of excessive scarring of the pelvis. When anatomic reconstruction is not possible, ureterocalicostomy (anastomosis of the ureter to the lower pole calyx) is an option. The renal capsule should be preserved to cover the lower pole of the kidney. If not enough capsule is available, omentum can be used to avoid stenosis at the calicoureteral anastomosis (Carl and Stark, 1997).

Upper and middle ureteric strictures can be managed by excision of the diseased segment, and, with adequate mobilization, a primary tension-free ureteroureterostomy can be performed. Alternatively, lysis of adhesions and intubation (Davis intubated ureterotomy) may be done. Lower ureter strictures requiring surgery are best managed by complete excision of the entire affected ureteral segment back to healthy ureteric mucosa that has good blood supply. The resultant gap is bridged with a tension-free, well-vascularized anastomosis to healthy bladder (ureteroneocystostomy). Various procedures exist to bring the bladder closer to the ureteric end. Simple mobilization of the lateral attachments of the bladder on the contralateral side, accompanied by division of the superior vesical artery, may provide 2 to 3 cm of length to bridge a small gap. In patients with good bladder capacity, a psoas hitch may also be performed. Care must be taken to avoid the genitofemoral and femoral nerves when placing these sutures. A well-performed psoas hitch can bridge a gap of up to 5 cm. A Boari flap is another method of bridging a longer gap of 10 to 15 cm and may be performed in combination with a psoas hitch (Sankari, 2007). It is important to note that a poorly executed Boari flap can compromise bladder capacity. Contracted bladders from TB cystitis may not have sufficient surface area and elasticity to allow flap creation. Finally, ileal interposition (ileal ureteric replacement) can be done in patients with multiple or recurrent strictures when the native ureter is no longer an adequate conduit (Goel and Dalela, 2008).

Bladder Surgery. Augmentation cystoplasty and bladder substitution are options in the management of the tuberculous contracted bladder. First described in the 19th century for a tuberculous contracted bladder, augmentation is indicated when frequency, nocturia, urgency, pain, and hematuria become intolerable—typically when bladder capacity is less than 100 mL (Gupta et al, 2008b). For severely contracted bladders, ileocecum or sigmoid segments are most suitable. When only half the bladder is diseased, ileum is often used. Other segments used in augmentation include stomach and cecum. The general rules of incorporating the bowel into the urinary tract apply, such as thoroughly evaluating renal function, reconfiguring a low-pressure reservoir (de Figueiredo et al, 2006), performing patient education, and conducting long-term follow-up. Thimble bladders with capacity less than 20 mL are best managed by orthotopic bladder substitution (Hemal and Aron, 1999). Complications of either bladder augmentation or substitution include mucus production, electrolyte derangements, and secondary bacterial infection.

Urethral Procedures. Bladder neck contracture is best managed endoscopically by transurethral incision of the contracture. Urethral strictures are also managed endoscopically and often require repeated procedures. Tuberculous urethral fistulae are treated by initiation of medical therapy and suprapubic bladder drainage. Delayed reconstruction is preferred. Drainage of a seminal vesicle tuberculous cavity into the bladder by cold knife incision has been reported (Dewani et al, 2006).

Genital Surgery. Extirpative surgery for genital TB is considered only for patients in whom medical therapy has failed. When the epididymis is infected with sparing of the testis, every effort should be made to perform an epididymectomy alone without orchiectomy. Preserving testicular blood supply is important during dissection of the epididymis. Initiating dissection at the globus minor after ligation of the vas facilitates excision. If the testes are infected, a scrotal orchiectomy can be done. Involvement of the vas deferens by TB is usually distal to the external ring, and ligation at the level of the ring is possible and sufficient.

Monitoring for Tuberculosis Relapse

Even with optimized treatment, as with any infection, TB can relapse in 2% to 6% of pulmonary TB patients, particularly within the first year after treatment (CDC, 2003). A second, longer, or different drug course is then required. GU TB patients may relapse at a higher rate than pulmonary TB patients, in 6.3% to 22% of cases, even after 12 months of medical therapy (Figueiredo and Lucon, 2008). The extensively diseased kidney can contain innumerable foci of tubercle bacilli. Difficulty in achieving complete sterilization of all foci with antituberculous drugs may be the reason for the higher relapse rate. Viable bacilli have been identified in the kidneys even after 9 months of treatment (Figueiredo and Lucon, 2008). In all patients with recurrent TB, extra effort should be exerted to isolate the organism for drug susceptibility testing. Pulmonary TB patients are usually followed for 2 years after completing treatment; for GU TB patients, some investigators have recommended 10 years of follow-up, because the average time of relapse was 5.3 years (Gokce et al, 2002).

Management of Genitourinary Tuberculosis in Special Situations

Each of the special situations that follow require special handling of the antituberculous regimen because of side effects, interactions, and drug toxicities. Expert advice should be sought from infectious diseases specialists or physicians experienced in the treatment of TB.

Multidrug-Resistant and Extensively Drug-Resistant Tuberculosis

Persons with MTBC strains that are resistant to both INH and rifampin (the two most important first-line agents) have MDR-TB. Worldwide, approximately 3.7% of newly diagnosed patients and 20% of previously treated patients have MDR-TB (CDC, 2013b). Treatment is complicated by the need to use regimens longer than 18 months. The cure rate is 50% to 60% compared with 94% to 97% in patients with drug-susceptible TB (CDC, 2009). Among patients with MDR-TB, 9% have additional drug resistance, qualifying as extensively drug-resistant tuberculosis (XDR-TB) (CDC, 2013b). XDR-TB is resistant to INH, rifampin, any fluoroquinolone, and at least one of the injectable second-line aminoglycosides (amikacin, kanamycin, or capreomycin). XDR-TB is exceedingly difficult to cure, with complicated regimens involving five or six drugs for 2 years or more. As a result, the cure rate of patients with XDR-TB is only 30% to 50% (CDC, 2013c)

Pregnancy and Lactation

Women of childbearing age should be advised to avoid pregnancy while being treated for active TB. If the diagnosis is discovered during pregnancy, prompt therapy should be initiated because the risk to the fetus from TB outweighs the risk of adverse drug effects. Treatment consists of INH, ethambutol, rifampin, and pyridoxine, for 9 months. Pyrazinamide is avoided because the effects on the fetus are unknown. Postpartum, women may breastfeed their infants because drug concentrations in breast milk are too low to cause toxicity.

Human Immunodeficiency Virus Infection

HIV infection increases the risk of active TB 30-fold. With HIV and TB coinfection, each disease accelerates the other. All TB patients should be tested for HIV. Among HIV-positive persons in the world, almost 25% of deaths are due to TB (WHO, 2013). This is reminiscent of TB mortality rates in 18th- and 19th-century Europe.

Extrapulmonary, and consequently, GU TB may be more common in HIV-positive patients. In a small study in India, GU TB was found postmortem in 49% of AIDS patients (Lanjewar et al, 1999). In HIV-positive patients, GU TB can be more disseminated, with more lymph node enlargement and bilateral renal disease. Usually, less caseation, necrosis, and fibrosis are present because a competent immune system is necessary for the vigorous inflammatory process that leads to fibrosis and scarring. As a result, among patients with GU TB, stenosis of the collecting system occurs less frequently (12.5% vs. 93.8% in HIV-negative persons), and there is a lower incidence of bladder contracture (12.5% vs. 65.3% in HIV-negative persons with GU TB) (Figueiredo et al, 2009). Despite the lower incidence of obstructive cicatricial lesions, GU TB in HIV-positive persons is associated with high mortality.

TB treatment in HIV-positive patients should not be delayed. Treatment guidelines are similar to those for persons without HIV infection. Short-course chemotherapy for 6 months is effective, and 9 months of treatment is no longer routinely recommended. Instead, duration of treatment is determined by the usual factors: disease location and severity, drugs tolerated, and response. During the continuation phase of therapy, however, HIV-positive patients should undergo daily or thrice-weekly administration, and nothing less frequent. Drug interactions with antiretrovirals can be complex and need to be considered. The rifamycins (rifampin and to a lesser degree rifabutin) may decrease serum levels of antivirals to suboptimal levels. Dose increases may be needed as a result (Kaplan et al, 2009).

Renal Transplant Recipients

Renal allograft TB is rare. Infection usually occurs in kidney transplant patients within 6 months of transplantation but can occur as late as 7 years after. The shorter interval from infection to presentation may be a result of the immunosuppression required for the graft or of preexisting TB in the donor kidney. Because patients are seen very early in the disease process, no changes are usually visible on imaging. Furthermore, the immunosuppression prevents much of the pathology that is part of the natural course of GU TB. Diagnosis is difficult because many of the symptoms and findings of GU TB are absent. Fever is the usual presenting symptom. Urinary symptoms are present in only 20% of cases (el-Agroudy et al, 2003). Chest x-ray findings are abnormal but not specific in 55% of patients. Regardless of chest x-ray findings, 56% of patients have positive sputum cultures. In one study, urine AFB culture was positive in 100% of patients (Dowdy et al, 2001). Many patients are diagnosed after graft nephrectomy with histopathology (Lorimer et al, 1999).

Treatment is complicated by drug interactions between the rifamycins and the immunosuppressive drugs, necessitating frequent monitoring of serum drug levels and dosage adjustments. Rifamycin-free regimens are possible but lengthen the duration of treatment to at least 12 to 18 months. Complications in transplant patients include graft rejection, disseminated TB, and death in up to 36% of patients (Dowdy et al, 2001).

PARASITIC INFECTIONS OF THE UROGENITAL TRACT

A number of parasitic infections affect the urogenital tract. Although urologists practicing in nonendemic areas may encounter patients with urogenital parasitic infections only rarely, it is nevertheless critical for physicians to understand these diseases to facilitate appropriate diagnosis and therapy of affected individuals. Parasitic infections relevant to urology include urogenital schistosomiasis, filariasis, amebiasis, enterobiasis, and echinococcosis.

Schistosomiasis

More than 200 million people globally are infected by *Schistosoma* species. The three species of primary medical importance are *Schistosoma mansoni* (found primarily in Africa, the Arabian Peninsula, and South America), *Schistosoma japonicum* (China and Southeast Asia), and *Schistosoma haematobium* (Africa and the Arabian Peninsula). Whereas *S. mansoni* and *S. japonicum* primarily affect the liver and GI tract, *S. haematobium* infection primarily affects the GU tract and is the focus of this chapter. Urogenital schistosomiasis is a disease featuring a complex parasite life cycle, multifaceted human disease, and close ecologic links to the environment. *S. haematobium* likely has co-evolved with humans and nonhuman primates for millennia; as a result, even ancient civilizations realized the constellation of signs and symptoms associated with urogenital schistosomiasis.

History

The presence of schistosome antigens in Egyptian mummies (circa 3500 BCE), including more recent mummies with confirmed *S. haematobium* eggs in tissues (Deelder et al, 1990), confirms that urogenital schistosomiasis has been with *Homo sapiens* for millennia. Indeed, the Egyptians recognized this infection and named it "A-a-a disease," which was depicted hieroglyphically by a penis dripping with bloody urine (Hanafy et al, 1974; Shokeir and Hussein, 1999). Later, the German pathologist Theodor Bilharz, performing autopsies in Cairo in 1852, found worms in mesenteric veins and linked them to eggs found in human urine and stool.

Biology and Life Cycle

Human infection is initiated by the penetration of *S. haematobium* cercariae through (even intact) skin that is in contact with infested fresh water (Fig. 17-8). The average life span of cercariae is 1 day.

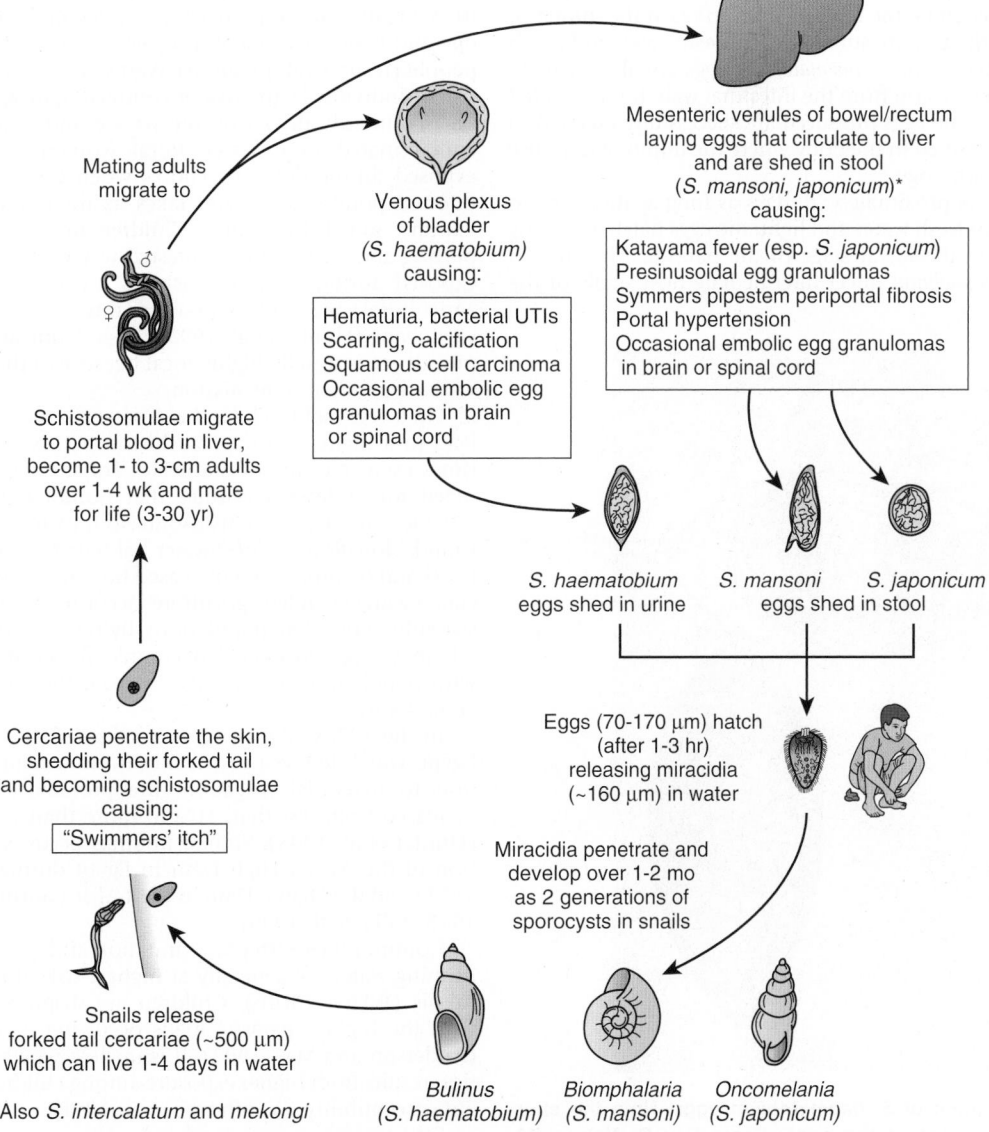

Figure 17-8. Life cycle of a schistosome. UTIs, urinary tract infections. (From King CH. Schistosomiasis. In: Guerrant RL, Walker DH, Weller PF, editors. Tropical infectious diseases, principles, pathogens, and practice. 2nd ed. Philadelphia: Churchill Livingstone; 2006. p. 1341–8.)

Penetration success rates fall off quickly within hours of cercarial shedding from the intermediate snail host (King, 2006).

After penetration, schistosomes transform from free-living cercariae into obligate parasites called *schistosomulae*, by first shedding their tails over approximately 90 to 120 minutes and then undergoing a series of structural changes (Melo and Pereira, 1985). The transformed schistosomulae migrate to the lungs via the bloodstream or lymphatics, and then the liver via the venous circulation (Wilson, 2009). Migration out of the skin and into the lungs takes several weeks (Rheinberg et al, 1998; Wilson, 2009).

The juvenile schistosomes then arrive at the liver sinusoids via the venous circulation, where they begin blood feeding. Soon thereafter, the now-mature worms preferentially migrate to the venous plexus of the bladder and other pelvic organs, where they live an average of 3 to 5 years. The developmental period from cercaria to adult worm ranges from 80 to 110 days. After worm pairing, males clasp the females in a ventral groove termed the *gynecophoric canal*, using their muscular bodies to help females pump host blood into their mouths and secreting chemical signals to stimulate oviposition (Gupta and Basch, 1987).

Eggs are laid by adult female worms in the pelvic venous circulation. Human schistosomes are very fecund, with egg-laying rates of hundreds to thousands of eggs per female per day. *S. haematobium* eggs are ovoid, measuring approximately 140 μm long and featuring a terminal spine (Loker, 1983; Ratard and Greer, 1991) (Fig. 17-9). Eggs must penetrate the endothelium to reach the lumen of bladder to exit via the urinary stream, reach fresh water, and hatch to become miracidia. Some *S. haematobium* eggs are also excreted into the feces after expulsion from the intestinal wall. It is estimated that less than half of the eggs produced are successfully excreted in urine. The rest are retained in the body where the immune response causes significant pathology.

Eggs can survive approximately 20 days as long as they remain wet. On contact with fresh water and light, the eggs hatch, releasing miracidia, which are the larval stage of the parasite. The ciliated miracidia of *S. haematobium* infect intermediate host snails of the *Bulinus* genus. *Bulinus* snails prefer slow-flowing freshwater habitats and are able to withstand low-oxygen conditions.

The typical life span of a miracidium is 6 hours. If during this brief period a *Bulinus* snail is encountered, the miracidia will penetrate the snail tissue and form a primary sporocyst. After several days, 20 to 40 daughter sporocysts are generated by the primary sporocyst. These eventually mature into 200 to 400 cercariae (per sporocyst), which are released back into water. The prepatent period (the time between initial penetration of the snail by a miracidium and release of the first cercariae) varies with water temperature; at temperatures below 15° C or greater than 35° C, no cercariae are shed (Pflüger et al, 1984).

Epidemiology

The geographic distribution of urogenital schistosomiasis is dependent on the tropical conditions required by *S. haematobium* and its specific snail hosts. Consequently, *S. haematobium* is endemic throughout much of sub-Saharan Africa and in portions of North Africa and the Middle East. Approximately 112 million people worldwide have urogenital schistosomiasis (van der Werf et al, 2003). Up to 150,000 people die annually from *S. haematobium*–induced obstructive renal failure alone. It has been calculated that in a 2-week period in 2003, 70 million and 32 million individuals in sub-Saharan Africa experienced *S. haematobium*–induced hematuria and dysuria (respectively), and that major bladder wall pathology and major hydronephrosis were present in 18 and 10 million people (respectively) (van der Werf et al, 2003).

For individuals, the risk of contracting urogenital schistosomiasis is primarily driven by the nature and length of contact with contaminated fresh water. Rural women and children can be exposed during domestic chores when they use *S. haematobium*–infested ponds, rivers, and lakes as their water supply (e.g., for laundry and dishwashing). Children may also be infected while playing and swimming in infested water. Men and women can be exposed during freshwater fishing, washing cars, and working in agricultural areas with high–water-intensity crops such as rice and sugar cane (Hunter et al, 1993). In endemic areas, schistosomiasis prevalence is usually highly focal because of the localized nature of water-dependent transmission.

On a regional level, land-use patterns and ecologic changes can lead to a higher burden of schistosomiasis in some areas, sometimes even resulting in outbreaks. For instance, it has been recognized for at least a century that building dams and irrigation schemes can increase schistosomiasis transmission by creating year-round, slow-flowing, freshwater habitats for the intermediate snail hosts and by promoting increased human population density associated with expanded agriculture. Accordingly, data from Africa consistently show that populations living near dams and irrigation schemes have a greater risk of contracting schistosomiasis compared with populations living distantly from these schemes (Steinmann et al, 2006).

In the 1930s after the construction of the Aswan Low Dam in Egypt, which led to a conversion from ancient, flood-based irrigation to perennial irrigation, the prevalence of schistosomiasis increased from less than 11% to more than 75% in some regions (Hunter et al, 1993). Similar findings occurred after the construction of the Aswan High Dam in Egypt during the 1960s (Malek, 1975) and the Diama Dam in West Africa during the 1980s (Malek, 1975; Talla et al, 1990).

Communities with poor sanitation and a lack of access to clean, running water are generally at highest risk of harboring schistosomiasis (WHO, 2014b). Children are disproportionately affected, with the highest parasite loads occurring in those aged 5 to 15 (Anderson and May, 1992). It is unclear whether this age distribution results from higher exposure among children or a higher inherent susceptibility (Woolhouse et al, 1991).

Schistosomiasis is associated with poverty for a number of reasons. First, the aquatic snails that harbor the larval forms of schistosomes are distributed within tropical and subtropical developing countries, whereas they are not present in developed nations

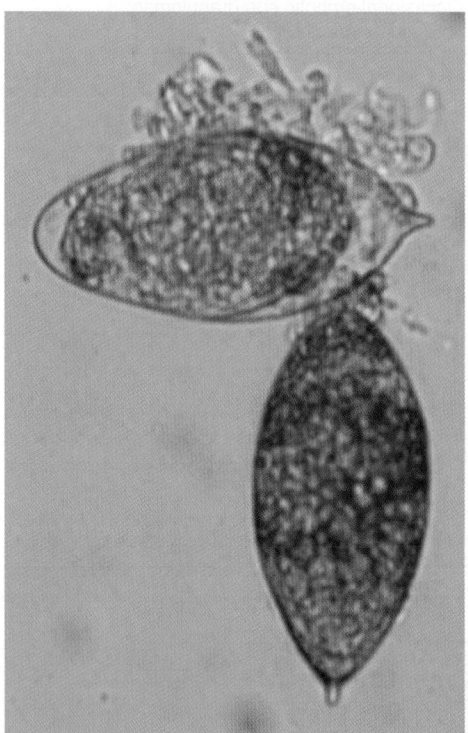

Figure 17-9. Micrograph of *S. haematobium* eggs. Note the characteristic terminal spines of the eggs. (From Ray D, Nelson TA, Fu CL, et al. Transcriptional profiling of the bladder in urogenital schistosomiasis reveals pathways of inflammatory fibrosis and urothelial compromise. PLoS Negl Trop Dis 2012; 6(11):e1912.)

in temperate zones. Second, inadequate sanitation exacerbates the schistosomiasis problem because the schistosome life cycle requires an influx of eggs from human excreta into surface fresh waters. Moreover, prolonged contact with surface fresh water is promoted by lack of safe water supplies, leading to higher risk of infection (Soares Magalhães et al, 2011). Finally, schistosomiasis contributes to the perpetuation of poverty. Chronic infection adversely affects childhood growth, development, and learning, as well as worker productivity (Bonds et al, 2010).

Pathogenesis and Pathology

Cercarial skin penetration is facilitated by secreted molecules such as proteases, which initiate the cellular and humoral responses to schistosome infection (Curwen et al, 2006). However, likely as a result of the parasite strategy of modulating the host immune response from the moment of first contact, brief cercarial penetration does not typically induce an immune response beyond localized skin inflammation (Jenkins et al, 2005). Regardless, repeated exposure to schistosomulae can lead to hypersensitization and the development of a maculopapular rash.

During subsequent maturation into adult worms, schistosomulae begin to generate a double lipid bilayer outer surface (the tegument), which allows them to evade an immunopathologic response and remain in the host for years, facilitating chronic infection. As the survival of the worm within the host depends significantly on the tegument, numerous mechanisms are employed for immune evasion, including host antigenic mimicry, continual membrane turnover, immunomodulatory proteins and proteases, host-evading biophysical properties of the tegument, and modulation of expression of surface antigens (Abath and Werkhauser, 1996).

Because it is difficult to study the natural pathogenesis of egg-associated disease in humans, much of our knowledge stems from autopsy studies and animal models. In contrast to the relatively silent immune response to worms, the main immunopathologic responses raised against S. haematobium are triggered by oviposition in the walls of the bladder and other pelvic organs. With heavy worm burdens, egg deposition in the pelvic organs leads to granuloma development and eventual fibrosis, often obstructing the flow of blood or urine. Granulomas are characterized by a mixed leukocytic infiltration, including eosinophils, plasma cells, and lymphocytes. Because of continuous oviposition, all stages of granulomas are simultaneously present in individuals with chronic infection. Composite, coalescing granulomas are common, secondary to S. haematobium egg deposition in clusters. Grossly, granulomatous inflammation can form bulky, hyperemic, and polypoid masses projecting into the bladder lumen (Fig. 17-10). Other factors that have been shown to influence the host immune response and resulting disease severity include host genetics, in utero sensitization to parasitic antigens, and coinfection by other microbes or parasites (Pearce and MacDonald, 2002; Eriksson et al, 2007; Grant et al, 2011). S. haematobium eggs appear to rapidly induce bladder expression of type 2 inflammation–associated genes and suppress transcription of urothelial barrier function–related genes (Fu et al, 2012; Ray et al, 2012). These findings suggest that the parasite and human host may share the goal of expelling eggs from the bladder wall, across a temporarily lowered urothelial barrier, and out into the urinary stream.

Although S. haematobium has tropism for the pelvic organs, some oviposition occurs in the portal tract. As a result, portal hypertension occurs when eggs are swept into the liver, clog presinusoidal capillaries, induce granuloma formation, and consequently block the hepatic vasculature. Alternatively, embolized eggs can cause granulomatous and fibrotic portal areas and the dilation of collateral portosystemic shunts, permitting the lodging of eggs in these vessels and the formation of pipestem fibrosis (Symmer fibrosis) (Aubry et al, 1980). Hepatosplenomegaly is one clinical manifestation of Symmer fibrosis, although susceptibility to its development depends largely on the variability of individual immune responses. In addition to portal involvement, migration of worm pairs to the pulmonary vessels can result in oviposition in the lungs. In general,

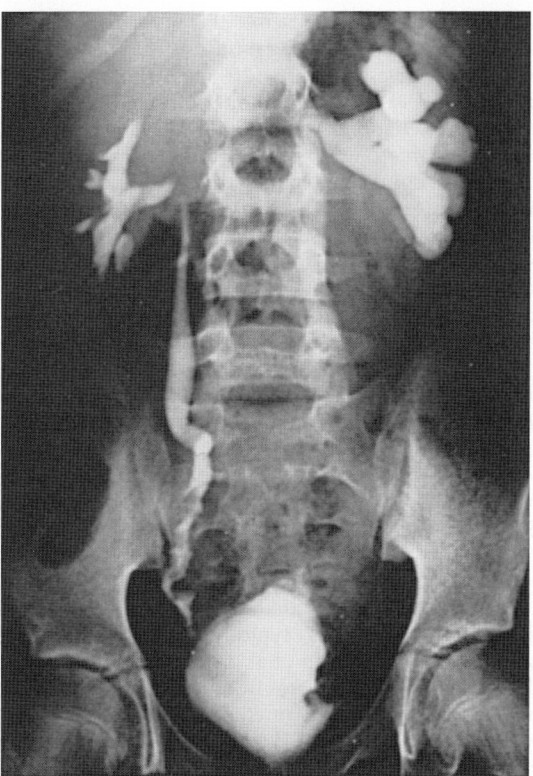

Figure 17-10. Intravenous urogram in an Egyptian boy shows scalloping of the bladder and right lower ureter by schistosomal polypoid lesions.

pulmonary schistosomiasis develops only in very severe cases of infection and when pathogenesis in other organs (i.e., pelvic) has already occurred (Borgstein, 1964). When pulmonary oviposition occurs, eggs may obstruct the lung vasculature and lead to pulmonary fibrosis, pulmonary hypertension, and/or cor pulmonale (Bedford et al, 1946).

Naturally acquired immunity to urogenital schistosomiasis exists; some individuals maintain negative urine egg counts for at least 5 years despite never having received anthelmintics in the face of continual exposure to S. haematobium (McManus and Loukas, 2008). The resistance of these individuals to reinfection has been attributed to the involvement of both a T-helper type 1 (Th1) and a Th2 cytokine response, whereas chronically infected individuals exclusively mount a Th2 response (McManus and Loukas, 2008). In some individuals the activity of potentially protective immunoglobulin E (IgE) antibodies may be blocked by IgG4 antibodies generated against worm and egg antigens, possibly hampering the development of protective immunity to schistosomiasis (Hagan et al, 1991).

Because levels of IgE antibodies to worm antigens have been observed to increase with age (Roberts et al, 1993), many workers have suggested an immune-mediated development of resistance. This age-dependent trend, however, could be a result of either behavioral or immunologic changes, because studies in endemic communities have ascertained a general decline in contact with infected water with increasing age (Dalton and Pole, 1978). Nevertheless, recent analyses suggest that even when exposure to infected water is controlled for, age may play a role in the development of resistance.

Eggs that are not promptly expelled from pelvic organs calcify, including those in the bladder and ureters. The accumulation of eggs results in decreased compliance of the urinary tract and increases upper tract pressures. In turn, this promotes the development of urinary stasis, hydronephrosis, and hydroureter (Cheever et al, 1975). The extent of organ calcification can often be identified through radiologic imaging and is roughly correlated with the tissue burden of calcified eggs (Cheever et al, 1975). The anatomic level of obstruction involves the ureteral meatus (1%), interstitial ureter (10% to 30%), juxtavesical ureter (20% to 60%), lower third of the ureter (15% to 50%), or a contiguous combination of these areas (30% to 60%) (Gelfand, 1948; Smith et al, 1977b; Al-Shukri and Alwan, 1983). Three patterns of hydroureter are associated with urogenital schistosomiasis: segmental (i.e., cylindric or fusiform), tonic, and atonic (Smith et al, 1977a). About one quarter of obstructive uropathy cases involve segmental ureteral dilation, with 80% of those cases occurring in the lower ureter. The dilations occur above areas of concentric ureteral muscular replacement by fibrosis and "sandy patches." It is unusual for segmental lesions to cause significant hydronephrosis. Up to 30% of obstructive uropathy is caused by tonic hydroureter. This is characterized by dilated, tortuous, thick-walled, and trabeculated ureters with marked ureteral muscular hypertrophy and impaired peristalsis. Typically the entire ureter proximal to an obstructive lesion is involved, generating a functional stenosis. This is often accompanied by significant hydronephrosis, which is reversible if the obstruction is relieved (Smith et al, 1977a). Atonic hydroureters are found in the remaining patients with obstructive uropathy. These ureters are markedly dilated, very tortuous, and thin walled; lack peristalsis; and are associated with atrophic, fibrotic ureteral muscle.

Schistosomal hydroureter typically precedes hydronephrosis (Lehman et al, 1973; Cheever et al, 1978). Left untreated, schistosomal hydronephrosis progresses from worsening renal pelvic dilation to medullary atrophy to medullary effacement and cortical atrophy (Smith et al, 1974, 1977b). This pathophysiologic sequence accounts for the abrogation of tubular function (especially concentrating ability) before compromise of glomerular function (Lehman et al, 1971, 1973).

Patients with chronic S. haematobium are at increased risk of bacterial urinary tract superinfections, possibly because the bacteria can affix to the tegument of adult worms, or secondary to urinary stasis or immunomodulation. Patients infected with S. haematobium are also at higher risk for bladder cancer, especially squamous cell carcinoma. The relationship between S. haematobium and bladder cancer is perhaps the strongest of any helminthic infection–cancer association. This association is supported by both epidemiologic studies (particularly in Egypt) and experimental models (Mostafa et al, 1999). Rates of bladder cancer are linked with duration and severity of infection and are associated with a mortality rate as high as 10.8 per 100,000 males in Egypt (Mustacchi, 2003).

Female genital schistosomiasis (FGS) remains poorly understood. Sequestration of eggs in the female reproductive tract results in the formation of fibrotic nodules, or sandy patches, in the uterus, cervix, and lower genital tract (Badawy, 1962) (Fig. 17-11). Little is known about the mechanism through which S. haematobium generates female genital disease aside from the increased vascularization of the female genital mucosa that occurs as a result of the presence of eggs (Jourdan et al, 2011).

Other bladder sequelae of long-term S. haematobium infection include the development of urothelial hyperplasia, squamous metaplasia, urothelial dysplasia, and eventually urothelial or squamous cell carcinoma. Bladder cancer is the final pathologic sequela of schistosomiasis. Schistosomal bladder cancer features an early onset (40 to 50 years) and is often squamous cell carcinoma (60% to 90%) or adenocarcinoma (5% to 15%) (Cheever et al, 1978; Lucas, 1982; Al-Shukri et al, 1987; Thomas et al, 1990; Bedwani et al, 1998). Over 40% of schistosomiasis-associated bladder squamous cell carcinomas are well differentiated and verrucous and feature an overall good prognosis. Tumors are found on the posterior wall about half of the time and on the lateral wall approximately 30% of the time. Exophytic neoplasms account for roughly two thirds of schistosomal bladder cancers, and the remainder are ulcerative endophytic tumors. Mass drug administration (MDA) campaigns in Egypt have been associated with an overall reduction of bladder neoplasms from 28% to 12% and a shift from squamous cell carcinomas to transitional cell carcinomas (Gouda et al, 2007). Although transitional cell carcinomas of the bladder are less frequently associated with S. haematobium infection (Michaud, 2007),

some epidemiologists believe that the relatively high rate of smoking in schistosomiasis-endemic regions may further increase the risk of bladder cancer, possibly synergistically with S. haematobium infection (Bedwani et al, 1998). However, some unselected autopsy series from the same regions have reported similar frequencies of bladder cancers in patients without schistosomiasis (Smith et al, 1977a; Cheever et al, 1978).

Egg deposition into the bladder wall has been implicated as a major factor in carcinogenesis, and S. haematobium has been classified as a Class I agent (carcinogenic to humans) by the International Agency for Research on Cancer within WHO (International Agency for Research on Cancer, 2011).Vascular endothelial growth factor (VEGF) is increased in the bladder early after S. haematobium egg exposure (Fu et al, 2012; Ray et al, 2012; Salem et al, 2012). VEGF may promote tumor vasculogenesis and facilitate carcinogenesis and/or cancer progression. One potential pathway of schistosomal bladder oncogenesis may be initiated when papillomas merge with the basal transitional epithelium, forming benign fibroepithelial papillary growths. After successive episodes of inflammation and fibrosis, some of the urothelial cells may sequester together (or expand clonally) and form potentially precancerous lesions, including squamous metaplasia (Mustacchi, 2003). Molecular profiling of the mouse bladder indicates that S. haematobium egg exposure induces transcriptional alterations in bladder carcinogenesis–related signaling pathways (Ray et al, 2012). Bacterial urinary tract coinfections may also contribute to S. haematobium–associated bladder carcinoma, given that S. haematobium increases the ability of bacteria to reduce nitrates to nitrosamines, which can alkylate proteins and nucleic acids (Grisham and Yamada, 1992). Resulting mutations in oncogenes (i.e., p53) may then contribute to neoplasia (Mustacchi, 2003).

Clinical Manifestations

Acute schistosomiasis encompasses the transient human responses to cercarial penetration and the longer-lasting responses to schistosome tissue migration and maturation. Chronic schistosomiasis results from the immune response to protracted oviposition, often lasting for years and leading to organ damage. As a result, clinically apparent chronic schistosomiasis is limited to long-term residents of endemic areas, who are continually reinfected, have long-term, high worm burdens, and are re-exposed to eggs. As with most human helminths, Schistosoma species cannot complete their life cycle nor replicate in the human host. Thus, in tourists or short-term visitors who are exposed once to the parasite, even in the absence of efficacious chemotherapy, adult worms die of senescence within 3 to 5 years, limiting subsequent pathology.

Acute Schistosomiasis. The first clinical manifestation of schistosomiasis is often an itchy maculopapular rash (cercarial dermatitis), usually within 1 to 2 days of cercarial penetration. The rash usually resolves before travelers have returned from endemic areas, making the diagnosis more difficult (Stuiver, 1984).

Acute schistosomiasis is seen 2 to 8 weeks later in some patients during their primary infection (although it is silent in many). The well-known eponym for acute schistosomiasis, "Katayama fever," is derived from early descriptions of the syndrome in the Katayama Valley in Japan; it occurs most commonly with heavy primary S. japonicum infections, less commonly with S. mansoni, and rarely with S. haematobium. The initial signs and symptoms of Katayama fever include fever, dry cough, fatigue, headache, diarrhea, eosinophilia, neck pain, and urticaria (Jauréguiberry et al, 2010). Acute schistosomiasis is seen rarely among people living in endemic areas (Meltzer et al, 2006). Because the signs and symptoms of acute schistosomiasis are nonspecific, cases often remain undiagnosed or confused with other endemic diseases such as malaria or enteric fever (Jensen et al, 1995).

Because acute schistosomiasis may be clinically silent, all individuals with exposure to potentially infested water should be aware of the possibility of infection, with considerations for accurate diagnosis and treatment based on these factors (Jauréguiberry et al, 2010).

Chronic Schistosomiasis. Adult *S. haematobium* worm pairs shed eggs into the bladder wall, beginning about 8 to 12 weeks after infection. This is sometimes heralded by painless, recurrent hematuria, dysuria, or urinary frequency (Mahmoud, 2001). In some highly endemic cultures, hematuria in males is seen as a sign of puberty and can be sufficiently severe as to result in anemia (Wilkins et al, 1985). Proteinuria is also often associated with urogenital schistosomiasis. Hematuria is a consistent and specific enough sign of infection that it is used as a primary diagnostic technique in endemic areas. However, given the many other possible causes of hematuria, urogenital schistosomiasis is often unsuspected and misdiagnosed in infected travelers returning to their nonendemic home countries (Raglio et al, 1995).

Long-term urogenital schistosomiasis results in fibrosis that may obstruct urinary drainage and result in organ dysfunction. Egg deposition in the ureters and subsequent granuloma, polyp, and ulcer formation increases the risk of hydronephrosis and hydroureter caused by impaired peristalsis of the walls of the renal pelvis and ureter, which in turn can result in obstruction, and vesicoureteral reflux. Recovery of renal function may be achieved through anthelmintic therapy in shorter-term infections, whereas surgical repair of the ureter or urinary diversion may be necessary during late-stage or more severe disease (Mahmoud, 2001).

FGS is another form of chronic schistosomiasis and occurs in 33% to 75% of females with *S. haematobium* infection as a result of egg deposition into the fallopian tubes, cervix, vagina, vulva, ovaries, and/or uterus (Kjetland et al, 2012). Friable mucosal lesions (sandy patches) can result, which often bleed on contact during pelvic examinations or sexual intercourse (Hotez and Fenwick, 2009). Dyspareunia, pelvic and abdominal pain, vaginal bleeding and discharge, urinary frequency, and infertility are common but resemble signs and symptoms of urinary tract infections (UTIs) and sexually transmitted diseases of other causes, so FGS is often misdiagnosed and left untreated (Hotez and Fenwick, 2009).

Men can carry high numbers of *S. haematobium* eggs in the ejaculatory ducts and seminal vesicles, and blood and/or schistosome eggs may be present in the ejaculate before they are detectable in the urine. Patients with involvement of these urogenital structures often have a testicular mass or scrotal pain. Egg burdens of the epididymis, ovaries, and fallopian tubes are generally higher than those of the testes, uterus, and vagina (Cheever et al, 1977, 1978; Helling-Giese et al, 1996a).

As infection progresses, a late, chronic, active stage develops when tissue egg burdens peak. Chronic suprapubic and pelvic pain with associated urinary urgency, frequency, and incontinence are classic for the schistosomal contracted bladder (Duvie, 1986). Frequently the trigone appears normal or somewhat hyperemic and edematous, whereas the remainder of the detrusor muscle is thickened and indurated, as is the entire bladder wall. Functional bladder capacity can be as low as 50 mL in adults.

Over years, active infection becomes more quiescent, and oviposition and egg excretion occur at a lower rate and symptoms are dampened. Over 30% of light infections become asymptomatic in some endemic regions (Rutasitara and Chimbe, 1985). In spite of this, clinically silent obstructive uropathy may evolve throughout this period as fibrosis replaces polypoid lesions and the bladder and ureters undergo sometimes irreversible damage. As a result, severe hydroureteronephrosis can develop insidiously.

Infected individuals can enter a chronic inactive phase, in which viable eggs are no longer detected in urine or tissues. Signs and symptoms at this stage are caused by sequelae and complications of the immune reaction to the calcified, dead eggs rather than the schistosomal infection itself. Unfortunately, among patients with schistosomal obstructive uropathy, 40% to 60% present to urologists at this end stage (Smith and Christie, 1986). In heavily endemic regions, poorly or nonfunctioning kidneys are common in patients who are asymptomatic. About half of patients will develop bacterial urinary tract coinfections superimposed on their schistosomal obstructive uropathy. The bacteria associated with urogenital schistosomiasis are the same organisms that cause UTIs in patients without schistosomiasis. There is evidence that these coinfections

may occur more readily because of parasite immunomodulation of the host (Hsieh et al, 2014). Some series have noted an association of chronic or recurring UTIs caused by *Salmonella*, often associated with intermittent bacteremia in some patients with urogenital schistosomiasis (King, 2001). This association suggests that *Salmonella* bacteriuria in this setting may actually be "spillover" of bacteremia into the urinary stream. *Salmonella* organisms reside in the apical invaginations of the schistosome tegument, where they are sheltered from host defenses and antibiotics. Awareness of this association can lead to treatment of both infections with good response. Antibiotics alone do not fully resolve this process.

Another manifestation of urogenital schistosomiasis is the development of bladder urothelial ulcers (Smith et al, 1977a). On presentation, acute schistosomal ulcers rarely are in the active stage, when necrotic polyps slough into the urine and leave behind a urothelial ulcer. The more common chronic bladder ulcer is a late sequela of heavy infection. This lesion is associated with a constant burning sensation and intense suprapubic and pelvic pain. The majority of these patients exhibit gross hematuria and pyuria.

Eosinophilia is very common during acute schistosomiasis and is seen even during chronic infection. During chronic infection the eosinophilia is usually low grade, and although neither sensitive nor specific for schistosomiasis, its presence can be a clue that a parasitic infection such as schistosomiasis may be present. Exceptions to this usual sequence of acute and chronic infection may occur and sometimes manifest in the form of ectopic pulmonary schistosomiasis, neuroschistosomiasis, and FGS.

Diagnosis

Finding *S. haematobium* eggs in urine or stool remains the gold standard for diagnosis of active infection, although eggs do not appear until oviposition begins 8 to 12 weeks after initial infection. Because maximal egg shedding in the urine peaks at noon, urine samples should be ideally collected between 9 AM and 3 PM for examination (Doehring et al, 1983, 1985). Urine samples can be concentrated to increase sensitivity and detect low-intensity infections. If eggs are not found in the urine or stool but clinical suspicion remains high and serology is consistent with exposure, tissue biopsy can be considered. A rectal snip biopsy should be performed before a bladder biopsy, because eggs are common in the rectal mucosa and the risk of a bladder biopsy–related complication (e.g., infection, perforation) is avoided. A squash preparation of the biopsy specimen between glass slides is superior to histopathologic analysis, because it is more sensitive and allows determination of egg viability. In potential cases of FGS, microscopic inspection of biopsy samples from lesions on the vulva, vagina, or cervix may result in egg identification and diagnosis (Helling-Giese et al, 1996b). Visual and dipstick-based detection of gross or microscopic hematuria and urine turbidity are also used to indirectly diagnose urogenital schistosomiasis, although these methods are less sensitive and specific and best combined with already-established diagnostic tools; they are most commonly used in the developing world as part of control and elimination campaigns (Adesola et al, 2012).

Serologic tests that combine a Falcon assay screening test–enzyme-linked immunosorbent assay (FAST-ELISA) with a Western blot analysis are available at the CDC (Wilson et al, 1995; Al-Sherbiny et al, 1999). Together, the assays are over 90% sensitive and specific for *S. haematobium* infection. When the diagnosis is suspected but eggs are not present, serology can be useful, but it does not distinguish between acute and chronic infection because antibody titers remain positive even after curative chemotherapy. Other serologic assays are also available at commercial laboratories. Patients generally first become antibody positive about 4 to 6 weeks after infection (Schwartz et al, 2005).

Ultrasonography can also be useful and may demonstrate bladder or ureteral wall thickening, polypoid lesions, hydroureter, hydronephrosis, urinary tract calcifications, and even bladder carcinoma (Kardorff and Döhring, 2001). Plain abdominal radiographs may reveal urinary tract calcifications; a calcified bladder, which may resemble a fetal head in the pelvis, is characteristic of chronic

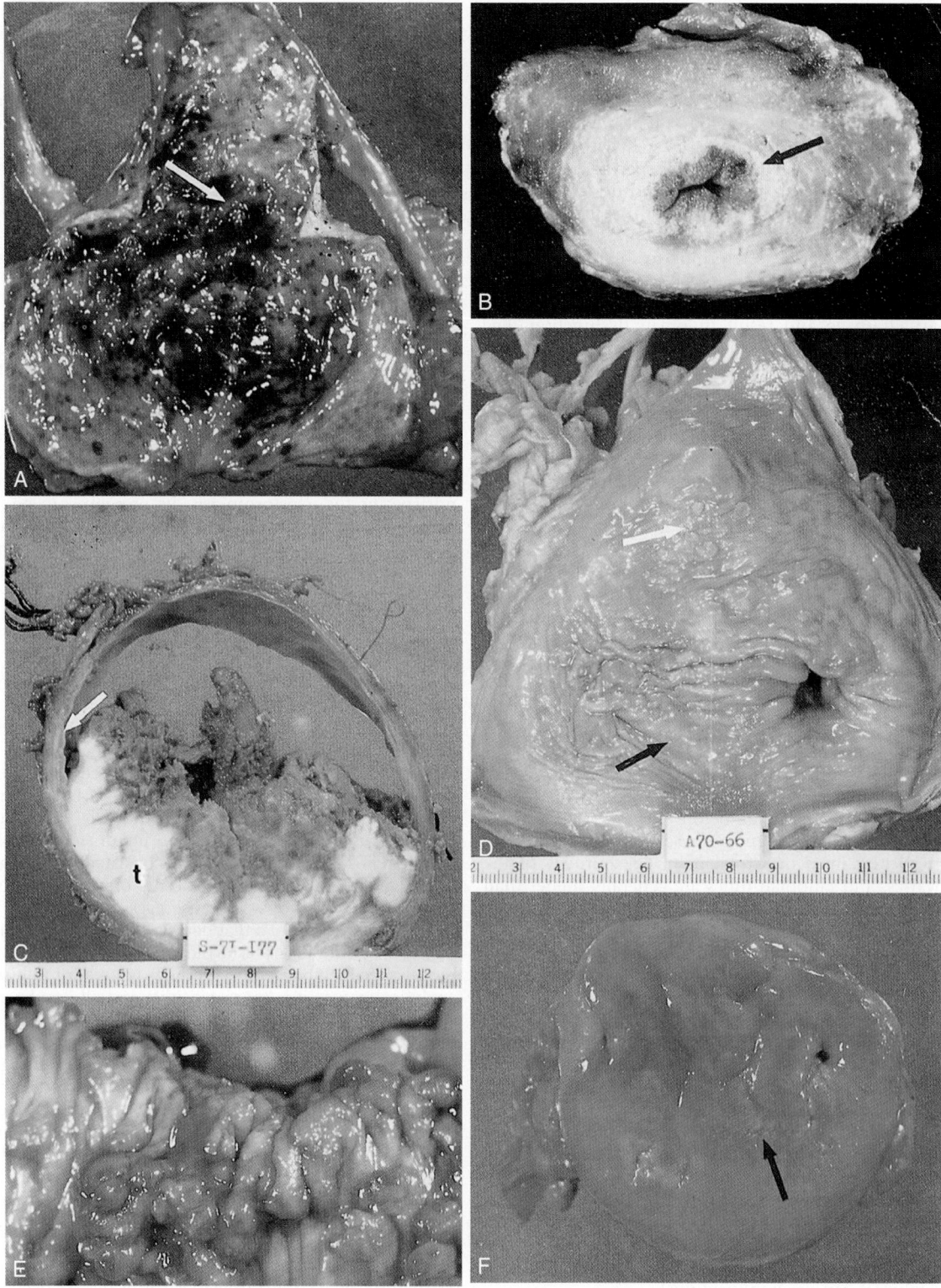

urogenital schistosomiasis (Fig. 17-12). The prostate, seminal vesicles, posterior urethra, distal ureters, and, occasionally, colon may also demonstrate calcifications.

The earliest radiographic changes on IVU appear to be striations in the ureters and renal pelvis (Hugosson, 1987). Ureteral calcification is typically intramural, and the ureters are dilated. This differs from the calcifications seen in TB, which form casts of nondilated

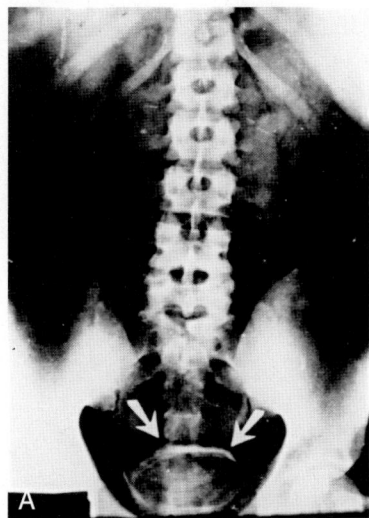

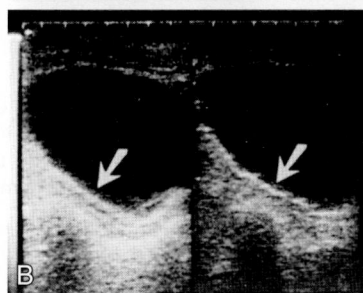

Figure 17-12. Bladder calcification in a 30-year-old Egyptian farmer. A, Plain x-ray film of the abdomen shows a rim of calcification surrounding the urinary bladder *(arrows)*. B, Abdominal ultrasound study shows a bright line surrounding the bladder with a definite dark rim behind it *(arrows)*. (A and B, Courtesy G. Thomas Strickland, MD. From Abdel-Wahab MF, Ramzy I, Esmat G, et al. Ultrasonography for detecting *Schistosoma haematobium* urinary tract complications: comparison with radiographic procedures. J Urol 1992;148:346.)

ureters. Other findings on IVU include hydronephrosis, hydroureter, nonfunctioning kidney, ureteral stenosis, and bladder and ureteral filling defects caused by polypoid lesions. Similar lesions can also be identified through US. With IVU, delayed films are often necessary in the presence of severe obstructive uropathy to discern distended ureters and kidneys. Postvoid views may reveal bladder neck obstruction with retention. Combining IVU with fluoroscopy can differentiate between tonic and atonic ureters (Abdel-Halim et al, 1985) and identify nonstenotic, immobile ureters.

CT can detect both obstructive uropathy and calcified lesions in the colon and urinary tract (Jorulf and Linstedt, 1985), a potential advantage over IVU. MRI does not yet seem to provide enough diagnostic superiority to warrant widespread use (Kohno et al, 2008). Fluoroscopic voiding cystourethrography can detect vesicoureteral reflux, which occurs in 25% of infected ureters. Cystourethroscopy may reveal mucosal lesions in the bladder (Fig. 17-13). Retrograde fluoroscopic pyelography during cystourethroscopy may reveal important details regarding ureteral anatomy and drainage.

Antigen detection or PCR may be a more sensitive means of diagnosis. Serum or urine samples from infected individuals can be tested for the presence of circulating anodic antigens (CAAs) and circulating cathodic schistosome antigens (CCAs). CAAs and CCAs are specific for active infection because they are released only by viable adult worms and have the added benefit of producing quantitative measurements useful for determining infection severity (Kremsner et al, 1994; Agnew et al, 1995). Moreover, the development of an ELISA reagent strip test for urine samples has allowed for point-of-care detection of CCAs that is more user-friendly and field applicable (van Dam et al, 2004). However, in some hands the CCA test completely failed to detect *S. haematobium* infection (versus more than 80% sensitivity and specificity for detection of *S. mansoni* infection) (Stothard et al, 2006), and it is relatively expensive for wide-scale use in the developing world.

By far the most sensitive method for diagnosing urogenital schistosomiasis from urine or even stool samples is PCR (Obeng et al, 2008; ten Hove et al, 2008). PCR is also highly sensitive and specific for diagnosing FGS from vaginal lavage samples, although detection may vary based on patient age and length of infection (Kjetland et al, 2009). Unfortunately, PCR is difficult to use in the developing world and in the field because it requires highly trained technicians and the use of organic solvents and commercial kits. Still, in the context of transmission control and disease surveillance, especially in settings of low-intensity transmission, PCR is a useful option.

Globally, many cases of urogenital schistosomiasis remain undetected and untreated because most are diagnosed only through direct egg detection rather than more sensitive methods. The need for more reliable and accessible diagnostic tools is thus particularly important for the development of more effective schistosomiasis control strategies in the developing world.

Figure 17-11. Macroscopic appearance of human urinary schistosomiasis. A, Urinary bladder opened with an anterior Y incision. The posterior and apical walls have many erythematous, granular, sessile, and pedunculated polyps *(arrow)*, characteristic of the early active stage of urinary schistosomiasis. B, Coronal section through the apex of a formalin-fixed urinary bladder. The lamina propria has been expanded and is replaced by a yellow-tan, finely granular, sandy patch *(arrow)*, which is characteristic of chronic inactive foci. Small sandy patches are sprinkled through the fibrotic, atrophic detrusor muscle, even in perivesical fat. The more superficial erythematous portion of the lamina propria contains some viable eggs with granulomatous response (chronic active stage of urinary schistosomiasis). C, Coronal section through the middle of a urinary bladder after formalin inflation and fixation. The lamina propria *(arrow)* has been replaced by a concentric sandy patch, most prominent at the margin of the exophytic, moderately differentiated squamous cell carcinoma. The bladder wall is attenuated except for the tumor (t). No evidence of recent oviposition was found in the lower urinary tract (chronic inactive stage of urinary schistosomiasis, usually found with the bilharzial bladder cancer syndrome). D, Urinary bladder opened with anterior Y incision shows several features of severe chronic inactive urinary schistosomiasis. The entire lamina propria has been replaced by a sandy patch. Foci of epidermization are seen at or near the white arrow. The left ureteral orifice *(right)* is markedly dilated (the so-called golf-hole ureter of schistosomal uropathy). The right ureteral orifice *(point of black arrow)* is markedly stenotic. E, Rectosigmoid colon with polyposis. Numerous sessile and pedunculated polyps are visible. Many are erythematous, indicative of active oviposition with granuloma formation. Some have necrotic hemorrhagic tips. F, Mucosal surface of partial cystectomy specimen (4- to 5-cm ellipse) from a patient with the chronic inactive stage of the disease. There is a stellate chronic schistosomal ulcer. Despite the inactivity of the disease, these ulcers may bleed profusely. Pale mucoid flecks at the margin of the ulcer *(arrow)* are areas of adenoid (goblet cell) metaplasia.

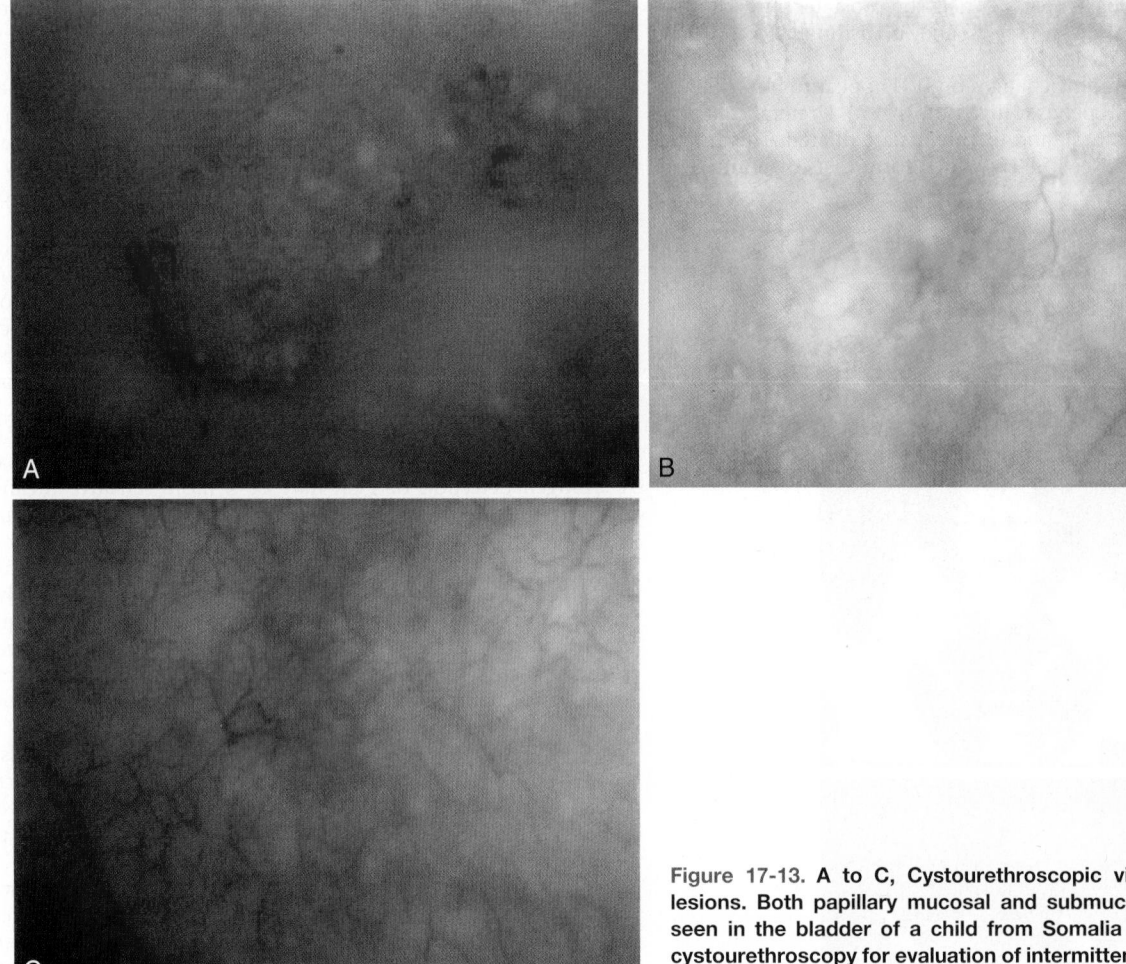

Figure 17-13. **A to C, Cystourethroscopic views of bladder lesions. Both papillary mucosal and submucosal lesions are seen in the bladder of a child from Somalia who underwent cystourethroscopy for evaluation of intermittent hematuria and dysuria. (Courtesy Craig Peters, MD.)**

Treatment

Medical Management. Praziquantel (PZQ) is currently the only WHO-recommended drug for schistosomiasis (WHO, 2014a) and has replaced metrifonate and oxamniquine as the main therapeutic agent. Although dependence on a single drug increases the potential for parasitic resistance, PZQ's efficacy, widespread availability, and low toxicity are favorable factors, and there has been little incentive for the development of alternative drugs. Two 20-mg/kg oral doses of PZQ are given on the same day, 6 to 8 hours apart (or alternatively, one 40- or 60-mg/kg dose) for *S. haematobium* infections. Corticosteroids are often added for the treatment of acute schistosomiasis (Katayama fever).

As measured by egg reduction and cure rate, PZQ's efficacy is 60% to 90% (Danso-Appiah et al, 2008; Doenhoff et al, 2008). Even in those not cured, the worm burden is likely substantially reduced, which significantly decreases the chances of development of further infectious sequelae. After treatment of a patient with PZQ, it is reasonable to monitor egg counts in urine and stool specimens and to perform serial ultrasonographic studies of the urogenital tract to assess response to drug therapy. Repeat PZQ courses can be given if there is a concern for persistent infection.

PZQ has a favorable pharmacokinetic and side effect profile. The most common side effects (abdominal pain, nausea, headache, and dizziness) are typically mild, generally occur within 3 to 4 hours after administration, and resolve spontaneously. Most patients experience few or no side effects (N'Goran et al, 2003). However, PZQ pills are large and bitter tasting, making oral administration difficult to tolerate, especially for children (Meyer et al, 2009). Perhaps because of its FDA classification as a Pregnancy Category B

drug (deemed safe in lactating and pregnant women based only on animal studies), many chemotherapy programs exclude pregnant and lactating women. However, there are few reports of adverse effects of PZQ among the millions of pregnant women treated with PZQ (Olds, 2003).

PZQ is less efficacious against schistosomulae than adult worms, which might partly explain the lower cure rates in areas with high rates of schistosomiasis transmission and reinfection. In addition, it means that PZQ cannot be used to abort infection shortly after exposure. Multiple PZQ doses administered several weeks apart can ensure that juvenile schistosomes missed by the first administration are eradicated after maturation (Doenhoff et al, 2008).

Whether schistosomes are developing resistance to PZQ is debatable. Most large studies conducted on *S. haematobium*–infected individuals suggest little drug resistance in endemic areas (King et al, 2000; Guidi et al, 2010). However, there have been reports of PZQ failures in the treatment of travelers or military personnel returning from endemic areas (Doenhoff et al, 2008). Even if resistance to PZQ is not already evolving, it could occur in the future. It is hoped that use of alternative drugs and combination of drug treatment programs with environmental control programs (snail control and sanitation improvement) may lower transmission and reduce the use of PZQ enough to prevent this.

Artemisinin and its analogues (artemether and artesunate, currently in use as antimalarials) are chemoprophylactic alternatives to PZQ because they specifically target the schistosomular stage of *S. haematobium*. Artemether and artesunate are 90% to 97% efficacious in preventing schistosomiasis but are poor treatments for established infections. Combined administration of PZQ and artemisinin derivatives results in lower infection rates than PZQ alone and thus offers a valuable tool for MDA programs, especially in areas of high transmission and reinfection rates. However, a major concern regarding the use of artemesinins in this manner is the induction of malaria resistance to artemisinin derivatives. Because of this, widespread PZQ–artemisinin derivative combination therapy should not be used in schistosomiasis-malaria co-endemic areas (Liu et al, 2011).

Surgical Management. The efficacy and ease of PZQ therapy for urogenital schistosomiasis, together with the possible reversibility of early-stage disease (Richter et al, 1996; Richter, 2000), mean that in most patients trials of medical therapy should be undertaken before elective surgical approaches (Cioli et al, 1995). In general, surgery is reserved for complications that have not responded to adequate medical treatment within a reasonable follow-up period and for those settings in which immediate surgical intervention is necessary. For example, severe bladder hemorrhage is one common cause for urgent surgical intervention.

Prostatitis and prostatic enlargement are uncommon in schistosomiasis. Accordingly, numerous autopsy studies have failed to demonstrate evidence of anatomic bladder outlet obstruction (Smith et al, 1974; Cheever et al, 1977, 1978). However, clinical studies consistently report cystoscopic (Fam, 1964), urodynamic (Sabha and Nilsson, 1988), and elevated postvoid residual urine volumes, which are evidence of functional bladder outlet obstruction that occasionally requires surgical intervention in patients with severe inactive urinary schistosomiasis (Abdel-Halim et al, 1985). *S. haematobium* infection–associated scrotal induration, pain, and enlargement associated with epididymitis can lead to surgery being performed for the suspicion of a testicular tumor.

Surgery is indicated for irreversibly contracted bladders; procedures include vesical denervation, urinary diversion, ileocystoplasty, and hydrodistention. Any treatment, however, must be performed in conjunction with medical chemotherapy. Chronic, deep bladder ulcers may necessitate a partial cystectomy, because fulguration rarely produces either symptomatic relief or ulcer healing. Urothelial hyperplasia is strongly associated with severe urogenital schistosomiasis, whereas urothelial dysplasia and metaplasia commonly accompany schistosomal bladder cancer (Khafagy et al, 1972). Treatment of bladder cancer secondary to schistosomiasis is typically surgical and discussed elsewhere (see Chapters 92 to 96).

The most frequent sequelae of urinary schistosomiasis result from ureteral involvement causing obstructive uropathy (Lehman et al, 1973; Smith et al, 1974; Cheever et al, 1978; Smith and Christie, 1986). Hydroureter and hydronephrosis are linked to the intensity of *S. haematobium* infection. **Because ureteral obstruction observed during schistosomiasis is most often caused by concentric or hemiconcentric polypoid lesions that "girdle" the ureteral muscle in the intramural and adjacent extravesical ureter, it often responds well to medical management alone.** Complete resolution of deteriorated renal function caused by active infection–associated obstructive uropathy responds within 1 to 2 months of PZQ chemotherapy (Lehman et al, 1973). Chemotherapy not only reverses schistosomal obstructive uropathy but can also prevent it, even in persons who are continually reinfected (Subramanian et al, 1999). However, in late, chronic, active and inactive urinary schistosomiasis, anatomic obstruction may be less amenable to chemotherapeutic cure.

Anatomic ureteral stenosis, with or without calculi, has been identified in up to 80% of patients with ureteral obstruction (Lehman et al, 1973; Smith et al, 1977b; Al-Shukri and Alwan, 1983; El-Nahas et al, 2003). **When residual ureteral stenosis persists after chemotherapy, it is usually amenable to surgical intervention. Depending on the location and extent of the stricture, procedures involving dilatation or excision have been employed.** Balloon dilatation is efficacious with anatomic stenosis (Jacobsson et al, 1987), but mechanical dilatation is frequently plagued by recurrent stenosis (Wishahi, 1987). When the ureteral meatus, intramural ureter, ureterovesical junction, or distal ureter is involved, options to reconstruct a functional valve include a variety of plastic operations. Most of these procedures

are variants of the Politano-Leadbetter operation (Politano and Leadbetter, 1958; Leadbetter and Leadbetter, 1961). Although the procedures are highly efficacious for some patients (Smith et al, 1977b; Al-Shukri and Alwan, 1983), other authors have noted that restenosis can occur (Umerah, 1981).

In long or multifocal lesions of the ureter, excision of the affected portion may leave an inadequate residual ureter for reimplantation or simple ureteroureterostomy; in these patients, surgeons have successfully employed the Boari flap, ileal conduit, suprapubic intravesical ureterostomy (in which the obstructed ureteral segment is bypassed with use of a peritoneal dialysis catheter and drained into the bladder), and replacement of the ureter with ileal segments, taking care to maintain an isoperistaltic direction of the ileal segment (Abdel-Halim, 1980, 1984; Al-Shukri and Alwan, 1983; Abu-Aisha et al, 1985). Isolated meatal stenosis of the ureter may be amenable to simple meatoplasty (Al-Shukri and Alwan, 1983). When a ureter is hopelessly obstructed and cannot be reconstructed, long-term nephrostomy drainage is another option.

Prognosis

Approximately 112 million people are infected with *S. haematobium*, but **most have mild infections and a good prognosis. The morbidity and mortality of urogenital schistosomiasis is determined by the overall intensity of infection and genetic polymorphisms for relevant immune response genes** (Kouriba et al, 2005; He et al, 2008; Isnard and Chevillard, 2008; Isnard et al, 2011; Ouf et al, 2012). In regions of low *S. haematobium* prevalence, such as Nigeria, essentially no schistosomiasis-related mortality is observed and the frequency and severity of schistosomal obstructive uropathy are low. In contrast, when Egypt had a prevalence of 50%, schistosomiasis contributed to mortality in 10% of *S. haematobium*–infected individuals (Smith et al, 1974; Cheever et al, 1978). **Among patients with severe disease, mortality approached 50% in 2 to 5 years** (Lehman et al, 1970).

Patients who die of schistosomal obstructive uropathy (bilateral end-stage hydronephrosis or unilateral hydronephrosis with contralateral nonschistosomal end-stage renal disease) are typically in their 20s and have heavy total egg burdens. Patients who develop the complications of pyelonephritis and urothelial cancer are commonly older than age 40, consistent with time- and intensity-related pathology (Christie et al, 1986; Smith and Christie, 1986).

The prognosis for patients with urinary tract lesions has dramatically improved with PZQ therapy. In children with obstructive polyps, the uropathy usually completely resolves within 2 to 6 weeks of treatment. For patients with chronic obstructive uropathy from sandy patches and fibrosis, the prognosis is less clear. Some individuals tolerate advanced obstructive uropathy with little, if any, deterioration in renal function. **Schistosomal obstructive uropathy, urolithiasis, bladder outlet obstruction, and bacterial cystitis all predispose to pyelonephritis.** Bacterial superinfection can be life-threatening and should be treated aggressively and promptly. Finally, for **those who develop a bladder malignancy, their prognosis is dependent on the aggressiveness of their tumor.**

Prevention and Control

Travelers to endemic areas should be advised to avoid contact with potentially infested fresh water (streams, rivers, ponds, and lakes). Fast-flowing water can still harbor *S. haematobium*. Heating water to more than 125° F for 5 minutes kills the cercariae, as does chlorination and allowing the water to stand for more than 2 days in a setting free of snails. Since the advent of PZQ in the late 1970s and its subsequent mass distribution beginning in the 1980s, schistosomiasis has become relatively simple and affordable to treat, but it remains difficult to control. For the past three decades, control efforts have focused heavily on reducing morbidity using periodic, typically annual targeted mass drug treatments with PZQ, a strategy advocated by WHO. However, when access to safe water is not available, rural poor communities are subject to vicious cycles of infection, treatment, and reinfection, making more frequent PZQ administration necessary. Sanitation improvements, health education, and snail control are approaches used to break the cycle of transmission, by slowing or halting the influx of eggs into the aquatic habitat, decreasing individual exposure, and reducing the availability of snail intermediate hosts, respectively. Although PZQ is inexpensive, the cost-effectiveness of chemotherapy fluctuates widely among MDA settings as a result of variations in the number of doses of PZQ given per person, variability in transportation and delivery costs, and the potential to take advantage of preexisting public health control programs or other infrastructure (Brooker et al, 2008). The per-person cost in control campaigns is typically under U.S. $0.50—although even this modest cost, at sufficient scale, may exceed the available resources of many endemic countries (Hotez et al, 2009). Fortunately, a number of pharmaceutical companies and foundations are donating PZQ for use in MDA campaigns.

Because asexual reproduction in the snail host allows the parasite to amplify rapidly, sanitation programs and drug treatment campaigns must reduce egg input into the environment by nearly 90% before a substantial decrease in transmission can be achieved (Woolhouse, 1992). Reductions in snail populations, in contrast, can theoretically effect proportional decreases in disease transmission risk (Woolhouse, 1992). However, considering that adult worms can live for years in the human host, without concurrent mass treatment snail population control alone would need to persist for many years to eliminate transmission. Thus, integrated campaigns focusing on three aims (treating human patients, reducing contact of humans and their wastes with infested water, and controlling snails) offer the most promise.

Other control efforts include mollusciciding (Zhang and Jiang, 2011; Knopp et al, 2012, 2013), biologic control using snail predators or competitors (Roberts and Kuris, 1990; Mkoji et al, 1999; Pointier and Jourdane, 2000; Allen and Victory, 2003; Coelho et al, 2004; Sokolow et al, 2014), and vaccine development (although an efficacious vaccine currently remains out of reach) (Bethony et al, 2008; Gray et al, 2010). Water, sanitation, and hygiene ("WASH") programs are also, once again, taking center stage and feature many additional benefits beyond potential schistosomiasis reduction (Soares Magalhães et al, 2011; Giné Garriga and Pérez Foguet, 2013).

Schistosomiasis has been eliminated in 10 countries to date (Iran, Japan, Lebanon, Malaysia, Martinique, Montserrat, Morocco, Thailand, Tunisia, and Turkey) (Amarir et al, 2011; Rollinson et al, 2013). At the 65th WHO World Health Assembly (May 2012), resolution WHA65.21 was passed, calling on the global community to "make available the necessary and sufficient means and resources … to intensify control programmes in most disease-endemic countries and initiate elimination campaigns, where appropriate" (WHO, 2012). Representing a shift from morbidity control to a new focus on elimination, this marks an exciting and hopeful milestone in the global fight against schistosomiasis.

KEY POINTS: SCHISTOSOMIASIS

- *S. haematobium* worms can survive in human hosts for years to decades. A careful travel and social history is crucial to identify potential exposures, correlate them with urogenital symptoms, and determine the need to perform specific diagnostic assays.
- Praziquantel therapy of early stage urogenital schistosomiasis can reverse inflammatory lesions, including fibrosis, of the urinary tract caused by the host response to eggs deposited in tissues.
- The gold standard for diagnosis of active urogenital schistosomiasis is the identification of eggs in urine, stool, or bladder or rectal biopsy specimens. Serologic and PCR-based assays are highly sensitive but may not distinguish between active and resolved infection, and are impractical in endemic regions.

Filariasis

The filariae are vector-borne tissue nematodes. Human pathogens in this group include the agents of **lymphatic filariasis** (LF), *Onchocerca volvulus*, and *Loa loa*.

LF is caused by the mosquito-borne helminths *Wuchereria bancrofti*, *Brugia malayi*, and *Brugia timori*. The symptoms of LF range from acute lymphatic inflammation to chronic lymphatic dilation with hydrocele, lymphedema, and elephantiasis of the limbs.

Organisms

W. bancrofti, *B. malayi*, and *B. timori* are threadlike nematodes. Infective (third-stage) larvae are transmitted to humans by mosquito bites. After entering humans, larvae migrate to central lymphatic vessels and eventually mature (over 6 to 9 months) into adult male or female worms. Adults (approximately 20 to 100 mm × 0.2 mm) are considerably larger than microfilariae (approximately 200 µm × 10 µm) (Fig. 17-14). Adult worms live primarily in the afferent lymphatics, especially in the lower extremities (inguinal, iliac, and periaortic lymphatics), and (for *W. bancrofti* only) male genitalia (epididymis, spermatic cord, testicles). Adult worms live approximately 5 to 7 years.

After mating with males, female worms release large numbers of microfilariae. In most endemic areas, *W. bancrofti* and *Brugia* microfilaremia peaks in the middle of the night as an adaptation to facilitate transmission, coinciding with peak local mosquito vector activity. In some parts of the Pacific, the periodicity of *W. bancrofti* is diurnal rather than nocturnal. After mosquito ingestion, microfilariae mature over 10 to 14 days into infective third-stage larvae.

W. bancrofti and *Brugia* species harbor an obligate rickettsia-like endosymbiont (*Wolbachia*). These endosymbionts are involved in embryogenesis, and antimicrobial therapy (e.g., doxycycline) kills them, resulting in decreased microfilariae release and suppressed larval molting (Hoerauf et al, 2001).

Epidemiology

Globally, 120 million people are infected with LF. Over 90% of infections are caused by *W. bancrofti*, mostly in sub-Saharan Africa, South and Southeast Asia, and the western Pacific. In the Americas, *W. bancrofti* is endemic only to Haiti, the Dominican Republic, Guyana, and Brazil. Infection with *B. malayi* is limited to Asia and several Pacific islands (e.g., Indonesia and the Philippines). *B. timori* infection occurs only in southeastern Indonesia. Within a given

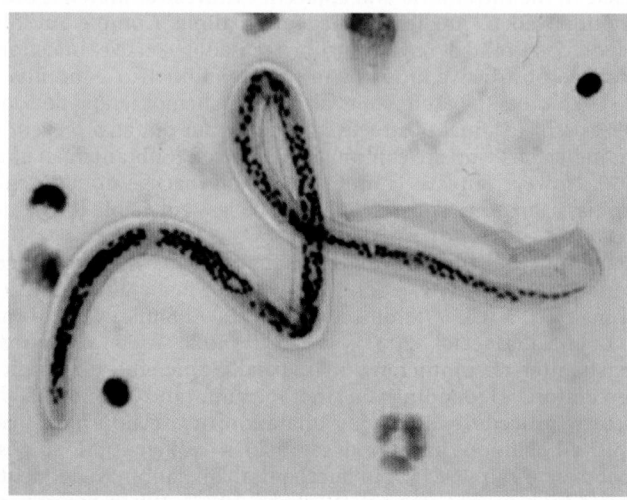

Figure 17-14. Microfilaria of *Wuchereria bancrofti* in peripheral blood. (Courtesy Division of Parasitic Diseases and Malaria, Centers for Disease Control and Prevention.)

geographic area, the distribution of LF is often quite heterogeneous. Several genera of mosquitoes are capable of transmission, including *Anopheles* (rural Africa and the Pacific), *Culex* (urban areas, especially India), *Aedes aegypti* in some Pacific islands, and others.

Although varying among different locales and mosquito vectors, transmission of LF is relatively inefficient, and obstructive lymphatic disease is generally seen only in persons repeatedly infected over many years (i.e., usually long-term residents of endemic areas). In endemic communities, prevalence increases from childhood through the third or fourth decade of life, after which it remains fairly constant (because of the gradual accumulation of adult-stage worms in the population over time). Lymphedema and genital disease are rare before age 10 but increase in prevalence with age. Overall, about one third of infected persons have clinically overt disease. The likelihood of developing clinical manifestations is particularly high in India, Papua New Guinea, and Africa, whereas it is lower in the Americas (Kazura et al, 1997).

Pathology and Clinical Manifestations

The initial immune response to infective larvae and early adult worms is mostly proinflammatory (involving both Th1 and Th2 T-cell responses). The contribution of humoral immunity includes an increase in filaria-specific IgE titers. Eosinophil-mediated killing of microfilariae also likely plays a role. With the onset of microfilaremia, T-cell responses decrease, mediated by IL-10, IgG4-blocking antibodies, and antigen-specific suppressor T cells. Whether protective immunity develops has been difficult to determine, but groups of individuals have remained infection free despite long-term exposure in highly endemic settings (Steel et al, 1996).

Clinical manifestations in infected patients vary greatly, ranging from subclinical infection to severe disfigurement of the limbs and genitalia. Damage from established infection is cumulative because of progressive scarring and lymphatic obstruction. Medical therapy does not readily reverse such damage but can prevent further progression in patients with active LF infection. Although rarely fatal, LF can cause severe disability and among parasitic infections is responsible for the third highest number of disability-adjusted life years (DALYs) lost globally.

The mechanisms leading to lymphedema have been poorly established. However, parasite-derived factors are at least partly responsible for initial lymphatic dilatation, with subsequent contributions from secondary bacterial infections and inflammatory responses to dying or dead parasites. *Wolbachia* endosymbionts also appear to drive a proinflammatory response. Lesions vary from nodular inflammation to suppuration, histologically appearing as granulomas around worms, sometimes with tissue eosinophils (Fig. 17-15). A vicious cycle can result, with acute attacks worsening lymphedema, predisposing to more secondary infections, worsening lymphedema, and so on; episodic filarial inflammation eventually abates, leaving obliterated lymphatics surrounded by scar tissue. Elephantiasis or hydrocele is then the end stage in some patients.

Subclinical Infection. Most LF-infected persons have few overt clinical manifestations, even with high-grade microfilaremia. However, though the infection is clinically asymptomatic, virtually all persons with patent *W. bancrofti* or *B. malayi* infection have at least some subclinical disease (e.g., dilated lymphatics, scrotal lymphangiectasia, microscopic hematuria, or proteinuria). Eosinophilia is also very common with most forms of LF.

Acute Adenolymphangitis. Acute adenolymphangitis (ADL) is often the first clinical manifestation of LF, consisting of fever, lymphadenitis, lymphangitis, and edema that usually lasts days to a week. The lymphangitis is retrograde (extending peripherally), which distinguishes it from bacterial lymphangitis. Although all four extremities can be involved in both bancroftian and brugian filariasis, the genital lymphatics are affected almost exclusively by *W. bancrofti* infection. This can result in funiculitis, epididymitis, scrotal pain, tenderness, and lymph scrotum (ruptured lymphatic vesicles on the scrotal skin that yield a whitish discharge and secondary bacterial infections).

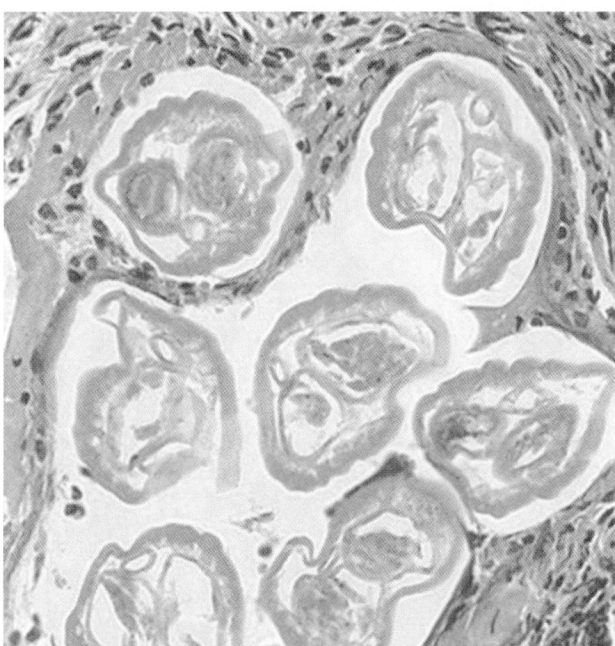

Figure 17-15. Section of an adult *Brugia* organism in a lymph node. (Courtesy Division of Parasitic Diseases and Malaria, Centers for Disease Control and Prevention.)

Another acute manifestation, **dermatolymphangioadenitis** (DLA), is characterized by fever, chills, myalgias, and headache. Edematous inflammatory plaques occur, as well as hyperpigmentation, vesicles, and ulcers, often at the site of an inciting skin injury. Inflammation progresses proximally and is thought to be secondary to bacterial infections.

Lymphedema. Lower or upper extremity edema is the most common chronic manifestation of LF, with lower extremity edema being the more prevalent. Bancroftian filariasis typically involves the entire limb, whereas brugian filariasis usually involves only the leg below the knee. Although both lower extremities are often affected, asymmetrical involvement is most common. The overlying skin may exude serous fluid. Breast involvement can also occur in females.

Genitourinary Manifestations. Male genital involvement is very common with bancroftian filariasis but uncommon with *Brugia* infection. The prevalence of female genital involvement has not been well established, although anecdotal evidence suggests that it is uncommon (Nutman and Kazura, 2011). Genital disease is not usually experienced until at least the teenage years. Acute painful episodes of (usually unilateral) epididymitis or funiculitis accompanied by fever and malaise can last several days and are one of the most common consequences of bancroftian filariasis.

Funiculoepididymitis. Funiculoepididymitis is characterized by palpable cordlike swellings and edema. Although the condition is usually self-limited, recurrences and the subsequent development of chronic lymphedema are common. Filarial funiculitis rarely results in sterility or orchitis, because the spermatic cord usually remains uninvolved. This manifestation is often mistaken for malignancy, and many patients undergo surgery as a result (including orchiectomy). Varicocele may complicate inflammation, increasing pain and swelling. Bacterial superinfection is a rare but severe complication, with exquisite pain and septic thrombophlebitis often present.

Hydroceles. Chronic disease of the male genitals often results in hydroceles, which can be very large (Fig. 17-16). In endemic areas, differentiation of filarial from nonfilarial hydrocele is difficult, and parasites are rarely detected in the hydrocele fluid. Hydrocele accompanied by nodules in the cord or epididymis and a history of travel to or residence in an endemic area suggests LF. A thick,

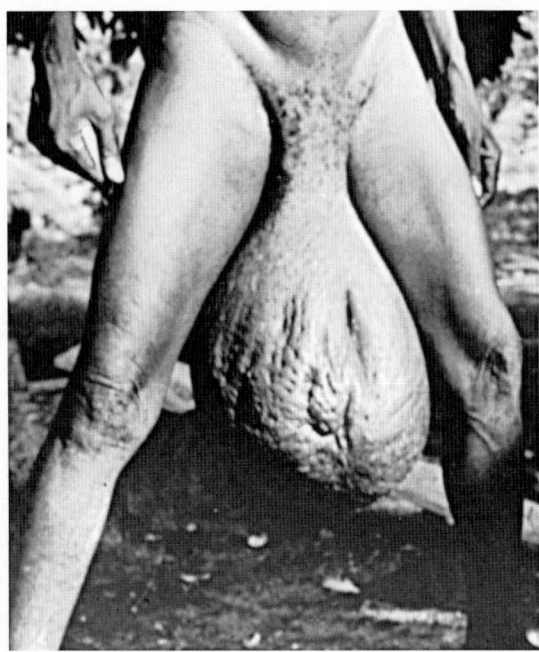

Figure 17-16. Huge hydrocele and scrotal elephantiasis. (Courtesy Dr. B. H. Kean. From Zaiman H. A pictorial presentation of parasites, Valley City, ND.)

fibrous tunica, especially with cholesterol or calcium deposits, also suggests LF.

Hydroceles are usually painless unless complicated by acute epididymitis or funiculitis. The scrotal skin may also be thickened and brawny as a result of lymphedema, with oozing lymph. Patients with filarial hydrocele rarely experience bacterial superinfection, although those with elephantiasis and lymph scrotum are often superinfected.

Scrotal and Penile Elephantiasis. Mild scrotal edema is not unusual during early infection or with established hydrocele. Conversely, penile edema is unusual, and massive enlargement of the scrotum or penis occurs late, largely in individuals with poor access to medical care. Genital elephantiasis rarely arises from causes other than LF.

Chyluria. Chyluria occurs when GU tract lymphatics are damaged, resulting in lymph passage into the urine and massive fat and protein loss. Although rare, this can result in serious nutritional consequences. It usually occurs earlier in the natural history of filariasis than genital elephantiasis. Chyluria is usually intermittent and may spontaneously remit.

Tropical Pulmonary Eosinophilia. Tropical pulmonary eosinophilia (TPE) is a syndrome characterized by paroxysmal cough and wheezing (usually nocturnal), fever, adenopathy, high-grade eosinophilia, and elevated IgE levels. It is caused by an allergic response to microfilarial antigens and is seen most commonly in South and Southeast Asia. Chest radiographs range from normal to diffuse reticulonodular infiltrates, and pulmonary function tests show restrictive (and sometimes obstructive) defects. If done, lung biopsy reveals an eosinophilic interstitial pneumonitis. Microfilaremia is usually absent.

Diagnosis

In residents of endemic areas, lymphedema or male genital disease is epidemiologically more likely a result of LF than a similar presentation in the developed world (assuming no other cause of secondary edema is present). Still, tuberculosis, *S. haematobium* infection (urogenital schistosomiasis), and gonorrhea may also produce funiculoepididymitis and are in the differential diagnosis. In addition, nonfilarial hydrocele is common in both tropical and

nontropical areas. However, hydrocele occurs at an earlier age and with greater frequency in filariasis-endemic areas.

For parasitologic confirmation, it is difficult to visualize adult worms directly because they are localized in the lymphatics; they are usually seen only via histologic examination of surgical or biopsy specimens (in which visualizing adult worms is diagnostically definitive but insensitive). However, ultrasound examination of lymphatics has at least 80% sensitivity in some settings, in part because live adult worms have a distinctive pattern of movement (the "filaria dance sign") (Amaral et al, 1994). Online examples can be found at www.youtube.com/watch?v=ER1BFx4_qGc, http://www.filariajournal.com/content/2/1/3/figure/F1?highres=y, and www.youtube.com/watch?v=d3KWh6xqQm0. Plain radiographs may reveal calcifications, which are also suggestive of LF in the appropriate clinical setting.

Microfilariae can be found in blood and occasionally in other body fluids; they are best detected by a Giemsa-stained blood smear. The timing of blood collection should be based on the periodicity of the microfilariae in the geographic location involved (highest at midnight in most cases). Microfilaremia is found in only 30% to 40% of all infections, and definitive diagnosis in amicrofilaremic cases can be more difficult. Detection of circulating *W. bancrofti* antigens is one means to detect such infections, and this can be done with both an ELISA and a point-of-care immunochromatographic card test (ICT). Recently, a new ICT (the Alere Filariasis Test Strip) has shown better sensitivity in field conditions than the BinaxNOW Filariasis ICT, which has been in use for the past 10 to 20 years (Weil et al, 2013). There are currently no tests for circulating antigens in brugian filariasis. PCR-based assays for *W. bancrofti* and *B. malayi* in blood are very sensitive but are not yet widely available.

Antibody-based assays for diagnosing LF have traditionally suffered from poor specificity. IgG4 antibodies are less cross-reactive to nonfilarial helminth antigens and thus are more specific. Specificity has also been improved with species-specific antigens for both brugian and bancroftian infection. A dipstick antibody test has been developed for brugian filariasis (Weil et al, 2011).

Patients with so-called burned-out infections (e.g., those who have received antiparasitic therapy or who departed endemic areas years previously and in whom the worms have now died) often have lasting damage (i.e., lymphedema, genital disease, and other clinical manifestations). In these patients, negative testing for microfilaremia and circulating antigens does not exclude the possibility that their lesions could be a result of LF. However, such patients are usually LF antibody positive.

Radionuclide lymphoscintigraphic imaging reliably demonstrates lymphatic abnormalities in patients with LF. Although helpful in documenting the degree of damage associated with infection, this is not useful for differentiating LF from other causes of lymphatic disease.

Treatment

Because most patients with microfilaremia have at least subclinical disease, treatment is recommended for both symptomatic and asymptomatic individuals with microfilaremia. Diethylcarbamazine (DEC, 2 mg/kg orally three times a day) is the treatment of choice for active LF (microfilaremia, antigen positivity, or live adult worms on ultrasound). A 1-day course appears to be as effective as the traditional 12-day regimen for most patients (CDC, 2013a), although those with TPE should receive a 2- to 3-week course. DEC kills microfilariae but has only modest activity against adult worms, and in the United States is available only through the CDC (phone: 404-718-4745). DEC should not be given to persons from areas co-endemic for onchocerciasis or *L. loa* (e.g., West and Central Africa) unless these infections have been excluded because of potentially serious side effects related to the killing of these parasites by DEC. Alternatives for LF include albendazole and ivermectin. Albendazole (400 mg orally twice daily for 21 days) has both microfilaricidal and macrofilaricidal activity, but the activity of ivermectin (150 to 400 µg/kg orally once) is limited mostly to microfilariae.

Side effects of DEC include fever, chills, arthralgias, headaches, nausea, and vomiting. In heavily infected patients, painful skin nodules, lymphadenitis, and epididymitis may occur as a reaction to dying parasites or *Wolbachia* endosymbionts, usually days to weeks after initiation of therapy. Ivermectin has a side effect profile similar to DEC when used for LF; it also must be used with caution if co-infection with *L. loa* is possible. Albendazole (when used in single-dose regimens; see later) has relatively few side effects when used for LF.

Doxycycline (200 mg daily) augments the suppression of micro-filaremia induced by antifilarial drugs and has some macrofilari-cidal activity. Prolonged courses (4 to 8 weeks) render adult worms sterile (Kappagoda et al, 2011). Individuals treated with doxycycline can experience substantial improvements in lymphedema and hydrocele. These benefits are seen even in lymphedema patients without active infection, suggesting that the benefit of doxycycline extends beyond the macrofilaricidal and anti-*Wolbachia* activity of this drug (Mand et al, 2012). The prolonged course is problematic for administration in the developing world, and doxycycline cannot be given to pregnant women or young children. However, in the United States a 6-week treatment course of this drug is a reasonable consideration in properly selected patients.

In persons with chronic lymphedema, prevention of secondary bacterial infections, good hygiene, elastic stockings, elevation, and physiotherapy are important for morbidity control. Anti-parasitic therapy in these patients should be reserved for those with active infection. Surgical correction is challenging and often unnecessary. Lymphatic-venous and nodal-venous anastomoses for elephantiasis have been somewhat successful in decreasing leg swelling, as has reconstructive surgery for genital involvement. The long-term effects of these intensive surgical techniques have not been determined.

Genital elephantiasis is rarely amenable to surgery, and lymph-adenectomy may further compromise lymph drainage and worsen symptoms. In some cases of funiculoepididymitis, surgery, such as decompression or excision of filarial nodules, might be indicated to preserve the testis and spermatic cord. When funiculoepididymi-tis is recurrent, painful, and deforming or complicated by blood vessel involvement, more radical surgery is warranted. Drainage of hydroceles provides immediate relief, although recurrence is common in the absence of medical and definitive surgical therapy. Hydrocelectomy is often indicated for large or symptomatic hydro-celes. Excision of the intact hydrocele sac is the procedure of choice; alternatively, inversion with partial excision can be considered. When identified, leaking or dilated lymphatic vessels should be sutured or excised. Small hydroceles that do not enlarge usually do not require surgery. Reconstruction of the scrotum or vulva, with removal of redundant tissue, can also provide symptomatic relief to selected patients.

Prevention and Control

Individual protection against LF infection involves avoidance of infected mosquitoes through personal protective measures and long-lasting insecticide–treated bednets (LLINs); LLINs have recently been shown to be a valuable tool for the control and elimi-nation of LF (Reimer et al, 2013). Elimination of microfilariae within communities can interrupt transmission because patent microfilaremia is necessary for mosquitoes to transmit the infection from person to person. However, because chemotherapy does not kill all of the adult worms, it is necessary to continue intermittent administration of antiparasitic drugs for many years, until the adult worms die of senescence. This strategy can be effective for *W. ban-crofti* elimination (Molyneux, 2009) but is more challenging in *Brugia*-endemic areas because animals also serve as reservoirs of infection for the latter. MDA campaigns (involving distribution of single annual doses of albendazole plus either DEC or ivermectin, which have a sustained microfilaricidal effect, to most of the popu-lation) are the mainstay of control programs in Africa (albendazole/ivermectin) and elsewhere (albendazole/DEC). These campaigns have been successful in control and elimination of LF, especially in

many of the endemic middle-income countries of Asia, Latin America, and the Pacific.

Onchocerciasis, also known as **river blindness**, is a filarial infec-tion caused by *O. volvulus*. The infection is transmitted by *Simulium* black flies; 99% of onchocerciasis cases are found in Africa, with limited foci in Latin America and the Arabian Peninsula. About 37 million people are infected globally (Taylor et al, 2010). As with LF, transmission is inefficient and highly focal. Adult worms live in subcutaneous nodules (mean life span, 9 to 10 years) and release microfilariae that travel through the skin (and eye). *O. volvulus* adults also harbor *Wolbachia* endosymbionts. Infection classically causes dermatitis, keratitis, and chorioretinitis, with blindness as an end result after many years, from corneal scarring. Diagnosis is confirmed by microscopically examining skin snips for microfilar-iae, finding adult worms in subcutaneous nodules, or seeing micro-filariae in the anterior chamber of the eye via slit lamp. Antibody and antigen detection tests are less well developed than for LF.

In late stages, *Onchocerca* infection may produce "hanging groin" or scrotal elephantiasis as a result of recurrent lymphadenitis and loss of skin elasticity. Histology demonstrates atrophy and fibrosis of inguinal lymph nodes with subcutaneous edema and fibrosis. Onchocerciasis is also occasionally accompanied by massive ingui-nal lymphadenopathy.

Ivermectin is the treatment of choice (150 µg/kg orally once, repeated every 6 to 12 months until patient is asymptomatic), although it kills only microfilariae. Ivermectin must be used with caution if coinfection with *L. loa* is possible. Adverse effects include fever, rash, dizziness, pruritus, myalgias, arthralgias, and lymph-adenopathy, mostly caused by dying filariae and *Wolbachia*. Six weeks of doxycycline (200 mg/day orally) kills more than 60% of adult female worms and sterilizes most of the remainder (Hoerauf, 2011). DEC should not be administered to persons infected with onchocerciasis because blindness and systemic toxic-ity can result from the resulting ocular and systemic inflammatory responses.

Loaiasis is caused by *L. loa*, a filarial infection that is limited to Central and West Africa and transmitted by *Chrysops* flies. Adult worms migrate in subcutaneous tissues, and microfilariae circulate diurnally in the blood. *L. loa* does not harbor *Wolbachia*. Most infected persons have asymptomatic eosinophilia; some have urti-caria, migratory subcutaneous lesions, and visible worms migrating across the conjunctivae *(eye worms)*. Hematuria and proteinuria occur in 30% of patients; lymphadenitis and hydrocele also rarely occur. DEC (2 to 3 mg/kg orally three times a day for 14 to 21 days) is effective against loaiasis, although multiple courses may be neces-sary (Klion and Nutman, 2011). Treatment can cause pruritus, arthralgias, migratory swellings, fever, eye worms, diarrhea, and renal failure. Patients with detectable microfilaremia (particularly more than 2500 to 8000 microfilariae per milliliter) are at risk of treatment-associated encephalopathy, which may be ameliorated by pretreatment apheresis. Albendazole (200 mg orally twice daily for 3 weeks) is associated with a lower risk of encephalopathy than DEC and may be safer in patients with high-grade parasitemia (Kappagoda et al, 2011).

Other Nonfilarial Genitourinary Parasites

Echinococcosis

Echinococcus granulosus is a cestode (tapeworm) that causes cystic echinococcosis. Infection results from ingestion of food or water contaminated with *Echinococcus* eggs or contact with infected dogs. Prevalence is high in pastoral communities, particularly in South America, the Mediterranean littoral, Eastern Europe, the Middle East, East Africa, Central Asia, China, Russia, and Australia. After infection the parasites encyst, usually in the liver or (less com-monly) in the lungs. Although rare, cysts can grow ectopically in almost any organ in the body, with the kidneys being the third most common organ affected after the liver and lungs (<2% to 3% of cases) (Moscatelli et al, 2013). Initially, cysts are asymp-tomatic, but over time they enlarge (1 to 2 cm/yr) and eventually cause pain or a palpable abdominal mass; hydatiduria and renal colic occur in a minority of patients. Renal function is usually unaffected. Imaging shows a thick-walled, fluid-filled spheric cyst, often with a calcified wall; the appearance helps define the stage of the disease and, in turn, management strategies. Serologic testing is adjunctive for diagnosis, with a sensitivity of only 60% to 90%. Although use of percutaneous puncture, aspiration, injection, and reaspiration (PAIR) is a good therapeutic option for liver cysts, this is not done for renal cysts, for which the only options are surgical resection or antiparasitic chemotherapy. Albendazole (400 mg orally twice per day for 1 to 6 months) is the recommended medical therapy (Kappagoda et al, 2011). Surgical excision is indicated in some patients because of the size or location of the lesions. Cyst rupture can cause anaphylaxis. Some evidence suggests that PZQ plus albendazole preoperatively and postoperatively may minimize secondary seeding and metastatic infection (Bygott and Chiodini, 2009).

Enterobiasis

Enterobius vermicularis (pinworm) causes enterobiasis, which occurs worldwide (common in both temperate and tropical countries). The worms live in the proximal colon and migrate to the perianal region to lay eggs, which become infectious after 6 hours. Transmission is mainly person to person, often via fecal-oral contamination of hands or fomites. Although most infections are asymptomatic, perianal pruritus can be severe. Rarely, pinworms can also migrate ectopically, including through the vagina, uterus, and fallopian tubes and into the peritoneal cavity of females. Dead worms and eggs incite granulomas and adhesions. Vulvar and cervical granulomas, salpingitis, oophoritis, tubo-ovarian abscess, appendicitis, and peritonitis can result. Epididymal involvement and inguinal hernias have been rarely reported in men (Moore and McCarthy, 2011).

Treatment with single-dose albendazole (400 mg orally) or mebendazole (100 mg orally) is highly effective. Alternatives include ivermectin (200 µg/kg orally once). Household and other close contacts should be treated, and treatment should be repeated after 2 weeks because of frequent reinfection and autoinfection (Kappagoda et al, 2011).

Amebiasis

Entamoeba histolytica, a protozoan transmitted by the fecal-oral route, is most common in tropical regions. Most infected persons remain asymptomatic, but 10% develop symptoms in other organs, including the kidneys. Cutaneous amebiasis can also occur, with painful ulcers often involving the perianal area and genitals (Peterson et al, 2011). Treatment is with tinidazole (2 g orally per day for 3 days) or metronidazole (750 mg orally three times a day for 10 days), followed by paromomycin (8 to 12 mg/kg orally three times a day for 7 days) or iodoquinol (650 mg orally three times a day for 20 days) (Kappagoda et al, 2011).

Trichomoniasis

Trichomonas vaginalis is a common sexually transmitted protozoan. See Chapter 15 for details.

REFERENCES

The complete reference list is available online at www.expertconsult.com.

SUGGESTED READINGS

TUBERCULOSIS

American Thoracic Society. Diagnostic Standards and Classification of Tuberculosis in Adults and Children. This official statement of the American Thoracic Society and the Centers for Disease Control and Prevention was adopted by the ATS Board of Directors, July 1999. This statement was endorsed by the Council of the Infectious Diseases Society of America, September 1999. Am J Respir Crit Care Med 2000a;161 (4 Pt 1):1376–95.

Centers for Disease Control and Prevention (CDC). Treatment of tuberculosis, American Thoracic Society, CDC, and Infectious Diseases Society of America. MMWR Recomm Rep 2003;52(RR-11):1–77.

Figueiredo AA, Lucon AM. Urogenital tuberculosis: update and review of 8961 cases from the world literature. Rev Urol 2008;10(3):207–17.

Goel A, Dalela D. Options in the management of tuberculous ureteric stricture. Indian J Urol 2008;24(3):376–81.

Gupta NP, Kumar A, Sharma S. Reconstructive bladder surgery in genitourinary tuberculosis. Indian J Urol 2008b;24(3):382–7.

Hemal AK. Laparoscopic retroperitoneal extirpative and reconstructive renal surgery. J Endourol 2011;25(2):209–16.

Merchant S, Bharati A, Merchant N. Tuberculosis of the genitourinary system—Urinary tract tuberculosis: Renal tuberculosis—Part I. Indian J Radiol Imaging 2013a;23(1):46–63.

Sakula A. Robert Koch: centenary of the discovery of the tubercle bacillus, 1882. Thorax 1982;37(4):246–51.

SCHISTOSOMIASIS

Doenhoff MJ, Cioli D, Utzinger J. Praziquantel: mechanisms of action, resistance and new derivatives for schistosomiasis. Curr Opin Infect Dis 2008;21:659–67.

Drugs for parasitic infections. 3rd ed. New Rochelle (NY): The Medical Letter; 2013.

Elliott DE. Schistosomiasis. Pathophysiology, diagnosis, and treatment. Gastroenterol Clin North Am 1996;25:599–625.

Fu CL, Odegaard JI, Herbert DR, et al. A novel mouse model of *Schistosoma haematobium* egg–induced immunopathology. PLoS Pathog 2012;8(3): e1002605.

Gryseels B, Polman K, Clerinx J, et al. Human schistosomiasis. Lancet 2006;368:1106–18.

Hsieh YJ, Fu CL, Hsieh MH. Helminth-induced interleukin-4 abrogates invariant natural killer T cell activation-associated clearance of bacterial infection. Infect Immun 2014;82(5):2087–97.

International Agency for Research on Cancer. *Schistosoma haematobium*. In: A review of human carcinogens: biological agents. Geneva: World Health Organization; 2011. p. 377–90.

King C. Schistosomiasis. In: Guerrant RL, Walker DH, Weller PF, editors. Tropical infectious diseases: principles, pathogens, and practice. 2nd ed. Philadelphia: Saunders; 2006. p. 1341–8.

Mahmoud AAF. Schistosomiasis. London: Imperial College Press; 2001.

Meltzer E, Artom G, Marva E, et al. Schistosomiasis among travelers: new aspects of an old disease. Emerg Infect Dis 2006;12:1696–700.

Mustacchi P. Schistosomiasis. In: Kufe D, Pollack R, Weichselbaum R, editors. Cancer medicine. 6th ed. Hamilton (Ontario, Canada): BC Decker; 2003.

Ray D, Nelson TA, Fu CL, et al. Transcriptional profiling of the bladder in urogenital schistosomiasis reveals pathways of inflammatory fibrosis and urothelial compromise. PLoS Negl Trop Dis 2012;6(11):e1912.

Shokeir AA, Hussein M. The urology of Pharaonic Egypt. BJU Int 1999; 84:755–61.

Stuiver PC. Acute schistosomiasis (Katayama fever). Br Med J (Clin Res Ed) 1984;288:221–2.

van der Werf MJ, de Vlas SJ, Brooker S, et al. Quantification of clinical morbidity associated with schistosome infection in sub-Saharan Africa. Acta Trop 2003;86(2–3):125–39.

OTHER PARASITIC INFECTIONS

Kappagoda S, Singh U, Blackburn BG. Antiparasitic therapy. Mayo Clin Proc 2011;86:561–83.

Taylor MJ, Hoerauf A, Bockarie M. Lymphatic filariasis and onchocerciasis. Lancet 2010;376:1175–85.

18   Basic Principles of Immunology and Immunotherapy in Urologic Oncology

Charles G. Drake, MD, PhD

Immunotherapy is emerging as an important treatment modality for multiple tumor types, including melanoma, lung cancer, and kidney cancer (Drake et al, 2014b). What is often forgotten as the field moves forward is the prominent role that immunotherapy has long played in bladder cancer (Brandau and Suttmann, 2007). In fact, the use of bacille Calmette-Guérin (BCG) in bladder cancer provides an ideal framework through which to understand immunotherapy for genitourinary (GU) cancers, although there are still many unanswered questions regarding its mechanism of action. In addition to BCG, which is a relatively nonspecific agent, immunotherapy for GU cancer has also involved the concept of inducing a specific anticancer immune response via a cancer vaccine. Vaccine approaches for prostate cancer and kidney cancer will be discussed at some length; more detailed clinical information is included in specific chapters dedicated to treatment. Finally, recent clinical and laboratory data support a novel approach to immunotherapy: in many patients, it appears that antigen-specific immune responses to cancer are restrained by a specific set of molecules expressed on CD4 and CD8 tumor-infiltrating lymphocytes (TILs) (Pardoll, 2012). These "checkpoint" molecules are critically important in restraining an antitumor immune response, so treatment with monoclonal antibodies blocking specific checkpoint molecules such as CTLA-4 (cytotoxic T-lymphocyte antigen–4) and PD-1 (programmed death–1) can lead to objective clinical responses (i.e., tumor shrinkage) in approximately 30% of patients with kidney cancer. These checkpoint molecules will be introduced, and some early clinical data highlighted as well.

BASIC IMMUNOLOGY

The Innate Immune System

For didactic purposes, the immune system is often parsed into two basic divisions, the **innate** and the **adaptive.** Evolutionarily, the innate immune system is the older of the two, and it is present in all vertebrate organisms. Functionally, the innate system recognizes its targets through repeated patterns associated with pathogens. These pathogen-associated molecular patterns (PAMPs) are recognized by a series of receptors related to Toll molecules in *Drosophila,* and are known as *Toll-like receptors* (TLRs) (Medzhitov and Janeway, 2000). The binding of PAMPs to TLRs is a fundamental immunologic mechanism though which the organism recognizes "danger."

Urologists who treat bladder cancer with intravesical BCG employ these innate immune immunologic mechanisms clinically; peptidoglycans in the BCG cell wall are canonical PAMPs, which bind to the Toll-like receptor TLR2 on innate immune cells resident in the bladder wall, serving to activate them and to initiate a cascading immune response (Brandau and Suttmann, 2007).

The initial immune cell that responds to an invading pathogen (or to instilled BCG) is most likely a tissue-resident macrophage (Table 18-1). Their name is derived from the Greek *makros* ("large") and *phagos* ("to eat"); macrophages are large cells that have evolved to engulf and destroy pathogens. Recognition of PAMPs by tissue-resident macrophages leads to their activation and subsequent secretion of chemical messengers known as *cytokines* and *chemokines* (see later), which in turn recruit and activate additional immune cells important in controlling a local infection. Again, BCG therapy for bladder cancer provides an excellent example, as both recognition by macrophages and the adherence of bacteria to urothelial cells lining the bladder results in the secretion of a series of chemokines and cytokines (Fig. 18-1). Some of these secreted cytokines attract a second cell type of major importance in the innate immune system, the neutrophil (also known as a *polymorphonuclear neutrophil* [PMN]). PMNs are the most abundant immune cell in the periphery and comprise approximately 60% of the white cells in the blood. These cells have a half-life measured in hours in the peripheral blood but can survive for days when present in the tissue at a site of infection or inflammation. In that sense, PMNs are the major cellular constituent of pus, and the hallmark of acute inflammation. One remarkable feature of neutrophil biology is their ability to emigrate from the circulation into tissues; this occurs when they squeeze between cells in the vascular endothelium as they follow a chemokine concentration gradient toward an area of infection within tissues. The hypersegmented configuration of their nucleus likely helps in this process by presenting a less formidable structural barrier to deformation. Like macrophages, neutrophils synthesize a variety of secretory granules that are released on PAMP recognition and that serve to facilitate destruction of an invading pathogen.

Cytokines and Chemokines

Cytokines and chemokines are small-molecule chemical messengers through which epithelial cells communicate with key cells in the immune system, and through which cells in the immune system

TABLE 18-1 Selected Cell Types Involved in the Immune Response to Genitourinary Cancers

CELL TYPE	IMMUNOLOGIC ROLE
Epithelial or urothelial cell	Secrete type I interferons as well as chemokines in response to stress, inflammation, viral infection, or danger signals mediated by pathogen-associated molecular patterns (PAMPs).
Macrophage	An innate immune cell that engulfs both pathogens and dead or dying cells. Secretes cytokines and chemokines to amplify or initiate an immune response.
Neutrophil (polymorphonuclear neutrophil ([PMN])	The most numerous of all innate immune cells in the peripheral blood, critically important in controlling bacterial infections. A collection of neutrophils (pus) is a characteristic of acute inflammation.
Dendritic cell (DC)	The cell type that bridges the innate and adaptive immune systems by presenting antigens (peptides) from dead or dying cells or debris to T cells in the lymph node. Like macrophages, DCs are activated by "danger" signals transmitted through PAMPs, or by cytokines in the microenvironment.
CD4 T cell	A "helper" T cell; can help CD8 T cells to kill or B cells to secrete antibodies.
CD8 T cell	A "killer" T cell; once activated, serially lyses specific targets.
Regulatory T cell (Treg)	A subset of CD4 T cells characterized by expression of the transcription factor FoxP3. Major role is to downregulate an ongoing immune response. In cancer, this is generally a detrimental function.

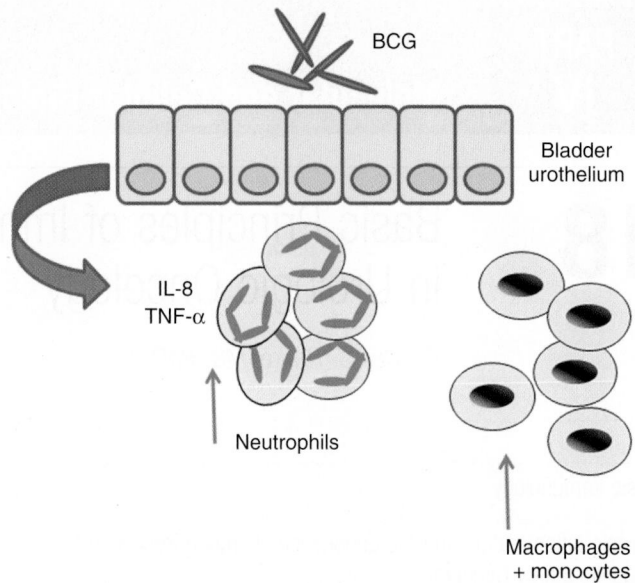

Figure 18-1. **Activation of the innate immune system by bacille Calmette-Guérin (BCG). IL-8, interleukin-8; TNF-α, tumor necrosis factor-α. (Modified from Brandau S, Suttmann H. Thirty years of BCG immunotherapy for non-muscle invasive bladder cancer: a success story with room for improvement. Biomed Pharmacother 2007;61:299–305.)**

communicate with one another. There are a large number of such molecules, and their nomenclature can be confusing. However, these molecules have a critical role in both acute and chronic inflammation, in the innate immune response, and in the adaptive immune response to cancer, so understanding a few key players is important. In this regard, the term *cytokine* is a rather general one, referring to any small immunologically relevant molecule secreted by a cell. Because many (but not all) of these molecules are involved in the migration of cells, the name derives from *cyto* ("cell") and *kinesis* ("movement"). Typical cytokines include the type I interferons (IFN-α and IFN-β), which are produced by virally infected or otherwise stressed epithelial cells. Immunologically, type I IFNs render epithelial cells more sensitive to immunologic attack, by increasing their recognition by cells of the adaptive immune system, and also by directly facilitating epithelial cell death through a number of mechanisms. As discussed later, intravesical instillation of IFN-α has been evaluated in a number of clinical trials in bladder cancer, with encouraging but somewhat mixed results (Askeland et al, 2012).

The term *chemokine* refers to a subset of cytokines whose primary function is to induce the migration of immune cells along a concentration gradient. The prototypic example is CXCL8, which can be secreted by most epithelial cell types, including bladder urothelium, in response to inflammatory signals. CXCL8 is a powerful chemoattractant for neutrophils and is likely important in the immune response to BCG in bladder cancer patients. The final subset of cytokines worth reviewing is a series of molecules originally described as facilitating communication between leukocytes, the interleukins. Interleukins were numbered in the order of their discovery, leading to an unfortunately complex situation in which an interleukin's designation usually has very little to do with its functional role or cell of origin. Interleukin-1 (IL-1), for example, is really more of an innate cytokine than an interleukin; it is secreted from stressed epithelial cells, serves to attract a variety of immune cells, and in the systemic circulation is one of the primary mediators of an elevated temperature in response to infection. On the other hand, there are two discrete sets of cytokines associated with a broad polarization in the adaptive (T cell–mediated) immune response. These are termed the "Th1" and "Th2" family of cytokines (Tables 18-1 and 18-2; Fig. 18-2). These cytokines are secreted by CD4 (helper) T cells in response to various stimuli and are critically important in polarizing the immune system in one of several broad directions (Weaver et al, 2006). In bladder cancer, these patterns of response are especially important, because a Th1 response is associated with a successful response to BCG treatment whereas a Th2 response is associated with BCG failure (de Reijke et al, 1996; Thalmann et al, 2000; Saint et al, 2001, 2002). Mechanistically, this skewing occurs as naive CD4 helper cells are activated (see Fig. 18-2). In an environment rich in IL-12, they differentiate into Th1 CD4 T cells and in turn secrete IL-2, tumor necrosis factor-α (TNF-α), and IFN-γ. These Th1 cytokines, in turn, help to activate CD8 (killer) T cells and are important in a successful antitumor response. Conversely, when naive CD4 T cells recognize their targets in the context of IL-4, they differentiate into a phenotype associated with chronic inflammation and antibody production and in turn secrete IL-4, IL-5, IL-10, and IL-13. It is interesting to note that in bladder cancer these cytokines can be detected systemically after BCG treatment, so elevated serum IL-2 after treatment is associated with a favorable outcome. These are important data, showing that the immune effects of BCG are not merely local and illustrating the point that activation of the immune system in a single organ can have detectable effects throughout the entire organism.

TABLE 18-2 Selected Cytokines, Chemokines, and Interleukins Involved in the Immune Response to Genitourinary Cancers

CYTOKINE	CELL OF ORIGIN	ROLE
TYPE I INTERFERONS		
IFN-α	Urothelial cells Epithelial cells Macrophages	A type I interferon typically secreted by virally infected cells or cells sensing "danger" through Toll-like receptor (TLR) engagement. Upregulates class I MHC and antigen processing, rendering cells more susceptible to immunologic attack.
IFN-β	Urothelial cells Epithelial cells Macrophages	Similar to IFN-α, another type I interferon.
CHEMOKINES		
CXCL8	Urothelial cells Epithelial cells	A chemokine that is a powerful chemoattractant for neutrophils.
IL-1	Epithelial cells Macrophages	Like IL-8, also attracts other immune cells such as monocytes from the circulation.
SLC	Stromal cells in lymph nodes	Also known as CXCL21, SLC serves to attract activated dendritic cells and T cells into the lymph nodes. It is sensed by the receptor CCR-7.
INTERLEUKINS AND Th1 AND Th2 POLARIZATION		
IL-12	Dendritic cells	A Th1-inducing cytokine; when naive CD4 T cells are activated in the presence of IL-12, they differentiate into Th1 cells.
IL-4	Dendritic cells Natural killer T cells	A Th2 cytokine; when naive CD4 T cells are activated in the presence of IL-4, they differentiate into Th2 cells.
IL-2, TNF-α, IFN-γ	Th1 cells (CD4 T cells)	Canonical cytokines secreted by Th1 cells; associated with a favorable response to BCG in bladder cancer. These cytokines are also associated with inducing CD8 (killer) T-cell function.
IL-4, IL-5, IL-10, IL-13	Th2 cells (CD4 T cells)	Canonical cytokines secreted by Th2 cells; associated with an unfavorable response to BCG in bladder cancer. These cytokines are also associated with the induction of antibody production.

BCG, bacille Calmette-Guérin; IFN, interferon; IL, interleukin; MHC, major histocompatibility complex; SLC, secondary lymphoid chemokine; TNF, tumor necrosis factor.

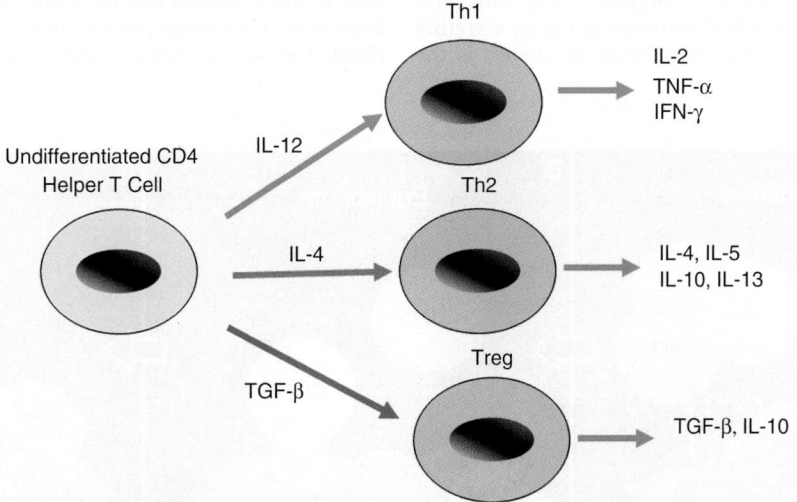

Figure 18-2. CD4 T-cell polarization and the Th1 and Th2 families of cytokines. IL, interleukin; TGF, transforming growth factor; TNF, tumor necrosis factor. (Modified from Weaver CT, Harrington LE, Mangan PR, et al. Th17: an effector CD4 T cell lineage with regulatory T-cell ties. Immunity 2006;24:677–88.)

The Adaptive Immune System

The adaptive immune system consists of CD4 (helper) T cells, CD8 (killer) T cells, and B cells. These cells are recruited into an immune response in response to activation of the innate immune system. They are important in two key facets of the immune response—its specificity and its ability to "remember" antigen encounters and respond more robustly when an antigen is encountered again in the future. Before we expound on those properties, it is important to understand how information from the innate immune system is transferred to the adaptive immune system. This transfer depends on a unique cell type known as the *dendritic cell* (DC), which serves as a bridge between an innate and an adaptive immune response. DCs get their name from their long and fine cytoplasmic projections, which microscopically resemble nerve cells. Functionally, DCs are scattered throughout the peripheral tissues, as exemplified by Langerhans cells in the skin. They spend the majority of their life span at rest, continually sampling their microenvironment, taking in fluid and protein antigens through the process of pinocytosis. In the absence of an activating or "danger" signal, DCs remain in situ and in a quiescent state. A danger signal can come in the form of cytokines such as TNF-α secreted from innate immune cells such as macrophages, or through direct contact with bacterial products through pattern receptors (TLRs) on DCs. When DCs are activated, a remarkable transition takes place. First, they cease taking in antigens, because their new role will be to present the antigens they have already taken up to T and B cells. Therefore their dendrites are retracted and the cells develop a more compact morphology. Second, they upregulate cell surface molecules important for presenting the antigens they are carrying to T cells. These include major histocompatibility complex molecules, which bind 9 to 12 amino acid peptide antigens in their grooves for interacting with specific receptors on T cells (TCRs), as well as a set of molecules designed to optimally stimulate T cells; these are called *costimulatory molecules* and include B7-1, B7-2, and others. Finally, DCs must solve a spatial problem: resting lymphocytes (T cells and B cells) reside in the secondary lymphoid structures—that is, in the lymph nodes—whereas resting DCs are situated in the tissues. Thus, DCs must migrate into the lymphatic system and enter into the lymph nodes through afferent lymphatic vessels. This is accomplished via chemotaxis; activated DCs follow a gradient of secondary lymphoid chemokine (SLC) using a receptor known as CCR7 into the lymph nodes. Once in the lymph nodes, DCs interact with (and activate) specific CD4, CD8, and B lymphocytes, facilitating the transfer of information from the innate to the adaptive immune system.

Thus, a CD4 T cell is activated when an antigen-presenting DC presents its cognate (specific) peptide antigen (usually 11 amino acids long) in the context of a class II major histocompatibility complex (MHC) molecule. These are helper cells; they either help CD8 T cells to become fully activated and exert their lytic function or assist B cells in making antibodies. As described earlier, CD4 T-cell responses fall into several basic categories, including a Th1 response, which serves to fully activate CD8 (killer cells), and a Th2 response, which serves to help B cells mature into antibody-secreting plasma cells. An additional CD4 T-cell subtype of interest is the

regulatory T cell (Treg). These cells suppress adaptive immune responses and appear to play a role in preventing a successful adaptive Th1- or CD8-driven anticancer response (Curiel, 2008). The origin of Tregs is complex; a population of "natural" Tregs arises de novo in the course of T-cell development in the thymus, and a second population is "induced" when naive CD4 T cells recognize their antigen in a microenvironment that is low in proinflammatory signals and rich in transforming growth factor-β (TGF-β) (see Fig. 18-2). The relative contribution of these two types of Tregs to the progression of GU cancers in humans is unclear; however, recent laboratory data point to a critical role for natural, thymus-derived Tregs (Savage et al, 2013).

Perhaps the most fascinating adaptive immune cell is the CD8 T cell. These cells recognize their specific cognate antigen 9 amino-acid long peptides in the context of class I MHC, which is present on almost all cell types but which is upregulated in the context of inflammation and on virally infected cells. When a specific CD8 T cell recognizes its target, it secretes a series of molecules that result in destruction of that cell type. This killing process is remarkably specific; in the autoimmune disease type 1 diabetes, CD8 T cells can lyse beta cells in the pancreas while leaving immediately adjacent alpha cells completely intact. The mechanism of killing is also exquisite; CD8 T cells employ multiple molecular mechanisms to induce their target cells to commit suicide—that is, to undergo programmed cell death or apoptosis. Finally, CD8 T cells are serial killers, able to lyse multiple specific targets in a sequential manner. As discussed later, the major goal of cancer vaccines is to activate antigen-specific CD8 T cells and to thereby eliminate an evolving tumor.

The Immune Editing Hypothesis

Before moving forward with a discussion of how the immune system may be manipulated to treat GU cancers, it is worthwhile to consider the immune system's baseline role in either the promotion or the elimination of cancer. With the exception of certain virally mediated tumors that occur most commonly in immunocompromised individuals, most human cancers develop in immunologically intact hosts. As tumorigenesis proceeds from low-grade or localized disease to distant metastases, an interaction between the host immune system and the tumor mass occurs. This process has been well characterized in a number of animal models and can be divided into three distinct stages (Dunn et al, 2004) (Fig. 18-3). In

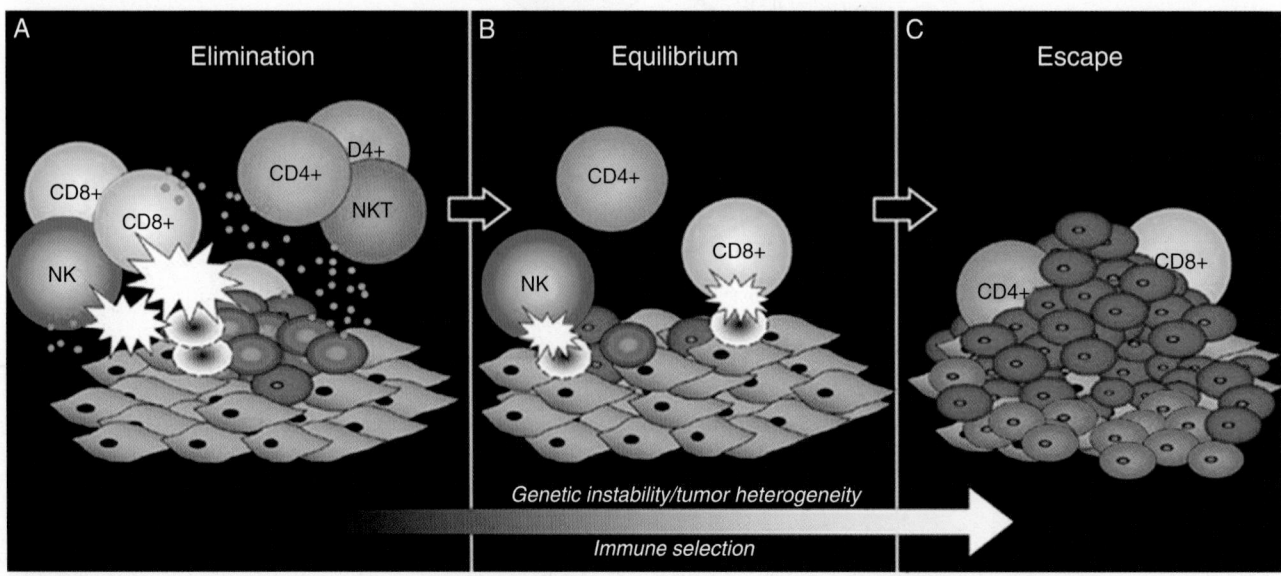

Figure 18-3. **A-C, The immune editing hypothesis. NK, natural killer; NKT, natural killer T cell. (From Dunn GP, Old LJ, Schreiber RD. The immunobiology of cancer immunosurveillance and immunoediting. Immunity 2004;21:137–48.)**

the first stage of the process, early tumors are recognized by the immune system in a productive, proactive way, leading to **elimination** of small, clinically undetectable masses. Elimination is most likely mediated by a concerted effort between the innate (macrophages and DCs) and the adaptive immune system. As tumors progress, they acquire genetic and epigenetic alterations that render an antitumor immune response less efficacious. Therefore in the next phase of tumor–immune system interactions, tumors are able to exist in a sort of **equilibrium** with the host immune response, with progression slowed by an ongoing immune response, but in which tumors can no longer be successfully eliminated. Equilibrium may persist for a significant period of time, and some tumors may remain in the equilibrium stage for the life of the host. Eventually, though, many tumors proceed to **escape** the host immune response and become clinically apparent. The molecular mechanisms involved in the escape phase are multiple and include downregulation of tumor antigens against which a host response is directed (Drake et al, 2006), downregulation of MHC molecules, and the induction or expansion of Tregs that actively inhibit an immune response. The three phases of tumor-host interactions (elimination, equilibrium, and escape) collectively form the immune editing hypothesis, which serves as a valuable framework through which to understand the immune response to cancer. Indeed, subversion of a productive host antitumor response is now designated as one of the hallmarks of cancer (Hanahan and Weinberg, 2011).

KEY POINTS: BASIC IMMUNOLOGY

- An immune response begins with an innate response that is swift but relatively nonspecific then progresses to include the adaptive immune system, which is characterized by both specificity and memory.
- For an antitumor immune response, a Th1 response dominated by IFN-γ, IL-2, and TNF-α is desired.
- CD4+ regulatory T cells (Tregs) inhibit an adaptive immune response.
- The immune editing hypothesis explains how early tumors can be recognized and eliminated by the immune system, whereas clinically evident tumors must escape immune recognition to evolve.

CHRONIC INFLAMMATION AND THE ENDOGENOUS IMMUNE RESPONSE TO GENITOURINARY CANCERS

Although the immune editing hypothesis would leave one with the impression that antitumor immune responses are, in general, beneficial, those data need to be considered along with a great deal of apparently contradictory data suggesting that inflammation can promote tumor progression (Balkwill et al, 2005; de Visser et al, 2006). Human and animal studies indicate that inflammation has a clear role in the development of bladder cancer (Michaud, 2007) and likely plays a role in the development of prostate cancer, as well (De Marzo et al, 2007).

Chronic Inflammation and the Immune Response to Bladder Cancer

Among the various GU malignancies, bladder cancer provides the strongest evidence for a link between chronic inflammation and carcinogenesis (Michaud, 2007). The evidence linking inflammatory schistosomiasis infections to bladder cancer is particularly robust, and *Schistosoma haematobium* has been classified as a known carcinogen by the International Agency for Research on Cancer. Epidemiologically, countries with high rates of endemic infection have high rates of bladder cancer, and high levels of infestation are

associated with a squamous cell phenotype (Mostafa et al, 1999). Other sources of bladder inflammation that have been linked to carcinogenesis include chronic urinary tract infections (Kantor et al, 1984), chronic indwelling catheters (Groah et al, 2002), and cystitis induced by cyclophosphamide treatment (Talar-Williams et al, 1996). The cellular and molecular mechanisms by which chronic bladder infection leads to cancer have not been fully elucidated but likely involve mechanisms similar to those described in other cancers (Mantovani et al, 2008)—that is, dysfunctional (M2) macrophages that produce immune suppressive cytokines, a subset of myeloid cells that suppress an active immune response (myeloid suppressor cells [MSCs]) (Ostrand-Rosenberg and Sinha, 2009), and a polarization of the adaptive immune response toward a Th2 and Treg phenotype.

Once bladder tumors develop, the immune editing hypothesis (see Fig. 18-3) would suggest that early tumors might be recognized by the immune system and eliminated. That hypothesis is supported by data showing that CD8 T-cell infiltration correlates with outcome in patients with muscle-invasive bladder cancer (Sharma et al, 2007). Obviously a successful CD8-mediated antitumor response does not occur in all patients, and recent data describe an important mechanism by which bladder tumors may "escape" immune recognition (Sharpe et al, 2007; Zou and Chen 2008; Pardoll, 2012). This occurs through the interaction between immune checkpoint molecules expressed on cancer-specific T cells and their checkpoint ligands, expressed on either tumor cells or tumor-associated macrophages (Fig. 18-4). This interaction is profoundly inhibitory to T-cell efficacy, attenuating proliferation as well as effector function. In this regard, several tissue-based studies showed that the epithelial cells in bladder cancer express the immune checkpoint ligand PD-L1 (Inman et al, 2007; Nakanishi et al, 2007; Xylinas et al, 2014). In the first of these studies, PD-L1 expression was noted in approximately 15% to 35% of patients, and expression was associated with increased tumor grade (Nakanishi et al, 2007). It is interesting to note that in these patients, PD-L1 expression was more closely associated with prognosis than was World Health Organization (WHO) grade, pointing to a functional role for PD-1/PD-L1 interaction in bladder cancer progression. A second, related, study confirmed the relationship between PD-L1 expression and high-grade tumors and further demonstrated that PD-L1 expression was associated with tumor infiltration by immune cells (Inman et al, 2007). This group also showed that PD-L1 was highly expressed in BCG-induced granulomas in patients progressing on therapy, suggesting a possible escape mechanism. Mechanistically, these data support a model known as "adaptive immune resistance" (Fig. 18-5), which explains how PD-L1 expression may be a critical mechanism by which tumors evade the immune response (Topalian et al, 2012a). In this model, mutations arising as a tumor progresses lead to an adaptive immune response, characterized by CD8 T-cell recognition. These CD8 T cells migrate to the tumor, and in the course of their effector function they secrete the cytokine IFN-γ. IFN-γ is a powerful inducer of PD-L1 expression in both tumor cells and epithelial cells, and it is these induced PD-L1 molecules on tumor cells that interact with PD-1 on the infiltrating CD8 T cells to effectively curtail their antitumor effector function. These data would suggest that a monoclonal antibody that blocks either PD-1 or PD-L1 could potentially lead to objective tumor responses in patients with bladder cancer—a hypothesis that is currently being tested in several ongoing phase 1 and phase 2 trials.

The Immune Microenvironment in Kidney Cancer

Unlike with bladder and prostate cancer, a link between chronic inflammation and kidney cancer is less clear and is only weakly suggested by the associations of kidney cancer with proinflammatory risk factors such as smoking or obesity (Chow et al, 2010). Regarding the adaptive immune response to kidney cancer, data are somewhat conflicting as to whether CD4 T-cell infiltration is a positive or negative prognostic feature in renal cell carcinoma (RCC) patients. One early study reported that CD4 T-cell infiltration is associated with an improved outcome (in the context of IFN-α

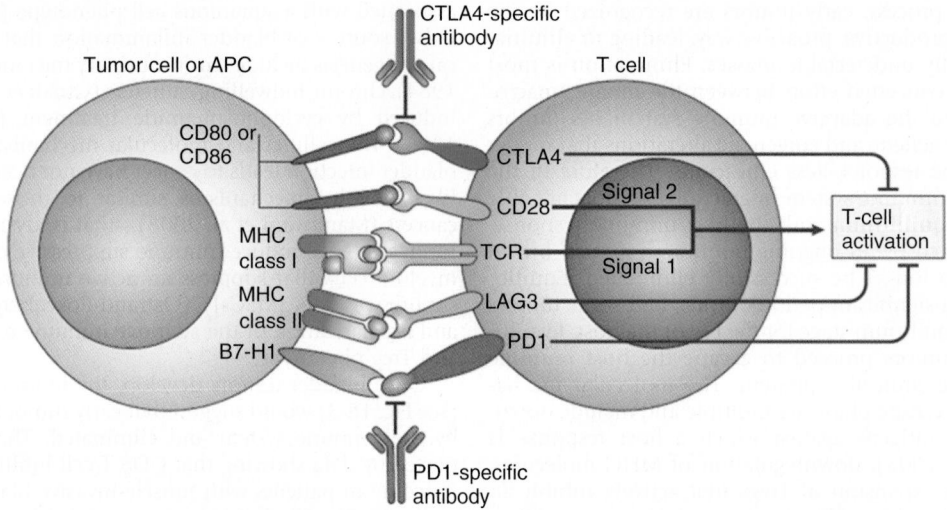

Figure 18-4. Immune checkpoint molecules. APC, antigen-presenting cell; MHC, major histocompatibility complex. **(From Drake CG. Prostate cancer as a model for tumour immunotherapy. Nat Rev Immunol 2010;10:580–93.)**

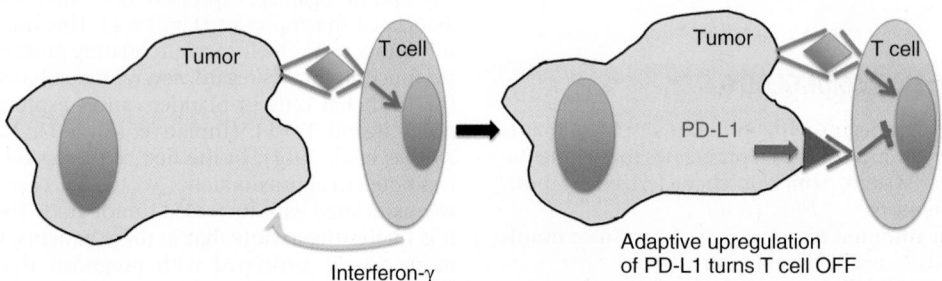

Figure 18-5. Adaptive immune resistance.

treatment) (Igarashi et al, 2002), but a more recent study suggested the opposite correlation (Hotta et al, 2011). Because neither study specifically examined whether the CD4 TILs were of the regulatory phenotype, differences in the number and/or function of CD4 Tregs could potentially explain that apparent contradiction. In this regard, as is the case in many other tumor types, tumor infiltration with Tregs has been described in RCC (Attig et al, 2009), and an association between both distant relapse and decreased overall survival with Treg infiltration has been reported in patients with clear cell RCC (Kang et al, 2013). Kidney tumors are also commonly infiltrated with CD8 T cells, suggesting an ongoing and potentially effective antitumor response, and the clonal nature of these infiltrating cells suggests an antigen-specific response (Sittig et al, 2013). As is the case for bladder cancer (Sharma et al, 2007), infiltration with proliferating CD8 T cells has been associated with an improved outcome in RCC (Nakano et al, 2001). Also similar to findings with bladder cancer, adaptive immune resistance is likely to play an important role in immune escape in kidney cancer, because PD-L1 expression has been associated with poor outcome (Thompson et al, 2007). Not unexpectedly, the CD8 T cells that infiltrate RCC express PD-1, suggesting that blocking PD-1 or PD-L1 in RCC could lead to clinical benefit. Several recent clinical trials support this concept, as is further described later.

Chronic Inflammation and the Immune Response to Prostate Cancer

Long before the appearance of clinical symptoms, the prostate microenvironment is frequently infiltrated by several types of inflammatory cells including innate cells such as macrophages and adaptive cells such as T and B cells. This baseline inflammation is likely tumor promoting, and accumulating data from several groups support a model in which chronic prostatic inflammation drives the development of cancer (De Marzo et al, 2007). Multiple lines of evidence support this hypothesis. First, chronic inflammation in the prostate gland is frequently focused in the peripheral zone, the region in which more than 90% of tumors arise (McNeal et al, 1988). Second, epidemiologic studies show that Western nations, in which chronic prostatic inflammation is endemic, have a significantly increased incidence of prostate cancer as compared with Asian populations, in which inflammation is less prevalent (Sfanos and De Marzo, 2012). Finally, and perhaps most convincing, are data surrounding a prostatic lesion known as *prostatic inflammatory atrophy* (PIA) (De Marzo et al, 1999), a region characterized by flattened but proliferating epithelial cells and associated inflammatory cells. Morphologic studies showed that regions of PIA are located geographically proximal to high-grade prostatic intraepithelial neoplasia (PIN) lesions (Putzi and De Marzo, 2000), suggesting a possible etiologic link between PIA and the eventual development of cancer.

The adaptive T-cell environment of prostate cancer seems to be dominated by Tregs, which have been described both in the gland itself (Miller et al, 2006; Fox et al, 2007; Sfanos et al, 2008) and in the periphery (Yokokawa et al, 2008). A role for Tregs may extend even to metastatic lesions; recent studies by the Zhao group showed an increased prevalence of functional Tregs in the bone marrow of patients with prostate cancer (Zhao et al, 2012). In keeping with the notion of immunosuppression in prostate cancer, surprising data from both humans (Kiniwa et al, 2007) and animals

(Shafer-Weaver et al, 2009) suggest that in prostate cancer, CD8 T cells can also have a regulatory phenotype. In perhaps the most convincing of these studies, the McNeel group was able to show that regulatory CD8 T cells in the peripheral blood were sufficiently suppressive to mask an antigen-specific T-cell response driven by vaccination (Olson et al, 2012). Finally, as in other GU cancers, there is some evidence that the PD-1/PD-L1 axis may restrain an adaptive T-cell response to prostate cancer, because the CD8 T cells that infiltrate the prostate gland are clearly PD-1 positive (Sfanos et al, 2009). However, PD-1 blockade as a therapeutic maneuver for prostate cancer may be diminished by the finding that the tumor cells themselves do not appear to express PD-L1, suggesting either an intrinsic inability to upregulate the molecule or an absence of productive (IFN-γ) mediated inflammation. Taken together, these data suggest that prostate cancer develops in an environment characterized by chronic inflammation as well as a nonproductive adaptive CD4 and CD8 T-cell response (Bronte et al, 2005; Gannon et al, 2009).

> ## KEY POINTS: CHRONIC INFLAMMATION AND THE ENDOGENOUS IMMUNE RESPONSE TO GENITOURINARY CANCERS
>
> - Bladder cancer may be promoted by chronic inflammation initiated by infection or other stimuli.
> - In kidney cancer, there is good evidence for an ongoing adaptive, T cell–mediated response, but that response is, in general, nonproductive.
> - Prostate cancer may also be initiated through chronic inflammation.
> - Expression of immune checkpoint molecules on TILs may attenuate the adaptive immune response to GU tumors.

IMMUNOTHERAPY FOR GENITOURINARY CANCERS

Bacille Calmette-Guérin in Bladder Cancer

The mechanism of action of BCG provides an excellent framework through which to understand the course of an induced immune response, an understanding that will be useful in appreciating the mechanisms of other immunotherapy modalities described later (Brandau and Suttmann, 2007) (Fig. 18-6). The process begins with the instillation of 1 to 5×10^8 viable mycobacteria into the bladder. Most of these will be washed out with the first postinstillation void, but a significant fraction will adhere to the urothelial cells lining the bladder via a fibronectin attachment protein (Kavoussi et al, 1990). Repeated patterns (PAMPs) on the bacteria stimulate the urothelial cells to secrete cytokines, likely through the Toll-like receptors TLR-2 and TLR-4. Direct activation of resident macrophages and DCs by BCG components is also likely but has been less well described. The BCG-stimulated urothelial cells initiate a cascading immune response by secreting the chemokine IL-8 (among many others), and IL-8 is a powerful neutrophil attractant. TNF-α is also secreted, and in this setting this Th1 family cytokine recruits and activates macrophages. A few hours after BCG instillation, a wave of neutrophils migrates into bladder wall (de Boer et al, 1991). This wave of neutrophils is characteristic of acute inflammation, and neutrophils clear residual bacilli by secreting cytotoxic granules in addition to releasing a series of cytokines that help activate DC to potentiate the eventual involvement of the adaptive immune system. The next step in this inflammatory cascade occurs over several weeks as an adaptive immune response, primarily CD4 T cell driven, is recruited to the bladder. Although the precise mechanisms through which CD4 T cells are involved have not been well documented in bladder cancer, this most likely occurs in the same manner as it does in other immune responses: DCs are activated by neutrophil- and urothelial cell–derived cytokines (in addition to bacterial products) and traffic to the draining lymph nodes, where they present antigens to CD4 T cells to activate specific lymphocytes. The antigenic targets of CD4 T cells during BCG therapy for bladder cancer have not been well described but likely include bacterial

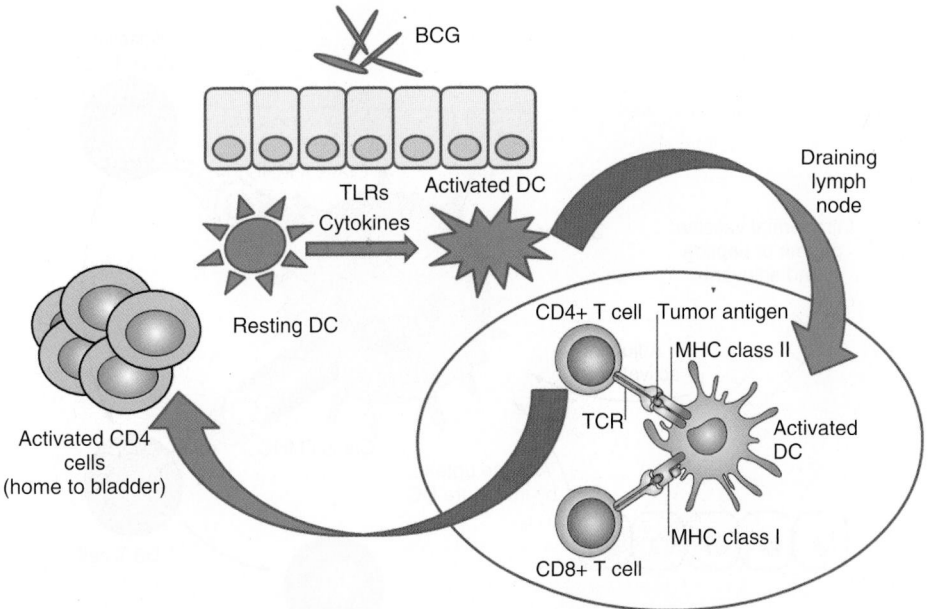

Figure 18-6. Bacille Calmette-Guérin (BCG) and an adaptive immune response. DC, dendritic cell; MHC, major histocompatibility complex; TCR, T-cell receptor; TLRs, Toll-like receptors. (Modified from Brandau S, Suttmann H. Thirty years of BCG immunotherapy for non-muscle invasive bladder cancer: a success story with room for improvement. Biomed Pharmacother 2007;61:299–305; and Drake CG. Prostate cancer as a model for tumour immunotherapy. Nat Rev Immunol 2010;10:580–93.)

antigens as well as tissue- and tumor-specific antigens. Nevertheless, an adaptive immune response has been demonstrated to be required for successful BCG therapy of bladder cancer in laboratory studies (Ratliff et al, 1987), and the presence of CD4 T cell–rich granulomas in BCG-treated patients provides evidence that this may be the case in humans as well (Prescott et al, 1992). As mentioned earlier, the adaptive immune response is capable of generating long-lived memory T cells, which may persist for the life of a vaccinated patient. The generation of memory CD4 cells by BCG treatment of bladder cancer has not been well studied in patients, but their induction is strongly suggested by the significant fraction (approximately 50%) of patients whose non–muscle invasive disease remains in remission for years after BCG therapy. In summary, successful immunotherapy for bladder cancer represents a typical immune response, initially characterized by activation and involvement of the innate immune system (neutrophils and macrophages), which then transitions to an adaptive immune response driven by CD4 T cells polarized to secrete Th1 cytokines (IL-2, TNF-α, and IFN-γ), followed by eventual consolidation in the form of long-lived T-cell memory.

CANCER VACCINES

Like BCG, a "cancer vaccine" also aims to raise a T-cell response against cancer (Fig. 18-7). When a vaccine is injected into the skin, the components of the vaccine known as *pathogen-associated molecular patterns* (Medzhitov and Janeway, 2000) activate resting DCs and program them to migrate to a local lymph node. Thus, in general a vaccine incudes some component(s) intended to activate DCs, although the precise substances employed vary among different vaccines. Another common term for these activating components is *adjuvant*, because they "add" immunogenicity to the protein or peptide components of a vaccine. The other key component of a vaccine is a target protein or proteins that are expected to be relatively overexpressed in a tumor relative to normal tissue. The choice of vaccine antigen(s) is somewhat empirical and, like adjuvant choice, varies widely among approaches. Once a resting DC has been loaded with antigen, has been activated, and has migrated to

a lymph node—it then displays fragments of antigen in the form of small peptides. Cellular recognition of these small peptide fragments (antigens) is complex; as introduced earlier, these peptides are not presented alone, but instead are bound within a genetically diverse set of host molecules collectively encoded by a set of genes within the MHC. Specific receptors on CD4 and CD8 T cells recognize a structure composed of both MHC molecules and a specific peptide. To increase specificity, simple recognition (a good fit) is insufficient for full T-cell activation; T cells must also receive additional costimulatory signals provided by mature DCs to proliferate and acquire effector function. In the case of CD8 T cells, the principal hoped-for effector function is the ability to lyse target cells expressing the same MHC-peptide complex that served to activate them—that is, their target antigen. For CD4 T cells, a Th1 response is desired. Once fully activated, CD8 T cells leave the lymph node and travel widely through the host in search of their targets. In the case of therapeutic cancer vaccines, the hoped-for goal is a clinically apparent reduction in tumor burden.

Vaccines for Kidney Cancer

Although an in-depth discussion of all the cancer vaccine approaches in GU cancers is beyond the scope of this chapter, several vaccines are highlighted. The chosen examples illustrate key immunologic principles, as well as the clinical challenges inherent in developing immunotherapy. In that regard, one interesting vaccine approach for kidney cancer focuses on targeting multiple, carefully selected antigens with a fairly simple adjuvant. To select relevant antigens, resected kidney tumors from a series of patients expressing the common class I MHC allele HLA-A2 were isolated, and the cell surface peptides residing in class I MHC molecules were eluted and analyzed with use of mass spectrometry (Walter et al, 2012). This approach identified a set of nine tumor-associated peptides, which were used to design a vaccine incorporating granulocyte-macrophage colony-stimulating factor (GM-CSF) as an adjuvant (Immatics Biotechnologies, Tübingen, Germany). GM-CSF is a strong inducer of DC migration, but perhaps less robust than several of the TLR agonists in terms of inducing DC activation. In the phase 1 study of this agent (IMA901), 28 patients with RCC were enrolled; because

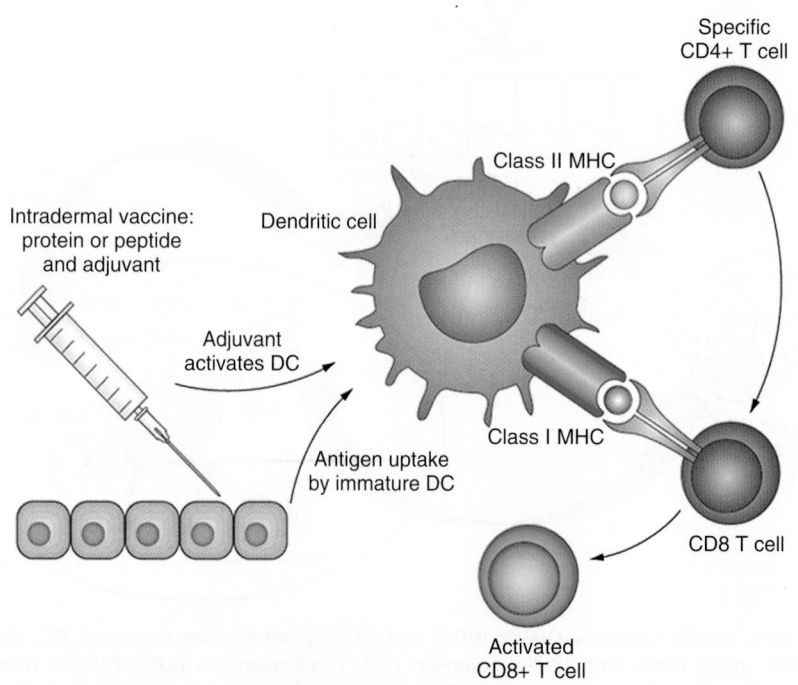

Figure 18-7. Cancer vaccines. DC, dendritic cell; MHC, major histocompatibility complex. (From Drake CG, Lipson EJ, Brahmer JR. Breathing new life into immunotherapy: review of melanoma, lung and kidney cancer. Nat Rev Clin Oncol 2014b;11:24-37.)

the peptides in the vaccine are presented only by the MHC class I allele HLA-A2, patients were required to be A2 positive. These patients received up to eight multipeptide vaccinations, each preceded by GM-CSF as an adjuvant. The vaccine was well tolerated, with no grade 3 or 4 adverse events reported. At a 3-month follow-up point, a single patient showed a partial response, 16 patients had disease progression, and 11 had stable disease. Immune responses to the targeted peptides were detected in several of the treated patients (Walter et al, 2012). To improve the clinical activity of this kidney cancer vaccine, investigators made use of well-established data showing that low doses of the alkylating agent cyclophosphamide have vaccine-potentiating immune effects (North, 1982); these effects are at least partially mediated by the depletion of the Tregs that turn off an immune response(Machiels et al, 2001; Wada et al, 2009). In a randomized phase 2 trial, 68 HLA-A2–positive patients with RCC were randomly assigned either to vaccine or to vaccine preceded by a single immunomodulatory dose of intravenous cyclophosphamide (300 mg/m^2). As noted in many other cancer vaccine trials, objective tumor regressions were rare, with a single confirmed partial response among 64 patients. Subsequent immunologic analyses showed an increased T-cell response to the targeted peptides and verified that low-dose cyclophosphamide depletes Tregs in humans. There was a trend toward improved overall survival in the vaccine plus low-dose cyclophosphamide arm (hazard ratio [HR] 0.57, $P = .090$), but this was not statistically significant. Despite these less than optimal phase 2 results, a randomized phase 3 trial was initiated in which IMA901 was added to a first-line tyrosine kinase inhibitor in patients with metastatic RCC (NCT01265901). Enrollment of 330 patients to this trial was completed in 2012. A second illustrative vaccine approach involves autologous vaccines, in which antigens are derived from a patient's individual tumor lysate or whole cells. Such vaccines have been tested in RCC and lung cancer (Simons et al, 1997; Eager and Nemunaitis, 2005), but autologous vaccine approaches are complicated by the variability and complexity in generating a vaccine from variable amounts of patient material. To overcome these challenges, a novel approach was developed, whereby a vaccine was generated using RNA extracted from patient-derived tumor material rather than tumor lysate or cells (AGS-003, Argos Therapeutics, Durham, NC). With this approach, substantial quantities of vaccine can be manufactured using a relatively small amount of resected tumor. Rather than relying on the patient's endogenous DCs (which are often defective or dysfunctional) (Gabrilovich et al, 1997), the AGS-003 vaccine uses autologous DCs generated ex vivo through maturation of immature monocytes in the presence of the cytokines IL-4 and GM-CSF (Palucka et al, 2005). To manufacture AGS-003, patients undergo leukapheresis, and DCs are cultured. Simultaneously, tumor RNA is prepared and used to transfect those autologous DCs to generate a mature, cell-based vaccine, which is then frozen and stored for repeated intranodal injections. In a phase 2 trial using the AGS-003 vaccine, the incorporation of sunitinib, a standard therapy for RCC, was shown to result in proimmunogenic properties (Figlin et al, 2012). A phase 3 trial of AGS-003 is currently in progress; this trial will randomly assign 600 patients with metastatic high-risk RCC to receive either ongoing treatment with the standard-of-care tyrosine kinase inhibitor sunitinib, or one cycle (6 weeks) of sunitinib followed by AGS-003 coadministered along with sunitinib (NCT01582672). The primary end point of the study is progression-free survival (PFS), and enrollment has not yet been completed. Taken together, these two vaccine approaches for kidney cancer illustrate some basic principles of cancer vaccines but highlight the notion that vaccination alone is unlikely to achieve objective clinical responses in the majority of patients treated.

Vaccines for Prostate Cancer

As highlighted earlier, an adaptive immune response depends on DCs, and a cancer vaccine, like any other vaccine, depends on the presence of a population of host DCs that are numerically and functionally competent. As noted previously, this is often not the case in cancer patients, in whom DCs are dysfunctional

(Gabrilovich, 2004). One approach to overcoming DC dysfunction is to generate new DCs outside of the patient's tolerogenic environment. In prostate cancer, this approach is exemplified by Sipuleucel-T, which was the first cancer vaccine approved by the U.S. Food and Drug Administration (FDA) for the treatment of patients with a solid tumor (Kantoff et al, 2010a). Sipuleucel-T is individually manufactured for each patient with prostate cancer in a process that includes multiple steps. Briefly, patients undergo leukapheresis; peripheral blood mononuclear cells (PBMCs) are extracted and then incubated with PAP2024, a fusion protein that links the antigen prostatic acid phosphatase (PAP) to GM-CSF. After approximately 36 hours of incubation, cells are washed and resuspended for infusion back into the patient. In this approach, the GM-CSF serves as the adjuvant that helps to activate DCs. The process is repeated three times at 2-week intervals (Sonpavde et al, 2012). Of interest, the final Sipuleucel-T product is heterogeneous and includes mature antigen-presenting cells (APCs) as well as other cell types, including T cells, B cells, and natural killer cells (Sonpavde et al, 2012). Once infused, the autologous ex vivo–activated APCs are thought to prime PAP-specific CD4+ and CD8+ T cells in a manner similar to a classical vaccine-mediated prime-boost regimen, in which the first infusion primes the immune system and subsequent infusions boost the response (Drake, 2010). Recently, a combined analysis of immunologic data from several phase 3 trials of Sipuleucel-T (D9901, D9902A, and IMPACT) was completed (Sheikh et al, 2013). These combined data demonstrated that APC activation in the infused product occurred with the initial dose and increased with subsequent doses. Furthermore, antigen-specific T-cell activity (proliferation) was detectable in preculture cells obtained at weeks 2 and 4 (but not week 0). Finally, T-cell activation–associated cytokines were also noted in the second and third doses of Sipuleucel-T, supporting the idea that the first infusion of activated, antigen-loaded APCs primes T cells in patients in vivo. These results also show that the second and third doses of Sipuleucel-T are biologically different from the first and that each dose contains progressively more activated APCs and possibly a greater proportion of antigen-specific T cells with the capacity to recognize and kill prostate cancer cells. Finally, the authors demonstrated a positive correlation between overall survival and cumulative APC activation and antigen-specific immune responses. Taken together, these analyses showed that Sipuleucel-T induces an antigen-specific immune response and that the response appears to be associated with a survival benefit in treated patients.

A second prostate cancer vaccine that has reached late stages of clinical development is ProstVac-VF (Bavarian Nordic, Washington, DC) (Madan et al, 2009). This vaccine approach is quite different from the peptide- or cell-based vaccines discussed previously and relies on the incorporation of a target antigen into a virus to specifically activate the immune system (Fig. 18-8). The antigen chosen for this approach is prostate-specific antigen (PSA), and the viral backbone comes from poxviruses, which are related to the vaccine used in the successful worldwide eradication of smallpox. This technology has been honed over several decades, and the iteration in a phase 3 trial includes a number of important modifications designed to optimize immunogenicity. First, the vaccine involves a heterologous prime-boost regimen, in which the initial vaccine is based on a modified vaccinia Ankara (MVA) backbone, followed by a series of booster vaccines with a fowlpox backbone. This is necessary because the immune response to the MVA backbone is quite robust, so boosting with an identical vaccine is limited by the host's immune antibody response to the viral backbone itself. To further increase immunogenicity, the vaccine was engineered to incorporate a triad of costimulatory molecules designed to generate DCs with an enhanced potential for T-cell activation (Hodge et al, 1999). Finally, and similar to IMA901 in RCC, administration of GM-CSF at the vaccination site is used to help recruit local DCs and enhance antigen presentation. In patients, poxvirus vectors most likely infect epithelial cells, a proportion of which undergo cell death. Cellular debris, including encoded antigens, are then taken up by nearby immature DCs, which, when appropriately activated, can present these antigens to CD4+ and CD8+ T cells in a

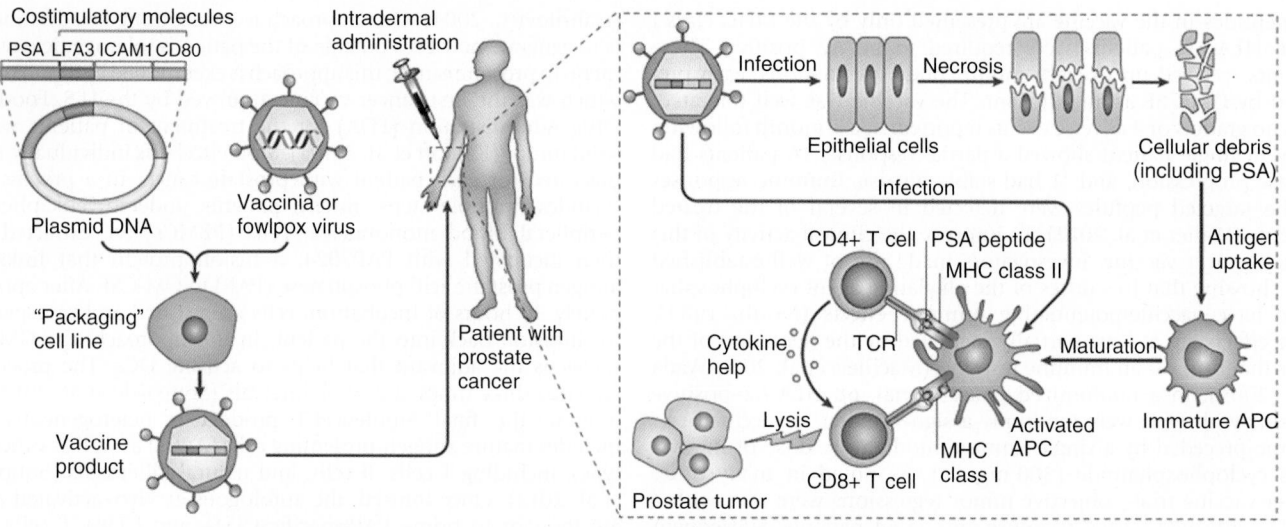

Figure 18-8. Virus-based cancer vaccines (ProstVac VF). APC, antigen-presenting cell; MHC, major histocompatibility complex; PSA, prostate-specific antigen; TCR, T-cell receptor. (From Drake CG. Prostate cancer as a model for tumour immunotherapy. Nat Rev Immunol 2010;10:580–93.)

proinflammatory context (Drake, 2010). Direct infection of DCs, particularly the Langerhans cells in the skin, is another mechanism by which poxvirus vectors can prime an immune response (Drake, 2010). The end result of ProstVac treatment is postulated to be activation and proliferation of PSA-specific CD8 and CD4 T cells, which was demonstrated in early correlative studies. In contrast to Sipuleucel-T (Sheikh et al, 2013), ProstVac-VF doesn't appear to prime much of an antibody response; indeed, antibodies specific for PSA have not been reported with this agent. Based on a potential survival benefit shown in a randomized phase 2 trial (Kantoff et al, 2010b), an international randomized phase 3 trial of ProstVac-VF was initiated (NCT01322490). This trial has enrolled 1200 patients and randomized them to placebo, ProstVac-VF plus subcutaneous GM-CSF, or ProstVac-VF alone. The primary end point of the trial is overall survival, and enrollment was limited to men with asymptomatic or minimally symptomatic metastatic castration-resistant prostate cancer (mCRPC) who are chemotherapy naive.

Genitourinary Tumors

GVAX Prostate (Aduro BioTech, Berkeley, CA) is a cell-based immunotherapy based on irradiated allogeneic tumor cell lines genetically engineered to secrete GM-CSF (Dranoff et al, 1993). The product uses two prostate carcinoma cell lines: the androgen-sensitive line LNCaP, as well as the castration-resistant line PC3 (Simons and Sacks, 2006). The immunologic concept underlying whole-cell vaccines such as this is that these cells may provide a source of multiple tumor- and tissue-specific antigens, at least some of which will correlate with those expressed in an individual patient's tumor. So, like IMA901 in kidney cancer, GVAX vaccines are considered polyvalent. However, unlike IMA901, the precise antigens recognized when a prostate cancer patient is treated with GVAX are not known. The theoretic advantage to polyvalent vaccines such as GVAX prostate (or AGS-003 in RCC) is that it is possible that the inclusion of multiple antigens might prevent tumors from escaping immune pressure by downregulating the expression of any one tumor-associated antigen. The major disadvantage of cell-based vaccines is that they are relatively difficult to monitor immunologically, because the key target antigens are not known for any particular patient. Mechanistically, GVAX prostate is thought to function in a manner similar to ProstVac-VF: irradiated cells are administered intradermally, where they undergo necrosis and are taken up by resident DCs attracted by secreted GM-CSF. After uptake of cellular debris and processing, antigens are presented to host

CD4 and CD8 T cells in draining lymph nodes in the context of host MHC molecules on the APCs. This process, called *cross-presentation*, has been demonstrated to occur in the clinic (Thomas et al, 2004). Although phase 2 trials failed to demonstrate clear clinical benefit, two randomized phase 3 trials were launched. The first of these was a 626-patient trial in which men with asymptomatic mCRPC were randomized 1:1 to GVAX Prostate or to chemotherapy with standard doses of docetaxel administered every 3 weeks (Higano et al, 2009). The primary end point of the trial was overall survival, but the trial was halted prematurely based on an unplanned and underpowered futility analysis. Thus, it remains unknown whether GVAX Prostate provides a survival advantage in men with early-stage mCRPC. A second trial, comparing the combination of GVAX Prostate and chemotherapy versus docetaxel chemotherapy alone was initiated, but enrollment was halted based on a reported imbalance in deaths, with an interim analysis showing 67 deaths in the GVAX plus chemotherapy arm, versus 47 in the chemotherapy-alone arm. The trial was permanently closed on the basis of that "imbalance," but follow-up data showed that, in a final analysis, there was no statistical imbalance in deaths, with 85 on the combination arm and 76 in the chemotherapy-alone arm. Taken together, the two GVAX trials support the safety of these cell-based vaccines in prostate cancer, but unfortunately no conclusions can be drawn about efficacy because both trials were halted before meeting prespecified enrollment criteria. An interesting facet of both trials is the choice of chemotherapy as a comparator arm; no large randomized clinical trial of immunotherapy in GU cancer either before or after this has chosen chemotherapy as a comparator, and these data, although clearly incomplete, suggest that comparing a cancer vaccine with chemotherapy is challenging.

IMMUNE CHECKPOINT BLOCKADE IN GENITOURINARY CANCERS

As discussed earlier, most tumors have evolved multiple mechanisms to evade immune-mediated destruction (Drake et al, 2006), and one of the most important of these mechanisms involves T-cell expression of one or more of a series of molecules that effectively limit T-cell proliferation and killing capacity (Chen 2004; Keir et al, 2008; Pardoll, 2012). Collectively these molecules are referred to as *immune checkpoints*; perhaps the best known of them is CTLA-4 (Hoos et al, 2010). Critically important preclinical studies using transplantable murine colon carcinoma and fibrosarcoma lines showed that blocking CTLA-4 with a monoclonal antibody permits antitumor T cells to acquire effector function (Leach et al, 1996), a finding that has recently been borne out in randomized phase 3 studies in patients with metastatic melanoma. In two large, randomized phase 3 trials involving a total of 1178 patients, blocking CTLA-4 with the monoclonal antibody ipilimumab (Bristol-Myers Squibb, Princeton, NJ) resulted in a significant survival benefit. In the first of these studies, which enrolled previously treated patients, the median overall survival with single-agent ipilimumab was 10.1 months versus 6.4 months for patients treated with a peptide vaccine on the control arm (Hodi et al, 2010). In the second of these studies, which enrolled treatment-naive patients and randomized them to either ipilimumab plus chemotherapy with dacarbazine or dacarbazine alone, median overall survival was 11.2 months versus 9.1 months. Long-term follow-up from the first trial showed that approximately 15% of treated patients were alive 5 years after enrollment. As reviewed elsewhere, CTLA-4 blockade is moving forward in lung cancer and other tumor types (Drake et al, 2014b). Because the immune checkpoint molecule CTLA-4 likely evolved to protect self-tissues from autoimmunity, it is not surprising that clinical trials of anti–CTLA-4 (including the pivotal phase 3 trials) were associated with an approximate 20% incidence of grade 3 and 4 immune-related adverse events (IRAEs), including colitis and dermatitis (Attia et al, 2005; Blansfield et al, 2005; Weber 2009; Lipson and Drake 2011). As introduced earlier, blocking a second immune checkpoint, PD-1, has also led to objective responses in melanoma, kidney cancer, and, perhaps somewhat surprisingly, lung cancer (Brahmer et al, 2010; Topalian et al, 2013). Toxicity rates for the two agents are difficult to compare because PD-1 blocking antibodies have only recently entered phase 3 development. Nonetheless, the rate of grade 3 and 4 adverse events does seem to be lower with PD-1 blockade than with CTLA-4 blockade (Topalian et al, 2012b, 2013), possibly because the PD-1/PD-L1 pathway acts more peripherally than the CTLA-4/B7-1 pathway, which likely operates in the lymph nodes (Ribas, 2012). In contrast to the cancer vaccines discussed earlier, objective tumor regression and long-term complete responses have occasionally been observed with either PD-1 or CTLA-4 blockade (Lipson et al, 2013). Although it remains unclear why cancer vaccines rarely generate objective tumor shrinkage, accumulating clinical data suggest that current vaccines are likely unable to effectively circumvent the multiple immunosuppressive mechanisms operative in the tumor microenvironment (Drake et al, 2006).

Bladder Cancer

Because bladder cancers frequently express PD-L1, blocking PD-1 and/or PD-L1 in that disease would seem a logical approach. Currently the PD-1 blocking antibody pembrolizumab (Merck, Whitehouse Station, NJ) and the PD-L1 blocking antibody MPDL-3280A (Genentech, South San Francisco, CA) are both in early-phase trials, but no mature data on response rates have yet been reported.

Kidney Cancer

In addition to multiple trials in melanoma, CTLA-4 blockade has also been tested in patients with metastatic RCC; a phase 2 trial conducted mostly at the National Cancer Institute (NCI) treated 61 patients with 3-mg/kg doses of ipilimumab every 3 weeks, or with a single 3-mg/kg loading dose followed by 1-mg/kg doses every 3 weeks. In this trial sequential cohorts were assessed, with no planned comparative analyses (Yang et al, 2007). Partial responses were observed in 5 out of 40 patients receiving the higher dose. As expected, grade 3 or 4 IRAEs were observed in 33% of patients; this appears to be a higher rate than that observed in melanoma patients, but likely reflects the continuous every-third-week administration regimen. It is interesting to note that a clear association between immune-related toxicity and responses was observed in this trial. At this time, single-agent CTLA-4 blockade is not under study in RCC, most likely because of competition from the plethora of targeted agents for kidney cancer, both FDA approved and in clinical trials.

Because RCC is usually considered to be an immune-sensitive tumor type, the observation of single-agent objective responses in RCC patients treated with single-agent anti–PD-1 in phase 1 trials was not completely unexpected. Indeed, a patient with advanced RCC showed a stable partial response for over 4 years in the first-in-human dose-escalation study (Brahmer et al, 2010). Perhaps more noteworthy, this sustained partial response eventually evolved into a documented complete response, and the patient had remained off treatment for longer than 5 years at last follow-up (Lipson et al, 2013). This initial indication of clinical activity for PD-1 blockade in RCC was supported by data from the more dose-intense phase 1b trial discussed previously (Drake et al, 2013). Here, the objective response rate was 30% to 35%, with an additional 10% of patients showing stable disease. Based on the activity seen in phase 1 trials, several phase 1 and 2 studies of PD-1 blockade using nivolumab in RCC were initiated. One interesting trial was a dose-ranging study (NCT01354431); this trial enrolled a total of 150 patients, randomized into treatment cohorts at doses of 0.3 mg/kg, 2 mg/kg, and 10 mg/kg, treated every 3 weeks (in contrast to the once every-2-week administration in the phase 1b study). Accrual to that trial has been completed, but final data have not yet been reported. A second trial (NCT01358721) mirrors that design but incorporates pretreatment and post-treatment biopsies in an effort to discover predictive biomarkers for PD-1 blockade in RCC. Because treatment with the tyrosine kinase inhibitor sunitinib appears to confer antitumor immune modulating effects (Finke et al, 2008), a phase 1 study combining PD-1 blockade with either of the tyrosine kinase inhibitors pazopanib and sunitinib was initiated; that study is currently ongoing (NCT01472081). Most important from a clinical standpoint is a potentially pivotal, randomized phase 3 study (NCT01668784); that study, which has completed accrual, randomized 820 previously treated RCC patients in a 1:1 ratio to receive either nivolumab at a dose of 3 mg/kg every 2 weeks or to standard second-line therapy with the mammalian target of rapamycin (mTOR) inhibitor everolimus given at a dose of 10 mg once daily. The primary end point of the study is overall survival. Overall, the clinical experience with immune checkpoint blockade in RCC has been thus far favorable, with a measurable rate of objective responses and a tolerable toxicity profile. Still, without randomized phase 3 data the overall clinical impact of these agents has yet to be determined.

Prostate Cancer

As was the case for RCC, immune checkpoint blockade using anti–CTLA-4 (ipilimumab) was evaluated in a number of early-phase studies in men with prostate cancer. These data were recently summarized by Slovin and colleagues and show that treatment is associated with a PSA response rate of approximately 15% to 20%, but with few objective (radiographic) responses (Slovin et al, 2013). In several of these studies, a low dose of radiation therapy (RT) was tested in an effort to "release antigen" and potentiate an immune response. However, in the small dataset accumulated to date, there was no evidence for such an effect; for example, the PSA response rate in patients treated with a dose of 10 mg/kg of ipilimumab was 12% in the presence of RT versus 25% without. Despite this relatively low PSA response rate and little evidence that low-dose RT applied to a single lesion in men with metastatic disease improved the PSA response rate to ipilimumab, a phase 3 trial combining RT and ipilimumab was launched in men with mCRPC who had progressed on or after treatment with docetaxel chemotherapy. This trial enrolled approximately 800 men and randomized them to a single low-dose treatment of RT alone versus RT followed by ipilimumab at a dose of 10 mg/kg every 3 weeks × 4, with every-3-month maintenance for men who were not progressing. The primary outcome of this trial was overall survival, and results were recently reported (Drake et al, 2014a). The trial did not meet its primary overall survival end point, with a median overall survival of 11.2 months in the ipilimumab group versus 10.0 months for placebo. The prespecified secondary end point of PFS was met, with a PFS of 4.0 months in the ipilimumab group versus 3.1 months in the placebo group (HR = 0.070, $P < .001$). These data provide additional evidence that ipilimumab may have clinical activity in prostate cancer but are clearly insufficient for regulatory approval. Retrospective analyses of the phase 3 data showed that men with more favorable disease characteristics (no visceral metastases, normal alkaline phosphatase, normal hemoglobin) appeared to potentially benefit from treatment, although post hoc analyses of that sort require verification in a prospective trial. One fascinating finding in these post hoc analyses was that men with visceral benefit appeared to derive absolutely no benefit from ipilimumab treatment, whereas in men with bone-only disease there was a clear suggestion of clinical benefit. The precise mechanisms underlying this dichotomy are unclear, but it may reflect a different immune microenvironment in bone versus soft tissue metastases in prostate cancer. Relevant to those findings, a second phase 3 trial in the prechemotherapy setting has also completed enrollment; that trial specifically excluded men with soft tissue disease, perhaps boding well for its success. In summary, these data suggest that ipilimumab may have some activity in mCRPC, but the results of the second phase 3 trial will be required for that clinical question to be answered in a definitive manner.

PD-1 blockade has also been evaluated in a small number of patients with mCRPC, the majority of whom were heavily pretreated (Brahmer et al, 2010; Topalian et al, 2012b). These data were, in general, disappointing; no objective responses were noted in approximately 20 men. Biologically, the lack of response to PD-1 blockade in prostate cancer might be explained by the notion that prostate cancer cells do not appear to express PD-L1, although the majority of CD8 T cells that infiltrate the gland do express PD-1 (Sfanos et al, 2009). Taken together, immune checkpoint blockade will likely play an important role in treating RCC and possibly in bladder cancer—but additional combinatorial efforts will almost certainly be required for achievement of objective responses in men with later-stage prostate cancer.

KEY POINTS: IMMUNOTHERAPY FOR GENITOURINARY CANCERS

- BCG therapy for bladder cancer stimulates both the innate and adaptive immune systems and is a prototype for successful cancer immunotherapy.
- Cancer vaccines have been evaluated in both kidney and prostate cancer, and a single vaccine (Sipuleucel-T) is FDA approved for metastatic prostate cancer.
- Cancer vaccines are usually well tolerated but result in few objective clinical responses.
- Blocking immune checkpoints with monoclonal antibodies shows significant clinical promise in both kidney cancer and bladder cancer, but for unclear reasons appears to be less effective in prostate cancer.

CONCLUSIONS

Cancer immunotherapy is a rapidly advancing field of both clinical and preclinical study, and progress in this area has been especially strong in the case of GU cancers. A more robust understanding of both basic immunology and immune resistance to tumors has driven recent progress, and a large number of trials are ongoing.

One should not lose sight of the fact that BCG immunotherapy for bladder cancer was one of the first immune-based treatments to enter into routine clinical practice in any cancer type. As discussed in other chapters, the future of immunotherapy will most likely involve combination approaches, anchored in immune checkpoint blockade but weaving in RT, conventional chemotherapy, and perhaps initial immune activation via cancer vaccines.

REFERENCES

The complete reference list is available online at www.expertconsult.com.

SUGGESTED READINGS

Balkwill F, Charles KA, Mantovani A. Smoldering and polarized inflammation in the initiation and promotion of malignant disease. Cancer Cell 2005;7:211–7.

Brandau S, Suttmann H. Thirty years of BCG immunotherapy for non-muscle invasive bladder cancer: a success story with room for improvement. Biomed Pharmacother 2007;61:299–305.

De Marzo AM, Platz EA, Sutcliffe S, et al. Inflammation in prostate carcinogenesis. Nat Rev Cancer 2007;7:256–69.

Drake CG. Prostate cancer as a model for tumour immunotherapy. Nat Rev Immunol 2010;10:580–93.

Drake CG, Jaffee E, Pardoll DM. Mechanisms of immune evasion by tumors. Adv Immunol 2006;90:51–81.

Dunn GP, Old LJ, Schreiber RD. The immunobiology of cancer immunosurveillance and immunoediting. Immunity 2004;21:137–48.

Gabrilovich D. Mechanisms and functional significance of tumour-induced dendritic-cell defects. Nat Rev Immunol 2004;4:941–52.

Gannon PO, Poisson AO, Delvoye N, et al. Characterization of the intraprostatic immune cell infiltration in androgen-deprived prostate cancer patients. J Immunol Methods 2009;348:9–17.

Hanahan D, Weinberg RA. Hallmarks of cancer: the next generation. Cell 2011;144:646–74.

Hodi FS, O'Day SJ, McDermott DF, et al. Improved survival with ipilimumab in patients with metastatic melanoma. N Engl J Med 2010;363:711–23.

Kantoff PW, Higano CS, Shore ND, et al. Sipuleucel-T immunotherapy for castration-resistant prostate cancer. N Engl J Med 2010a;363:411–22.

Kantoff PW, Schuetz TJ, Blumenstein BA, et al. Overall survival analysis of a phase II randomized controlled trial of a poxviral-based PSA-targeted immunotherapy in metastatic castration-resistant prostate cancer. J Clin Oncol 2010b;28:1099–105.

Madan RA, Arlen PM, Mohebtash M, et al. Prostvac-VF: a vector-based vaccine targeting PSA in prostate cancer. Expert Opin Investig Drugs 2009;18:1001–11.

Medzhitov R, Janeway C Jr. Innate immune recognition: mechanisms and pathways. Immunol Rev 2000;173:89–97.

Michaud DS. Chronic inflammation and bladder cancer. Urol Oncol 2007;25:260–8.

Ostrand-Rosenberg S, Sinha P. Myeloid-derived suppressor cells: linking inflammation and cancer. J Immunol 2009;182:4499–506.

Palucka AK, Laupeze B, Aspord C, et al. Immunotherapy via dendritic cells. Adv Exp Med Biol 2005;560:105–14.

Pardoll DM. The blockade of immune checkpoints in cancer immunotherapy. Nat Rev Cancer 2012;12:252–64.

Ribas A. Tumor immunotherapy directed at PD-1. N Engl J Med 2012; 366:2517–9.

Savage PA, Malchow S, Leventhal DS. Basic principles of tumor-associated regulatory T cell biology. Trends Immunol 2013;34:33–40.

Slovin SF, Higano CS, Hamid O, et al. Ipilimumab alone or in combination with radiotherapy in metastatic castration-resistant prostate cancer: results from an open-label, multicenter phase I/II study. Ann Oncol 2013; 24(7):1813–21.

Topalian SL, Hodi FS, Brahmer JR, et al. Safety, activity, and immune correlates of anti-PD-1 antibody in cancer. N Engl J Med 2012b;366:2443–54.

19 Molecular Genetics and Cancer Biology

Mark L. Gonzalgo, MD, PhD, Karen S. Sfanos, PhD, and Alan K. Meeker, PhD

Despite decades of intensive biomedical research, cancer remains a significant cause of morbidity and mortality worldwide. This situation is due in part to the complexity inherent in this disease, which is not truly a single disease at all but well over 100 separate subtypes, all grouped together under the single term "cancer."

In the United States alone, cancer strikes more than half a million people annually and is currently the second leading cause of death; if more recent trends continue, it is poised to become the leading cause of death in the near future. According to statistics reported in 2013, genitourinary (GU) malignancies comprise 29% (n = 480,240) of all cancer cases in the United States (nonmelanoma skin cancers excluded) and 15% (n = 88,270) of all cancer deaths (Siegel et al, 2013). However, significant advances have been made in the diagnosis and treatment of certain GU cancers. For example, the cure rate for testicular cancer now approaches 100% (Einhorn, 2002; Horwich et al, 2006). Testicular cancer is unusual in its responsiveness to therapy and is relatively uncommon. There has been less success with the more prevalent GU malignancies such as prostate, bladder, and renal cancers—the first (prostate), sixth (bladder), and eighth (renal) most common cancers (Siegel et al, 2013). However, mortality figures for these malignancies have shown a slow but steady decline over the past decade, and these trends are likely to continue and even to accelerate in the future.

Much of the current understanding of cancer is the direct result of the molecular biology revolution that developed rapidly following the elucidation of the molecular structure of DNA by Watson and Crick in 1953. In subsequent years, the field of molecular genetics has complemented and greatly expanded on knowledge gleaned by other disciplines, such as biochemistry and cell biology, providing important insights at the molecular level regarding the abnormalities present in cancer cells. More recent years have seen a tremendous expansion in the tools available for studying the genetic basis of human cancer, including whole genome and whole "exome" (the coding regions of the genome) sequencing efforts that have become relatively affordable and routine. A great deal is now known concerning the numerous molecular signaling pathways that provide both positive and negative regulatory signals, which in normal cells stringently control cell proliferation such that any losses in cell number are precisely counterbalanced, maintaining tissue and organ homeostasis—processes that go awry in cancer cells. Renegade populations of autonomously proliferating cells represent a serious threat to survival of the organism, particularly to large, long-lived species such as humans, and we have evolved multiple barriers to prevent such outbreaks from occurring. Incipient cancer cells must overcome several hurdles on the way to becoming fully malignant—a multistep process that takes many years to decades to complete. Cancer cells need to acquire at least eight key attributes to make the transition from a normal cell to a malignant one, including (1) genetic instability and mutation, (2) autonomous growth, (3) insensitivity to internal and external antiproliferative signals, (4) resistance to apoptosis and other forms of induced cell suicide, (5) unlimited cell division potential, (6) the ability to induce new blood vessel formation (angiogenesis), (7) locally invasive behavior that uniquely distinguishes malignant from benign neoplasms, and (8) evasion of the immune system. In addition, cancer cells need to deal with various cellular stresses that are by-products of their abnormal physiology and increase their energy metabolism required to fuel autonomous growth and unlimited replication. Also, tumor-associated inflammation may drive the development of early preneoplastic lesions into invasive cancers and promote tumor progression. Finally, many cancers develop an additional, lethal attribute—the ability to leave the site of the primary tumor to colonize and thrive in distant organs or tissues as metastases (Hanahan and Weinberg, 2000; Solimini et al, 2007; Luo et al, 2009; Hanahan and Weinberg, 2011).

This chapter outlines fundamental concepts of molecular genetics that are directly related to human cancer in general, with an emphasis on GU malignancies in particular. Spurred by more recent technologic advances such as high-throughput DNA sequencing, knowledge of the molecular genetics of cancer is rapidly expanding, providing new insights that are just beginning to be successfully exploited for use in novel diagnostic, prognostic, and therapeutic applications.

TUMOR SUPPRESSOR GENES AND ONCOGENES

For a detailed description of basic molecular genetics (DNA, RNA and transcription, protein synthesis, chromosomes, and gene structure) see the Expert Consult website.

Tumor Suppressor Genes

Tumor suppressor genes negatively regulate cellular growth and play a critical role in the normal processes of the cell cycle. These genes are also important for DNA repair and cell signaling. The absence of tumor suppressor gene function may lead to dysregulation of normal growth control and malignancy. **Loss of function of both copies (alleles) of a tumor suppressor gene is typically required for carcinogenesis.** This functional loss can occur via (1) homozygous gene deletion; (2) loss of one allele and mutational inactivation of the second allele; (3) mutational events involving both alleles; or (4) loss of one allele and epigenetic inactivation of the second allele, often involving DNA methylation, which suppresses expression

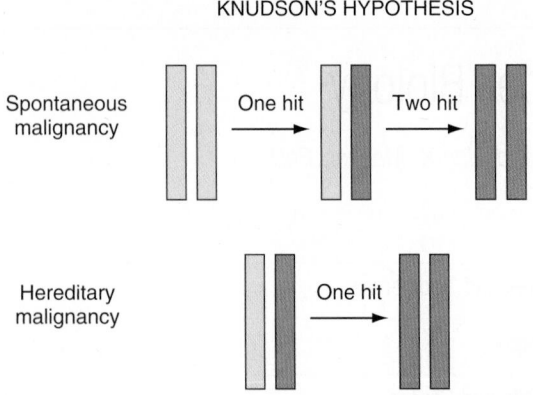

KNUDSON'S HYPOTHESIS

Figure 19-6. Knudson's hypothesis was that inactivation of the same gene was responsible for both sporadic and hereditary malignancies. Patients with sporadic tumors had two normal copies of the gene, and the sporadic tumors required inactivation of both copies of the gene. Patients with hereditary tumor syndromes were born with only one functioning copy of the gene of interest, and the hereditary tumors required inactivation of only one copy.

of the gene. Classic tumor suppressor genes discussed later in this chapter are the retinoblastoma gene (*RB1*) and the *TP53* gene (see Cell Cycle Deregulation).

The "two-hit" hypothesis was first proposed in cases of retinoblastoma, which required mutations in both alleles for disease manifestation (Knudson, 1971). This requirement is due to the fact that if just one allele is inactivated, the remaining allele could produce sufficient amounts of the correct protein to maintain the normal state (Fig. 19-6). However, specific types of mutations in certain genes may not follow this two-hit rule and can function in a dominant negative capacity when mutated, inhibiting the function of the normal protein from the unaltered allele. An example is when two or more of the same protein molecules act together (e.g., dimerization), as is the case for TP53 (Baker et al, 1990). Alternatively, deletion or mutation of a single allele may result in insufficient protein production (haploinsufficiency) causing an increased carcinogen susceptibility as in the case of the *CDKN1B* (p27Kip1) gene (Fero et al, 1998).

Oncogenes

Oncogenes are positively associated with cellular proliferation and are the mutated form of normal genes (proto-oncogenes). Two oncogenes that have been found to be overexpressed in various cancers include *MYC* and *MET* (Wong et al, 1986; Bottaro et al, 1991). The proto-oncogene *MYC* encodes an early-response gene product that is a transcription factor responsible for regulating cellular proliferation. Amplification of *MYC* is a frequent event in prostate cancer, and expression of *MYC* in human prostate epithelial cells has been associated with immortalization (Gil et al, 2005).

Hepatocyte growth factor acts through a receptor that is encoded by the proto-oncogene *MET* (Bottaro et al, 1991). Increased expression of *MET* has been reported in renal cell carcinoma (RCC) and is more frequent in higher grade cancers (Pisters et al, 1997). Missense mutations of the *MET* proto-oncogene may also result in constitutive activation of the MET protein in tumors associated with hereditary RCC (Schmidt et al, 1997).

Mechanisms by which a proto-oncogene can be converted to an activated oncogene are via (1) mutation of the proto-oncogene resulting in an active form of the gene product, (2) gene amplification, and (3) chromosomal rearrangement. A mutation occurring within the protein coding sequence of a gene can lead to a continuous proliferation signal from the mutant protein. For example, mutation of the proto-oncogene *ERBB*, which encodes

for the epidermal growth factor receptor (EGFR), results in expression of a receptor that is constitutively active (Downward et al, 1984). Errors that occur during chromosomal replication may result in gene amplification and aneuploidy. Such an increase in gene copy number often results in an increased number of mRNA transcripts and overproduction of the corresponding protein. For example, certain types of bladder cancer overexpress *MYC* by this mechanism (Christoph et al, 1999). Immunohistochemical (IHC) staining of bladder cancer specimens has demonstrated overexpression of MYC protein in more than half of papillary and invasive tumors (Schmitz-Drager et al, 1997). Finally, chromosomal structural rearrangements such as translocation events can result in the formation of an oncogene; for example, genetic rearrangement leads to the fusion of a portion of the *TMPRSS2* gene and the *ERG* oncogene in a large proportion of prostate cancers (Tomlins et al, 2005).

KEY POINTS: TUMOR SUPPRESSOR GENES AND ONCOGENES

- Mutations in DNA can lead to changes in protein function or expression that increase the potential for cancer initiation, progression, or metastasis.
- Tumor suppressor genes normally negatively regulate and control cellular growth. Oncogenes normally promote cell growth.
- Loss of tumor suppressor gene function can occur primarily by (1) homozygous deletion, (2) loss of one allele and mutational inactivation of the second allele, (3) mutational events involving both alleles, and (4) loss of one allele and epigenetic inactivation of the second allele.
- Certain tumor suppressor genes do not follow the "two-hit" hypothesis and may be inactivated via dominant negative mutations or haploinsufficiency.
- Proto-oncogenes can be converted to oncogenes by (1) mutation of the proto-oncogene resulting in an activated form of the gene, (2) gene amplification, and (3) chromosomal rearrangement.

CELL CYCLE DEREGULATION

Apart from development and growth, **cell division is tightly regulated such that the production of new cells precisely balances loss of cells during normal wear and tear, maintaining tissue and organ homeostasis.** In contrast to single-celled eukaryotes, individual human cells are not allowed to make autonomous decisions regarding their proliferation. Rather, **a complex series of external growth inhibitory and growth stimulatory signals are integrated by the cell, resulting in either cell division or quiescence. In cancer, activated oncogenes and inactivated tumor suppressor genes alter the balance between these signals such that net proliferation is continuously favored.**

Quiescent cells are considered to be out of cycle, in a reversible state known as "G_0" that is the default state for most cells. When signaled to proliferate, cells activate their **cell cycle** machinery, initiating an **orderly, unidirectional series of events resulting in duplication of the cell's genome during the DNA synthetic phase (S phase), followed by segregation of each genomic complement to each of two resulting daughter cells, a process referred to as mitosis (M phase).** These two critical phases are **separated by two so-called "gap" phases (G_1 and G_2).** Throughout the cell cycle, which takes approximately 24 hours to complete, each step depends on completion of the prior step before progressing further (Hartwell et al, 1974). In addition, **checkpoint mechanisms closely monitor DNA integrity and certain critical cell cycle events. If problems are detected (e.g., DNA damage), the cell cycle is paused to allow for repair** (Hartwell and Weinert, 1989). **If repair is impossible,** normal cells often commit cellular suicide through an active process termed *apoptosis*. Many oncogenes and tumor suppressors exert their effects by interfering with cell cycle checkpoints and apoptotic pathways, allowing cancer cells to divide continuously and accumulate. Loss of ability to respond appropriately to damaged DNA is particularly dangerous because it fosters genetic instability, a key attribute of cancer cells. Loss of DNA damage checkpoint controls results in an increased mutation rate, accelerating the mutation of cancer-associated genes and contributing to carcinogenesis and disease progression (Bartek et al, 1999).

Additional details of the eukaryotic cell cycle (cyclin-dependent kinases and cyclins, cell cycle entry, the retinoblastoma protein and the restriction point, S phase, mitosis, and cell cycle checkpoints) can be found on the Expert Consult website.

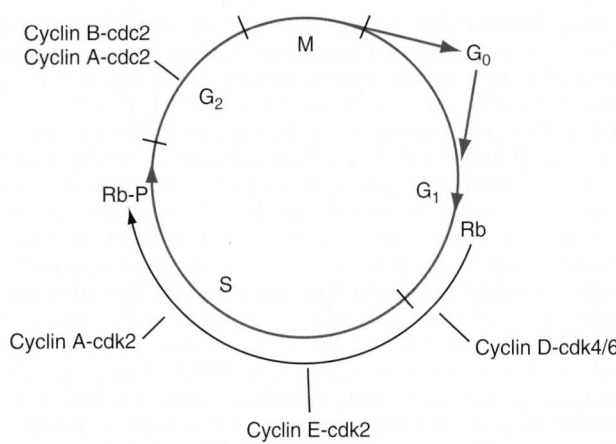

Figure 19-7. Schematic drawing of the cell cycle. Sequential activation of cyclin-cdk complexes is critical to the orderly progression of replication of the cell.

Retinoblastoma Protein and Genitourinary Malignancies

The retinoblastoma susceptibility protein, RB1 (formerly pRb), plays a central role in controlling the R-point—a decision point in late G_1 beyond which an irreversible commitment to divide is made. The inappropriate, continuous proliferation of cancer cells is largely due to a loss of R-point control, typically the result of functional inactivation of the RB1 pathway (Pardee, 1989). *RB1* gene mutations have been identified in approximately one third of bladder tumors (Horowitz et al, 1990), and reintroduction of the *RB1* gene into bladder carcinoma cell lines has been found to inhibit cell growth in vitro and tumor formation in vivo (Takahashi et al, 1991). Altered expression of RB1 protein also has been identified in approximately one third of bladder carcinomas (Logothetis et al, 1992), and altered expression has been correlated with higher stage disease and decreased patient survival (Cordon-Cardo et al, 1992).

Prostate carcinoma has not been as strongly linked to *RB1*. Although *RB1* mutations are present in 10% to 30% of prostate cancer specimens (Bookstein et al, 1990; Kubota et al, 1995), decreased expression is not consistently identified with high-risk patients or recurrent disease (Kibel and Isaacs, 2000). In other studies, no correlation was found between expression and grade or stage (Ittmann and Wieczorek, 1996), but Theodorescu and colleagues (1997) reported that low RB1 protein expression correlated with decreased disease-specific survival in univariate and multivariate analysis.

Renal carcinoma has not been clearly linked to *RB1*. *RB1* is rarely inactivated in renal carcinoma cell lines or tumors (Ishikawa et al, 1991). Analysis of clinical specimens has not demonstrated a clear association between prognosis and *RB1* expression (Lipponen et al, 1995).

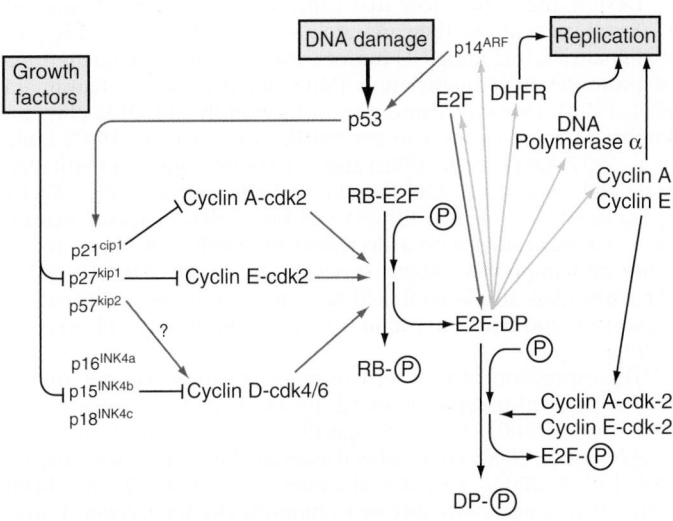

Figure 19-8. Schematic representation of the stimulatory and inhibitory cascade at the G_1/S boundary. This finely tuned system takes advantage of multiple negative and positive feedback loops.

Cyclin-Dependent Kinase Inhibitors

The temporal sequencing of events occurring throughout the cell cycle is affected by cyclin-dependent kinases (cdks), a highly conserved set of protein kinases (Meyerson et al, 1992). The cdks phosphorylate specific protein substrates involved in executing the phase-specific activities of the cell cycle. The enzymatic activities of the cdks depend on cyclins, so named because their abundances are tightly linked to specific phases of the cell cycle, during which they physically associate with and activate the enzymatic activity of the cdks (Fig. 19-7) (De Bondt et al, 1993; Jeffrey et al, 1995). Another group of proteins termed *cyclin-dependent kinase inhibitors* (CDKIs) bind to and directly inhibit cdk activity or their activating phosphorylations (Peter and Herskowitz, 1994; Sherr and Roberts, 1995). Although cyclins play major regulatory roles in orchestrating cdk activities, cdks are subject to additional levels of control, and these processes are commonly altered in cancer cells. CDKIs belong to either of two different classes, the Cip/Kip family, which includes the proteins CDKN1A (p21), CDKN1B (p27), and CDKN1C (p57), and the INK4 (*inhibit cdk4*) family, which includes INK4B (p15), INK4A (p16), INK4C (p18), and INK4D (p19). The Cip/Kip proteins have broad actions, able to inhibit multiple cyclin-cdk complexes throughout the cell cycle (Clurman and Porter,

1998). The INK4 proteins are more restricted in their activities, inhibiting cdk4-containing and cdk6-containing complexes; they are critical regulators of the R-point and the G_1/S transition because they can block RB1 phosphorylation (Fig. 19-8). **The cell uses increased expression and accumulation of CDKIs as a means of halting the cell cycle in response to various stresses.** For example, p21 expression is increased in response to DNA damage (el-Deiry et al, 1993). CDKIs function in nonstress situations as well. For example, p27 levels are high in quiescent cells, and all of the Cip/Kip proteins appear to play some role in maintenance of the G_0 state in terminally differentiated cells (Halevy et al, 1995; Matsuoka et al, 1995; Parker et al, 1995).

Among the INK4 family, inactivating mutations and abnormal gene promoter methylation of p15 and p16 have been strongly implicated in cancer in general (Kamb et al, 1994; Hirama and Koeffler, 1995) and specifically in GU malignancies (Cairns et al, 1995; Herman et al, 1995). The best studied of the INK4 proteins is p16. The p16 protein binds to cdks 4 and 6 and inhibits their interaction with cyclin D1 that normally mediates passage through the G_1 phase of the cell cycle by phosphorylation of the RB1 protein (Serrano et al, 1993). The *INK4A* gene encoding p16 was initially found to be mutated and deleted in a wide variety of tumors including bladder and kidney (Kamb et al, 1994). Subsequent analysis demonstrated that **inactivation often occurs by DNA hypermethylation at the** *INK4A* **promoter**—an alternative, epigenetic method of gene inactivation (Merlo et al, 1995).

The *INK4A* gene is frequently inactivated by deletion in bladder carcinomas (Cairns et al, 1995; Williamson et al, 1995). Despite its proximity, the *INK4B* gene was ruled out as the primary tumor suppressor at this site because it was not within the deletion interval. A study by Orlow and colleagues (1999) found that deletion and methylation of the gene encoding p16 occurred frequently in superficial bladder carcinoma, but only deletions that affect genes encoding both p16 and p14, which are located at the same locus, correlated with a decrease in disease-free survival. In contrast to bladder cancer, mutational inactivation of INK4 family members appears to be rare in prostate carcinoma. However, inactivation of *INK4A* by promoter hypermethylation has been implicated in prostate cancer. Herman and associates (1995, 1996) demonstrated *INK4A* hypermethylation in 60% of prostate cancer cell lines, whereas *INK4B* was rarely inactivated. However, these results are tempered by the fact that silencing of the *INK4A* gene by promoter hypermethylation often occurs during the establishment of cell lines in vitro.

Despite the critical role that Cip/Kip family members play in G_1/S cell cycle arrest, they are rarely mutated in a wide variety of malignancies, including GU tumors, and there are only rare reports of promoter hypermethylation (Shiohara et al, 1994; Kawamata et al, 1995). However, expression of this family of CDKIs plays an important role in cancer in general (Catzavelos et al, 1997; Loda et al, 1997; Yatabe et al, 1998) and in GU carcinomas in particular. Stein and associates (1998) found increased expression of *CDKN1A* (p21) in 64% of bladder tumors and found that increased expression was associated with a decreased probability of tumor recurrence and improved patient survival. Decreased *CDKN1B* (p27) expression has also been linked to increasing tumor grade, pathologic stage, and poor survival in bladder carcinoma (Del Pizzo et al, 1999).

The expression of *CDKN1A* in prostate cancer has not shown a clear correlation with advanced disease or poor outcome (Kibel and Isaacs, 2000). However, specific genetic polymorphisms in *CDKN1A* and *CDKN1B* have been associated with advanced disease (Kibel et al, 2003), and altered expression of *CDKN1B* has been implicated in aggressive disease in multiple studies. Cordon-Cardo and colleagues (1998) examined radical prostatectomy specimens and found that absent or low *CDKN1B* production by immunohistochemistry was an independent risk factor for decreased disease-free survival by multivariate analysis. Cote and coworkers (1998) found that decreased *CDKN1B* nuclear staining correlated not only with decreased disease-free survival but also overall survival in patients undergoing radical prostatectomy, whereas Freedland and colleagues (2003) found that patients with *CDKN1B*-positive cells in the prostate needle biopsy specimen had a 2.5-fold increased risk of biochemical recurrence (prostate-specific antigen [PSA] relapse).

The relevance of *CDKN1B* to prostate cancer is also supported by studies of mouse models. For example, mice deficient in *CDKN1B* develop prostate hyperplasia, confirming the potential importance of this gene in prostate tissue homeostasis (Cordon-Cardo et al, 1998). Other studies have shown that mice deficient in both *CDKN1B* and *PTEN* have a high incidence of prostate cancer (Di Cristofano et al, 2001).

TP53 Tumor Suppressor

The TP53 tumor suppressor protein is a key player in cell cycle checkpoints, responding to DNA damage by signaling cell cycle arrest and repair of the damage (Fig. 19-9). If the DNA damage cannot be repaired, TP53 may trigger cell death (apoptosis). *TP53* is the most commonly mutated gene in cancer and plays a prominent role in GU malignancies. Alterations to *TP53* in regard to GU cancers are discussed in detail in the following sections.

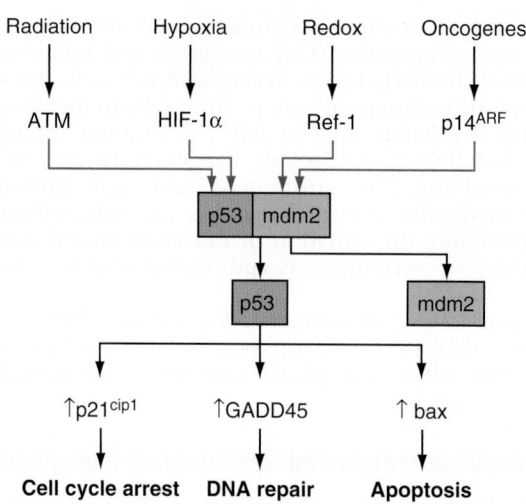

Figure 19-9. *TP53* plays a central role in the cell's response to extracellular stimuli. Radiation, hypoxia, redox reactions, and oncogenes all can increase *TP53* activity through different mechanisms. In response, the cell initially stops dividing and then attempts to repair the DNA damage. If it fails to repair the DNA, it undergoes apoptosis (programmed cell death). These functions are mediated through transcriptional activation of various genes, some examples of which are indicated in the figure.

KEY POINTS: CELL CYCLE DEREGULATION

- The cell cycle consists of an ordered, unidirectional series of events, the main goal of which is to replicate the cell's genome and partition one copy into each of two resulting daughter cells.
- The cell cycle is divided into four phases; G_1, S, G_2, and M. The transition from G_1 into S phase is critically dependent on phosphorylation of the RB1 tumor suppressor protein. Mutations in *RB1* are common in urologic malignancies.
- Phase-specific phosphorylation of substrate proteins by cdks orchestrates progression through the cycle.
- The activities of cdks depend on their association with specific cyclin proteins. Cyclins accumulate and are rapidly degraded in a phase-specific manner, ensuring the proper sequencing and irreversibility of key events throughout the cell cycle.
- Primary points of cell cycle control are the G_1/S and G_2/M checkpoints. Checkpoints employ CDKIs to pause the cell cycle in response to various signals, including DNA damage, cell-cell contact, cytokine release, and hypoxia.
- The TP53 tumor suppressor protein is a key player in cell cycle checkpoints, responding to DNA damage by signaling cell cycle arrest and repair of the DNA damage. If the DNA damage cannot be repaired, TP53 may trigger cell death (apoptosis).
- *TP53* is the most commonly mutated gene in cancer and plays a prominent role in GU malignancies.
- Defects in cell cycle checkpoints lead to unregulated cell proliferation and genetic instability.

DNA METHYLATION

The covalent modification of the C-5 position of cytosine by a methyl group is mediated by DNA methyltransferase, resulting in the formation of 5-methylcytosine, an epigenetic modification of DNA that occurs in vertebrates and is essential for normal embryonic development (Jones, 1986; Bird, 1992). Methylation of cytosine occurs primarily at the CpG palindrome in DNA. The presence of 5-methylcytosine at CpG dinucleotides has resulted in a significant depletion of this sequence from the genome during the course of vertebrate evolution (Schorderet and Gartler, 1992). This reduction in frequency of CpG dinucleotides in the genome is the result of spontaneous deamination of 5-methylcytosine to thymine (Rideout et al, 1990; Sved and Bird, 1990). Certain areas of the genome do not show a depletion of the CpG dinucleotides and contain the expected frequency of this sequence. These regions are referred to as CpG islands; although CpG islands constitute approximately 1% of vertebrate genomes, they account for approximately 15% of the total number of CpG dinucleotides in DNA (Bird, 1986; Gardiner-Garden and Frommer, 1987). CpG islands are typically located upstream of many ubiquitous housekeeping and tissue-specific genes. CpG island methylation affects the levels of gene transcription (Cedar, 1988). Hypermethylation of CpG islands usually results in transcriptional downregulation, whereas hypomethylation of these regions may increase gene expression.

CpG islands located in the promoter regions of tumor suppressor genes are normally unmethylated. Abnormal methylation of these regions may result in a progressive reduction in gene expression, altering normal cellular growth control in favor of proliferation. Methylation of CpG islands may lead to decreased gene expression by mechanisms including changes in local chromatin structure, inhibition of transcription factor binding, or exclusion of transcriptional machinery from methylated promoter DNA (Bird and Wolffe, 1999). The epigenetic properties of methylation may affect gene activity without altering the DNA sequence and represent an alternative means of gene inactivation apart from gene mutation or deletion.

Changes in global levels and regional patterns of DNA methylation are among the earliest and most frequent events known to occur in human cancer (Jones and Baylin, 2002). Alterations in DNA methylation have a direct impact on mutational and epigenetic components that may contribute to neoplastic transformation. **Three major pathways by which DNA methylation may result in genetic dysregulation in human cancer include (1) inherent mutational effects of 5-methylcytosine, (2) epigenetic effects of promoter methylation on gene transcription, and (3) potential gene activation and induction of chromosomal instability by DNA hypomethylation** (Gonzalgo and Jones, 1997; Jones and Gonzalgo, 1997).

DNA Methylation and Prostate Cancer

Glutathione-S-transferases belong to a superfamily of enzymes responsible for detoxification of a wide range of xenobiotics. These enzymes catalyze the nucleophilic attack of reduced glutathione on potentially damaging electrophilic compounds. **Aberrant methylation of the CpG island at the glutathione-S-transferase pi (GSTP1) locus is the most frequent somatic genome alteration reported in prostate cancer** (Lee et al, 1994; Jerónimo et al, 2001). Methylation of GSTP1 has been detected in greater than 90% of prostate carcinomas and approximately 70% of prostatic intraepithelial neoplasia (PIN) lesions, but it is not present in normal prostate tissue or benign prostatic hyperplasia (Lee et al, 1994). In normal prostate tissue, expression of GSTP1 is limited to basal cells, but it can be upregulated in columnar epithelial cells exposed to oxidative stress. Increased levels of DNA methylation have also been associated with worse clinical outcomes in patients with prostate cancer (Maruyama et al, 2002).

The ras association domain family protein 1 isoform A (RASSF1A) gene is located on chromosome 3p21. RASSF1A is a tumor suppressor gene that is frequently altered in various human cancers. Abnormal methylation of RASSF1A has been reported to occur in 60% to 70% of prostate carcinomas (Kuzmin et al, 2002). Loss of heterozygosity (LOH) of the 3p21 region is associated with methylation and silencing of the remaining RASSF1A allele during tumorigenesis. Methylation RASSF1A has been observed more frequently in higher grade prostate cancers compared with less aggressive tumors (Liu et al, 2002).

Genome-wide methylation analyses were conducted in prostate cancer more recently, and the results indicated that there are widespread changes in methylation patterns (both hypermethylation and hypomethylation) that occur in both gene-associated and conserved intergenic regions. Although interindividual heterogeneity in DNA methylation patterns was observed among patients with prostate cancer, in individuals with metastatic prostate cancer, DNA methylation alterations were highly conserved across all of their metastases, suggesting that DNA methylation alterations undergo clonal selection (Yegnasubramanian et al, 2011; Aryee et al, 2013).

Role of DNA Methylation in Bladder Cancer

Mutations of the TP53 gene are present in more than half of all human malignancies. Many of the mutational hot spots found in the TP53 gene occur at CpG dinucleotides that are normally methylated, implicating 5-methylcytosine as an endogenous mutagen in the genome (Rideout et al, 1990; Greenblatt et al, 1994; Tornaletti and Pfeifer, 1995). Mutational inactivation of TP53 is a frequent event in urothelial dysplasia, carcinoma in situ (CIS), and invasive bladder cancer (Spruck et al, 1994).

The contribution of DNA methylation to these mutational events varies depending on the type of bladder cancer and the etiologic agent believed to be responsible for tumor formation (Jones et al, 1998). Urothelial carcinomas in Western countries and Japan have relatively few mutations at CpG sites, suggesting that DNA methylation may not play a major role in inducing these changes. In contrast, a higher frequency of mutations at CpG dinucleotides consistent with 5-methylcytosine deamination is observed in patients with squamous cell carcinoma and urothelial carcinoma with a history of exposure to phenacetin or arsenic (Jones et al, 1998). These observations highlight the potential mutagenic effects of DNA methylation on the genome and the contribution of methylation to TP53 inactivation during bladder carcinogenesis.

INK4A (p16) Methylation in Bladder Cancer

Inactivation of the INK4A gene may occur by various mechanisms, including deletion, mutation, and promoter methylation (Spruck et al, 1994; Gonzalez-Zulueta et al, 1995; Herman et al, 1995). Mutation or deletion of one INK4A allele and concurrent methylation of the remaining allele results in complete loss of functional activity. Methylation of INK4A has been reported in 27% to 60% of primary urothelial carcinomas (Chan et al, 2002; Chang et al, 2003). Such epigenetic changes are among the earliest molecular events associated with transformation and may precede morphologic alterations in cellular architecture.

The first detailed study investigating the effects of INK4A promoter methylation on transcriptional activity was performed in bladder cancer cells, where a reduction in INK4A expression was associated with higher levels of methylation in the upstream promoter region. Methylation of specific CpG sites in the INK4A promoter was shown to result in significant downregulation of transcriptional activity of the gene (Gonzalgo et al, 1998). Administration of the demethylating agent 5-aza-2'-deoxycytidine (5-Aza-CdR) was capable of reactivating INK4A expression in bladder cancer cells that were previously shown to contain methylated alleles of the gene. Methylation in exon 2 of the INK4A gene is also a frequent occurrence in various cancers and is an excellent marker for transformation, although the presence of methylation in this region of the INK4A gene does not affect INK4A transcription in bladder cancer cells (Gonzalgo et al, 1998).

Hypermethylation of Other Genes in Bladder Cancer

The E-cadherin (CDH1) gene encodes a transmembrane glycoprotein that modulates calcium-dependent intercellular adhesion in epithelial tissues. Methylation of the CpG island located in the CDH1 promoter is associated with decreased gene expression in high-grade urothelial carcinoma, including disease associated with CIS (Graff et al, 1995; Horikawa et al, 2003). CDH1 methylation has also been reported in histologically normal urothelium; however, many of these cases were from patients older than 70 years of age and may be related to a potential link between methylation and aging (Ahuja and Issa, 2000; Bornman et al, 2001). Lower levels of CDH1 expression may increase β-catenin/T-cell factor/lymphocyte enhancer factor signaling activity and proliferation in urothelial carcinomas (Maruyama et al, 2002; Thievessen et al, 2003).

Methylation of *RASSF1A* has been reported in 97% of primary bladder tumors, suggesting that epigenetic inactivation of this gene may play an important role in bladder carcinogenesis (Lee et al, 2001). High tumor grade, nonpapillary growth pattern, and muscle-invasive disease are associated with *RASSF1A* promoter methylation in bladder cancer (Maruyama et al, 2001).

Hypomethylation in Bladder Cancer

Global DNA hypomethylation is also a frequent event in tumorigenesis (Jones and Baylin, 2002). **Hypomethylation may result in genomic instability via alterations in chromatin structure, increased genetic recombination between repetitive elements, or derepression of retrotransposons** (Baylin et al, 2001). Methylation of CpG sites is normally maintained by the enzymatic activities of DNA methyltransferase 1 (*DNMT1*), whereas de novo methylation of CpG sites is mediated by DNA methyltransferases 3A and 3B (*DNMT3A, DNMT3B*) (Jones and Baylin, 2002). **One important role for methylation is genomic imprinting, which results in monoallelic gene expression without altering the genetic sequence.** Loss of imprinting is a reduction in the methylation of the normally methylated allele that can lead to activation of the normally silent copy of a growth-promoting gene (Feinberg and Tycko, 2004). This phenomenon has been reported for the human insulin-like growth factor-2 gene (*IGF2*) in various cancers (Woodson et al, 2004; Sakatani et al, 2005).

Methylation of long interspersed nuclear element (L1 LINE) sequences is reduced in bladder cancer cell lines and primary tumors compared with normal bladder mucosa (Jürgens et al, 1996). However, DNA methyltransferase expression did not correlate with methylation status of cell lines, and methyltransferase activity was reduced in quiescent cells suggesting that aberrant expression of *DNMT1* does not account for the altered methylation patterns found in urothelial carcinoma (Jürgens et al, 1996). Decreased *DNMT1* expression and induction of *DNMT3A* and *DNMT3B* in bladder cancer have also been reported (Kimura et al, 2003). These data suggest that downregulation of *DNMT1* expression may be at least partly responsible for hypomethylation of repetitive elements in bladder cancer.

KEY POINTS: DNA METHYLATION

- Methylation occurs specifically at CpG dinucleotides in the genome. The presence of 5-methylcytosine in DNA can result in spontaneous deamination to thymine and the formation of C→T transition mutations.
- DNA methylation can affect gene function by subsequent mutational events or epigenetic mechanisms. Methylation of CpG islands associated with the promoter region of genes may result in suppression of gene expression.
- Loss of promoter methylation of normally methylated genes can lead to inappropriate gene expression (e.g., expression of oncogenes).

DNA DAMAGE AND REPAIR

Cancer is fundamentally a genetic disease. Alterations in numerous genes provide the malignant cell the means to activate cancer-associated pathways and inactivate tumor suppressive barriers, making possible the acquisition of the key set of attributes associated with the cancer phenotype. **The intrinsic accuracy of DNA polymerase coupled with associated error-correction mechanisms keeps the error rate during DNA replication to an astonishingly low estimated value of approximately three incorrect** bases per cell division—in a genome of more than 3 billion bases! However, these processes are not perfect, and cancer-causing changes occur in oncogenes and tumor suppressor genes via epigenetic, mutational, and copy number alterations (CNAs), in addition to epigenetic abnormalities. Many of these genetic changes are thought to result from various endogenous (e.g., mitochondrial respiratory by-products) and exogenous (e.g., chemicals, radiation) DNA-damaging agents that constantly assault the genome (Ames and Gold, 1991, 1998). To counter these threats, cells employ a plethora of defensive mechanisms, including free radical scavengers such as α-tocopherol, vitamin C, carotenoids, bilirubin, and urate as well as protective enzymes such as superoxide dismutases, glutathione peroxidases, and glutathione transferases, which serve to detoxify a wide range of carcinogens (Mates and Sanchez-Jimenez, 1999; Finkel and Holbrook, 2000). Loss of expression, owing to promoter hypermethylation, of the glutathione-*S*-transferase pi enzyme encoded by the *GSTP1* gene is observed in most prostate cancer cases (Lee et al, 1994; Lin et al, 2001), and more recent studies have found associations between genetic polymorphisms in glutathione-*S*-transferases and the risk of biochemical recurrence in patients with prostate cancer (Nock et al, 2009). Epidemiologic and retrospective studies on prostate cancer risk have found a protective effect for selenium, which is used as a cofactor by glutathione peroxidases (Lowe and Frazee, 2006; Colli and Amling, 2009), raising hope that dietary intervention might be protective against prostate cancer. However, a large clinical trial showed no benefit for dietary supplementation with selenium (Hatfield and Gladyshev, 2009), and it now appears that observed protective effects of selenium may be limited to men with low baseline selenium levels. Results from other clinical chemoprevention trials in prostate cancer have been similarly disappointing (Gaziano et al, 2009).

In addition to DNA damage prevention, the cell employs a host of DNA repair systems. The set of pathways dealing with DNA damage recognition and repair is **referred to as the DNA damage response (DDR)** and encompasses a plethora of genes. The DDR includes the replication machinery itself (with its associated proofreading capability) and the many components of specific DNA repair systems, such as base excision repair, nucleotide excision repair, double-stranded break repair, and mismatch repair described in detail further on (Loeb, 1998; Schmutte and Fishel, 1999).

As previously mentioned, **the cell cycle and the DDR are closely integrated. In response to DNA damage, the first step is to arrest the cell cycle so that the DNA can be repaired. There is substantial overlap between the initiators of DNA repair and cell cycle arrest** (Kastan and Bartek, 2004). For example, ATM and ATR kinases are both activated in response to DNA damage, and both activate TP53, CHK1, and other proteins critical to cell cycle arrest (Bartek and Lukas, 2003).

Considering the number of genetic changes calculated to be required for cancer development as well as the large number of changes actually observed in cancer cells and taking into account the very low spontaneous mutation rates in normal human cells, Loeb concluded that the spontaneous mutation rate is insufficient to explain the number of mutations observed in most human cancers. Loeb hypothesized that early in the process of tumorigenesis, preneoplastic cells might develop defects in one or more of the genes responsible for the fidelity of DNA replication (Loeb et al, 1974; Loeb, 1991; Cheng and Loeb, 1993). Such a defect would lead to an increased mutation rate resulting in a so-called mutator phenotype. This hypothesis gains further support from the fact that most cells in proliferating tissues, such as epithelial tissues, the source of most human cancers, are relatively short-lived, being eliminated either by cell shedding or by apoptosis. The target population of cells at risk for becoming cancerous is far less than the total number of cells in the body, yet cancers are common. In addition, cells with a "hypermutable" phenotype are often more difficult to treat because the selection pressure of therapy may rapidly select tumor cells with mutations conferring resistance (Tlsty et al, 1989).

The term *mutator phenotype* was originally used to refer to defects in the DNA replication and repair proteins, resulting in small-scale errors in the DNA sequence, such as single base substitutions, deletions, and duplications. Despite (or perhaps because of) the many potential targets for mutator genes, few such genes have been found to be consistently mutated in significant proportions of common human cancers, a notable exception being the mismatch repair pathway. Mismatch repair defects are the underlying cause of hereditary nonpolyposis colorectal cancer (Aaltonen et al, 1993) and have been reported in 15% of sporadic colon cancers (Liu et al, 1995).

Although defects in DNA repair genes in sporadic malignancies, including GU tumors, have been identified, Loeb's concept of the mutator phenotype, as originally stated, has yet to be fully evaluated, and it currently appears that it may not be a major player in the development of most common sporadic human cancers. However, if one broadens the mutator concept to include systems involved in *chromosomal* stability, it may become widely applicable. At any rate, the current consensus is that genetic instability of *some* sort is required for cancer development.

Additional information on DNA repair mechanisms (nucleotide excision repair, base excision repair, mismatch repair, DNA double-stranded break repair, nonhomologous end joining) can be found on the Expert Consult website.

KEY POINTS: DNA DAMAGE AND REPAIR

- DNA damage does not often lead to malignancy because the cell possesses multiple repair mechanisms.
- Defects in DNA repair facilitate the accumulation of the mutations critical for tumor formation and progression.
- NER is a major defense against DNA damage caused by ultraviolet radiation and chemical exposure.
- BER repairs DNA damage caused by spontaneous deamination of bases, radiation, oxidative stress, alkylating agents, and replication errors.
- MMR removes nucleotides mispaired by DNA polymerase.
- Double-stranded break repair is a major defense again DNA damage caused by ionizing radiation, free radicals, and chemicals.
- Many syndromes that involve inherited defects in DNA repair exhibit marked increases in cancer susceptibility, strongly linking genomic instability and cancer.

GENOMIC ALTERATIONS

Although the ultimate source of genetic instability in cancer is still unclear, **research by many different groups on several different tumor types has strongly implicated genetic instability as an important determinant of tumorigenesis** (Loeb, 1991; Hartwell, 1992). As mentioned previously, although important in specific instances, such as inherited cancer susceptibility syndromes, deficiencies in genes involved in the replication, maintenance, and repair of DNA have not yet been shown to play a major direct role in the genesis of most sporadic human cancers. **More recent studies on numerous human cancers found that the genomes of each cancer have numerous mutations (on average 33 to 66 somatic mutations in solid tumors) in gene coding sequences that are predicted to alter significantly the corresponding protein products** (Vogelstein et al, 2013). **Comprehensive sequencing efforts coupled with statistical methods to predict the effects of individual mutations have revealed that approximately 140 genes, when mutated, can "drive" tumorigenesis (e.g., "driver" genes). Most tumors contain only two to eight such driver mutations,** whereas the remaining mutations in any particular cancer case are considered "passengers" that do not confer a selective growth advantage (Sjoblom et al, 2006; Wood et al, 2007; Vogelstein et al, 2013).

Apart from the sequence alterations predicted to arise from the original mutator phenotype concept, *chromosomal* instability leads to gross changes in chromosome number and structure or both. The spectrum and severity of such chromosomal alterations may differ for different tumor types. For instance, **hematologic malignancies often manifest with simple diploid or near-diploid karyotypes with only one or very few detectable, often balanced, chromosomal rearrangements.** However, as a class, these cancers account for only about 10% of all human cancers. **In stark contrast, the presence of large variations in chromosome numbers and complex structural rearrangements as well as intratumoral variation in these aberrations are hallmarks of most human solid tumors,** which represent the bulk of human malignancies. Important exceptions include certain tumors deficient in MMR. **In prostate cancer as well as most human tumor types and transplantable tumor models, the extent of chromosomal abnormalities correlates with disease severity and aggressiveness,** pointing to a role for these changes in cancer progression—spanning from premalignant lesions to localized primary tumors to metastatic disease to which patients typically succumb (Brothman et al, 1990; Lundgren et al, 1992; Sandberg, 1992; Isaacs et al, 1995; Bostwick et al, 1996). For example, in a study that used a computational method to infer aneuploidy based on gene expression data of genes that are located in adjacent chromosomal regions, greater levels of aneuploidy were found to confer worse survival (Carter et al, 2006). Likewise, a study on prostate cancer performed unsupervised hierarchical clustering of copy number alterations (CNAs) in 218 tumor samples and found that tumors with the highest number of genome-wide CNAs had a significantly accelerated time to biochemical recurrence (Taylor et al, 2010).

The chromosomal changes seen in solid tumors can be broken down into two main classes: changes in the number of whole chromosomes and changes in chromosomal structure. Numerical chromosomal alterations can be subdivided further into changes in the numbers of specific individual chromosomes, aneusomies (e.g., monosomies and trisomies), and changes in the number of copies of the entire diploid set of chromosomes, ploidy changes (e.g., tetraploidy, octaploidy). Possible mechanisms responsible for such numerical changes include nondisjunction, endoreduplication (an abrupt doubling of the chromosome complement without cell division), cytokinesis defects, and cell fusion events. Likewise, structural changes can be subdivided into several distinct types of chromosomal aberrations as listed in Box 19-2. An additional mechanism

---

BOX 19-2 Gross Chromosomal Abnormalities Frequently Observed in Cancer

NUMERICAL ABNORMALITIES

Aneuploidies

Abnormal numbers of whole chromosome complement (e.g., triploidy, tetraploidy)

Losses or gains of single chromosomes (e.g., monosomy, trisomy)

STRUCTURAL ABNORMALITIES

Rearrangements

Inversions

Translocations (either balanced or unbalanced)

Chromothripsis

Chromosomal fusions

End-to-end fusion = dicentric chromosome

Intrachromosomal fusion = ring chromosome

Deletions (from small segments up to entire chromosome arms)

Duplications, amplifications

Double minutes (often containing amplified sequences)

Isochromosomes (loss of one chromosomal arm, replaced by duplication of the remaining arm)

Complex (various combinations of the above-listed abnormalities)

for genomic rearrangement, termed *chromothripsis* (literally meaning "chromosome shattering"), has been described that was initially extrapolated from genomic sequencing studies on cancer cells (Stephens et al, 2011). Chromothripsis is evidenced by a large number (possibly hundreds) of chromosomal rearrangements in confined chromosomal regions that have occurred after apparent shattering and rejoining of a chromosomal region in a sometimes disordered fashion.

As previously mentioned, cancer-associated chromosomal changes were recognized in the 1900s by Boveri, who proposed that such abnormalities might be involved in cancer causation. Much later, Klein (1981) suggested that chromosomal rearrangements affect the expression of cancer-related genes located near the observed chromosomal breakpoints. This hypothesis has been validated over the ensuing years, in large part as a result of studies on what were observed to be consistent chromosomal changes found in hematologic malignancies and soft tissue sarcomas, eventually leading to the isolation and cloning of the resident genes involved (Nowell, 1994). Over the years, painstaking dissection of chromosomal regions that are repeatedly found to undergo alteration in specific tumor types or subtypes has led to the discovery of hundreds of individual cancer-associated genes. Typically, genomic loci that are frequently lost tend to harbor tumor suppressor genes, whereas loci exhibiting copy number gains (e.g., gene amplification) point toward oncogenes (Snijders et al, 2005). Examples of genes frequently amplified in cancers include members of the *MYC*, *RAS*, *EGFR*, and *FGF* gene families as well as cell cycle regulatory genes such as *CCND1* (cyclin D gene), *CDK4*, and *HDM2*. **Gene amplifications in cancer are usually seen either as multiple small extrachromosomal copies, called *double minutes*, or as amplified regions within chromosomes, so-called homogeneous staining regions** (Cowell, 1982).

Specific Chromosomal Rearrangements in Genitourinary Malignancies

Recurrent Gene Rearrangements in Prostate Cancer

Although they are much less frequently observed in common adult solid tumors, recurrent translocations do occur, often amid the backdrop of countless chromosomal abnormalities (Sandberg, 1985). **One of the most exciting more recent findings in prostate cancer research has been the discovery of recurrent structural rearrangements in most prostate cancer cases, primarily involving oncogenic ETS transcription factor family members.** The initial report by Tomlins and coworkers in 2005 described the use of a novel bioinformatic approach that led to the identification of recurrent gene fusions between the upstream regulatory region of the androgen-regulated gene *TMPRSS2* and *ERG*, an ETS family member previously known to be involved in Ewing sarcoma and various leukemias. These two genes reside 3 Mb apart on chromosome 21 (*TMPRSS2*, 21q22.3; *ERG*, 21q22.2), and detailed molecular analysis revealed that in most rearranged cases (approximately two thirds), the gene fusion occurs via deletion of the intervening sequence, with the remaining fusions resulting from more complex, translocation-type rearrangements (Tomlins et al, 2005; Perner et al, 2007). In either case, **the net result is to place a known oncogenic transcription factor under the control of an androgen-regulated promoter, resulting in androgen-driven expression of the fusion transcript** (Wang et al, 2008a). As expected, increased *ERG* transcription and ERG protein expression are positively correlated with presence of the gene fusion. In addition to various splice variants, there are multiple forms of the genomic rearrangement, the most common one being a fusion between exon 1 of *TMPRSS2* and exon 4 of *ERG*. **These gene rearrangements can be readily detected, either by assaying for the presence of the fusion transcripts by reverse-transcription polymerase chain reaction (PCR) or by assaying for the rearrangement directly by multiprobe, multicolor fluorescence in situ hybridization (FISH). Such approaches are currently being evaluated for potential use in noninvasive diagnostic applications (e.g., in urine or blood).**

More recently, detection of ERG protein expression by immunostaining has been shown to be an excellent surrogate marker for chromosomal rearrangements involving the *ERG* gene, providing a simpler method for their detection (Park et al, 2010; Chaux et al, 2011; Falzarano et al, 2011).

Since the publication of the initial report by Tomlins and coworkers, several large retrospective studies have been performed assessing these fusions in localized prostate cancers in PSA-screened cohorts. These studies confirmed the initial finding and found the prevalence of the *TMPRSS2-ERG* fusion in prostate cancer to be 40% to 60%, making this one of the most common somatic genetic alterations in prostate cancer (Mehra et al, 2007; Nam et al, 2007; Perner et al, 2007; Tu et al, 2007; Wang et al, 2008a; Gopalan et al, 2009b; Mosquera et al, 2009). One anatomic exception is cancer originating in the transition zone of the prostate, which appears to lack *TMPRSS2-ERG* gene rearrangements completely (Guo et al, 2009a).

As assessed by FISH in tissue sections, the *TMPRSS2-ERG* fusion has not been observed in benign prostate epithelial or stromal cells, although it has been reported to be present in high-grade prostatic intraepithelial neoplasia (PIN), the presumptive precursor lesion for prostate adenocarcinoma, at frequencies between 15% and 20%, which is about one half the frequency observed in localized PSA-detected cancers (Cerveira et al, 2006; Perner et al, 2007; Mosquera et al, 2008; Han et al, 2009). This finding implies that, at least in a subset of cases, the rearrangement may be an early event in prostate tumorigenesis. **With the important exceptions of transition zone cancers and high-grade PIN, the prevalence and high degree of specificity of the *TMPRSS2-ERG* fusion for prostate cancer makes this a potentially useful biomarker for diagnosis and disease monitoring, one that could be used in conjunction with current markers such as serum PSA that have limited specificity.** The detection of *TMPRSS2-ERG* fusion-driven ERG overexpression in prostate biopsy specimens from men found to have only high-grade PIN was shown to be predictive of cancer diagnosis on subsequent biopsy (Park et al, 2014), and multiple studies have demonstrated the utility of *TMPRSS2-ERG* detection in the blood or urine either alone or in combination with the non–protein-coding RNA prostate cancer antigen 3 (PCA3) in enhancing the sensitivity of prostate cancer diagnosis (Hessels et al, 2007; Tomlins et al, 2011; Leyten et al, 2014).

Apart from the promising potential of *TMPRSS2-ERG* as a diagnostic prostate cancer marker, it is unclear at the present time if additional clinical information might be provided by determining a patient's *TMPRSS2-ERG* gene fusion status. **The prognostic significance of fusion status in prostate cancer remains uncertain.** Although several studies have reported associations between *TMPRSS2-ERG* rearrangement and various indicators of disease aggressiveness, including higher stage, presence of metastases, and disease-specific death (Demichelis et al, 2007; Mehra et al, 2007; Nam et al, 2007; Perner et al, 2007; Rajput et al, 2007; Attard et al, 2008a; Cheville et al, 2008; Barwick et al, 2010; Leyten et al, 2014), several other published studies failed to observe such associations (Yoshimoto et al, 2006; Lapointe et al, 2007; Tu et al, 2007; Dai et al, 2008; Rouzier et al, 2008; Albadine et al, 2009; Darnel et al, 2009; Gopalan et al, 2009b; Lotan et al, 2009; Fine et al, 2010). A large prospective study of 1180 men treated by radical prostatectomy found that the presence of the *TMPRSS2-ERG* rearrangement was not predictive of recurrence or mortality but was associated with tumor stage (Pettersson et al, 2012). Studies examining the prognostic capabilities of *TMPRSS2-ERG* positivity in predicting treatment outcomes to androgen deprivation (Leinonen et al, 2010), abiraterone (Danila et al, 2011), or radiotherapy (Dal Pra et al, 2013) showed no association. In addition, one study reported a link between gene fusion and *favorable* prognosis (Saramaki et al, 2008), and Petrovics and colleagues (2005) reported that higher levels of *ERG* mRNA expression appeared to be positively associated with disease-free survival. Another study reported that *ERG* gene copy number gain without the presence of the gene fusion is prognostic for recurrence after radical prostatectomy (Toubaji et al, 2011). The precise reasons for these conflicting results are not apparent. Numerous variables differ among many of these studies, including the nature of the study cohort, sample size, method of cancer detection, how the tissues were obtained, intratumoral heterogeneity in the presence of the fusion (Minner et al, 2013), how the gene fusions were detected (e.g., PCR or FISH), length of patient follow-up, and the clinical end points assessed. Further research in this area is warranted for better resolution of these issues.

Following the report of *TMPRSS2-ERG* rearrangements, further study revealed additional gene fusions in prostate cancer. The *TMPRSS2* gene can fuse to other ETS family member genes including *ETV1*, *ETV4*, and *ETV5* (Tomlins et al, 2005, 2006; Helgeson et al, 2008). These additional translocations are much rarer than the *TMPRSS2-ERG* rearrangement, which is estimated to represent greater than 90% of all fusions involving ETS genes in prostate cancer (Kumar-Sinha et al, 2008). In addition, fusions involving upstream fusion partners other than *TMPRSS2* have been found, including the fusions *SLC45A3-ETV5*, *SLC45A3-ERG*, *HNRPA2B1-ETV5*, and *SLC45A3-ELK4*; however, these are also relatively rare (Tomlins et al, 2007; Attard et al, 2008a, 2008b; Hermans et al, 2008; Maher et al, 2009; Rickman et al, 2009). Although the fusion events in prostate cancer are typically driven by genomic rearrangements, the *SLC45A3-ELK4* fusion was later found to be due to RNA cis-splicing events between these two genes (which are located adjacent to each other on chromosome 1 band q32) with no alterations to the DNA sequence (Zhang et al, 2012). To date, additional low-frequency gene fusions have been identified in prostate cancer that involve non-ETS family members, such as *CDKN1A*, *CD9*, *IKBKB*, the oncogene *PIGU*, the tumor suppressor *RSRC2*, and members of the RAF pathway (*BRAF*, *RAF1*) (Palanisamy et al, 2010; Pflueger et al, 2011; Ren et al, 2012). These studies have been facilitated by next-generation RNA sequencing (RNA-seq or whole "transcriptome" shotgun sequencing) technologies that unbiasedly sequence all RNA species in a sample, with an analysis that is not limited to "annotated" sequences. The results of RNA-seq studies indicate that some of the fusion events that occur in prostate cancer may be "private events" (e.g., occurring in only one patient), implying that the frequency and range of fusion events in prostate cancer may be far greater than what is currently understood (Pflueger et al, 2011).

Recurrent Gene Rearrangements in Renal Cancer

A novel subtype of RCC, MiTF/TFE family translocation carcinomas, has been described that features chromosomal translocations involving one of two members of the microphthalmia transcription factor (MiTF) family (Hemesath et al, 1994; Argani and Ladanyi, 2005). The first involves the *TFE3* gene on chromosome Xp11.2, which translocates to one of several partner genes including *PRCC* (1q21), *ASPL* (17q25), *PSF* (1p34), *NonO* (Xq12; rearranged via inversion), and an unknown gene at 3q23 (Sidhar et al, 1996; Weterman et al, 1996; Argani et al, 2001a, 2001b; Argani and Ladanyi, 2005; Argani et al, 2005; Martignoni et al, 2009). These translocations place the *TFE3* gene under the control of strong promoters that then drive inappropriate expression of *TFE3* (or a *TFE3*-containing fusion protein). In these cancers, TFE3 protein is readily detectable in the nucleus by IHC staining with anti-*TFE3* antibody, aiding in diagnosis. TFE3 RCCs are primarily found in children and adolescents and account for most pediatric cases of RCC (Argani and Ladanyi, 2005). Activation of the *MET* proto-oncogene may play a role with *TFE3* in these tumors (Tsuda et al, 2007), which is of interest because these tumors display papillary histologic architecture, and mutations in the *MET* gene are the underlying cause of hereditary papillary RCC (Jeffers et al, 1997).

A second class of MiTF/TFE family translocation carcinomas contains a specific translocation between the *TFEB* gene on 6p21 and the *ALPHA* gene on 11q12 (Argani et al, 2005). Similar to the Xp11 translocation RCCs, this entity is also most commonly found in children and adolescents and shares many other features with the *TFE3* translocation tumors. In addition to IHC staining for TFE3 and TFEB proteins, it was demonstrated that these tumors are also marked by staining for the protein cathepsin K, a shared transcriptional target gene of these transcription factors (Martignoni et al,

2009). The use of such markers or PCR to detect these specific gene fusions may have clinical importance because, as the cathepsin K example shows, these tumors likely are controlled by a different transcriptional program than conventional RCC, and therapeutic targets used against these cancers may not be effective against translocation RCCs.

Recurrent Gene Rearrangements in Testicular Cancer

In testicular germ cell tumors (TGCTs), gain of the short arm of chromosome 12 is a nearly universal finding, with the notable exception of the rare spermatocytic seminoma subtype (Atkin and Baker, 1982; Rodriguez et al, 1993; Rosenberg et al, 1998; Verdorfer et al, 2004). In most cases (approximately 80%), this finding occurs through a structural rearrangement producing an isochromosome 12p—that is, a version of chromosome 12 consisting of 2 p arms and no q (long) arm. In the remaining cases, 12p material is gained through more complex chromosomal rearrangements (Rosenberg et al, 2000; Ottesen et al, 2003; Looijenga et al, 2007). More detailed analyses have revealed amplification of specific regions on 12p, including the area 12p11-12p13. One common region of amplification at 12p11.2-12p12.1 contains 22 potential genes, including *KRAS*, a promising candidate TGCT gene, which also undergoes activating mutations in TGCTs (Moul et al, 1992; Olie et al, 1995; Rodriguez et al, 2003; Zafarana et al, 2003; Goddard et al, 2007). An additional region of interest lies at 12p13.31, where the so-called stem cell cluster region is located. This region contains several stem cell–related genes including *CD9*, *EDR1*, *GDF3*, *SCNN1A*, *NANOG*, and *STELLAR*, which exhibit coordinate overexpression (Clark et al, 2004; Korkola et al, 2006).

Other Genomic Alterations in Genitourinary Malignancies

Apart from chromosomal translocations, which are primarily specific changes in the spatial organization of the genome, an overall derangement of the chromosomal complement is nearly universal in human cancer, particularly in carcinomas—cancers that originate from epithelial cells and represent most adult GU malignancies. Such abnormalities are wide-ranging, affecting the genome at multiple scales, including losses and gains of entire chromosomes or chromosomal arms as well as deletions and amplifications of large and small chromosomal regions. These changes are generically referred to as CNAs. In addition to mutations, structural rearrangements, and epigenetic changes, CNAs are yet another reflection of the underlying genomic instability in cancer cells, resulting in the large number of genetic changes required for malignant transformation. This instability generates a great degree of genetic heterogeneity. For instance, when metaphase chromosomes of tumor cells are examined during karyotypic analysis, a bewildering array of chromosomal aberrations is typically observed, such that no two karyotypes within a given cancer cell population are exactly the same. However, within this seemingly random assortment of alterations, some changes are seen in multiple different cells and multiple tumor samples, providing a strong indication that a gene or genes located in the region undergoing recurrent alteration is involved in the pathogenesis of the disease. Over the past several decades, using ever more sophisticated and higher resolution molecular methods, many such changes have been cataloged and candidate cancer genes have been identified. Two general approaches are used here. In the first, inherited (germline) defects in genes that cause hereditary cancer predisposition syndromes are sought, often by performing genetic linkage analysis in affected and nonaffected family members in an attempt to find genetic loci that track in a mendelian fashion with disease status. Several familial cancer predisposition syndromes are now understood in significant detail, some featuring GU malignancies and others not (Tables 19-1 and 19-2). In the second approach, various techniques are employed to discover disease-associated genes in sporadic cancers that lack a strong familial component (caused by somatic rather than germline genetic alterations). The detection of CNAs in a particular gene (or region containing the gene)

TABLE 19-1 Tumor Syndromes Associated with Genitourinary Malignancies

SYNDROME	TUMOR	CHROMOSOME(S)	GENE(S)	(FUNCTION)
Wilms tumor	Wilms tumor	11p13	WT1	(Transcriptional repressor)
Beckwith-Wiedemann	Wilms tumor	11p15	CDKN1C	(Cell cycle regulator)
von Hippel-Lindau	Clear cell renal carcinoma Pheochromocytoma	3p25	VHL	(Transcriptional elongation and ubiquitination)
Hereditary papillary renal cancer	Papillary renal carcinoma	7q31	MET	(Receptor tyrosine kinase)
Birt-Hogg-Dube	Papillary renal carcinoma Oncocytoma	17p11.2	FLCN	(Unknown function)
MEN type 2	Pheochromocytoma	10q11	RET	(Receptor tyrosine kinase)
Hereditary nonpolyposis colorectal cancer	Upper tract transitional cell carcinoma	2p22, 3p21.3, 2p18, 2q31-q33, 7p22, 14q24.3	MSH2, MLH1, MSH6, PMS1, PMS2, MLH3	(DNA mismatch repair)
Hereditary prostate cancer	Prostate cancer	1q24-25, 1p36, 1q42-43, 8p22-23, 17p11, 20q13, Xq27-28	RNASEL, MSR1, ELAC2	(Endoribonuclease, macrophage specific receptor, cell cycle regulator)

MEN, multiple endocrine neoplasia.

TABLE 19-2 Selected Tumor Syndromes Not Strongly Associated with Genitourinary Malignancies

SYNDROME	PRIMARY TUMOR	CHROMOSOME(S)	GENE(S)	(FUNCTION)
Familial retinoblastoma	Retinoblastoma	13q14	RB	(Transcriptional regulation)
Li-Fraumeni	Sarcoma, breast carcinoma	17p13, 22q12	TP53, hCHK2	(Transcription factor, serine kinase)
Familial adenomatous polyposis	Colorectal carcinoma	5q21	APC	(Regulates β-catenin activity)
Familial breast carcinoma	Breast carcinoma	17q21, 13q12	BRCA1, BRCA2	(DNA double-stranded break repair)
Cowden disease	Breast carcinoma	10q23	PTEN	(Phosphatase; PI3K antagonist)
MEN type 1	Pancreatic islet cell carcinoma	11q13	MEN1	(Transcription factor)

MEN, multiple endocrine neoplasia; PI3K, phosphatidylinositol-3′-kinase.

coupled with mutations in the other allele is persuasive evidence for that gene functioning as a disease-relevant oncogene (with activating mutations) or tumor suppressor gene (featuring inactivating mutations or promoter methylation). In the case of cancer-related genes identified in hereditary predisposition syndromes, one hopes that alterations of genes discovered in familial forms of the disease are also relevant to their more common sporadic counterparts. In many instances, this has been found to be the case; for example, gene abnormalities linked to certain familial forms of kidney cancer are also involved in sporadic forms of the disease. In the following sections, we describe some of the recurrent genetic changes identified in familial and sporadic forms of GU malignancies.

Hereditary Prostate Cancer

Family history is one of the strongest risk factors for prostate cancer (Steinberg et al, 1990), and criteria defining a hereditary form of the disease have been established (Carter et al, 1993). Twin studies have estimated a heritable risk for prostate cancer of approximately 50% (Page et al, 1997; Lichtenstein et al, 2000). Traditional linkage analysis is well suited to identify highly penetrant genetic alterations (Fig. 19-12). The overall low yield and irreproducibility seen in hereditary prostate cancer (HPC) linkage studies has led to the conclusion that rather than being caused by a few high-impact genes, HPC is instead likely to depend on

alterations in many genes, each of which has only a modest effect (Easton et al, 2003; Schaid, 2004).

Initial genome-wide searches in HPC families uncovered evidence for susceptibility loci on chromosomes 1q, 4q, 5p, 7p, 13q, and Xq (Smith et al, 1996). The first strong candidate locus, HPC1, was localized to the region 1q24.25 (Gronberg et al, 1997) and a gene, RNASEL, was later identified at this locus (Carpten et al, 2002; Rokman et al, 2002). Although this linkage was replicated in some studies, it was not confirmed in others (Cooney et al, 1997; McIndoe et al, 1997; Eeles et al, 1998; Bergthorsson et al, 2000). Similarly, a failure to confirm linkage consistently has plagued other candidate HPC loci and genes as well, highlighting the difficulty in conducting such studies. Because prostate cancer is a relatively common disease, HPC families are contaminated with sporadic cases ("phenocopies"). It has become apparent that familial prostate cancer may lack the type of high-risk susceptibility genes such as BRCA1 or BRCA2 that are clearly linked to hereditary forms of breast and ovarian cancers (Simard et al, 2003). Among other considerations, these facts underline the need for large, well-defined HPC cohorts, making genetic studies difficult to perform. One large HPC cohort of 175 pedigrees identified a region in chromosome 17q21-22 near BRCA1 with linkage to prostate cancer susceptibility (Lange et al, 2003). This region has subsequently become one of the most intensively investigated regions of the genome for HPC susceptibility. More recently, targeted next-generation sequencing of exons in 202 genes on chromosome 17q21-22 from germline DNA

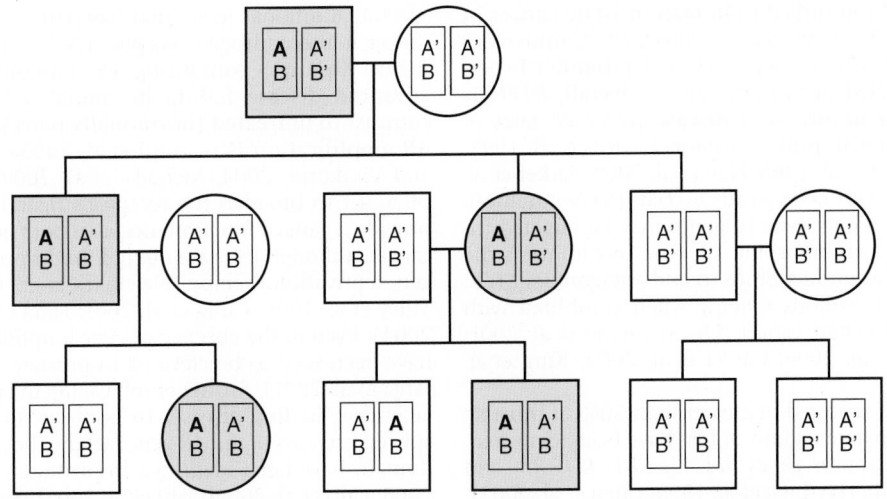

Figure 19-12. The familial tumor syndrome is passed from generation to generation. Genotyping demonstrates that the polymorphic marker A *(marked in bold)* is passed also from generation to generation in concert with the phenotypic disease. Presumably, a gene responsible for the syndrome is located near marker A. Linkage analysis is complicated by incomplete penetrance (not all members of the family with the allele get the disease), phenocopies (family members who have sporadic disease), inability to get DNA from all family members, and the large number of markers being simultaneously analyzed.

of unrelated patients with prostate cancer from families that were selected for linkage to the 17q22-22 region identified a variant in the *HOXB13* gene (*HOXB13* G84E) that significantly increased the risk of HPC (Ewing et al, 2012). The carrier frequency of the G84E allele was found in 0.1% of men without prostate cancer and 1.4% of men with prostate cancer. The frequency of the allele was much higher in men with early-onset, familial prostate cancer (3.1%) compared with men with late-onset, nonfamilial prostate cancer (0.6%) (Ewing et al, 2012). Although the carrier rate of the G84E allele is rare, the strong linkage to prostate cancer risk may warrant genetic testing for the variant, similar to testing that is currently performed for *BRCA1* or *BRCA2* in hereditary breast and ovarian cancers. Other candidate HPC susceptibility genes include *ELAC2* (*HPC2*), macrophage scavenger receptor-1 (*MSR-1*), and *PODXL* (Tavtigian et al, 2001; Xu et al, 2002a; Nupponen et al, 2004; Casey et al, 2006). It is intriguing that two of the HPC candidates, *RNASEL* and *MSR-1*, are both associated with functions of the immune response because inflammation is currently considered a likely contributor to the pathogenesis of prostate cancer (De Marzo et al, 2007; Sfanos and De Marzo, 2012).

Sporadic Prostate Cancer

In sporadic prostate cancer, initial studies found recurrent changes involving losses of genetic material at 6q, 7q, 8p, 10q, 13q, 16q, 17p, 17q, and 18q; however, in most cases, the precise genes involved have yet to be identified (Karan et al, 2003). **Changes in chromosome 8, typically loss of the p arm and gain of the q arm, or portions of these arms, are the most frequently observed genetic alterations.** At least two to three separate regions are deleted on 8p, implying the existence of multiple tumor suppressor genes. **The region 8p22 is commonly deleted, with frequencies of 32% to 65% reported in primary tumors and 65% to 100% in metastases. *MSR-1* lies in this region,** and sequence variants in *MSR-1* have been found to be associated with increased disease risk; however, mutations in *MSR-1* have not been reported in sporadic prostate cancers (Xu et al, 2002a; Nupponen et al, 2004; Wiklund et al, 2009). **Another promising candidate tumor suppressor gene on 8p is the prostate-restricted homeobox gene *NKX3.1* at 8p21** (He et al, 1997). Mice engineered with a loss of a single allele of *NKX3.1* develop prostate hyperplasia and PIN, an example of haploinsufficiency, wherein a phenotypic effect is observed secondary

to the loss of a single allele (Bhatia-Gaur et al, 1999; Abdulkadir et al, 2002).

The most common chromosomal abnormality found in advanced prostate cancer (e.g., hormone-refractory lymph node metastases) **is 8q gain, often involving the entire chromosomal arm leading to isochromosome 8q formation,** and it is correlated with disease progression and resistance to hormone deprivation or blockade (Alers et al, 2000; Isaacs, 2002; van Dekken et al, 2003). **The proto-oncogene *MYC* at 8q24 is a likely candidate gene on 8q,** but the observed gains are large, and more work is required to assess this possibility properly. Elevated expression of another gene in this region, *EIF3S3*, has been documented in cancer compared with benign prostatic hyperplasia (Savinainen et al, 2004). Mouse models lend support for a linkage to *MYC*; transgenic mice with forced prostate-specific expression of human *MYC* develop PIN and invasive adenocarcinomas (Ellwood-Yen et al, 2003). Amplification at the *MYC* locus has been reported in some human prostate cancers and is associated with a poor prognosis (Jenkins et al, 1997; Sato et al, 1999).

Chromosome 7 abnormalities are also frequently observed in prostate cancer. Aneusomy of the entire chromosome (trisomy 7) has been reported in both PIN and cancer and has been associated with advanced stage and a poor prognosis (Arps et al, 1993; Macoska et al, 1993; Alcaraz et al, 1994; Zitzelsberger et al, 1994; Qian et al, 1995). Apart from whole chromosome gains, losses involving 7q31.1 have been documented, suggesting a tumor suppressor resides here (Zenklusen et al, 1994; Takahashi et al, 1995). A potential candidate tumor suppressor gene in this region is caveolin (*CAV1*), whose expression is reportedly decreased in cancer (Bender et al, 2000; Wiechen et al, 2001). However, positive IHC staining for caveolin has been associated with *poor* prognosis, and its role in prostate cancer remains unclear (Yang et al, 1999; Tahir et al, 2001). Another attractive candidate gene in this region is *EZH2*, which codes for a histone methyltransferase involved in gene silencing. In microarray analyses, *EZH2* has been found to be overexpressed in prostate cancer metastases, and its expression in primary tumors is associated with disease (PSA) recurrence (Varambally et al, 2002; Rhodes et al, 2003; Lapointe et al, 2004).

Chromosome 10 also undergoes alteration in prostate cancer, with deletions observed at 10p11.2 and 10q23-q24 (Ittmann, 1996; Trybus et al, 1996). **The tumor suppressor gene *PTEN*, a phosphatidylinositol-3′ (PI3) kinase antagonist, maps to this**

second region and has been linked to human prostate cancer in many studies (Li et al, 1997a; Ayala et al, 2004). *PTEN* undergoes homozygous (both copies) deletion, LOH, and promoter hypermethylation and is mutated in prostate cancer. **Overall, *PTEN* is more frequently altered in advanced disease** (reported rates of 60% to 100%) compared with primary tumors (Cairns et al, 1997; Pesche et al, 1998; Whang et al, 1998; Han et al, 2009; Sarker et al, 2009). The frequency of *PTEN* LOH greatly exceeds *PTEN* mutation, and it is suggested that another gene or genes may be targeted for deletion in this region of chromosome 10. One possibility is the *MXI1* gene, whose protein product binds to and antagonizes *MYC*. In mice, *PTEN* deficiency exhibits synergy when combined with other mouse models of prostate cancer (Di Cristofano et al, 2001; Kim et al, 2002; Chen et al, 2006; Carver et al, 2009; King et al, 2009).

LOH on 13q has been reported in greater than 50% of prostate cases examined. Three separate regions of loss have been identified, containing the potential cancer genes *BRCA2*, *RB1*, *EDNRB*, and *KLF5* (Cooney et al, 1996b; Hyytinen et al, 1999; Chen et al, 2003). High rates of *RB1* loss (up to 80%) have been reported in advanced cancers (Cher et al, 1996); however, the *RB1* mutation rate is relatively low, and RB1 expression is not well correlated with the gene dosage or disease status (Bookstein et al, 1990; Kubota et al, 1995; Ittmann and Wieczorek, 1996; Kibel and Isaacs, 2000). However, Theodorescu and associates (1997) reported that low RB1 protein expression was correlated with decreased disease-specific survival in univariate and multivariate analysis.

Losses on 16q have been observed with reported frequencies ranging from 30% to 56% of prostate cancer cases, being more commonly seen in advanced cancer and associated with a poor prognosis (Carter et al, 1990; Bergerheim et al, 1991; Suzuki et al, 1996; Elo et al, 1997; Li et al, 1999). A common region of loss at 16q22-q24 contains two likely candidate genes, the *CDH1* gene at 16q22.1 that codes for the calcium-dependent cell-cell adhesion protein E-cadherin (Morton et al, 1993; Umbas et al, 1994; Murant et al, 2000; Rubin et al, 2001), and the *ATBF1* gene at 16q22, coding for an AT-sequence binding transcription factor (Sun et al, 2005). Loss of *CDH1* has been associated with metastatic prostate cancer; however, IHC staining studies have produced mixed results, and reports of mutation or LOH of E-cadherin are lacking; *CDH1* may not be the primary target of the 16q deletion. The *ATBF1* gene has been reported to be mutated in 40% of prostate cancers (Sun et al, 2005).

Reports of LOH on 6q range from 30% to 50%, with a minimal region of loss at 6q14-q22. No strong candidate gene has been identified in this region (Cooney et al, 1996a; Hyytinen et al, 2002).

Allelic losses of a region on 17p that includes the *TP53* gene have been documented but are infrequent in primary prostate cancer compared with more advanced disease (Brooks et al, 1996). This matches findings of mutational analyses in which *TP53* mutations are rarely found in primary tumors but are reported in 40% of advanced disease (Visakorpi et al, 1992; Bookstein et al, 1993; Navone et al, 1993). A recurrent region of loss on 17q is located near the *BRCA1* gene at 17q21; however, the identified common area of loss does not include this critical tumor suppressor gene (Brothman et al, 1995; Williams et al, 1996).

Deletions on 18q are mainly observed in advanced prostate cancer. A common region of deletion encompasses the known cancer-related genes *DCC*, *SMAD2*, and *SMAD4* (Ueda et al, 1997; Yin et al, 2001).

Loss of the cell cycle regulatory gene *CDKN2A* on 9p21, which encodes the CDKI p16, has been reported in 20% of prostate cancers and at twice this frequency in advanced disease (Cairns et al, 1995; Jarrard et al, 1997). As discussed previously, this locus also contains the p14 and p15 genes, making it difficult to pinpoint the exact target or targets of genetic loss in this region. Reduced expression and LOH of another CDKI gene, *CDKN1B* on 12p13.1-p12, which encodes the p27 protein, are also found in prostate cancer and are associated with more advanced disease (Guo et al, 1997; Kibel et al, 1998; Yang et al, 1998).

One additional locus that has particular relevance for prostate cancer is the androgen receptor (*AR*) gene located on Xq12. **The region Xq11-q13 containing *AR* is amplified in 30% of cases of advanced disease failing hormonal ablation therapy, in stark contrast to untreated (hormonally naive) cases that do not show *AR* amplification** (Visakorpi et al, 1995a; Chen et al, 2004; Linja and Visakorpi, 2004; Mellado et al, 2009). *AR* mutations, which often act to broaden the receptor's ligand specificity or otherwise provide a gain of function, occur in both advanced and lower stage cancer, although they are rarely found in cases untreated by androgen deprivation therapy (Newmark et al, 1992; Taplin et al, 1995; Tilley et al, 1996; Culig et al, 2001; Hara et al, 2003; Gottlieb et al, 2004). Even in the absence of gene amplification, AR protein levels have been seen to be elevated in prostate cancer (Latil et al, 2001; Linja et al, 2001), further emphasizing the importance of AR hyperactivation in this disease. In addition to mutation, alternatively spliced versions of the *AR* gene lacking the androgen ligand-binding domain have been identified in prostate cancer cells (Dehm et al, 2008; Guo et al, 2009b; Hu et al, 2009). Such *AR* splice variants are active in the absence of bound ligand and may contribute to the emergence of prostate cancer refractory to androgen ablative therapies.

Subsequent studies using the comparative genomic hybridization (CGH) technique, in which competitive reactions between differentially labeled tumor-derived versus normal-derived genomic DNA highlight regions lost or gained in the tumor sample, have largely confirmed as well as extended the genomic alterations previously uncovered using LOH analysis. These CGH studies indicate that the number of different alterations is increased in advanced disease and that losses are more frequent than gains in early stages of the disease, with gains and genetic amplifications more commonly seen in advanced hormone-refractory disease (Visakorpi et al, 1995b; Cher et al, 1996; Nupponen and Visakorpi, 2000). Sun and coworkers (2007) reviewed all published prostate cancer CGH studies and found that, overall, 13 regions were found to be altered in at least 10% of prostate cancer cases, with 8 regions showing deletion and 5 regions showing copy number gain. An additional six regions (three with gains, three with losses) were found to be altered in greater than 10% of advanced cancers. In agreement with earlier studies, 8p was the most frequent region of genomic loss (with a peak at 8p21.3), being observed in one third of all cases and one half of cases of advanced disease. Likewise, 8q was gained most often (bimodal peaks at 8q22.2 and 8q24.13), being observed in one quarter of all cases and one half of cases of advanced disease (Sun et al, 2007). The other regions commonly lost, in decreasing order of frequency, included 13q21.q31, 6q14.1-q21, 16q13-q24.3, and 18q12.1-q23; regions exhibiting gain included 7q11.21-q32.3, Xq11.1-q23, 17q24.1-q25.3, and 3q26.23-q33. Also in keeping with the general observation that more aggressive and advanced cancers typically harbor more genetic abnormalities than their lower grade and lower stage counterparts, advanced prostate cancers displayed twofold to threefold more CNAs.

The application of modern high-resolution methods for assessing CNA, such as representational oligonucleotide microarray analysis and single nucleotide polymorphism (SNP) mapping arrays, will vastly improve our ability to detect CNA, particularly smaller alterations below the resolution limit of CGH, as well as aid in the identification of the resident oncogenes and tumor suppressor genes (Lucito et al, 2003; Sebat et al, 2004; Slater et al, 2005; Zhao et al, 2005; Liu et al, 2006).

High-density SNP microarrays have been used in genome-wide association studies (GWAS), high-resolution association studies between common DNA sequence variants (SNPs) and prostate cancer risk. In contrast to the more traditional linkage analyses of the past, the new platform is amenable to very large cohorts and is better able to detect genetic variations with small to moderate effects on disease risk (Risch and Merikangas, 1996; Jorgenson and Witte, 2007; Manolio, 2010). To date, several GWAS have been published on prostate cancer, resulting in the identification of more than 70 germline variants (SNPs) that are associated with the risk of developing prostate cancer (Amundadottir et al, 2006; Duggan et al, 2007; Gudmundsson et al, 2007; Haiman et al, 2007; Witte, 2007; Eeles et al, 2008; Gudmundsson et al, 2008; Thomas et al, 2008; Breyer et al, 2009; Eeles et al, 2009; Yeager et al, 2009; Nakagawa et al, 2012; Eeles et al, 2013). With larger meta-analyses being conducted worldwide, the number of prostate cancer SNPs is expected to increase to greater than 100 in the near future (Nakagawa, 2013). Most of the SNPs are not located in or even near genes previously shown to be involved in prostate cancer pathogenesis. Three independent loci were identified on 8q24, all contained within a 1-Mb DNA segment; however, no genes have been identified yet to account for these risk alleles (Cheng et al, 2008). A systematic review of replication studies in prostate cancer susceptibility loci identified from GWAS found that the 8q24 region continues to be the most implicated in prostate cancer risk and among different racial cohorts (Ishak and Giri, 2011). Although the *MYC* gene is in this vicinity, it is still 200 kb away from the nearest SNP, and its relevance, if any, remains uncertain. In contrast to the loci identified in earlier linkage studies in HPC families, the risk alleles identified in these GWAS have been independently confirmed. As predicted, the risk attributable to each locus is small to modest; however, because of the large cohorts studied, each association is highly statistically significant, and each has been shown to confer risk independent of the other loci. These risk alleles act in a fairly additive fashion (Kote-Jarai et al, 2008; Sun et al, 2008; Zheng et al, 2008; Witte, 2009). The clinical utility of using SNP "panels" for prostate cancer risk assessment is currently being investigated (Nam et al, 2009; Zheng et al, 2009; Chatterjee et al, 2013). However, **although men in the top decile in terms of number of combined risk alleles have a twofold to fourfold increased risk for prostate cancer compared with the bottom decile, the numbers of men harboring such large numbers of risk alleles is small, and these SNPs are unlikely to have utility for population screening purposes.** An important facet to these studies is that so far most of these prostate cancer risk alleles do not appear to be associated specifically with risk for aggressive disease (Kader et al, 2009; Wiklund et al, 2009). The lack of strong prognostic markers is a key shortcoming in the field that desperately needs to be resolved. **Most current GWAS used case-control designs. New case-case studies comparing aggressive versus nonaggressive disease will likely be required to uncover new SNPs informative for disease aggressiveness. It is thought that the recently identified SNPs are more likely related to prostate cancer initiation rather than progression.** One such study that compared SNP frequencies among patients with prostate cancer who were defined as having aggressive versus nonaggressive disease identified a region of 17p12 (TT genotype of SNP rs4054823) that was consistently higher among patients with more aggressive disease (Xu et al, 2010). The SNP in 17p12 resides in a region that does not contain any known genes; at the present time, the molecular mechanism by which it is associated with aggressive disease remains unknown. **Another approach that has had some early success in other cancers is to use gene expression array data to develop "gene signatures" able to predict aggressive behavior** (Cheville et al, 2008; Mucci et al, 2008; Setlur et al, 2008).

More recent rapid advances in next-generation sequencing technologies, allowing for whole genome sequencing and whole exome sequencing of multiple tumor samples at a time, have enabled comprehensive analyses of the complete landscape of genomic alterations (e.g., SNPs, CNAs, chromosomal rearrangements) present in human prostate cancer. One such study that conducted massively parallel sequencing of tumor and matched genomic DNA from seven patients with Gleason grade 7 or higher tumors identified a median of 3866 putative somatic base mutations (range 3192 to 5865) covering approximately 80% of the genome per tumor with a 10-fold higher mutation rate in CpG dinucleotides than in all other genomic positions (Berger et al, 2011). Of the somatic mutations identified, a median of 20 mutations per tumor that cause a change in amino acid sequence were found to occur within protein-coding genes. Specific genes found to be mutated in multiple tumors included the scaffold protein *SPTA1*; a modulator of

the transcriptional regulator DAXX called *SPOP*; chromatin modifiers *CHD1*, *CHD5*, and *HDAC9*; and members of the heat shock protein (HSP1) stress response complex *HSPA2*, *HSPA5*, and *HSP90AB1*. In addition to somatic mutations, a median of 90 chromosomal rearrangements were identified per tumor genome (range 43 to 213), all of which produced balanced translocations without genomic loss and with the generation of "chimeric" chromosomes. Additional genes found to be specifically targeted by mutation or rearrangements were the tumor suppressor *PTEN* and the PTEN-interacting protein *MAGI2*. In a separate study of whole exome sequencing of 112 prostate tumor and normal pairs, mutations in *SPOP* were again detected, and this was found to be the most frequently mutated gene (Barbieri et al, 2012). Barbieri and colleagues found that *SPOP* mutations occurred in the tumors that lacked ETS family gene rearrangements, possibly defining a new molecular subtype of prostate cancer. Additional recurrent mutations were identified in the forkhead transcription factor gene *FOXA1* and *MED12*, a protein involved in transcription initiation. As exome sequencing becomes increasingly more routine, attention has turned to the possibility of performing rapid high-throughput sequencing of patient samples that can inform therapeutic decisions on men with a new diagnosis of advanced prostate cancer (Roychowdhury et al, 2011).

In addition to novel gene fusions that have been identified via RNA-seq analyses, numerous novel noncoding RNA (ncRNA) species have been identified in prostate cancer samples. Much of the focus of ncRNA species in prostate cancer to date has been on microRNA (miRNA) species, which are small (approximately 22 nucleotides) molecules that function in gene silencing and may be linked to prostate cancer aggressiveness, may promote the development of castration resistance, or may serve as markers of prostate cancer stem cells (Bolton et al, 2014). Multiple novel long noncoding RNA (lncRNA) transcripts that may play a functional role in prostate carcinogenesis have also been discovered; lncRNAs are distinguished from small ncRNA species (e.g., miRNAs, small interfering RNAs, and small nucleolar RNAs) in that they are typically greater than 200 nucleotides in length. Although they do not encode for functional peptides, lncRNAs play a role in gene regulation and other cellular processes (Ulitsky and Bartel, 2013). One of the most clinically advanced biomarkers of prostate cancer, *PCA3* (also known as *DD3*), happens to be an lncRNA (Bussemakers et al, 1999). RNA-seq performed on a cohort of 102 prostate tissues and cell lines identified 106 unannotated intergenic RNAs that were differentially expressed between prostate cancer and benign prostate samples (Prensner et al, 2011). One of the top upregulated transcripts, an lncRNA called *PCAT-1*, was markedly upregulated in metastases and was found to act as a target of the Polycomb Repressive Complex 2 (PRC2). *PCAT-1* is located on chromosome 8q24—discussed previously in regard to susceptibility loci in prostate cancer—and is approximately 725 kb upstream of the c-*MYC* oncogene. Another lncRNA identified in this study, *SChLAP1*, was found in a follow-up study to antagonize chromatin remodeling complex activity and serve as a prognostic indicator of poor prostate cancer outcome (Prensner et al, 2013).

Renal Cancer

RCCs include a spectrum of subtypes and can be subdivided into at least five different categories: clear cell RCC (ccRCC), which account for most adult cases (70% to 80%); papillary RCC, which accounts for most of the remaining adult cases (10% to 20%); chromophobe RCC; collecting duct RCC; and the MiTF/TFE family translocation carcinomas described earlier. In addition, there are more than four inherited forms of RCC. **The genes discovered to have germline mutations that cause these familial forms of the disease have been found to play important roles in sporadic RCC as well** (Coleman, 2008).

Patients with von Hippel-Lindau disease are predisposed to numerous tumor types, notably ccRCC (Coleman, 2008). The finding of consistent losses of 3p in this disease led to the identification of the *VHL* gene located at 3p25-p26; germline mutation of this gene causes VHL disease (Zbar et al, 1987; Tory et al, 1989; Latif et al, 1993; Stolle et al, 1998). **When the *VHL* gene was identified, its status was assessed in sporadic (nonfamilial) RCC, where it was found to be mutated in more than half of sporadic ccRCC cases** (Gnarra et al, 1994; Shuin et al, 1994). To date, more than 300 different *VHL* mutations have been cataloged, and ccRCC cases not harboring *VHL* mutations often undergo LOH (deletion) or silencing of the gene by promoter hypermethylation. Altogether, most ccRCCs have compromised *VHL*. **The VHL protein normally functions as part of a multiprotein complex with elonginB, elonginC, Cul-2 (cullin-2), and Rbx1 (ring box-1), which exhibits E3 ubiquitin ligase activity and targets subunits of the hypoxia-inducible factor-1 (HIF-1) transcription factor for ubiquitination and subsequent proteosomal destruction** (Kibel et al, 1995; Iliopoulos et al, 1996; Pause et al, 1997; Kamura et al, 1999; Kaelin, 2002). **HIF-1 functions as a master regulator of the cellular response to low oxygen levels.** Under normal conditions, specific proline amino acid residues in the two HIF-1 subunits, HIF-1 alpha and HIF-1 beta, are hydroxylated by the oxygen-dependent proline hydroxylase enzymes *EGLN1-3*. This oxygen-dependent modification signals ubiquitination of HIF-1, and HIF-1 is rapidly turned over (Maxwell et al, 1999; Bruick and McKnight, 2001; Ivan et al, 2001; Jaakkola et al, 2001). **Under conditions of oxygen deprivation (hypoxia), the prolyl hydroxylases fail to act, and HIF-1 is spared and accumulates, allowing its translocation to the nucleus where it activates numerous target genes,** including the glucose transporter *GLUT-1*, the proangiogenic growth factors *PDGF* and *VEGF*, the chemokine *CXCL-1* and its receptor *CXCL4*, transforming growth factor-α, and the hepatocyte growth factor receptor MET (Wykoff et al, 2001; Igarashi et al, 2002; Hu et al, 2003; Staller et al, 2003; Linehan et al, 2007). That the HIF-1 pathway is activated in ccRCC is supported by the highly vascular nature of these tumors and the fact that expression of HIF-1 target genes is found to be elevated. **In ccRCC, the loss of VHL function leads to a state of "pseudohypoxia," in which the cells respond as if they are being starved for oxygen.**

Several of the genes activated by HIF-1 have been singled out for therapeutic targeting, and positive results in clinical trials have led to U.S. Food and Drug Administration (FDA) approval of some of these agents (Linehan, 2002; Hansel and Rini, 2008). For example, the monoclonal anti–vascular endothelial growth factor (VEGF) antibody bevacizumab and the small molecule kinase inhibitors sunitinib and sorafenib, which inhibit both VEGF and platelet-derived growth factor, all have shown improvements in progression-free survival in clinical trials for metastatic RCC, leading in the latter two cases to FDA approval (Hansel and Rini, 2008).

The VHL/sporadic ccRCC example epitomizes the potential for translational application of cancer molecular genetics. Work began with studies on a familial cancer, which were translated to the sporadic form of the disease, culminating in the rational design of therapeutic agents against revealed molecular targets, having a positive impact in the clinic.

A second familial form of RCC is hereditary papillary renal carcinoma, the cause of which has been pinpointed to activation of the proto-oncogene tyrosine kinase c-Met, which is the cell surface receptor for hepatocyte growth factor (Jeffers et al, 1997). *MET* is located at 7q31-q34, which is notable because most sporadic papillary RCC cases show trisomy of chromosome 7 (Kovacs, 1993). In addition, activating mutations, typically affecting the tyrosine kinase domain and leading to a constitutively active receptor, have been found in sporadic cases (Schmidt et al, 1997).

A third type of hereditary RCC predisposition is Birt-Hogg-Dube (BHD) syndrome. Individuals with BHD syndrome most commonly develop chromophobe RCC, but other forms such as ccRCC, papillary RCC, and benign oncocytomas are also observed (Pavlovich et al, 2002, 2005). The *BHD* gene underlying the disease is located at 17p11.12 and codes for the protein folliculin (Schmidt et al, 2001). A spectrum of disruptive mutations and gene deletions supports a tumor suppressor gene function for folliculin (Khoo et al, 2002; Nickerson et al, 2002; Schmidt et al, 2005; Vocke et al, 2005). The precise function of this protein has not been elucidated,

although evidence indicates it affects both the ERK and Akt/mTOR signaling pathways (Baba et al, 2008).

A fourth, rare familial RCC subtype is hereditary leiomyomatosis renal cell carcinoma (HLRCC), featuring an aggressive form of papillary RCC (Kiuru and Launonen, 2004; Merino et al, 2007; Sudarshan et al, 2007). The cause of HLRCC has been traced to the Fumarate Hydratase gene at 1q42.3-q43, whose protein product acts to convert fumarate to malate in the Krebs cycle. The HIF-1 pathway is again implicated in RCC tumorigenesis because the resulting accumulation of fumarate acts as a competitive inhibitor of the prolyl hydroxylases *EGLIN1-3*, preventing modification of HIF-1 subunits, prolonging their half-lives and leading to a pseudohypoxic state, as was the case for mutated *VHL*. In support of this pathogenetic scheme, increased expression of VEGF and a high microvessel density have been found in HLRCC tumors (Isaacs et al, 2005; Pollard et al, 2005).

In 2011, a germline missense substitution was discovered in microphthalmia-associated transcription factor (*MITF*, another member of the MiTF family discussed earlier in regard to MiTF/TFE family translocation carcinomas) that conferred a greater than five-fold increase in risk of developing RCC, melanoma, or both types of cancer (Bertolotto et al, 2011). The germline substitution in codon 318 (E318K) was found to impair SUMOylation of MITF, leading to transcriptional activation of genes that function in the hypoxia pathway (*HIF1A*, *CCR7*, *HMOX1*), the importance of which in RCC has already been discussed.

Bladder Cancer

Although first-degree relatives of patients with bladder cancer are at increased risk of developing the disease, high-risk families are very rare and lack clear mendelian inheritance patterns, precluding classic linkage analysis. Bladder cancer is not considered a familial disease. Instead, it has been proposed that many susceptibility genes likely exist with small to moderate effects on disease risk (Aben et al, 2006; Kiemeney, 2008). More recent attention has turned to the use of GWAS, which are better suited to the discovery of low-penetrance susceptibility loci. The first such studies have been published, and reported susceptibility loci include 8q24.21, near the *MYC* proto-oncogene; 3q28, associated with the *TP53* relative *TP63*; and 5p15.33, which is near the *HTERT* gene coding for the cancer-associated telomere maintenance enzyme telomerase (Kiemeney et al, 2008, 2009; Rafnar et al, 2009; Wang et al, 2009a). Gain of 5p15.33 had previously been identified as being associated with bladder cancer progression (Yamamoto et al, 2007), and reduced or absent TP63 expression has been associated with disease progression and poor prognosis (Urist et al, 2002; Koga et al, 2003). An additional GWAS reported by Wu and coworkers (2009b) found a missense variant in the prostate stem cell antigen (PSCA) gene to be associated with bladder cancer risk in whites and was subsequently shown in a GWAS by Wang and associates (2010) to be associated with bladder cancer risk in a Chinese population. The rs2294008 variant of PSCA has also been shown to be significantly associated with gastric cancer in both Japan and China (Sakamoto et al, 2008; Matsuo et al, 2009; Wu et al, 2009a). This mutation is predicted to result in truncation of the first nine amino acids of the PSCA protein, and earlier studies reported that PSCA mRNA and protein levels are increased in bladder cancer compared with normal urothelium, with mRNA expression serving as an independent predictor of recurrence in superficial bladder cancer (Amara et al, 2001; Elsamman et al, 2006; Wang et al, 2010). Recent years have seen an explosion in large-scale GWAS in Europe and the United States that have now accounted for at least 11 extensively replicated urinary bladder cancer susceptibility loci: 1p13.3 (*GSTM1*), 2q37.1 (*UGT1A* cluster), 3q28 (*TP63*), 4p16.3 (*TMEM129* and *TACC3-FGFR3*), 5p15.33 (*HTERT-CLPTM1L*), 8p22 (*NAT2*), 8q24.21 (*MYC*), 8q24.3 (*PSCA*), 18q12.3 (*SLC14A1*), 19q12 (*CCNE1*), and 22q13.1 (*CBX6*, *APOBEC3A*) (García-Closas et al, 2005; Kiemeney et al, 2008; Rafnar et al, 2009; Wu et al, 2009b; Kiemeney et al, 2010; Rothman et al, 2010; García-Closas et al, 2011; Moore et al, 2011; Rafnar et al, 2011; Tang et al, 2012). Additional loci have been reported more recently on 3q26.2 and 11p15.5 as well as two suggested regions on 20p12.2 and 6q22.3 (Figueroa et al, 2014). Pathway analysis of five GWAS conducted on bladder cancer cases and controls of European background found the genetic variants associated with bladder cancer to belong to three fundamental cellular processes: metabolic detoxification, mitosis, and clathrin-mediated vesicles (Menashe et al, 2012).

Most (75% to 85%) bladder cancer and cancer-associated lesions seen in the clinic are of superficial type (stages pTa, pTis, pT1). Recurrences after therapy are frequent, requiring diligent surveillance by urine cytology and cystoscopy resulting in frequent resections. In addition, the risk of progression is high. Accurate assessment of risk for recurrence and progression to muscle-invasive disease is critical, and current predictive schemes based on histopathologic features are suboptimal. It is hoped that information at the molecular level will help improve current methods of risk stratification.

Much work has been done to identify genetic alterations in bladder cancer. In general, observed changes fall into two groups: changes that are mostly unrelated to clinical subtype (e.g., changes in chromosome 9 and *RAS* mutations) and changes that are related to specific grades or stages of the disease (e.g., *FGFR3* mutations in superficial pTa disease, *TP53* and *RB1* alterations in muscle-invasive disease) (Knowles, 2008).

Greater than half of urothelial cell carcinomas of all grades show chromosome 9 alterations; these are commonly losses of the entire chromosome or entire chromosomal arms. LOH events of more restricted regions are also seen, leading to the current consensus that there are multiple tumor suppressor genes located on both chromosomal arms (Tsai et al, 1990; Cairns et al, 1993; Linnenbach et al, 1993). In otherwise near-diploid tumors, complete loss of one copy (monosomy 9) is the only karyotypic abnormality seen (Gibas et al, 1984; Fadl-Elmula et al, 2000). **The region at 9p21 containing the genes for the CDKI proteins INK4B (p15) and INK4A (p16), which suppress the RB1 pathway, as well as harboring the TP53-stabilizing gene p14ARF is a strong candidate for bladder cancer tumor suppressor gene locus.** This region commonly undergoes LOH or homozygous deletion in bladder cancers, including low-grade and low-stage tumors (Devlin et al, 1994; Orlow et al, 1995; Williamson et al, 1995; Berggren et al, 2003), and mutations have been associated with high-grade disease and tumor progression (Orlow et al, 1999).

At least three different regions of loss have been mapped on 9q, and candidate bladder cancer tumor suppressor genes have been proposed including the patched gene, *PTCH*, at 9q22, which shows mutations and LOH in up to 40% of cancers (McGarvey et al, 1998; Aboulkassim et al, 2003); the region termed DBC1 at 9q32-q33, which exhibits deletion and silencing in approximately 50% of cases (Habuchi et al, 1998; Nishiyama et al, 1999); and 9q34, which exhibits LOH and contains the gene *TSC1* (tuberous sclerosis gene 1), a strong candidate bladder tumor suppressor gene owing to the finding of *TSC1* mutations in conjunction with LOH (Hornigold et al, 1999; Adachi et al, 2003; Knowles et al, 2003). The *TSC1* gene encodes the protein hamartin, which is a phosphorylation target of Akt and functions in negative regulation of mechanistic target of rapamycin (mTOR), a downstream target of the PI3 kinase pathway that is also dysregulated in bladder cancer via inactivation of the PI3 kinase antagonist *PTEN* as well as mutational activation of the p110 catalytic subunit of PI3 kinase, *PIK3CA* (Cairns et al, 1998; Aveyard et al, 1999; Wang et al, 2000).

Noninvasive (superficial, pTa) papillary urothelial cell carcinoma represents a major bladder cancer subgroup at diagnosis. Apart from changes involving chromosome 9, these tumors appear relatively stable with respect to chromosomal structural changes, with losses and gains reported for approximately 12 different chromosomal locations, most in 20% or less of cases examined (Koed et al, 2005; Knowles, 2008). More subtle genetic alterations in oncogenes and tumor suppressor genes also occur with varying frequencies. As reviewed by Knowles (2008), activating mutations in the *RAS* family of proto-oncogenes (H-RAS, K-RAS, and N-RAS) have been reported in 15% of cases; mutations in

PIK3CA have been reported in 16% of cases; and amplification/overexpression of *CCND1* and *HDM2* have been reported in 10% to 20% and approximately 30% of cases, respectively.

In addition to oncogene activation, inactivation of several tumor suppressor genes by either deletion or promoter hypermethylation has been reported in superficial papillary urothelial cell carcinoma. These genes include several genes on chromosome 9 such as *CDKN2A* (p16), affected in 30% to 60% of cases; *PTCH*, the *DBC1* locus; and *TSC1*, each reportedly affected in 60% of cases (Knowles, 2008).

The most frequently altered tumor suppressor gene in superficial stage Ta disease is the fibroblast growth factor receptor 3 (FGFR3), with mutation frequencies approaching 90% of cases reported (Cappellen et al, 1999; Billerey et al, 2001; Sibley et al, 2001; Tomlinson et al, 2007). The most common *FGFR3* mutation is a serine-to-cysteine mutation at amino acid 249, which has been shown to cause constitutive ligand-independent receptor activation secondary to induced receptor dimerization via intermolecular Cys-Cys disulfide bonding (Li et al, 2006). **The frequency of FGFR3 mutations is much lower in higher stage, invasive bladder cancers, and mutations are lacking in the superficial Tis stage (CIS) lesions, which have a high propensity for recurrence and progression to invasive disease.** In addition, in stage Ta disease, there is a strong inverse correlation between mutation and tumor grade (Billerey et al, 2001). The high preferential prevalence of *FGFR3* mutations in stage Ta disease suggests an association with low-risk bladder cancer (Tomlinson et al, 2007). In this respect, it is noteworthy that *FGFR3* mutations are also associated with benign tumors of the skin (seborrheic keratoses) (Logie et al, 2005; Hafner et al, 2006). In a prospective study, Hernandez and colleagues (2006) concluded that *FGFR3* mutations are associated with a subgroup of tumors having a good prognosis, and Burger and associates (2008) reported *FGFR3* status is useful in risk stratification for patients with high-grade non–muscle-invasive urothelial cell carcinoma. Finally, there are indications that *FGFR3* mutations and *RAS* family mutations are mutually exclusive (Jebar et al, 2005; Logie et al, 2005; Hafner et al, 2006). These findings may be rationalized by considering that FGFR3 itself is known to activate the RAS/RAF/MEK/ERK pathway (Choi et al, 2001). Likewise, reports of mutational exclusivity have been made regarding *FGFR3* and *TP53*, which is mutated in only about 5% of stage pTa cases and is associated with higher grade disease (Bakkar et al, 2003; Zieger et al, 2005). In stage pT1 disease, the frequency of *FGFR3* mutations is lower, and *TP53* mutation frequency is higher; in contrast to stage pTa disease, these mutations are not necessarily mutually exclusive (Bakkar et al, 2003; van Rhijn et al, 2004; Tomlinson et al, 2007).

Although the frequency of chromosome 9 alterations and *RAS* family mutations is comparable across all grades and stages of bladder cancer, **muscle-invasive urothelial carcinomas (stage pT2 and higher) exhibit more genetic alterations (both qualitatively and quantitatively) than lower stage disease, in keeping with the general observation that more aggressive cancers tend to exhibit evidence of greater genetic instability than their less aggressive counterparts.** Invasive bladder tumors exhibit a wide range of CNAs across virtually every chromosome, although the gene targets of these changes are largely unknown at the present time (Koed et al, 2005). In a similar vein, Blaveri and colleagues (2005) used cluster analysis of array CGH data to separate bladder tumors of differing stages and grades successfully from one another. In addition, a quantitative measure of the fraction of genome altered was shown to be inversely related to patient survival time in cases with muscle-invasive cancer (Blaveri et al, 2005). Ploidy, another reflection of genomic instability, has been found to be associated with progression from noninvasive to invasive bladder cancer (Holmang et al, 2001). Mutational inactivation of *TP53* is seen in greater than 40% of invasive pT2 tumors, in sharp contrast to the low mutational rate seen in pTa disease, where *TP53* mutation is associated with risk for progression (Fujimoto et al, 1992; Spruck et al, 1994; Uchida et al, 1995; George et al, 2007). Likewise, inactivation of *RB1*, either by LOH or through *INK4A* inactivation, is common in invasive bladder cancer but is infrequent in stage pTa tumors (Cairns et al, 1991;

Benedict et al, 1999; Chatterjee et al, 2004; Shariat et al, 2004). Loss of the region of 10q harboring the *PTEN* tumor suppressor gene is also more frequent in muscle-invasive bladder cancer than in lower stage pTa tumors (Cappellen et al, 1997; Kagan et al, 1998; Aveyard et al, 1999).

Genetic Alterations in Precursor Lesions to Bladder Neoplasia

Urothelial hyperplasias with flat or papillary histomorphology have been proposed to be precursors of low-grade bladder cancers, although this concept is controversial (Chow et al, 2000). In support, Hartmann and associates (1999) reported that, when present, genetic alterations (assayed at 9q21, 9q22, and 17p13) in hyperplasias were also found in superficial papillary tumors from the same patient. Genetic studies on hyperplasias have reported moderate to high frequencies of chromosome 9 alterations, whereas other genetic changes that are associated with aggressive forms of bladder cancer are reportedly infrequent (Chow et al, 2000). Dysplastic urothelial lesions have been found to have frequent changes of chromosome 9 and frequent aneuploidy, and approximately half are *TP53* mutated (Hartmann et al, 2002; Mallofre et al, 2003). The prevalence of changes seen in low-grade intraurothelial neoplasia was lower than that observed in high-grade (CIS) lesions (Hartmann et al, 2002). CIS lesions (pTis) are aggressive, high-grade precursor lesions, exhibiting high rates of recurrence and progression to invasive disease. In contrast to superficial papillary lesions, CIS exhibits frequent (50% to 70%) genetic alterations (LOH) of 4q, 8p, 11p, 13q, and 14q, in addition to several other chromosomal alterations observed at lower but still significant frequencies (Rosin et al, 1995). CIS lesions may be subdivided into primary lesions, which are isolated without associated cancer, and cancer-associated secondary lesions. It has been reported that chromosome 9 changes are infrequent in primary lesions, whereas most secondary lesions exhibit deletions on chromosome 9 (Spruck et al, 1994; Billerey et al, 2001; Hartmann et al, 2002; Hopman et al, 2002).

As expected, given their aggressive nature, *FGFR3* mutation rates are low in CIS, whereas the *TP53* pathway shows frequent alterations. *TP53* mutation occurs in more than half of CIS lesions and is correlated with strong nuclear TP53 staining by IHC (Hartmann et al, 2002; Hopman et al, 2002). Nuclear *TP53* expression in transitional cell carcinoma has been associated with increased risk of recurrence and death, independent of tumor grade, stage, and lymph node status in patients with transitional cell carcinoma (Lipponen, 1993; Sarkis et al, 1993; Esrig et al, 1994).

Genetic Alterations in Normal and Benign Bladder Urothelium

Given the propensity of bladder cancer to recur, plus the fact that it is often multifocal, it has been proposed that there may be genetic changes in broad areas of the urothelium. Such a hypothesis would be in keeping with the "field cancerization" concept (also known as "field effect"), first put forward by Slaughter and associates in 1953 to help explain the multifocal nature and high local recurrence rates of cancers of the oral cavity as well as the finding of histologically abnormal epithelium in areas adjacent to cancer. These authors proposed that multiple cancer foci arose within a wider field of abnormal epithelium that had been preconditioned by some prior carcinogenic insult, a process they termed *field cancerization*. Genetic changes have been detected in samples of histologically normal-appearing urothelium obtained from surgical samples from patients with cancer. For example, Muto and colleagues (2000) found shared instances of LOH as well as promoter hypermethylation of the *INK4A* gene between normal-appearing areas and tumor areas from the same case. Likewise, Stoehr and coworkers (2005) performed LOH analyses on a large number of cases in which normal-appearing epithelium was isolated by laser capture microdissection. These authors also reported cancer-associated genetic changes in the normal-appearing urothelium, which in some cases matched the changes found in concurrent cancers in the same case (Stoehr et al, 2005). However, caution is warranted when assessing such results given the possibility of contamination of the normal areas sampled by small multifocal cancer lesions or by pagetoid spread of tumor cells (Junker et al, 2003). A study by (Obermann and colleagues (2004) using interphase FISH in tissue sections detected losses involving chromosome 9 in normal-appearing cells, which, from a technical standpoint, should be effective at excluding possible confounding microscopic foci of cancer cells.

Inverted papillomas of the urinary bladder are considered benign entities. In keeping with this benign status, they exhibit infrequent LOH at cancer-associated chromosomal loci as well as infrequent (<10%) mutations of *FGFR3* (Sung et al, 2006; Eiber et al, 2007). In contrast to inverted papillomas, papillary urothelial neoplasia of low malignant potential exhibits high rates (85%) of *FGFR3* mutation (van Rhijn et al, 2002)—a genetic alteration that, as described earlier, is strongly associated with bladder tumors of low stage and low grade. However, a study by Cheng and associates (2004) found frequent LOH at several loci that typically undergo LOH in advanced stages (pT2 or higher).

Molecular Genetics–Based Assays for Bladder Cancer Detection and Surveillance

The large amount of data concerning common genetic alterations in bladder cancer has been exploited to aid in detecting the presence of bladder cancer. One widely used test termed UroVysion (Abbott Molecular/Vysis, Abbott Laboratories, Abbott Park, IL) is a multiplex, multicolor FISH-based assay that features a cocktail of four hybridization probes that assess the status of four chromosomes (Bubendorf et al, 2001; Halling, 2003). Probes specific for the centromeres of chromosomes 3, 7, and 17 provide information on cancer-associated gains of these chromosomes; the fourth probe is specific for 9p21, which harbors the p14 and p16 genes that are often deleted in bladder cancers. This test, approved by the FDA in 2005, is used in conjunction with standard urine cytology in diagnosing suspected cases and monitoring for local recurrence in patients with previous diagnosis and treatment (Halling et al, 2000; Hajdinjak, 2008). In addition, the test may have utility in monitoring response in patients with superficial bladder cancer treated with intravesical bacillus Calmette-Guérin therapy (Kipp et al, 2005) and may be useful in distinguishing inverted papillomas from urothelial carcinoma with inverted growth pattern (Jones et al, 2007).

At the present time, there are six FDA-approved urine-based molecular tests for bladder cancer focused on either genetic or immunochemical targets, and many other potential markers are under development (van Rhijn et al, 2005; Herman et al, 2008; Zwarthoff, 2008; Sullivan et al, 2009). **However, although these tests improve on standard urine cytology, they do not supplant it.** Finally, Wang and colleagues (2009b) reported the development of a quantitative PCR gene signature for predicting progression in cases of non–muscle-invasive bladder cancer.

Testicular Cancer

TGCTs possess many unique features (Oosterhuis and Looijenga, 2005). These cancers appear to originate from totipotent stem cells, with evidence strongly supporting TGCT initiation in utero, whereby abnormal primordial germ cells (PGCs) or gonocytes are blocked in their differentiation, remaining dormant until puberty. This theory is supported by expression in TGCT of markers closely associated with PGCs, including placental alkaline phosphatase (PLAP), the stem cell factor tyrosine kinase receptor KIT (c-kit), and the transcription factors POU5F1 (Oct3/4) and NANOG that are involved in maintenance of pluripotency or "stemness." The presumptive common precursors to TGCT are the intratubular germ cell neoplasia unclassified (ITGCNU), which closely resemble PGCs, sharing many of the same markers (PLAP, KIT, POU5F1) (Skakkebaek et al, 1987). ITGCNU, also traditionally referred to as

CIS, although this nomenclature is technically inaccurate, have a very high rate of progression to invasive disease, estimated to be essentially 100% if allowed sufficient time (Linke et al, 2005).

TGCTs are classified into two main categories: seminomas and nonseminomas. A third type, so-called spermatocytic seminomas, are extremely rare and are not discussed here (Ulbright, 1993). **Similar to the TGCT precursor ITGCNU, seminomas closely resemble PGCs/gonocytes, both morphologically and in their expression of molecular markers** (positive expression of PLAP, KIT, POU5F1, NANOG, STELLAR, SOX17) (Sperger et al, 2003; de Jong et al, 2008). **Nonseminomatous TGCTs resemble embryonic and extraembryonic tissues that have undergone varying extents of differentiation.** Nonseminomas include four subtypes. Embryonal carcinomas are similar in many respects to embryonic stem cells, or perhaps primitive ectoderm, and express POU5F1, NANOG, and STELLAR as well as SOX2 (Gopalan et al, 2009a). Extraembryonic differentiation is apparent in yolk sac tumors and choriocarcinomas, whereas somatic tissue differentiation is found in teratomas.

Besides their unique pathogenesis, TGCTs are unique in their responsiveness to treatment modalities that induce DNA damage (e.g., ionizing radiation and cisplatin-based chemotherapy). Most patients are currently curable, including patients with advanced disseminated disease (Einhorn, 2002). This extreme sensitivity to DNA damage is thought to be related to the origins of TGCTs; their normal stem cell counterparts are poised to undergo apoptosis in response to DNA damage, and **most TGCTs maintain wild-type *TP53* and apparently intact DDR** (Kersemaekers et al, 2002; Gorgoulis et al, 2005; Bartkova et al, 2007). Responsiveness to therapy in TGCT is inverse to responses seen in most other cancers—that is, sensitivity decreases with increasing differentiation state, such that ITGCNU are eliminated with low-dose radiation, whereas teratomas exhibit resistance to radiation and chemotherapy.

Family history is a strong risk factor for the development of TGCT, stronger than that found in most other cancers (Forman et al, 1992; Westergaard et al, 1996; Czene et al, 2002; Mai et al, 2010). Despite this fact, initial reports of an association between specific losses on Yq and risk were not confirmed later (Krausz and Looijenga, 2008). Genetic polymorphisms in CAG tract length, which codes for polyglutamine repeats in the androgen receptor, were assessed but were not found to be associated with disease risk (Rajpert-De Meyts et al, 2002; Giwercman et al, 2004; Garolla et al, 2005). **Linkage analyses and more recent GWAS have not revealed evidence for major TGCT-related genetic loci, implying instead the existence of multiple loci having modest influence** (Lutke Holzik et al, 2005; Crockford et al, 2006; Rapley, 2007). **However, in two GWAS, Kanetsky and colleagues (2009) and Rapley and associates (2009) reported that common genetic variants at 5q31.3 near sprouty 4 (*SPRY4*, an inhibitor of the mitogen-activated protein kinase signaling pathway) and in the *KITLG* gene region (c-KIT ligand, also known as stem cell factor or steel factor) on 12q22 are significantly associated with TGCT risk,** including both seminomas and nonseminomas. Rapley and associates (2009) additionally identified a susceptibility locus on chromosome 6 in an intron of *BAK1*, a gene that promotes apoptosis.

Spontaneous (as opposed to inherited) genetic alterations have been cataloged in TGCTs. Apart from aneuploidy, relatively few genetic changes or gene mutations are found in TGCTs, giving an overall picture of a relatively low level of genetic instability, which may be due largely to the aforementioned intact DDR and predominately wild-type *TP53* status in these cancers (Bignell et al, 2006; Greenman et al, 2007). One recurrent, nearly universal genetic alteration in TGCTs (excluding the rare spermatocytic seminomas) is the previously described gain of 12p, which may involve the *KRAS* gene or genes such as *NANOG* and *STELLAR* located in the stem cell cluster region at 12p13.31. Additional evidence for *KRAS* involvement in TGCTs includes reports of activating mutations in 40% of cases as well as increases in expression in concert with increased gene copy number. *BRAF* mutations have also been identified in TGCTs but are seen to be mutually exclusive to K-Ras overexpression (McIntyre et al, 2005b; Sommerer et al, 2005).

Other changes that have been reported in sporadic TGCTs include gains of material on chromosomes 1, 5, 7, and X and losses on chromosome 18 in both ITGCNU and invasive cancer. Also, losses from chromosomes 4 and 13 plus gain of chromosome 2p are more restricted to invasive cancers (Summersgill et al, 2001).

In seminomas, recurrent gains of 4q12, 16p13, and Xq22 plus losses of 3q29, 11q12.1, and 14q13.2 have been reported (Goddard et al, 2007). The *KIT* gene, whose protein product is a receptor tyrosine kinase also known as CD117, is located at 4q12. *KIT* amplifications have been reported in 24% of seminomas, and gene-specific amplifications have been reported in 17%, but these changes were lacking in nonseminomas and ITGCNU (McIntyre et al, 2005a). Also, mutations in c-kit represent the most common somatic mutations found in seminomas (25% of cases) but are rarely found in nonseminomas (Forbes et al, 2006; Coffey et al, 2008). Despite the apparent lack of c-kit gene amplifications in ITGCNU, activating mutations in *KIT* have been reported, and IHC staining is positive for this entity as well as seminomas, although positive staining is not seen in nonseminomas or spermatocytic seminomas (Tian et al, 1999; Przygodzki et al, 2002; Looijenga et al, 2003; Kemmer et al, 2004; Goddard et al, 2007).

Gains of 17q11.2-q21 have been reported in TGCTs, and this region contains the *ERBB2* receptor tyrosine kinase gene as well as the *GRB7* adapter protein gene. *ERBB2* ties into the RAS pathway, whereas *GRB7* binds to and likely regulates KIT, ERBB2, and RAS and is reportedly overexpressed in TGCTs and ITGCNU precursor (Kraggerud et al, 2002; Skotheim et al, 2003).

The above-described results create an emerging picture of derangement of growth-stimulatory protein kinase signaling pathways in TGCT, including activations in the RAS and KIT pathways in most seminomas and nonseminomas (Kemmer et al, 2004; Sommerer et al, 2005). In keeping with the fact that **both RAS and KIT activate the PI3 kinase/AKT pathway,** activated Akt has also been observed (Kemmer et al, 2004). In addition, **the PI3 kinase antagonist PTEN is reported to be frequently inactivated by either mutation or deletion in both seminomas and nonseminomas,** further suggesting an important role for activated PI3 kinase/AKT pathway in TGCTs (Di Vizio et al, 2005; Teng et al, 1997).

Normal PGCs undergo programmed erasure of DNA CpG methylation marks and a loss of imprinting. IHC studies using an anti-5-methylcytosine antibody to assess global methylation status in situ confirmed and extended prior reports focusing on specific loci. The newer studies found very low to absent 5-methylcytosine in most ITGCNU and seminomas compared with robust detection of 5-methylcytosine in nonseminomas (Peltomaki, 1991; Smiraglia et al, 2002; Zhang et al, 2005; Netto et al, 2008). These results are supportive of a model for TGCT pathogenesis in which ITGCNU is derived from retained abnormal PGCs that have matured to the point of 5-methylcytosine erasure but before the point in normal PGC development where epigenetic marks are reestablished via de novo DNA methylation. Such observed changes in global methylation do not rule out the existence of hypermethylation at specific gene promoters. For instance, epigenetic silencing of specific genes, such as the tumor suppressor *RASSF1A*, has been reported in seminoma (Koul et al, 2002; Honorio et al, 2003).

TELOMERES AND TELOMERASE

As we have seen, **cancer cells exhibit marked genetic, morphologic, and behavioral heterogeneity, a reflection of their underlying genetic complexity and instability.** In addition, **most cancers display a strong positive association with increasing age.** As discussed previously, it has been persuasively argued that an increase over the extremely low baseline mutation rate (a mutator phenotype) is needed for accrual of sufficient mutations to bring about malignant transformation (Loeb, 1991).

Cancer genomes exhibit clear evidence of genetic instability; however, defective DNA maintenance and repair genes do not appear to be major contributors to the development of most sporadic cancers. The source of the genetic instability involved in most cancers has been unclear; this has been particularly true of chromosomal instability, a nearly ubiquitous feature of carcinomas. Although alterations in chromosome number may arise via defects in centrosomes or the mitotic spindle checkpoint, little information exists regarding the origins of structural chromosomal abnormalities (Pihan et al, 2003; Roh et al, 2003). **An attractive candidate for the source of chromosomal instability in cancer is telomere dysfunction. Telomeres may provide a common link between genetic instability, cellular proliferation, and aging** (Shay, 1997; DePinho, 2000).

Telomeres and Chromosomal Instability

Telomeres are structures composed of specialized repetitive DNA complexed with telomere-specific binding proteins, located at the ends of every human chromosome where they function to stabilize and protect the ends (Blackburn, 1991). Telomeric DNA is noncoding and consists of tandem repeats of the 6-base pair sequence TTAGGG (Moyzis et al, 1988; Meyne et al, 1989). In normal human cells, telomere lengths typically range from 6 to 12 kb per chromosome. **Telomeres that are too short are dysfunctional ("uncapped"), causing chromosomal destabilization** (Karlseder, 2003; Saldanha et al, 2003).

Telomeres are dynamic and shorten by approximately 100 base pairs each time a cell divides because of inability of DNA polymerases to replicate terminal DNA sequences completely (Harley et al, 1990; Lindsey et al, 1991). **Telomere length is inversely correlated with the number of times a cell has divided** (Hastie et al, 1990; Levy et al, 1992). Telomere shortening may also occur as a result of unrepaired single-strand breaks caused by oxidative damage to telomeric DNA (Kruk et al, 1995; von Zglinicki et al, 2000). Conversely, telomeres may be elongated through the action of the telomere synthetic enzyme telomerase or, uncommonly, via a telomerase-independent genetic recombination mechanism termed *alternative lengthening of telomeres* (ALT) (Greider and Blackburn, 1985; Reddel et al, 2001; Heaphy et al, 2011).

Chromosomes with short, dysfunctional telomeres are prone to fusion, leading to the formation of dicentric chromosomes that mis-segregate or break in mitosis during anaphase. The newly generated chromosomal breaks are themselves fusogenic, perpetuating a cycle of chromosome fusion and breakage (McClintock, 1941; Lo et al, 2002). In this way, critically short telomeres initiate chromosomal instability (Artandi and DePinho, 2000; Feldser et al, 2003; Vukovic et al, 2007). **Numerous studies support the link between telomere dysfunction and chromosomal instability in human cancers.** For example, in head and neck tumors, chromosomes bearing severely short telomeres are associated with chromosomal fusions, rearrangements, anaphase bridges, and multipolar mitoses (Gisselsson et al, 2000).

Telomere Shortening Acts as a Tumor Suppressive Mechanism in Normal Cells

Normal cells closely monitor their telomere lengths. Moderate telomere shortening either signals entry into an irreversible cell cycle arrest termed *replicative senescence* or initiates programmed cell death—responses thought to have evolved as tumor suppressive barriers against abnormal clonal expansion and the development of excessive telomere shortening that would accompany further cell division were it to be allowed to continue (Wright and Shay, 2001). **Progressive telomere shortening acts as a "mitotic clock" counting down cell divisions and signaling cell cycle exit when one or more telomeres reach a threshold length** (Harley et al, 1990).

Forced expression of the enzyme telomerase in presenescent cells counteracts telomere shortening, preventing replicative senescence and endowing the cells with unlimited cell division potential or "immortalization" (Bodnar et al, 1998; Vaziri and Benchimol, 1998). In normal somatic human cells, telomerase activity is stringently repressed, and telomere length will decrease in proliferating cells and can be used as a signal to halt further expansion. **Although the precise mechanisms by which short telomeres trigger senescence and apoptosis are still under study, evidence implicates the tumor suppressors *TP53* and *RB1* as being involved in the response to shortened telomeres** (Vaziri and Benchimol, 1999). Abrogation of this telomere length checkpoint allows continued cell division and, in the absence of telomerase, severe telomere shortening beyond the minimum length required for proper telomere function, causing telomere uncapping and chromosomal destabilization (Counter et al, 1992).

Telomere shortening presents two important barriers to incipient cancer cells. First, moderate shortening instigates the senescence cell cycle exit or apoptosis. Second, extreme telomere shortening causes chromosomal instability that, although it increases the mutation rate, also tends to result in genetic abnormalities lethal to the cell (Fig. 19-13).

Cancers and Premalignant Lesions Possess Abnormally Short Telomeres

Most human cancer tissues and cancer-derived cell lines examined to date have been found to contain abnormally short telomeres (Hastie et al, 1990; Mehle et al, 1996; Takagi et al, 1999; Furugori et al, 2000; Remes et al, 2000). For example, using a Southern blot technique for bulk telomere length assessment in radical prostatectomy specimens, Sommerfeld and colleagues (1996) and Koeneman and colleagues (1998) observed substantial telomere shortening in primary prostate cancer tissues compared with matched adjacent normal-appearing and benign proliferative (benign prostatic hyperplasia) areas. Likewise, results from direct telomere length assessment in archival tissue samples using telomere-specific FISH revealed significantly shorter telomeres in prostate cancer cells compared with their normal epithelial cell counterparts within the same tissue samples (Meeker et al, 2002a).

When examined using high-resolution telomere-specific FISH, **premalignant lesions, including lesions of bladder and prostate cancer, tend to have abnormally short telomeres** (van Heek et al, 2002; Meeker and Argani, 2004; Meeker et al, 2004; Hansel et al, 2006; Kawai et al, 2007). This finding indicates that **telomere loss occurs early in the disease process**, at the intraepithelial neoplasia stage, **strongly implying a causal role for telomere shortening in carcinogenesis through the initiation of chromosomal instability** (O'Shaughnessy et al, 2002). In the prostate, the premalignant precursor is high-grade PIN (Bostwick and Cheng, 2012), most of which (93%) is found to harbor abnormally short telomeres by FISH (Meeker et al, 2002b). In this study, telomere shortening in high-grade PIN foci was restricted to the *luminal* secretory epithelial cells only, whereas the underlying basal epithelial cells and surrounding stromal cells displayed normal telomere lengths. In a separate study, Vukovic and coworkers (2003) reported significant telomere shortening in 63% of high-grade PIN lesions, with a

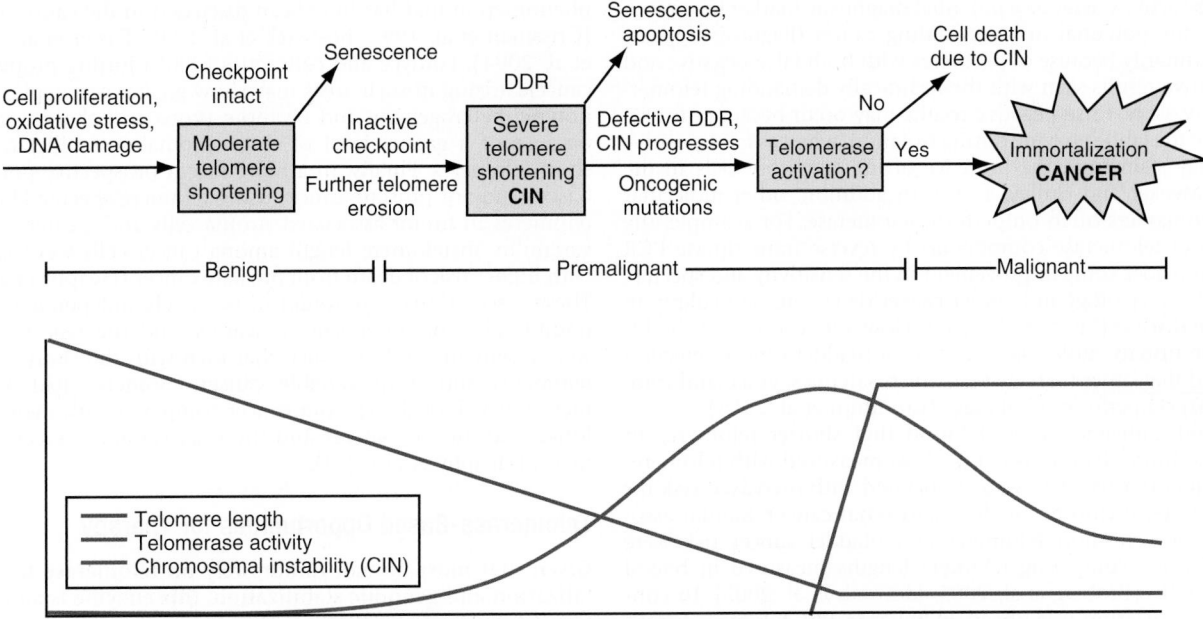

Figure 19-13. Contributions of telomere loss and telomerase activation to oncogenesis. Bypass of the normal telomere length–sensitive cell senescence checkpoint allows severe telomere loss, which initiates chromosomal instability (CIN). Defective DNA damage response (DDR) allows CIN to continue, generating potentially oncogenic mutations but also producing intolerable levels of genomic damage. Transformed cells may proceed through this second barrier by activating telomerase, which stabilizes the telomeres and provides an unlimited proliferative potential ("immortalization").

higher rate of telomere shortening (80%) reported for foci situated near (within 2 mm) adenocarcinoma within the same tissue sample. Studying a cohort of men with a diagnosis exclusively of high-grade PIN in prostate needle biopsy specimens, Joshua and associates (2007) reported an association between short telomeres in the PIN lesions or surrounding stromal cells and eventual diagnosis of prostate cancer as well as time to diagnosis.

Because most PIN lesions are not thought to progress to invasive cancers, intact telomere-based replicative senescence or apoptosis checkpoints may represent a critical bottleneck restraining the outgrowth of most PIN lesions. Even if incipient cancer cells manage to abrogate these checkpoints, as described subsequently, they would still need to activate telomerase to avoid intolerable levels of genetic instability and provide an immortalized phenotype.

Telomerase Activity Restabilizes Chromosomes and Allows Unlimited Cellular Replication

Although dysfunctional telomeres may help initiate cancer formation, if left unchecked, continued telomere shortening in premalignant lesions and cancers would cause increasing levels of genetic instability ultimately becoming lethal to the tumor. Cancer cells overcome this problem by restabilizing their telomeres, primarily through activation of the enzyme telomerase, a specialized reverse transcriptase that adds back telomere DNA repeats to chromosome ends (Greider and Blackburn, 1987). Telomerase provides at least two critical functions to the tumor cell—quelling chromosomal instability and supplying the capacity for unlimited replication ("immortalization") (Shay and Wright, 1996; Greider, 1998). Research has revealed that maintenance of telomere length appears to be a necessary step for human cells to become malignant, confirming the long-held belief that cellular immortalization is a key attribute of cancer cells (Hahn et al, 1999; Elenbaas et al, 2001). Although telomerase activity appears to be

the preferred way cancer cells stabilize their telomeres, 10% to 15% of cancer cases in human patients lack detectable telomerase activity. At least a subset of these, particularly certain central nervous system tumors and some cancers of mesenchymal origin, maintain their telomeres via a telomerase-independent genetic recombination pathway known as ALT (Reddel, 2003; Heaphy et al, 2011). With the exceptions of nonseminomatous TGCTs (15%), chromophobe RCC (9%), and small cell carcinoma of the bladder (23%), ALT is rarely if ever observed in common GU malignancies (Heaphy et al, 2011). However, almost all tissue samples assayed for ALT so far have been from primary tumors. Despite a lack of ALT in more than 1000 primary prostate cancers examined, ALT was found in all distant metastases assayed in a single patient with lethal prostate cancer. In this case, detailed genomic analysis indicated that ALT was acquired during the transition from local to disseminated growth, raising the possibility that ALT may play a role in advanced disease (Haffner et al, 2013).

Several studies have reported on telomerase activity in clinical prostate samples with positivity ranging from 47% to 100%, whereas normal and benign prostatic hyperplasia tissues taken from prostates without evidence of cancer are typically negative for telomerase activity (Kim et al, 1994; Sommerfeld et al, 1996; Engelhardt et al, 1997; Kallakury et al, 1997; Lin et al, 1997; Koeneman et al, 1998; Zhang et al, 1998; Wullich et al, 1999; Caldarera et al, 2000; Kamradt et al, 2003). Although two of these studies found a positive correlation between either the presence or the level of telomerase activity and tumor grade, four other studies found no correlation with grade, stage, or preoperative PSA levels. However, the number of cases in many of these studies was small.

Telomerase Activity as a Potential Diagnostic Marker

The high prevalence and relatively strong activity found in prostate cancers compared with normal tissue, plus the very high sensitivity of the standard telomerase activity assay, led to evaluation of the telomerase activity assay as a potential diagnostic marker for cancer. However, the potential utility of aiding cancer diagnosis appears limited primarily because of problems with both false-negative and false-positive results seen with the technically demanding telomerase activity assay. False-negative results may occur because of inactivation of the labile enzyme during isolation, whereas false-positive results may stem from the presence of inflammatory cells in the sample (Meeker and Coffey, 1997). In addition, other molecular cancer biomarkers often outperform telomerase. For example, the detection of telomerase components by reverse transcriptase PCR in urine provides some improvement in the sensitivity and specificity over urine cytology in bladder cancer detection, particularly in low-grade disease (Eissa et al, 2007). However, a review of the literature on urinary molecular markers for bladder cancer detection concluded that other markers (e.g., microsatellites, FISH, and cytokeratin 20) outperform telomerase (van Rhijn et al, 2005).

Wu and colleagues (2003) **found that shorter telomeres in peripheral blood leukocytes (PBLs)**, as measured with telomere-specific quantitative PCR, **were associated with increased risk for many cancers, including bladder and renal cancer.** Similar associations between short telomeres and bladder cancer risk were observed when comparing telomere lengths measured in buccal cells and PBLs (Broberg et al, 2005; McGrath et al, 2007). **In contrast, no association was observed between PBL telomere length and prostate cancer risk in a study by Mirabello and coworkers** (2009). The variations in the PBL telomere lengths measured in these studies are thought to be due to inherited interindividual differences in telomere lengths modified by changes occurring postnatally, perhaps as a result of diet and lifestyle factors.

Potential Prognostic Value of Telomere Length in Prostate Cancer

Telomere shortening has been found to be predictive of poor prognosis in several cancers, including cancers of the lung, endometrium, and breast and neuroblastoma (Smith and Yeh, 1992; Hiyama et al, 1995a; Hiyama et al, 1995b; Griffith et al, 1999; Bisoffi et al, 2006). A potential link between telomere length and prostate cancer prognosis was first reported by Donaldson and associates (1999). In this retrospective case-control study, both biochemical recurrence and overall survival were significantly correlated with tumor telomere content, a surrogate for telomere length. Specifically, all seven patients who underwent prostatectomy whose tumor telomeric DNA contents were less than that of control samples (placental DNA) showed evidence of biochemical recurrence (elevated PSA) within 10 years after surgery (Donaldson et al, 1999). Of the nine patients in this study with short tumor telomeres, seven died within 10 years, in contrast to 100% 10-year survival for patients with normal-to-long tumor telomeres. Additionally, these patients showed no evidence of biochemical recurrence. Potential drawbacks of this study include a small sample size (18 patients; only 7 of 9 men in the short telomere category underwent surgery) and the fact that it was unknown whether the deaths observed were due specifically to prostate cancer. In a more recent retrospective study using 77 prostatectomy samples and a more sensitive chemiluminescent slot blot assay, (Fordyce et al, 2002), it was reported that less-than-normal telomere content in primary prostate cancers was associated with recurrence, independent of patient age, grade (Gleason sum), and regional lymph node status (Fordyce et al, 2005). The magnitude of the relative hazard for disease recurrence associated with low telomere content (relative hazard = 5.02) was on par with that of Gleason grade and nodal status. A positive correlation was found between telomere content of the tumor and telomere content of the surrounding normal-appearing prostate tissue within the same prostatectomy samples. An association was also found between telomere content of these normal-appearing prostate tissues and 72-month recurrence-free survival. The authors postulated that telomere loss in morphologically normal tissue represents areas at heightened risk of experiencing genetic instability; this is reminiscent of the so-called field effect

phenomenon that has long been discussed in the cancer literature (Crissman et al, 1993; Bostwick et al, 1998; Foster et al, 2000; Yu et al, 2004). Fordyce and colleagues (2005) further proposed that cancers arising in such areas may show greater genotypic and phenotypic heterogeneity and be more prone to behave aggressively because of a greater level of chromosomal instability caused by short telomeres. Finally, in a more recent prospective population-based study of prostate cancer using telomere-specific FISH, short telomeres in tumor-associated stroma cells and greater cell-to-cell variability in telomere length among cancer cells were associated with higher risk of death from prostate cancer (Heaphy et al, 2013). These associations were found to be largely independent of other traditional poor prognostic indicators, and the risk associations were essentially additive, such that men with the shortest stromal telomeres and most variable cancer telomeres had a 14-fold increased risk of dying from cancer compared with men with the longest stromal telomeres and the least variable cancer cell telomeres (Heaphy et al, 2013).

Telomerase-Based Opportunities for Therapy

Given that most human tumors rely on telomerase for immortalization and genomic stabilization, this enzyme is an attractive target for anticancer therapy. There are two overall strategic paradigms for therapeutic targeting of telomerase in cancer. The first involves taking advantage of the tumor's dependence on telomerase enzymatic activity for survival. This strategy includes approaches aimed at directly inhibiting telomerase enzymatic activity or blocking its expression. The second approach attempts to exploit the fact that the telomerase gene (*HTERT*) promoter is selectively active in cancer cells, for example, by using the telomerase promoter to drive oncolytic virus or gene therapy vectors to limit their replication or expression to tumor cells or by directing immunotherapy against cells expressing hTERT protein.

Many of these approaches have undergone preclinical testing using prostate cancer cell lines and xenografts, and some are currently in early clinical trials. One point of concern with antitelomerase therapies has to do with the question of selectivity of action against tumor cells over normal telomerase-positive cells, such as the stem cells of the hematopoietic system and cells within tissues with high turnover rates. This question is of particular importance for approaches in which telomerase-positive cells are actively targeted for destruction, including immunotherapy, gene therapy, and oncolytic viral therapies. Work to date describing the treatment of human tumor xenografts in mice in general has not produced major toxicity in normal tissues.

KEY POINTS: TELOMERES AND TELOMERASE

- Telomeres contain stretches of terminal, noncoding, repetitive DNA that cap the ends of each chromosome, stabilizing them.
- Telomere DNA repeats are progressively lost as cells divide and as a result of oxidative DNA damage at the telomeres.
- Normal cells monitor their telomere lengths and permanently exit the cell cycle (cellular senescence) or commit suicide (apoptosis) in tumor suppressive responses to telomere shortening. This telomere length checkpoint involves *TP53* and *RB1*.
- Loss of telomere length checkpoints leads to critical telomere shortening, which initiates chromosomal instability contributing to cancer initiation.
- Most cancers and premalignant lesions have abnormally short telomeres.
- Most cancers express the enzyme telomerase, which restabilizes the telomeres and allows unlimited cell division potential (immortalization), making telomerase an attractive therapeutic target.

APOPTOSIS

Apoptosis, also known as programmed cell death, is a tightly regulated process used by multicellular organisms to eliminate unwanted cells. Apoptosis is used in tissue remodeling during development and in the immune system to eliminate self-reactive T cells (Kerr et al, 1972; Ashkenazi and Dixit, 1998). **Apoptosis contrasts sharply with necrosis, a nonprogrammed form of cell death** in which cells that are acutely injured (e.g., by physical trauma) swell and burst, abruptly releasing their contents, which act as potent inducers of the inflammatory response. **Apoptosis is a more orderly, energy-requiring process in which the contents of the dying cell are degraded and neatly packaged into so-called apoptotic bodies, which are engulfed by neighboring cells or macrophages—a process that does not elicit a strong inflammatory response** (Fadok et al, 1992).

Apoptosis and Cancer

In contrast to unicellular organisms, cancer poses a risk to multicellular life forms, and various potentially tumorigenic abnormalities can signal a cell to eliminate itself as a potential threat via apoptosis. For example, if a cell sustains DNA damage (potentially mutagenic) but fails to make repairs, it will be eliminated and replaced from the organism's pool of undamaged cells. Aberrations of apoptosis can be detrimental, and failure of dividing cells to initiate apoptosis contributes to cancer (Ashkenazi and Dixit, 1998).

Abnormalities in the apoptotic machinery have implications for malignancy beyond the ability of an individual cell to respond appropriately to cell physiologic stresses such as DNA damage. First, **the apoptosis cascade is critical to the immune system's ability to eliminate cancer cells by inducing them to undergo apoptosis** (Nagata, 1997); this has clear implications for both the organism's intrinsic immunosurveillance for malignancy and the tumor's response to extrinsic immunotherapy. Second, because cytotoxic cancer therapies also depend in large part on inducing apoptosis, **defects in the apoptosis cascade can profoundly influence tumor responses to chemotherapy and radiotherapy** (Walton et al, 1993; Minn et al, 1995; Thornberry and Lazebnik, 1998).

Apoptosis Is an Evolutionarily Conserved Process

Apoptosis is tightly regulated by an evolutionarily conserved system of positive and negative signals, the balance of which determines whether the cell will undergo apoptosis. These signals ultimately converge on an important family of proteases named *caspases* ("cysteine proteases with aspartic acid specificity"), key components of the apoptotic machinery (Thornberry, 1998). Caspases, of which there are at least 13, are **broadly categorized as either initiator caspases (e.g., caspase-8, caspase-9, and caspase-10) or executioner caspases (e.g., caspase-3, caspase-6, and caspase-7). Caspases are synthesized as larger, inactive forms called procaspases, which require specific proteolytic cleavage to become active proteases themselves.** Often a procaspase is activated by another caspase, setting in motion a sequential, amplifying, proteolytic cascade. **Initiator caspases begin the cascade, which ultimately leads to activation of executioner caspases downstream. Once activated, the executioner caspases attack several intracellular protein targets.** Executioner caspases cleave antiapoptotic proteins, such as Bcl-2 and Bcl-X$_L$, which not only destroys their antiapoptotic function but releases pro-apoptotic carboxyl-terminal fragments, further stimulating cell death (Wolf and Green, 1999). Executioner caspases target proteins critical to cell survival. Cleavage of DNA repair and replication proteins, such as DNA-PK$_{cs}$ and replication factor C, leads to nuclear dysregulation. Nuclear structural proteins, such as lamins NuMa and SAF-A, are fragmented, contributing to dissolution of the nucleus and nuclear condensation, a hallmark of cells undergoing apoptosis. Proteolysis of cytoskeletal proteins such as keratin and actin leads to destruction of the internal structural integrity of the cell. Lastly, cleavage of proteins critical to cell-cell interaction, such as

beta-catenin and focal adhesion kinase, precipitates the specific and irreversible phenotypic changes associated with apoptosis (Orth et al, 1996; Wen et al, 1997; Wolf and Green, 1999). **The end result is a stereotypic death in which the cytoplasm shrinks, the cell membrane blebs, and the nuclear chromatin condenses. The entire apoptotic process can be completed in 60 minutes** (Thornberry and Lazebnik, 1998).

Additional details of the intrinsic and extrinsic apoptotic pathways can be found on the Expert Consult website.

Role of TP53 in Apoptosis

In addition to the key roles played by TP53 in cell cycle arrest and DNA damage repair, TP53 can also induce apoptosis (May and May, 1999). TP53-induced apoptosis is mediated through the Bcl-2 family, via the intrinsic pathway, and dysregulation of this apoptotic pathway has direct relevance to the etiology of cancer. TP53-induced apoptosis is mediated by transcriptional activation of genes that initiate the apoptotic cascade and inhibition of genes that block the cascade (Miyashita et al, 1994; Miyashita and Reed, 1995; Oda et al, 2000). TP53-induced apoptosis is dependent on the Apaf-1/caspase-9 activation pathway (Soengas et al, 1999). Although the Bcl-2 family member Bax has been implicated as the primary factor responsible for TP53 induction of this cascade (Miyashita and Reed, 1995), Bax is not essential for TP53-dependent apoptosis (Knudson et al, 1995). It is possible that inhibition of Bcl-2 (Miyashita et al, 1994) or upregulation of the pro-apoptotic Bcl-2 family member noxa may still allow cells lacking Bax to undergo TP53-dependent apoptosis (Oda et al, 2000). **Considering the role of** *TP53* **in multiple tumor suppressive pathways (DNA damage response, cellular senescence, and apoptosis), it is not surprising that it is so frequently mutated in cancer.**

Apoptosis and Genitourinary Malignancies

Because the inability of a tumor cell to undergo apoptosis is a hallmark of malignancy, multiple groups have attempted to characterize the apoptotic response of GU malignancies. Because cells undergoing apoptosis exhibit a stereotypic death, global analysis of apoptosis is possible using assays designed to detect key hallmarks of the apoptotic process, such as the fragmentation of DNA characteristic of the process as well as assays designed to detect abnormalities in specific apoptotic proteins.

Global Defects in Apoptosis

Both high-grade PIN and prostate carcinoma have significantly higher levels of apoptosis than normal prostatic epithelium. The level of apoptotic activity is relatively low compared with other malignancies and is opposed by increased replication. Many prostate cancer cells can be induced to undergo apoptosis in response to androgen withdrawal, which represents a frontline therapy for patients with advanced disease (Kyprianou et al, 1990; Isaacs, 1994; Denmeade and Isaacs, 1996; Tu et al, 1996). However, not all of a patient's cancer cells succumb because recurrences inevitably arise. As the tumor progresses to androgen independence, it is unclear if the androgen-resistant cells have an increased or decreased rate of apoptosis because studies have demonstrated both in hormone-refractory disease (Berges et al, 1995; Koivisto et al, 1997). The conflicting data may reflect both the tumor's dynamics and the effect of therapy. There is a clear survival advantage for the advanced cancer cell that can protect itself from apoptosis. However, **a rapidly growing, infiltrative, advanced tumor, which is outgrowing its blood supply and mutating its DNA, may have a high apoptotic rate despite protective mechanisms the tumor's cells have acquired.**

Studies of apoptosis in bladder carcinoma have demonstrated an association with aggressive high-grade advanced disease but not with decreased disease-free survival (Lipponen and Aaltomaa, 1994; King et al, 1996). External-beam radiation therapy has been associated with a modest improvement in survival for tumors with high apoptotic rates. This improved survival may reflect the fact that external-beam radiation therapy requires an intact apoptotic mechanism to be effective (Rodel et al, 2000).

As previously mentioned, **most TGCTs maintain intact DDR and wild-type *TP53* and display high cure rates in response to therapies that induce DNA damage** (Einhorn, 2002; Kersemaekers et al, 2002; Gorgoulis et al, 2005; Bartkova et al, 2007).

Individual members of the apoptotic machinery have been frequently studied. However, all studies are limited by an inability to assay all elements of the apoptotic machinery simultaneously and to assess globally the ability of the tumor to undergo programmed cell death.

TP53 **mutations and abnormalities in expression are among the most frequent in cancer and have been identified in prostate, bladder, and renal cancers** (Hollstein et al, 1991; Sidransky et al, 1991; Reiter et al, 1993). Abnormalities in *TP53* cause dysregulation of the cell cycle and DNA repair mechanisms in addition to apoptosis and are covered in more detail in Cell Cycle Deregulation.

Bcl-2 family members have been studied in GU malignancies. **Elevated levels of Bcl-2 have been identified in most hormone-refractory prostate tumors, reflecting the tumor's relative resistance to apoptosis in the advanced state** (McDonnell et al, 1992; Colombel et al, 1993). Both increased and decreased levels of Bcl-2 have been identified in localized prostate tumors, and a few studies have found a correlation with grade, stage, and progression (Byrne et al, 1997; Lipponen and Vesalainen, 1997; Theodorescu et al, 1997). Other antiapoptotic members of the Bcl-2 gene family, Bcl-X_L and Mcl1, may also be linked to prostate carcinoma (Krajewska et al, 1996). Analysis of bladder carcinoma has demonstrated similar results. Bcl-2 levels are higher in more aggressive bladder carcinoma, but expression of Bcl-2 had no effect on treatment outcome (King et al, 1996; Rodel et al, 2000). As noted earlier, phosphorylation of Bad by Akt can also tilt the scales toward cell survival, especially in concert with elevated levels of Bcl-2. Akt activation is commonly seen in many urologic malignancies and can result from loss of the tumor suppressor *PTEN*; mutation and constitutive activation of PI3 kinase; or activation of tyrosine kinase receptors such as HER2/NEU, EGFR, and insulin-like growth factor receptor.

Other Bcl-2 family members have not been as well studied. Loss of Bax expression is apparently an uncommon mechanism for the development of prostate carcinoma (Krajewska et al, 1996; Johnson and Hamdy, 1998), but it may play a role in progression of localized bladder carcinoma (Ye et al, 1998).

Deficiencies in signal transduction pathways leading to apoptosis play a role in the initiation and progression of malignancy. It is unclear if expression analysis of the apoptotic machinery will provide additional prognostic information than that provided by traditional histochemical analysis. However, it is clear that effective chemotherapy and radiation therapy are largely dependent on apoptosis. In addition, in the future the apoptotic machinery may be manipulated using novel ligands that bind to death receptors and promote *TP53*-independent cancer cell death.

Alternative Regulators of Apoptosis in Genitourinary Malignancies

In addition to the classic regulators of apoptosis, numerous other pathways for cell survival and death have been uncovered that play key roles in urologic cancer. Some of these pathways are being actively explored as targets for cancer therapy. The Vancouver group mapped out a detailed gene profile of prostate tumors treated with neoadjuvant hormonal ablation therapy to identify key regulators of cell death and survival after castration. In addition to Bcl-2, which is upregulated in surviving cancer cells, they also reported on clusterin and Hsp27. **Clusterin, or TRPM2 (testosterone repressed prostate message–2), is upregulated both in patient samples after hormone ablation and in the Shionogi and CWR-22 xenograft models of hormone-sensitive tumors.** Although its precise

function is unknown, a large body of evidence suggests that clusterin is induced by stress and functions to stabilize the cell during periods of stress (Miyake et al, 2000). In this model, clusterin is believed to act like heat shock proteins, whose role as a protein chaperone is also to stabilize client proteins. Clusterin is activated by HSP1. Functional evidence of the role of clusterin comes from studies in which clusterin is either overexpressed or knocked down using antisense strategies. In the first scenario, clusterin expression promotes hormone-refractory cell growth and prevents androgen withdrawal–induced apoptosis. In the second scenario, treatment of hormone-refractory cells with antisense clusterin promotes apoptosis (July et al, 2002; Miyake et al, 2004; Gleave and Miyake, 2005). This same group of investigators also reported that the heat shock protein HSP27 is frequently overexpressed in hormone-refractory prostate cancers. Similar experiments using overexpression and antisense strategies have suggested that targeting HSP27 may influence the course of hormone-refractory cancers, in particular in combination with cytotoxic chemotherapies (Rocchi et al, 2004).

Another family of cellular signaling molecules that play a role in the regulation of cell survival and apoptosis is the sphingolipids. Sphingolipids are one of three major constituents of the cell membrane, alongside phospholipids and cholesterol. Sphingolipid generation is regulated by a large cast of enzymes, notably the sphingomyelinases, ceramide synthase, and the ceramidases. Ceramide is produced from sphingomyelin by sphingomyelinase and from sphinganine by ceramide synthase. Ceramidases degrade ceramide and lead to formation of sphingosine and sphingosine-1-phosphate. Ceramide is a potent pro-apoptotic molecule that can promote apoptosis through the classic mitochondrial activation of caspases or through a nonclassic caspase-independent form of apoptosis (Kolesnick and Fuks, 2003). Sphingosine-1-phosphate, in contrast, is a powerful antiapoptotic molecule that may modulate the degree of apoptosis similar to a rheostat (Maceyka et al, 2002).

The importance of ceramide to GU tumors is that it appears to be a key modulator of radiation-induced tissue damage and apoptosis. Similar to clusterin and other heat shock proteins, ceramide appears to be a critical mediator of stress response in cells, in this case promoting apoptosis as opposed to cell survival. Studies supporting the role of ceramide in radiation-induced apoptosis are manifold, including studies demonstrating the direct cell death signal induced by exogenous treatment of cells with ceramide, studies of radiation response in mouse knockout models, and studies of radiation response in the presence and absence of inhibitors of sphingolipid metabolism. It is hoped that therapeutics that increase ceramide production and promote apoptosis can be developed. The role of sphingolipid-1-phosphate has also emerged from these studies, and work from several investigators suggests that this molecule is a promising target for cancer therapy (Gulbins and Kolesnick, 2003; Kester and Kolesnick, 2003; Perry and Kolesnick, 2003).

STEM CELLS AND CANCER

Stem cells are found in multicellular organisms and are characterized by the ability of self-renewal through mitotic cell division and differentiation into a diverse range of specialized cell types. **Common properties of stem cells include the ability of self-renewal, generation of cellular progeny, localization within specialized niches, and the ability to give rise to all cell types within an organ.** For example, human prostate stem cells are believed to be localized within the basal epithelium and give rise to a hierarchy of progenitor cells that may differentiate into secretory or neuroendocrine cells (Burger et al, 2005; Xin et al, 2005).

Studies suggest that neoplastic cells mimic normal tissue development and may arise from and are dependent on a small population of stem cells. **The cancer stem cell hypothesis argues that cancers arise from transformation of stem or progenitor cells that are capable of multilineage differentiation.** Cancer stem cells may account for only a small percentage of any tumor, but this

KEY POINTS: APOPTOSIS

- Apoptosis is a rapid, orderly programmed form of cell death that is used by multicellular organisms to eliminate unwanted cells.
- Apoptosis is believed to play an important role in tumor suppression because many of the signals that induce apoptosis arise from potentially tumorigenic cell stresses such as DNA damage.
- Cancer is characterized by interruptions in the normal process of apoptosis, resulting in inappropriate cell survival.
- Apoptosis is mediated by a conserved family of proteases known as caspases. Initiator caspases start caspase proteolytic cascades terminating in the activation of executioner caspases that target several cellular proteins.
- Two main apoptotic pathways have been identified. In the intrinsic pathway, Bcl-2 family members modulate the release of cytochrome *c* from the mitochondria, which participates in the activation of initiator caspases. The extrinsic pathway activates caspases in response to signals from extracellular "death receptors."
- In addition to its functions in cell cycle arrest and DNA repair, *TP53* plays a key role in apoptosis.
- Bcl-2 is a classic inhibitor of the mitochondrial pathway of apoptosis and is overexpressed in some GU malignancies.
- Therapeutic response often depends on the integrity of apoptotic pathways in the cancer cells. Most TGCTs retain intact DDR, wild-type *TP53*, and apoptotic responses, providing high cure rates with DNA-damaging agents.
- Novel agonists and antagonists of apoptosis, such as ceramide and clusterin, may successfully be controlled to combat cancer.

this group of cells, and blockade of CD47 resulted in macrophage engulfment of bladder cancer stem cells in vitro. This finding suggests a potential role for therapeutic targeting of CD47 and the T-IC subpopulation in bladder cancer (Chan et al, 2009). To date, numerous other putative cancer stem cell populations have been identified in bladder cancer, including CK17+/67LR+/CAECAM− cells, embryonic stem cell marker *POU5F1*+ cells, and high aldehyde dehydrogenase activity (ALDH^{hi}) cells (van der Horst et al, 2012).

KEY POINTS: STEM CELLS AND CANCER

- Stem cells are defined by their ability to differentiate along multiple lineages and their immortality.
- Cancer is believed to be a stem cell disease in which a small population of cancer stem cells maintains the larger tumor.
- Cancer may ultimately be eradicated by targeting only the cancer stem cell.

REFERENCES

The complete reference list is available online at www.expertconsult.com.

SUGGESTED READINGS

Ames BN, Gold LS. The causes and prevention of cancer: the role of environment. Biotherapy 1998;11:205–20.

Blackburn EH. Telomeres. Trends Biochem Sci 1991;16:378–81.

DePinho RA. The age of cancer. Nature 2000;408:248–54.

Fearon ER. Human cancer syndromes: clues to the origin and nature of cancer. Science 1997;278:1043–50.

Feinberg AP. The epigenetics of cancer etiology. Semin Cancer Biol 2004;14:427–32.

Greider CW. Telomerase activity, cell proliferation, and cancer. Proc Natl Acad Sci U S A 1998;95:90–2.

Guttmacher AE, Collins FS. Genomic medicine—a primer. N Engl J Med 2002;347:1512–20.

Hahn WC, Counter CM, Lundberg AS, et al. Creation of human tumour cells with defined genetic elements. Nature 1999;400:464–8.

Hanahan D, Weinberg RA. The hallmarks of cancer. Cell 2000;100:57–70.

Hanahan D, Weinberg RA. Hallmarks of cancer: the next generation. Cell 2011;144:646–74.

Hartwell L, Weinert T, Kadyk L, et al. Cell cycle checkpoints, genomic integrity, and cancer. Cold Spring Harb Symp Quant Biol 1994;59:259–63.

Jones PA, Baylin SB. The fundamental role of epigenetic events in cancer. Nat Rev Genet 2004;3:415–28.

Jones PA, Baylin SB. The epigenomics of cancer. Cell 2007;128:683–92.

Kaelin WG Jr. Molecular basis of the VHL hereditary cancer syndrome. Nat Rev Cancer 2002;2:673–82.

Kastan MB, Bartek J. Cell-cycle checkpoints and cancer. Nature 2004;432:316–23.

Massague J. G1 cell-cycle control and cancer. Nature 2004;432:298–306.

Rebbeck TR, Spitz M, Wu X. Assessing the function of genetic variants in candidate gene association studies. Nat Rev Genet 2004;5:589–97.

Reya T, Morrison SJ, Clarke MF, et al. Stem cells, cancer, and cancer stem cells. Nature 2001;414:105–11.

Sancar A, Lindsey-Boltz LA, Unsal-Kacmaz K, et al. Molecular mechanisms of mammalian DNA repair and the DNA damage checkpoints. Annu Rev Biochem 2004;73:39–85.

Sjoblom T, Jones S, Wood LD, et al. The consensus coding sequences of human breast and colorectal cancers. Science 2006;314:268–74.

Vogelstein B, Papadopoulos N, Velculescu VE, et al. Cancer genome landscapes. Science 2013;339:1546–58.

Watson J, Crick F. Molecular structure of nucleic acids: a structure for deoxyribose nucleic acid. Nature 1953;171:737–8.

small population of cells is critical for tumor survival. The most readily accepted experimental demonstration of cancer stem cells relies on serial transplantation of tumor cell populations isolated based on one or numerous putative cancer stem cell markers into immune-deficient mice or three-dimensional culture systems and recapitulation of the heterogeneous primary tumor. Using this experimental strategy, initial evidence to support the cancer stem cell hypothesis was discovered in leukemia, breast cancer, and neurologic cancers. For example, a CD44+/CD24^{low}/− population of cells in primary breast tumors was specifically capable of new tumor formation when engrafted into nude mice (Al-Hajj et al, 2003; Dontu et al, 2003). Similar reports in glioblastoma suggest that a CD133+ population is the putative stem cell (Singh et al, 2003; Dirks, 2005). One challenge in cancer stem cell research is the lack of any one marker that is exclusively expressed by cancer stem cells. For any given tumor type, typically many different markers can be identified that confer a cancer stem cell phenotype, and absence of the marker does not always imply that a cell is not a cancer stem cell. For example, in glioblastoma, both CD133+ and CD133− cell populations have been shown to possess cancer stem cell–like properties (Beier et al, 2007).

A tumor-initiating cell (T-IC) subpopulation has also been identified in human bladder cancer. This group of cells was found to express CD44+/CK5+/CK20− markers similar to normal bladder basal cells (Chan et al, 2009). The bladder T-IC subpopulation was also capable of forming xenograft tumors in vivo that recapitulated characteristics of the original tumor. CD47 was highly expressed in

20 Principles of Tissue Engineering

Anthony Atala, MD

Regenerative Medicine: Strategies for Tissue and Organ Reconstitution

Biomaterials and Vascularization for Genitourinary Regenerative Medicine

Sources of Cells for Therapy

Regenerative Medicine of Urologic Structures

The field of urology was the earliest to gain from the advent of transplantation, with the kidney being the first entire organ to be replaced in a human, in 1955 (Guild et al, 1955). In the early 1960s, Murray, who later received the Nobel Prize for his work, performed a nonrelated kidney transplantation from a non–genetically identical patient into another. This transplant, which overcame the immunologic barrier, marked a new era in medical therapy and opened the door for use of transplantation as a means of therapy for different organ systems. However, lack of good immunosuppression and the ability to monitor and control rejection, as well as a severe organ donor shortage, opened the door for other alternatives.

As times evolved, synthetic materials were introduced to replace or rebuild diseased tissues or parts in the human body. The advent of new manmade materials, such as tetrafluoroethylene (Teflon) and silicone, opened a new field that included a wide array of devices that could be applied for human use. Although these devices could provide for structural replacement, the functional component of the original tissue was not achieved.

Simultaneous with this development was an increased body of knowledge of the biologic sciences that included new techniques for cell harvesting, culture, and expansion. The areas of cell biology, molecular biology, and biochemistry were advancing rapidly. Studies of the extracellular matrix (ECM) and its interaction with cells and with growth factors and their ligands led the way to a further understanding of cell and tissue growth and differentiation. The concept of cell transplantation took hold in the research arena and culminated with the first human bone marrow cell transplant in the 1970s.

In the 1970s, a natural evolution occurred wherein researchers started to combine the fields of devices and materials sciences with cell biology, in effect starting a new field called *tissue engineering*. As more scientists from different fields came together with the common goal of tissue replacement, the field of tissue engineering became more formally established. Tissue engineering was defined as "an interdisciplinary field which applies the principles of engineering and life sciences towards the development of biological substitutes that aim to maintain, restore or improve tissue function" (Atala and Lanza, 2001). The first use of the term *tissue engineering* in the literature can be traced to a reference dealing with corneal tissue in 1985 (Wolter et al, 1985).

The field of stem cells also received a large boost with the discovery of mouse embryonic stem cells in the early 1980s (Martin, 1981). However, the field remained relatively dormant until the description of human embryonic stem cells (hESCs) in 1998 (Thomson et al, 1998). The description of these cells led to one of the most contested ethical debates in the field of medicine. Just a year later, in 1999, the world awoke to the startling media announcement of the creation of the first cloned mammal, a sheep named Dolly (Wilmut et al, 1997). Although cloning, or nuclear transfer, had been done in amphibians and other animal models for years, this accomplishment in a mammal showed once again that concepts believed to be scientifically prohibitive were indeed possible.

The fields of cell transplantation, tissue engineering and nuclear transfer all had one unifying concept—the regeneration of living tissues (organs). Thus in 1999, William Haseltine, then the Scientific Founder and Chief Executive Officer of Human Genome Sciences, coined the term *regenerative medicine*, in effect bringing all these areas under one defining field (Haseltine, 1999). Soon the first online journal in the field, *Regenerative Medicine*, was founded, along with the Regenerative Medicine Society.

Organ transplantation remains a mainstay of treatment for patients with severely compromised organ function. Despite initiatives to increase the availability of transplant organs, however, the number of patients in need of treatment far exceeds the organ supply, and this shortfall is expected to worsen as the global population ages. One alternative treatment approach is regenerative medicine. In the last two decades, scientists have attempted to grow native and stem cells, engineer tissues, and design treatment modalities using regenerative medicine techniques for virtually every tissue of the human body. This chapter reviews some of the progress that has been achieved in the field of genitourinary regenerative medicine.

REGENERATIVE MEDICINE: STRATEGIES FOR TISSUE AND ORGAN RECONSTITUTION

Regenerative medicine follows the principles of cell transplantation, materials science, and engineering toward the development of biologic strategies that can restore and maintain normal function. Regenerative medicine strategies usually fall into one of three categories: cell-based therapies; the use of biomaterials (scaffolds) alone, wherein the body's natural ability to regenerate is used to orient or direct new tissue growth; and the use of scaffolds seeded with cells to create tissue substitutes.

SOURCES OF CELLS FOR THERAPY

Stem Cells

The cells used for regenerative medicine can be autologous or heterologous, and from either native or stem cell sources. In general, there are three broad categories of stem cells obtained from living tissue that are used for cell therapies. Embryonic stem cells are obtained through the aspiration of the inner cell mass of a blastocyst or a single cell from this mass. Fetal and neonatal amniotic fluid and placenta may contain multipotent cells that may be useful in cell therapy applications. Cord blood cells have potency mainly limited to hematopoietic lineages, although differentiation to other cell types has also been reported. Adult stem cells, on the other hand, are usually isolated from organ or bone marrow biopsy specimens. Stem cells are defined as having three important properties: the ability to self-renew, the ability to differentiate into a number of different cell types, and the ability to easily form clonal populations (populations of cells derived from a single stem cell). Many techniques for generating stem cells have been studied over the past

TABLE 20-1 Summary of Alternate Methods for Generating Pluripotent Stem Cells

METHOD	ADVANTAGES	LIMITATIONS
Somatic cell nuclear transfer	Customized stem cells Has been shown to work in nonhuman primates	Requires oocytes Has not been shown to work in humans
Single-cell embryo biopsy	Patient specific to embryo Does not destroy or create embryos Has been done in humans	Allogeneic cell types Is not known if single cells are totipotent Requires coculturing with a previously established human embryonic stem cell line
Arrested embryos	Cells obtained from discarded embryos Has been done in humans	Allogeneic cell types Quality of cell lines might be questionable
Altered nuclear transfer	Customized stem cells	Ethical issues surround embryos with no potential Modified genome Has not been done with human cells
Reprogramming	Customized stem cells No embryos or oocytes needed Has been done with human cells	Retroviral transduction Oncogenes

few decades. Some of these techniques have yielded promising results, but others require further research. The main techniques are discussed in detail later, and their advantages and limitations are summarized in Table 20-1.

Embryonic Stem Cells

In 1981 pluripotent cells were found in the inner cell mass of the human embryo, and the term *human embryonic stem cell* was coined (Martin, 1981). These cells are able to differentiate into all cells of the human body, excluding placental cells (only cells from the morula are totipotent—that is, able to develop into all cells of the human body). These cells have great therapeutic potential; their use is limited mostly by their biologic properties.

An ethical controversy surrounding stem cells was initiated in 1998 with the creation of hESCs derived from discarded embryos. hESCs were isolated from the inner cell mass of a blastocyst (an embryo 5 days after fertilization) using an immunosurgical technique. Given that some cells cannot be expanded ex vivo, hESCs could be an ideal resource for regenerative medicine because of their fundamental properties: the ability to self-renew indefinitely and the ability to differentiate into cells from all three embryonic germ layers, from skin to neurons. In addition, as further evidence of their pluripotency, embryonic stem cells can form embryoid bodies, which are cell aggregations that contain all three embryonic germ layers while in culture, and can form teratomas in vivo (Itskovitz-Eldor et al, 2000). These cells have demonstrated longevity in culture and can maintain their undifferentiated state for at least 80 passages when grown using current published protocols (Thomson et al, 1998). However, the clinical application of

embryonic stem cells is limited because they represent an allogeneic resource and thus have the potential to evoke an immune response. In addition, by definition the cells form teratomas, which may be problematic when treating patients. In October 2010, a phase 1 clinical trial was begun to assess the safety of hESC-derived oligodendrocyte progenitors for patients with thoracic spinal cord injuries. Unfortunately, the trial was discontinued in November 2011 (Frantz, 2012). hESC-derived retinal pigment epithelium has also been used in patients with macular degeneration and dystrophy (Schwartz et al, 2012). It might seem that we have waited too long to see hESCs in the clinic. However, this has been accomplished with incredible speed when it is considered that hESCs were first isolated just in 1998 (Atala, 2012).

A major objection to hESC research by some is that it results in the destruction of embryos. A method of isolating these cells without destroying the embryo would be advantageous. Three methods have been established experimentally for the generation of embryonic stem cell lines using alternate techniques whereby the embryos are not destroyed; these include performing a single-cell embryo biopsy (Chung et al, 2006), obtaining cells from arrested embryos (Zhang et al, 2006a), and using altered nuclear transfer (Hurlbut, 2005; Meissner and Jaenisch, 2006).

A description of these techniques appears on the Expert Consult website.

Therapeutic Cloning (Somatic Cell Nuclear Transfer)

SCNT, or therapeutic cloning, entails the removal of an oocyte nucleus in culture, followed by its replacement with a nucleus derived from a somatic cell obtained from a patient. Activation with chemicals or electricity stimulates cell division up to the blastocyst stage.

It is important to differentiate between the two types of cloning that exist—reproductive cloning and therapeutic cloning. Both involve the insertion of donor DNA into an enucleated oocyte to generate an embryo that has identical genetic material to its DNA source. However, the similarities end there. In reproductive cloning, the embryo is implanted into the uterus of a pseudopregnant female to produce an infant that is a clone of the donor. A prominent example of this type of cloning resulted in the birth of a sheep named Dolly in 1997 (Wilmut et al, 1997). However, there are many ethical concerns surrounding such practices, and as a result, reproductive cloning has been banned.

Although therapeutic cloning also produces an embryo that is genetically identical to the donor, this process is used to generate blastocysts that are explanted and grown in culture rather than in utero. Embryonic stem cell lines can then be derived from blastocysts, which are allowed to grow only up to a 100-cell stage. At this time the inner cell mass is isolated and cultured, resulting in embryonic stem cells that are genetically identical to the patient. This process is detailed in Figure 20-1. It has been shown that nuclear-transferred embryonic stem cells derived from fibroblasts, lymphocytes, and olfactory neurons are pluripotent and can generate live pups after injection into blastocysts. This shows that cells generated by SCNT have the same developmental potential as blastocysts that are fertilized and produced naturally (Hochedlinger et al, 2002; Eggan et al, 2004; Brambrink et al, 2006). In addition, the embryonic stem cells generated by SCNT are perfectly matched to the patient's immune system and no immunosuppressants would be required to prevent rejection should these cells be used in regenerative medicine applications.

Although embryonic stem cells derived from SCNT contain the nuclear genome of the donor cells, mitochondrial DNA (mtDNA) contained in the oocyte could lead to immunogenicity after transplantation. To assess the histocompatibility of tissue generated using SCNT, the nucleus of a bovine skin fibroblast was microinjected into an enucleated oocyte (Lanza et al, 2002). Although the blastocyst was implanted (reproductive cloning), the purpose was to generate renal, cardiac, and skeletal muscle cells, which were then harvested, expanded in vitro, and seeded onto biodegradable scaffolds. These scaffolds were then implanted into the donor steer

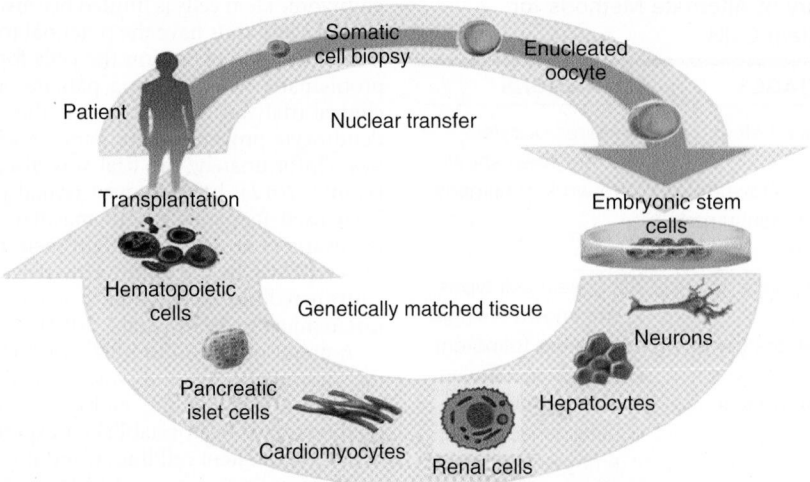

Figure 20-1. Therapeutic cloning strategy and its application to the engineering of tissues and organs.

from which the cells were cloned to determine if the cells were histocompatible. Analysis revealed that cloned renal cells showed no evidence of T-cell response, suggesting that rejection will not necessarily occur in the presence of oocyte-derived mtDNA. This finding represents a step forward in overcoming the histocompatibility problem of stem cell therapy.

Although promising, SCNT has certain limitations that require further improvement before its clinical application, in addition to the ethical considerations regarding the potential of the resulting embryos to develop into cloned embryos if implanted into a uterus. In addition, this technique has not been shown to work in humans to date. The initial failures and fraudulent reports of nuclear transfer in humans reduced enthusiasm for human applications (Simerly et al, 2003; Hwang et al, 2004, 2005), although nonhuman primate embryonic stem cell lines have been generated by SCNT of nuclei from adult skin fibroblasts (Byrne et al, 2007; Mitalipov, 2007).

Reprogramming (Induced Pluripotent Stem Cells)

Reprogramming is a technique that involves de-differentiation of adult somatic cells to produce patient-specific pluripotent stem cells, eliminating the need to create embryos. Cells generated by reprogramming would be genetically identical to the somatic cells (and therefore to the patient who donated these cells) and would not be rejected. Yamanaka was the first to discover that mouse embryonic fibroblasts (MEFs) and adult mouse fibroblasts could be reprogrammed into an "induced pluripotent state (iPS)" (Takahashi et al, 2006). These iPS cells possessed the immortal growth characteristics of self-renewing embryonic stem cells, expressed genes specific for embryonic stem cells, and generated embryoid bodies in vitro and teratomas in vivo. When iPS cells were injected into mouse blastocysts, they contributed to a variety of cell types. However, although iPS cells selected in this way were pluripotent, they were not identical to embryonic stem cells. Unlike with embryonic stem cells, chimeras made from iPS cells did not result in full-term pregnancies. Gene expression profiles of the iPS cells showed that they possessed a distinct gene expression signature that was different from that of embryonic stem cells. In addition, the epigenetic state of the iPS cells was somewhere between that found in somatic cells and that found in embryonic stem cells, suggesting that the reprogramming was incomplete.

These results were improved by Wernig and Jaenisch in July 2007 (Wernig et al, 2007). In this study, DNA methylation, gene expression profiles, and the chromatin state of the reprogrammed cells were similar to those of embryonic stem cells. Teratomas induced by these cells contained differentiated cell types representing all

three embryonic germ layers. Most important, the reprogrammed cells from this experiment were able to form viable chimeras and contribute to the germline-like embryonic stem cells, suggesting that these iPS cells were completely reprogrammed.

A major advance has been the reprogramming of human cells (Takahashi et al, 2007; Yu et al, 2007). Yamanaka generated human iPS cells that are similar to hESCs in terms of morphology, proliferation, gene expression, surface markers, and teratoma formation. Yamanaka received the Nobel Prize in Medicine for this work in 2012. Thompson's group showed that retroviral transduction of the stem cell markers *OCT4*, *SOX2*, *NANOG*, and *LIN28* could generate pluripotent stem cells. Recently the cells have been noted to have the potential to be reversed to a ground state of pluripotency (Gafni et al, 2013). Since the discovery of iPS cells, work surrounding these cells has grown exponentially, with more than 6000 peer-reviewed papers listed in MEDLINE by 2014. The cells have shown great promise in the understanding of human disease, as well as the use of these cells for therapy. Like embryonic stem cells, the iPS cells also form teratomas, and this has limited their therapeutic potential, with no human trials to date. Direct in vivo reprogramming also leads to the formation of teratomas (Abad et al, 2013). Nonetheless, the potential of reprogramming remains exciting.

Perinatal Stem Cells

Various sources of perinatal stem cells have been reported, with varied potency. Umbilical cord blood is collected at the time of birth and provides a source of undifferentiated cells that may be banked at the time of birth to be available for autologous and allogeneic cell therapy. Umbilical cord blood stem cells were first used clinically in 1989 (Gluckman et al, 1989). Since then, the cells have been used in more than 25,000 patients worldwide. The cells are more immature than adult bone marrow stem cells (Tursky et al, 2012). Cord blood stem cells are mostly used for hematopoietic applications (Kurtzberg, 1996).

Early stem cell populations can be obtained from Wharton jelly, which surrounds the cord (Romanov et al, 2003; Hass et al, 2011). The cells are mesenchymal in origin, although limited multipotentiality has been demonstrated. The cells have not been used clinically.

The most recent perinatal stem cell type described was derived from both the amniotic fluid and placenta. The isolation of multipotent human and mouse amniotic fluid and placental–derived stem (AFPS) cells that are capable of extensive self-renewal and give rise to cells from all three germ layers was reported in 2007 (De Coppi et al, 2007b). AFPS cells represent a class of stem cells with properties somewhere between those of embryonic and adult stem cell types; they are more agile than adult stem cells but less so than embryonic stem cells. Unlike embryonic and induced pluripotent stem cells, however, AFPS cells do not form teratomas, and if preserved for self-use, avoid the problems of rejection. The cells could be obtained either from amniocentesis or chorionic villous sampling in the developing fetus or from the placenta at the time of birth. The cells can be directed into all three germ layers, and they expand readily. Amniotic fluid stem cells have been used experimentally to treat bladder dysfunction (De Coppi et al, 2007a). Many different stem cell types can be obtained from the amniotic fluid or the placenta. There are more than 2500 references in the literature to studies involving these cells. The cells have varied properties and applications, depending on the specific source (Murphy and Atala, 2013).

Adult Stem Cells

Adult stem cells, especially hematopoietic stem cells from the bone marrow, are the best understood cell type in stem cell biology (Ballas et al, 2002). These cells have been used for decades for hematopoietic disorders. However, adult stem cell research remains an area of intense study, as the potential of these cells for therapy may be applicable to myriad degenerative disorders. Within the past decade, adult stem cell populations have been found in many adult tissues other than the bone marrow and the gastrointestinal tract, including the brain (Taupin, 2006; Jiao et al, 2008), skin (Jensen et al, 2008), and muscle (Crisan et al, 2008). **Many types of adult stem cells have been identified in organs throughout the body and are thought to serve as the primary repair entities for their corresponding organs** (Weiner, 2008) (Fig. 20-2). The discovery of such tissue-specific progenitors has opened up new avenues for research.

A notable exception to the tissue specificity of adult stem cells is the mesenchymal stem cell, also known as the *multipotent adult progenitor cell*. This cell type is also derived from bone marrow stroma (Devine, 2002; Jiang et al, 2002). Such cells can differentiate in vitro into numerous tissue types (Caplan, 2007; da Silva Meirelles et al, 2008). Some cells, such as those of the liver, pancreas, and nerve, have very low proliferative capacity in vitro, and the functionality of some cell types is reduced after the cells are cultivated. Isolation of cells has also been problematic because stem cells are present in extremely low numbers in adult tissue (Hristov et al, 2008; Mimeault et al, 2008). Bone marrow stem cells have been differentiated to both bladder urothelium and muscle (Anumanthan et al, 2008; Tian et al, 2010). The cells have also been used in experimental animal models for the enhancement of bladder function and regeneration (Soler et al, 2012; Sharma et al, 2013).

Adipose-derived stem cells that could give rise to multiple lineages were first reported in 2001 (Zuk et al, 2001). The cells have been used for differentiation into urologic cells such as bladder smooth muscle (Jack et al, 2009; Zhang et al, 2012b) and urothelium (Zhang et al, 2013). The adipose-derived cells have also been used experimentally to improve bladder function (Zhang et al, 2012a; Song et al, 2013). Urine-derived stem cells have also been proposed for genitourinary reconstruction (Zhang et al, 2008; Bharadwaj et al, 2013).

Although the clinical usefulness of adult stem cells is currently limited, great potential exists for future use of such cells in tissue-specific regenerative therapies. The advantage of adult stem cells is that they can be used in autologous therapies, thus avoiding any complications associated with immune rejection. Composite adult cell populations from many sources, including bone marrow, fat, and fragments of peripheral blood have been used more extensively in patients for multiple indications more recently. These cells are currently being tested for urologic applications, such as erectile or voiding dysfunction. The mechanisms behind their mode of action need to be further elucidated.

Native Targeted Progenitor Cells

In the past, one of the limitations of applying cell-based regenerative medicine techniques to organ replacement was the inherent difficulty of growing certain human cell types in large quantities. Native targeted progenitor cells, or native cells, are tissue specific unipotent cells derived from most organs. The advantage of these cells is that they are already programmed to become the cell type needed, without any extra-lineage differentiation. By noting the location of the progenitor cells, as well as by exploring the conditions that promote differentiation and/or self-renewal, it has been possible to overcome some of the obstacles that limit cell expansion in vitro. One example is the urothelial cell. Urothelial cells could be grown in the laboratory setting in the past, but only with limited success. It was believed that urothelial cells had a natural senescence that was hard to overcome. Several protocols have been developed over the last two decades that have improved urothelial growth and expansion (Cilento et al, 1994; Liebert et al, 1997; Scriven et al, 1997; Puthenveettil et al, 1999). A system of urothelial cell harvesting was developed that does not use any enzymes or serum and has a large expansion potential. Using these methods of cell culture, it is possible to expand a urothelial strain from a single specimen that initially covers a surface area of 1 cm^2 to one covering a surface area of 4202 m^2 (the equivalent area of one football field) within 8 weeks (Cilento et al, 1994).

An additional advantage in using native cells is that they can be obtained from the specific organ to be regenerated, expanded, and used in the same patient without rejection, in an autologous manner. Bladder, ureter, and renal pelvis cells can equally be harvested, cultured, and expanded in a similar fashion. Normal human bladder epithelial and muscle cells can be efficiently harvested from surgical material and extensively expanded in culture, and their differentiation characteristics, growth requirements, and other biologic properties can be studied (Liebert et al, 1991; Cilento et al, 1994; Tobin et al, 1994; Harriss, 1995; Freeman et al, 1997; Liebert et al, 1997; Fauza et al, 1998; Lobban et al, 1998; Solomon et al, 1998; Nguyen et al, 1999; Puthenveettil et al, 1999; Rackley et al, 1999). Major advances in cell culture techniques have been made within the past several decades, and these techniques make the use of autologous cells possible for clinical application. However, even now, not all human cells can be grown or expanded in vitro. Liver, nerve, and pancreas are examples of human tissues for which the technology is not yet advanced to the point where these cells can be grown and expanded.

When cells are used for tissue reconstitution, donor tissue is dissociated into individual cells, which are either implanted directly into the host or expanded in culture, attached to a support matrix, and reimplanted after expansion.

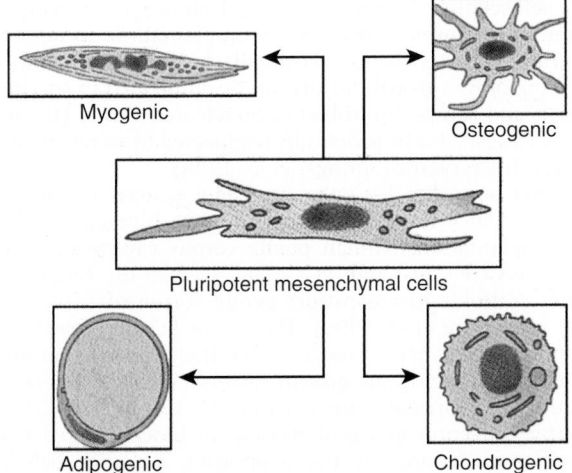

Figure 20-2. Schematic diagram of pluripotential stem cell lineages that can be derived from postnatal tissue.

BIOMATERIALS AND VASCULARIZATION FOR GENITOURINARY REGENERATIVE MEDICINE

For regenerative medicine purposes, there are clear advantages to use of degradable, biocompatible materials that can function as cell delivery vehicles and/or provide the structural parameters needed for tissue replacement. **Biomaterials in regenerative medicine function as an artificial ECM and elicit biologic and mechanical functions of native ECM found in tissues in the body.** Native ECM brings cells together into tissue, controls the tissue structure, and regulates the cell phenotype (Alberts et al, 1994). Biomaterials facilitate the localization and delivery of cells and/or bioactive factors (e.g., cell adhesion peptides, growth factors) to desired sites in the body; define a three-dimensional space for the formation of new tissues with appropriate structure; and guide the development of new tissues with appropriate function (Kim et al, 1998). Direct injection of cell suspensions without biomaterial matrices has been used in some cases (Ponder et al, 1991; Brittberg et al, 1994), but it is difficult to control the localization of transplanted cells. In addition, the majority of mammalian cell types are anchorage dependent and will die if not provided with a cell-adhesion substrate.

Design and Selection of Biomaterials

The design and selection of the biomaterial is critical in the development of engineered genitourinary tissues. The biomaterial must be capable of controlling the structure and function of the engineered tissue in a predesigned manner by interacting with transplanted cells and/or host cells. In general, the ideal biomaterial should be biocompatible, promote cellular interaction and tissue development, and possess proper mechanical and physical properties.

The selected biomaterial should be biodegradable and bioresorbable to support the reconstruction of a completely normal tissue without inflammation. Such behavior of the biomaterials avoids the risk of inflammatory or foreign-body responses that may be associated with the permanent presence of a foreign material in the body. The degradation rate and the concentration of degradation products in the tissues surrounding the implant must be at a tolerable level (Bergsma et al, 1995).

The biomaterials should provide an appropriate regulation of cell behavior (e.g., adhesion, proliferation, migration, differentiation) to promote the development of functional new tissue. Cell behavior in engineered tissues is regulated by multiple interactions with the microenvironment, including interactions with cell-adhesion ligands (Hynes, 1992) and with soluble growth factors (Deuel, 1997). Cell adhesion–promoting factors (e.g., Arg-Gly-Asp [RGD]) can be presented by the biomaterial itself or incorporated into the biomaterial to control cell behavior through ligand-induced cell receptor signaling processes (Barrera et al, 1993; Cook et al, 1997). The biomaterials provide temporary mechanical support sufficient to withstand in vivo forces exerted by the surrounding tissue and maintain a potential space for tissue development. The mechanical support of the biomaterials should be maintained until the engineered tissue has sufficient mechanical integrity to support itself (Atala, 2007). This potentially can be achieved by an appropriate choice of mechanical and degradative properties of the biomaterials (Kim et al, 1998).

The biomaterials need to be processed into specific configurations. A large ratio of surface area to volume is often desirable to allow the delivery of a high density of cells. A high-porosity, interconnected pore structure with specific pore sizes promotes tissue ingrowth from the surrounding host tissue. Several techniques, such as electrospinning, have been developed that readily control porosity, pore size, and pore structure (Lee et al, 2007; Yoo et al, 2007; Choi et al, 2008; Lee et al, 2008a, 2008b, 2008c, 2010).

In general, three classes of biomaterials have been used for engineering of genitourinary tissues: naturally derived materials, such as collagen; acellular tissue matrices, such as bladder submucosa and small-intestinal submucosa; and synthetic polymers, such as polyglycolic acid (PGA), polylactic acid (PLA), and poly(lactic-co-glycolic acid) (PLGA). These classes of biomaterials have been tested with regard to their biocompatibility with primary human urothelial and bladder muscle cells (Pariente et al, 2001). Naturally derived materials and acellular tissue matrices have the potential advantage of biologic recognition. Synthetic polymers can be produced reproducibly on a large scale with controlled properties of strength, degradation rate, and microstructure. Combination scaffolds have also been used (Engelhardt et al, 2011).

Additional information on the general types of biomaterials used can be found on the Expert Consult website.

Vascularization

The goals in regenerative medicine include the replacement of damaged, injured, or missing body tissues with biologic-compatible substitutes. **A limiting factor for the engineering of tissues is that cells cannot be implanted in volumes exceeding 3 mm^3 (Folkman and Hochberg, 1973). Nutrition and gas exchange are limited by this maximal diffusion distance. If cells were implanted in volumes exceeding 3 mm^3, only the cells on the surface would survive, and the central cell core would undergo necrosis resulting from a lack of vascularity.** Therefore a critical obstacle in regenerative medicine is the ability to maintain large masses of cells alive, on transfer from the in vitro culture conditions into the host, in vivo (Mooney and Mikos, 1999). To achieve the goals of engineering large complex tissues, and possibly internal organs, vascularization of the regenerating cells is essential.

Formation of new blood vessels and capillaries is composed of two different processes: vasculogenesis, the in situ assembly of capillaries from undifferentiated endothelial cells (ECs), and angiogenesis, the sprouting of capillaries from preexisting blood vessels.

More information on these two processes is included on the Expert Consult website.

The understanding of the angiogenic process and the isolation of potent and specific angiogenic growth factors has encouraged the use of these factors therapeutically (Loges et al, 2009; Phelps and Garcia, 2009). Efforts have been aimed at incorporating the knowledge acquired in angiogenesis of ischemic tissues into practical approaches to vascularize bioengineered tissues (Stosich et al, 2009). Bioengineered tissues are usually supported by scaffolds of biocompatible matrices made from natural or artificial sources (Hubbell et al, 1991). Successful vascularization is dependent on the porosity of the supporting matrix. A positive correlation between the pore size of poly(L-lactic acid) (PLLA) implants and the rate of vascularization has been observed (Mikos et al, 1993).

Three approaches have been used for vascularization of bioengineered tissue: (1) incorporation of angiogenic factors in the bioengineered tissue; (2) seeding ECs with other cell types in the bioengineered tissue; and (3) prevascularization of the matrix before cell seeding. Angiogenic growth factors may be incorporated into the bioengineered tissue before implantation, to attract host capillaries and to enhance neovascularization of the implanted tissue. Angiogenic growth factors can be embedded in specific biomaterials and can be controlled to be released slowly (Eiselt et al, 1998). Cells can also be genetically engineered to secrete high levels of angiogenic proteins (Springer et al, 1998).

Another approach for enhancing angiogenesis employed cultured ECs, which are incorporated into the bioengineered tissue before implantation. Human penile corpus cavernosum–derived smooth muscle cells and ECs were seeded on biodegradable polymer scaffolds to reconstruct penile corporeal tissue in vitro and in vivo (Park et al, 1999). The use of ECs improved the formation of the engineered tissue. In another study the addition of both ECs and angiogenic growth factors (VEGF) accelerated the formation of engineered muscle tissue (De Coppi et al, 2005). An alternative direction in vascularization of bioengineered tissue is the prevascularization of the supporting polymer before cell seeding. In this manner, the bioengineered tissue will be organized around the vascular network, providing sufficient tissue perfusion (Fontaine et al, 1995).

Despite the successes in bioengineering tissues consisting of thin layers of cells such as skin, a major challenge for regenerative medicine in the future is the production of larger organs with more complex structures, such as the kidney. Tissues with a large mass of cells require a vascular network of arteries, veins, and capillaries to deliver nutrients to each cell. The development of efficient methods to vascularize bioengineered tissues is critical for a successful outcome. There are many obstacles to overcome before large entire tissue-engineered solid organs are produced. Recent developments in angiogenesis research may provide important knowledge and are essential.

REGENERATIVE MEDICINE OF UROLOGIC STRUCTURES

Urethra

Various strategies have been proposed over the years for the regeneration of urethral tissue. Woven meshes of PGA without cells (Bazeed et al, 1983; Olsen et al, 1992) and with cells (Atala, et al, 1992) were used to regenerate urethras in various animal models. Naturally derived collagen-based materials such as bladder-derived acellular submucosa (Chen et al, 1999), acellular urethral submucosa (Sievert et al, 2000), and collagen gels (Micol et al, 2012) have also been tried experimentally in various animal models for urethral reconstruction.

The bladder submucosa matrix (Chen et al, 1999) proved to be a suitable graft for repair of urethral defects in rabbits. The neourethras demonstrated a normal urothelial luminal lining and organized muscle bundles. These results were confirmed clinically in a series of patients with a history of failed hypospadias reconstruction wherein the urethral defects were repaired with human bladder acellular collagen matrices (Atala et al, 1999). The neourethras were created by anastomosing the matrix in an onlay fashion to the urethral plate. The size of the created neourethra ranged from 5 to 15 cm. After a 3-year follow-up, three of the four patients had a successful outcome with regard to cosmetic appearance and function (Fig. 20-4). One patient who had a 15-cm neourethra created

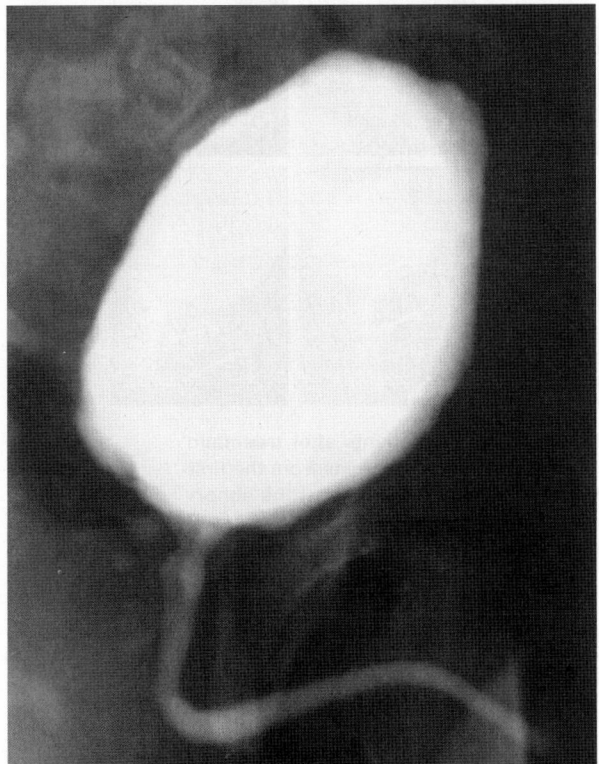

Figure 20-4. Urethrogram 6 months after surgery in a patient who had a portion of his urethra replaced as an onlay with the use of an acellular bladder submucosa matrix.

developed a subglanular fistula. The acellular collagen-based matrix eliminated the necessity of performing additional surgical procedures for graft harvesting, and both operative time and the potential morbidity from the harvest procedure were decreased. Similar results were obtained in pediatric and adult patients with primary urethral stricture disease using the same collagen matrices (El-Kassaby et al, 2003). Another study in 30 patients with recurrent stricture disease showed that a healthy urethral bed (two or fewer prior urethral surgeries) was needed for successful urethral reconstruction using acellular collagen-based grafts (El-Kassaby et al, 2008). A clinical trial using tubularized nonseeded small intestinal submucosa (SIS) for urethral stricture repair was performed in eight evaluable patients. Two patients with short inflammatory strictures maintained urethral patency. Stricture recurrence developed in the other six patients within 3 months of surgery (le Roux, 2005). Many pediatric and adult patients with urethral disease have been successfully treated in an onlay manner with collagen-based matrices. One of the advantages of this method over nongenital tissue grafts used for urethroplasty is that the material is "off the shelf." This eliminates the necessity of additional surgical procedures for graft harvesting, which may decrease operative time, as well as the potential morbidity from the harvest procedure.

The techniques previously described, involving the use of nonseeded acellular matrices, were applied experimentally and clinically in a successful manner for onlay urethral repairs. However, when tubularized urethral repairs were attempted experimentally, adequate urethral tissue regeneration was not achieved and complications ensued, such as graft contracture and stricture formation (De Filippo et al, 2002). Autologous rabbit bladder epithelial and smooth muscle cells were grown and seeded onto preconfigured tubular matrices. Entire urethra segments were resected and urethroplasties were performed with tubularized collagen matrices either seeded with cells or without cells. The tubularized collagen matrices seeded with autologous cells formed new tissue that was histologically similar to native urethra. Use of the tubularized collagen matrices without cells led to poor tissue development, fibrosis, and stricture formation (Orabi et al, 2013). These findings were confirmed clinically. In a pilot series of patients published in *The Lancet*, five patients with urethral injuries secondary to motor vehicle accidents had a small tissue biopsy specimen retrieved starting in 2004. The cells were expanded in vitro and seeded in two layers, muscle and epithelia, on tubularized scaffolds that were implanted surgically (Fig. 20-5). The tubularized engineered urethras were able to show adequate anatomy, both by urethroscopy and with urethrography (see Fig. 20-5), and function long term, currently with follow-up exceeding 10 years (Raya-Rivera et al, 2011). In another series of five patients, tissue-engineered oral mucosa was seeded in cadaveric dermis, mainly with fibroblasts and keratinocytes. All patients required instrumentation postoperatively because of strictures, but they all had the diagnosis of lichen sclerosis (Bhargava et al, 2008). Other cell types have also been tried experimentally in acellular bladder collagen matrices, including foreskin epidermal cells and oral keratinocytes (Fu et al, 2007; Li et al, 2008). VEGF gene-modified urothelial cells have also been used experimentally for urethral reconstruction (Guan et al, 2008).

The normal wound healing response to injury has been studied extensively, and this knowledge has been helpful in maximizing success for the engineering of tissues. At the time of tissue injury, cell ingrowth is initiated from the wound edges to cover the tissue defect. The cells from the edges of the native tissue are able to traverse short distances without any detrimental effects. If the wound is large, more than a few millimeters in distance or depth, increased collagen deposition, fibrosis, and scar formation ensue. Matrices implanted in wound beds are able to lengthen the distances that cells can traverse without initiating an adverse fibrotic response. However, these distances are also limited. The maximum distance that adjacent cells from the wound edge have to travel to create normal tissue over a biologic matrix is approximately 1 cm (Dorin et al, 2008). Tissue defects greater than 1 cm that are treated with a matrix alone, without cells, usually have increased collagen deposition, increased

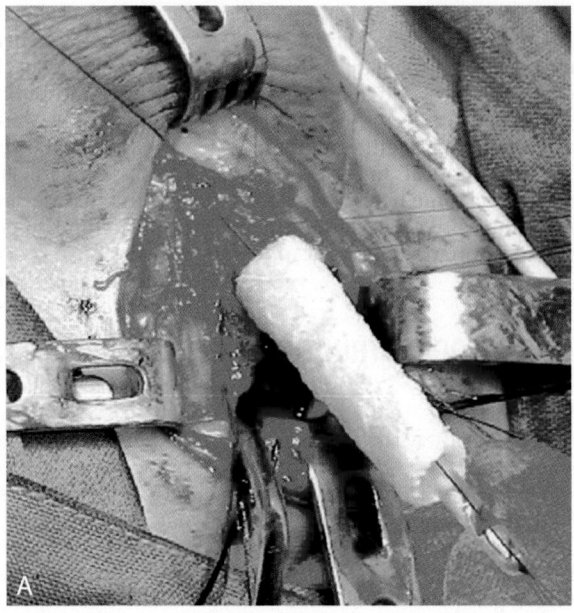

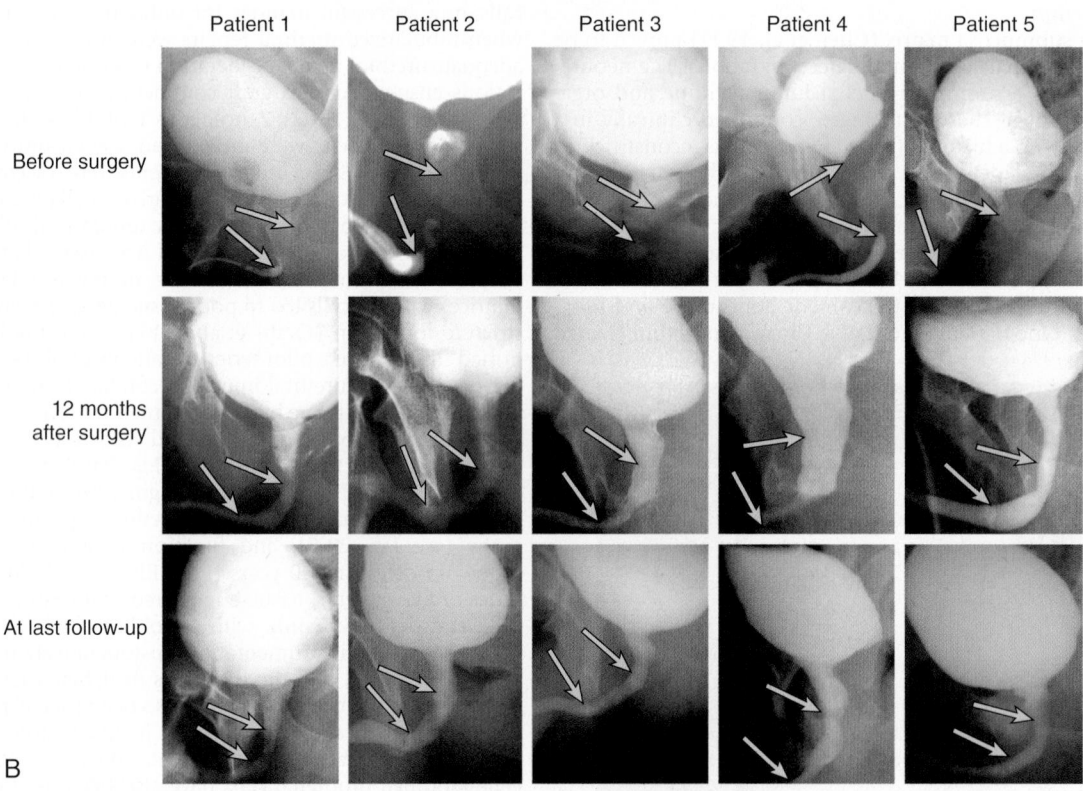

Figure 20-5. **Tissue urethra implantation and clinical outcome in five patients after traumatic injury. A,** An autologous cell-seeded graft sutured to the normal urethral margins from the first patient. **B,** Voiding cystourethrograms of five patients before surgery (*arrows* show the abnormal margins), 12 months after surgery (*arrows* show margins of tissue-engineered urethras), and at last follow-up to 7 years after surgery (*arrows* show margins of tissue-engineered urethras).

fibrosis, and scar formation. Cell-seeded matrices implanted in wound beds are able to further lengthen the distance for normal tissue formation without initiating an adverse fibrotic response. Studies in the field of regenerative medicine have shown that very large defects, greater than 30 cm, can be successfully treated using cell-seeded scaffolds. This explains the described experimental and clinical results noted with urethral repair. Nonseeded matrices are able to replace urethral segments when used in an onlay fashion because of the short distances required for tissue ingrowth. However, if a tubularized urethral repair is needed, the matrices need to be seeded with autologous cells to avoid the risk of stricture formation and poor tissue development.

Bladder

Currently, gastrointestinal segments are commonly used as tissues for bladder replacement or repair. However, gastrointestinal tissues are designed to absorb specific solutes, whereas bladder tissue is designed for the excretion of solutes. **When gastrointestinal tissue is in contact with the urinary tract, multiple complications may ensue, such as infection, metabolic disturbances, urolithiasis, perforation, increased mucus production, and malignancy** (McDougal, 1992). Because of the problems encountered with the use of gastrointestinal segments, numerous investigators have attempted alternative reconstructive procedures for bladder replacement or repair. These include autoaugmentation (Cartwright and Snow, 1989a, 1989b) and ureterocystoplasty (Adams et al, 1998). In addition, alternate methods for bladder reconstruction have been explored, such as the use of tissue expansion (Lailas et al, 1996; Satar et al, 1999) and regenerative medicine with cell transplantation.

Matrices for Bladder Regeneration

Over the last few decades, several bladder wall substitutes have been used in attempts at regeneration, with both synthetic and organic materials. Synthetic materials that have been tried in experimental and clinical settings include polyvinyl sponge, Teflon, collagen matrices, Vicryl (PGA) matrices, and silicone. Most of these attempts failed because of mechanical, structural, functional, or biocompatibility problems. **Usually, permanent synthetic materials used for bladder reconstruction succumb to mechanical failure and urinary stone formation, and use of degradable materials leads to fibroblast deposition, scarring, graft contracture, and a reduced reservoir volume over time** (Atala, 1995, 1998).

There has been a resurgence in the use of various collagen-based matrices for tissue regeneration. Nonseeded allogeneic acellular bladder matrices have served as scaffolds for the ingrowth of host bladder wall components. The matrices are prepared by mechanically and chemically removing all cellular components from bladder tissue (Probst et al, 1997; Yoo et al, 1998b). The matrices serve as vehicles for partial bladder regeneration, and relevant antigenicity is not evident.

Cell-seeded allogeneic acellular bladder matrices were used for bladder augmentation in dogs (Yoo et al, 1998b). Biomaterials preloaded with cells before their implantation showed better tissue regeneration compared with biomaterials implanted with no cells, in which tissue regeneration depended on ingrowth of cells from the surrounding tissue. The acellular collagen matrices can be enhanced with growth factors to improve bladder regeneration (Kikuno et al, 2009).

SIS, a biodegradable, acellular, xenogeneic collagen-based tissue-matrix graft, was first described in the early 1960s as an acellular matrix for tissue replacement in the vascular field (Rotthoff et al, 1964, 1969). The matrix is derived from pig small intestine in which the mucosa is mechanically removed from the inner surface and the serosa and muscular layer are removed from the outer surface. Animal studies have shown that the nonseeded SIS matrix used for bladder augmentation is able to regenerate in vivo (Kropp et al, 1996). Histologically, the transitional layer was the same as that of the native bladder tissue but, as with other nonseeded collagen matrices used experimentally, the muscle layer was not fully developed. In vitro contractility studies performed on SIS-regenerated dog bladders showed a decrease in maximal contractile response by 50% from that of normal bladder tissues.

Bladder augmentation using laparoscopic techniques was performed on minipigs with porcine bowel acellular tissue matrix, human placental membranes, or porcine SIS. At 12 weeks' postoperatively the grafts had contracted down to 60% of their original sizes, and histologically the grafts showed predominantly only mucosal regeneration (Portis et al, 2000). Hemicystectomy and bladder replacement with SIS showed muscle at the graft periphery and center but it consisted of small fused bundles with significant fibrosis at 1 year. Compared with primary bladder closure after hemicystectomy, no advantage in bladder capacity or compliance was documented (Landman et al, 2004).

In multiple studies using various materials as nonseeded grafts for cystoplasty, the urothelial layer was able to regenerate normally, but the muscle layer, although present, was not fully

developed (Kropp et al, 1996; Sutherland et al, 1996; Probst et al, 1997; Yoo et al, 1998b; Jayo et al, 2008b; Zhang, 2008). Studies involving acellular matrices that may provide the necessary environment to promote cell migration, growth, and differentiation are being conducted (Chun et al, 2007). With continued bladder research in this area, these matrices may have a clinical role in bladder replacement in the future.

Regenerative Medicine for Bladder Using Cell Transplantation

Regenerative medicine with selective cell transplantation may provide a means to create functional new bladder segments (Atala, 1997). The success of cell transplantation strategies for bladder reconstruction depends on the ability to use donor tissue efficiently and to provide the right conditions for long-term survival, differentiation, and growth. Various cell sources have been explored for bladder regeneration. Native cells are currently preferable because they can be used without rejection (Cilento et al, 1994). Amniotic fluid– and bone marrow–derived stem cells can also be used in an autologous manner and have the potential to differentiate into bladder muscle (De Coppi et al, 2007b; Shukla et al, 2008) and urothelium (Anumanthan et al, 2008). Embryonic stem cells also have the potential to differentiate into bladder tissue (Oottamasathien et al, 2007).

Formation of Bladder Tissue

Human urothelial and muscle cells can be expanded in vitro, seeded onto polymer scaffolds, and allowed to attach and form sheets of cells. The cell-polymer scaffold can then be implanted in vivo. Histologic analysis indicated that viable cells were able to self-assemble back into their respective tissue types, and would retain their native phenotype (Atala et al, 1993b). These experiments demonstrated, for the first time, that composite layered tissue-engineered structures could be created de novo.

It has been well established for decades that the bladder is able to regenerate generously over free grafts. Urothelium is associated with a high reparative capacity (de Boer et al, 1994). Bladder muscle tissue is less likely to regenerate in a normal fashion. Both urothelial and muscle ingrowth are believed to be initiated from the edges of the normal bladder toward the region of the free graft (Baker et al, 1958; Gorham et al, 1989). Usually, however, contracture or resorption of the graft has been evident. The inflammatory response toward the matrix may contribute to the resorption of the free graft. It was hypothesized that building the three-dimensional structure constructs in vitro, before implantation, would facilitate the eventual terminal differentiation of the cells after implantation in vivo and would minimize the inflammatory response toward the matrix, thus avoiding graft contracture and shrinkage. A dog study demonstrated a major difference between matrices used with autologous cells (tissue-engineered matrices) and those used without cells (Yoo et al, 1998b). **Matrices implanted with cells for bladder augmentation retained most of their implanted diameter, as opposed to matrices implanted without cells for bladder augmentation, in which graft contraction and shrinkage occurred. The histomorphology demonstrated a marked paucity of muscle cells and a more aggressive inflammatory reaction in the matrices implanted without cells.**

To better address the functional parameters of tissue-engineered bladders, a canine animal model was designed that required a subtotal cystectomy with subsequent replacement with a tissue-engineered organ (Oberpenning et al, 1999).Cystectomy-only and nonseeded controls maintained average capacities of 22% and 46% of preoperative values, respectively. An average bladder capacity of 95% of the original precystectomy volume was achieved in the cell-seeded tissue-engineered bladder replacements. These findings were confirmed radiographically (Fig. 20-6). Histologically, the nonseeded scaffold bladders presented a pattern of normal urothelial cells with a thickened fibrotic submucosa and a thin layer of muscle

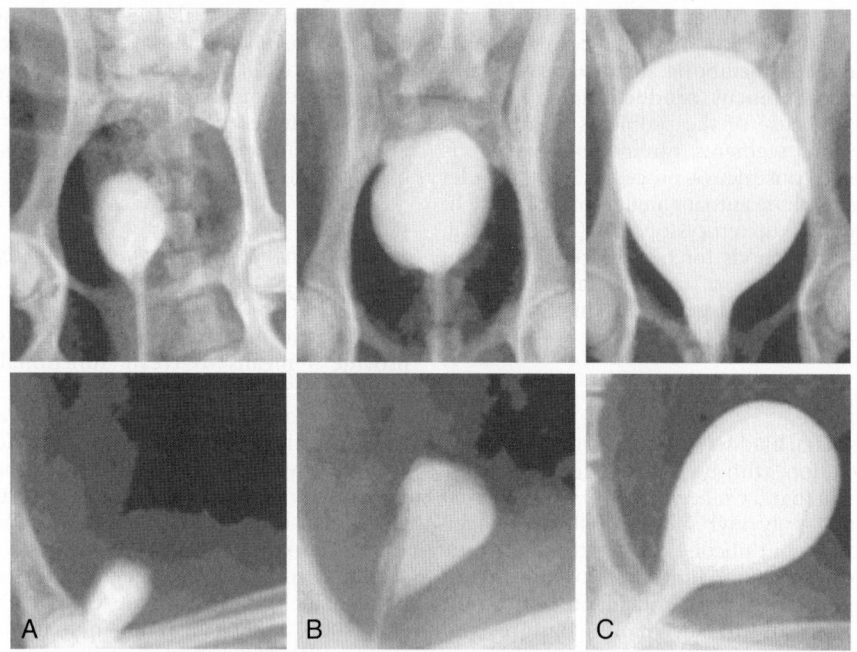

Figure 20-6. Radiographic cystograms in beagles 11 months after subtotal cystectomy without reconstruction (A); with reconstruction using a polymer without cells (B); and with reconstruction with a polymer and cell-seeded tissue-engineered organ (C). Organs after trigone-sparing cystectomy retained a small reservoir. Tissue-engineered neobladders showed a normal configuration and a larger capacity than the trigones grafted with polymer only.

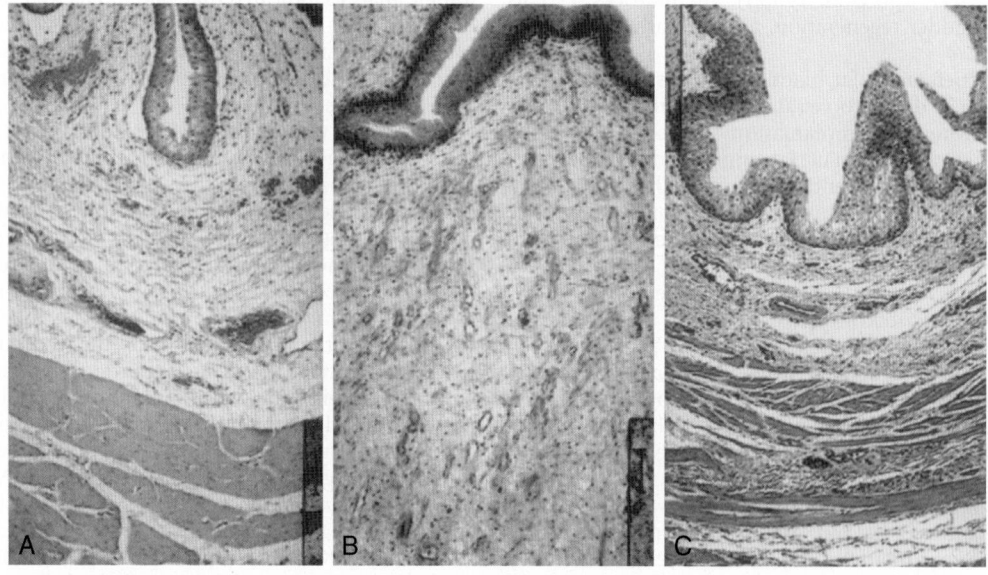

Figure 20-7. Hematoxylin and eosin staining shows histologic results 6 months after surgery (original magnification, ×250). A, Normal canine bladder. B, The bladder dome of the bladder reconstructed with cell-free polymer consists of normal urothelium over a thickened layer of collagen and fibrotic tissue; only scarce muscle fibers are apparent. C, The tissue-engineered neo-organ has a histomorphologically normal appearance. A trilayered architecture consisting of urothelium, submucosa, and smooth muscle is evident.

fibers. The retrieved tissue-engineered bladders showed a normal cellular organization, consisting of a trilayer of urothelium, submucosa, and muscle (Fig. 20-7). These studies, performed with PGA-based scaffolds, have been repeated by other investigators, showing similar results in large numbers of animals long term (Jayo et al, 2008a, 2008b). However, not all scaffolds perform well if a large portion of the bladder needs replacement. In a study using SIS for subtotal bladder replacement in dogs, both the unseeded and cell-seeded experimental groups showed graft shrinkage and poor results (Zhang et al, 2006b). The type of scaffold used is critical for the success of these technologies. The use of bioreactors, wherein mechanical stimulation is started at the time of organ production, has also been proposed as an important parameter for success (Farhat and Yeger, 2008; Bouhout et al, 2011).

A clinical experience involving engineered bladder tissue for cystoplasty reconstruction was conducted starting in 1998. A small

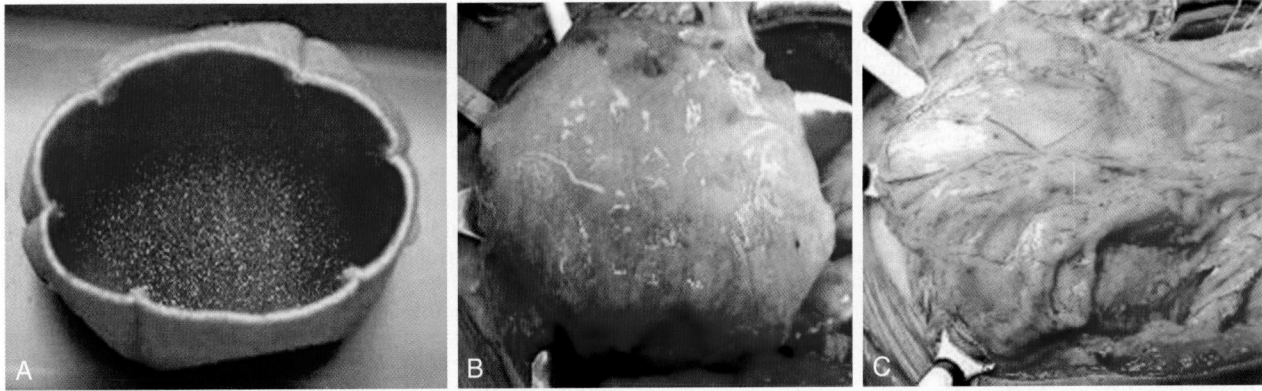

Figure 20-8. Construction of engineered bladder. A, Scaffold material seeded with cells for use in bladder repair. B, The seeded scaffold is anastomosed to native bladder with running 4-0 polyglycolic sutures. C, Implant covered with fibrin glue and omentum.

pilot study of seven patients was reported, using a collagen scaffold seeded with cells either with or without omentum coverage, or a combined PGA-collagen scaffold seeded with cells and omental coverage (Fig. 20-8). The patients who underwent reconstruction with the engineered bladder tissue created with the PGA-collagen cell-seeded scaffolds with omental coverage showed increased compliance, decreased end-filling pressures, increased capacities, and longer dry periods over time (Atala et al, 2006). Although the experience is promising in terms of showing that engineered tissues can be implanted safely, it is just a start in terms of accomplishing the goal of engineering fully functional bladders. This was a limited clinical experience, and the technology is not yet ready for wide dissemination; further experimental and clinical studies are required. FDA phase 2 studies have now been completed.

From the aforementioned studies it is evident, as with the urethral studies, that the use of cell-seeded matrices is superior to the use of nonseeded matrices for the creation of engineered bladder tissues. Although advances have been made with the engineering of bladder tissues, many challenges remain. Current research in many centers is aimed at the development of biologically active and "smart" biomaterials that may improve tissue regeneration. Also, similar engineering techniques are now being used for patients with bladder cancer, who are having engineered urinary conduits implanted after cystectomy (Hyndman et al, 2012). Stem cells derived from fat can be differentiated into smooth muscle for the conduits, thus avoiding native cells from bladder cancer patients (Basu et al, 2012).

Bladder Cell Therapies

Both urinary incontinence and vesicoureteral reflux are common conditions affecting the genitourinary system for which injectable therapy within the bladder may be useful. The ideal substance for the endoscopic treatment of reflux and incontinence should be injectable, nonantigenic, nonmigratory, volume stable, and safe for human use (Kershen et al, 1999). Toward this goal, long-term studies were conducted to determine the effect of injectable chondrocytes in vivo (Atala et al, 1993a). This system was adapted for the treatment of reflux in a porcine model (Atala et al, 1994).

The first human application of cell-based regenerative medicine technology for urologic applications occurred with the injection of chondrocytes for the correction of vesicoureteral reflux in children and for urinary incontinence in adults. Phase 1 trials showed an approximate success rate of 80% at both 3 and 12 months postoperatively (Bent et al, 2001). Patients with vesicoureteral reflux were treated at 10 centers throughout the United States. The patients had a similar success rate as with other injectable substances in terms of cure. The overall success rate in 29 children (47 ureters) was 86%. At 1-year follow-up, reflux correction was maintained in 70% of the

ureters. Chondrocyte formation was not noted in patients who had treatment failure (Diamond et al, 1999).

With cell therapy techniques, the use of autologous smooth muscle cells was explored for both urinary incontinence and vesicoureteral reflux applications (Cilento et al, 1995). In vivo experiments were conducted in minipigs, and reflux was successfully corrected. The potential use of injectable, cultured myoblasts for the treatment of stress urinary incontinence has been investigated in animal models (Chancellor et al, 2000; Yokoyama et al, 2000; Cannon et al, 2003; Lee et al, 2003; Strasser et al, 2004; Kwon et al, 2006; Mitterberger et al, 2007b). Intrinsic muscle precursor cells have also been shown to play an active role in the regeneration of injured striated urethral sphincter (Yiou et al, 2003a, 2003b). A canine model of irreversible urethral sphincter injury was also created to test these technologies (Eberli et al, 2008, 2012).

Other cell types have also been used for urinary incontinence. The use of amniotic fluid–derived stem cells has been tested experimentally (Chun et al, 2012; Kim et al, 2012a). The use of lipoaspirate cells has also been proposed for the treatment of urinary incontinence. The lipoaspirate cells were injected into mice bladders and urethras, and regenerated muscle tissue (Jack et al, 2005; Fu et al, 2010; Zhao et al, 2011). The cells were used in the clinical setting in patients in an autologous manner in a pilot study with adequate results (Yamamoto et al, 2012).

Several clinical trials using myoblast injection have been conducted in patients with stress urinary incontinence (Mitterberger et al, 2007a). The authors compared the effectiveness and tolerability of ultrasonography-guided injections of autologous cells with those of endoscopic injections of collagen for stress incontinence in 63 patients, showing improved results for the patients receiving the myoblasts. However, controversy surrounding the trial ensued and the paper was retracted. In another trial, myoblasts isolated from the abdominal wall vasculature were injected in a series of bladder exstrophy patients with urinary incontinence. The authors reported that 88% of patients were socially dry, described as daytime dryness lasting more than 3 hours. The patients were also on a pelvic floor electrical stimulation and pelvic floor exercise program (Kajbafzadeh et al, 2008). Another study described the use of autologous muscle-derived stem cell injection to treat stress urinary incontinence. After 1 year, one of eight women achieved total continence and five reported improvement (Carr et al, 2008). A 24% success rate was obtained in a patient trial using myoblasts delivered with ultrasound guidance (Blaganje and Lukianović, 2012). Activity has increased in the area of cell therapy for urinary incontinence in the last several years. Further trials and follow-up will be needed to determine long-term efficacy.

Cell therapy studies have also been conducted for radiation cystitis. Bone marrow cells have been injected in rats (Imamura et al, 2012). Both amniotic fluid and bone marrow stem cells have been used to ameliorate bladder dysfunction in a Parkinson animal model (Soler et al, 2012). Also, recently, mechanisms are being elucidated for the regeneration of bladder stem cells in situ—for example, with a Hedgehog and Wnt feedback system (Shin et al, 2011). These studies are certain to advance with the generation of small molecules and pharmacologic agents for regenerative medicine (Lu and Atala, 2013).

Ureters

Various strategies have been used to engineer ureteral tissues experimentally, but these have not yet been implanted in patients.

Additional information on regenerative medicine efforts in the ureter appears on the Expert Consult website.

Male Genital and Reproductive Tissues

Reconstructive surgery is required for a wide variety of pathologic penile conditions, including penile carcinoma, trauma, severe erectile dysfunction, and congenital conditions such as ambiguous genitalia, hypospadias, and epispadias. One of the major limitations of genital reconstructive surgery is the availability of sufficient autologous tissue. Nongenital autologous tissue sources have been used for decades. Phallic reconstruction was initially attempted in the late 1930s, with rib cartilage used as a stiffener for patients with traumatic penile loss (Frumpkin, 1944; Goodwin and Scott, 1952). This method, involving multiple staged surgeries, was soon discouraged because of the unsatisfactory functional and cosmetic results. Silicone rigid prostheses were popularized in the 1970s and have been used widely (Small et al, 1975; Bretan, 1989). However, biocompatibility issues have been a problem in selected patients (Thomalla et al, 1987; Nukui et al, 1997).

Research has also been performed looking at the possibility of creating prostheses with cells; this information appears on the Expert Consult website.

Reconstruction of Penile Corpora

One of the major components of the phallus is corporeal smooth muscle. The creation of autologous functional and structural corporeal tissue de novo would be beneficial. Initial experiments showed that cultured human corporeal smooth muscle cells may be used in conjunction with biodegradable polymers to create corpus cavernosum tissue de novo (Kershen et al, 2002). When grown on collagen, corporeal cavernosal ECs formed capillary structures that created complex three-dimensional capillary networks. In a subsequent study, human corporeal smooth muscle cells and ECs seeded on biodegradable polymer scaffolds were able to form vascularized cavernosal muscle when implanted in vivo (Park et al, 1999). A naturally derived acellular corporeal tissue matrix that possesses the same architecture as native corpora was developed. Acellular collagen matrices were derived from processed donor rabbit corpora using cell lysis techniques. Human corpus cavernosal muscle and ECs were derived from donor penile tissue, and the cells were expanded in vitro and seeded on the acellular matrices. The matrices were covered with the appropriate cell architecture 4 weeks after implantation (Falke et al, 2003). The use of these tissue-derived matrices as cell-delivery scaffolds allowed for the development of adequate structural and vascular corpora cavernosa constructs.

To look at the functional parameters of the engineered corpora, acellular corporeal collagen matrices were obtained from donor rabbit penis and autologous corpus cavernosal smooth muscle, and ECs were harvested, expanded, and seeded on the matrices. An entire cross-sectional segment of protruding rabbit phallus was excised, leaving the urethra intact, and the cell-seeded matrices were interposed into the excised corporeal space. Functional and structural parameters (cavernosography, cavernosometry, mating behavior, and sperm ejaculation) were followed, and histochemical, immunocytochemical, and Western blot analyses were performed up to 6 months after implantation. The engineered corpora cavernosa achieved adequate structural and functional parameters (Kwon et al, 2002). This technology was further confirmed when the entire

rabbit phallus corpora were removed and replaced with the engineered scaffolds seeded with both corporeal endothelial and smooth muscle cells (Fig. 20-9). The experimental corporeal bodies demonstrated intact structural integrity by cavernosography and showed similar pressure by cavernosometry when compared with normal controls (Fig. 20-10). The control rabbits without cells failed to show normal erectile function throughout the study period. Mating activity in the animals with the engineered corpora appeared normal by 1 month after implantation. The presence of sperm was confirmed during mating, and sperm was present in all the rabbits with the engineered corpora. The female rabbits mated with the animals implanted with engineered corpora and also conceived and delivered healthy pups. Animals implanted with the matrix alone were unable to demonstrate normal mating activity and failed to ejaculate into the vagina. Grossly, the corporeal implants with cells showed continuous integration of the graft into native tissue. Histologically, sinusoidal spaces and walls, lined with endothelium and smooth muscle, were observed in the engineered grafts. Grafts without cells contained fibrotic tissue and calcifications with sparse corporeal elements. Each cell type was identified immunocytochemically and by Western blot analyses. The engineered corporeal tissues were able to contract and relax in response to electric field and pharmacologic stimulation, and the contractile response reached levels similar to normal corpora by 6 months after implantation (Chen et al, 2010).

The aforementioned series of studies demonstrates that penile corpora cavernosa tissue can be engineered. The engineered tissue is able to achieve adequate structural and functional parameters sufficient for erection, copulation, ejaculation, conception, and delivery experimentally. Further studies will be needed to confirm the long-term functionality of these organs. In addition, further studies are needed to show that human structures can also be engineered.

Penile Cell Therapy

Various cell therapies have been proposed and used experimentally for erectile dysfunction. ECs have been used in animal models to reverse erectile dysfunction (Gou et al, 2011). Mesenchymal stem cells have been used either alone or in combination with matrices (Lin et al, 2011; Kim et al, 2012b), showing an improvement in function in mice. The delivery of human bone marrow–derived stem cells to the periprostatic region in rats led to improved response after the cells were injected in the corpora (Qiu et al, 2011; You et al, 2013). Muscle-derived stem cells showed the prevention of erectile dysfunction after cavernosal injury in rats (Kovanecz et al, 2012). Adipose-derived cells have also been used in rodents, showing reversal of corporeal damage, with or without growth factors (Orabi et al, 2012; Qiu et al, 2012; Ryu et al, 2012; Liu et al, 2013). Similar cells have also been used to treat Peyronie disease (Castiglione et al, 2013). Various cell populations are making a transition into the clinic. Long-term studies will be needed to gauge the full impact of these therapies.

Testis

Leydig cells are the major source of testosterone production in males. Patients with testicular dysfunction require androgen replacement for somatic development. Conventional treatment for testicular dysfunction consists of periodic intramuscular injections of chemically modified testosterone or, more recently, skin patch applications. However, long-term nonpulsatile testosterone therapy is not optimal and can cause multiple problems, including erythropoiesis and bone density changes.

A system was designed wherein Leydig cells were microencapsulated for controlled testosterone replacement. Microencapsulated Leydig cells offer several advantages, such as serving as a semipermeable barrier between the transplanted cells and the host's immune system, as well as allowing for the long-term physiologic release of testosterone. Purified Leydig cells were isolated and encapsulated in an alginate-poly-L-lysine solution. The encapsulated Leydig cells

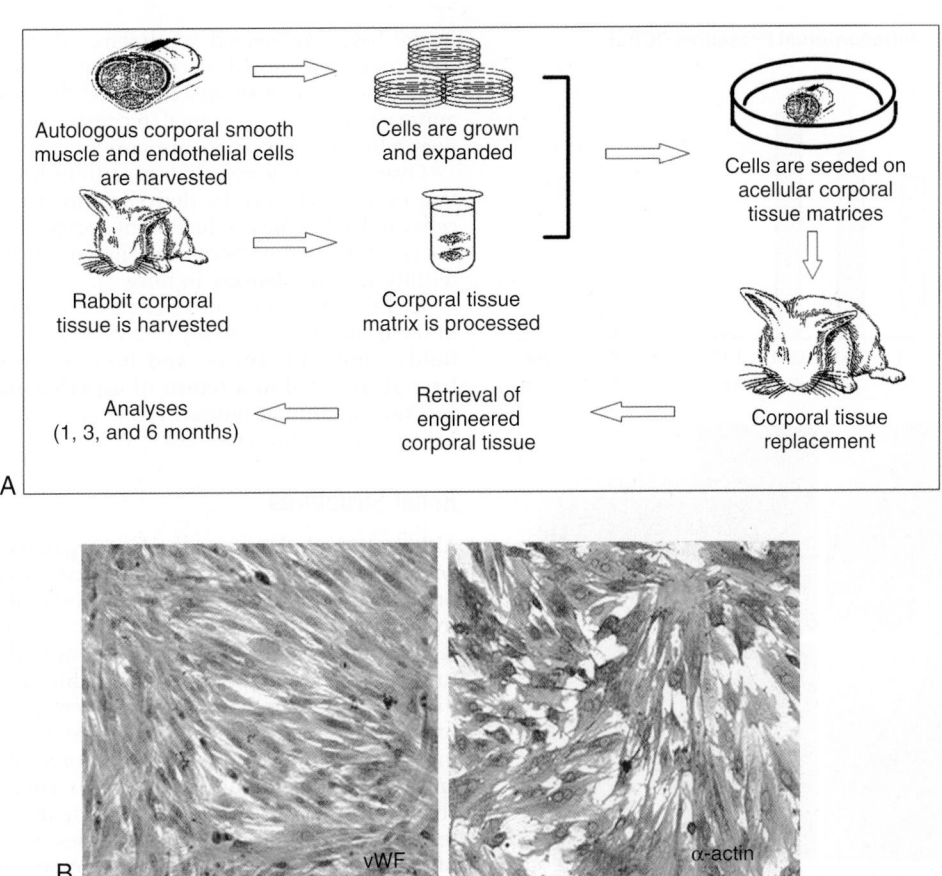

Figure 20-9. Isolation and culture of autologous corporeal cavernosal cells for tissue engineering. **A,** Overall study design. **B,** Culture expanded endothelial cells *(left)* show positive expression of cell-specific marker von Willebrand factor (vWF) protein, and smooth muscle cells show expression of smooth muscle–specific α-actin *(right)*.

were injected into castrated animals, and serum testosterone was measured serially; the animals were able to maintain testosterone levels in the long term (Machluf and Atala, 1998). These studies suggest that microencapsulated Leydig cells may be able to replace or supplement testosterone in situations where anorchia or testicular failure is present. A novel technique to isolate Leydig stem cells and to study Leydig cell development has also been described (Lo et al, 2004). The successful transplantation of functional Leydig stem cells into a hypogonadal recipient showed that the de novo synthesis of testosterone is possible.

Further studies showed that testicular prostheses created with chondrocytes in bioreactors could be loaded with testosterone. The prostheses were implanted in athymic mice with bilateral anorchia, and testosterone was released long term, maintaining the androgen level at a physiologic range (Raya-Rivera et al, 2008). One could envision combining the Leydig cell technology previously described with engineered prostheses for the long-term functional replacement of androgen levels.

The ability to have spermatogenesis for infertility purposes has been a major area of interest in the last several decades. The introduction of spermatogonial stem cell transplanation in mice opened new avenues to the field of male infertility treatment (Brinster and Zimmermann, 1994). Since the discovery of the feasibility of spermatogonial stem cell isolation and autotransplanation, it has been demonstrated in several species including nonhuman primates. The first successful isolation of human spermatogonial stem cells in 2002 showed that the cells were able to colonize and survive for 6 months in mice recipient testes (Nagano et al, 2002). The same group had been able to show the restoration of fertility in mice with the transplantation of male germline stem cells (Ogawa et al, 2000). Sertoli cells, the main component of the testicular germ cell niche,

were also able to restore fertility in mice (Kanatsu-Shinohara et al, 2005). More recently, succesful autologous and allogeneic spermatogonial stem cell transplantation was demonstrated in adult and prepubertal macaque testes that were previously rendered infertile with alkylating chemotherapy (Hermann et al, 2012). **In vitro propagation of human spermatogonial stem cells from both adult and pubertal testes has been established** (Sadri-Ardekani et al, 2009). In these systems, human spermatogonial stem cells are supported by a feeder layer from the same patient's testicular somatic cells. Human spermatogonial stem cells could be maintained in vitro for more than 15 weeks (Sadri-Ardekani et al, 2011). Optimization of this culture system based on FDA regulations and current good tissue practice (CGTP) requirements is imperative before use in a clinical application.

Female Genital and Reproductive Tissues

Congenital malformations of the uterus may have profound implications clinically. Patients with cloacal exstrophy and intersex disorders may not have sufficient uterine tissue present for future reproduction. The possibility of engineering functional uterine tissue using autologous cells was investigated (Wang et al, 2003). Autologous rabbit uterine smooth muscle and epithelial cells were harvested, grown, and expanded in culture. These cells were seeded onto preconfigured uterine-shaped biodegradable polymer scaffolds, which were then used for subtotal uterine tissue replacement in the corresponding autologous animals. On retrieval 6 months after implantation, histologic, immunocytochemical, and Western blot analyses confirmed the presence of uterine tissue components. Biomechanical analyses and organ bath studies showed that the functional characteristics of these tissues were similar to those of

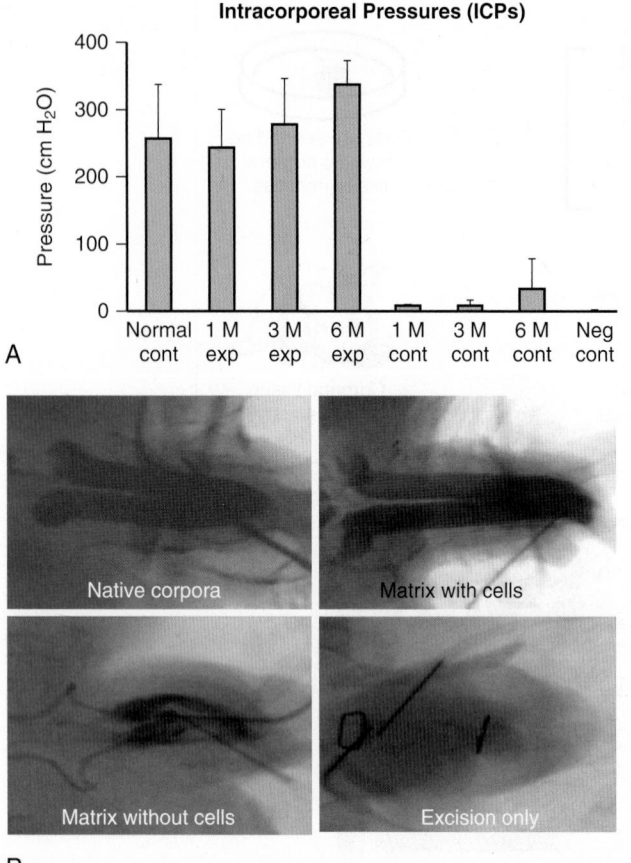

Intracorporeal Pressures (ICPs)

A

B

Figure 20-10. Cavernosometry and cavernosography. A, Caverno-sometry shows that all rabbits implanted with the bioengineered corpora after complete pendular penile corporeal excision had sufficient intracorporeal pressure (ICP) to attain erection (n = 12). The levels of ICP were comparable to native corpora (n = 12). **B,** Caver-nosography shows a homogeneous appearance of corpora in the bioengineered group (n = 12) similar to the native corpora (n = 16), numerous filling defects in the unseeded control group (n = 12), and major filling gaps in the negative control group (n = 3).

normal uterine tissue. Breeding studies using these engineered uteri are currently being performed.

Similarly, several pathologic conditions, including congenital malformations and malignancy, can adversely affect normal vaginal development or anatomy. Vaginal reconstruction has traditionally been challenging because of the paucity of available native tissue.

Many techniques and materials can be used successfully for vaginal reconstruction, The most common surgical reconstructive approach involves creating a canal by dissecting the potential neo-vaginal space and subsequently lining the pelvic canal with a graft. Multiple materials have been used to line the surgically created cavity, including mostly full- or split-thickness skin grafts, but also cellulose (Dornelas et al, 2012), decellularized matrices derived from skin or intestinal mucosa (Ding et al, 2013; Zhu et al, 2013), and vaginal epithelia (Panici et al, 2007).

The feasibility of engineering vaginal tissue with cells in vivo was also investigated (De Filippo et al, 2003). Vaginal epithelial and smooth muscle cells of female rabbits were harvested, expanded, and seeded onto biodegradable polymer scaffolds, and the cell-seeded constructs were then implanted into both athymic mice ex situ and rabbits as a full replacement of the organ. Functional studies in the tissue-engineered constructs showed similar properties to those of normal vaginal tissue. When these constructs were used for autologous total vaginal replacement in a rabbit model, patent functional vaginal structures were noted

in the tissue-engineered specimens, whereas the non–cell-seeded structures were noted to be stenotic (De Filippo et al, 2008) (Fig. 20-11). These studies indicated that a regenerative medicine approach to clinical vaginal reconstruction would be a realistic possibility. Clinical trials are currently being conducted.

Ovarian tissue is essential for fertility. Recent studies have shown that ovarian cells can be derived from stem cell populations. The cells can lead to the production of oocytes and embryos (Choi et al, 2011). Implanted oocytes have shown full functionality, including fertility and live delivery in mice.

Cell therapies have also been used to enhance the functionality of the ovary experimentally in animal models. **Adipose-, amniotic fluid–, umbilical cord–, and bone marrow–derived stem cells have all resulted in a return of experimentally damaged ovarian function in animal models** (Fu et al, 2008; Abd-Allah et al, 2013; Lai et al, 2013; Sun et al, 2013; Wang et al, 2013).

Renal Structures

Although the kidney was the first organ to undergo substitution with an artificial device and the first successfully transplanted organ (Guild et al, 1955), **current modalities of treatment are far from satisfactory.** Dialysis remains the most common treatment for renal failure. Renal tissue is arguably one of the most difficult tissues to replicate in the laboratory. The kidney is a complex organ, and the unique structural and cellular heterogeneity present within this organ creates many challenges. The system of nephrons and collecting ducts within the kidney is composed of multiple functionally and morphologically distinct segments. For this reason, appropriate conditions must be provided to ensure the long-term survival, differentiation, and growth of many types of cells. Efforts in the area of kidney tissue regeneration have focused on the development of reliable cell sources (Prockop, 1997; Kale et al, 2003; Lin et al, 2003; Ikarashi et al, 2005; Lin et al, 2005; Yokoo et al, 2005). Moreover, optimal growth conditions have been extensively investigated to provide adequate enrichment to achieve stable renal cell expansion systems (Milici et al, 1985; Carley et al, 1988; Humes et al, 1992; Schena, 1998).

Isolation of particular cell types that produce specific factors may be a good approach for selective cell therapies. For example, renal cells that produce erythropoietin have been isolated in culture, and these cells could eventually be used to treat anemia that results from end-stage renal failure (AbouShwareb et al, 2008; Gyabaah et al, 2012). These cells have also been used to improve renal function in a model of chronic kidney disease (Yamaleyeva et al, 2012). Defined primary cells from the kidney have been studied extensively and used to reconstitute human function (Guimaraes-Souza et al, 2012). More ambitious approaches involve working toward the goal of total renal function replacement. To create kidney tissue that would deliver full renal function, a culture containing all of the cell types comprising the functional nephron units should be used. Optimal culture conditions to nurture renal cells have been extensively studied, and cells grown under these conditions have been reported to maintain their cellular characteristics (Lanza et al, 2002). Cells obtained through the initial process of nuclear transfer have been retrieved and expanded from cloned tissue. Moreover, renal cells placed in a three-dimensional culture environment are able to reconstitute into renal structures. In vitro generated kidney constructs were implanted in the renal capsule region in rats, and they vascularized and formed glomeruli (Joraku et al, 2009).

Recent investigative efforts in the search for a reliable cell source have been expanded to stem and progenitor cells. Use of these cells for tissue regeneration is attractive because of their ability to differentiate and mature into specific cell types needed. This is particularly useful when primary renal cells are unavailable as a result of extensive tissue damage. Bone marrow–derived human mesenchymal stem cells have been shown to be a potential source because of their ability to differentiate into several cell lineages (Ikarashi et al, 2005). The creation of adequate experimental models of renal failure has been critical for the testing of various cell therapies (Wang et al, 2013). Bone marrow–derived cells have been shown to

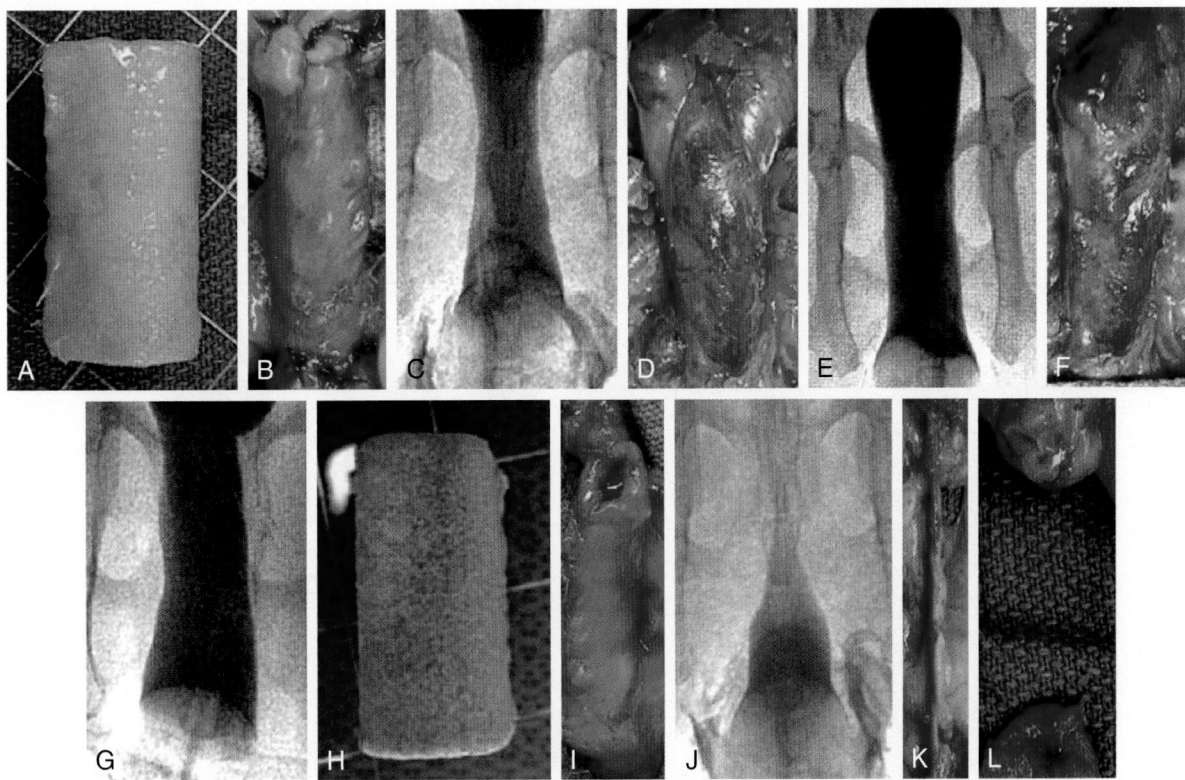

Figure 20-11. Appearance of tissue-engineered neovaginas. A, Tubular polymer scaffold after cell seeding and 1 week in vitro culture, before implantation in vivo. B, D, and F indicate gross appearance and C, E, and G show vaginography of cell-seeded constructs 1, 3, and 6 months postimplantation, respectively. H, Unseeded control scaffold before implantation. I, K, L, Gross appearance of unseeded construct at 1, 3, and 6 months postimplantation. J, Vaginography of unseeded graft at 1 month.

participate in kidney development when they are placed in a rat embryonic niche that allows for continued exposure to a repertoire of nephrogenic signals (Yokoo et al, 2005). The major cell source of kidney regeneration was found to originate from intrarenal cells in an ischemic renal injury model (Lin et al, 2005). Systemic administration of bone marrow–derived mesenchymal stem cells in mice has led to prevention of kidney damage in various animal models (Humphreys and Bonventre, 2008; Lin, 2008; Morigi et al, 2010). Autologous bone marrow cells have been used clinically for the treatment of allograft rejection after transplantation in a pilot study (Reinders et al, 2013). Other trials are also currently underway with bone marrow–derived stem cells and with primary renal cells, and it is still early to define the outcomes.

Other stem cell types, such as hESCs (Lin, 2006; Bruce et al, 2007), induced pluripotent stem cells (Osafune, 2010; Song et al, 2012), and human amniotic fluid and placental stem cells (Perin et al, 2007; Hauser et al, 2010) can also lead to renal differentiation and reversal of renal injury in animal models. Developmental approaches to kidney regeneration have also been studied, but these are mostly research-driven approaches without a direct clinical pathway.

Additional information can be found on the Expert Consult website.

Regenerative Medicine Approaches to Kidney Regeneration

The ability to grow and expand renal cells is one of the essential requirements in engineering tissues. The feasibility of achieving renal cell growth, expansion, and in vivo reconstitution using regenerative medicine techniques has been investigated (Atala et al, 1991). Donor rabbit kidney cells including distal tubules, glomeruli, and proximal tubules were plated separately in vitro and after expansion were seeded onto biodegradable PGA scaffolds.

Histologic examination demonstrated progressive formation and organization of the nephron segments within the polymer fibers with time. These results demonstrated that renal-specific cells can be successfully harvested and cultured and can subsequently attach to artificial biodegradable polymers. However, it was unclear whether the tubular structures reconstituted de novo from dispersed renal elements or if they merely represented fragments of donor tubules that survived the original dissociation and culture processes intact. Further investigation was conducted to examine the process (Fung et al, 1996). Mouse renal cells were harvested and expanded in culture. Subsequently, single isolated cells were seeded on biodegradable polymers and implanted into immune-competent syngeneic hosts. Renal epithelial cells were observed to reconstitute into tubular structures in vivo. Sequential analyses of the retrieved implants over time demonstrated that renal epithelial cells first organized into a cordlike structure with a solid center. Subsequent canalization into a hollow tube could be seen by 2 weeks. Histologic examination with nephron segment-specific lactins showed successful reconstitution of proximal tubules, distal tubules, loop of Henle, collecting tubules, and collecting ducts. These results showed that single suspended cells are capable of reconstituting into tubular structures, with homogeneous cell types within each tubule.

In a subsequent study mouse renal cells were harvested, expanded in culture, and seeded onto a tubular device constructed from polycarbonate (Yoo et al, 1996). The tubular device was connected at one end to a Silastic catheter that terminated into a reservoir. The device was implanted subcutaneously in athymic mice. Histologic examination of the implanted device demonstrated extensive vascularization as well as formation of glomeruli and highly organized tubulelike structures that were consistent with proximal and distal tubular cells and the cells of the thin ascending loop of Henle. The fluid collected from the reservoir suggested that the tubules are

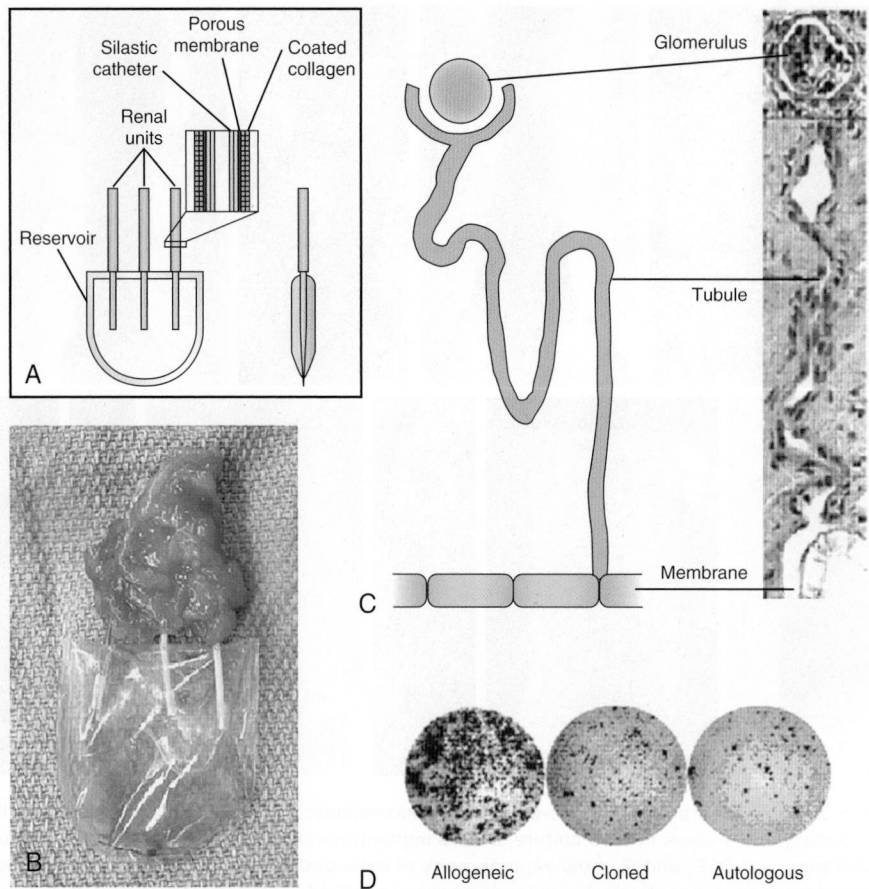

Figure 20-12. Production of kidney tissue by therapeutic cloning and regenerative medicine. A, Illustration of the tissue-engineered renal unit. **B,** Renal unit seeded with cloned cells, 3 months after implantation, showing the accumulation of urinelike fluid. **C,** There was a clear unidirectional continuity between the mature glomeruli, their tubules, and the polycarbonate membrane. **D,** ELISpot analyses of the frequencies of T cells that secrete interferon-γ after primary and secondary stimulation with allogeneic renal cells, cloned renal cells, or nuclear donor fibroblasts.

capable of unidirectional secretion and concentration of uric acid. The creatinine assay performed on the collected fluid showed an 8.2-fold increase in concentration as compared with serum. These results demonstrated that single cells from multicellular structures can become organized into functional renal units that are able to excrete high levels of solutes through a urinelike fluid (Yoo et al, 1996).

To determine whether renal tissue could be formed using an alternative cell source, nuclear transplantation (therapeutic cloning) was performed to generate histocompatible tissues, and the feasibility of engineering syngeneic renal tissues in vivo using these cloned cells was investigated (Lanza et al, 2002). Nuclear material from bovine dermal fibroblasts was transferred into unfertilized enucleated donor bovine eggs. Renal cells from the cloned embryos were harvested, expanded in vitro, and seeded onto three-dimensional renal devices. The devices were implanted into the back of the same steer from which the cells were cloned, and were retrieved 12 weeks later. This process produced functioning renal units (Fig. 20-12). Urine production and viability were demonstrated after transplantation back into the nuclear donor animal. Chemical analysis suggested unidirectional secretion and concentration of urea nitrogen and creatinine. Microscopic analysis revealed formation of organized glomeruli and tubular structures. Immunohistochemical and reverse-transcriptase polymerase chain reaction (RT-PCR) analysis confirmed the expression of renal messenger (m)RNA and proteins. These studies demonstrated that cells derived from nuclear transfer can be successfully harvested, expanded in culture, and transplanted

in vivo with the use of biodegradable scaffolds on which the single suspended cells can organize into tissue structures that are genetically identical to those of the host. These studies were the first demonstration of the use of therapeutic cloning for regeneration of tissues in vivo.

A naturally derived tissue matrix with existing three-dimensional kidney architecture would be preferable to the artificial matrix used in the aforementioned experiments because it would allow for transplantation of a larger number of cells, resulting in greater renal tissue volumes. Thus, an acellular collagen-based kidney matrix, which is similar to the native renal architecture, was developed. A subsequent study investigated whether these collagen-based matrices could accommodate large volumes of renal cells and form kidney structures in vivo (Amiel et al, 2000). Renal cells seeded on the matrix adhered to the inner surface and proliferated to confluency by 7 days after seeding. Renal tubular and glomerulus-like structures were observed 8 weeks after implantation. More recent data has confirmed that the creation of larger kidney structures using decellularized kidney matrices and repopulated with cells is possible (Orlando et al, 2012; Sullivan et al, 2012; Arenas-Herrera et al, 2013).

Summary

Regenerative medicine efforts continue to expand in the field of urology and are currently being undertaken for every type of tissue and organ within the urinary system. Most of the efforts expended in the genitourinary field have occurred within the last several decades. Regenerative medicine strategies involve the use of biomaterials alone, as has been accomplished clinically in patients with urethral disease; biomaterials with cells, as is currently being tested clinically with bladder, urethral, and vaginal tissues; and cell therapies alone, as those applied clinically for erectile dysfunction, Peyronie disease, bladder dysfunction, urinary incontinence, and renal disease. The number of patients and the indications now amenable to regenerative medicine therapies keep increasing. Regenerative medicine is a multidisciplinary field that requires expertise in a wide variety of scientific disciplines, including cell and molecular biology, physiology, pharmacology, chemical engineering, biomaterials, nanotechnology, and clinical sciences. Although modest clinical success has been achieved to date in specific areas, technologies need to be further defined in terms of best patients to treat, because the field continues to be in its infancy. Long-term studies are still essential to ensure safety and efficacy before these technologies have widespread clinical application.

KEY POINTS

- New advances in the ability to expand cells in vitro and to use smart biomaterials and new techniques for vascularization are allowing more complex organs to be engineered.
- Tissue injury can be repaired with minimal fibrosis by the natural wound-healing response for small defects, by the use of nonseeded matrices for defects up to 1 cm from any edge, and by the use of cell-seeded matrices for defects larger than 1 cm.
- Stem cells may provide large repositories of different cell types for tissue and organ repair. Embryonic and induced pluripotent stem cells differentiate easily but may form tumors and may necessitate immunosuppression. Fetal stem cells replicate readily and do not form tumors but may be more limited than embryonic stem cells in their differentiation potential. Adult stem cells may not form tumors or necessitate immunosuppression, but they may not replicate readily.
- Both tissue engineering approaches and injectable cell therapy approaches are being used clinically. The types of cells used, the regenerative medicine strategies applied, the number of patients treated, and the indications for treatment continue to expand.

REFERENCES

The complete reference list is available online at www.expertconsult.com.

SUGGESTED READINGS

Bent AE, Tutrone RT, McLennan MT, et al. Treatment of intrinsic sphincter deficiency using autologous ear chondrocytes as a bulking agent. Neurourol Urodyn 2001;20:157–65.

Carr LK, Steele D, Steele S, et al. 1-year follow-up of autologous muscle-derived stem cell injection pilot study to treat stress urinary incontinence. Int Urogynecol J Pelvic Floor Dysfunct 2008;19:881–3.

Diamond DA, Caldamone AA. Endoscopic correction of vesicoureteral reflux in children using autologous chondrocytes: preliminary results. J Urol 1999;162:1185.

Kassaby EA, Yoo J, Retik A, et al. A novel inert collagen matrix for urethral stricture repair. J Urol 2000;308S:70.

Raya-Rivera A, Esquiliano DR, Yoo JJ, et al. Tissue-engineered autologous urethras for patients who need reconstruction: an observational study. Lancet 2011;377:1175–82.

21 Surgical, Radiographic, and Endoscopic Anatomy of the Male Reproductive System

Parviz K. Kavoussi, MD, FACS

Testis	Prostate
Epididymis	Urethra
Vas Deferens	Penis
Seminal Vesicles and Ejaculatory Ducts	Scrotum

A fundamental comprehension of male genital anatomy is necessary for understanding normal reproduction as well as pathology and treatment options. This chapter provides a general anatomic framework of the surgical, radiographic, and endoscopic anatomy of the normal male reproductive system. As this chapter is dedicated solely to the anatomy of the male reproductive system, please refer to Chapter 68 for further description of pelvic anatomy including bones, soft tissue, circulation, and innervation of the pelvis not directly related to reproduction.

TESTIS

Gross Structure

The testicles are paired organs within the scrotum that include both reproductive and endocrine functions. It is common for the right testis to be lower hanging compared to the left in approximately 85% of men. **The dimensions of the normal testis include a length of 4 to 5 cm, a width of 3 cm, and a depth of 2.5 cm; and the testis normally has a volume of 15 to 25 mL.** The organ is ovoid in shape and white in color (Prader, 1966; Tishler, 1971). There is a small pedunculated or sessile body at the upper pole of the testis, which is known as the appendix testis. A tough capsule envelops the testis, composed from external to internal of the visceral tunica vaginalis, the tunica albuginea, and the tunica vasculosa, before reaching the parenchyma of the testis. The tunica albuginea is composed of smooth muscle cells that pass through collagenous tissue (Langford and Heller, 1973). It is believed that these smooth muscle cells provide the testicular capsule with some ability to contract and may impact arterial flow into the testis. They may also promote the flow of seminiferous tubule fluid on its way out of the testis (Schweitzer, 1929; Rikmaru and Shirai, 1972; Davis and Horowitz, 1978). The attachment to the epididymis is on the posterolateral aspect of the testis (Figs. 21-1 and 21-2).

Microanatomic Architecture

The tunica albuginea invaginates into the testis to form the mediastinum testis, where vessels and ducts traverse the testicular capsule. The mediastinum testis sends septa that attach to the inner surface of the tunica albuginea to form 200 to 300 cone-shaped lobules, each of which contains one or more convoluted seminiferous tubules. Each lobule contains a centrifugal artery. Seminiferous tubules are coiled and long, with both ends typically ending in the rete testis. The seminiferous tubules contain germ cells and supporting cells including Sertoli cells, fibrocytes, and myoid cells of the basement membrane. Each seminiferous tubule is U-shaped, but if a seminiferous tubule were stretched out from its convoluted form, each would measure nearly 1 m in length. **Each seminiferous tubule in the normal testis contains developing germ cells. The testosterone-producing Leydig cells are interdispersed in the loose tissue around the seminiferous tubules.** The interstitial tissue includes Leydig cells, mast cells, macrophages, nerves, blood vessels, and lymphatic vessels. This interstitial tissue makes up a total of 20% to 30% of the testicular volume (Setchell and Brooks, 1988). Sertoli cells line the seminiferous tubules and rest on the tubular basement membrane. The cellular characteristics of Sertoli cells include a low mitotic index, prominent nucleoli, and nuclei with irregular shapes. There are strong tight junctions between the Sertoli cells, which compartmentalize the seminiferous tubular space into adluminal and basal spaces. The seminiferous tubules straighten out and become tubuli recti toward the apex of each lobule, where they enter the mediastinum testis and anastomose with a network of tubules lined by flattened epithelia. This tubular network is the rete testis and forms 12 to 20 efferent ductules that anastomose into the caput of the epididymis. At this point, the efferent ductules convolute, enlarge, and form conical lobules. Each lobule produces a duct that drains into a single epididymal duct. The epididymal duct would be approximately 6 m in length if it were stretched out. It winds within the epididymis to form the body and the tail of the epididymis, all of which are surrounded by a fibrous sheath. The thickening and straightening of the duct forms the vas deferens as it reaches the tail of the epididymis (Figs. 21-3 and 21-4).

Arterial Supply

There are three arterial supplies to the testis: the testicular (internal spermatic) artery, the artery of the vas deferens (deferential artery), and the cremasteric (external spermatic) artery (Harrison and Barclay, 1948). **The testicular artery is the main blood supply to the testis and its diameter is greater than the deferential and**

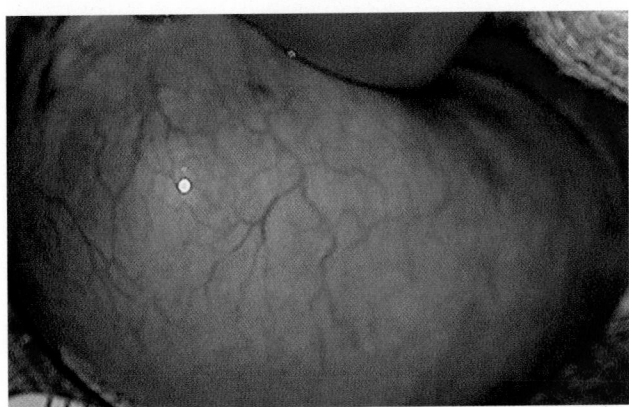

Figure 21-1. **The appearance of the testis with its shiny tunica albuginea layer.**

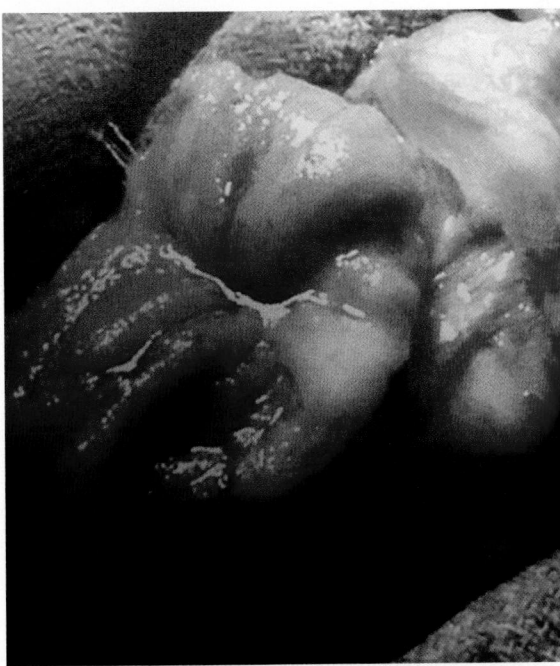

Figure 21-2. **The appearance of the testicular parenchyma when bivalved. The white nodule at the right inferior margin represents a sarcoid nodule.**

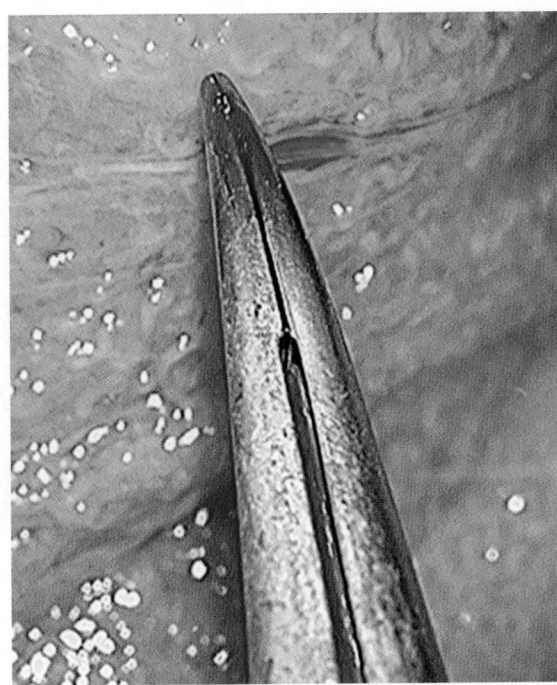

Figure 21-3. **Appearance of the seminiferous tubules under magnification.**

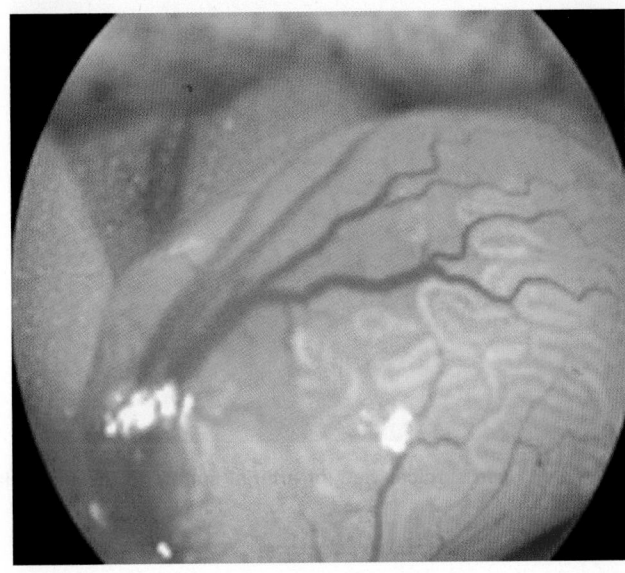

Figure 21-4. **Microbeads injected retrograde through the rete testis into the seminiferous tubules demonstrating the tubular structure. This is a mouse testis that has very similar architecture to the human testis. (Courtesy Jeffrey Lysiak, PhD.)**

cremasteric arteries combined (Raman and Goldstein, 2004). The testicular artery arises from the abdominal aorta and descends in the intermediate stratum of the retroperitoneum to enter the internal inguinal ring. From its aortic origin, it crosses the psoas muscle and the ureter to reach the inguinal ring to enter the spermatic cord. As the testicular artery descends toward the testis, it branches into an internal artery and an inferior testicular artery and into a capital artery to the caput epididymis. There may be variation at the level of this branching, which has been found to occur within the inguinal canal in 31% to 88% of cases (Beck et al, 1992; Jarow et al, 1992). In 56% of cases, a single artery enters the testis. In 31% of cases, there are two branches, and in 13% there are three or more branches of this artery (Kormano and Suoranta, 1971). Arterial anastomosis occurs at the head of the epididymis, allowing for a rich blood supply between the testicular and capital arteries. At the tail of the epididymis, arterial anastomoses are formed between the testicular, epididymal, cremasteric, and vasal arteries. The testicular arteries pass into the mediastinum testis and supply the tunica vasculosa in the anterior portion of the upper pole of the testis and the anterior, medial, and lateral portions of the lower pole of the testis. Therefore, care must be taken not to devascularize the testis by passing a traction suture through the lower pole, as well as by performing testis biopsies in the medial or lateral surfaces of the upper pole to minimize the risk of vascular injury. The middle of the testis has fewer vessels than the upper or lower poles. The deferential artery derives from the internal iliac artery or from the superior vesical artery. The cremasteric artery derives from the inferior epigastric artery and primarily supplies the tunica vaginalis, but it has branches going to the testis. Centrifugal arteries, which are the individual arteries supplying the seminiferous tubules, pass within the septa containing the seminiferous tubules and branch into arterioles that ultimately become intertubular and peritubular capillaries (Muller, 1957). Although in the case of testicular artery

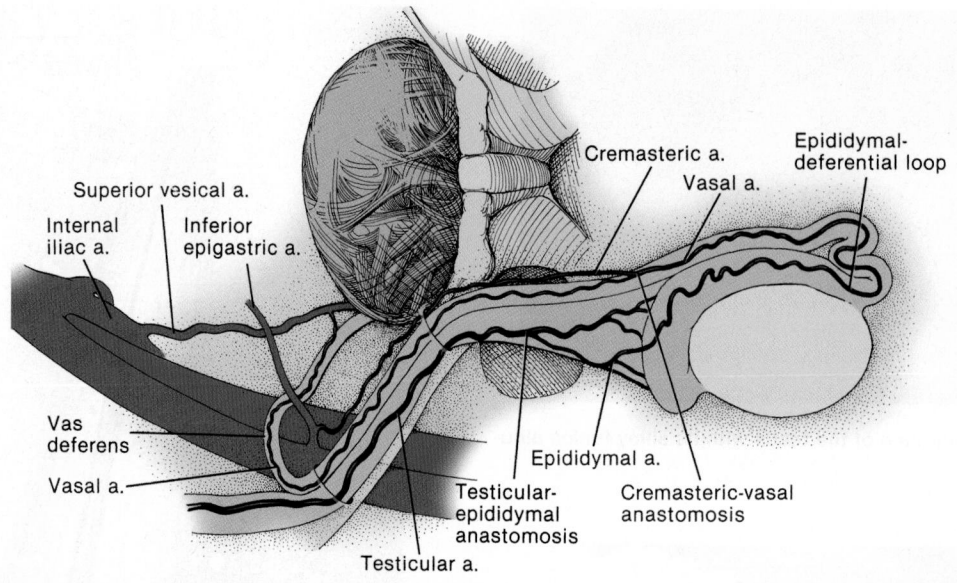

Figure 21-5. Collateral arterial circulation to the testis. (From Hinman F Jr. Atlas of urosurgical anatomy. Philadelphia: Saunders; 1993. p. 497.)

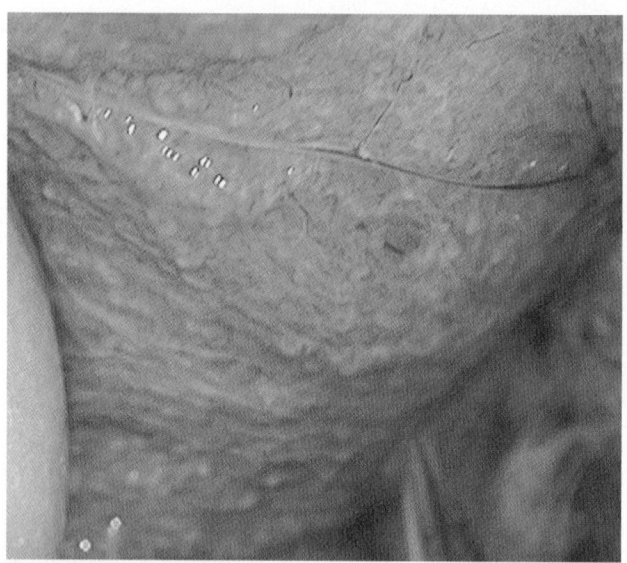

Figure 21-6. Microsurgical view of arterial supply to the testicular parenchyma.

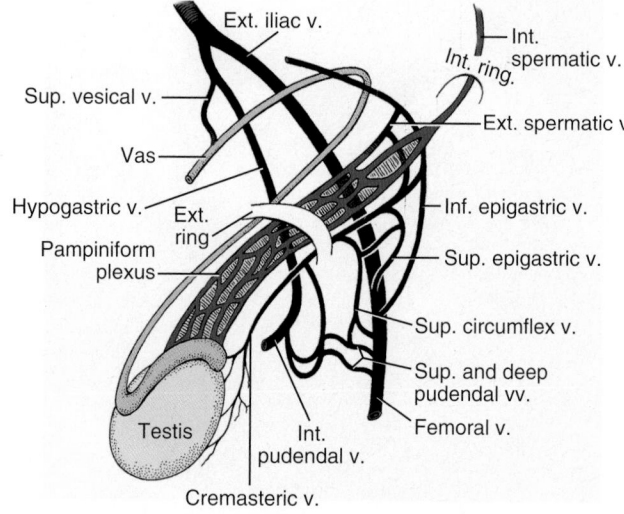

Figure 21-7. Venous drainage of the testis and epididymis. Note connections between the pampiniform plexus and the saphenous, internal iliac, and external iliac veins.

ligation, the deferential and cremasteric arteries can potentially provide adequate blood supply to the testis, atrophy and/or azoospermia has resulted from testicular artery ligation in adults and children. Men who have undergone vasectomy deserve special attention in preserving the testicular artery in future surgeries such as varicocelectomy because of the risk of having had the deferential artery compromised at the time of vasectomy (Lee et al, 2007) (Figs. 21-5 and 21-6).

Venous Drainage

Unlike most other venous patterns in the human body, veins within the testis do not travel with their corresponding arteries. Small parenchymal veins either drain into a group of veins near the mediastinum testis, or they drain into veins on the surface of the testis (Setchell and Brooks, 1988). These two groups of veins anastomose with each other and the deferential veins to form the pampiniform plexus. The pampiniform plexus is a network of testicular veins that anastomose as they ascend surrounding the testicular artery. This

allows for a countercurrent heat exchange that cools the blood flow within the testicular artery. Ultimately, these veins join one another to form two or three veins at the level of the inguinal canal, and then they form one vein that ascends to drain into the inferior vena cava on the right and into the renal vein on the left side. There may be variations where the testicular veins can anastomose with the external pudendal, cremasteric, and vasal veins; this can allow varicocele ablations to result in recurrence (Figs. 21-7 and 21-8).

Lymphatic Supply

Lymphatic channels from the testis drain into the para-aortic and interaortocaval lymph nodes. These lymphatic channels ascend within the spermatic cord after leaving the testis (Hundeiker, 1969).

Nerve Supply

Visceral innervation to the testis and epididymis arise in the renal and aortic plexuses and course alongside the gonadal vessels. This is autonomic innervation, as the testis does not have

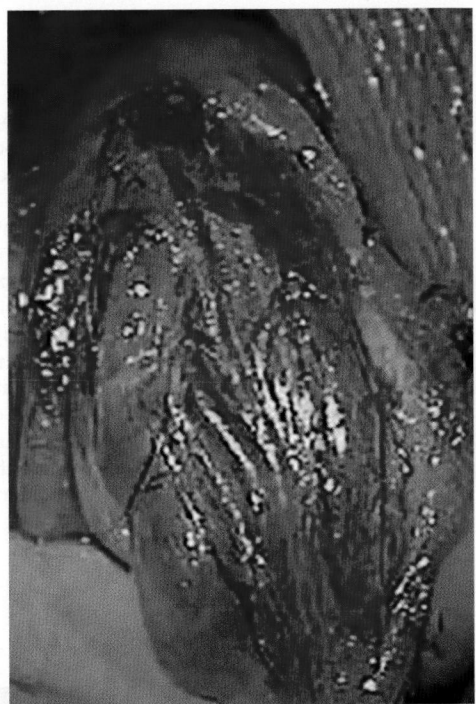

Figure 21-8. Microsurgical view of the veins of the pampiniform plexus during varicocele ligation through a subinguinal approach.

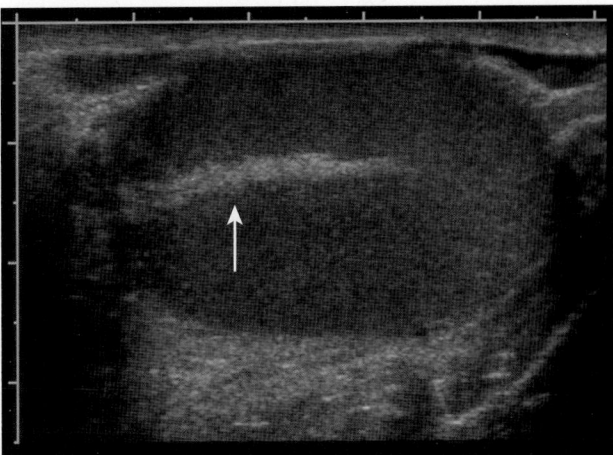

Figure 21-9. Testis ultrasound image demonstrating rete testis (arrow).

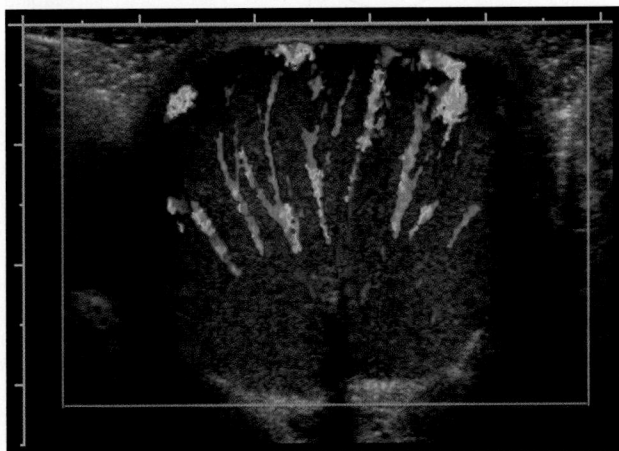

Figure 21-10. Doppler ultrasound image of testis demonstrating spokelike radiation of testicular vessels originating from the mediastinum testis.

any known somatic innervation (Mitchell, 1935). The pelvic plexus, in association with the vas deferens, offers additional gonadal afferent and efferent nerves (Rauchenwald et al, 1995). Three distinct anatomic distributions of nerves have been isolated within the spermatic cord, and are thought to be the primary contributors in men with chronic orchialgia. These include a perivasal complex, posterior periarterial/lipomatous complex, and intracremasteric complex (Parekattil et al, 2013). Some afferent and efferent nerves cross over to the contralateral pelvic plexus (Taguchi et al, 1999). This may account for pathology in one testis impacting the function of the contralateral testis, which has been reported with varicoceles and testicular tumors. **The genital branch of the genitofemoral nerve primarily supplies sensation to the parietal and visceral tunica vaginalis and the overlying scrotum.** These nerves travel along the testicular artery to reach the testis. These nerves ramify within the tunica albuginea, but do not enter the seminiferous tubules. Nerves are absent from the seminiferous epithelium.

Blood-Testis Barrier

The fluid passing from the seminiferous tubules and exiting from the testis has been found to have a substantially different fluid composition than that of blood plasma or lymphatics. This suggests that compounds do not freely diffuse to and from the tubules, indicating that a barrier exists, which is known as the blood-testis barrier (Setchell and Waites, 1975). There are extremely strong, tight junctions between Sertoli cells, which provide an intracellular barrier that allows for spermatogenesis in an immune privileged site. This is the barrier known as the blood-testis barrier (Ewing et al, 1980). This accounts for the anatomic component of the blood-testis barrier. The functional component will be further discussed in Chapter 22.

Ultrasonography

Ultrasonography is the primary imaging modality used to interrogate the scrotum and its contents. Scrotal ultrasound uses high-frequency transducers (7.5 to 10 MHz), grey scale real-time techniques, as well as color flow and power Doppler. The patient is

placed in the supine position and a coupling gel is used with the transducer probe on the scrotal skin. The normal scrotal wall is 3 to 4 mm thick and is hypoechoic. An anechoic area between the echogenic scrotal wall and testicle is commonly visualized, which represents a small amount of physiologic fluid between the visceral and parietal layers of the tunica vaginalis. The mediastinum testis is visualized posteriorly as an echogenic band parallel to the epididymis. It may have variable lengths and thicknesses dependent on each patient's physiology (Dogra et al, 2003). **The echo pattern of the normal testis is fine, uniform, with a medium-level echo pattern.** Sonographically, the normal testis measures approximately 5 cm × 3 cm × 2 cm (Dogra et al, 2001). Color Doppler can identify testicular vessels in the majority of patients (Spirnak and Resnick, 2002). Waveforms from intratesticular arteries and testicular capsular arteries demonstrate consistently low-impedance patterns with high levels of diastolic flow. This represents the lower vascular resistance of the testis. Supratesticular arteries are also sonographically identifiable and show low-impedance waveforms from the testicular, deferential, and cremasteric arteries (Middleton et al, 1989) (Figs. 21-9 and 21-10).

EPIDIDYMIS

Gross Structure

The epididymis is a duct or tubule that is attached to the postero-lateral aspect of the testis and is nearest to the testis at its upper

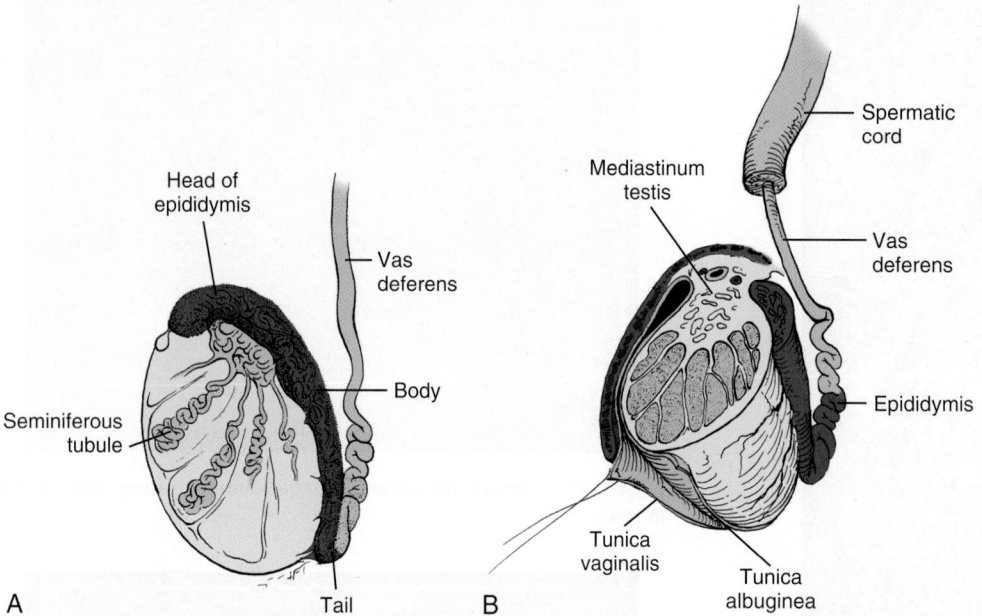

Figure 21-11. **Testis and epididymis. A,** One to three seminiferous tubules fill each compartment and drain into the rete testis in the mediastinum. Twelve to 20 efferent ductules become convoluted in the head of the epididymis and drain into a single coiled duct of the epididymis. The vas is convoluted in its first portion. **B,** Cross section of the testis, showing the mediastinum and septations continuous with the tunica albuginea. The parietal and visceral tunica vaginalis are confluent where the vessels and nerves enter the posterior aspect of the testis.

KEY POINTS: TESTIS

- The seminiferous tubules contain developing germ cells.
- The Leydig cells produce testosterone.
- There are three arterial supplies to the testis including the testicular artery, deferential artery, and cremasteric artery.
- Lymphatic channels from the testis drain into the para-aortic and interaortocaval lymph nodes.
- The nerves contributing to chronic orchialgia include a perivasal complex, posterior periarterial/lipomatous complex, and intracremasteric complex.
- Tight junctions between Sertoli cells comprise the anatomic component of the blood-testis barrier.
- Ultrasonography is the primary imaging modality for intrascrotal content.

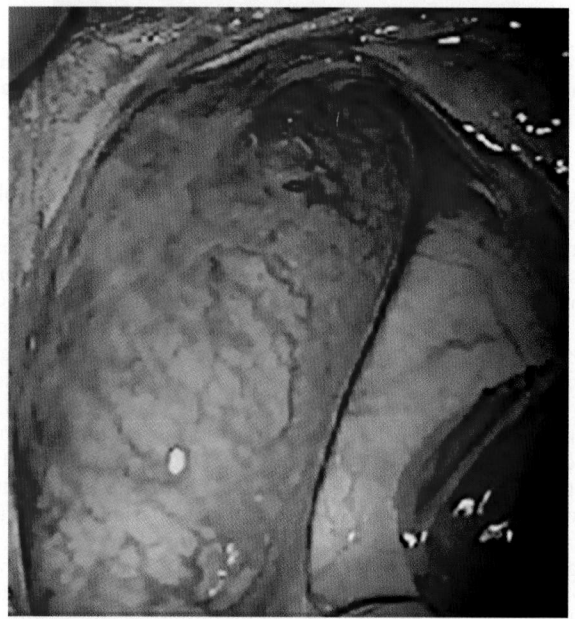

Figure 21-12. **Gross microsurgical appearance of the epididymal caput and corpus.**

pole. Its lower pole is connected to the testis with fibrous tissue. The epididymis is comma shaped. The epididymis is tightly coiled and encapsulated within the tunica vaginalis sheath and would measure 3 to 4 m in length if stretched out (Von Lanz and Neuhaeuser, 1964; Turner et al, 1978). Septa form by extensions of the tunica vaginalis sheath into interductal spaces that divide the duct into histologically characteristic areas (Kormano and Reijonen, 1976). The three areas are characterized as the caput (head), the corpus (body), and the cauda (tail) of the epididymis. Eight to 12 ductuli efferentes from the testis comprise the caput epididymis. The caput epididymis is connected to the testis by multiple efferent ducts. The tightly coiled duct, which makes up the epididymis, is continuous with the vas deferens at the most distal portion of the cauda epididymis. Adjacent to the testis, this duct is irregularly shaped and comparatively large. The duct becomes more narrow and concentric near the junction with the ductus epididymis. The duct diameter remains unchanged throughout the corpus epididymis. The diameter of the duct enlarges and becomes irregular in shape in the cauda epididymis. The duct then progresses distally to form the vas deferens. A cystic body on the upper pole of the caput epididymis, which may be pedunculated or sessile, is known as the appendix of the epididymis (Figs. 21-11, 21-12, and 21-13).

Microanatomic Architecture

There are two primary types of cells throughout the epididymis: principal cells and basal cells (Holstein, 1969; Vendrely, 1981).

From caput to cauda, the height of the epithelium decreases, whereas the diameter of the ductus and lumen increases. There are stereocilia that shorten progressively from the proximal to the distal epididymis. In the proximal epididymis, these stereocilia measure 120 μm in height and decrease to 50 μm in the distal epididymis. The principal cells contain elongated nuclei that are commonly clefted, and they contain one or two nucleoli. As the principal cells have absorptive and secretive functions, the apex of each of these cells contain multiple coated pits, membranous vesicles, multivesicular bodies, micropinocytic vesicles, and an extensive Golgi apparatus (Vendrely and Dadoune, 1988). There is a much larger number of principal cells in the epididymal epithelium than the number of basal cells that exist there. The basal cells are interdispersed between the principal cells. The basal cells are tear-shaped. They are positioned on the basal lamina and are 25 μm in length as they reach up toward the lumen. As opposed to the morphology of the principal cells, which varies throughout the epididymis, the basal cells' shape remains relatively consistent throughout the entirety of the

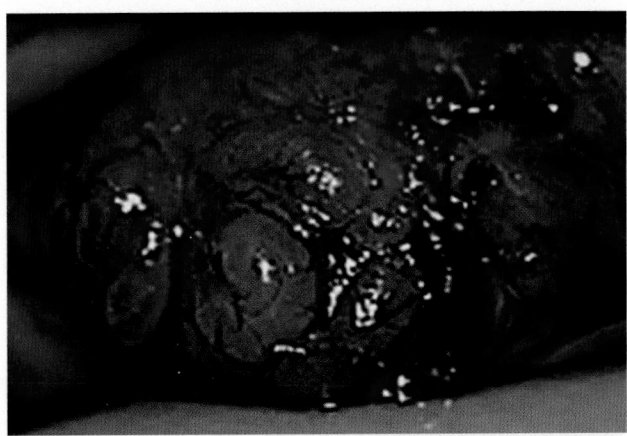

Figure 21-13. Microsurgical appearance of the epididymal duct after being stained with methylene blue.

epididymis. The basal cells are believed to be derived from macrophages and to be precursors of principal cells. There is a fair amount of variability in the nature of the epithelium of the epididymis, which is dependent on the region. There is a clear transition from a low to a high cuboidal epithelium where the rete testis and ductuli efferentes meet. The ductuli efferentes contain ciliated and nonciliated cells and the epithelium appears uneven (Holstein, 1969). The epithelium of the proximal ductuli efferentes primarily consists of nonciliated cells with extending apices thought to be for secretory function. The ciliated cells conduct sperm cells from the efferent duct to the epididymis, and they are widely dispersed throughout the epithelium (Vendrely, 1981). Junctional complexes join ciliated and nonciliated cells together at their apices, suggesting a blood-epididymis barrier (Suzuki and Nagano, 1978; Turner, 1979; Hoffer and Hinton, 1984). In the ductuli efferentes, the proximal corpus epididymis, and the distal caput epididymis there are contractile cells around the tubule in a loose, two-to-four cell–deep layer (Baumgarten et al, 1971). Nexuslike junctions connect these contractile cells to one another and each cell contains myofilaments. These cells are larger and appear like thin smooth muscle cells in the distal corpus epididymis, where they have fewer intracellular junctions. Thick smooth muscle cells are found in the cauda epididymis. The smooth muscle cells are organized in three layers. The cells have a longitudinal orientation in the two outer layers and a circular orientation in the central layer. The thickness of the distal contractile layer progressively increases as it forms the vas deferens.

Arterial Supply

A branch of the testicular artery supplies the caput and corpus epididymis. This arterial branch then further divides to supply the superior and inferior epididymal branches (Macmillan, 1954). **The deferential artery also provides vascular supply to the epididymis.** Branches from the deferential artery supply the cauda epididymis. As with the testis, the deferential and cremasteric arteries also supply the epididymis and can compensate for a ligated testicular artery. The connective tissue sheaths forming septa in the epididymis are the entry points for arterial supply within the epididymis. The coiled vessels ultimately straighten to form the microvascular bed within the epididymis (Kormano and Reijonen, 1976). The density of the microvasculature decreases progressively, with the caput containing the highest density of microvasculature and the more distal segments containing lower density (Clavert et al, 1981).

Venous Drainage

The corpus and cauda epididymis have their venous drainage through the vena marginalis of Haberer, draining into the

pampiniform plexus via the vena marginalis testis, or through deferential or cremasteric veins (Macmillan, 1954).

Lymphatic Supply

Similar to that of the testis, the caput and corpus epididymis have their lymphatic drainage through channels that travel with the internal spermatic vein, draining to the preaortic nodes. Lymphatic channels from the cauda epididymis join those leaving the vas deferens to drain ultimately into the external iliac nodes.

Nerve Supply

The superior portion of the hypogastric plexus and the pelvic plexus yield the intermediate and inferior spermatic nerves, respectively, which innervate the epididymis (Mitchell, 1935). Fibers from the sympathetic nervous system sparsely innervate the proximal portion of the epididymis as well as the ductuli efferentes (Baumgarten and Holstein, 1967; Baumgarten et al, 1971). These fibers form a peritubular plexus that is adjacent to the vasculature. The corpus epididymis includes sparse numbers of nerve fibers, and the density of nerve fibers increases progressively traveling toward the cauda epididymis. The density of fibers begins to increase at the midcorpus of the epididymis and the progressive increase in fibers is associated with the progressive proliferation of smooth muscle cells (Baumgarten et al, 1971).

Ultrasonography

The epididymis can be visualized ultrasonographically in its posterolateral position to the testis. **The epididymis appears either hyperechoic or isoechoic in comparison to the testis** (Spirnak and Resnick, 2002). Compared to the testis, the caput epididymis is typically isoechoic, the corpus epididymis is hypoechoic, and the vas deferens is anechoic (Puttemans et al, 2006). The epididymis is typically homogeneous, with well-defined echoes surrounding the epididymis that represent the fascial lining (Black and Patel, 1996). By sonographic measurement, the normal caput epididymis diameter measures between 10 mm and 12 mm and the normal corpus epididymis measures between 2 mm and 5 mm (Pezzella et al, 2013). In 98% of men, the caput epididymis is above the upper pole of the testis, with the corpus epididymis typically lateral to the testis. The corpus epididymis is posterior to the body of the testis in 6% of men. The epididymis is inverted with the caput epididymis inferior to the lower pole of the testis in 2.4% of men (Puttemans et al, 2006). The appendix epididymis can be identified as an isoechoic structure attached to the caput epididymis (Black and Patel, 1996). Vascular flow is detectable with pulsed Doppler and color Doppler in all regions of the epididymis in nonpathologic states. The mean resistive index throughout the normal epididymis is approximately 0.55 (Keener et al, 1997) (Fig. 21-14).

> ### KEY POINTS: EPIDIDYMIS
>
> - The two primary cell types throughout the epididymis are principal cells and basal cells.
> - The arterial supply to the caput and corpus epididymis is from a branch of the testicular artery and the cauda is supplied from deferential arterial branches.

VAS DEFERENS
Gross Structure

The vas deferens, also known as the ductus deferens, extends from the distal end of the cauda epididymis. It is tubular and its embryologic origin is the mesonephric (wolffian) duct. The vas deferens is tortuous for 2 to 3 cm as it leaves the epididymis (the convoluted vas deferens). From the cauda epididymis to its termination at the

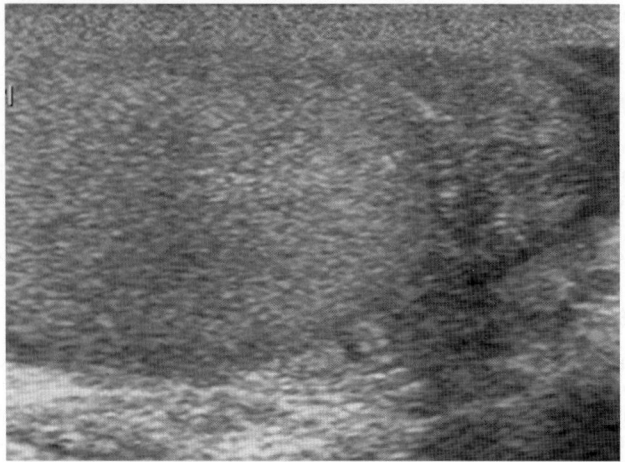

Figure 21-14. Ultrasound imaging of the caput epididymis, which appears hyperechoic to the testis and is at the right of the testis on this image.

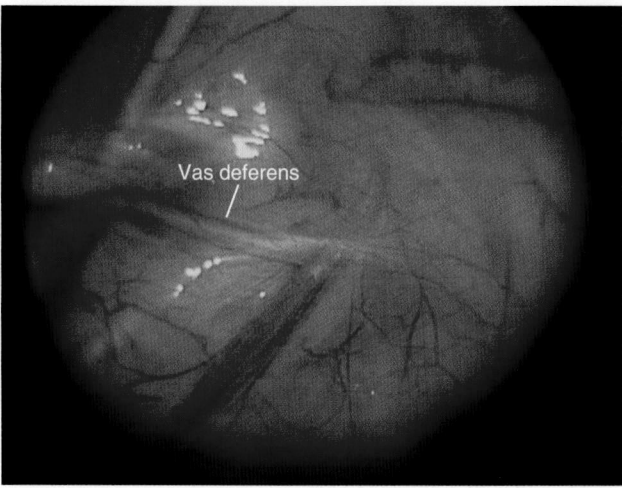

Figure 21-16. Laparoscopic visualization of the vas deferens.

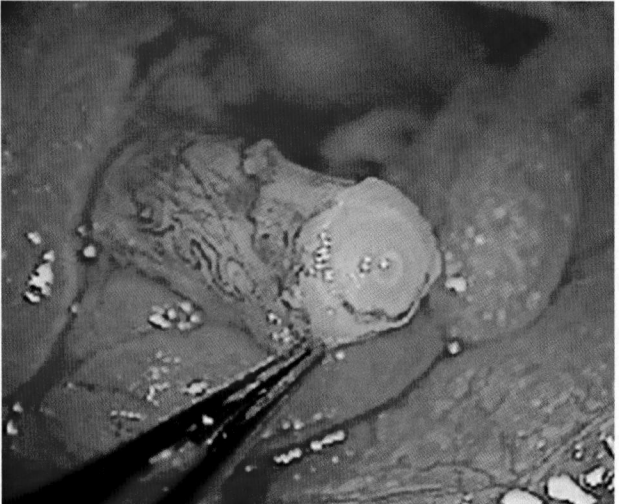

Figure 21-15. Microsurgical appearance of the transected vas deferens at the time of vasovasostomy.

ejaculatory duct, the vas deferens measures between 30 and 35 cm in length. **The vas deferens travels posteriorly along the spermatic cord, behind the vessels in the cord. The vas deferens passes through the inguinal canal and enters the pelvis lateral to the epigastric vessels.** On entering the pelvis, after passing through the internal inguinal ring, the vas deferens separates from the testicular vessels. The vas deferens ultimately reaches the posterior base of the prostate after traveling medial to the pelvic sidewall. The vas deferens is compartmentalized into five different regions. The first is the epididymal segment within the tunica vaginalis, which does not have a sheath. The second is the segment within the scrotum. The third segment is that within the inguinal canal. The fourth is the retroperitoneal segment, and the fifth is the ampulla of the vas deferens (Lich et al,1978). **The lumen of the vas deferens ranges between 0.2 and 0.7 mm in diameter, depending on the segment.** The outer diameter of the vas deferens ranges between 1.5 and 2.7 mm (Middleton et al, 2009) (Figs. 21-15 and 21-16).

Microanatomic Architecture

There is an outer adventitial connective tissue layer surrounding the vas deferens that contains blood vessels and small nerves. Within this connective tissue layer, smooth muscle cells comprise the thick wall of the vas deferens. These smooth muscle cells are organized as an inner and outer longitudinal layer, a middle circular layer, and a pseudostratified columnar epithelial layer with nonmotile stereocilia as the inner lining, known as its mucosa (Neaves, 1975; Paniagua et al, 1981). The epithelial cell height decreases progressively throughout the length of the vas deferens from the testis to the seminal vesicle. There are three types of tall, thin columnar cells, as well as basal cells, comprising the pseudostratified epithelium of the vas deferens (Hoffer, 1976; Paniagua et al, 1981). Principal cells, pencil cells, and mitochondria-rich cells comprise the columnar cells that extend from the epithelial base to the lumen. The columnar cells have irregularly shaped convoluted nuclei and have stereocilia. In the proximal vas deferens, principal cells are the predominant cell type. Traveling more distally throughout the vas deferens, more pencil cells and mitochondria-rich cells are present. The muscular layer of the vas deferens progressively decreases from proximal to distal.

Arterial Supply

The superior vesical artery gives off the deferential artery, which supplies the vas deferens (Sjostrand, 1965).

Venous Drainage

The venous drainage of the scrotal vas deferens is via the deferential vein, which drains into the pampiniform plexus. The pelvic vas deferens' venous drainage is to the pelvic venous plexus.

Lymphatic Supply

Lymphatic drainage from the vas deferens travels to the external and internal iliac nodes.

Nerve Supply

The vas deferens receives sympathetic and parasympathetic innervation (Sjostrand, 1965). The sympathetic adrenergic nerves travel via the presacral nerve from the hypogastric nerve (Batra and Lardner, 1976; McConnell et al, 1982). All three layers of the vas deferens tunica muscularis contain adrenergic fibers, but the greatest density of these nerve fibers is found in the outer longitudinal layer (McConnell et al, 1982). Other types of neurotransmitters have been identified within neurons such as somatostatin, galanin, enkephalin, neuropeptide Y, vasoactive intestinal peptide, and nitric oxide. The function of these neurotransmitters in the vas deferens is not well understood (Dixon et al, 1998).

Vasogram

The vasogram was previously considered to be the radiographic test of choice to evaluate the prostate, ejaculatory duct, and seminal vesicles in the infertile male. The vasogram has been replaced by transrectal ultrasonography for the most part, and the vasogram is only used in conjunction with reconstructive surgery (Honig, 1994).

KEY POINTS: VAS DEFERENS

- The lumen of the vas deferens ranges between 0.2 and 0.7 mm in diameter, depending on the segment.
- The superior vesical artery gives off the deferential artery, which supplies the vas deferens.
- A vasogram should only be performed in conjunction with reconstructive surgery.

SEMINAL VESICLES AND EJACULATORY DUCTS

Gross Structure

The seminal vesicles are paired, viscous organs that are positioned posterior to the bladder and prostate. The seminal vesicle is a lateral outpouching of the vas deferens. It has the capacity for 3 to 4 mL of volume and the nonobstructed seminal vesicle typically measures 5 to 7 cm in length and 1.5 cm in width. The seminal vesicle is a single tube that is highly coiled, and it forms several outpouchings and would measure 15 cm in length if stretched out. The joining of the seminal vesicle with the vas deferens creates the ejaculatory duct. The smooth muscle sheaths from the seminal vesicle and the vas deferens combine with the capsule of the prostate at the prostatic base. The seminal vesicles' excretory duct joins the duct of the ampullary vas deferens as it enters the prostate.

The ejaculatory ducts are positioned at the junction of the vas deferens and the seminal vesicle. The ejaculatory ducts are paired visceral organs. **They ultimately empty through the verumontanum into the prostatic urethra.** The ejaculatory duct is divided into three distinct anatomic regions. These include the extraprostatic region (proximal), intraprostatic region (mid), and the distal region, which joins the lateral aspect of the verumontanum to empty into the prostatic urethra (Nguyen et al, 1996). In contrast to the first two regions, the third distal region is not surrounded by an outer muscular layer and does not form an anatomic sphincter at the ejaculatory duct orifice at the verumontanum (Nguyen et al, 1996).

Microanatomic Architecture

The seminal vesicle has a columnar epithelium with goblet cells. The seminal vesicle tube is surrounded by a thin layer of smooth muscle cells, which is enveloped by a loose adventitia. The three layers comprising the tubule of the seminal vesicle include an inner mucous membrane, a collagenous middle layer, and the outer circular and longitudinal muscle layers. The muscle layers account for 80% of the thickness of the wall of the seminal vesicle (Nguyen et al, 1996). The thin, folded mucosa of the seminal vesicle is comprised of nonciliated, pseudostratified cuboidal or columnar cells. The ejaculatory ducts have similar microanatomic architecture to the seminal vesicles, but they do not have the outer circular muscle layer that is found in the seminal vesicle (Nguyen et al, 1996). The inner epithelial layer of the ejaculatory duct is composed of simple and pseudostratified columnar cells in a folded pattern.

Arterial Supply

The arterial supply to the seminal vesicle originates from the superior vesical artery, which branches into the vesiculodeferential

artery. The vesiculodeferential artery supplies the anterior surface of the seminal vesicle in proximity to its tip. The internal iliac artery and inferior vesical artery provide additional arterial supply to the seminal vesicle via the prostatovesicular branch (Clegg, 1955). Variations of arterial supply include the prostatovesicular branch originating from the pudendal artery or the superior vesical artery. Arterial supply to the ejaculatory duct arises from branches of the inferior vesical artery.

Venous Drainage

The venous drainage of the seminal vesicle follows the arterial supply draining through the vesiculodeferential veins and the inferior vesical plexus to the pelvic venous plexus.

Lymphatic Supply

The lymphatic drainage from the seminal vesicle is to the internal iliac nodes (Mawhinney and Tarry, 1991).

Nerve Supply

Seminal vesicle parasympathetic innervation originates from the pelvic plexus with the sympathetic nervous system contributing fibers from the hypogastric nerves and the superior lumbar nerves (Kolbeck and Steers, 1993). The pelvic plexus innervates the ejaculatory ducts.

Transrectal Ultrasonography

The seminal vesicles can be imaged by transrectal ultrasonography, as they are positioned posteriorly at the base of the prostate. The seminal vesicles appear hypoechoic, compared to the prostate, and are crescent-shaped, paired, and symmetrical. The normal seminal vesicle measures 2 cm in width and 4.5 to 5.5 cm in length. They can be visualized as oriented horizontally in the transverse plane. Hypoechoic fatty tissue can be seen separating the seminal vesicles from the base of the prostate. The ejaculatory ducts may occasionally be seen by transrectal ultrasonography and they appear hypoechoic as they enter the prostate posteriorly.

Computed Tomography

Computed tomography (CT) can image the seminal vesicles. The mean measurements by CT of the seminal vesicles are 3 cm in length and 1.5 cm in width. No significant change is seen by CT in seminal vesicle length on the basis of age. However, the width of the seminal vesicle is smaller in men of increasing age. The pudendal venous plexus can be identified by CT as small punctuate densities along the lateral aspect of the seminal vesicle (Silverman et al, 1985).

Magnetic Resonance Imaging

Magnetic resonance imaging (MRI) of the normal seminal vesicles demonstrate similar signal intensity to that of the bladder or muscle on T1 imaging. The seminal vesicles demonstrate a higher signal intensity than the surrounding fat on T2 imaging (King et al, 1989; Secaf et al, 1991) (Fig. 21-17; also see Fig. 21-16).

KEY POINTS: SEMINAL VESICLES AND EJACULATORY DUCTS

- The nonobstructed seminal vesicle typically measures 5 to 7 cm in length and 1.5 cm in width.
- The ejaculatory ducts empty through the verumontanum into the prostatic urethra.
- Transrectal ultrasound, CT, and MRI can image the seminal vesicles.

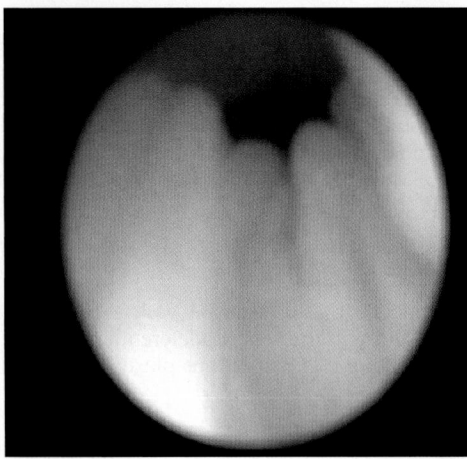

Figure 21-17. Endoscopic view into the os of the ejaculatory duct transurethrally.

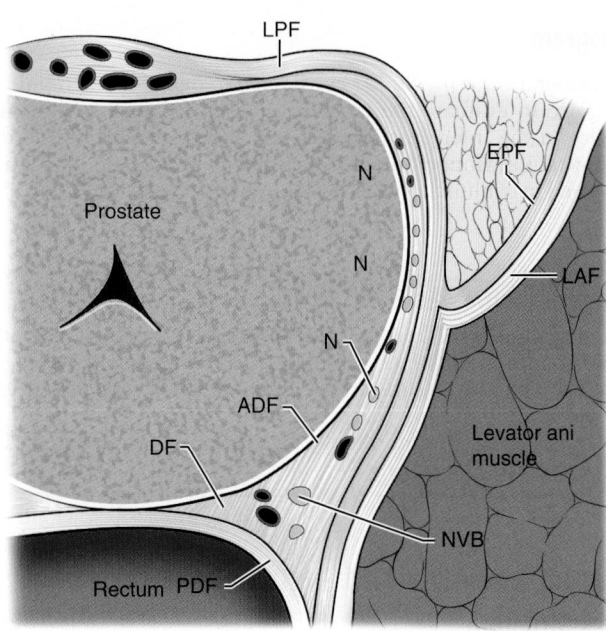

Figure 21-18. Cross section of prostate with prostatic fascial layers outlined, including the lateral prostatic fascia (LPF), endopelvic fascia (EPF), levator ani fascia (LAF), Denonvilliers fascia (DF), anterior lamina of Denonvilliers fascia (ADF), posterior lamina of Denonvilliers fascia (PDF), neurovascular bundle (NVB), and lateral nerves (N). (From Walz J, Graefen M, Huland H. Basic principles of anatomy for optimal surgical treatment of prostate cancer. World J Urol 2007;25:31–8.)

PROSTATE

Gross Structure

The normal prostate gland is ovoid in shape and measures 3 cm in length, 4 cm in width, and 2 cm in depth; it has a weight of 18 to 20 g. It is homologous to the Skene glands in females. The prostate is composed of glandular elements and fibromuscular stroma. The prostate is positioned just inferior to the bladder. The prostatic urethra travels through the prostate gland. **The base of the prostate is at the bladder-prostate junction and the narrowed apex is the most inferior portion of the prostate gland, reaching the urogenital diaphragm.** The prostate is palpable approximately 4 cm from the anus on digital rectal examination. **The apex of the prostate is continuous with the striated urethral sphincter.** The prostate is comprised of an anterior surface, a posterior surface, and lateral surfaces, and these are in relationship to the prostatic urethra traversing the prostate. A collagen, elastin, and smooth muscle capsule envelops the prostate. The capsule measures 0.5 mm in thickness posteriorly and laterally on average. There is no true prostatic capsule at the apex of the prostate, where normal prostate glands are seen blending into the striated muscle of the urethral sphincter. Similarly, there is no true capsule at the base separating the prostate from the bladder, where the detrusor muscle's outer longitudinal fibers fuse with the fibromuscular capsule of the prostate (Epstein, 1989). The prostate capsule blends with the continuation of the endopelvic fascia on the anterior and anterolateral aspects of the prostate. The prostate is fixed to the pubic bone anteriorly by the puboprostatic ligaments near the apex of the prostate. The superficial branch of the dorsal vein is positioned in the retropubic fat outside the prostatic fascia. It drains into the dorsal vein complex. The levator ani's pubococcygeal portion hugs the lateral aspects of the prostate and is related to its overlying endopelvic fascia. The prostate capsule and the pelvic fascia separate below the parietal and visceral endopelvic fascia juncture (arcus tendineus fascia pelvis). Fatty, areolar tissue and the lateral branches of the dorsal vein complex take up the space of this separation between the prostate capsule and the pelvic fascia. **The cavernosal nerves travel within the parietal pelvic fascia, also known as the lateral prostatic fascia, posterolateral to the prostate.** As more anatomic attention has been taken with higher-magnification robotic techniques at the time of radical prostatectomy, the lateral prostatic fascia has been defined in greater detail in an effort to preserve the cavernosal nerves. Nerve bundles have been identified traveling along the prostate laterally and anterior to the previously defined neurovascular bundle (Eichelberg et al, 2007; Raychaudhuri and Cahill, 2008) (Fig. 21-18).

The prostate has been divided into distinct anatomic zones. These zones can be identified with transrectal ultrasonography. The transition zone is the smallest of the zones of the prostate. The ducts of the transition zone begin at the angle dividing the preprostatic and the prostatic urethra, and they travel beneath the preprostatic sphincter to course along its lateral and posterior sides. The transition zone comprises 5% to 10% of the glandular tissue of the normal prostate. The transition zone is separated from the rest of the glandular compartments of the prostate by a distinct fibromuscular band. Benign prostatic hyperplasia most commonly occurs in the transition zone. The central zone ducts are positioned circumferentially, surrounding the openings of the ejaculatory ducts. This zone expands toward the base of the bladder, surrounding the ejaculatory ducts, in the shape of a cone. The central zone comprises 25% of the glandular tissue of the prostate. The glands of the central zone are thought to be of wolffian duct origin, as they differ immunohistochemically and structurally from the other glands of the prostate (McNeal, 1988). **The peripheral zone of the prostate is the largest zone. Seventy percent of the glandular tissue of the prostate is comprised of the peripheral zone.** The peripheral zone makes up the posterior and lateral aspects of the prostate gland. The ducts of the peripheral zone drain into the prostatic sinus along the entire length of the postsphincteric prostatic urethra. Seventy percent of prostate cancers are found in the peripheral zone. The nonglandular anterior fibromuscular stroma is found extending from the bladder neck to the striated sphincter, and it may comprise up to one third of the mass of the prostate. It is composed of collagen, smooth and striated muscle, and elastin. It is anatomically continuous with the anterior visceral fascia, the anterior preprostatic sphincter, and the prostatic capsule.

The prostate is also compartmentalized clinically, based on digital rectal examination and cystoscopic appearance. A central sulcus divides the two lateral lobes of the prostate and a middle lobe. The middle lobe may become hyperplastic and may extend into the bladder neck with age (Fig. 21-19).

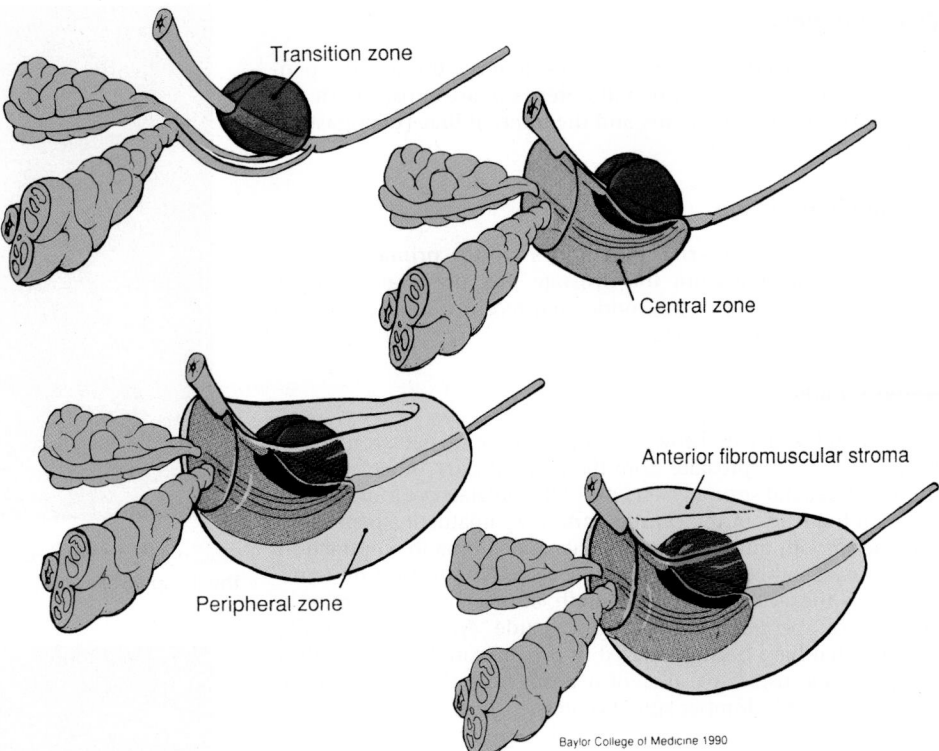

Figure 21-19. **Zonal anatomy of the prostate as described by McNeal (1988). The transition zone surrounds the urethra proximal to the ejaculatory ducts. The central zone surrounds the ejaculatory ducts and projects under the bladder base. The peripheral zone constitutes the bulk of the apical, posterior, and lateral aspects of the prostate. The anterior fibromuscular stroma extends from the bladder neck to the striated urethral sphincter. (© 1990, Baylor College of Medicine.)**

Microanatomic Architecture

Seventy percent of the prostate's composition is glandular elements, whereas 30% is made up of fibromuscular stroma. The epithelial cells of the prostate glands are cuboidal or columnar. These secretory epithelial cells are terminally differentiated, have a low proliferative index, and measure 10 to 20 µm in height (De Marzo et al, 1998). These epithelial cells have abundant secretory granules and are organized in rows with their apices projecting into the lumen and their bases attached to a basement membrane (Knox et al, 1994). The nuclei of the cells are at their base, below the Golgi apparatus. The luminal apices have microvilli. The epithelial cells line the periphery of the acinus and secrete into the acinus, which drain into ducts to the urethra ultimately. The tubuloalveolar glands have simple branching patterns. Flattened, undifferentiated basal cells line each acinus beneath the epithelial cells. A thin layer of connective tissue and stromal smooth muscle surrounds each acinus. The secretory cells have scattered, terminally differentiated, nonproliferating neuroendocrine cells between them. Two types of neuroendocrine cells have been identified in the prostate. One is a closed cell with dendritelike processes that extend toward epithelial cells and basal cells in its proximity. The other type of neuroendocrine cell type seen is an open one with microvilli extending into the lumen (di Sant'Agnese and De Mesy Jensen, 1984; Abrahamsson, 1999; Vashchenko and Abrahamsson, 2005). The stroma is composed of smooth muscle, which is rich in α-actin, myosin, and desmin, and it is also composed of collagen and is continuous with the prostatic capsule. At the junction of the prostate gland, the prostatic urethra, the transitional cells of the prostatic urethra's epithelium, may extend into prostatic ducts. The preprostatic (internal urethral) sphincter encloses the small periurethral prostatic glands without periglandular smooth muscle, and these glands are positioned between fibers of longitudinal smooth muscle. Posterior to the prostate, microscopic smooth muscle bands fuse with Denonvilliers fascia after extending from the posterior aspect of the prostatic capsule. There is a plane of loose, areolar tissue between Denonvilliers fascia and the rectum.

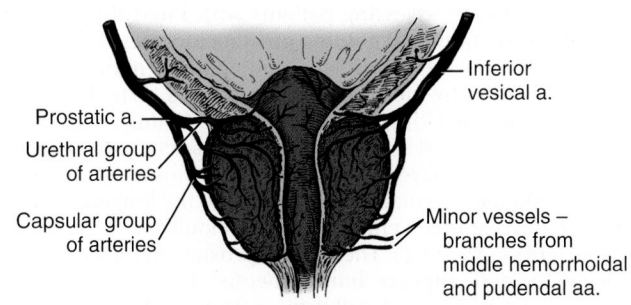

Figure 21-20. **Arterial supply of the prostate. (Modified from Flocks RH. The arterial distribution within the prostate gland: its role in transurethral prostatic resection. J Urol 1937;37:527.)**

Arterial Supply

The inferior vesical artery is the typical arterial supply to the prostate. The inferior vesical artery branches into urethral arteries that enter the prostatovesical junction posterolaterally and course in a perpendicular route to the urethra. They travel toward the bladder neck with the largest branches posteriorly, approaching the bladder neck in the one o'clock to five o'clock positions and the seven o'clock to eleven o'clock positions. They then supply the urethra after making a caudal turn to run parallel to the urethra. These branches supply the urethra, the periurethral glands, and the transition zone of the prostate (Flocks, 1937). The inferior vesical artery also branches into the capsular artery. The capsular artery yields small branches that supply the anterior prostatic capsule. The capsular branches enter the prostate at 90-degree angles and provide arterial supply to the glandular tissues, coursing along the reticular bands of the stroma. The majority of the inferior vesical artery travels posterolateral to the prostate to form the neurovascular bundles coursing with the cavernous nerves, terminating at the pelvic diaphragm. Branches from the internal pudendal artery and the middle rectal (hemorrhoidal) artery also contribute a supply to the prostate (Fig. 21-20).

Venous Drainage

The prostate includes abundant venous drainage through the periprostatic plexus. **The periprostatic plexus anastomoses with the deep dorsal vein of the penis and the internal iliac (hypogastric) veins.**

Lymphatic Drainage

The obturator and internal iliac nodes are the primary sites of lymphatic drainage from the prostate. The presacral group or, infrequently, the external iliac nodes may receive a small portion of the initial lymphatic drainage.

Nerve Supply

The cavernous nerves provide sympathetic and parasympathetic innervation to the prostate from the pelvic plexus. Innervations to the glandular and stromal elements of the prostate are found traveling with branches of the capsular artery. Sympathetic fibers innervate the smooth muscle of the capsule and stroma for contraction. The parasympathetic nerves promote secretory function by terminating in the acini. Prostate smooth muscle relaxation may be affected by peptidergic and nitric oxide synthase–containing neurons that have been identified in the prostate (Burnett, 1995). The pelvic plexuses carry afferent neurons from the prostate to the pelvic and thoracolumbar spinal centers.

Transrectal Ultrasonography of the Prostate

Transrectal ultrasonography of the prostate provides multiple diagnostic utilities including assessing prostate volume, locating focal abnormalities, assessing patients with infertility with suspicion of obstruction, and guiding prostate biopsies. The prostate is imaged with biplane, multiplane, and end-fire endorectal transducer probes with a frequency ranging from 6 to 8 MHz. The patient should be positioned either in the lateral decubitus or the dorsal lithotomy position, and a well-lubricated transrectal probe is gently passed into rectum above the anal verge. The prostate and seminal vesicles should be systematically examined in the longitudinal and transverse orientations. Pertinent images should be recorded and labeled (Terris et al, 1992). **The normal prostate has a stipple grey echogenicity and appears homogeneous.** The capsule appears echogenic, continuous, and well defined. **The zonal compartments can be identified.** A distinct layer of echogenic fibrous tissue separates the zones. The prostate presents a semilunar shape and appears symmetrical in the transverse orientation. The peripheral zone has a homogeneous, fine echo pattern. The periurethral tissue is centrally positioned and appears hypoechoic. The relation of the prostate to the surrounding structures such as the seminal vesicles, bladder neck, and prostatic urethra can be identified in the longitudinal orientation. The urethra will appear curved within the central portion of the prostate.

The prostate volume can be measured using transrectal ultrasonography with an accuracy of within 5% of its true weight (Hastak et al, 1982). Transverse and longitudinal orientations are used to measure the length, width, and height of the prostate. An ellipsoid formula is then used to estimate the volume of the prostate: Volume = $\frac{1}{3}\pi$ × length × width × height (Roehrborn et al, 1986) (Fig. 21-21).

Magnetic Resonance Imaging of the Prostate

MRI of the prostate has been used to provide high-quality, clear images. MRI's direct multiplanar imaging has allowed for detailed demonstration of prostate anatomy (Dooms and Hricak, 1986). Zonal anatomy can be more clearly demonstrated by MRI using 0.5 cm slices. The peripheral zone showed higher signal intensity than the other zones and can be well visualized in the coronal, sagittal, and transverse planes. The central zone was well visualized in the coronal and sagittal planes and was of low signal intensity.

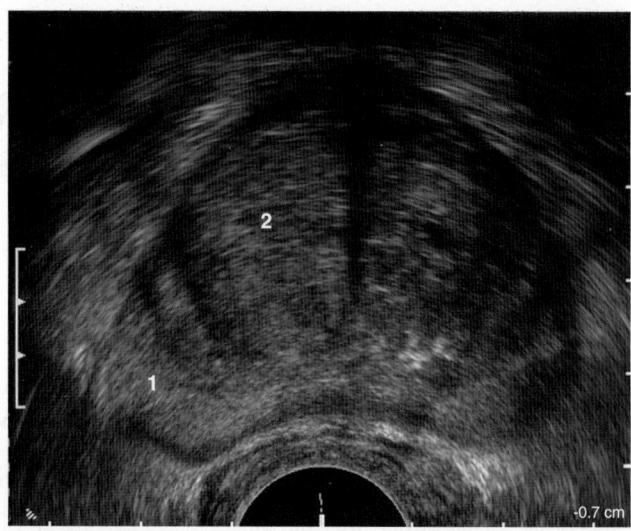

Figure 21-21. Transrectal ultrasound of the prostate demonstrating the peripheral zone (1) and the transition zone (2).

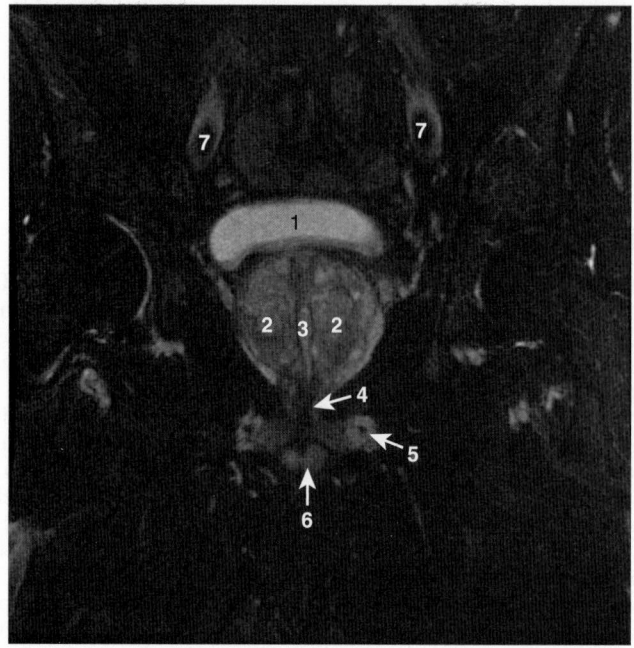

Figure 21-22. Axial T2-weighted magnetic resonance image of the male pelvis through the prostate gland and adjacent structures. 1, Urinary bladder; 2, lateral lobes of prostate; 3, verumontanum; 4, striated urethral sphincter; 5, inferior pubic ramus; 6, corpus spongiosum in cross section; 7, external iliac artery.

The transition zone showed similar MR parameters to the central zone (Hricak et al, 1987). **Zonal anatomy is best demonstrated by T2-weighted images** (Gevenois et al, 1990). Using a specific pulse sequence, the periprostatic venous plexus can be imaged (Poon et al, 1985). The endorectal surface coil has been used to enhance resolution (Schnall and Pollack, 1990). The use of MRI of the prostate has become more frequent for use with pathologic processes (Fig. 21-22).

URETHRA

The urethra is contained within the vascular corpus spongiosum and the glans penis. **The normal urethral diameter is 8 to 9 mm.** Anatomists have organized the urethra into multiple different

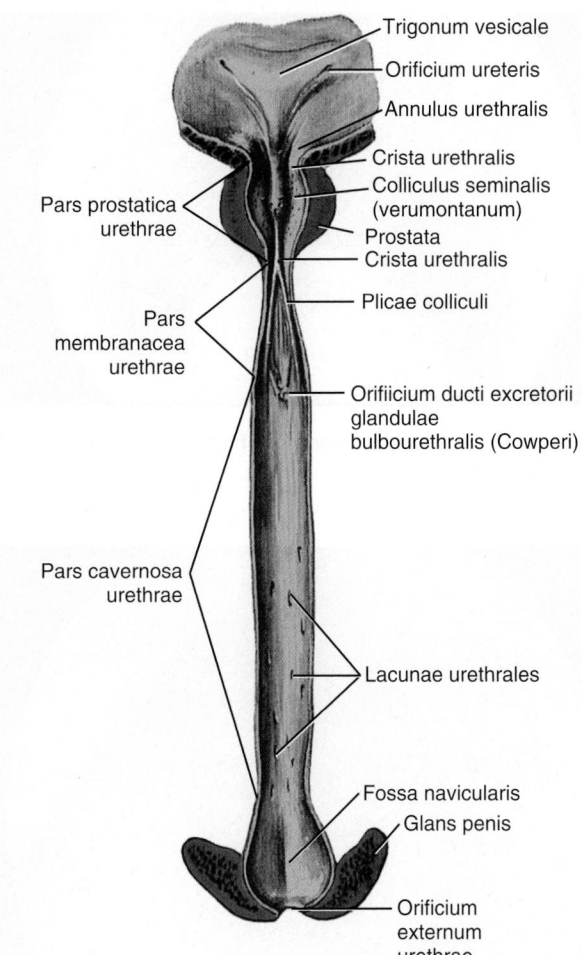

Figure 21-23. Posterior wall of the male urethra. (From Anson BJ, McVay CB. Surgical anatomy. 6th ed. Philadelphia: Saunders; 1984. p. 833.)

segmental divisions. It has been categorized in two broad segments: the anterior urethra and the posterior urethra. **The anterior urethra begins at the perineal membrane and continues distally to the urethral meatus. The posterior urethra begins distal to the bladder neck and the transition to the anterior urethra is made at the perineal membrane.** The segments have been further divided to characterize urethral anatomy more precisely. **The urethral epithelium is transitional in type until the urethral epithelium becomes squamous where it traverses the glans penis.** The submucosa contains smooth muscle, connective tissue, and elastic tissue. The glands of Littre are in the submucosa and their ducts empty into the urethral lumen. **The arterial supply to the urethra is from the internal pudendal artery whose bulbourethral branches supply the urethra, the corpus spongiosum, as well as the glans penis. The venous drainage from the urethra drains to the pudendal plexus, which drains into the internal pudendal vein. The lymphatics from the urethra drain to the internal iliac (hypogastric) and common iliac nodes** (Fig. 21-23).

Prostatic Urethra

The prostatic urethra travels the length of the prostate and is in greater proximity to the anterior surface of the prostate. A urethral crest extends inward from the posterior midline of the prostatic urethra and is present throughout the length of the prostatic urethra. This urethral crest is no longer present at the level of the striated sphincter. All glandular elements of the prostate drain into prostatic sinuses, which are positioned on either side of the urethral crest (McNeal, 1972). The urothelium of the prostatic urethra is made up of transitional epithelial cells. This transitional urothelium may extend into prostatic ducts. An angle at the midpoint of the prostatic urethra turns 35 degrees anteriorly and separates the prostatic urethra into anatomically and functionally distinct segments. These are termed the preprostatic (proximal) and prostatic (distal) segments of the prostatic urethra. This angle may range from zero to 90 degrees depending on variable anatomy (McNeal, 1972, 1988). All glandular elements of the prostate open into the prostatic urethra past the urethral angle. **The verumontanum is formed by the widening and protrusion of the urethral crest from the posterior wall. The prostatic utricles orifice appears like a slit at the apex of the verumontanum.** The utricles orifice is cystoscopically visible and measures 6 mm. **The prostatic utricle is a müllerian remnant.** The two small openings of the ejaculatory ducts are located on either side of the utricular orifice. After forming

at the juncture of the vas deferens and seminal vesicles, the ejaculatory ducts travel approximately 2 cm through the prostate surrounded by circular smooth muscle, until they finally open into the distal prostatic urethra. The preprostatic sphincter is made up of thickened circular smooth muscle, synonymous with the internal urethral sphincter in the proximal segment. The prostatic segment is innervated by motor somatic fibers with an absence of any autonomic innervation (Figs. 21-24 and 21-25).

Membranous Urethra

On average the membranous urethra measures 2 to 2.5 cm in length and spans between the prostatic apex and the perineal membrane (Myers, 1991). A thin, smooth muscle layer spans across the membranous urethra. An outer layer of circularly arranged striated muscle in the shape of a horseshoe near the prostatic apex is found on the anterior surface of the urethra. The striated muscle reaches from the base of the bladder and the anterior aspect of the prostate extending the complete length of the membranous urethra. This signet ring–shaped striated sphincter is broad based and narrows as it courses through the urogenital hiatus of the levator ani to reach the prostatic apex. The posterior portion of the striated sphincter inserts into the perineal body throughout its length (Strasser et al, 1998). The striated sphincter is anterior to the dorsal vein complex and lateral to the levator ani. The band of fibrous tissue that suspends the urethra from the pubis anteriorly and that forms the suspensory ligament of the penis posteriorly, is made up of connective tissue from deep within the anterior and lateral walls. The striated sphincter's lumen consists of a pseudostratified columnar epithelium. There is a vascular submucosa that is surrounded by

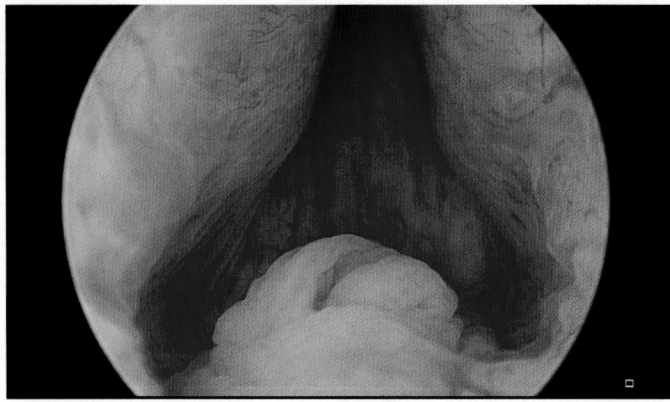

Figure 21-24. Cystoscopic appearance of the verumontanum. (Courtesy David Leavitt, MD.)

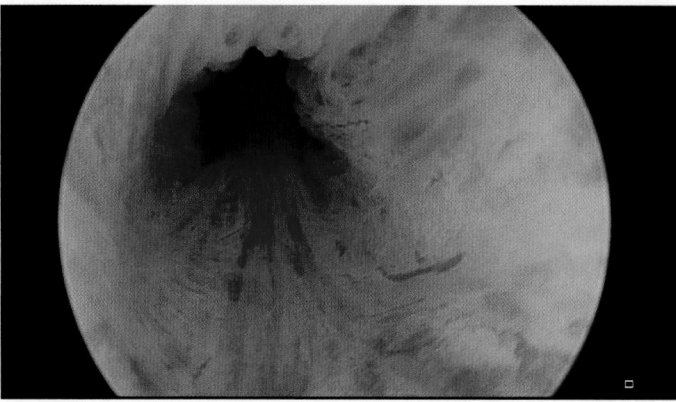

Figure 21-26. Cystoscopic appearance of the striated sphincter. (Courtesy David Leavitt, MD.)

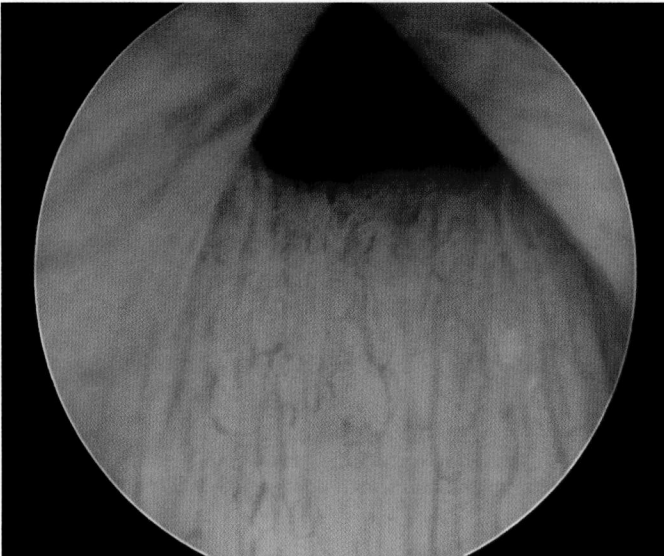

Figure 21-25. Cystoscopic appearance of the bladder neck. (Courtesy David Leavitt, MD.)

the longitudinal and circular urethral smooth muscle, which is the intrinsic component of the external sphincter (Raz et al, 1972). The pudendal nerve supplies innervation to the striated sphincter (Tanagho et al, 1982). A branch of the sacral plexus that travels along the surface of the levator ani provides another source of somatic innervation to the sphincter (Hollabaugh et al, 1997). The cavernous nerves are believed to supply autonomic innervation to the intrinsic smooth muscle of the membranous urethra (Steiner et al, 1991). The urethral stroma contains longitudinally organized collagen fibers and elastin fibers (Hickey et al, 1982). Lymphatic drainage from the membranous urethra travels in front of the prostate to join lymphatic channels draining the anteroinferior bladder. These channels terminate in the anterior or medial retrofemoral nodes and the middle node of the medial group of the external iliac nodes. Innervation is solely by motor somatic fibers without autonomic innervation. The ventral root of S3, with some contribution from S2, provides the somatic supply. The supply branches to the pelvic (splanchnic) nerve and passes to the pelvic (inferior hypogastric) plexus. Sensory innervation from the striated sphincter travels through the pudendal nerves via S2, and to a lesser extent S3, to travel to the node of Onuf centrally (Fig. 21-26).

Penile Urethra

The penile urethra, also known as the pendulous urethra and the spongy urethra, as it is surrounded by the corpus spongiosum,

comprises the urethra distal to the membranous urethra. The urethra is often subdivided even further at the junction of the membranous and penile urethra, and is termed the bulbomembranous urethra. This region comprises a 2-cm length of urethra within the urogenital diaphragm as well as being within the striated urethral sphincter and the first few proximal centimeters of the bulbous urethra, just distal to the sphincter within the penile bulb. The bulbospongy urethra begins a few centimeters distal to the membranous urethra and extends distally to the level of the suspensory ligament. The lumen widens to form the urethral bulb. The bulbourethral glands, also known as Cowper glands, empty into this region at the three o'clock and nine o'clock positions. The bulbourethral glands themselves are located more proximally on either side of the membranous urethra. The penile urethra measures approximately 15 cm in length in its entirety from the suspensory ligament to the meatus. It is positioned more dorsally than ventrally within the corpus spongiosum. The bulb and the fossa navicularis are the two segments of urethral lumen widening; otherwise the luminal diameter is relatively consistent throughout. The mucosa of the penile urethra includes a transitional epithelium until it reaches the fossa navicularis. The muscle layer is made up of an inner longitudinal, a middle circular, and an inconsistently characterized outer longitudinal stratum. The glands of Littre are composed of small mucus-secreting cells that lubricate the urethra before ejaculation, and they empty into orifices on the posterior wall of the penile urethra. The glands of Littre are rich in goblet cells and enter the spongy tissue between the vascular spaces and the trabeculae. **The penile urethra receives arterial supply from a branch of the internal pudendal artery, which enters at the level of the penile bulb, and is known as the bulbourethral artery.** Venous drainage of the bulbar urethra is by bulbar veins that drain into the prostatic plexus, which is the internal pudendal vein. The penile urethral lymphatics drain through a lymphatic network that is associated with the mucous membrane. These lymphatic channels course longitudinally but anastomose transversely and obliquely. The lymphatic channels drain proximally into trunks at the bulbomembranous urethra. The bulbomembranous lymphatic drainage may be variable. Some lymphatic drainage travels along the urethral artery or artery of the bulb, whereas others drain to the medial retrofemoral node after traveling behind the symphysis pubis. The penile urethral sensory innervation runs through submucosal axons that pass centrally through the dorsal nerve of the penis (Fig. 21-27).

Fossa Navicularis

The glanular portion of the urethra is known as the fossa navicularis, where its caliber dilates when compared to the urethra proximal to the fossa navicularis. It narrows again at the urethral meatus. **Unlike the transitional epithelium of the remainder of the urethra, the urethral mucosa that traverses the glans penis is a**

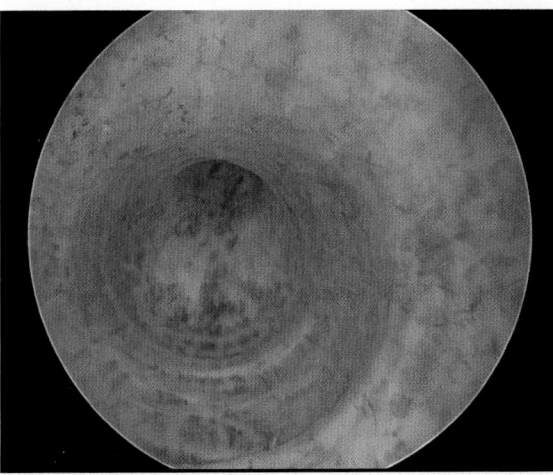

Figure 21-27. Cystoscopic appearance of the bulbar urethra. (Courtesy David Leavitt, MD.)

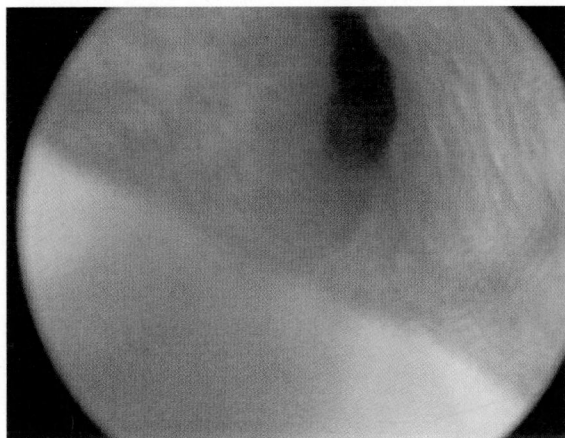

Figure 21-28. Cystoscopic appearance of the fossa navicularis.

squamous epithelium. These cells become keratinized near the meatus. The epithelium is separated from the smooth muscle of the spongy tissue by loose connective tissue, and a muscularis mucosa is absent. There are multiple pockets on the dorsal and lateral surfaces of the fossa navicularis. The lacuna magna (Morgagni) is a large pocket opening on the roof of the fossa navicularis (Figs. 21-28, 21-29, and 21-30).

KEY POINTS: URETHRA

- The urethra is contained within the corpus spongiosum and the glans penis.
- The anterior urethra begins at the perineal membrane and continues distally to the urethral meatus.
- The posterior urethra begins distal to the bladder neck and the transition to anterior urethra is made at the perineal membrane.
- The urethral epithelium is transitional in type until the urethral epithelium becomes squamous where it traverses the glans penis at the fossa navicularis.
- The arterial supply to the urethra is from the internal pudendal artery whose bulbourethral branches supply the urethra, the corpus spongiosum, and glans penis.
- The verumontanum is formed by the widening and protrusion of the urethral crest from the posterior wall.
- The prostatic utricles (müllerian remnants) orifice appears like a slit at the apex of the verumontanum.

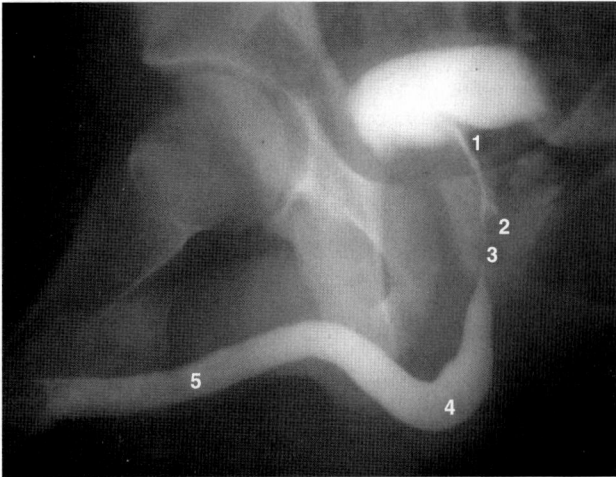

Figure 21-29. Retrograde urethrogram of the male urethra demonstrating urethral anatomy. 1, Prostatic urethra; 2, verumontanum, into which enter the ejaculatory ducts; 3, membranous urethra, note physiologic narrowing of urethral luminal diameter resulting from external striated sphincter; 4, bulbar urethra; 5, pendulous urethra.

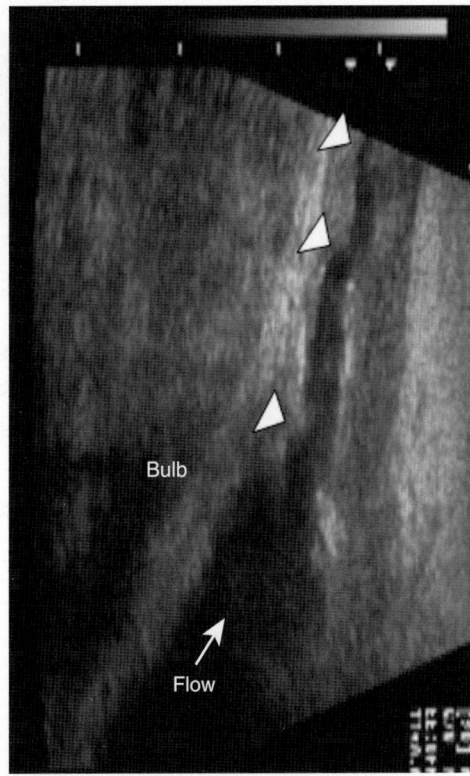

Figure 21-30. Urethral ultrasonography has been used to assist in assessing the urethra in a noninvasive fashion. The *arrowheads* indicate the direction of urine flow during voiding in a normal urethra without stricture. (Courtesy Jonathan Rhee, MD.)

PENIS

Structure

The gross structures of the penis can be divided into distinct anatomic compartments. The paired corpora cavernosa, which are the erectile bodies, prolongate proximally as the crus and attach to the pubic arch. The urethra travels through the corpus spongiosum, with its proximal segment known as the bulb. The glans

penis is an expansion of the corpus spongiosum. The superior surface of the penis during erection is known as the dorsum and the inferior surface during erection, containing the urethra, is known as the ventrum. The major portion of the body of the penis is formed by the corpora cavernosa as they join beneath the pubis (penile hilum). **A septum separates the corpora cavernosa but is permeable distally to allow for free communication between their vascular spaces.** The tunica albuginea is the tough connective tissue layer that envelops the corpora cavernosa and is primarily collagenous. With erection, the outer longitudinal layers and inner circular fibers of the tunica albuginea are tightly stretched, and in the flaccid state they form an undulating meshwork (Goldstein et al, 1982). Smooth muscle bundles traversing the corpora cavernosa form endothelial-lined cavernous sinuses. Myoendothelial junctions, which are cellular extensions through the internal elastic lamina, have been identified as connecting the vascular smooth muscle cells to the endothelial cells. Gap junctions have been identified at the point of cell-to-cell contact in the myoendothelial junction (Kavoussi et al, 2010). The corpus spongiosum tapers and

travels ventrally to the corpora cavernosa, distal to the bulb. The glans penis is the most distal expansion of the corpus spongiosum. The shaft of the penis and the base of the glans are separated by the corona. The corpora cavernosa are surrounded by Buck fascia dorsally. Buck fascia splits to surround the corpus spongiosum ventrally. The fundiform ligament of the penis is composed of collagenous and elastic fibers from the rectus sheath blending with and surrounding Buck fascia. The suspensory ligament of the penis is made up of deeper fibers from the pubis. Deep to the muscles of the corpora cavernosa, the tunica albuginea and the Buck fascia fuse (Uhlenhuth et al, 1949). Buck fascia joins the base of the glans at the corona distally. The penile shaft skin is very elastic and its only glandular elements are the smegma-producing glands, located at the base of the corona. The penile skin is very mobile as its dartos fascia backing is very loosely attached to Buck fascia. In uncircumcised men, the prepuce (foreskin) is the penile skin as it folds over the glans and attaches below the corona. The glans penis skin is immobile as it is attached to the tunica albuginea below it (Figs. 21-31 and 21-32).

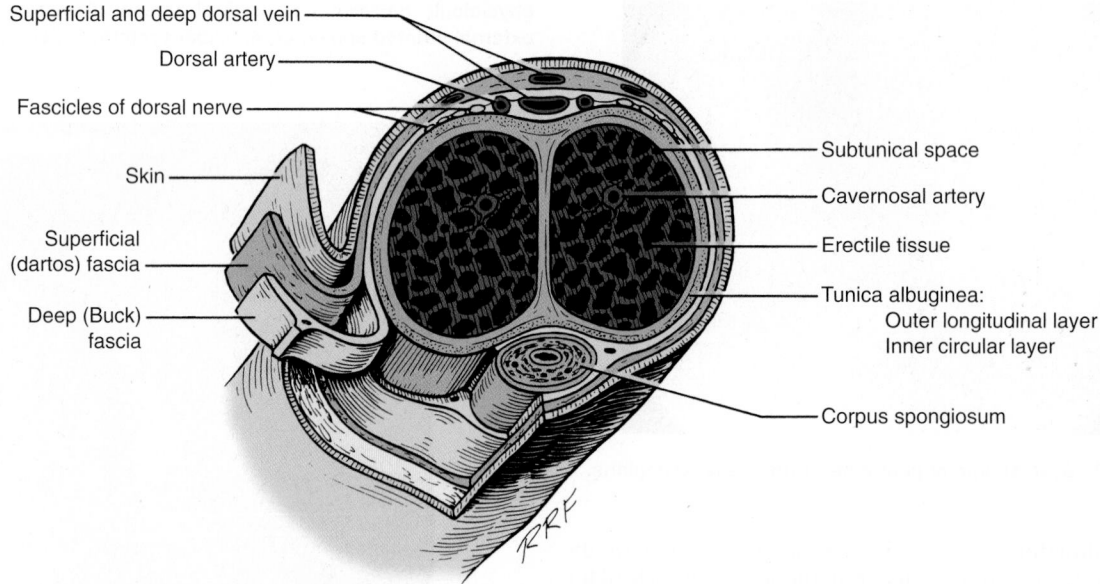

Figure 21-31. **Cross section of the penis, demonstrating the relationship between the corporal bodies, penile fascia, vessels, and nerves. (From Devine CJ Jr, Angermeier KW. Anatomy of the penis and male perineum. AUA Update Series 1994;13:10–23.)**

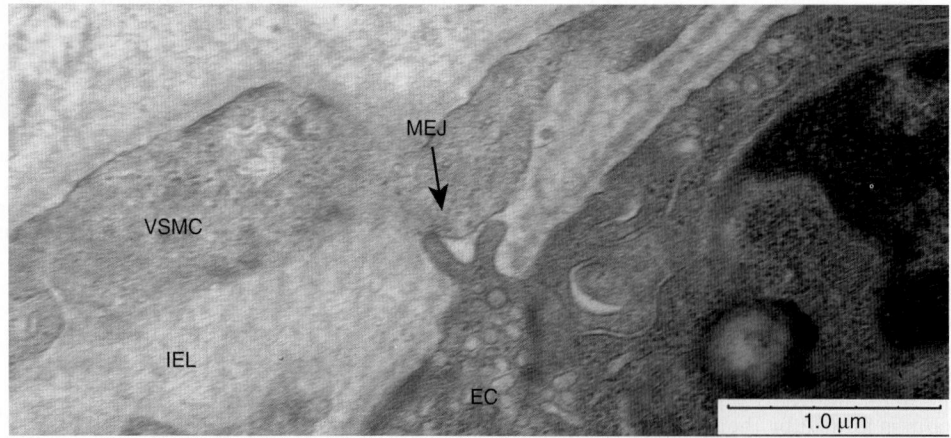

Figure 21-32. **Electron microscopy of a myoendothelial junction (MEJ) in human corpus cavernosal tissue. The MEJ is extending from the endothelial cell (EC) through the internal elastic lamina (IEL) to communicate with the vascular smooth muscle cell (VSMC).**

Arterial Supply

There is a superficial arterial system supplying the penis, which originates from the external pudendal arteries, and a deep arterial system that arises from each side from the internal pudendal arteries. The pudendal artery branches into a deep artery, supplying the corpora cavernosa, a dorsal artery, and the bulbourethral artery. Above the perineal membrane, the common penile artery travels in the Alcock canal, and it supplies the corpora cavernosa via three branches. The bulbourethral artery penetrates the perineal membrane where it enters the corpus spongiosum from above at its posterolateral border. This provides arterial supply to the corpus spongiosum, glans, and urethra. The cavernosal artery penetrates the corpus cavernosum in the penile hilum to nearly the center of the erectile tissue. It provides straight and helicine arteries that supply the cavernous sinuses. After it travels between the crus and the pubis, the dorsal artery of the penis supplies the dorsal surfaces of the corporeal bodies. The dorsal artery travels between the dorsal vein and the dorsal penile nerve, and they all attach to the underside of Buck fascia. The dorsal artery travels distally toward the glans and supplies cavernous branches and circumferential branches to the urethra and the corpus spongiosum (Devine and Angermeier, 1994). There can be a great deal of variability in penile arteries (Bare et al, 1994). A single cavernosal artery may supply both corpora cavernosa or it may be completely absent. In some cases, an accessory pudendal artery may supplement or completely take the place of branches of the common penile artery (Breza et al, 1989). The arterial supply to the penile skin is from the external pudendal branches of the femoral vessels. These vessels run longitudinally in the dartos fascia layer and provide a rich blood supply after entering the base of the penis (Fig. 21-33).

Venous Drainage

The superficial dorsal vein lies external to Buck fascia, whereas the deep dorsal vein is beneath Buck fascia and runs between dorsal arteries. A number of venous channels anastomose at the base of the glans to form the dorsal vein of the penis. **The dorsal vein travels between the corporeal bodies, in a groove, and drains into the preprostatic plexus.** In the distal two thirds of the penile shaft, the circumflex veins from the corpus spongiosum course around the corpora cavernosa to enter the deep dorsal vein perpendicularly. There are typically 3 to 10 circumflex veins. The cavernous sinuses form intermediary venules that empty into the subtunical capillary plexus. Emissary veins from these plexuses travel obliquely between the layers of the tunica and drain into the circumflex veins dorsolaterally. Emissary veins form two to five cavernous veins in the

proximal third of the penis, joining on the dorsomedial surface of the corpora cavernosa. These veins travel between the bulb and crura at the hilum of the penis. They receive branches from the bulb and the crura and empty into the internal pudendal veins.

Lymphatic Supply

Lymphatics from the skin of the penis drain to the superficial inguinal and subinguinal lymph nodes. **Penile shaft lymphatics converge on the dorsum and ramify to both sides of the groin to drain into inguinal lymph nodes.** Lymphatics from the glans run deep to Buck fascia dorsally to drain to the superficial and deep inguinal nodes bilaterally. Some studies have suggested direct lymphatic channels from the glans to pelvic nodes as well as studies proposing lymphatic drainage through sentinel nodes positioned medial to the superficial epigastric veins. These models have been challenged (Catalona, 1988).

Nerve Supply

Sensory innervation of the penis is through the dorsal nerves. These nerves richly supply the glans. The dorsal nerves travel alongside the dorsal arteries. Small branches of the perineal nerve supply the ventrum of the penis as distally as the glans (Uchio et al, 1999). The somatic nerve supply originates from spinal nerves S2, S3, and S4 via the pudendal nerve. The pudendal nerve passes through the Alcock canal and continues as the dorsal nerve of the penis. The cavernous nerves supply sympathetic and parasympathetic innervation from the pelvic plexus to the corporeal bodies after penetrating them to ramify in the erectile tissue (Fig. 21-34).

Cavernosogram

Cavernosograms were primarily used historically to assist in the diagnosis of venous leak erectile dysfunction. Radiopaque contrast is injected into the corporal body with plain film imaging. This is not a commonly used diagnostic test any longer, but it is occasionally used at the time of penile fracture repair (Fitzpatrick and Cooper, 1975; Mydlo et al, 1998) (Fig. 21-35).

KEY POINTS: PENIS

- The paired erectile bodies are known as the corpora cavernosa.
- The glans penis is an expansion of the corpus spongiosum.
- A permeable septum separates the corpora cavernosa for free communication between their vascular spaces.
- The superficial arterial system to the penis originates from the external pudendal arteries, and a deep arterial system arises from the internal pudendal arteries.
- The dorsal vein runs between the corporeal bodies and drains into the preprostatic plexus.
- Penile shaft lymphatics converge on the dorsum and ramify to both sides of the groin to drain into inguinal lymph nodes.
- Sensory innervation of the penis is through the dorsal nerves, and the somatic nerve supply originates from spinal nerves S2, S3, and S4 via the pudendal nerve.

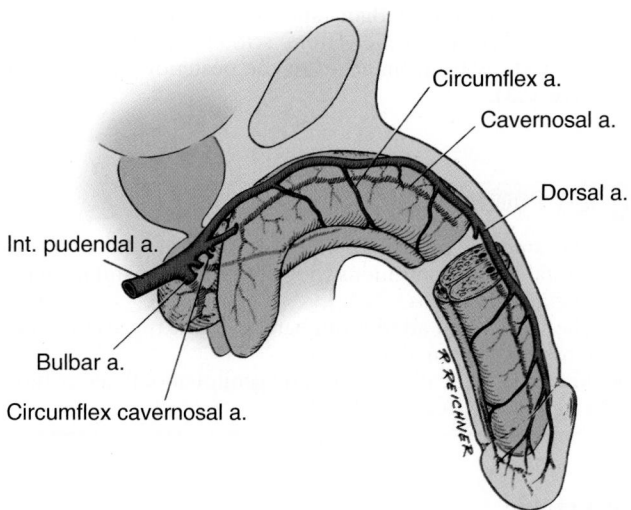

Figure 21-33. Arterial supply of the penis.

Circumflex a.
Cavernosal a.
Dorsal a.
Int. pudendal a.
Bulbar a.
Circumflex cavernosal a.

SCROTUM

Gross Structure

The scrotal skin is hair bearing, pigmented, with abundant sebaceous and sweat glands, and has an absence of fat. It is variable

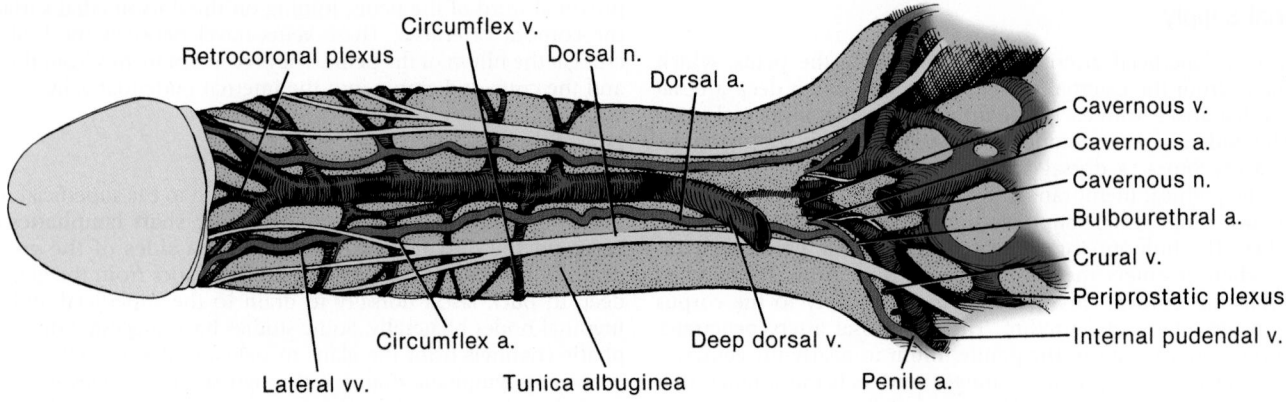

Figure 21-34. **Dorsal penile arteries, veins, and nerves. (From Hinman F Jr. Atlas of urosurgical anatomy. Philadelphia: Saunders; 1993. p. 445.)**

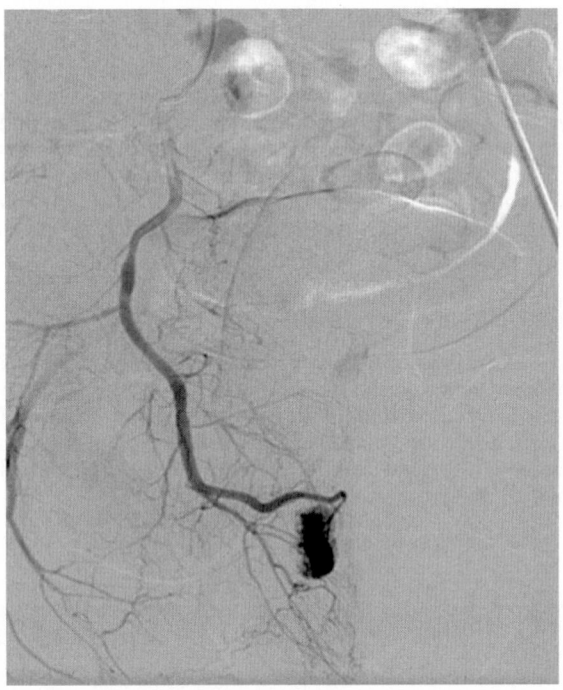

Figure 21-35. **Angiogram of arteriocorporeal fistula in patient with nonischemic priapism showing filling of the right corpus cavernosum.**

and may be folded with transverse rugae or it may appear loose and shiny. Its appearance depends on the tone of the underlying dartos smooth muscle. The median raphe runs longitudinally in the midline from the urethral meatus to the anus. Deep to the raphe, the scrotum is divided by a septum into two compartments, each containing a testis. The smooth muscle of the dartos fascia underlying the skin is continuous with Colles, Scarpa, and the dartos fascia of the penis. The spermatic fasciae are layers of the abdominal wall that extend to form parts of the scrotal wall. The external oblique extends to form the external spermatic fascia, which attaches to the borders of the external inguinal ring. The internal oblique extends to form the cremaster muscle and fascia, which attach to the inguinal ligament laterally, to the iliopsoas laterally, and to the pubic tubercle medially. The transversalis fascia continues to become the internal spermatic fascia in the scrotum. A peritoneal derivative known as the parietal and visceral tunica vaginalis surrounds the testis with a mesothelium-lined pouch. The tunica vaginalis is continuous with the testis posterolaterally at its mesentery, where it is attached to the scrotal wall. The gubernaculum fixes the testis at its inferior pole (Fig. 21-36).

Arterial Supply

The external pudendal arteries supply the anterior wall of the scrotum. **The arteries run parallel to the rugae and do not cross the median raphe.** The posterior aspect of the scrotum has arterial supply from perineal branches. Arterial supply to the spermatic fascia is from the cremasteric, testicular, and deferential branches.

Venous Drainage

The external pudendal veins drain the anterior scrotal wall. The veins run parallel to the rugae and do not cross the median raphe.

Lymphatic Supply

Scrotal lymphatics do not cross the median raphe and drain into the superficial inguinal nodes on the ipsilateral side.

Nerve Supply

Branches of the ilioinguinal and genitofemoral nerves innervate the anterior scrotal wall. The nerves run parallel to the rugae and do not cross the median raphe. The posterior aspect of the scrotum receives innervation from scrotal branches of perineal nerves as well as from branches of the posterior femoral cutaneous nerve (S3).

KEY POINTS: SCROTUM

- The smooth muscle of the dartos fascia underlying the scrotal skin is continuous with Colles, Scarpa, and the dartos fascia of the penis.
- The scrotal wall arteries run parallel to the rugae and do not cross over the median raphe.
- Branches of the ilioinguinal and genitofemoral nerves innervate the anterior scrotal wall.

REFERENCES

The complete reference list is available online at www.expertconsult.com.

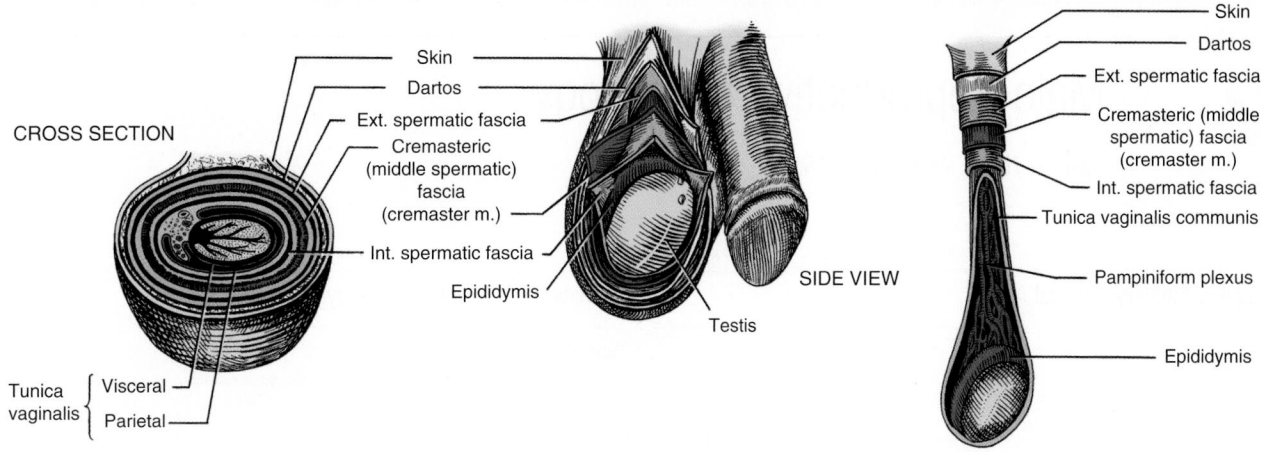

Figure 21-36. Scrotum and its layers. (From Pansky B. Review of gross anatomy. 6th ed. New York: McGraw-Hill; 1987.)

SUGGESTED READINGS

Breza J, Aboseif SR, Orvis BR, et al. Detailed anatomy of penile neurovascular structures: surgical significance. J Urol 1989;141(2):437–43.

Clegg EJ. The arterial supply of the human prostate and seminal vesicles. J Anat 1955;89(2):209–16.

Devine CJ Jr, Angermeier KW. Anatomy of the penis and male perineum. AUA Update Series 1994;13:10–23.

Dogra VS, Gottlieb RH, Oka M, et al. Sonography of the scrotum. Radiology 2003;227(1):18–36.

Epstein J. The prostate and seminal vesicles. New York: Raven; 1989.

McNeal JE. The prostate and prostatic urethra: a morphologic synthesis. J Urol 1972;107(6):1008–16.

Setchell BP, Brooks DI. Anatomy, vasculature, innervation and fluids of the male reproductive tract. New York: Raven Press; 1988.

22 Male Reproductive Physiology

Paul J. Turek, MD, FACS, FRSM

Hypothalamic-Pituitary-Gonadal Axis

Testis

Epididymis

Ductus (Vas) Deferens

Seminal Vesicle and Ejaculatory Ducts

Spermatozoa

Summary

The male reproductive axis of hormones and organs is an efficient, well-orchestrated, and precisely managed biologic system that has evolved over millions of years. It is responsible for reproductive tract formation and development, fertility potential at puberty, and the maintenance of adult maleness. This chapter explores our current understanding of this complex system by defining the anatomy and physiology of its components, including the hypothalamic-pituitary-gonadal (HPG) hormonal axis, spermatogenesis and androgen production within the testicle, and maturation and transport of sperm in the ductal system. In addition, new concepts in genetic infertility, stem cell science, and ejaculatory physiology are explained. Through such rigorous intellectual dissection, the true beauty and sophistication of the reproductive process is appreciated.

HYPOTHALAMIC-PITUITARY-GONADAL AXIS

The HPG axis plays a critical role during development and adulthood in four physiologic processes: (1) **phenotypic gender** development during embryogenesis, (2) **sexual maturation** at puberty, (3) testis endocrine function—**testosterone production,** and (4) testis exocrine function—**sperm production.**

Basic Endocrine Concepts

Two types of hormones mediate communication in the reproductive axis: peptide and steroid. **Peptide hormones are small, secretory proteins that act through cell surface receptors.** Hormone signals are transduced by one of several second-messenger pathways (Fig. 22-1). Ultimately, most peptide hormones induce phosphorylation of proteins that alter cell function. Examples of peptide hormones are luteinizing hormone (LH) and follicle-stimulating hormone (FSH). In contrast, **steroid hormones are derived from cholesterol. They are not stored in secretory granules; consequently, steroid secretion directly reflects rates of hormone production.** In plasma, these hormones are usually bound to carrier proteins, and because they are lipophilic, steroid hormones are cell membrane permeable. After binding to intracellular receptors, steroids are translocated to nuclear DNA recognition sites and regulate target gene transcription. Examples of reproductive axis steroid hormones are testosterone and estradiol.

Hormonal signaling within the HPG axis is hierarchically governed by a free-running pulse generator within the hypothalamus. The amplitude and frequency with which hormone secretions occur within the reproductive axis determine downstream organ responsiveness. Feedback control is the principal mechanism through which hormonal regulation occurs in the HPG axis (Fig. 22-2). With feedback control, a hormone can regulate the synthesis and action of itself or of another hormone. **In the HPG axis, negative feedback activity is primarily responsible for minimizing perturbations and maintaining homeostasis.**

Components of the Reproductive Axis

Hypothalamus

As the integrative center of the HPG axis, the hypothalamus receives neuronal input from the amygdala, thalamus, pons, retina, olfactory cortex, and many other areas (see Fig. 22-2). The pulse generator for the cyclic secretion of pituitary hormones, **the hypothalamus is anatomically linked to the pituitary gland by both a portal vascular system and neuronal pathways.** By avoiding the systemic circulation, the portal vascular system allows direct delivery of hypothalamic hormones to the anterior pituitary.

The most important hypothalamic hormone for reproduction is gonadotropin-releasing hormone (GnRH) or luteinizing hormone–releasing hormone (LHRH), a 10–amino acid peptide generated in the neuronal cell bodies in the preoptic and arcuate nuclei. Currently, the only known function of GnRH is to stimulate the secretion of LH and FSH from the anterior pituitary. GnRH has a plasma half-life of approximately 5 to 7 minutes and is almost entirely removed on the first pass through the pituitary either by receptor internalization or enzymatic degradation. GnRH secretion results from integrated input from the effects of stress, exercise, and diet from higher brain centers, gonadotropins secreted from the pituitary, and circulating gonadal hormones. Substances known to regulate GnRH secretion are listed in Table 22-1. In Kallman syndrome, characterized by congenital hypogonadotropic hypogonadism, the GnRH precursor neurons fail to migrate normally, with a subsequent absence of hypothalamic GnRH secretion (Bick et al, 1992; Dode et al, 2003). Affected individuals have delayed puberty or infertility owing to lack of testosterone production.

GnRH output exhibits several types of rhythmicity: seasonal, on a time scale of months and peaking in the spring; circadian, resulting in higher testosterone levels during the early morning hours; and pulsatile, with GnRH peaks occurring every 90 to 120 minutes on average. The importance of pulsatile GnRH secretions in normal HPG axis function is aptly demonstrated by the ability of exogenous GnRH agonists (e.g., leuprolide acetate) to stop testicular testosterone production by changing pituitary exposure to GnRH from a cyclic to a constant pattern.

Anterior Pituitary

Located within the bony sella turcica of the skull, the pituitary has two lobes: posterior and anterior. The posterior lobe, or

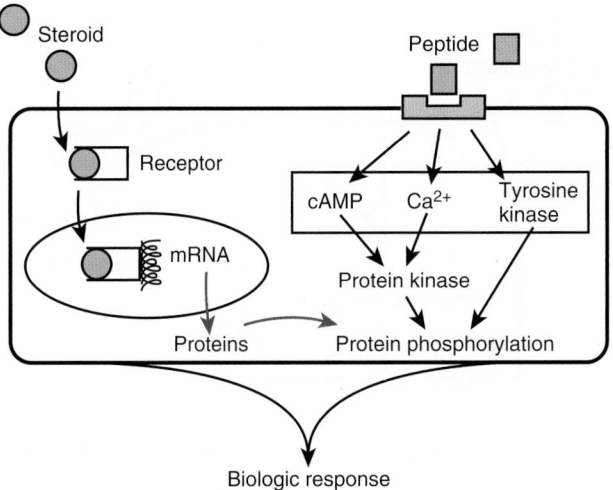

Figure 22-1. Two kinds of hormone classes mediate intercellular communication in the reproductive hormone axis: peptide and steroid. (Modified from Turek PJ. Male infertility. In: Tanagho EA, McAninch JC, editors. Smith's urology. 16th ed. Stamford [CT]: Appleton & Lange; 2008.)

TABLE 22-1 Substances That Modulate Gonadotropin-Releasing Hormone (GnRH) Secretion

GnRH MODULATOR	TYPE OF FEEDBACK	EXAMPLES
Opioids	Negative	β-Endorphin
Catecholamines	Variable	Dopamine
Peptide hormones	Negative	FSH, LH
Sex steroids	Negative	Testosterone
Prostaglandins	Positive	PGE₂
Insulin	Positive	Insulin
Kisspeptins	Positive	Kisspeptin (puberty)
Leptins	Positive	Leptin

FSH, follicle-stimulating hormone; LH, luteinizing hormone; PGE$_2$, prostaglandin E$_2$.

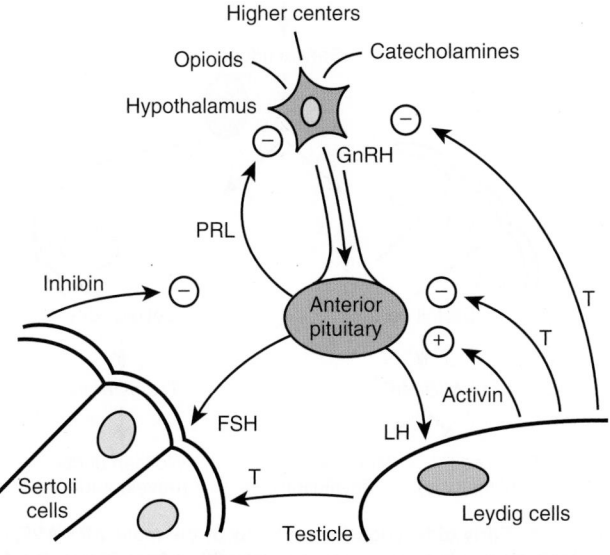

Figure 22-2. Diagram of the hypothalamic-pituitary-testis hormonal axis. +, Positive feedback; −, negative feedback; FSH, follicle-stimulating hormone; GnRH, gonadotropin-releasing hormone; LH, luteinizing hormone; PRL, prolactin; T, testosterone. (Modified from Turek PJ. Male infertility. In: Tanagho EA, McAninch JC, editors. Smith's urology. 16th ed. Stamford [CT]: Appleton & Lange; 2008.)

neurohypophysis, secretes two hormones, oxytocin and vasopressin, and is driven by neural stimuli. In contrast, **the anterior pituitary, or adenohypophysis, is regulated by blood-borne factors and is the site of action of GnRH** (see Fig. 22-2). GnRH stimulates the production and release of FSH and LH by a calcium flux–dependent mechanism. The sensitivity of pituitary gonadotrophs for GnRH varies with an individual's age and hormonal status. **LH and FSH are the primary pituitary hormones that regulate testis function.** They are glycoproteins composed of two polypeptide chain subunits, termed α and β, each coded by a separate gene. The α subunit of each hormone is identical and is similar to that of all other pituitary hormones; biologic and immunologic activities are conferred by the unique β subunit. Both subunits are required for endocrine activity. Sugars linked to these peptide subunits, consisting of oligosaccharides with sialic acid residues, differ in content between FSH and LH and likely account for differences in their plasma clearance rates. Secretory pulses of LH vary in frequency from 8 to 16 pulses in 24 hours and vary in amplitude by onefold to threefold. These pulse patterns closely reflect GnRH release. **Both androgens and estrogens regulate LH secretion through negative feedback.** On average, FSH pulses occur approximately every 1.5 hours and vary in amplitude by 25%. The FSH response to GnRH is more difficult to assess than that of LH for two reasons: (1) FSH has a smaller amplitude response and a longer serum half-life, and (2) **the gonadal proteins inhibin and activin may affect FSH secretion and are thought to account for the relative secretory independence of FSH from GnRH secretion.**

FSH and LH are only known to act in the gonads. They activate adenylate cyclase, which leads to increases in intracellular cyclic adenosine monophosphate (cAMP). In the testis, LH stimulates steroidogenesis within Leydig cells by inducing the mitochondrial conversion of cholesterol to pregnenolone and testosterone. **FSH binds to Sertoli cells and spermatogonial membranes within the testis and is the major stimulator of seminiferous tubule growth during development. FSH is essential for the initiation of spermatogenesis at puberty.** In the adult, the major physiologic role of FSH is to stimulate quantitatively normal levels of spermatogenesis.

A third anterior pituitary hormone, prolactin, can also affect the HPG axis and fertility. Prolactin is a large, globular protein of 199 amino acids (23 kD) that is responsible for milk synthesis during pregnancy and lactation in women. No human mutations have been found in either the human prolactin gene or its receptor (Goffin et al, 2002). **The normal role of prolactin in men is less clear, but it may increase the concentration of LH receptors on Leydig cells and sustain normal, high intratesticular testosterone levels. It may also potentiate the effects of androgens on the growth and secretions of the male accessory sex glands** (Wennbo et al, 1997; Steger et al, 1998). Normal prolactin levels may be important to maintain libido. Although low prolactin levels are not necessarily pathologic, hyperprolactinemia abolishes gonadotropin pulsatility by interfering with episodic GnRH release. In addition, the anterior pituitary contains cells that secrete other glycoprotein hormones: adrenocorticotropic hormone (ACTH), growth hormone (GH), and thyroid-stimulating hormone (TSH). These glycoprotein hormones can also have significant effects on male reproduction.

Testis

Normal male virility and fertility require the collaboration of the exocrine and endocrine testis (see Fig. 22-2). The interstitial compartment, composed mainly of Leydig cells, is responsible for steroidogenesis. The seminiferous tubules produce spermatozoa.

Normal testosterone production in men is approximately 5 g/day, and secretion occurs in a damped, irregular, pulsatile

manner (nyctohemeral). Testosterone is metabolized into two major active metabolites in target tissue: (1) the major androgen **dihydrotestosterone (DHT)** from the action of 5α-reductase, and (2) the estrogen **estradiol** through the action of aromatases. DHT is a much more potent androgen than is testosterone. In most peripheral tissues, testosterone reduction to DHT is required for androgen action, but in the testis and skeletal muscle, conversion to DHT is not essential for hormonal activity.

The primary site of FSH action is on Sertoli cells within seminiferous tubules. In response to FSH, Sertoli cells produce androgen-binding protein (ABP), transferrin, lactate, ceruloplasmin, clusterin, plasminogen activator, prostaglandins, and growth factors. Through these FSH-mediated factors, seminiferous tubule growth is stimulated during development, and sperm production is initiated during puberty. It is interesting to note that mice FSH knockout studies suggest that FSH is not essential for spermatogenesis, because affected mice can be fertile (Levallet et al, 1999). In humans, it is thought that FSH is required for normal spermatogenesis (Tapanainen et al, 1997).

The testis also produces the protein hormones inhibin and activin (Itman et al, 2006). Inhibin is a 32-kD protein made by Sertoli cells that inhibits FSH release from the pituitary. Within the testis, **inhibin production is stimulated by FSH and acts by negative feedback at the pituitary or hypothalamus. Activin, a testis protein with close structural homology to transforming growth factor-β (TGF-β),** exerts a stimulatory effect on FSH secretion. Activin receptors are found in a host of extragonadal tissues, suggesting that this hormone may have growth factor or regulatory roles in the body.

Negative feedback suppression of GnRH release by testosterone occurs through androgen receptors (ARs) in hypothalamic neurons and in the pituitary. **In studies of genetic mutations, it is clear that both testosterone and estrogen participate in negative feedback** (Shupnik and Schreihofer, 1997). Steroid negative feedback results mainly from AR binding to testosterone, with a smaller contribution from estradiol binding. **Testosterone feedback occurs mainly at the hypothalamus, whereas estrogen feedback is mainly in the pituitary** (Santen, 1975). It also appears that although testosterone is the primary regulator of LH secretion, estradiol (along with inhibin from Sertoli cells) is the predominant regulator of FSH secretion (Hayes et al, 2001).

Development of the Hypothalamic-Pituitary-Gonadal Axis

Sex determination is genetically determined in humans. **A critical gene for sex determination is *SRY* (sex-determining region Y gene) on the short arm of the Y chromosome.** The *SRY* gene product is a protein with a high mobility group box (HMG) sequence, a highly conserved DNA-binding motif that kinks DNA. This DNA bending effect alters gene expression, leading to testis formation and subsequently to the male phenotype. However, the *SRY* gene does not act in isolation to determine human sex. *DAX1*, a nuclear hormone receptor gene, can alter *SRY* activity during development by suppressing genes downstream to *SRY* that would normally induce testis differentiation. A second gene, *WNT4*, largely confined to the adult ovary, may also serve as an "antitestis" gene. The discovery of these genes has significantly altered theories of sex determination. In the past, the female genotype was considered the "default," *SRY*-negative, developmental pathway. **It is now clear that genes such as *WNT4* and *DAX1* can proactively induce female gonadal development, even in the presence of *SRY*** (DiNapoli and Capel, 2008).

Once gonadal sex is determined, Leydig cells make **testosterone,** which induces development of the **internal genitalia** (Fig. 22-3). Leydig cells also synthesize **insulin-like growth factor-3** to promote **transabdominal testis migration** into the scrotum. **DHT** masculinizes the genital anlage to form the **external genitalia** (see Fig. 22-3). In addition, Sertoli cells within the developing testis synthesize **müllerian-inhibiting substance (MIS, or antimüllerian hormone [AMH]),** which prevents the müllerian duct from developing into uterus and fallopian tubes and keeps the early germ

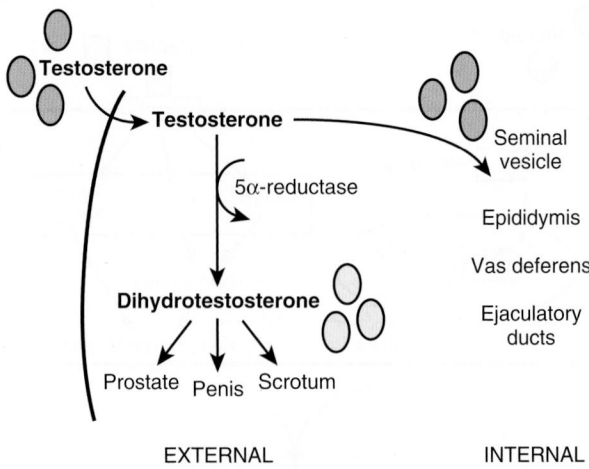

Figure 22-3. Diagram of internal and external genitalia development. Testosterone is the main androgenic steroid responsible for the developing male internal genitalia, whereas dihydrotestosterone is the main androgen responsible for development of male external genitalia.

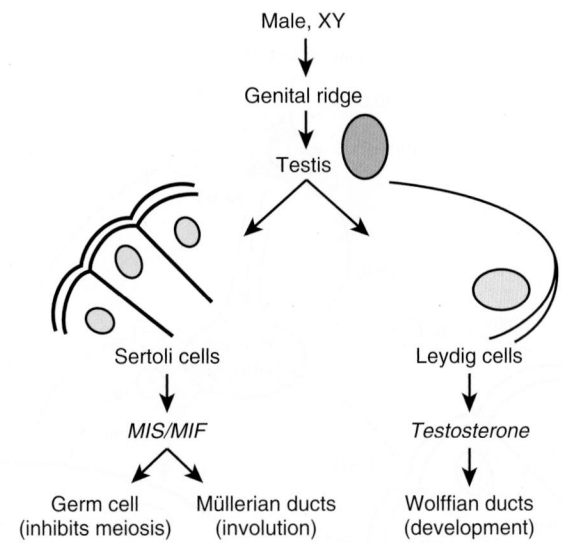

Figure 22-4. Early differentiation pathway of the male. *MIS/MIF*, müllerian inhibiting substance or factor. (Modified from Turek PJ. Male infertility. In: Tanagho EA, McAninch JC, editors. Smith's urology. 16th ed. Stamford [CT]: Appleton & Lange; 2008.)

cells quiescent in the testis (Fig. 22-4). In general, deficiencies in these developmental pathways result in either birth defects or intersex disorders.

The hormonal feedback relationships within the HPG axis become established during gestation. **The expression of kisspeptin protein is in part responsible for activating GnRH neurons and triggering GnRH release.** In addition, SF-1, an orphan nuclear receptor, is secreted by developing Sertoli cells and contributes to HPG axis development (Val et al, 2003). After the withdrawal of placental steroids at birth, there is a period of high gonadotropin secretion in the neonate. Subsequently, as axis sensitivity to gonadotropins increases, FSH and LH secretions fall to the low levels characteristic of childhood. Puberty begins with GnRH pulsing, leading gonadotropins to increase to adult levels and subsequently to increase sex hormones. **The hypothalamic capacity to generate GnRH pulses arises at puberty, usually starting around the 12th year in males.** Puberty begins at critical growth, weight, and nutritional rates for boys and girls and is likely initiated by kisspeptin, melatonin, and leptin (Clement et al, 1998). The adipocyte hormone leptin is the body's regulatory signal governing the size of the fat stores, and there is increasing evidence that leptin modulates hypothalamic and pituitary activity (Caprio et al, 1999; Kiess et al, 1999; Quinton et al, 1999).

Aging and the Hypothalamic-Pituitary-Gonadal Axis

A progressive decline in testosterone and sperm production occurs with age, such that men in the seventh decade have mean plasma testosterone levels 35% lower than young men (Vermeulen et al, 1995). The consequence of this is a phenomenon that has been variously termed **male menopause, male climacteric, andropause, or, more appropriately, partial androgen deficiency in the aging male (PADAM).** The changes to the seminiferous epithelium with age include decreases in seminiferous tubule volume and length. **An age-related decrease in sperm production in older testes appears to stem from decreased germ cell proliferation rather than increased cellular degeneration. Correspondingly, FSH levels also increase with age, with mean values threefold higher in older than younger men.** The cause of the age-related decline in HPG axis function is multifactorial. Testosterone production is reduced because of fewer Leydig cells and more testosterone-binding proteins. Diurnal variation of testosterone secretion is also lost in elderly men. With age, there is also evidence for a blunted HPG feedback response to low testosterone (despite generally high levels of gonadotropins) and to GnRH stimulation. Finally, normal pulsatile GnRH release is replaced by irregular pulses that are less effective in stimulating gonadotropin release (Mulligan et al, 1997). A combination of these effects is likely responsible for diminished HPG axis function with age.

KEY POINTS: HYPOTHALAMIC-PITUITARY-GONADAL AXIS

- Normal testosterone and sperm production depends on the pulsatile secretion of hypothalamic GnRH and LH and FSH from the anterior pituitary gland.
- Regulation of HPG axis hormones occurs primarily through negative feedback.
- The determination of maleness is derived from the *SRY* gene on the Y chromosome. However, developmental genes such as *WNT4* and *DAX1* are considered antitestis genes and can proactively induce female gonadal development.
- Changes to the HPG axis with paternal age include lower testosterone levels, blunted axis feedback, and irregular hormone pulsatility.

TESTIS

Gross Architecture

The testis is a white, ovoid organ that is normally 15 to 25 mL in volume (Prader, 1966) and has a length of 4.5 to 5.1 cm (Tishler, 1971; Winter and Faiman, 1972). The tunica albuginea has smooth muscle cells that course through predominantly collagenous tissue (Langford and Heller, 1973). Smooth muscle cells may impart contractile capability to the capsule (Rikmaru and Shirai, 1972), may affect blood flow into the testis (Schweitzer, 1929), and promote the flow of seminiferous tubule fluid from the testis (Davis and Horowitz, 1978).

The testis parenchyma is divided into compartments by septa. Each septum divides seminiferous tubules into lobes that each contain a centrifugal artery. **Individual seminiferous tubules harbor developing germ cells. Interstitial tissue is composed of Leydig cells, mast cells, macrophages, nerves, and blood and lymph vessels. In humans, interstitial tissue comprises 20% to 30% of total testicular volume** (Setchell and Brooks, 1988). The

relationship between seminiferous tubules and interstitial tissue anatomy is demonstrated in Figure 22-5. Seminiferous tubules are long, highly coiled, and looped. Both ends terminate in the rete testis. **The combined length of the 600 to 1200 tubules in the human testis is estimated to be 250 meters** (Lennox and Ahmad, 1970) (Fig. 22-6). The "hub" of the testis, also termed the **rete testis,** coalesces to form 6 to 12 **ductuli efferentes** that carry testicular fluid and spermatozoa into the **caput epididymis** (see Fig. 22-6).

The arterial supply to the testis and epididymis is derived from three sources: the internal spermatic artery, the deferential (vasal) artery, and the external spermatic (or cremasteric) artery (Harrison and Barclay, 1948). The internal spermatic artery arises from the abdominal aorta and is intimately associated with the pampiniform plexus of veins. The vascular arrangement within the pampiniform plexus, with the counterflowing artery and veins, facilitates the exchange of heat and small molecules. For example, testosterone passively diffuses from veins to the artery in a concentration-limited manner (Bayard et al, 1975). **The counter-current heat exchange supplies arterial blood to the testis that is 2° C to 4° C lower than the rectal temperature in normal men** (Agger, 1971). A loss of the temperature differential is associated with testicular dysfunction in men with varicocele (Goldstein and Eid, 1989) and cryptorchidism (Marshall and Edler, 1982). As the spermatic cord is commonly dissected during varicocele repair, it is surgically relevant to know that a single artery is observed in 50% of spermatic cords, with two arteries in 30% and three arteries in 20% of cases (Beck et al, 1992).

Inferior to the scrotal pampiniform plexus and near the mediastinal testis, the spermatic artery is highly coiled and branches before entering the testis. Extensive interconnections, especially between the internal spermatic and deferential arteries, allow maintenance of testis viability even after division of the internal spermatic artery (Fig. 22-7). From angiographic studies, a single artery enters the testis in 56% of cases; two branches enter in 31% of cases, and three

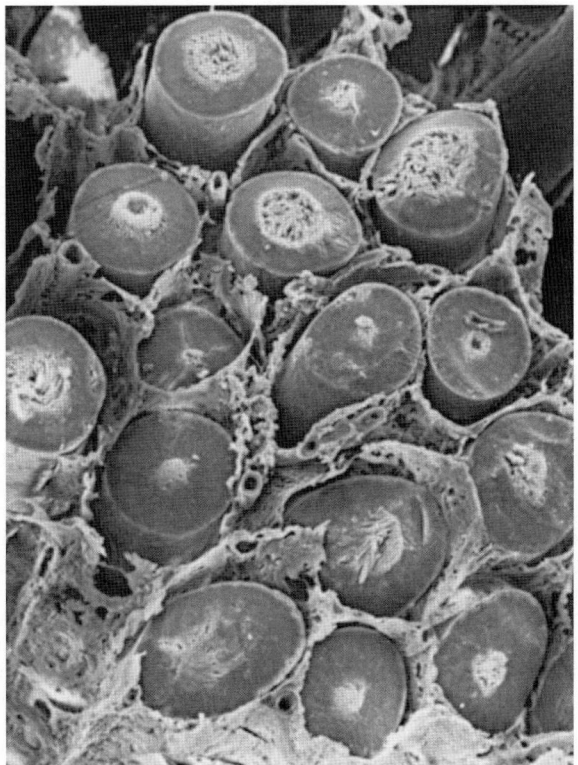

Figure 22-5. Scanning electron micrograph of the cut surface of the human testis. Note the relationship of interstitial tissue to seminiferous tubules. (From Christensen AK. Leydig cells. In: Greep RO, Astwood EB, editors. Handbook of physiology. Washington [DC]: American Physiology Society; 1975. p. 57–94.)

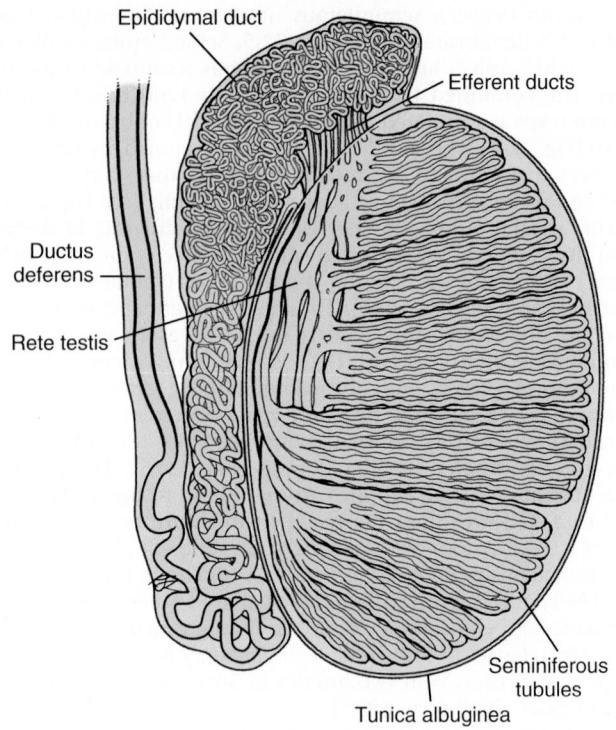

Figure 22-6. Drawing of the human testis showing the seminiferous tubules (250 meters in length), epididymis (3 to 4 meters in length), and vas deferens. (Based on Hirsh AV. The anatomical preparations of the human testis and epididymis in the Glasgow Hunterian Collection. Hum Reprod Update 1995;1:515–21.)

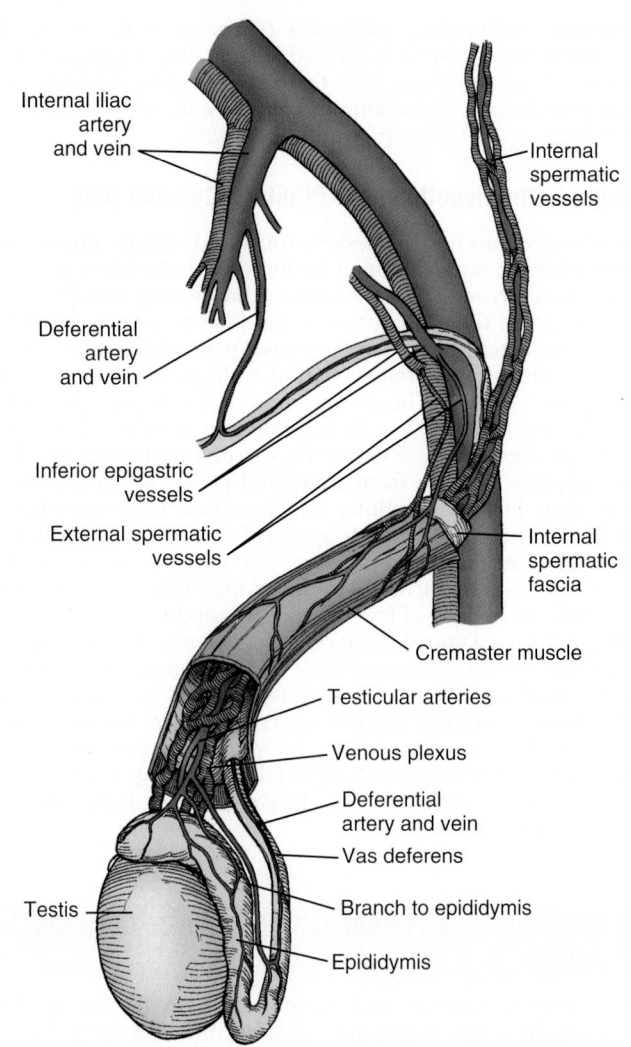

Figure 22-7. Schematic illustration of interconnections between internal spermatic, external spermatic (cremasteric), and deferential vessels in the peritesticular region and spermatic cord.

or more branches in 13% of testes (Kormano and Suoranta, 1971). In men with a single testicular artery, its interruption can result in testicular atrophy (Silber, 1979). The testicular arteries penetrate the tunica albuginea and then travel inferiorly along the posterior surface of the testis within the parenchyma. Branching arteries pass anteriorly over the testicular parenchyma. Major testicular artery branches also travel over the inferior pole of the testis, pass anteriorly, and branch out over the surface of the testis. The location of these vessels is clinically important, because they may be injured during orchiopexy or testis biopsy procedures (Jarow, 1991; Schlegel and Su, 1997). **The midsection of the testis has relatively fewer vessels compared with superior or inferior areas.** Individual arteries to the seminiferous tubules, termed *centrifugal arteries*, travel within the septa, which contain tubules. Centrifugal artery branches give rise to arterioles that supply individual intertubular and peritubular capillaries (Muller, 1957). The intertubular capillaries are located within the columns of interstitial tissue, whereas the ladder-like capillaries running near the seminiferous tubule are called *peritubular capillaries*. Through this vascular complex, the human testis is provided with 9 mL of blood per 100 g of tissue per minute (Pettersson et al, 1973).

Veins within the testis are unusual in that they do not run with the corresponding intratesticular arteries. Small parenchymal veins empty either into the veins on the testis surface or into a group of veins near the mediastinum testis that travels along the rete testis (Setchell and Brooks, 1988). These two sets of veins join together with deferential veins to form the pampiniform plexus as they ascend into the scrotum. Pampiniform plexus veins are thin walled, which likely contributes to the passive diffusion of testosterone and heat with the closely associated spermatic artery.

The testis has no known somatic innervation. It receives autonomic innervation primarily from the intermesenteric nerves and renal plexus (Mitchell, 1935). These nerves run along the testicular artery into the testis. It appears that testicular adrenergic innervation

is restricted primarily to small blood vessels that supply Leydig cell clusters that may regulate Leydig cell steroidogenesis (Baumgarten et al, 1968; Turnbull and Rivier, 1997). It is thought that vascular tone in the testis may involve regulation at several levels (Linzell and Setchell, 1969), including autoregulation of capsular arteries (Davis et al, 1990), regional variation based on local metabolic need and governed by peptides such as atrial natriuretic peptide (Collin et al, 1997), and assisted transport of molecules such as LH across the vascular endothelium (Milgrom et al, 1997). Indeed, these observations suggest a highly specialized function for the microvasculature of the testis (see review by Desjardins [1989]).

Prominent lymphatics can be observed within the spermatic cord (Hundeiker, 1971). Obstruction of these ducts results in dilation of the testis interstitium but not the seminiferous tubules, suggesting that the interstitial space is drained by lymphatics, but the seminiferous tubules are not. **Lymphatic obstruction can also result in hydrocele formation, a known complication of varicocelectomy and herniorrhaphy procedures.** The sperm-containing intratubular fluid that bathes Sertoli cells flows from the seminiferous tubules into the rete testis and subsequently into the caput epididymis. This fluid, isosmotic with plasma, is thought to be mainly of seminiferous tubule origin (Setchell and Brooks, 1988). **Reabsorption of this fluid within the rete testis and efferent ductules is regulated by estrogens (Lee et al, 2000).** Tubular fluid composition is markedly different from blood plasma or lymphatics, suggesting that substances are not freely diffusible into and out of the tubules (Setchell and Waites, 1975). This has led to the concept of a "blood-testis barrier" to be discussed later.

Testis Cytoarchitecture

Interstitium

Leydig Cells. The testis interstitium contains blood vessels, lymphatics, fibroblasts, macrophages, mast cells, and Leydig cells (Fig. 22-8). **Leydig cells are responsible for the bulk of testicular steroid production.** Leydig cells differentiate from mesenchymal

precursor cells by the 7th week of gestation. The activation of Leydig cell steroidogenesis correlates with the onset of androgen-dependent differentiation of the male reproductive system. Although Leydig cells express steroidogenic enzymes before becoming responsive to LH (El-Gehani et al, 1998; Majdic et al, 1998), they also differentiate from precursors under the influence of LH and placental-derived human chorionic gonadotropin (hCG) and from the effect of local paracrine factors such as insulin-like growth factor-1 (IGF-1) (Huhtaniemi and Pelliniemi, 1992; Teerds and Dorrington, 1993; Le Roy et al, 1999). **At 2 to 3 months after birth, a second wave of Leydig cell differentiation occurs in response to pituitary gonadotropin production, briefly elevating**

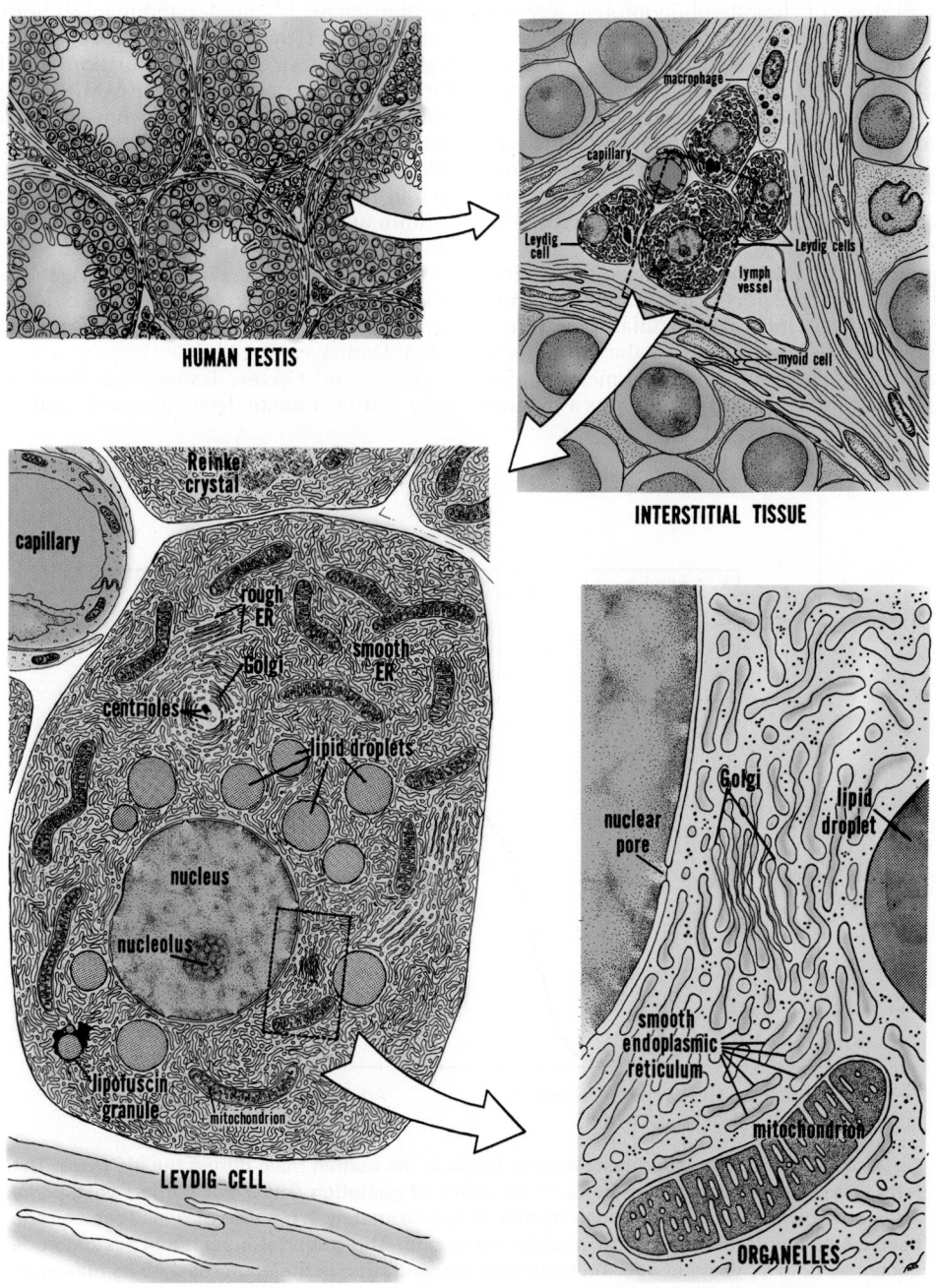

Figure 22-8. Fine structure of human Leydig cells. Leydig cells occur in clusters in the interstitium between seminiferous tubules *(upper left)*. Interstitial tissue *(upper right)* contains macrophages and fibroblasts and capillaries and lymph vessels. The most abundant organelle within the Leydig cell cytoplasm is the smooth endoplasmic reticulum *(lower left)*. Organelles seen in greater detail *(lower right)*. (From Christensen AK. Leydig cells. In: Greep RO, Astwood WB, editors. Handbook of physiology. Baltimore: Williams & Wilkins; 1975. Copyright 1975, American Physiological Society, Bethesda, MD.)

testosterone levels. Androgen produced during the early male neonate's life is thought to hormonally imprint the hypothalamus, liver, and prostate such that they respond appropriately to androgen stimulation later in life. **After reactivation of the HPG axis at puberty, stereologic analysis has revealed that a single testis from a young adult contains approximately 700 million Leydig cells** (Kaler and Neaves, 1978).

Testosterone. Testosterone, synthesized from cholesterol, is the **principal steroid produced by the testis** (Lipsett, 1974). Numerous C18, C19, and C21 steroids are also produced (Lipsett, 1974; Ewing and Brown, 1977). Cholesterol must be transported into Leydig cell mitochondria, where the cholesterol side-chain cleavage enzyme converts it to pregnenolone. The three main sources of cholesterol in the Leydig cell are (1) external, from blood-borne lipoprotein and internalization of cholesterol-lipoprotein receptor complexes, (2) de novo synthesis from acetate, and (3) stored cholesterol esters in lipid droplets. Maintenance of cholesterol stores is part of normal Leydig cell function; LH stimulation evokes cholesterol mobilization through cholesterol esterase activity. Pregnenolone is transported out of the mitochondrial membrane into the smooth endoplasmic reticulum, where it is converted into testosterone. Testosterone diffuses across the cell membrane and is trapped within the extracellular fluid and blood plasma by steroid-binding proteins.

Cholesterol transport to the inner membrane of the mitochondrion is regulated by two transport proteins: steroid acute regulatory protein (StAR) and peripheral benzodiazepine receptor (PBR). LH binding elicits StAR synthesis in the Leydig cell, which then threads through the outer mitochondrial membrane to facilitate cholesterol transport (Stocco, 2000). PBR forms a channel for cholesterol in the mitochondrial membrane (Culty et al, 1999), but it is not clear whether PBR functionally interacts with StAR (West et al, 2001).

The four major enzymes participating in testosterone biosynthesis from pregnenolone are cholesterol side-chain cleavage enzyme, 3β-hydroxysteroid dehydrogenase, cytochrome P450 17α-hydroxylase/C17-20-lyase, and 17β-hydroxysteroid dehydrogenase. The enzymology, chromosomal locations, and molecular genetics of these enzymes are well described (Payne and Hales, 2004). Mutations in the genes encoding these enzymes have been described and the resulting disorders of androgen biosynthesis are a relatively rare cause of sexual ambiguity in chromosomally normal males (Miller, 2002).

Control of Testosterone Synthesis. The control of Leydig cell steroidogenesis is complex and involves both pituitary and nonpituitary factors (Payne and Youngblood, 1995). **The most important regulator of testosterone production is LH. After binding LH, through the second messenger cAMP, Leydig cells initiate transport of cholesterol into mitochondria.** Pituitary peptides other than LH (e.g., FSH and prolactin) modify the response to LH (Ewing, 1983). Other, nonpituitary factors capable of modifying steroid production by Leydig cells include **GnRH** (Sharpe, 1984); **inhibin and activin** (Bardin et al, 1989); **epidermal growth factor (EGF), IGF-1, and TGF-β** (Ascoli and Segaloff, 1989; Saez et al, 1991); prostaglandins (Eik-Nes, 1975); and adrenergic stimulation (Eik-Nes, 1975). Moreover, direct inhibition of Leydig cell steroidogenesis may also occur through **estrogens and androgens** (Ewing, 1983; Darney et al, 1996).

Testosterone Cycles. Testosterone blood levels change dramatically during human fetal, neonatal, and adult life. Figure 22-9

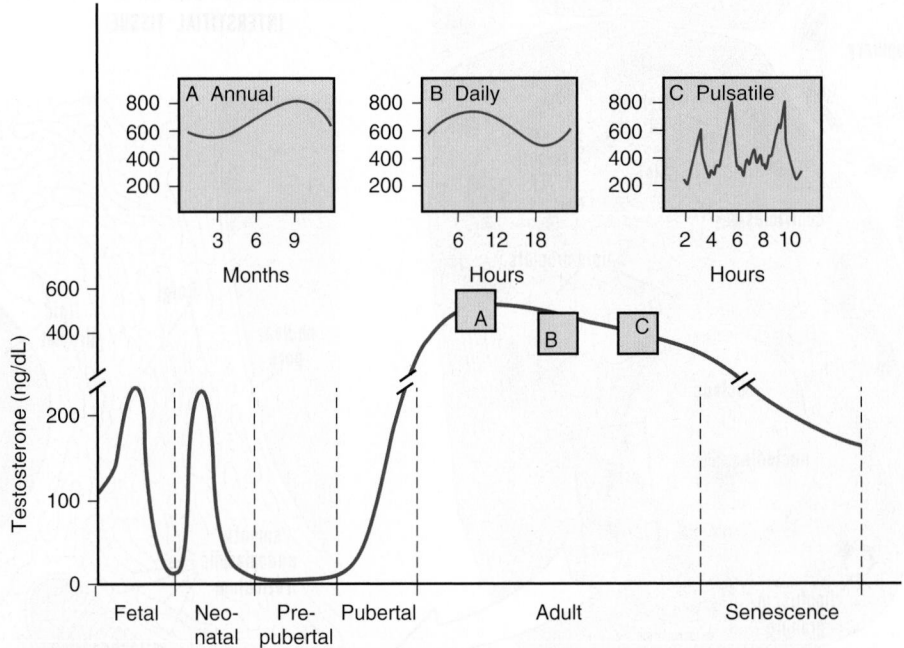

Figure 22-9. Peripheral blood testosterone levels in the human male during the life cycle. The fetal testosterone peak occurs at 12 to 18 weeks of gestation *(lower left corner; gestational age not shown).* The neonatal peak occurs at approximately 2 months of age. Testosterone declines to low levels during the prepubertal period. The pubertal increase in testosterone occurs at 12 to 17 years of age. Testosterone concentration in the adult reaches its maximum during the second or third decade of life and then declines slowly. Testosterone declines dramatically during senescence. *Inset A* shows the annual rhythm in testosterone concentration in the human male. The peak and nadir occur in the fall and spring, respectively. *Inset B* shows the daily rhythm in testosterone concentration. The peak and nadir occur in the morning and evening, respectively. *Inset C* shows the frequent and irregular fluctuations in testosterone concentration. (From Ewing LL, Davis JC, Zirkin BR. Regulation of testicular function: a spatial and temporal view. In: Greep RO, editor. International review of physiology. Baltimore: University Park Press; 1980. p. 41.)

shows that a testosterone peak occurs in the human fetus at 12 to 18 weeks of gestation. Another testosterone peak occurs at approximately 2 months of age. A third testosterone peak occurs during the second or third decade of life. After this, there is a plateau, and then a slow decline with age. Superimposed on this, there are annual and daily rhythms of testosterone production (see Fig. 22-9, *insets A and B*) and irregular daily fluctuations in testosterone (see Fig. 22-9, *inset C*). These temporal changes in testosterone production during human life reflect a complex interaction between the pituitary gland and testis. **The testosterone peaks correspond temporally to four developmental events: (1) the differentiation and development of the fetal reproductive tract, (2) the neonatal organization or "imprinting" of androgen-dependent target tissues, (3) the masculinization of the male at puberty, and (4) the maintenance of growth and function of androgen-dependent organs in the adult.** This topic has been reviewed thoroughly by Swerdloff and Heber (1981).

Seminiferous Tubules

The seminiferous tubules consist of germ cells and supporting cells and are a unique environment for gamete production. Support cells include Sertoli cells and fibrocyte and myoid cells of the basement membrane. The germ cells include a slowly dividing stem cell population, more rapidly proliferating spermatogonia and spermatocytes, and metamorphosing spermatids.

Sertoli Cells. The seminiferous tubules are lined with Sertoli cells that rest on the tubular basement membrane and extend cytoplasmic ramifications into its lumen (Fig. 22-10). The ultrastructural features of Sertoli cells are well described (Bardin et al, 1994). They have irregularly shaped nuclei, prominent nucleoli, and a low mitotic index and exhibit unique **tight junctional complexes** between adjacent Sertoli cells. **These tight junctions are the strongest intercellular barriers in the body. They divide the seminiferous tubule space into basal (basement membrane) and adluminal (lumen) compartments** (see Fig. 22-10). This anatomic arrangement forms the basis for the **blood-testis barrier** and allows spermatogenesis to occur in an immunologically privileged site. **Sertoli cells serve as nurse cells for spermatogenesis, nourishing developing germ cells within and between Sertoli cell cytoplasmic projections. The undifferentiated spermatogonia are near the basement membrane of the tubule, whereas the more advanced spermatocytes and spermatids are near the luminal surface.** Thus the Sertoli cell is a polarized epithelium in which the base approximates the plasma environment, and its apex harbors an environment unique to the seminiferous tubule (Ewing et al, 1980).

Sertoli cells nurture germ cell development by **(1) providing a specialized adluminal microenvironment, (2) supporting germ cells through gap junctions between Sertoli and germ cells, and (3) allowing migration of developing germ cells within the tubule** (see Fig. 22-10). The tight junctions between Sertoli cells are constantly remodeled to allow "opening" and "closing" necessary for germ cell interaction and migration (Mruk and Cheng, 2004). Ligand-receptor complexes, such as c-kit and kit ligand, are likely involved in mediating communication between germ and Sertoli cells. Sertoli cells also participate in germ cell phagocytosis and produce and secrete fluid and important effector molecules. ABP is one of earliest described Sertoli cell secretory products (Hansson and Djoseland, 1972). ABP is an intracellular carrier of androgen within the Sertoli cell. **By binding testosterone, ABP maintains high levels of androgen (50-fold higher than serum) within the seminiferous tubules.** Testosterone also plays an important role in the regulation of Sertoli cell function, including ABP production (Griswold et al, 1988). Inhibin is Sertoli cell derived and plays an important regulatory role in the negative feedback loop of FSH secretion. Inhibin B is emerging as an important endocrine marker of Sertoli cell function in the male infertility evaluation.

As keepers of the immunologic sanctuary in the testis, Sertoli cells maintain a germ cell microenvironment entirely distinct from that of plasma. As such, Sertoli cells secrete numerous other products including extracellular matrix components (lamin, collagen type IV, and collagen type I) and proteins such as ceruloplasmin, transferrin, glycoprotein 2, plasminogen activator, somatomedin-like substances, T proteins, H-Y antigen, clusterin, cyclic proteins, growth factors, and somatomedin (Mruk and Cheng, 2004). Steroids, such as DHT, testosterone, androstenediols, 17β-estradiol, and numerous other C21 steroids are also produced by Sertoli cells (Ewing et al, 1980; Mather et al, 1983). Although the function of many Sertoli cell and peritubular-derived substances is unclear, further research should enlighten our understanding of how Sertoli cells orchestrate and support spermatogenesis.

Germ Cells. Within the human seminiferous tubule, germ cells give rise to approximately 123×10^6 (range, 21 to 374×10^6) spermatozoa daily (Amann and Howards, 1980). This equates to the production of about 1200 sperm per heartbeat. Within the seminiferous tubule, germ cells are arranged in a highly ordered sequence from the basement membrane to the lumen. **Morphologic analysis of the various germ cells reveals at least 13 recognizable germ cell types in the human testis** (Clermont, 1963; Heller and Clermont, 1964) (Fig. 22-11). Each cell type is thought to represent a different step in the spermatogenic process. Proceeding from the least to the most differentiated, based on morphologic appearance, they have been named **dark type A spermatogonia (Ad); pale type A spermatogonia (Ap); type B spermatogonia (B); preleptotene (R), leptotene (L), zygotene (Z), and pachytene (P) primary spermatocytes; secondary spermatocytes (II); and Sa, Sb, Sc, Sd$_1$, and Sd$_2$ spermatids.** The tight junctions maintain spermatogonia and early spermatocytes within the basal compartment and all subsequent germ cells in the adluminal compartment.

Peritubular Structure

The human seminiferous tubule is surrounded by several layers of peritubular tissue (Hermo et al, 1977) (Fig. 22-12). The outer adventitial layer consists of fibrocytes. In the middle layer are myoid cells interspersed with connective tissue lamellae. The inner layer consists of a collagen matrix. In humans the peritubular myoid cells are thought to have contractile function (Toyama, 1977). Myoid cells actively secrete extracellular matrix components fibronectin and collagen type I, and produce the inner collagenous layer (Tung et al, 1984). Myoid cells may also affect Sertoli cell function and are known to associate with Sertoli cells in a precise mesenchymal-epithelial interaction. Skinner and coworkers (1988) isolated a paracrine factor produced by myoid cells, P-Mod-S (peritubular modifies Sertoli), that profoundly affects Sertoli cell synthetic and differentiation functions in vitro. Human peritubular cells have also been shown to secrete testosterone and may influence Sertoli cell activity (Cigorraga et al, 1994).

Blood-Testis Barrier

Dyes and other substances, when injected into the bloodstream of animals, will rapidly appear throughout all body tissues but fail to penetrate regions of the brain and testis. This led to the concept of the existence of a blood-testis barrier. **More appropriately termed the "blood–seminiferous tubule barrier," it has two components: an anatomic or mechanical element and functional elements.** The mechanical barrier is created, in part, by muscle-like myoid cells that surround seminiferous tubules (Dym and Fawcett, 1970; Fawcett et al, 1970). Regulation of molecular traffic also occurs at the level of capillary endothelial cells. However, the most important component of this barrier is the synaptic tight junctions between Sertoli cells that preclude the passage of large molecules and lymphocytes. These anatomic elements of the barrier are necessary but not sufficient for maintaining the immunologic "sanctuary" status within the tubule, because they are not observed in other protected areas of the reproductive tract (Tung et al, 1971; Brown et al, 1972).

Thus, although the mechanical barrier contributes to the isolation of the testis, other "functional" components must also exist to suppress the normal immune response. Several mechanisms likely work in concert to protect sperm from destruction. First, lymphocytes are excluded from anatomically vulnerable regions in the

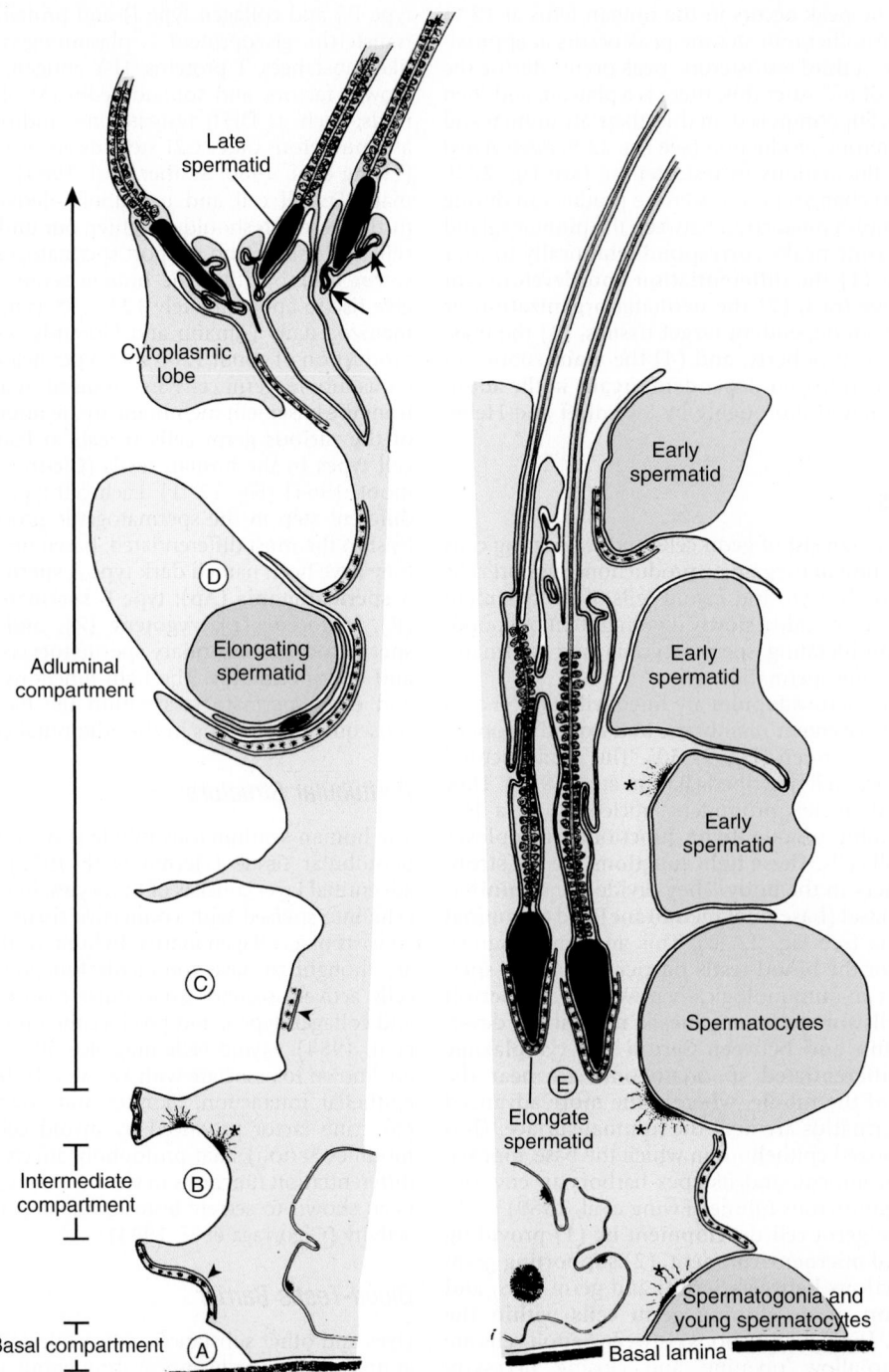

Figure 22-10. Representation of the tree-shaped Sertoli cell with a thickened central portion, or "trunk," and more delicate processes, or "limbs." Note the basal, intermediate, and adluminal compartments of the seminiferous epithelium. *A,* Spermatogonia and early spermatocytes share positions on the basal lamina and are enveloped by adjacent Sertoli cells that join to form tight junctional complexes (site of blood-testis barrier). *B,* Sertoli cells form junctional complexes both above and below leptotene-zygotene spermatocytes as they translocate from the basal to adluminal compartments. *C,* The spermatocytes enter the adluminal compartment when Sertoli tight junctions dissociate. *D,* The elongating spermatid is situated within a narrow recess of the Sertoli cell trunk. *E,* As the spermatid elongates further, the cell becomes lodged within the body of the Sertoli cell. The advanced spermatid moves toward the lumen of the epithelium in preparation for spermiation. Only the sperm head remains in intimate contact with the Sertoli cell. Specialized cell-to-cell contacts: *asterisks,* desmosome-gap junction complex; *arrowheads,* ectoplasmic specializations; *isolated arrows,* tubulobulbar complexes. (From Russell L. Sertoli-germ cell interactions: a review. Gamete Res 1980;3:179.)

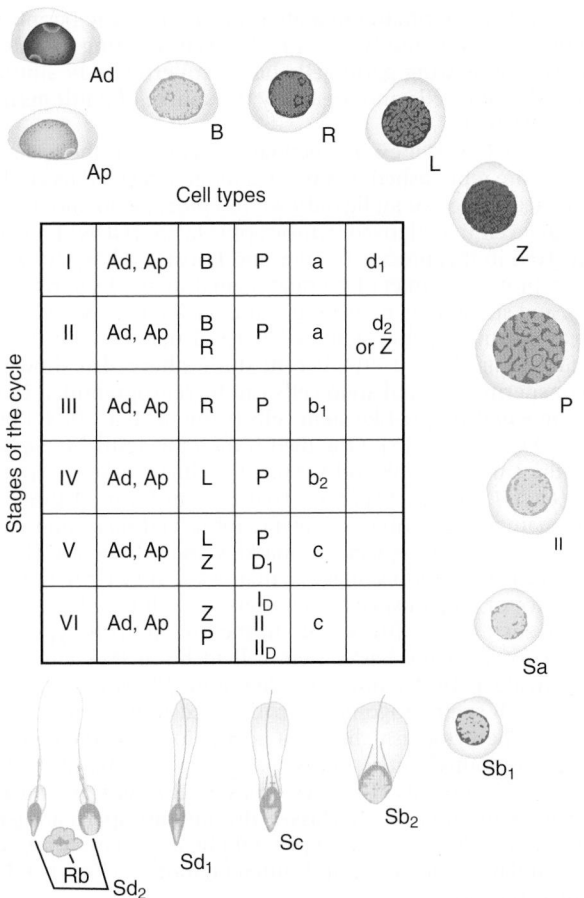

Cell types

Stages of the cycle						
I	Ad, Ap	B	P	a	d₁	
II	Ad, Ap	B R	P	a	d₂ or Z	
III	Ad, Ap	R	P	b₁		
IV	Ad, Ap	L	P	b₂		
V	Ad, Ap	L Z	P D₁	c		
VI	Ad, Ap	Z P	I_D II II_D	c		

Figure 22-11. The steps of spermatogenesis in man. Ad, dark type A spermatogonium; Ap, pale type A spermatogonium; B, type B spermatogonium; II, secondary spermatocyte; L, leptotene spermatocyte; P, pachytene spermatocyte; R, resting or preleptotene primary spermatocyte; Rb, residual body; Sa(a), Sb₁ (b₁), Sb₂ (b₂), Sc (c), Sd₁ (d₁), Sd₂ (d₂), spermatids; Z, zygotene spermatocyte. The table shows cells that make up the six stages of the "cycle" of the seminiferous epithelium (I to VI): D₁, diakinesis; ID and IID, first and second maturation divisions of spermatocytes. (Modified from Clermont Y. Renewal of spermatogonia in man. Am J Anat 1966;118:509.)

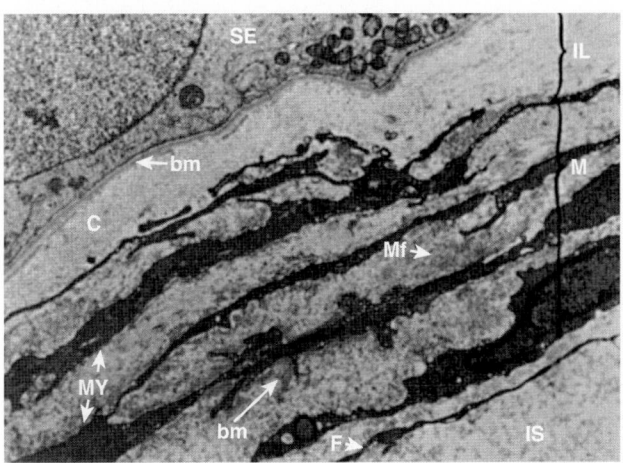

Figure 22-12. Low-power electron micrograph of human peritubular testis tissue. Peritubular tissue lies between the basement membrane (bm) of the seminiferous epithelium (SE) and the interstitial tissue (IS). Peritubular tissue has three zones: the inner lamella (IL); the myoid layer (M), containing myoid cells (MY) with abundant microfibrils (Mf); and an adventitial layer containing fibroblasts (F). (From Hermo L, Lalli M, Clermont Y. Arrangement of connective tissue elements in the walls of seminiferous tubules of man and monkey. Am J Anat 1977;148:433–46.)

germinal epithelium (Mahi-Brown et al, 1988). Second, these vulnerable regions harbor mainly T-suppressor cells (el-Demiry et al, 1985; Anderson and Hill, 1988). Owing to deficiencies in antigen–human leukocyte antigen association, there may be a lack of sperm antigen presentation to lymphocytes, impairing the immune response (Jenkins et al, 1987; Anderson and Hill, 1988). There is also evidence to suggest that immunologic tolerance plays a role in the functional blood-testis barrier. The leading theory proposes that within the anatomically weaker areas (rete testis, efferent tubule, epididymis) of the barrier, there is a small, continuous leak of sperm antigens (Tung, 1980). This leak generates T-suppressor cells and immune tolerance, similar to desensitization protocols for common environmental allergens. However, with larger antigenic challenges, a true immune response results (Turek, 1997). Cytokines may contribute to immune tolerance, including interferon-γ, soluble Fc receptor, and TGF-β (Perussia et al, 1987; Ben-Rafael and Orvieto, 1992; Turek, 1997). In addition, androgens have mild immunosuppressive activity and may regulate immunity (Diemer et al, 2003).

Why does the blood-testis barrier exist? Since it develops at spermarche during puberty (Kormano, 1967), it is likely important for meiosis. In addition, it may immunologically isolate developing male gametes that are not recognized as self by the adult male immune system. In this sense, the value of a blood-testis barrier is fully realized after puberty, because foreign "antigens" on postmeiotic germ cells exist only after spermarche. A testicular insult such as biopsy, torsion, or trauma will not induce anti-sperm antibodies if it occurs before puberty. After puberty, however, immunologic infertility is a known risk (Turek, 1997). Clinically, the blood-testis barrier may also limit chemotherapy access to cancer cells sequestered behind it and result in isolated cancer recurrence within the testis.

Spermatogenesis

Spermatogenesis is a remarkably complex and specialized process of DNA reduction and germ cell metamorphosis. Older studies have estimated that the entire process in humans requires approximately 64 days (Clermont, 1972). However, an in vivo kinetic study in healthy men revealed that the total time to produce an ejaculated sperm ranges from 42 to 76 days, suggesting that the duration of spermatogenesis can vary widely among individuals (Misell et al, 2006) (Fig. 22-13). Spermatogenesis involves (1) a proliferative phase as spermatogonia divide to replace their number (self-renewal) or differentiate into daughter cells that become mature gametes; (2) a meiotic phase when germ cells undergo a reduction division, resulting in haploid (half the normal DNA complement) spermatids; and (3) a spermiogenesis phase in which spermatids undergo a profound metamorphosis to become mature spermatozoa. (For excellent reviews, see Steinberger [1976] and de Kretser and Kerr [1988].)

A cycle of spermatogenesis involves the division of primitive spermatogonial stem cells into subsequent germ cells. Several cycles of spermatogenesis coexist within the germinal epithelium at any one time, and they are described morphologically as stages. If spermatogenesis is viewed from a single fixed point within a seminiferous tubule, six recognizable cellular associations or stages are predictably observed in humans (Heller and Clermont, 1964) (see Fig. 22-11). In addition, there is also a specific organization of spermatogenic cycles within the tubular space, termed *spermatogenic waves*. The best evidence suggests that human spermatogenesis exists in a spiral or helical cellular arrangement that ensures sperm production is a continuous and not a pulsatile process (Schulze, 1989) (Fig. 22-14).

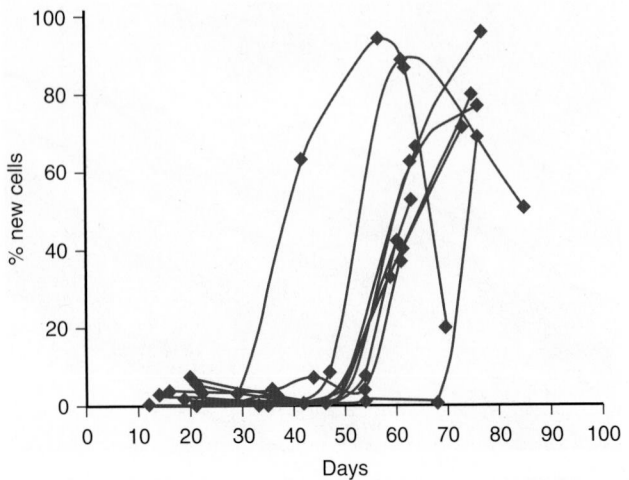

Figure 22-13. Time to make and ejaculate human sperm. Combined spermatocyte labeling curves for 11 individuals with normal semen quality who ingested 50 mL of ^2H_2O twice daily for 3 weeks. New ejaculated sperm was found as early as 42 days after ingestion of label, and there was considerable interindividual variation in the time to make and ejaculate sperm. (From Misell LM, Holochwost D, Boban D, et al. A stable isotope/mass spectrometric method for measuring the kinetics of human spermatogenesis in vivo. J Urol 2006;175:242–6.)

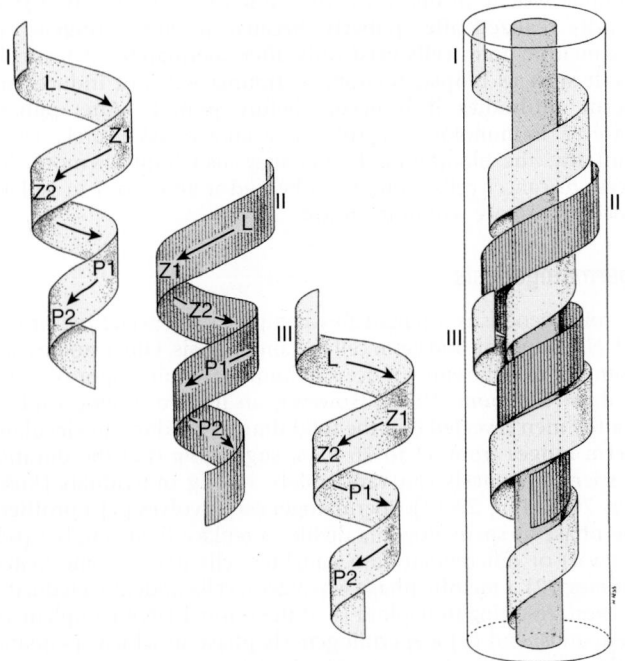

Figure 22-14. Helical configuration of seminiferous tubule epithelial cycles in man, forming overlapping waves of spermatogenesis that keep sperm production constant. (From Schulze W, Rehder U. Organization and morphogenesis of the human seminiferous epithelium. Cell Tissue Res 1984;237:395–407.)

Testis Stem Cell Migration, Renewal, and Proliferation

Testis Stem Cell Migration. During early prenatal development, **primordial germ cells** migrate to the gonadal ridge and associate with Sertoli cells to form primitive testicular cords (Witschi, 1948). These primitive germline stem cells are termed **gonocytes** after the gonad differentiates into a testis by forming seminiferous cords.

They are called **spermatogonia** after migration to the periphery of the tubule (Gondos and Hobel, 1971). **It is interesting to note that these early migrating germ cells have properties very similar to embryonic stem cells and are likely the source of adult germ cell tumors** (Ezeh et al, 2005).

Testis Stem Cell Renewal. Spermatogonia within the testis stem cell niche are replenished in a process termed *stem cell renewal*. The growth factor receptor kit ligand/c-kit receptor system and the niche factor glial cell line–derived neurotrophic factor (GDNF) appear to be involved in this process (Oatley and Brinster, 2008). In fact, the c-kit receptor is a marker of spermatogonial stem cells in rats (Dym, 1994), and spermatogenesis in the rat is a c-kit–dependent process, whereas spermatogonial stem cell renewal may be c-kit independent (Yoshinaga et al, 1991). **Recent studies have also shown that human spermatogonial stem cells can be reprogrammed in vitro to become embryonic-like stem cells** (Conrad et al, 2008; Kossack et al, 2009) (Fig. 22-15). Obtained from adult testis biopsy specimens, the embryonic-like cells express distinct markers of pluripotency (*OCT-4, SOX-2, STELLAR, GDF-3*), can form all three germ layers, maintain a normal karyotype, form teratomas, and express appropriate levels of epigenetic markers and telomerase (Kossack et al, 2009). This finding suggests that in the future the testis may be a source of patient-specific stem cells for cell-based therapy.

Testis Stem Cell Proliferation. In the human, pale type A (Ap) spermatogonia in the basal, stem cell niche of the seminiferous tubule divide at 16-day intervals (Clermont, 1972) to form B spermatogonia. B spermatogonia are committed to become spermatocytes, but the cytoplasm between spermatogonial daughter cells remains conjoined after mitosis, forming cytoplasmic bridges between adjacent cells. These **cytoplasmic bridges are observed between germ cells of all classes throughout spermatogenesis** (Ewing et al, 1980). These bridges could be important for synchronized cellular proliferation and differentiation and for regulation of gene expression.

Meiosis

Somatic cells replicate by mitosis, in which genetically identical daughter cells are formed. **Germ cells replicate by meiosis, in which the genetic material is halved to allow reproduction.** Meiosis generates genetic diversity, providing a richer source of material on which natural selection can act. Cell replication by mitosis is a precise, well-orchestrated sequence of events involving duplication of the genetic material (chromosomes), breakdown of the nuclear envelope, and equal division of the chromosomes and cytoplasm into daughter cells. **The essential difference between mitotic and meiotic replication is that a single DNA duplication step is followed by only one cell division in mitosis, but two cell divisions in meiosis (four daughter cells).** Consequently, daughter cells contain only half of the chromosome content of parent cells. Thus a diploid ($2n$) parent cell becomes a haploid (n) gamete. Other major differences between mitosis and meiosis are outlined in Table 22-2. Research has shown that small RNA molecules (small RNAs), including small interfering RNAs (siRNAs), microRNAs (miRNAs), and piwi-interacting RNAs (piRNAs), are important regulators of gene germ cell expression at the post-transcriptional or translation level (Tolia and Joshua-Tor, 2007; He et al, 2009).

Spermatogenesis begins with type B spermatogonia dividing mitotically to form primary spermatocytes within the adluminal compartment. **Mature spermatocytes are the first germ cells to undergo meiosis** (Kerr and de Kretser, 1981). In this process, a meiotic division is followed by a typical mitotic reduction division, resulting in daughter cells with a haploid chromosome complement. In addition, as a consequence of chromosomal recombination, each daughter cell contains different genetic information. The resultant cell is the Sa spermatid (see Fig. 22-11).

Chromosomal recombination, the defining feature of mammalian meiosis, ensures that haploid gametes differ genetically from their adult precursors and is the real engine of genetic diversity and evolution. During meiotic prophase, formation of a synaptonemal complex with pairing of homologous (maternal and

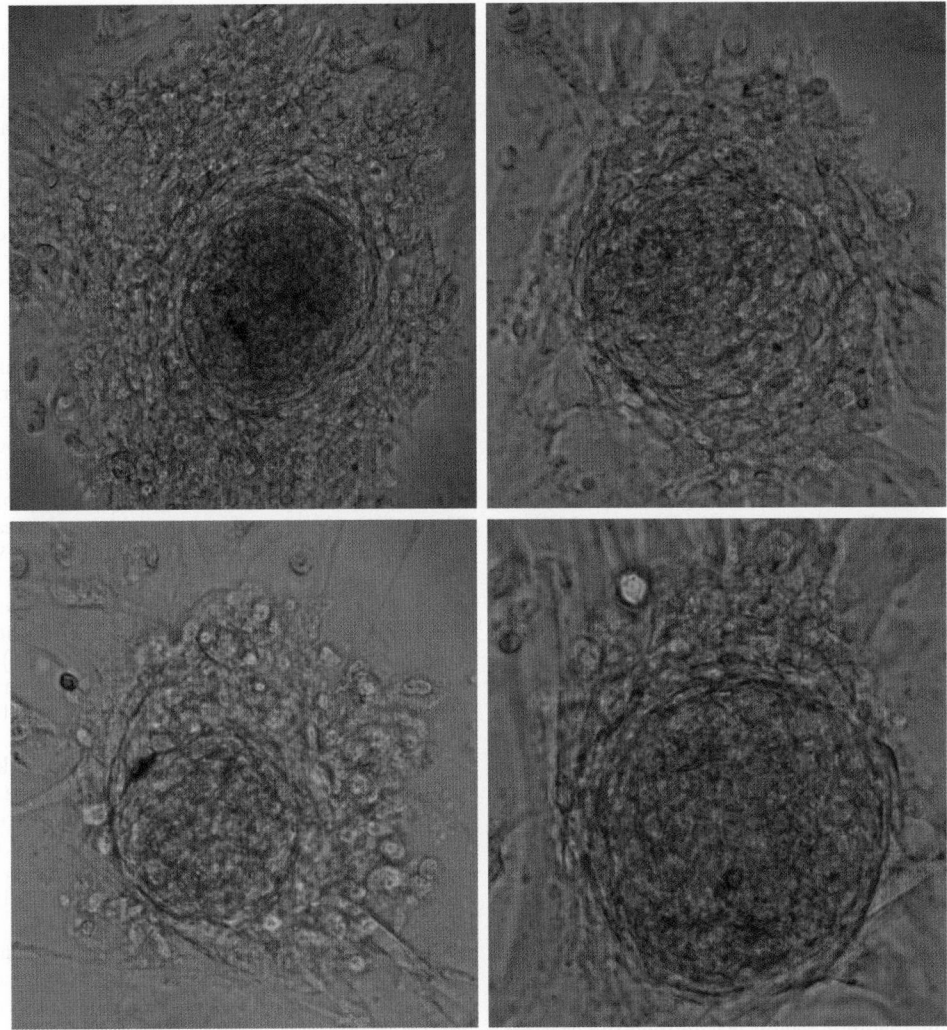

Figure 22-15. Microphotograph of four different colonies of adult testis spermatogonial-derived stem cells. Cell clusters are the result of reprogramming of adult spermatogonia in culture conditions used for human embryonic stem cells (HESCs). They exhibit the typical cobblestone appearance of HESCs and are functionally multipotent.

paternal) chromosomes occurs, along with physical interaction and exchange of DNA through reciprocal sites of crossing over (**chiasmata**) between homologs. Recent research has shown that defects in the fidelity of recombination within human male germ cells can cause azoospermia and male infertility (Walsh et al, 2009). **In one study, 10% of nonobstructive azoospermic men had significant defects in recombination compared with men with normal spermatogenesis** (Gonsalves et al, 2004). In addition, among men with maturation arrest pattern on testis biopsy, faulty recombination was observed in about half of cases, providing evidence that faulty recombination is linked to poor sperm production (Gonsalves et al, 2004). Variations in recombination also have implications for sperm aneuploidy, because alterations in crossover position are risk factors for chromosomal nondisjunction. **Indeed, evidence suggests that the correlation of faulty recombination and sperm aneuploidy in azoospermic men is strong enough to explain the higher rate of chromosomal abnormalities in offspring conceived with in vitro fertilization (IVF) and intracytoplasmic sperm injection (ICSI)** (Sun et al, 2008).

Spermiogenesis

During spermiogenesis, round Sa spermatids mature into spermatozoa (see Fig. 22-11). During this maturation sequence, cell division does not occur, but there are extensive changes to the spermatid

TABLE 22-2 Essential Differences: Mitosis and Meiosis

MITOSIS	MEIOSIS
Occurs in somatic cells	Occurs in sexual cells
One cell division, two daughter cells	Two cell divisions, four daughter cells
Chromosome number maintained	Chromosome number halved
No pairing, chromosome homologs	Synapse of homologs, prophase I
No crossovers	More than one crossover per homolog pair
Centromeres divide, anaphase	Centromeres divide, anaphase II
Identical daughter genotype	Genetic variation in daughter cells

nucleus and cytoplasm. **These include the loss of cytoplasm, migration of cytoplasmic organelles, formation of the acrosome from the Golgi apparatus, formation of the flagellum from the centriole, nuclear compaction to about 10% of former size, and reorganization of mitochondria around the sperm midpiece**

(Kerr and de Kretser, 1981). The nucleus of the round spermatid changes from spheric to asymmetrical as chromatin condenses. Many cellular elements contribute to the reshaping process, including chromosome structure, associated chromosomal proteins, the perinuclear cytoskeletal theca layer, the manchette of nuclear microtubules, subacrosomal actin, and Sertoli cell interactions. With completion of spermatid elongation, the Sertoli cell cytoplasm retracts around the developing sperm, stripping it of all unnecessary cytoplasm and extruding it into the tubule lumen. The mature sperm has remarkably little cytoplasm and is produced in massive quantities—up to 300 per gram of testis per second.

Sertoli Cell–Germ Cell Interaction

A complex network of cell-cell interactions exists within the testis between Leydig cells and Sertoli cells, between Leydig cells and peritubular cells, between Sertoli and peritubular cells, and between Sertoli cells and germ cells. Several Sertoli cell–germ cell associations in mammalian testes are illustrated in Figure 22-10 (Russell and Clermont, 1976; Romrell and Ross, 1979; Skinner, 1995). In addition, there are factors that can reversibly disrupt the blood-testis barrier, including TGF-β3 and tumor necrosis factor-α (TNF-α). These substances act by reducing the levels of occludin and zonula occludens-1 (ZO-1) in the barrier through a p38 mitogen-activated protein (MAP) kinase signaling pathway (Xia et al, 2009). This represents only a piece of the remarkably complex and highly interactive process that characterizes spermatogenesis.

Genetics

Genetic causes of abnormal spermatogenesis have been identified as point mutations in single genes inherited in mendelian fashion (e.g., cystic fibrosis), and as chromosomal disorders in which segments of (or entire) chromosomes have structural or numerical abnormalities. The reader is referred to Turek and Reijo Pera (2002) for a comprehensive review of such disorders. The postulation that deletions in the long arm of the Y chromosome cause azoospermia was made over three decades ago (Tiepolo et al, 1976). Based on cytogenetic analysis, this theoretic region was termed the *azoospermia factor* (AZF). **Currently, the positional patterns of deletions (termed *microdeletions*) in the AZF region are used to subdivide this region into AZFa, AZFb, and AZFc subregions** (Vogt et al, 1996). **Regional deletions of the Y chromosome, termed *Yq microdeletions*, occur in 6% to 8% of severely oligospermic men and in 15% of azoospermic men** (Reijo et al, 1996). Taken together, such deletions are the most commonly defined molecular cause of male infertility (Kostiner et al, 1998).

There is emerging literature addressing the prognostic value of specific AZF deletions. In contrast to partial and complete AZFc-deletion patients, in whom sperm is often found on semen analysis or testis biopsy, the chance of finding ejaculated or testis sperm in men with complete AZFa or AZFb deletions is highly unlikely (Hopps et al, 2003). Complete AZFa deletions are associated with germ cell aplasia or Sertoli cell–only histology. In general, complete AZFb deletions are associated with maturation arrest at the primary spermatocyte (early) or spermatid (late) stages. AZFc deletions are associated with hypospermatogenesis or a Sertoli cell–only pattern with foci of spermatogenesis. Sperm have been detected in ejaculates of men with presumed and confirmed partial AZFa and AZFb deletions (Foresta et al, 2001). Similarly, ejaculated sperm in men with AZFa + b, and AZFb + c deletions (presumably partial deletions) has also been reported, but the finding of AZFa – c deletions has been associated with azoospermia and no sperm on testis biopsy.

More recently, it has become clear that the **X chromosome** is also important for spermatogenesis, first postulated in rodent studies. In 2001, Wang and colleagues reported on a systematic search for genes expressed exclusively in mouse spermatogonia (Wang et al, 2001). Twenty-five genes were identified by complementary DNA (cDNA) subtraction, of which 10 localized to the X chromosome, suggesting that the X chromosome may have a key role in premeiotic stages of spermatogenesis. A recent comparison of the mouse and human X chromosomes suggests that this chromosome may lead a double life and contribute significantly to both human male and female fertility (Mueller et al, 2013). Mutation studies of X-linked genes in male infertility patients have identified the *SOX3* gene (sex determining region Y box 3) and the *FATE* gene as two potential candidate fertility genes (Olesen et al, 2003; Raverot et al, 2004). In the future, mutations in these and other X chromosome genes have the potential to define many currently unexplained cases of male infertility.

Genetics and Paternal Age

Age-Related Sperm Chromosomal Anomalies. The aneuploidy status and polyploidy status of sperm were first investigated owing to concern that advanced paternal age was associated with increased cases of trisomy, especially trisomy 21 or Down syndrome, in offspring. With fluorescence in situ hybridization (FISH) technology, subtle paternal-age effects on sperm aneuploidy are now evident. **The paternal age effect appears to increase the fraction of sperm with sex chromosomal aneuploidies** (Wyrobek et al, 1996). **However, there is little evidence to support a paternal age–related increase in aneuploid births, except for possibly trisomy 21 and disomy 1 (very rare).** Examining sperm chromosome structural abnormalities, Martin and Rademaker (1987) found that a significant linear relationship exists between paternal age and the frequency of structural anomalies in sperm ($r = 0.63$). **One explanation for this association may be that continued cell division during spermatogenesis places germ cells at risk for chromosomal injury, especially with advanced paternal age.** Except for reciprocal translocations, however, there is little evidence to indicate that this association leads to an increased frequency of offspring with de novo structural chromosomal anomalies.

Age-Related Sperm Genetic Mutations. Single gene defects in sperm result from errors in DNA replication. To date, it has been difficult to assess the presence or absence of such defects in sperm. However, the effect of advanced paternal age on conditions in offspring associated with single-gene deletions is clear. These disorders are listed in Box 22-1 and consist of autosomal dominant diseases that have known associations with advanced paternal age. They are termed *sentinel phenotypes* because they are disorders of significant

---

BOX 22-1 Genetic Disorders in Offspring Associated with Advanced Paternal Age

Achondroplasias
Aniridia
Apert syndrome
Bilateral retinoblastoma
Crouzon syndrome
Fibrodysplasia ossificans
Hemophilia A
Lesch-Nyhan syndrome
Marfan syndrome
Neurofibromatosis
Oculodentodigital syndrome
Polycystic kidney disease
Polyposis coli
Progeria
Treacher Collins syndrome
Tuberous sclerosis
Waardenburg syndrome
Schizophrenia (postulated)
Bipolar disorder (postulated)
Autism (postulated)

frequency and low fitness, and stem from highly penetrant mutations. **One mechanism for the development of new single-gene mutations with age implicates the characteristic and continuous process of spermatogonial cell division in spermatogenesis.** By puberty, 30 cell divisions of spermatogonia have occurred, resulting in a large pool of undifferentiated cells. After puberty, 23 divisions per year occur in these cells. **The simple fact that the spermatogonia of older men have undergone numerous cell divisions may make them more likely to harbor errors in DNA transcription, the source of single-gene defects.** Formal risk estimates exist for the contribution of advanced paternal age to autosomal dominant mutations: In men younger than 29 years, the risk of a mutation occurring in offspring is 0.22 per 1000 births. This risk doubles (0.45 per 1000) at paternal ages 40 to 44, and then climbs to 3.7 per 1000 births at ages older than 45 (Friedman, 1981).

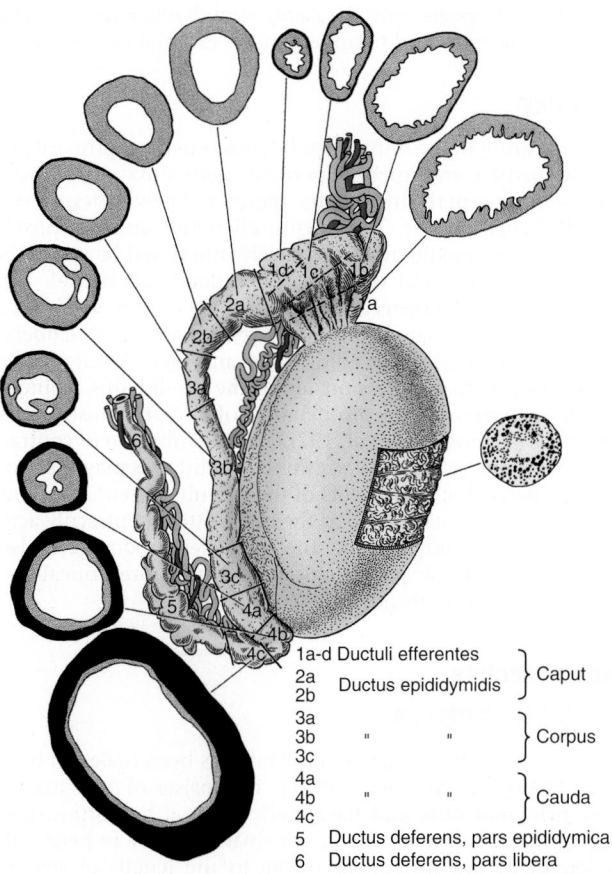

1a-d	Ductuli efferentes	} Caput
2a	Ductus epididymidis	
2b		
3a		} Corpus
3b	" "	
3c		
4a		} Cauda
4b	" "	
4c		
5	Ductus deferens, pars epididymica	
6	Ductus deferens, pars libera	

Figure 22-16. Drawing of the human epididymis showing regionalization of the ductal epithelium and muscle layer. Epididymal segment locations are shown in cross section and are identified by number. (From Baumgarten HG, Holstein AF, Rosengren E. Arrangement, ultrastructure, and adrenergic innervation of smooth musculature of the ductal efferentes, ductus epididymidis, and ductus deferens in man. Z Zellforsch Mikrosk Anat 1971;120:37.)

KEY POINTS: TESTIS

- The testis contains 250 meters of seminiferous tubules and 700 million Leydig cells in the young adult.
- Spermatogenesis occurs in stages, cycles, and waves to ensure constant sperm production.
- Genes on the X, as well as the Y, chromosome govern spermatogenesis and contribute to male infertility.
- With paternal age, there are increases in structural chromosomal abnormalities in sperm and autosomal dominant mutations leading to sentinel phenotypes in offspring.

EPIDIDYMIS

Gross Architecture

The epididymis is a comma-shaped organ located along the posterolateral surface of the testis. **Passage through the epididymis induces many changes to newly formed sperm, including gains in functional motility, and alterations in surface charge, membrane proteins, immunoreactivity, phospholipids, fatty acid content, and adenylate cyclase activity. These changes improve cell membrane structural integrity, increase fertilization ability, and improve motility.** Spermatozoa within the testis have very poor or no motility. They become progressively motile and functional only after traversing the epididymis. The transit time of sperm through the epididymis is thought to take 12 days in humans (Johnson and Varner, 1988).

The epididymis is a tubule or duct that is 3 to 4 meters in length and is tightly coiled and encapsulated within the sheath of connective tissue of the tunica vaginalis (Lanz and Neuhauser, 1964; Turner et al, 1978). Extensions from the sheath enter interductal spaces and form septa that divide the duct into histologically characteristic regions (Kormano and Reijonen, 1976). **Anatomically, these are classically divided into three regions: caput or head, corpus or body, and cauda or tail** (Fig. 22-16). The caput epididymis consists of 8 to 12 ductuli efferentes from the testis. The lumen of the ductuli efferentes is large and somewhat irregular in shape near the testis, becoming narrow and oval near the junction with the ductus epididymis. Distal to this junction, the duct diameter increases slightly and thereafter remains constant in the corpus epididymis. In the bulky cauda epididymis, the tubule diameter enlarges substantially and acquires an irregular shape. Progressing distally, the tubule gradually assumes the characteristic appearance of the vas deferens.

Vascular and Lymph Supply

In humans, the caput and the corpus epididymis receive arterial blood from a branch of the testicular artery (see Fig. 22-7). It subsequently divides into superior and inferior epididymal branches (MacMillan, 1954). The epididymis also receives blood from

branches of the deferential arteries (artery of the vas deferens), and collateral vessels connect the deferential artery to the testicular blood supply. The cauda epididymis is supplied by branches of the deferential artery. **The deferential and cremasteric arteries serve as collateral sources to the epididymis, when the main testicular artery is obstructed or ligated.** The arterial branches within the epididymis enter along septa formed from the connective tissue sheath. These vessels coil extensively before transforming into the straight vessels of the microvascular bed (Kormano and Reijonen, 1976). Microvascularization density varies significantly along the length of the epididymis, with the proximal caput containing the densest subepithelial capillary network, and the more distal segments harboring less dense vascularization. From animal studies, the epididymal capillary network is under hormonal control. For example, in rabbits, bilateral hormonal castration results in progressive deterioration and eventual disappearance of the epididymal capillary network (Clavert et al, 1981). It is not clear whether vascularization in the human epididymis is similarly controlled.

According to MacMillan (1954), venous drainage from the corpus and cauda epididymis joins to form the vena marginalis epididymis of Haberer. These veins drain into the pampiniform plexus through the vena marginalis testis, or through the cremasteric or deferential veins. Lymphatic drainage of the epididymis occurs through two routes (Wenzel and Kellermann, 1966). Lymph from the caput and corpus epididymis is removed through the same route as that described for the testis. These vessels course beside the internal spermatic vein and ultimately terminate in the preaortic nodes. Lymph vessels from the cauda epididymis join those draining the vas deferens and terminate in the external iliac nodes.

Innervation

The innervation of the human epididymis is derived primarily from the intermediate and inferior spermatic nerves that arise from the superior portion of the hypogastric plexus and pelvic plexus, respectively (Mitchell, 1935). The ductuli efferentes and the proximal segments of the epididymis are sparsely innervated by sympathetic fibers (Baumgarten and Holstein, 1967; Baumgarten et al, 1968). In these regions, the fibers are observed in a peritubular plexus and are principally associated with blood vessels. Many more fibers are observed in the midcorpus epididymis, and their density increases progressively with progression along the epididymis, coincident with the appearance and proliferation of smooth muscle cells in these areas (Baumgarten et al, 1971). The distribution of contractile cells and sympathetic nerves within the epididymis may explain the rhythmic peristaltic movements of the ductuli efferentes and initial epididymal segments, as well as the intermittent contractile activity of the cauda epididymis and the vas deferens during emission (Risely, 1963). These physiologic contractions are critical to the movement of sperm through the epididymis.

Cytoarchitecture

Epididymal Epithelium

The histology of the human epididymis has been reviewed by Holstein (1969) and Vendrely (1981). It consists of two main cell types: **principal cells and basal cells** (seen at low ultrastructural magnification in Figure 22-17). Principal cells vary in height along the length of the epididymis owing to the length of stereocilia (microvilli, not cilia). In general, tall stereocilia (120 μm) are found in the proximal epididymis, and smaller or shorter stereocilia (50 μm) are observed in more distal regions. The nuclei in principal cells are elongated and often possess large clefts and one or two nucleoli. Consistent with the idea that principal cells carry out both absorptive and secretive processes, their cellular apices have numerous coated pits, micropinocytotic vesicles, multivesicular bodies, irregularly shaped membranous vesicles, and an extensive Golgi apparatus. Because these cytologic features vary along the length of the epididymis, it suggests that there is varying absorptive and secretory capacity along the length of the duct (Vendrely and Dadoune, 1988).

There are far fewer basal cells than principal cells lining the epididymal epithelium, and they are dispersed among the more numerous principal cells. Tear-shaped basal cells rest on the basal lamina and extend toward the lumen, their apices forming threads between adjacent principal cells. They are thought to be derived from macrophages. Unlike the principal cells, the morphology of basal cells remains relatively constant throughout the epididymal duct. They are thought to be the precursors of principal cells.

The epithelium of the epididymis exhibits regional differences along its length. Within the epididymis proper, the epithelium is pseudostratified and consists of principal and basal cells as described earlier. Proximally, at the junction of the rete testis and ductuli efferentes, there is a distinct transition from a low to a high cuboidal epithelium. The epithelium in the ductuli efferentes consists of ciliated and nonciliated cells (Holstein, 1969). The ciliated cells conduct sperm from the efferent ducts into the epididymis. The nonciliated cells with protruding apices are likely secretory in nature and predominate in the proximal ductuli efferentes (Vendrely, 1981). Other nonciliated cells have microvilli suggestive of resorptive activity and predominate in the distal ductuli efferentes. Both nonciliated and ciliated cells are joined apically through junctional complexes. This suggests the existence of a blood-epididymis barrier analogous to the blood-testis barrier (Suzuki and Nagano, 1978; Hoffer and Hinton, 1984). **Although not as dense as the blood-testis barrier, the blood-epididymis barrier extends from the caput to the cauda epididymis and may play an important role**

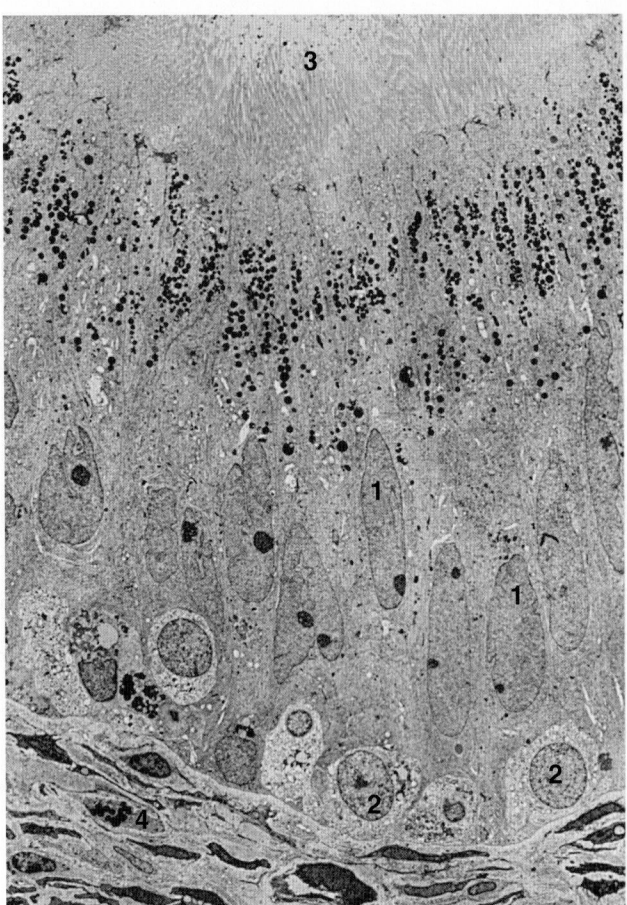

Figure 22-17. Electron micrograph of a human epididymis in cross section. Major components of the luminal epithelium are principal cells (1), basal cells (2), stereocilia (3), and myofilaments (4). Magnification approximately ×1800. (From Holstein AF. In: Hafez ESE, editor. Human semen and fertility regulation in men. St. Louis: Mosby; 1976.)

in influencing the composition of fluid within different segments of the epididymal lumen (Turner, 1979).

Epididymal Contractile Tissue. Peripheral to the basal lamina of the ductuli efferentes and the epididymal tubule are various contractile cells (Baumgarten et al, 1971) (see Fig. 22-17). In the ductuli efferentes (distal regions of the caput and the proximal corpus epididymis), the contractile cells form a loose layer, two to four cells deep, around the tubule. These cells contain myofilaments and are connected by numerous nexus-like junctions. In the distal corpus epididymis, there are larger contractile cells with fewer nexus-like intracellular junctions that resemble smooth muscle cells. In the cauda epididymis, the thin contractile cells are replaced by thick smooth muscle cells that form three layers—the outer two layers oriented longitudinally and the central layer circularly. This distal contractile layer increases in thickness as it forms the vas deferens. The contractile tissue throughout the epididymis is likely involved in sperm transport.

Epididymal Function

Described variations in the anatomy and histology of the epididymal tubule from the caput to cauda regions suggest that the epididymis is actually several different functional tissues (Vendrely, 1981). It is clear that sperm transport and storage, fertilizing ability, and motility maturation are several consequences of epididymal passage. This is addressed more fully in reviews by Robaire and Hermo (1988) and Moore and Smith (1988).

Sperm Transport

Sperm transport through the human epididymis has been calculated to take from 2 to 12 days (Johnson and Varner, 1988). **Sperm transit time through the caput-corpus epididymis is roughly similar to the transit time through the cauda epididymis and is more likely related to daily testicular sperm production rather than a man's age or the frequency of ejaculation** (Amann, 1981; Johnson and Varner, 1988). In one study, sperm epididymal transit time averaged 2 days in men with a high daily rate of sperm production, compared with 6 days in men with low daily sperm production (Johnson and Varner, 1988). Although the frequency of sexual activity does not affect sperm transit time through the caput and corpus epididymis, "recent emissions" can reduce transit time through the cauda epididymis by 68% (Amann, 1981).

Because normal human testicular sperm are immotile as they enter the epididymis, and remain relatively immotile within the caput, **mechanisms other than sperm motility must exist to transport sperm through the epididymis.** Animal studies have been very revealing in this regard (Bedford, 1975; Hamilton, 1977; Courot, 1981; Jaakkola and Talo, 1982; Jaakkola, 1983). Initially, sperm are carried into the ductuli efferentes by rete testis fluid, and **fluid flow is facilitated by fluid resorption by ductal epithelial cells mediated by the estrogen receptor.** Motile cilia and myoid cell contractions within the ductuli efferentes also assist with sperm movement. **Within the epididymis proper, the principal mechanism responsible for sperm transport is likely the spontaneous, rhythmic contraction of the contractile cells surrounding the epididymal duct.**

Sperm Storage

After migrating through the caput and corpus epididymis, sperm are retained in the cauda epididymis for varying lengths of time, depending on the frequency of sexual activity. In men 21 to 55 years of age, **an average of 155 to 209 million sperm are present in each epididymis** (Amann, 1981; Johnson and Varner, 1988), **and approximately half are stored in the caudal region.**

Spermatozoa stored in the cauda epididymis, unlike testicular sperm, are capable of progressive motility and are able to fertilize eggs. The exact amount of time that sperm can remain fertile within the epididymis is unclear, but animal studies have shown that sperm can remain viable for several weeks after vas deferens ligation (Hammond and Asdell, 1926; Young, 1929). However, it is also clear that sperm fertility measured in vivo diminishes when sperm are maintained in the epididymis for prolonged periods of time (Cooper and Orgebin-Crist, 1977; Cuasnicu and Bedford, 1989). In humans, sperm aging as a result of extended epididymal transit time and prolonged storage may contribute to reduced fertility (Johnson and Varner, 1988).

The exact fate of unejaculated epididymal sperm is unknown. In animals, sperm are lost through spontaneous seminal discharge, through oral self-cleaning (Martan, 1969), in urine (Lino et al, 1967), or by epididymal reabsorption (Amann and Almquist, 1961). Phagocytosis of spermatozoa by macrophages (spermiophages) within the epididymal lumen has been observed in humans after ligation of the vas deferens (Alexander, 1972). However, whether this mechanism can remove large numbers of spermatozoa from the epididymis of unvasectomized men is unclear.

Sperm Maturation

Sperm Motility. Sperm gain an increased capacity for motility with migration through the epididymis. This is observed as both a change in the pattern of motility and as an increase in the proportion of sperm exhibiting "mature" motility patterns. Bedford and coworkers (1973) first observed that the majority of sperm from the ductuli efferentes, when placed in culture medium, are immotile or show only weak, twitching movement. Occasionally, they also observed sperm showing "immature" tail movements characterized by "thrashing" beats in wide arcs that result in little

forward progression. The proportion of sperm with this immature motility pattern increased within the initial epididymal segment. However, in the corpus region, the proportion of sperm exhibiting this motility pattern decreased. Within the corpus region, there was an increase in the fraction of sperm with a "mature" motility pattern characterized by high-frequency, low-amplitude beats that result in progressive motility (Fig. 22-18). Within the cauda epididymis, more than 50% of sperm had a mature motility pattern, with the remainder either immotile or showing the immature motility patterns described earlier. Moore and colleagues (1983) also formally demonstrated the increased capacity of human sperm to show progressive forward motility with epididymal transit. When placed in buffer in vitro, increasing proportions of sperm were motile as they progressed from the efferent ducts to the caput, proximal corpus, distal corpus, and cauda epididymis (Fig. 22-19).

The relative importance of overall epididymal contact time versus region-specific maturation to gains in mature sperm motility patterns is unknown. Animal studies indicate that motility maturation may, in part, be an intrinsic sperm process that occurs independent of specific epididymal interactions. For example, although hamster and rabbit sperm are in general immotile within the caput epididymis, motile sperm are found in this region (albeit developing motility far more slowly and persisting for shorter periods than in the normal system) after epididymal duct ligation within the corpus region (Orgebin-Crist, 1969; Horan and Bedford, 1972). Human studies in obstructed patients with congenital absence of the vas deferens or epididymal obstruction also frequently report poor motility in spermatozoa aspirated from the distal epididymis, and better sperm motility in the proximal epididymis (Silber, 1989; Matthews et al, 1995). When combined, **these observations suggest that spermatozoa are able to develop motility based on contact time with the proximal epididymal epithelium.** However, this maturation process may not be the same as that which occurs through sperm interaction with the epididymis during migration through all ductal regions.

Sperm Fertility. Testicular sperm are incapable of fertilizing eggs unless injected into them with micromanipulation (Orgebin-Crist, 1969; Bedford, 1974; Yanagimachi, 2005). In most animals, the ability of sperm to fertilize eggs is acquired gradually as the sperm pass through the distal epididymis (see Fig. 22-19). Indeed, it has

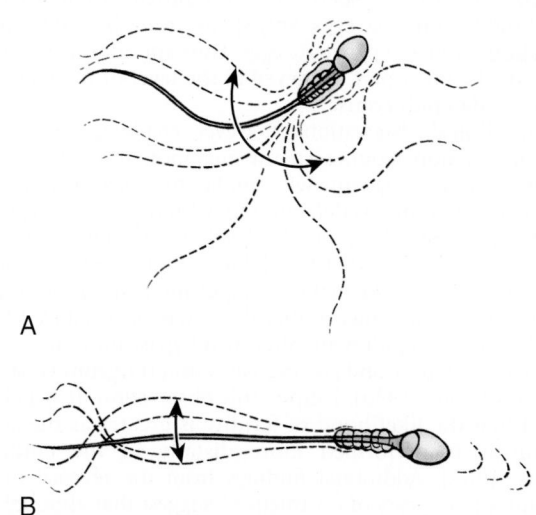

A

B

Figure 22-18. **Patterns of tail movement of human epididymal sperm. A, The pattern shown by sperm taken from the proximal epididymis is characterized by high-amplitude, low-frequency beats producing little forward movement. B, In contrast, tail movement in a large proportion of sperm from the cauda epididymis is characterized by low-amplitude, rapid beats with forward progression. (From Bedford JM, Calvin HI, Cooper GW. The maturation of spermatozoa in the human epididymis. J Reprod Fertil 1973;18:199–213.)**

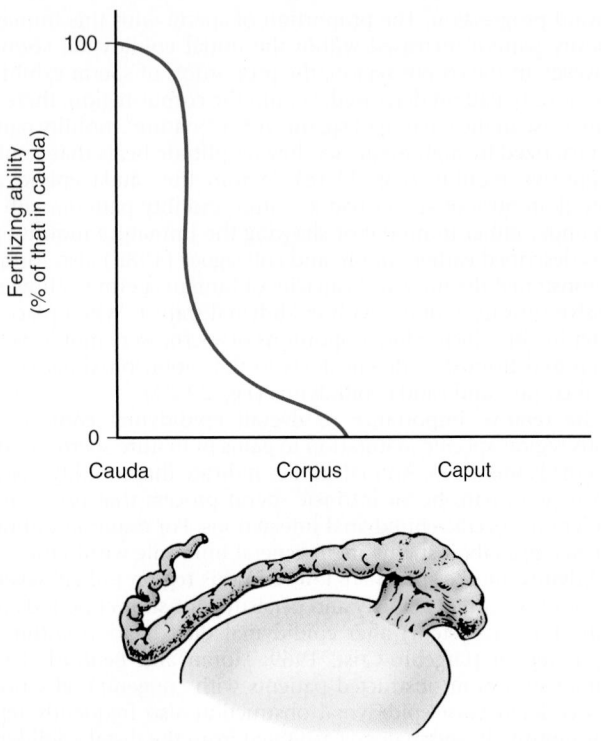

Figure 22-19. Sperm fertility maturation in the human epididymis. Sperm fertilizing ability was assessed using zona pellucida–free hamster eggs and by changes in motility. (From Bedford JM. The bearing of epididymal function in strategies for in vitro fertilization and gamete intrafallopian transfer. Ann N Y Acad Sci 1988;541:284–91.)

been shown in rabbits that sperm from the caput, corpus, and cauda epididymis can fertilize 1%, 63%, and 92% of rabbit eggs, respectively (Orgebin-Crist, 1969). Human in vitro experiments using zona pellucida–free hamster eggs have corroborated these findings (Moore et al, 1983). In a study that assessed the fertilizing capacity of human epididymal sperm, Hinrichsen and Blaquier (1980) demonstrated that although sperm from the proximal epididymis are able to bind to zona-free eggs, only sperm from the cauda epididymis can both bind and penetrate eggs. **Thus sperm fertility maturation is, for the most part, achieved at the level of the late corpus or early cauda epididymis.**

Recent clinical observations, however, challenge the idea that fertility maturation requires sperm migration through the entire epididymis. Indeed, patients with epididymal obstruction or congenital absence of the vas deferens can achieve natural pregnancies after vasoepididymostomy at the level of the ductuli efferentes (Schoysman and Bedford, 1986; Silber, 1989). This suggests that obstruction induces proximal skewing of the maturation sequence along the epididymal duct or that there may be a reduced flow of sperm through the epididymis after such bypass procedures, allowing more contact time and sperm maturation (Orgebin-Crist, 1969; Turner and Roddy, 1990). Despite this observation, **it is generally believed that the likelihood of fertility is greater as the surgical anastomosis is performed more distally in the epididymis** (Thomas, 1987). Additional findings from the reversal of older vasectomies (>15 years of obstruction) suggest that although postoperative ejaculated sperm concentrations are maintained after reversals with prolonged obstructive intervals, sperm motility is significantly decreased. This indicates that acquired epididymal dysfunction resulting from prolonged blockage may play an important role in the fertility potential of men after vasectomy reversal (Mui et al, 2014).

Sperm Biochemical Changes. Sperm undergo many biochemical changes with passage through the epididymis (Brooks, 1983). **Epididymal sperm transit induces a net negative surface membrane charge** (Bedford et al, 1973), **and sperm membrane sulfhydryl groups oxidize to disulfide bonds, improving sperm structural rigidity necessary for progressive motility and egg penetration** (Bedford et al, 1973; Reyes et al, 1976). Other post-testicular modifications of sperm membranes include changes in sperm lectin-binding properties (Courtens and Fournier-Delpech, 1979; Olson and Danzo, 1981), phospholipid and lipid content (Nikolopoulou et al, 1985), glycoprotein composition (Brown et al, 1983), immunoreactivity (Tezón et al, 1985), and iodination characteristics (Olson and Danzo, 1981). **Overall, these membrane modifications during epididymal passage may enhance sperm adherence to the egg zona pellucida** (Orgebin-Crist and Fournier-Delpech, 1982; Blobel et al, 1990). Sperm also undergo numerous metabolic changes during epididymal transit (Dacheux and Paquignon, 1980). These include an increased capacity for glycolysis (Hoskins et al, 1975), changes in intracellular pH and calcium content, modification of adenylate cyclase activity (Casillas et al, 1980), and alterations in cellular phospholipid and phospholipid-like fatty acid content (Voglmayr, 1975).

Regulation of Epididymal Function

Sperm changes within the epididymis are likely influenced by fluids and secretions within the epididymal lumen (Robaire and Hermo, 1988; Blaquier et al, 1989). The biochemical composition of epididymal fluid differs from that of serum and also shows regional differences in osmolarity, electrolyte content, and protein composition (Robaire and Hermo, 1988). These differences are likely the consequence of variations in vascularization, blood-epididymis barrier activity, and selective absorption and secretion of substances such as glycerylphosphorylcholine (GPC), carnitine, and sialic acids along the epididymal duct. Proteins within epididymal fluid that are known to have physiologic effects on sperm in vitro include forward motility protein (Brandt et al, 1978), sperm survival factor (Morton et al, 1978), progressive motility sustaining factor (Sheth et al, 1981), sperm motility-inhibiting factor (Turner and Giles, 1982), acidic epididymal glycoprotein (Pholpramool et al, 1983), and the EP2-EP3 proteins that induce sperm binding to zona pellucida (Cuasnicu et al, 1984; Blaquier et al, 1988). Thus, variations in epididymal tubule fluid characteristics play an important role in sperm maturation during epididymal transit. It is not surprising, then, that the epididymis is a potentially important source of sperm dysfunction and male infertility.

Epididymal function is hormonally regulated. Testosterone and DHT are found in very high concentrations within the epididymis and do not show regional gradients in androgen levels (Leinonen et al, 1980). This suggests the importance of androgens for epididymal function (Brooks and Tiver, 1983). In animals, castration results not only in the loss of androgen-dependent epididymal proteins but also losses in epididymal weight, changes in luminal histology, and alterations in the synthesis and secretion of epididymal fluid GPC, carnitine, and sialic acid. Ultimately, the castrated epididymis loses the ability to sustain sperm motility, fertility maturation, and sperm storage capacities, processes that are reversed with androgen replacement.

Compared with other accessory sex glands, the epididymis requires relatively higher levels of androgen to maintain its structure and function (Prasad and Rajalakshmi, 1976). **Androgen effects on the epididymis are mediated mainly through DHT, the primary androgen in epididymal tissue extracts** (Pujol et al, 1976), and/or 5α-androstane-3α, 17β-diol (3α-diol) (Orgebin-Crist et al, 1975). Indeed, this is corroborated by the fact that the enzymes Δ4-5α-reductase (catalyzes DHT formation from testosterone) and 3α-hydroxysteroid dehydrogenase (converts DHT to 3α-diol), which produce testosterone metabolites, are also found in the human epididymis (Kinoshita et al, 1980; Larminat et al, 1980). It may also help to explain the recent observation that the clinical use of 5α-reductase inhibitors is associated with impaired semen quality (Amory et al, 2007).

Epididymal function is also influenced by temperature (Foldesy and Bedford, 1982; Wong et al, 1982). Chronic exposure of the epididymis to elevated temperatures, for example by placing them within the abdomen, results in the loss of sperm storage and electrolyte transport functions. The effect of temperature on epididymal function may help explain how varicocele and cryptorchidism affect male infertility. Abnormalities in epididymal myoid cell contractility may also influence epididymal function. In the rat, partial surgical denervation of the epididymis results in an abnormal accumulation of sperm within the cauda epididymis and a decrease in the swimming speed of sperm (Billups et al, 1990). These findings have implications for infertility from neuropathic causes such as spinal cord injury and diabetes mellitus.

KEY POINTS: EPIDIDYMIS

- The epididymis consists of principal cells with absorptive and secretory function, basal cells derived from macrophages, and contractile cells that facilitate sperm transport.
- During epididymal passage, sperm mature by gaining progressive motility and the ability to bind to and penetrate the egg zona pellucida.
- Epididymal function is temperature and androgen (mainly DHT) dependent, important considerations for cryptorchidism, varicocele, and 5α-reductase use.

DUCTUS (VAS) DEFERENS

Gross Architecture

The vas deferens is a tubular organ derived from the mesonephric (wolffian) duct. In humans, the vas deferens is 30 to 35 cm long, beginning at the cauda epididymis and terminating in the ejaculatory duct, medial to the seminal vesicle and posterior to the prostate. It is classically divided into five regions: (1) the sheathless epididymal segment contained within the tunica vaginalis, (2) the scrotal segment, (3) the inguinal segment, (4) the retroperitoneal or pelvic portion, and (5) the ampulla (Lich et al, 1978). In cross section, the vas deferens consists of an outer adventitial connective tissue sheet containing blood vessels and small nerves, a muscular coat that consists of a middle circular layer surrounded by inner and outer longitudinal muscle layers, and an inner mucosal layer with an epithelial lining (Neaves, 1975). The outer diameter of the vas deferens varies from 1.5 to 3 mm, and the lumen of the unobstructed vas deferens varies from 200 to 700 μm in diameter (Middleton et al, 2009).

The vas deferens receives its blood supply from the deferential artery, a branch of the superior vesical artery. Venous drainage corresponds to arterial supply. The vas deferens receives innervation from both the sympathetic and the parasympathetic nervous systems (Sjostrand, 1965). The cholinergic supply does not appear important for motor activity of the vas deferens (Baumgarten et al, 1975). There is a rich supply of sympathetic adrenergic nerves derived from hypogastric nerve coursing via the presacral nerve (Batra and Lardner, 1976; McConnell et al, 1982). Adrenergic nerve fibers have been observed in all three layers of the vas muscularis, with the greatest concentration in the outer longitudinal layer (McConnell et al, 1982). The vas deferens also receives a short adrenergic nerve (Sjostrand, 1965) and has an abundance of ligand-gated, purinergic receptors in its smooth muscle membranes, suggesting sympathetic and purinergic cotransmission in sperm transport and ejaculation (Gur et al, 2007). Neurons containing other neurotransmitters, including neuropeptide Y, enkephalin, galanin, somatostatin, vasoactive intestinal polypeptide, and nitric oxide, have also been identified; however, their role in vas deferens function is unknown (Dixon et al, 1998). It is interesting to note that observations from human vas deferens specimens obtained at vasovasostomy after vasectomy show a marked reduction in the density of muscular noradrenergic and subepithelial secretomotor nerves in testicular compared with abdominal segments. These changes may influence subsequent sperm transport processes, and hence procedural success, after vasectomy reversal (Dixon et al, 1998).

Cytoarchitecture

The human vas deferens is lined by pseudostratified epithelium (Paniagua et al, 1981). The height of the epithelium decreases along the length of the vas deferens from the testis to the seminal vesicle. In addition, the longitudinal epithelial folds are simpler near the testis and become more complex distally. The pseudostratified epithelium vasal lining is composed of basal cells and three types of tall, thin columnar cells (Hoffer, 1976; Paniagua et al, 1981). The columnar cells, extending from the epithelial base to the lumen, include principal cells, but also pencil cells and mitochondria-rich cells. All columnar cells exhibit stereocilia and irregular convoluted nuclei. Principal cells are the most frequent columnar cell type in the proximal vas deferens, whereas both pencil cells and mitochondria-rich cells increase in density distally. The thickness of the total muscle layer gradually decreases along the length of the vas deferens. This complex cytoarchitecture strongly suggests that the vas deferens is more than simply a passive conduit for sperm transport.

Vas Deferens Function

Sperm Transport

Sperm transport through the vas deferens is influenced by several physiologic processes. First, **the human vas deferens exhibits spontaneous motility** (Ventura et al, 1973). **It also has the capacity to respond when stretched** (Bruschini et al, 1977). **Finally, fluid within the vas deferens can be propelled into the urethra by strong peristaltic contractions elicited either by electrical stimulation of the hypogastric nerve** (Bruschini et al, 1977) or by adrenergic neurotransmitters (Bruschini et al, 1977; Lipshultz et al, 1981). This suggests that immediately before emission, with sympathetic stimulation, sperm is rapidly transported from the distal epididymis through the vas deferens to the ejaculatory duct. **This rapid transport is consistent with the vas deferens having the highest muscle-to-lumen ratio (approximately 10:1) of any hollow viscus in the body.**

Sperm reserves in the vas deferens have been estimated at **approximately 130 million, suggesting that a significant proportion of human ejaculated sperm is stored in the vas deferens** (Amann and Howards, 1980). In addition, vasal sperm quality, as assessed from fertile men at the time of vasectomy, is very similar to that of the ejaculate, with 71% motility and 91% viability (Bachtell et al, 1999). In the rabbit, it has been shown that during sexual rest, epididymal sperm are transported through the vas deferens and leak into the urethra in small amounts (Prins and Zaneveld, 1979, 1980a, 1980b). This suggests that the vas deferens is involved in ridding the epididymis of excess, stored sperm. On sexual stimulation, rabbit sperm are transported through the vas deferens similar to humans. **After sexual stimulation, however, the vas deferens contents are propelled proximally toward the epididymis because the distal vas deferens contracts with greater amplitude, frequency, and duration than the proximal segment** (Prins and Zaneveld, 1980a). Notably, with prolonged sexual rest, excess epididymal sperm are once again transported distally, supporting the idea that the vas deferens is important for sperm transport and for maintenance of epididymal sperm reserves.

Absorption and Secretion

Based on its cytoarchitecture, the human vas deferens likely has both absorptive and secretory functions (Hoffer, 1976; Paniagua et al, 1981). The principal cells are typical of cells that synthesize and secrete glycoproteins (Bennett et al, 1974; Gupta et al, 1974). The stereocilia, apical blebbing, and primary and secondary lysosomes within principal cells are also characteristic of cells involved in absorptive function (Friend and Farquhar, 1967; Murakami et al, 1988). Lastly, spermiophagy by epithelial cells in the ampullary vas deferens has been observed with scanning electron microscopy in both men and monkeys (Murakami et al, 1988). **It is important to note that normal vas deferens function is likely to be androgen dependent because the vas deferens actively converts testosterone to DHT** (Dupuy et al, 1979). Castration causes atrophy of—and testosterone treatment, restoration of—monkey vas cytoarchitecture (Dinakar et al, 1977), and spontaneous and α- and β-adrenergic–stimulated contractions of the rat vas deferens are altered by castration (Borda et al, 1981). Thus, although once thought to be a simple muscular conduit for sperm, the vas deferens is now viewed as a complex reproductive organ.

SEMINAL VESICLE AND EJACULATORY DUCTS

Gross Architecture and Cytoarchitecture

Seminal Vesicle

In the adult, the seminal vesicles are paired, elongated, hollow viscous organs located posterior to the prostate and bladder. Each seminal vesicle is 5 to 7 cm long and up to 1.5 cm wide. Each seminal vesicle actually consists of a tubule that is 15 cm long and highly coiled and convoluted. **The tubule itself is composed of three layers: The inner lining is a moist and folded mucous membrane; the middle layer is largely collagenous; and the outer layer consists of circular and longitudinal muscle layers that constitute 80% of the wall thickness** (Nguyen et al, 1996). The mucosa of the seminal vesicle, mainly nonciliated, pseudostratified columnar or cuboidal cells, is notable for many thin, complicated folds that produce numerous crypts. The excretory duct of the seminal vesicle opens into the ampullary vas deferens as it enters the prostate gland.

The blood supply to the seminal vesicle arises from the internal iliac artery and inferior vesicular artery through the prostatovesicular branch (Clegg, 1955). The prostatovesicular artery can also arise from the superior vesicular artery or from the pudendal artery. Most commonly, the prostatovesicular artery has anterior and posterior branches that supply the respective surfaces of the seminal vesicle. The lymphatic drainage of the seminal vesicle is through the internal iliac lymph nodes. The seminal vesicles are innervated through sympathetic nerves from the superior lumbar and hypogastric nerves. Parasympathetic innervation occurs through the pelvic plexus.

Ejaculatory Ducts

The ejaculatory ducts are paired, collagenous, tubular structures that commence at the junction of the vas deferens and seminal vesicle, course through the prostate, and empty into the prostatic urethra at the verumontanum. Histologically, the ejaculatory ducts are a continuation of the seminal vesicle, except that the outer circular muscle layer does not extend into the ducts (Nguyen et al, 1996). There are three distinct anatomic regions to the ejaculatory duct: the proximal, extraprostatic portion; the middle intraprostatic segment; and a short distal segment incorporating the lateral aspect of the verumontanum in the urethra (Nguyen et al, 1996) (Fig. 22-20). Although the ejaculatory duct contains an outer muscular layer in its extraprostatic and intraprostatic segments, as the duct courses distally the outer muscular layer dissipates, and **there is no valvelike, muscular "sphincter" at the ejaculatory duct orifice,** as was once thought (Nguyen et al, 1996) (Fig. 22-21). Instead, urinary reflux is prevented and ejaculatory continence is maintained by the acute angle of duct insertion into the urethra. The inner epithelial layer of the ejaculatory ducts is also complex and folded and consists of simple and pseudostratified columnar cells. The ejaculatory ducts receive their blood supply from branches of the inferior vesical artery and are innervated through the pelvic plexus.

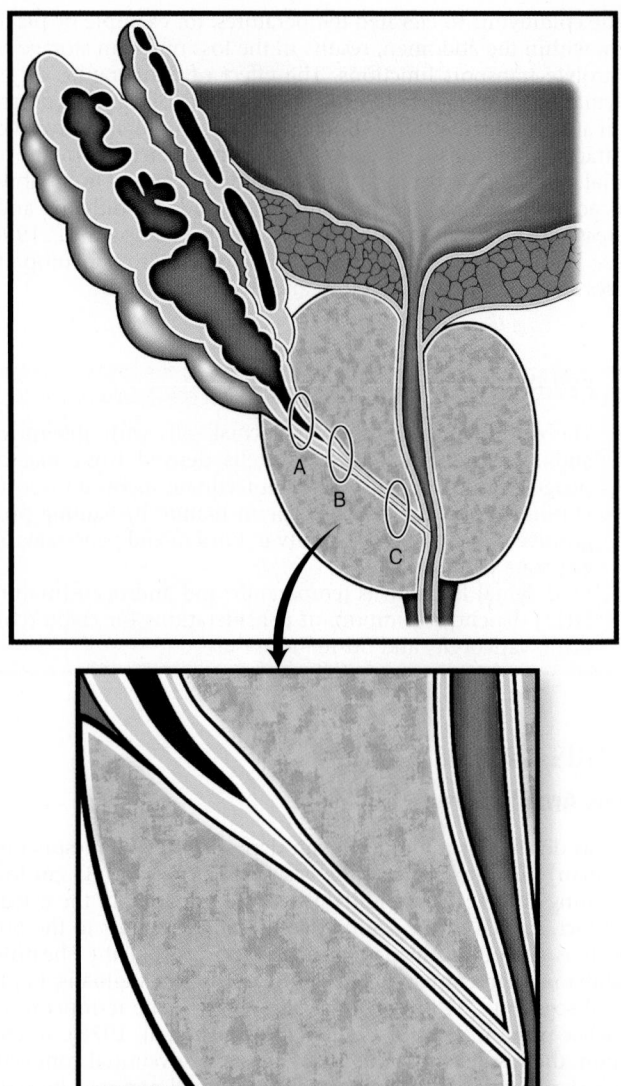

Figure 22-20. Schematic anatomy of the human ejaculatory duct complex. *A,* Proximal; *B,* intraprostatic or middle; and *C,* distal ejaculatory duct regions. The *inset* shows how the muscle layer thins out in the middle segment. (From Nguyen HT, Etzell J, Turek PJ, et al. Normal human ejaculatory duct anatomy: a study of cadaveric and surgical specimens. J Urol 1996;155:1639–42.)

Seminal Vesicle and Ejaculatory Duct–Unit Function

Animal studies suggest that the seminal vesicle and ejaculatory ducts are functionally similar to the bladder and urethra (Turek et al, 1998). **The seminal vesicle is a contractile, compliant, smooth muscular organ with dynamic properties analogous to those of the bladder, and the ejaculatory ducts serve as a urethra-like conduit.** This theory allows the classification of ejaculatory duct obstruction into **two types of disorders, analogous to bladder outlet obstruction: (1) obstruction resulting from physical blockage of the ducts, similar to bladder outlet obstruction, and (2) "functional" obstruction of the seminal vesicle, similar to voiding dysfunction caused by bladder myopathy.** In addition, this has implications for the diagnosis of ejaculatory duct disorders because "static" anatomic imaging, such as transrectal ultrasonography, may not be sufficient to differentiate between these disorders, and medications and conditions (such as diabetes) might predispose the system to seminal vesicle dysfunction (Smith et al, 2008).

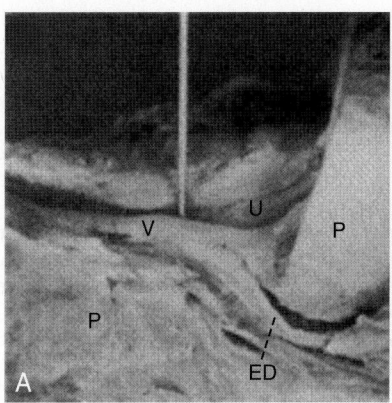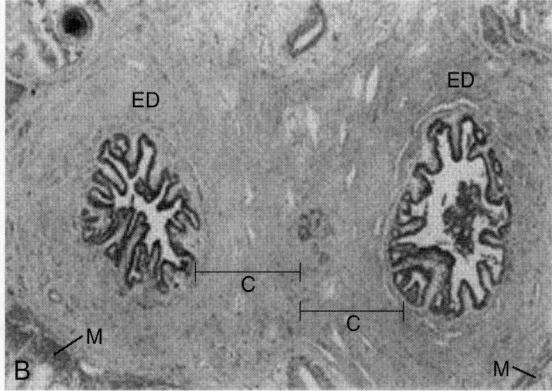

Figure 22-21. Human ejaculatory duct gross and microscopic anatomy from cadaver specimens. A, Sagittal section through the midline with pin in ejaculatory duct orifice and ejaculatory duct (ED) and veru (V), urethra (U), and prostate (P) visible. B, Microphotograph of the paired ejaculatory ducts in the middle intraprostatic segment showing the thick collagenous layer (C) surrounding the mucosa with a thin, outer muscular layer (M). (From Nguyen HT, Etzell J, Turek PJ, et al. Normal human ejaculatory duct anatomy: a study of cadaveric and surgical specimens. J Urol 1996;155:1639–42.)

Seminal Vesicle Function

The seminal vesicles secrete a significant proportion (80%) of the seminal fluid, and these secretions are found in later fractions of the ejaculate, after the sperm-rich epididymal and prostatic secretions. After ejaculation, sperm pass into and through the female cervical mucus and subsequently the uterus to enter the oviduct, where fertilization occurs. During residence in the female reproductive tract, sperm must undergo capacitation before oocyte fertilization. During capacitation, the acrosome reaction and development of hyperactivated motility occurs (Yanagimachi, 1994). It is not clear if prostatic or seminal vesicle secretions contribute to capacitation.

In fact, the exact physiologic role of seminal vesicle fluid is not clear, although in rodents it functions as a plug or barrier that reduces the chances for sperm from a subsequent male to fertilize the oocyte. Before ejaculation, semen is a liquid, and after all components mix with the seminal vesicle secretions, it coagulates. The major component of the coagulum is **semenogelin I, a 52-kD protein expressed exclusively in the seminal vesicles** (Robert et al, 1999). **Through coagulating semen, seminal vesicle secretions may promote sperm motility, increase stability of sperm chromatin, and suppress immune activity in the female reproductive tract.** The best-elucidated function of **human semen** appears to be its ability to **provide antioxidative protection to sperm.** Semen is rich in antioxidant enzymes, including glutathione peroxidase, superoxide dismutase, and catalase (Yeung et al, 1998). In addition, the antioxidant molecules taurine, hypotaurine, and tyrosine are present in high concentrations (van Overveld et al, 2000). Lipofuscin granules from dead epithelial cells give seminal vesicle secretions a yellow-white color. In addition, seminal vesicle secretions are alkaline and contain fructose, mucus, vitamin C, flavins, phosphoryl choline, and prostaglandins. High fructose levels provide nutrient energy for the sperm when studied in vitro. The mixing of seminal vesicle with prostatic secretions results in human semen having a mildly alkaline pH. **Acidic ejaculate (pH <7.2) is associated with blockage or absence of seminal vesicles** (Turek, 2005).

SPERMATOZOA

Anatomy and Physiology

The human spermatozoon is approximately 60 μm in length and is divided into three morphologic sections: head, neck, and tail (Fig. 22-22). The oval **sperm head,** about 4.5 μm long and 3 μm wide, contains a nucleus with highly compacted **chromatin** and an

> **KEY POINTS: VAS DEFERENS, SEMINAL VESICLE, AND EJACULATORY DUCTS**
>
> - The vas deferens is of wolffian (mesonephric) duct origin and serves to transport sperm from the cauda epididymis to the ejaculatory duct during seminal emission.
> - The seminal vesicle and ejaculatory duct unit is analogous to the bladder and urethra and is subject to both physical blockage and functional disorders that result in infertility.

acrosome, a membrane-bound organelle that harbors enzymes required for penetration of the outer vestments of the egg before fertilization (Yanagimachi, 1978). The **sperm neck** maintains the connection between the sperm head and tail. It consists of the **connecting piece** and **proximal centriole.** The **axonemal complex** extends from the proximal centriole through the sperm tail. The **tail** harbors the **midpiece, principal piece, and endpiece** (Zamboni, 1992). The midpiece is 7 to 8 μm long and is the most proximal segment of the tail, terminating in the annulus. It contains **the axoneme,** with its characteristic microtubule arrangement, and surrounding **outer dense fibers** (Fig. 22-23). It also contains the **mitochondrial sheath,** which is helically arranged around the outer dense fibers. The outer dense fibers, rich in disulfide bonds, are not contractile proteins but are thought to provide the sperm tail with the elastic rigidity necessary for progressive motility (Oko and Clermont, 1990). Similar in structure to the midpiece, the principal piece has several columns of outer dense fibers that are replaced by the fibrous sheath. The fibrous sheath consists of **longitudinal columns** and **transverse ribs.** The sperm terminates in the endpiece, the most distal segment of the sperm tail, and contains axonemal structures and the fibrous sheath. Except for the endpiece region, the sperm is enveloped by a highly specialized plasma membrane that regulates the transmembrane movement of ions and other molecules (Friend, 1989).

The spermatozoon is a remarkably complex metabolic and genetic machine. The 75 sperm mitochondria that surround the axoneme contain enzymes required for oxidative metabolism and produce adenosine triphosphate (ATP), the primary energy molecule for the cell. Mitochondria are organelles that produce cellular energy and can also cause apoptotic cell death through the release of cytochrome *c*. Mitochondria are composed of outer and inner membranes. The inner membrane forms deep folds into the matrix, called the cristae, which make the surface area of the inner membrane larger than that of the outer membrane. Five distinct respiratory chain complexes span the width of the inner membrane and are necessary for oxidative phosphorylation: nicotinamide adenosine diphosphate (NADPH) dehydrogenase, succinate dehydrogenase, cytochrome *bc1*, cytochrome *c* oxidase, and ATP synthase complexes. Contained within the matrix are citric acid cycle, fatty acid, and amino acid oxidative enzymes; newly made ATP; mitochondrial DNA (mtDNA); and ribosomes.

Human mitochondria contain DNA (mtDNA) that is distinct from sperm nuclear DNA. mtDNA consists of a circular, histone-free chromosome of 16,569 base pairs of DNA arranged in a single heavy and single light strand and **encodes respiratory-chain–complex subunit proteins, mitochondrial rRNAs, and tRNAs used for protein synthesis.** These genes have no introns. mtDNA is also far more susceptible to mutations than is nuclear DNA (estimated 40 to 100 times higher). Reasons for this may include the fact that mitochondria are near respiratory-chain complexes and may be easily attacked by reactive oxygen species. **In addition, mtDNA is not coated with protective histones, and mitochondria have very limited DNA repair mechanisms** (Hirata et al, 2002). **The fact that mitochondria rapidly accumulate mutations suggests the necessity of degrading all paternal mtDNA in the fertilized egg.** This degradation is likely mediated by the small proteolytic polypeptide ubiquitin, which regulates proteolysis in many tissues (Sutovsky et al, 1999).

From animal studies, it is clear that the plasma membrane covering the sperm-head region harbors specialized proteins that participate in sperm-egg interaction (Saling, 1989). Indeed, carbohydrate-binding proteins on the sperm membrane interact with the species-specific ZP3 protein in the egg zona pellucida, resulting first in sperm binding to the zona and subsequently to induction of the acrosome reaction (Shabanowitz, 1990). Another sperm membrane protein, PH30, is present on testicular sperm, is modified during sperm migration through the epididymis, and functions as a fusion protein between the sperm and egg membranes at fertilization (Primakoff et al, 1987; Blobel et al, 1990).

Physiologically, the axoneme is the true motor assembly and requires 200 to 300 proteins for proper function. Among these, the "9 + 2" pattern of outer and inner doublets of microtubules is the best-understood component (see Fig. 22-23). The dynein proteins extend from one microtubule doublet to the adjacent doublet and form both the inner and outer arms of the axoneme. **The sperm axoneme contains the enzymes and structural proteins necessary for the chemical transduction of ATP into mechanical movement and motility.** Dynein is a large (2000 kD), Mg^{2+}-stimulated ATPase responsible for ATP-generated microtubule sliding that causes axonemal bending and, ultimately, sperm flagellar movement. The dynein structure has two or three globular, outer (heavy) chain heads (500 kD) joined to a common stem. The heads control movement along the microtubules. The inner (light) chain arms (14 to 120 kD) are the primary effectors of movement and are associated with the radial spokes of the dynein assembly. Sperm with outer arm mutants have reduced motility, and those with inner arm mutants have no motility. Radial links or spokes connect a microtubule of each doublet to the central inner doublet and consist of

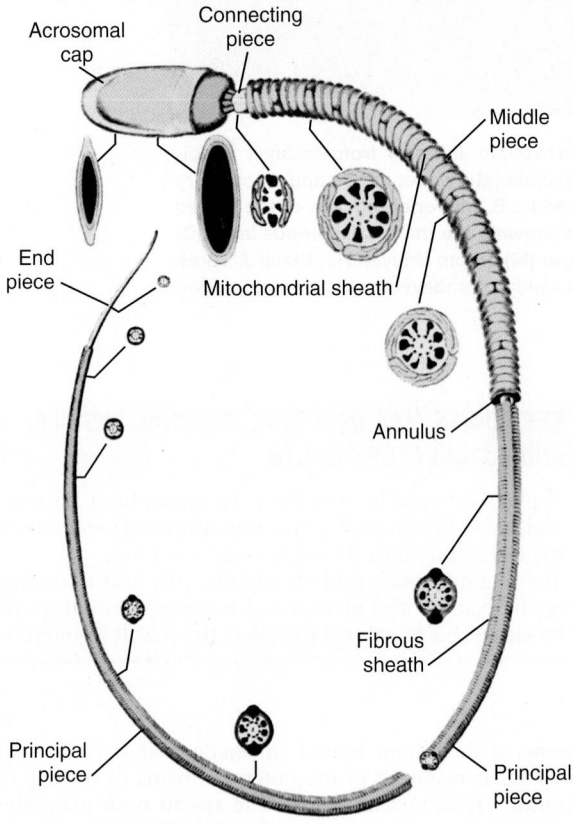

Figure 22-22. **Diagram of a typical mammalian spermatozoon. The plasma membrane is omitted to illustrate the major cellular components. Cross-sectional insets show the orientation of the internal cell structures. (From Fawcett DW. The mammalian spermatozoon. Dev Biol 1975;44:394–436.)**

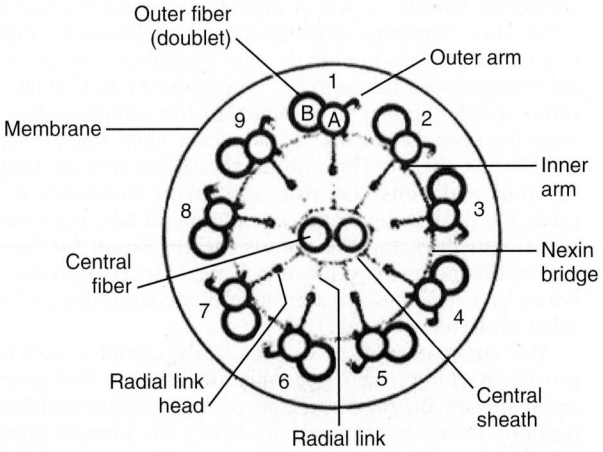

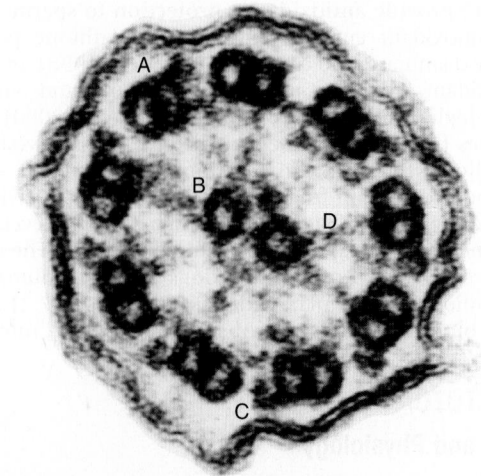

Figure 22-23. **The "9 + 2" sperm axonemal structure. *Left,* Schematic cross section of axoneme, demonstrating microtubule arrangement. *Right,* Electron micrograph of axoneme. A, outer doublet; B, inner central doublet; C, outer dynein arm; D, radial link.**

a complex of proteins. The central inner doublet is surrounded by a ringlike helical sheath to which the radial links from the outer doublets are attached. Tektins are proteins associated with the outer microtubular doublets, and nexin links are proteins that connect the outer doublets to one another and maintain the cylindric axonemal shape.

The phenotype of defective sperm structure has been recognized as ciliary dyskinesia. Although infertility is the rule with ciliary dyskinesias, ejaculated sperm can be motile and sperm concentrations can be normal. With ICSI, clinical pregnancies and live births have been reported after use of affected sperm (Cayan et al, 2001). Because the inheritance is usually recessive, normal offspring are likely. In general, patients suspected of harboring sperm structural defects exhibit severely compromised sperm motility (<10%). Sperm electron microscopy can reveal ultrastructural or functional sperm abnormalities. Sperm structural abnormalities are currently categorized by Chemes (2000) as follows:

1. **Nonspecific flagellar anomalies.** This is the most frequent flagellar anomaly underlying severely low motility and shows a structural phenotype of random, heterogeneous, microtubular alterations. These anomalies can arise from correctable disorders such as varicocele, reactive oxygen species, and gonadotoxin exposure. There is no evidence of familial occurrence.

2. **Dysplasia of the fibrous sheath.** This condition is a systematic sperm abnormality, usually associated with near-complete or total immotility. It has a more homogenous and distinctive phenotype characterized by sperm fibrous sheath, axonemal, and periaxonemal distortions. A subset of these patients exhibit the classic ciliary dyskinesia (formerly *immotile cilia syndrome*), in which sperm immotility is associated with respiratory disease and dextrocardia. There is a strong familial incidence, suggesting that such conditions are genetic in origin.

KEY POINTS: SPERM

- Sperm are ciliated cells that possess a "9 + 2" axonemal structure that allows motility.
- It is estimated that 200 to 300 genes regulate sperm motility.
- Sperm motility defects, termed *ciliary dyskinesias,* are common and can be either correctable (nonspecific flagellar anomalies) or genetic (dysplasia of the fibrous sheath).
- Human sperm mtDNA is a circular, histone- and intron-free DNA ring that encodes for respiratory-chain–complex proteins and is very susceptible to mutations.

SUMMARY

Spermatogenesis is a remarkably intricate and complex process that is driven by precisely regulated secretions of GnRH, LH, and FSH from the HPG axis. Perturbations in this hormonal milieu are common causes of male infertility. Sperm production in the testis functions optimally at 2°C to 4°C below body temperature and generates a mature human sperm in 64 days. Well-integrated cycles and waves of spermatogenesis ensure that human sperm production is constant at about 1200 sperm per second. Spermatogenesis is an androgen-dependent process that occurs with very high intratesticular testosterone levels. The product of spermatogenesis, the spermatozoa, leave the testis as immotile cells with limited capacity to fertilize oocytes. After epididymal transit, sperm are typically motile and capable of fertilization. During ejaculation, sperm are rapidly transported through the ejaculatory ducts into the urethra from the distal epididymis. The ejaculate itself supports sperm metabolism and motility, serves as an antioxidant, and serves as a barrier to exclude subsequent gamete deposits from gaining access to the egg.

REFERENCES

The complete reference list is available online at www.expertconsult.com.

SUGGESTED READINGS

Akre O, Richiardi L. Does a testicular dysgenesis syndrome exist? Hum Reprod 2009;24:2053–60. [*An excellent and critical review of the TDS concept*].

Cornwall GA. New insights into epididymal biology and function. Hum Reprod Update 2009;15:213–27. [*Up-to-date review of epididymal biology*].

De Jonge CJ, Barratt CL, editors. The sperm cell: production, maturation, fertilization, regeneration. New York: Cambridge University Press; 2006 [*An up-to-date review of mammalian and human sperm biology, genetics, and function*].

DiNapoli L, Capel B. SRY and the standoff in sex determination. Mol Endocrinol 2008;22:1–9. [*A review of the new theory of sex determination in which "testis genes" coexist with "antitestis genes"*].

Itman C, Mendis S, Barakat B, et al. All in the family: TGF-beta family action in testis development. Reproduction 2006;132:233–46. [*An excellent review of HPG axis factors inhibin and activin*].

Masters V, Turek PJ. Ejaculatory physiology and dysfunction. Urol Clin North Am 2001;28:363. [*Review of the fundamentals of the physiology and pathology of ejaculation*].

Payne AH, Hales DB. Overview of steroidogenic enzymes in the pathway from cholesterol to active steroid hormones. Endocr Rev 2004;25:947–70. [*Review of the complex biology of steroid hormone production*].

Robaire B, Hinton BT, editors. The epididymis: from molecules to clinical practice: a comprehensive survey of the efferent ducts, the epididymis and vas deferens. New York: Kluwer Academic and Plenum; 2002 [*Easily the most comprehensive basic science text on the biology of the epididymis and vas deferens*].

Skinner MK, Griswold MD, editors. Sertoli cell biology. San Diego: Elsevier; 2005 [*State-of-the-art update on Sertoli cells and male reproduction*].

Smith JF, Turek PJ. Ejaculatory duct obstruction. Urol Clin North Am 2008;35:221–7. [*Comprehensive review of the biology, physiology, and pathology of the seminal vesicle and ejaculatory duct complex*].

Turek PJ. Male infertility. In: Tanagho EA, McAninch JC, editors. Smith's urology. 17th ed. Stamford (CT): Lange Clinical Medicine; 2007 [*Basic review of human meiosis*].

Turek PJ, Reijo Pera RA. Current and future genetic screening for male infertility. Urol Clin North Am 2002;29:767–92. [*Comprehensive review of genetic associations with male infertility*].

Walker WH. Molecular mechanisms of testosterone action in spermatogenesis. Steroids 2009;74:602. [*Up-to-date review of the hormone biology of spermatogenesis*].

23 Integrated Men's Health: Androgen Deficiency, Cardiovascular Risk, and Metabolic Syndrome

J. Kellogg Parsons, MD, MHS, FACS, and Tung-Chin Hsieh, MD

Androgen Deficiency: An Evidence-Based Approach

Cardiovascular Disease and Testosterone

Metabolic Syndrome and Urologic Diseases

ANDROGEN DEFICIENCY: AN EVIDENCE-BASED APPROACH

Introduction

Testosterone is an essential male hormone. In utero, it serves a paramount role in the proper development of male genital organs. At puberty, it is important for the initiation of spermatogenesis and secondary sexual characteristics. During adulthood, testosterone continues to serve as a predominant circulating androgen, and the male hormonal reproductive axis is a finely controlled system with exquisite control of its biologic effects.

Lessons from androgen deprivation therapy (ADT) for prostate cancer have shown the detrimental effects of androgen deficiency (AD) on overall male health. **AD has been associated with mortality in men and a significant decrease in quality of life, from sexual dysfunction to metabolic and musculoskeletal complications** (Basaria, 2008). With an aging population, AD in the aging male, known as late-onset hypogonadism (LOH), has become a topic of increasing interest throughout the world.

Gonadal function decline has been recognized as part of normal male aging. **It is estimated that testosterone levels in men older than 40 years decrease at a rate of 1% to 2% per year** (Bremner et al, 1983). **However, unlike female menopause, which is a universal process associated with aging, the exact rate of decline and presenting symptoms are highly variable in men.** At the same time, biochemical measurements among assays also produce nonuniform reference ranges because of assay sensitivity variation, making diagnosis difficult (Lazarou et al, 2006).

Heightened awareness of AD has led to the development of many treatment options for LOH. Literature is limited regarding the long-term outcomes of LOH. **Despite the wide recognition and adaptation to intervention, debate is ongoing regarding the benefit, and, most importantly, the risks associated with treatment** (Conners and Morgentaler, 2013). Although more appears to be known about the aging female, men's health is a rapidly evolving field, and most physicians are actively engaged in bridging the significant knowledge and skill gaps in caring for the aging male population.

Definition

The International Society for the Study of the Aging Male has defined AD syndrome as "a biochemical syndrome associated with advancing age and characterized by a deficiency in serum androgen levels with or without a decreased genomic sensitivity to androgen. It may result in significant alterations in the quality of life and adversely affects the function of multiple organ systems" (Morales and Lunenfeld, 2002). Precise definition of LOH has yet to be established in the literature, despite the fact that Professor Brown-Sequard

first reported it in the nineteenth century (Brinkmann, 2011). Without novel diagnostic markers, neither biochemical nor clinical parameters alone are sufficient for identifying affected individuals.

Epidemiology

According to data from the Organization for Economic Cooperation and Development and Centers for Disease Control and Prevention, U.S. life expectancy was 78.7 years in 2011 (76 for U.S. men and 81 for U.S. women). This represents a 9-year increase from the 1960s, and this increase is consistent with other observed trends in industrialized countries and signifies trends in the aging population around the world. Diseases associated with aging are now integral to the future of medicine, with AD playing an important role in men's health. The true prevalence of AD in the adult male is unknown because of differing definitions in the literature.

The **Hypogonadism in Males study** was a cohort analysis: Morning serum testosterone levels were obtained from men age 45 years and older who were visiting primary care practices in the United States (Mulligan et al, 2006). **Using 300 ng/dL as a threshold for biochemical AD, the overall prevalence was 38.7%. A total of 52.4% of obese and 50% of diabetic men's testosterone values were found to be below the AD threshold.** Even though AD symptoms were assessed, only the biochemical definition of AD was used in the study.

Studies that incorporated symptoms along with biochemical testing include Massachusetts Male Aging Study (MMAS) and the European Male Aging Study (EMAS). MMAS was a longitudinal cohort study: Men aged 40 to 70 years with three or more AD signs or symptoms were included (Araujo et al, 2004). **Using a cut-off of total testosterone less than 200 ng/dL, the prevalence of AD was 6% and 12.3% at an approximate follow-up of 8.8 years.** Researchers reported a crude incidence rate of 12.3 per 1000 person-years, or approximately 481,000 cases of AD in U.S. men aged 40 to 69 years.

In EMAS, the observed prevalence for AD was 2.1% in men aged 40 to 79 years (Wu et al, 2010). Men were categorized as having AD if their serum testosterone was below the threshold of less than 11 nmol/L (approximately 320 ng/dL) and three sexual symptoms were present (erectile dysfunction, decreased libido, and decreased frequency of morning erection). Without accounting for hypogonadal symptoms, the biochemical AD prevalence was 17% in the cohort.

The prevalence of AD associated with systemic disease is higher than for the normal aging process and is well documented (Box 23-1). Since the 1970s, AD has been described in acute illness associated with surgery, stroke, traumatic brain injury, myocardial infarction, respiratory illness, and burns (Kalyani et al, 2007). As many as 90% of men with a total of 15% or more body burns have

---

BOX 23-1 Systemic Illnesses Associated with Androgen Deficiency

Burn injury
Traumatic brain injury
Respiratory illness
Surgical stress
Chronic opioid exposure
Chronic liver disease
Human immunodeficiency virus
Diabetes
Stroke
Myocardial infarction
Sepsis
Cancer
Chronic renal failure
Rheumatoid arthritis
Chronic obstructive pulmonary disease
Obesity

From Kalyani RR, Gavini S, Dobs AS. Male hypogonadism in systemic disease. Endocrinol Metab Clin North Am 2007;36:333–48.

---

been found to be AD (Vogel et al, 1985). Both free and total testosterone values decline rapidly 24 hours after injury and reach a nadir on average at day 11 (Lephart et al, 1987). Mean testosterone level among intensive-care patients has also been suggested to be a predictor for mortality: Surviving patients were shown to have significantly higher testosterone levels than nonsurvivors (Luppa et al, 1991).

Before highly active antiretroviral therapy (HAART), the prevalence of AD ranged from 30% to 50% in men suffering from acquired immunodeficiency syndrome (AIDS)–wasting (Crum et al, 2005). Currently, it still occurs in 20% to 25% of human immunodeficiency virus (HIV)-infected men undergoing HAART. Using a threshold of testosterone concentrations less than 300 ng/dL, AD is associated with AIDS-wasting syndrome and a decline in quality of life.

AD from chronic opioid exposure was first described in 1976 (Cicero et al, 1976). Testosterone levels can reach castration levels (reduced by >85% when compared to controls) within 24 hours after administration of a single opioid (Aloisi et al, 2005). Unlike other opiate-induced side effects, AD persists throughout treatment. In addition to its influence on sexual function, other physiologic changes such as fatigue, muscle wasting, osteoporosis, and changes in pain were also observed (Aloisi et al, 2009).

Testicular dysfunction is present in pretreatment and post-treatment oncologic patients. Approximately one third of patients with Hodgkin disease exhibit oligospermia and up to 70% of men experience abnormal semen parameters (Shekarriz et al, 1995). In testicular cancer, more than 50% of men have oligospermia before treatment (Meirow and Schenker, 1995). Although the exact mechanism of testicular dysfunction is unclear, both central and direct effects on the testis have been suggested (Kalyani et al, 2007).

About two thirds of men undergoing hemodialysis for end-stage renal disease (ESRD) show testosterone values in the AD range (Johansen, 2004). In nondialyzed men with chronic kidney disease, AD was associated with endothelial dysfunction and cardiovascular (CV) events (Yilmaz et al, 2011). In a cohort study of ESRD men, AD is independently associated with inflammation, CV comorbidity, and mortality (Carrero et al, 2011). **Renal transplantation appears to reverse the hormonal abnormalities associated with ESRD** (Prem et al, 1996). Further long-term study on the efficacy and safety of testosterone therapy (TT) in men with renal dysfunction is still warranted.

Physiology

Transport and Metabolism of Testosterone

After testosterone is excreted into circulation, the majority of testosterone is bound to plasma proteins. The primary androgen-binding proteins are sex hormone binding globulin (SHBG) and albumin. **The majority of testosterone is bound to albumin (54% to 68%); slightly less is bound to SHBG (30% to 44%), and only 0.5% to 3% remains unbound or as free testosterone** (Pardridge, 1986). **SHBG is produced by the liver and avidly binds to testosterone, rendering it biologically unavailable.** Albumin's association with testosterone is much weaker; albumin-bound testosterone and the unbound testosterone compose what is termed *bioavailable testosterone*. These bioavailable testosterone molecules have the ability to enter target organs, bind to the androgen receptor (AR), and initiate protein synthesis.

Testosterone metabolism is important to maintain proper balance between production and to achieve appropriate androgen levels in the target organs. **Testosterone metabolism occurs primarily in the liver** (Luetjens and Weinbauer, 2012). Extratesticular aromatization results in the conversion of androstenedione to estrone with subsequent reduction to estradiol. The half-life of testosterone in plasma is only about 12 minutes; estrogen influences testosterone's effects by acting either synergistically or antagonistically. Bioavailable estrogen and testosterone are strongly associated with high bone turnover, low bone mineral density, and risk of osteoporotic fractures. The imbalance of the testosterone-to-estrogen ratio is thought to be responsible for the development of impaired glucose tolerance and insulin resistance in the setting of aromatase-deficient men (Maffei et al, 2004).

Testosterone gives rise to 5α–dihydrotestosterone (DHT) through 5α-reduction, mainly in the target organs. Although testosterone and DHT both bind to the same intracellular AR, they produce distinct biologic responses. Two isoforms of 5α-reductase have been identified in humans. Type 1 5α-reductase has been localized in the nongenital skin, liver, brain, prostate, and testis, whereas type 2 is mainly active in the classical androgen-dependent tissues, such as the epididymis, genitalia, seminal vesicle, testis, and prostate but also in liver, uterus, breast, hair follicles, and placenta (Luetjens and Weinbauer, 2012). **DHT is responsible for normal sexual development and virilization in men and when combined with transactivation of AR leads to prostate gene transcription and growth** (Penning et al, 2000).

A functional AR is crucial for the optimal action of the androgens. The AR is a ligand-activated transcription factor present in all tissues responsive to testosterone or DHT. The human AR gene was cloned and mapped to Xq11-12 more than 20 years ago (Chang et al, 1988). The N-terminal domain harbors two polymorphic repeats, including a polyglutamine repeat of 9-36 residues and a polyglycine repeat of 10-27 glycine residues, and the length of these repeats affects AR transactivation and sensitivity (Werner et al, 2006). The length of trinucleotide repeats cytosine, adenosine, and guanosine (CAG) has been implicated in various disease processes relating to hyperandrogenicity and hypoandrogenicity. The contribution of CAG repeat polymorphism to prostate cancer has been well described; either to age of onset (Latil et al, 2001) or to the general risk development (Balic et al, 2002). The longer the CAG repeat in the AR gene translates to decreased androgen sensitivity, the earlier the onset of the AD is observed and the more severe the symptoms of AD are (Dejager et al, 2002).

Etiology. **AD can be a result of testicular failure (primary hypogonadism), or it can be caused by the disruption at the hypothalamic–pituitary–gonadal (HPG) axis level (secondary hypogonadism).** It is important to identify defects in the central level, as it can be a consequence of pituitary pathology, which can be restored by hormonal stimulation in most patients with secondary hypogonadism (Table 23-1). The pathophysiology of these disorders is characterized by alteration of secretion or action of gonadotropin-releasing hormone (GnRH), resulting in impairment

TABLE 23-1 Forms of Hypogonadism

PRIMARY HYPOGONADISM	
DISEASE	**CAUSES OF DEFICIENCY**
Maldescended or ectopic testis	Failure of testicular descent, 85% idiopathic
Orchitis	Viral or bacterial etiology
Congenital anorchia (bilateral in 1 in 20,000 males, unilateral 4 times as often)	Probably intrauterine torsion
Acquired anorchia	Traumatic, torsion, inflammation, orchiectomy
Secondary testicular dysfunction	Medication, systemic disease, radiotherapy, or toxin exposure
46,XY disorders of sexual development (male pseudohermaphroditism)	Enzymatic defects of steroid biosynthesis
47,XXY syndrome	Nondisjunction in paternal meiosis
Gonadal dysgenesis	Genetic mutations
Leydig cell hypoplasia	Luteinizing hormone receptor mutation
Noonan syndrome	Autosomal dominant congenital disorder

From Dohle GR, Arver S, Bettocchi C, et al. Guidelines on male hypogonadism, <http://www.uroweb.org/gls/pdf/17_Male_Hypogonadism_LR.pdf>; 2013 [accessed 04.11.14].

of pituitary luteinizing hormone (LH) and follicle-stimulating hormone (FSH) secretion (Pitteloud et al, 2010).

As men age, testosterone serum levels progressively decrease (Harman et al, 2001). Despite the recognition of this phenomenon since the nineteenth century, the exact mechanism is yet to be elucidated. **Circulating LH concentrations do not decline as men age** (Harman and Tsitouras, 1980), **suggesting that reduced testosterone results from primary gonadal hypofunction rather than changes at the hypothalamic-pituitary levels.**

Reduction in testosterone levels might be caused by a reduced number of Leydig cells or by reduced androgenic activity of the cells. AD is also observed with aging in rodents. In the Brown Norway rat strain, similar hormonal changes were observed with aging, and they were studied extensively as models of aging testis (Chen et al, 1994). The number of Leydig cells per testis has been shown to remain unchanged, suggesting that changes in the steroidogenic machinery of the individual cells and not their reduced number are responsible for the declining serum testosterone concentrations. Furthermore, Leydig cells from aged Brown Norway rats have been shown to produce less cAMP and testosterone in response to LH when compared to young rats (Chen et al, 2002). Consistent with animal studies, the administration of human chorionic gonadotropin (hCG) has been shown to stimulate testosterone production to a lesser extent in older than in younger men (Liu et al, 2005), suggesting reduced responsiveness of Leydig cells to LH. Although serum LH levels do not change significantly with age, age-related changes in LH frequency and amplitude have been reported (Bonavera et al, 1997), and these changes could affect Leydig cell testosterone production.

In the setting of systemic illness, alterations in both HPG axis and testicular function have been demonstrated. HPG axis suppression was observed after acute injury: Significant falls of FSH and LH along with testosterone and estradiol were found in both genders (Woolf et al, 1985; Bonavera et al, 1997). In addition to declining

LH levels, decreased pulsatility of LH release in burn patients has also been found, suggesting another plausible mechanism for central hypogonadism (Semple et al, 1987). The degree of HPG suppression is related to the severity of illness in critically ill patients. Both APACHE (Acute Physiology and Chronic Health Evaluation) score and degree of burns in patients were shown to correlate with degree of AD (Kalyani et al, 2007). Severity of head trauma also correlated with AD, and patients who presented with the lowest Glasgow Coma Scale score displayed the lowest levels of baseline and peak FSH and testosterone (Dimopoulou et al, 2004).

Other illnesses also exhibit suppression of the HPG axis. Central hypogonadism is more common in HIV-positive patients. Malnutrition with acute and chronic illness can cause significant weight loss and can disrupt the HPG axis (Dobs et al, 1996). Cytokines have also been implicated in the AD of HIV-infected men: Interleukin (IL)-1 was shown to inhibit gonadotropin release and LH binding to Leydig cells, and tumor necrosis factor can also affect HPG axis (Mylonakis et al, 2001). Naturally occurring opiates (endorphins) inhibit GnRH, and the direct suppressive effect of chronic opioid exposure on the pituitary and testis was proposed (Blank et al, 1986). Uremia also diminishes the amplitude of pulsatile LH release leading to secondary hypogonadism (Palmer, 1999).

Many mechanisms of testicular injury from systemic illness have been demonstrated. Both the germinal epithelium and Leydig cells of the adult testis are more highly predisposed to cytotoxic damage than the prepubertal testis. In a cohort study of patients undergoing high-dose chemotherapy for a variety of hematologic malignancies, one third of the patients showed evidence of Leydig cell dysfunction and 90% of patients experienced germinal epithelial failure (Howell et al, 1999). Single-dose irradiation as low as 0.1 Gy can cause testicular dysfunction, and doses greater than 0.8 Gy result in azoospermia (Rowley et al, 1974). Factors affecting impairment and recovery of testicular function after cytotoxic therapy include the agent used, the dose received, and the maturation of testis at the time of insult (Pryzant et al, 1993). Testicular atrophy from opportunistic infections was also suggested; nonspecific interstitial inflammation and fibrosis were observed in 32% of AIDS patients during autopsy examination (De Paepe and Waxman, 1989). A serum factor present in uremia also exhibits inhibition of LH receptor resulting in decreased Leydig cell sensitivity to LH (Handelsman and Dong, 1993). In alcoholic liver disease, primary testicular failure resulting from defective morphology of Leydig cells caused by ethanol can occur even before any clinical sign and symptom of AD are present (Gursoy et al, 2004).

Systemic illness can also affect testosterone metabolism and transport. The prevalence of AD in chronic liver disease is unknown. Liver failure and other systemic illnesses are associated with elevated levels of sex hormone-binding globulin (SHBG) in liver failure, leading to the overestimation of bioavailable testosterone. Therefore a direct assay for free testosterone might be used in the initial evaluation of the patient's endocrine status, because AD is a

---

KEY POINTS: EPIDEMIOLOGY AND PHYSIOLOGY

- The true prevalence of AD in the adult male is unknown as a result of inconsistent definitions used in the literature. Population-based studies suggest the prevalence to be between 2.1% and 38.7%.
- The prevalence of AD in men suffering from systemic diseases is significantly higher than those not evincing these diseases. Physicians caring for these patients need to be aware of the increased prevalence and need to offer appropriate screening.
- AD can be a result of primary testicular failure or can be caused by the disruption at the HPG axis. Testosterone metabolism and transport can also be affected by systemic illnesses.
- A functional AR is critical for the action of androgens. AR polymorphism likely contributes to the clinical symptomatology, treatment response, and adverse reaction to therapy.

TABLE 23-2 Comparison of Available Questionnaires

AGING MALE SYMPTOM	ANDROGEN DEFICIENCY IN AGING MALE	MASSACHUSETTS MALE AGING STUDY
1. General well-being	1. Low libido	1. Age
2. Musculoskeletal symptoms	2. Lack of energy	2. Diabetes mellitus
3. Sweating	3. Decrease in strength	3. Asthma
4. Sleep problems	4. Loss of height	4. Sleep quality
5. Tiredness	5. Decreased enjoyment of life	5. Smoking habit
6. Irritability	6. Sadness	6. Headache
7. Nervousness	7. Sexual problems	7. Sexual problems
8. Anxiety	8. Reduced sports performance	8. Managing ability
9. Lacking vitality	9. Tiredness after dinner	9. Height and weight
10. Decreased muscular strength	10. Reduced work performance	
11. Depression		
12-13. Burnt-out feelings		
14. Reduction of beard growth		
15. Decreased sexual performance		
16. Reduced nocturnal erections		
17. Low libido		

From Corona G, Rastrelli G, Forti G, Maggi M. Update in testosterone therapy for men. J Sex Med 8:639–54.

Diagnosis

Diagnosis of AD poses several challenges in men. Clinical signs and symptoms are often nonspecific, and modification by age, comorbid illness, severity and duration of AD, variation in androgen sensitivity, and previous TT can all lead to variable presentation. Multiple questionnaires were developed to screen and quantify the severity of AD in aging men (Table 23-2). Researchers at Saint Louis University first developed the **Androgen Deficiency in Aging Male (ADAM)** in 2000 (Morley et al, 2000). The standard ADAM questionnaire consists of 10 "yes or no" questions concerning symptoms of AD without severity of symptoms. The report initially presented a sensitivity of 88% and specificity of 60% in identifying men with serum biochemical AD as defined by bioavailable free testosterone that was less than 90 ng/dL. However, it was shown to be less specific at 60% in a study of Spanish men older than 50 years of age (Martinez-Jabaloyas et al, 2007). A modification of the original ADAM by quantifying each of the 10 symptoms into a Likert scale of 1 to 5 was shown to improve the questionnaire's correlation with biochemical AD in a group of men with prostate cancer (Mohamed et al, 2010). The **Aging Male Symptom (AMS) scale** consists of a battery of 17 questions graded on a Likert scale of 1 to 5, which allows one to quantify the degree of improvement in AD symptoms after therapy. However, similar to standard ADAM, AMS lacks specificity. In a study of 1174 men with AD who were undergoing treatment for TT, authors found a sensitivity of 96% but a specificity of only 30% (Moore et al, 2004). The questionnaire from MMAS is mainly a risk questionnaire using a combination of symptom and epidemiologic findings. It was validated against AD as defined by serum total testosterone less than 12.1 nmol/L (Smith et al, 2000), with a sensitivity of 60% and specificity of 59% (Morley et al, 2006). These questionnaires mainly serve as screening tools; their usefulness in diagnosing and evaluating treatment efficacy remains to be determined.

Men with suspicious signs or symptoms or at risk for AD need confirmatory biochemical testing before the diagnosis is made. **We do not yet know the exact biochemical threshold serum testosterone concentration below which symptoms of AD and adverse outcomes occur** (Table 23-3). Age, target tissue, and androgen sensitivity all can affect threshold of testosterone levels producing various symptoms. The average testosterone threshold corresponding to the lower limit of the normal range for young men, approximately 300 ng/dL (10.4 nmol/L), was shown to be associated with

significant risk factor for osteoporosis and for spinal fracture, and it is a predictor of mortality in men (Grossmann et al, 2012).

TABLE 23-3 Biochemical Definition of Hypogonadism Proposed by Various International Societies

	TOTAL TESTOSTERONE CONCENTRATION		
	nmol/L	ng/mL	ng/dL
EAA, ISA, ISSAM	Mild <12	<3.40	<340
EAU, ASA, ISSM	Severe <8	<2.31	<231
ES*	<10.4	<3.00	<300
AACE	7	<2.00	<200

*Pituitary imaging is required in the presence of severe secondary hypogonadism (total testosterone < 5.2 nmol/L or 150 ng/dL).

AACE, American Association of Clinical Endocrinologists; ASA, American Society of Andrology; EAA, European Academy of Andrology; EAU, European Association of Urology; ES, Endocrine Society; ISA, International Society of Andrology; ISSAM, International Society for the Study of the Aging Male; ISSM, International Society of Sexual Medicine.

From Corona G, Rastrelli G, Forti G, Maggi M. Update in testosterone therapy for men. J Sex Med 8:639–54.

greater likelihood of experiencing clinical symptoms (Zitzmann et al, 2006).

Serum testosterone levels peak in the morning and vary significantly as a result of circadian and circannual rhythm (Bremner et al, 1983). Most normal ranges for testosterone levels are established using morning blood samples, therefore diagnostic biochemical measurement for AD should be performed in the morning. Even though the effect of circadian rhythm is blunted with aging, a substantial fraction of men older than 65 years who had low serum testosterone levels in the afternoon was shown to have normal testosterone concentrations in the morning (Brambilla et al, 2007). It is important to confirm low testosterone concentrations in men with initial testosterone level less than the biochemical threshold range. In a cohort study of men aged 30 to 79 years, the day-to-day intraindividual variation in the level of testosterone exceeded the approximate 25% difference in half the men (Brambilla et al, 2007). **Serum total testosterone concentration represents both protein-bound and unbound testosterone in circulation.** Bioavailable testosterone refers to unbound testosterone and albumin-bound testosterone that is readily dissociable. Free or bioavailable testosterone concentrations should be measured when total testosterone levels are at the lower limit

BOX 23-2 Conditions Associated with Abnormal Sex Hormone Binding Globulin (SHBG)

CONDITIONS ASSOCIATED WITH DECREASED SHBG CONCENTRATIONS

Obesity
Nephrotic syndrome
Hypothyroidism
Use of glucocorticoids, progestins, and androgenic steroids
Acromegaly
Diabetes mellitus

CONDITIONS ASSOCIATED WITH INCREASED SHBG CONCENTRATIONS

Aging
Hepatitis and cirrhosis
Hyperthyroidism
Use of anticonvulsants
Use of estrogens
Human immunodeficiency virus

From Bhasin S, Cunningham GR, Hayes FJ, et al. Testosterone therapy in men with androgen deficiency syndromes: an Endocrine Society clinical practice guideline. J Clin Endocrinol Metab 2010;95:2536–59.

of the normal range or when altered SHBG levels are suspected (Box 23-2). It is also important to assess gonadotropins and prolactin during confirmatory testing to exclude secondary hypogonadism. If abnormality of the HPG axis is suspected, magnetic resonance imaging (MRI) of the central nervous system is indicated.

Total testosterone concentrations can be measured by three methods: radioimmunoassay, immunometric assay, or liquid chromatography tandem mass spectrometry. In most laboratories, automated immunoassays for total testosterone are performed using chemiluminescence detection. A major problem exists when the standard reference range for the adult male does not correspond to values reported by clinical laboratories (Bhasin et al, 2008). There are significant variations among assay techniques and among different laboratories. An external quality-control program by the College of American Pathologists has shown that the interlaboratory variation of a control sample is in a range between 215 and 348 ng/dL (7.5 and 12 nmol/L) with coefficients of variation among laboratories using the same method ranging between 5.1% and 22.7% (Wang et al, 2004). Using liquid chromatography tandem mass spectrometry as the standard, both radioimmunoassay techniques and automated immunoassay techniques performed within the clinically acceptable limits of ±20% of the reference method in more than 60% of the samples at differentiating the eugonadal from the AD male with established reference ranges for the particular laboratory. However, with their lack of precision at low testosterone levels, the tested assays cannot be used to measure testosterone accurately in females or prepubertal subjects.

Equilibrium dialysis is the gold standard for measuring free testosterone; however, it is costly and is often unavailable in local laboratories. Many analog methods are frequently used in place of equilibrium dialysis, but these methods are heavily affected by SHBG levels and are often inaccurate (Rosner et al, 2007). Routine free testosterone testing using analog measurement is not recommended by the American Endocrine Society. Many calculations were developed to estimate free testosterone concentrations from total testosterone, SHBG, and albumen. The calculated free testosterone values are dependent on the quality of total testosterone and SHBG assays. Because calculations are systematically different from equilibrium dialysis measurements, a significant variability exists in the calculated free testosterone estimates (Sartorius et al, 2009).

Diagnosis for AD in men should begin with a general health evaluation to assess for clinical signs, symptoms, systemic illness, and medications that might contribute to transient depression of testosterone levels. Confirmatory biochemical testing should be performed to support any clinically suspected cases. Gonadotropins and prolactin evaluation is crucial to identify alteration of the HPG axis, and an appropriate imaging study should also be performed. Urologists must become familiar with the limitation of the biochemical assays and the reference range of their local laboratory. Health care providers must exercise clinical judgment in selecting appropriate patients for treatment, because no single modality is capable of providing an accurate diagnosis of AD (Fig. 23-1).

KEY POINTS: DIAGNOSIS

- All men suspected of having AD need to undergo confirmatory biochemical testing.
- The exact biochemical threshold testosterone concentration that correlates with symptoms of AD or adverse outcomes has yet to be elucidated.
- The gold-standard biochemical assay for testosterone is often unavailable; physicians need to be familiar with their local laboratory's protocol and the limitations of different methodologies.
- If testosterone levels are below or at the lower limit of the accepted normal values, a repeat confirmatory morning test along with an assessment of the pituitary function are required.
- In men with abnormal gonadotropins (secondary hypogonadism), MRI of the pituitary might be indicated.

Treatment

The goal of AD treatment is to restore physiologic testosterone levels in AD men while alleviating symptomatic AD. Given the nonspecific clinical presentation of AD, physicians must counsel patients on lifestyle modifications in addition to TT. Increased physical activity, reduction of total caloric intake, and tobacco cessation have all been shown to reduce the risk of cardiovascular disease (CVD) and are part of the first-line management of metabolic syndrome based on American Heart Association recommendations (Grundy et al, 2005). Only by combining lifestyle changes with the restoration of androgen balance can the optimal health of the aging male be achieved.

Randomized controlled studies have shown that TT provides several positive improvements in body composition, metabolic control, and psychological and sexual parameters. For a group of elderly men with stable congestive heart failure, those patients receiving long-acting TT in addition to optimal medical therapy experienced improved exercise capacity (peak oxygen consumption), quadriceps isometric strength, insulin sensitivity, and baroreflex sensitivity compared to the placebo-controlled group (Caminiti et al, 2009). In a meta-analysis of randomized placebo-controlled trials, intramuscular (IM) TT was associated with an 8% gain in lumbar bone mineral density score with mixed results on femoral neck bone mineral density (Tracz et al, 2006). Cohort studies on long-acting TT have demonstrated a clear decrease in waist circumference, a significant reduction in trunk adipose composition and body mass index (BMI), and improvement of lipid profile after 1 year of therapy (Saad et al, 2007; Haider et al, 2010). In a multicenter prospective study, AD men receiving long-acting TT showed a significant improvement in the International Index of Erectile Function (IIEF) score for libido, intercourse satisfaction, and overall satisfaction at 6 weeks of therapy (Moon du et al, 2010). Meta-analysis of randomized, placebo-controlled trials showed that TT in patients with borderline biochemical AD was associated with minimal improvement in erectile function (95% confidence interval [CI] 0.03 to 0.65), nonsignificant effect on libido (95% CI −0.01

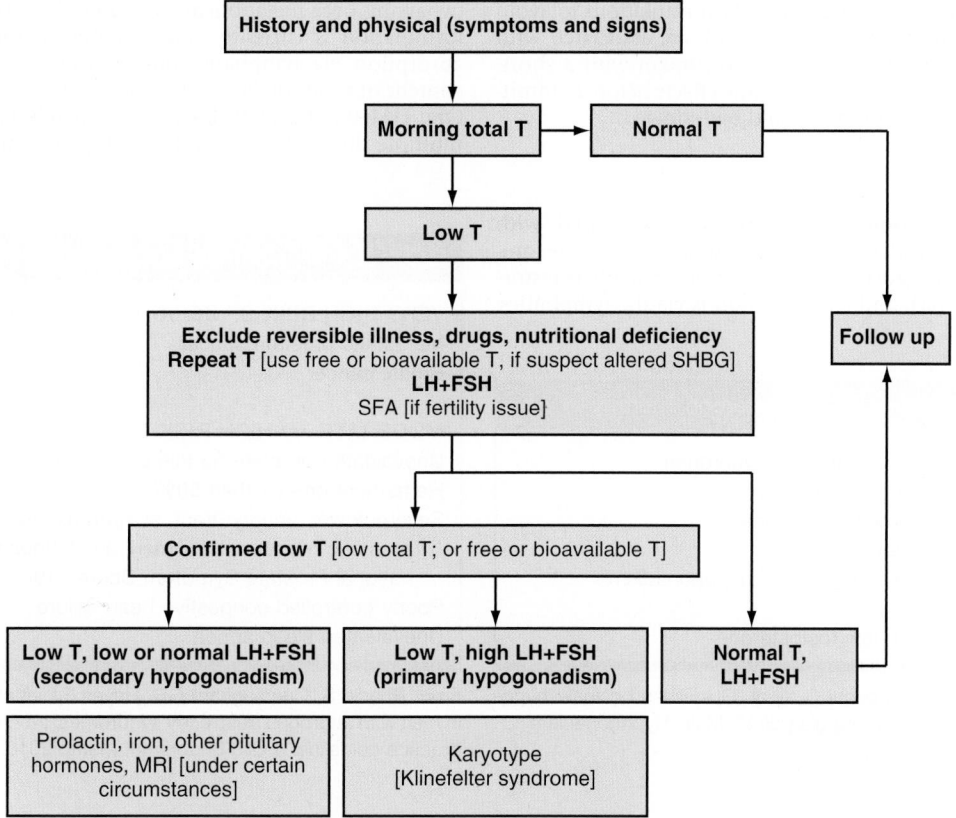

Figure 23-1. Approach for the evaluation for suspected androgen deficiency: endocrine guideline. FSH, follicle-stimulating hormone; LH, luteinizing hormone; MRI, magnetic resonance imaging; SFA, sperm fine-needle aspiration; SHBG, sex hormone binding globulin; T, testosterone. (Modified from Bhasin S, Cunningham GR, Hayes FJ, et al. Testosterone therapy in men with androgen deficiency syndromes: an Endocrine Society clinical practice guideline. J Clin Endocrinol Metab 2010;95:2536–59.)

to 0.83), and no effect on overall sexual satisfaction (Bolona et al, 2007). In a randomized, placebo-controlled study of AD men with metabolic syndrome, long-acting TT administration significantly improved depressive symptoms (−2.5 points, Beck depression inventory), AD symptoms (−7.4 points, AMS), and sexual function (+3.1 points, IIEF) after 30 weeks of therapy as compared to the control group (Giltay et al, 2010). In placebo-controlled, randomized trials of aging men, TT failed to showed significant improvement in cognitive function (Blackman et al, 2002; Kenny et al, 2004).

Randomized controlled studies also demonstrated the benefit of TT in patients suffering from systemic diseases. In a study of 70 HIV-positive men with symptomatic and biochemical confirmation of AD, biweekly IM TT was shown to improve libido, fatigue, depressive mood, and muscle mass compared to the placebo group (Rabkin et al, 2000). In a small randomized study of asthmatic men receiving long-term glucocorticoid treatment, TT increased bone density of the lumbar spine by 5% compared to no change in the placebo group after 1 year of therapy (Reid et al, 1996). In a double-blinded, placebo-controlled trial of men with severe burn (40% to 70% of body surface), patients treated with a testosterone analogue, Oxandrolone, were found to decrease significantly both weight and net nitrogen loss while improving donor-site wound healing compared to the placebo group (Demling and Orgill, 2000).

Administration of native testosterone either orally or parenterally results in absorption by portal circulation and rapid metabolism by the liver, and only a small concentration reaches the systemic circulation (Qoubaitary et al, 2005). Advancement in chemical modification using esterification results in a series of testosterone analogues with improved bioavailability and pharmacokinetics (Corona et al, 2011) (Fig. 23-2).

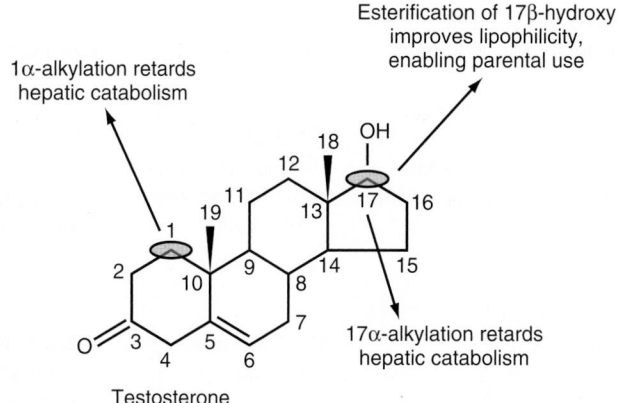

Figure 23-2. Biochemical structure of testosterone and potential site of modification: chemical structure of testosterone and possible site of structural modification to improve its bioavailability and pharmacokinetics. (Modified from Corona G, Rastrelli G, Forti G, et al. Update in testosterone therapy for men. J Sex Med 2011;8:639–54.)

TT is indicated in AD men who are demonstrating a decline in muscle mass and strength, a reduction of bone mineral density, and a decrease in sexual function (Boxes 23-3 and 23-4). TT is safe, and several preparations are available: oral, buccal, transdermal, IM injections, and subcutaneous implantation (Table 23-4 and Box 23-5). TT's goal and aim is to restore biochemical testosterone levels in a range for healthy young men. Physicians need to be aware of the pharmacology of different TT formulations to avoid undertreatment and overtreatment when both are associated with increased adverse events. The principle of treatment with a short-acting formulation to assess efficacy and side effects before commitment to a long-acting preparation should be followed.

Oral Preparations

Oral alkylated testosterone preparations are associated with hepatoxicity; use is considered obsolete and is no longer recommended. The only oral testosterone formulation available is testosterone undecanoate (TU), and its absorption is via the lymphatics,

bypassing liver metabolism to enable delivery (Seftel, 2007). This formulation is currently not available in the United States. The absorption via lymphatic route is highly dependent on the fat content of food intake: It must be taken with at least 20 mg of fat. Oral TU has a short half-life (approximately 4 hours) and it requires multiple dosing (2 to 3 times daily), resulting in irregular serum

---

BOX 23-3 Indications for Testosterone Therapy

Delayed puberty (idiopathic, Kallmann syndrome)
Klinefelter syndrome with hypogonadism
Sexual dysfunction with low testosterone
Low bone mass in hypogonadism
Adult men with signs and symptoms of hypogonadism
Hypopituitarism
Testicular dysgenesis with low testosterone

From Dohle GR, Arver S, Bettocchi C, et al. Guidelines on male hypogonadism, <http://www.uroweb.org/gls/pdf/17_Male_Hypogonadism_LR .pdf>; 2013 [accessed 04.11.14].

BOX 23-4 Contraindications for Testosterone Therapy

VERY HIGH RISK OF SERIOUS ADVERSE OUTCOMES
Metastatic prostate cancer
Breast cancer

MODERATE TO HIGH RISK OF ADVERSE OUTCOMES
Unevaluated prostate nodule or induration
Hematocrit greater than 50%
Severe lower urinary tract symptoms associated with benign prostatic hypertrophy (American Urological Association International Prostate Symptom Score >19)
Poorly controlled congestive heart failure
Unevaluated sleep apnea

From Bhasin S, Cunningham GR, Hayes FJ, et al. Testosterone therapy in men with androgen deficiency syndromes: an Endocrine Society clinical practice guideline. J Clin Endocrinol Metab 2010;95:2536–59.

TABLE 23-4 Available Testosterone Therapy Preparations

COMPOUND	DOSAGE	ADVANTAGES	DISADVANTAGES
ORAL AGENTS			
Testosterone undecanoate	120-240 mg, 2-3 times daily	Oral, adjustable dose	Variable testosterone levels and clinical response, must be taken with meals containing at least 20 g of lipids
INTRAMUSCULAR AGENTS			
Testosterone enanthate	200 mg every 1-2 wk	Low cost	Wide fluctuation in testosterone levels, multiple injections, increased risk for polycythemias
Testosterone cypionate	100-200 mg every 1-2 wk		
Testosterone propriate	100 mg every 2 days		
Testosterone undecanoate	750-1000 mg every 10-14 wk	Efficient testosterone normalization, long lasting, improved compliance	Injection site pain, requires injection training
SUBUTANEOUS AGENTS			
Surgical implants	450-700 mg every 4-6 mo	Efficient testosterone normalization, long lasting, improved compliance	Invasive placement, risk of extrusion and site infections
CONTROLLED-RELEASE BUCCAL FORMULATION			
Testosterone buccal	30 mg, twice daily	Oral	Mucosal irritation, twice daily administration
TRANSDERMAL AGENTS			
Testosterone patches	5-10 mg daily	Simple administration, mimics circadian rhythm	Skin irritation, daily administration, hygiene issues
Testosterone gel 1%-2%	40-80 mg daily	Efficient testosterone normalization, flexible doses, simple administration	Skin irritation, daily administration, possible transference during contact
Underarm Testosterone 2% solution	60-120mg daily		
Testosterone gel 1.62%	20.25-81 mg daily		

From Isidori AM, Buvat J, Corona G, et al. A critical analysis of the role of testosterone in erectile function, from pathophysiology to treatment—a systematic review. Eur Urol 2014;65:99–112.

BOX 23-5 Monitoring after Initiation of Testosterone Therapy

1. Evaluate the patient every 3 to 6 months after treatment initiation and then annually to assess symptom response and assess adverse effects.
2. Monitor testosterone level 3 to 6 months after treatment initiation with goal to raise serum testosterone level into the mid-normal range.
   Injectable formulations: Measure serum testosterone level midway between injections.
   Transdermal patch: Assess testosterone level 3 to 12 hours after application.
   Transdermal gels: Assess testosterone level any time after 1 week of treatment.
   Buccal testosterone: Assess testosterone level immediately before or after application.
   Oral agent: Monitor testosterone level 3 to 5 hours after ingestion.
   Testosterone pellets: Measure testosterone levels at the end of the dosing interval.
3. Check hematocrit at baseline, at 3 to 6 months, and then annually.
   If Hct is greater than 54%, stop therapy until Hct decreases to a safe level.
4. Measure bone mineral density of lumbar spine and/or femoral neck after 1 to 2 years of testosterone therapy in men with osteoporosis or low-trauma fracture.
5. Perform DRE and check PSA before initiation of therapy, at 3 to 6 months, and then in accordance with prostate cancer screening guidelines.
6. Additional urologic workup is indicated if there is abnormal DRE, elevation of PSA, worsening lower urinary tract symptoms, or an AUA/IPSS greater than 19.
7. Evaluate formulation-specific adverse effects at each visit.
   Buccal: alterations in taste and examination of gum and oral mucosa for irritation
   Injectable: fluctuations in symptom, fluid retention
   Testosterone patches: irritation at the application site
   Testosterone gels: Advise patient to cover the application sites with clothing, local hygiene before skin-to-skin contact with women or child. Serum testosterone levels are maintained when application site is washed 4 to 6 hours after application.
   Testosterone pellet: Check for signs of infection, fibrosis, or pellet extrusion.

AUA/IPSS, American Urological Association International Prostate Symptom Score; DRE, digital rectal examination; Hct, hematocrit; PSA, prostate-specific antigen.
From Bhasin S, Cunningham GR, Hayes FJ, et al. Testosterone therapy in men with androgen deficiency syndromes: an Endocrine Society clinical practice guideline. J Clin Endocrinol Metab 2010;95:2536–59.

testosterone levels throughout the day. Oral TU has the advantages of flexible dosage, self-administration, and immediate decrease in testosterone serum concentrations after cessation of therapy.

Transbuccal Preparation

A sustained-release mucoadhesive system offers an alternative preparation for oral TT. Transbuccal administration allows the absorption of testosterone through oral mucosa bypassing liver metabolism. Softening and molding the tablet to the shape of the gum work to apply the system, and this tablet must be removed after 12 hours to avoid local irritation. This formulation was shown to restore testosterone to the physiologic levels while demonstrating efficacy similar to other testosterone formulations (Pfeil and Dobs, 2008).

Transdermal Preparations

A variety of transdermal formations is current available. They are normally to be used daily and they deliver consistent serum testosterone levels into the circulation during treatment. Available transdermal testosterone patches are frequently associated with local skin reactions and decreased compliance rate (Seftel, 2007). The patches can be scrotal and nonscrotal, and they can either include or not include enhancers to increase the skin absorption.

Transdermal testosterone gels were first introduced in the United States in 2000. The recommended starting dose is 50 mg/5 g per day, which provides the delivery of approximately 50 mg/day into circulation. The formulations are either 1% or 2% hydroalcoholic testosterone gels capable of continuous delivery of testosterone for 24 hours after a single daily application. **When transdermal gels are applied, testosterone is rapidly absorbed into the stratum corneum, which forms a reservoir and serves as a rate-controlling membrane** (Corona et al, 2011). It is recommended that testosterone gel be applied on intact dry skin over the shoulders, upper arms, axilla, abdomen, or inner thigh area. Dose adjustment might be needed after therapy because skin absorption is variable among men. Testosterone gels show an improved safety profile with a significant decrease in skin adverse reaction compared to the testosterone patch (Wang et al, 2000). **Transference to others during close contact with the skin's surface is a potential adverse event when using testosterone gels.** This risk can be avoided by wearing clothing or by removing the residue of gel on the skin by local hygiene or by showering after the mandatory residence time (2 to 4 hours based on the preparation).

Injectable Preparations

Injectable 17β-hydroxyl esters are available in oil depot formulation. When administered into the muscle, testosterone is absorbed directly into the bloodstream. The frequency of injections is based on their half-lives. The propionate-testosterone ester is not widely used because of its short-term formulation, requiring 2 or 3 fractionated doses weekly. Cypionate and enanthate-testosterone esters are injected every 2 weeks. **After administration of injectable preparations, supraphysiologic levels of serum testosterone are reached after 24 hours, followed by a gradual decline to AD levels throughout the following 10 to 14 days** (Matsumoto, 1994). The "peak and valley" variation in serum testosterone concentration is often paralleled by variations of well-being and hypogonadal symptom recurrence. It is postulated that the wide fluctuation in testosterone concentrations contributes to the frequent side effects, including polycythemia, requiring dose adaptation, temporary interruption of therapy, and/or phlebotomy.

A longer-lasting injection preparation of TU is available, although not in the United States. It is administered into the gluteal muscle every 12 weeks following a 6-week loading dose. Testosterone is gradually released into systemic circulation at a consistent normal physiologic level while avoiding complications associated with the fluctuation of testosterone levels. Randomized, placebo-controlled studies have validated the clinical efficacy and the ability to maintain therapeutic testosterone levels of injectable TU (Caminiti et al, 2009; Corona et al, 2011).

Subcutaneous Implant Preparation

The testosterone pellet is the only long-acting testosterone formulation approved for the treatment of male AD in the United States, and it is also available as a different preparation in Europe and Australia. The crystalline testosterone pellets are inserted into subcutaneous tissue under local anesthesia, with complications of infection or pellet extrusion. **Serum testosterone reaches supraphysiologic levels approximately 1 month after implantation, with a gradual decline during the following 3 to 6 months** (Kelleher et al, 2004). It offers the longest duration of action among the currently available TT preparations with a steady-state delivery in a multi-institution observational study (McCullough et al, 2012). The convenience of long-acting testosterone preparations has the potential to increase patient compliance, although long-term data on the testosterone pellet are still to be determined. In a randomized, crossover study comparing long-acting TT (testosterone pellet vs. injectable TU), patients preferred the injectable formulation despite no difference in clinical efficacy (Fennell et al, 2010). It should be noted that both formulations from the study are not available in the United States.

Any patient undergoing TT requires scheduled follow-up. **During the first year of therapy, men should be monitored at 3- to 6-month intervals and at least annually thereafter** (see Box 23-5). A complete clinical and andrologic evaluation is mandatory at each visit. **Biochemical assessment of hormonal levels along with hematocrit (Hct) and prostate-specific antigen (PSA) are mandatory. Metabolic parameters can also be measured (e.g., lipid profile), whereas liver function testing is no longer required using the available testosterone formulations.**

Complications and Controversies

Erythrocytosis

Testosterone appears to stimulate erythropoiesis. ADT and AD are both risk factors for anemia. In men with chronic kidney disease, AD was shown to be associated with reduced responsiveness to erythropoiesis-stimulating agents (Carrero et al, 2012). Despite the known association, the underlying mechanism of testosterone's role in erythropoiesis is poorly understood. One potential mechanism of action of testosterone is by improvement of iron bioavailability. Weekly administration of IM TT appeared to suppress hepcidin, an iron-regulating protein, resulting in erythrocytosis in a dose- and age-dependent manner (Bachman et al, 2010). **Elderly men are at increased risk for developing post-treatment erythrocytosis.** DHT has also been implicated at testosterone-induced erythrocytosis. In a randomized, placebo-controlled trial, men who received topical DHT experienced asymptomatic increases of Hct despite a decrease in serum testosterone concentrations, requiring the discontinuation of treatment per protocol (Idan et al, 2010).

Erythrocytosis is the most common side effect of TT with variable prevalence based on testosterone formulations; injection therapy is associated with a greater risk of erythrocytosis as compared to topical preparations. Comparing the testosterone patch with IM injections, the rate of erythrocytosis, as defined by Hct greater than 52%, was 15.4% and 43.8%, respectively (Dobs et al, 1999). **Increased blood viscosity can aggravate vascular disease in the coronary, cerebrovascular, or peripheral vascular circulation, particularly in the elderly with pre-existing conditions** (Jonathan, 2002). Therefore men receiving TT need to be monitored for erythrocytosis and appropriate measures: Dose reduction, withholding of therapy, therapeutic phlebotomy, or blood donation needs to be instituted in appropriate cases.

Benign Prostatic Hyperplasia

Androgen is important for the development of prostate tissue. Chemical or surgical castration results in the reduction of prostate volume. TT poses as a theoretic risk in men with known lower urinary tract symptoms (LUTS) relating to benign prostatic hyperplasia (BPH). **Studies have shown a significant increase in prostate volume; measurement by transrectal sonography was associated with TT during the first 6 months of treatment** (Pechersky et al, 2002). However, the increase in prostate volume did not translate into worsening LUTS. **Multiple studies failed to demonstrate a significant increase in BPH-related voiding symptoms,** measured by International Prostate Symptom Score (IPSS), urine

flow rates, postvoid residual volumes or complications, such as urinary retention, in men undergoing TT as compared to placebo-controlled groups (Fernandez-Balsells et al, 2010). **Severe LUTS (IPSS >20) is a relative contraindication to TT and patients should consider evaluation and treatment before initiation of therapy.** Urinary symptoms should be assessed as part of follow-up monitoring of men undergoing TT.

Prostate Cancer

Advancement in the understanding of androgen's effect on the prostate is the basis of modern ADT for prostate cancer. TT trials have shown a rise in serum PSA levels, which heightened the concern for the development of prostate cancer (Slater and Oliver, 2000). A collaborative analysis of 18 prospective studies showed no association between serum androgen concentrations and risk of prostate cancer (Roddam et al, 2008). **Prospective trials on TT did not show an increase in the incidence of prostate cancer or the risk for prostate biopsy compared to placebo groups** (Fernandez-Balsells et al, 2010). TT has emerged as a strategy for sexual function rehabilitation following treatment of prostate cancer. Multiple retrospective cohort studies of TT following prostate cancer treatment demonstrated an improvement in the recovery of sexual function without an increased rate of biochemical recurrence compared to matched controls (Pastuszak et al, 2013).

To date, no definitive evidence suggests that TT has a causative role in prostate cancer or that raising serum testosterone levels by exogenous TT increases the risk for prostate cancer. Both prostate cancer and AD are diseases of aging. Therefore a baseline measurement of PSA and a digital rectal examination should be performed during the evaluation of AD. Men with abnormal PSA or abnormal digital rectal examination require appropriate workup and counseling before TT. Careful monitoring of prostate pathology is critical after TT. Prostate biopsy is indicated in the presence of suspected prostate cancer following the established guidelines for eugonadal men.

Lipid Profile. Data on the relation of TT and lipid profile are inconsistent. Supertherapeutic dosage of androgens appears to lower high-density lipoprotein (HDL) levels (Singh et al, 2002). **Multiple prospective studies using TT to restore testosterone in physiologic levels have shown either no change or minimal reduction in HDL** (Whitsel et al, 2001). **Both total cholesterol and low-density lipoprotein (LDL) levels were also unchanged or reduced compared to pretreatment levels.** Transdermal preparation appears to have lesser effects on the lipid profile compared to injectable TT. In a double-blinded placebo-controlled study, there was no significant difference in serum lipids and apolipoprotein between healthy men receiving transdermal testosterone and a placebo group during 36 months of treatment (Snyder et al, 2001). Available data suggest that TT within a physiologic range is not associated with detrimental changes of the lipid profile.

Testicular Hypofunction

Testicular size and consistency often diminish after TT. Exogenous testosterone administration leads to excess negative feedback of the HPG axis, which results in suppression of endogenous testosterone production and spermatogenesis. An international multicenter male contraceptive study conducted by the World Health Organization showed that weekly administration of 100 mg IM testosterone enanthate in healthy men resulted in 98% suppression of spermatogenesis to severe oligospermic (<3 million sperm per mL) or azoospermic level (World Health Organization, 1996). **Recovery after TT cessation usually occurs in 12 to 15 months, although normal spermatogenesis is not always observed** (Gu et al, 2003). Despite existing literature on exogenous testosterone as male contraception, many physicians are unaware of the effect of exogenous testosterone on fertility. A survey of practicing urologists showed that 25% of respondents would use exogenous testosterone for the treatment of male infertility (Ko et al, 2012).

Strategies such as pretreatment sperm cryopreservation or concomitant administration of hCG have been shown to preserve spermatogenesis in men undergoing TT (Hsieh et al, 2013). **Be cautious when initiating TT in men who still desire to preserve fertility.** Physicians need to offer detailed counseling, monitoring of spermatogenesis, and appropriate strategy to preserve fertility.

Other Adverse Reactions

TT was shown to be associated with the development of sleep apnea (Attal and Chanson, 2010). This phenomenon generally occurs in men undergoing high-dosage TT with other identifiable risk factors for sleep apnea. Upper airway anatomy is unaffected by TT, suggesting a potential central mechanism of altered breathing during sleep rather than anatomical obstruction.

Dermatologic reactions are more common with transdermal patches (up to 66%) than with gel preparations (approximately 5%) (Wang et al, 2000). IM injections can cause local pain, ecchymosis, erythema, swelling, hematoma, abscess, or furuncles (von Eckardstein and Nieschlag, 2002). Acne, oily skin, changes in body hair, and flushing have also been observed but are generally well tolerated.

Fluid retention is uncommon and is generally mild. However, caution is needed when initiating TT in men with congestive heart failure or renal insufficiency.

Gynecomastia is a rare complication after TT. It is related to increased serum estradiol levels from aromatization of testosterone and is often managed by dose adjustment of TT.

Testosterone Therapy for Erectile Dysfunction

Erectile dysfunction (ED) has emerged as an important independent risk factor for CVD, and sexual dysfunction is the most specific symptom of LOH (Isidori et al, 2014). **Population-based studies have shown that the prevalence of AD in men experiencing ED ranges from 23% to 47%** (Kohler et al, 2008). **The association between ADT and sexual dysfunction is well documented but the role of TT as a monotherapy for ED is less clear.**

Testosterone is responsible for normal genital development, and the literature supports its role in erectile physiology. In the central nervous system, testosterone was shown to stimulate the release of excitatory neurotransmitters such as dopamine, oxytocin, and nitric oxide, which control sexual dimorphic development and mating behavior (Hull et al, 1999). Peripherally, testosterone modulates multiple components involved in erectile function: structure, function, and innervation of smooth muscle cells, endothelial function of penile vessels, and fibroelastic properties of the corpus cavernosum (Isidori et al, 2014). Unfortunately many available data derived from animal castration models, which are very different from AD in men, generate uncertainty, further complicated by the limited available human data.

Combination therapy with phosphodiesterase type 5 inhibitors (PDE5-I) and TT is a highly debated topic. PDE5-I monotherapy is effective at improving erection but is often inadequate in addressing other domains of sexual dysfunction, such as decreased libido, for the AD men. The concept of salvage therapy for nonresponders of PDE5-I was examined in a multicenter, double-blind, placebo-controlled study of 173 men (Buvat et al, 2011). Administration of topical TT resulted in additional beneficial effect only in AD men with total testosterone below the threshold of 10.4 nmol/L (300 ng/dL). The concept of combination therapy was further tested in a large randomized trial to address whether TT includes any additional benefit in AD men whose erectile function is already maximized by a PDE5-I (Spitzer et al, 2012). The study definitively confirmed that TT does not provide additional benefit when erectile function is already restored by PDE5-I. However, the study was not powered to assess the role of salvage therapy, because the overall number of PDE5-I failures was low.

In young men with symptomatic AD, TT should be the first-line treatment with high likelihood of improvement in all domains of sexual function, and PDE5-I can be added if necessary. In elderly men with ED, PDE5-I should be first-line therapy with optimization of comorbid conditions. In the case of nonresponders, TT should be reserved only in men with biochemical confirmation of AD. Available evidence shows that there are no major safety concerns with combination therapy.

KEY POINTS: TESTOSTERONE THERAPY FOR ERECTILE DYSFUNCTION

- ED along with sexual dysfunction is the most specific predictor of AD.
- Testosterone acts peripherally to modulate multiple components responsible for normal erection.
- When erection is restored by PDE5-I, the addition of TT does not result in further benefit of erectile function.
- For ED refractory to PDE5-I, TT has the potential to improve the efficacy of therapy only in men with biochemical AD (<300 ng/dL).

CARDIOVASCULAR DISEASE AND TESTOSTERONE

CVD is the leading cause of death in most developed countries, with an estimated 17.3 million deaths worldwide per year (Laslett et al, 2012). The lifetime risk of coronary heart disease (CAD) at age 40 is one in two for men and one in three for women (Lloyd-Jones et al, 2004). Although mortality has decreased considerably in recent years, CVD and its complications remain highly prevalent and are significant burdens to the health system (Smolina et al, 2012). The American Heart Association projected that costs of CVD care would triple from $272.5 billion in 2010 to an estimated $818.1 billion in 2030 (Laslett et al, 2012). Men are at greater risk for CVD than premenopausal women, suggesting a possible influence of sex hormones (Yang and Reckelhoff, 2011).

Both CVD and AD are diseases of aging; they share many risk factors such as age, obesity, diabetes, alcohol consumption, and chronic diseases. **The association between AD and CVD has become evident in observational studies** (Araujo et al, 2011). **ADT is associated with an increased risk for CV events in patients with prostate cancer** (Levine et al, 2010). Prospective studies demonstrated that ADT increases CVD by affecting various risk factors: increased body weight, decreased insulin sensitivity, altered lipid profile, and increased fat mass. Two population-based studies reported that ADT is associated significantly with CAD and sudden cardiac death or life-threatening arrhythmia (Saigal et al, 2007). Data from the Cancer of the Prostate Strategic Urologic Research Endeavor also showed a significantly increased risk of CV death in men who underwent radical prostatectomy and received ADT compared with those undergoing surgery alone (Tsai et al, 2007). Endogenous testosterone has been suggested as CV-protective or as a secondary risk predictor of other processes, although the mechanism is still unclear.

Men with LOH commonly exhibit coexisting CVD risk factors; the safety of TT is often questioned, given the known adverse reaction of polycythemia. In 2004, the Institute of Medicine reviewed the evidence on TT and concluded that "there is not clear evidence of benefit for any of the health outcomes examined" (Xu et al, 2013). A randomized, placebo-controlled study on TT in elderly men with limitations in mobility was discontinued early because of an increase in CV-related events in the treatment arm despite showing an improvement in musculoskeletal parameters (Basaria et al, 2010). The generalizability of the results was often questioned, however, because the study population was elderly men (mean age of 74 years) with serious chronic illnesses. The number of CV adverse events was small and the trial was not originally designed to analyze CV outcomes. Meta-analysis of randomized studies on the adverse events associated with TT yielded mixed results on CV events and mortality (Fernandez-Balsells et al, 2010; Xu et al, 2013).

A retrospective study of 8709 male veterans showed a 29% increased risk of CV events in men undergoing TT (Vigen et al, 2013). However, the study was criticized for many flaws: improper patient exclusion, unbalanced comparison, and unusual complexity of statistical analysis. Another cohort study using a health care database (Truven Health MarketScan) suggested the risk of myocardial infarction doubled within 90 days after initiation of TT (Finkle et al, 2014). Researchers used prescription claim information, which does not accurately reflect initiation of TT when known patient compliance issues are considered. Additional statistical modeling was applied to the weighted data. Definitive assessment of CV risk associated with TT must await an ongoing large randomized, controlled trial.

Coronary Artery Disease

Traditionally, AD is not considered a risk factor for CAD. An earlier longitudinal case control study reported no significant difference in testosterone between low-risk men who developed CAD and those who did not (Heller et al, 1983). **A growing body of evidence suggests a link between low endogenous testosterone levels and CAD.** Several studies have demonstrated that patients with CAD as diagnosed by coronary angiography have lower levels of testosterone compared to control subjects (Chute et al, 1987; Sieminska et al, 2003; Cao et al, 2010). In addition to total testosterone, a significantly lower level of bioavailable testosterone was also found in patients with catheterization-proven CAD (Rosano et al, 2007).

In addition, **the degree of AD has been reported as having an inverse relationship to the severity of CAD.** Epidemiologic evidence reported a fivefold decrease in the risk of severe atherosclerotic CAD between the lowest and the highest quartiles of total testosterone (Chute et al, 1987). Four small studies have demonstrated independently that in men with CAD, lower levels of endogenous testosterone are associated with more severe CAD (Phillips et al, 1994; Rosano et al, 2007; Hu et al, 2011; Li et al, 2012). This correlation between low testosterone and CAD severity has also been demonstrated in both men and postmenopausal women with CAD (Phillips et al, 1997; Kaczmarek et al, 2003). Men with myocardial infarctions and ischemia have been reported as having lower testosterone and an increased estradiol-to-testosterone ratio when compared to controls (Sewdarsen et al, 1986; Lichtenstein et al, 1987).

Several population-based studies examined the association between mortality secondary to CVD and levels of total testosterone. Although some researchers found significantly greater CV mortality associated with lower testosterone concentrations, others did not (Oskui et al, 2013). A meta-analysis showed a trend toward increased CV mortality associated with lower levels of total testosterone, but statistical significance was not reached (Araujo et al, 2011). An analysis of 2416 Swedish men demonstrated that levels of endogenous total testosterone were significantly inversely associated with risk of adverse CV events (Ohlsson et al, 2011). Men in the fourth quartile of total testosterone showed significant improvement in event-free survival for both major adverse CAD events. Several studies also analyzed the association between bioavailable testosterone and CV mortality, and all indicated that a higher risk of CV mortality was associated with lower levels of bioavailable testosterone (Laughlin et al, 2008; Malkin et al, 2010; Menke et al, 2010).

Cerebral Vascular Disease

AD has also been implicated in the development of cerebral vascular disease. Low levels of total testosterone and bioavailable testosterone have been reported as predictive of an increased incidence of cerebral vascular accidents or transient ischemic attack, even after adjusting for conventional risk factors for cerebral vascular disease (Yeap et al, 2009). Multiple studies have demonstrated that low testosterone concentration is associated with increased carotid intimal-media thickness (IMT), which serves as a measure of cerebrovascular atherosclerosis (De Pergola et al, 2003; Fukui

et al, 2003; van den Beld et al, 2003). Several population-based studies reported an inverse association between total testosterone levels and carotid artery IMT that was present after excluding men with cerebral vascular disease; this relationship, however, was not independent of BMI (Svartberg et al, 2006; Debing et al, 2008). Similarly, a cross-sectional analysis of the Tromso cohort demonstrated an inverse association between testosterone levels and total carotid plaque area (Vikan et al, 2009). In studies without association with total testosterone, low levels of bioavailable testosterone were associated with carotid artery IMT after adjusting for age, BMI, and known cerebral vascular disease risk factors (Tsujimura et al, 2012). The association between testosterone and cerebral vascular disease appeared to be gender specific. No association was observed for free testosterone or total testosterone with carotid IMT in young to middle-aged women (Calderon-Margalit et al, 2010) or with progression of carotid IMT and adventitial diameter in perimenopausal women (El Khoudary et al, 2012).

Proposed Mechanism of Testosterone's Action on the Cardiovascular System

Endothelial Dysfunction

Endothelial dysfunction is the first step in the formation of atherosclerotic lesions. Testosterone has been demonstrated as having a protective effect on endothelial function (Fu et al, 2008). Testosterone has been inversely correlated with vascular cell adhesion molecule-1, which is produced by endothelial cells and is upregulated when endothelial cells undergo inflammatory and malignant stimulation. Investigators reported that hypogonadal men exhibited lower levels of endothelial progenitor cells), which are important in endothelial regeneration, and higher levels of an osteocalcin-positive subpopulation of endothelial progenitor cells, which are highly correlated with atherosclerosis progression, compared to eugonadal men (Foresta et al, 2010). Finally, testosterone has been shown to reduce significantly endoplasmic reticulum stress and superoxide generation in human umbilical vein endothelial cells, both of which have been implicated in atherosclerosis; however, when combined with aromatase inhibitors, the protective effect of testosterone was lost, suggesting an estradiol-mediated mechanism (Haas et al, 2012).

The antianginal and anti-ischemial effects of TT have been recognized since the late 1930s (Oskui et al, 2013). TT in AD men suffering from CAD has proven effective in increasing time to 1-mm ST-segment depression with an exercise stress test (Rosano et al, 1999; English et al, 2000). Although testosterone's vasodilatory effects are well recognized, the exact mechanism of action has yet to be elucidated. Testosterone has been reported to induce endothelium-independent relaxation of numerous vascular beds including human internal mammary arteries and radial arteries (Yildiz et al, 2005b). Both in vivo animal models and in vitro models provided evidence that testosterone induces coronary vasodilation by modulating the activity of ion channels. This direct relaxation response to testosterone has been attributed to conductance of non–adenosine triphosphate sensitive potassium channel (Yue et al, 1995), adenosine triphosphate–sensitive potassium channel (Seyrek et al, 2007), and large conductance calcium-activated potassium channel opening action (Yildiz et al, 2005a). Testosterone has also been reported to induce vasodilation by reducing calcium influx into vascular smooth muscle by acting as a selective and potent inhibitor of L-type calcium channels at physiologic levels and as an inhibitor of testosterone-type channels at supraphysiologic levels (Scragg et al, 2004).

Contrarily, other studies have suggested an endothelium-dependent mediated mechanism behind testosterone's vasodilatory effect (Ong et al, 2000; Kang et al, 2002). Both acute and long-term administration of testosterone in men with CAD have been shown to increase brachial artery flow–mediated reactivity, which induces shear stress release of nitric oxide and subsequently leads to vasodilation. This relation has also been demonstrated in postmenopausal women (Montalcini et al, 2007).

Arterial wall stiffness is an independent predictor of CVD risk. Low testosterone levels have been associated with endothelial dysfunction (Laurent et al, 2006). This inverse relationship has been demonstrated using both pulse pressure and pulse wave velocity as reflections of arterial wall stiffness (Fukui et al, 2007; Corona et al, 2009). Interestingly, the association between testosterone and CVD mortality was lost in male hemodialysis patients after adjusting for pulse wave velocity, suggesting that endothelial dysfunction may be a possible explanation of testosterone's inverse association with CVD (Kyriazis et al, 2011). Contrarily, long-term (8-week) administration of testosterone increased myocardial perfusion in unobstructed coronary arteries and decreased radial and aortic augmentation indexes, indicating decreased arterial wall stiffness; however, no effect was observed on global perfusion or on endothelial function (Webb et al, 2008).

Inflammation

Atherosclerosis is mediated by an ongoing inflammatory response, which is induced by cytokines and other inflammatory markers. Cytokines cause cellular and local arterial wall inflammation and may lead to vascular smooth muscle apoptosis, degradation of the fibrin cap, and plaque rupture, thereby leading to platelet adhesion, thrombus formation, and ultimately angina or myocardial infarction (Malkin et al, 2003). An elevation in inflammatory markers or cytokines has been identified to be predictive of outcomes in patients with CVD (Libby et al, 2002). In a cross-sectional study, inflammatory markers, macrophage inflammatory protein 1-α, 1-β, and tumor necrosis factor-α, have been negatively associated with total testosterone levels in young healthy men, suggesting a low-grade inflammatory state (Bobjer et al, 2013).

TT was reported to suppress the expression of high-sensitivity C-reactive protein and IL-6 in patients who underwent coronary artery stent implantation, leading to the hypothesis that testosterone's anti-inflammatory property could potentially attenuate major CV events (Guler et al, 2006). In a randomized, placebo-controlled, crossover study of AD men, TT reduced levels of proinflammatory cytokines tumor necrosis factor-α and IL-1β while suppressing levels of cytokine IL-10 (Malkin et al, 2004). However, the inverse relationship between cytokines and testosterone was not identified in AD men with congestive heart failure and in diabetic males compared to eugonadal controls (Pugh et al, 2005; Hernandez-Mijares et al, 2010).

Coagulation

The effect of testosterone on clotting factors including fibrinogen and plasminogen activator inhibitor-1 (PAI-1) has been studied previously. Fibrinogen is a known risk factor for CVD as well as an inflammatory biomarker (Danesh et al, 2005); it increases CVD risk through its effects on atherogenesis, thrombogenesis, and ischemia by the mechanism of increasing plasma and blood viscosity (Kaptoge et al, 2007). It was shown that endogenous testosterone levels were negatively correlated with fibrinogen (Phillips et al, 1994). In a study comparing patients with prostate cancer on ADT to healthy controls, patients on ADT presented with elevated levels of fibrinogen (Ziaran et al, 2013). In addition to fibrinogen, PAI-1, another risk factor for ischemic heart disease, was also negatively correlated with endogenous testosterone levels (Yang et al, 1993; Phillips et al, 1994).

Contrarily, a double-blinded, randomized placebo-controlled trial of testosterone supplementation in men with chronic stable angina demonstrated no changes in fibrinogen or PAI-1, suggesting that testosterone supplementation does not affect blood coagulation status (Smith et al, 2005). Moreover, a study comparing chemically or surgically castrated males to eugonadal controls showed that castrated men had less platelet thromboxane A2 (TXA2) receptors, suggesting that the inhibition of testosterone production may attenuate platelet aggregation responses (Ajayi and Halushka, 2005).

> ### KEY POINTS: CARDIOVASCULAR DISEASE AND TESTOSTERONE
>
> - Increased awareness has been dedicated to the interplay between testosterone and various aspects of CV health. Existing literature suggests that lower levels of endogenous testosterone are associated with higher rates of all-cause and CV mortality.
> - Negative correlation has been demonstrated among endogenous testosterone and severity of CAD, congestive failure, and IMT of the vasculature (Oskui et al, 2013).
> - Normal testosterone levels play an important role in maintaining CV health.
> - Exogenous TT in men with AD improves myocardial ischemia, exercise capacity, and CV risk factors.
> - Current available guidelines do not recommend offering AD screening to patients with heart disease, nor do they recommend supplementing TT to improve outcome.
> - Results from the Effects of Testosterone Replacement on Atherosclerosis Progressions in Older Men with Low Testosterone Levels trial have the potential to clarify any long-term adverse consequences and the role of exogenous testosterone in the survival of patients with heart disease.

METABOLIC SYNDROME AND UROLOGIC DISEASES

Introduction

Metabolic syndrome (MetS) is a constellation of clinical factors—including obesity, insulin resistance, hypertension (HTN), and abnormal serum lipid concentrations—associated with an increased risk of incident CVD and diabetes mellitus (DM). Other terms applied to this cluster include the obesity dyslipidemia syndrome, syndrome X, and the deadly quartet. The global prevalence and incidence of MetS have increased substantially since the mid-2000s, particularly in the developed world.

Epidemiologic studies have shown strong associations of MetS and its individual components with increased risks of developing a host of benign and malignant urologic diseases. These observations show novel pathways in the etiology of urologic diseases, underscore the links of urologic conditions with overall health, and suggest new interventions for their prevention and treatment.

These data also have promoted the idea of "men's health," which, broadly speaking, represents the integration of male urologic care with the prevention and treatment of systemic CVD. However, the concept of men's health is an evolving paradigm with no clearly defined clinical parameters. In the absence of robust randomized clinical trial data and evidence-based guidelines, there are currently few, if any, clearly defined roles for the evaluation or treatment of MetS in the practical management of urology patients.

Definition and Epidemiology

Disagreement exists about the exact diagnostic criteria of MetS. At least five separate organizations have issued definitions, all of which contain the same five basic components (Table 23-5).

The National Cholesterol Education Program (Adult Treatment Panel [ATP] III) issued guidelines in 2001, which the American Heart Association/National Heart, Lung, and Blood Institute updated in 2005. This statement, one of the most commonly used, **currently defines MetS as a condition in which at least three of the following factors are present:**
- *Abdominal obesity*
  Defined as a waist circumference greater than or equal to 88 cm in women and greater than or equal to 102 cm in men

TABLE 23-5 Metabolic Syndrome Definitions

	WHO (1998)	EGIR (1999)	AACE (2003)	IDF (2005)	NCEP ATP III (2005 REVISION)
Required component	IR (IGT, IFG, T2DM, or additional evidence of IR)	Hyperinsulinemia* (plasma insulin >75th percentile)	IR (IGT or IFG)	CO (WC)†	None
Criteria	Required component and ≥2/5 below	Required component and ≥2/4 below	Required component and any below, based on clinical judgment	Required component and ≥2/4 below	≥3/5 below
Obesity	WHR >0.9 (M), >0.85 (F), or BMI >30 kg/m²	WC ≥94 cm (M), ≥80 cm (F)	BMI ≥25 kg/m²	—	WC >102 cm (M), >88 cm (F)
Hyperglycemia (mg/dL)	+	+	+	Fasting glucose ≥100	Fasting glucose ≥100 or Rx
Dyslipidemia (mg/dL)	TG ≥150 or HDL-C <35 (M), <39 (F)	TG ≥150 or HDL-C <39	TG ≥150 and HDL-C <40 (M), <50 (F)	TG ≥150 or Rx HDL <40 (M), <50 (F), or Rx	TG ≥150 or Rx HDL <40 (M), 50 (F), or Rx
Hypertension (mm Hg)	>140/90	>140/90 or Rx	>130/85	>130 (S), >85 (D) or Rx	>130 (S), >85 (D) or Rx
Other criteria	Microalbuminuria‡	—	Other features of IR§	—	—

*In patients without T2DM.
†Values are population dependent.
‡Urinary albumin excretion of 20 µg/min or albumin-to-creatinine ratio of greater than or equal to 30 mg/g.
§This includes family history of T2DM, polycystic ovary syndrome, sedentary lifestyle, advancing age, and ethnic groups susceptible to T2DM.
+, criteria fulfilled with required component; AACE, American Association of Clinical Endocrinologists; BMI, body mass index; CO, central obesity; D, diastolic; EGIR, European Group for the Study of Insulin Resistance; F, female; HDL, high-density lipoprotein; IDF, International Diabetes Foundation; IFG, impaired fasting glucose; IGT, impaired glucose tolerance; IR, insulin resistance; M, male; NCEP ATP III, National Cholesterol Education Program Adult Treatment Panel III; Rx, pharmacologic intervention for that criterion; S, systolic; T2DM, type 2 diabetes mellitus; TG, triglycerides; WC, waist circumference; WHO, World Health Organization; WHR, waist-to-hip ratio.

- *Elevated blood glucose*
  Fasting plasma glucose greater than or equal to 100 mg/dL or drug treatment for elevated blood glucose
- *Elevated blood pressure*
  Blood pressure greater than or equal to 130/85 mm Hg or drug treatment for elevated blood pressure
- *Elevated triglycerides*
  Serum triglycerides greater than or equal to 150 mg/dL or drug treatment for elevated triglycerides
- *Decreased HDL cholesterol*
  Serum HDL cholesterol less than 50 mg/dL in women and less than 40 mg/dL in men or drug treatment for decreased HDL cholesterol

Epidemiology of Metabolic Syndrome

MetS is common, and there is evidence that its prevalence is substantially increasing. Among 8814 U.S. adults participating in the third National Health and Nutrition Examination Survey (NHANES III, 1988 to 1994) the overall prevalence of MetS as defined by the 2001 ATP III criteria was 22%. **Prevalence increased steadily with age**; Mexican-Americans had the highest age-adjusted prevalence (31.9%). The age-adjusted prevalence for men (24.0%) was similar to women (23.4%) (Ford et al, 2002). An updated analysis among 1677 participants from NHANES 1999 to 2000 demonstrated that the overall prevalence had increased to 26.7% ($P = .043$), a trend driven primarily by a 23.5% increase in prevalence among women (Ford et al, 2004).

Similarly, among 3323 adult participants in the Framingham Heart Study, the baseline prevalence of MetS as defined by the 2005 revised ATP III criteria was 26.8% in men and 16.6% in women. After 8 years of follow-up, there was an age-adjusted 56% increase in prevalence among men and a 47% increase among women (Wilson et al, 2005).

Metabolic Syndrome and Clinical Urology

Although an emerging body of knowledge links MetS to the development of urologic diseases, and familiarity with these concepts is important, practical applications of these data to urologic practice are currently limited. At least two clinical issues remain unresolved with respect to MetS and the care of the urology patient.

First, because the management of MetS-related conditions primarily rests with cardiologists, endocrinologists, and primary care physicians, how urologists should approach urologic diseases in the context of MetS is currently unclear. Pathophysiologic links of MetS with urologic diseases, and a small number of clinical trials, imply that treating systemic manifestations of MetS will mitigate their effects on urologic conditions. Yet weight loss, lipid control, and other medical interventions do not typically fall within the purview of urologic practice; and without substantial changes in current care delivery paradigms, it is unlikely that urologists will oversee these therapies independent of other health care providers.

Second, because ED and male LUTS are potential markers for occult CVD (Thompson et al, 2005), some investigators have proposed that urologists routinely screen for CVD. This endeavor, too, is one that urologists do not normally pursue. Moreover, CVD screening is a discipline for which most urologists typically lack formal training, and it is therefore fraught with as-yet-unanswered practical, medical, and medicolegal questions.

Metabolic Syndrome, Benign Prostatic Enlargement, and Male Lower Urinary Tract Symptoms

MetS and its individual components have been associated with increased risks of benign prostatic enlargement (BPE) (formerly known as benign prostatic hyperplasia [BPH]) and male LUTS. Definitions of BPE in the literature are heterogeneous and include radiographically determined prostate enlargement, decreased urinary flow rates, history of noncancer prostate surgery, physician diagnosis, and urinary symptoms.

LUTS describes a distinct phenotype of a group of disorders affecting the prostate and bladder that share a common clinical manifestation. In its evidenced-based report, the International Consultation on Urological Diseases (2012) used the term "LUTS" to classify the diagnosis, treatment, and study of these conditions. LUTS has also become the preferred term for studying urinary symptoms in populations. Most studies use the IPSS or the American Urological Association Symptom Index (AUASI) to quantify the severity of symptoms; older studies focused on specific symptoms, including nocturia and frequency.

Metabolic Syndrome and Cardiovascular Disease

A systematic review and meta-analysis of 8 studies involving more than 5400 men observed significant direct associations of a diagnosis of MetS with increased prostate volume (Gacci et al, 2015).

Other studies have shown that men with cardiac disease or who are receiving treatment for cardiac disease (and thus have a high likelihood of having at least one component of MetS) are at significantly increased risks of physician-diagnosed BPE and LUTS (De Nunzio et al, 2012).

Correlation between Metabolic Syndrome and Prostatic Diseases

Obesity

Increased adiposity is associated with increased ultrasound- and MRI-determined prostate volume as measured by body weight, BMI, and waist circumference. In the Baltimore Longitudinal Study of Aging (BLSA) cohort, each 1 kg/m^2 increase in BMI corresponded to a 0.41 mL increase in prostate volume, and obese (BMI ≥35 kg/m^2) participants had a 3.5-fold increased risk of prostate enlargement compared to nonobese (BMI <25 kg/m^2) participants (P trend = .06) (Parsons et al, 2006; Raheem and Parsons, 2014).

Obesity has been associated with increased risks of symptomatic BPE and LUTS in several different populations, including the U.S. Health Professionals Follow-up Study (n = 26,000), a study group in China (n = 500), a 7-year prospective analysis of the U.S. Prostate Cancer Prevention Trial (PCPT) (n = 4770), NHANES III (n = 2800), the second Nord-Trøndelag Health Study (HUNT-2) (n = 21,700), and the Prostate Study Group of the Austrian Society of Urology (n = 1500). Other studies have shown that obesity increases the risks of BPE surgery, initiation of BPE medical therapy, and LUTS (Raheem and Parsons, 2014).

Obesity also attenuates the efficacy of the 5α-reductase inhibitors (5ARI) finasteride and dutasteride, which decrease serum concentrations of DHT, prevent clinical progression of BPE and LUTS, and prevent incident-symptomatic BPE. An analysis of the PCPT showed that obesity diminished the efficacy of finasteride for preventing symptomatic BPE. Similarly, a secondary analysis of the Reduction by Dutasteride of Prostate Cancer Events (REDUCE) trial concluded that obesity enhanced prostate volume growth and weakened the magnitude of prostate volume reduction by dutasteride. These observations likely highlight a balance between 5ARI-driven prostate volume reduction and obesity-driven prostate volume growth (Parsons, 2010, 2011; Raheem and Parsons, 2014).

Diabetes and Disruptions in Glucose Homeostasis

Higher serum concentrations of insulin-like growth factor-1 and insulin-like growth factor binding protein-3 were consistently associated with increased risks of BPE diagnosis and BPE surgery. **DM, increased serum insulin, and elevated fasting plasma glucose have been associated with increased prostate volume and prostate enlargement, clinical diagnosis of BPE, BPE surgery, and LUTS in many different cohorts** cumulatively involving tens of thousands of men (Sarma et al, 2009; Parsons, 2010, 2011; Raheem and Parsons, 2014).

Diabetes and Disruptions in Glucose Homeostasis: The Epidemiology of Diabetes Interventions and Complications Study

The Epidemiology of Diabetes Interventions and Complications (UroEDIC) follow-up study of the Diabetes Control and Complications Trial (DCCT) was a post hoc analysis of 591 men enrolled in a randomized clinical trial comparing intensive to conventional glycemic control in type 1 DM (Van Den Eeden et al, 2009). The aim was to determine whether intensive glycemic control reduces LUTS severity in men with type 1 DM. Intensive treatment consisted of insulin administered three or more times daily by injection or by infusion pump coupled with rigorous monitoring of blood glucose levels. No associations were observed between LUTS, as measured by the AUASI, and intensive glycemic control. However, because these men were younger (mean age 45 years) and had type 1 rather than type 2 DM, these data may not apply to the broader population of older diabetic men with LUTS.

Elevated Blood Pressure

Associations of HTN with BPE and LUTS remain unclear. There have been at least six studies among men with HTN, three of which observed an increased risk of LUTS, one of which noted an increased risk of BPE surgery, and two of which observed no risk.

Elevated Triglycerides and Decreased High-Density Lipoprotein

Studies of BPE and LUTS with serum triglycerides and HDL are also conflicting. There have been at least six studies, including three showing positive and three showing null associations (Hammarsten et al, 1998; Zucchetto et al, 2005; Gupta et al, 2006; Lekili et al, 2006; Nandeesha et al, 2006; Parsons et al, 2008; Parsons, 2011).

Metabolic Syndrome and Urinary Incontinence

MetS and some of its features, primarily obesity, were linked to a higher risk of urinary incontinence in women.

Metabolic Syndrome

One study of 400 women in Turkey observed an increased, albeit unadjusted, risk of stress urinary incontinence (SUI) in those with MetS compared to those without it in both the pre- and postmenopausal groups (P = .001 and P < .001, respectively) (Octuntemur et al, 2014).

Obesity

Multiple studies have noted strong associations of obesity with urinary incontinence in women across different populations. In a cross-sectional analysis of Taiwanese women, those who were obese (BMI >27 kg/m^2) had a more than threefold (odds ratio [OR] 3.38, 95% CI 1.94 to 6.98, P < .001) increased adjusted risk of incontinence (stress, urge, or mixed) compared to those of normal weight (BMI ≤24 kg/m^2) (Tsai and Liu, 2009).

In a study of more than 19,000 Chinese women, waist circumference greater than or equal to 80 cm was associated with an increased adjusted risk of SUI (OR 1.38, 95% CI 1.25 to 1.52) (Zhu et al, 2009); in another study by the same investigators that measured BMI, overweight (OR 1.31, 95% CI 1.12 to 1.55) and obese (OR 1.44, 95% CI 1.21 to 1.72) women were more likely to report SUI (Zhu et al, 2008).

In a randomized clinical trial of women with type 2 DM—the Action for Health in Diabetes (Look AHEAD) study—obese (BMI

>35 kg/m²) women were more likely to experience both SUI and overall incontinence (Phelan et al, 2009). In a randomized clinical trial of hormone replacement in postmenopausal women—the Heart and Estrogen/progestin Replacement Study (HERS)—BMI and waist-to-hip ratio were each directly associated with SUI risk; BMI was also associated with mixed incontinence (Brown et al, 1999).

In a survey of 6000 women living in the Pacific Northwest region of the United States, BMI greater than or equal to 30 kg/m² was associated with an increased risk of self-reported urinary incontinence (OR 2.39, 95% CI 1.99 to 2.87) (Melville et al, 2005). Finally, in a cross-sectional analysis of nearly 4000 women in southern California, obesity was associated with SUI in both nondiabetic (OR 2.62, 95% CI 2.09 to 3.30) and diabetic (OR 3.67, 95% CI 2.48 to 5.43) participants (Lawrence et al, 2007).

Obesity: Weight Loss and Urinary Incontinence

SUI in women is one of the few urologic conditions for which level I evidence exists favoring an intervention that, by targeting a feature of MetS, improves the urologic condition. The Program to Reduce Incontinence by Diet and Exercise (PRIDE) trial randomized overweight or obese women who experienced 10 or more incontinence episodes per week to either an intensive 6-month behavioral weight loss intervention or a structured educational program. Women in the behavioral intervention group lost more weight and showed significant improvements in SUI (but not urge incontinence) compared to those in the education group (Subak et al, 2009). Two systematic reviews also concluded that weight loss improves SUI in women (Hunskaar, 2008; Imamura et al, 2010).

Based on these data, the 2012 European Association of Urology Guidelines on Urinary Incontinence concluded that evidence in support of weight loss as an effective lifestyle intervention for incontinence was Grade A, and the recommendations also encouraged "obese women suffering from any urinary incontinence to lose weight (>5%)" (http://www.uroweb.org/gls/pdf/18_Urinary_Incontinence_LR.pdf). The extent to which urologists and other health care providers have adopted this recommendation, and routinely use weight loss as a first-line intervention for incontinence in obese women, is unknown. The American Urological Association guidelines have not as yet addressed the topic of lifestyle interventions and urinary incontinence (www.auanet.org).

Diabetes and Disruptions in Glucose Homeostasis

In the southern California study, nonobese women with type 2 DM were 80% more likely to report SUI (OR 1.81, 95% CI 1.09 to 3.00) (Lawrence et al, 2007). In HERS, DM was associated with a 49% increased risk of urge incontinence (OR 1.49, 95% CI 1.11 to 2.00) and a 32% increased risk of mixed incontinence (OR 1.04, 95% CI 1.11 to 2.00) (Brown et al, 1999).

Metabolic Syndrome and Urinary Stones

MetS has been associated with an increased risk of urinary lithiasis. Putative causal factors include decreased urine pH, hypercalciuria, hyperuricosuria, and hyperoxaluria (Gorbachinsky et al, 2010).

Metabolic Syndrome

Studies have shown robust associations of MetS with an increased prevalence of urinary stones in U.S., European, and Southeast Asian populations. In the U.S. NHANES, the prevalence of self-reported history of kidney stones in an analytic cohort of 14,870 men and women increased substantially with the presence of increased MetS components, with a prevalence of 3%, 7.5%, and 9.8% in participants with 0, 3, and 5 components, respectively. Multivariable adjustment showed further that the presence of greater than or equal to 2 components significantly increased the odds of kidney stones, and that the presence of greater than or equal to 4 components increased the odds approximately twofold (West et al, 2008).

In a study of a screened Korean population (n = 34,895), those with MetS showed a 25% increase in the multivariable adjusted odds (OR 1.25, 95% CI 1.03 to 1.50) in kidney-stone prevalence as detected with computed tomography or ultrasound.

Finally, in an Italian study (n = 2132) of hospitalized patients, MetS was associated with a twofold adjusted risk in the prevalence of ultrasound-detected kidney stones (OR 2.62, 95% CI 1.50 to 4.64) (Rendina et al, 2009).

Obesity

Increased waist circumference and BMI have been independently associated with an increased risk of urinary stones. In an analysis that combined the U.S. Health Professionals Follow-up Study (n = 45,988 men), the Nurses' Health Study I (n = 93,758), and the Nurses' Health Study II (n = 101,877), male participants with a BMI greater than or equal to 30 kg/m² showed a 33% increased risk of incident stone disease compared to those with a BMI of 21 kg/m² to 22.9 kg/m² (relative risk [RR] 1.33, 95% CI 1.08 to 1.63; $P < .001$ for trend). For the same categories of BMI in older and younger women, the increased risks were 90% (RR 1.90, 95% CI 1.61 to 2.25; $P < .001$ for trend) and more than twofold (RR 2.09, 95% CI 1.77 to 2.48; $P < .001$ for trend), respectively. Waist circumference was also positively associated with an increased risk of stones in both men ($P = .002$ for trend) and women ($P < .001$) (Taylor et al, 2005b).

In a study of 95,598 patients in a U.S. health administrative database, obesity was associated with a significantly increased risk of kidney-stone diagnosis at all stratifications comparing obese to nonobese patients. The odds generally increased with increasing BMI. Compared to men with BMI less than 20, those with a BMI of 45.0 to 49.9 had more than a threefold risk of stone diagnosis (OR 3.18, 95% CI 1.61 to 6.29; $P < .0009$) (Semins et al, 2010).

In the aforementioned Korean study, the adjusted odds for kidney stones increased with an increasing quintile of waist circumference ($P < .001$).

Diabetes and Disruptions in Glucose Homeostasis

In another analysis combining more than 200,000 participants in the Health Professionals Follow-up Study and Nurses' Health Studies I and II, DM was associated with an increased adjusted prevalence of stone disease in all groups, with increased risks of 38% (RR 1.38, 95% CI 1.06 to 1.79) in older women, 67% (RR 1.67, 95% CI 1.28 to 2.20) in younger women, and 31% (RR 1.31, 95% CI 1.11 to 1.54) in men.

Similarly, in a prospective analysis of the same cohorts, the adjusted stone incidence was greater in female participants with DM compared to those without: a 29% (1.29, 95% CI 1.05 to 1.58) and a 60% (1.60, 95% CI 1.16 to 2.21) increased risk in older and younger women, respectively. Although there was no association of DM with incident kidney-stone risk in men (RR 0.81, 95% CI 0.59 to 1.09), men with kidney stones at baseline were 49% more likely to develop incident DM (RR 1.49, 95% CI 1.29 to 1.72) than those without kidney stones, as were both older (1.33, 95% CI 1.18 to 1.50) and younger (1.48, 95% CI 1.14 to 1.91) women, respectively.

These investigators speculated that the association of stone disease with incident DM was potentially linked to subclinical insulin resistance (Taylor et al, 2005a).

Elevated Blood Pressure

In the Korean study, participants with HTN showed a 47% increased adjusted risk of kidney stones (1.47, 95% CI 1.25 to 1.71) compared to participants without HTN, and the multivariable-adjusted odds for kidney stones increased with increasing quintile of blood pressure ($P < .001$).

In a study of Italian male factory workers, those with HTN showed an unadjusted increased risk of a history of kidney stones compared to those without HTN (OR 2.11, 95% CI 1.17 to 3.81), which was even higher in men with treated HTN (OR 3.16, 95% CI

1.75 to 5.71). Men with treated HTN also had an increased, if slightly attenuated, age-adjusted kidney-stone risk (OR 2.63, 95% CI 2.23 to 3.10) (Cappuccio et al, 1990).

In a prospective study of the same population followed for 8 years, those with HTN at baseline were approximately twice as likely to develop kidney stones (Cappuccio et al, 1999).

Other studies have shown that nephrolithiasis is a risk factor for the development of HTN, suggesting that these associations are bidirectional (Madore et al, 1998a, 1998b).

Metabolic Syndrome and Erectile Dysfunction

The presence of MetS, each of the five individual components of MetS, and CVD all substantially increase the risk of ED. Several different etiologies are likely involved, including but not necessarily limited to the following: inhibition of nitric oxide synthase pathways; MetS-associated hypogonadism; atherosclerosis-mediated vasculopathy; disruption of autonomic signaling pathways; and promotion of corporal cavernosal fibrosis (Gorbachinsky et al, 2010).

Metabolic Syndrome and Cardiovascular Disease

Multiple studies worldwide have included observations showing a significantly increased prevalence of ED among men with a diagnosis of MetS, including a German health screening project of 2371 men (P = .01), a case control analysis of Italian men (P = .03), a cohort of 393 Turkish men (P < .001), a separate cohort of 268 Turkish men (P < .001), and a primary case-based population of 3921 Canadian men (Esposito et al, 2005; Grover et al, 2006; Bal et al, 2007; Heidler et al, 2007).

Moreover, ED appears to be an independent risk factor for incident CVD. In a study of more than 8063 men greater than or equal to age 55 years who were randomized to the placebo arm of the PCPT, those with incident ED experienced a 25% increased adjusted risk of incident CVD (defined as myocardial infarction or surgical treatment of coronary artery disease, angina, cerebrovascular accident, transient ischemic attack, congestive heart failure, or nonfatal cardiac arrhythmia requiring treatment) compared to those without ED (hazard ratio [HR] 1.25, 95% CI 1.02 to 1.53). Men with either incident or prevalent ED experienced a 45% increased adjusted risk (HR 1.45, 95% CI 1.25 to 1.69). The magnitudes of these risks were similar to those observed for current smoking or a family history of myocardial infarction (Thompson et al, 2005).

Similar conclusions were reported in other studies (Montorsi et al, 2006; Inman et al, 2009). ED has also been associated with subclinical atherosclerosis (Chiurlia et al, 2005), endothelial dysfunction (Yavuzgil et al, 2005), and reduced brachial artery vasodilation (Kaiser et al, 2004).

Nevertheless, although these data thus implicate ED as an independent risk factor for clinically significant CVD, the validity of routinely using ED for CVD screening has not been defined (Alhathal and Carrier, 2011; Ewane et al, 2012), and formal guidelines as yet do not exist.

Obesity

Obesity—including central obesity as measured by waist circumference—was one of the first modifiable risk factors linked to ED (Derby et al, 2000; Feldman et al, 2000; Bacon et al, 2003; Fung et al, 2004; Carvalho et al, 2013).

Obesity: Weight Loss, Exercise, and Erectile Dysfunction

Similar to SUI in obese women, level I evidence indicates that a lifestyle intervention aimed at weight loss improves erectile function in obese men. In an Italian randomized clinical trial, 110 obese men (BMI ≥30 kg/m^2) aged 35 to 55 years with ED as determined by IIEF score and without DM, HTN, or hyperlipidemia were randomized to either an intensive weight loss intervention of caloric reduction and exercise or a control state that provided general

information about healthy food choices and exercise. After 2 years, men in the intervention group had lost more weight, were more physically active, and reported significantly larger increases in IIEF score than those in the control group. Moreover, in multivariate analyses, changes in BMI (P = .02) and physical activity (P = .02) were independently associated with changes in IIEF score (Esposito et al, 2004).

It is not clear to what extent these data are applied in the clinical management of ED. The American Urological Association Guidelines for the Management of Erectile Dysfunction did not formally address the use of weight loss or other lifestyle interventions in the management of ED (www.auanet.org).

Diabetes and Disruptions in Glucose Homeostasis

Although diabetes is a well-established risk factor for ED (Feldman et al, 1994, 2000; Maiorino et al, 2014), data have also shown links between ED and prediabetic states characteristic of MetS. In a cohort of Argentinian men, ED was associated with an increased risk of insulin resistance, defined as homeostasis model assessment greater than or equal to 3 (P = .04) (Knoblovits et al, 2010). Similarly, in a cohort of Chinese patients, ED was also associated with insulin resistance, defined as quantitative insulin sensitivity check index less than or equal to 0.357 (Chen et al, 2013).

Elevated Blood Pressure

Men with HTN are more likely to experience ED than those without HTN (Feldman et al, 1994; Saigal et al, 2006).

Metabolic Syndrome and Male Infertility

MetS and its components are associated with an increased risk of infertility. Several factors may potentially contribute to male infertility in the setting of MetS and its components, including associations of obesity with spermatic DNA damage, low ejaculate volume, and diminished sperm motility, volume, and count; associations of type 2 DM with lower sperm motility, semen volume, and ejaculatory dysfunction; and associations of MetS with hypogonadism (Fig. 23-3) (Gorbachinsky et al, 2010).

Obesity

A systematic review and meta-analysis of BMI and sperm count, which included 21 studies and 13,077 men, reported the conclusion that compared to men of normal weight, overweight (OR 1.28, 95% CI 1.06 to 1.55) and obese (OR 2.04, 95% CI 1.59 to 2.62) men were more likely to have oligozoospermia or azoospermia (Sermondade et al, 2013).

In a Norwegian study of 26,303 planned pregnancies, overweight (BMI 25 to 29.9 kg/m^2) and obese (BMI 30 to 34.9 kg/m^2) men were 20% (OR 1.20, 95% CI 1.04 to 1.38) and 36% (OR 1.36, 95% CI 1.13 to 1.63) more likely, respectively, to report infertility, defined as a need for up to 12 months to achieve pregnancy or a need for infertility treatment (Nguyen et al, 2007).

Similarly, in a prospective Japanese study of 74 healthy men, those with higher BMI were 20% less likely (HR 0.80, 95% CI 0.67 to 0.95) to father a child during a median follow-up period of 20 months (Ohwaki et al, 2009).

Finally, among an analytic sample of 1329 men enrolled in the U.S. Agricultural Health Study, a 3-unit increase in BMI was associated with a 12% increased adjusted risk (OR 1.12, 95% CI 1.01 to 1.25) of infertility, defined as not conceiving after 12 or more months of unprotected intercourse, regardless of whether or not a pregnancy subsequently occurred (Sallmén et al, 2006).

Diabetes and Disruptions in Glucose Homeostasis

In a cross-sectional study of 857 men in Qatar, those with type 2 DM were more likely to be diagnosed with infertility (P = .003).

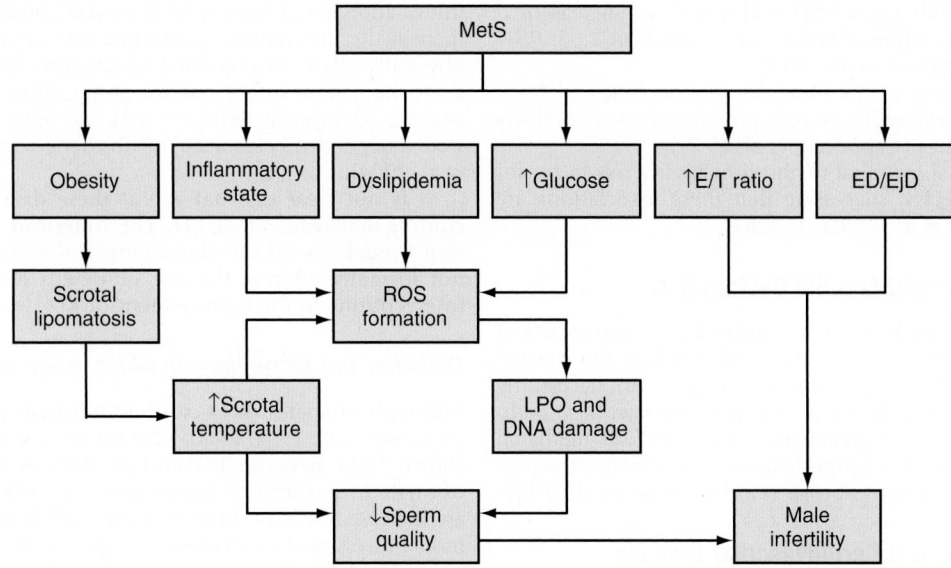

Figure 23-3. Possible mechanisms of male infertility in metabolic syndrome (MetS). DNA, deoxyribonucleic acid; ED/EjD, erectile dysfunction/ejaculatory dysfunction; E/T, estrogen/testosterone; LPO, lipid peroxidation; ROS, reactive oxygen species. (Modified from Gorbachinsky I, Akpinar H, Assimos G. Metabolic syndrome and urologic diseases. Rev Urol 2010;12: e157–e180.)

However, in reaching this conclusion, these investigators did not provide specific definitions for infertility nor did they control for potential confounders such as obesity. Indeed, the men with type 2 DM were more likely to be obese (*P* = .073), and in a multivariable-adjusted subgroup analysis of men with type 2 DM, obesity was strongly associated with infertility (OR 3.36, 95% CI 1.81 to 6.23), suggesting that obesity may have confounded the association of DM with infertility in these men (Bener et al, 2009).

Metabolic Syndrome and Urologic Cancers

Associations of MetS with urologic cancers are beginning to emerge, with epidemiologic studies indicating that some aspects of MetS may influence the natural histories of prostate, kidney, and bladder cancer. However, some of these data are conflicting, and not all risk patterns are entirely clear.

Prostate Cancer

The findings for prostate cancer are perhaps the most puzzling, with studies showing MetS associated with both increased and decreased risks of incident prostate cancer. In addition, obesity increases the risk of incident high-grade disease and biochemical recurrence after primary therapy, but decreases the risk of incident low-grade disease. DM decreases the risk of incident disease. Some investigators have speculated that these contradictory observations result from differential effects of different MetS components on the pathogenesis of prostate cancer (Buschemeyer and Freedland, 2007; De Nunzio et al, 2012).

Kidney Cancer

The most extensively studied MetS factor for kidney cancer is obesity, which has been associated with increased risks of disease prevalence and incidence (Chow et al, 2010; Ljungberg et al, 2011; Hakimi et al, 2013). In addition to obesity, at least one study—a cohort analysis of 560,388 men and women from Norway, Austria, and Sweden—indicated an increased risk of incident renal cell carcinoma with increased systolic or diastolic blood pressure, blood glucose, triglycerides, and a composite metabolic score that assessed the combined effects of adiposity, blood pressure, glucose, and triglycerides (Häggström et al, 2013).

Bladder Cancer

Several studies have focused on obesity, DM, and bladder cancer. A meta-analysis of 11 cohort studies noted a modest, but significant, increased risk of bladder cancer incidence and prevalence for obesity (Qin et al, 2013). A meta-analysis combining 36 studies observed an increased risk of bladder cancer among diabetics, with an overall increased risk of 35% compared with nondiabetics (RR 1.35, 95% CI 1.17 to 1.56), although men predominantly drove the risk (Zhu et al, 2013).

KEY POINTS: METABOLIC SYNDROME AND UROLOGIC DISEASES

- MetS is a constellation of clinical factors associated with an increased risk of incident CVD and diabetes.
- At least three of the following factors must be present to render a diagnosis of MetS:
  - Abdominal obesity
  - Elevated blood glucose
  - Elevated blood pressure
  - Elevated serum triglycerides
  - Decreased HDL cholesterol
- Men's health integrates male urologic care with the prevention and treatment of systemic CVD. It is an evolving paradigm with no clearly defined clinical parameters.
- There are no formal guidelines for the evaluation or treatment of MetS in the practical management of urologic conditions.
- MetS and its components are associated with increased risks of the following urologic conditions:
  - BPE and male LUTS
  - Female urinary incontinence
  - Urinary stones
  - ED
  - Male factor infertility
  - High-grade prostate cancer
  - Kidney cancer
  - Bladder cancer
- Weight loss improves continence in obese women with SUI.
- Weight loss improves erectile function in obese men with ED.

REFERENCES

The complete reference list is available online at www.expertconsult.com.

SUGGESTED READINGS

"ANDROGEN DEFICIENCY: AN EVIDENCE-BASED APPROACH" AND "CARDIOVASCULAR DISEASE AND TESTOSTERONE"

Basaria S, Coviello AD, Travison TG, et al. Adverse events associated with testosterone administration. N Engl J Med 2010;8(363):109–22.

Bhasin S, Cunningham GR, Hayes FJ, et al. Testosterone therapy in men with androgen deficiency syndrome: an Endocrine Society clinical practice guideline. J Clin Endocrinol Metab 2010;95:2536–69.

Corona G, Rastrelli G, Forti G, et al. Update in testosterone therapy for men. J Sex Med 2011;8:639–54.

Isidori AM, Buvat J, Corona G, et al. A critical analysis of the role of testosterone in erectile function, from pathophysiology to treatment—a systematic review. Eur Urol 2014;65:99–112.

Kalyani RR, Gavini S, Dobs AS, et al. Male hypogonadism in systemic disease. Endocrinol Metab Clin N Am 2007;36:333–48.

Wang C, Nieschlag E, Swerdloff R, et al. Investigation, treatment, and monitoring of late-onset hypogonadism in males: ISA, ISSAM, EAU, EAA and ASA recommendations. Eur Urol 2009;55:121–30.

"METABOLIC SYNDROME AND UROLOGIC DISEASES"

De Nunzio C, Aronson W, Freedland SJ, et al. The correlation between metabolic syndrome and prostatic diseases. Eur Urol 2012;61(3):560–70.

Gorbachinsky I, Akpinar H, Assimos DG. Metabolic syndrome and urologic diseases. Rev Urol 2010;12:e157–80.

Parsons JK. Modifiable risk factors for benign prostatic hyperplasia and lower urinary tract symptoms: new approaches to old problems. J Urol 2007;178:395–401.

24 Male Infertility

Craig Stuart Niederberger, MD, FACS

EPIDEMIOLOGY

The disease of infertility affects approximately 15% of couples, rendering nearly one of six childless (World Health Organization [WHO], 1991). Multiple sources of bias historically have served to distort assessment of the contribution of each gender to infertility, but we can reasonably expect men to contribute equally to women when it comes to whose gametes are faulty (Tielemans et al, 2002). Hence, accurate evaluation and treatment of the man becomes of great importance in addressing a significant health care issue.

Unfortunately, much of infertility care for men is delivered outside of well-established reimbursement systems, frustrating accurate calculation of epidemiologic metrics (Meacham et al, 2007). Fortunately, the American Society for Reproductive Medicine's professional group, the Society for Assisted Reproductive Technologies (SART), compels in vitro fertilization (IVF), clinics to report outcomes in a systematic fashion, allowing limited evaluation of the impact of male infertility. However, this assessment is through the lens of women seeking the most evolved technology for female reproductive care and necessarily skews the appraisal of the incidence and prevalence of the male contribution to the disease.

The Urologic Diseases in America (UDA) Project included collection of male reproductive epidemiologic data from a variety of sources, which, albeit sparse, allowed for some limited analysis of the parameters of the disease of male infertility (Meacham et al, 2007). Considering ambulatory surgery for conditions associated with male infertility, it is unsurprising that men aged 25 to 34 years had higher usage with an average rate of 126 per 100,000 compared with men aged 35 to 44 with 83 per 100,000 and those aged 45 and older at 20 per 100,000 (Meacham et al, 2007). Thus, younger men represent over half of male infertility cases, and nearly one in 11 cases occurs in men in the fifth decade and older (Meacham et al, 2007). Considering geographic distribution in the United States, men living in the West had lower use of ambulatory surgery compared with those in the Northeast and Midwest (29 per 100,000, 104 per 100,000 and 72 per 100,000, respectively) (Meacham et al, 2007).

From an economic perspective, the UDA Project estimated total expenditures for treating primary male infertility at 17 million U.S. dollars (USD) in the year 2000, clearly an underestimate because of the delivered care absent from traditional databases (Meacham et al, 2007). Because a significant amount of male reproductive medical care delivery involves assisted technologies for the female partner, accounting for this care the assessed total cost is a sizable 18 billion USD (Meacham et al, 2007).

Complicating epidemiologic assessment is the fact that the primary assay for male infertility, the semen analysis, is a poor predictor with a low receiver operating characteristic (ROC) curve area for all available parameters (Guzick et al, 2001) Consequently, men with some presence of sperm on semen analysis may be inaccurately judged to be fertile and omitted from accurate accrual in a tabulation of insufficient reproductive potential.

HISTORY

The production and delivery of the male gamete requires high orchestration among endocrine, immune, and neural systems, passage through intricately constructed anatomy, complex orchestrated sequences of gene expression and chromosomal structural events, and the proper embryologic and postnatal development of all systems. It is consequently unsurprising that myriad disparate conditions contribute to male reproductive dysfunction. Table 24-1 enumerates percentages of final diagnoses made in one infertility clinic (Sigman et al, 2009). As will become clear in this chapter, the percentages in Table 24-1 for each condition are highly variable depending on how the individual conditions are assessed in published studies, and the data contained within the table are an indictment of how poorly male reproductive information is systematically collected. However, the table does demonstrate the wide variety of diagnoses associated with male infertility. To address all potential possibilities, the practitioner must approach inquiring about past history in a methodical fashion. For the sake of efficiency, the patient may complete a form at home or in the waiting area before the physician encounter.

Reproductive health is an unusual aspect of medicine in that two patients are required for a positive outcome. Several consequences arise from this unique circumstance, the first being that a probabilistic approach to diagnosing infertility is necessary. In the best circumstances, with intercourse timed to menstruation and a rigorous calculation of optimal timing including assessment of quality of cervical mucus and measurement of basal body temperature, cumulative pregnancy rates for all tracked subjects in one well-conducted study were 38% at one cycle, 68% at three cycles, 81% at six cycles, and 92% at 12 cycles (Gnoth et al, 2003). For those who ultimately became pregnant, the cumulative pregnancy rates were 42% at one cycle, 75% at three cycles, 88% at six cycles, and 98% at 12 cycles (Gnoth et al, 2003). Hence, a couple seeking treatment for infertility a month or two after discontinuing contraceptive measures should be counseled to continue to try for a few more months unless other significant conditions exist. **A minority of**

TABLE 24-1 Distribution of Final Diagnoses from a Male Infertility Clinic

CATEGORY	NUMBER	%
Immunologic	121	2.6%
Idiopathic	1535	32.6%
Varicocele	1253	26.6%
Obstruction	720	15.3%
Normal female factor	503	10.7%
Cryptorchidism	129	2.7%
Ejaculatory failure	95	2.0%
Endocrinologic	70	1.5%
Drug or radiation	64	1.4%
Genetic	56	1.2%
Testicular failure	52	1.1%
Sexual dysfunction	32	0.7%
Pyospermia	25	0.5%
Cancer	20	0.4%
Systemic disease	15	0.3%
Infection	10	0.2%
Torsion	5	0.1%
Ultrastructural	5	0.1%
TOTAL	4710	100.0%

From Sigman M, Lipshultz LI, Howards SS. Office evaluation of the sub-fertile male. In: Lipshultz LI, Howards SS, Niederberger CS, editors. Infertility in the male. 4th edition. New York: Cambridge University Press; 2009. p. 153–76.

couples who have not conceived after six cycles may still do so, and it is reasonable to initiate an evaluation after 6 months with the understanding that some couples will still conceive shortly afterward. It is useful to communicate to patients the probabilistic nature of reproduction by describing each month of trying as rolling a die or flipping a coin.

An important question to ask is how often the couple is having intercourse. In general, semen parameters peak after 1 or 2 days of abstinence and then decline (Levitas et al, 2005). Often in an attempt to accumulate sperm, men wait long periods before attempting to impregnate their partners. Data suggest that not only is this practice unhelpful, it actually results in poorer sperm quality (Levitas et al, 2005). **For an optimal characterization of semen, a man should be instructed to wait 1 or 2 days after an ejaculation to submit a specimen for semen analysis** (Levitas et al, 2005). **However, for increasing the probability of conception and pregnancy, intercourse every day around the time of ovulation is likely the best strategy** (Scarpa et al, 2007).

Another consequence of the fact that two patients are required for a positive outcome in this unique area of medicine is that consideration of the female partner's age is a critical component in judging reproductive potential and planning therapeutic strategies. Whereas the effects of male age on reproductive potential remain to be fully elucidated, advancing male age appears to affect bulk seminal parameters and sperm DNA packaging to only a limited degree, allowing a male to father children well into his later years (Henkel et al, 2005; Hellstrom et al, 2006; Moskovtsev et al, 2006; Schmid et al, 2007; Sloter et al, 2007; Yang et al, 2007; Cocuzza et al, 2008a; Colin et al, 2010; Silva et al, 2012). For the woman, age is a critical predictor of reproductive potential, especially when artificial reproductive technologies are used (te Velde and Pearson, 2002; Balasch and Gratacós, 2012). **On average, female fecundity declines precipitously after age 35** (Balasch and Gratacós, 2012). In some geographic regions, female fertility appears to decline more rapidly than others (Zargar et al, 1997). Hence, determining the female partner's age and assessing it in the context of her locale are essential aspects of the reproductive history.

An important general question to ask is whether the man and his partner have previously conceived children, or if each has with other partners, and the age or ages of the offspring. Proven fertility at some point in time demonstrates a functioning reproductive system after puberty, which eliminates a number of concerns regarding congenital issues.

The typical enumeration of systemic diseases and past surgeries in taking the reproductive history reveals a number of conditions associated with reproductive dysfunction. Diabetes mellitus and multiple sclerosis interfere with normal coordinated ejaculatory function, as does spinal cord injury (Vinik et al, 2003; Kafetsoulis et al, 2006; Tepavcevic et al, 2008). **Even before spermatotoxic chemotherapy, cancer itself appears to negatively affect spermatogenesis, especially if the cancer is of testicular origin** (de Bruin et al, 2009). It is interesting to note that azoospermia may reveal cancer, and the physician considering a man with no sperm on semen analysis should regard testis cancer as a a possible cause (Mancini et al, 2007). Surgeries such as transurethral resection of the prostate and minimally invasive therapies for prostatic enlargement are associated with ejaculatory dysfunction (Jaidane et al, 2010; Elshal et al, 2012). As discussed elsewhere in this text, retrograde ejaculation of varying degrees may occur after retroperitoneal lymph node dissection for testis cancer, depending on the type of dissection and the clinical context within which the dissection occurs.

Herniorrhaphy may result in obstruction of the vas deferens (Shin et al, 2005; Hallén et al, 2011, 2012; Tekatli et al, 2012). Mesh in particular appears to incite a dense foreign body inflammatory response that may entrap the vas deferens even if the placement of mesh is not be immediately adjacent to the vas (Maciel et al, 2007; Hallén et al, 2011, 2012; Tekatli et al, 2012). If vasal occlusion is the sole cause of infertility, then both vasa must be occluded, an expectedly infrequent event. However, occlusion of one vasa from herniorrhaphy with contralateral spermatogenic dysfunction of another source may serve as a cause of infertility in the male.

Aside from the typical questions regarding medical and surgical history, answers to a number of questions specifically related to male reproduction may elucidate causes of infertility. If the practitioner is not using a history form, a helpful mnemonic is *TICS*, as if one is ticking off items on a list. *T* stands for toxins, *I* for infectious disease, *C* for childhood history, and *S* for sexual history.

Spermatotoxicity

In the *TICS* mnemonic, *T* is for toxins. A variety of substances interfere with spermatogenesis, mature sperm function, and sperm delivery. Many common medications, prescribed and over the counter, can be associated with male reproductive dysfunction.

Endocrine Modulators

Medications may affect the ratio of estrogen to androgen through a variety of mechanisms, including a molecular similarity to estrogen, increased estrogen synthesis, increased aromatase activity, dissociation of steroids from sex hormone-binding globulin (SHBG), decreased testosterone synthesis, competitive and noncompetitive binding to steroid receptors, decreased synthesis of adrenal steroids, and induction of hyperprolactinemia (Bowman et al, 2012). **Some of the more commonly encountered agents warranting inquiry include the antiandrogens bicalutamide, flutamide, and nilutamide; the antihypertensive spironolactone; the antiretroviral protease inhibitors such as indinavir; the nucleoside reverse transcriptase inhibitors such as stavudine; corticosteroids, especially in adolescence; and exogenous estrogen** (Bowman et al, 2012).

Although a source of debate, the 5α-reductase inhibitors finasteride and dutasteride appear to have only limited spermatogenic suppressive effects if at all (Overstreet et al, 1999; Amory et al, 2007). Occasional anecdotal case reports suggest that sperm parameters dramatically improve in an individual man after discontinuation of a 5α-reductase inhibitor, but the substantial interassay variability of semen parameters calls into question whether these effects could simply be the result of chance (Chiba et al, 2011).

Primarily through conversion to estradiol by aromatase and consequent inhibition of luteinizing hormone (LH) secretion by the pituitary, exogenous testosterone acts to decrease intratesticular testosterone synthesis and reduce spermatogenesis (Grimes et al, 2012). Agents with androgenic properties similarly diminish sperm production (de Souza and Hallak, 2011). In fact, investigators have studied testosterone and androgenic steroids as potential targets for male contraception since the 1970s (WHO Task Force, 1990; Gu et al, 2009; Grimes et al, 2012; Ilani et al, 2012). In general, these studies have a duration of 2 years or less of application of testosterone or androgenic steroid and demonstrate reversibility with return to sperm in the ejaculate after approximately 4 months or more of discontinuation of the contraceptive agent (WHO Task Force, 1990; Gu et al, 2009; Grimes et al, 2012; Ilani et al, 2012). However, whether and when spermatogenesis returns after longer periods of use is unknown.

Recreational Drugs

Although data are conflicting, most studies suggest that cannabis decreases plasma testosterone in a dose-dependent and duration-dependent manner (Gorzalka et al, 2010). More robust data associate chronic alcohol intake with decreases in androgens and sperm parameters (Villalta et al, 1997; Pasqualotto et al, 2004). Heavy chronic alcohol intake also appears to increase aromatization of testosterone to estradiol (Purohit, 2000). Investigators have observed that more moderate use of alcohol may decrease intracytoplasmic sperm injection (ICSI) outcomes (Braga et al, 2012).

Early studies suggested worsening of bulk seminal parameters with cigarette smoking (Stillman et al, 1986). **Although the results of subsequent studies associating smoking and bulk parameters were conflicting, more recent cross-sectional analysis has supported deterioration of seminal parameters in a dose-dependent manner, arguing more strongly that cigarette smoking impairs male reproductive potential** (Ramlau-Hansen et al, 2007). Investigators observed that cigarette smoking increased seminal oxidative stress parameters and decreased metrics of sperm DNA quality (Pasqualotto et al, 2008b; Taha et al, 2012). An abnormal ratio of protamines 1 and 2 was observed in smokers with evidence of atypical protamine 2 expression, pointing to DNA packaging as directly compromised by tobacco use (Hammadeh et al, 2010). The negative effects of cigarette smoking on sperm bulk parameters and DNA quality appear to be especially acute in the presence of a clinical varicocele, suggesting the possibility of additive toxicity (Fariello et al, 2012b). Researchers studied effects of an aryl hydrocarbon receptor ligand present in cigarette smoke and found that it induced apoptosis in fetal testis in a manner that was preventable with an aryl hydrocarbon receptor antagonist, providing evidence that maternal smoking may affect the reproductive potential of male offspring (Coutts et al, 2007). Consistent with these laboratory findings, epidemiologic data associated maternal cigarette smoking to smaller testes, lower sperm counts, and alterations in sex hormones in the adult male offspring (Jensen et al, 2005; Ravnborg et al, 2011). It is interesting to note that epidemiologic evidence supports that the secondary sex ratio, the ratio of boys to girls born, is altered in mothers who smoke (Beratis et al, 2008). One explanation is that cigarette smoking alters circulating testosterone concentrations in pregnant women (James, 2002).

Antihypertensives

 Please see the Expert Consult website for details.

Antipsychotics

The most common mechanism of action for antipsychotic drugs is antagonism of dopamine, which causes loss of libido as a side effect in the majority of patients (Stimmel and Gutierrez, 2006). Another proposed reason for diminished libido with use of antipsychotics is elevation of prolactin levels, which appears to be most acute for risperidone and to a lesser extent olanzapine (Melkersson, 2005). As discussed elsewhere in this text, selective serotonin reuptake inhibitors (SSRIs) are commonly associated with anorgasmia and delayed or absent ejaculation (Clayton and Montejo, 2006; Stimmel and Gutierrez, 2006).

Opioids

Opioid analgesics suppress LH release primarily through hypothalamic-mediated mechanisms and consequently reduce testosterone synthesis (Subirán et al, 2011). Experimental evidence in animals demonstrates endogenous opioid peptides, their precursors, and their receptors in various testis cell types (Subirán et al, 2011). Endogenous opioid peptides are primarily synthesized by Leydig and Sertoli cells and inhibit Sertoli cell function, via autocrine and paracrine mechanisms (Subirán et al, 2011). Hence, not only can opioids induce the hypogonadotropic hypogonadism commonly observed in chronic use, they may also diminish spermatogenesis directly in the testis (Brennan, 2013; Subirán et al, 2011). Evidence suggests that discontinuation of opioid analgesics may be associated with rapid return of androgen, perhaps as early as within 1 month (Brennan, 2013). **With the widespread prescribing of opioid analgesics, their use as a cause of hypogonadotropic hypogonadism should be suspected in all such hypoandrogenic men.**

Antibiotics

Please see the Expert Consult website for details.

Cytotoxic Chemotherapeutics

Because chemotherapeutic agents are most effectively applied to suppress a briskly proliferating population of cells, and the pathway of male gamete development primarily involves a rapidly dividing stem cell cohort, it is unsurprising that medical therapies directed toward cancers impair spermatogenesis. Alkylating agents such as the nitrogen mustard cyclophosphamide have been long identified to impair sperm production (Vaisheva et al, 2007). These spermatogenic suppressive effects were noted to be dose and time dependent, with lower doses and shorter durations of therapy leading to reversible dysfunction but ultimate return to male fertility potential, and higher doses and longer durations of therapies resulting in permanently impaired fertility (Vaisheva et al, 2007). Other chemotherapeutic agents commonly used in conjunction with cyclophosphamide to treat non-Hodgkin lymphoma, including doxorubicin, vincristine, and prednisone, have all been reported to impair spermatogenesis as individual agents (Vaisheva et al, 2007). Likewise, investigators reported that cisplatin, etoposide, and bleomycin were associated with diminished sperm parameters in a dose- and time-dependent manner (Gandini et al, 2006).

One concern of both patients and physicians is how much chemotherapy damages the DNA of sperm (Robbins, 1996; Spermon et al, 2006; Stahl et al, 2006; Delbes et al, 2007; O'Flaherty et al, 2008; Tempest et al, 2008; O'Flaherty et al, 2010; Smit et al, 2010). Evidence suggests that sperm DNA damage can be detected at least up to 2 years after chemotherapy, arguing that cryopreservation of sperm before treatment with cytotoxic chemotherapeutic agents is preferable to awaiting the return of sperm after chemotherapy (Tempest et al, 2008). The question is whether sperm is "safe" to use after a discrete amount of time after the induction of chemotherapeutic agents that might mutate cellular DNA in a way that may be translated through the germ line into offspring. An informed answer to that question based on well-conducted clinical trials is not yet available. This lack of knowledge frustrates male reproductive specialists who counsel patients on whether their own biologic material or donor sperm would be the best choice after cytotoxic chemotherapy. **Questions about sperm DNA integrity and mutagenicity after chemotherapy serve as a second reason to encourage men undergoing such oncologic therapy to cryopreserve** sperm before induction, because cryopreservation presents a well-established means for fertility preservation in the setting of cancer (Anger et al, 2003; Meseguer et al, 2006; Crha et al, 2009). Proper cryopreservation of sperm results in long-term potential for reproductive success, and patients may be assured that should they store sperm in this way, it will be available when they need it (Rofeim and Gilbert, 2005). Although many patients may recover sperm in the ejaculate after cytotoxic chemotherapy, and it is very possible that, after a period as yet to be determined, ejaculated sperm after chemotherapy will be safe for conception, many men do not develop sufficient ejaculated sperm for fertility. These men do use cryopreserved sperm if available to successfully father offspring (Meseguer et al, 2006).

Systemic application of antitumor medication is not necessarily the only form of chemotherapy that may alter fertility potential. Investigators noted in a small series of young men that local instillation of bacille Calmette-Guérin into the bladder for superficial transitional cell carcinoma resulted in a significant decrease in sperm concentration and motility (Raviv et al, 2005).

A special case arises in peripubertal boys undergoing cytotoxic chemotherapy for cancer. Oncologists are often in a rush to apply lifesaving therapy, and parents may be uncomfortable discussing topics such as masturbation for semen collection with their children. However, if oncologic therapy is successful, it is precisely these patients with a potentially long life expectancy who would benefit from sperm cryopreservation as an option for future fertility. Peripubertal boys are capable of producing semen samples suitable for cryopreservation, and it is entirely feasible to obtain an ejaculate suitable for storage (van Casteren et al, 2008; Menon et al, 2009). The urologist need simply be comfortable enough to discuss the advantages of fertility preservation and the methods to achieve it.

Anti-Inflammatory Agents

Please see the Expert Consult website for details.

Phosphodiesterase V Inhibitors

Please see the Expert Consult website for details.

Environmental Toxicants

Please see the Expert Consult website for details.

Thermal Toxicity

For reasons not entirely clear but engendering much speculation, mammals evolved so that the scrotal container of the testis was housed outside the body cavity, keeping its contents at a temperature considerably cooler than that of the internal organs (Setchell, 1998; Thonneau et al, 1998). **Scrotal temperature in humans is maintained to be 2° C to 4° C below core body temperature by mechanisms including a counter-current heat exchange between a central set of linear arteries directing blood toward the testis and a plexus of veins surrounding the arteries draining blood back toward the vena cava** (Setchell, 1998; Thonneau et al, 1998). Many investigators have exhaustively studied the effects of heat on spermatogenesis in animals, observing depopulation of germ cells, perturbations in the various spermatogenic cell types, and apoptosis within specific cell types (Setchell, 1998; Absalan et al, 2010). Cryptorchidism provides a model by which the effects of heat can be studied on sperm production: increasing testis temperature to that of the abdominal cavity significantly impairs spermatogenesis (Setchell, 1998).

The degree to which scrotal temperature can be raised without affecting male fertility remains an open question. Clothing, physical activity, and body posture such as whether the legs are crossed or not in a sitting position all change scrotal temperature to an incremental degree, but whether that translates to alterations in spermatogenesis is purely speculative at this point (Jung et al, 2005; Mieusset et al, 2007). Researchers observed an increase in scrotal temperature on the order of a half a degree Celsius with prolonged sitting on heated car seats, and speculated that such an effect may be additive to the intrascrotal temperature rise that occurs when sitting (Jung et al, 2008). One study observed that when a man was naked, mean scrotal temperature was significantly lower on the left than on the right, but when he was clothed, the temperature was significantly higher on the left than on the right (Bengoudifa and Mieusset, 2007). Clothing may thus confer a greater differential increase in left scrotal temperature than right scrotal temperature (Bengoudifa and Mieusset, 2007).

A number of studies associate occupational exposure resulting in a significant increase in intrascrotal temperature with detrimental effects on sperm (Thonneau et al, 1998; De Fleurian et al, 2009). However, other researchers have observed no significant negative effects on sperm in fertile men exposed to high heat at work, and postulated that in the normal state, compensatory mechanisms protect the testis when a prolonged rise in ambient temperature occurs (Momen et al, 2010).

Laptop computers radiate heat, and researchers have studied the effects of these devices on scrotal temperature. In one study, under controlled conditions, having a laptop computer resting on the lap for 1 hour raised the scrotal temperature an average 2.6° C on the left and 2.8° C on the right side (Sheynkin et al, 2005). However, simply sitting without a laptop raised the scrotal temperature an average of 2.1° C (Sheynkin et al, 2005). Whether the extra approximately half-degree Celsius imparts significant damage to spermatogenesis remains an open question. However, investigators have observed that a man sitting with his legs apart and for shorter periods of time experiences less of an increase in scrotal temperature (Sheynkin et al, 2011).

Radiation

Testes directly exposed to ionizing radiation suffer germ cell loss and Leydig cell dysfunction (Clermont, 1972; Castillo et al, 1990; Bahadur and Ralph, 1999; Gandini et al, 2006; Green et al, 2010). In one survey of boys with acute lymphoblastic leukemia who underwent testicular irradiation at 12, 15, and 24 Gray (Gy), all became azoospermic, but those receiving less than 24 Gy had normal testosterone production (Castillo et al, 1990). The investigators observed elevated gonadotropins and noted that this finding indicated the possibility of subclinical Leydig cell damage (Castillo et al, 1990). **In a survey of childhood cancer survivors, chances of having future offspring were lessened by radiation doses to the testes of 7.5 Gy and above** (Green et al, 2010). The testis need not be directly irradiated for spermatogenic impairment to occur; if the radiation field is proximal to the testis and the dose is sufficient, sperm production may be diminished even if the testis is shielded (Gandini et al, 2006).

With widespread use of radiofrequency devices for telecommunications and wireless networks, investigators have questioned the effects of this band of the electromagnetic spectrum on sperm (Erogul et al, 2006; Agarwal et al, 2008b; Baste et al, 2008; Falzone et al, 2008; Agarwal et al, 2009). Researchers observed negative effects on sperm motility parameters, viability, and reactive oxygen species (ROS) generation after electromagnetic radiation generated by 850- and 900- MHz cell phone transmission systems in vitro (Erogul et al, 2006; Falzone et al, 2008; Agarwal et al, 2009). However, in vitro exposure of sperm to electromagnetic radiation does not account for the distance and material, including biologic tissues, that separate a cell phone transceiver and sperm during common use. To address a more typical usage scenario, investigators have used epidemiologic data to gauge potential in vivo effects. In one questionnaire-based study of Norwegian sailors exposed to high-power electromagnetic fields in a military environment, researchers noted a significant linear relationship between increasing exposure and reported infertility (Baste et al, 2008). It is interesting to note that the offspring's sex ratio at birth also revealed a linear relationship, with a decreasing ratio of boys to girls with higher degrees of exposure to electromagnetic radiation (Baste et al, 2008). Researchers in another epidemiologic study divided men into four groups based on cell phone talking time: no use; less than 2 hours per day; 2 to 4 hours per day; and more than 4 hours per day (Agarwal et al, 2008b). The investigators observed that semen analyses in the four groups of increasing cell phone use revealed a linear decrease in sperm count, motility, viability, and normal morphology (Agarwal et al, 2008b).

Infections and Inflammation

In the *TICS* mnemonic, *I* stands for infectious and inflammatory disease leading to male reproductive dysfunction. Infections of the testis, epididymis, prostate, and urethra may lead to male infertility through anatomic and functional means (Kasturi et al, 2009). Common organisms affecting the prostate include *Escherichia coli, Pseudomonas aeruginosa,* and *Klebsiella, Proteus,* and *Enterococcus* species (Kasturi et al, 2009). Typical epididymal organisms include *Neisseria gonorrhoeae, Chlamydia trachomatis,* and *E. coli* (Kasturi et al, 2009). Infectious urethral organisms in the context of impaired male reproduction include *N. gonorrhoeae, C. trachomatis, Mycoplasma* species, and *Trichomonas vaginalis* (Kasturi et al, 2009). Although relatively infrequently encountered, infections of the testis may include the Rubulavirus mumps, Coxsackievirus B, *N. gonorrhoeae, C. trachomatis, E. coli, P. aeruginosa,* and *Klebsiella, Staphylococcus,* and *Streptococcus* species (Kasturi et al, 2009). Mumps orchitis is typically so painful and bizarre to the person so affected that even at a very young age, a boy with mumps traveling into his testis is unlikely to forget the event. Infrequently encountered in modern industrialized nations, *Mycobacterium tuberculosis* may affect any reproductive organ and cause scarring of the vas deferens and epididymis (Niederberger, 2011).

Infectious consequences may be anatomic, such as urethral infection leading to stricture, or functional, impairing sperm (Kasturi et al, 2009). Functional alterations may derive from direct effects of the infectious organism on sperm or through induction of immunologic responses in any male reproductive organ, leading to sperm dysfunction (La Vignera et al, 2011). As an example of direct effects, investigators observed that incubating sperm with increasing concentrations of *C. trachomatis* serovar E elementary bodies was associated with degradation of sperm DNA in a time-dependent manner (Satta et al, 2005). **Although in vitro laboratory experiments have also demonstrated a negative effect of *E. coli* on sperm, the majority of bacteria including *E. coli* have limited or no effects on sperm motility in vivo** (Diemer et al, 2003; Lackner et al, 2006). Whereas bacteria may coexist with sperm without significant pathologic consequence, sexually transmitted organisms may play a more virulent role (Bezold et al, 2007). The differential effects on sperm of common bacteria and sexually transmitted infectious agents remain far from clear.

Viruses proffer a potentially unique negative direct effect on sperm by integration into a man's genome and vertical transmission through his germ line (La Vignera et al, 2011). **Although viral nucleic material appears to be present in the seminal plasma, neither hepatitis C nor human immunodeficiency virus appear to be correlated with a direct negative effect on sperm function** (Garrido et al, 2005). Human papillomavirus was associated with impairment of bulk seminal parameters, and in vitro treatment of sperm in the laboratory with heparinase III appeared to diminish viral load without significantly altering functional semen parameters (Garolla et al, 2012).

Researchers have studied a wide variety of indirect negative effects of infection on sperm including through leukocytosis, ROSs, interleukins 1, 6, and 8, interferon-γ, macrophage migration inhibitory factor, tumor necrosis factor-α, epididymal macrophages, and dendritic cells (La Vignera et al, 2011). It is logical that any part of the immune system may lose self-recognition of sperm or in the presence of an active infection overwhelm sperm defenses.

Evidence suggests that noninfectious or postinfectious inflammatory processes of the prostate may lead to sperm alterations and male infertility, but the degree to which inflammation alters male reproductive potential beyond what infection imparts remains unknown (Schoor, 2002; Wagenlehner et al, 2008; Ausmees et al,

2013). One putative mechanism by which nonbacterial prostatitis may lead to male infertility is through seminal leukocytosis or pyospermia and the release of ROSs resulting in sperm damage (Schoor, 2002). Other possible means of sperm dysfunction via prostatic inflammation include generation of antisperm antibodies and biochemical alterations in prostatic ions such as zinc, magnesium, calcium, or selenium (Schoor, 2002). Prostatitis may itself damage sperm by inducing ROSs without leukocytosis as an intermediary (Pasqualotto et al, 2000; Schoor, 2002).

Childhood Diseases

The *C* in *TICS* stands for childhood diseases. Maladies of early development include anatomic maldevelopment leading to obstruction or misdirection of the male gamete as it traverses the journey from the testis to the female reproductive tract and disorders that lead to disturbed sperm production or to conditions that damage mature sperm.

Pediatric Surgery

Hydroceles and hernias repaired during childhood are associated with a low but discrete incidence of complications causing vasal obstruction (Lao et al, 2012). In one large series, the rate of testis atrophy after pediatric inguinal hernia was 0.3% (Ein et al, 2006). As hernias repaired during adolescence often include surgical mesh, vasal occlusion as a result of inflammation associated with this material should be considered in an infertile man with such a procedure in his surgical history (Shin et al, 2005; Hallén et al, 2011, 2012; Lao et al, 2012; Tekatli et al, 2012). Other surgical procedures during childhood may also affect future reproductive status. In earlier series, investigators associated scarring from posterior urethral valve ablation with male reproductive dysfunction, but in more recent series, fertility complications with urethral valve surgery are rarely observed (Caione and Nappo, 2011). Older procedures for restoring bladder neck anatomy in children were associated with retrograde ejaculation, but these surgeries are rarely performed today (Sigman et al, 2009).

Testis Torsion

For males 25 years and younger, testis torsion is more than three times more common than testis cancer, with an estimated incidence of 4.5 cases per 100,000 per year (Mansbach et al, 2005; Mellick, 2012). It is interesting to note that contralateral testicular biopsy findings are abnormal in 57% to 88% of males when torsion occurs, which suggests either that unnoticed torsion is damaging the testis before torsion becomes clinically evident or that some underlying pathology is present that manifests both as abnormal scrotal anatomy and as spermatogenic dysfunction (Visser and Heyns, 2003). **Approximately half of men with torsion will develop adverse spermatogenic effects** (Visser and Heyns, 2003). Overall after torsion, 36% to 39% of men will have sperm concentrations below 20 million/mL (Visser and Heyns, 2003). Because torsion is a traumatic event that disrupts intratesticular architecture including the tight junctions between the Sertoli cells that comprise the blood-testis barrier, it is unsurprising that up to 11% of men will develop antisperm antibodies after torsion (Visser and Heyns, 2003).

Cryptorchidism

As described elsewhere in this text, during the fifth week of gestation, cells destined to become gonads arise in the posterior abdominal wall of the developing embryo (Lewis and Kaplan, 2009). A complex set of highly orchestrated sequenced events occurs, including differentiation of the various testis cell types, organization into what will ultimately become histologic compartments within the testicle, and development of the outer container of the testis and its connection to the distal organs where sperm will be ultimately routed (Lewis and Kaplan, 2009). The most overt anatomic change is migration of germ cells from the posterior abdominal wall toward the nascent inguinal canals and eventually into the scrotum, resulting in an extra-abdominal localization of the male gonads (Lewis and Kaplan, 2009). This process does not conclude until the third trimester (Lewis and Kaplan, 2009). Researchers have identified multiple regulatory triggers in animal models that direct descent of the testis, including the insulin-like 3 (*INSL3*) gene, the relaxin/insulin-like family peptide receptor 2 (*LGRF8*) gene, antimüllerian hormone (AMH), and members of the *HOX* gene family such as *HOX10* (Hughes and Acerini, 2008; Lewis and Kaplan, 2009). Dysfunction of certain of these genes may result primarily in arresting the mechanical journey of the germ cells, whereas aberrant expression of others may be involved in the processes of both spermatogenesis and descent, causing infertility in ways beyond the thermal toxicity to which undescended testes are subject in later reproductive life. **Androgens are required to induce regression of the cranial suspensory ligament during the fourth month of gestation to allow descent of the testis** (Hughes and Acerini, 2008; Lewis and Kaplan, 2009). Failure of any of these processes impedes descent of the testis into the scrotum, resulting in cryptorchidism, which is widely known to be associated with impaired reproductive potential in later life (Sigman et al, 2009).

Undescended testes occur in up to 4% of newborn boys at term (Barthold and González, 2003). The prevalence of cryptorchid testes decreases to less than 1.5% by 1 year of age (Barthold and González, 2003; Chung and Brock, 2011). Cryptorchidism concordance analysis in twins and siblings indicates a pattern of maternal inheritance, but also suggests that the intrauterine environment plays an important role (Jensen et al, 2010). In most series, the incidence of unilateral cryptorchidism is usually around twice that of bilateral undescended testes (Barthold and González, 2003). The distinction is important, because prognosis is related to whether cryptorchidism is unilateral or bilateral. The reproductive prognosis in later life is similar in men with no history of cryptorchidism and in those with a unilateral undescended testis who underwent orchidopexy as a child, regardless of age at surgery or the size of the undescended testis (Lee et al, 2001; Miller et al, 2001). **In one large epidemiologic study of men who had orchidopexy during childhood, successful rates for those attempting paternity with a history of surgically treated unilateral cryptorchidism were 96% compared with a control population, but only 70% for those who had bilateral cryptorchidism** (Lee, 2005). In that study, men with bilateral cryptorchidism had levels of the Sertoli cell product and marker of spermatogenesis inhibin B that were nearly one third of the levels in controls, compared with men with unilateral undescended testes repaired in childhood, who had inhibin B levels approximately two thirds that of controls (Lee, 2005). Differences in testosterone concentrations were less than those of inhibin B, arguing that fertility impairment caused by cryptorchidism is less based in Leydig cell steroidogenesis than in dysfunction of the seminiferous epithelium (Lee, 2005). Congruent with the identified differences in inhibin B between men with neither, one, or both testes undescended, researchers observed that sperm density on semen analysis is lower in men who had surgical repair of bilateral cryptorchidism than in those with a unilateral undescended testis, which in turn is lower than in men with normally descended testes (Lee, 1993; Lee and Coughlin, 2001; Moretti et al, 2007). With transmission electron microscopy, investigators also found a greater number of ultrastructural defects in men who had cryptorchidism surgically treated as a child compared with controls, and sperm from men with bilateral undescended testes had more defects than from those with unilateral disease (Moretti et al, 2007).

Conclusive data associating the timing of orchidopexy with reproductive outcomes in later life remain elusive. It is widely recognized that surgical correction of undescended testes after puberty likely has minimal effect on bulk semen analysis parameters (Grasso et al, 1991). However, the age before puberty at which orchidopexy results in optimal effect in reproductive potential has not been definitively established. Regression analysis demonstrated

that serum testosterone concentrations in men were negatively correlated to increasing age at orchidopexy, indicating that Leydig cell function is better spared by earlier age of surgical correction for cryptorchidism (Lee, 2005). Conventional wisdom contended that full germ cell development is arrested and remains quiescent before puberty, implying that orchidopexy performed at any earlier age would have similar outcomes. However, maturational alterations may occur in the hypothalamic, pituitary, and testicular endocrine axis much earlier than adolescence (Hadziselimovic, 2002). Likewise, a transition from the spermatogonial cell types of the fetal germ cell reservoir to that of the adult occurs at a very early age (Hadziselimovic, 2002).

Studies of men undergoing testis sperm extraction with the intent for use in ICSI and who had cryptorchidism and orchidopexy at an earlier time offer some information about the optimal timing of surgical correction of undescended testes, although results are conflicting. In an early study of 30 azoospermic men who had bilateral cryptorchidism, no correlation was found between the age at bilateral orchidopexy and the rate of successful surgical sperm retrieval, which was 73% overall (Negri et al, 2003). In a later study of 42 azoospermic men in whom all but two had bilateral cryptorchidism, no significant differences in surgical sperm retrieval rate were observed comparing men who had orchidopexy up to 10 years of age (61.9%) and men whose testes were brought into the scrotum after 10 years of age (57.1%) (Wiser et al, 2009). However, in an early study of 38 azoospermic men with 30 having had bilateral cryptorchidism, the successful surgical retrieval of sperm in 94% for men who had orchidopexy up to 10 years, 43% for 11 to 20 years, and 44% for older than 20 years, was statistically different at the selected threshold of 10 years (*P* < .01) (Raman and Schlegel, 2003). Congruent with these results, in 79 azoospermic men, 62% having had bilateral orchidopexy and 20.3% having had unilateral orchidopexy (with 17.7% unknown), ROC curve analysis revealed age at orchidopexy to have the second greatest area under the curve (AUC) after testosterone in discriminating successful surgical sperm retrieval (Vernaeve et al, 2004). **It consequently appears prudent to recommend orchidopexy before 10 years of age from a reproductive perspective, recognizing that cryptorchid boys who pass that threshold still may have sperm surgically retrieved for use in ICSI later in life.**

Testes that change in position after descent and those that are nearly but not fully descended present special challenges in assessing potential alterations in reproductive potential. Numerous reports clearly document testes as being descended that are later observed to have ascended to varying degrees (Gracia et al, 1997; Barthold and González, 2003). Whereas most appear to ascend to a location distal to the inguinal canal, clinicians have reported ascent as high as to an intra-abdominal position (Gracia et al, 1997; Barthold and González, 2003). Unfortunately, the fertility potential for these patients has not yet been systematically studied, and their reproductive prognosis must be considered unknown at present. For men with retractile testes, limited data suggest that although sperm are often observed in the ejaculate in a man, sperm density is lower than would be expected in a man with normal fertility, approaching that of men with a history of cryptorchidism (Caroppo et al, 2005).

Testicular Dysgenesis Hypothesis

Please see the Expert Consult website for details.

Genetics

What is currently known of the genetic basis of male infertility will be discussed systematically later in this chapter. A good reproductive history should include whether any blood relatives experienced difficulty conceiving offspring. The evaluating physician should also inquire as to the presence in the patient's family of genetic syndromes known to be related to reproductive dysfunction such as cystic fibrosis and other entities detailed in the latter part of this chapter (Anguiano et al, 1992).

Sexual History

The *S* in *TICS* is for the sexual history. Although it may seem intuitive that a couple would engage in a sufficient frequency of intercourse when attempting to conceive, lifestyle or proclivities may intervene and interfere. As discussed previously in this chapter, optimum timing for intercourse appears to be daily around the time of ovulation (Scarpa et al, 2007). Some women accurately predict the periovulatory period by symptoms, the so-called mittelschmerz (O'Herlihy et al, 1980). However, many women mistake bodily sensations as ovulation, and symptoms alone cannot reliably be used to assess optimal timing for intercourse. **Because ovulation is detectable by basal body temperature or home hormonal kits *after* it has occurred, a couple should be encouraged if possible to record the day of ovulation for two or three menstrual cycles, and begin daily intercourse several days before the earliest recorded day.** Such a method is impractical for women with advanced age, as it delays potential reproductive therapies. In the setting of advanced maternal age, more aggressive strategies in collaboration with the female fertility specialist should be considered.

Lubricants commonly used during sexual activity such as K-Y Jelly, Keri Lotion, Astroglide, and others are associated with impaired sperm motility (Sigman et al, 2009). Saliva should also be considered toxic to sperm (Sigman et al, 2009). Researchers incubated a variety of lubricants with sperm and observed that the isotonic preparation Pre-Seed did not result in a significant decrease in sperm motility or chromatin integrity as assessed by an acridine orange–based sperm chromatin structure assay (Agarwal et al, 2008a). In that study, FemGlide, Replens, and Astroglide lubricants resulted in a significant decrease in motility, and FemGlide and K-Y Jelly resulted in a significant decline in sperm chromatin quality (Agarwal et al, 2008a). Laboratory investigators have also provided evidence that use of Pre-Seed during semen collection for analysis does not affect assessment of bulk seminal parameters, sperm membrane functional integrity, levels of ROSs, total antioxidant capacity (TAC), and DNA integrity (Agarwal et al, 2013).

The urologist should inquire about erectile function, because obviously if intercourse is impeded or impossible, sperm will not be deposited successfully in the vaginal vault near the cervical os. The physiology, evaluation, and treatment of erectile dysfunction are discussed extensively elsewhere in this text.

The psychological weight of having a diagnosis of infertility and the stress of therapy are significant (Schanz et al, 2005; Volgsten et al, 2008). One metric of whether infertility is exerting an adverse psychological effect on the male is frequency of intercourse, which may be altered in up to half of men being treated for infertility and is associated with libido and sexual satisfaction (Ramezanzadeh et al, 2006). A revealing question for a man undergoing male reproductive evaluation is whether the frequency of coitus has changed during the process.

Men and women adapt to the stress of infertility in different ways with different coping mechanisms (Peterson et al, 2006). Men tend to distance themselves and problem solve, whereas women are more likely to seek social support (Peterson et al, 2006). Men and women may consequently interpret their partner's natural adaptive strategy as problematic when in fact it is simply a different means of coping. **A common misconception is that men conflate fertility with masculinity, which in fact happens only infrequently** (Fisher et al, 2010).

Stress itself may impair semen quality, creating a vicious circle for men experiencing infertility and its related psychological distress (Gollenberg et al, 2010). Fortunately, evidence suggests that once men have entered into reproductive medical therapy including IVF with their partners, the diagnosis of male infertility does not disturb psychological well-being and well-adjusted relationships (Holter et al, 2007). The clinician treating male reproductive dysfunction should consider referral to a qualified psychologist to ease the transition from the fearsome diagnosis of infertility to the many effective therapies that are available. If the discussion is couched in terms of problem solving, many men are very willing to engage in psychological counseling.

> ### KEY POINTS: MALE REPRODUCTIVE HISTORY
>
> - The most important determinant of a couple's reproductive potential is maternal age.
> - Many conditions may affect male reproductive function. The examining physician may organize the male reproductive history into toxicants, infectious processes, childhood conditions, and sexual history.

PHYSICAL EXAMINATION

General Physical Examination

Because male infertility may be related to many systemic and genetic conditions, the general physical examination often yields clues as to the source of reproductive dysfunction. Male and female faces are morphologically distinct, and female facial characteristics alert the examining physician to potential sex chromosomal and androgenization disorders (Velemínská et al, 2012). Alterations in secondary sexual characteristics such as facial, truncal, axillary, and pubic hair suggest inadequate androgenization (Sigman et al, 2009). If androgenization is significantly impaired through puberty, a high-pitched voice may result (Sokol, 2009). An overabundance of endogenous or therapeutically induced estradiol may lead to gynecomastia (Sigman et al, 2009). If testosterone production during puberty is so low that closure of the epiphyses of the long bones of the extremities fails to occur, typical body morphology will include an arm span 5 cm longer than the patient's height and a lower body segment as defined by pubic-to-heel distance more than 5 cm longer than the upper body segment as measured from the crown to the pubis (Sokol, 2009).

With the lack of virilization at the anticipated time of puberty, Klinefelter syndrome is classically detailed in textbooks as resulting in gynecomastia, a eunuchoid appearance, and tall height for age (Oates and Lamb, 2009). However, it should be noted that many men with a 47,XXY karyotype do not display the typical body morphology and habitus so described.

Obesity should be noted because substantial evidence associates it with male reproductive dysfunction. **It is well established that obese men have elevated estradiol as a result of peripheral conversion from testosterone by an overabundance of adipose cells that contain the enzyme aromatase** (Hammoud et al, 2006; Aggerholm et al, 2008; Chavarro et al, 2010; Hammoud et al, 2010b; Hofny et al, 2010). A TTTA aromatase polymorphism appears to be particularly related to increasing estradiol with increasing body mass, and those with the polymorphism are most likely to experience decreasing estradiol when they lose weight (Hammoud et al, 2010b). **Serum testosterone is also well known to be lower in obese men** (Hammoud et al, 2006). Four main causes are hypothesized: negative feedback of estradiol on the hypothalamic-pituitary axis resulting in decreased LH release; increased leptin; insulin resistance; and sleep apnea (Hammoud et al, 2006; Hofny et al, 2010). It should be noted that although some studies correlate increasing obesity with decreased LH, others do not, and the mechanism of reduced testosterone in obese men may be unrelated to gonadotropins (Hammoud et al, 2006; Aggerholm et al, 2008; Pauli et al, 2008; Hofny et al, 2010; Paasch et al, 2010; Teerds et al, 2011).

SHBG is typically reduced in obese men, in general ascribed to increased circulating insulin in obesity (Hammoud et al, 2006; 2008; Pauli et al, 2008; Teerds et al, 2011). The consequence of lowered SHBG is that bioavailable testosterone may be greater than what total testosterone predicts, and an obese man may be more androgenized than expected on superficial laboratory assessment.

Researchers observed an inverse correlation between serum inhibin B concentrations and body mass index (BMI) in men but not prepubertal boys (Winters et al, 2006). The association between decreasing inhibin B and increasing obesity in men potentially indicates decreased Sertoli cell number, and that the relationship is not seen before puberty suggests that obesity exerts its negative effect on Sertoli cells during puberty (Winters et al, 2006).

Although these kinds of studies have associated obesity with altered male hormones that consequently result in infertility through an endocrine effect, researchers have also implicated increased BMI with decreased paternity in investigations that suggest that the adverse effects of obesity on male reproduction may be independent of the endocrine system (Pauli et al, 2008; Stewart et al, 2009). Some evidence suggests that only extreme obesity negatively affects male fertility through an endocrine pathway (Chavarro et al, 2010). Other published studies have observed a relationship only between sperm motility and BMI, but not an association with sperm concentration, suggesting that obesity may primarily interfere with epididymal function that imparts motility to sperm (Martini et al, 2010). Some studies indicate that obesity may degrade sperm DNA integrity and mitochondrial activity, whether through the final common pathway of the endocrine system or another hormonal-independent mechanism (Fariello, et al, 2012a). Although this evidence suggests that the endocrine system is a probable target for impairment of reproductive effects in the male, it is likely that the full elucidation of the means by which excess adiposity exerts its effects on male reproduction is beyond such a singular process.

Male Reproductive Physical Examination

Fortunately for the examining physician, much of the male reproductive system is located outside of the body cavity, where it can be easily palpated. Because much of the male reproductive physical examination is most effectively performed with the patient standing, it is important to put the patient both at ease and before a low examining table or chair, as some men will develop syncope during palpation of the scrotum. Asking a man about his work often serves to distract him from the male genital examination (Niederberger, 2011).

If the partner of the patient is present during the history, she may relate valuable information. However, the patient may also feel reluctant to divulge specific facts of reproductive significance before his partner, and the physical examination presents an opportunity to tactfully ask her to leave the room to allow the man time to discuss issues with his physician privately (Niederberger, 2011).

Examining the Scrotum

Visual observation of the scrotum may be revealing. One or both sides may be hypoplastic, indicating an absence of the scrotal contents since birth (Niederberger, 2011). One side may be substantially larger than the other, suggesting a reactive hydrocele or tumor. A varicocele may be so large as to be visible. Finally, proximity to the thighs in a large or obese male may indicate an insufficient difference between intrascrotal and body temperature.

Examining the Testis and Epididymis

The examiner first palpates the testis and epididymis through the scrotum, noting any abnormalities. The epididymis is typically difficult to appreciate; if it is easily palpated, it is likely engorged, which suggests obstruction. Segmentation of the epididymis is also worthwhile to note: If the portion near the upper pole is easy to discern but the lower pole is not, wolffian ductal development may have been incomplete (Lewis and Kaplan, 2009).

Testis size is well established to correlate with sperm production and is consequently an important assessment in the physical examination of the infertile male (Takihara et al, 1987; Bujan et al, 1989). The size of the testis may be assessed by calipers often referred to as the *Seager orchidometer* (Fig. 24-1) (Niederberger, 2011). **The long axis of the testis is gently grasped between the jaws of the calipers, and a measurement of 4.6 cm or less is associated with spermatogenic impairment** (Schoor et al, 2001). A second method to ascertain testis size is to compare the examiner's palpation findings with a string of ellipsoids of increasing size with marked

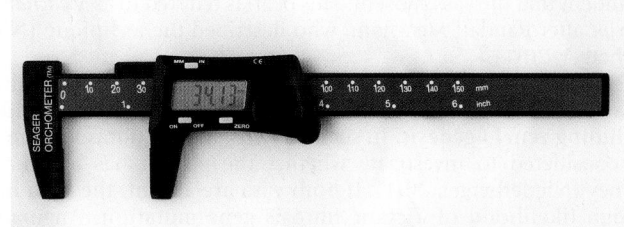

Figure 24-1. **Caliper (Seager) orchidometer.**

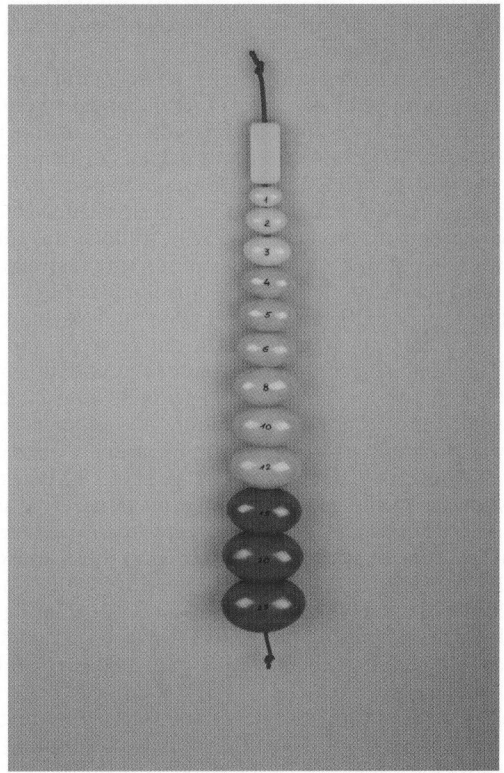

Figure 24-2. **Prader orchidometer. (Courtesy Erler Zimmer GmbH and Co. KG, Germany.)**

volumes as shown in Figure 24-2 (Niederberger, 2011). **A volume of 20 mL or less is considered low** (Sigman et al, 2009). Finally, testis volume may be more directly measured by ultrasonography of the scrotum (Sakamoto et al, 2007a, 2007b; Abdulwahed et al, 2013). However, it is unclear the degree to which the incremental increase in accuracy that testis ultrasound adds to that obtained by the caliper or Prader orchidometer translates to clinically useful information (Sakamoto et al, 2007a).

Examining the Spermatic Cord

Palpation of the spermatic cord yields two features of reproductive significance: whether the vas deferens is palpable, and whether a varicocele is present. The vas is a firm cordlike structure differentiated from vasculature within the spermatic cord by the compressibility of the vessels. Because the veins within the cord may be mistaken for the vas on manual examination of the upper scrotum, absence of the vas can be a difficult physical sign to identify. **For the clinician with experience in vasectomy, one useful method of identifying whether the structure is absent is to search for the vas as if performing the first step of a vasectomy, bringing it to the surface of the skin.** If what is presumed to be the vas disappears from the examiner's fingers three times, the clinician can be confident that the vas is absent. This pearl is referred to as *Meacham's maxim* after Randall Meacham, who described the technique (Niederberger, 2011).

Unilateral absence of the vas deferens suggests the possibility of a complete lack of wolffian ductal development on that side, including renal agenesis. In such patients, a renal ultrasound may be considered to investigate whether the patient has a solitary kidney (Niederberger, 2011). **If both vasa are absent, the man has a high likelihood of a cystic fibrosis gene mutation** (Anguiano et al, 1992). In such patients, laboratory genetic assessment of the cystic fibrosis transmembrane conductance regulator gene sequence is indicated (Lyon and Miller, 2003; Bombieri et al, 2011). Because investigators have noted renal agenesis in 11% of men with congenital bilateral absence of the vas deferens (CBAVD), renal ultrasound may also be considered to investigate whether a solitary kidney is present (Schlegel et al, 1996).

In addition to assessing the presence, absence, and continuity of the vas deferens, the clinician examining the upper scrotum views its surface to determine if a plexus of varicose veins arising from the spermatic cord is visible and then gently palpates to identify whether a varicocele may be felt. Although sporadic reports before 1955 described cases in which surgery on varicocele yielded evidence of improved reproductive potential, W. Selby Tulloch was the first to systematically report a series of cases of infertile men undergoing high ligation of a varicocele and subsequent improvement in sperm counts (Tulloch, 1955). Lawrence Dubin and Richard Amelar studied varicocele and its treatment in larger series and broadly educated urologic surgeons on its pathology and the merits of therapy (Dubin and Amelar, 1975; Nagler and Grotas, 2009).

The varicocele is the most commonly encountered nonductal surgically addressable pathologic entity potentially affecting male reproductive potential (Nagler and Grotas, 2009). **In general, incidence estimates in the general population range from one fifth to one sixth, whereas most studies suggest the incidence of varicocele in infertile males to be between one third and one half** (Pryor and Howards, 1987; Fretz and Sandlow, 2002; Nagler and Grotas, 2009). That not all men with varicocele are infertile remains one of the most perplexing problems in male reproductive medicine today; the choice of therapy for a particular man with a varicocele is challenging.

Clinical studies of varicocele have used multiple grading systems to describe the severity of the entity, further complicating the task of the evaluating physician (Nagler and Grotas, 2009; Williams, 2011). Most systems use three or four grades, usually with the first being a varicocele that cannot be palpated but can be detected only by radiographic evaluation, typically ultrasound (Nagler and Grotas, 2009; Williams, 2011). Some systems differentiate varicoceles that can be palpated only during the Valsalva maneuver (Nagler and Grotas, 2009). Because the majority of studies concur that treatment of subclinical varicoceles does not significantly improve male reproductive potential, a sensible grading system would include these entities, which are best left untreated, to differentiate them from those that ought to be addressed with therapy (Niederberger, 2011). Likewise, the difference between varicoceles that can be seen and those that can only be felt is clinically obvious, and a reasonable grading system would differentiate the two (Niederberger, 2011). As the clinical significance of those varicoceles that can only be appreciated with the Valsalva maneuver is uncertain, a rational grading system would not include this feature as a major discriminator. Hence, **the modern evidence-based clinical grading system for varicocele includes grade I, which is not palpable or visible and can only be detected by radiographic evaluation such as Doppler ultrasound; grade II, which is palpable but not visible; and grade III, a varicocele that is so large as to be visible by the examining physician through the rugae of the scrotum** (Niederberger, 2011).

Examining the Phallus

In the typical setting of intercourse, semen must be deposited proximal to the cervical os for optimal chance of reproduction. Consequently, any abnormality of the phallus that may prevent placement of the semen at that locale should be noted by the examining physician. These abnormalities include phimosis, meatal displacement in hypospadias or epispadias, and significant penile curvature (Niederberger, 2011).

Examining the Prostate and Seminal Vesicles

In general, examination of the prostate and seminal vesicles does not add a significant amount of information to the evaluation of the infertile male, and if the patient is sufficiently apprehensive about digital rectal examination, it may be prudently omitted. Should rectal examination be performed, the clinician notes the size of the prostate, as it may be aplastic or hypoplastic in cases of congenital malformation or significant hypoandrogenism (Niederberger, 2011). **The seminal vesicles cannot typically be palpated; if they are palpable, it is an abnormal finding suggesting engorgement and possible ejaculatory ductal obstruction** (Niederberger, 2011).

KEY POINTS: MALE REPRODUCTIVE PHYSICAL EXAMINATION

- Obesity impairs male reproductive potential by endocrine-dependent and endocrine-independent mechanisms.
- Testis size directly reflects spermatogenic mass.
- Unilateral absence of the vas deferens suggests a wolffian ductal anomaly; bilateral absence is associated with mutations in the gene responsible for cystic fibrosis. In both, renal agenesis may result.

LABORATORY EVALUATION OF MALE INFERTILITY

Like other aspects of urology, much can be learned about the condition of male infertility from blood tests, in this case, primarily of the endocrine system. Also similar to other urologic fields, genomic assessment of male reproductive function is a burgeoning area of research and increasing clinical usefulness. However, the laboratory inquiry into male infertility also includes a way of directly appraising the severity of the condition by observing the male gametes in the semen analysis. These three general laboratory assessments comprise the laboratory evaluation of male infertility: the endocrine evaluation, analysis of semen, and genomic assessment.

Endocrine Evaluation

As spermatogenesis is highly dependent on intratesticular testosterone synthesis, it is unsurprising that hypoandrogenism is associated with male infertility. Testosterone levels in men vary widely, and most investigators use either 280 ng/dL or 300 ng/dL as a threshold for adequate androgenization in a man (Petak et al, 2002; Sokol, 2009). Approximately 45% of men with azoospermia caused by spermatogenic dysfunction are observed to have testosterone less than 300 ng/dL, and serum testosterone below that threshold is found in 43% of men with oligospermia and 35% of men in an infertility clinic with sperm density greater than the threshold of 20 million/mL specified in the fourth edition of the WHO laboratory manual for the examination and processing of human semen (Sussman et al, 2008). Because 90% of men with sperm density of 22 million/mL or less will not have conceived with their partners within 1 year, many with sperm density less than that value are expected to have pathologic reproductive dysfunction, and consequently in approximately one third it is likely related to endocrinopathy (WHO, 2010). **Androgenization should therefore be assessed by laboratory evaluation in all men presenting for infertility including those in whom sperm density is greater than 20 million/mL.** An upper limit of sperm density has not been established above which endocrine dysfunction is unlikely to be discovered; clinicians may reasonably use the 50th percentile value in the fourth edition of the WHO manual of 73 million/mL with time to pregnancy within 1 year as a guide, suggesting that a full endocrine evaluation is not necessary (WHO, 2010).

Testosterone circulates in three main forms: tightly bound to SHBG; loosely bound to protein, primarily albumin; and unbound or free (Matsumoto and Bremner, 2011). The forms inducing cellular activity are free and loosely bound, together comprising what is referred to as *bioavailable testosterone* (Matsumoto and Bremner, 2011). In the healthy man, 30% to 44% of circulating testosterone is bound to SHBG, 54% to 68% is loosely bound to albumin, and 0.5% to 3.0% is unbound (Matsumoto and Bremner, 2011). **Using a threshold of 300 ng/dL for testosterone and the lower limit of 54.5% for percent bioavailable testosterone, a reasonable lower limit for the concentration of bioavailable testosterone would consequently be 164 ng/dL.**

SHBG is altered in a variety of medical conditions and states such as obesity and aging (Box 24-1) (Bhasin et al, 2010). The clinician cannot rely on total testosterone to gauge bioavailable testosterone, and because obtaining an accurate laboratory assessment of free testosterone can be difficult, a practical method of determining bioavailable testosterone is to calculate it from total testosterone, SHBG, and albumin (Vermeulen et al, 1999). Internet-based and smartphone calculators are available; as of this writing, the International Society for the Study of the Aging Male hosts a calculator at www.issam.ch/freetesto.htm, and a calculator for iOS devices may be found at http://itunes.apple.com/us/app/bioavailable-testosterone/id308770722.

In young, healthy men, total serum testosterone exhibits a circadian rhythm, with a peak in the early morning and trough levels in the late afternoon (Plymate et al, 1989). SHBG displays an opposing circadian rhythm in men of all ages, with a peak in the late afternoon and a trough in the early morning (Plymate et al, 1989). **Consequently, bioavailable testosterone demonstrates a marked circadian rhythm in young, healthy men, with a peak in the early morning and trough in the late afternoon** (Plymate et al, 1989). In older men, total testosterone and its circadian rhythm are attenuated, and the circadian rhythm and concentration of bioavailable testosterone are substantially diminished (Plymate et al, 1989). To standardize sampling of total and bioavailable testosterone in all men, assays are typically performed in the morning, although the necessity of such timing is more important in younger men.

In the case of hypoandrogenism, a pituitary or testicular source is identified by assessing LH (Niederberger, 2011). If testicular Leydig cell dysfunction is the cause, LH is elevated to varying degrees (Niederberger, 2011). In the case of pituitary dysfunction, LH is decreased (Niederberger, 2011). The clinician may assess LH after total or bioavailable testosterone returns with a low value, or, for efficiency, both assays may be performed simultaneously. Because testosterone and LH are released in a pulsatile fashion, borderline results may be investigated further by obtaining three morning samples at 20-minute intervals (Sokol, 2009). Historically, clinicians pooled these samples for a single measure, but three separate assay results may be determined and arithmetically averaged.

The Sertoli cell products inhibin B and activin regulate pituitary follicle-stimulating hormone (FSH) by respectively inhibiting and stimulating its release (Caroppo, 2011). Because the Sertoli cells are regulated by robust paracrine interaction with germ cells, with depopulation of the latter, inhibin levels decrease and FSH consequently increases (Niederberger, 2011). Clinicians have consequently used FSH as an indirect assessment of germ cell mass, with higher concentrations of FSH indicating increasing germ cell dysfunction and depopulation (Niederberger, 2011). **Combined with testis size as measured by caliper orchidometer, FSH is an accurate predictor of whether azoospermia is a result of obstruction or spermatogenic dysfunction: 96% of men with obstructive azoospermia had FSH assay values of 7.6 IU/L or less and testis long axis greater than 4.6 cm, whereas 89% of men with azoospermia caused by spermatogenic dysfunction had FSH values greater than 7.6 IU/L and testis long axis 4.6 cm or less** (Schoor et al, 2001). In the case of male reproductive dysfunction in which sperm is present in the ejaculate, the odds ratio of abnormal sperm concentration increased markedly at an FSH value of 4.5 IU/L, suggesting another threshold that the clinician may use to assess male reproductive dysfunction (Gordetsky et al, 2011).

Assays of inhibin B are clinically available, and investigators have investigated whether measuring inhibin B directly is a more accurate assessment of spermatogenic function than the indirect assay of FSH (Kumanov et al, 2006; Muttukrishna et al, 2007; van Beek et al, 2007; Myers et al, 2009; Jørgensen et al, 2010; Grunewald et al, 2013). In general, these studies include analyses of correlation between inhibin B or FSH and sperm parameters or testis parameters measured by physical examination. Many studies observe greater accuracy with measuring inhibin B than with FSH in these correlations, and some data suggest that lower ranges of inhibin B allow improved correlation (Kumanov et al, 2006; van Beek et al, 2007; Myers et al, 2009; Grunewald et al, 2013). **However, the incremental improvement in accuracy is typically small, and inhibin and FSH both provide clinically useful markers of spermatogenic function** (Myers et al, 2009). The clinician may consequently use either marker based on cost and availability.

Like inhibin B, AMH is a member of the transforming growth factor-β (TGF-β) family synthesized by Sertoli cells, and investigators have studied its use as an assay in assessing spermatogenic function (Fénichel et al, 1999; Fujisawa et al, 2002; Muttukrishna et al, 2007). Although results from pilot studies are encouraging, reported data sets remain small, and use of AMH is considered primarily experimental.

Aromatase enzymes convert cholesterol-based molecules such as testosterone to estrogens and are found in many organ systems including testis, adipose tissue, liver, and brain (Kim et al, 2013). Estradiol is consequently measurable in men, and investigators have proposed that elevated estradiol adversely affects male reproductive potential (Raman and Schlegel, 2002; Gregoriou et al, 2012; Schlegel, 2012). **A ratio of total testosterone to estradiol below 10:1 is suggested to indicate reproductive dysfunction** (Raman and Schlegel, 2002; Gregoriou et al, 2012; Schlegel, 2012).

The pituitary hormone prolactin is known to inhibit gonadotropins and suppress testosterone production in men, and it may be elevated in pituitary hyperplasia, adenoma, or tumors (Sokol, 2009). Clinically significant disease of the pituitary is typically associated with symptoms such as visual field changes, headache, or erectile dysfunction (Niederberger, 2011). Prolactin assay should be considered when these symptoms accompany male infertility, especially if total or bioavailable testosterone is low. However, the

---

BOX 24-1 Conditions Associated with Altered Sex Hormone-Binding Globulin (SHBG) Concentrations

CONDITIONS ASSOCIATED WITH DECREASED SHBG

Obesity
Nephrotic syndrome
Hypothyroidism
Glucocorticoids, progestins, and androgenic steroid therapy
Acromegaly
Diabetes mellitus

CONDITIONS ASSOCIATED WITH INCREASED SHBG

Aging
Hepatic cirrhosis and hepatitis
Hyperthyroidism
Anticonvulsant therapy
Estrogen therapy
Human immunodeficiency virus disease

Modified from Bhasin S, Cunningham GR, Hayes FJ, et al. Testosterone therapy in men with androgen deficiency syndromes: an Endocrine Society clinical practice guideline. J Clin Endocrinol Metab 2010;95:2536–59.

incidence of clinically significant prolactinoma is very low in infertile males, with only four detected in 1035 men in one large screening study, and prolactin need not be routinely included in the initial endocrine evaluation of an infertile man (Sigman and Jarow, 1997). Prolactin is commonly a labile assay; should it be found to be elevated, repetition of the test is warranted (Niederberger, 2011). Assessment of other pituitary hormones such as thyroid-stimulating hormone, adrenocorticotropic hormone, or growth hormone is indicated if a space-occupying pituitary lesion is suspected or found on imaging examination (Sokol, 2009). Likewise, should signs of other endocrine disease, such as exophthalmos, striations, moon facies, or facial bony changes, be observed, thyroid hormone, cortisol, or growth hormone assays may be entertained. However, they need not be included in the initial screening evaluation of an infertile man. **A reasonable initial laboratory screen to assess an endocrine basis for male reproductive dysfunction should be performed in the morning and includes total testosterone, SHBG, and albumin to calculate bioavailable testosterone; LH and FSH to gauge pituitary function; and estradiol to evaluate aromatization.**

Men with a history of congenital adrenal hyperplasia (CAH) may develop testicular adrenal rest tumors and infertility later in life (Pierre et al, 2012; Aycan et al, 2013). In these patients, serum 17-hydroxyprogesterone, Δ4-androstenedione, renin, and testosterone can be used to assess response to therapy (Pierre et al, 2012).

Evaluation of Semen

Reproduction is a probabilistic system: The more viable sperm that begin their journey in the female reproductive tract, the greater the chance that one will penetrate and fertilize the ovum. In this sense, there is only one definitive result of a semen analysis, and that is the condition in which no sperm are present; only in that case can a man be absolutely considered sterile.

In 1951, the physiologist John MacLeod published the first stringent statistical assessment comparing what could be observed under the light microscope in semen from men who had successfully impregnated their partners versus semen of men who had not done so (MacLeod, 1951). MacLeod applied a descriptive statistical approach, computing cumulative probability histograms for each observable parameter and determining quartiles for each of the two groups of men (MacLeod, 1951). Basic parameters studied included the concentration of sperm, their movement, and their shape (MacLeod, 1951). What is immediately evident from MacLeod's seminal publication is that the histograms for sperm parameters from fertile and infertile men are largely overlapping, meaning that a substantial range of values for any parameter do not discriminate between male fertility and infertility (MacLeod, 1951). MacLeod sensibly approached this problem by considering lower sperm parameter values to be more appropriate thresholds for suggesting male infertility; however, values above these lower thresholds do not confirm fertility (MacLeod, 1951). This proved to be very difficult to grasp in clinical implementation, and the field of reproductive medicine is rife with the assumption that should a parameter be above a threshold—for example, sperm concentration greater than 20 million/mL—then the man is established to be fertile, which is incorrect. The only conclusion that may be drawn from such a comparison is that should the parameter be lower than the threshold, the man is likely to be infertile; the converse is not necessarily true.

One general approach to the problem of an assay for which the values representing disease and health are overly coincident is to establish two thresholds, beyond which health or disease is probable, and within which no predictive statement can be made. In one study to develop two such sets of thresholds for semen analysis, investigators applied the computational method classification and regression tree (CART) analysis to semen analyses from fertile men and those whose wives were undergoing intrauterine insemination (IUI) and for whom female infertility had been largely excluded (Guzick et al, 2001). **As an example, for sperm concentration, 13.5 million/mL was found to be the lower parameter, and 48.0 million/mL was identified as the upper parameter** (Guzick et al, 2001). Using these parameters, the clinician would counsel a man whose sperm concentration was less than 13.5 million/mL that he was likely infertile, and one with a concentration greater than 48.0 million/mL that he was likely fertile. Should the man's concentration be greater than 13.5 million/mL and less than 48.0 million/mL, no assessment of fertility potential could be accurately made.

Bulk Semen Parameters and the World Health Organization Criteria

Building on the original work by MacLeod and deriving consensus from a group of experts, WHO established criteria for semen analysis parameters in its laboratory manual for the examination and processing of human semen (Cooper et al, 2010; WHO, 2010; Niederberger, 2011; Murray et al, 2012). For the first four editions of the manual, criteria were set both by expert panel and survey data, and included such thresholds as sperm density of 20 million/mL, which would be judged as a reasonable number below which a man should be considered likely infertile (Cooper et al, 2010; WHO, 2010; Niederberger, 2011; Murray et al, 2012). The problems with such a set of criteria are manifestly evident: fertile men may be found below the thresholds and infertile men above.

The fifth edition of the WHO laboratory manual departed from the previous four by emphasizing the statistical description of the population of men on which it was based (Cooper et al, 2010; WHO, 2010). Values for percentiles of semen parameters from men whose partners became pregnant within 1 year of discontinuation of contraceptives are tabulated, allowing the clinician to compare an infertile patient's results with a fertile cohort (Table 24-2)

TABLE 24-2 Bulk Semen Analysis Parameter Percentiles

PERCENTILE	2.5	95% CI	5	95% CI	10	25	50	75	90	95	97.5
Semen volume (mL)	1.2	(1.0-1.3)	1.5	(1.4-1.7)	2	2.7	3.7	4.8	6	6.8	7
Sperm concentration (million/mL)	9	(8-11)	15	(12-16)	22	41	73	116	169	213	259
Total number (million/ejaculate)	23	(18-29)	39	(33-46)	69	142	255	422	647	802	928
Total motility (%)	34	(33-37)	40	(38-42)	45	53	61	69	75	78	81
Progressive motility (%)	28	(25-29)	32	(31-34)	39	47	55	62	69	72	75
Normal forms (%)	3	(2.0-3.0)	4	(3.0-4.0)	5.5	9	15	24.5	36	44	48
Vitality (%)	53	(48-56)	58	(55-63)	64	72	79	84	88	91	92

CI, confidence interval.

Modified from Cooper TG, Noonan E, von Eckardstein S, et al. World Health Organization reference values for human semen characteristics. Hum Reprod Update 2010;16(3):231–45.

(Cooper et al, 2010; WHO, 2010). Two limitations of such an approach are clear: First, the data are derived from a fertile population and not an infertile one, and second, the clinician cannot rely on descriptive statistics to predict outcomes. Nonetheless, the manual's tables offer the physician useful comparative information that would be otherwise unavailable in evaluating and treating infertile men.

Somewhat confusingly, the fifth edition of the manual published alongside the full percentile table a separate list of the 5th percentiles and their 95% confidence intervals (CIs) (Cooper et al, 2010; WHO, 2010). For example, the 5th percentile value for sperm density is 15 million/mL with a 95% CI range of 12 to 16 million/mL (Cooper et al, 2010; WHO, 2010). Although the authors of the companion publication to the manual very clearly describe the problems inherent in using thresholds derived from descriptive statistics of a fertile male population, the enumeration of the 5th percentile values has appeared to spur their use as new thresholds. The best use of the tables in the fifth edition of the manual would be for the urologist to present to a man alongside the patient's own parameters as a reference for an ultimately fertile population, but clinical reality dictates that both physicians and patients are interested in defining what represents infertility to consider when medical or surgical therapy is appropriately invoked. Communicating the 5th percentile value as one that likely represents infertility and the 50th percentile as typical for a man conceiving with his wife within 1 year is reasonable practice for clinical urology. As an example, for sperm density, that would be lower than 15 million/mL suggesting infertility, and 73 million/mL as typical (Cooper et al, 2010; WHO, 2010).

To complicate matters, semen analysis parameters are highly variable, and investigators typically recommend a minimum of two analyses separated by 2 to 3 weeks for assessment (Centola, 2011). Although data exist to the contrary, most investigators observe a linear decline in bulk seminal parameters with increasing days of abstinence, and variability in abstinence may be responsible for variability in semen analysis results (Levitas et al, 2005; Keel, 2006; Elzanaty, 2008). Consequently, the physician evaluating a man for his reproductive potential should ensure that the duration of abstinence before an ejaculated specimen is as constant as possible. **Historically, men were instructed to wait 2 to 5 days after an ejaculation to submit a sample for semen analysis** (WHO, 2010; Centola, 2011). **More recent studies suggest that a single day of abstinence is optimal for assessing bulk seminal parameters** (Levitas et al, 2005; Elzanaty, 2008).

A nontoxic wide-mouthed glass or plastic cup is used to collect the semen sample (WHO, 2010). In the case of religious or cultural stipulations that do not allow collection by masturbation, a special nontoxic condom may be used (WHO, 2010).

The physical and chemical characteristics of a semen sample are first assessed before microscopic examination. Ejaculated semen first forms a coagulum, and the sample is allowed to liquefy for 30 minutes before evaluation (Centola, 2011). Viscosity is assessed by aspiration into a pipette and measuring the length of the drop that forms, which should be no longer than 2 cm (WHO, 2010; Centola, 2011). The sample is then inspected visually for coloration. A normal ejaculate is white or light gray; a yellow or green hue may indicate infection, jaundice, or vitamins or medication; brown is often observed in spinal cord–injured men; and red suggests blood (WHO, 2010; Centola, 2011).

Historically, semen pH was reported, but its measurement is no longer recommended because environmental conditions may alter it, and the original intent of using pH to gauge whether obstruction exists is hampered by the vast difference in size between a hydrogen ion and sperm head (Centola, 2011). For bulk seminal parameters describing microscopic features, a specialized slide with a compartment with defined volume such as a hemocytometer or Makler counting chamber is typically used (Centola, 2011).

Semen Volume. Often unreported by laboratories infrequently performing semen analysis, semen volume is of significant clinical importance (Niederberger, 2011). Conditions causing seminal hypovolemia include anatomic factors, such as ejaculatory ductal

obstruction or hypoplasia of the prostate and seminal vesicles as may occur in severe androgen deficiency or CBAVD; functional issues, such as in retrograde ejaculation; neurologic conditions, such as in spinal cord injury, diabetes mellitus, or multiple sclerosis; and pharmacologic factors, which may occur in men prescribed α-adrenergic blocking agents such as tamsulosin (Sigman et al, 2009; Niederberger, 2011). The 5th percentile for volume according to the fifth edition of the WHO laboratory manual is 1.5 mL with a 95% CI of 1.4 to 1.7 mL, and the 2.5th percentile is 1.2 mL with a 95% CI of 1.0 to 1.3 mL (WHO, 2010). **For practical purposes, the most frequently used threshold value for volume is 1.0 mL to initiate evaluation for seminal hypovolemia** (Niederberger, 2011).

Aspermia, dry ejaculate, and *anejaculation* refer to the condition in which no fluid is discharged from the urethra during male orgasm (Sigman et al, 2009). It is caused by the same conditions associated with seminal hypovolemia (Sigman et al, 2009; Niederberger, 2011). **If aspermia or seminal hypovolemia is observed, a postejaculatory urinalysis is performed to identify retrograde ejaculation, and some form of investigation such as transrectal ultrasonography (TRUS) is conducted to evaluate whether ejaculatory ductal obstruction may be present** (Sigman et al, 2009; Niederberger, 2011). For postejaculatory urinalysis, the patient is instructed to void before ejaculation for a semen analysis and then to urinate after collection of the semen sample into separate containers (Sigman et al, 2009). The urine is reconstituted by centrifugation and the number of sperm in the pellet is counted (Sigman et al, 2009). A small number of sperm in the urine is of little consequence if the number of sperm in the antegrade sample is large. In general, if the number of sperm in the urine nears or exceeds that in the antegrade specimen, retrograde ejaculation is considered clinically significant (Sigman et al, 2009).

Seminal hypervolemia with an ejaculate volume exceeding 5 mL is a rare condition (Sigman et al, 2009). It is proposed to interfere with male reproduction by diluting sperm (Sigman et al, 2009). If a too-large seminal volume is of concern, the sperm may be reconstituted by processing into a smaller volume, and IUI performed (Sigman et al, 2009; Centola, 2011).

Sperm Density. Sperm density or concentration is typically recorded in millions per milliliter. The term *oligospermia* refers to low sperm density, and *cryptozoospermia* denotes sperm so few as to be difficult to reliably measure (Niederberger, 2011). The 5th percentile for sperm density according to the fifth edition of the WHO laboratory manual is 15 million/mL with a 95% CI of 12 to 16 million/mL, and the 50th percentile is 73 million/mL (Cooper et al, 2010; WHO, 2010). Previous editions of the WHO laboratory manual included a threshold for sperm density of 20 million/mL, and it was common in the past for practitioners to define oligospermia as lower than that value. With the descriptive tabulation of sperm parameters in the fifth edition of the WHO manual, oligospermia is more appropriately defined in a clinical context: A man with a single semen sample demonstrating 10 million/mL who has had no difficulty impregnating his wife may not be oligospermic, whereas one with small testes, an elevated FSH, and densities on several semen analyses ranging from 20 to 25 million/mL may be reasonably considered oligospermic. **As previously written, a large CART analysis revealed 13.5 million/mL to be a lower parameter for sperm density and 48.0 million/mL to be an upper parameter** (Guzick et al, 2001). In CART analysis, the ROC AUC for sperm density was 0.60, indicating relatively poor discriminating ability between fertile and subfertile subgroups (Guzick et al, 2001).

Total sperm count or number is calculated by multiplying semen volume and sperm density and is typically recorded in millions (Niederberger, 2011). The 5th percentile for total sperm number according to the fifth edition of the WHO laboratory manual is 39 million with a 95% CI of 33 to 46 million, and the 50th percentile is 255 million (Cooper et al, 2010; WHO, 2010).

Sperm Motility. Sperm motility is assessed optimally within 30 minutes of liquefaction and refers to a percentage of sperm observed with defined motion (WHO, 2010). Low motility is termed *asthenospermia* (Niederberger, 2011). The fifth edition of the WHO manual classifies motility into three categories—progressive, nonprogressive, and immotility—replacing the four categories of older grading systems (a through d, where a and b indicated "rapid" and "slow" progressive motility) (WHO, 2010). *Progressive motility* is defined as sperm "moving actively, either linearly or in a large circle, regardless of speed," and nonprogressive motility as "all other patterns of motility with an absence of progression" (WHO, 2010). The 5th percentile for progressive motility according to the fifth edition of the WHO laboratory manual is 32% with a 95% CI of 31% to 34%, and the 50th percentile is 55% (Cooper et al, 2010; WHO, 2010). **CART analysis revealed 32% to be a lower parameter for sperm motility and 63% to be an upper parameter** (Guzick et al, 2001). In CART analysis, the ROC AUC for sperm motility was 0.59, revealing low discriminating ability for this parameter (Guzick et al, 2001).

Sperm Morphology. Human sperm is highly pleomorphic with more bizarrely shaped sperm in any man's ejaculate than those with configuration anticipated to successfully penetrate and fertilize an ovum (Niederberger, 2011). An overabundance of abnormal forms is termed *teratozoospermia* (Niederberger, 2011). Earlier editions of the WHO manual described fairly generous criteria as characterizing an acceptably shaped sperm, and even then, the majority of sperm were classified as misshapen in a normal semen analysis (Niederberger, 2011). **In an attempt to improve the predictive capability of sperm morphology, Kruger proposed a grading system in which several aspects of sperm were assessed, and if any one was out of range, the sperm was counted as abnormal** (Kruger et al, 1987; van der Merwe et al, 2005). This system is variably referred to as "strict" morphology, "Kruger" morphology, and "Tygerberg" morphology, and as a result of the more stringent criteria defining a normal sperm, thresholds in the range of 5% typically characterize a normal ejaculate (van der Merwe et al, 2005). The fifth edition of the WHO manual adopted strict morphology as its assessment of sperm shape (WHO, 2010). The 5th percentile for normal morphologic forms according to the fifth edition is 4% with a 95% CI of 3.0% to 4.0%, and the 50th percentile is 15% (Cooper et al, 2010; WHO, 2010). CART analysis revealed 9% to be a lower parameter for strict morphology and 12% to be an upper parameter (Guzick et al, 2001). In CART analysis, the ROC AUC for sperm motility was 0.66, as with the bulk parameters of density and motility revealing low discriminating capacity (Guzick et al, 2001).

The clinical predictive value of strict morphology is questionable. Although limited data suggest that the parameter may be associated with embryo formation, the majority of studies support that strict morphology is unassociated with sperm nuclear integrity and that it does not predict natural conception or IVF outcomes (Keegan et al, 2007; Dubey et al, 2008; Avendaño et al, 2009; Dayal et al, 2010; French et al, 2010; Sripada et al, 2010; Morbeck et al, 2011). To complicate matters, evidence suggests that as laboratory technicians have learned to inspect each sperm more closely for eccentricities of shape, an increasing number of men are described as having lower percentages of sperm with normal morphology (Morbeck et al, 2011). The practical implication of this trend is that currently many men who seek evaluation are identified as having isolated teratozoospermia and are likely to have adequate reproductive potential.

Conditions exist in which specific biologic defects are associated with the majority of sperm. For example, should the acrosome fail to form, the preponderance of sperm will have small, round heads, a disorder referred to as *globozoospermia* (WHO, 2010). During spermiation, if the basal plate does not attach to the nucleus opposite the acrosome, the heads are absorbed (WHO, 2010). This defect results in only tails observed and is termed *pinhead sperm* (WHO, 2010). Undoubtedly, these relatively uncommon specific morphologic conditions affect male reproductive potential.

Please see the Expert Consult website for further details.

Sperm Vitality. *Vitality* refers to the portion of sperm that are metabolically active living cells (WHO, 2010; Niederberger, 2011). *Necrospermia* is the condition describing a large number of nonliving sperm (Niederberger, 2011). **The assessment of whether or not sperm are living is essential if near or total asthenospermia is observed to discriminate whether the lack of motility is a result of cell death or of dysfunction of molecular processes involved in sperm motion** (Niederberger, 2011; WHO, 2010). If the test is purely diagnostic and the sperm are not to be used in IVF, it is performed by staining with eosin Y and with or without nigrosin (WHO, 2010; Niederberger, 2011). A metabolically active sperm excludes the eosin Y dye, whereas a dead one cannot and absorbs the pigment (WHO, 2010; Niederberger, 2011). Nigrosin darkens the background and increases the contrast between it and the live sperm heads, allowing them to be identified more easily (WHO, 2010). The 5th percentile for sperm vitality according to the fifth edition of the WHO laboratory manual is 58% with a 95% CI of 55% to 63%, and the 50th percentile is 79% (Cooper et al, 2010; WHO, 2010).

A method of assessing sperm vitality in a nondestructive manner amenable to subsequent use in IVF is the hypo-osmotic swelling (HOS) test (Jeyendran et al, 1984). When incubated in hypo-osmotic medium, the tails of live sperm with unimpaired membranes swell within 5 minutes, allowing for identification of viable gametes (WHO, 2010).

Please see the Expert Consult website for further details.

Secondary Semen Assays

The haploid male gamete expresses different surface antigens than the remainder of diploid cells in the male body and consequently must be protected from the immune system by tight junctions between Sertoli cells (Walsh and Turek, 2009). Should this "blood-testis barrier" be disrupted, sperm exposed to the immune system may incite an immune response of varying severity involving secretory and humoral immunoglobulins and affecting multiple regions of the surface of the sperm cell (Walsh and Turek, 2009). **Conditions observed to be associated with antisperm antibody formation include vasectomy, testis trauma, orchitis, cryptorchidism, testis cancer, and varicocele** (Walsh and Turek, 2009).

Leukocytes may be harmful to sperm, with evidence suggesting that production of ROSs may be the destructive mechanism (Pasqualotto et al, 2000; Agarwal et al, 2006; Lackner et al, 2006; Desai et al, 2009; Domes et al, 2012; Aktan et al, 2013). Moderate levels of leukocytes in semen may be physiologic, and may even be beneficial for sperm function (Barraud-Lange et al, 2011).

Use of an assay for antisperm antibodies should be entertained if agglutination of sperm is observed or if sperm motility is decreased, especially if conditions associated with antisperm antibodies exist (Walsh and Turek, 2009; WHO, 2010; Brannigan, 2011; Niederberger, 2011). Two types of assays for antisperm antibodies are available; those that test for immunoglobulins on the surface of sperm are referred to as *direct* tests, and those that measure antibodies in fluid such as seminal plasma or serum are *indirect* assays (WHO, 2010; Brannigan, 2011). **Direct assays are preferred for clinical relevance, because antibodies in plasma or serum may not correlate to sperm surface binding** (Walsh and Turek, 2009; Brannigan, 2011; Niederberger, 2011). Owing to its large size, immunoglobulin M (IgM) is present in very low quantities if at all in semen, and consequently IgG and IgA are the primary assay targets (Walsh and Turek, 2009; Brannigan, 2011; Niederberger, 2011).

Two direct assays are available, the mixed antiglobulin reaction (MAR) test and the immunobead assay (WHO, 2010; Brannigan, 2011). The MAR test uses latex beads coated with an anti-IgG or anti-IgA "bridging" antibody incubated with sperm, whereas the direct immunobead test involves polyacrylamide beads coated with rabbit immunoglobulins against human IgG or IgA (WHO, 2010; Brannigan, 2011). **In both cases, after incubation the technician identifies the presence of antisperm antibodies by association of moving particles proximal to motile sperm, and thus some amount of sperm motion is essential for these assays; complete asthenospermia renders direct antisperm antibody assays unable to be performed** (WHO, 2010; Brannigan, 2011; Niederberger, 2011). The direct immunobead test is more laborious than the MAR assay but yields more precise information (WHO, 2010).

The WHO laboratory manual loosely specifies 50% as a threshold for both the MAR and immunobead tests and notes that reference values are not established, leaving the interpretation of these assays to the physician considering the degree and localization of antisperm antibody binding and the clinical context (WHO, 2010). Sperm head binding is considered to be of greater clinical significance than tail binding (Niederberger, 2011).

Pyospermia Assays. Under phase contrast microscopy without staining, leukocytes and immature germ cells are indistinguishable (Brannigan, 2011). Consequently, when faced with a report indicating an abundance of cells resembling leukocytes observed only with phase contrast microscopy, the evaluating physician cannot accurately diagnose pyospermia (Brannigan, 2011). Fortunately, laboratory testing to evaluate the presence of leukocytes is not difficult. The Papanicolaou stain may be used to differentiate leukocytes from immature germ cells based on nuclear morphology (WHO, 2010). **The current consensus threshold for leukocytes according to the WHO laboratory manual is 1 million/mL** (WHO, 2010). Should pyospermia be excluded, the patient can be reassured that the presence of immature germ cells is common and not of pathologic significance (Brannigan, 2011).

Tertiary and Investigational Sperm Assays

The limitations of bulk seminal parameters spawned myriad additional means to assess sperm structure and function in hopes of better diagnosing male reproductive dysfunction, applying therapies, and predicting outcomes in techniques such as IVF. Most are promising, but few are even close to proven. Many provide insight into the biologic processes involved in reproduction, but similarly designed studies report conflicting results when these assays are applied to clinical problems. Emphasizing a lack of consensus on how they are to be used clinically, the fifth edition of the WHO manual details these assays in its "research procedures" chapter (WHO, 2010). The prudent practitioner will continue to follow the literature as it evolves and use these assays clinically should a clear consensus emerge regarding usefulness.

Sperm DNA Integrity Assays. Sperm DNA molecular and spatial organization is highly specific to cells of the male gamete. Sperm DNA is six times more compact than in somatic cells, and it is arranged with protamines to form tightly linear side-by-side sheets (Ward and Coffey, 1991). Investigators have hypothesized that fragmentation or disturbances in DNA arrangement lead to aberrations in sperm function, fertilization, implantation, and pregnancy. Conflicting data and opinions abound in testing this hypothesis, indicating that our understanding of the role of sperm DNA quaternary structure is limited, the assays available are imperfect, or both. In general, there are two types of test methods that assess DNA structural integrity (Sakkas and Alvarez, 2010). In one, DNA fragmentation is measured directly (Sakkas and Alvarez, 2010). In general, this type of assessment is preferred by andrology laboratories at present because it appears to more effectively correlate with clinical outcomes (Sakkas and Alvarez, 2010). In the other, DNA is denatured before analysis (Sakkas and Alvarez, 2010). In a comprehensive meta-analysis, higher rates of miscarriage were associated with an overall approximately double risk ratio with increasing sperm DNA fragmentation, but different assays yielded markedly different risk strengths (Robinson et al, 2012).

TUNEL Assay. The terminal deoxynucleotidyl transferase dUTP nick end labeling (TUNEL) assay represents a general method in widespread use in molecular biology to assess DNA fragmentation by labeling the terminal end of nucleic acid strands with a fluorescent marker, and it was adopted in the andrology laboratory with various modifications to detect sperm head DNA fragmentation (Gavrieli et al, 1992; Mitchell et al, 2011). Figure 24-3 details one method. In panels A and B, a fluorescent stain that binds to DNA regions rich in adenine and thymine, 4′,6-diamidino-2-phenylindole (DAPI), identifies sperm heads containing packed DNA. Panel A is a brightfield image that allows sperm tails to be seen, confirming that the area under scrutiny is a sperm. Panel B is a fluorescent image, allowing comparison with TUNEL-positive sperm, which are

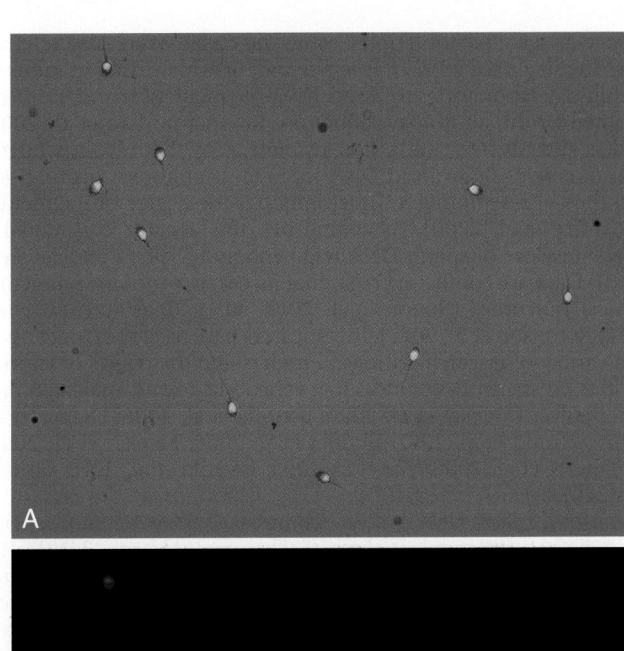
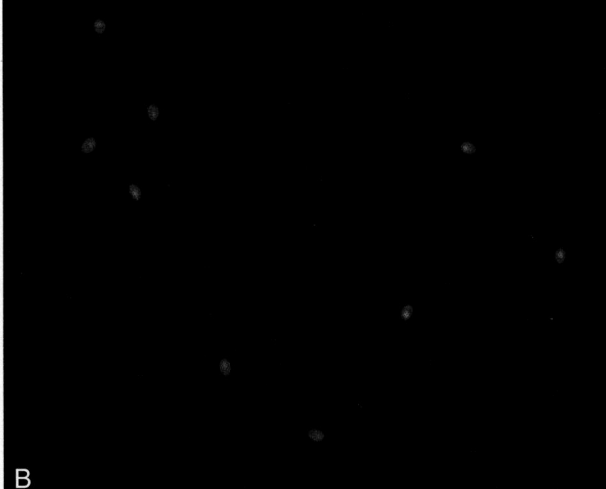
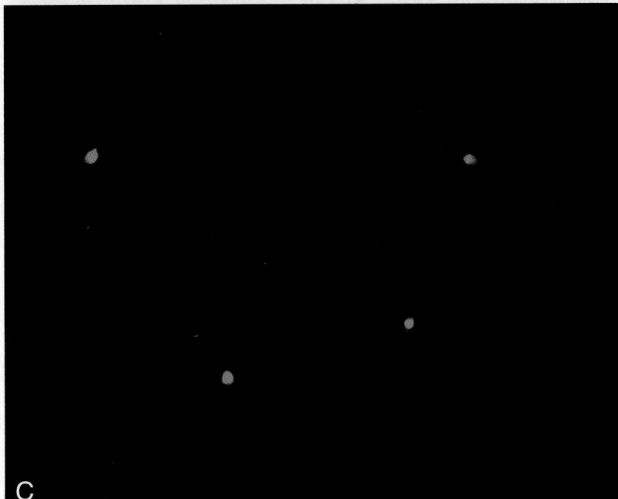

Figure 24-3. **TUNEL assay. Bright field is shown in A. Sperm heads by fluorescence are demonstrated in B. TUNEL-positive sperm are identified in C.**

identified in panel C. In general, results are reported as a DNA fragmentation index (DFI), which is calculated as the ratio of TUNEL-positive sperm to all sperm and expressed as a percentage. **TUNEL is considered a direct measure of sperm DNA fragmentation, and in a meta-analysis of miscarriage rates, TUNEL had the highest associated risk ratio at nearly four** (Sakkas and Alvarez, 2010; Robinson et al, 2012).

Comet Assay. Like the TUNEL assay, the comet assay, also referred to as the *single-cell gel electrophoresis assay,* is widely used in molecular biology laboratories to assess DNA fragmentation and has been adopted in the andrology laboratory for sperm (Tice et al, 2000; Sakkas and Alvarez, 2010). It is a simple assay that involves migration of single sperm head DNA in an electrophoretic agarose gel, and the tail resembling a comet indicates the degree of fragmentation (Tice et al, 2000). At neutral pH, this assay is considered a direct measure of sperm DNA fragmentation (Sakkas and Alvarez, 2010). Data are conflicting regarding its use as a tool for predicting clinical outcomes (Simon et al, 2010, 2011; Ribas-Maynou et al, 2012; Robinson et al, 2012). Investigators have used the comet assay in a variety of research settings to understand the effects of various entities on sperm DNA, including varicocele, toxins, male age, and testis cancer (Meeker et al, 2004; Bertolla et al, 2006; Delbes et al, 2007; Schmid et al, 2007; Blumer et al, 2008; Meeker et al, 2008; O'Flaherty et al, 2008; Wu et al, 2009; Lacerda et al, 2011; Fariello et al, 2012b).

Denatured Sperm DNA Assays. A number of assays denature sperm DNA before structural analysis (Sakkas and Alvarez, 2010). The comet assay performed in acidic or alkaline conditions denatures DNA, and like the comet assay, the sperm chromatin dispersion (SCD) assay allows visual identification of individual sperm head DNA structure by dispersion on agarose followed by nucleic acid staining (Fernández et al, 2003; Sakkas and Alvarez, 2010). The most established assay for sperm head DNA structure is the Sperm Chromatic Structure Assay (SCSA) (SCSA Diagnostics, Brookings, SD) (Evenson and Melamed, 1983; Evenson and Jost, 2000; Larson et al, 2000; Boe-Hansen et al, 2006; Chohan et al, 2006). The SCSA does not identify individual sperm but rather a population of cells by flow cytometry after denaturation in acidic conditions followed by staining with acridine orange (Evenson and Jost, 2000; Larson et al, 2000). Graphic analysis of flow cytometric data yields several outcome parameters for SCSA, with the DFI and high DNA stainability (HDS) being the two reported in common clinical use (Evenson and Jost, 2000; Larson et al, 2000). Although a number of studies have associated human reproductive outcomes with SCSA reported values, many failed to find statistically valid correlations (Evenson and Jost, 2000; Larson et al, 2000; Payne et al, 2005; Boe-Hansen et al, 2006; Bungum et al, 2007, 2008; Lin et al, 2008). In a meta-analysis of miscarriage rates, SCSA had a risk ratio of 1.47 with a 95% CI of 1.04 to 2.09, indicating a weak likely association.

Reactive Oxygen Species. Naturally occurring chemical reactions generate highly reactive molecules with unpaired electrons termed *free radicals.* Free radicals produced from oxidative reactions are referred to as *reactive oxygen species.* ROSs are involved in multiple physiologic processes important to sperm function, but investigators theorize that if present in excess, seminal ROSs may cause reproductive dysfunction (Agarwal et al, 2006, 2008c; Desai et al, 2009). TAC may be quantified in seminal fluid, and one popular method of quantifying how ROSs may affect sperm function is calculation of a ROS-TAC score (Rice-Evans and Miller, 1994; Sharma et al, 1999). Researchers have assessed ROS activity in aging, prostatitis, varicocele, lubricants, radiation, smoking, toxins, and obesity (Pasqualotto et al, 2000; Smith et al, 2005; Cocuzza et al, 2008a, 2008b; Farombi et al, 2008; Pasqualotto et al, 2008a; Agarwal et al, 2009; Hsu et al, 2009; Palmer et al, 2012; Taha et al, 2012; Agarwal et al, 2013).

Acrosome Reaction. *Please see the Expert Consult website for details.*

Sperm Mucous Interaction. *Please see the Expert Consult website for details.*

Sperm Ovum Interaction. *Please see the Expert Consult website for details.*

Sperm Ultrastructural Assessment. MSOME involving sperm head morphologic inspection with high-power Nomarski differential interference contrast optics that magnify the field over 6000× is discussed in the section on sperm morphology in this chapter. Although electron microscopy is widely used in scientific research on the male gamete, it also has a place in the clinical assessment of the infertile male (Chemes and Rawe, 2003). **Sperm motility is dependent on the ultrastructural arrangement of microtubules in the tail with a peripheral array of nine pairs and a central two microtubules connected by dynein arms** (Chemes and Rawe, 2003). **This "9 + 2" architecture is shared with cilia, and genetic disorders affecting it can manifest as respiratory pathology associated with male reproductive dysfunction, referred to as the** *immotile cilia syndrome, primary ciliary dyskinesia* **(PCD), or** *Kartagener syndrome* (Eliasson et al, 1977; Guichard et al, 2001; Chemes and Rawe, 2003). Kartagener syndrome results in sperm that are nearly totally or completely immotile but metabolically active (Peeraer et al, 2004). Semen samples with less than 10% motility and vitality demonstrated by testing may be investigated with electron microscopy to assess tail ultrastructural defects (Zini and Sigman, 2009). Electron microscopy is not available in all andrology laboratories.

Genomic Assessment

As odd as it may be to imagine that genes passed from parent to male offspring may be responsible for a condition that, if left untreated, would prevent those genes from being passed to future generations, evidence suggests that genetics plays a significant role in male reproductive dysfunction (Oates and Lamb, 2009). Known genetic conditions associated with the male sex are detailed in later sections of this chapter. In this section, clinically available assays are described.

Karyotype

Staining chromosomes with dyes binding to various moieties of the chemical structure of DNA resulting in banding patterns represents the classic means of cytogenetic analysis of chromosomes (Swansbury, 2003). Fluorescence in situ hybridization (FISH) uses fluorescent probes hybridizing to determined sequences on chromosomes, allowing for identification of specific regions or entire chromosomes depending on the specificity of the probe (Swansbury, 2003). One advantage of FISH is that it offers the ability to investigate the cytogenetics of both somatic and germ cells, which may differ beyond the expected halving of chromosomes (Martin, 2008). Other techniques, such as the spectral karyotype (SKY), use combinatorial methods to visualize all chromosomes in multiple colors (Swansbury, 2003). **The American Urological Association Best Practice Statement on the Optimal Evaluation of the Infertile Male recommends that genetic testing including karyotype be performed in all males with azoospermia caused by spermatogenic dysfunction and in those with severe oligospermia defined as less than 5 million sperm/mL** (Jarow et al, 2010). However, as numerical and structural chromosomal anomalies vary by geographic region, and obtaining a karyotype may represent a significant expense to the patient, the treating physician may judge whether this assay is indicated in his or her patient population.

Y Chromosome Microdeletion Testing

The Y chromosome is one of the smallest in humans at approximately 60 mega base pairs (Mb) (Tilford et al, 2001; Navarro-Costa, 2012). It is the determinant of the male gender and is the only chromosome passed directly from father to son (Navarro-Costa, 2012). It consists of a male-specific region with no homologous chromosomal mate and a pseudoautosomal region (Graves et al, 1998; Tilford et al, 2001; Navarro-Costa, 2012). In an elegant series of cytogenetic analyses for the time, **Tiepolo and Zuffardi determined in 1976 that a region in the long arm of the Y chromosome was critical to the formation of sperm in man, which became known as** *AZF* **(azoospermia factor)** (Tiepolo and Zuffardi, 1976; Chandley et al, 1989).

The portion of the Y chromosome that does not recombine represents approximately 95% of its sequence (Tilford et al, 2001). About one third of this nonrecombinant region consists of palindromic inner sequences present at least twice in forward and reverse reading frames referred to as *amplicons* (Tilford et al, 2001). This sequence structure is believed to substitute in part in place of sexual recombination in repair of the Y chromosome but may also engender a particular fragility in increasing the likelihood of the loss of segments, or microdeletions (Oates and Lamb, 2009). Based on the work of Tiepolo and Zuffardi, investigators observed microdeletions of three regions on the Y chromosome to be commonly associated with azoospermia or oligospermia, which were termed *AZFa, AZFb,* and *AZFc* (Oates and Lamb, 2009). Once thought to be separate and distinct regions, AZFb and AZFc overlap, whereas AZFa is distant and isolated (Jobling and Tyler-Smith, 2003). The *DAZ* genes, believed to be integrally associated with spermatogenesis, are housed within the AZFc region (Saxena et al, 2000). Investigators have also referred to the proximal portion of AZFc as *AZFd*, but the usefulness of isolating this subregion remains unclear (Müslümanoğlu et al, 2005).

Some microdeletions of AZFc appear to be associated with spermatogenic impairment but not failure (Mulhall et al, 1997; Oates et al, 2002). Likewise, the clinical relevance of analysis of AZFc subregions such as gr/gr is unclear, because sperm may be present in the ejaculate and in the testis (Lardone et al, 2007; Wu et al, 2007; Giachini et al, 2008; Stouffs et al, 2008; Visser et al, 2009). However, evidence strongly suggests that AZFa and AZFb microdeletions cause significant pathology of the testis resulting in diminishing low likelihood of sperm retrieval by surgery (Hopps et al, 2003). **It is reasonable practice to recommend Y chromosomal microdeletion assessment to azoospermic men before surgical sperm extraction to counsel them on the likelihood of retrieval** (Jarow et al, 2010). However, it is also reasonable to omit testing based on the relative rarity of AZFa and AZFb microdeletions in clinical practice.

Genomic Sequence Assessment

A variety of technologies such as DNA microarrays allow multiple single nucleotide polymorphisms (SNPs) and mutations associated with known diseases to be screened for and reported (Schena et al, 1995; Hunter et al, 2008; Lazarin et al, 2013). These reports can be used to identify whether parents are carriers for a large number of genetic diseases and the probability of affected offspring. Whole genome sequencing as a clinical tool is also under current development (Moorthie et al, 2013). Although these technologies may ultimately be used to diagnose underlying causes of male reproductive dysfunction, use as general screening tools in evaluating male infertility is not yet warranted.

Cystic Fibrosis Transmembrane Conductance Regulator Mutation Assessment

The relationship between alterations in the cystic fibrosis transmembrane conductance regulator (CFTR) and maldevelopment of the vas is discussed in the section on developmental disorders in this chapter. This section describes what testing is available.

The protein encoded by CFTR forms a channel for chloride ions and possibly bicarbonate and may serve to regulate transport of other ions (Hampton and Stanton, 2010). More than 1600 CFTR mutations have been identified, and they may be mild or severe, defined by whether the full cystic fibrosis disease phenotype results from the mutation (Ratbi et al, 2007; Oates and Lamb, 2009; Hampton and Stanton, 2010; Bombieri et al, 2011; Yu et al, 2012). **The most common severe mutation is ΔF508, which results from deletion of three base pairs that consequently remove the amino acid phenylalanine typically at position 508 of the encoded protein** (Hampton and Stanton, 2010). A high incidence of patients harbor more than one mutation; approximately 46% have two (Yu et al, 2012). **A severe mutation such as ΔF508 on each allele will result in a child with cystic fibrosis, making screening imperative for both the prospective father and mother for those suspected of harboring genetic alterations in CFTR.**

Currently available CFTR screening panels typically include 25 to 40 of the most common mutations. Because a subset of known mutations is screened for, a negative result still carries a defined risk. Testing is commercially available for all known mutations but is expectedly more expensive. CFTR mutation prevalence varies by ethnicity and geography (Hamosh et al, 1998; Boyd et al, 2004; Foresta et al, 2005; Schulz et al, 2006; Ratbi et al, 2007; Havasi et al, 2010; Li et al, 2010; Bombieri et al, 2011). Consequently, the clinician should take into account location and ethnicity in interpreting results. Typically, CFTR screening panel reports are stratified by ethnicity.

KEY POINTS: LABORATORY EVALUATION OF MALE INFERTILITY

- Endocrine assessment of male reproductive status includes total testosterone, the portion of testosterone not bound to SHBG, estradiol, and the pituitary gonadotropins LH and FSH.
- The semen analysis represents a probabilistic assessment of male reproductive potential. Aside from azoospermia, no specific threshold applied to any parameter absolutely discerns infertility from fertility.
- The differential diagnosis for men with semen volumes less than 1.0 mL includes ejaculatory ductal obstruction, retrograde ejaculation, and vasal and accessory sex gland maldevelopment such as that occurring with CBAVD.
- Sperm vitality staining differentiates complete asthenospermia from necrospermia. Common laboratory staining methods differentiate pyospermia from immature germ cells.
- A preponderance of sperm with round heads, a condition referred to as *globozoospermia*, indicates deficient acrosome formation. The treatment is IVF with ICSI.
- Disruption in the blood-testis barrier formed by tight junctions between Sertoli cells results in antisperm antibodies, which have varying clinical significance depending on the degree of binding to sperm heads.
- Genetic screening of the CFTR in men with CBAVD and their partners identifies the presence of severe mutations such as ΔF508 that may result in clinically overt cystic fibrosis in offspring.

IMAGING IN THE EVALUATION OF MALE INFERTILITY

Radiographic or ultrasonographic imaging is infrequently needed in the diagnosis of male reproductive dysfunction and should be ordered cautiously. Likely benign conditions such as testicular microlithiasis may be detected, resulting in patient distress and often unnecessary additional testing (Dagash and MacKinnon, 2007). The following descriptions of imaging in the evaluation of male reproductive dysfunction should not be interpreted as indicated in typical screening.

Scrotal Ultrasonography

Evaluation of the infertile male includes a detailed manual examination of the scrotum and its contents. As with the scrotal physical examination for any urologic evaluation, abnormalities may be detected that warrant scrotal ultrasonography for further investigation. In Figure 24-4, color duplex Doppler ultrasonography demonstrates a varicocele. Panel A reveals the varicocele to be adjacent to the testis, and the colored areas in panel B demonstrate the direction of flow. The diameter of the largest vein can be measured and reported.

Ultrasonography of the spermatic cord may be indicated if the evaluating physician is uncertain whether a varicocele is present on palpation (Nagler and Grotas, 2009). However, the varicoceles so identified are often so small as to be of questionable clinical

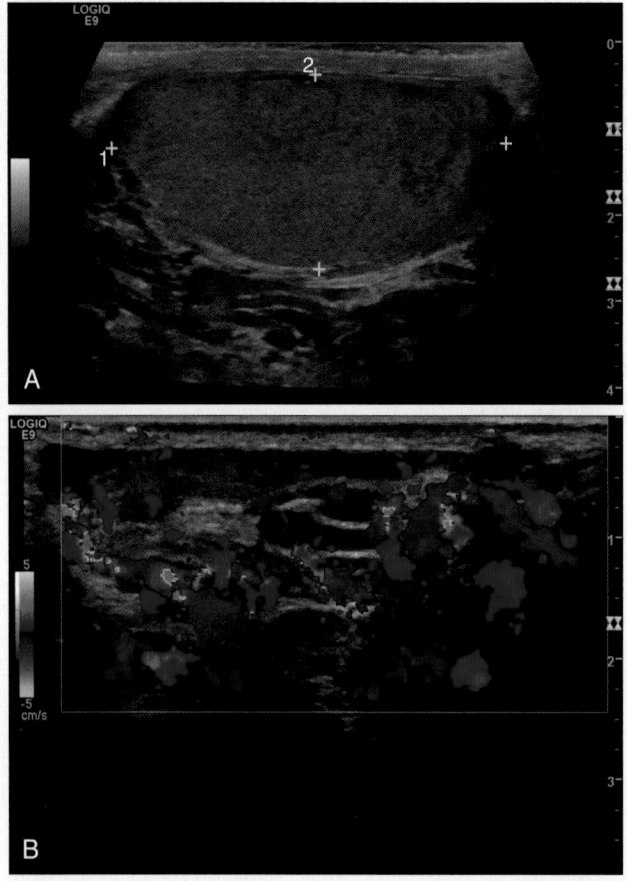

Figure 24-4. Color duplex Doppler ultrasonography of scrotum demonstrating varicocele. Dilated veins adjacent to the testis are exhibited in A, and directional flow in the vessels is revealed in B.

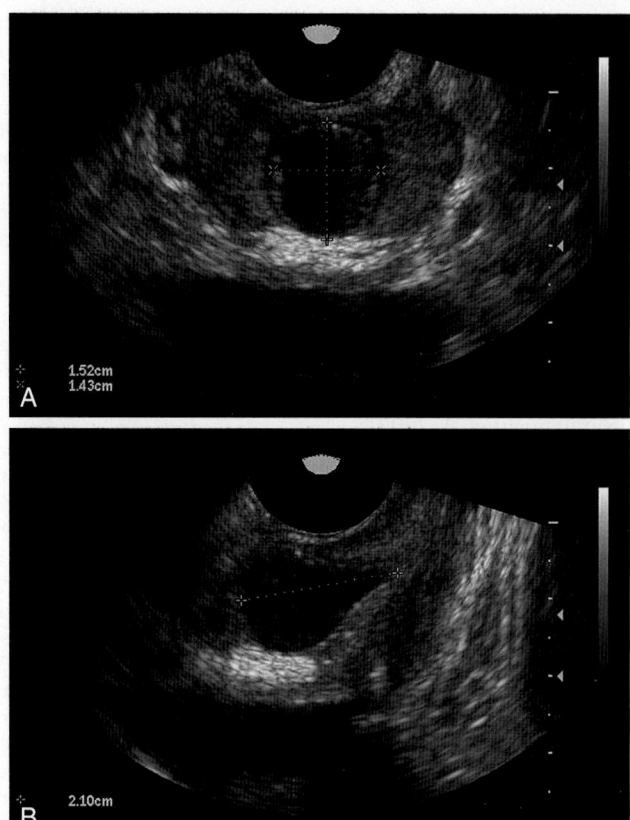

Figure 24-5. Transrectal ultrasonography revealing an intraprostatic cyst. A is transverse, and B is longitudinal. (Courtesy Marcelo Vieira.)

significance. Varicoceles become palpable at approximately 2.7 to 3.6 mm in diameter, and surgical treatment of varicoceles smaller than 3.5 mm that are not palpable on physical examination but observed on ultrasound does not result in improved seminal outcomes (Eskew et al, 1993; Hoekstra and Witt, 1995; Jarow et al, 1996; Schiff et al, 2006). **Consequently, the most rational approach based on whether identification of a varicocele is likely to affect treatment outcomes is not to rely on ultrasound as a necessary diagnostic tool.**

Direction of flow may be assessed by color Doppler ultrasound, and investigators have reported that reversal of flow is a positive prognostic sign that surgical treatment of varicocele may result in improved seminal parameters (Hussein, 2006; Schiff et al, 2006). At this time, insufficient numbers of men with nonpalpable varicoceles that are identified with reversal of flow are reported in studies investigating surgical treatment to conclude that color Doppler ultrasound is indicated as a screening modality for infertile men.

In conjunction with TRUS, investigators have observed sensitivity of 75% and specificity of 72% for diagnosing azoospermia caused by spermatogenic dysfunction and sensitivity of 29.8% and specificity of 87% for diagnosing azoospermia caused by obstruction (Abdulwahed et al, 2013). However, given the high accuracy in differentiating azoospermia caused by spermatogenic dysfunction versus obstruction yielded by measuring testis longitudinal axis and assaying serum FSH, it seems more prudent and cost-effective not to use ultrasonography in an attempt to diagnose the cause of azoospermia in men with adequate seminal volumes.

Vasography

Contrast vasography in the direction of the abdomen allows determination of patency of the vas deferens from the scrotum to the ejaculatory ducts (Ammar et al, 2012). It is currently rarely performed because image modalities such as TRUS and magnetic resonance imaging (MRI) have superseded it; it is invasive and may result in scar tissue formation in the vasal lumen and obstruction; and injection of saline into the vasal lumen during intended vasal reconstructive procedures with the manual feedback of whether fluid flows easily or backflow occurs offers similar information. **Fluid, contrast or otherwise, should never be injected into the vasal lumen in the direction of the epididymis because it will rupture the delicate epididymal tubules.** Should backflow be identified during intraoperative saline vasography, a monofilament suture such as 4-0 polypropylene may be inserted into the vasal lumen, advanced until resistance is encountered, and then withdrawn and the distance measured to determine the location of the obstruction.

Venography

Please see the Expert Consult website for details.

Transrectal Imaging

The diagnosis of ejaculatory ductal obstruction is considered when azoospermia in conjunction with low seminal volume is encountered (Niederberger, 2011). The earliest and still currently the most prevalent method of investigating whether ejaculatory ductal obstruction in present is TRUS (Jarow, 1996; Niederberger, 2011). **TRUS imaging evidence of ejaculatory duct obstruction includes an anteroposterior seminal vesicle diameter of greater than 1.5 cm with or without a midline prostatic cyst** (Jarow, 1996; Niederberger, 2011; Ammar et al, 2012). Figure 24-5 demonstrates an intraprostatic cyst, with panel A exhibiting the transverse view and panel B the longitudinal view. Unfortunately, although TRUS is convenient and common, its specificity is low compared with other modalities for identifying whether or not obstruction is

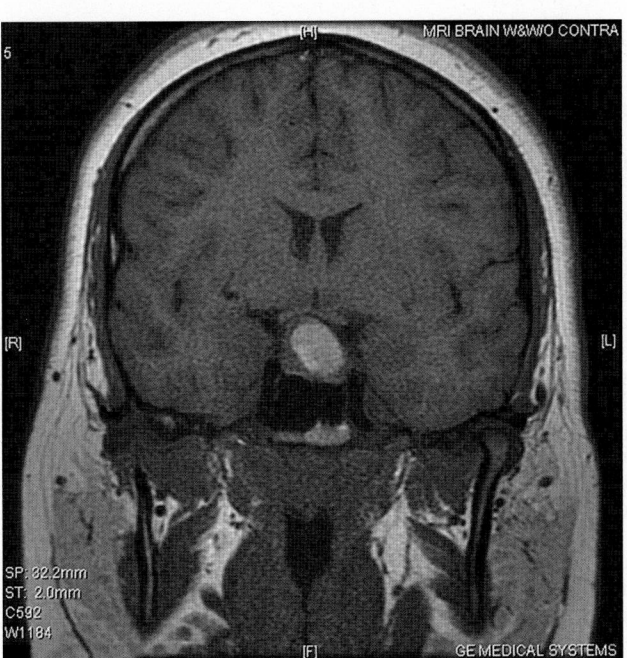

Figure 24-6. Large pituitary macroadenoma revealed by cranial magnetic resonance imaging.

present (Purohit et al, 2004). These other assessments include radiographic imaging after injection of contrast directly into the seminal vesicles, or vesiculography; aspiration of the seminal vesicles to determine whether sperm is present; and injection of diluted indigo carmine or methylene blue dye into the seminal vesicles and observation by cystoscopy of whether the colored dye flows from the ductal orifices at the verumontanum, a technique referred to as *chromotubation* (Purohit et al, 2004). In a small series, vesiculography and chromotubation were more accurate than TRUS by a margin of 25% (Purohit et al, 2004). However, these techniques are more invasive and expensive, and an incremental improvement in diagnostic accuracy compared with TRUS if conclusively demonstrated in larger studies may not justify the additional risk and cost.

Please see the Expert Consult website for further details.

Abdominal Imaging

Please see the Expert Consult website for details.

Cranial Imaging

Cranial MRI allows assessment of whether hyperprolactinemia is associated with an anatomic pituitary lesion (Niederberger, 2011). MRI may distinguish between microadenomas and macroadenomas and may assist in judging whether medical or surgical therapy is indicated (Johnsen et al, 1991). Figure 24-6 demonstrates a cranial MRI revealing a large pituitary macroadenoma.

KEY POINT: IMAGING

- Imaging can reveal sequelae of genetic conditions such as congenital absence of the vas deferens and renal aplasia, and it can differentiate reasons for seminal hypovolemia such as ejaculatory ductal obstruction, but it is infrequently necessary to establish diagnoses such as varicocele or spermatogenic dysfunction.

TESTIS HISTOPATHOLOGY

Please see the Expert Consult website for details.

ASSISTED REPRODUCTION

Please see the Expert Consult website for details.

DIAGNOSES AND THERAPIES

The understanding of the pathophysiology of male reproductive dysfunction has expanded in past years but remains manifestly incomplete. The difficulties inherent in the probabilistic nature of reproduction and its assessment pose challenges to the physician evaluating and consequently treating male infertility, but sufficient information is known for the treating physician to make reasoned assumptions about whether a pathologic explanation involving the man exists, its likely basis, and plausible therapy. This section reviews discrete diagnoses and possible medical therapies.

Genetic Syndromes

With the completion of sequencing of the human genome in 2004, knowledge of how the genes involved in human reproduction conspire to create fully formed and viable sperm will follow (International Human Genome Sequencing Consortium, 2004). As discussed in the section of this chapter describing genomic sequence assessment, broad panels are available that identify carrier risk of known genetic diseases, and whole genomic sequencing is under development. However, current use of the former and use of the latter, should it become immediately available, as general screening tools for male reproductive dysfunction are hampered by the lack of an understanding of how the majority of the genetic mechanisms involved in spermatogenesis function in concert to produce viable sperm. A certain number of genetic associations are known to be involved in male infertility, and these are detailed in subsequent sections. In this section, general genetic causes of male fertility involving chromosomal number, structure, and epigenetic mechanisms are discussed.

Chromosomal Numerical Disorders

The presence of a supernumerary X chromosome yielding 47,XXY, or Klinefelter syndrome, is the most commonly identified genetic cause of male infertility (Oates and Lamb, 2009; Sigman, 2012; Groth et al, 2013). A 47,XXY genotype is observed in 1 in 500 to 1000 live births, and in over 95% of affected adults results in azoospermia, small testes, and elevated gonadotropin levels (Maiburg et al, 2012; Groth et al, 2013). Approximately 75% of children have learning disabilities, and 63% to 85% of men have low testosterone levels (Groth et al, 2013). **Body morphology features such as increased height are observed in only 30% of Klinefelter males, and consequently the condition cannot be excluded by physical examination and physical inspection alone** (Groth et al, 2013). Increased incidence of other disorders related to the testis such as mediastinal germ cell tumors is documented in men with Klinefelter syndrome, suggesting broader testicular effects (Sokol, 2012).

A nonmosaic 47,XXY karyotype is observed in 80% to 90% of men with Klinefelter syndrome (Maiburg et al, 2012). The remainder are mosaic 46,XY/47,XXY or have additional or structurally abnormal X chromosomes (Maiburg et al, 2012). In the man, approximately 8% have sperm in the ejaculate, and the remainder are azoospermic (Oates, 2012). Within the testis, approximately half of men with Klinefelter syndrome have sufficient mature sperm amenable to surgical sperm retrieval for use with IVF and ICSI (Oates, 2012). **Early age at diagnosis appears to offer a more favorable prognosis** (Mehta and Paduch, 2012).

Until recently, fertility management of men with Klinefelter syndrome was limited to diagnosing the condition with karyotype analysis, assessing whether sperm was present in the ejaculate, and attempting to extract sperm from the testis if it was not. Many of these men are identified shortly after puberty with low testosterone levels and prescribed exogenous testosterone alone, suppressing native spermatogenesis if present. Citing the progressive decline in spermatogenesis over time, investigators have argued for aggressive management including surgical extraction of sperm at early to mid puberty before initiation of therapy with exogenous testosterone (Mehta and Paduch, 2012). This approach is primarily investigational at this time.

Structural Chromosomal Anomalies

As discussed in the section detailing Y chromosome microdeletion testing, investigators observed three regions on the Y chromosome, designated AZFa, AZFb, and AZFc, to be associated with azoospermia or oligospermia (Oates and Lamb, 2009). **Microdeletions of AZFc currently have unclear clinical significance, whereas AZFa and AZFb microdeletions are nearly always associated with absence of retrievable sperm from the testis** (Mulhall et al, 1997; Oates et al, 2002; Hopps et al, 2003; Lardone et al, 2007; Wu et al, 2007; Giachini et al, 2008; Stouffs et al, 2008; Visser et al, 2009). **AZFa microdeletions have particular clinical significance, as spatially the AZFa region appears to be localized distinctly from AZFb and AZFc, with the latter two overlapping** (Oates and Lamb, 2009).

Other structural anomalies of the Y chromosome may be identified by karyotypic analysis (Oates and Lamb, 2009). Two terminal breaks in both chromosome arms and subsequent fusion may lead to a ring Y chromosome, or r(Y), with variable phenotype depending on the amount of chromosomal material lost (Arnedo et al, 2005). Karyotypic anomalies in somatic chromosomes may also be associated with infertility (Mau-Holzmann, 2005).

Epigenetic Anomalies

Not only must the DNA sequence be intact for successful function of the male gamete, the DNA must be tightly coiled and packaged (O'Flynn O'Brien et al, 2010). As discussed in the section describing denatured sperm DNA assays, investigators have constructed various methods of interrogating sperm DNA structure with unclear prognostic outcomes at present. Other components of sperm DNA packaging may yield future diagnostic tools; for example, animal studies revealed that premature translation of protamine 1 resulted in postmeiotic maturational arrest in mouse spermatogenesis, and protamine 2 deficiency led to sperm DNA damage and embryo demise (Lee et al, 1995; Cho et al, 2003). In humans, evidence links protamine 2 precursors and the protamine 1–protamine 2 ratio to sperm DNA quality and IVF outcomes (Aoki et al, 2006; Torregrosa et al, 2006; de Mateo et al, 2009). Histones also offer a future target for clinical assessment. They are highly specifically localized along human sperm DNA, and researchers have observed histone variants to relate to fertility in bulls (Hammoud et al, 2009; de Oliveira et al, 2013).

DNA methylation allows coordination of gene expression in somatic cell development (Boissonnas et al, 2013). Once thought to be of little consequence in sperm, this epigenetic modification is now considered to play key roles in spermatogenesis and embryogenesis (Molaro et al, 2011; Carrell, 2012; Boissonnas et al, 2013). The pattern of gene promoter methylation is substantially different in somatic and sperm cell DNA and may have future clinical applicability in the assessment of male reproductive potential (Molaro et al, 2011).

Testicular Causes

The testis essentially consists of two compartments, the seminiferous tubules that house the developing male gametes and the interstitial spaces between the tubules, inhabited by Leydig cells. Both are required for sperm production, which then must conclude with transit of the male gamete outward. Testicular causes of male reproductive dysfunction may consequently be considered to derive from pathology in the production of sperm in the seminiferous epithelium or in the synthesis of testosterone by Leydig cells, or obstruction in the microductal system transporting sperm toward the ejaculatory ducts.

Spermatogenic Dysfunction

As discussed in the section describing testis histopathology, dysfunction in the seminiferous epithelium may be globally described as hypospermatogenesis, which indicates a decrease in sperm production; maturation arrest, which represents halting of the sequence of steps of the male gamete at some point through premeiotic, meiotic, and postmeiotic development; and Sertoli cell–only syndrome, which denotes a complete depopulation of spermatogonial cells. The molecular mechanisms leading to completion of spermatogenesis are still under investigation, and in the future it is likely that genomic, proteomic, and metabolomic markers will become available for clinical use to diagnose specific causes of spermatogenic dysfunction (Kovac et al, 2013). At present, the primary means of assessing deficiencies in spermatogenesis is histopathologic inspection. As previously described, should azoospermia be present, in 89% of cases spermatogenic dysfunction is identified as the cause with an FSH value greater than 7.6 IU/L and the testis long axis 4.6 cm or less (Schoor et al, 2001).

Another form of spermatogenic pathology arises in the testis and impedes sperm in the ejaculate. In the seminiferous epithelium, Sertoli cell tight junctions protect haploid germ cells from circulating immunologic cells, forming a blood-testis barrier (Brannigan, 2011). **Pathologic conditions that disrupt this blood-testis barrier may expose the immunologically protected spermatids and spermatozoa to antibody formation, which may cause sperm agglutination, impeded sperm motility, and reduced fertilizing potential** (Brannigan, 2011). These conditions include obstruction in the male reproductive tract such as that occurring after vasectomy; inflammation associated with orchitis, prostatitis, or sexually transmitted disease; exposure to heat with varicocele, cryptorchidism, or external sources such as hot tubs; trauma and testis torsion; and genetic associations including thymic maldevelopment and the HLA-B28 haplotype (Walsh and Turek, 2009). Assays for antisperm antibodies are detailed in the section describing the laboratory evaluation of semen.

For treatment of antisperm antibodies, simple measures include use of condoms and washing sperm. Neither has good evidence to substantiate its use (Walsh and Turek, 2009). Washing may remove unbound antibodies, but those that matter remain bound to sperm (Walsh and Turek, 2009). More direct treatments include immunosuppression with corticosteroids and ART. Two controlled trials of corticosteroids offer conflicting results, with one demonstrating improved fertility and the other not (Haas and Manganiello, 1987; Hendry et al, 1990). Whether because of a lack of compelling evidence or because of more direct results, IVF and ICSI have become common treatment for antisperm antibodies.

Steroidogenic Dysfunction

The terms hypergonadotropic hypogonadism, primary hypogonadism, and primary hypoandrogenism refer to impaired testosterone synthesis caused by Leydig cell dysfunction (Sokol, 2009). **This entity is typically identified by elevated LH levels and decreased circulating testosterone** (Sokol, 2009). However, Leydig cell dysfunction may exist concurrently with pituitary insufficiency, and these men will have decreased testosterone concentrations and variable LH levels that do not reflect the typical increase associated with primary Leydig cell insufficiency (Sokol, 2009). Increasing age is a condition associated with decreasing androgen and blunted pituitary response (Feldman et al, 2002; Sokol, 2009).

An absolute requirement for spermatogenesis is intratesticular steroidogenesis, which appears to be especially important for the postmeiotic maturation of sperm (Caroppo, 2011). Men with Klinefelter syndrome often have lower levels of circulating testosterone, but impaired Leydig cell function may not be the only mechanism responsible for a phenotype that resembles those of hypoandrogenic males (Sokol, 2009; Oates, 2012). Investigators have reported evidence of Leydig cell dysfunction in humans associated with mutations in the LH receptor gene and in FSH receptor–deficient mice, and as the genes responsible for steroidogenesis become clinically available for assessment in humans, it is anticipated that more cases of Leydig cell dysfunction with genetic causes will be identified (Latronico et al, 1996; Baker et al, 2003). Other potential clinical causes of Leydig cell dysfunction include orchitis, cytotoxic chemotherapy, and exposure to environmental toxicants (Skakkebaek et al, 2001; Sokol, 2009).

There is currently no accepted therapy for hypoandrogenism caused by Leydig cell insufficiency (Sokol, 2009). Exogenous testosterone is not indicated, because insufficient testicular testosterone concentrations are achieved for spermatogenesis, and pituitary LH release is suppressed (Niederberger, 2011). **Should azoospermia be associated with low testosterone concentrations and significantly elevated LH levels, if the patient desires paternity, the treatment is surgical sperm extraction.**

Microductal Obstruction

Either by congenital or acquired means, the epididymis or scrotal vas deferens may be obstructed. If obstruction is bilateral, azoospermia typically results. As discussed in the section describing the endocrine evaluation, the physician may use the FSH level combined with the testis longitudinal axis as measured by calipers to predict whether azoospermia is associated with obstruction; 96% of men with obstructive azoospermia had FSH concentration of 7.6 IU/L or less and testis long axis greater than 4.6 cm (Schoor et al, 2001). Figure 24-11 illustrates an algorithm for the evaluation of azoospermia. Microductal obstruction may also be unilateral: in that case, bulk seminal parameters may be reduced or not depending on the function of the contralateral testis. Should unilateral obstruction be present with adequate spermatogenesis present in the ipsilateral testis and the existence of spermatogenic pathology in the contralateral testis, impaired bulk seminal parameters may result and microductal reconstruction may be indicated.

As discussed in the section describing evaluation of the surgical history of an infertile male, herniorrhaphy especially with mesh may result in obstruction of the vas deferens in the inguinal canal (Shin et al, 2005; Maciel et al, 2007; Hallén et al, 2011, 2012; Tekatli et al, 2012). If both vasa are occluded, azoospermia likely results.

Pituitary Dysfunction

The pituitary hormones LH and FSH regulate spermatogenesis: LH directs Leydig cell steroidogenesis; and FSH controls spermatogenesis via the Sertoli cells (Caroppo, 2011). If by intrinsic dysfunction or external pathology LH, FSH, or both are suppressed, spermatogenesis suffers.

Hypogonadotropic Hypogonadism

Hypogonadotropic hypogonadism refers to the condition of decreased pituitary hormonal secretion. **Kallmann described anosmia associated with decreased pituitary function, and the syndrome bears his name** (Kallmann and Schoenfeld, 1944). The incidence of the syndrome is approximately one in 10,000 males, and the mode of inheritance is most frequently autosomal recessive, but autosomal-dominant and X-linked recessive patterns are also observed (Bhagavath et al, 2006; Sokol, 2009). Investigators have identified associations with Kallmann syndrome and the *KAL1* gene encoding anosmin-1 responsible for neurotropic growth factors during embryogenesis, the *GNRHR* gene encoding gonadotropin-releasing hormone (GnRH) receptor, the pituitary-specific transcription factor PIT1, the PIT1-related transcription factor PROP1, the G protein–coupled Kisspeptin receptor GPR54, the homeobox genes *HESX1*, *LEX3*, and *LEX4*, and others (Dattani et al, 1998; Wu et al, 1998; de Roux et al, 2003; Kim et al, 2003; Sobrier et al, 2004; Bhagavath et al, 2006; Newbern et al, 2013). Researchers noted approximately 10% of men with Kallmann syndrome to harbor mutations in either the *GNRHR* or *KAL1* gene (Bhagavath et al, 2006).

Treatment includes replacement of LH with human chorionic gonadotropin (hCG) and replacement of FSH with recombinant FSH (rFSH) or hMG, which exhibits both LH and FSH-like activity (Sokol, 2009). Treatment with hCG alone may initiate spermatogenesis; if hMG or rFSH is prescribed, after spermatogenesis returns, these agents may be withdrawn after several months of therapy (Sokol, 2009). Men who are identified as having Kallmann syndrome later in life when reproductive interests occur have often been prescribed exogenous androgen since adolescence. These men may require gonadotropin therapy for 1 to 2 years before sperm becomes evident in the ejaculate. Typical doses for intramuscular or subcutaneous hCG are 1500 to 5000 international units two to three times weekly to a maximum of 10,000 international units per week and are titrated to serum testosterone results (Sokol, 2009; Hussein et al, 2013). The dose of hMG is 75 international units two to three times weekly, typically administered subcutaneously (Sokol, 2009).

Rarely, men may have isolated decreased secretion of either LH or FSH (Giltay et al, 2004; Sokol, 2009). Isolated LH deficiency was termed the "fertile eunuch syndrome" and characterizes men who have features of hypoandrogenism owing to low levels of LH but who produce sperm as a result of adequate FSH (Sokol, 2009). Conversely, men with isolated FSH deficiency have suppressed spermatogenesis but adequate androgenization (Giltay et al, 2004).

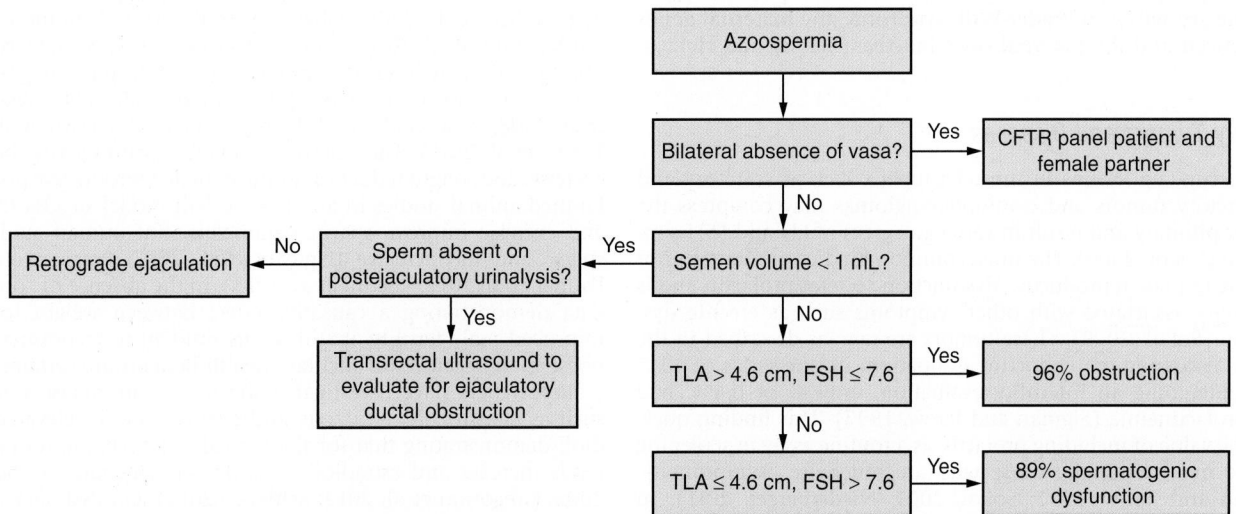

Figure 24-11. **Algorithm for evaluation of azoospermia. CFTR, cystic fibrosis transmembrane conductance regulator; FSH, follicle-stimulating hormone; TLA, testis longitudinal axis measured by caliper orchidometer.**

Treatment of these uncommon conditions includes replacement with the appropriate gonadotropin (Giltay et al, 2004; Sokol, 2009). Men may also infrequently have isolated hypothalamic GnRH deficiency (Nachtigall et al, 1997). Treatment includes GnRH administration by a subcutaneous portable mini-infusion pump every 2 hours, and, as with treatment for Kallmann syndrome, long-term courses of at least 6 months' duration may be required (Nachtigall et al, 1997).

Kallmann and the associated syndromes of hypogonadotropic hypogonadism are the most severe forms of conditions resulting in diminished pituitary hormonal secretion. **Incomplete forms with hypoandrogenism associated with serum LH concentrations above those observed with Kallmann syndrome but lower than expected for the diminished testosterone are common** (Bhaga-vath et al, 2006). For these men, pituitary stimulation with anti-estrogenic agents such as clomiphene or tamoxifen or with aromatase inhibitors such as anastrozole or letrozole may restore testosterone levels and possibly improve spermatogenesis (Raman and Schlegel, 2002; Siddiq and Sigman, 2002; Hussein et al, 2005; Ioannidou-Kadis et al, 2006; Whitten et al, 2006; Sussman et al, 2008; Katz et al, 2012; Moskovic et al, 2012; Hussein et al, 2013; Roth et al, 2013). The initial dose of clomiphene citrate is typically 25 mg every day or 50 mg every other day and is increased by titrating to serum testosterone to a maximum of 100 mg daily (Hussein et al, 2005; Sussman et al, 2008; Hussein et al, 2013). In some studies, the titration target is restoration of normal androgen levels; in others, it is elevated at 600 to 800 ng/dL (Hussein et al, 2005; Sussman et al, 2008; Hussein et al, 2013). The typical dose of anastrozole is 1 mg daily (Raman and Schlegel, 2002).

Prader-Willi syndrome is characterized by failure to thrive in infancy associated with a poor suck reflex followed by loss of satiety in early childhood, which may lead to marked obesity if poorly controlled (Cassidy and Driscoll, 2009). Its incidence is approximately 1 in 15,000 to 30,000 (Cassidy and Driscoll, 2009). Features associated with the syndrome include hypogonadism, small testes, dysmorphic facies, growth hormone deficiency with short stature and small hands and feet, pain insensitivity, and cognitive disorders such as obsessive-compulsive traits (Bervini and Herzog, 2013). Researchers have suspected that the association of growth hormone deficiency and hypogonadism with the syndrome derive from hypothalamic dysfunction, but the precise pathophysiology is still uncertain (Bervini and Herzog, 2013). Prader-Willi syndrome is typically caused by the loss of expression of genes located on human chromosome 15q11-q13 by means of failed imprinting, which is the epigenetic phenomenon that allows genes on only one chromosome to be active (Bervini and Herzog, 2013). **In the healthy state, the genes located on the maternal chromosome 15q11-q13 are silenced, and those on the paternal chromosome are active; in Prader-Willi syndrome, the maternal genes are silenced and the paternal ones inactive** (Bervini and Herzog, 2013).

Pituitary Tumors and Diseases

Space-occupying lesions in the sella turcica such as secretory and nonsecretory tumors and craniopharyngiomas may compress the anterior pituitary and result in varying degrees of LH and FSH suppression (Sokol, 2009). The most common kind of pituitary tumor resulting in male reproductive dysfunction secretes prolactin and is commonly associated with other symptoms such as erectile dysfunction (Sokol, 2009). These tumors are rare; as described in the section discussing the endocrine evaluation, in one series of 1035 men undergoing an infertility evaluation, only 4, or 0.4%, had hyperprolactinemia (Sigman and Jarow, 1997). This finding questions the value of including prolactin as a routine assay in screening infertile men, especially those who are otherwise asymptomatic (Sigman and Jarow, 1997; Sokol, 2009; Niederberger, 2011). **In general, mild elevations of prolactin in the range of 20 to 50 µg/L do not warrant further evaluation; if prolactin is significantly elevated, cranial MRI is indicated** (Niederberger, 2011). The dopamine agonists bromocriptine and cabergoline may be prescribed for prolactin-secreting adenomas for which surgery is not indicated, with cabergoline exhibiting fewer side effects (Klibanski, 2010).

Other Pituitary Lesions

Diseases infiltrating the pituitary may also suppress its secretion of hormones, including granulomata of infection, sarcoidosis, and histiocytosis (Sokol, 2009). Deposition of iron by hemachromatosis or repeated blood transfusions may also invoke hypogonadotropic hypogonadism (Sokol, 2009). Systemic diseases such as morbid obesity, chronic malnutrition, and type 2 diabetes may also be associated with hypogonadotropic hypogonadism (Dhindsa et al, 2004; Sokol, 2009). Treatment of these disorders is aimed at ameliorating the underlying condition.

Extrapituitary Endocrine Modulators

As described in the section discussing the role of investigating endocrine modulators when taking the history of an infertile man, exogenous androgenic agents, especially testosterone, suppress pituitary gonadotropins (Grimes et al, 2012). Also discussed in that section are cannabis, antipsychotics, opioids, and environmental toxicants, which inhibit pituitary function via estrogenic and dopaminergic pathways (Carlsen et al, 1992; Stimmel and Gutierrez, 2006; Gorzalka et al, 2010; Subirán et al, 2011). Treatment is directed toward removing the offending agent when possible. CAH, especially in milder forms that manifest clinically in adolescence or adult life, may be associated with hypogonadotropic hypogonadism (Reisch et al, 2011). A high incidence of testicular adrenal rest tumors adds to the reproductive dysfunction present in these men (Claahsen-van der Grinten et al, 2008; Reisch et al, 2011). Fertility may be restored with corticosteroid therapy (Claahsen-van der Grinten et al, 2007). However, side effects such as weight gain and skin changes from the lengthy application of therapy required to address the long duration of spermatogenesis may prove problematic (Claahsen-van der Grinten et al, 2007).

Extratesticular Endocrine Dysfunction

Because estradiol inhibits gonadotropin release, conditions that increase its concentration may lead to hypogonadotropic hypogonadism. These include the pharmacologic agents described in the section discussing medications that alter the ratio of estrogen to androgen through a variety of means (Bowman et al, 2012). When possible, use of another agent may improve fertility. As described in the section discussing the general physical examination of the infertile male, elevated estradiol is associated with obesity by the mass of adipose cells containing aromatase (Hammoud et al, 2006; Aggerholm et al, 2008; Chavarro et al, 2010; Hammoud et al, 2010b; Hofny et al, 2010). Multiple factors are suspected to associate obesity with male infertility, and hypogonadotropic hypogonadism may or may not be involved (Hammoud et al, 2006; Aggerholm et al, 2008; Pauli et al, 2008; Hofny et al, 2010; Paasch et al, 2010; Teerds et al, 2011). The question remains regarding whether diet, exercise, and weight reduction improve male reproductive potential. Limited animal studies in an obese rodent model suggest that diet and exercise improve sperm parameters, but human studies are sparse and inconclusive (Nguyen et al, 2007; Braga et al, 2012; Palmer et al, 2012; Luconi et al, 2013). In the absence of conclusive data demonstrating a causative effect between weight loss and improved male fertility, it still seems prudent to recommend it in obese men because the ancillary health benefits are certain.

Researchers have investigated the use of aromatase inhibitors such as anastrozole, letrozole, and testolactone for elevated estradiol, demonstrating that for the typical male patient, testosterone levels increase and estradiol levels decline (Raman and Schlegel, 2002; Gregoriou et al, 2012; Schlegel, 2012). Limited data support that sperm parameters may concurrently improve (Raman and Schlegel, 2002; Gregoriou et al, 2012; Schlegel, 2012). As described in the section discussing the endocrine evaluation of male infertility, researchers have proposed that a testosterone-to-estradiol ratio in nanograms per deciliter (ng/dL) to picograms per milliliter (pg/mL) of less than 10:1 indicates aromatase overactivity that would benefit from inhibitory therapy (Raman and Schlegel, 2002; Gregoriou et al, 2012; Schlegel, 2012). Prescribers should be cautious in the long-term use of aromatase inhibitors, because bone density in the male may be estradiol dependent, and long-term studies of this class of drug in men are lacking (Khosla et al, 2001; Kim et al, 2013).

Mutations in the androgen receptor *(AR)* gene located on the long arm of the X chromosome at banding region Xq11-12 lead to a spectrum of disorders from complete testicular feminization to male infertility (Dowsing et al, 1999; Davis-Dao et al, 2007; Sokol, 2009). Male reproductive dysfunction appears to be related to a longer cytosine-adenine-guanine (CAG) repeat length in exon one of the *AR* gene (Dowsing et al, 1999; Davis-Dao et al, 2007; Sokol, 2009). **Male infertility associated with AR insensitivity is characterized by increased testosterone, estradiol, and LH to variable degrees with typical FSH levels; significantly elevated testosterone in the presence of impaired male fertility should consequently raise the suspicion of AR resistance** (Sokol, 2009). High-dose testosterone therapy may result in improved spermatogenesis, but data on this form of treatment are limited (Tordjman et al, 2014). Pregnancy may be achieved by ICSI with ejaculated sperm or that derived by surgical extraction from the testis (Massin et al, 2012; Tordjman et al, 2014).

Because dihydrotestosterone regulates the anatomic development of external male genitalia, mutations in the gene encoding isozyme 2 of 5α-reductase located on the short arm of chromosome 2 at banding region 2p23 result in a spectrum ranging from a female to a male phenotype (Johnson et al, 1986; Thigpen et al, 1993; Sokol, 2009). Phenotypic females with 5α-reductase 2 mutations may harbor testes with intact spermatogenesis (Johnson et al, 1986; Thigpen et al, 1993). No medical treatment is currently available for this disorder. Pregnancies have been successfully attained with ICSI from sperm from men with 5α-reductase-2 deficiency (Matsubara et al, 2010; Kang et al, 2011).

Developmental Disorders

Anatomic development that results in aberrant genital formation may manifest in later life as male infertility. Main areas of maldevelopment include the testes, the external genitalia, and the reproductive microductal system.

Intersex or Disorders of Sexual Development

Previously, intersex was divided into categories such as male pseudohermaphroditism, female pseudohermaphroditism, true hermaphroditism, and mixed or complete gonadal dysgenesis, with true hermaphrodites having components of both ovaries and testes (Oates and Lamb, 2009; Ono and Harley, 2013). Disorders of sex development (DSDs) are increasingly being understood as the consequence of specific aberrant genes, and the current nomenclature used to describe intersex now includes the karyotype, a clinically descriptive term, and the molecular basis of the disorder if it is known (Ono and Harley, 2013). An example of an intersex description using this nomenclature might be "46,XY DSD complete gonadal dysgenesis with SF1 mutation" (Ono and Harley, 2013). Genes identified to be involved in DSD are too numerous to be listed here, and the reader is referred to Ono and Harley for a current review (Ono and Harley, 2013). In general, the genes involved in DSDs that manifest as male infertility do so by developmental anatomic abnormalities, abnormal or absent spermatogenesis, general endocrinopathy, or encoding for defective endocrine receptors and target complexes (Oates and Lamb, 2009; Ono and Harley, 2013).

Hypospadias and Epispadias

Aberrant anatomic location of the urethra in hypospadias or epispadias may result in deposition of semen too distal in the vaginal vault (Niederberger, 2011). These men may have adequate bulk seminal parameters, and if screening semen analysis is performed before physical examination of the man, the diagnosis may be missed. Hypospadias appears to have both genetic and environmental causes, with genetic polymorphisms playing a predominant role rather than isolated gene defects (Macedo et al, 2012). The pathophysiology of epispadias is different from that of hypospadias, and it is typically considered on the spectrum of bladder-exstrophy-epispadias complex (BEEC) disorders (Rasouly and Lu, 2013).

Cryptorchidism

The basis of cryptorchidism and the relationship of the disorder to male reproductive function is detailed in the section of this chapter describing childhood diseases in the reproductive history of the infertile male. The most significant feature related to the prognosis of cryptorchidism is whether the condition is unilateral or bilateral (Lee et al, 2001; Miller et al, 2001; Lee, 2005).

Microductal Aplasia

The vas deferens may fail to develop on one side or both. The distinction is significant, as the pathophysiologic basis of each is different.

Congenital Unilateral Absence of the Vas Deferens. As described in the section detailing the physical examination of the infertile male, unilateral absence of the vas deferens implies that wolffian, or mesonephric, ductal development on the ipsilateral side was aberrant. As these ducts become in embryogenesis the epididymis, vas deferens, and ejaculatory duct, the proximal and distal portions may be malformed or absent as well (Lewis and Kaplan, 2009). The most important consideration if unilateral absence of the vas is observed is that because renal development is coupled with wolffian ductal development, a solitary absent vas deferens may signal renal agenesis (Niederberger, 2011).

Congenital Bilateral Absence of the Vas Deferens. Oates and colleagues reported in the early 1990s that males with CBAVD had a high frequency of genetic sequence abnormalities associated with cystic fibrosis (Anguiano et al, 1992). **Coupled with the observation that in nearly all men with cystic fibrosis the vasa are absent bilaterally, these findings suggested that CBAVD is frequently a phenotype for a spectrum of disorders involving mutations in the gene responsible for cystic fibrosis** (Anguiano et al, 1992). As described in the section discussing genomic sequence assessment in the laboratory evaluation of the infertile male, that gene encodes a predominantly chloride ion channel termed the *cystic fibrosis transmembrane conductance regulator,* and currently more than 1600 mutations in the gene have been identified, which vary in the severity of the phenotype from CBAVD to cystic fibrosis (Ratbi et al, 2007; Oates and Lamb, 2009; Hampton and Stanton, 2010; Bombieri et al, 2011; Yu et al, 2012).

It is currently believed that two genetic causes of CBAVD exist: one that results from mutations in CFTR, and another that results from alterations in as-yet-unidentified other genes involved in mesonephric ductal development (Oates and Lamb, 2009). CFTR mutations represent a spectrum of disease severity; should both alleles harbor severe mutations, cystic fibrosis results, and if one or both alleles contain the milder forms, CBAVD may occur (Ratbi et al, 2007; Oates and Lamb, 2009; Hampton and Stanton, 2010; Bombieri et al, 2011; Yu et al, 2012). As described in the section detailing genomic sequence assessment, the most common mutation is ΔF508, which is severe (Hampton and Stanton, 2010). **The carrier frequency for cystic fibrosis gene mutations is high—approximately 1 in 20 in persons of Northern European descent—and it is consequently important to investigate the CFTR status of the female partner of a man identified to have CBAVD in addition to his genetic evaluation** (Oates and Lamb, 2009). Symptoms such as chronic sinus or respiratory infections may be overlooked if mild, and the urologist diagnosing CBAVD might be the first to uncover an indolent form of cystic fibrosis (Oates and Lamb, 2009).

Spermatogenesis in men with CBAVD is typically normal, and ICSI with surgically extracted sperm is typically effective (Kamal et al, 2010). Genetic counseling taking into account the CFTR genetic assessment of the affected man and his female partner allows for the couple to understand the likelihood of cystic fibrosis in offspring and the implications of carrier status, and it may be performed by the urologist or a clinical geneticist.

Varicocele

The diagnosis of varicocele was discussed in the section detailing the physical examination of the infertile man: why imaging such as ultrasound is most rationally not recommended for the screening evaluation of a varicocele is discussed in the section describing imaging.

That most men with varicocele have sperm present on semen analysis has proved to be one of the most confounding aspects of its diagnosis and treatment. As discussed in the section describing the semen analysis, the results of this assay are assessed in a probabilistic context with substantial variability, making analytical statements concerning its effect on male reproductive potential difficult. Taking into account confounding factors involving the female partner that are often opaque and difficult to control in analyses, determining the effect of a varicocele on pregnancy, miscarriage, and birth becomes intractable. However, substantial evidence links varicocele to spermatogenic dysfunction and impaired male reproductive potential.

Because the left internal spermatic vein drains into the left renal vein approximately 8 to 10 cm superior to the entry of the right internal spermatic vein draining into the vena cava, the hydrostatic column of blood on the left predisposes that side to incompetence in its venous valves more so than on the right (Shafik and Bedeir, 1980; Gat et al, 2005; Masson and Brannigan, 2014). **As a result, varicose veins in the pampiniform plexus are more common on the left than on the right** (Gat et al, 2005; Masson and Brannigan, 2014). The incidence of bilateral varicoceles depends on the techniques involved in detection, with over 80% observed to be bilateral on contact thermography, Doppler sonography, and venography in one series (Gat et al, 2004). Whether these bilateral varicoceles so identified are clinically significant remains an open question. **One clinical consequence of the infrequency of solitary right varicoceles is that should one be identified, renal pathology such as tumor should be considered, especially if the right-sided varicocele is of abrupt onset** (Masson and Brannigan, 2014).

Varicoceles likely arise as most varicose veins do by intravenous valvular incompetence (Wishahi, 1991; Gat et al, 2005). Genetics may predispose to a valvular defect, as investigators have noted an increased incidence of varicoceles in first-degree relatives of men with a known varicocele (Raman et al, 2005).

Substantial evidence correlates the presence of palpable varicoceles to male reproductive dysfunction. Bulk seminal parameters are poorer in men with varicocele than in the fertile population (WHO, 1992; Al-Ali et al, 2010). Testis size, which reflects the mass of spermatogenesis, is smaller in men with varicocele, and investigators have documented progressive atrophy associated with the condition (Lipshultz and Corriere, 1977; Sakamoto et al, 2008; Patel and Sigman, 2010).

Most studies investigating how varicocele exerts deleterious effects on male reproductive function consider the primary event to be an increase in intratesticular temperature secondary to interruption in the counter-current heat exchange provided in the pampiniform plexus with opposing flow vectors in a central arterial system and surrounding veins (Zorgniotti and MacLeod, 1973; Goldstein and Eid, 1989; Masson and Brannigan, 2014). The proposed mechanisms by which male fertility is impaired by this effect mainly include DNA fragmentation and apoptosis, oxidative stress, predisposition to aneuploidy, and intracellular metabolic and ionic changes (Benoff et al, 2004; Smith et al, 2005; Baccetti et al, 2006; Bertolla et al, 2006; Enciso et al, 2006; Lima et al, 2006; Zucchi et al, 2006; Shiraishi and Naito, 2007; Agarwal et al, 2008c; Blumer et al, 2008; Pasqualotto et al, 2008a; Ghabili

et al, 2009; Wu et al, 2009; Abd-Elmoaty et al, 2010; El-Domyati et al, 2010).

Ejaculatory Dysfunction

Disorders of ejaculation may be anatomic, functional, or neuropathic in origin, resulting in absence of emission, resistance, or misdirection. The three main categories of ejaculatory dysfunction encountered in a clinical setting include ejaculatory ductal obstruction, retrograde ejaculation, and anejaculation.

Ejaculatory Ductal Obstruction

The ejaculatory ducts are primarily intraprostatic structures that originate at the terminus of the seminal vesicles and serve as their extensions but without their musculature, functioning within the prostate as simple conduits (Nguyen et al, 1996). The ampulla of the vas enters the prostate medially and at an acute angle with the terminating limb of the seminal vesicle (Nguyen et al, 1996). The intraprostatic conduit ends angled at the verumontanum, which contains two layers of longitudinal muscular bundles extending into the urethra (Nguyen et al, 1996).

Obstruction of the ejaculatory ducts is infrequent and is the cause of azoospermia in less than 5% of men without sperm in the ejaculate (Wosnitzer and Goldstein, 2014). It may occur at any point along the transit of the ducts within the prostate and result from infection, inflammation, prior surgery, or compression by congenital cysts (Wosnitzer and Goldstein, 2014). As detailed in the section discussing the semen analysis, an evaluation for ejaculatory ductal obstruction is indicated when the seminal volume is less than 1.0 mL. As noted in the section describing imaging to evaluate for ejaculatory ductal obstruction, techniques to investigate it include TRUS, MRI, chromotubation, and hydraulic pressure measurements. If clinically significant ejaculatory ductal obstruction is suspected and if the position of the obstruction is amenable to surgery, treatment is surgical resection.

Retrograde Ejaculation

Ejaculation is a multiphasic event that includes coordinated neural activity and muscular contraction and relaxation (Jefferys et al, 2012; Phillips et al, 2014). Afferent genital stimulation and cognitive ideation initiate the process, which induces emission through sympathetic stimulation of the bladder neck, vasal ampullae, seminal vesicles, and prostate (Jefferys et al, 2012; Phillips et al, 2014). **Essential to antegrade ejaculation, the bladder neck must first close while temporal neural sequencing first causes closure of the external sphincter to create a high pressure compartment that is emptied with its subsequent opening** (Shafik, 1995).

Failure of sufficient resistance at the bladder neck during generation of the high-pressure system within the prostatic urethra may redirect emission into the bladder, causing retrograde ejaculation. Pathologic causes include congenital abnormalities of or surgery to the bladder neck, spinal cord or neural injury during trauma or retroperitoneal lymph node dissection, diabetes mellitus, or idiopathic causes (Jefferys et al, 2012). **Like ejaculatory ductal obstruction, retrograde ejaculation is infrequent and is established as the diagnosis in less than 2% of infertile men** (Jefferys et al, 2012).

As detailed in the section discussing the semen analysis, an evaluation for ejaculatory ductal obstruction is indicated when the seminal volume is less than 1.0 mL and includes a postejaculatory urinalysis, which is considered significant if the number of sperm in the urine nears or exceeds that in the antegrade specimen (Sigman et al, 2009). **Primary treatment modalities include retrieval of retrograde ejaculated sperm and increasing resistance at the bladder neck with sympathomimetic agents.** In both cases, the sperm so obtained is processed for use in IUI or IVF. If retrieval is to be attempted, the urine is typically first alkalinized with oral bicarbonate or diluted by oral fluid intake, and then the voided urine or a catheterized specimen is obtained after masturbation and orgasm (Jefferys et al, 2012). Investigators have also described ejaculation on a full bladder with successful results (Crich and Jequier, 1978; Templeton and Mortimer, 1982). **Clinicians may also use sympathomimetic agents such as synephrine, pseudoephedrine, ephedrine, or phenylpropanolamine, with approximately one in four patients achieving antegrade ejaculation** (Jefferys et al, 2012). Researchers have described other therapy such as anticholinergic agents, acupuncture, and surgery, but these should be considered investigational (Jefferys et al, 2012).

Anejaculation

Anejaculation refers to lack of seminal emission and projectile ejaculation, and it must be distinguished from anorgasmia, in which the absence of an ejaculation has a cerebral cause (Brackett et al, 2009). Conditions that result in anejaculation are primarily neurologic and include retroperitoneal lymph node dissection, pelvic surgery, multiple sclerosis, transverse myelitis, congenital neural tube defects, diabetes mellitus, and spinal cord injury (Brackett et al, 2009; Phillips et al, 2014).

For patients with sufficient peripheral neural function, neurostimulation with penile vibratory devices or application of current with a rectal electrode, or electroejaculation, may result in sufficient sperm for IUI or IVF (Brackett et al, 2009; Phillips et al, 2014). **For men with spinal cord injuries at a level of T6 or above, stimulation may cause autonomic dysreflexia, an uninhibited sympathetic reflex accompanied by headache, diaphoresis, hypertension, bradycardia, and diaphoresis, which may be life-threatening.** Autonomic dysreflexia can be addressed before stimulation by treatment with nifedipine and during the procedure with monitoring of cardiac activity and blood pressure (Brackett et al, 2009; Phillips et al, 2014).

The sperm achieved by stimulation in patients with spinal cord injury is typically characterized by adequate count but impaired motility (Brackett et al, 2009). Evidence supports impairment of sexual accessory gland function, a noxious seminal plasma milieu, and immunopathic mechanisms as causative (Brackett et al, 2009).

Stimulation with penile vibratory devices serves as first-line therapy, with electroejaculation used if the former is unsuccessful (Brackett et al, 2009). If electroejaculation does not yield sperm or if other factors prevent its use, surgical extraction is indicated (Brackett et al, 2009).

Structural Sperm Abnormalities

As discussed in the section describing evaluation of sperm morphology, the majority of sperm in fertile men are eccentrically shaped, and associating the typical variation of sperm shape to clinical relevance in a quantifiable manner has proved challenging. Investigators have characterized certain infrequent discrete structural abnormalities with overt clinical manifestations.

Evidence suggests genetic bases and consequences for two rare types of specific sperm head abnormalities, globozoospermia and macrocephaly. In globozoospermia, the majority of the sperm lack acrosomal caps, rendering the heads spheric rather than ovoid. Investigators have associated globozoospermia in humans with mutations in the genes *SPATA16* at chromosome band 3q26.32, *PICK1* at 22q12.3-q13.2, and *DPY19L2* at 12q14.2 (Perrin et al, 2013). Both *SPATA16* and *PICK1* localize to proacrosomal granules that are involved in formation of the acrosome during spermatogenesis (Perrin et al, 2013). **It is debatable whether higher rates of aneuploidy are present in patients with globozoospermia or teratozoospermia in general; however, for men in whom nearly all sperm have enlarged heads, multiple tails, and abnormal acrosomes, a very high rate of aneuploidy is found** (Machev et al, 2005; Sun et al, 2006). The treatment for globozoospermia is IVF with ICSI; owing to the high rate of aneuploidy in sperm associated with macrocephaly and multiple tails, ICSI is not recommended (Machev et al, 2005; Sun et al, 2006; Perrin et al, 2013).

As discussed in the section describing the ultrastructural assessment of sperm, *primary ciliary dyskinesia* refers to a rare condition in which the microtubular architecture of cilia is disrupted (Boon et al,

2013). Because structures such as the sperm tail share similar microtubular construction with cilia, conditions that affect this architecture frequently result in a variety of other clinical manifestations such as immotile sperm, congenital heart disease, chronic respiratory and otolaryngologic infections, and laterality defects (Ferkol and Leigh, 2012). PCD occurs in 1 in 15,000 to 30,000 live births and is typically inherited in an autosomal recessive manner, with occasional X-linked inheritance reported (Ferkol and Leigh, 2012; Boon et al, 2013). Investigators have associated numerous genetic mutations with PCD, with mutations in dynein axonemal heavy chain 5 (DNAH5) and intermediate chain 1 (DNAI1) accounting for 38% of patients with the condition (Hildebrandt et al, 2011; Zariwala et al, 2011; Davis and Katsanis, 2012; Ferkol and Leigh, 2012; Boon et al, 2013). ICSI may achieve pregnancy in cases of PCD (Peeraer et al, 2004).

Empirical Treatment

Please see the Expert Consult website for details.

> **KEY POINTS: DIAGNOSES AND THERAPIES**
>
> - Klinefelter syndrome, characterized by 47,XXY, is the most commonly identified genetic cause of male infertility. Bodily morphologic features cannot reliably exclude the presence of the condition.
> - The clinical evaluation of a man identified with CBAVD includes CFTR assessment of both him and his female partner to determine risk of cystic fibrosis in offspring.
> - Severe hypogonadotropic hypogonadism may be associated with anosmia and is treated with gonadotropin replacement. Less severe forms are more common, and patients may respond to antiestrogenic agents or aromatase inhibitors.

REFERENCES
The complete reference list is available online at www.expertconsult.com.

SUGGESTED READINGS

Anguiano A, Oates RD, Amos JA, et al. Congenital bilateral absence of the vas deferens. A primarily genital form of cystic fibrosis. JAMA 1992;267: 1794–7.

Dubin L, Amelar RD. Varicocelectomy as therapy in male infertility: a study of 504 cases. Fertil Steril 1975;26:217–20.

Jarow JP, Sigman M, Kolettis PN, et al. The evaluation of the azoospermic male: AUA best practice statement. Linthicum (MD): American Urological Association Education and Research; 2011.

Lipshultz LI, Howards SS, Niederberger CS. Infertility in the male. 4th ed. New York: Cambridge University Press; 2009.

MacLeod J. Semen quality in 1000 men of known fertility and in 800 cases of infertile marriage. Fertil Steril 1951;2:115–39.

Meacham RB, Joyce GF, Wise M, et al. Male infertility. J Urol 2007;177: 2058–66.

Niederberger CS. An introduction to male reproductive medicine. New York: Cambridge University Press; 2011.

Niederberger CS. Current management of male infertility. Urol Clin North Am 2014;41(1).

Sigman M. A meta-analysis of meta-analyses. Fertil Steril 2011;96:11–4.

Sigman M, Kolettis PN, McClure RD, et al. The optimal evaluation of the infertile male: AUA best practice statement. Linthicum (MD): American Urological Association Education and Research; 2011.

Tilford CA, Kuroda-Kawaguchi T, Skaletsky H, et al. A physical map of the human Y chromosome. Nature 2001;409:943–5.

Vermeulen A, Verdonck L, Kaufman JM. A critical evaluation of simple methods for the estimation of free testosterone in serum. J Clin Endocrinol Metab 1999;84:3666–72.

World Health Organization (WHO). World Health Organization laboratory manual for the examination and processing of human semen. Geneva: World Health Organization; 2010.

25 Surgical Management of Male Infertility

Marc Goldstein, MD, DSc (Hon), FACS

Since the 10th edition of this book was published, the indications for and techniques of surgery for male infertility have been significantly refined, resulting in substantially increased success in the management of male-factor infertility. These advances include (1) increasing use of genetic and molecular biologic markers (see Chapters 22 and 24) to better select patients for surgical treatment; (2) improved techniques for microsurgical reconstruction for obstruction; (3) the use of varicocelectomy for enhancement of spermatogenesis in azoospermic or severely oligospermic men (Inci et al, 2013; Kirac et al, 2013), for prevention of future infertility and androgen deficiency in young men, and for treatment of androgen deficiency in men of all ages (Tanrikut et al, 2011); and (4) refined microsurgical techniques for sperm retrieval combined with in vitro fertilization (IVF) with intracytoplasmic sperm injection (ICSI) for men with nonobstructive azoospermia. Even **men with nonobstructive azoospermia caused by Klinefelter syndrome, once regarded as hopeless cases, can now father biologic offspring with assisted reproductive techniques** (Tournaye et al, 1996; Palermo et al, 1998; Ramasamy et al, 2009).

Use of transrectal high-resolution ultrasound as well as scrotal ultrasound with color flow Doppler has substantially improved our diagnostic and therapeutic abilities. Not only does transrectal ultrasound of the seminal vesicles provide diagnostic information, but ultrasound-guided aspiration of the seminal vesicles allows retrieval of sperm to be used for IVF with ICSI (Jarow, 1996). Power Doppler may allow identification of pockets of sperm production in the testis, which may help guide sperm retrieval in men with nonobstructive azoospermia (Har-Toov et al, 2004; Herwig et al, 2004; Tunc et al, 2005). Experimental use of multiphoton tomography in animals and human tissue has potential to further refine our ability to identify sperm in testes (Najari et al, 2012).

IVF with ICSI has expanded our ability to treat even the most severe forms of male-factor infertility such as unreconstructable reproductive tract obstruction and nonobstructive azoospermia. It is, however, a costly procedure and an intense process for the female partner, with associated risks of complications including ovarian hyperstimulation and multiple gestations, as well as complications of the procedures for oocyte retrieval. Furthermore, because ICSI bypasses all natural biologic barriers, it raises realistic concerns of passing genetic abnormalities to the offspring (Kim et al, 1998; Foresta et al, 2005) and is associated with an increased incidence of birth defects in resultant children (Davies et al, 2012). On the other hand, recent analyses clearly indicate that **specific treatments for male-factor infertility, such as microsurgical reconstruction for obstructive azoospermia and varicocelectomy for impaired testis function, in properly selected patients remain the safest and most cost-effective ways of managing infertile men** (Kolettis and Thomas, 1997; Pavlovich and Schlegel, 1997; Marmar et al, 2007; Lee et al, 2008; Smit et al, 2010). Specific treatment aimed at correcting or enhancing male infertility can upgrade a couple from intensive levels of assisted reproduction to simpler methods such as intrauterine insemination (IUI) or even to naturally conceived pregnancies (Samplaski et al, 2013).

For men with unreconstructable obstruction as well as men with nonobstructive azoospermia, surgical retrieval of sperm to achieve fertilization, pregnancy, and live birth with IVF and ICSI is a feasible management option. The development and recent refinement of the various techniques of surgical sperm retrieval, from testes, epididymides, or seminal vesicles, with percutaneous or open surgical approaches, have expanded the armamentarium of urologists treating infertile men. In particular, use of the operating microscope to evaluate and identify individual seminiferous tubules more likely to contain sperm has significantly improved the success of testicular sperm extraction (TESE) (Schlegel, 1999; Dabaja and Schlegel, 2013) while minimizing morbidity significantly (Tsujimura et al, 2002; Ramasamy et al, 2005).

The use of microsurgical techniques has also been extended to varicocelectomy. Varicoceles have long been known to be associated with male infertility and have now clearly been shown to result in progressive, duration-dependent testicular injury (Russell, 1957; Lipshultz and Corriere, 1977; Nagler et al, 1985; Sigman and Jarow, 1997). **Furthermore, microsurgical varicocelectomy, previously reserved only for men with oligospermia, has now been applied to men with nonobstructive azoospermia, resulting in induction of spermatogenesis and successful return of sperm to the ejaculate in many patients** (Matthews et al, 1998; Kim et al, 1999; Pasqualotto et al, 2003, 2006; Ishikawa et al, 2008; Youssef et al, 2009). Although varicocelectomy has historically been reserved for the treatment of infertile men and varicocele-induced pain, there is an emerging concept of **early repair of varicoceles to prevent both future infertility and Leydig cell dysfunction.** Substantial evidence has accumulated suggesting that varicocele adversely affects Leydig cell function, resulting in lower serum testosterone levels when compared with age-matched controls without varicocele (Tanrikut et al, 2011). Varicocelectomy can halt and even partially reverse this decline (Castro-Magana et al, 1989; Su et al, 1995; Cayan et al, 1999; Tanrikut et al, 2011). **In selected men, varicocelectomy may be an effective treatment for symptomatic, age-related androgen deficiency, a condition increasingly referred to as *andropause* or *testosterone deficiency syndrome* (TDS). Thus, with safer and more effective microsurgical techniques, early varicocelectomy has expanded the urologist's role from that of** salvaging remaining testicular function to that of preventing future infertility and TDS.

When surgery for male infertility is undertaken, only rarely is the life (or death) of the patient at stake. What is at stake when the surgery described in this chapter is undertaken is new life, with the potential for altering not only the quality of a couple's life but the future of our species. The responsibilities assumed by the surgeon in these circumstances demand the utmost in judgment and skill. **Many of the procedures described in this chapter are among the most technically demanding in all of urology.** Acquisition of the skills required to perform them demands intensive laboratory training in microsurgery and a thorough knowledge of the anatomy and physiology of the male reproductive system. **Attempting such surgery only occasionally and without proper training would be doing a terrible disservice to the patient and his partner.**

SURGICAL ANATOMY

The scrotal contents are unique in their accessibility for physical examination, imaging modalities, and surgical intervention. The success of surgery for male infertility and scrotal disorders is predicated on selection of the correct operation and the most appropriate surgical approach. The details of the history and careful physical examination followed by confirmatory, judiciously selected laboratory and imaging procedures are presented in Chapter 24. When surgical intervention for diagnostic or therapeutic purposes is indicated, a thorough understanding of the anatomy (see Chapter 21) and physiology (see Chapter 22) of the male reproductive system is requisite for planning and carrying out a surgical procedure with the highest probability of success and lowest morbidity.

The key points of surgical anatomy are discussed in the following sections.

Testicular Blood Supply (Box 25-1)

The main blood supply to the testis is from the testicular (internal spermatic) artery arising directly from the aorta. A second blood supply comes from the artery of the vas deferens (deferential artery), which derives from the hypogastric (internal iliac) artery or the superior vesical artery (also a branch of the hypogastric). The third blood supply, primarily to the tunica vaginalis, but with branches going to the testes, comes from the cremasteric (external spermatic) artery, which derives from the inferior epigastric artery. **The testicular artery is the main blood supply to the testes.** Its diameter exceeds the diameter of the deferential (vasal) artery and the cremasteric artery combined (Raman and Goldstein, 2004). Although the vasal and cremasteric arteries can provide adequate blood

---

BOX 25-1 Blood Supply to Testis, Epididymis, and Vas Deferens

TESTIS
Testicular (internal spermatic) artery from aorta (main blood supply)
Deferential artery from internal iliac (hypogastric) artery and superior vesical artery
Cremasteric (external spermatic) artery from inferior epigastric artery

EPIDIDYMIS
Superior epididymal artery derived from testicular artery
Inferior epididymal artery derived from vasal (deferential) artery

VAS DEFERENS
Seminal vesical end: deferential artery
Testicular end: deferential artery and inferior epididymal artery

---

supply to the testes in the event that the testicular artery is ligated, especially in children, **atrophy and/or azoospermia has resulted from testicular artery ligation both in adults and in children.** Experience with the one-stage Fowler-Stephens operation for orchiopexy, in which the testicular artery is intentionally ligated, indicates that 20% to 40% of such testes atrophy, although the rate of atrophy is lower in the staged procedure.

Special attention should be paid to men who have undergone vasectomy, in whom the vasal artery has likely been compromised. In these men, maintaining the integrity of the testicular artery in any future operations, such as varicocelectomy, is critical (Lee et al, 2007b).

Epididymal Blood Supply (see Box 25-1)

The epididymis has a rich blood supply. The superior and the medial epididymal arteries derive from the testicular artery. The blood supply to the cauda (inferior pole) of the epididymis derives from the vasal (deferential) artery. The two main blood supplies to the epididymis, running superiorly and inferiorly, form an extensive interconnection such that if the vasal artery is ligated from previous vasectomy, the blood supply to the epididymis from the testicular artery is more than adequate. In addition, in preparation for vaso-epididymostomy or vasovasostomy, the epididymis can be intentionally dissected off the testis and mobilized to the caput (see the discussion of long-term follow-up, evaluation, and results), with the inferior and medial epididymal arteries intentionally ligated without adverse consequence. **As long as the superior epididymal artery remains intact, the blood supply to the epididymis will be adequate.**

Blood Supply of the Vas Deferens (see Box 25-1)

The vas deferens obtains its blood supply from two sources. The seminal vesical (abdominal) end of the vas derives its blood supply from the deferential (vasal) artery. The testicular end of the vas receives additional blood supply from the inferior epididymal arterial interconnections, which extend onto the vas deferens. The two blood supplies to the vas deferens freely anastomose with each other. **After vasectomy, if the vasal vessels are ligated, the testicular end of the vas receives all of its blood supply from branches of the testicular artery and epididymal artery, whereas the seminal vesical (abdominal) end of the vas receives all of its blood supply from the deferential artery. The vas deferens receives no blood supply from the surrounding cremaster muscle or from any blood vessels from the spermatic cord. Therefore, if the vas deferens is sectioned or obstructed in two different locations, the intervening segment will fibrose owing to lack of blood supply. Therefore, two simultaneous vasovasostomies cannot be safely performed on the same vas if the vasal vessels have been interrupted in both locations.**

Anatomy of the Excurrent Ducts

Sperm and testicular fluid exit the testes through 7 to 11 tiny efferent ducts. These ducts become convoluted when they exit the testes and form the caput of the epididymis (see Chapters 21 and 41). At that level, they freely anastomose with one another. They all coalesce at the distal caput to form a single epididymal tubule from the caput-corpus junction all the way to the vas deferens. Therefore, **if the epididymis is accidentally injured or ligated distal to the caput, the entire system on that side will be completely obstructed.** This is an important consideration when performing epididymal surgery or surgery near the epididymis. **Hydrocelectomy** is a common surgical procedure that can result in **iatrogenic injury to the epididymis.** In long-standing large hydroceles, the epididymis is often splayed out and difficult to identify. Use of an operating microscope and transillumination of the hydrocele sac help avoid injury to the epididymis, vas, and testicular blood supply (Dabaja and Goldstein, 2014). **Generous margins from the epididymis should be allowed when performing hydrocelectomy** (see Chapter 21 and 41).

Orchiopexy for torsion can also result in inadvertent injury to the epididymis. **A single stitch through an epididymal tubule in the corpus or cauda will result in complete obstruction** of that side. Because there are multiple lobules at the levels of the caput, **puncture of a single tubule for sperm aspiration can be safely performed at the most proximal region of the caput** without significantly compromising the flow of sperm into the corpus. Multiple punctures of many tubules at the caput, or any puncture distal to the caput, however, can cause obstruction (Zhang et al, 2013).

Ejaculatory Ducts

The left and right ejaculatory ducts enter the prostatic urethra at the level of the utricle. Obstruction of ejaculatory ducts can lead to azoospermia. Transurethral resection (TUR) of the ejaculatory ducts (TURED) can relieve the obstruction. TURED should not be considered a benign procedure, as it is occasionally associated with significant morbidity (see the section on TURED). Normally, the ejaculatory ducts contain a valvelike mechanism that prevents reflux of urine into the ejaculatory duct. **After TURED, a significant percentage of men develop reflux of urine up the excurrent ductal system** (Vazquez-Levin et al, 1994) **causing chemical and/or bacterial epididymitis.**

TESTIS BIOPSY

Indications

The indications for testis biopsy are detailed in Chapter 24. Briefly, **testis biopsy is indicated in azoospermic men with testis of normal size and consistency, palpable vasa deferentia, and normal serum follicle-stimulating hormone (FSH) levels, and a negative serum antisperm antibody assay** (Lee et al, 2009). Under these circumstances, **biopsy will distinguish obstructive from nonobstructive azoospermia.** In men with **congenital absence of vasa and normal serum FSH levels,** biopsy always reveals spermatogenesis (Goldstein and Schlossberg, 1988) and **biopsy is not necessary** before definitive sperm aspiration and IVF with ICSI. **Diagnostic biopsy should usually be performed bilaterally irrespective of the size discrepancy of the two testes.** Good spermatogenesis is sometimes found in small, firm testes, and biopsies of large, healthy testes may reveal maturation arrest.

The ability to achieve pregnancy with only a single testicular sperm has turned biopsy into a potentially therapeutic, as well as diagnostic, procedure. Even men with markedly elevated serum FSH levels and small, soft testes, in whom testicular failure is certain, often harbor rare mature sperm in their testes. These sperm can be extracted using techniques described later in this chapter and used for IVF with intracytoplasmic injection of testicular sperm.

The recently discovered heterogeneity of the testes of men with nonobstructive azoospermia coupled with the ability of testicular sperm to acquire motility (Jow et al, 1993) has resulted in changes in the techniques of testis biopsy. **Examination of fresh, unfixed tissue for the presence of sperm with tails** and possible motility, **and examination of multiple samples if sperm are not found initially, is now recommended. Furthermore, optimal care requires the availability, at the time of biopsy, of an andrology laboratory capable of processing and cryopreserving any sperm found at the time of biopsy.**

Open Testis Biopsy: Microsurgical Technique

Open biopsy remains the gold standard because it provides an optimal amount of tissue both for accurate diagnosis and for retrieval of sperm for IVF (Rosenlund et al, 1998; Schlegel, 1999; Dardashti et al, 2000). Open testis biopsy may be performed using either general, spinal, or local anesthetic. Local anesthesia of just the skin and tunicas without a cord block is uncomfortable; local anesthesia with spermatic cord block can be effective and comfortable. However, there are limitations to the cord block. In animal studies, the incidence of accidental damage to the testicular artery

during blind cord block is 5% (Goldstein et al, 1983). In addition, if there has been previous scrotal surgery with scar or adhesions and if more extensive dissection and manipulation may be required, I prefer to use general or spinal anesthetic.

The surgeon's goal when performing a testis biopsy is to provide an optimal tissue sample, avoid trauma to the specimen, and avoid injury to the epididymis or testicular blood supply. Open biopsy under magnification (preferably with an operating microscope) satisfies these requirements.

An assistant stretches the scrotal skin tightly over the anterior surface of the surface of the testis and confirms that the epididymis is posterior. Bilateral 1-cm transverse scrotal incisions within the scrotal skin folds provide good exposure with a minimum of scrotal bleeding. Alternatively, a single vertical incision in the median raphe may be used. The incision is carried through the skin and dartos muscle, and the tunica vaginalis is opened. **If the anatomy is distorted from previous surgery, the epididymis cannot be clearly palpated posteriorly, or the tunica albuginea cannot be clearly identified, the incision should be enlarged and the testis delivered.** The edges of the tunica vaginalis are held open with hemostats, and any bleeding vessels are cauterized. **Use of loupes or, better yet, the operating microscope allows ready identification of a spot on the tunica albuginea relatively free of visible surface vessels.** The wound should be dry before incision of the tunica albuginea to prevent saturation of the biopsy with blood. A 3- to 4-mm incision is made in the tunica albuginea with a 15-degree microknife (Fig. 25-1A). Small crossing vessels are cauterized with bipolar cautery and divided before excision of a pea-sized sample of seminiferous tubules with razor sharp iris scissors (Fig. 25-1B). **When handling testis biopsy material for permanent fixation, avoid crushing tissue in any way (including with forceps) because this may traumatize and distort the testicular architecture.** The specimen is then deposited directly into either Bouin, Zenker, or collidine buffered glutaraldehyde solution. **Formalin fixation** results in distortion of testicular histology and **should not be used for testis biopsy.** A "touch-prep" is made by blotting the cut surface of the testis several times with a glass slide (Fig. 25-1C) and adding a drop of saline, lactated Ringer solution, or human tubal fluid with IVF medium and a coverslip. Examination under high power using a light microscope with or without phase contrast will reveal the presence of sperm with tails and allow assessment of motility (Fig. 25-1D). If no sperm are found in the touch-prep, a second specimen may be cut for a wet "squash prep." In this case, the specimen is placed on a slide, a drop of saline is added, and the specimen is crushed under a coverslip (Jow et al, 1993). If no sperm are found, the tunica is closed with two or three interrupted sutures of 5-0 Vicryl (Fig. 25-1E), and biopsy of another area is performed through the same skin incision. As described later in this chapter, **use of an operating microscope providing 10× to 25× magnification may allow selective sampling of larger seminiferous tubules more likely to contain sperm** (Schlegel, 1999). **If sperm are identified,** the slide as well as additional **tissue removed are sent for cryopreservation** in the andrology laboratory. **The location of the biopsy site where sperm were found is noted and the tunica albuginea is closed with two or three interrupted sutures of 6-0 nylon. This facilitates identification of sites of spermatogenesis for future TESE for IVF with ICSI.**

The tunica vaginalis is closed with 5-0 monofilament nonabsorbable suture for hemostasis. Use of a nonabsorbable suture facilitates identification of the biopsy site if sperm were found at that site and subsequent TESE is required at the time of IVF with ICSI. The skin is closed with subcuticular 5-0 Monocryl. The wounds are covered with Bacitracin ointment and a fluff-type dressing secured with a snug scrotal support. Antibiotics are unnecessary.

Percutaneous Testis Biopsy

Percutaneous testis biopsy using the same 14-gauge biopsy gun used for prostatic biopsy **is a blind procedure and could result in unintentional injury to either the epididymis or the testicular artery. This technique should not be used when previous surgery**

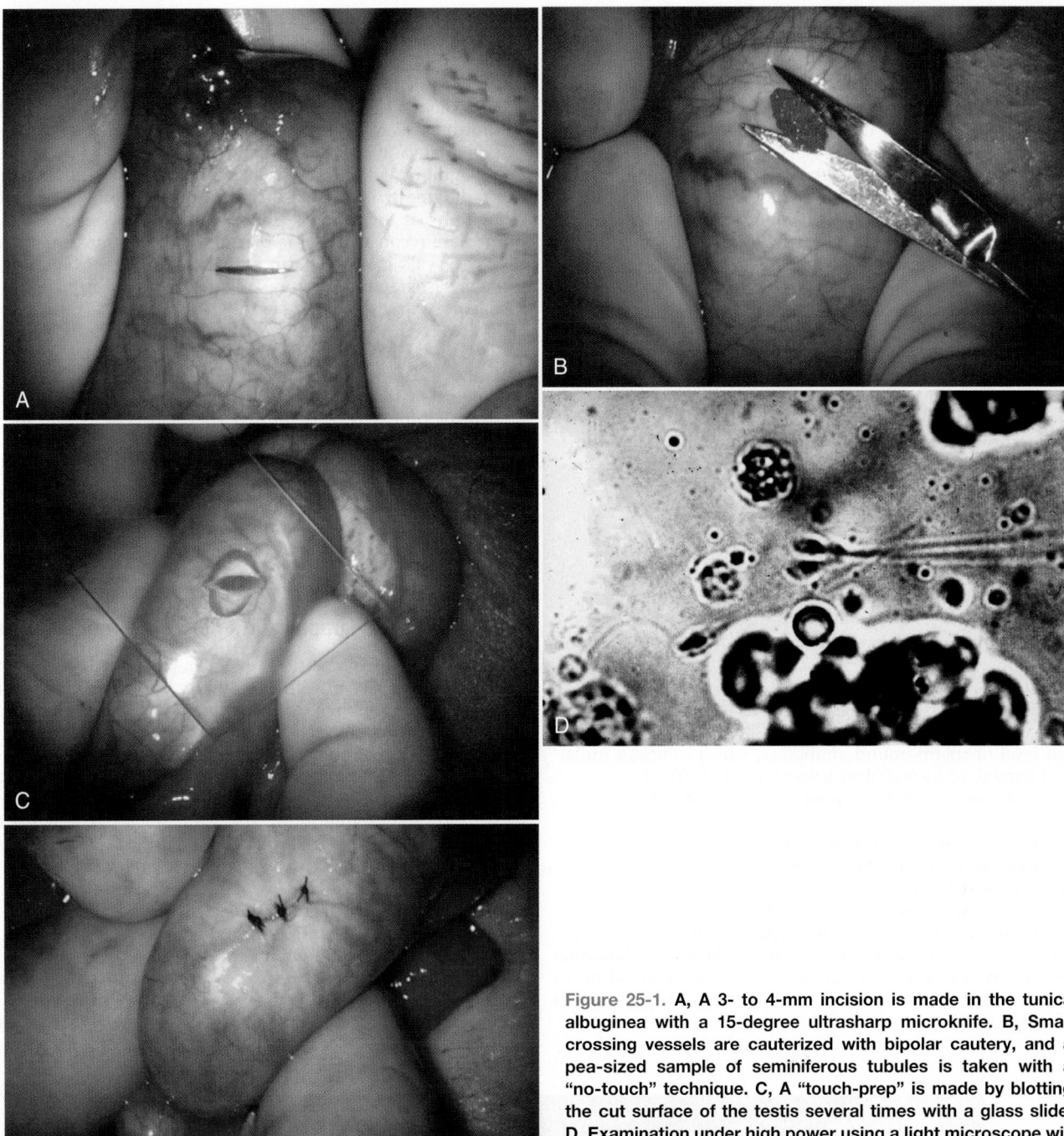

Figure 25-1. **A,** A 3- to 4-mm incision is made in the tunica albuginea with a 15-degree ultrasharp microknife. **B,** Small crossing vessels are cauterized with bipolar cautery, and a pea-sized sample of seminiferous tubules is taken with a "no-touch" technique. **C,** A "touch-prep" is made by blotting the cut surface of the testis several times with a glass slide. **D,** Examination under high power using a light microscope will reveal the presence of sperm and allow assessment of motility. **E,** The biopsy site is closed with two or three interrupted sutures of 6-0 nylon or Prolene.

has resulted in scarring and obliteration of normal anatomy. Fine-needle aspiration usually yields specimens that contain few tubules with poorly preserved architecture. When performed with the patient under local anesthesia, a cord block is necessary to minimize pain. The technique of percutaneous biopsy is described later in this chapter. As a therapeutic tool for sperm retrieval, **percutaneous biopsy or aspiration is most useful for fresh sperm retrieval for IVF with ICSI in men with obstructive azoospermia and normal spermatogenesis.**

Percutaneous Testicular Aspiration

Testicular aspiration performed with a 23-gauge needle or angiocath sheath (Marmar and Benoff, 2005) is probably less invasive

and less painful than percutaneous biopsy but usually yields few tubules with poorly preserved architecture. Although flow cytometric evaluation of this material can distinguish haploid from diploid cells and therefore confirm the presence or absence of late stages of spermatogenesis (Chan et al, 1984), direct wet examination of the aspirate for sperm and assessment of motility provide the most practical clinical information. Three or four aspirations can be performed until sperm are identified. In cases of obstructive azoospermia, these sperm can be used for IVF with ICSI (Craft et al, 1995) when sperm cannot be retrieved from the epididymis (see the section discussing TESE). Fine-needle aspiration has a significantly lower yield of sperm than open microsurgical TESE (micro-TESE) in men with nonobstructive azoospermia.

Complications of Testis Biopsy

Carefully performed, testis biopsy is associated with few complications (Schlegel and Su, 1997; Dardashti et al, 2000). **The most serious complication associated with testis biopsy is inadvertent biopsy of the epididymis.** If histologic evaluation of the biopsy material reveals epididymis with sperm within the epididymal tubule, obstruction of the epididymis at the site of the biopsy is certain. If, however, there are no sperm within the epididymal tubules, the patient is either obstructed above the level of the epididymal biopsy site or has primary seminiferous tubular failure and no harm has been done.

The most common complication of testis biopsy is hematoma. Hematomas can be quite large and may require drainage. Use of magnification to avoid vessels and bipolar cautery for hemostasis will help prevent this complication. Proper closure of the well-vascularized tunica vaginalis with a continuous 5-0 suture will minimize bleeding and adhesions.

With the rich blood supply of the scrotum and its contents, wound infection is rare in the absence of hematoma, and antibiotics are unnecessary.

VASOGRAPHY

Indications

The absolute indications for vasography are as follows:
1. Azoospermia, plus
2. **Complete spermatogenesis with many mature spermatids on testis biopsy,** plus
3. **At least one palpable vas**
   Relative indications for vasography are as follows:
1. Severe oligospermia with normal testis biopsy
2. High level of sperm-bound antibodies, which indicates unilateral, bilateral, or partial obstruction (Lee et al, 2009)
3. Low semen volume and very poor sperm motility (partial ejaculatory duct obstruction)
   Vasography should answer the following questions:
1. **Are there sperm in the vasal fluid?**
2. **Is the vas obstructed?**
   If the testis biopsy reveals many sperm, then:
1. **Absence of sperm in vasal fluid indicates** obstruction on the testicular side of the vasotomy site, most likely an **epididymal obstruction.** Vasography is done in this case with saline or indigo carmine to confirm patency of the seminal vesical (distal) end of the vas before vasoepididymostomy.

2. **Copious vasal fluid containing many sperm indicates vasal or ejaculatory duct obstruction,** and formal contrast vasography is performed as described later to document the exact location of the obstruction.
3. **Copious thick white fluid without sperm in a dilated vas indicates secondary epididymal obstruction** in addition to a potential vasal or ejaculatory duct obstruction.
   Vasography with radiographic contrast media and intraoperative radiography is rarely indicated. There is no need to perform vasography at the time of testis biopsy for azoospermia unless immediate reconstruction is planned and the touch or wet prep biopsy reveals mature sperm with tails. If not meticulously performed, vasography can cause stricture or even obstruction at the vasography site, which can complicate subsequent reconstruction (Howards et al, 1975b; Poore et al, 1997). In addition, vasography is of no value in making the diagnosis of epididymal obstruction, and the majority of nonvasectomy related obstructions are epididymal.

If testis biopsy reveals normal spermatogenesis and the vasa are palpable, vasography, if necessary, should be performed only at the time of definitive repair of obstruction. General anesthesia provides the most flexibility for scrotal exploration, vasography, and repair of obstruction. Although local anesthesia can provide adequate analgesia, patients are often unable to lie still through several hours of microsurgery. Long-acting hypobaric spinal or continuous epidural anesthesia can be a satisfactory alternative.

Technique of Vasography and Interpretation of Findings

Inguinal hernia repair, particularly when performed on children, is known to be associated with vasal injury leading to obstruction. If there is no previous inguinal incision and the side of obstruction is unknown, the testis is delivered through a high vertical scrotal incision (see the discussion of surgical scrotal approaches). The vas deferens is identified and isolated at the junction of the straight and convoluted portions of the vas deferens. Using an operating microscope and 10× magnification, the vasal sheath is longitudinally incised and the vasal vessels are carefully preserved (Fig. 25-2A).

A clean segment of bare vas is delivered and surrounded with a vessel loop. A straight clamp is placed beneath the vas to act as a platform. Under 25× magnification, a 15-degree microknife is used to hemitransect the vas until the lumen is revealed (Fig. 25-2B). **Any fluid exuding from the lumen is placed on a slide, mixed with a drop of saline, and sealed with a coverslip for microscopic examination. If the vasal fluid is devoid of sperm with repeated sampling** after milking the epididymis and convoluted vas, **epididymal**

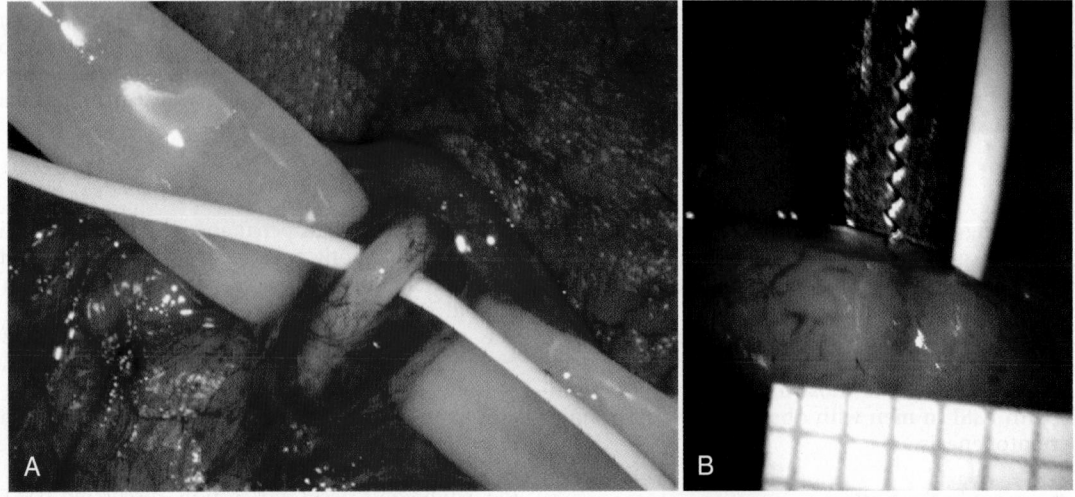

Figure 25-2. A, With use of an operating microscope and 10× magnification, the vasal sheath is longitudinally incised and vasal vessels are carefully preserved. **B,** Under 25× magnification, a 15-degree microknife is used to hemitransect the vas until the lumen is revealed.

obstruction is present. The end of the vas toward the seminal vesicles is then cannulated with a 24-gauge angiocatheter sheath and is injected with 1 mL of lactated Ringer solution with a 1-mL tuberculin syringe to confirm its patency (Fig. 25-3). If the Ringer solution passes easily, formal vasography is not necessary. If further proof of patency of the vas deferens is desired, 1 mL of 50% dilute indigo carmine may be injected and the bladder catheterized. The presence of blue-green dye in the urine confirms patency of the vas. Indigo carmine diluted 50/50 with Ringer solution is preferred instead of methylene blue because even at low concentrations methylene blue kills sperm and renders them useless for cryopreservation or for immediate IVF and ICSI (Chang et al, 1998; Sheynkin et al, 1999b; Wood et al, 2003). **If motile sperm are found in the vas, the testicular end should be gently barbotaged with 0.2 mL of human tubal fluid medium, and the fluid processed by the andrology laboratory for sperm cryopreservation for potential future use for IVF and ICSI. This should be done before injection with indigo carmine or x-ray contrast material** (Sheynkin et al, 1999b).

If a large amount of fluid is found in the vasal lumen and microscopic examination reveals the presence of sperm, the obstruction is toward the seminal vesical end of the vas. In these cases, the vas is usually markedly dilated. A 2-0 Prolene suture can be passed toward the seminal vesical end of the vas and a clamp

placed on the Prolene when the suture passes no further. This is particularly useful for delineating the site of inguinal obstruction from prior groin surgery. If the obstruction is proximal to the inguinal scar, formal vasography is performed by passing a No. 3 whistle-tip ureteral catheter toward the seminal vesical end of the vas. A 16-Fr Foley catheter is placed in the bladder and the balloon is filled with 5 mL of air. Placing the balloon on gentle traction before vasography prevents reflux of contrast into the bladder, which can obscure detail (Fig. 25-4). The air-filled balloon also identifies the location of the bladder neck relative to any obstruction. After the vasa have been cannulated, vasograms are performed with the injection of 0.5 mL of water-soluble contrast media (Fig. 25-5). **If vasography reveals obstruction at the site of the ejaculatory ducts** (Fig. 25-6), **indigo carmine is injected in both vasa to facilitate TURED** (see the section on diagnosis of TURED). If both vasa are visualized after injection of contrast into only one vas (Fig. 25-7), it means that both vasa empty into a single cavity, usually a midline ejaculatory duct cyst.

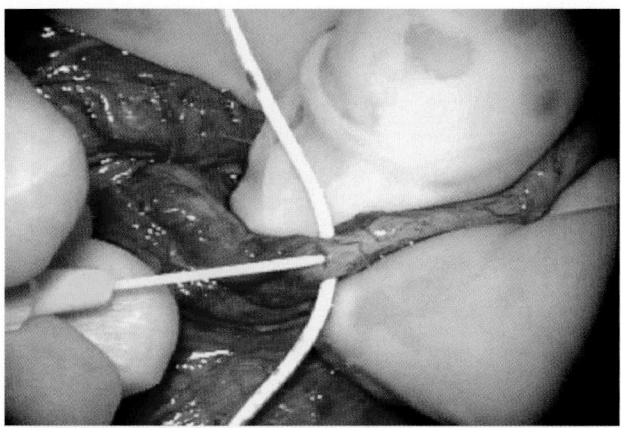

Figure 25-3. The end of the vas toward the seminal vesicles is cannulated with a 24-gauge angiocatheter, and then injected with 1 mL of lactated Ringer solution with a 1-mL tuberculin syringe to confirm its patency.

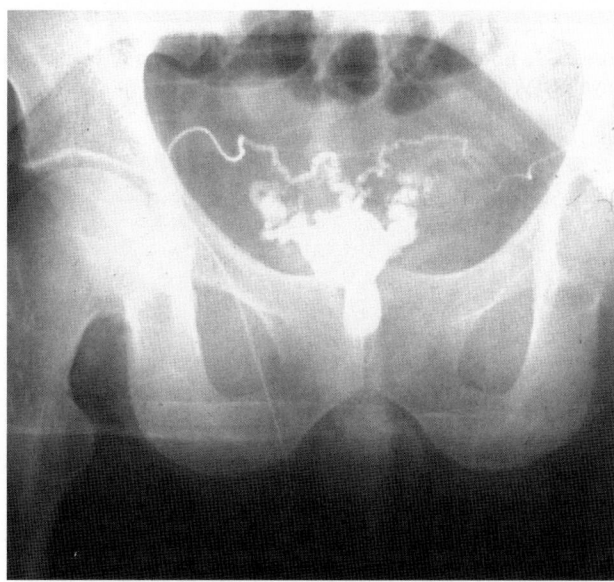

Figure 25-5. Vasograms are performed with 0.5 mL of water-soluble contrast media.

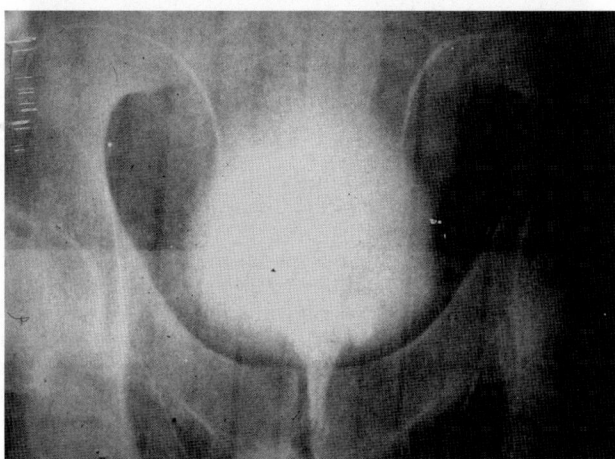

Figure 25-4. Placing the balloon on gentle traction before vasography prevents reflux of contrast into the bladder, which can obscure detail.

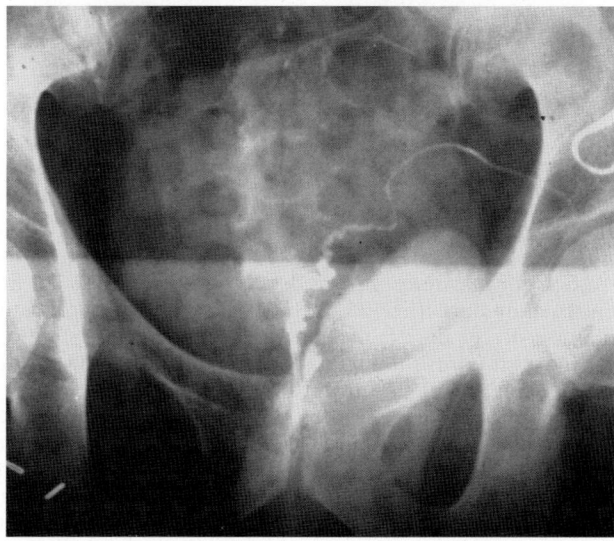

Figure 25-6. Vasography reveals obstruction at the site of the ejaculatory ducts.

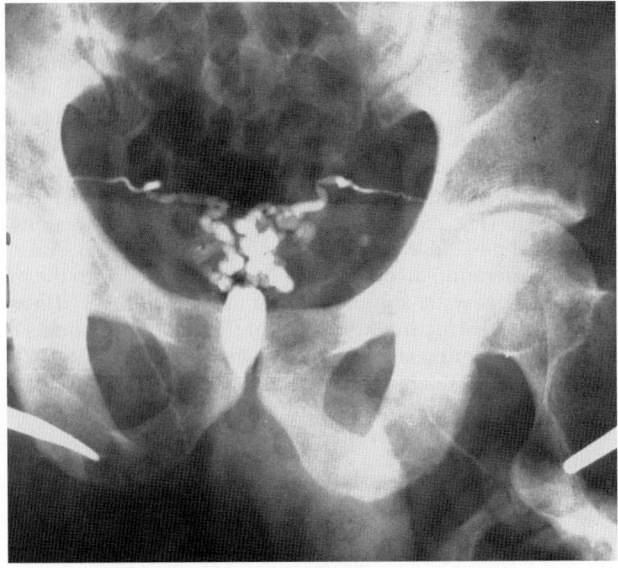

Figure 25-7. **Both vasa are visualized after injection of contrast into one vas only, revealing distal obstruction.**

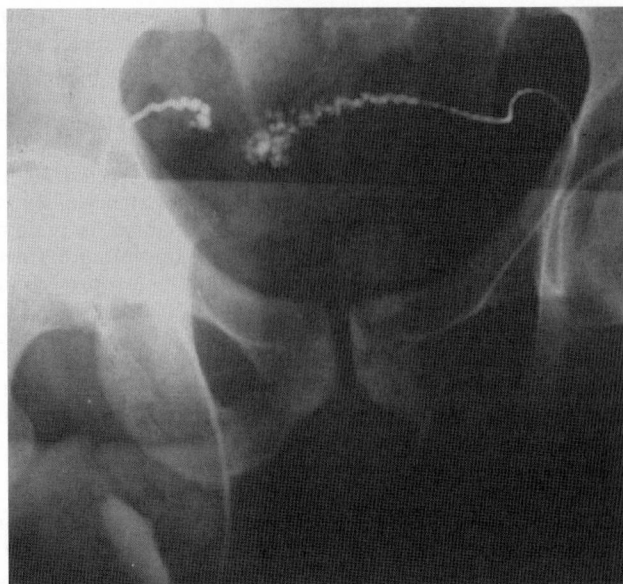

Figure 25-9. **Vasogram demonstrating partial absence of the vas deferens.**

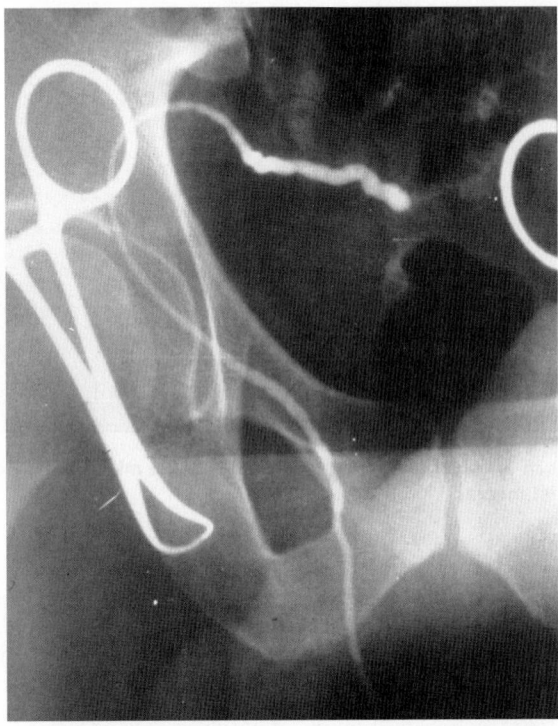

Figure 25-8. **Vasography reveals a blind-ending vas deferens far from the ejaculatory duct.**

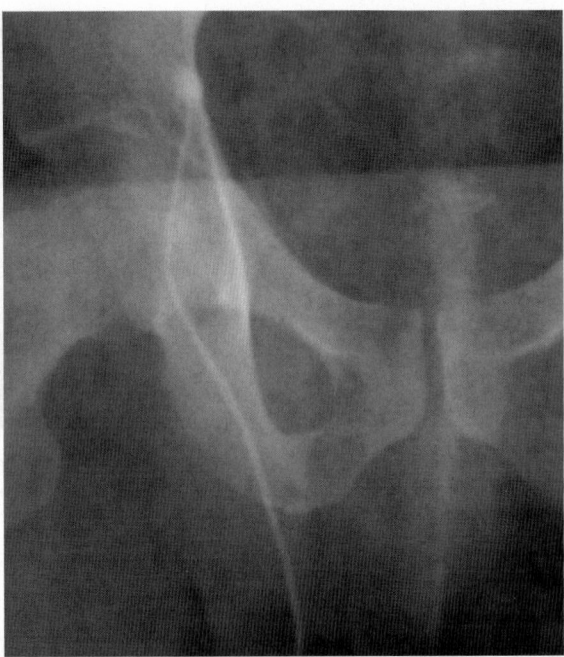

Figure 25-10. **Vasography reveals an obstruction in the inguinal region.**

Vasography may reveal the vas deferens ending blindly, far from the ejaculatory ducts (Fig. 25-8). This finding indicates congenital partial absence of the vas deferens, and these patients should be tested for cystic fibrosis mutations (see Chapter 24). If this is found bilaterally (Fig. 25-9), reconstruction is impossible, but vasal or epididymal sperm can be aspirated into standard laboratory pipettes (see the section on microsurgical epididymal sperm aspiration techniques) and cryopreserved for future IVF with ICSI. If vasography reveals obstruction in the inguinal region (Fig. 25-10), either inguinal vasovasostomy or crossed transseptal vasovasostomy, using the contralateral unobstructed vas (see the section on crossed vasovasostomy), may be performed. **The hemitransected vasography sites are carefully closed microsurgically** using two or three interrupted

10-0 monofilament nylon sutures for the mucosa and 9-0 for the muscularis and adventitia (see the discussion of the microsurgical multilayer microdot method).

If the vasal fluid reveals no sperm and vasography confirms patency of the seminal vesical end of the vas, the vas is completely transected, and the seminal vesical end is prepared for vasoepididymostomy (see later). If the vasal fluid reveals many sperm and vasography is normal, then retrograde ejaculation, lack of emission, or aperistalsis of the vas (Tiffany and Goldstein, 1985; Tillem and Mellinger, 1999) is the cause of the azoospermia.

Fine-Needle Vasography

Exposure of the vas in its straight portion may allow vasography to be performed with a fine needle, obviating the need for hemitransection of the vas. Dewire and Thomas (1995) used a 30-gauge lymphangiogram needle attached to Silastic tubing. When the sensation of puncture of the lumen is detected, 50% water-soluble contrast is injected to confirm patency radiographically. This has proven to be a difficult technique for even experienced microsurgeons to master. Accurate evaluation of vasal fluid for sperm is difficult because it is so scant. If barbotage with saline or lactated Ringer solution reveals the presence of sperm, then epididymal obstruction has been excluded and contrast can be injected. Collection of vasal sperm for cryopreservation is difficult with this technique. Percutaneous vasography through the scrotal skin has been successfully performed in China (Li, 1980) using the same ringed percutaneous fixation clamp as for the no-scalpel vasectomy. After fixation of the vas beneath the scrotal skin, the vas lumen is punctured with a 22-gauge sharp needle and cannulated with a 24-gauge blunt needle through which vasography is performed. This technique is even more difficult than the direct vision technique with a fine needle.

Complications of Vasography

Stricture

Multiple attempts at percutaneous vasography using sharp needles can result in stricture or obstruction at the vasography site. Imprecise closure of a vasotomy can also result in stricture and obstruction (Howards et al, 1975a; Poore et al, 1997). Use of non–water-soluble contrast agents may also result in stricture, and these agents should not be used for vasography.

Injury to the Vasal Blood Supply

If the vasal blood supply is injured at the site of vasography, vasovasostomy proximal to the vasography site may result in ischemia, necrosis, and obstruction of the intervening segment of vas.

Hematoma

Bipolar cautery should be used for meticulous hemostasis to prevent hematoma in the perivasal sheath.

Sperm Granuloma

Leaky closure of a vasography site may lead to the development of a sperm granuloma, which can result in stricture or obstruction of the vas. The microsurgical technique for closure of vasography sites is identical to that for vasovasostomy described later in this chapter.

Transrectal Vasography and Seminal Vesiculography

If transrectal ultrasound reveals markedly dilated seminal vesicles and/or a midline müllerian duct cyst in a man with obstructive azoospermia, transrectal aspiration followed by instillation of indigo carmine mixed with radiographic contrast is a useful diagnostic maneuver (Jarow, 1994; Katz et al, 1994; Riedenklau et al, 1995; Eisenberg et al, 2008).

The same bowel preparation and antibiotic coverage used for transrectal prostate biopsy is employed. The fine-needle aspirate is examined for sperm. If sperm are present, it means that at least one vas and epididymis are patent. One-half milliliter of indigo carmine is diluted with 1.5 mL of 50% water-soluble contrast and instilled. If a flat plate reveals a potentially resectable lesion, TURED is performed (see later). Visualization of blue dye effluxing from the ejaculatory ducts or an unroofed cyst aids in determining the adequacy of the resection (Cornel et al, 1999).

This technique obviates the need for formal open scrotal vasography in men with transrectally accessible lesions. If sperm are found in the aspirate, TUR may immediately be undertaken without violating the scrotum. Sperm-laden aspirates may be frozen for future IVF with ICSI if surgery fails.

If no sperm are found in the aspirated fluid, it suggests that secondary epididymal obstruction exists. Simultaneous TURED and vasoepididymostomy is rarely successful. In the face of both ejaculatory duct obstruction and bilateral epididymal obstruction, the best option would be epididymal sperm aspiration for cryopreservation for future IVF and ICSI.

KEY POINTS: VASOGRAPHY

- Perform vasography only if testicular biopsy confirms spermatogenesis consistent with obstructive azoospermia.
- Perform vasography only at the time of planned reconstruction.
- Always sample vasal fluid first to allow cryopreservation of motile sperm if found.
- Use indigo carmine instead of methylene blue to confirm patency.
- Formal vasography with x-ray contrast is needed only to locate obstructions proximal to the internal inguinal ring.
- If transrectal ultrasound reveals dilated seminal vesicles and/or a midline (müllerian duct) cyst, transrectal fine-needle aspiration followed by instillation of contrast and indigo carmine should be performed. If motile sperm are found, they should be cryopreserved.

VASOVASOSTOMY

The number of American men who undergo vasectomy has remained stable at about 500,000 per year, as has the divorce rate of 50%. Surveys suggest that 2% to 6% of vasectomized men will ultimately seek reversal. Furthermore, obstructive azoospermia can be the result of iatrogenic injuries to the vas deferens, usually from hernia repair, in 6% of azoospermic men (Sheynkin et al, 1998a; Shin et al, 2005).

Preoperative Evaluation

Before attempted surgical reconstruction of the reproductive tract, adequate spermatogenesis should be documented. A prior history of natural fertility prevasectomy is usually adequate.

Physical Examination

Testis. Small or soft testes suggest impaired spermatogenesis and predict a poor outcome.
Epididymis. An indurated irregular epididymis often predicts secondary epididymal obstruction, necessitating vasoepididymostomy.
Sperm Granuloma. A sperm granuloma at the testicular end of the vas suggests that sperm have been leaking at the vasectomy site. This vents the high pressures away from the epididymis and is associated with a better prognosis for restored fertility regardless of the time interval since vasectomy (Wosnitzer and Goldstein, 2013).
Vasal Gap. When a very destructive vasectomy has been performed, most of the scrotal straight vas may be absent or fibrotic and the patient should be advised that inguinal extension of the scrotal incision will be necessary to mobilize adequate length of vas to enable a tension-free anastomosis.
Scars from Previous Surgery. Operative scars in the inguinal or scrotal region should alert surgeon to the possibility of iatrogenic inguinal obstruction (hernia repair) or vasal or epididymal obstruction (hydrocelectomy, orchiopexy) (Sheynkin et al, 1998a; Hopps and Goldstein, 2006).

Laboratory Tests

1. Semen analysis with centrifugation and examination of the pellet for sperm should be performed preoperatively.

Complete sperm with tails are found in 10% of preoperative pellets a mean of 10 years after vasectomy (Lemack and Goldstein, 1996). **Under these circumstances sperm are certain to be found in the vas on at least one side, indicating a favorable prognosis for restored fertility.** Men with a low semen volume should have a transrectal ultrasound to investigate the possibility of an additional ejaculatory duct obstruction.

2. Serum and antisperm antibody studies: **The presence of serum antisperm antibodies corroborates the diagnosis of obstruction and the presence of active spermatogenesis** (Lee et al, 2009).

3. Serum FSH: Men with small soft testes should have serum FSH measured. An elevated FSH predicts impaired spermatogenesis and a poorer prognosis.

4. Prostate-specific antigen (PSA): Vasectomy reversal candidates over age 40 should have serum PSA measured.

Anesthesia

General anesthesia is preferred. Slight movements are greatly magnified by the operating microscope and disturb performance of the anastomosis. In cooperative patients regional or even local anesthesia with sedation can be used if the vasal ends are easily palpable, a sperm granuloma is present, and/or the time interval since vasectomy is short, decreasing the likelihood of secondary epididymal obstruction. When large vasal gaps are present, extensions of the incisions high into the inguinal canal may be necessary. Furthermore, if vasoepididymostomy is necessary, the operating time could exceed 4 or 5 hours. **Local anesthesia limits the options available to the surgeon.** Hypobaric spinal anesthesia with long-acting agents such as bupivacaine (Marcaine) can provide 4 to 5 hours of anesthesia time and has the advantage of eliminating lower body motion. Epidural anesthesia with an indwelling catheter can be equally effective.

Surgical Approaches

Scrotal Incision

Bilateral high vertical scrotal incisions provide the most direct access to the obstructed site in cases of vasectomy reversal. Length is usually a problem on the abdominal end but not on the testicular end. Mark the location of the external inguinal ring (Fig. 25-11). **If the vasal gap is large or the vasectomy site is high, this incision can easily be extended toward the external ring.** If the vasectomy site is low, it is easy to pull up the testicular end. This incision should be made at least 1 cm lateral to the base of the penis. **The testis should be delivered with the tunica vaginalis left intact.** This provides excellent exposure of the entire scrotal vas deferens and, if necessary, the epididymis.

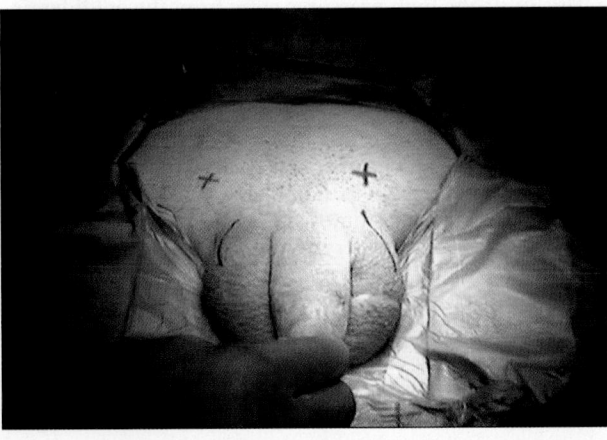

Figure 25-11. **The Xs mark the locations of the external ring. Incisions are marked on the hemiscrotums.**

Inguinal Incision

An inguinal incision is the preferred approach in men when obstruction of the inguinal vas deferens from prior herniorrhaphy or orchiopexy is strongly suspected. Incision through the previous scar usually leads directly to the site of obstruction. If the obstruction turns out to be scrotal or epididymal, it is a simple matter to deliver the testis through the inguinal incision or through a separate scrotal incision to perform the anastomosis.

Preparation of the Vasa

The vas is grasped above and below the site of obstruction with two Babcock clamps. Penrose drains replace the Babcock clamps and facilitate the dissection. The vasal vessels and periadventitial sheath are included. **Transillumination of the periadventitial sheath** by proper adjustment of the operating light **allows clear visualization of the blood vessels, which facilitates dissection of the periadventitial sheath and prevents damage to the vasal vessels.** The vas is mobilized enough to allow a tension-free anastomosis. To preserve good blood supply **the vas should not be stripped of its sheath.** The obstructed segment and, if present, sperm granuloma at the vasectomy site should be dissected out and excised. By staying right on the vas and/or sperm granuloma during this dissection, the surgeon reduces the risk of injuring the testicular artery. **Injury to adjacent cord structures, especially the testicular artery, is likely to result in testicular atrophy because the vasal artery has usually been interrupted at the vasectomy site.**

When large vasal gaps are present, a gauze-wrapped index finger is used to bluntly separate the cord structures from the vas. Blunt finger dissection through the external ring will free the vas to the internal inguinal ring if additional abdominal side length is necessary. These maneuvers will leave all the vasal vessels intact. **When the vasal gap is extremely large, additional length can be achieved by dissecting the entire convoluted vas free of its attachments to the epididymal tunica (Fig. 25-12),** allowing the testis to drop upside down. These maneuvers can provide an additional 4 to 6 cm of length. To maintain the integrity of the vasal vessels, this dissection is best performed using magnifying loupes or the

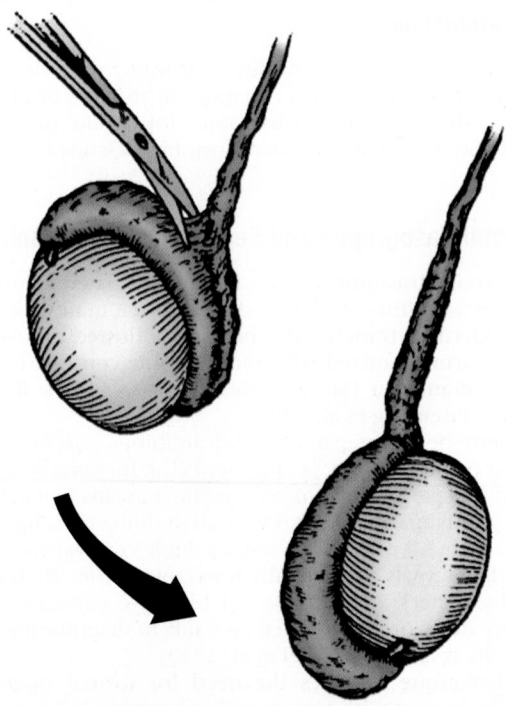

Figure 25-12. **An additional 4 to 6 cm of length can be obtained by dissecting the epididymis off the testis from the vasoepididymal junction to the caput epididymis.**

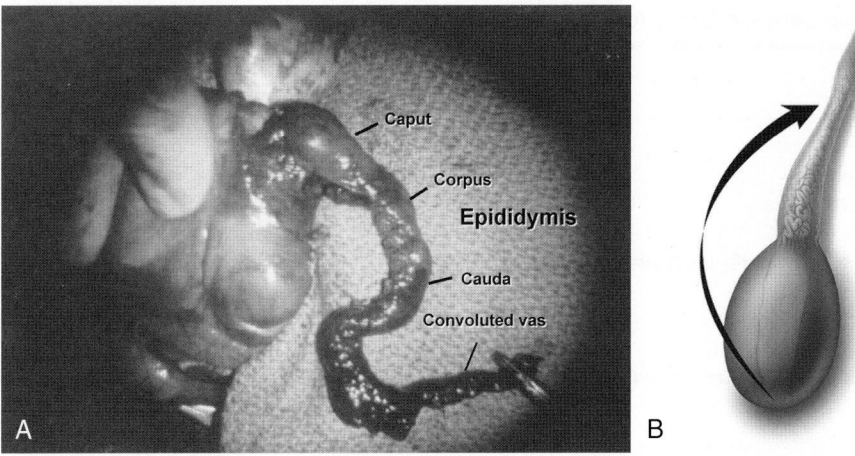

Figure 25-13. **A and B, An additional 4 to 6 cm of length can be obtained by dissecting the epididymis off the testis from the vasoepididymal junction to the caput epididymis.**

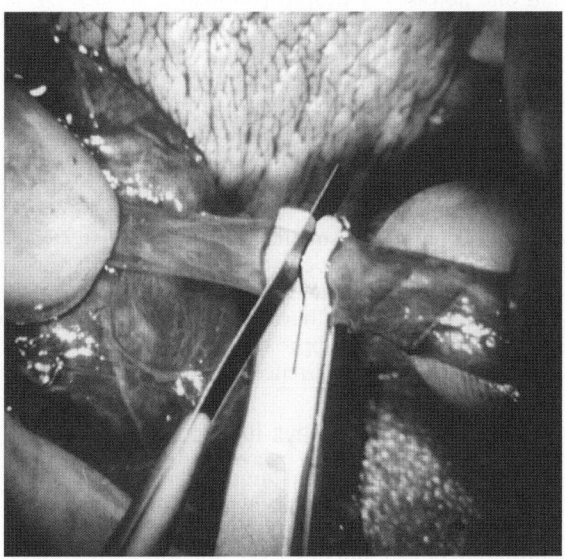

Figure 25-14. **An ultrasharp knife drawn through a slotted 2-, 2.5-, or 3-mm diameter nerve-holding clamp (Accurate Surgical and Scientific Instrument Corp., Westbury, NY) yields a perfect 90-degree cut.**

operating microscope under low power. If the amount of vas removed is so large that even these measures fail to allow a tension-free anastomosis, the incision can be extended to the internal inguinal ring, the floor of the inguinal canal cut, and the vas rerouted under the floor, as in a difficult orchiopexy. An additional 4 to 6 cm of length can be obtained by dissecting the epididymis off the testis from the vasoepididymal (VE) junction to the caput epididymis (Fig. 25-13). The superior epididymal vessels are left intact and provide adequate blood supply to the testicular end of the vas. With this combination of maneuvers, up to 10-cm gaps can be bridged.

After the vasa have been freed, the testicular end of the vas is cut transversely. An ultrasharp knife drawn through a slotted 2-, 2.5- or 3-mm diameter nerve-holding clamp (Accurate Surgical and Scientific Instrument Corp., Westbury, NY) yields a perfect 90-degree cut (Fig. 25-14). The cut surface of the testicular end of the vas deferens is inspected under 15× to 25× magnification. **A healthy white mucosal ring should be seen and should spring back immediately after gentle dilation. The muscularis should appear smooth and soft. A gritty-looking muscularis layer indicates the presence of scar or fibrotic tissues.** The cut surface should look like a bull's eye with the three vasal layers distinctly visible. Healthy bleeding

should be noted from both the cut edge of the mucosa and the surface of the muscularis. If the blood supply is poor or the muscularis is gritty, the vas is recut until healthy tissue is found. The vasal artery and vein are then clamped and ligated with 6-0 nylon. Small bleeders are controlled with microbipolar forceps set at low power. Once a patent lumen has been established on the testicular end, the vas is milked and a clean glass slide is touched to its surface. The vasal fluid is immediately mixed with a drop or two of saline or lactated Ringer solution and preserved under a coverslip for microscope examination. The abdominal end of the vas deferens is prepared in a similar manner and the lumen gently dilated with a microvessel dilator and cannulated with a 24-gauge angiocatheter sheath. Injection of saline or Ringer lactate confirms its patency. After injection of Ringer solution and a test dilation the vas is recut to obtain a fresh surface. **A minimum of instrumentation of the mucosa should be performed.**

After preparation, the ends of the vasa are stabilized with a Microspike approximator clamp (Goldstein, 1985) to remove all tension before the anastomosis is performed. Isolating the field through a slit in a rubber dam prevents microsutures from sticking to the surrounding tissue. A sterile tongue blade covered with a large Penrose drain is placed beneath the ends of the vasa to provide a platform on which to perform the anastomosis.

When to Perform Vasoepididymostomy

The gross appearance of fluid expressed from the testicular end of the vas is usually predictive of findings on microscopic examination (Table 25-1). If microscopic examination of the vasal fluid reveals the presence of sperm with tails, vasovasostomy is performed. If no fluid is found, a 24-gauge angiocatheter sheath is inserted into the lumen of the testicular end of the vas and barbotaged with 0.1 mL of saline while the convoluted vas is vigorously milked. The barbotage fluid is expressed onto a slide and examined. **Men with large sperm granulomas often have virtually no dilation of the testicular end of the vas and little or no fluid initially; however, with barbotage and vigorous milking, invariably sperm can be found in this scant fluid.** If there is no sperm granuloma, and the vas is absolutely dry and spermless after multiple samples have been examined, vasoepididymostomy is indicated. If the fluid expressed from the vas is found to be thick, white, water insoluble, and toothpaste-like in quality, microscope examination rarely reveals sperm. Under these circumstances, the tunica vaginalis is opened and the epididymis inspected. If clear evidence of obstruction is found—that is, an epididymal sperm granuloma with dilated tubules above and collapsed tubules below—vasoepididymostomy is performed. **When in doubt, or if not very experienced with vasoepididymostomy, vasovasostomy should be performed.** However, only 15% of men with bilateral absence of sperm in the

TABLE 25-1 Relationship between Gross Appearance of Vasal Fluid and Microscopic Findings

VASAL FLUID APPEARANCE	MOST COMMON FINDINGS ON MICROSCOPIC EXAMINATION	SURGICAL PROCEDURE INDICATED
Copious, crystal clear, watery	No sperm in fluid	Vasovasostomy
Copious, cloudy thin, water soluble	Usually sperm with tails	Vasovasostomy
Copious, creamy yellow, water soluble	Usually many sperm heads, occasional sperm with short tails	Vasovasostomy
Copious, thick white toothpaste-like, water insoluble	No sperm	Vasoepididymostomy
Scant white thin fluid	No sperm	Vasoepididymostomy
Dry spermless vas; no granuloma at vasectomy site	No sperm	Vasoepididymostomy
Scant fluid, granuloma present at vasectomy site	Barbotage fluid reveals sperm	Vasovasostomy

vasal fluid after barbotage and an intensive search will have sperm return to the ejaculate after vasovasostomy (Sheynkin et al, 2000).

When copious, crystal clear, water-like fluid squirts out from the vas and no sperm are found in this fluid, a vasovasostomy is performed because the likelihood is that sperm will return to the ejaculate after vasovasostomy is performed.

Multiple Vasal Obstructions

If saline injection reveals that the abdominal end of the vas deferens is not patent, a 2-0 nylon or polypropylene suture is gently threaded into the vas lumen to determine the site of obstruction. If the obstruction is within 5 cm of the original vasectomy site, the abdominal end of the vas deferens may be dissected to this site and excised. The incision should then be extended inguinally to free the vas up extensively toward the internal inguinal ring. The testicular end then should also be freed up to the VE junction. If the site of the second obstruction is so far from the vasectomy site that two vasovasostomies are necessary, a single crossed vasovasostomy should be performed to yield one good system (see the section on crossed vasovasostomy). If this is not possible, vasal or epididymal sperm is aspirated into micropipettes and cryopreserved for future IVF with ICSI (see the section on sperm retrieval techniques). Simultaneous vasovasostomies at two separate sites will usually lead to devascularization of the intervening segment with fibrosis and necrosis.

Varicocelectomy and Vasovasostomy

When men undergoing vasovasostomy or vasoepididymostomy are found to have significant varicoceles on physical examination, it is tempting to repair the varicoceles at the same time. When varicocelectomy is properly performed, all spermatic veins are ligated and the only remaining avenues for testicular venous return are the vasal veins. In men who have had vasectomy and are seeking reversal, the vasal veins are likely to be compromised from either the original vasectomy or the reversal itself. Furthermore the integrity of the vasal artery in those men is also likely to be compromised. Varicocelectomy in such men requires preservation of the testicular artery as the primary remaining testicular blood supply as well as preservation of some avenue for venous return.

Microscopic varicocelectomy can ensure preservation of the testicular artery in most cases. Deliberate preservation of small cremasteric or perivasal veins provides venous return. In one series of 570 men seeking vasectomy reversal, 19 had large varicoceles (20 left, 7 bilateral). Microsurgical varicocelectomy was performed at the same time as vasovasostomy. The cremasteric veins and the fine network of veins adherent to the testicular artery were left intact for venous return and to minimize the chances of injury to the testicular artery. Postoperatively, 5 of 26 varicoceles recurred (19%) (Goldstein, 1995). This compares with a recurrence rate of less than 1% in 3500 varicocelectomies I performed in nonvasectomized men in whom the vasal vessels were intact and the cremasteric veins and

periarterial venous network were ligated. However, Mullhall and colleagues performed a series of simultaneous microsurgical vasovasostomies and varicocelectomies without intentionally preserving the cremasteric and periarterial network. They reported a low recurrence rate and no cases of atrophy (Mulhall et al, 1997). It is interesting to note that the increase in recurrences when the cremasteric veins and periarterial venous network were left intact suggests that these veins contribute to a significant proportion of varicocele recurrences.

If varicocelectomy is performed at the same time as vasovasostomy or vasoepididymostomy, it is important that a microscope be used and the testicular artery preserved. Another approach, especially when the female partner is young, is to do the vasovasostomy or vasoepididymostomy first. The semen quality is then assessed postoperatively. If necessary, varicocelectomy can be safely performed 6 months or more later when venous and arterial channels have formed across the anastomotic line. This two-stage delayed approach has been completed a dozen times with no atrophy or recurrence.

Anastomotic Techniques: Keys to Success

All successful vasovasostomy techniques depend on adherence to surgical principles that are universally applicable to anastomoses of all tubular structures. These include the following.
1. **Accurate mucosa-to-mucosa approximation**
   In human vasovasostomy, the lumen on the testicular side is usually dilated, often to a diameter two to five times that of the abdominal side. Techniques that work well with lumina of equal diameters may be less successful when applied to lumina of markedly discrepant diameters.
2. **Leakproof anastomosis**
   Sperm are highly antigenic and provoke an inflammatory reaction when they escape from the normally intact lining of the excurrent ducts of the male reproductive tract. Extravasated sperm adversely influence the success of vasovasostomy (Hagan and Coffey, 1977). Unlike blood vessel anastomoses, in which platelets and clotting factors seal the gaps between sutures, vasal and epididymal fluid contain no platelets or clotting factors, so the water-tightness of the anastomosis is entirely dependent on the mucosal sutures.
3. **Tension-free anastomosis**
   When an anastomosis is performed under tension, sperm may appear in the ejaculate for several months after surgery. Ultimately, sperm counts and motility will decrease and azoospermia may ensue. At re-exploration only a thin fibrotic band is found at the anastomotic site. This can be prevented by adequately freeing up the vasa and placing reinforcing sutures in the sheath of the vas.
4. **Good blood supply**
   If the cut vas exhibits poor blood supply, it should be recut until healthy bleeding is encountered. If extensive resection is necessary, additional length should be obtained using the techniques previously described.

5. **Healthy mucosa and muscularis**

If the mucosa or cut surface of the vas exhibits poor distensibility after dilation, peels away from the underlying muscularis, or shreds easily, then the vas should be cut back until healthy mucosa is found. Surgeons should be aware that if needle electrocautery was used in vasectomy, the area of damage to the mucosa and muscularis by the electric current may extend far beyond the tip of the needle cautery. If the muscularis is found to be fibrotic or gritty, the vas must be recut until healthy tissue is found.

6. **Good atraumatic anastomotic technique**

If multiple surgical errors occur during the procedure, such as inadvertent cutting of the mucosa with the needles when placing sutures, tearing through of sutures, or back-walling of the mucosa, the anastomosis should be resected and redone immediately.

Setup

An operating microscope providing variable magnification from 6× to 32× is used. A diploscope providing identical fields for both surgeon and assistant is preferred. Foot pedal controls for a motorized zoom and focus leave the surgeon's hands free.

Both surgeon and assistant should be comfortably seated on microsurgical chairs that stabilize the chest and arms. This dramatically improves stability and accuracy. An inexpensive alternative is a simple rolling stool with a round bean bag (meditation pillow) taped on top for padding. Two armboards placed on both sides of the surgeon and built up to the appropriate height with folded blankets taped to the boards provide excellent arm support. **A right-handed surgeon should sit at the patient's right side** so that the forehand stitch is always on the smaller, more difficult abdominal side lumen.

Microsurgical Multilayer Microdot Method

The microsurgical multilayer microdot method of vasovasostomy can handle lumina of markedly discrepant diameters in the straight or convoluted vas. **The microdot technique ensures precise suture placement by exact mapping of each planned suture. The microdot method separates the planning from the placement** (Goldstein et al, 1998; Dabaja et al, 2013). This allows focus on only one task at a time and results in substantially improved accuracy.

A microtip marking pen (Devon Skin Marker Extra Fine No. 151) is used to map out planned needle exit points. **Exactly six mucosal sutures are used for every anastomosis** because it is easy to map out and always results in a leakproof closure even when the lumen diameters are markedly discrepant.

Immediately after drying of the cut surface of the testicular end of the vas with a Weck-Cel, a dot is made at the 3 o'clock position halfway between the mucosal ring and the outer edge of the muscle layer. A line is extended out from this dot to serve as a reference point. The second dot is made at the 9 o'clock position, and a line is extended from this dot as well. Additional dots are placed at the 11, 1, 5, and 7 o'clock positions for a total of six. The abdominal end of the vas is marked in the same way to exactly match the testicular end (Fig. 25-15). Monofilament 10-0 nylon sutures, double-armed with 70-micron diameter taper-point needles bent into a fish hook configuration (available from Sharpoint and Ethicon), are used. **Double-armed sutures allow inside-out placement** (Fig. 25-16), **eliminating the need for manipulation of the mucosa and the possibility of back-walling.** If the mucosal rings are not sharply defined, the cut surfaces of the vasal ends are stained with indigo carmine to highlight the mucosa (Sheynkin et al, 1999b). The anastomosis is begun with the placement of three 10-0 mucosal sutures anteriorly (Fig. 25-17). **The small abdominal side lumen is gently and momentarily dilated with a microvessel dilator just before placement of the sutures.** For accurate mucosal approximation, only a small amount of mucosa is included, but one third to one half the muscle wall thickness. **Exactly the same amount of tissue is included in the bites on each side. The needle**

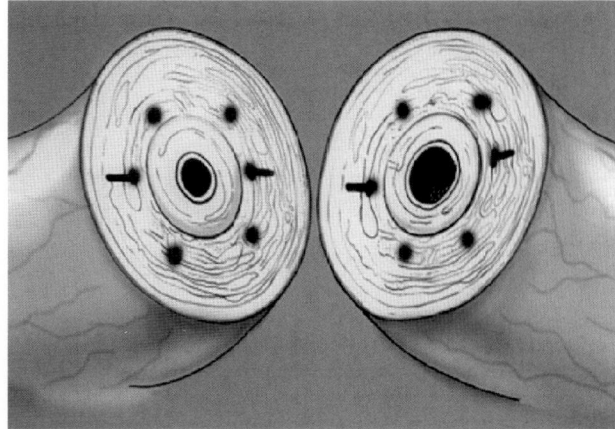

Figure 25-15. The abdominal end of the vas is marked in the same way to exactly match the testicular end.

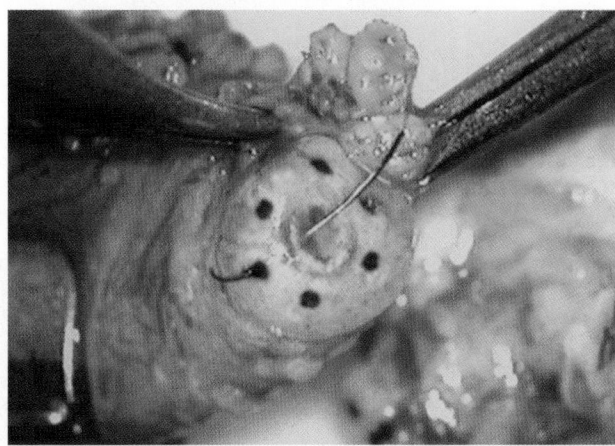

Figure 25-16. Double-armed sutures allow inside-out placement.

should exit through the center of each dot. After placement, the three mucosal sutures are tied. Two 9-0 monofilament nylon deep muscularis sutures are placed exactly between the previously placed mucosal sutures, just above but not through the mucosa (Fig. 25-18), and then are tied. These sutures seal the gaps between the mucosal sutures without trauma to the mucosa from the larger 100-micron diameter cutting needle required to penetrate the tough vas muscularis and adventitia. The vas is rotated 180 degrees (Fig. 25-19), and three additional 10-0 sutures are placed through each microdot and then tied to complete the mucosal portion of the anastomosis (Fig. 25-20). Just before the last mucosal suture is tied, the lumen is irrigated with heparinized Ringer solution to prevent the formation of clot in the lumen. After completion of the mucosal layer (Fig. 25-21), four more 9-0 deep muscularis sutures are placed exactly between each mucosal suture, just above but not penetrating the mucosa. Four to six 9-0 nylon interrupted sutures are placed between each muscular suture. This is a purely adventitial layer that covers the underlying mucosal suture. The anastomosis is finished by approximation of the vasal sheath with six to eight interrupted sutures of 8-0 nylon, completely covering the anastomosis and relieving it of all tension (Fig. 25-22).

Anastomosis in the Convoluted Vas

Vasovasostomy performed in the convoluted portion of the vas deferens is technically more demanding than anastomoses in the straight portion. **Fear of cutting back into the convoluted vas to obtain healthy tissue may lead surgeons to complete an**

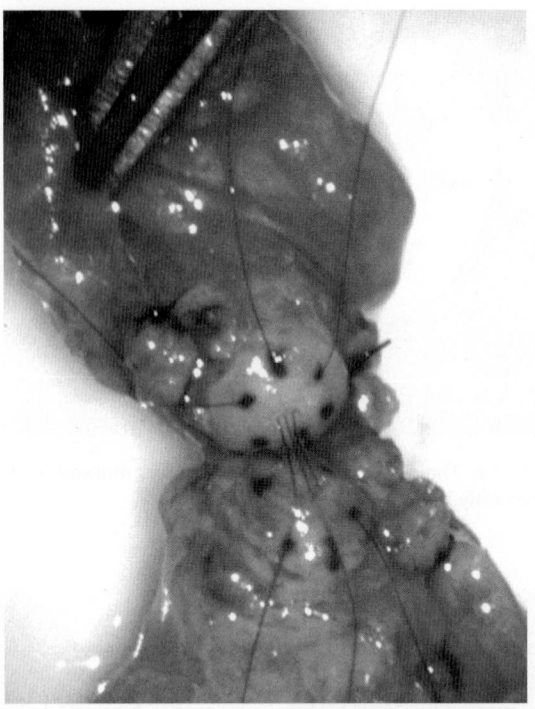

Figure 25-17. **The anastomosis is begun with the placement of three 10-0 mucosal sutures anteriorly.**

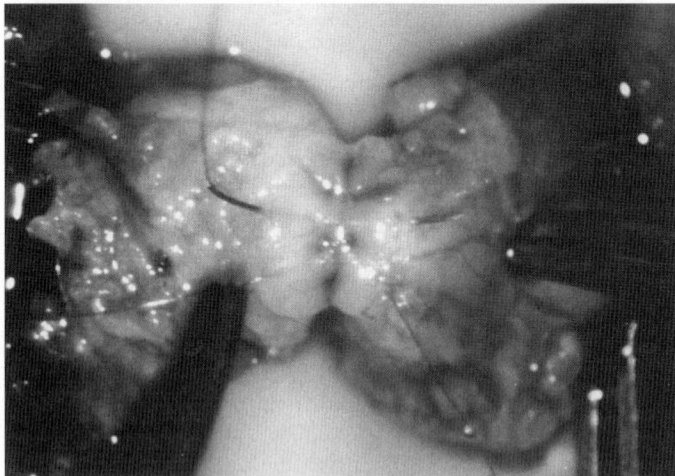

Figure 25-18. Place two 9-0 monofilament nylon deep muscularis sutures exactly between the previously placed mucosal sutures, just above but not through the mucosa.

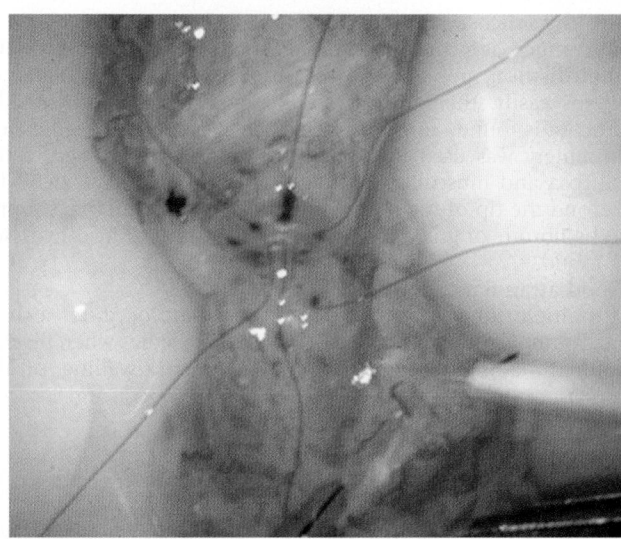

Figure 25-19. **Rotate the vas 180 degrees, then place three more 10-0 sutures through the remaining microdots.**

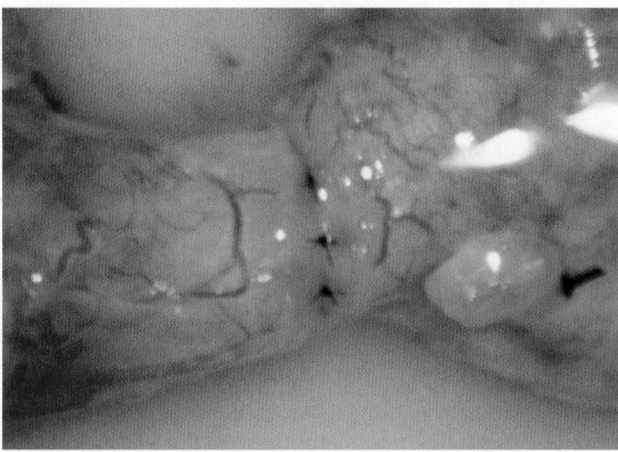

Figure 25-20. **The mucosal layer is complete.**

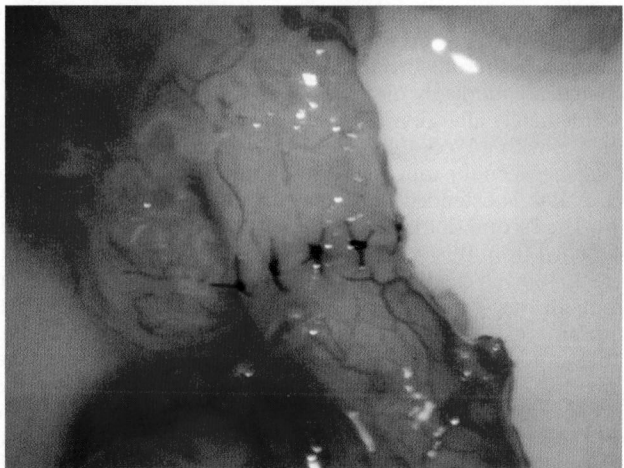

Figure 25-21. **Additional sutures are placed between the mucosal sutures, completing the anastomosis.**

anastomosis in the straight portion when the testicular end of the vas has poor blood supply, unhealthy or friable mucosa, or gritty fibrotic muscularis. Adherence to the following principles will enable anastomosis in the convoluted vas to succeed as often as those in the straight portion.

1. **A perfect transverse cut yielding a round ring of mucosa and a lumen directed straight down is essential.** A very oblique lumen with a thin flap of muscle and mucosa on one side is not acceptable (Fig. 25-23). The vas should be recut at 0.5-mm intervals until a perfect cut with good blood supply and healthy tissue is obtained. Use of a slotted nerve clamp 2.5 or 3 mm in diameter and an ultrasharp knife facilitates this part of the procedure (see Fig. 25-14). Often the vas must be recut two or three times until a satisfactory cut is obtained.

2. **The convoluted vas should not be unraveled.** This disturbs the blood supply at the anastomotic line.

3. The sheath of the convoluted vas may be carefully dissected free of its attachments to the epididymal tunica (see Fig. 25-12). This will minimize disturbance of its blood supply and provide the necessary length to perform a tension-free anastomosis.

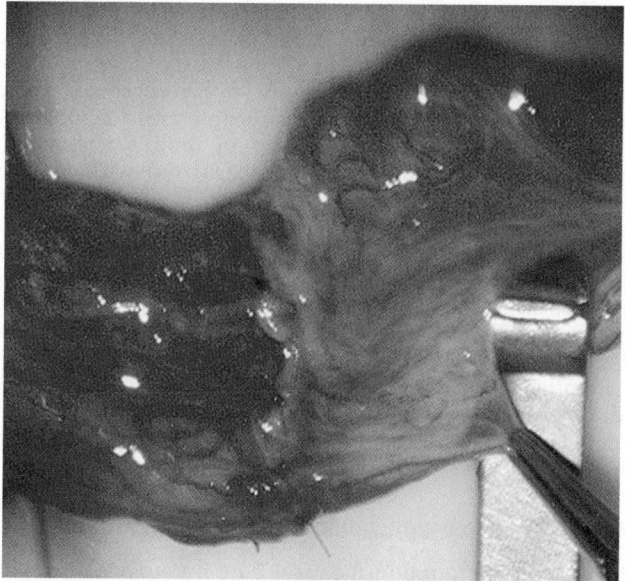

Figure 25-22. **Finish the anastomosis by approximating the vasal sheath with six interrupted sutures of 8-0 nylon, completely covering the anastomosis and relieving it of all tension.**

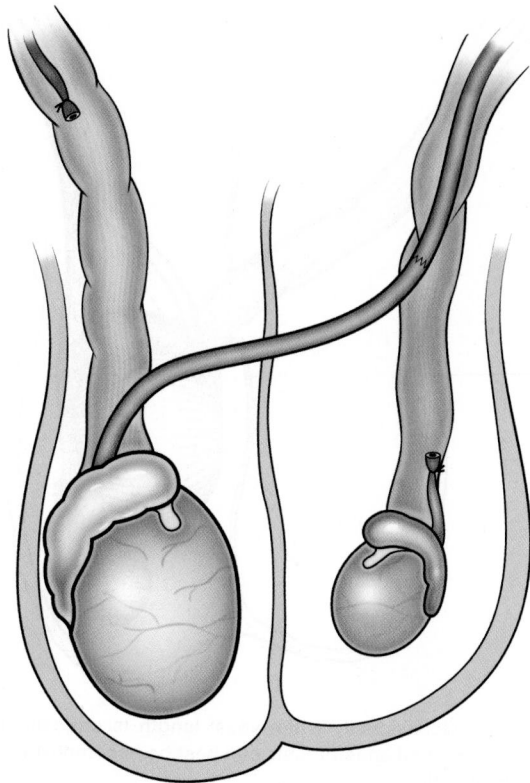

Figure 25-24. **A crossed vasovasostomy can be done in patients with a unilateral atrophic testis.**

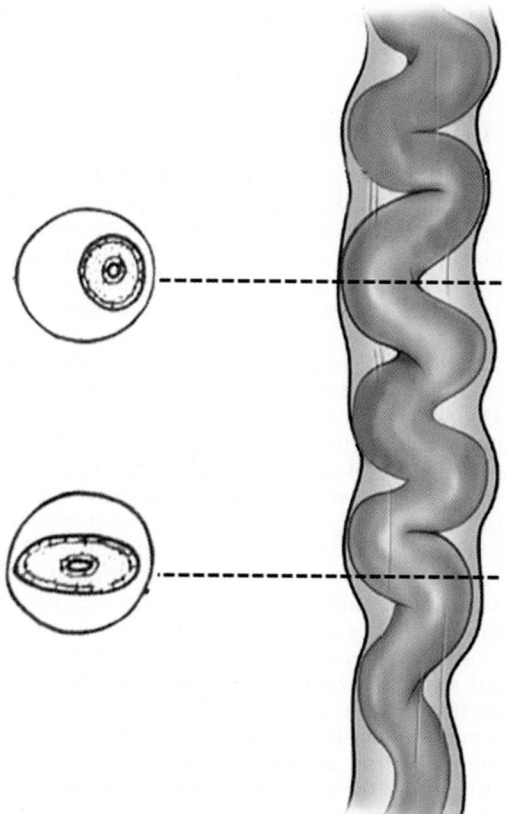

Figure 25-23. **A very oblique lumen with a thin flap of muscle and mucosa on one side is not acceptable.**

4. Care must be taken to avoid taking large bites of the muscularis and adventitial layers on the convoluted side to prevent inadvertent perforation of adjacent convolutions.
5. Reinforce the anastomosis by approximating the vasal sheath of the straight portion to the sheath of the convoluted portion with six interrupted sutures of 7-0 nylon. This will remove all tension from the anastomosis.

Crossed Vasovasostomy

Crossed vasovasostomy is a useful procedure that often provides an easy solution for otherwise difficult problems (Lizza et al, 1985; Hamidinia, 1988; Sheynkin et al, 1998a). **Crossover is indicated in the following circumstances:**
1. **Unilateral inguinal obstruction of the vas deferens associated with an atrophic testis on the contralateral side. A crossover vasovasostomy should be performed to connect a healthy testicle to the contralateral unobstructed vas.**
2. **Obstruction or aplasia of the inguinal vas or ejaculatory duct on one side and epididymal obstruction on the contralateral side.**

It is preferable to perform one anastomosis with a high probability of success (vasovasostomy) than two operations with a much lower chance of success (e.g., unilateral vasovasoepididymostomy and contralateral TURED).

Technique (Fig. 25-24)

Transect the vas attached to the atrophic testis at the junction of its straight and convoluted portion and confirm its patency with a Ringer or indigo carmine vasogram. Dissect the contralateral vas with the normal testis toward the inguinal obstruction. Clamp and transect it as high up as possible with a right angle clamp. Cross the testicular end of the vas through a capacious opening made in the scrotal septum and proceed with vasovasostomy as described earlier. This procedure is much easier than inguinal vasovasostomy, which requires finding both ends of the vas within the dense scar of a previous inguinal operation.

Transposition of the Testis

Occasionally when vasal length is critically short, a tension-free crossed anastomosis can best be accomplished by testicular transposition (Fig. 25-25). The spermatic cord is always longer than the vas.

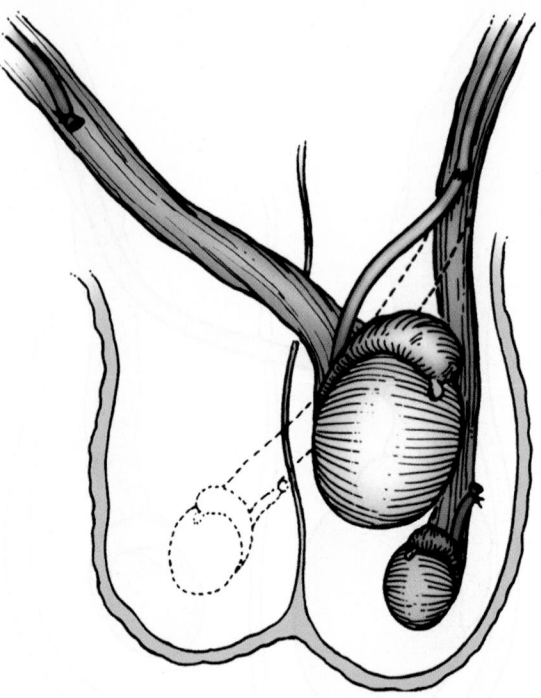

Figure 25-25. Occasionally when vasal length is critically short, a tension-free crossed anastomosis can best be accomplished by testicular transposition.

The testes will comfortably cross through a generous opening in the septum and sit nicely in the contralateral scrotal compartment.

Wound Closure

If the vasal dissection was extensive, Penrose drains are brought out the dependent portion of the right and left hemiscrota and fixed in place with sutures and safety pins, preferably before the anastomosis is begun. Placement of drains at the end of the procedure may potentially disturb the anastomosis. The dartos layer is approximated with interrupted 4-0 absorbable sutures and the skin with subcuticular sutures of 5-0 Monocryl. The wound heals with a fine scar. The use of through-and-through skin closures, which give an unacceptable "railroad track" scar, should be avoided. **Virtually all of our procedures are performed on an ambulatory basis.** If drains were placed, the patients are given detailed instructions (with explicit drawings) on how to remove the drains the next morning.

Postoperative Management

Sterile fluff gauze dressings are held in place with a snug-fitting scrotal supporter. Only perioperative antibiotics are used. Patients are discharged with a prescription for acetaminophen with codeine. They shower 48 hours after surgery. **They wear a scrotal supporter at all times (except in the shower), even when sleeping, for 6 weeks postoperatively. Thereafter, a scrotal supporter is worn during athletic activity until pregnancy is achieved.** Desk work is resumed in 3 days. No heavy work or sports are allowed for 3 weeks. **No intercourse or ejaculation is allowed for 3 weeks postoperatively.** Semen analyses are obtained at 1, 3, and 6 months postoperatively and every 6 months thereafter. If azoospermia persists at 6 months, a redo vasovasostomy or vasoepididymostomy will be necessary.

Postoperative Complications

The most common complication is hematoma. In 2500 operations, seven small hematomas occurred. None required surgical drainage. Most were walnut sized and perivasal. They take 6 to 12 weeks to resolve. Wound infection has not occurred. Late complications include sperm granuloma at the anastomotic site (approximately 5%). This usually is a harbinger of eventual obstruction. Late stricture and obstruction are disappointingly common (see later). **Progressive loss of motility followed by decreasing counts indicates stricture.** Our recent change from Prolene to **nylon sutures** (Sheynkin et al, 1999a), **use of the microdot system to prevent leaks, extensive dissection of the vas until healthy mucosa and muscularis are identified, constant attention to the preservation of good blood supply, and generous use of scrotal support until pregnancy is established have reduced the incidence of late obstruction from 12%** (Matthews et al, 1995) **to 5%** (Kolettis and Thomas, 1997) **at 18 months after surgery.** Because of the risk of late stricture and obstruction, we strongly encourage cryopreservation of semen specimens as soon as motile sperm appear in the ejaculate.

Long-Term Follow-up Evaluation after Vasovasostomy

When sperm are found in the vasal fluid on at least one side at the time of surgery, the anastomotic technique described results in appearance of sperm in the ejaculate in 99.5% of men (Goldstein et al, 1998; Dabaja et al, 2013). Pregnancy has occurred in 52% of couples followed for at least 2 years and 63% when female factors are excluded, with outcomes dependent on the time since vasectomy and female partner age (Kolettis et al, 2003; Boorjian et al, 2004; Kolettis et al, 2005; Gerrard et al, 2007; Wosnitzer and Goldstein, 2013).

SURGERY OF THE EPIDIDYMIS

Detailed knowledge of epididymal anatomy and physiology (presented in Chapters 21 and 22) is essential before undertaking surgery of this delicate but important structure. Sperm motility and fertilizing capacity progressively increase during passage through the 200-micron diameter, 12- to 15-foot long, tightly coiled single tubule. When the epididymis is obstructed and functionally shortened after vasoepididymostomy, even very short lengths of epididymis are able to adapt and allow some sperm to acquire motility and fertilizing capacity (Silber, 1989a; Jow et al, 1993). Adaptation may gradually continue for up to 2 years after surgical reconstruction, with progressive improvement in the fertility and motility of sperm. Nevertheless, preservation of the greatest possible length of functional epididymis is most likely to result in the best sperm quality after vasoepididymostomy (Schoysman and Bedford, 1986; Schlegel and Goldstein, 1993). Furthermore, because the wall of the epididymis is thinnest in the caput region and gradually thickens, because of the increasing numbers of smooth muscle cells in its more distal (inferior) end, anastomoses are technically easier to perform and more likely to succeed in its distal regions. **Because the corpus and cauda epididymis is a single tubule with a very small diameter, injury or occlusion of a tubule anywhere along its length will lead to total obstruction of outflow at that level.** For these reasons, **magnification, with loupes for macrodissection and with the operating microscope for anastomosis, is essential for performing all epididymal surgery.**

Fortunately, the epididymis is blessed with a rich blood supply derived from the testicular vessels superiorly and the deferential vessels inferiorly (see the earlier section on testicular blood supply and Chapter 21). Because of the extensive interconnections among these branches, either the testicular or deferential branches (but not both) to the epididymis may be divided without compromising epididymal viability.

Conversely, because the epididymal branches of the testicular artery are medial to and separate from the main testicular artery and veins, surgical procedures may be performed on the epididymis without compromise to testicular blood supply.

TABLE 25-2 Comparison of Three Common Techniques for Vasoepididymostomy

TECHNIQUES	ADVANTAGES	DISADVANTAGES
Intussusception (longitudinal intussusception vasoepididymostomy)	Two sutures placed longitudinally in the dilated epididymal tubule provide four points of fixation. Virtually bloodless anastomosis.	Cannot assess tubular fluid for sperm before anastomosis setup.
End-side	Virtually bloodless anastomosis. Epididymal fluid can be examined before anastomosis.	Difficult suture placement to a collapsed tubule.
End-end	Epididymal fluid can be examined before anastomosis. Easy and rapid identification of the level of obstruction in the epididymis. Allows upward mobilization of epididymis to bridge a large vasal gap.	Difficult hemostasis on transected epididymis. Difficult to identify the proper tubule for anastomosis. Difficult outer layer closure. Vasal blood supply from inferior epididymal artery is sacrificed.

Vasoepididymostomy

Before the development of microsurgical techniques, accurate approximation of the vasal lumen to that of a specific epididymal tubule was not possible. Vasoepididymostomy was performed by aligning the vas deferens adjacent to a slash made in multiple epididymal tubules and hoping a fistula would form. Results with this primitive technique were poor. Microsurgical approaches allow accurate approximation of the vasal mucosa to that of a single epididymal tubule (Silber, 1978), resulting in marked improvement in the patency and pregnancy rates (Schlegel and Goldstein, 1993; Chan et al, 2005). **Microsurgical vasoepididymostomy, however, is the most technically demanding procedure in all of microsurgery.** In virtually no other operation are results so dependent on technical perfection. **Microsurgical vasoepididymostomy should be attempted only by microsurgeons who perform the procedure frequently.**

Indications

The indications for vasoepididymostomy at the time of vasectomy reversal are reviewed in the earlier section on vasovasostomy. For obstructive azoospermia not caused by vasectomy, **vasoepididymostomy is indicated when the testis biopsy reveals complete spermatogenesis and scrotal exploration reveals the absence of sperm in the vasal lumen with no vasal or ejaculatory duct obstruction.** The preoperative evaluation is identical to that described earlier for vasovasostomy.

Microsurgical End-to-Side Vasoepididymostomy

End-to-side techniques of vasoepididymostomy have the advantage of being minimally traumatic to the epididymis and relatively bloodless (Table 25-2) (Wagenknecht et al, 1980; Krylov and Borovikov, 1984; Fogdestam et al, 1986; Thomas, 1987; Chan et al, 2005; Schiff et al, 2005). The end-to-side technique does not disturb the epididymal blood supply. When the level of epididymal obstruction is clearly demarcated by the presence of markedly dilated tubules proximally and collapsed tubules distally, the site at which the anastomosis should be performed is readily apparent. The end-to-side approach has the advantage of allowing accurate approximation of the muscularis and adventitia of the vas deferens to a precisely tailored opening in the tunica of the epididymis. This is the preferred technique when vasoepididymostomy is performed simultaneously with inguinal vasovasostomy because it is possible to preserve the vasal blood supply deriving from epididymal branches of the testicular artery (Fig. 25-26). This provides blood supply to the segment of vas intervening between the two anastomoses. Maintenance of the deferential artery's contribution to the testicular blood supply is also important in situations in which the integrity of the testicular artery is in doubt owing to prior surgery

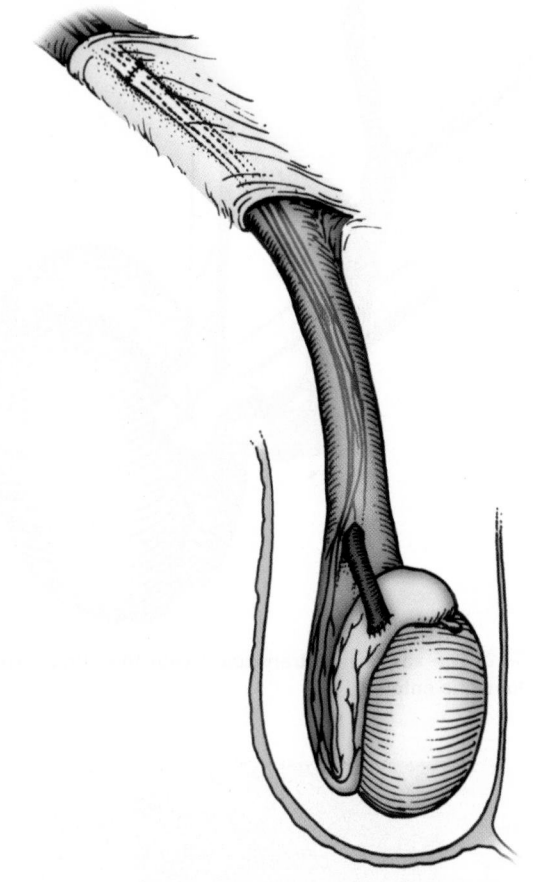

Figure 25-26. A diagram of a finished vasoepididymostomy.

such as orchiopexy, nonmicroscopic varicocelectomy, or hernia repair.

The testis is delivered through a 3- to 4-cm high vertical scrotal incision. The vas deferens is identified, isolated with a Babcock clamp, and then surrounded with a Penrose drain at the junction of the straight and convoluted portions of the vas deferens. Under 8× to 15× magnification provided by the operating microscope, the vasal sheath is longitudinally incised with a microknife, and a bare segment of vas stripped of its carefully preserved vessels is delivered. The vas is hemitransected with the ultrasharp knife until the lumen is entered (Fig. 25-27). **The vasal fluid is sampled. If microscopic examination of this fluid reveals the absence of sperm, the diagnosis of epididymal obstruction is confirmed.** Patency of the vas and ejaculatory ducts is confirmed by cannulating the abdominal end of the vas with a 24-gauge angiocatheter sheath and gently injecting lactated Ringer solution with a 1-mL tuberculin syringe (see Fig. 25-3). Further confirmation of patency may be obtained by injecting indigo carmine, catheterizing the bladder, and observing blue-tinged urine. The vas is then completely transected with use of a 2.5-mm slotted nerve clamp (see Fig. 25-27) and the vas is prepared as for vasovasostomy as described earlier.

After the tunica vaginalis has been opened, the epididymis is inspected under the operating microscope. An anastomotic site is selected above the area of suspected obstruction, proximal to any visible sperm granulomas, where dilated epididymal tubules are clearly seen beneath the epididymal tunica (Fig. 25-28). A relatively avascular area is grasped with sharp jeweler's forceps and the epididymal tunica tented upward. **A 3- to 4-mm buttonhole is made in the tunica with microscissors to create a round opening that matches the outer diameter of the previously prepared vas deferens.** The epididymal tubules are then gently dissected with a combination of sharp and blunt dissection until dilated loops of tubule are clearly exposed (Fig. 25-29). **If the level of obstruction is not clearly delineated, after the buttonhole opening has been made in the tunic, a 70-μm diameter tapered needle from the 10-0 nylon microsuture is used to puncture the epididymal tubule beginning as distal as possible; fluid from the puncture site is examined under the 400-power magnification bench microscope. When sperm are found, the puncture sites are sealed with microbipolar forceps, a new buttonhole is made in the epididymal tunic just proximal, and the tubule is prepared as described previously.**

The vas deferens is drawn through an opening in the tunica vaginalis and secured in proximity to the anastomotic site with two to four interrupted sutures of 6-0 polypropylene placed through the vasal adventitia and the tunica vaginalis. **The vasal lumen should reach the opening in the epididymal tunica easily, with length to spare.** The posterior edge of the epididymal tunica is then approximated to the posterior edge of the vas muscularis and adventitia with two to three interrupted sutures of double-armed 9-0 nylon (Fig. 25-30). This is done in such a way as to bring the vasal lumen in close approximation to the epididymal tubule selected for anastomosis.

Classic End-to-Side Technique

Under 25× to 32× magnification, with use of small curved microscissors or a 15-degree microknife, an opening about 0.3 to 0.5 mm

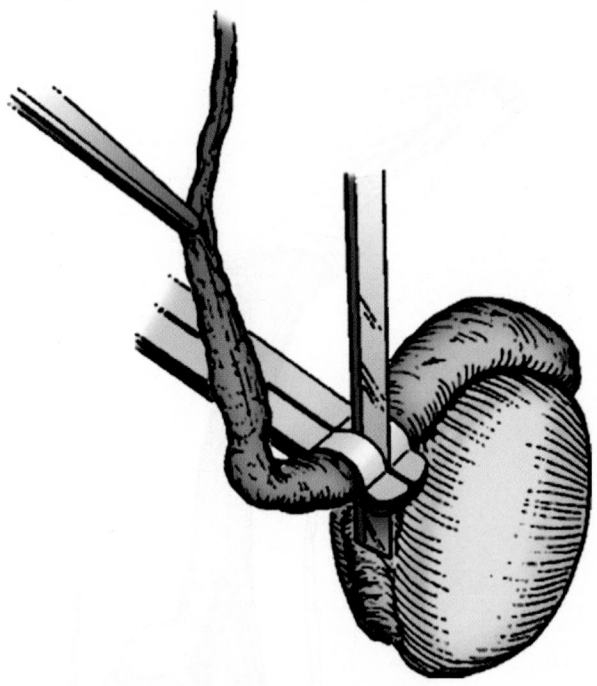

Figure 25-27. The vas is hemitransected with the ultrasharp knife until the lumen is entered.

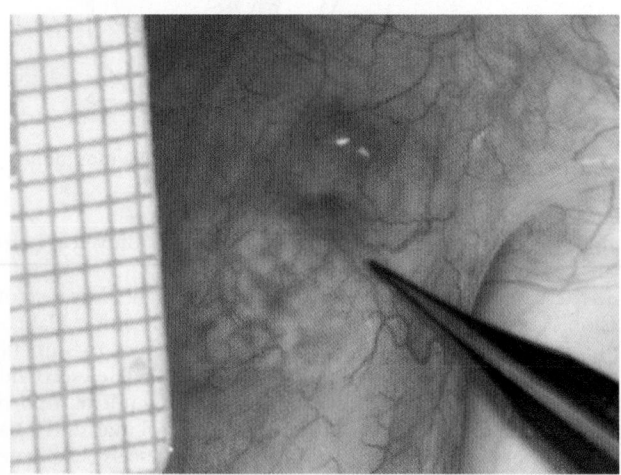

Figure 25-28. An anastomotic site is selected above the area of suspected obstruction, proximal to any visible sperm granulomas, where dilated epididymal tubules are clearly seen beneath the epididymal tunica.

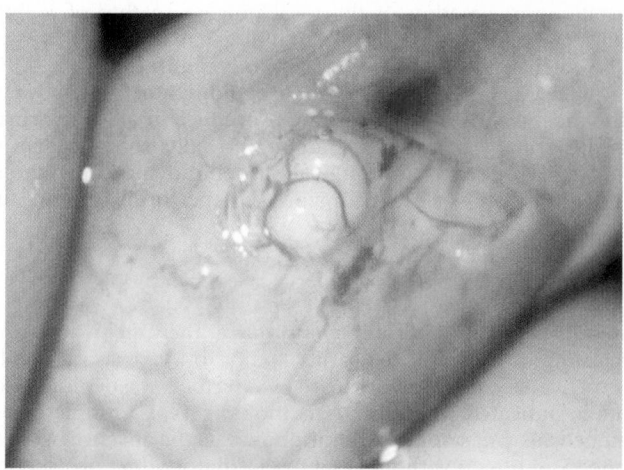

Figure 25-29. The epididymal tubules are then gently dissected with a combination of sharp and blunt dissection until dilated loops of tubule are clearly exposed.

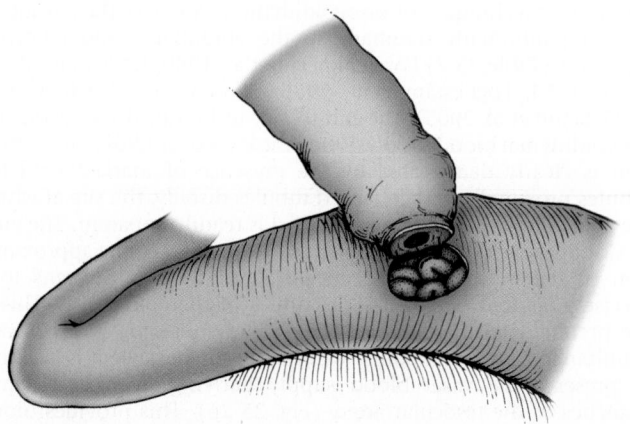

Figure 25-30. The posterior edge of the epididymal tunica is then approximated to the posterior edge of the vas muscularis and adventitia with two to three interrupted sutures of double-armed 9-0 nylon.

in diameter is made in the selected tubule. Epididymal fluid is touched to a slide, diluted with saline or Ringer solution, and inspected under the microscope for sperm. If no sperm are found, the opening in the tubule is closed with 10-0 sutures, the vas detached, and the tunica incision closed with 9-0 nylon. The procedure is then repeated more proximally in the epididymis.

Once sperm have been identified, they are aspirated into glass capillary tubes and flushed into media for cryopreservation (Fig. 25-31; see the section on the open tubule technique later in this chapter) (Matthews et al, 1995). **Indigo carmine solution is dripped on the cut tubule to outline the mucosa.** Methylene blue kills sperm instantly even when diluted, rendering the sperm useless for cryopreservation (Sheynkin et al, 1999b). Indigo carmine, diluted 50%, is safe for sperm. The posterior mucosal edge of the epididymal tubule is approximated to the posterior edge of the vasal mucosa with two interrupted 10-0 monofilament nylon sutures double-armed with fish hook 70-micron diameter tapered needles (Fig. 25-32). The lumen is irrigated with Ringer solution just before placement of each suture to keep the epididymal lumen open. The lumen is irrigated with heparinized saline just before the last mucosal suture is tied, to prevent clots from obstructing the lumen. Unlike with blood vessels, there are no platelets and fibrinogen to seal a leaky anastomosis and no clot lysis factor to dissolve clots. After these mucosal sutures are tied, the anterior mucosal anastomosis is completed with two to four additional 10-0 sutures.

The outer muscularis and adventitia of the vas are then approximated to the cut edge of the epididymal tunica with 6 to 10 additional interrupted sutures of 9-0 nylon double-armed with 100-micron diameter needles (Fig. 25-33). The vasal sheath is secured to the epididymal tunica with three to five sutures of 9-0 nylon. The testis and epididymis are gently returned to the tunica vaginalis, which is closed with 5-0 Vicryl. Penrose drains are usually not necessary. The scrotum is closed as previously described for vasovasostomy.

Two-Stitch Longitudinal Intussusception Vasoepididymostomy Technique

The original intussusception technique described by Berger (1998) used three double-armed 10-0 sutures placed in the epididymal tubule in a triangular fashion and a 9-0 needle to tear an opening in the middle of the triangle. **We now use a two-stitch longitudinal intussusception (LIVE) technique for all vasoepididymostomies.**

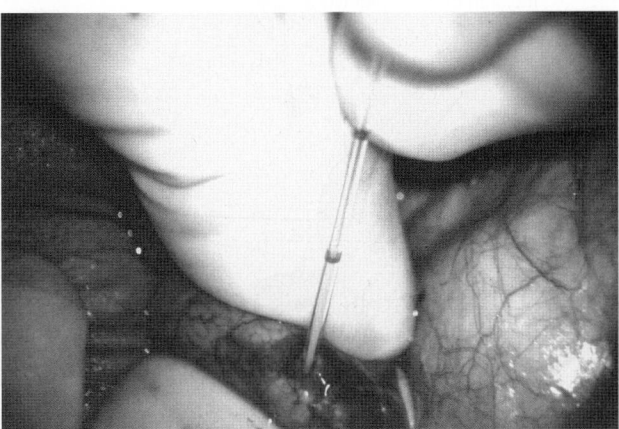

Figure 25-31. Once sperm have been identified, they are aspirated into glass capillary tubes and flushed into media for cryopreservation.

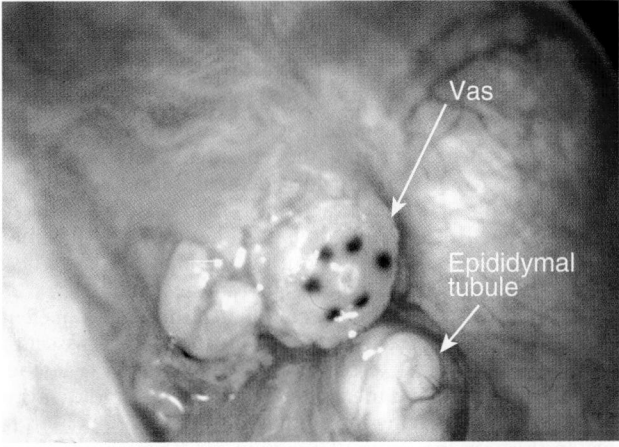

Figure 25-32. The posterior mucosal edge of the epididymal tubule is approximated to the posterior edge of the vasal mucosa with two interrupted 10-0 monofilament nylon sutures double-armed with fish-hook 70-micron diameter tapered needles.

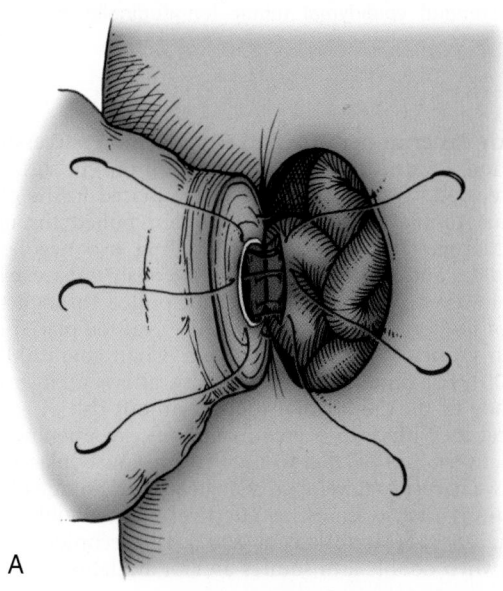

A

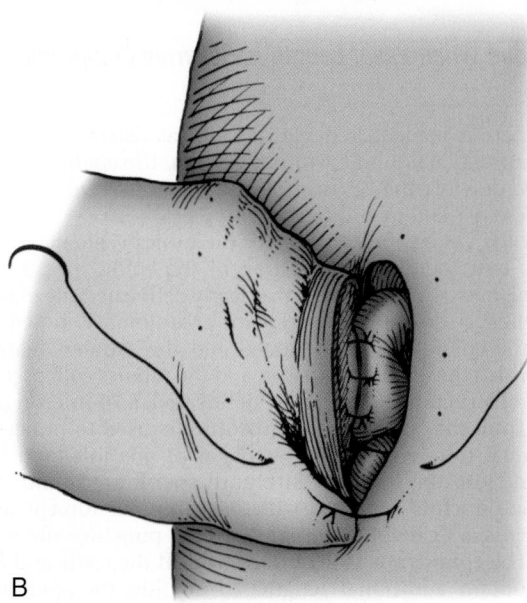

B

Figure 25-33. A and B, The outer muscularis and adventitia of the vas are then approximated to the cut edge of the epididymal tunica with 6 to 10 additional interrupted sutures of 9-0 nylon double-armed with 100-micron diameter needles.

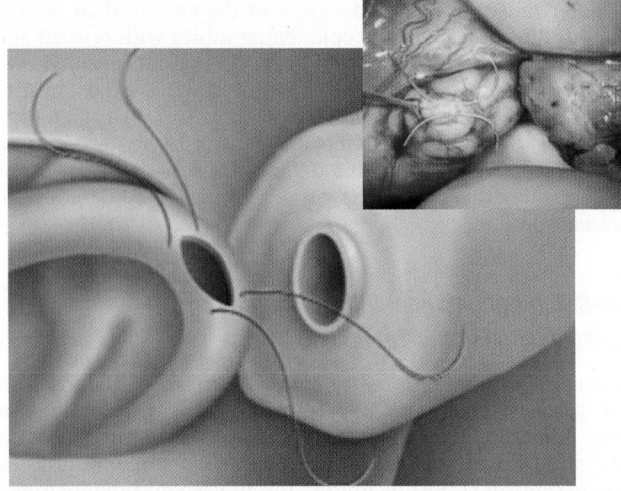

Figure 25-34. With this method, four microdots are marked on the cut surface of the vas deferens and two parallel sutures are placed in the distended epididymal tubule longitudinally, but not pulled through.

It is much easier to perform and is even more successful. With this method, four microdots are marked on the cut surface of the vas deferens and two parallel sutures are placed in the distended epididymal tubule longitudinally, but not pulled through (Fig. 25-34). Marmar (2000) suggests mounting two needles in the needle holder and placing them simultaneously transversely in the tubule. However, if the needles are not pulled through to avoid leakage of fluid and tubular collapse, they can be placed one at a time with greater control and accuracy (Chan et al, 2005; Schiff et al, 2005). Longitudinal placement also allows a larger opening to be made in the epididymal tubule without risk of completely transecting it. With a 15-degree microknife, an opening is made exactly between and parallel to the two previously placed sutures. Of note, we have also developed a single-arm technique of vasoepididymostomy that is almost as effective as the double-arm technique (Fig. 25-35) (Monoski et al, 2007). This technique may prove valuable when double-arm sutures are not available.

Technique When Vasal Length Is Severely Compromised
(Fig. 25-36)

When there is inadequate length of the vas deferens to reach the dilated epididymal tubule without tension, the epididymis can be dissected down to the VE junction and then dissected off the testes as in the older end-to-end operation.

After the vas has been prepared, the tunica vaginalis is opened and the testis delivered. Inspection of the epididymis under the operating microscope may reveal a clearly delineated site of obstruction. Often, a discrete yellow sperm granuloma is noted, above which the epididymis is indurated and the tubules dilated and below which the epididymis is soft and the tubules collapsed. **If the level of obstruction is not clearly delineated, a 70-micron tapered needle from the 10-0 nylon microsuture is used to puncture the epididymal tubule beginning as distal as possible, and fluid is sampled from the puncture site until sperm are found. At that level the puncture is sealed with microbipolar forceps and the epididymis is ligated just proximal to the puncture site with 6-0 nylon. The epididymis is then dissected off the testis and flipped up to obtain additional length.** To do this, the epididymis is encircled with a small Penrose drain at the level of obstruction and, under 2.5× loupe magnification, dissected off the testis for 3 to 5 cm, yielding sufficient length to perform the anastomosis. Usually a nice plane can be found between the epididymis and testis, and injury to the epididymal blood supply can be avoided by staying

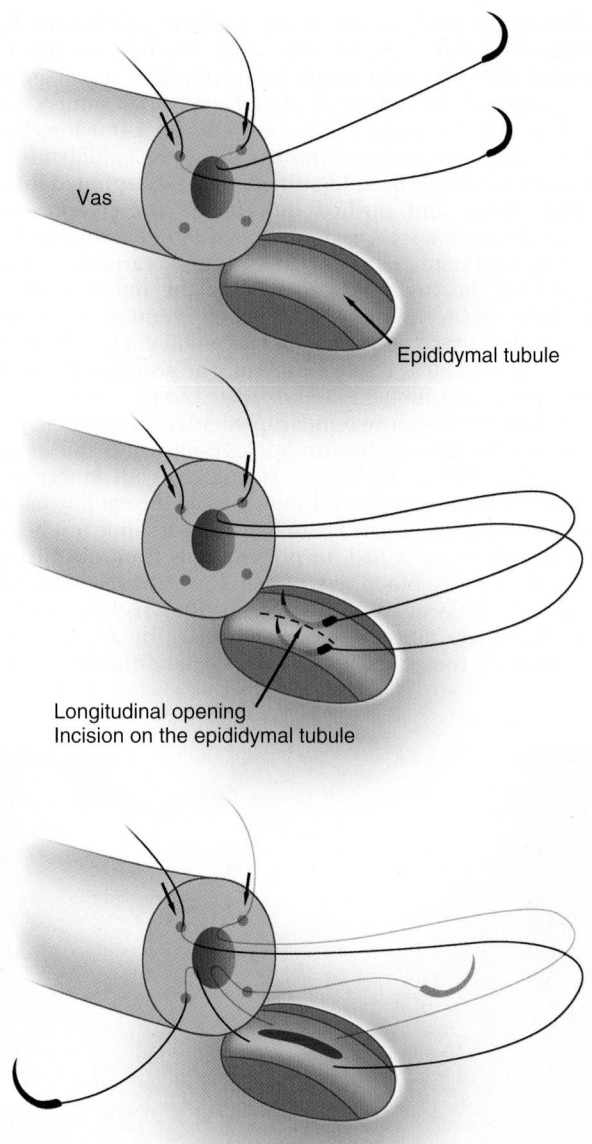

Figure 25-35. Of note, we have also developed a single-arm technique of vasoepididymostomy that is almost as effective as the double-arm technique.

right on the tunica albuginea of the testis. The inferior and, if necessary, middle epididymal branches of the testicular artery are ligated and divided to free an adequate length of epididymis. The superior epididymal branches entering the epididymis at the caput are always preserved and can provide adequate blood supply to the entire epididymis. The tunica vaginalis is then closed over the testis with 5-0 Vicryl. This prevents drying of the testis and thrombosis of the surface testicular vessels during the anastomosis. The dissected epididymis remains outside the tunica vaginalis.

If the epididymis is indurated and dilated throughout its length, the epididymis is dissected to the VE junction. This dissection is often facilitated by first dissecting the convoluted vas to the VE junction from below and then, after encircling the epididymis with a Penrose drain, dissecting the epididymis to the VE junction from above. In this way the entire VE junction can be freed up. This will allow preservation of maximal epididymal length in cases of distal obstruction near the VE junction. After the epididymis has been dissected off the testis and flipped up, a two-stitch end-to-side intussusception anastomosis is performed as described earlier.

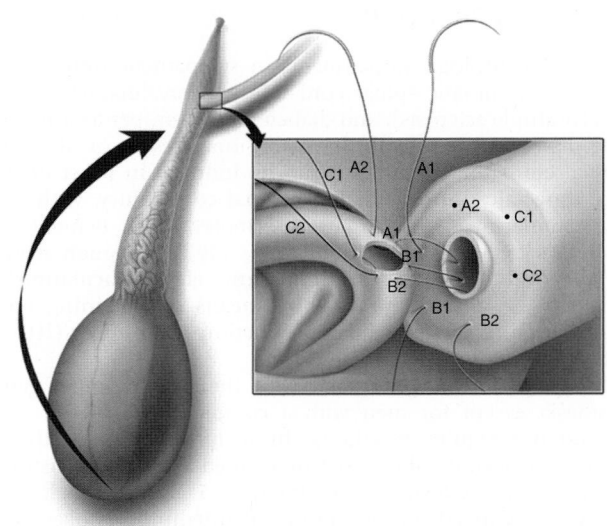

Figure 25-36. In addition, if vasal length is compromised, the epididymis can be dissected to the caput by ligating the inferior and medial epididymal vessels and flipping the epididymis up, providing additional length. A1, A2, B1, B2, C1, and C2 indicate needle exit points.

Long Term Follow-up: Evaluation and Results

Microsurgical vasoepididymostomy in the hands of experienced and skilled microsurgeons will result in the appearance of sperm in the ejaculate in 50% to 85% of men. Patency rates with the intussusception technique can exceed 80% (Berger, 1998; Brandell and Goldstein, 1999; Marmar, 2000). With the classic end-to-side or older end-to-end method, the patency rate is about 70%, and 43% of men with sperm will impregnate their partners after a minimum follow-up of 2 years (Schlegel and Goldstein, 1993; Pasqualotto et al, 1999). With the intussusception technique, patency rates are 70% to 90% (Kolettis and Thomas, 1997; Chan et al, 2005; Schiff et al, 2005). Regardless of technique, pregnancy rates are higher the more distally the anastomosis is performed (Silber, 1989b). **With the older end-to-end or end-to-side methods, at 14 months after surgery 25% of initially patent anastomoses have shut down** (Matthews et al, 1995). **With the intussusception technique, the late shut-down rates appear to be less than 10%,** but long-term follow-up with this technique has not been reported. **Nevertheless, we recommend banking sperm both intraoperatively** (Matthews and Goldstein, 1996) **and as soon as they appear in the ejaculate postoperatively after vasoepididymostomy, regardless of technique used.** In men with very low counts or poor sperm quality postoperatively and men who remain azoospermic, the sperm intraoperatively cryopreserved can be used for IVF with ICSI. Persistently azoospermic men without cryopreserved sperm can opt for either a redo vasoepididymostomy and/or microscopic epididymal sperm aspiration combined with IVF and ICSI (see the section on sperm retrieval techniques).

TRANSURETHRAL RESECTION OF THE EJACULATORY DUCTS

Ejaculatory duct obstruction is usually a congenital anomaly that represents the opposite end of the spectrum of excurrent ductal system anomalies that begins with congenital complete absence of the vas deferens and most of the epididymis. When the aplastic segment occurs at the terminal end of the vas, where the ejaculatory duct enters the urethra, it is potentially correctable by TUR (Paick et al, 2000; Schroeder-Printzen et al, 2000; Kadioglu et al, 2001; Ozgok et al, 2001; Yurdakul et al, 2008).

Occasionally, ejaculatory duct obstruction results from chronic prostatitis or extrinsic compression of the ejaculatory ducts by prostate or seminal vesical duct cysts (Cornel et al, 1999; Paick et al, 2000; Kadioglu et al, 2001). Higher ejaculatory duct pressures have been directly measured in men with ejaculatory duct obstruction (Eisenberg et al, 2008).

Diagnosis

The work-up leading to the diagnosis of probable ejaculatory duct obstruction is covered in Chapter 24. Briefly, ejaculatory duct obstruction is suspected in azoospermic or severely oligospermic and/or asthenospermic men with at least one palpable vas deferens, a low semen volume, acidic semen pH, and negative, equivocal, or low semen fructose levels. If these men have normal serum levels of FSH and testis biopsy reveals normal spermatogenesis, the diagnosis of ejaculatory duct obstruction is entertained.

Digital rectal examination may reveal a midline cystic structure. **Transrectal sonography is key to the diagnosis and treatment of ejaculatory duct obstruction.** A midline cystic lesion or dilated ejaculatory ducts and seminal vesicles can be visualized sonographically. As described in the section on transrectal vasography and seminal vesiculography earlier in this chapter, **transrectal ultrasound-guided aspiration of the cystic or dilated ejaculatory ducts or seminal vesicles is performed** (Jarow, 1994). **The aspirate is examined microscopically; if motile sperm are found, they are cryopreserved and 2 to 3 mL of indigo carmine diluted with water-soluble radiographic contrast is instilled. If a radiograph confirms a potentially resectable lesion, TURED is performed without the need for prior vasography** because the presence of sperm in the seminal vesicles indicates that at least one epididymis is patent and that the cyst or dilated ejaculatory duct communicates with a nonobstructed vas. The instillation of indigo carmine assists in localizing the opening of the ejaculatory duct and confirms when resection has successfully opened the obstructed system. **Transrectal sonography with aspiration should be performed immediately before anticipated surgery and uses the same bowel preparation and antibiotic prophylaxis as for transrectal prostate biopsy.**

If no sperm are found in the aspirate, vasography, as described in the earlier section on technique of vasography and interpretation of findings, is necessary. **If no sperm are found in either vas when the vasotomy is made and vasography reveals ejaculatory duct obstruction, it is best to abandon attempts at reconstruction and simply perform microsurgical epididymal sperm aspiration and cryopreservation for future IVF and ICSI. Performance of simultaneous vasoepididymostomy and TURED has never worked in my experience.** If ejaculatory duct obstruction is confirmed by vasography using a 50% water-soluble contrast medium and sperm are present in the vasa, the 3-Fr whistle tip ureteral vasography stents are left in place so that a dilute indigo carmine solution can be injected by the assistant to aid resection.

Technique

Cold knife incision alone almost always leads to reobstruction. The resectoscope, with the 24-Fr cutting loop, is engaged with a finger placed in the rectum providing anterior displacement of the posterior lobe of the prostate. The ejaculatory ducts course between the bladder neck and the verumontanum and exit at the level of and along the lateral aspect of the verumontanum (Fig. 25-37). **Resection of the verumontanum will often reveal the dilated ejaculatory duct orifice or cyst cavity. Resection should be carried out in this region with great care to preserve the bladder neck proximally, the striated sphincter distally, and the rectal mucosa posteriorly.** Efflux of indigo carmine from dilated orifices confirms adequate resection. **Avoid excessive coagulation.** If formal vasography was performed, the hemivasotomies are carefully closed using microsurgical technique. A Foley catheter is left overnight and the patient receives an additional 7 days of oral antibiotics.

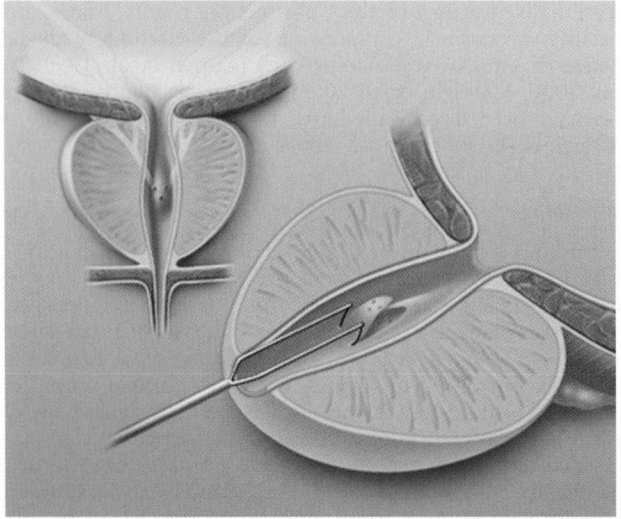

Figure 25-37. The ejaculatory ducts course between the bladder neck and the verumontanum and exit at the level of and along the lateral aspect of the verumontanum.

Complications

Reflux

Reflux of urine into the ejaculatory ducts, vas, and seminal vesicles occurs after a majority of resections. This can be documented by voiding cystourethrography or measurement of semen creatinine levels (Malkevich et al, 1994). Contamination of semen by urine impairs sperm quality.

Epididymitis

Reflux can lead to acute and chronic epididymitis. Recurrent epididymitis often results in epididymal obstruction. The incidence of epididymitis after TUR is probably underestimated. Symptomatic chemical epididymitis may occur from refluxing urine. Chronic low-dose antibacterial suppression, such as that used for vesicoureteral reflux, may be necessary until pregnancy is achieved. If epididymitis is chronic and recurrent, vasectomy or even epididymectomy may be necessary.

Retrograde Ejaculation

Even when care has been taken to spare the bladder neck, retrograde ejaculation is common after TUR. Pseudoephedrine 120 mg orally 90 minutes before ejaculation or Ornade Spansules (chlorpheniramine and phenylpropanolamine) twice a day for a week may prevent this. If this is not successful, sperm can be retrieved from alkalinized urine and used for either IUI or IVF with ICSI.

Results

TURED results in increased semen volume about two thirds of the time and appearance of sperm in the ejaculate in about 50% of previously azoospermic men. Pregnancy rates are based on case reports and small series (Goldwasser et al, 1985; Paick et al, 2000; Ozgok et al, 2001; Fuse et al, 2003; Yurdakul et al, 2008). If viable sperm appear in the ejaculate but the quality is poor, IVF with ICSI is recommended and currently yields delivery rates of up to 38.5% per attempt. Because of the potential for serious complications, TUR should be performed only in azoospermic men or in severely oligoasthenospermic men and only after the male and female partners have stated they are unwilling to undergo IVF and have been fully apprised of the risks of TUR.

ELECTROEJACULATION

Men with neurologic impairments in sympathetic outflow, such as seen in traumatic spinal cord injury, demyelinating neuropathies (multiple sclerosis), and diabetes after retroperitoneal lymph node dissection, frequently have abnormalities in or absence of seminal emission. Ejaculation can be induced in most of these men, especially those with high spinal cord injury, with vibratory stimulation (Schellan, 1968; Brindley, 1981; Bennett et al, 1987; Brackett et al, 1997; Ohl et al, 1997). For men who do not respond to vibratory stimulation, electroejaculation has proven to be a safe and effective means of obtaining motile sperm suitable for assisted reproduction techniques (IUI, IVF with ICSI).

The procedure is performed with the patient under general anesthesia except for men with a complete spinal cord injury, who do not require anesthesia. In men with a high thoracic spinal cord lesion (above T6) or in men with prior history of autonomic dysreflexia, pretreatment, 15 minutes before the procedure, with 20 mg of sublingual nifedipine is used. These men should have intravenous access and their blood pressure and pulse should be monitored every 2 minutes before, during, and for 20 minutes after electroejaculation. In the event of a sympathetic outflow (autonomic dysreflexia), termination of the procedure should be sufficient to break the response; however, intravenous access allows for delivery of sympatholytic agents should they become necessary.

Before placing the patient in the lateral decubitus position, the bladder is catheterized and emptied. A 12-Fr or 14-Fr Silastic catheter lubricated with a small amount of mineral oil is used because common lubricants are spermicidal. Ten milliliters of buffer (HEPES-BSA) is instilled into the bladder. Before the electroejaculation sequence, a digital rectal examination and anoscopy are performed. A rectal probe with three large horizontal stripes is well lubricated, inserted with the electrodes facing anteriorly, and applied against the posterior aspect of the prostate and seminal vesicles. The probe is connected to a variable output power source which simultaneously records probe temperature through a thermistor in the rectal probe. Electrostimulation is started at 3 to 5 volts and increased in 1-volt increments with each stimulation (Ohl et al, 2001). An assistant records probe temperatures, number of stimulations to full erection, and ejaculation, and collects the ejaculate in a sterile wide mouth plastic container. The number of stimulations and maximum voltage required are variable and the ejaculate may be retrograde. If probe temperature rises rapidly or above 40° C, stimulation is suspended until the temperature falls below 38° C or the probes are changed. At the completion of stimulation, anoscopy is again performed to check for rectal injury. The bladder is recatheterized to obtain any retrograde-ejaculated sperm. The specimens are then delivered to the laboratory for processing. A second electroejaculation sequence can be immediately performed under the same anesthetic to obtain additional sperm.

With this technique, sperm can be recovered in more than 90% of men. Overall pregnancy rates of up to 40% can be achieved after multiple cycles with IUI. Use of IVF with ICSI will yield 50% live delivery rates for a single (albeit costly) procedure if motile sperm are obtained.

SPERM RETRIEVAL TECHNIQUES

Men with congenital absence or bilateral partial aplasia of vas deferens or those with failed or surgically unreconstructable obstructions can now be treated through use of sperm retrieval techniques in conjunction with IVF (Table 25-3) (Temple-Smith et al, 1985; Silber et al, 1990; Schlegel et al, 1994; Craft et al, 1995; Sheynkin et al, 1998b; Janzen et al, 2000; Levine et al, 2003; Qiu et al, 2003; Anger et al, 2004). These techniques are also useful for intraoperative retrieval of sperm during reconstructive procedures such as vasoepididymostomy, which have significant failure rates. The intraoperatively retrieved sperm may be used immediately if the female

TABLE 25-3 Surgical Techniques for Sperm Retrieval

	ADVANTAGES	DISADVANTAGES
MESA (microsurgical epididymal sperm aspiration)	Microsurgical procedure allows lower complication rate. Epididymal sperm has better motility than testicular sperm. Large number of sperm can be harvested for cryopreservation of multiple vials in a single procedure.	Requires anesthesia and microsurgical skills. Not indicated for nonobstructive azoospermia.
PESA (percutaneous epididymal sperm aspiration)	No microsurgical skill required. Local anesthesia. Epididymal sperm has better motility than testicular sperm.	Complications include hematoma, pain, and vascular injury to testes and obstruction of the epididymis. Variable success in obtaining sperm. Smaller quantity of sperm obtained than with MESA. Not indicated for nonobstructive azoospermia.
TESA (testicular sperm aspiration)	No microsurgical skill required. Local anesthesia. Can be used for obstructive azoospermia.	Immature or immotile testicular sperm. Small quantity of sperm obtained. Poor results in nonobstructive azoospermia. Complications include hematoma, pain, and vascular injury to testes and epididymis.
TESE (testicular sperm extraction)	Low complication rate if performed microsurgically. Preferred technique for nonobstructive azoospermia.	Requires anesthesia and microsurgical skills.

partner has been prepared for IVF or may be cryopreserved for a future IVF with ICSI cycle in the event the reconstructive surgery is unsuccessful. Sperm obtained from chronically obstructed systems usually have poor motility and decreased fertilizing capacity. **The use of ICSI combined with IVF is essential regardless of the count and motility of the aspirated sperm.**

Microsurgical Epididymal Sperm Aspiration Techniques

Open Tubule Technique

The technique described here can be used for either intraoperative sperm retrieval at the time of vasoepididymostomy or as an isolated procedure in men with congenital absence of the vas or unreconstructable obstructions (Matthews and Goldstein, 1996; Nudell et al, 1998). A median raphe approach through two small transverse scrotal incisions within the scrotal skin folds is made. After delivery of the testis, the tunica vaginalis is opened and the epididymis inspected under 16× to 25× magnification using the operating microscope. The epididymal tunica is incised over a dilated tubule as described previously for vasoepididymostomy. Meticulous hemostasis is obtained using bipolar cautery. A dilated tubule is isolated and incised with a 15-degree microknife. The fluid is touched to a slide, a drop of human tubal fluid media is added, a coverslip is placed, and the fluid examined. If no sperm are obtained, the epididymal tubule and tunica are closed with 10-0 and 9-0 monofilament nylon sutures, respectively, and an incision is made more proximally in the epididymis or even at the level of the efferent ductules until motile sperm are obtained.

As soon as motile sperm are found, a dry micropipette (5 μL; Drummond Scientific, Broomall, PA) is placed adjacent to the effluxing epididymal tubule (Fig. 25-38). A standard hematocrit pipette is less satisfactory but can be used if micropipettes are not available. **Sperm are drawn into the micropipette by simple capillary action.** Negative pressure, as is generated by action of an in-line syringe, should not be applied during sperm recovery because this could disrupt the delicate epididymal mucosa. Two micropipettes may be employed simultaneously to increase speed of sperm recovery.

The highest rate of flow is observed immediately after incision of the tubule. Progressively better quality sperm are often found after the initial washout. **Gentle compression of the testis and epididymis enhances flow from the incised tubule.** With patience, 10 to 20 μL of epididymal fluid can be recovered.

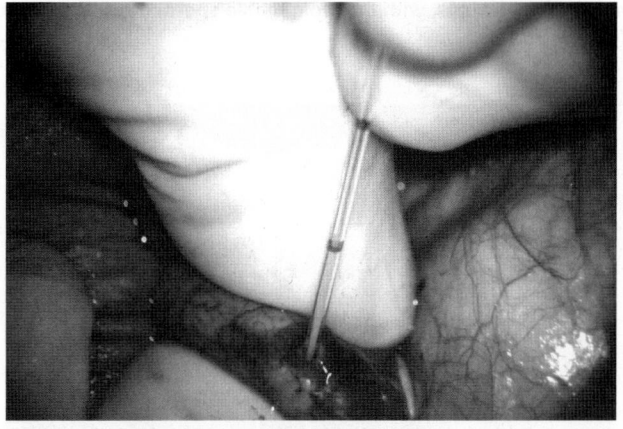

Figure 25-38. As soon as motile sperm are found, a dry micropipette (5 μL; Drummond Scientific Co., Broomall, PA) is placed adjacent to the effluxing epididymal tubule.

The micropipette is connected to a short (3 to 5 cm) segment of medical grade silicone tubing (American Scientific Products, McGaw Park, IL). Alternatively, the tubing attached to a 25-gauge butterfly needle may be used. A 20-gauge needle fitted to a Luer-tip syringe is then placed in line. The fluid is flushed with IVF medium (0.5 to 1.0 mL) into a sterile container. Once a micropipette has been used, it is discarded. Residual fluid in the pipette will disrupt capillary action. A typical procedure requires 4 to 12 micropipettes. The sperm bank should be instructed to cryopreserve the aspirate in multiple vials (aliquots) so that several IVF cycles may be attempted if required (Janzen et al, 2000; Anger et al, 2004).

Experience with the technique has revealed that, paradoxically, in obstructed systems sperm motility is better more proximal in the epididymis, with the most motile sperm often found in the efferent ductules (Fig. 25-39). Motility immediately after aspiration and consequently fertilization rates are highest in men who have the longest length of epididymal tubule available. Even when packed with debris distally, the epididymal tubule may be capable of secreting substances that can diffuse proximally and benefit sperm motility and fertilizing capacity.

With use of ICSI, ongoing pregnancy or delivery rates exceeding 60% have been achieved with this technique using either

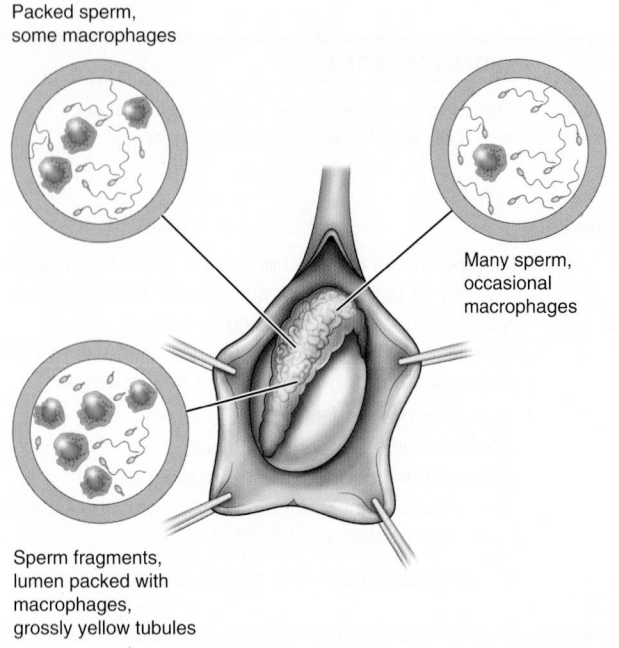

Packed sperm,
some macrophages

Many sperm,
occasional
macrophages

Sperm fragments,
lumen packed with
macrophages,
grossly yellow tubules

Figure 25-39. Experience with the technique has revealed that, paradoxically, in obstructed systems sperm motility is better more proximal in the epididymis, with the most motile sperm often found in the efferent ductules.

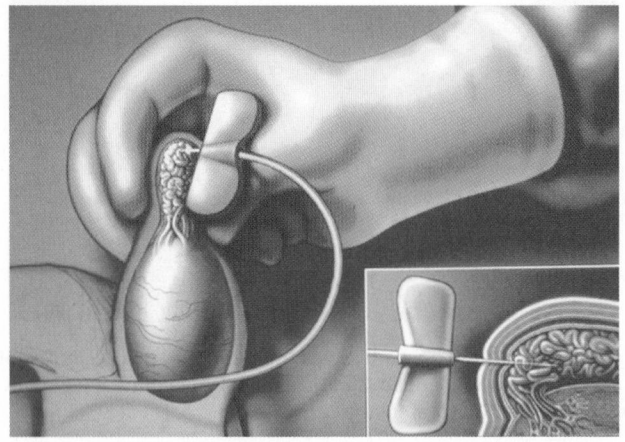

Figure 25-40. Percutaneous puncture of the epididymis with a fine needle.

fresh or cryopreserved epididymal sperm (Schlegel et al, 1995; Nudell et al, 1998). **Epididymal sperm aspiration can be done electively, with the cryopreserved sperm used for multiple future IVF cycles** (Janzen et al, 2000; Anger et al, 2004).

Percutaneous Epididymal Sperm Aspiration

Percutaneous puncture of the epididymis with a fine needle (Fig. 25-40) has been successfully used to obtain sperm and achieve pregnancies (Shrivastav et al, 1994; Craft and Tsirigotis, 1995; Levine et al, 2003; Qiu et al, 2003; Lin et al, 2004). The technique is less reliable than open retrieval, and the small quantities of sperm obtained are sometimes inadequate for cryopreservation. Reported pregnancy rates are half those achieved with open techniques (Sheynkin et al, 1998b). It can also potentially obstruct the epididymis in men in whom future vasoepididymostomy is considered. In view of the enormous costs and effort involved in IVF, epididymal sperm retrieval under direct vision is the preferred technique (Zhang et al, 2013).

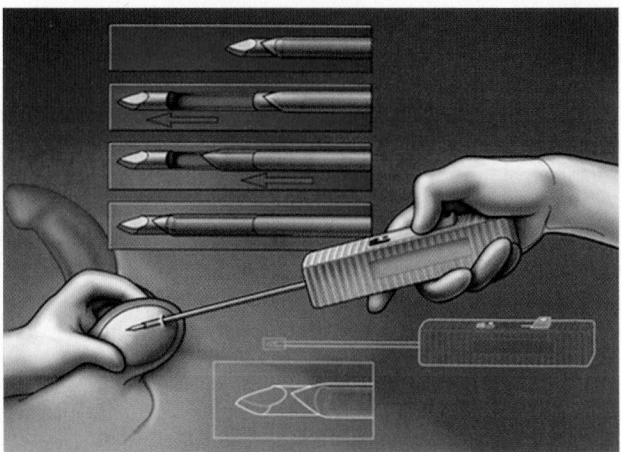

Figure 25-41. Percutaneous core biopsy; uses the same 14-gauge biopsy gun as prostate biopsy.

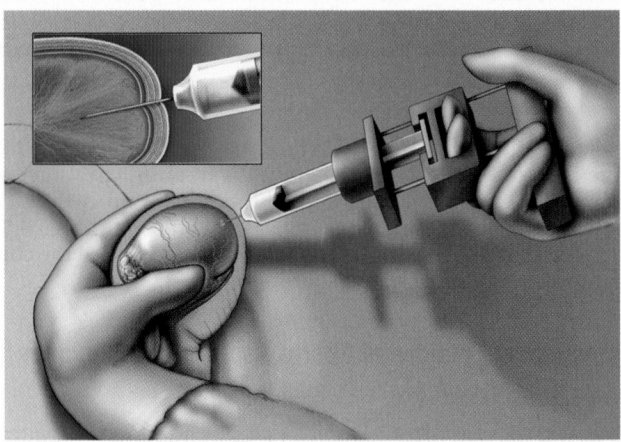

Figure 25-42. Percutaneous aspiration (testicular sperm aspiration) with a high-suction glass syringe and a 23-gauge needle. This is the least invasive procedure but requires 10 to 20 passes to obtain an adequate yield.

Testicular Sperm Extraction

The indications for TESE are as follows:
1. **Failure to find sperm in the epididymis** in the presence of the spermatogenesis or complete absence of the epididymis.
2. **Nonobstructive azoospermia** (Schlegel et al, 1997; Tsujimura et al, 2002; Ramasamy et al, 2013a, 2013b).
   Testicular sperm has been retrieved via one of three techniques:
3. **Open microsurgical TESE,** preferably with an operating microscope (micro-TESE), which allows retrieval of the largest number of sperm with potential for cryopreservation; this **is the best technique in men with nonobstructive azoospermia.**
4. Percutaneous core biopsy; uses the same 14-gauge biopsy gun used for prostate biopsy (Fig. 25-41).
5. Percutaneous aspiration (testicular sperm aspiration [TESA]) with a high-suction glass syringe and a 23-gauge needle. This is the least invasive procedure but often requires 10 to 20 passes to obtain an adequate yield (Fig. 25-42) (Rajfer and Binder, 1989; Harrington et al, 1996; Friedler et al, 1997; Sheynkin et al, 1998b; Mercan et al, 2000; Carpi et al, 2005).

The percutaneous methods are most appropriate in men with normal spermatogenesis and obstructive azoospermia when adequate numbers of sperm can be retrieved in a small amount of tissue (Craft et al, 1995). The pros and cons of these three methods are discussed in the section on testis biopsy, earlier in this chapter.

Microsurgical Testicular Sperm Extraction

The use of an operating microscope for standard open diagnostic testes biopsy allows identification of an area in the tunica albuginea free of blood vessels (Fig. 25-43), minimizing the risk of injury to testicular blood supply and allowing a relatively blood-free biopsy specimen (Dardashti et al, 2000). Using the microscope for testis biopsy, Schlegel (1999) discovered that in men with nonobstructive azoospermia, some of the tubules were larger than others. **The larger tubules are more likely to yield sperm.** Previous studies had revealed that testicular biopsy specimens in men with nonobstructive azoospermia display considerable heterogeneity. Examination of permanently fixed biopsy specimens that display heterogeneity reveals that **tubules with spermatogenesis are of considerably larger diameter than tubules that are Sertoli cell only. This difference can be readily observed under the operating microscope** (Fig. 25-44).

Technique. With the patient under general or regional anesthetic, the testes are exposed through either a single midline median raphe incision or two transverse incisions within the skin lines and between the scrotal blood vessels. The testes is delivered into the wound. The tunica vaginalis is opened and the operating microscope is brought into the field. Under 10× magnification,

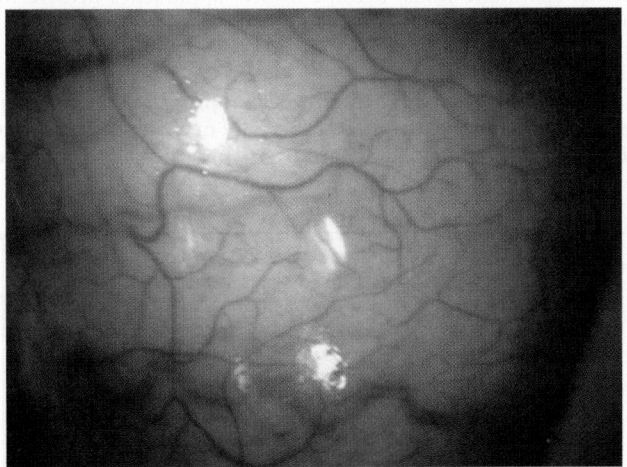

Figure 25-43. The use of an operating microscope for standard open diagnostic testes biopsy allows identification of an area in the tunica albuginea free of blood vessels.

an avascular plane is identified on the anterior surface of the tunica albuginea. Using a 15-degree microknife, a generous transverse incision is made between the blood vessels through the tunica albuginea. Small blood vessels that are seen coursing across the incision are coagulated with the microbipolar cautery before they are incised. This yields a blood-free field. The seminiferous tubules are observed. **Sertoli cell–only tubules tend to be thin, white, and stringy. Tubules with active spermatogenesis are larger, plumper, and somewhat yellow.** With a micro needle holder or microbipolar forceps, the seminiferous tubules are dissected in an attempt to identify larger tubules. If such a tubule is found, sharp curved iris scissors are used to selectively excise these tubules. The sample is placed in human tubal fluid medium, microdissected, and immediately examined by an andrology laboratory technician present in the operating room. After sperm have been found, hemostasis is obtained with the microbipolar cautery. The incision in the tunica albuginea is closed with a 6-0 nylon suture. The testis is returned to the tunica vaginalis, which is closed with a continuous suture of 5-0 Vicryl. If necessary, the opposite testis is explored.

Results. With use of the microdissection technique, sperm have been identified in 50% of men explored. (Schlegel, 1999; Dabaja and Schlegel, 2013). In men in whom sperm are found, a pregnancy rate of 45%, with a live delivery rate of almost 40%, has been achieved at Cornell using IVF with ICSI. The spontaneous abortion rate is 19%. The high rate of spontaneous abortion is probably a result of the increased incidence of chromosomal abnormalities and DNA damage in the sperm of men with nonobstructive azoospermia (Rucker et al, 1998). Even in severe cases of congenital or acquired testicular failure, as in Sertoli cell–only syndrome (Ramasamy et al, 2013a), postchemotherapy azoospermia (Chan et al, 2001), and nonmosaic (47,XXY) Klinefelter syndrome (Palermo et al, 1998; Ramasamy et al, 2009), sperm have been found and pregnancy and live births achieved (Table 25-4).

Postmortem Sperm Retrieval

Postmortem sperm retrieval and cryopreservation (but no pregnancies) were initially reported by Rothman in 1980 and involved removal and mincing of the epididymis. The retrieved sperm can be frozen and subsequently used to attempt to achieve pregnancy. Pregnancy has now been achieved with sperm retrieved postmortem using IVF with ICSI (reviewed in Benshushan and Schenker, 1998; Tash et al, 2003; Dostal et al, 2005).

Retrieval of sperm from the vas can be performed using the technique described for vasectomy (see earlier). Once the vas has

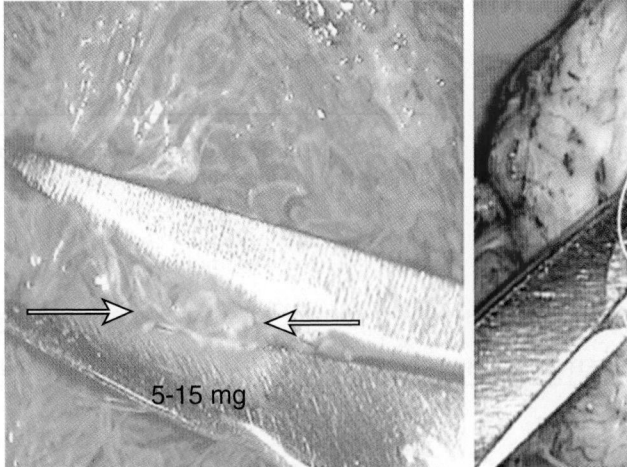
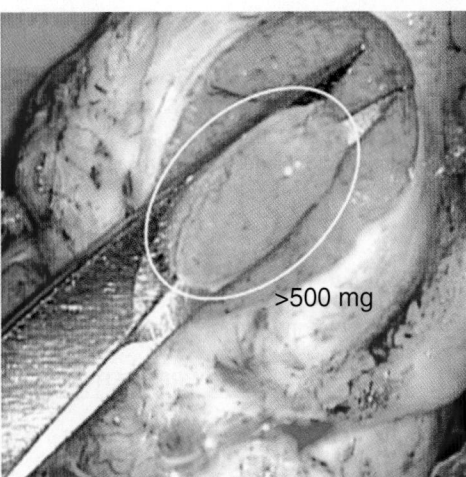

5-15 mg

>500 mg

Figure 25-44. Tubules with spermatogenesis are of considerably larger diameter than tubules that are Sertoli cell only. This difference can be readily observed under the operating microscope.

been delivered, a hemivasotomy is made with a 15-degree microknife (as described in the section on technique of vasography and interpretation of findings). The testicular end of the vas is cannulated with a 22-gauge angiocatheter and the vas irrigated with a 0.2-mL volume of human tubal fluid medium while the convoluted vas and epididymis are massaged.

The ethical appropriateness of such retrieval is the most important issue surrounding its use, and current guidelines require the patient to have given permission for sperm retrieval and use before death (Trinkoff and Barone, 2013).

VARICOCELECTOMY

Varicocele is by far the most commonly performed operation for the treatment of male infertility. **Varicocele is found in approximately 15% of the general population, 35% of men with primary infertility, and 75% to 81% of men with secondary infertility.** Animal and human studies have demonstrated that **varicocele is associated with a progressive and duration-dependent decline in testicular function** (Russell, 1957; Lipshultz and Corriere, 1977; Nagler et al, 1985; Harrison et al, 1986; Kass and Belman, 1987; Hadziselimovic et al, 1989; Chehval and Purcell, 1992; Gorelick and Goldstein, 1993; Witt and Lipshultz, 1993).

Repair of varicocele will halt any further damage to testicular function (Kass and Belman, 1987; Gorelick and Goldstein, 1993) and in a large percentage of men will result in improved spermatogenesis (Dubin and Amelar, 1977; Schlegel and Goldstein, 1992; Marmar et al, 2007) as well as enhanced Leydig cell function (Su et al, 1995; Tanrikut et al, 2011). The potentially important role of urologists in preventing future infertility and/or androgen deficiency underscores the importance of using a varicocelectomy technique that minimizes the risk of complications and recurrence. Table 25-5 summarizes the pros and cons of various methods of varicocele repair.

Scrotal Operations

A variety of surgical approaches have been advocated for varicocelectomy. The earliest recorded attempts at repair of varicocele date to antiquity and involved external clamping of the scrotal skin, including the enlarged veins. In the early 1900s an open scrotal approach was used, involving the mass ligation and excision of the varicosed plexus of veins. At the level of the scrotum, however, the pampiniform plexus of veins are intimately entwined with the coiled testicular artery. Therefore, **scrotal operations are to be avoided because damage to the arterial supply of the testis frequently results in testicular atrophy and further impairment of spermatogenesis and fertility.**

Retroperitoneal Operations

Retroperitoneal repair of varicocele involves incision at the level of the internal inguinal ring (Fig. 25-45), splitting of the external and internal oblique muscles, and exposure of the internal spermatic artery and vein retroperitoneally near the ureter. This approach has the advantage of isolating the internal spermatic veins proximally, near the point of drainage into the left renal vein. At this level, only one or two large veins are present, and in addition the testicular artery has not yet branched and is often distinctly separate from the internal spermatic veins. Retroperitoneal approaches involve ligation of the fewest number of veins. This approach is still a commonly used method for the repair of varicocele, especially in children.

A disadvantage of a retroperitoneal approach is the high incidence of varicocele recurrence, especially in children and adolescents, when the testicular artery is intentionally preserved.

TABLE 25-4 Testicular Sperm Extraction Outcomes by Diagnosis

CONDITION	RETRIEVAL
Klinefelter syndrome	68%
AZFc deletions	70%
Sertoli cell only	30%
Postchemotherapy	53%
Cryptorchidism (postorchiopexy)	74%
Maturation arrest	40%
AZFa, AZFb deletions	0%

AZF, azoospermia factor (Y chromosome gene).
Data from Chan et al, 2001; Hopps et al, 2003b; Raman and Schlegel, 2003; Hung et al, 2007; Ramasamy and Schlegel, 2007; Ramasamy et al, 2009.

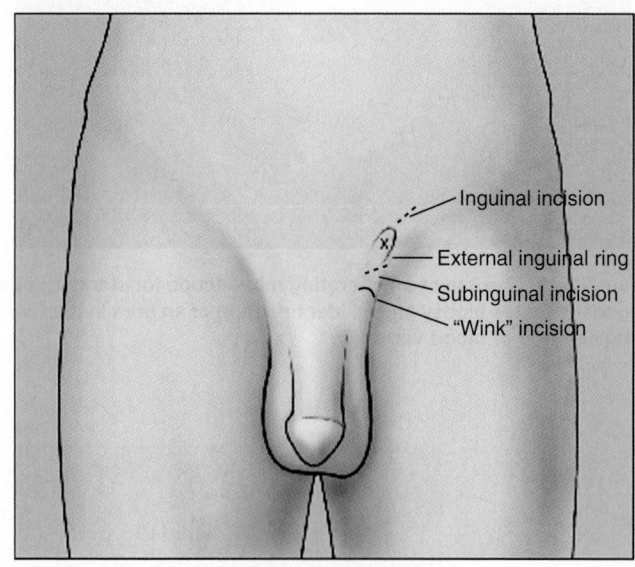

Figure 25-45. Retroperitoneal repair of varicocele involves incision at the level of the internal inguinal ring.

- Inguinal incision
- External inguinal ring
- Subinguinal incision
- "Wink" incision

TABLE 25-5 Techniques of Varicocelectomy

TECHNIQUE	ARTERY PRESERVED	HYDROCELE (%)	FAILURE (%)	POTENTIAL FOR SERIOUS MORBIDITY
Retroperitoneal	No	7	15-25	No
Conventional inguinal	No	3-30	5-15	No
Laparoscopic	Yes	12	3-15	Yes
Radiographic	Yes	0	15-25	Yes
Microscopic inguinal or subinguinal	Yes	0	0.5-1.0	No

Recurrence rates after retroperitoneal varicocelectomy are in the range of 15% (Homonnai et al, 1980; Rothman et al, 1981; Watanabe et al, 2005). Failure is usually the result of preservation of the periarterial plexus of fine veins (venae comitantes) along with the artery. These veins have been shown to communicate with larger internal spermatic veins. If left intact they may dilate and cause recurrence. Less commonly, failure is a result of the presence of parallel inguinal or retroperitoneal collaterals, which may exit the testis and bypass the ligated retroperitoneal veins, rejoining the internal spermatic vein proximal to the site of ligation (Sayfan et al, 1981; Murray et al, 1986). Dilated cremasteric veins (Sayfan et al, 1980) and scrotal collaterals (Kaufman et al, 1983) are also causes of varicocele recurrence and cannot be identified with a retroperitoneal approach. Positive identification and preservation of the 1.0- to 1.5-mm testicular artery via the retroperitoneal approach are difficult, especially in children in whom the artery is small. The operation involves working in a deep hole, and because at this level the internal spermatic vessels cannot be delivered into the wound, they must be dissected and ligated in situ in the retroperitoneum. In addition, the difficulty of positively identifying and preserving lymphatics while using this approach results in postoperative hydrocele formation after 7% to 33% of retroperitoneal operations (Szabo and Kessler, 1984). The incidence of recurrence appears to be higher in children, with rates of 15% to 45% reported in adolescents (Gorenstein et al, 1986; Levitt et al, 1987; Reitelman et al, 1987). Kass reports that **recurrence can be markedly reduced in children and adolescents by intentional ligation of the testicular artery** (Kass and Marcol, 1992). This ensures ligation of the periarterial network of fine veins. Although reversal of testicular growth failure has been documented with intentional testicular artery ligation at the time of retroperitoneal repair in children, **the effect of artery ligation on subsequent spermatogenesis is uncertain.** In adults, bilateral artery ligation has been documented to occasionally cause azoospermia and testicular atrophy. At least, **it is inarguable that testicular artery ligation will not enhance testicular function.**

Laparoscopic Varicocelectomy

Laparoscopic repair is in essence a retroperitoneal approach, and many of the advantages and disadvantages are similar to those of the open retroperitoneal approach (Donovan and Winfield, 1992; Hagood et al, 1992; Enquist et al, 1994; Hirsch et al, 1998; Riccabona et al, 2003; Watanabe et al, 2005).

With use of the laparoscope, the internal spermatic vessels and vas deferens can be clearly visualized through the laparoscope as they course through the internal inguinal ring. **The magnification provided by the laparoscope allows visualization of the testicular artery** (Kobori et al, 2013). **With experience, the lymphatics may be visualized and preserved as well** (Glassberg et al, 2008). With laparoscopic varicocelectomy the internal spermatic veins are ligated at the same level as with the retroperitoneal (Palomo) approach described previously in the section on retroperitoneal operations. Laparoscopic varicocelectomy should allow preservation of the testicular artery in a majority of patients, as well as preservation of lymphatics. The incidence of varicocele recurrence would be expected to be similar to that associated with the open retroperitoneal operations. These recurrences would be the result of collaterals joining the internal spermatic vein near its entrance to the renal vein, or entering the renal vein separately.

Most series of laparoscopic varicocelectomy report a recurrence rate of 2.9% to 4.5% (May et al, 2006; Glassberg et al, 2008; Barroso et al, 2009), but up to 17% in some (Al-Said et al, 2008). An artery ligation but lymphatic-sparing laparoscopic technique has markedly reduced the incidence of postoperative hydrocele formation in children (Glassberg et al, 2008). The potential complications of laparoscopic varicocelectomy (injury to bowel, vessels, or viscera; air embolism; peritonitis) are significantly more serious than those associated with the open techniques. Furthermore, laparoscopic varicocelectomy requires a general anesthetic. The microsurgical techniques described next can be performed with local or regional

anesthesia and use an incision of 2 to 3 cm for unilateral repair. This is often no greater than the sum of incisions used for a laparoscopic approach. Postoperative pain and recovery from the laparoscopic technique are the same as those associated with subinguinal varicocelectomy (Hirsch et al, 1998). In the hands of an experienced laparoscopist, the approach is a reasonable alternative for the repair of bilateral varicoceles (Donovan and Winfield, 1992; Diamond et al, 2009; Mendez-Gallart et al, 2009; Tong et al, 2009.)

Microsurgical Inguinal and Subinguinal Operations: Preferred Approaches

Subinguinal varicocelectomy is currently the most popular approach. It has the advantage of allowing the spermatic cord structures to be pulled up and out of the wound so that the testicular artery, lymphatics, and small periarterial veins may be more easily identified. In addition, **an inguinal or subinguinal approach allows access to external spermatic and even gubernacular veins** (Kaufman et al, 1983), which may bypass the spermatic cord and result in recurrence if not ligated. Lastly, an inguinal or subinguinal approach allows access to the testis for biopsy or examination of the epididymis for obstruction or repair of hydrocele (Dabaja and Goldstein, 2014).

Traditional approaches to inguinal varicocelectomy involve a 5-cm incision made over the inguinal canal, opening of the external oblique aponeurosis, and encirclement and delivery of the spermatic cord. The cord is then dissected and all the internal spermatic veins are ligated (Dubin and Amelar, 1977). The vas deferens and its vessels are preserved. An attempt is made to identify and preserve the testicular artery and, if possible, the lymphatics. In addition, the cord is elevated, and any external spermatic veins that are running parallel to the spermatic cord or perforating the floor of the inguinal canal are identified and ligated. Compared with retroperitoneal operations, conventional nonmagnified inguinal approaches lower the incidence of varicocele recurrence but do not alter the incidence of either hydrocele formation or testicular artery injury. **Conventional inguinal operations are associated with an incidence of postoperative hydrocele formation varying from 3% to 15% with an average incidence of 7%** (Szabo and Kessler, 1984). Analysis of the hydrocele fluid has clearly indicated that hydrocele formation after varicocelectomy is a result of ligation of the lymphatics (Szabo and Kessler, 1984). The incidence of testicular artery injury during nonmagnified inguinal varicocelectomy is unknown. Case reports, however, suggest that this complication may be more common than realized. It can result in testicular atrophy, and if the operation is performed bilaterally, azoospermia may ensue in a previously oligospermic man. Furthermore, Starzl and his transplant group reported a 14% incidence of testicular atrophy and 70% incidence of hydrocele formation when the spermatic cord was divided and only the vas and vasal vessels were preserved (Penn et al, 1972).

The introduction of **microsurgical technique** to varicocelectomy **has resulted in a substantial reduction in the incidence of hydrocele formation** (Goldstein et al, 1992; Marmar and Kim, 1994; Matthews et al, 1998; Cayan et al, 2000). This is **because the lymphatics can be more easily identified and preserved.** Furthermore, the use of **magnification enhances the ability to identify and preserve the 0.5- to 1.5-mm testicular artery, thus avoiding the complications of atrophy or azoospermia.**

Advocates of nonmicrosurgical techniques contend that the deferential (vasal) artery and, if preserved, the cremasteric artery will provide adequate blood supply to the testes to prevent atrophy. However, anatomic studies have shown that the diameter of the testicular artery is greater than the diameter of the deferential artery and cremasteric artery combined (Raman and Goldstein, 2004). **The testicular artery is the main blood supply to the testis.** Experience with the one-stage Fowler and Stephens orchiopexy, in which the testicular artery is intentionally ligated, reveals that a substantial percentage of such procedures result in an atrophic testis. Also, animal models indicate that artery preservation varicocelectomy results in improved testicular ultrastructure whereas artery ligation resulted in further deterioration of ultrastructure (Zheng et al, 2008). At the very least, it is inarguable that **ligation of the testicular artery is unlikely to enhance testicular function.**

Anesthesia

If the testis is delivered as described later, regional or light general anesthesia is preferred. If only the cord is delivered, local anesthesia with a 50%-50% combination of 0.25% bupivacaine and 1% lidocaine is satisfactory with adjunctive intravenous heavy sedation. After infiltration of the skin and subcutaneous tissues the cord is infiltrated before delivery. Blind cord block carries with it a small risk of inadvertent testicular artery injury (Goldstein et al, 1983). A 30-gauge needle should therefore be used for cord block to minimize the risk of injury and hematoma.

Inguinal and Subinguinal Approaches

The introduction of the subinguinal approach, just below the external inguinal ring (Marmar et al, 1985), obviates the necessity for opening any fascial layer and is associated with less pain and a rapid recovery comparable to laparoscopic procedures. At the subinguinal level, however, significantly more veins are encountered, the artery is more often surrounded by a network of tiny veins that must be ligated, and the testicular artery has often divided into two or three branches, making arterial identification and preservation more difficult (Hopps et al, 2003a).

Subinguinally, the arterial pulsations are often dampened by compression on the edge of the external ring, making its identification somewhat more difficult than when the external oblique is opened. Table 25-6 summarizes the criteria for performing the operation inguinally (external oblique opened) versus subinguinally (fascia intact). **In general, it is best to use a subinguinal approach in men with a history of any prior inguinal surgery.** Under these circumstances the cord is usually stuck to the undersurface of the external oblique, and opening the fascia risks injury to the cord. A subinguinal approach is easier in obese men in whom opening and closing the fascia is difficult through a small incision. A subinguinal approach is easier in men with high, lax, capacious external rings and in men with long cords and low-lying testes. In these men the level of the external ring is fairly proximal to the testis, and opening the fascia will not result in a significant diminution in the number of veins to be ligated or in the branching of the testicular artery.

I recommend always opening the external oblique in prepubertal children without prior inguinal surgery. In children the testicular artery is very small and systemic blood pressure is low, making identification of the artery very difficult in a subinguinal approach. The fascia could also be opened in men with a solitary testis in whom preservation of the artery is critical. Exposure of the cord more proximally (at the inguinal level) allows identification of the artery before it has branched, where clear pulsations are more readily observed.

Consider opening the fascia in men with prior failed subinguinal varicocelectomy to dissect proximal to the prior scarred ligation area. The microdissection will be quicker and easier. A subinguinal operation is significantly more difficult than a high inguinal operation and should be used only by surgeons who perform the operation frequently. Less experienced microsurgeons should start out doing inguinal operations because it is easier. **An inguinal operation is used when simultaneous ipsilateral hernia repair is performed.**

Before the incision is made the location of the external inguinal ring is determined by invagination of the scrotal skin and is marked. The size of the incision is determined by the size of the testis when delivery of the testis (see later) is planned. Atrophic testes can be delivered through a 2- to 2.5-cm incision. Larger testes require a 3-cm incision. The incision is made within the Langer lines to minimize scarring.

If the decision is made to perform an inguinal operation and thus to open the fascia, the incision is begun at the external ring and extended laterally 2 to 3.5 cm along the Langer lines (Fig. 25-46). If the operation is to be performed subinguinally, the incision is placed in the skin lines right over the external ring (Fig. 25-47).

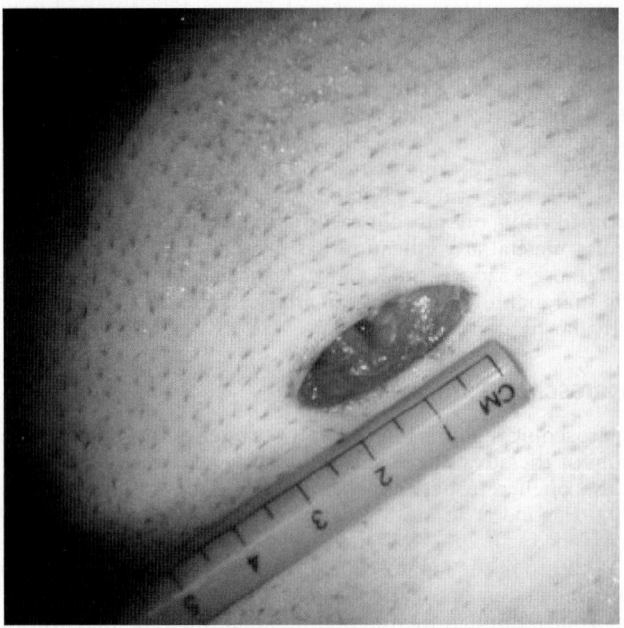

Figure 25-46. **If the decision is made to perform an inguinal operation and thus to open the fascia, the incision is begun at the external ring and extended laterally 2 to 3.5 cm along the Langer lines.**

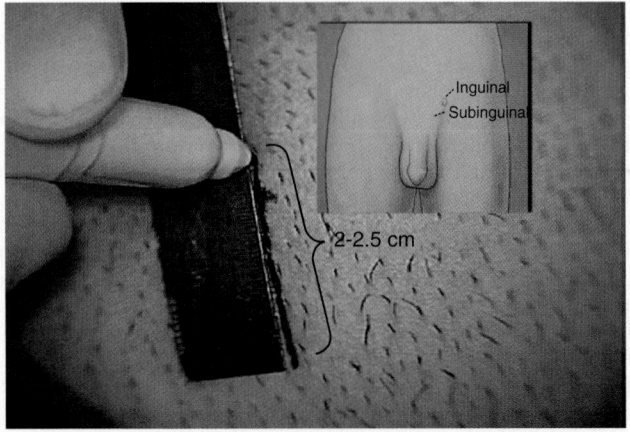

Figure 25-47. **If the operation is to be performed subinguinally, the incision is placed in the skin lines just below the external ring.**

TABLE 25-6 Indications for Inguinal (External Oblique Opened) Versus Subinguinal (Fascia Intact) Varicocelectomy

INGUINAL	SUBINGUINAL
Prepubertal children	Prior inguinal surgery
Solitary testis	Obesity
Tight, low external ring	Lax, capacious external ring
	High external ring
Short cord, high-lying testis	Long cord with low-lying testis
Less experienced with microsurgical repair	Very experienced with microsurgical repair

The Camper fascia and Scarpa fascia are divided with the electrocautery between the blades of a Crile clamp. The superficial epigastric artery and vein, if encountered, are retracted or alternately may be clamped, divided, and ligated.

If an inguinal approach is selected, the external oblique aponeurosis is cleaned and opened the length of the incision to the external inguinal ring in the direction of its fibers. A 3-0 absorbable suture placed at the apex of the external oblique incision facilitates later closure.

The spermatic cord is grasped with a Babcock clamp and delivered through the wound. The ilioinguinal and genital branches of the genitofemoral nerve are excluded from the cord, which is then surrounded with a large Penrose drain. If a subinguinal incision was made, the Camper and Scarpa fascia are incised as described earlier. An index finger is introduced into the wound and along the cord into the scrotum. The index finger is then hooked under the external inguinal ring, retracting it cephalad. A small Richardson retractor is slid along the back of the index finger and retracted caudad over the cord toward the scrotum (Fig. 25-48). The spermatic cord will be revealed between the index finger and retractor. The assistant grasps the cord with a Babcock clamp and delivers it through the wound. The cord is surrounded with a large Penrose drain.

Dissection of the Cord

The operating microscope is then brought into the field. Under 6× to 10× magnification the external spermatic fascia is opened with a

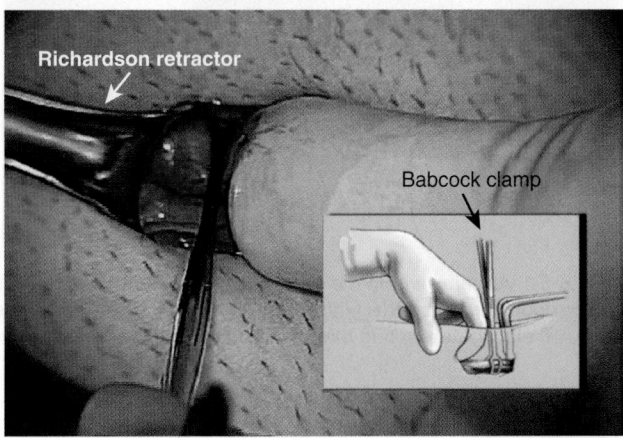

Figure 25-48. A small Richardson retractor is slid along the back of the index finger and retracted caudad over the cord toward the scrotum.

Bovie electrocautery instrument in the direction of the cremasteric fibers to avoid injury to the cremasteric arteries. A 5-0 Vicryl suture is placed at the apex of the opening to facilitate later closure. The relatively avascular internal spermatic fascia is opened with scissors as high as possible and held open with the straight mosquito forceps (Fig. 25-49). The magnification is increased to 10× to 25× and, after irrigation with 1% papaverine solution, the cord is inspected for the presence of pulsations revealing the location of the testicular artery. **Micro-Doppler is extremely useful in identifying arteries** (Fig. 25-50). **Once the testicular artery has been identified, it is dissected free of all surrounding tissue, tiny veins, and lymphatics, using a fine-tipped nonlocking micro needle holder and microforceps.** The artery is encircled with a vessel loop for positive identification and gentle retraction (Fig. 25-51). The suspected artery is tested by elevating the artery with the tips of the micro needle holder until it is completely occluded and then slowly lowering it until a pulsating blush of blood appears just over the needle holder. If the artery is not immediately identified, the cord is carefully dissected beginning with the largest veins. The veins are stripped clean of adherent lymphatics (Fig. 25-52) and the undersides of the largest veins inspected for an adherent artery. **In approximately 50% of patients the testicular artery is adherent to the undersurface of a large vein** (Beck et al, 1992). All veins within the cord, with the exception of the vasal veins, are doubly ligated either with hemoclips (Fig. 25-53) or by passing two 4-0 silk ligatures, one black and one white, beneath the vein (Fig. 25-54). These are then tied, and the vein is divided. Medium hemoclips are used for veins 5 mm or larger, small auto-hemoclips for veins 1 to 5 mm, and 4-0 silk for veins smaller than 2 mm. **The use of an automatic clip applier** (Ligaclip small size, Ethicon, Somerville, NJ) **significantly reduces operating time.** Bipolar cautery can be used for veins smaller than 0.5 mm. The vasal veins are preserved, providing venous return. If the vas deferens is accompanied by dilated veins greater than 2.5 mm in diameter, they are dissected free of the vasal artery and ligated. The vas deferens is always accompanied by two sets of vessels. **As long as at least one set of deferential veins remains intact, venous return will be adequate.** At the completion of the dissection, the cord is run over the index finger and inspected to verify that all veins have been identified and ligated. Small veins adherent to the testicular artery are dissected free and ligated or, if smaller than 1 mm, cauterized using a bipolar unit with a jeweler's forcep tip, and divided. Cremasteric arteries are found (usually between and adherent to two cremasteric veins) and preserved in at least 90% of patients. Recent studies using power Doppler imaging in men with nonobstructive azoospermia undergoing TESE have found that tubules containing sperm are most likely to be found in areas of the testis with the greatest blood supply. Therefore, logic would dictate that preservation of maximum testicular blood supply, including both testicular and cremasteric arteries, would be

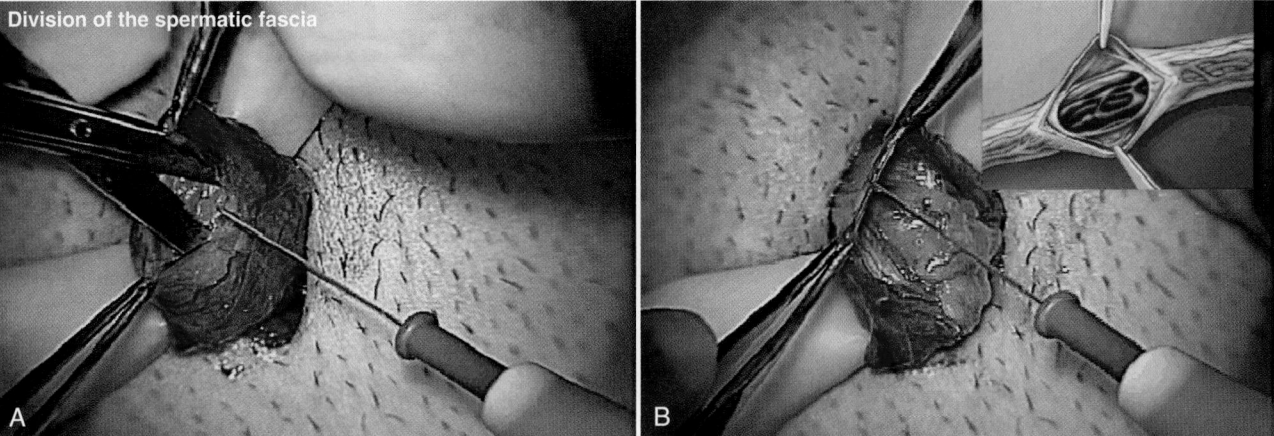

Figure 25-49. A and B, The operating microscope is then brought into the field. Under 4× to 6× magnification, the external and internal spermatic fasciae are opened.

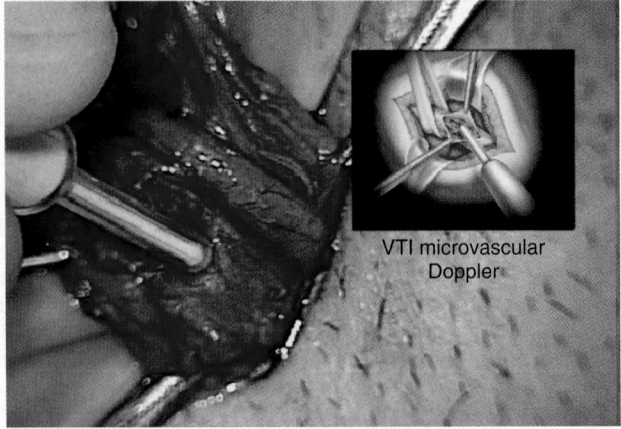

Figure 25-50. **Micro-Doppler is extremely useful in identifying arteries.**

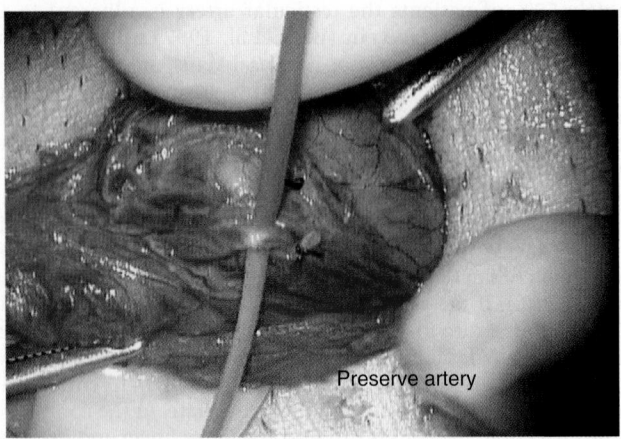

Figure 25-51. **The artery is encircled with a vessel loop for positive identification and gentle retraction.**

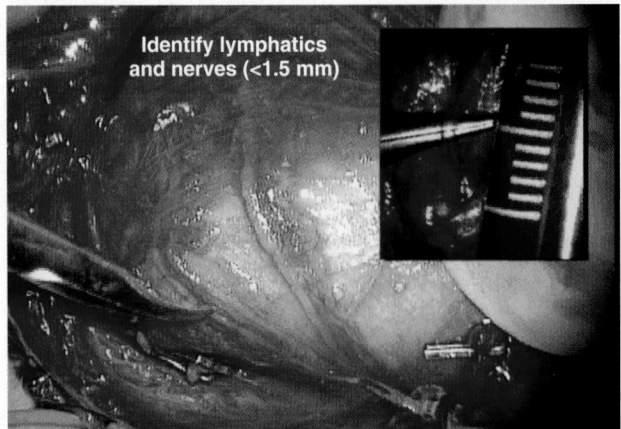

Figure 25-52. **If the artery is not immediately identified, the cord is carefully dissected, beginning with the largest veins. The veins are stripped clean of adherent lymphatics.**

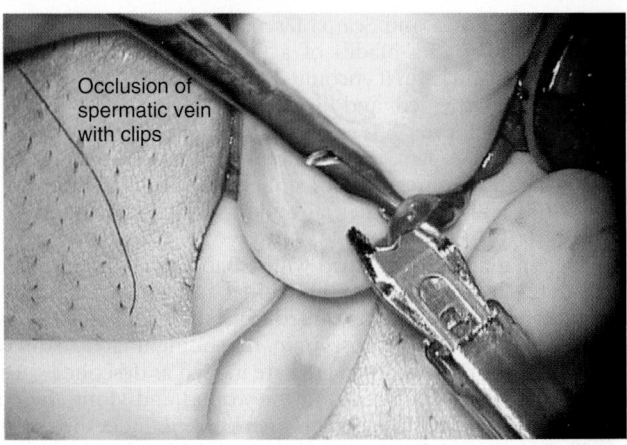

Figure 25-53. **All veins within the cord, with the exception of the vasal veins, are doubly ligated, either with hemoclips or by passing two 4-0 silk ligatures, one black and one white, beneath the vein (see Fig. 25-54).**

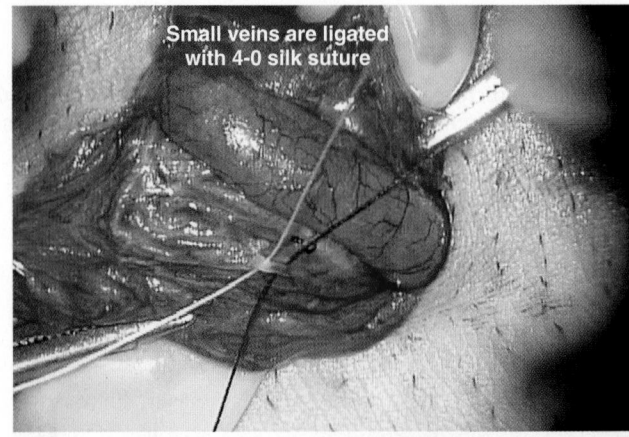

Figure 25-54. **All veins within the cord, with the exception of the vasal veins, are doubly ligated, either with hemoclips (see Fig. 25-53) or by passing two 4-0 silk ligatures, one black and one white, beneath the vein.**

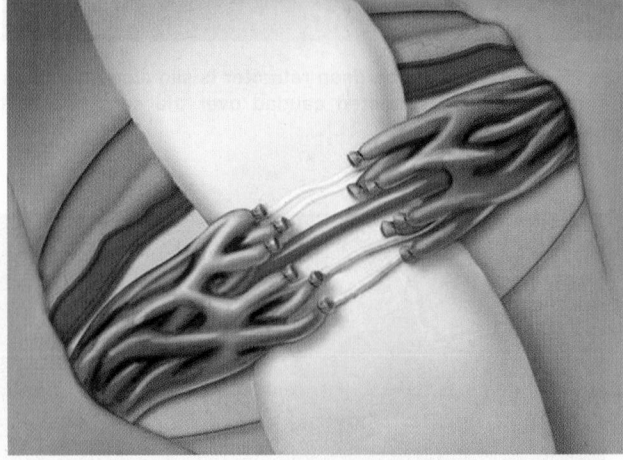

Figure 25-55. **At the completion of the dissection, only the testicular arteries, cremasteric arteries, lymphatics, and vas deferens with its vessels remain.**

beneficial to testicular function. **At the completion of the dissection, only the testicular arteries, cremasteric arteries, lymphatics, and vas deferens with its vessels remain** (Fig. 25-55). Dissection is not deemed complete until a run through the cord reveals no additional internal or external spermatic veins. Each time a vein is found and ligated, any remaining veins will dilate up.

Delivery of the Testis

Delivery of the testis through a small inguinal or subinguinal incision guarantees direct visual access to all possible avenues of testicular venous drainage. Delivery of only the cord allows

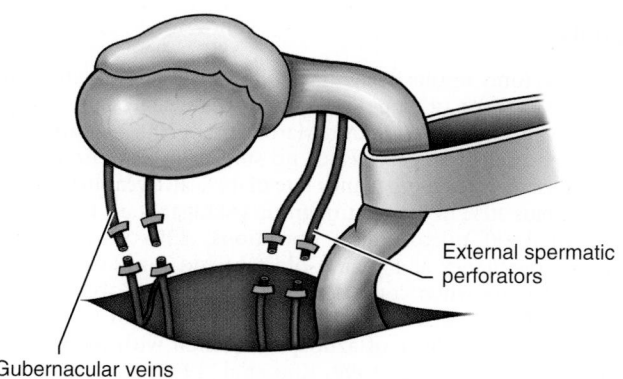

Figure 25-56. All external spermatic veins are identified and doubly ligated with hemoclips and divided.

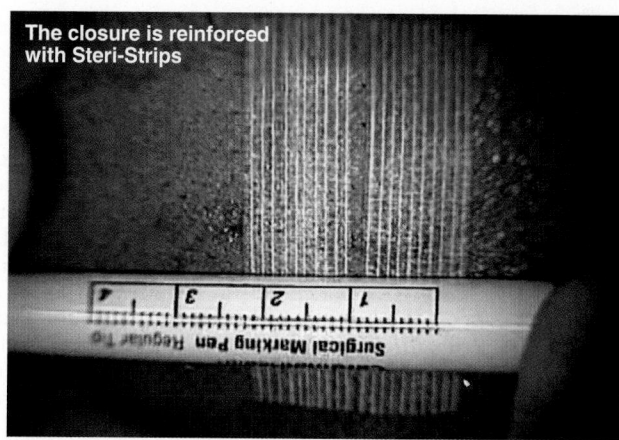

Figure 25-57. Scarpa and Camper fasciae are reapproximated with a single or continuous 3-0 plain catgut suture, and the skin is approximated with a 5-0 monofilament absorbable subcuticular suture, reinforced by two or three Steri-Strips.

access to most external spermatic collaterals but may miss those close to the testis and will not allow access to scrotal or gubernacular collaterals, which have been demonstrated radiographically to be the cause of 10% of recurrent varicoceles (Kaufman et al, 1983). With gentle upward traction on the cord and upward pressure on the testis through the invaginated scrotum, the testis is easily delivered through the wound. All external spermatic veins are identified and doubly ligated with hemoclips and divided (Fig. 25-56). The gubernaculum is inspected for the presence of veins exiting from the tunica vaginalis. These are either cauterized or doubly clipped and divided. **When this step is completed, all testicular venous return must be within the Penrose-surrounded cord.**

Hydroceles are found in 15% of testes associated with varicoceles. **As little as 3 mL of hydrocele fluid can significantly alter testicular temperature regulation** (Wysock et al, 2009). If a hydrocele is noted when the testis is delivered, it is repaired. Small ones may be treated with excision of a segment of the hydrocele sac and cauterization of the edges. Larger hydroceles are treated with either a bottleneck or excision technique. **The temporary high venous pressure immediately after varicocelectomy can make good hemostasis difficult to achieve after excisional hydrocelectomy. Therefore, there should be no hesitation to use a scrotal Penrose drain placed in the dependent portion of the scrotum for 24 hours after combined varicocelectomy and excisional hydrocelectomy.** The testis is then returned to the scrotum and the Penrose drain is left beneath the cord structures.

The external oblique aponeurosis, if opened, is reapproximated with continuous suturing using the previously placed 3-0 suture. The Scarpa and Camper fasciae are reapproximated with a single or continuous 3-0 plain catgut suture, and the skin is approximated with a 5-0 monofilament absorbable subcuticular suture reinforced by two or three Steri-Strips (Fig. 25-57). A scrotal supporter is applied and stuffed with fluff-type dressings. The patient is discharged on the day of surgery with a prescription for Tylenol with codeine. Light work may be resumed in 2 or 3 days.

If any large external or gubernacular veins are ligated after delivery of the testis, the cord is again run over the index finger to search for veins that may dilate after gubernacular or external spermatic veins are ligated. The external spermatic fascia is closed with interrupted 5-0 Vicryl, facilitated by the previously placed suture at the apex of the external spermatic fascia.

Radiographic Occlusion Techniques

Intraoperative venography has been used to visualize the venous collaterals, which if left unligated may result in varicocele recurrence (Sayfan et al, 1981; Belgrano et al, 1984; Levitt et al, 1987; Zaontz and Firlit, 1987). Intraoperative venography does reduce the incidence of varicocele recurrence, but the two-dimensional view afforded often does not enable the surgeon to identify the location of all collaterals.

Radiographic coil occlusion of the internal spermatic veins has been successfully used for varicoceles (Lima et al, 1978; Walsh and White, 1981; Weissbach et al, 1981). These techniques are performed under a local anesthetic through a small cut-down incision over the femoral vein. The recurrence rate after balloon occlusion was originally 11% and more recently was reportedly as low as 4% (Kaufman et al, 1983; Mitchell et al, 1985; Murray et al, 1986; Matthews et al, 1992). Failure to successfully cannulate small collaterals and external spermatic veins and scrotal collaterals results in recurrence. **Venographic placement of a balloon or coil in the internal spermatic vein is successfully accomplished in 75% to 90% of attempts** (White et al, 1981; Morag et al, 1984; Winkelbauer et al, 1994; Sivanathan and Abernethy, 2003); **therefore a significant number of men undergoing attempted radiographic occlusion will ultimately require a surgical approach.** In addition, the radiographic techniques take 1 to 3 hours to perform compared with 25 to 45 minutes for surgical repair. Although rare, serious complications of radiographic balloon or coil occlusion have included migration of the balloon or coil into the renal vein, resulting in loss of a kidney, pulmonary embolization of the coil or balloon (Matthews et al, 1992), femoral vein perforation or thrombosis, and anaphylactic reaction to radiographic contrast medium. Antegrade scrotal sclerotherapy via cannulation of a scrotal vein has been used in Europe (Tauber and Johnsen, 1994; Ficarra et al, 2002; Minucci et al, 2004). The recurrence rate is similar to that of balloon or coil techniques. Long-term follow-up is not available, and the consequence of escape of the sclerosing agent into the renal vein and vena cava is unknown. In addition, the larger the varicocele, the higher the failure and recurrence rate with this technique. **We have seen many men referred with late (2 to 5 years) recurrence after radiographic occlusion. On presentation they typically have slow-filling veins that become prominent at the end of the day. Initial cursory physical examination can miss these recurrences. I believe these recurrences are likely the result of recanalization through the coils because, unlike with surgical repair, the veins are not ligated and divided.** Although often initially successful, I believe that radiographic occlusion is less durable than microsurgical ligation.

Complications of Varicocelectomy

Hydrocele

Hydrocele formation is the most common complication reported after nonmicroscopic varicocelectomy. The incidence of this complication varies from 3% to 33%, with an average incidence of about 7%. Analysis of the protein concentration of hydrocele fluid indicates that **hydrocele formation after varicocelectomy is caused by lymphatic obstruction** (Szabo and Kessler, 1984). At least half of postvaricocelectomy hydroceles grow to a size large enough to warrant surgical excision as a result of the discomfort and growth of the hydrocele to a large size. The effect of hydrocele formation on sperm function and fertility is uncertain. It is known that men with varicocele have significantly elevated intratesticular temperatures (Zorgniotti et al, 1979; Goldstein and Eid, 1989), and this appears to be an important pathophysiologic phenomenon mediating the adverse effects of varicocele on fertility (Saypol et al, 1981). The development of a large hydrocele creates an abnormal insulating layer that surrounds the testis. This may impair the efficiency of the counter-current heat exchange mechanism and therefore obviate some of the benefits of varicocelectomy (Wysock et al, 2009).

Use of magnification to identify and preserve lymphatics can virtually eliminate the risk of hydrocele formation after varicocelectomy (Goldstein et al, 1992; Marmar and Kim, 1994; Glassberg et al, 2008). The management of postvaricocelectomy hydrocele is identical to that for other hydroceles (see Chapter 41).

Testicular Artery Injury

The diameter of the testicular artery in humans is 1.0 to 1.5 mm. The testicular artery supplies two thirds of the testicular blood supply, and the vasal and cremasteric arteries the remaining one third (Raman and Goldstein, 2004). Microdissections of the human spermatic cord have revealed that the testicular artery is closely adherent to a large internal spermatic vein in 40% of men. In another 20% of men the testicular artery is surrounded by a network of tiny veins (Beck et al, 1992). During the course of cord dissection for varicocelectomy the artery may go into spasm and even in its unconstricted state is often difficult to positively identify and preserve. **Injury or ligation of the testicular artery carries with it the risk of testicular atrophy and/or impaired spermatogenesis.** Starzl's transplant group (Penn et al, 1972) reported a 14% incidence of frank testicular atrophy when the testicular artery was purposely ligated. The actual incidence of testicular artery ligation during varicocelectomy is unknown, but some studies suggest it is common (Wosnitzer and Roth, 1983). Animal studies have indicated that the risk of testicular atrophy after testicular artery ligation varies from 20% to 100% (MacMahon et al, 1976; Goldstein et al, 1983). In humans, atrophy after artery ligation is probably less likely a result of the contribution of the cremasteric as well as vasal arterial supply (Raman and Goldstein, 2004). **In children the potential for neovascularization and compensatory hypertrophy of the vasal and cremasteric vessels is probably greater than in adults, making atrophy after testicular artery ligation less likely.** Use of magnifying loupes, or preferably an operating microscope and/or a fine-tipped Doppler probe, facilitates identification and preservation of the testicular artery and therefore minimizes the risk of testicular injury. Radiographic balloon or coil occlusion techniques also eliminate this risk.

Varicocele Recurrence

The incidence of varicocele recurrence after surgical repair varies from 0.6% to 45% (Barbalias et al, 1998; Lemack et al, 1998; Cayan et al, 2000; Al-Kandari et al, 2007). Recurrence is more common after repair of pediatric varicoceles. Radiographic studies of recurrent varicoceles visualize periarterial, parallel inguinal, or midretroperitoneal collaterals or, more rarely, transscrotal collaterals (Kaufman et al, 1983). **Retroperitoneal operations miss parallel inguinal and scrotal collaterals.** Nonmagnified inguinal operations have a lower incidence of varicocele recurrence but fail to address the issue of scrotal collaterals or small veins surrounding the testicular artery. The microsurgical approach with delivery of the testis lowers the incidence of varicocele recurrence to less than 1% compared with 9% with use of conventional inguinal techniques (Goldstein et al, 1992; Marmar and Kim, 1994).

Results

Varicocelectomy results in significant improvement in semen analysis in 60% to 80% of men. Reported pregnancy rates after varicocelectomy vary from 20% to 60% (Marmar et al, 2007). A randomized controlled trial of surgery versus no surgery in infertile men with varicoceles revealed a pregnancy rate of 44% at 1 year in the surgery group versus 10% in the control group (Madgar et al, 1995). In our series of 1500 microsurgical operations, 43% of couples had achieved pregnancy at 1 year (Goldstein and Tanrikut, 2006) and 69% at 2 years when couples with female factors were excluded. **Microsurgical varicocelectomy results in return of sperm to the ejaculate in up to 50% of azoospermic men with palpable varicoceles** (Matthews et al, 1998; Kim et al, 1999; Pasqualotto et al, 2006; Lee et al, 2007a; Ishikawa et al, 2008).

The results of varicocelectomy are also related to the size of the varicocele. **Repair of large varicoceles results in a significantly greater improvement in semen quality than repair of small varicoceles** (Steckel et al, 1993; Jarow et al, 1996). In addition, large varicoceles are associated with greater preoperative impairment in semen quality than small varicoceles, and overall pregnancy rates consequently are similar regardless of varicocele size. Some evidence suggests that the younger the patient is at the time of varicocele repair, the greater the improvement after repair and the more likely the testis is to recover from varicocele-induced injury (Kass et al, 1987). Varicocele recurrence, testicular artery ligation, or postvaricocelectomy hydrocele formation are often associated with poor postoperative results. **In infertile men with low serum testosterone levels, microsurgical varicocelectomy alone results in substantial improvement in serum testosterone levels** (Su et al, 1995; Cayan et al, 1999; Younes, 2003; Rosoff et al, 2009; Tanrikut et al, 2011).

Summary

Varicocele is an extremely common entity, present in 15% of the male population. Varicoceles are found in approximately 35% of men with primary infertility but 75% to 81% of men with secondary infertility. Mounting evidence clearly demonstrates that varicocele causes progressive duration-dependent injury to the testis. Larger varicoceles appear to cause more damage than small varicoceles, and, conversely, repair of large varicoceles results in greater improvement of semen quality. **Varicocelectomy can halt the progressive duration-dependent decline in semen quality found in men with varicoceles.** The earlier the age at which varicocele is repaired, the more likely is recovery of spermatogenic function. **Varicocelectomy can also improve Leydig cell function, resulting in increased testosterone levels** (Su et al, 1995; Cayan et al, 1999; Younes, 2003; Tanrikut et al, 2011).

The most common complications after varicocelectomy are hydrocele formation, testicular artery injury, and varicocele persistence or recurrence. **The incidence of these complications can be reduced by using microsurgical techniques, inguinal or subinguinal operations, and exposure of the external spermatic and scrotal veins.** Use of these advanced techniques of varicocelectomy provides a safe, effective approach to elimination of varicocele, preservation of testicular function, and, in a substantial number of men, an increase in semen quality and likelihood of pregnancy, as well as increase in serum testosterone in men with androgen deficiency.

ORCHIOPEXY IN ADULTS

It is well known that cryptorchidism is associated with a high incidence of infertility even when unilateral. Long hot baths and saunas in humans, on a regular basis, have been shown to impair spermatogenesis. Elevated testicular temperature is also thought to be the primary pathophysiologic feature of varicocele (Zorgniotti, 1980; Saypol et al, 1981; Goldstein and Eid, 1989; Wright et al, 1997). Spermatogenesis is exquisitely temperature sensitive. Both

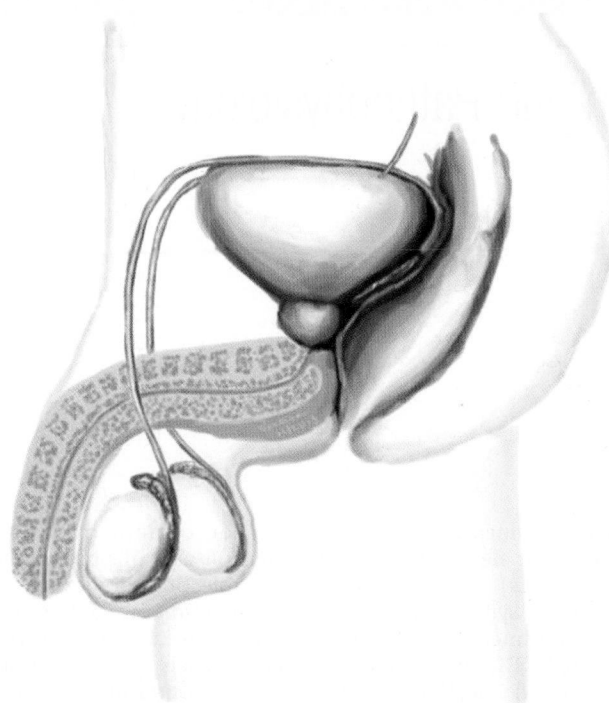

Figure 25-58. Instead of the testes being side by side, an ectopic testis is one behind the other, almost in the perineum.

animal and human studies have shown that artificial elevation of testicular temperature results in impaired spermatogenesis (Shin et al, 1997; Perez-Crespo et al, 2008; Shiraishi et al, 2010). It will also preserve testicular hormonal function. The technique of orchiopexy in adults is identical to that employed for children. Even with a normal contralateral testis, orchiopexy is worthwhile to bring down a unilateral undescended testis to, if possible, a scrotal location where it can be examined. Leydig cell function in undescended testis can be retained. Orchiopexy in adults with bilateral undescended testes can induce spermatogenesis and allow pregnancy (Shin et al, 1997). Even **a solitary cryptorchid testis, when properly placed in the scrotum, can provide enough testosterone to obviate the need for hormone replacement. When orchiopexy is performed in adults, regular self-examination and yearly sonography are mandatory.**

Retractile or Ectopic Testes in Adults

Retractile testes in boys are usually not surgically repaired if the testes can be manually manipulated to stay down in the scrotum either in the office or under anesthesia. The fate of persistently retractile testis in adults is unknown. A subset of infertile men have retractile testis (Caucci et al, 1997). The semen analyses of these men often demonstrate a typical stressed pattern similar to those of men with varicoceles. These men, however, do not have palpable varicoceles. They all have at least one and frequently both testes that retract out of the scrotum and into the abdomen and remain there for an hour or more a day. In some men these testes remain in the abdomen virtually all the time, except when in a warm shower or under anesthesia. It is likely that these testes will suffer from impaired temperature regulation and impaired spermatogenesis. Scrotal orchiopexy can improve the semen quality and fertility of some of these men. Some men have ectopic testis, in which instead of the testes being side by side, one testis is behind the other (Fig. 25-58), almost in the perineum. This is also likely to elevate testis temperature.

When scrotal orchiopexy is performed for retractile or ectopic testis in adults, a dartos pouch operation should be performed. Simple suture orchiopexy of the tunica albuginea of the testis to the dartos, as is performed sometimes to prevent torsion, will not prevent retraction of these testes into the groin. Creation of a dartos pouch will keep the testis well down in the scrotum and permanently prevent retraction. **This is also the most reliable and safest technique for the prevention of testicular torsion** (Redman and Barthold, 1995).

A 3- to 4-cm transverse incision is made in the low scrotal skin folds overlying the testis. **The incision is kept very superficial, just through the dermis and not into the dartos. A large pouch must be created to accommodate the adult testis.** The place of dissection is above the dartos and just below the skin, which is kept thin.

After a capacious pouch is created, the dartos and underlying tunica vaginalis are vertically incised and the testis delivered. The cremasteric fibers overlying the spermatic cord are divided and ligated to minimize the tendency of the testis to retract. The opening in the dartos is closed around the cord (but not too tightly) to prevent the testis from falling out of the pouch. The cut edge of the everted tunica is approximated to the opening in the dartos with interrupted synthetic monofilament absorbable sutures. This allows placement of the testis in the pouch without the need for fixation sutures in the tunica albuginea (Redman and Barthold, 1995). The skin is closed over the testis with interrupted sutures of 4-0 chromic catgut. This technique obviates the risk of inadvertent injury to and bleeding from the testicular artery, which courses just under the tunica albuginea (Jarow, 1990).

ACKNOWLEDGMENT

I thank Vanessa L. Dudley and Philip Shihua Li, MD, for their immeasurable assistance in the preparation of this manuscript.

Please visit the accompanying website at www.expertconsult.com to view videos associated with this chapter.

REFERENCES

The complete reference list is available online at www.expertconsult.com.

SUGGESTED READINGS

Dabaja A, Goldstein M. Microsurgical hydrocelectomy: rationale and technique. Urol Practice 2014;1(4):189–93.

Goldstein M, Tanrikut C. Microsurgical management of male infertility. Nat Clin Pract Urol 2006;3(7):381–91.

Marmar JL, Agarwal A, Prabakaran S, et al. Reassessing the value of varicocelectomy as a treatment for male subfertility with a new meta-analysis. Fertil Steril 2007;88(3):639–48.

Matthews GJ, Matthews ED, Goldstein M. Induction of spermatogenesis and achievement of pregnancy after microsurgical varicocelectomy in men with azoospermia and severe oligoasthenospermia. Fertil Steril 1998; 70(1):71–5.

Pasqualotto FF, Lucon AM, Hallak J, et al. Induction of spermatogenesis in azoospermic men after varicocele repair. Hum Reprod 2003; 18(1):108–12.

Schiff J, Chan P, Li PS, et al. Outcome and late failures compared in 4 techniques of microsurgical vasoepididymostomy in 153 consecutive men. J Urol 2005;174(2):651–5, quiz 801.

Schlegel PN. Testicular sperm extraction: microdissection improves sperm yield with minimal tissue excision. Hum Reprod 1999;14(1):131–5.

Sigman M, Jarow JP. Ipsilateral testicular hypotrophy is associated with decreased sperm counts in infertile men with varicoceles. J Urol 1997;158(2):605–7.

Tanrikut C, Goldstein M, Rosoff JS, et al. Varicocele as a risk factor for androgen deficiency and effect of repair. BJU Int 2011;108:1480–4.

26 Physiology of Penile Erection and Pathophysiology of Erectile Dysfunction

Tom F. Lue, MD, ScD (Hon), FACS

Physiology of Penile Erection

Pathophysiology of Erectile Dysfunction

Perspectives

"The penis does not obey the order of its master, who tries to erect or shrink it at will. Instead, the penis erects freely while its master is asleep. The penis must be said to have its own mind, by any stretch of the imagination."

– Leonardo da Vinci

PHYSIOLOGY OF PENILE ERECTION

Historical Aspects

The first description of erectile dysfunction (ED) dates from about 2000 BC and was set down on Egyptian papyrus. Two types were described: natural ("the man is incapable of accomplishing the sex act") and supernatural (evil charms and spells). Later, Hippocrates reported many cases of male impotence among the rich inhabitants of Scythia and ascribed it to excessive horseback riding. Aristotle stated that three branches of nerves carry spirit and energy to the penis and that erection is produced by the influx of air (Brenot, 1994). His theory was well accepted until Leonardo da Vinci (1504) noted a large amount of blood in the erect penis of hanged men and cast doubt on the concept of the air-filled penis. However, da Vinci's writings were kept secret until the beginning of the 20th century (Brenot, 1994). Nevertheless, in 1585, in *Ten Books on Surgery* and the *Book of Reproduction*, Ambroise Paré gave an accurate account of penile anatomy and the concept of erection. He described the penis as being composed of concentric coats of nerves, veins, and arteries and of two ligaments (corpora cavernosa), a urinary tract, and four muscles. "When the man becomes inflamed with lust and desire, blood rushes into the male member and causes it to become erect," Paré wrote. The importance of retaining blood in the penis was stressed by Dionis (1718; quoted by Brenot, 1994), who attributed this to the muscles cramping the veins at the proximal end, and by Hunter (1787), who thought that venous spasm prevented the exit of blood.

Modern investigations of penile hemodynamics began in the 1970s with xenon washout and cavernosography studies in human volunteers exposed to audiovisual sexual stimuli. These studies yielded conflicting results: Shirai and associates (1978) concluded that penile venous flow is increased during erection, but markedly increased arterial flow compensates for this; Wagner (1981) also demonstrated increased arterial flow but concluded that venous drainage is decreased during erection.

Much of the current understanding of erectile physiology was gained in the 1980s and 1990s. In addition to the role of smooth muscle in regulating arterial and venous flow, the three-dimensional structure of the tunica albuginea and its role in venous occlusion were elucidated. An important breakthrough in the understanding of neural influences was the identification of nitric oxide (NO) as the major neurotransmitter for erection and of phosphodiesterases (PDEs) for detumescence. The role of endothelium and nitric oxide synthase (NOS) in regulating smooth muscle tone and of the intercellular links affected by gap junctions has been uncovered. The importance of ion channels (potassium and calcium) and Rho/Rho-kinase pathways in contraction and relaxation of smooth muscle also has been shown. In regard to pathophysiology, changes in smooth muscle, nerve endings, endothelium, and the fibroelastic framework associated with many diseases have been identified. These developments are discussed in detail in this chapter.

Functional Anatomy of the Penis

The penis is composed of three cylindrical structures: the paired corpora cavernosa and the corpus spongiosum (which houses the urethra), covered by a loose subcutaneous layer and skin. Its flaccid length is controlled by the contractile state of the erectile smooth muscle and the amount of blood in the sinusoids and varies considerably, depending on emotion and outside temperature. In one study, penile length, measured from the pubopenile junction to the meatus, was 8.8 cm flaccid, 12.4 cm stretched, and 12.9 cm erect, with neither age nor the size of the flaccid penis accurately predicting erectile length (Wessells et al, 1996). In another study, Sparling (1997) concluded that about 15% of men have a downward curve during erection, erect angle is below horizontal in one quarter, and shorter erect lengths (from 4.5 to 5.75 inches) occur in 40% of men. Since then, more studies have been reported from several countries (Awwad et al, 2005) (Table 26-1). Regarding penile morphology and erection, one study showed that, during erection, the penile buckling forces are dependent not only on intracavernous pressures but also on penile geometry and erectile tissue properties. The authors concluded that in patients with normal penile hemodynamics but without adequate rigidity, structural causes should be investigated (Udelson et al, 1998).

Tunica Albuginea

The tunica affords great flexibility, rigidity, and tissue strength to the penis (Hsu et al, 1992) (Fig. 26-1). **The tunical covering of the corpora cavernosa is a bilayered structure with multiple sublayers. Inner-layer bundles support and contain the cavernous tissue and are oriented circularly. Radiating from this inner layer are intracavernous pillars that act as struts to augment the septum and provide essential support to the erectile tissue. Outer-layer bundles are oriented longitudinally, extending from the glans penis to the proximal crura; they insert into the inferior pubic rami but are absent between the 5 o'clock and the 7 o'clock positions. Less abundant are oblique-oriented fibers that connect the two main layers. In contrast, the corpus spongiosum lacks an**

TABLE 26-1   Penile Length in Adults

FIRST AUTHOR	YEAR OF REPORT	NO. SUBJECTS	AGE IN YEARS (RANGE)	FLACCID LENGTH (cm)	STRETCHED OR ERECT LENGTH (cm)	COUNTRY
Kinsey	1948	2770	20-59	9.7	15.5 (E)	United States
Bondil	1992	905	17-91	10.7	16.74 (S)	France
Wessells	1996	80	21-82	8.85	12.45 (S), 12.89 (E)	United States
Ponchietti	2001	3300	17-19	9	12.5 (S)	Italy
Ajmani	1985	320	17-23	8.16	NA	Nigeria
Schneider	2001	111	18-19	8.6	14.48 (E)	Germany
		32	40-68	9.22	14.18 (E)	
Awwad	2005	271 (N)	17-83	9.3	13.5 (S)	Jordan
		109 (ED)	22-68	7.7	11.6 (S)	

E, erect length; ED, erectile dysfunction; N, normal; NA, not available; S, stretched length.
Modified from Awwad Z, Abu-Hijleh M, Basri S, et al. Penile measurements in normal adult Jordanians and in patients with erectile dysfunction. Int J Impot Res 2005;17:191–5.

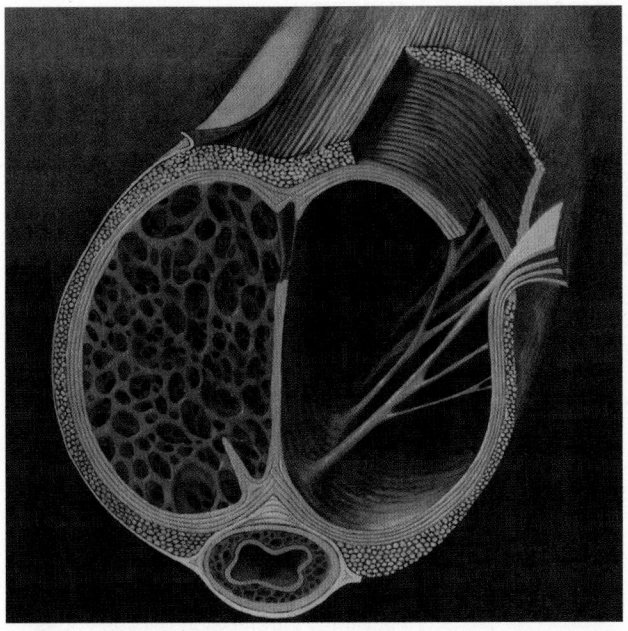

Figure 26-1. Artist's cross-sectional drawing of the penis, depicting the inner circular and outer longitudinal layers of the tunica albuginea and the intracavernous pillars. The longitudinal layer is absent in the ventral groove housing the corpus spongiosum. (From Lue TF, Akkus E, Kour NW. Physiology of erectile function and dysfunction. Campbell's Urology Update 1994;12:1–10.)

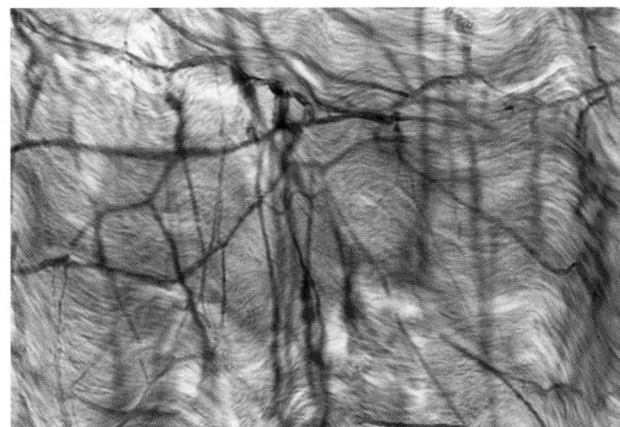

Figure 26-2. Micrograph of the human tunica albuginea, showing the interwoven elastic fibers and the finer collagen fibers (Hart stain ×100).

outer layer or intracorporeal struts, ensuring a low-pressure structure during erection.

The tunica is composed of elastic fibers that form an irregular, latticed network on which the collagen fibers rest (Fig. 26-2). The detailed histologic composition of the tunica varies with anatomic location and function. Emissary veins run between the inner and outer layers of the tunica for a short distance, often piercing the outer bundles obliquely. However, the cavernous artery and the branches of the dorsal artery that give additional blood supply to the corpus cavernosum take a more direct route and are surrounded by a periarterial soft-tissue sheath, which protects the arteries from occlusion by the tunica albuginea during erection.

The outer tunical layer appears to play an additional role in compression of the emissary veins during erection. It also determines, to a large extent, the variability in tunical thickness and strength (Hsu et al, 1992). Between the 6 o'clock and 7 o'clock positions, the tunical thickness is 0.8 ± 0.1 mm; at the 9 o'clock

position, 1.2 ± 0.2 mm; and at the 11 o'clock position, 2.2 ± 0.4 mm. At the 3 o'clock, 5 o'clock to 6 o'clock, and 1 o'clock positions, the measurements are nearly identical in mirror-image fashion. (Differences at specific locations have been found to be statistically significant.)

The stress on the tunica before penetration of a test object has been measured as $1.6 \pm 0.2 \times 10^7$ N/m^2 between the 6 o'clock and 7 o'clock positions, $3.0 \pm 0.3 \times 10^7$ N/m^2 at the 9 o'clock position, and $4.5 \pm 0.5 \times 10^7$ N/m^2 at the 11 o'clock position. **The strength and thickness of the tunica correlate in a statistically significant fashion with location. The most vulnerable area is located on the ventral groove (between the 5 o'clock and 7 o'clock positions), where the longitudinal outer layer is absent; most prostheses tend to extrude here** (Hsu et al, 1994).

The tunica albuginea is composed of fibrillar collagen (mostly type I but also type III) in organized arrays interlaced with elastin fibers. Although collagen has a greater tensile strength than steel, it is unyielding. In contrast, elastin can be stretched up to 150% of its length. The elastin content allows tunical expansion and helps to determine stretched penile length.

External penile support consists of two ligamentous structures: the fundiform and suspensory ligaments. The fundiform ligament arises from Colles fascia and is lateral, superficial, and not adherent to the tunica albuginea of the corpora cavernosa. The suspensory ligament arises from Buck fascia and consists of two lateral bundles and one median bundle, which circumscribe the dorsal vein of the penis. Its main function is to attach the tunica albuginea of the corpora cavernosa to the pubis, and it provides support for the mobile portion of the penis (Hoznek et al, 1998). In patients with congenital deficiency or in whom this ligament has been severed in "penile elongation" surgery, the erect penis may be unstable or droop.

Corpora Cavernosa, Corpus Spongiosum, and Glans Penis

The corpora cavernosa comprise two spongy, paired cylinders contained in the thick envelope of the tunica albuginea. Their proximal ends, the crura, originate at the undersurface of the puboischial rami as two separate structures but merge under the pubic arch and remain attached up to the glans. **The septum between the two corpora cavernosa is incomplete in men but is complete in some species such as dogs.**

The corpora cavernosa are supported by a fibrous skeleton that includes the tunica albuginea, the septum, the intracavernous pillars, the intracavernous fibrous framework, and the periarterial and perineural fibrous sheath (Goldstein and Padma-Nathan, 1990; Hsu et al, 1992). Within the tunica are the interconnected sinusoids separated by smooth muscle trabeculae surrounded by elastic fibers, collagen, and loose areolar tissue. The terminal cavernous nerves and helicine arteries are intimately associated with the smooth muscle. Each corpus cavernosum is a conglomeration of sinusoids, larger in the center and smaller in the periphery. In the flaccid state, the blood slowly diffuses from the central to the peripheral sinusoids, and the blood gas levels are similar to those of venous blood. During erection, the rapid entry of arterial blood to both the central and the peripheral sinusoids changes the intracavernous blood gas levels to those of arterial blood (Sattar et al, 1995).

The structure of the corpus spongiosum and glans is similar to that of the corpora cavernosa except that the sinusoids are larger. The tunica is thinner in the spongiosum (with only a circular layer [see earlier]) and is absent in the glans (Table 26-2).

Arteries

The source of penile blood is usually the internal pudendal artery, a branch of the internal iliac artery (Fig. 26-3A). **In many instances, however, accessory arteries exist, arising from the external iliac, obturator, and vesical and femoral arteries, and they may constitute the dominant or only arterial supply to the corpus cavernosum in some men** (Breza et al, 1989). In a study of 20 fresh human cadavers, Droupy and colleagues (1997) reported three patterns of penile arterial supply: type I, arising exclusively from internal pudendal arteries (in 3 of 20 samples); type II, arising from both accessory and internal pudendal arteries (in 14 of 20 samples); and type III, arising exclusively from accessory pudendal arteries (in 3 of 20 samples). **Nehra and colleagues (2008) studied 79 consecutive patients with a history of ED and noted that 35% had an accessory pudendal artery, typically arising from the obturator artery. In these men, the accessory pudendal was the dominant blood supply in 54% and the only corporeal blood supply in 11%. The importance of accessory pudendal artery preservation during radical prostatectomy was demonstrated by Mulhall and colleagues (2008), who reported more rapid recovery of sexual function in men who underwent artery-sparing radical prostatectomy.**

The internal pudendal artery becomes the common penile artery after giving off a branch to the perineum. The three branches of the penile artery are the dorsal, bulbourethral, and cavernous. Distally, they join to form a vascular ring near the

TABLE 26-2 Penile Components and Their Function during Penile Erection

COMPONENT	FUNCTION
Corpora cavernosa	Support corpus spongiosum and glans
Tunica albuginea (of corpora cavernosa)	Contains and protects erectile tissue Provides rigidity of the corpora cavernosa Participates in veno-occlusive mechanism
Smooth muscle	Regulates blood flow into and out of the sinusoids
Ischiocavernosus muscle	Pumps blood distally to hasten erection Provides additional penile rigidity during rigid erection phase
Bulbocavernosus muscle	Compresses the bulb to help expel semen
Corpus spongiosum	Pressurizes and constricts the urethral lumen to allow forceful expulsion of semen
Glans	Acts as a cushion to lessen the impact of penis on female organs Provides sensory input to facilitate erection and enhance pleasure Facilitates intromission because of its cone shape

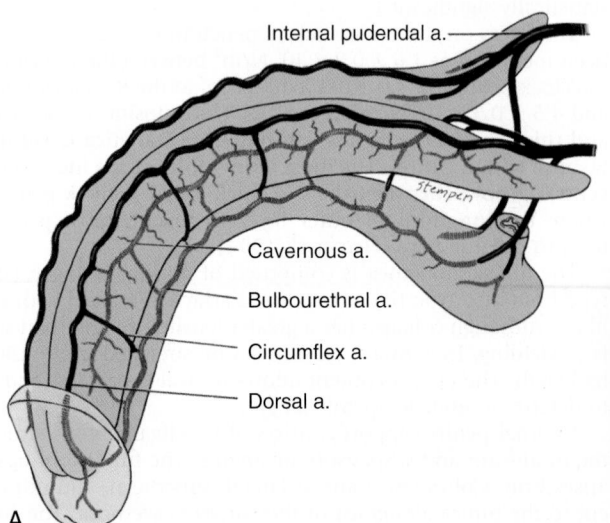

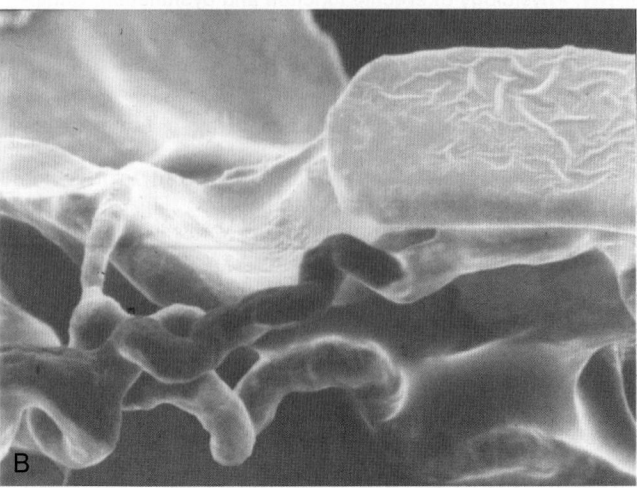

Figure 26-3. A, Penile arterial supply. **B,** Scanning electron micrograph of a human penile cast showing helicine arteries opening directly into the sinusoids without intervening capillaries.

glans. The dorsal artery is responsible for engorgement of the glans during erection. The bulbourethral artery supplies the bulb and corpus spongiosum. The cavernous artery effects tumescence of the corpus cavernosum and enters it at the hilum of the penis, where the two crura merge. It gives off many helicine arteries along its course, which supply the trabecular erectile tissue and the sinusoids (Fig. 26-3B). These helicine arteries are contracted and tortuous in the flaccid state and become dilated and straight during erection. Diallo and associates (2013) noted that in four of their five cadaveric specimens, the dorsal artery sent two to four penetrating branches to join the cavernous artery and supply blood to the distal one third of the penis. The bulbourethral and urethral arteries are situated outside the tunica albuginea of the corpus spongiosum on the lateral and dorsal sides. Anastomosis of the cavernous and urethral arteries occurs outside the tunica of the spongiosum.

Veins

The venous drainage from the three corpora originates in tiny venules leading from the peripheral sinusoids immediately beneath the tunica albuginea. These venules travel in the trabeculae between the tunica and the peripheral sinusoids to form the subtunical venous plexus before exiting as the emissary veins (Fig. 26-4A). Outside the tunica albuginea, venous drainage is as follows.

Skin and Subcutaneous Tissue. Multiple superficial veins run subcutaneously and unite near the root of the penis to form a single (or paired) superficial dorsal vein, which drains into the saphenous veins. Occasionally, the superficial dorsal vein may also drain a portion of the corpora cavernosa.

Pendulous Penis. The emissary veins from the corpus cavernosum and spongiosum drain dorsally to the deep dorsal, laterally to the

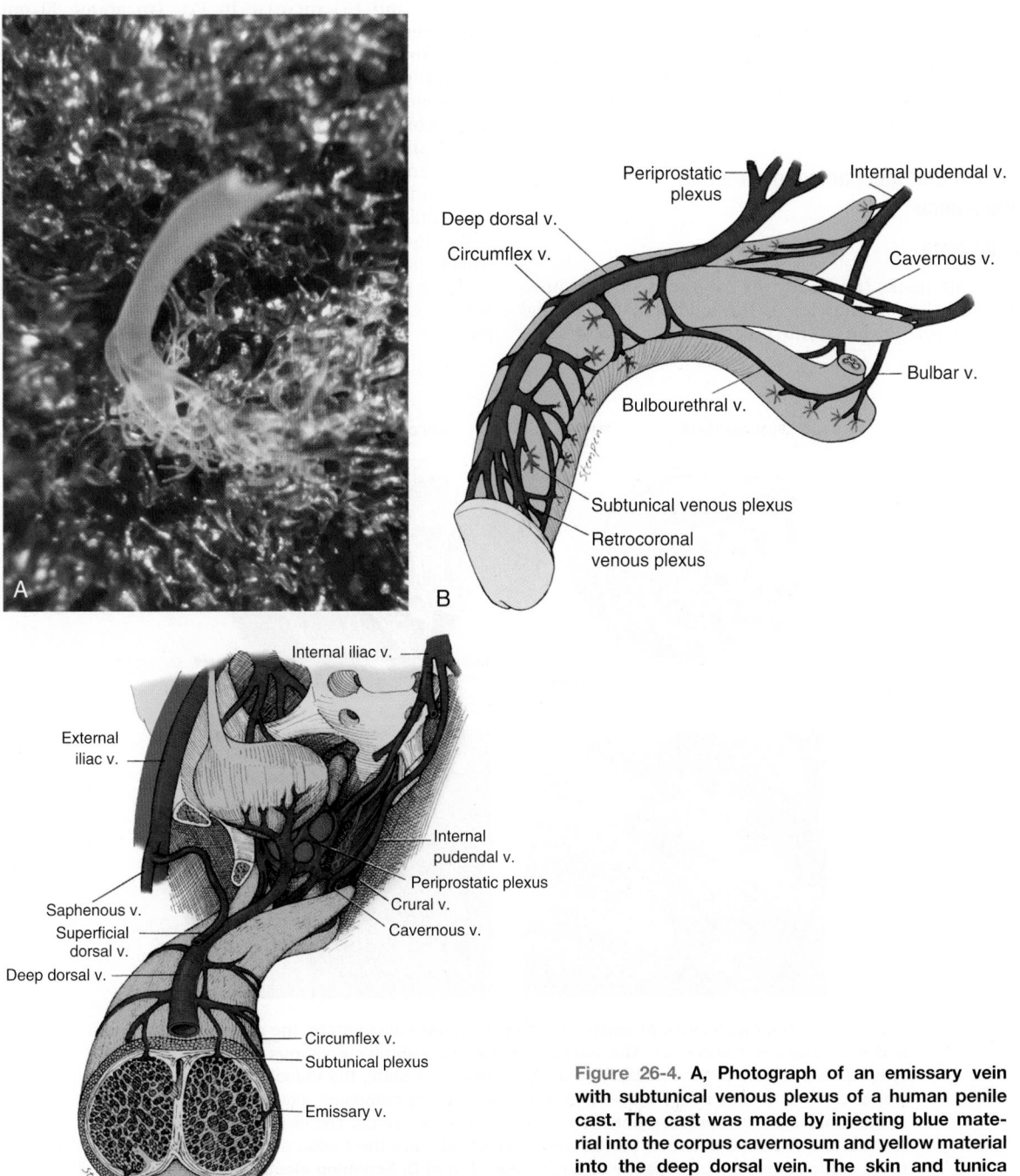

Figure 26-4. **A, Photograph of an emissary vein with subtunical venous plexus of a human penile cast. The cast was made by injecting blue material into the corpus cavernosum and yellow material into the deep dorsal vein. The skin and tunica albuginea were then digested away with potassium hydroxide solution. B and C, Penile venous drainage.**

circumflex, and ventrally to the periurethral veins. Beginning at the coronal sulcus, multiple venous channels coalesce to form the deep dorsal vein, which is the main venous drainage of the glans penis and distal two thirds of the corpora cavernosa. Usually a single vein, but sometimes more than one deep dorsal vein, runs upward behind the symphysis pubis to join the periprostatic venous plexus. There are also small venous channels accompanying the paired dorsal artery. Periarterial veins also travel longitudinally to join the dorsal vein or Santorini plexus proximally (Hsu et al, 2003). These become enlarged after the deep dorsal vein is ligated and may be the cause of recurrent leakage in venogenic ED (Chen et al, 2005). **Infrapubic Penis.** Emissary veins draining the proximal corpora cavernosa join to form cavernous and crural veins. These join the periurethral veins from the urethral bulb to form the internal pudendal veins.

The veins of the three systems communicate variably with each other. Variations in the number, distribution, and termination of these venous systems are common (Fig. 26-4B and C). In fresh cadavers, Hsu and coworkers (2012) determined the following percentage of venous flow from the corpora: deep dorsal vein, 65%; cavernous vein, 11.9%; periarterial vein, 11.4%; others, 15.6%. The study was performed in cadavers, and the cavernous vein is not the same as described by others.

Hemodynamics and Mechanism of Erection and Detumescence

Corpora Cavernosa

The penile erectile tissue, specifically the cavernous smooth musculature and the smooth muscles of the arteriolar and arterial walls, plays a key role in the erectile process. **In the flaccid state,** these smooth muscles are tonically contracted, allowing only a small amount of arterial flow into the corpora. The blood partial pressure of oxygen (PO_2) is about 35 mm Hg (Sattar et al, 1995). The flaccid penis is in a moderate state of contraction, as evidenced by further shrinkage in cold weather and after phenylephrine injection.

Sexual stimulation triggers release of neurotransmitters from the cavernous nerve terminals. This release of neurotransmitters results in relaxation of these smooth muscles and the following events (Fig. 26-5): (1) dilation of the arterioles and arteries by increased blood flow in the diastolic and systolic phases; (2) trapping of the incoming blood by the expanding sinusoids; (3) compression of the subtunical venous plexuses between the tunica albuginea and the peripheral sinusoids, reducing venous outflow; (4) stretching of the tunica to its capacity, which occludes the emissary veins between the inner circular and outer longitudinal layers and further decreases venous outflow; and (5) increase in PO_2 (to about 90 mm Hg) and intracavernous pressure (around 100 mm Hg), which raises the penis from the dependent position to the erect state (the full-erection phase). A further pressure increase (to several hundred millimeters of mercury) can occur with reflex contractions of the ischiocavernosus muscles (rigid-erection phase) during sexual stimulation.

The angle of the erect penis is determined by its size and attachment to the puboischial rami (the crura) and the anterior surface of the pubic bone (the suspensory and funiform ligaments). In men with a long heavy penis or a loose suspensory ligament, the penis usually points downward, even with full rigidity.

Three phases of detumescence were reported in an animal study (Bosch et al, 1991). The first entails a transient intracorporeal pressure increase, indicating the beginning of smooth muscle

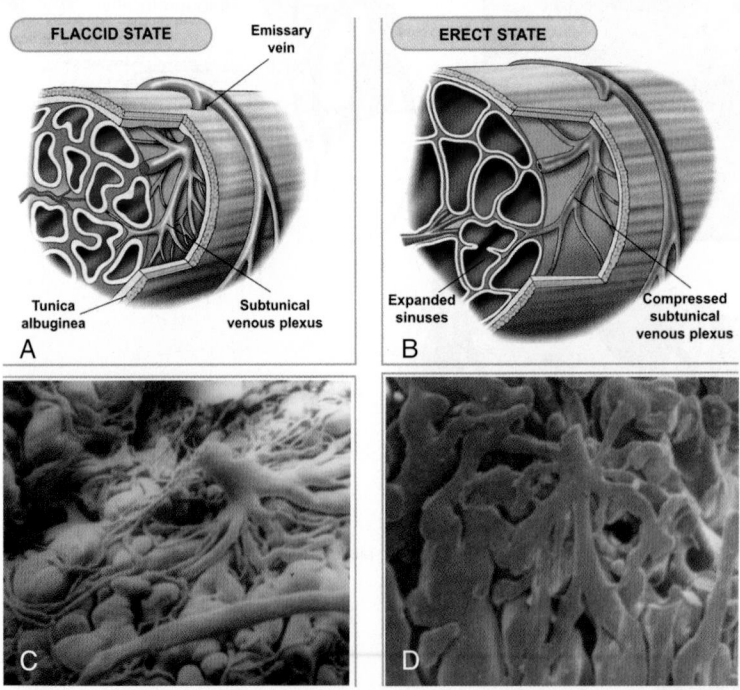

Figure 26-5. The mechanism of penile erection. **A,** In the flaccid state, the arteries, arterioles, and sinusoids are contracted. The intersinusoidal and subtunical venous plexuses are wide open, with free flow to the emissary veins. **B,** In the erect state, the muscles of the sinusoidal wall and the arterioles relax, allowing maximal flow to the compliant sinusoidal spaces. Most of the venules are compressed between the expanding sinusoids. The larger venules are sandwiched and flattened between the distended sinusoids and the tunica albuginea. This effectively reduces the venous capacity to a minimum. **C and D,** Scanning electron micrographs of casts of a canine subtunical venous plexus in the flaccid (**C**) and erect (**D**) states. (A and B, From Lue TF, Giuliano F, Khoury S, et al. Clinical manual of sexual medicine: sexual dysfunction in men. Paris: Health Publications; 2004.)

contraction against a closed venous system. The second phase shows a slow pressure decrease, suggesting a slow reopening of the venous channels with resumption of the basal level of arterial flow. The third phase shows a fast pressure decrease with fully restored venous outflow capacity.

Erection involves sinusoidal relaxation, arterial dilation, and venous compression (Lue et al, 1983). The importance of smooth muscle relaxation has been demonstrated in animal and human studies (Saenz de Tejada et al, 1989a; Ignarro et al, 1990). To summarize the hemodynamic events of erection and detumescence, seven phases have been observed in animal experiments that reflect the changes in and the relationship between penile arterial flow and intracavernous pressure (Fig. 26-6).

Corpus Spongiosum and Glans Penis

The hemodynamics of the corpus spongiosum and glans penis differ from those of the corpora cavernosa. During erection, the arterial flow increases in a similar manner; however, the pressure in the corpus spongiosum and glans is only one third to one half that in the corpora cavernosa because the tunical covering, which is thin over the corpus spongiosum and virtually absent over the glans, ensures minimal venous occlusion. During the full-erection phase, partial compression of the deep dorsal and circumflex veins between Buck fascia and the engorged corpora cavernosa contributes to glanular tumescence, although the spongiosum and glans essentially function as a large arteriovenous shunt during this phase. In the rigid-erection phase, the ischiocavernosus and bulbocavernosus muscles forcefully compress the spongiosum and penile veins, resulting in further engorgement and increased pressure in the glans and spongiosum (Table 26-3).

Neuroanatomy and Neurophysiology of Penile Erection

Spinal Centers and Peripheral Pathways

The innervation of the penis is both autonomic (sympathetic and parasympathetic) and somatic (sensory and motor) (Fig. 26-7). From the neurons in the spinal cord and peripheral ganglia, the sympathetic and parasympathetic nerves merge to form the cavernous nerves, which enter the corpora cavernosa and corpus spongiosum to modulate the neurovascular events during erection and detumescence. The somatic nerves are primarily responsible for

sensation and the contraction of the bulbocavernosus and ischiocavernosus muscles.

Autonomic Pathways. The sympathetic pathway originates from the 11th thoracic to the 2nd lumbar spinal segments and passes through the white rami to the sympathetic chain ganglia. Some fibers travel through the lumbar splanchnic nerves to the inferior mesenteric and superior hypogastric plexuses, from which fibers travel in the hypogastric nerves to the pelvic plexus. In humans, the T10 to T12 segments are most often the origin of the sympathetic fibers, and the chain ganglia cells projecting to the penis are located in the sacral and caudal ganglia (de Groat and Booth, 1993).

The parasympathetic pathway arises from neurons in the intermediolateral cell columns of the second, third, and fourth sacral spinal cord segments. The preganglionic fibers pass in the pelvic nerves to the pelvic plexus, where they are joined by the sympathetic nerves from the superior hypogastric plexus. The cavernous nerves are branches of the pelvic plexus that innervate the penis. Other branches innervate the rectum, bladder, prostate, and sphincters. The cavernous nerves are easily damaged during radical excision of the rectum, bladder, and prostate. A clear understanding of the course of these nerves is essential to the prevention of iatrogenic ED (Walsh et al, 1990). Human cadaveric dissection has revealed medial and lateral branches of the cavernous nerves (the former accompanying the urethra and the latter piercing the urogenital diaphragm 4 to 7 mm lateral to the sphincter) and multiple communications between the cavernous and dorsal nerves (Paick et al, 1993) (Fig. 26-8). In addition to the cavernous nerve proper, pelvic ganglion cells exist in and along the nerve components and pelvic viscera. These are seen at the bladder/prostate junction, the dorsal aspect of the seminal vesicles, and along the prostate. Takenaka and colleagues (2005) reported

TABLE 26-3 Comparison of Corpus Spongiosum and Glans Penis

	CORPUS SPONGIOSUM	GLANS PENIS
Tunica albuginea	Thin (circular layer only)	Absent
Main blood supply	Bulbal and spongiosal arteries	Dorsal artery
Venous occlusion during erection	No	No
Compression by skeletal muscle	Yes (ischiocavernosus, bulbocavernosus)	No

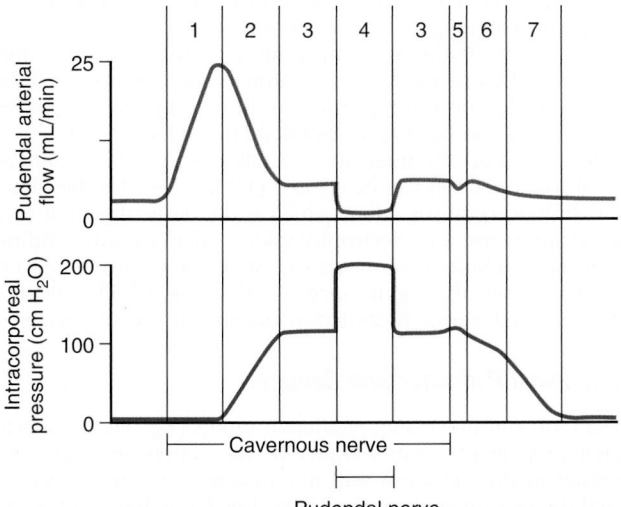

Figure 26-6. **Blood flow and intracavernous pressure changes during the seven phases of penile erection and detumescence: 0, flaccid; 1, latent; 2, tumescence; 3, full erection; 4, rigid erection; 5, initial detumescence; 6, slow detumescence; 7, fast detumescence.**

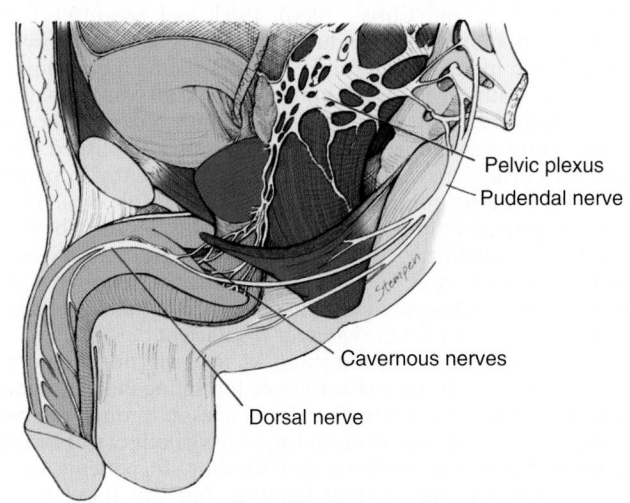

Figure 26-7. **Penile neuroanatomy.**

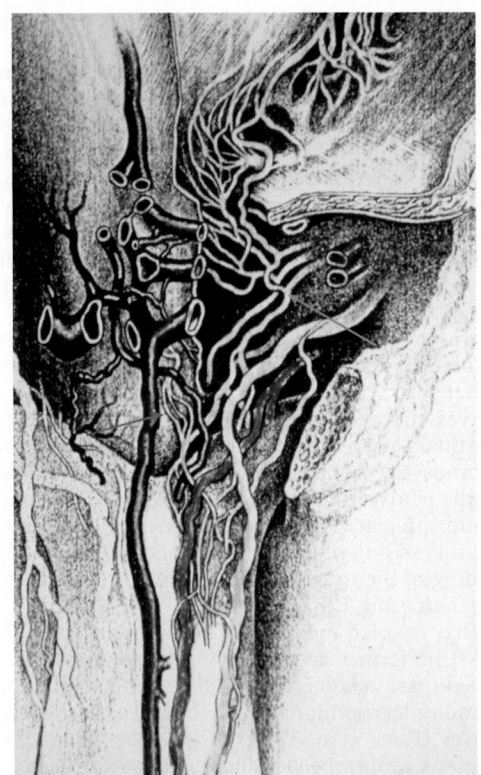

Figure 26-8. Drawing from a human cadaveric dissection shows the medial *(red arrow)* and lateral *(green arrow)* bundles of the cavernous nerve distal to the prostate. (From Paick JS, Donatucci EF, Lue TF. Anatomy of cavernous nerves distal to prostate: microdissection study in adult male cadavers. Urology 1993;42:145–9, with permission from Excerpta Medica, Inc.)

individual variations in distribution of these extramural ganglion cells in the male pelvis, which may complicate nerve-sparing efforts.

Stimulation of the pelvic plexus and the cavernous nerves induces erection, whereas stimulation of the sympathetic trunk causes detumescence. This clearly implies that the sacral parasympathetic input is responsible for tumescence, and the thoracolumbar sympathetic pathway is responsible for detumescence. In experiments with cats and rats, removal of the spinal cord below L4 or L5 reportedly eliminated the reflex erectile response, but placement with a female in heat or electrical stimulation of the medial preoptic area (MPOA) produced marked erection (Giuliano et al, 1996; Sato and Christ, 2000). Paick and Lee (1994) also reported that apomorphine-induced erection is similar to psychogenic erection in the rat and can be induced via the thoracolumbar sympathetic pathway in case of injury to the sacral parasympathetic centers. Many men with sacral spinal cord injury retain psychogenic erectile ability even though reflexogenic erection is abolished. These cerebrally elicited erections are found more frequently in patients with lower motoneuron lesions below T12 (Courtois et al, 1999); no psychogenic erection occurs in patients with lesions above T9. The efferent sympathetic outflow is suggested to be at the levels T11 and T12 (Chapelle et al, 1980). These authors also reported that in patients with psychogenic erections, lengthening and swelling of the penis are observed, but rigidity is insufficient.

It is possible that for production of rigid erection in normal men, cerebral impulses travel as follows: inhibiting the sympathetic pathway and decreasing norepinephrine release; through the parasympathetic pathway, releasing NO and acetylcholine; and through the somatic pathway, releasing acetylcholine. In patients with a sacral cord lesion, the cerebral impulses can still travel via the sympathetic pathway to inhibit norepinephrine release, and NO and acetylcholine can still be released through synapse with postganglionic parasympathetic and somatic neurons. Because the number of these synapses is less than in men with an intact sacral spinal cord, the resulting erection will not be as strong.

Somatic Pathways. The somatosensory pathway originates at the sensory receptors in the penile skin, glans, and urethra and within the corpus cavernosum. There are numerous afferent terminations in the human glans penis: free nerve endings and corpuscular receptors in a ratio of 10:1. The free nerve endings are derived from thin myelinated A_δ and unmyelinated C fibers and are unlike any other cutaneous area in the body (Halata and Munger, 1986). The nerve fibers from the receptors converge to form bundles of the dorsal nerve of the penis, which joins other nerves to become the pudendal nerve. The latter enters the spinal cord via the S2-S4 roots to terminate on spinal neurons and interneurons in the central gray region of the lumbosacral segment (McKenna, 1998). Activation of these sensory neurons sends messages of pain, temperature, and touch by means of spinothalamic and spinoreticular pathways to the thalamus and sensory cortex for sensory perception.

Kozacioglu and associates (2014) reported a detailed study of the dorsal nerve. They noted that the dorsal nerve of the penis is composed of two to six branches, and in 16 of 22 adult cadaveric specimens, branches perforating the tunica albuginea to the corpus cavernosum were noted. The dorsal nerve of the penis previously was regarded as purely somatic; however, nerve bundles testing positive for NOS, which is autonomic in origin, have been demonstrated in humans by Burnett and colleagues (1993) and in rats by Carrier and colleagues (1995). These NOS-positive nerve bundles in the dorsal nerve are reduced after damage of the cavernous nerve near the rat prostate. Giuliano and coworkers (1993) have also shown that stimulation of the sympathetic chain at the L4-L5 level elicits an evoked discharge on the dorsal nerve and that stimulation of the dorsal nerve evokes a reflex discharge in the lumbosacral sympathetic chain of rats. These findings demonstrate that the dorsal nerve has somatic and autonomic components that enable it to regulate erectile and ejaculatory functions.

The Onuf nucleus in the second to fourth sacral spinal segments is the center of somatomotor penile innervation. These nerves travel in the sacral nerves to the pudendal nerve to innervate the ischiocavernosus and bulbocavernosus muscles. **Contraction of the ischiocavernosus muscles produces the rigid-erection phase. Rhythmic contraction and compression of the bulbocavernosus muscle on the proximal corpus spongiosum helps semen expulsion, provided that the external sphincter is relaxed and the urethral lumen is compressed by the engorged spongiosum.** In animal studies, direct innervation of the sacral spinal motoneurons by brainstem sympathetic centers (A5-catecholaminergic cell group and locus ceruleus) has been identified (Marson and McKenna, 1996). This adrenergic innervation of pudendal motoneurons may be involved in rhythmic contractions of perineal muscles during ejaculation. Oxytocinergic and serotoninergic innervation of lumbosacral nuclei controlling penile erection and perineal muscles in male rats has also been demonstrated (Tang et al, 1998).

Depending on the intensity and nature of genital stimulation, several spinal reflexes can be elicited (Table 26-4). The best known is the bulbocavernosus reflex, which is the basis of genital neurologic examination and electrophysiologic latency testing. Although impairment of bulbocavernosus and ischiocavernosus muscles may impair erection, the significance of obtaining a bulbocavernosus reflex in overall sexual dysfunction assessment is controversial.

Supraspinal Pathways and Centers

Integration and processing of afferent inputs (e.g., visual, olfactory, imaginative, genital stimulation) in the supraspinal centers are essential in the initiation and maintenance of penile erection. A spinal transection study at the T8 level by Hubscher and associates (2010) revealed that ascending bilateral projections in the dorsal, dorsolateral, and ventrolateral white matter of the spinal cord convey information from the male external genitalia to the medullary reticular formation. The authors postulate that these multiple spinal pathways may correspond to different functions, including

TABLE 26-4 Spinal Reflexes Involved in Stimulation of Penile Dorsal Nerve

STIMULATION	SPINAL CENTER	EFFERENT	EFFECT
Noxious, abrupt stimulation	Sacral motor neurons	Pudendal nerve (motor)	Bulbocavernous reflex
Low-intensity continuous (e.g., vibratory, manual)	Sacral parasympathetic neurons and interneurons	1. Pelvic nerves 2. Cavernous nerve	1. Bladder inhibition and closure of bladder neck 2. Penile erection
High-intensity continuous	Sacral motor and parasympathetic Thoracolumbar sympathetic neurons	Pudendal, pelvic, and cavernous nerves	Ejaculation

TABLE 26-5 Brain Centers Involved in Sexual Function

LEVEL	REGION	FUNCTION
Forebrain	Medial amygdala Stria terminalis	Control sexual motivation
	Pyriform cortex	Inhibits sexual drive (hypersexuality when destroyed)
	Hippocampus	Involved in penile erection
	Right insula and inferior frontal cortex Left anterior cingulate cortex	Increased activity during visually evoked sexual stimulation (sexual arousal)
Hypothalamus	Medial preoptic area	Ability to recognize a sexual partner, integration of hormonal and sensory cues
	Lateral preoptic area	Control nocturnal penile tumescence in rats
	Paraventricular nucleus	Facilitates penile erection (via oxytocin neurons to lumbosacral spinal autonomic and somatic efferents)
Brainstem	Nucleus paragigantocellularis	Inhibits penile erection (via serotonin neurons to lumbosacral spinal neurons and interneurons)
	A5-catecholaminergic cell group Locus ceruleus	Major noradrenergic center
Midbrain	Periaqueductal gray	Relay center for sexually relevant stimuli

functions processing affective, pleasure, and motivational; nociception; and mating-specific (e.g., for erection and ejaculation) inputs. In animal studies, the central supraspinal systems controlling sexual arousal are localized predominantly in the limbic system (e.g., olfactory nuclei, MPOA, nucleus accumbens, amygdala, and hippocampus) and hypothalamus (paraventricular and ventromedial nuclei). In particular, the medial amygdala, MPOA, paraventricular nucleus (PVN), periaqueductal gray, and ventral tegmentum are recognized as key structures in the central control of the male sexual response (Andersson, 2011; Melis and Argiolas, 2011).

In humans, positron emission tomography (PET) and functional magnetic resonance imaging (fMRI) have allowed a greater understanding of brain activation during human sexual arousal by demonstrating increases in regional cerebral blood flow or changes in regional cerebral activity during a particular moment in time. Generally, in young heterosexual men, sexual arousal is triggered with sexually explicit pictures or videos. Scanned brain images taken during arousal are compared with images taken in response to sexually neutral media (e.g., documentaries or humorous video clips). Centers of activation and deactivation can be demonstrated. Although the simplicity of these study designs is elegant, multiple factors are involved in sexual arousal—especially when triggered by visual clues. The authors of these studies have placed many necessary conditions in experiments in an attempt to standardize the methods and participants; however, the complexity of human emotion and sexual response is extremely difficult to regulate (Table 26-5).

Kühn and Gallinat (2011) performed a quantitative meta-analysis of 11 fMRI studies that compared brain activity in response to erotic visual stimuli versus neutral visual stimuli. The meta-analysis identified a neural network that constitutes a core circuit of male sexual arousal in humans and consists of the following components: cognitive (parietal cortex, anterior cingulate gyrus, thalamus, insula), emotional (amygdala, insula), motivational (precentral gyrus, parietal cortex), and physiologic (hypothalamus/thalamus, insula).

Using fMRI, detailed comparisons of brain activation in response to visual sexual stimuli have also been performed on varied groups. Stoléru and colleagues (2003) compared healthy men with men with hypoactive sexual desire disorder and reported that the left gyrus rectus, a portion of the medial orbitofrontal cortex, remained activated in the latter group in contrast to its deactivation in healthy men. This region is believed to mediate inhibition of motivated behavior, and its continued activation may help explain the pathophysiology of hypoactive sexual desire disorder. Montorsi and colleagues (2003) compared men with psychogenic ED and potent control subjects after the administration of apomorphine. During visual sexual stimulation, the men with psychogenic ED evidenced extended activation of the cingulated gyrus, frontal mesial, and frontal basal cortex, suggesting an underlying organic cause for psychogenic ED. However, fMRI images obtained after apomorphine were similar to the images of the potent control subjects. Apomorphine caused additional activation of foci in the patients with psychogenic ED (seen in the nucleus accumbens, hypothalamus, and mesencephalon), and it was significantly greater in the right hemisphere than in the left. This greater right-sided activation is a common finding in sexually evoked brain activation studies.

Brain scanning with PET and fMRI has become a powerful tool in the study of central activation of sexual arousal, with many brain regions of activation demonstrated in these studies (Table 26-6). Psychogenic ED, premature ejaculation, sexual deviations, and orgasmic dysfunction are just a few conditions that may accompany alterations in higher brain function and perhaps now can be studied. As we begin to understand brain function with normal sexual response and arousal, the causes of dysfunction may be elucidated.

The structures discussed earlier are responsible for the three types of erection: psychogenic, reflexogenic, and nocturnal. **Psychogenic erection is a result of audiovisual stimuli or fantasy. Impulses from the brain modulate the spinal erection centers (T11-L2 and S2-S4) to activate the erectile process. Reflexogenic erection is produced by tactile stimulation of the genital organs. The impulses reach the spinal erection centers; some then follow the ascending tract, resulting in sensory perception, whereas others activate the autonomic nuclei to send messages via the cavernous nerves to the penis to induce erection. This type of erection is preserved in patients with upper spinal cord injury. Nocturnal erection occurs mostly during rapid eye movement (REM) sleep.** PET scanning of humans in REM sleep shows increased activity in the pontine area, the amygdalae, and the anterior cingulate gyrus but decreased activity in the prefrontal and parietal cortex. The mechanism that triggers REM sleep is located in the pontine reticular formation; the cholinergic neurons in the lateral pontine tegmentum are activated, whereas the adrenergic neurons in the locus ceruleus and the serotoninergic neurons in the midbrain raphe are silent. In a brain stimulation study in rats, the sites for eliciting erection during REM sleep were located in the dorsal and intermediate parts of the lateral septum, whereas the ventral part of the lateral septum was the most effective site for eliciting erections during wakefulness (Gulia et al, 2008).

The brain centers activated during orgasm and ejaculation have also been studied. Holstege and colleagues (2003) used PET to measure increases in regional cerebral blood flow during ejaculation versus sexual stimulation without orgasm in heterosexual volunteers. Manual penile stimulation was performed by the volunteer's female partner. Primary brain activation was found in the mesodiencephalic transition zone (including the ventral tegmental area), an area frequently activated with "reward" behaviors and with injection of opioids such as heroin. Other activated mesodiencephalic structures included the midbrain lateral central tegmental field; the zona incerta; the subparafascicular nucleus; and the ventroposterior, midline, and intralaminar thalamic nuclei. Increased activation was also observed in the lateral putamen and adjoining parts of the claustrum. Neocortical activity was found in Brodmann areas 7/40, 18, 21, 23, and 47, exclusively on the right side. Conversely, in the amygdala and adjacent entorhinal cortex, a decrease in activation was observed. Remarkably strong increases in blood flow were observed in the cerebellum. These findings corroborate the notion that the cerebellum plays an important role in emotional processing. Although activation of these particular areas is of great interest, further studies are necessary to understand completely the neurobiology of orgasm, ejaculation, and sexual satisfaction in men (Table 26-7).

Neurotransmitters

Peripheral Neurotransmitters and Endothelium-Derived Factors

Flaccidity and Detumescence. α-**Adrenergic nerve fibers and receptors have been demonstrated in the cavernous trabeculae and surrounding the cavernous arteries, and norepinephrine has generally been accepted as the principal neurotransmitter to keep the penis in the flaccid state** (Andersson, 2011; Diederichs et al, 1990). Both α_1-adrenergic and α_2-adrenergic receptors have been demonstrated in human corpus cavernosum tissue (Prieto, 2008). Research findings support a functional predominance of postjunctional α_1-adrenergic receptors for contraction and of prejunctional α_2-adrenergic receptors for downregulating not only release of norepinephrine but also NO (Prieto, 2008). Norepinephrine, released from adrenergic nerves, stimulates adrenergic receptors in the penile vessels and corpus cavernosum, producing a contraction that involves Ca^{2+} entry through calcium channels as well as calcium sensitization mechanisms mediated by protein kinase C, tyrosine kinases, and Rho-kinase (Andersson, 2011).

Endothelin-1, synthesized by endothelium, is a more potent vasoconstrictor than epinephrine and has been suggested to be a mediator for detumescence (Holmquist et al, 1990; Saenz de Tejada et al, 1991a). Endothelin-1 induces slowly developing, long-lasting contractions in different smooth muscles of the penis: corpus cavernosum, cavernosal artery, deep dorsal vein, and penile circumflex veins. Endothelin also potentiates the constrictor effects of catecholamines on trabecular smooth muscle (Christ et al, 1995b). Two receptors for endothelin, endothelin-A and endothelin-B, mediate the biologic effects of endothelin in vascular tissue: Endothelin-A receptors mediate contraction, whereas endothelin-B receptors induce relaxation.

TABLE 26-6 Common Brain Activation Regions with Visual Sexual Stimuli*

BRAIN ACTIVATION REGIONS	FUNCTIONAL ASSOCIATION
Bilateral inferior temporal cortex (right > left)	Visual association area
Right insula	Processes somatosensory information with motivational states
Right inferior frontal cortex	Processes sensory information
Left anterior cingulate cortex	Controls autonomic and neuroendocrine function
Right occipital gyrus	Visual processing
Right hypothalamus	Male copulatory behavior
Left caudate (the striatum)	Processes attention and guides responsiveness to new environmental stimuli

*These regions demonstrate activation with visual sexual stimuli in multiple studies.

TABLE 26-7 Brain Centers of Orgasm

	BRAIN AREAS	RELEVANCE
Increased activity: primary area	Mesodiencephalic transition zone (including the ventral tegmental area)	"Reward" center also activated by opioid
Increased activity: secondary areas	Midbrain lateral central tegmental field, the zona incerta, subparafascicular nucleus, ventroposterior, midline, and intralaminar thalamic nuclei Lateral putamen and adjoining parts of the claustrum Brodmann areas 7/40, 18, 21, 23, and 47, exclusively on the right side	
Increased activity: other area	Cerebellum	Emotional processing
Deceased activity	Amygdala and adjacent entorhinal cortex	

Several constrictor prostanoids, including prostaglandin I_2 (PGI_2), prostaglandin $F_{2\alpha}$ ($PGF_{2\alpha}$), and thromboxane A_2 (TXA_2), are synthesized by the human cavernous tissue. In vitro studies demonstrated that prostanoids are responsible for the tone and spontaneous activity of isolated trabecular muscle (Christ et al, 1990). Functional characterization of prostanoid receptors in human trabecular and arterial penile smooth muscle revealed that only thromboxane A_2 (TP) receptors mediate contractile effects of prostanoids in these tissues (Angulo et al, 2002). Also, it has been observed in vitro that constrictor prostanoids, simultaneously released with NO, attenuate the dilator effect of NO (Azadzoi et al, 1992; Minhas et al, 2001).

The renin-angiotensin system (RAS) may also play a significant role in the maintenance of penile smooth muscle tone. The RAS comprises two major arms: a vasoconstrictor/proliferative arm, in which the main mediator is angiotensin II acting on angiotensin (AT1) receptors, and a vasodilator/antiproliferative arm in which the major effector is angiotensin-(1-7) acting via the G protein–coupled receptor Mas (Sousa et al, 2010). The mediators and receptors of both arms have been demonstrated in the corpus cavernosum. The RAS system may have a dual role in erectile function: pro-detumescence mediated by the angiotensin II–AT1 axis and pro-erection mediated by the angiotensin-(1-7)–Mas axis. Uckert and associates (2012) have also reported a decrease in cavernous blood level of neuropeptide Y during sexual arousal and suggested that neuropeptide Y may contribute to maintenance of a flaccid penis. In addition, the endothelium has been shown to release potent vasoconstrictors, including endoperoxides, TXA_2, and superoxide anions.

The current consensus holds that the maintenance of the intracorporeal smooth muscle in a semicontracted (flaccid) state likely results from three factors: intrinsic myogenic activity (Andersson and Wagner, 1995); **adrenergic neurotransmission; and endothelium-derived contracting factors such as angiotensin II, $PGF_{2\alpha}$, and endothelin-1. Detumescence after erection may be a result of cessation of NO release, the breakdown of cyclic guanosine monophosphate (cGMP) by PDEs, and/or sympathetic discharge during ejaculation.**

Erection. Acetylcholine has been shown to be released with electrical field stimulation of human erectile tissue (Blanco et al, 1988). Traish and colleagues (1990) reported the density of muscarinic receptors in cavernous tissue to range from 35 to 65 fmol/mg protein and in endothelial cell membrane from 5 to 10 fmol/mg protein. However, intravenous or intracavernous injection of atropine failed to abolish erection induced in animals by electrical neurostimulation (Stief et al, 1989a) and in men by erotic stimuli (Wagner and Uhrenholdt, 1980). **Although acetylcholine is not the predominant neurotransmitter, it contributes indirectly to penile erection by presynaptic inhibition of adrenergic neurons and stimulation of NO release from endothelial cells** (Saenz de Tejada et al, 1989a).

Most researchers now agree that **NO released from nonadrenergic/noncholinergic neurotransmission and from the endothelium is the principal neurotransmitter mediating penile erection. NO increases the production of cGMP, which relaxes the cavernous smooth muscle** (Ignarro et al, 1990; Kim et al, 1991; Burnett et al, 1992; Rajfer et al, 1992; Trigo-Rocha et al, 1993; Andersson, 2011). **The consensus is that NO derived from neuronal nitric oxide synthase (nNOS) in the nitrergic nerves is responsible for the initiation, whereby NO from endothelial nitric oxide synthase (eNOS) contributes to the maintenance of smooth muscle relaxation and erection** (Hurt et al, 2002). (For a more detailed discussion of NO, see specific Nitric Oxide sections.)

Aside from its role in releasing vasoconstrictors, the endothelium can also release factors that induce smooth muscle relaxation, including carbon monoxide (CO), endothelium-derived hyperpolarizing factor (EDHF), prostacyclin (PGI_2), and endothelin (which may induce relaxation via activation of endothelin-B receptors).

Interactions among Nerves and Neurotransmitters. Acetylcholine, by acting on the presynaptic receptors on adrenergic neurons,

has been shown to modulate the release of norepinephrine (Saenz de Tejada et al, 1989b), which also can be inhibited by PGE_1 (Molderings et al, 1992). In the human corpus cavernosum, noradrenergic responses are under nitrergic control. Conversely, adrenergic neurons, through prejunctional α_2 receptors, can also regulate the release of NO.

Several studies have demonstrated that the interaction between the two systems also occurs in the smooth muscle (Brave et al, 1993; Angulo et al, 2001a). The NO–cGMP–protein kinase G (PKG)-I pathway can lead to inhibition at several sites on the noradrenergic contractile pathway in the vascular smooth muscle, impairing inositol 1,4,5-triphosphate (IP3) production by phospholipase C (Hirata et al, 1990), IP3 receptor activity (Schlossmann et al, 2000), and the RhoA/Rho-kinase pathway (Sauzeau et al, 2000). However, interaction sites have not yet been identified in penile smooth muscle. A nitrergic-noradrenergic imbalance owing to defective nitrergic neurotransmission has been implicated in penile tissue from patients and in animal models with ED (Christ et al, 1995a; Cellek et al, 1999). Similar to the interaction between nitrergic and noradrenergic pathways, vasoconstrictive actions of endothelin have been shown to be inhibited by NO during erection (Mills et al, 2001).

Numerous factors have been reported to increase NOS activity and NO release, including molecular oxygen, androgen, long-term administration of L-arginine, and repeated intracavernous injection of PGE_1 (Kim et al, 1993; Escrig et al, 1999; Marin et al, 1999). Decreased NOS activity has been associated with castration, denervation, hypercholesterolemia, and diabetes mellitus. Interaction of different types of NOS may also occur. For example, nNOS activity has been shown to decrease and inducible nitric oxide synthase (iNOS) levels to increase after injection of transforming growth factor (TGF)-$\beta1$ into the penis (Bivalacqua et al, 2000), and eNOS levels are reportedly significantly higher in nNOS-knockout mice (Burnett et al, 1996).

In a study of neurotransmitters in human corpus cavernosum and spongiosum, Hedlund and colleagues (2000b) reported that vesicular acetylcholine transporter, vasoactive intestinal polypeptide (VIP), and nNOS are found in the same nerve terminals. Tyrosine hydroxylase–positive nerves do not contain vesicular acetylcholine transporter, VIP, or NOS. Heme oxygenase (HO) enzymes HO-1 and HO-2 and eNOS are localized to the endothelium. Interaction of these neurotransmitters may modify the effect of parasympathetic and sympathetic activation on penile function.

Role of Caveolae. Caveolae are invaginated microdomains of plasma membrane that are rich in eNOS and caveolins as well as cholesterol, sphingolipids, and glycosylphosphatidylinositol-linked proteins. In addition, caveolae contain numerous other signaling proteins, such as receptors with seven-transmembrane domains, G proteins, adenylyl cyclase, phospholipase C, protein kinase C, calcium pumps, and calcium channels. Decreased caveolin-1 expression has been reported in the cavernous smooth muscle of aged rats (Bakircioglu et al, 2001). Linder and colleagues (2006) demonstrated that penile erection requires association of soluble guanylyl cyclase with endothelial caveolin-1 in rat corpus cavernosum. Shakirova and colleagues (2009) reported that nerve-mediated relaxation of penile tissue from caveolin-1-deficient mice was impaired. Caveolin-1 in both the cavernous smooth muscle and the endothelium is decreased after bilateral cavernous nerve injury (Becher et al, 2009). In a rat model with diabetes induced by fructose and streptozotocin, Elçioglu and associates (2010) reported attenuation of erectile responses in both diabetic groups, an enhanced expression of caveolin-1, and a decrease in the eNOS activity with a concomitant decrease in NO synthesis. These reports strongly suggest that the caveolae and caveolin are involved in the regulation of penile function.

Central Neurotransmitters and Neuropeptides. Numerous **neurotransmitters and neuropeptides have been implicated in regulation of sexual function. The major ones are dopamine, oxytocin, NO, norepinephrine, serotonin (5-hydroxytryptamine [5-HT]), and prolactin. In general, dopaminergic and adrenergic**

receptors promote sexual function, and 5-HT receptors inhibit it (Foreman and Wernicke, 1990). Androgens also have an important role in modulating the effect of the transmitters.

Dopamine. There are many dopaminergic systems in the brain with ultrashort, intermediate, and long axons. The cell bodies are located in the ventral tegmentum, substantia nigra, and hypothalamus. One of these dopaminergic systems, the tuberoinfundibular system, secretes dopamine into the portal hypophysial vessels to inhibit prolactin secretion (Ganong, 1999a). Five different dopamine receptors have been cloned (D_1 to D_5), and several of these exist in multiple forms (Ganong, 1999b). **In men, apomorphine, which stimulates both D_1 and D_2 receptors, induces erection that is unaccompanied by sexual arousal** (Danjou et al, 1988). Neuroscientists have discovered that dopamine receptors (D_2, D_3, and D_4), nNOS, and oxytocin are coexpressed in the cell bodies of oxytocinergic neurons in the PVN and MPOA (Xiao et al, 2005; Baskerville et al, 2009). In male rats, injection of dopaminergic agonists to the PVN to stimulate D_2, but not D_3 or D_4, receptors, increases Ca^{2+} influx in cell bodies of oxytocinergic neurons. This increases the production of NO, which activates oxytocinergic neurotransmission in extrahypothalamic brain areas and spinal cord, leading to penile erection and yawning. The stimulation of D_4 receptors also increases Ca^{2+} influx and NO production leading to penile erection but not yawning. Nevertheless, D_4 receptors seem to play only a modest role in the pro-erectile effect (Melis and Argiolas, 2011).

Dopamine agonist in the form of sublingual apomorphine is available for the treatment of ED in many countries, but its utility is limited because of emetic side effects.

Oxytocin. Oxytocin is a neural hormone secreted by the neurons into the circulation. Oxytocin is found in the posterior pituitary gland, but because it is also found in the neurons projecting from the PVN to the brainstem and spinal cord, it can also function as a neurotransmitter. The blood level is increased during sexual activity in humans and animals. Oxytocin is a potent inducer of penile erection when injected into the central nervous system (CNS). In rats, the most sensitive brain area for the pro-erectile effect of oxytocin is the PVN of the hypothalamus. Oxytocin release after stimulation of dopamine receptors in the PVN influences the appetitive and reinforcing effects of sexual activity (Succu et al, 2007). As mentioned earlier, neurons in the paraventricular area contain NOS, and because NOS inhibitors prevent apomorphine-induced and oxytocin-induced erection, it is evident that oxytocin acts on neurons whose activity is dependent on certain levels of NO (Vincent and Kimura, 1992; Melis and Argiolas, 2011).

Nitric Oxide. NO mediates penile erection at the level of the PVN (Melis et al, 1998) and at other levels of the neural pathway supporting sexual response. The presence of NO and the soluble guanylyl cyclase needed to generate cGMP is seen throughout the human brain. The NO/cGMP pathway (see later) is affected by aging in the brain and offers a potentially significant but unexplored site for mediating the deleterious effects of age on sexual function (Ibarra et al, 2001). Reduced nNOS protein within the PVN leading to blunting of the erectile response has been reported in streptozotocin-induced diabetic rats (Zheng et al, 2007). In animals, testosterone increases NOS in the MPOA. NO increases basal and female-stimulated dopamine release, which facilitates copulation and genital reflexes. In rodents, dopamine receptor agonist–induced erections were abolished by castration, and testosterone replacement restored erectile function (Hull et al, 1999).

Serotonin. Neurons containing 5-HT have their cell bodies in the midline raphe nuclei of the brainstem and project to a portion of the hypothalamus, limbic system, neocortex, and spinal cord (Ganong, 1999a). At the present time, 5-HT receptors 1 to 7 have been cloned and characterized. Within the $5\text{-}HT_1$ group are the $5\text{-}HT_1$ A, B, D, E, and F subtypes. Within the $5\text{-}HT_2$ group are the $5\text{-}HT_2$ A, B, and C subtypes. There are two $5\text{-}HT_5$ subtypes, $5\text{-}HT_{5A}$ and $5\text{-}HT_{5B}$ (Ganong, 1999b). **General pharmacologic data indicate that 5-HT pathways inhibit copulation, but 5-HT may have both facilitatory and inhibitory effects on sexual function, depending on the receptor subtype, the receptor location, and the species investigated** (de Groat and Booth, 1993). Andersson

and Wagner (1995) summarized the results of administration of selective agonists and antagonists as follows: $5\text{-}HT_{1A}$ receptor agonists inhibit erectile activity but assist ejaculation, stimulation of $5\text{-}HT_{2C}$ receptors cause erection, and $5\text{-}HT_2$ agonists inhibit erection but assist seminal emission and ejaculation. Also, Steers and de Groat (1989) showed increased firing of the cavernous nerve and erection when *m*-chlorophenylpiperazine, a $5\text{-}HT_{2C}$ receptor agonist, was given to rats. Applying a novel $5\text{-}HT_{2C}$ receptor agonist (YM348) and antagonist SB242084, Kimura and colleagues (2006) confirmed the pro-erectile effect of the $5\text{-}HT_{2C}$ receptor stimulation in rats. In rats, 5-HT, dopamine, oxytocin, and melanocortin pathways are known to be involved in the induction of penile erections. Kimura and colleagues (2008) suggested that $5\text{-}HT_{2C}$ receptors in the lumbosacral spinal sites mediate not only dopamine–oxytocin–5-HT action but also melanocortin effects on penile erections and that the 5-HT pathway is located downstream from the melanocortin and the dopamine-oxytocin pathways.

5-HT is believed to be an inhibitory transmitter in the control of sexual drive (Foreman et al, 1989). Suppressed libido has been reported in patients taking fenfluramine, a 5-HT-releasing agent, but elevated libido occurred in patients taking buspirone, a 5-HT neuron suppressor (Buffum, 1982).

Norepinephrine. The cell bodies of the norepinephrine-containing neurons are located in the locus ceruleus and the A5-catecholaminergic cell group in the pons and medulla. The axons of these noradrenergic neurons ascend to innervate the paraventricular, supraoptic, and periventricular nuclei of the hypothalamus, thalamus, and neocortex. They also descend into the spinal cord and the cerebellum. **Central norepinephrine transmission seems to have a positive effect on sexual function.** In humans and rats, inhibition of norepinephrine release by clonidine, an α_2-adrenergic agonist, is associated with a decrease in sexual behavior, and yohimbine, an α_2-receptor antagonist, has been shown to increase sexual activity (Clark et al, 1985). β-Blockers have also been implicated in sexual dysfunction, probably because of their central side effects such as sedation, sleep disturbances, and depression.

Melanocortins. Melanocortin-4 receptor (MC4R), implicated in the control of food intake and energy expenditure, also modulates erectile function and sexual behavior. Evidence supporting this notion is based on several findings, as follows: (1) A highly selective nonpeptide MC4R agonist augments erectile activity initiated by electrical stimulation of the cavernous nerve in wild-type, but not MC4R-null, mice; (2) copulatory behavior is enhanced by administration of a selective MC4R agonist and is diminished in mice lacking MC4R; (3) reverse transcriptase polymerase chain reaction and non–polymerase chain reaction–based methods demonstrate MC4R expression in the rat and human penis and rat spinal cord, hypothalamus, brainstem, and pelvic ganglion (major autonomic relay center to the penis) but not in rat primary corpus cavernosum smooth muscle cells; and (4) in situ hybridization of glans tissue from the human and rat penis reveals MC4R expression in nerve fibers and mechanoreceptors in the glans. Collectively, these data implicate MC4R in the modulation of penile erectile function and provide evidence that MC4R-mediated pro-erectile responses may be activated through neuronal circuitry in spinal cord erectile centers and somatosensory afferent nerve terminals of the penis (Van der Ploeg et al, 2002).

Prolactin. **Increased levels of prolactin suppress sexual function in men and experimental animals. In rats, high levels of prolactin decrease the genital reflex and disturb copulatory behavior** (Rehman et al, 2000). **It is suggested that the mechanism of action of prolactin is through inhibition of dopaminergic activity in the MPOA and decreased testosterone. In addition, prolactin may have a direct effect on the penis through its contractile effect on the cavernous smooth muscle** (Ra et al, 1996). In a study of sexual activity of married men with ED, men with sexual inactivity were noted to have a significantly higher mean prolactin level (Paick et al, 2006) (Table 26-8).

γ-Aminobutyric Acid. γ-Aminobutyric acid (GABA) activity in the PVN provides a mechanism to balance (inhibit) pro-erectile signaling. Systemic administration or intrathecal injection at the

TABLE 26-8   Central Neurotransmitters and Their Function

NEUROTRANSMITTER	RECEPTOR AND FUNCTION
Dopamine	D1 and D4 receptor—enhances erection
	D2 receptor—enhances seminal emission
Serotonin (5-HT)	5-HT—inhibits sex drive and spinal sexual reflex
	5-HT1A—inhibits erection, facilitates ejaculation
	5-HT2C—enhances erection
Norepinephrine	Enhances sexual function
γ-aminobutyric acid	Inhibits erectile signals
Opioids	Inhibit penile erection
Cannabinoids	Inhibit sexual function
Oxytocin	Enhances appetitive and reinforcing effects of sexual activity
Nitric oxide	Mediates erection at paraventricular nucleus
Melanocortins	MCR4—enhances erection
Prolactin	Suppresses sexual function

lumbosacral level of the GABA$_B$ receptor agonist baclofen decreased the frequency of erections in rats (Bitran and Hull, 1987). Activation of GABA$_A$ receptors in the PVN reduced penile erection and yawning in male rats induced by apomorphine, *N*-methyl-D-aspartate, and oxytocin (Melis and Argiolas, 2002).

Opioids. Endogenous opioids are known to affect sexual function, but the mechanism of action is unclear. Injection of small amounts of morphine into the MPOA assists sexual behavior in rats. However, larger doses inhibit penile erection and yawning induced by oxytocin or apomorphine. It is suggested that endogenous opioids may exert an inhibitory control on central oxytocinergic transmission (Argiolas, 1992). Injection of morphine into the PVN of the hypothalamus prevents noncontact penile erections and impairs copulation in rats. It is speculated that intracellular NO may be involved in this process (Melis et al, 1999).

Cannabinoids. Cannabinoid CB$_1$ receptor activation inhibits sexual function by modulating the paraventricular oxytocinergic neurons, which mediate erection. Antagonism of CB$_1$ receptors in the PVN of male rats induces penile erection, which seems to involve glutamic acid and NO (Melis et al, 2004, 2006).

Smooth Muscle Physiology

In contrast to many other smooth muscles, corpus cavernosum smooth muscle is in a contracted state most of the time. In a study of myosin isoforms in smooth muscle cells in the corpus cavernosum, DiSanto and colleagues (1998) reported that their overall composition is between that in aorta and bladder smooth muscles, which generally express toniclike and phasiclike characteristics, respectively. Spontaneous contractile activity of cavernous smooth muscle has been recorded in vitro and in vivo. In a study in men, Yarnitsky and colleagues (1995) found two types of electrical activity recorded from the corpus cavernosum: spontaneous and activity induced. Berridge (2008) proposed that the rhythmic contractions of corpus cavernosum smooth muscle depend on an endogenous pacemaker driven by a cytosolic Ca^{2+} oscillator that releases Ca^{2+} from the sarcoplasmic reticulum periodically. This cytosolic oscillator can be modulated by neurotransmitters and hormones.

Molecular Mechanism of Smooth Muscle Contraction

Smooth muscle contraction is controlled by two major factors: cytosolic calcium concentration and Rho-kinase signaling (Berridge, 2008). Smooth muscle contraction can occur with or without change in membrane potential (Somlyo and Somlyo 2000; Berridge, 2008).

Cytosolic Free Calcium. Smooth muscle contraction is regulated by intracellular free calcium (Ca^{2+}) acting through calmodulin. Calcium-bound calmodulin undergoes a conformational change, increasing its affinity for myosin light chain (MLC) kinase. MLC kinase is activated by binding of the calcium-calmodulin complex, leading to phosphorylation of the serine-19 residue of regulatory MLC$_{20}$. In the presence of adenosine triphosphate (ATP), this phosphorylation enables actin to activate the myosin ATPase and initiates cross-bridge cycling. Hydrolysis of ATP by ATPase supplies the energy for the contractile process (Fig. 26-9). The muscle contractile process ends when MLC$_{20}$ is dephosphorylated (inactivated) by myosin light chain phosphatase (MLCP). MLCP is a holoenzyme consisting of a type 1 phosphatase (PP1c), a myosin-targeting subunit (MYPT1), and a 20-kD subunit of unknown function (Hersch et al, 2004; Ito et al, 2004).

Rho Kinase Signaling Pathway (Calcium Sensitization Pathway). Theoretically, MLCP inhibition may lead to enhanced smooth muscle contraction. This is also termed the *calcium sensitization pathway*. The activity of MLCP can be modulated by Rho/Rho-kinase signaling (Fig. 26-10). Agonist activation causes dissociation of RhoA from Rho-guanine dissociation inhibitor and activates Rho-kinase. Phosphorylation of the regulatory subunit of MLCP by Rho-kinase inhibits phosphatase activity and enhances the contractile response (Hirano, 2007). RhoA and Rho-kinase are expressed in penile smooth muscle (Rees et al, 2002; Wang et al, 2002). The emerging consensus is that phasic contraction of penile smooth muscle is regulated by an increase in cytosolic Ca^{2+} and that tonic contraction is governed by the calcium-sensitizing pathways (Cellek et al, 2002). Several studies suggest that NO regulates RhoA/Rho-kinase activity (Bivalacqua et al, 2007; Priviero et al, 2010), and Chitaley and coworkers (2001) reported that Rho-kinase antagonism stimulated rat penile erection.

Latch State: A Unique Characteristic of Smooth Muscle Contraction. Smooth muscle has the ability to maintain tension for prolonged periods with minimal energy expenditure. This efficiency has been termed the **latch** state and is critical for sustaining the "basal" tone of the smooth muscle. It has been proposed that dephosphorylated myosin remains bound to actin in the high-affinity state to help stabilize the latch state. Others have proposed that calponin participates in the latch state by simultaneously binding actin and myosin to stabilize cross-bridge interactions and slow the rate of detachment (Szymanski, 2004).

Pathways Involving Inositol 1,4,5-Triphosphate, 1,2-Diacylglycerol, and Protein Kinase C. Vasoconstrictor agonists such as norepinephrine (α_1-adrenergic receptors), endothelin-1 (endothelin-A receptors), angiotensin II (AT1 receptors), prostaglandin F$_{2\alpha}$ (FP receptors), and TXA$_2$ (TP receptors) bind their respective receptors to activate Gq, which stimulates phospholipase C beta. This membrane-bound enzyme hydrolyzes phosphatidylinositol 4,5-bisphosphate to liberate IP$_3$ and 1,2-diacylglycerol. IP$_3$ binds to specific receptors (IP$_3$ receptor) on the smooth endoplasmic reticulum to stimulate the release of Ca^{2+} from intracellular stores. Binding of IP$_3$ to these receptors not only activates the channel but also increases the sensitivity of the IP$_3$ receptor to Ca^{2+} and assists **calcium-induced calcium release**.

Another mechanism of increased intracellular Ca^{2+} is by permitting entry of extracellular Ca^{2+} through **receptor-operated channels** without a change in membrane potential (Large, 2002). Norepinephrine, endothelin, vasopressin, and angiotensin II cause the opening of Ca^{2+}-permeable, nonselective cation channels.

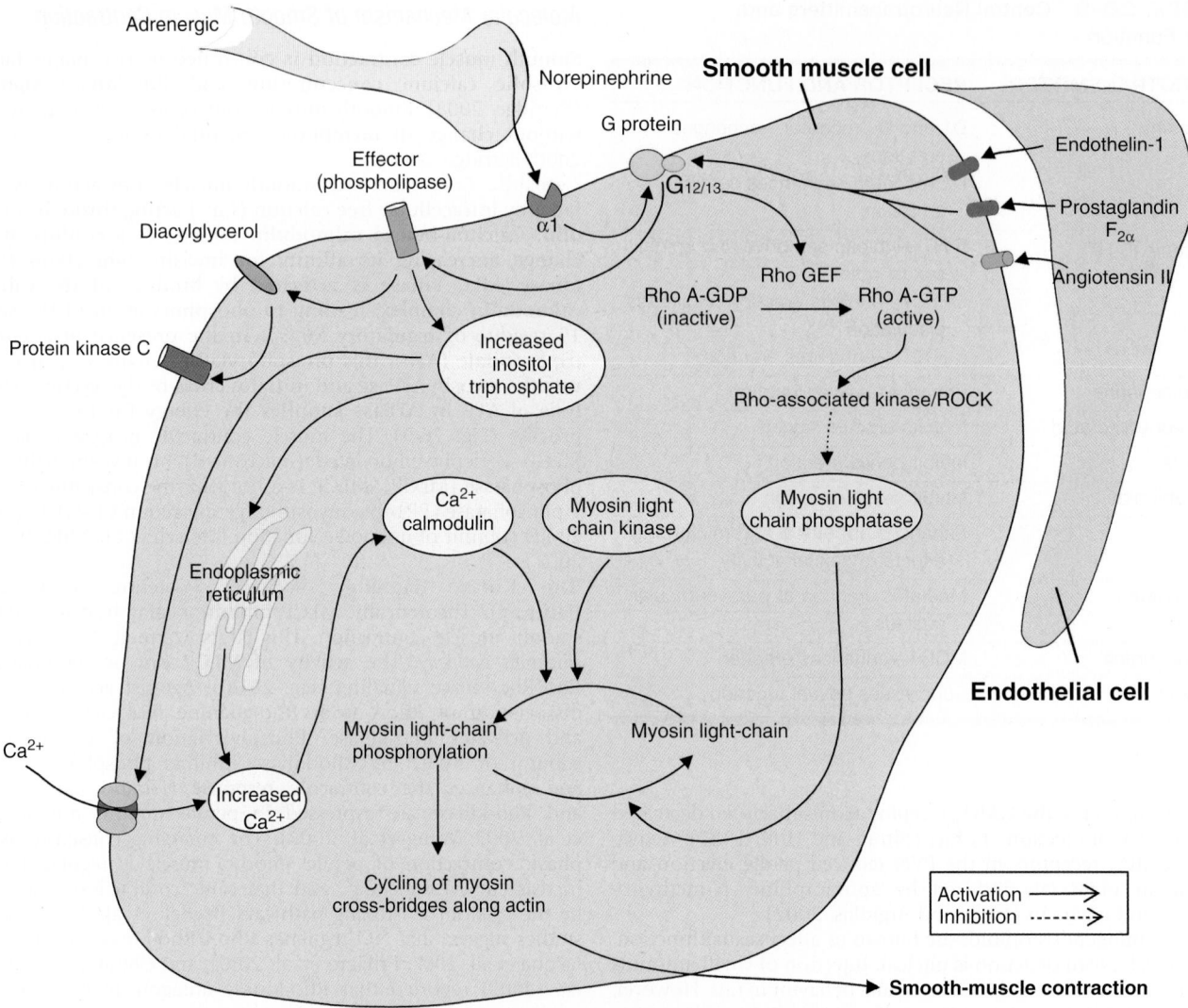

Figure 26-9. Molecular mechanism of penile smooth muscle contraction. Norepinephrine from sympathetic nerve endings and endothelins, angiotensin II, and prostaglandin $F_{2\alpha}$ from the endothelium activate receptors on smooth muscle cells to initiate the cascade of reactions that eventually result in elevation of intracellular calcium concentrations, activation of Rho-kinase, and smooth muscle contraction. Protein kinase C is a regulatory component of the Ca^{2+}-independent, sustained phase of agonist-induced contractile responses. GDP, guanosine diphosphate; GEF, guanine nucleotide exchange factor; GTP, guanosine triphosphate.

Molecular Mechanism of Smooth Muscle Relaxation

After contraction, relaxation of the muscle follows a decrease of free Ca^{2+} in the sarcoplasm. Calmodulin dissociates from MLC kinase and inactivates it. Myosin is dephosphorylated by MLCP and detaches from the actin filament, and the muscle relaxes (Fig. 26-11) (Walsh, 1991).

Another mechanism of smooth muscle relaxation is through cyclic adenosine monophosphate (cAMP) and cGMP, which are the two major second messengers involved in smooth muscle relaxation. They activate cAMP-dependent and cGMP-dependent protein kinases, which phosphorylate certain proteins and ion channels, resulting in (1) opening of the potassium channels and hyperpolarization; (2) sequestration of intracellular calcium by the endoplasmic reticulum; and (3) inhibition of voltage-dependent calcium channels, blocking calcium influx. The consequence is a decrease in cytosolic free calcium and smooth muscle relaxation.

Cyclic Guanosine Monophosphate–Signaling Pathway. Signaling molecules in the cGMP pathway include NO, CO, hydrogen sulfide (H_2S), and natriuretic peptides.

Nitric Oxide. Because of its small size, NO can diffuse inside its target cell, where it interacts with molecules that contain iron in either a heme or an iron-sulfur complex. The most physiologically relevant receptor for NO is soluble guanylyl cyclase (sGC), and the NO-sGC-cGMP pathway is responsible for the vasorelaxation effect of many endothelium-dependent vasodilators, including histamine, estrogens, insulin, corticotropin-releasing hormone, nitrovasodilators, and acetylcholine. This pathway is also principally responsible for physiologic penile erection.

Synthesis of NO is catalyzed by NOS, which converts L-arginine and oxygen to L-citrulline and NO. NOS exists as three isoforms in mammals: nNOS and eNOS are preferentially expressed in neurons/nerves and endothelial cells, respectively, and iNOS is expressed in virtually all cell types. All three NOS isoforms have been identified in the corpus cavernosum, with nNOS and eNOS being considered responsible for initiating and sustaining erection, respectively (Hurt et al, 2002; Musicki et al, 2009). A variant of nNOS (penile nNOS) has been identified as two distinct isoforms in the penis of rats and mice (Magee et al, 1996). eNOS has an indispensable role in penile erection, and its activity and bioavailability are regulated by multiple mechanisms,

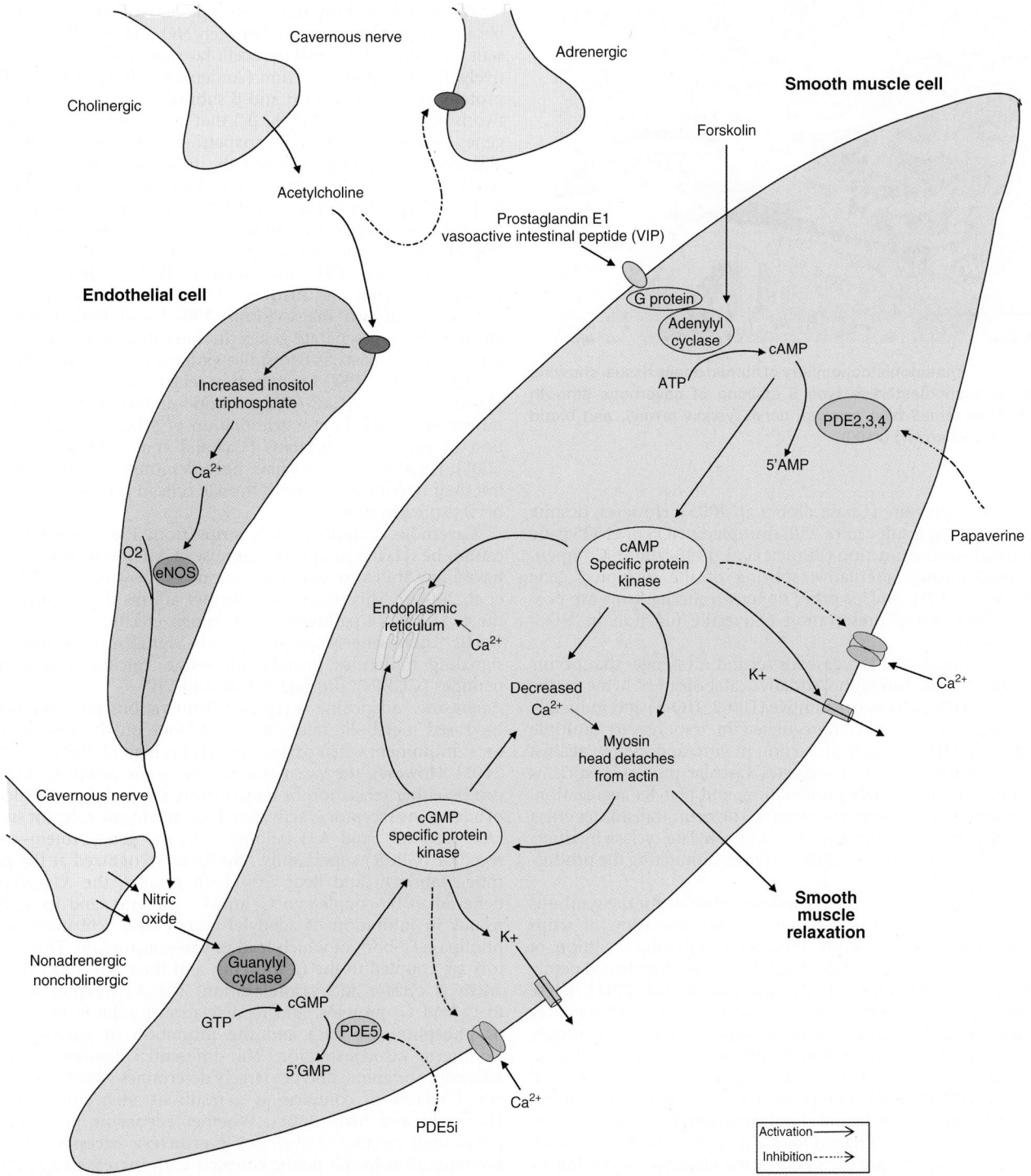

Figure 26-10. **Molecular mechanism of penile smooth muscle relaxation. The intracellular second messengers mediating smooth muscle relaxation, cyclic adenosine monophosphate (cAMP) and cyclic guanosine monophosphate (cGMP), activate their specific protein kinases, which phosphorylate certain proteins to cause opening of potassium channels, closing of calcium channels, and sequestration of intracellular calcium by the endoplasmic reticulum. The resultant decrease in intracellular calcium leads to smooth muscle relaxation. Sildenafil inhibits the action of phosphodiesterase (PDE) type 5 and increases the intracellular concentration of cGMP. Papaverine is a nonspecific phosphodiesterase inhibitor. ATP, adenosine triphosphate; eNOS, endothelial nitric oxide synthase; GTP, guanosine triphosphate.**

such as eNOS phosphorylation, eNOS interaction with regulatory proteins and contractile pathways, and actions of reactive oxygen species. Endothelial NO availability may be altered in vasculogenic ED. Downregulation of nNOS expression has been found in the corpus cavernosum of aging rats (Carrier et al, 1997),

castrated rats (Penson et al, 1996), and diabetic rats (Rehman et al, 1997).

Gene transfer of nNOS or eNOS to the penis has been shown to augment erectile responses in aging rats (Champion et al, 1999; Magee et al, 2002), and gene transfer of iNOS has enhanced

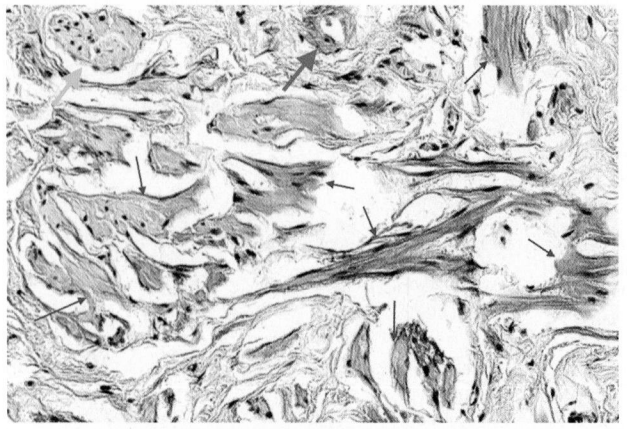

Figure 26-11. Immunohistochemistry of human penile tissue, showing positive phosphodiesterase type 5 staining of cavernous smooth muscle fibers *(small blue arrows)*, nerve *(yellow arrow)*, and blood vessel wall *(red arrow)* (×100).

intracavernous pressure (Chancellor et al, 2003). However, despite these encouraging results, mice with disrupted nNOS or eNOS gene have normal erectile function (Burnett et al, 1996, 2002). Compensatory mechanisms, alternative splicing of the disrupted gene (Ferrini et al, 2003), and/or other unknown mechanisms are possibly involved in the preservation of erectile function in NOS-knockout mice.

Carbon Monoxide. CO is a gaseous second messenger that occurs in biologic systems during the oxidative catabolism of heme by the HO enzyme. HO exists as constitutive (HO-2, HO-3) and inducible (HO-1) isoforms. HO-1 is upregulated in response to multiple stress stimuli. HO-1 confers protection in vitro and in vivo against oxidative cellular stress. CO regulates vascular processes, such as vessel tone, smooth muscle proliferation, and platelet aggregation, and may function as a neurotransmitter. The neurotransmitter effect of CO is dependent on the activation of guanylate cyclase by direct binding to the heme moiety of the enzyme, stimulating the production of cGMP.

Hydrogen Sulfide. L-Cysteine is a natural substrate for the synthesis of H_2S. Exogenous H_2S or L-cysteine causes relaxation of strips of human corpus cavernosum. Intracavernosal administration of either H_2S, sodium hydrosulfide (NaHS), or L-cysteine elicited penile erection in rats (d'Emmanuele di Villa Bianca et al, 2011). These observations indicate that a functional L-cysteine/H_2S pathway may be involved in mediating penile erection in men and some mammals.

Natriuretic Peptides. The natriuretic peptide family is involved in the regulation of cardiovascular homeostasis and consists of atrial (ANP), brain (BNP), and C-type (CNP) natriuretic peptides (Matsuo, 2001). ANP and BNP are ligands for the natriuretic peptide receptor NPR-A, whereas CNP is a ligand for the natriuretic peptide receptor NPR-B. Both receptors are members of the guanylyl cyclase family and are also called GC-A and GC-B.

The effects of ANP, BNP, and CNP on cGMP production and smooth muscle relaxation in isolated human and animal corpus cavernosum and in cultured cavernous smooth muscle cells have been investigated (Kim et al, 1998; Kuthe et al, 2003; Sousa et al, 2010). The results indicate that CNP is the most potent natriuretic peptide and that it relaxes the isolated cavernous smooth muscle by binding to NPR-B. However, whether CNP and NPR-B play a role in physiologic erection remains to be seen.

Guanylyl Cyclase. In mammals, seven membrane-bound (particulate) guanylyl cyclase isoforms (GC-A to GC-G) and one soluble isoform (sGC) have been identified (Andreopoulos and Papapetropoulos, 2000). Although the membrane-bound guanylyl cyclase system is not known to play a role in physiologic erection, expression of GC-B in human and rat corpus cavernosum and induction of cavernous smooth muscle relaxation by CNP (ligand for GC-B) have been demonstrated (Guidone et al, 2002; Kuthe et al, 2003).

The soluble isoform sGC plays a pivotal role in erectile function because it provides the link between NO and cGMP, which represent the extracellular and intracellular signaling molecules, respectively, in physiologic erection (Andersson, 2001). A heterodimeric protein, sGC consists of α and β subunits, each of which exists in two isoforms ($α_1$, $α_2$, and $β_1$, $β_2$) that are encoded by two separate genes (Andreopoulos and Papapetropoulos, 2000). Nimmegeers and associates (2008) assessed the functional importance of the sGCα1β1 isoform in corpus cavernosum from male sGCα1 (−/−) and wild-type mice and concluded that the sGCα1β1 isoform is involved in corpus cavernosum smooth muscle relaxation in response to NO and NO-independent sGC stimulators.

Protein Kinase G. PKG, also called cGMP-dependent kinase, is the principal receptor and mediator for cGMP signals. In mammals, PKG exists in two major forms, PKG-I and PKG-II, which are encoded by two separate genes. In smooth muscle, only PKG-I is expressed and exists as two splice variants (PKG-Iα and PKG-Iβ).

cGMP and/or PKG-I may induce relaxation via activation of the plasma membrane Ca^{2+}-ATPase pump, inhibition of IP_3 generation, inhibition of Rho-kinase, stimulation of MLCP, and phosphorylation of heat shock proteins (Carvajal et al, 2000; Lincoln et al, 2001). These mechanisms have been demonstrated in various cells, but their relevance to smooth muscle cells in genital tissues has not been explicitly shown.

Cavernous smooth muscle strips from PKG-I knockout mice cannot be relaxed by agents that raise cGMP levels, and these mice have a low ability to reproduce, presumably owing to ED (Hedlund et al, 2000a). This observation further affirms the essential role of the cGMP/PKG-I pathway in physiologic erectile function.

Cyclic Adenosine Monophosphate–Signaling Pathway. cAMP-signaling molecules include adenosine, calcitonin gene–related peptides (CGRPs), prostaglandins, and VIP.

Adenosine. Adenosine is released from various cells as a result of increased metabolic rates, and its actions on the vasculature are most prominent when oxygen demand is high (Tabrizchi and Bedi, 2001). However, the vascular response to the action of adenosine can be either relaxation or constriction, depending on which type of adenosine receptor is activated. Four adenosine receptor subtypes (A1, A2$_A$, A2$_B$, and A3) belonging to the gene protein–coupled receptor (GPCR) superfamily have been recognized at the present time (Tabrizchi and Bedi, 2001). In general, the A1 receptor is believed to be coupled to G_i and G_o proteins, and its activation results in inhibition of adenylyl cyclase and activation of phospholipase C, both of which lead to vasoconstriction. The A2 receptors are coupled to the G_s proteins, and their activation stimulates adenylyl cyclase and vasorelaxation. The A3 receptor is coupled to G_i and G_q proteins, and its activation results in the activation of phospholipase C/D and the inhibition of adenylyl cyclase, leading to vasoconstriction. The differential distribution of these adenosine receptor subtypes largely determines whether a particular vessel relaxes or contracts as a result of adenosine stimulation (Tabrizchi and Bedi, 2001). Whether adenosine plays a role in physiologic erection is unclear. **Nevertheless, excessive adenosine accumulation in the penis, coupled with increased A2$_B$ receptor signaling, contributes to priapism in two independent lines of mutant mice. One is adenosine deaminase–deficient mice (the animals display spontaneously prolonged penile erection), and the other is sickle cell disease transgenic mice, a well-accepted animal model for priapism (Bivalacqua et al, 2009; Dai et al, 2009).**

Calcitonin Gene–Related Peptide Family. CGRP, amylin, and adrenomedullin are members of the CGRP family. These short-chain peptides are potent vasodilators released from perivascular nerve fibers. They act through the calcitonin receptor–like receptor, which belongs to the GPCR superfamily (Conner et al, 2002).

In rats, CGRP levels in the penis, bladder, kidney, testis, and adrenal gland were found to increase gradually up to maturity and then rapidly decline (Wimalawansa, 1992). In patients with ED given CGRP via intracavernous injection, a dose-related increase in penile arterial inflow (and erection) occurred (Stief et al, 1991). Adenovirus-mediated gene transfer of CGRP also enhanced erectile responses in aged rats, apparently through an increase of cAMP levels in the corpora cavernosa (Bivalacqua et al, 2001).

Prostaglandins. Prostaglandins are a family of eicosanoids capable of initiating numerous biologic functions. The prime mode of prostaglandin action is through specific prostaglandin receptors that all belong to the GPCR family. There are at least nine known prostaglandin receptor subtypes in mice and humans and several additional splice variants with divergent carboxyl termini (Narumiya and FitzGerald, 2001). Four of the subtypes (EP1 to EP4) bind PGE_2, two (DP1 and DP2) bind PGD_2, and the other three subtypes (FP, IP, and TP) bind $PGF_{2\alpha}$ (FP), PGI_2 (IP), and TXA_2 (TP). On the basis of signaling attributes, the prostaglandin receptors are classified into three types. The "relaxant" receptors IP, DP1, EP2, and EP4 are coupled to an α_s-containing G protein and are capable of stimulating adenylyl cyclase to increase intracellular cAMP. The "contractile" receptors EP1, FP, and TP are coupled to an α_q-containing G protein, which activates phospholipase C instead of adenylyl cyclase. These contractile receptors do not signal through the cAMP pathway, and their signaling outcome is an increase of intracellular calcium. The EP3 receptor is also a contractile receptor, but it is coupled to an α_i-containing G protein that inhibits adenylyl cyclase to result in a decrease of cAMP formation.

Animal and human corpora cavernosa produce several prostaglandins including $PGF_{2\alpha}$, PGE_2, PGD_2, PGI_2, and TXA_2 (Moreland et al, 2001). In studies in isolated human penile tissue, different PGs have been shown to elicit different effects in human corpus cavernosum, corpus spongiosum, and cavernous artery (Hedlund and Andersson, 1985). Although $PGF_{2\alpha}$, PGI_2, and TXA_2 contract the corpus cavernosum and corpus spongiosum, PGE_1 and PGE_2 (but not PGI_2) relax the corpus cavernosum and spongiosum that have been precontracted with noradrenaline or $PGF_{2\alpha}$. Although PGI_2 is the predominant vasorelaxant in blood vessels, its action in the erectile tissue is either contractile or neutral. This disparity in the action of PGI_2 between blood vessels and the erectile tissue and the difference between the effects of PGI_2 and PGE_1 and PGE_2 in the erectile tissue are most likely due to differences in the distribution of prostaglandin receptors. Other studies have shown that in the corpus cavernosum, the relaxant effects of prostanoids are mediated by EP2 and/or EP4 receptors (for PGE_1 and PGE_2) but not IP receptor (for PGI_2) (Angulo et al, 2002).

Although the production of prostaglandins and the expression of prostaglandin receptors in the erectile tissue have been clearly demonstrated, their roles in physiologic erection are still undefined. **The erectogenic effects of PGE_1 as a pharmaceutic agent have been extensively documented. First described in 1998, intracavernous injection of PGE_1 is one of the safest and most effective treatments for ED** (Stackl et al, 1988). Transurethral application is an alternative.

Vasoactive Intestinal Peptide. The human or animal penis is richly supplied with nerves containing VIP and VIP-related peptides such as pituitary adenylate cyclase–activating polypeptide. Most of these nerves also contain immunoreactivity to NOS, and colocalization of NOS and VIP within nerves innervates the penises of both animals and humans (Andersson, 2001). Two subtypes of VIP receptors, VPAC1 and VPAC2, belonging to the GPCR family have been cloned from human and rat tissues. VPAC2, but not VPAC1, messenger RNA has been identified in cultured rat cavernous smooth muscle cells (Guidone et al, 2002). In dogs, intracavernous VIP injection has been found to induce penile erection (Juenemann et al, 1987b); in men, it has not produced rigid erection, but success rates are improved when VIP is combined with papaverine and phentolamine (Kiely et al, 1989). However, it has been shown that VIP release is not essential for neurogenic relaxation of human cavernous smooth muscle (Pickard et al, 1993), and the physiologic role of VIP in penile erection has not been resolved.

Adenylyl Cyclase. Signaling molecules in the cAMP pathway bind to and activate specific cytoplasmic membrane receptors that, through their coupled G proteins, activate adenylyl cyclases. To date, nine membrane-bound isoforms and one soluble form of mammalian adenylyl cyclase have been cloned and characterized (Patel et al, 2001). Although different membrane-bound adenylyl cyclases

are regulated differently, they all are stimulated by the GTP-bound form of the G_a subunit, and all (except AC9) are stimulated by forskolin.

In rabbits with alloxan-induced diabetes, cAMP formation in the corpus cavernosum in response to forskolin has been shown to be reduced. This suggests impaired adenylyl cyclase function in diabetes mellitus (Sullivan et al, 1998).

Protein Kinase A. Protein kinase A (PKA), also called cAMP-dependent kinase, is the principal receptor for cAMP, and it mediates most of the cellular effects of cAMP by phosphorylating a wide variety of downstream targets in the cytoplasmic and nuclear compartments (Johnson et al, 2001). PKA is composed of two regulatory (R) and two catalytic (C) subunits that form a tetrameric holoenzyme R_2C_2. Binding of cAMP to the R subunits causes the holoenzyme to dissociate into an $R_2(cAMP)_4$ dimer and two free catalytically active C subunits. The presence of multiple C subunit genes further adds to the diversity and complexity of the various holoenzyme complexes, which differ in biochemical and functional properties as well as patterns of expression and localization. These differences among the isozymes contribute to the broad specificity of PKA in a wide variety of physiologic processes in response to cAMP signaling.

More than 100 different cellular proteins have been identified as physiologic substrates of PKA, with more than 90% (135 of 145) being phosphorylated at serine and the remainder at threonine (Shabb, 2001). The predominant target sequence (>50%) is Arg-Arg-X-Ser, in which Ser is the phosphate acceptor. Three PKA substrate proteins have been identified in penile tissue: PDEs, cAMP-responsive element-binding protein, and ATP-sensitive potassium (K_{ATP}) channel.

Cross-Activation. Increased levels of intracellular cAMP and cGMP cause the activation of *cAMP-dependent* and *cGMP-dependent protein kinases* (PKA and PKG). Each cyclic nucleotide–dependent kinase can be activated by either cAMP or cGMP, although cross-activation requires an approximately 10-fold higher concentration of cyclic nucleotide (Walsh, 1994). Although PKA and PKG may phosphorylate numerous common substrates, several lines of evidence indicate that the activation of PKG by cGMP and cAMP is the predominant mechanism by which cyclic nucleotides decrease intracellular Ca^{2+} to cause vascular smooth muscle relaxation (Lincoln et al, 1990; Jiang et al, 1992; Komalavilas and Lincoln, 1996).

Phosphodiesterase. In each episode of cyclic nucleotide signaling, the increase of intracellular cAMP or cGMP concentration is typically twofold to threefold baseline (Francis et al, 2001). Decline occurs rapidly and often during the continued presence of the signaling hormone (Francis et al, 2001). Termination of cyclic nucleotide signals is principally carried out by PDEs, which catalyze the hydrolysis of cAMP and cGMP to AMP and GMP, respectively. Feedback mechanisms that increase PDE activities and/or expression by the increased cyclic nucleotide level assist cyclic nucleotide degradation (Corbin et al, 2000; Lin et al, 2001a, 2001b).

The superfamily of mammalian PDEs consists of 11 families (PDE1 to PDE11) that are encoded from 21 distinct genes (Lin et al, 2003; Montorsi et al, 2004). Each PDE gene usually encodes more than one isoform through alternative splicing or from alternative gene promoters. PDE1, PDE3, PDE4, PDE7, and PDE8 are multigene families, whereas PDE2, PDE5, PDE9, PDE10, and PDE11 are unigene families. PDE1, PDE2, PDE3, PDE10, and PDE11 hydrolyze cAMP and cGMP; PDE4, PDE7, and PDE8 hydrolyze cAMP; and PDE5, PDE6, and PDE9 hydrolyze cGMP.

With the exception of PDE6, which is specifically expressed in photoreceptor cells, all PDEs have been identified in the corpus cavernosum (Küthe et al, 2001). However, there is ample evidence that **PDE5 is the principal PDE for the termination of cavernous cGMP signaling** (Fig. 26-12), and inhibition of the cGMP-catalytic activity by PDE5 inhibitors is highly effective in treating ED.

PDE3 also appears to play a role in erection, as demonstrated by the erectogenic effect of a PDE3-specific inhibitor, milrinone (Kuthe et al, 2002). Although direct inhibition of PDE5 is the main mechanism through which sildenafil exerts its erectogenic effect, it has been shown that sildenafil also significantly increases cAMP

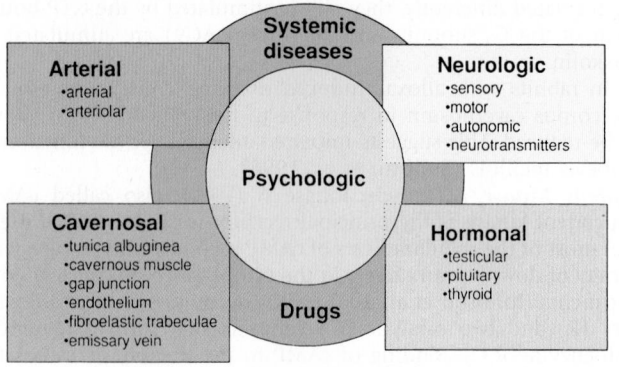

Figure 26-12. Functional classification of impotence. It is unlikely for impotence in an individual patient to derive solely from one source. Most cases have a psychogenic component of varying degree, and systemic diseases and pharmacologic effects can be concomitant and causative. (Modified from Carrier S, Brock G, Kour NW, et al. Pathophysiology of erectile dysfunction. Urology 1993;42:468–81, with permission of Excerpta Medica, Inc.)

concentration in isolated human cavernous tissue strips (Stief et al, 2000). This effect is thought to involve PDE3 because cGMP, which is accumulated as a result of PDE5 inhibition by sildenafil, is capable of preventing cAMP degradation by competing for the same catalytic sites on the PDE3 molecules (Francis et al, 2001). This attenuating effect of cGMP on the cAMP-catalytic activity of PDE3 is also believed to explain why inhibition of PKG could suppress the relaxing effect of forskolin in isolated human cavernous smooth muscle (Uckert et al, 2004).

Ion Channels. In general, there are four major types of ion channels: (1) external ligand-gated, which open to a specific extracellular molecule (e.g., acetylcholine); (2) internal ligand-gated, which open or close in response to an intracellular molecule (e.g., ATP); (3) voltage-gated, which open in response to a change in membrane potential (e.g., sodium, potassium, and calcium channels); and (4) mechanically gated, which open in response to mechanical pressure.

Smooth muscle has neither a T-tubule system nor a well-developed sarcoplasmic reticulum. Extracellular calcium plays an important role, and calcium must enter the cytoplasm through the plasma membrane during an action potential. Three transmembrane proteins are known to regulate calcium inflow and outflow: Calcium channels are the major inflow regulators, whereas the calcium-sodium exchanger and calcium-ATPase regulate calcium exit from muscle cells. The presence of voltage-dependent L-type calcium channels (long-duration current, slow calcium channel) in isolated cavernous smooth muscle and cultured muscle cells has been documented. Christ and colleagues (1993a) reported that both calcium influx through calcium channels and mobilization of intracellular calcium stores are involved during phenylephrine-induced and endothelin-induced contraction.

Studies have shown at least four types of potassium channel subtypes in the cavernous smooth muscle: (1) calcium-sensitive potassium channel (e.g., maxi-K); (2) metabolically regulated potassium channels (K_{ATP}); (3) delayed rectifier; and (4) fast transient A current (Christ et al, 1993a; Fan et al, 1995). The calcium-sensitive potassium channels may be involved in cAMP-mediated smooth muscle relaxation. Decreased intracytosolic potassium and altered potassium conductance have been shown to occur in corpus cavernosum smooth muscle treated with acetylcholine and sodium nitroprusside (Seftel et al, 1996). The movement of positively charged K^+ out of the cell causes hyperpolarization and relaxation of smooth muscle (Andersson, 2001).

Calcium-activated chloride channels on the smooth muscle cells of corpus cavernosum are thought to be involved in the maintenance of spontaneous tone and the contractile response to adrenaline and other agonists (Fan et al, 1999; Chu and Adaikan, 2008).

Hyperpolarization of Smooth Muscle Cells. Hyperpolarization causes closure of voltage-dependent calcium channels, a decrease in the intracellular free calcium concentration, and relaxation of the smooth muscle. One of the hyperpolarization mechanisms is through the opening of potassium channels. The opening of ATP-sensitive K^+ channels (K_{ATP}) and Ca^{2+}-activated K^+ channels (K_{Ca}) causes hyperpolarization and relaxation of vascular smooth muscle. These two types of channels are present in human corpus cavernosum smooth muscle (Christ et al, 1993b), and pharmacologic stimulation of K_{ATP} channels induces penile smooth muscle relaxation (Venkateswarlu et al, 2002). PNU-83757, an opener of K_{ATP} channels, has been shown to induce erection when administered intracavernously to patients with ED (Vick et al, 2002). The opening of large-conductance K_{Ca} channels, also known as *maxi-K*, has been found to hyperpolarize and relax human corpus cavernosum (Spektor et al, 2002). The opening of K^+ channels can be stimulated by PKA, PKG, or cGMP.

Hyperpolarization of penile smooth muscle is also important in endothelium-dependent relaxation of human penile arteries, in which significant relaxation remains despite blockade of NO and prostaglandin synthesis (Angulo et al, 2003b). This activity has been attributed to EDHF, which opens K_{Ca} channels and produces hyperpolarization and vasodilation. The nature of EDHF remains undetermined.

Molecular Oxygen as a Modulator of Penile Erection. The P_{O_2} level of cavernous blood in the flaccid state is similar to that of venous blood (≈35 mm Hg). During erection, the large inflow of arterial blood increases P_{O_2} to approximately 90 mm Hg (Sattar et al, 1995). Molecular oxygen is a substrate, together with L-arginine, for the synthesis of NO by NOS. In the flaccid state, the low oxygen concentration inhibits NO synthesis; during erection, the higher level of substrate induces NO synthesis. It has been estimated that the minimal concentration of oxygen in the cavernous bodies necessary to reach full NOS activity is 50 to 60 mm Hg (Kim et al, 1993).

Similarly, prostaglandin H synthase is also an oxygenase (cyclooxygenase) and uses oxygen as substrate for the synthesis of prostanoids. Production of PGE_1 has been shown to be inhibited in flaccidity and stimulated during erection. Endothelin synthesis is also modulated by oxygen: A low oxygen concentration promotes production, whereas a high concentration inhibits it.

Intercellular Communication. During erection and detumescence, communication should exist among cavernous smooth muscles to mediate synchronized relaxation and contraction (Christ et al, 1991). **Several studies have demonstrated the presence of gap junctions in the membrane of adjacent muscle cells. These intercellular channels allow exchange of ions such as calcium and second-messenger molecules** (Christ et al, 1993a). The major component of gap junctions is connexin-43, a membrane-sparing protein of less than 0.25 μm that has been identified between smooth muscle cells of human corpus cavernosum (Campos de Calvalho et al, 1993). Cell-to-cell communication through these gap junctions most likely explains the synchronized erectile response, although their pathophysiologic impact is still unclear.

Intracavernous Tissue Architecture

The trabeculae of the corpora cavernosa provide the structural support and regulatory mechanism for the endothelial-lined sinusoidal spaces as well as the conduit for blood vessels and nerves. Relaxation of the trabeculae allows the expansion and filling of the sinusoids by the incoming blood, whereas "recoil" of the trabeculae expels blood to the emissary veins and returns the penis to a flaccid state. In 24 men undergoing penile prosthesis implantation for severe ED, Nehra and colleagues (1996) categorized the smooth muscle content of the corpus cavernosum into four groups—high (39% to 42%), intermediate (30% to 37%), low (13% to 29%), and normal (42% to 50%)—and reported that increasing degree of venous leakage correlates with decreasing muscle content. In specimens from six men who died of nongenital causes, Costa and colleagues (2006) showed that the major constituents of the trabeculae are collagen fibers (40.8%), smooth muscle (40.4%), and elastic fibers (13.2%). In seven men undergoing penile prosthesis implantation, the three components were composed of collagen fibers (41.6%), smooth muscle (42%), and elastic fibers (9.1%); the only significant change in men with ED compared with normal men was a reduction of elastic fibers. From these two reports, it seems likely that the histologic changes associated with ED consist primarily of decline in either smooth muscle or elastic fibers.

The complex architecture of the penis is maintained by the dynamic expression and interaction of numerous trophic factors. One is sonic hedgehog (SHH), which plays a key role in regulating vertebrate organogenesis, such as the growth of digits on limbs and organization of the brain. SHH remains important in adults. It controls cell division of adult stem cells and has been implicated in development of some cancers. SHH has been identified in the penis; inhibition of SHH in adult rats leads to rapid atrophy and disorganization of the corpus cavernosum (Podlasek et al, 2003, 2005). In addition, SHH has been shown to stimulate the expression of vascular endothelial growth factor (VEGF) and NOS in the penis (Podlasek et al, 2005) (Table 26-9).

KEY POINTS: SMOOTH MUSCLE PHYSIOLOGY

- Relaxation of the cavernous smooth muscle is the key to penile erection.
- NO released by nNOS contained in the terminals of the cavernous nerve initiates the erection process, whereas NO released from eNOS in the endothelium helps maintain erection.
- On entering the smooth muscle cells, NO stimulates the production of cGMP.
- cGMP activates PKG, which opens the potassium channels and closes the calcium channels.
- Low cytosolic calcium favors smooth muscle relaxation.
- The smooth muscle regains its tone when cGMP is degraded by PDE.

TABLE 26-9 Key Molecules Involved in Physiologic Regulation of Cavernous Smooth Muscle

CONTRACTION	
NAME	**FUNCTION**
High cytosolic calcium	Binds calmodulin to activate MLC kinase
MLC kinase	Converts MLC to active form, MLCP
Phosphorylated MLC (MLCP)	Cycling of myosin cross-bridges along actin results in muscle contraction
MLCP	Dephosphorylates MLCP to inactive form, MLC
Rho-kinase	Inhibits MLC phosphatase to enhance contraction (calcium sensitization pathway)

RELAXATION	
NAME	**FUNCTION**
Nitric oxide	Binds soluble guanylyl cyclase to produce cGMP
cGMP	Activates protein kinase G
Protein kinase G	Opens potassium channels and closes calcium channels
Low cytosolic calcium	Calcium dissociates from calmodulin, muscle relaxes

cGMP, cyclic guanosine monophosphate; MLC, myosin light chain; MLCP, myosin light chain phosphatase.

PATHOPHYSIOLOGY OF ERECTILE DYSFUNCTION

"The Penis Poem"
My nookie days are over, My pilot light is out.
What used to be my sex appeal, Is now my water spout.
Time was when, on its own accord, From my trousers it would spring.
But now I've got a full time job, To find the gosh darn thing.
It used to be embarrassing, The way it would behave.
For every single morning, It would stand and watch me shave.
Now as old age approaches, It sure gives me the blues.
To see it hang its little head, And watch me tie my shoes!!

– Willie Nelson

Incidence and Epidemiology

The increasing incidence of impotence with age was noted by Kinsey and colleagues in 1948: only 1 of 50 men at age 40 years, but 1 in 4 men by age 65. In 1990, Diokno and colleagues reported that 35% of married men 60 years old and older experienced erectile impotence.

Modern probability sampling techniques were used by two surveys obtaining prevalence data of ED in the United States: the Massachusetts Male Aging Study (MMAS) and the National Health and Social Life Survey (NHSLS). The **MMAS** consisted of 1709 non-institutionalized men between the ages of 40 and 70 years living in the greater Boston area first surveyed between 1987 and 1989 and resurveyed between 1995 and 1997 (Feldman et al, 1994; Johannes et al, 2000). Extensive physiologic measures, demographic information, and self-reported ED status (nine items related to potency on a questionnaire) were components of this report. The MMAS was the first cross-sectional, community-based, random-sample, multidisciplinary epidemiologic survey on ED and its physiologic and psychosocial correlates in men in the United States. **From the prevalence rates reported in the MMAS study, between the ages of 40 and 70 years, the probability of complete ED increased from 5.1% to 15%, the probability of moderate dysfunction increased from 17% to 34%, and the probability of mild dysfunction remained constant at about 17%.**

The **NHSLS** was a national probability survey of men (N = 1410) and women between the ages of 18 and 59 years living in households in the United States in 1992 (Laumann et al, 1999) and was principally a broad-ranging inquiry into sexual practices and beliefs within that age group. The survey collected only limited information on sexual function broadly defined. The following prevalence rates for ED were reported (responses to questions regarding obtaining and maintaining erection): 7% for ages 18 to 29 years, 9% for ages 30 to 39, 11% for ages 40 to 49, and 18% for ages 50 to 59.

Regarding worldwide prevalence of ED, 24 international studies were reported between 1993 and 2003 (Lewis et al, 2004). All studies that were stratified by age showed an increasing prevalence of ED. For men younger than age 40, the rate was 1% to 9%; from 40 to 59, it ranged from 2% to 9% to 20% to 30%, with some studies showing marked differences between the 40 to 49 and the 50 to 59 age groups. The 50 to 59 age groups showed the greatest range of reported prevalence rates. For the 60 to 69 age group, most of the world showed a high rate (20% to 40%), with some showing increases after age 65 except for the Scandinavian reports, in which the 70s and older were the time of major rate change. Almost all of the reports showed high prevalence rates for men in their 70s and 80s, ranging from 50% to 75%.

Incidence Studies

The MMAS (Johannes et al, 2000) is the only longitudinal study conducted in the United States (1987-1989 and 1995-1997). Analyses were performed on 847 of the 1297 men without ED at baseline (1987-1989) and with follow-up information from 1995 to 1997. The average age of these men at baseline was 52.2 years (range 40 to 69 years). **From this group of men, the crude incidence rate of impotence in white men in the United States was 25.9 cases/1000**

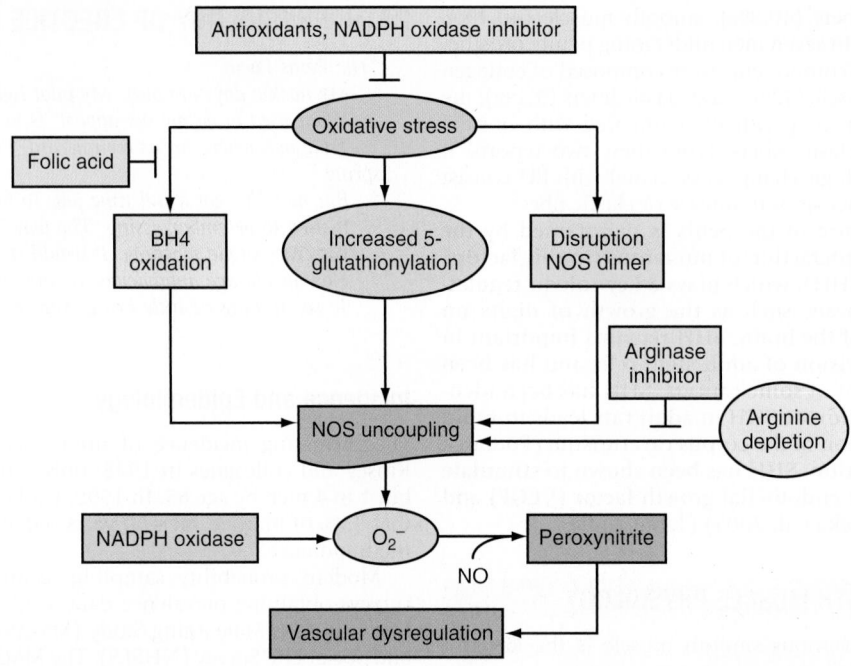

Figure 26-13. **Factors contributing to nitric oxide synthase (NOS) uncoupling and the potential inhibitors. BH4, tetrahydrobiopterin; NADPH, reduced nicotinamide adenine dinucleotide phosphate.**

man-years (95% confidence interval 22.5 to 29.9). The annual incidence rates increased with each decade (per 1000 man-years): 12.4 cases for 40 to 49 years, 29.8 cases for 50 to 59 years, and 46.4 cases for 60 to 69 years. Age-adjusted risk (per 1000 man-years) of ED was higher for men with diabetes mellitus (50.7 cases), treated heart disease (58.3 cases), and treated hypertension (42.5 cases). By using these data and the known population of the United States, it was estimated that, for white men, the new cases in the 40 to 69 age group would be 617,715 per year (Lewis et al, 2000). Rates reported from Europe and Brazil also suggest an incidence of 25 to 30 per 1000 man-years (Moreira et al, 2003; Schouten et al, 2005). A study using a validated questionnaire in a random sample of 2213 men conducted in Olmsted County, Minnesota, from 1996 to 2004 revealed that the five sexual function domains change together over time in this community-based cohort. Erectile function, ejaculatory function, and sexual drive decrease over time with greater rates of decline for older men. However, older men are less likely to perceive these declines as a problem and are less likely to express dissatisfaction referable to them (Gades et al, 2009).

Risk Factors

Common risk factor categories associated with sexual dysfunction include the following: general health status, diabetes mellitus, cardiovascular disease, concurrence of other genitourinary disease, psychiatric/psychological disorders, other chronic diseases, and sociodemographic conditions. In a study of race/ethnicity and socioeconomic status in 2301 men 30 to 79 years old from Boston, it was reported that men in the low socioeconomic status category had a greater than twofold increase in risk of ED (adjusted odds ratio 2.26, 95% confidence interval 1.39, 3.66). The increased risk of ED in black and Hispanic men in this study was thought to be associated with differences in socioeconomic status rather than biologic factors (Kupelian et al, 2008).

For ED, smoking, medications, and hormonal factors also serve as well-defined risk factors. In men, diabetes has been associated with a greater prevalence of decreased desire and orgasmic dysfunction as well as ED. A higher odds ratio is seen with insulin-dependent diabetes mellitus; diabetes present for more than 10

years; fair or poor control based on glycosylated hemoglobin; management by means other than diet; a history of diabetes-related arterial, renal, or retinal disease and neuropathy; and concurrent cigarette smoking. Endothelial dysfunction is a condition present in many cases of ED, and there are common etiologic pathways for other vascular disease states (Lewis et al, 2004).

Classification

Many classifications have been proposed (Fig. 26-13). Some are based on the cause (diabetic, iatrogenic, traumatic), and some are based on the neurovascular mechanism (failure to initiate [neurogenic], failure to fill [arterial], and failure to store [venous]) (Goldstein, personal communication, 1990). A classification recommended by the International Society of Impotence Research is shown in Box 26-1 (Lizza and Rosen, 1999).

Psychogenic

Previously, psychogenic impotence was believed to be the most common, thought to affect 90% of impotent men (Masters and Johnson, 1965). This belief has given way to the realization that **ED is usually a mixed condition that may be predominantly functional or physical.**

Sexual behavior and penile erection are controlled by the hypothalamus, limbic system, and cerebral cortex. Stimulatory or inhibitory messages can be relayed to the spinal erection centers to assist or inhibit erection. **Two possible mechanisms have been proposed to explain the inhibition of erection in psychogenic dysfunction: direct inhibition of the spinal erection center by the brain as an exaggeration of the normal suprasacral inhibition** (Steers, 2000) **and excessive sympathetic outflow or elevated peripheral catecholamine levels, which may increase penile smooth muscle tone to prevent its necessary relaxation.** Animal studies demonstrate that the stimulation of sympathetic nerves or systemic infusion of epinephrine causes detumescence of the erect penis (Diederichs et al, 1991a, 1991b). Clinically, higher levels of serum norepinephrine have been reported in patients with psychogenic ED than in normal controls or patients with vasculogenic ED (Kim and Oh, 1992).

ORGANIC
I. Vasculogenic
   A. Arteriogenic
   B. Cavernosal
   C. Mixed
II. Neurogenic
III. Anatomic
IV. Endocrinologic

PSYCHOGENIC
I. Generalized
   A. Generalized unresponsiveness
      1. Primary lack of sexual arousability
      2. Aging-related decline in sexual arousability
   B. Generalized inhibition
      1. Chronic disorder of sexual intimacy
II. Situational
   A. Partner-related
      1. Lack of arousability in specific relationship
      2. Lack of arousability owing to sexual object preference
      3. High central inhibition owing to partner conflict or threat
   B. Performance-related
      1. Associated with other sexual dysfunction (e.g., rapid ejaculation)
      2. Situational performance anxiety (e.g., fear of failure)
   C. Psychological distress or adjustment related
      1. Associated with negative mood state (e.g., depression) or major life stress (e.g., death of partner)

Bancroft and Janssen (2000) theorized that male sexual response depends on the balance between excitatory and inhibitory impulses within the CNS. One example is the high prevalence of sexual dysfunction/ED in men with psychiatric disorders. Mosaku and Ukpong (2009) surveyed patients (mean age 39.6, standard deviation 11.6 years) with a diagnosis of schizophrenia, bipolar affective disorder, recurrent depressive disorder, and/or substance use disorder with mean duration of illness of 10.24 years (standard deviation 8.2 years) who were attending a psychiatry clinic. In this population, the prevalence of ED was 83%; older age, unmarried status, use of medications, and the presence of comorbid medical conditions were significantly predictive of ED.

Neurogenic

It has been estimated that 10% to 19% of ED is neurogenic. If one includes iatrogenic causes and mixed ED, the prevalence is likely much higher. The presence of a neurologic disorder or neuropathy does not exclude other causes, and confirming that ED is neurogenic can be challenging. Because erection is a neurovascular event, **any disease or dysfunction affecting the brain, spinal cord, and cavernous or pudendal nerves can induce dysfunction.**

As discussed earlier, the MPOA, PVN, and hippocampus have been regarded as important integration centers for sexual drive and erection (Sachs and Meisel, 1988), and pathologic processes in these regions, such as **Parkinson disease, stroke, encephalitis, or temporal lobe epilepsy, are often associated with ED.** The effect of parkinsonism may result from the imbalance of the dopaminergic pathways (Chaudhuri and Schapira, 2009). **Other brain lesions associated with ED are tumors, dementias, Alzheimer disease, multiple system atrophy, and trauma.** In studies of sexual function in men after stroke, lack of sexual desire was found to be common (Jung et al, 2008). ED is more prevalent in patients who have cerebrovascular accident lesions in the thalamic area (Jeon et al, 2009).

In men with a **spinal cord injury,** the nature, location, and extent of the injury largely determine erectile function. In addition to ED, these men may have impaired ejaculation and orgasm. **Reflexogenic erection is preserved in 95% of patients with complete upper cord lesions but in only about 25% of patients with complete lower cord lesions** (Biering-Sørensen and Sønksen, 2001). Sacral parasympathetic neurons are important in the preservation of reflexogenic erection, although the thoracolumbar pathway may compensate for sacral loss through synaptic connections. In these patients, minimal tactile stimulation can trigger erection, albeit of short duration and requiring continuous stimulation. **Other disorders at the spinal level** (e.g., spina bifida, disk herniation, syringomyelia, tumor, transverse myelitis, and multiple sclerosis) **may affect the afferent or efferent neural pathway in a similar manner.**

Because of the close relationship between the cavernous nerves and the pelvic organs, the incidence of iatrogenic impotence from pelvic surgical procedures is reportedly high: radical prostatectomy, 43% to 100% (Walsh and Donker, 1982; Borchers et al, 2006), and abdominal perineal resection, 15% to 100% (Weinstein and Roberts, 1977).

An improved understanding of the neuroanatomy of the pelvic and cavernous nerves (Walsh and Donker, 1982) has resulted in modified surgery for cancer of the rectum, bladder, and prostate, producing a lower incidence of iatrogenic impotence. For example, the introduction of nerve sparing has reduced the incidence of impotence to 30% to 50% after radical prostatectomy (Catalona and Bigg, 1990; Quinlan et al, 1991) and less than 10% after radical rectal surgery (Liang et al, 2008).

In cases of **pelvic fracture,** ED can be a result of cavernous nerve injury or vascular insufficiency or both. In men with posterior urethral injury, early realignment has been associated with better potency preservation rate relative to delayed anastomosis (ED rate 34% vs. 42%) (Mouraviev et al, 2005). In **diabetics,** impairment of neurogenic and endothelium-dependent relaxation results in inadequate NO release (Saenz de Tejada et al, 1989a). Because autonomic penile innervation cannot be tested directly, clinicians should be cautious in diagnosing neurogenic ED. A corpus cavernosum electromyograph has been developed and refined for diagnosis of various conditions affecting the penis (including autonomic neuropathy), but the clinical utility of this device is still under investigation (Guiliano and Rowland, 2013).

A decrease in penile tactile sensitivity with increasing age was also reported by Rowland and colleagues (1993). Sensory input from the genitalia is essential to achieve and maintain reflexogenic erection, and the input becomes even more important when older people gradually lose psychogenic erection. Sensory evaluation should be an integral part of the evaluation for ED in all patients with or without an apparent neurologic disorder.

Endocrinologic

Hypogonadism is a frequent finding in impotent patients. Androgens influence the growth and development of the male reproductive tract and secondary sex characteristics; their effects on libido and sexual behavior are well established. In a review of published articles from 1975 to 1992, **Mulligan and Schmitt (1993) concluded that testosterone (1) enhances sexual interest, (2) increases the frequency of sexual acts, and (3) increases the frequency of nocturnal erection but has little or no effect on fantasy-induced or visually stimulated erections.** Granata and colleagues (1997) reported that the threshold level of testosterone for normal nocturnal erections is about 200 ng/dL. In a population-based, observational survey conducted in the Boston area, Araujo and colleagues (2007) reported a 5.6% prevalence of symptomatic androgen deficiency in men between the ages of 30 and 79 years, with older men at greater risk. Prevalence of symptoms was as follows: low libido, 12%; ED, 16%; osteoporosis/fracture, 1%; and two or more nonspecific symptoms, 20%. However, **many men with low testosterone levels are asymptomatic.** In a study of patients presenting with ED, Köhler and colleagues (2008) reported androgen deficiency symptoms in 47% of men with testosterone levels of less than 200 ng/dL, 33% of men with levels less than 300 ng/dL, 23% of men with levels less than 346 ng/dL, and 7% of men with levels less than 400 ng/dL. Age, the presence of uncontrolled diabetes, high total cholesterol, and anemia all correlated with significantly decreased testosterone levels in men with ED. In another report from the same group, waist circumference was noted to be the most important predictor of low testosterone and symptomatic androgen deficiency (Hall et al, 2008). In men with a body mass index (BMI) of more than 30 kg/m², total testosterone was subnormal in 57.5%, and free testosterone subnormal in 35.6%. Most of these men had isolated hypogonadotropic hypogonadism (Hofstra et al, 2008). In a comprehensive literature review, Traish and colleagues (2009) noted that low testosterone precedes elevated fasting insulin, glucose, and hemoglobin A_{1c} values in men who develop diabetes, suggesting that hypogonadism may be a sentinel event in the development of diabetes. **The authors further suggested that androgen deficiency is associated with insulin resistance, type 2 diabetes, metabolic syndrome, and increased deposition of visceral fat. Visceral fat may serve as an endocrine organ, producing inflammatory cytokines and promoting endothelial dysfunction and vascular disease.**

The mechanism of androgen's effect has been examined by several investigators. Beyer and González-Mariscal (1994) reported that testosterone and dihydrotestosterone (DHT) are responsible for male pelvic thrusting and estradiol or testosterone is responsible for female pelvic thrusting during copulation. Androgens have beneficial effects on endothelial cells and smooth muscle cells: Androgens promote endothelial cell survival, reduce endothelial expression of proinflammatory markers, and inhibit proliferation and intimal migration of vascular smooth muscle cells. Low androgen levels are associated with apoptosis of endothelial cells and smooth muscle cells. Low androgen levels also impair proliferation, migration, and homing of endothelial progenitor cells as well as myogenic differentiation of mesenchymal progenitor cells (Mirone et al, 2009; Traish and Galoosian, 2013). Testosterone and DHT may also relax penile artery and cavernous smooth muscle through their nongenomic effects (Waldkirch et al, 2008). In rats, castration has been reported to decrease arterial flow, induce venous leakage, and reduce the erectile response to stimulation of the cavernous nerve by about 50% (Mills et al, 1994; Penson et al, 1996). Castration also increases α-adrenergic responsiveness of penile smooth muscle (Traish et al, 1999). Clinically, many men receiving long-term androgen ablation therapy for prostate cancer have reported poor libido and ED.

Any dysfunction of the hypothalamic-pituitary axis can result in hypogonadism. Hypogonadotropic hypogonadism can be congenital or caused by a tumor or injury. Hypergonadotropic hypogonadism may result from a tumor, injury, surgery, or mumps orchitis.

Hyperprolactinemia, whether secondary to a pituitary adenoma or drugs, results in both reproductive and sexual dysfunction. Symptoms may include loss of libido, ED, galactorrhea, gynecomastia, and infertility. Hyperprolactinemia is associated with low circulating levels of testosterone, which appear to be secondary to inhibition of gonadotropin-releasing hormone secretion by the elevated prolactin levels (Leonard et al, 1989). In a study of subjects consulting for sexual dysfunction, prolactin in the lowest quartile levels was noted to be associated with metabolic syndrome and arteriogenic ED as well as with premature ejaculation and anxiety symptoms (Corona et al, 2009).

ED may also be associated with hyperthyroidism and hypothyroidism. Hyperthyroidism is commonly associated with diminished libido (which may be caused by the increased circulating estrogen levels) and less often with ED. In hypothyroidism, low testosterone secretion and elevated prolactin levels contribute to ED.

Arteriogenic

Atherosclerotic or traumatic arterial occlusive disease of the hypogastric-cavernous-helicine arterial tree can decrease the perfusion pressure and arterial flow to the sinusoidal spaces, increasing the time to maximal erection and decreasing the rigidity of the erect penis. In most patients with arteriogenic ED, the impaired penile perfusion is a component of the generalized atherosclerotic process. Common risk factors associated with arterial insufficiency include hypertension, hyperlipidemia, cigarette smoking, diabetes mellitus, blunt perineal or pelvic trauma, and pelvic irradiation (Feldman et al, 1994; Martín-Morales et al, 2001). Shabsigh and colleagues (1991) reported that abnormal penile vascular findings increased significantly as the number of risk factors for ED increased. On arteriography, bilateral diffuse disease of the internal pudendal, common penile, and cavernous arteries has been found in ED patients with atherosclerosis. Focal stenosis of the common penile or cavernous artery is most often seen in young patients who have sustained blunt pelvic or perineal trauma (Levine et al, 1990). **Long-distance cycling is also a risk factor for vasculogenic and neurogenic ED.** There is a significant relationship between cycling-induced perineal compression leading to vascular, endothelial, and neurogenic dysfunction in men and the development of ED (Sommer et al, 2010). **Nevertheless, ED does not commonly occur in men who engage in recreational bicycle riding** (Kim et al, 2011).

ED and cardiovascular disease share the same risk factors such as hypertension, diabetes mellitus, hypercholesterolemia, and smoking (Feldman et al, 1994; Martín-Morales et al, 2001). Lesions in the pudendal arteries are much more common in men with ED than in the general population of similar age. Natural remission and progression occur in a substantial number of men with ED. The association of BMI with remission and progression and the association of smoking and health status with progression offer potential avenues for facilitating remission and delaying progression using lifestyle intervention (Travison et al, 2007).

Cardiovascular Diseases. High prevalence of ED has been reported in men with coronary, cerebral, and peripheral vascular diseases (Bener et al, 2008; Chai et al, 2009). **Among men with coronary arterial disease, the prevalence of ED increases as the severity of coronary arterial lesions increases** (Montorsi et al, 2006). **Several studies reported an association between ED and cardiovascular disease.** The link between these conditions might reside in the interaction between androgens, chronic inflammation, and cardiovascular risk factors that determines endothelial dysfunction and atherosclerosis, resulting in disorders of penile and coronary circulation. Because penile artery size is smaller compared with coronary arteries, the same level of endothelial dysfunction causes a more significant reduction of blood flow in erectile tissues compared with that in coronary circulation. ED could be an indicator of systemic endothelial dysfunction (Gandaglia et al, 2014). In patients with chronic coronary disease who also had ED, onset of sexual dysfunction occurred before coronary artery disease onset in 93%, with a mean time interval of 24 months (range 12 to 36 months) (Montorsi et al, 2006). These data have led some authors to advocate screening for ED as a means to identify men at risk for cardiovascular disease (Gandaglia et al, 2014).

Hyperlipidemia. ED has been associated with a high prevalence of hyperlipidemia and coronary heart disease (Roumeguere et al, 2003). Hypercholesterolemia at baseline was also shown to be a predictor of subsequent ED over the course of 25 years in 570 male patients included in the Rancho Bernardo Study (Fung et al, 2004). A survey of 1899 men 30 to 79 years old in the Boston area did not show an association between untreated hyperlipidemia and ED (Hall et al, 2009).

The effect of hypercholesterolemia on erectile function has been studied in different experimental models. In hypercholesterolemic rabbits, examination of the corpus cavernosum ultrastructure revealed an early atherosclerotic process in the sinusoids (Kim et al, 1994). Although the endothelial NO/cGMP pathway is impaired in this model, neuronal vasodilation does not appear to be affected (Azadzoi et al, 1998). The NO/cGMP pathway effect likely is due to increased superoxide production (Kim et al, 1997) or endogenous NOS inhibitors such as NG-monomethyl-L-arginine monoacetate and asymmetrical dimethylarginine (ADMA).

L-Arginine supplementation reverses impairment of endothelium-dependent relaxation (Azadzoi et al, 1998). VEGF is an important angiogenic factor for maintenance of endothelial health. Ryu and colleagues (2006) reported that VEGF and VEGF receptor 2 are downregulated in the corporeal tissue of rats eating a 4% cholesterol diet for 3 months. Xie and colleagues (2005) noted that levels of VEGF mRNA are reduced with subsequent observation of impaired endothelium-dependent relaxation in rabbits fed with a 1% cholesterol diet.

In a more severe ischemic experimental model, rabbits underwent balloon de-endothelialization of the iliac arteries followed by a high-cholesterol diet (Azadzoi et al, 1992). The rabbits developed penile arterial insufficiency and veno-occlusive dysfunction owing to decreased expandability of the cavernous smooth muscle (Azadzoi et al, 1997; Nehra et al, 1998). Changes in iliac and penile vasculature were noted, associated with decreased NOS activity and reduced endothelium-dependent and neurogenic NO-mediated relaxation of the cavernous tissue (Azadzoi et al, 1999). As a result of the impaired NO activity, production of contractile thromboxane and prostaglandin increased, leading to potentiation of neurogenic contractions of the cavernous smooth muscle (Azadzoi et al, 1998, 1999).

In large arteries in rabbits, oxidized low-density lipoproteins inhibited endothelium-dependent NO-mediated relaxation (Murohara et al, 1994). Enhanced corpus cavernosum muscle contractility by oxidized low-density lipoproteins has also been reported by Ahn and colleagues (1999).

Obesity. In a U.S. study of community-dwelling men 65 years old and older, Garimella and associates (2013) reported prevalence of complete ED of 42% in men who completed MMAS scale (N = 4108). In sexually active men who completed the five-item International Index of Erectile Function (IIEF-5) questionnaire (N = 1659) the prevalence of moderate to severe ED was 56%. **In multivariate-adjusted analyses, high body weight, BMI, and total body fat percentage were independently associated with greater prevalence of moderate to severe and complete ED.**

Perivascular adipose tissue (PVAT) is recognized as an active contributor to vascular function. Adipocytes and stromal cells contained within PVAT are sources of molecules with varied paracrine effects on the underlying smooth muscle and endothelial cells, including adipokines, cytokines, reactive oxygen species, and gaseous compounds. In obesity and diabetes, the expanded PVAT contributes to vascular insulin resistance. PVAT-derived cytokines may influence key steps of atherogenesis. The physiologic anticontractile effect of PVAT is severely diminished in hypertension. Above all, a common denominator of PVAT dysfunction in all these conditions is immune cell infiltration, which triggers the subsequent inflammation, oxidative stress, and hypoxic processes to promote vascular dysfunction (Szasz et al, 2013).

Hypertension. Hypertension is an independent risk factor for ED (Feldman et al, 1994; Johannes et al, 2000), **and its consequent cardiovascular complications such as ischemic heart disease and renal failure are associated with even higher ED prevalence** (Feldman et al, 1994; Kaufman et al, 1994; Johannes et al, 2000). **However, in hypertension, the increased blood pressure itself does not impair erectile function; rather, the associated arterial biochemical and structural changes are thought to be the causes** (Hsieh et al, 1989; Behr-Roussel et al, 2005). In two analyses including more than 270,000 men with ED from a U.S. care claim database, the prevalence of hypertension in men with versus without ED was 41.2% versus 19.2%, respectively (Seftel et al, 2004; Sun and Swindle, 2005).

The potential determinants for ED in hypertensive men include older age, longer duration of disease, greater severity of hypertension, and the use of antihypertensive medications (Doumas et al, 2006). Arterial hypertension is characterized by altered vascular tone and increased vascular contractility resulting in high blood pressure. It is accompanied by proliferation, migration of vascular smooth muscle cells, and varying levels of inflammation of the arterial wall. The Rho-kinase pathway plays a crucial role in the regulation of arterial blood pressure (Nunes et al, 2010).

Endothelial dysfunction, oxidative stress, and autoimmune diseases are also potential causes of arterial disease and ED. The Toll-like receptor activation on cells of the vasculature in response to the release of damage-associated molecular patterns and the consequences of this activation on inflammation, vasoreactivity, and vascular remodeling has been proposed as a novel link between inflammation and hypertension (McCarthy et al, 2014). In addition, endoplasmic reticulum stress leading to endothelium-dependent contractile responses in aorta has been proposed as a cause of hypertension in a spontaneously hypertensive rat (SHR) model (Spitler et al, 2013). Increased activity of angiotensin II–mediated reduced nicotinamide adenine dinucleotide phosphate oxidase in hypertensive rats is suggested to be the cause of increased superoxide anions (Jin et al, 2008).

Mechanism of Vascular Erectile Dysfunction

Structural Changes. In arteriogenic ED, oxygen tension in corpus cavernosum blood is less than that in psychogenic ED (Tarhan et al, 1997). Formation of PGE_1 and PGE_2 is oxygen dependent, and in rabbit and human corpus cavernosum, increased oxygen tension was associated with elevation of PGE_2 and suppression of TGF-β1–induced collagen synthesis (Moreland et al, 1995; Nehra et al, 1999). A decrease in oxygen tension may diminish cavernous trabecular smooth muscle content and lead to diffuse venous leakage (Saenz de Tejada et al, 1991b; Nehra et al, 1998).

A narrowed lumen or increased wall/lumen ratio in the arteries contributes to increased peripheral vascular resistance in hypertension. Increased resistance has also been found in the penile vasculature of SHR—an alteration ascribed to structural changes of the arterial and erectile tissue (Gradin et al, 2006; Arribas et al, 2008). Mitochondrial damage (in smooth muscle and endothelial cells) and nerve degeneration have been described in SHR (Jiang et al, 2005). Partial success in the prevention or reversal of the structural changes has been described when rats were treated with a type 1 angiotensin II receptor (AT1) blocker; an AT1 blocker with a PDE5 inhibitor; and a selective β_1 blocker, nebivolol (Mazza et al, 2006; Toblli et al, 2006a, 2006b).

Enhanced Smooth Muscle Contraction and Vasoconstriction. In animal models, increased RhoA/Rho-kinase activity leading to increased contractility of the corporeal smooth muscle is proposed to contribute to ED in diabetes (Bivalacqua et al, 2004), hypercholesterolemia (Morikage et al, 2006), hypertension (Fibbi et al, 2008), hypogonadism (Vignozzi et al, 2007), and aging (Jin et al, 2006; Andersson, 2011). Park and coworkers (2006) found that the Rho/Rho-kinase pathway is substantially involved in the development of ED and pelvic atherosclerosis, both of which could be prevented by long-term treatment with fasudil, a Rho-kinase inhibitor.

Endothelin-1 levels are elevated in plasma of men with atherosclerosis, hypertension, and hypercholesterolemia. Men with organic ED have higher venous and cavernous blood levels of endothelin-1 as well (Nohria et al, 2003; El Melegy et al, 2005). Despite this, a pilot study using an endothelin-A receptor antagonist as a treatment for men with ED did not produce positive results (Kim et al, 2002). AT1 receptor antagonist and angiotensin-converting enzyme (ACE) inhibitor have shown promise in the treatment of men with ED and hypertension and men with ED and atherosclerosis, respectively (Speel et al, 2005; Baumhäkel et al, 2008).

Impaired Endothelium-Dependent Smooth Muscle Relaxation. Endothelial dysfunction has been proposed as the common link between cardiovascular disease and ED (Brunner et al, 2005). Impairment of endothelium-dependent flow-mediated dilation of the brachial artery has been reported in men with ED, and the degree of impairment correlates with the severity of ED (Kovacs et al, 2008). A plethysmography device designed to assess endothelium-dependent vasodilation of the penis did not find a correlation between brachial and penile arteries in men with ED (Vardi et al, 2009).

Endothelial progenitor cells are regenerative cells produced in bone marrow that migrate to peripheral vessels to repair endothelial defects. The number of endothelial progenitor cells is reduced in

TABLE 26-10 Vascular and Structural Changes Leading to Erectile Dysfunction

PENILE STRUCTURE	CHANGES IN ERECTILE DYSFUNCTION
Cavernous artery	Increased vascular resistance, narrow lumen
Smooth muscle	Increased tone (hypertonicity) Decreases muscle content Alteration of potassium channels and gap junctions
Erectile tissue	Fibrosis Impaired veno-occlusive mechanism
Endothelium	Impaired endothelium-dependent relaxation
Tunica albuginea	Alteration of elastic and collagen fibers
Neurotransmitters	Decreased nNOS, eNOS

eNOS, endothelial nitric oxide synthase; nNOS, neuronal nitric oxide synthase.

men with ED and coronary heart disease and in overweight men (Foresta et al, 2005; Baumhäkel et al, 2006; Esposito et al, 2009). Short-term and long-term administration of PDE5 inhibitors increases the number of circulating endothelial progenitor cells and improves endothelial and erectile function (Foresta et al, 2005, 2009).

In SHR, the relaxing effect of acetylcholine is blunted in corporeal strips (Behr-Roussel et al, 2003). Impairment of endothelium-dependent relaxation in arteries from SHR could be ascribed to angiotensin II (Rajagopalan et al, 1996), thromboxane, and superoxide (Cosentino et al, 1998) or to high blood pressure per se (Paniagua et al, 2000) (Table 26-10).

Cavernous (Venogenic)

Failure of adequate venous occlusion has been proposed as one of the most common causes of vasculogenic impotence (Rajfer et al, 1988). **Veno-occlusive dysfunction may result from various pathophysiologic processes, including degenerative tunical changes, fibroelastic structural alterations, insufficient trabecular smooth muscle relaxation, and venous shunts.**

Degenerative changes (e.g., Peyronie disease, old age, and diabetes) or traumatic injury to the tunica albuginea (e.g., penile fracture) can impair the compression of the subtunical and emissary veins (Gonzalez-Cadavid, 2009). **In Peyronie disease, the inelastic tunica albuginea may prevent the emissary veins from closing** (Metz et al, 1983). Chiang and colleagues (1992) postulated that a decrease in the elastic fibers of the tunica albuginea and an alteration in the tunica albuginea microarchitecture may contribute to impotence in some men. Changes in the subtunical areolar layer may impair the veno-occlusive mechanism, as is occasionally seen in patients after surgery for Peyronie disease (Dalkin and Carter, 1991).

Structural alterations in the fibroelastic components of the trabeculae, cavernous smooth muscle, and endothelium may result in venous leakage. Insufficient trabecular smooth muscle relaxation, causing inadequate sinusoidal expansion and insufficient compression of the subtunical venules, may occur in anxious individuals with excessive adrenergic tone or in patients with inadequate neurotransmitter release. It has been shown that alteration of an α adrenoceptor or a decrease in NO release may heighten smooth muscle tone and impair relaxation in response to endogenous muscle relaxant (Christ et al, 1990).

Acquired venous shunts—the result of operative correction of priapism—may cause persistent glans/cavernosum or cavernosum/spongiosum shunting.

Fibroelastic Component. Loss of compliance of the penile sinusoids associated with increased deposition of collagen and decreased elastic fiber may be seen in diabetes, hypercholesterolemia, vascular disease, penile injury, or old age. Sattar and colleagues (1994) reported significant differences in the mean percentage of penile elastic fibers: 9% in normal men, 5.1% in patients with venous leakage, and 4.3% in patients with arterial disease. In an animal model of vasculogenic ED, Nehra and colleagues (1998) demonstrated that cavernous expandability correlates with smooth muscle content and may be used to predict trabecular histology. Moreland and colleagues (1995) showed that PGE$_1$ suppresses collagen synthesis by TGF-β1 in human cavernous smooth muscle, which implies that intracavernous injection of PGE$_1$ may be beneficial in preventing intracavernous fibrosis.

Smooth Muscle. Because corporeal smooth muscle controls the vascular events leading to erection, a change in smooth muscle content and ultrastructure can be expected to affect erectile response. In a study of human penile tissue, Sattar and colleagues (1996) demonstrated a significant difference between the mean percentage of cavernous smooth muscle in normal potent men, stained with antidesmin (38.5%) or antiactin (45.2%), and that in a venogenic group (antidesmin, 27.4%; antiactin, 34.2%) or an arteriogenic group (antidesmin, 23.7%; antiactin, 28.9%). An in vitro biochemical study showed impaired neurogenic and endothelium-related relaxation of penile smooth muscle in impotent diabetic men (Saenz de Tejada et al, 1989a). In vasculogenic and neurogenic ED, the damaged smooth muscle can be a key factor, aggravating the primary cause (Mersdorf et al, 1991). Pickard and colleagues (1994) also showed impairment of nerve-evoked relaxation and α-adrenergic-stimulated contraction of cavernous muscle and reduced muscle content in men with venous or mixed venous/arterial impotence.

Ion channels are intimately involved in the biochemical events of muscle function. Fan and colleagues (1995) reported an alteration of the maxi-K$^+$ channel in cells from impotent patients and suggested that this might contribute to decreased hyperpolarizing ability, altered calcium homeostasis, and impaired smooth muscle relaxation. In animal studies, Jünemann and colleagues (1991) showed significant smooth muscle degeneration with loss of cell-to-cell contact in rabbits fed a high-cholesterol diet for 3 months. In a rabbit model of vasculogenic impotence, Azadzoi and colleagues (1997) demonstrated that veno-occlusive dysfunction could be induced by cavernous ischemia. Cavernous nerve injury may also affect cavernous smooth muscle relaxation, as demonstrated in neurotomized dogs (Paick et al, 1991).

Gap Junctions. Gap junctions, intercellular communication channels, are responsible for synchronization and coordination of the erectile response (Christ et al, 1991). In severe arterial disease, the presence of collagen fibers between cell membranes reduces or abolishes their contact (Persson et al, 1989). Suadicani and colleagues (2009) reported a significant decrease of gap junction protein connexin 43 in the corpus cavernosum in aged and streptozotocin-induced diabetic rats.

Endothelium. It is now recognized that the endothelium is an important source of not only NO but also many other signaling molecules, including EDHF, PGI$_2$, and hydrogen peroxide. In addition, the endothelium, via transferred chemical mediators, such as NO and PGI$_2$, and/or low-resistance electrical coupling through myoendothelial gap junctions, modulates flow-mediated vasodilation and influences mitogenic activity, platelet aggregation, and neutrophil adhesion. Disruption of endothelial function is an early indicator of the development of vascular disease (Triggle et al, 2012). Diabetes and hypercholesterolemia have been shown to alter the function of endothelium-mediated relaxation of the cavernous muscle (Azadzoi et al, 1991) and impair erection. In a study of cell junction proteins in hypercholesterolemic mice, Ryu and colleagues (2013) reported downregulation of endothelium-specific cell-to-cell junction proteins, including claudin-5, vascular endothelial-cadherin, and platelet endothelial cell adhesion molecule 1, as well as decreased endothelial content, which may contribute to ED in these mice.

Maintenance of Structural Integrity. SHH is one of three proteins in the mammalian hedgehog family, the others being desert hedgehog and Indian hedgehog. SHH plays a key role in regulating vertebrate organogenesis, such as in the growth of digits on limbs and organization of the brain. SHH is also important in adults. It controls cell division of adult stem cells and has been implicated in development of some cancers. SHH has been shown to regulate cavernous smooth muscle apoptosis in response to signals from cavernous nerve. In an animal model of neurogenic ED, SHH protein treatment of the penis prevents cavernous nerve injury–induced apoptosis and structural changes (Podlasek, 2009).

Markers of Erectile Function. Variable coding sequence protein A1 (Vcsa1) has been proposed as a marker of erectile function in rats. Vcsa1 is downregulated in animal models of neurogenic, diabetic, and aging-associated ED. The Vcsa protein product sialorphin is an endogenous neutral endopeptidase inhibitor. In humans, there are at least three homologues to the Vcsa1 gene (hSMR3A, hSMR3B, and PROL1). Downregulation of hSMR3A has been reported in men with ED (Davies and Melman, 2008).

Various cardiovascular risk factors have been associated with the onset and the severity of ED, including markers of endothelial function, thrombosis, and dyslipidemia. These markers can be used as a cardiometabolic risk profile in patients with ED. Although NO, ADMA, and endothelin and genetic polymorphisms hold some promise as biochemical markers of cardiovascular disease and ED, these are still in development (Lippi et al, 2012).

Drug-Induced

ED is common among older men and inevitably coexists with other conditions that are themselves risk factors for ED, such as depression, diabetes, and cardiovascular disease (Feldman et al, 1994). In addition, sexual symptoms related to medication can involve a combination of complaints concerning desire, arousal, and orgasm rather than being limited to impaired function. Self-reported and questionnaire data concerning ED as a side effect of medication should be interpreted with caution.

Antihypertensive Agents. Almost all antihypertensive drugs have ED listed as a potential side effect. Nevertheless, more recent well-designed controlled clinical trials have clarified some myths.

Diuretics. Thiazide diuretics are carbonic anhydrase inhibitors that alkalinize cells and cause vasodilation. The predominant activity of thiazide diuretics is to inhibit a directly coupled Na-Cl cotransporter along the distal convoluted tubule of the kidney. Acutely, when extracellular fluid volume depletion occurs because of salt wasting, cardiac output tends to decline, resulting in reactive vasoconstriction. However, on a long-term basis, cardiac output is regulated according to metabolic needs, and vasodilation supervenes, returning cardiac output toward baseline; this transforms hypotension from hypovolemic to vasodilatory (Ellison et al, 2009).

This class of drug has been extensively studied. Data from a large trial in the United Kingdom showed that twice as many men taking thiazides for mild hypertension reported ED than men taking propranolol or placebo—the most common reason for withdrawal from the bendrofluazide arm of the study ("Adverse reactions to bendrofluazide and propranolol for the treatment of mild hypertension," 1981).

Similar findings were documented from the Treatment of Mild Hypertension Study (TOMHS), where the prevalence of ED at 2 years in men taking low-dose thiazide was twice that of men taking placebo or alternative agents (Grimm et al, 1997). After 4 years of treatment, the prevalence of ED in the placebo group approached that of the thiazide group, a finding not fully explained by dropouts. It may be that thiazide therapy, rather than causing ED directly, unmasks it at an earlier stage. A study comparing sexual side effects of thiazide, placebo, or atenolol in hypertensive patients also found a higher rate of ED in the thiazide group, although this was ameliorated by weight loss (Wassertheil-Smoller et al, 1991). **The mechanism of diuretic-induced ED remains to be elucidated.**

β-Adrenergic Blockers. Receptor studies show that only 10% of adrenoceptors in the penile tissue are of the β type, and their stimulation is thought to mediate relaxation (Andersson and Wagner, 1995). **This response is attenuated in vitro by nonselective drugs such as propranolol, possibly via a prejunctional β$_2$-receptor effect** (Srilatha et al, 1999), **but not by cardiac-selective agents such as practolol.** β antagonists also exert an inhibitory effect within the CNS, perhaps leading to decreased sex hormone levels (Suzuki et al, 1988).

The differential effects of β-adrenoceptor antagonists on erectile function may be explained by whether they are general antagonists, are selective antagonists, or possess vasodilatory properties. **Nonselective drugs such as propranolol are associated with higher prevalence of ED** compared with prevalence of ED observed in patients treated with placebo or ACE inhibitors (Croog et al, 1986). Subsequent trials using **agents with higher selectivity for the β$_1$ adrenoceptor such as acebutolol have shown a substantial reduction in ED** with no difference between placebo and ACE inhibitor groups (Grimm et al, 1997). Carvedilol, a general β-adrenoceptor antagonist that also causes vasodilation by blocking α$_1$ adrenoceptors, has been associated with worsening sexual function (Fogari et al, 2001). Some more recently introduced β$_1$-adrenoceptor antagonists, such as nebivolol, have vasodilatory effects mediated by release of NO (Reidenbach et al, 2007). In crossover studies using nebivolol versus the selective β$_1$-adrenoceptor antagonists metoprolol and atenolol, nebivolol did not decrease sexual intercourse activity in hypertensive men and in some cases had positive effects on erectile function (Boydak et al, 2005; Brixius et al, 2007).

α-Adrenoceptor Blockers. Animal studies have demonstrated a positive effect on erection for α antagonists, particularly antagonists acting on the α$_1$ receptor, by increasing or prolonging the relaxant response of cavernous smooth muscle (Andersson and Wagner, 1995). In addition, prejunctional α$_2$ receptor activation modulates the release of noradrenaline, suggesting a putative relaxant role for α$_2$ blockers. In clinical observations, **drugs such as doxazosin,** used to treat hypertension (Grimm et al, 1997) or reduce urinary tract symptoms (Flack, 2002), **were not associated with complaints of ED** and had lower rates than in placebo groups. **Drugs stimulatory to the α$_2$ receptor, such as clonidine, result in diminished erectile function** clinically and experimentally by peripheral and central mechanisms (Srilatha et al, 1999). **Methyldopa,** a centrally acting drug, **has also been associated with ED** in controlled trials comparing it with placebo and other antihypertensive agents (Croog et al, 1988), and it may act by antagonizing hypothalamic α$_2$ adrenoceptors.

Angiotensin-Converting Enzyme Inhibitors. **ACE inhibitors lack any easily appreciated peripheral or central effect that would interfere with sexual function.** An in vivo experiment showed that the ACE inhibitor captopril did not cause any significant adverse effect on sexual function in awake normotensive rats (Srilatha et al, 1999). In three clinical studies of hypertension treatment comparing an ACE inhibitor with other agents and placebo, all found either no difference from placebo or improved sexual function over baseline compared with other agents (Croog et al, 1988; Suzuki et al, 1988; Grimm et al, 1997).

Angiotensin II Type 1 Receptor Antagonist. In studies of hypertensive or aging normotensive animals, the AT1 receptor antagonists (e.g., losartan, valsartan, candesartan) reverse structural changes in the penile vasculature and appear to conserve erectile function (Hale et al, 2001, 2002; Park et al, 2005; Hannan et al, 2006). In clinical cross-sectional studies, AT1 receptor antagonists, in contrast to other antihypertensive drugs, seem to improve erectile function (Doumas et al, 2006). In a crossover study comparing valsartan with the β-adrenoceptor antagonist carvedilol, valsartan had a beneficial effect on preexisting sexual dysfunction and had no adverse sexual effects during 12 months of treatment (Fogari et al, 2001). Treatment with losartan for 3 months has also been reported to improve sexual function (Llisterri et al, 2001).

Calcium Channel Blockers. Clinical studies of calcium channel blockers have demonstrated **no adverse effect on erection;** ejaculatory complaints, which may be due to decreased force of bulbocavernous muscles, seem short-lived (Suzuki et al, 1988). In the TOMHS study, there was no increase in ED in the amlodipine group compared with placebo (Grimm et al, 1997). Another study also showed no increase in the prevalence of ED when hypertension was treated with diltiazem alone or in combination with an ACE inhibitor (Cushman et al, 1998).

Aldosterone Receptor Antagonist. Spironolactone and eplerenone are mineralocorticoid-blocking agents used for their ability to block the epithelial and nonepithelial actions of aldosterone. Spironolactone is a nonselective mineralocorticoid receptor antagonist with moderate affinity for progesterone and androgen receptors. The latter property increases the likelihood of endocrine side effects, including loss of libido, gynecomastia, and impotence. Eplerenone is a next-generation aldosterone receptor antagonist selective for aldosterone receptors alone. It has less affinity for progesterone and androgen receptors (Sica, 2005).

Summary. Treatment of mild to moderate hypertension requires agents with an acceptable side-effect profile to minimize noncompliance. Thiazide diuretics are associated with higher rates of ED, although this may be reduced by combination therapy and weight loss. α_1-Blockers and angiotensin II receptor blockers tend to improve sexual functioning during treatment and may be useful when starting antihypertensive therapy in men with preexisting ED (Khan et al, 2002) (Table 26-11).

Psychotropic Medication. As with hypertension, the underlying disorder may be more relevant for ED than the medication. However, receptor complexity and interrelationship of pathways within the CNS make it extremely likely that neurons and ganglia involved in sexual functioning will be affected by psychotropic drugs, leading to functional changes that may be positive or negative. An example is the loss of sexual desire among nonmedicated patients with schizophrenia, whereas patients on antipsychotic drugs have shown greater desire but increased erectile and ejaculatory disturbance (Aizenberg et al, 1995).

Antipsychotics. Members of this class of drug have many effects on CNS receptors and may act peripherally. The therapeutic effect of antipsychotics is thought to relate to dopaminergic receptor blockade within the limbic and prefrontal areas of the brain. Their

unwanted effects are due to β-adrenergic blockade and anticholinergic properties and to antidopaminergic actions within the basal ganglia, causing extrapyramidal side effects that commonly produce sexual symptoms (Sullivan and Lukoff, 1990).

The occurrence of extrapyramidal effects differentiates older "typical" antipsychotics (frequent extrapyramidal effects) from newer "atypical" antipsychotics (less common extrapyramidal effects). This difference probably relates to differential affinities for particular classes of receptor (Strange, 2001) or avidity for particular areas of the cerebral cortex (Westerink, 2002). An additional effect of dopamine blockade, hyperprolactinemia, which also alters sexual function by reducing dopamine release in permissive cerebral centers, is more common with older "typical" agents (Smith and Talbert, 1986).

Animal experiments, chiefly in rats, show that D1 receptor activation in the MPOA of the hypothalamus facilitates erection through intermediary oxytocinergic and spinal cholinergic pathways. It is also possible that activation of D2 receptors in this area has the opposite effect (Zarrindast et al, 1992). Older agents such as haloperidol and flupenthixol have been shown to reduce apomorphine-induced erections in experimental animals by means of D1 receptor antagonism (Andersson and Wagner, 1995). In addition, systemic administration of antipsychotic agents in rabbits produced erection by a local nondopaminergic action, possibly involving antagonism of α_1 adrenoceptors (Naganuma et al, 1993). **The clinical effect of antipsychotics on sexual function varies according to their affinity for particular receptors.**

In a nonrandomized comparative study of antipsychotic medications, the prevalence of sexual dysfunction ranged from 40% to 70% (Wirshing et al, 2002). Newer agents such as clozapine showed a lower reduction in sexual desire, and the group taking risperidone had the greatest decrease in erectile frequency.

Antidepressants. Sexual side effects of antidepressants in men and women are varied but are important factors governing compliance because these drugs are commonly prescribed to younger and middle-aged adults. In a Cochrane review of 15 randomized trials, besides changing medications, addition of bupropion or a PDE5 inhibitor to an antidepressant seems to be an effective method to correct antidepressant-associated ED (Rudkin et al, 2004).

Tricyclics act by inhibiting the reuptake of catecholamines in the CNS. Their sexual side-effect profile is thought to relate to peripheral anticholinergic and β-adrenergic effects. It is also possible that they antagonize 5-HT receptors. Controlled clinical studies suggest that orgasmic disorders in both sexes are frequent, explaining the use of these drugs as inhibitors of ejaculation (Harrison et al, 1986; Monteiro et al, 1987).

Monoamine oxidase inhibitors are associated with higher rates of orgasmic dysfunction in controlled trials (Harrison et al, 1986), but the nature of the central or peripheral mechanisms involved is uncertain.

Selective serotonin reuptake inhibitors (SSRIs) are the class of drug commonly used to treat depression at the present time. They inhibit the reuptake of 5-HT into CNS neurons and can produce stimulatory effects on various 5-HT receptors. It is estimated that up to 50% of patients taking SSRIs experience a change in sexual function (Rosen et al, 1999; Keltner et al, 2002). Possible mechanisms include stimulation of 5-HT$_2$ and 5-HT$_3$ receptors, which may inhibit erectogenic pathways within the spinal cord (Tang et al, 1998); decreased dopamine release in the MPOA (Maeda et al, 1994); inhibition of NOS; and lower serum levels of luteinizing hormone, follicle-stimulating hormone, and testosterone (Safarinejad, 2008). A controlled clinical study suggested that the improvement in sexual function resulting from alleviation of clinical depression with use of SSRIs outweighed any negative effect (Michelson et al, 2001). However, other placebo-controlled randomized studies revealed increased sexual dysfunction, mainly anorgasmia, in the group treated with SSRIs (Labbate et al, 1998; Croft et al, 1999). Further studies have suggested that these adverse effects can be modified by cotreatment with other drugs such as sildenafil (Fava et al, 2006) or mianserin (Aizenberg et al, 1997).

SSRIs differ in their ability to cause ED. A high incidence has been observed in patients treated with paroxetine (Kennedy et al,

TABLE 26-11 Effect of Antihypertensive Agents on Sexual Function

AGENT	EFFECT	MECHANISM
Diuretics	ED (twice as common as placebo)	Unknown
β-Blocker (nonselective)	ED	Prejunctional α_2-receptor inhibition
β_1-Blocker (selective)	None	
α_1-Blocker	Decreases ED rate but may cause retrograde ejaculation	Failure of sympathetically induced closure of internal sphincter and proximal urethra during ejaculation
α_2-Blocker	ED	Inhibition of central α_2 receptor
Angiotensin-converting enzyme inhibitor	None	
Angiotensin II receptor blocker	Decreases ED rate	
Calcium channel blocker	None	

ED, erectile dysfunction.

2000), whereas a lesser impact has been reported with citalopram (Mendels et al, 1999). This difference suggests that mechanisms other than inhibition of serotonin reuptake may be involved, which is supported by a report that short-term or long-term administration of paroxetine, but not citalopram, caused ED in rats by inhibiting NO production (Angulo et al, 2001b). The inhibitory effects induced by short-term administration of paroxetine on erectile function in the rat can be prevented by inhibition of PDE5 with vardenafil (Angulo et al, 2003a).

Other Antidepressants. Animal experiments suggest that stimulation of 5-HT$_1$ receptors within the CNS modulates sexual function, with the 5-HT$_{1A}$ subtype increasing ejaculation and the 5-HT$_{1C}$ subtype improving erection. Recently developed antidepressants such as mirtazapine and nefazodone tend to have beneficial effects on sexual function, possibly by activating the 5-HT$_{1C}$ receptor, which augments sexual response (Stancampiano et al, 1994), although they may also antagonize the 5-HT$_{2C}$ receptor (Millan et al, 2000). The isolated reports of priapism seen with a prototype agent, trazodone, may be related to the 5-HT$_{1C}$ erectogenic effect seen with its primary metabolite, *m*-chlorophenylpiperazine, in experimental animals (Andersson and Wagner, 1995). In a clinical study, trazodone was shown to increase nocturnal erectile activity, despite reducing REM sleep (Ware et al, 1994).

Anxiolytics. Although not previously associated with ED, anxiolytics have been implicated in sexual problems by the MMAS study (Derby et al, 2001). Benzodiazepines are thought to potentiate the action of GABA in the reticular and limbic system, but they may also affect the serotonin and dopaminergic pathways. Experimental studies suggest that GABAergic drugs inhibit erection induced by apomorphine, a dopamine agonist (Zarrindast and Farahvash, 1994). A controlled clinical study demonstrated that a combination of lithium and benzodiazepine was associated with a significantly higher rate of sexual dysfunction than treatment with lithium alone (Ghadirian et al, 1992). More recent anxiolytic agents, such as bupropion, acting mainly by inhibiting dopamine reuptake, and buspirone, acting on 5-HT$_{1A}$ receptors, were not associated with sexual side effects in placebo-controlled trials (Coleman et al, 2001) and can be used to alleviate sexual symptoms caused by other antidepressant medication (Gitlin et al, 2002).

Anticonvulsants. Epileptic discharges may affect the function of the hypothalamic-pituitary axis and the level of hormones important for sexual function (Morris and Vanderkolk, 2005). Sexual function, bioavailable testosterone levels, and gonadal efficiency in men with epilepsy who take lamotrigine are comparable to control and untreated values and significantly greater than in men treated with carbamazepine or phenytoin (Herzog et al, 2004). Orgasmic dysfunction is common in patients who receive carbamazepine therapy, and loss of sexual desire is common in men treated with valproate (Kuba et al, 2006). There are reports of improved sexual function and hypersexuality in patients treated with lamotrigine (Gil-Nagel et al, 2006; Grabowska-Grzyb et al, 2006).

Antiandrogens

Androgens are believed to modify sexual behavior by modulating androgen receptors within the CNS. **Antiandrogens cause partial or near-complete blockade of androgen's action by inhibiting production of or antagonizing the androgen receptor.** The effects of androgen deficiency on sexual activity are variable, ranging from complete loss to normal function. Experimental studies in humans suggest that nocturnal erections during REM sleep are androgen dependent, whereas erections in response to visual sexual stimulation are independent (Andersson and Wagner, 1995). An additional peripheral effect has been suggested from animal experiments in which castration decreased NOS activity within the rat corpus cavernosum, leading to reduced erectile activity. Testosterone restored NOS activity, but treatment with finasteride prevented this recovery, suggesting that DHT may be the important androgen in penile tissue (Lugg et al, 1995).

The **5α-reductase inhibitors, finasteride and dutasteride, are the antiandrogens with the least effect on circulating** testosterone. In randomized placebo-controlled studies of patients given finasteride (5 mg daily) for prostatic symptoms, approximately **5% complained of decreased desire and ED compared with 1% in the placebo group** (Gormley et al, 1992). At the lower dose used to treat male-pattern alopecia (1 mg daily), no sexual dysfunction was seen (Tosti et al, 2001). However, persistent sexual dysfunction for months to years after discontinuation of finasteride for hair loss (Propecia; 1 mg) has been reported. The side effects include low libido, ED, decreased arousal, and difficulty with orgasm (Irwig and Kolukula, 2011).

More complete androgen ablation is achieved by competitive antagonism at the androgen receptor, preventing signal transduction of testosterone and DHT. Nonsteroidal drugs such as flutamide and bicalutamide have relatively pure effects on the androgen receptor. The steroidal antiandrogen cyproterone acetate also has inhibitory effects on the hypothalamus. These drugs are used in the palliative treatment of locally advanced and metastatic prostate cancer, either alone or in combination with a luteinizing hormone–releasing hormone (LHRH) agonist or antagonist. When used alone, nonsteroidal antiandrogens are associated with an increase in serum testosterone levels. When nonsteroidal antiandrogen is combined with an LHRH agonist or antagonist, the combination reduces testosterone to the castrate range. The main side effect is a reduction of sexual desire, which occurs in up to 70% (Iversen et al, 2001).

In a clinical trial with larger sample size and longer duration, treatment with bicalutamide alone resulted in a smaller decrease in sexual desire than did castration (Iversen et al, 2000). However, in another large controlled trial, treatment with either flutamide or cyproterone resulted in a gradual loss of sexual desire over 2 to 6 years in approximately 80% (Schroder et al, 2000). In a placebo-controlled study, half of patients receiving bicalutamide therapy experienced loss of erectile function, even at a low dose of 50 mg (Eri and Tveter, 1994).

The near-complete androgen deprivation achieved by medical castration with LHRH antagonist (immediate testosterone suppression) or agonists (with an initial surge of testosterone) results in a profound loss of sexual desire, which is usually accompanied by ED (Basaria et al, 2002). In a small study, nocturnal penile tumescence (NPT) monitoring before and after initiation of therapy provided objective confirmation (Marumo et al, 1999).

Miscellaneous Drugs

Many other drugs are suggested to have sexual side effects, in particular, ED in men, but these contentions are usually based on anecdotal case reports or postmarketing drug alerts rather than controlled trials.

Digoxin. In an experimental in vitro study with isolated human corpus cavernosum tissue, digoxin attenuated the relaxant response to acetylcholine and intrinsic nerve stimulation; this was linked to findings of reduced penile rigidity not seen in men given a placebo after visual sexual stimulation (Gupta et al, 1998). A randomized clinical study confirmed a negative effect on general sexual functioning linked to a decrease in plasma testosterone (Neri et al, 1987). However, other investigators did not find change in sex and adrenal hormone levels in men taking digitalis (Kley et al, 1984).

Statins. Statins are used to reduce lipid levels and are commonly used in men likely to have established risk factors for sexual dysfunction, particularly ED. In a single placebo-controlled trial, the rate of ED was twice as high (12% vs. 6%) in men taking a statin, despite improvement in other parameters of hyperlipidemic endothelial dysfunction (Bruckert et al, 1996). In another study of 93 men attending cardiovascular risk clinics, after 6 months of statin therapy, the mean IIEF scores were reduced from 21 to 6.5 (range 0 to 25; $P < .001$), and 22% experienced new-onset ED. The authors suggest that ED after statin therapy is more likely in patients with severe endothelial dysfunction secondary to established cardiovascular risk factors including age, smoking, and diabetes (Solomon et al, 2006). In contrast, in the large Scandinavian simvastatin survival study, 4444 patients with coronary arterial disease were randomly assigned to treatment with simvastatin or placebo for up to

6 years. ED was found in 28 placebo-treated patients (8 resolved) and in 37 simvastatin-treated patients (14 resolved) (Pedersen and Faergeman, 1999). The **underlying disease process appears to be the cause of ED in men treated with statins rather than the drug itself.**

Regarding sexual side effects, the most studied statin is atorvastatin. In clinical studies, atorvastatin has been reported to have the following positive effects: (1) improvement in nocturnal penile activity and mean scores on the Sexual Health Inventory in Men questionnaire from 14.2 to 20.7 in hyperlipidemic patients treated for 4 months (Saltzman et al, 2004); (2) when combined with the ACE inhibitor quinapril, positive effects on ED in men with established penile disease and suboptimal response to PDE inhibitors (Bank et al, 2006); (3) improvement in the response to sildenafil in men with ED not initially responsive to sildenafil (Herrmann et al, 2006); (4) when combined with sildenafil, improvement in erectile function recovery in men who had undergone bilateral nerve-sparing radical prostatectomy (Hong et al, 2007); and (5) positive effect on IIEF questionnaire scores in patients with hyperlipidemia followed for 12 months (Dogru et al, 2008).

Statins are classified as natural (lovastatin), semisynthetic (simvastatin), and synthetic (atorvastatin, cerivastatin) and are structurally heterogeneous. The statins may have different effects on sexual function, which remain to be elucidated.

Histamine H$_2$ Receptor Antagonists. Cimetidine and ranitidine were widely prescribed for prophylaxis and treatment of peptic ulcer disease. Case reports suggested that cimetidine was associated with ED. A single in vitro animal study suggested that H$_2$ receptor stimulation causes cavernous relaxation, possibly via endothelial release of NO (Andersson and Wagner, 1995).

Opiates. Long-term intrathecal administration of opiates results in hypogonadotropic hypogonadism and associated sexual dysfunction that can be restored with appropriate supplementation (Abs et al, 2000). However, administration of opioid antagonists to older men with ED was not found to improve erectile function measured objectively by NPT monitoring (Billington et al, 1990). Opioids have a generalized depressant effect on sexual function when directly administered to the MPOA in rat brain, but treatment with the opioid receptor antagonist naloxone had no sexual effect on healthy male volunteers (Andersson and Wagner, 1995).

Antiretroviral Agents. Hypogonadism and ED appear to be more common among men infected with human immunodeficiency virus (HIV) compared with age-matched men in the general U.S. population (Crum et al, 2005). **Sexual dysfunction seems to be a common event after the introduction of antiretroviral therapy.** The average prevalence is ED, 46%; decreased libido, 44%; ejaculatory disturbances, 39%; and orgasmic disorders, 27% (Collazos, 2007). These disturbances seemed to be more common in patients treated with protease inhibitors. Because these patients may have diseases involving several organ systems and may be taking multiple drugs, the precise mechanism is difficult to determine.

Tobacco. **Cigarette smoking may induce vasoconstriction and penile venous leakage because of its contractile effect on the cavernous smooth muscle** (Juenemann et al, 1987a). In an NPT study in cigarette smokers, Hirshkowitz and colleagues (1992) reported an inverse correlation between nocturnal erection (rigidity and duration) and the number of cigarettes smoked per day: Men who smoked more than 40 cigarettes had the weakest and shortest nocturnal erections. **The Boston Area Community Health (BACH) survey** used a multistage stratified random sample to recruit 2301 men, 30 to 79 years to, from Boston. The authors' report **indicates a dose-response association between smoking and ED with a statistically significant effect observed with 20 or more pack-years of exposure. Passive smoking is associated with a small, statistically insignificant increase in risk of ED comparable to approximately 10 to 19 pack-years of active smoking** (Kupelian et al, 2007). In an experiment to elucidate the mechanisms of ED associated with tobacco use, nicotine-free and tar-free cigarette smoke extract was injected subcutaneously into adult male rabbits once a day for 5 weeks. The authors reported impaired NO production from blunted NOS activity, downregulation of nNOS protein,

accumulation of endogenous NOS inhibitors, enhanced arginase activity, and upregulation of arginase I protein in cavernous tissue. Cigarette smoke extract also caused accumulation of endogenous NOS inhibitors secondary to impaired dimethylarginine dimethylaminohydrolase activity and decreased expression of dimethylarginine dimethylaminohydrolase I protein. These alterations may be relevant to ED after administration of cigarette smoke extract (Imamura et al, 2007).

Alcohol. Alcohol in **small amounts improves erection and sexual drive because of its vasodilatory effect and suppression of anxiety; however, large amounts can cause central sedation, decreased libido, and transient ED.** In the Western Australia Men's Health Study, Chew and colleagues (2009) reported that compared with never-drinkers, the age-adjusted odds of ED were lower among current, weekend, and binge drinkers and higher among ex-drinkers.

Chronic alcoholism may result in liver dysfunction, decreased testosterone and increased estrogen levels, and alcoholic polyneuropathy, which may also affect penile nerves (Miller and Gold, 1988). In an in vitro study of rabbits given 5% alcohol for 6 weeks, Saito and colleagues (1994) reported augmented smooth muscle contraction and relaxation to both electrical field stimulation and vasoconstrictors such as phenylephrine and potassium chloride, but not to sodium nitroprusside, suggesting changes in neurovascular function. In a study of subacute alcohol effect, mice were exposed to alcohol vapor for 7 or 14 days. The authors reported impaired endothelium-dependent relaxation of cavernous smooth muscle and damage of endothelium in the group of mice exposed for 14 days but not the group exposed for 7 days (Aydinoglu et al, 2008) (Table 26-12).

TABLE 26-12 Drug-Induced Erectile Dysfunction and Suggested Alternatives

CLASS	KNOWN TO CAUSE ERECTILE DYSFUNCTION	SUGGESTED ALTERNATIVES
Antihypertensives	Thiazide diuretics General β blockers	α-Blockers Calcium channel blockers Specific β-blockers Angiotensin-converting enzyme inhibitors Angiotensin II receptor antagonists
Psychotropics	Antipsychotics Antidepressants Anxiolytics	Newer anxiolytics (bupropion, buspirone)
Antiandrogen	Androgen receptor antagonists Luteinizing hormone–releasing hormone agonists 5α-Reductase inhibitors	
Opiates		
Antiretroviral agents		
Tobacco		Quit smoking
Alcohol	Large amount	Small amount

U.S. Community Survey of Prescription Drugs and Erectile Dysfunction. The BACH survey used a multistage stratified design to recruit a random sample of 2301 men 30 to 79 years old. To investigate the association of ED with commonly used medications, including antihypertensive agents, psychoactive agents, and pain and anti-inflammatory medications. ED was assessed using the IIEF-5 questionnaire. Multivariable analyses showed benzodiazepines and tricyclic antidepressants were associated with ED, whereas no association was observed for SSRIs/serotonin-norepinephrine reuptake inhibitors and atypical antipsychotics. The use of antihypertensive treatment, whether in monotherapy or in conjunction with others, and pain or anti-inflammatory medications was not associated with ED after accounting for confounding factors (Kupelian et al, 2013).

Aging, Systemic Disease, and Other Causes

Numerous studies have indicated a progressive decline in sexual function in "healthy" aging men. Masters and Johnson (1977) **noted many changes in older men, including greater latency to erection, less turgidity, loss of forceful ejaculation and decreased volume, and a longer refractory period.** Decreased frequency and duration of nocturnal erection with increasing age were reported in a group of men who had regular intercourse (Schiavi and Schreiner-Engel, 1988). **Other research has also indicated a decrease in penile tactile sensitivity with age** (Rowland et al, 1989). A heightened cavernous muscle tone may also contribute to the decreased erectile response in older men (Christ et al, 1990). In one study, a decrease in testosterone in aging impotent men in association with relatively normal gonadotropins was reported, suggestive of hypothalamic-pituitary dysfunction (Kaiser et al, 1988). **Vascular endothelial dysfunction is regarded as a primary phenotypic expression of normal human aging. This senescence-induced disorder is the likely culprit underlying the increased cardiovascular and metabolic diseases associated with aging.** Aging impairs endothelial function through reduced eNOS expression and action, accelerated NO degradation, increased PDE activity, inhibition of NOS activity by endogenous NOS inhibitors, increased production of reactive oxygen species, inflammatory reactions, decreased endothelial progenitor cell number and function, and impaired telomerase activity or telomere shortening (Toda, 2012).

Penile structural and functional changes have been documented in various animal studies. Costa and Vendeira (2008) reported progressive decline of smooth muscle content and increase in the caliber of vascular spaces in the corpus cavernosum with increasing age in Wistar rats. Suadicani and colleagues (2009) showed a significant decrease in gap junction protein connexin 43 and purinoceptor subtype P2X1R and an increase in purinoceptor subtype P2X7R in the corpus cavernosum of aging Fischer-344 rats. Ferrini and colleagues (2001a, 2001b) reported an increase of inducible NO, peroxynitrite formation, and elevation of apoptotic index in the corpus cavernosum and hypothalamic regions. The increased contractile property of the erectile tissue associated with aging may be due to elevated RhoA/Rho-kinase activity (Jin et al, 2006), enhanced renin-angiotensin system (Park et al, 2005), or impaired angiotensin-(1-7)-mediated relaxation (Yousif et al, 2007).

Diabetes Mellitus. Diabetes mellitus is a common chronic disease, affecting 0.5% to 2% of the worldwide population. The **prevalence of ED is three times higher in diabetic men (28% vs. 9.6%)** (Feldman et al, 1994), **occurs at an earlier age, and increases with disease duration,** being approximately 15% at age 30 and increasing to 55% at 60 years (McCulloch et al, 1980, 1984). ED among men with diabetes **is more frequent in men with coexisting neuropathy.** In a study of men presenting with ED, the authors found a twofold increase of hypogonadism in men with diabetes (24% vs. 12%) (Corona et al, 2006). **The presence of ED is associated with more than 14 times higher risk for silent coronary artery disease, higher major cardiovascular morbidity, and mortality in diabetic men** (Gazzaruso et al, 2004). This evidence indicates **the presence of ED in diabetic patients could predict future major cardiovascular events.** Diabetes mellitus may cause ED by

affecting one or a combination of the following: **psychological well-being, CNS function, androgen secretion, peripheral nerve activity, endothelial cell function, and smooth muscle contractility** (Dunsmuir and Holmes, 1996).

In 12% of diabetic men, deterioration of sexual function can be the first symptom. Duplex ultrasound after intracavernous injection has revealed a high prevalence (>75%) of penile arterial insufficiency among diabetic men with ED (Wang et al, 1993). Pathologic changes in the cavernous arteries (Michal, 1980), ultrastructural changes in the cavernous smooth muscle (Mersdorf et al, 1991), and impaired endothelium-dependent relaxation of the corporeal smooth muscle (Saenz de Tejada et al, 1989a) also have been noted in penile specimens from diabetic men with ED. Hirshkowitz and colleagues (1990) reported that impotent men with diabetes have fewer sleep-related erections, shorter tumescence time, diminished penile rigidity, decreased heart rate response to deep breathing, and lower penile blood pressure than age-matched nondiabetic men. Different severities of endothelial apoptosis between diabetic patients who are "responders" and "nonresponders" to sildenafil have also been reported (Condorelli et al, 2013).

Numerous type 1 and type 2 diabetic animal models have been used to study the basic mechanisms of diabetes-induced ED. In these animals, diabetes causes endothelial cell dysfunction, incompetent cavernous endothelial cell-cell junctions resulting in an increased prevalence of vascular disease (Ryu et al, 2013). Other effects include decreased nNOS, reduced activity of eNOS, oxidative stress, increased advanced glycation end products, decreased elastin, reduced VEGF, hypercontractility of cavernous erectile tissue, and decreased smooth muscle/collagen ratio leading to impairment of the veno-occlusive mechanism. Kilarkaje and associates (2013) reported that angiotensin II signaling is also involved in diabetes-induced structural changes and oxidative DNA damage in the corpus cavernosum of rats and that modulation of the signaling by captopril, losartan, and angiotensin-(1-7) restores the effects of diabetes mellitus. Activated Rho-kinase mediates diabetes-induced elevation of vascular arginase activation, and impaired corpora cavernosa relaxation has also been reported (Toque et al, 2013). Cellek and associates (2013) revisited the concept of "point of no return" in the course of diabetic ED and proposed that research focus on the role of vasa nervorum and advanced glycation end products. Summaries of mechanistic studies in humans and animal models, derived from the committee report of the Second International Consultation of Sexual Medicine (Saenz de Tejada et al, 2005), are shown in Tables 26-13 and 26-14.

Metabolic Syndrome. The metabolic syndrome includes glucose intolerance, insulin resistance, obesity, dyslipidemia, and hypertension. **Higher prevalence of ED (26.7%) in men with metabolic syndrome relative to control subjects (13%) has been reported. The prevalence of ED increases as the number of metabolic syndrome components increases** (Esposito et al, 2005). **In an analysis of the Baltimore Longitudinal Study of Aging, in which men were followed for a mean of 5.8 years, Rodriguez and colleagues (2007) confirmed that the prevalence of metabolic syndrome increases with age and is associated with lower androgen levels. They also found that lower total testosterone levels, along with lower sex hormone–binding globulin levels, predicts a higher incidence of metabolic syndrome. Men with metabolic syndrome have an increased prevalence of ED, reduced endothelial function score, and higher circulating concentrations of C-reactive protein compared with men without metabolic disorders** (Esposito et al, 2005). La Vignera and associates (2012) studied endothelial cell turnover by blood endothelial progenitor cells and endothelial microparticles and reported highest levels in men with both metabolic syndrome and arteriogenic ED, followed by men with metabolic syndrome without ED and then men without metabolic syndrome and ED. In a study of endothelial function in patients with metabolic syndrome and ED, Tomada and associates (2013) reported an imbalance of angiopoietins in patients with metabolic syndrome and ED and suggested that angiopoietins may be early markers of endothelial dysfunction in this population with higher cardiovascular risk. In insulin-resistant obese Zucker rats,

TABLE 26-13 Summary Findings of Studies in Diabetic Patients

FOCUS	FINDING
Anatomic	• More atheromatic lesions in large vessels and stenosis in pudendal and iliac arteries
Functional	• Decreased number and rigidity of nocturnal erections • Lower penile rigidity after intracavernous injection of vasodilators • High prevalence of penile arterial insufficiency studied with duplex ultrasound
CAVERNOUS TISSUE STUDIES	
Ultrastructural	• Decreased smooth muscle content, increased collagen, thickening of basal lamina, and loss of endothelial cells (more severe in men with diabetes)
Functional	• Reduced endothelial and neurogenic NO-mediated penile smooth muscle relaxation but not nitroprusside-induced relaxation (suggesting impaired NO release or synthesis) • Increased advanced glycation end products in cavernous tissue • Contractile response to α-adrenergic agonist is higher in type 1 but not type 2 diabetics • In human penile arteries, EDHF-mediated endothelium-dependent relaxation is significantly reduced in penile resistance arteries from diabetic patients • Exposure to hyperglycemia induces increased expression of collagen, decreased proliferation, and increased programmed cell death (apoptosis). Expression of tumor necrosis factor-α is also increased • Insulin is thought to enhance NOS activity by increasing transport of L-arginine into the cell and furnishing greater quantities of the essential cofactor NADPH. These effects are reversed in insulin deficiency or insulin resistance in diabetes • The inducible form (arginase II) of arginase, an enzyme that competes with NOS for the substrate L-arginine, is overexpressed in corpus cavernosum of diabetic patients, where inhibition of arginase restores NOS activity

EDHF, endothelium-derived hyperpolarizing factor; NADPH, reduced nicotinamide adenine dinucleotide phosphate; NO, nitric oxide; NOS, nitric oxide synthase.

TABLE 26-14 Summary Findings of Studies in Diabetic Animal Models

MODEL	FINDING
Streptozocin-induced diabetic rats or mice	• Increased activity of AC and GC, resulting in production of more cAMP and cGMP in response to PGE_1 and nitroprusside, respectively • Decreased endothelial and neurogenic NO-mediated cavernous muscle relaxation • Increased prostacyclin synthesis • Increased cavernous muscle tone owing to upregulation of ET-A receptors • Increased contractile prostaglandins and free oxygen radicals in hyperglycemic state, resulting in reduced response to acetylcholine (reversed by indomethacin and antioxidants) • Increased levels of oxygen free radicals and oxidative stress injury. Preventive treatment with an antioxidant prevented the appearance of endothelial dysfunction in cavernosal tissue, whereas restorative treatment with same antioxidant only partially reversed the impairment of endothelium-dependent relaxation • Increased glycated hemoglobin, which impairs endothelium-dependent relaxation in aorta and corpus cavernosum from diabetic rats. This effect is reversed by SOD, the scavenger of superoxide anions • Inhibition of AGE formation improves endothelium-dependent relaxation and restores erectile function in diabetic rats • Impaired responses attributable to EDHF in the vasculature of diabetic animals • Plasma concentration and vascular content of L-arginine are reduced in diabetic rats • NO-dependent selective nitrergic nerve degeneration in diabetes
Diabetic rabbit	• Production of cAMP in response to PGE_1 or forskolin is reduced after 6 months, but not 3 months • Increased glucose-induced production of PKC mediated by oxidative stress in rabbit corpus cavernosum smooth muscle cells • Oxidative stress interferes with endothelial function in diabetic erectile tissue. This is supported by the potentiating effect of SOD or the natural antioxidant, vitamin E, on endothelium-dependent relaxation of corpus cavernosum from rabbits

AC, adenylyl cyclase; AGE, advanced glycation end product; cAMP, cyclic adenosine monophosphate; cGMP, cyclic guanosine monophosphate; EDHF, endothelium-derived hyperpolarizing factor; ET-A, endothelin-A; GC, guanylyl cyclase; NO, nitric oxide; PGE_1, prostaglandin E_1; PKC, protein kinase C; SOD, superoxide dismutase.

Sánchez and coworkers (2012) reported uncoupling of nNOS in the dysfunctional nitrergic vasorelaxation of penile arteries (see Fig. 26-13).

Chronic Renal Failure. Sexual dysfunction is common in men with chronic renal failure. In a survey of 69 men on hemodialysis, only 55% were sexually active, and the predominant sexual dysfunctions were loss of or diminished sexual needs (84.7%), ED (44.5%), and inhibited or lack of ejaculation (51.5%) (Lew-Starowicz and Gellert, 2009). Similarly, ED was reported in 52% of men undergoing peritoneal dialysis (Lai et al, 2007). The presence of depressive symptoms, highly prevalent in hemodialysis patients, is an independent factor of sexual dysfunction in male hemodialysis patients (Peng et al, 2007). Significant improvement of sexual function has been reported after kidney transplantation (Tavallaii et al, 2009). Nevertheless, in a report of 182 men who had undergone kidney transplantation, Espinoza and colleagues (2006) noted that 49% of men continued to have ED; 33% of men had normal sexual function, and 18% had no sexual activity. **Many of the effects of uremia can potentially contribute to the development of ED, including disturbance of the hypothalamic–pituitary–testicular axis, hyperprolactinemia, accelerated atheromatous disease, and psychological factors** (Ayub and Fletcher, 2000).

Bagcivan and colleagues (2003) suggest that ED may be due to either **decreased production or reduced bioavailability of endogenous NO.** Evidence from animal models of chronic uremia suggests that a decrease in functional NO may be responsible for vascular side effects including ED.

Evidence of **autonomic neuropathy** as a factor contributing to ED in men with chronic renal failure comes from studies that found a high rate of abnormality in vascular and bulbocavernous reflexes, suggesting nerve dysfunction (Campese et al, 1982; Vita et al, 1999). Neuropathy is a common complication of end-stage kidney disease, typically manifesting as a distal symmetrical process with insidious onset progressing over months. Neuropathy has been estimated to occur in 60% to 100% of patients on dialysis. Nerves of uremic patients have been shown to exist in a chronically depolarized state before initiation of dialysis, with subsequent improvement and normalization of resting membrane potential after initiation of dialysis. The degree of depolarization correlates with serum K^+, suggesting that chronic hyperkalemic depolarization plays an important role in the development of nerve dysfunction in end-stage kidney disease (Krishnan and Kiernan, 2007). Investigation of cavernous vascular function in 20 men undergoing renal replacement therapy showed that 80% had both arterial insufficiency and veno-occlusive dysfunction (Kaufman et al, 1994). A link between impairment of the NO-cGMP pathway relating to failure of cavernous relaxation is provided by the finding of increased serum levels of ADMA in uremic patients (Kielstein and Zoccali, 2005).

Patients with severe pulmonary disease often fear aggravating dyspnea during sexual intercourse. Patients with angina, heart failure, or myocardial infarction can become impotent from anxiety, depression, or arterial insufficiency. HIV infection itself is the strongest predictor of ED, and many factors related to the infection—fear of virus transmission, changes in body image, HIV-related comorbidities, infection stigma, obligatory condom use—impair erectile function (Santi et al, 2014). In two large European studies, Corona et al (2012) reported that overt hyperthyroidism was associated with an increased risk of severe ED. Conversely, no association between primary hypothyroidism and ED was observed. Other systemic diseases, such as cirrhosis of the liver, scleroderma, chronic debilitation, and cachexia, are also known to cause ED.

Primary Erectile Dysfunction

Primary ED refers to a **lifelong inability to initiate and/or maintain erections beginning with the first sexual encounter. Although most cases are due to psychological factors, a few afflicted men have a physical cause resulting from maldevelopment of the penis or the blood and nerve supply. Primary psychological dysfunction is usually related to anxiety about sexual performance** stemming from adverse childhood events, traumatic early sexual experience, or misinformation. Endocrine abnormalities, particularly low testosterone levels, may also be implicated in primary ED, although decreased sex drive is likely to be the main symptom. Evidence to support these concepts is confined to observation studies with varying numbers of cases. The largest study described 67 patients, of whom 10 (15%) had a predominantly psychological cause (Stief et al, 1989b). Patients with physical abnormalities had a variety of neurologic, arterial, and veno-occlusive dysfunction.

Micropenis. Symmetrical hypoplasia of the phallus, micropenis, is often related to urethral developmental abnormalities such as hypospadias and epispadias (Reilly and Woodhouse, 1989) or endocrine deficiency. The erectile tissue in such cases often functions normally; sexual dysfunction usually relates to lack of penile length or the degree of chordee, rather than to ED (Woodhouse, 1998).

Vascular Abnormalities. Primary ED in the presence of an externally normal phallus is unusual. Authors have described structural abnormalities of the cavernous tissue, such as absence (Teloken et al, 1993) or replacement by fibrous tissue (Aboseif et al, 1992). Other authors have found vascular abnormalities, including hypoplasia of the cavernous arteries (Montague et al, 1995) or veno-occlusive dysfunction owing to aberrant cavernous venous drainage (Lue, 1999). The underlying cause of these congenital abnormalities is unknown. Treatment in most cases has been vascular surgery or implantation of a penile prosthesis.

KEY POINTS: OTHER CAUSES OF ERECTILE DYSFUNCTION

- Aging is the most important contributing factor to ED. The aging process can affect the central regulatory mechanism, hormonal and neural function, and penile structure.
- Diabetes mellitus and metabolic syndrome may affect multiple organ systems and cause premature aging of central and peripheral structures and molecules that regulate erectile process.
- The diseases that cause chronic renal failure may also cause ED, and the condition may persist despite successful renal transplantation.
- Primary ED may be due to psychogenic cause, inexperience, congenital arterial insufficiency, or abnormal venous channels.

KEY POINTS: PATHOPHYSIOLOGY

- The prevalence of ED increases with age and concomitant medical diseases. The incidence is about 25 to 30 cases per 1000 person-years.
- ED is a symptom of many underlying conditions and diseases.
- Any condition that affects penile nerve, artery, endothelium, smooth muscle, or tunica albuginea can cause ED.
- Endothelial dysfunction seems to be a common final pathway to ED in patients with hyperlipidemia, diabetes mellitus, hypertension, and chronic renal failure.
- Drugs most commonly associated with ED include antiandrogens, antidepressants, and antihypertensives.

PERSPECTIVES

The past two decades have seen a continuing explosion of new information on the physiology of penile erection and the pathophysiology of ED. These new discoveries not only enhance our understanding of the disease process but also provide a solid basis for improving diagnosis and treatment. We can expect that the application of new research tools and information in molecular biology, signal transduction, growth factors, microarrays, and stem cells will bring the investigation of erectile function and ED to an even higher level in the near future.

REFERENCES

The complete reference list is available online at www.expertconsult.com.

SUGGESTED READINGS

Andersson KE. Mechanisms of penile erection and basis for pharmacological treatment of erectile dysfunction. Pharmacol Rev 2011;63:811–59.

Feldman HA, Goldstein I, Hatzichristou DG, et al. Impotence and its medical and psychosocial correlates: results of the Massachusetts Male Aging Study. J Urol 1994;151:54–61.

Gandaglia G, Briganti A, Jackson G, et al. A systematic review of the association between erectile dysfunction and cardiovascular disease. Eur Urol 2014;65:968–78.

Gratzke C, Angulo J, Chitaley K, et al. Anatomy, physiology, and pathophysiology of erectile dysfunction. J Sex Med 2010;7(1 Pt 2):445–75.

Lue TF. Erectile dysfunction. N Engl J Med 2000;342:1802–13.

Montorsi F, Adaikan G, Becher E, et al. Summary of the recommendations on sexual dysfunctions in men. J Sex Med 2010;7:3572–88.

Nehra A, Jackson G, Miner M, et al. The Princeton III Consensus recommendations for the management of erectile dysfunction and cardiovascular disease. Mayo Clin Proc 2012;87:766–78.

27 Evaluation and Management of Erectile Dysfunction

Arthur L. Burnett II, MD, MBA, FACS

HISTORICAL PERSPECTIVE

Erectile dysfunction (ED) management has evolved into a mature clinical discipline in the past few decades, owing to steady, considerable progress made in the basic science, epidemiology, clinical investigation, and health services research within this dynamic field. The field has advanced from its well-notioned beginnings of psychoanalysis and sex therapy, accompanied by the use of aphrodisiacs, herbal supplements, and hormonal treatments, typifying the knowledge and approach to clinical practice in the 1970s, to an increasingly structured, balanced, and evidence-based process of clinical evaluation and intervention of the contemporary era (Table 27-1).

Well-grounded ED management principles, premised on the highest clinical standards of ethics, quality, safety, and cost-effectiveness, are now well accepted by the scientific and clinical community in sexual medicine. These "guidelines" have derived from rigorous and timely review, organization, and reassessments of the constantly evolving body of knowledge in this field performed by assorted consensus bodies representing the spectrum of international and interdisciplinary authorities in sexual medicine. Most notably, the International Consultations on Sexual Medicine (ICSM), cosponsored variously by the World Health Organization, International Consultation on Urological Diseases, American Urological Association, Société Internationale D'Urologie, and the International Society for Sexual Medicine, have served this role and have published topical proceedings (Jardin et al, 2000; Lue et al, 2004; Montorsi et al, 2010).

PUBLIC HEALTH SIGNIFICANCE

ED is a medical condition of major health significance, with implications that extend beyond treating the occasionally presenting patient who possesses a problem of seemingly non–life-threatening magnitude. **The value of properly assessing and managing ED relates not only to affected individuals and their partners but also to society as a whole, and its scope encompasses physical and mental wellness aspects related to addressing (or failing to address) the sexual dysfunction, concurrent disease management issues, as well as its socioeconomic burden.**

Epidemiology

Epidemiologic investigation, which specifies that study results are readily generalized to the overall male population, has provided powerful information regarding the nature, etiology, and prognostic ramifications of ED. **As the most thoroughly studied sexual dysfunction in the context of epidemiologic research, ED is estimated to carry an overall adult male (older than 20 years of age) prevalence rate of 10% to 20% worldwide, with the majority of studies reporting a rate closer to 20%** (Derogatis and Burnett, 2008; Lewis et al, 2010). It is acknowledged that an age correlation exists for the prevalence of ED, with a worldwide prevalence of 1% to 10% for men younger than the age of 40 years, as high as 15% for men age 40 to 49 years, as high as 30% for men age 50 to 59 years, as high as 40% for men 60 to 69 years, and 50% to 100% for men in their 70s and 80s (Lewis et al, 2010). It was estimated that there were more than 152 million men worldwide who experienced ED in 1995, with a projection of the prevalence reaching approximately 322 million men having ED by 2025 (Aytac et al, 1999). This trend is maintained irrespective of racial/ethnic background or geographic region.

Current data have also confirmed that the prevalence of ED mounts with the presence of comorbid medical conditions, which include type 2 diabetes mellitus, obesity, cardiovascular disease, hypertension, dyslipidemia, depression, and prostate disease/benign prostatic hyperplasia (Braun et al, 2000; Martin-Morales et al, 2001; Nicolosi et al, 2004; Rosen et al, 2004c; Saigal et al, 2006; Laumann et al, 2007; Selvin et al, 2007). This correlation has supported the premise that ED and comorbid medical conditions share pathophysiologic mechanisms, such as endothelial dysfunction, arterial occlusion, and systemic inflammation (Solomon et al, 2003; Montorsi et al, 2004; Billups, 2005; Ganz, 2005; Kloner, 2005; Guay, 2007).

Novel disease-risk relationships for ED have been described, likely also exhibiting such concomitant pathophysiologic mechanistic associations as endothelial dysfunction and systemic inflammation. These disease relationships include epilepsy (Keller et al, 2012b), sensorineural hearing loss (Keller et al, 2012a), open-angle glaucoma (Chung et al, 2012a), urinary calculi (Chung et al, 2011), psoriasis (Chung et al, 2012b), atopic dermatitis (Chung et al, 2012d), chronic periodontitis (Keller et al, 2012d), viral hepatitis (Chung et al, 2012c), varicocele (Keller et al, 2012c), and gastric ulcers (Keller et al, 2012e).

Although they are few in number, prospectively conducted longitudinal studies have documented the true incidence and disease-risk relationships for ED. In one study, a crude ED incidence rate was 25.9 cases/1000 man-years among men aged 40 to 69 years (Johannes et al, 2000). According to another study, incident ED statistics were 57% at 5 years and 65% at 7 years in men 55 years or older (Thompson et al, 2005). **Such studies have uniquely affirmed predictors for the development of ED, which include age, lower education, diabetes, cardiovascular disease, hypertension, cigarette smoking, cigar smoking, passive exposure to cigarette smoke, and overweight condition** (Feldman et al, 2000; Johannes et al, 2000; Inman et al, 2009).

643

TABLE 27-1 Evolution in the Management of Erectile Dysfunction

	DIAGNOSTICS	TREATMENTS	GUIDES
Pre-1970	Psychosexual history	Psychosexual therapy Herbal supplements	Studies of Masters and Johnson
1970s	Medical and psychosexual history Nocturnal penile tumescence testing	Penile prosthesis surgery Penile revascularization	International Conferences on Corpus Cavernosum Revascularization
1980s	Physical examination Endocrine evaluation Penile duplex ultrasonography, DICC	Oral medications Intracavernous pharmacotherapy Vacuum device therapy	Goal-directed management
1990s	Combined intracavernous injection and stimulation	Intraurethral pharmacotherapy Oral phosphodiesterase type 5 therapy	NIH Consensus Statement Process of Care Model
2000-Present	Biomarkers of vascular health neuroimaging	? Gene therapy ? Stemcell therapy ? Tissue engineering	ICUD algorithms (patient-centered approach) AUA Practice Guidelines (evidence-based approach)

AUA, American Urological Association; DICC, dynamic infusion cavernosometry and cavernosography; ICUD, International Consultation on Urological Diseases; NIH, National Institutes of Health.

However, the strength of the risk association is also gauged from the opposite analytic direction, and incident ED may indeed inform the risk of subsequent disease morbidity and mortality. This relationship has been best demonstrated so far with respect to cardiovascular disease. The placebo arm of the Prostate Cancer Prevention Trial found that ED is a sentinel for future risk of cardiovascular events, comparable to that of current cigarette smoking or a family history of myocardial infarction (Thompson et al, 2005). This study established that men with ED were 45% more likely than men without ED to experience a cardiac event after 5 years of follow-up (Thompson et al, 2005). In another population-based study of community-dwelling men followed longitudinally, ED was associated with an approximately 80% higher risk of subsequent coronary artery disease at 10 years (Inman et al, 2009). In a long-term follow-up (15 years) of the Massachusetts Male Aging Study (Feldman et al, 1994), ED was found to be positively associated with subsequent all-cause and cardiovascular disease mortality and constituted a risk in this regard similar to that of conventional risk factors, such as increased body mass index, diabetes, and hypertension (Araujo et al, 2009). It is an increasingly recognized and striking observation, made in epidemiologic studies demonstrating the risk association of ED with cardiovascular events, that the development of ED at a younger age heightens this particular risk (Chew et al, 2010; Miner et al, 2012; Vlachopoulos et al, 2013).

Recent meta-analyses of longitudinal studies have supported the findings of earlier reports and have provided relative risk estimates. A meta-analysis of seven prospective cohort studies provided adjusted relative risks for ED subjects compared with healthy subjects, calculating 1.47-fold increased cardiovascular disease events overall and 1.23-fold increased all-cause mortality (Guo et al, 2010). Another meta-analysis of 12 cohort studies calculated overall combined relative risk for men with ED compared with the reference group to be 1.48 with cardiovascular disease, 1.46 for coronary heart disease, 1.35 for stroke, and 1.19 for all-cause mortality (Dong et al, 2011). A further meta-analysis comprising 14 studies documented relative risk of 1.44 for cardiovascular mortality, 1.19 for myocardial infarction, 1.62 for cerebrovascular events, and 1.25 for all-cause mortality for men with ED versus those without ED (Vlachopoulos et al, 2013).

Besides a predictive relationship of cardiovascular disease based on incident ED, a similar relationship has been suggested with respect to carcinogenesis risk. The "Longitudinal Health Insurance Database" study in Taiwan showed that cancer risk was 1.42-fold higher in ED patients than in patients without ED during a 5-year follow-up, after adjusting for socioeconomic and comorbid health variables (Chung et al, 2011).

These compelling data regarding occurrence rates and risk factors for ED contribute greatly toward an understanding of the importance of this medical condition. **The subject of ED offers a veritable clinical barometer of overall male health status, and efforts geared toward advancing its management are immediately consequential for disease prevention, health promotion, and survival improvement.**

Health Policy

Sexual dysfunctions and ED specifically have taken on increasing importance with respect to their socioeconomic impact. **In addition to its medical comorbidity associations, ED is recognized to affect adversely quality of life, to decrease occupational productivity, and to increase the use of health care resources** (Krane et al, 1989; Litwin et al, 1998). Because of the heightened ease of use and availability of effective first-line treatments combined with a growing societal awareness of ED and an acceptance of its treatment, it is understandable that a trend toward increased use of health care services surrounding ED has been observed (Wessells et al, 2007; Polinski and Kesselheim, 2011).

ED can be included among a host of urologic diseases having a substantial burden on the public financially. Total expenditures for outpatient clinical management of ED (exclusive of pharmaceutical costs) in the United States in the year 2000 approximated $330 million, ranking it the ninth most costly among the most frequent urologic diagnoses (Litwin et al, 2005). By contrast, this cost was approximately $185 million in 1994 (Wessells et al, 2007). Individual-level expenditures on an annual basis associated with an ED diagnosis (inclusive of pharmaceutical costs) among affected 18- to 64-year-old males in the United States in 2002 were calculated to be $1107 (Wessells et al, 2007). The Congressional Budget Office estimate of government expense for ED drugs in 2005 was $2 billion for the subsequent 10 years (Polinski and Kesselheim, 2011). These data have enormous implications for governmental as well as nongovernmental agencies in the United States and worldwide, whose work must consider the practical distribution and fiscal allocation of health care services for ED. Some experts have accordingly urged an account of the medical necessity and cost of ED therapy when formulating grounds for insurance coverage (Polinski and Kesselheim, 2011). However, evidence points to rational coverage for ED therapy, and in fact a significantly lower use of this therapy has been shown as compared to ED prevalence (Hornbrook and Holup, 2011). Arguments support the fact that ED is not a frivolous indication for clinical intervention, having quality-of-life and well-being implications as well as importance with respect to health and life preservation.

MANAGEMENT PRINCIPLES

The approach to the evaluation and treatment of ED is most assuredly different from that of many other urologic diseases in several basic respects. The diagnosis of ED customarily involves an acknowledgment of the subjective complaint of erectile inability by the patient (or patient and partner), and extensive diagnostic procedures are generally not required to proffer the diagnosis. Additionally, current first-line intervention in the form of effective oral pharmacotherapy is easily prescribed and administered and is frequently successful for the majority of patients. **However, notwithstanding the semblance that the management of ED is fairly uncomplicated, it is a structured process that critically incorporates several clinical practice concepts for bringing the best therapeutic outcomes to patients.**

Early Detection

Epidemiologic and clinical investigation has suggested that many patients with ED retain adverse clinical conditions and also lifestyle factors (e.g., diabetes, cardiovascular disease, prostate disease, overweight condition, current cigarette smoking, and physical inactivity) that potentially compromise erectile function (Saigal et al, 2006; Laumann et al, 2007; Selvin et al, 2007; Lewis et al, 2010). The extent of these risk factors comprises an increased global cardiometabolic risk profile in patients with ED (Miner et al, 2012; Nehra et al, 2012). Calculated odds ratios underscore the extent to which various ED risk factors correlate with ED (Table 27-2). **These data support the contention that patients with identifiable ED risk factors likely experience the sexual dysfunction currently or will eventually develop it at some time. Clinical screening of such patients based on these indications is advantageous in allowing opportunities to diagnose and treat ED.**

Growing evidence has also suggested that a patient's genotype influences the risk of developing ED, consistent with proposals that both molecular and genetic mechanisms account for the ED phenotype (Andersen et al, 2011; Lippi et al, 2012). This concept fits with the perspective that genetically determined biomarkers will eventually be defined to assess ED risk profile as well as level of responsiveness to a specific ED therapy in the advancing era of precision medicine.

Medication use has also been associated with ED in up to 25% of presentations (Keene and Davies, 1999; Francis et al, 2007). The most commonly implicated classes of drug include antihypertensive drugs, such as thiazide diuretics and β-adrenoceptor antagonists, and psychotherapeutic drugs, particularly selective serotonin reuptake inhibitor (SSRI) antidepressants. Table 27-3 lists several drug classes commonly associated with ED. It is important to recognize that medications may affect other components of the male sexual response cycle including sexual desire, arousal, and orgasm, which secondarily hampers erectile function. Of additional importance, the assignment of causation of ED for any particular medication is conditional, requiring that an increased prevalence exists in the

TABLE 27-2 Major Erectile Dysfunction Risk Factors

CONDITION	MULTIVARIATE ADJUSTED ODDS RATIO
Diabetes mellitus	2.9
Hypertension	1.6
Cardiovascular disease	1.1
Hypercholesterolemia	1.0
Benign prostate enlargement	1.6
Obstructive urinary symptoms	2.2
Increased body mass index (>30 kg/m^2)	1.5
Physical inactivity	1.5
Current cigarette smoking	1.6
Antidepressant use	9.1
Antihypertensive use	4.0

From Francis ME, Kusek JW, Nyberg LM, Eggers PW. The contribution of common medical conditions and drug exposures to erectile dysfunction in adult males. J Urol 2007;178:591–6; and Selvin E, Burnett AL, Platz EA. Prevalence and risk factors for erectile dysfunction in the US. Am J Med 2007;120:151–57.

TABLE 27-3 Drugs Associated with Erectile Dysfunction

CLASS	SPECIFIC AGENTS
Antihypertensives	Thiazide diuretics, nonselective β-blockers
Antidepressants	Tricyclics; selective serotonin reuptake inhibitors
Antipsychotics	Phenothiazines
Antiandrogens	Nonsteroidal (flutamide); steroidal (cyproterone acetate); luteinizing hormone-releasing hormone analogues
Antiulcer drugs	Histamine H$_2$ receptor antagonists (cimetidine)
Cytotoxic agents	Cyclophosphamide, methotrexate
Opiates	Morphine

target population compared with the placebo group after stratification for known risk factors or compared to another drug with an equivalent therapeutic effect, and, further, a credible physiologic mechanism should be established experimentally (Sáenz de Tejada et al, 2005).

Goal-Directed Management

A goal-directed approach to the management of patients with ED has largely been practiced in the field throughout the decades since Lue's original description (Lue, 1990). The approach dictates that the diagnostic evaluation and therapeutic plan relates to the individual patient's presentation and manner of deriving satisfaction, in accordance with a patient-centered framework (Hatzichristou et al, 2010). **The basic aim of goal-directed management is to allow the patient or couple to make an informed selection of the preferred therapy for sexual fulfillment based on a sound understanding of all treatment options after completing a thorough discussion with the treating clinician. The approach recognizes that patients vary in their acceptance of their sexual disorders and in their interest in pursuing management. Their decisions accordingly follow individual preferences, needs, and expectations regarding management options.** Evaluations of this approach have affirmed its utility and demonstrated that patient therapeutic preferences accord with the least invasive forms of therapy (Jarow et al, 1996; Hanash, 1997).

Role of Partner Interview

The partner interview is a critical component in initiating management of ED. Partner interviews have been shown to impact diagnosis and treatment in as much as 58% of cases (Tiefer and Schuetz-Mueller, 1995; Chun and Carson, 2001). **The partner may be the source of important information that guides optimal intervention and response to therapy. The partner may share a new and different perspective on sexual issues affecting the couple, might provide insight into the quality of the couple's relationship, and might relate his/her role in the sexual dysfunction** (Speckens et al, 1995; Fisher et al, 2009). **The partner's involvement and attitude may also impact the patient's initiation of and adherence to therapy** (Jackson and Lue, 1998; Fisher et al, 2005).

An important additional consideration is that partners' well-being may be affected by the patients' ED conditions. Studies have shown that women partners of men with ED are themselves more likely to have sexual dysfunction or to cease sexual activity entirely (Ichikawa et al, 2004; Montorsi and Althof, 2004; Fisher et al, 2005; Sand and Fisher, 2007). This observation further prompts the facilitatory role of the partner in ED management, which maximizes the success of therapy and inherently the satisfaction of the couple.

In practice, and as necessary, additional office visits, during which the partner accompanies the patient and the patient communicates educational information to the partner, are recommended techniques for involving partners in ED management (Dean et al, 2008).

Cardiac Risk Assessment

The frequent coexistence of ED and cardiovascular disease, as established by clinical epidemiologic study and by basic science research, has steered ED management to include procedures that account for the ED patient's cardiovascular health risks. The Princeton Consensus Conferences, a multidisciplinary forum convened successively on three occasions since the early 2000s, have emphasized the link between sexual activity and cardiac risk and have pronounced that all men with ED, even in the absence of manifesting cardiac symptoms, should be regarded as having potential risks for cardiovascular disease (DeBusk et al, 2000; Kostis et al, 2005; Jackson et al, 2006b; Nehra et al, 2012).

According to the Princeton Consensus expert panel guidelines, ED patients are recommended to undergo a full medical assessment with stratification of cardiovascular risk as high, medium, or low (Fig. 27-1). **Patients classified as having a high risk would be those with unstable or refractory angina, a recent history of myocardial infarction, certain arrhythmias, or uncontrolled hypertension. For these patients, sexual activity with any particular ED therapy should be deferred until the cardiac condition is stabilized. Such patients should ideally undergo cardiologic referral for cardiovascular stress testing and subsequent risk-reduction therapy. Importantly, even patients at low risk for cardiovascular events should receive the minimum recommendations of cardiovascular disease management.** Basic intervention includes counseling for lifestyle modifications such as increased physical activity and improved weight control combined with regular health monitoring by the patient's general practitioner (Kostis et al, 2005). A more comprehensive approach specifies cardiovascular risk reduction and affirmation of exercise tolerance for sexual activity following noninvasive cardiovascular risk assessment that may involve a specialist or collaborative medical team having such expertise (Nehra et al, 2012).

Step-Care Approach

Practitioners of ED management have always sought a rational approach for implementing diagnostic and therapeutic options. The "Process of Care Model for Erectile Dysfunction" was proposed as a stepwise methodology, combining processes, actions,

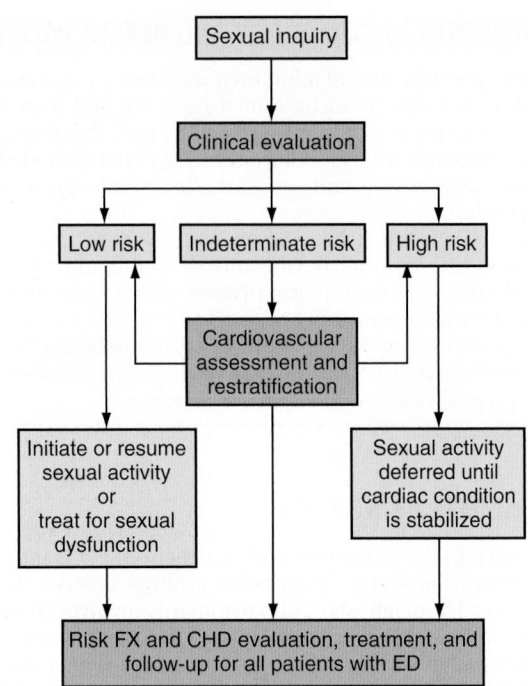

Figure 27-1. Algorithm for evaluation of the patient with cardiovascular disease recommended by the Second Princeton Panel. CHD, coronary heart disease; ED, erectile dysfunction; FX, factors.

and outcomes in the management of the ED patient (Process of Care Consensus Panel, 1999). It specified an algorithm for therapeutic decision making that takes into account patient needs and preferences (goal-directed management), although it was also based on specific criteria such as ease of administration, reversibility, relative invasiveness, and cost of therapies. This algorithm presented a strategy of staged therapy (i.e., first-, second-, and third-line interventions), which ranged from lifestyle modification to surgery. **In concept, the scheme has been borrowed and endorsed by other consensus panels that acknowledged the purpose of patient education and counseling along with medical therapies as initial forms of ED management in common practice** (Montague et al, 2005; Hatzichristou et al, 2010).

Shared Decision Making and Treatment Planning

The therapeutic plan may vary for every patient and couple and it ultimately depends on a host of factors including patient considerations as well as clinical indications and contraindications. **An informed decision-making process should dictate the best therapeutic option. It follows a balanced and thorough discussion led by the clinician of all treatment options, both medical and nonmedical, and their expected advantages and disadvantages. Perceived risks and benefits, which may be influenced by the individual clinical situation, should be weighed.** It is understood that the patient may appropriately select a preferred treatment option without necessarily adhering to a strictly prescribed succession of attempted therapies. Indeed, the patient may elect to defer treatment altogether. Whatever the patient (or couple) chooses, this option can then be pursued within the boundaries of safety, under the supportive partnership of his clinician.

Specialist Referral

The advent of effective oral pharmacotherapy for ED has enabled many primary practitioners to feel comfortable with managing the majority of clinical presentations of ED. At the same time, it is understood that situations arise in which the patient or primary practitioner may request the assistance of a consultant/specialist (e.g., cardiologist, endocrinologist, psychologist, or urologist) for further diagnostic evaluation and treatment beyond the boundaries of initial management (Process of Care Consensus Panel, 1999). Such referrals may be required for individuals with complicated or atypical presentations of ED, representing diagnostic challenges that exceed common clinical practices of nonspecialists. Specialized evaluation and management potentially offer improved therapeutic outcomes for these presentations.

Generally recommended indications for specialized evaluations and associated consultants are: failure of initial treatment, referred to a urologist; younger patients with a history of pelvic or perineal trauma, referred to a urologist; patients with significant penile deformity (e.g., Peyronie disease, congenital chordee), referred to a urologist; complicated endocrinopathies (e.g., secondary hypogonadism, pituitary adenoma), referred to an endocrinologist; complicated psychiatric or psychosexual disorders (e.g., refractory depression, hypoactive sexual desire), referred to a psychiatrist; presentations requiring vascular or neurosurgical intervention (e.g., aortic aneurysm, lumbosacral disk disease), referred to a vascular surgeon or neurosurgeon, respectively; medicolegal reasons (e.g., workman's compensation claims), referred to a urologist.

A caveat is that effort should be made at the time of referral to ensure that patients are fully informed about the rationale, costs, potential risks, and potential outcomes of the referral and possible additional procedures. This recommendation is made in accordance with the principles of patient-centered medicine, by which patients (and partners where possible) should be included in the decision-making process.

Follow-up Care

Follow-up care is an essential part of ED management and should not be overlooked. The objectives of this action are manifold. **A primary basis is to ensure continual success with the therapeutic outcome. It has been shown that treatment discontinuation occurs at high rates among patients who are not reassessed regularly** (Albaugh et al, 2002). Additional purposes are to reassess medical and psychosocial conditions adversely impacting ED and success of therapy, evaluate the need for dosage titration or treatment substitution, and monitor adverse drug interactions or drug-interaction effects. As always, follow-up attention offers educational opportunities for patient and partner with regard to addressing sexual health concerns as well as lending guidance for related health care matters.

DIAGNOSTIC EVALUATION

The cornerstone in the evaluation of ED involves a detailed case history, preferably taken from patient and partner, physical examination, and proper laboratory tests (Fig. 27-2). The diagnosis can be submitted based on an individual's report of consistent inability to attain and maintain an erection of the penis sufficient to permit satisfactory sexual intercourse (NIH Consensus Statement, 1992; Lewis et al, 2004). It is noteworthy that the original National Institutes of Health definition did not specify a parameter for the duration of symptoms to accept the diagnosis. Subsequent organizational statements did apply a 3-month interval as a minimal requirement diagnostically, except for cases of trauma or surgically induced ED (Lewis et al, 2004).

Sexual, Medical, and Psychosocial History

The comprehensive assessment of any sexual problem begins with the performance of a detailed case history including sexual, medical, and psychosocial components. The clinician may use brief checklists or questionnaires for the purpose of recognizing the problem and initiating its evaluation, although he/she should routinely perform a detailed interview to understand the nature of the sexual complaint. The sexual history component in particular should be elicited with utmost sensitivity, given the intrapersonal and interpersonal aspects of sexual dysfunction (Rosen et al, 2004d; Althof et al, 2013). Additional emphasis has been directed toward providing cultural competence when interacting with patients (Hatzichristou et al, 2010). **All discussion of sexual matters is done privately and confidentially, and the clinician is required to express trust and concern as well as a nonjudgmental manner that epitomizes the doctor-patient relationship.** The clinician should not assume that every patient is involved in a monogamous, heterosexual relationship. However, the situation may be presented whereby the partner can be interviewed, and this opportunity may be used, with the approval of the patient, to corroborate aspects of the clinical history and to confirm mutual therapeutic goals.

Sexual History

The sexual history is the central component of the clinical history and serves to confirm the patient's sexual dysfunction complaint of ED. **Objectives of the interview are also to delineate the problem according to such features as its onset, duration, conditions, severity, and etiology. The conditions of the problem are often**

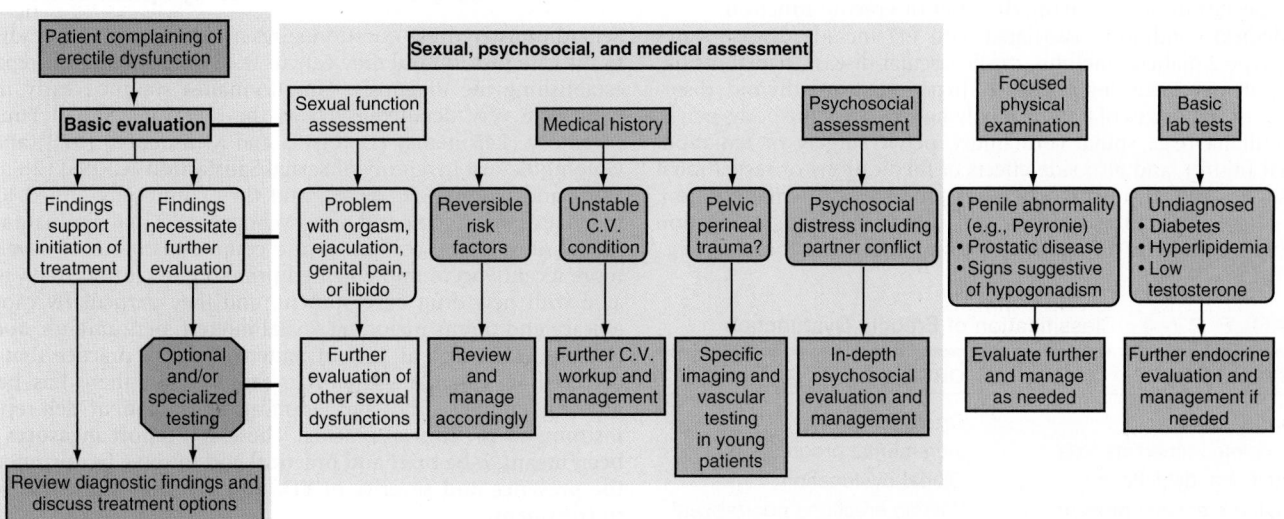

Figure 27-2. Diagnostic algorithm for erectile dysfunction (ED) recommended by the International Consultations on Sexual Medicine. C.V., cardiovascular.

determined by reviewing circumstances that facilitate or hinder erectile function. Circumstances for achievable erections include stimuli used during sexual encounters, erections on awakening, and the role of self-stimulation. Circumstances associated with erectile difficulty include performance anxiety, inability to perform with a designated partner, and motivational factors affecting lovemaking. Other pertinent issues include availability, interest and health of the partner, changes in medical status or other events relating to the onset of ED, and previous attempts to manage the problem by the patient or another caregiver.

The severity of ED can be defined as mild, moderate, or severe/complete, according to increasing degrees of loss of penile rigidity and the associated interference with sexual activity. For instance, mild ED may refer to a minimally decreased ability to attain and/or maintain an erection with intermittent satisfactory sexual performance, moderate ED may refer to a minimally decreased ability to attain and/or maintain an erection with infrequent satisfactory sexual performance, and severe ED may refer to a substantially decreased ability to attain and/or maintain an erection with rare or absent satisfactory performance.

The potential etiology of ED is commonly probed and may be categorized as psychogenic, organic, or mixed according to whether there is a presumed psychological or interpersonal determinant (psychogenic), a specific endocrinologic, neurologic, or cardiovascular cause (organic), or the coexistence of psychological or relationship factors and organic causes (mixed) (Table 27-4) (Ralph and McNicholas, 2000; Hatzichristou et al, 2010). It is accepted that many times ED cannot be fully dichotomized into psychogenic and organic categories. However, its characterization by a predominant etiologic basis may nonetheless facilitate therapeutic objectives. The interview should also assess whether ED is the primary source of the presenting complaint or secondary to some other aspect of the sexual response cycle (e.g., desire, ejaculation, orgasm) that may also relate to the clinical presentation (Rosen, 2004a). The association of decreased arousal, if present, may be explored as well and evaluated to determine whether it preceded or was incidental to the development of ED.

Medical History

The medical history primarily serves to identify and evaluate predictors and risk factors associated with ED. **The main objective is to explore the role of possibly related or underlying medical conditions and to ascertain the existence of comorbidities. Recognition of the association between medical conditions and ED not only may lend insight into the possible basis for the ED, which may guide the choice of therapy, but it may also specify reversible or treatable factors associated with ED that may be corrected with an expectation of improving the level of erectile function.**

Medical conditions associated with ED include disease states (e.g., type 2 diabetes mellitus, cardiovascular disease, hypertension, dyslipidemia, neurologic disease, hypogonadism, thyroid disorders), consequences of trauma involving aspects of the body, pelvis, or genitalia (e.g., spinal cord injury, pelvic surgery or radiation, sexual injury), and also side effects of medications or recreational substances that disturb biochemical processes of penile erection. Age is recorded, in accordance with the well-known association between aging and ED. It is important that comorbidities (e.g.,

depression, anxiety, anger) are registered because of their bidirectional relationship with ED.

Psychosocial History

The intake of psychosocial history is a necessary part of the clinical history. **The very best sexual performance most assuredly implies wellness of mind and body acting together, and unstable psychosocial circumstances of both intrapersonal and interpersonal contexts may adversely affect sexual function.** Accordingly, the presence and interaction of mental health problems, emotional stressors, and interpersonal relationship difficulties, both past and present, should be ascertained. Additional questions may be asked relating to occupational status, financial security, family life, and social support, which may also influence sexual function.

Physical Examination

The physical examination is a highly recommended component of the comprehensive assessment of sexual dysfunctions and complements the clinical case history (Ghanem et al, 2013). It may show possible etiologies for ED.

This evaluation consists of basic anthropometrics (i.e., height, weight, waist circumference), assessment of body habitus (appearance of secondary sexual characteristics), and examination of relevant body parts pertaining to cardiovascular, neurologic, and genital systems, with a particular focus on the external genitalia. The observation of a classically distinctive body habitus consistent with Kallman or Klinefelter syndrome or obvious physical signs of hypogonadism, such as gynecomastia and general poor masculine development, may suggest an endocrinologic basis for ED.

Findings of obesity, elevated blood pressure, or abnormal femoral or pedal pulses, all signs representative of cardiovascular disease, convey a potential vascular causation. Findings of abnormal genital and perineal sensation or bulbocavernosus reflex (squeezing of the glans penis resulting in contraction of the bulbocavernosus muscle detected by a finger in the anus) may indicate the presence of a peripheral neuropathy in association with a neurologic disorder or diabetes.

Detection of a penile deformity, such as micropenis, congenital chordee, or Peyronie disease-related fibrous plaques in the corpora cavernosa, supports the possibility that a physical impediment accounts for ED. Genital examination findings of abnormal position, size, and consistency of testes may also suggest hypogonadism and would indicate that ED exists on endocrinologic grounds.

Questionnaires and Sexual Function Symptom Scores

Self-administered ED questionnaires are extremely useful adjuncts to the case history, and they concur with the patient's self-report in establishing the diagnosis. Questionnaires supplied early in the field were very detailed, such as the Derogatis Sexual Function Inventory (245 items) (Derogatis and Melisaratos, 1979) and the Golombok Rust Inventory of Sexual Satisfaction (GRISS) (28 items) (Rust and Golombok, 1986), and they commonly aimed to differentiate psychogenic and nonpsychogenic ED or to evaluate sexual functioning in the context of the couple. Instruments developed more recently were implemented primarily in clinical trials associated with new drug development, and they particularly captured efficacy end points including sexual interest, performance, and satisfaction. However, as part of pattern shifts of practice that have occurred in ED management in recent years, there has been a growing emphasis on and application of patient self-reported instruments for clinical practice. **These self-report measures have been meant to be brief and practical and to serve in documenting the presence and severity of ED, and the responsiveness of ED to treatment.**

The most widely referenced instruments include the International Index of Erectile Function (IIEF) by Rosen and associates (1997), the Brief Male Sexual Function Inventory (BMSFI) by

TABLE 27-4 Classification of Erectile Dysfunction

PSYCHOGENIC	ORGANIC
Sudden onset	Gradual onset
Complete immediate loss	Incremental progression
Situational dysfunction	Global dysfunction
Waking erections present	Waking erections poor/absent

Modified from Ralph D, McNicholas T. UK management guidelines for erectile dysfunction. BMJ 2000;321:499–503.

O'Leary and colleagues (1995), the Center for Marital and Sexual Health Sexual Functioning Questionnaire by Glick and associates (1997), the Changes in Sexual Functioning Questionnaire by Clayton and associates (1997), and the Erectile Dysfunction Inventory of Treatment Satisfaction (EDITS) by Althof and colleagues (1999). The IIEF, which contains 15 items that address and quantify five domains: erectile function, orgasmic function, sexual desire, intercourse satisfaction, and overall satisfaction, is the most widely used questionnaire (Fig. 27-3). An abridged 5-item version of this instrument, the IIEF-5, has been useful to clinicians in routine clinical practice specifically for the evaluation of ED (Rosen et al, 1999a). The instrument classifies ED severity into five categories: severe

---

Patient Name: _____ MR#: _____ Date: _____

OVER THE PAST 4 WEEKS

1. How often were you able to get an erection during sexual activity?
   0 = No sexual activity
   1 = Almost never/never
   2 = A few times (much less than half the time)
   3 = Sometimes (about half the time)
   4 = Most times (much more than half the time)
   5 = Almost always/always

2. When you had erections with sexual stimulation, how often were your erections hard enough for penetration?
   0 = No sexual activity
   1 = Almost never/never
   2 = A few times (much less than half the time)
   3 = Sometimes (about half the time)
   4 = Most times (much more than half the time)
   5 = Almost always/always

3. When you attempted sexual intercourse, how often were you able to penetrate (enter)?
   0 = Did not attempt intercourse
   1 = Almost never/never
   2 = A few times (much less than half the time)
   3 = Sometimes (about half the time)
   4 = Most times (much more than half the time)
   5 = Almost always/always

4. During sexual intercourse, how often were you able to maintain your erection after you had penetrated (entered) your partner?
   0 = Did not attempt intercourse
   1 = Almost never/never
   2 = A few times (much less than half the time)
   3 = Sometimes (about half the time)
   4 = Most times (much more than half the time)
   5 = Almost always/always

5. During sexual intercourse, how difficult was it to maintain your erection to complete intercourse?
   0 = Did not attempt intercourse
   1 = Extremely difficult
   2 = Very difficult
   3 = Difficult
   4 = Slightly difficult
   5 = Not difficult

6. How many times have you attempted sexual intercourse?
   0 = No attempts
   1 = One to two attempts
   2 = Three to four attempts
   3 = Five to six attempts
   4 = Seven to ten attempts
   5 = Eleven or more attempts

7. When you attempted sexual intercourse, how often was it satisfactory to you?
   0 = Did not attempt intercourse
   1 = Almost never/never
   2 = A few times (much less than half the time)
   3 = Sometimes (about half the time)
   4 = Most times (much more than half the time)
   5 = Almost always/always

8. How much have you enjoyed sexual intercourse?
   0 = No intercourse
   1 = No enjoyment
   2 = Not very enjoyable
   3 = Fairly enjoyable
   4 = Highly enjoyable
   5 = Very highly enjoyable

9. When you had sexual stimulation or intercourse, how often did you ejaculate?
   0 = No sexual stimulation/intercourse
   1 = Almost never/never
   2 = A few times (much less than half the time)
   3 = Sometimes (about half the time)
   4 = Most times (much more than half the time)
   5 = Almost always/always

10. When you had sexual stimulation or intercourse, how often did you have the feeling of orgasm or climax?
    0 = No sexual stimulation/intercourse
    1 = Almost never/never
    2 = A few times (much less than half the time)
    3 = Sometimes (about half the time)
    4 = Most times (much more than half the time)
    5 = Almost always/always

11. How often have you felt sexual desire?
    1 = Almost never/never
    2 = A few times (much less than half the time)
    3 = Sometimes (about half the time)
    4 = Most times (much more than half the time)
    5 = Almost always/always

12. How would you rate your level of sexual desire?
    1 = Very low/none at all
    2 = Low
    3 = Moderate
    4 = High
    5 = Very high

13. How satisfied have you been with your overall sex life?
    1 = Very dissatisfied
    2 = Moderately dissatisfied
    3 = About equally satisfied and dissatisfied
    4 = Moderately satisfied
    5 = Very satisfied

14. How satisfied have you been with your sexual relationship with your partner?
    1 = Very dissatisfied
    2 = Moderately dissatisfied
    3 = About equally satisfied and dissatisfied
    4 = Moderately satisfied
    5 = Very satisfied

15. How do you rate your confidence that you could get and keep an erection?
    1 = Very low
    2 = Low
    3 = Moderate
    4 = High
    5 = Very high

Figure 27-3. International Index of Erectile Function Questionnaire.

(5 to 7), moderate (8 to 11), mild to moderate (12 to 16), mild (17 to 21), and no ED (22 to 25). The Male Sexual Health Questionnaire offers another instrument that assesses core components of male sexual function (i.e., desire, erection, ejaculation, satisfaction) and is useful in both clinical and research settings (Rosen et al, 2004b). The Sexual Experience Questionnaire is a brief but comprehensive tool for evaluating health-related quality-of-life concepts, and it comprises erection, individual satisfaction, and couple satisfaction domains (Mulhall et al, 2008).

A known limitation of self-administered questionnaires is that they do not distinguish an etiologic basis for ED, that is, they do not differentiate among the various causes of ED (Blander et al, 1999; Kassouf and Carrier, 2003). **Further, they may not sufficiently indicate the severity of ED that is evidenced on objective grounds** (Tokatli et al, 2006). Although the exact nature of the ED diagnosis arguably is not absolutely necessary to initiate ED treatment today with current management options, it is understood that further clinical evaluation with diagnostic tests may be required to discern the basis and extent of the ED by system (e.g., vascular, neurologic, endocrinologic) and take action that may be most effective and possibly corrective.

Cardiovascular Risk Assessment Tools

A trend in ED assessment is the application of cardiovascular disease-risk prediction models, which are used as scoring instruments to aid in the assessment of any man evaluated for ED (Nehra et al, 2013). **Such models as the Framingham Risk Score or an alternate global risk score, which incorporate such cardiovascular predictive variables as family history of coronary heart disease, body mass index, and metabolic laboratory biomarkers, offer a powerful initial step to characterize and possibly mitigate cardiovascular risk in this clinical setting.**

Laboratory Tests

Appropriate laboratory testing can be considered part of a systematic clinical evaluation for individuals presenting with ED (Ghanem et al, 2013). **Such evaluation may confirm or define etiologic medical conditions associated with the sexual dysfunction. At times, it may identify treatable conditions or previously undetected disease states that may contribute to ED.** A standardized panel of tests can be offered for the man presenting routinely with sexual dysfunction including ED. Further laboratory testing can be tailored to the clinical situation. Similarly, specialized endocrinologic assessment can be performed when indicated for select clinical presentations.

Recommended laboratory tests for men with sexual problems typically include serum chemistries, fasting glucose, complete blood count, lipid profile, and serum total testosterone. Total testosterone, measured from a morning-time blood draw, serves to screen androgenic status, and, if abnormally low, serum-free (or bioavailable) testosterone and luteinizing hormone (LH) should be measured. Prolactin measurement may also be done for hormonal assessment. Thyroid function tests may be performed at the clinician's discretion. Serum prostate-specific antigen (PSA) testing is performed as needed if there is a suspicion of prostate pathology that might be promoted by exogenously administered testosterone. Dipstick analysis of urine may show glucosuria, which suggests the diagnosis of diabetes.

SPECIALIZED EVALUATION AND TESTING

The implicit goal of specialized evaluations in medicine in general is to improve diagnostic accuracy and direct successful therapy based on the specific diagnosis. A similar principle applies to sexual medicine. However, at the present time, despite the availability of various technologies that may specify and define the causation for ED (i.e., vasculogenic, neurogenic, endocrinogenic, psychogenic), the treatment plan for this sexual dysfunction can often be formulated without performing extensive diagnostic testing. **Nonetheless,**

such testing is frequently applied for diagnostic precision, typically by specialists, particularly in settings of complex clinical presentations. Table 27-5 summarizes the most frequently used evidence-based test procedures for diagnostic evaluations of ED (Rosen et al, 2004d).

Vascular Evaluation

The vascular evaluation for ED conceptually connotes surveying the vascular requirements of the sexual organ for the erectile response: arterial blood inflow, blood engorgement, and blood retention within the corporeal structures. **From a diagnostic standpoint, the**

TABLE 27-5 Evidence-Based Tests for Organic Erectile Dysfunction and Recommendations

TEST	RECOMMENDATION*
VASCULAR	
Dynamic infusion cavernosometry and cavernosography (DICC)	B
Intracavernous injection pharmacotesting (ICI)	B
ICI and color duplex ultrasound	B
Arteriography	C
Computed tomography angiography	D
Magnetic resonance imaging (MRI)	D
Infrared spectrophotometry	D
Radioisotope penography	D
AUDIOVISUAL SEXUAL STIMULATION (AVSS)	
Independent or jointly with vascular testing	C
With or without: pharmacologic stimulation (oral, ICI)	C
NEUROPHYSIOLOGIC	
Nocturnal penile tumescence and rigidity (NPTR)	B
Erectiometer/rigidometer	D
Biothesiometry (vibratory thresholds)	C
Dorsal nerve conduction velocity	C
Bulbocavernosus reflex latency	B
Plethysmography/electrobioimpedance	D
Corpus cavernosum electromyography (CC-EMG)	C
MRI or positron emission tomography scanning of brain (during AVSS)	D

*Grades of recommendation:

A: At least one meta-analysis, systematic review, or randomized controlled trial with a low level of bias and directly applicable to the target population.

B: A body of evidence including high-quality systematic reviews of case-control or cohort studies directly applicable to the target population and demonstrating overall consistency of results.

C: A body of evidence including well-conducted case-control or cohort studies with a low risk of confounding, bias, or chance and a moderate probability that the relationship is causal, directly applicable to the target population, with overall consistency of results.

D: Nonanalytic studies (e.g., case reports, case series, expert opinion).
Modified from Harbour R, Miller J. A new system for grading recommendations in evidence-based guidelines. BMJ 2001;323:334–6; and Rosen RC, Hatzichristou D, Broderick G, et al. Clinical evaluation and symptom scales: sexual dysfunction assessment in men. In: Lue TF, Basson R, Rosen F, et al, editors. Sexual medicine: sexual dysfunctions in men and women. Paris: Health Publications; 2004. p. 173–220.

studies aim to assist in deriving the classic diagnoses of arterial impairment and veno-occlusive dysfunction. As for all diagnostic testing, hemodynamic tests of the penis require patient counseling regarding the purpose, alternatives, risks, and benefits of any procedure before its implementation.

Combined Intracavernosal Injection and Stimulation

The combined intracavernosal injection and stimulation (CIS) test serves as a first-line evaluation of penile blood flow because of its very basic manner of administration and assessment. **The test involves the intracavernosal injection of a vasodilatory drug or drugs as a direct pharmacologic stimulus, combined with genital or audiovisual sexual stimulation, and the erectile response is observed and rated by an independent assessor** (Donatucci and Lue, 1992; Katlowitz et al, 1993). **The test is designed to bypass neurologic and hormonal influences involved in the erectile response and allows the clinician to evaluate the vascular status of the penis directly and objectively.**

The clinician may decide the protocol for using vasodilator drugs. Alternative regimens include alprostadil alone (Caverject or Edex, 10 to 20 µg), a combination of papaverine and phentolamine (Bimix, 0.3 mL), or a mixture of all three of these agents (Trimix, 0.3 mL). The procedure requires a syringe with a ⅝-inch needle (27 to 29 gauge), which is inserted at the lateral base of the penis directly into the corpus cavernosum for medication delivery. After needle withdrawal, manual compression is applied to the injection site for 5 minutes to prevent local hematoma formation. The assessment is done periodically subsequently with rating of both rigidity and duration of response. Repeated dosing may be performed if the initial erectile response is poor. Return to penile flaccidity is required before allowing the patient to leave the office, and if detumescence does not occur spontaneously in approximately an hour after dosing, intracavernosal injection of a diluted phenylephrine solution (500 µg/mL) can be administered every 3 to 5 minutes until flaccidity returns.

A normal CIS test, based on the assessment of a sustainably rigid erection, is understood to signify normal erectile hemodynamics. Alternative diagnoses of psychogenic, neurogenic, or endocrinogenic ED may then be considered. However, it is known that false-positive results might occur in as many as 20% of patients with borderline arterial inflow (as defined by the measurement of 25 to 35 cm/s peak cavernous artery systolic flow on duplex ultrasonography) (Pescatori et al, 1994). False-negative results are also possible and occur most commonly because of patient anxiety, needle phobia, or inadequate dosage.

Duplex Ultrasonography (Gray Scale or Color-Coded)

Duplex ultrasound of the penis following pharmacostimulation or CIS represents second-line evaluation of penile blood flow. However, it is the most reliable and least invasive diagnostic modality for assessing ED. The test adds an imaging dimension and a quantification component to the evaluation of blood flow in the penis distinct from first-line evaluation, which relies on the assessor's judgment alone.

The technique consists of high-resolution (7.5 to 12 MHz) real-time ultrasonography and color-pulsed Doppler, which serves to visualize the dorsal and cavernous arteries selectively and to perform hemodynamic blood-flow analysis (Lue et al, 1989; Sikka et al, 2013). Scanning is applied to the surface of the penis and may include the entire penis from the crura in the perineum to the tip. Color-coded duplex ultrasonography indicates the direction of blood flow within vessels, with red designating direction toward the probe and blue designating direction away from the probe (Broderick and Arger, 1993; Herbener et al, 1994). Flow velocities are measured at baseline before injection and commonly every 5 minutes afterward up to 20 minutes. Cavernous arterial diameters may also be measured. Vascular anatomic communications between the paired cavernous arteries or between the dorsal and cavernous arteries should be noted (Fig. 27-4). Erection quality should also

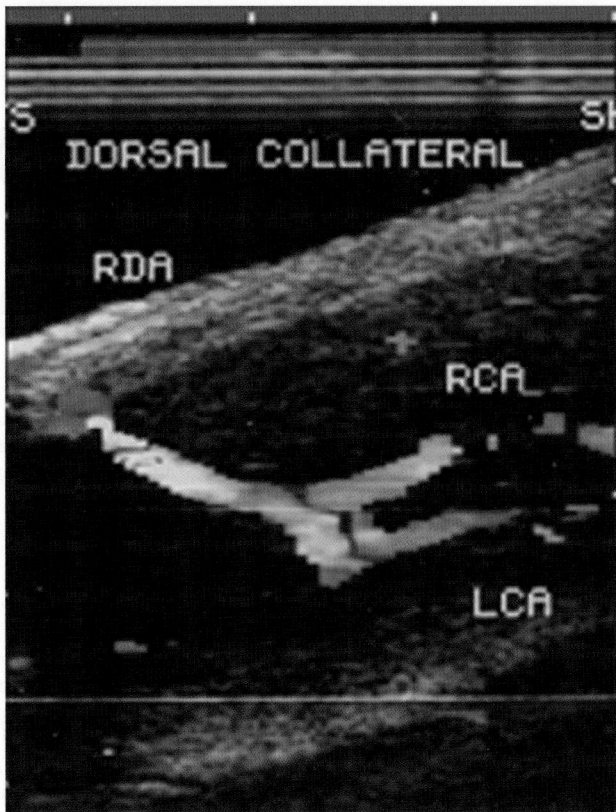

Figure 27-4. Collateral circulation connecting the right dorsal artery (RDA) to the right cavernous artery (RCA), and the left cavernous artery (LCA) is shown by color duplex ultrasonography in a longitudinal view.

be simultaneously assessed and rated. An observed poor erection, possibly associated with patient anxiety, should prompt vasodilator redosing as recommended for the CIS test.

A standard pattern of Doppler waveforms occurs with hemodynamic changes in corporeal pressure during progression to normal full erection (Fig. 27-5) (Schwartz et al, 1991). In the filling phase when sinusoidal resistance is low (within 5 minutes after vasodilator injection), the waveform increases in size consistent with high forward flow during both systole and diastole. As intracavernous pressure increases, diastolic velocities decrease. With full erection, the systolic waveforms sharply peak and may be slightly less than during full tumescence. At maximal rigidity, when intracavernous pressure exceeds systemic diastolic blood pressure, diastolic flow may be zero. The sonographic color pattern of the cavernous artery may demonstrate an impressive shift from red to blue in association with the reversal of diastolic flow.

Normative values have been described for peak systolic velocity (PSV) and diameter of the cavernous arteries during increases in arterial inflow to the penis. Early studies documented that the PSV of the cavernous arteries consistently exceeded 25 cm/s within 5 minutes of vasodilator injection in patients with nonarteriogenic causes of ED (i.e., psychogenic, neurogenic) (Lue et al, 1985; Mueller and Lue, 1988). Investigators subsequently confirmed mean PSV of cavernous arteries after pharmacostimulation to range from 35 cm/s to 47 cm/s in normal subjects (Benson and Vickers, 1989; Shabsigh et al, 1990). A cut point at 25 cm/s included a sensitivity of 100% and a specificity of 95% in patients with abnormal pudendal arteriography (Quam et al, 1989). Diameter changes of the cavernous artery after vasodilator injection were found to increase less than 75% and rarely to exceed 0.7 mm in patients with severe vascular ED (Lue and Tanagho, 1987; Mueller and Lue, 1988). Importantly, unlike PSV changes, a percentage of cavernous arterial vasodilation was not found to correlate well with findings on pudendal arteriography (Jarow et al, 1993).

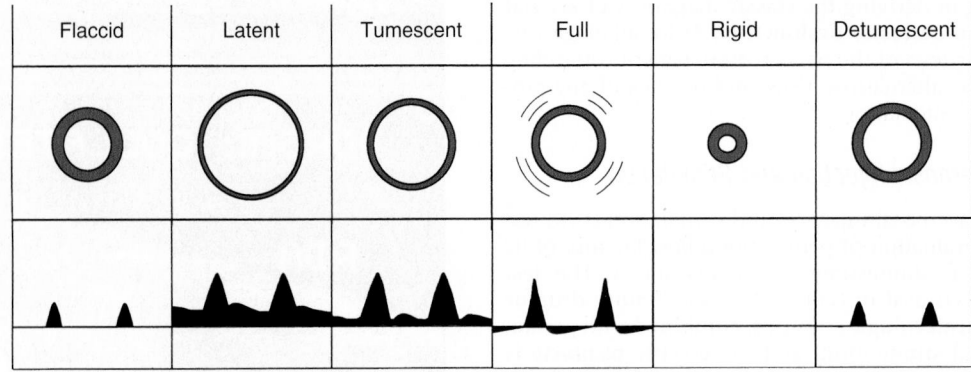

Flaccid	Latent	Tumescent	Full	Rigid	Detumescent

Figure 27-5. Artist's conception of the changes in diameter and flow waveform in the cavernous arteries induced by intracavernous injection of prostaglandin E_1 in a potent young man as demonstrated by duplex ultrasound. Forceful concentric pulsations are particularly noticeable during full erection.

Vascular arterial anatomic variants may confound the interpretation of duplex ultrasonography (Breza et al, 1989; Jarow et al, 1993). Early cavernous arterial branching or the presence of multiple such branches may affect blood-flow velocity determinations of the main cavernous artery. The presence of distal arterial perforators extending from the dorsal or spongiosal arteries also may alter the measurement of cavernous arterial blood-flow velocity. Accordingly, the clinician must recognize these variants to avoid making the incorrect diagnosis of arteriogenic ED. On the other hand, asymmetrical blood flow of the cavernous arteries may have diagnostic significance. The findings of dissimilar cavernous artery velocity measurements, which are greater than 10 cm/s between sides, or reversal of flow across a collateral may suggest a significant atherosclerotic lesion (Benson et al, 1993).

Duplex ultrasound measurements are informative for diagnosing vasculogenic ED (Rosen et al, 2004d). **Cavernous arterial insufficiency is suggested when PSV is less than 25 cm/s; a PSV consistently greater than 35 cm/s defines normal cavernous arterial inflow.** Cavernous artery acceleration time (i.e., PSV divided by systolic rise time) greater than 122 ms may also indicate this diagnosis. Cavernous veno-occlusive dysfunction, which refers to failure of erection maintenance despite adequate cavernous arterial inflow, is suggested by assorted sonographic parameters. Generally meaningful at 15 to 20 minutes after stimulatory onset, these parameters include persistent high systolic flow velocities (i.e., PSV >25 cm/s) and high end-diastolic flow velocities (EDV >5 cm/s), accompanied by rapid detumescence, following stimulatory onset. In addition, vascular resistive index (RI), based on the formula written as RI equals PSV minus EDV, which is then divided by PSV, has had tremendous diagnostic usefulness in this regard. The parameter is based on the concept that, as penile intracavernous pressure during erection achievement equals or exceeds diastolic pressure, diastolic flow in the corporeal bodies will approach zero and the value for RI will approach one. **An RI greater than 0.9 has been associated with normal penile vascular function, and that less than 0.75 is consistent with veno-occlusive dysfunction** (Naroda et al, 1996).

Several technical modifications of sonographic evaluation of the penis have been described. A portable Midus-pulsed Doppler unit connected to a laptop computer for in-office testing reliably records the Doppler waveform of the cavernous arteries despite the lack of a real-time ultrasound image (Metro and Broderick, 1999). Power Doppler offers an even more specialized technique to visualize distal ramifications of the main cavernous artery down to the level of arterioles (Sarteschi et al, 1998; Golubinski and Sikorski, 2002). A somewhat more invasive approach that evaluates the integrity of cavernosal arterial flow involves the measurement of the cavernous artery systolic occlusion pressure (CASOP) by a Doppler transducer during saline intracavernosal infusion (Rhee et al, 1995). As a variation on the stimulatory component of penile sonographic testing, a combination of an oral phosphodiesterase type 5 (PDE5) inhibitor in association with visual erotic stimulation has proven an effective, noninvasive method (Baçar et al, 2001; Speel et al, 2001). Sonographically measured postocclusive vasodilation of the cavernous arteries, which is believed to relate to the level of intact endothelial function in the penis, has been found diagnostic for organic ED (Virag et al, 2004). Cavernous artery intima-media thickness as demonstrated by high-resolution echo color Doppler ultrasound has been suggested as being more accurate than PSV in predicting vasculogenic ED (Caretta et al, 2009).

Dynamic Infusion Cavernosometry and Cavernosography

Cavernosometry and cavernosography, precisely referring to functional hemodynamic and radiographic assessments of the corpora cavernosa, represents third-line evaluation of the vascular integrity of the penis. **The testing is indicated for select patients who are suspected of having a site-specific vasculogenic leak resulting from perineal or pelvic trauma or who have had lifelong ED (primary ED). When used, it generally precedes consideration for corrective penile vascular surgery.**

The technique involves two needles inserted into the penis for simultaneous saline infusion and intracavernous pressure monitoring following intracavernosal pharmacologic injection (Glina and Ghanem, 2013). The testing requires complete trabecular smooth muscle relaxation to avoid erroneous results, and repeated and maximal pharmacologic dosing protocols are recommended (Hatzichristou et al, 1995). Measurements of maintenance flow rate, pressure drop, and CASOP are performed to verify complete smooth muscle relaxation (Fig. 27-6).

Dynamic infusion cavernosometry and cavernosography evaluates the penile venous outflow system. **The existence of veno-occlusive dysfunction is indicated by the failure to increase intracavernous pressure to the level of the mean systolic blood pressure with saline infusion or the demonstration of a rapid drop of intracavernous pressure after cessation of saline infusion** (Puyau and Lewis, 1983; Rudnick et al, 1991; Shabsigh et al, 1991; Motiwala, 1993). The flow rate required to maintain erection at an intracavernous pressure of more than 100 mm Hg is normally less than 3 to 5 mL/min, and the pressure decrease in 30 seconds from 150 mm Hg is normally less than 45 mm Hg. **Cavernosography follows cavernosometric evaluation and is intended to show the site of venous leakage** (Fig. 27-7). With normal veno-occlusive function, there should be opacification of the corpora cavernosa with minimal or no visualization of venous structures or corpus spongiosum. With impaired veno-occlusive function, leakage may be identified into such sites as the glans, corpus spongiosum, superficial dorsal veins, and cavernous and crural veins. More than one site is visualized in the majority of patients (Lue et al, 1986; Rajfer et al, 1988; Shabsigh et al, 1991).

Penile Angiography

Penile angiography essentially refers to an anatomic study of the arterial vasculature of the penis and also represents third-line evaluation of the penile vascular system. **It is commonly reserved for**

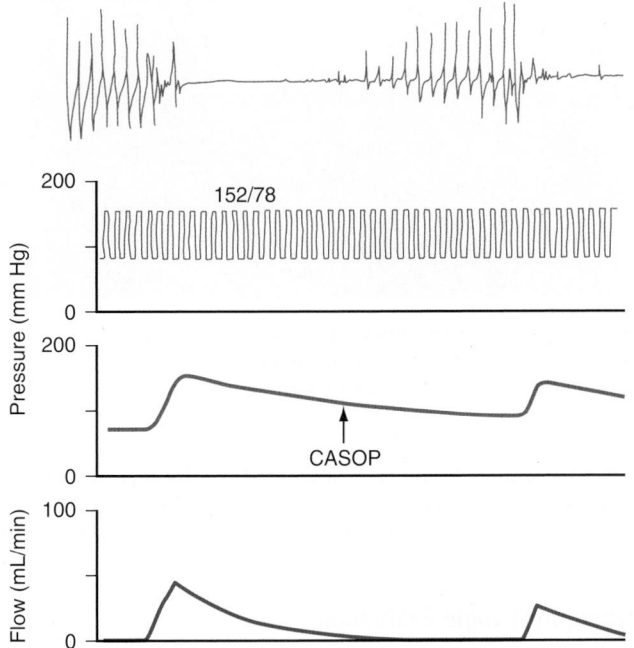

Figure 27-6. This tracing depicts four simultaneous variables obtained during the third phase of dynamic infusion cavernosometry and cavernosography. *Top to bottom:* Cavernosal artery flow recorded by using a continuous-wave Doppler ultrasound probe; systemic brachial systolic and diastolic arterial blood pressure (150/87 mm Hg); intracavernosal pressure, which varied from 70 to 160 mm Hg in this tracing; and intracavernosal heparinized saline inflow. The intracavernosal pressure at which the cavernosal artery pulsations returned, which is the effective cavernosal artery systolic occlusion pressure (CASOP), was 108 mm Hg. The gradient between the brachial and the cavernosal artery systolic occlusion pressures was 150 to 108, or 42 mm Hg, which is abnormal.

the young patient with ED secondary to a traumatic arterial disruption or the patient with a history of penile compression injury, who is being considered for penile revascularization surgery (Sikka et al, 2013).

The procedure involves selective cannulation of the internal pudendal artery and injection of radiographic contrast. The intracavernosal injection of a vasodilating agent is optimally used to induce maximal vasodilation of the penile arterial supply. The anatomy and radiographic appearance of the iliac, internal pudendal, and penile arteries are then evaluated and documented (Fig. 27-8). The inferior epigastric arteries are frequently studied as well to determine their suitability for use in surgical revascularization. It should be recognized that significant variation of the intrapenile arterial anatomy exists, challenging the angiographer to differentiate congenital variations from acquired abnormalities and to establish their clinicopathologic relevance (Bähren et al, 1988; Benson et al, 1993).

Historical and Investigational Studies of Penile Blood Flow

Penile Brachial Pressure Index

The penile brachial pressure index (PBI) test refers to the penile systolic blood pressure divided by the brachial systolic blood pressure. The technique involves applying a small pediatric blood pressure cuff to the base of the flaccid penis and measuring the systolic blood pressure with a continuous-wave Doppler probe. A PBI of 0.7 or less has been used to indicate arteriogenic ED (Metz and Bengtsson, 1981). **The technique has not been found valid because it does not assess the hemodynamic properties of a functionally relevant, induced erection, and thus it is not recommended for use** (Aitchison et al, 1990; Mueller et al, 1990).

Penile Plethysmography (Penile Pulse Volume Recording)

This test evaluates arterial pressure waveforms in the penis with an aggregate of the contributions of all penile vessels (Kedia, 1983). It requires the application of a 2.5- or 3-cm cuff connected to an air plethysmograph applied to the base of the penis, inflating the cuff to a pressure greater than brachial systolic pressure, and then decreasing the pressure by 10-mm Hg increments while recording pressure waveform tracings. Abnormal pressure waveforms by diagnostic criteria have been used to indicate vasculogenic ED (Doyle and Yu, 1986). **Because this study is performed in the flaccid penis, as is the PBI, its clinical relevance has been questioned.** Despite this concern, a technical modification that measures postischemic flow-mediated dilation was introduced as being

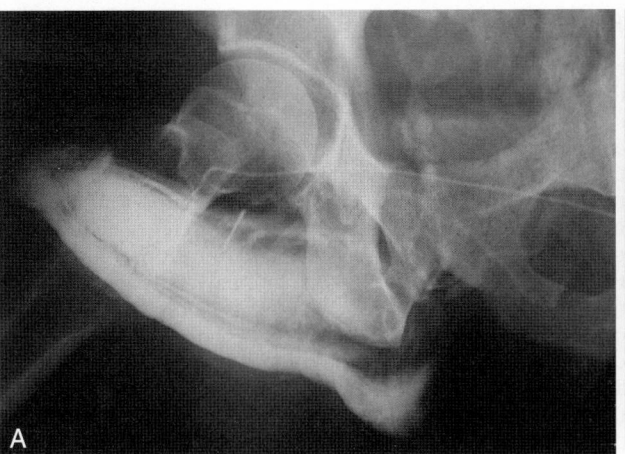
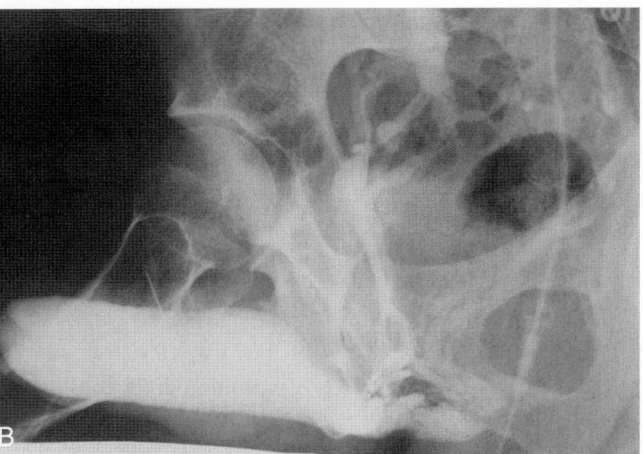

Figure 27-7. Pharmacologic cavernosography. A, In a patient 1 year after a penile fracture, a communication between the corpus cavernosum and the spongiosum is seen. **B,** In a 27-year-old man with primary impotence, venous leakage from the crura is seen.

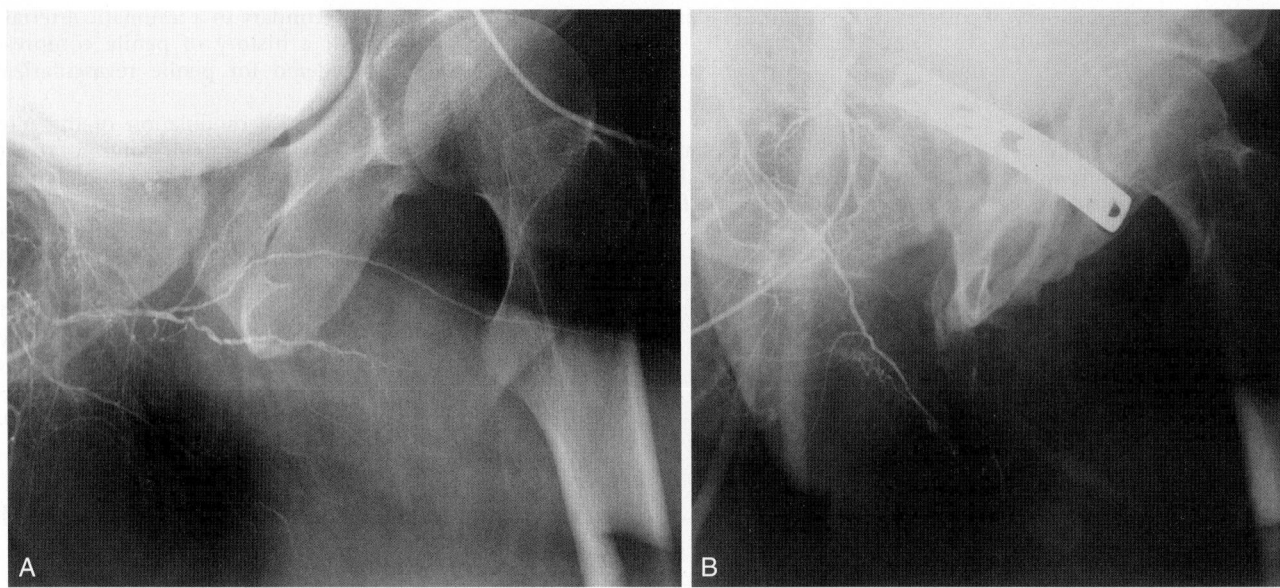

Figure 27-8. In this patient with a pelvic injury, pharmacologic penile arteriography (after intracavernous injection of 60 mg of papaverine) shows patent common penile, dorsal, and cavernous arteries (A) and nonvisualization of the common penile artery and its branches (B).

informative regarding penile vascular endothelial function (Dayan et al, 2005; Vardi et al, 2009).

Radioisotopic Penography

This test quantifies changes in penile blood volume after intracavernosal injection of a vasoactive agent using ^{99m}Tc-labeled red blood cells (Shirai et al, 1976). Extremely low flow is understood to mean arteriogenic ED (Smith et al, 1998). An evaluation comparing color duplex ultrasonography and radionuclide penography showed poor correlation (Glass et al, 1996).

Penile Magnetic Resonance Imaging

This test has significant potential applications for the assessment of anatomic details of the penis and penile microcirculation. Angiographic techniques may be combined with this test to evaluate the anatomic condition of the internal iliac and penile vasculature. Magnetic resonance angiography has been shown to correlate well with color duplex ultrasound testing (Stehling et al, 1997; John et al, 1999).

Penile Near Infrared Spectrophotometry

This test provides continuous, quantitative measurements of penile blood flow using a specialized near infrared spectrophotometry instrument (Burnett et al, 2000). It may be applied with an erectile stimulus and documents the hemodynamic phenomena of erection. Penile spectrophotometry has been further investigated in combination with intraurethral pharmacotherapy documenting blood-flow increase to the penis with this erectogenic modality (Padmanabhan and McCullough, 2007). Further investigation of this technique is needed to establish its clinical usefulness.

Cavernous Smooth Muscle Content

This test evaluates the smooth muscle composition of the corporeal tissue by light microscopic and computed morphometric assessment of biopsies of the penis and may serve adjunctively in the diagnosis of vasculogenic ED (Wespes et al, 1992). A reduced proportion of corporeal smooth muscle (and correspondingly increased collagen) has been observed in older men with veno-occlusive dysfunction (19% to 36% smooth muscle) and arteriogenic ED (10%

to 25%), compared with that of young, healthy men with normal erections and penile curvature (40% to 52%) (Wespes et al, 1991). In part because of its invasiveness, the test is controversial and thus it remains investigational at present.

Psychophysiologic Evaluation

The psychophysiologic evaluation of ED seeks to assess the erectile response by applying techniques that directly measure penile tumescence and rigidity. From the historical perspective of ED diagnostics, testing was applied primarily to differentiate psychogenic from organic ED. In general, the documentation of a full erection indicates functional integrity of the neurovascular axis regulating penile erection and thereby raises suspicion of a psychogenic etiology. There are several approaches to perform this evaluation. Importantly, the psychophysiologic evaluation does not currently represent first-line evaluation for ED, largely because of technical and cost limitations associated with current techniques. When considered to undergo any of these tests as part of a diagnostic plan, patients are counseled regarding the expected use, risks, and benefits of the tests.

Penile Tumescence and Rigidity Monitoring

Nocturnal penile tumescence (NPT) monitoring, which describes the study of erections that occur with nighttime sleep, was classically described as a technique offering the assessment of physiologic erectile ability (Wasserman et al, 1980). **As a standard, sleep laboratory nocturnal penile tumescence and rigidity (NPTR) testing applies nocturnal monitoring devices that measure the number of episodes, tumescence (circumference change by strain gauges), maximal penile rigidity, and duration of nocturnal erections** (Kessler, 1988). The conventional approach is to perform monitoring in conjunction with electroencephalography, electrooculography, and electromyography (EMG), with nasal airflow and oxygen saturation to document rapid eye movement (REM) sleep and the presence or absence of hypoxia (sleep apnea). It is important to note that documentation of REM sleep is undertaken because of the observation that true erectile phenomena occurring during sleep are associated with the REM sleep phase (Fisher et al, 1965). Sleep movement patterns are also monitored because periodic limb movement disorders are associated with abnormal NPT. Axial rigidity is measured along with photography of the erect penis when awakening the patient at maximal tumescence; a buckling device is applied to the tip of the penis to measure resistance (500 g minimum for vaginal penetration, 1.5 kg suggestive of complete rigidity) (Karacan et al, 1977). NPT has traditionally been performed during 2 to 3 nights to overcome the so-called first-night effect when REM sleep is inconsistent. Formal testing, which involves a specially equipped sleep laboratory staffed with trained observers, is costly. The monitoring of diurnal penile tumescence, in reference to monitoring performed during daytime napping, has served alternatively as an in-office evaluation (Morales et al, 1994).

Rigiscan (Timm Medical Technologies, Inc., Minneapolis, MN) is an automated, portable device used for NPTR, which combines the monitoring of radial rigidity, tumescence, number, and duration of erectile events (Bradley et al, 1985). The device employs two loops, one placed at the base of the penis and the other placed at the coronal sulcus (respectively, base and tip recording sites), and these loops record penile tumescence (circumference) and radial rigidity with timed, standardized constrictions of the loops. A baseline initialization is performed with the patient in the office, and then it is calibrated for home use. At home, registrations of penile rigidity are done every 3 minutes and increased to every 30 seconds when the base loop detects a circumference increase of greater than 10 mm (Fig. 27-9). **Recommended criteria for normal NPTR**

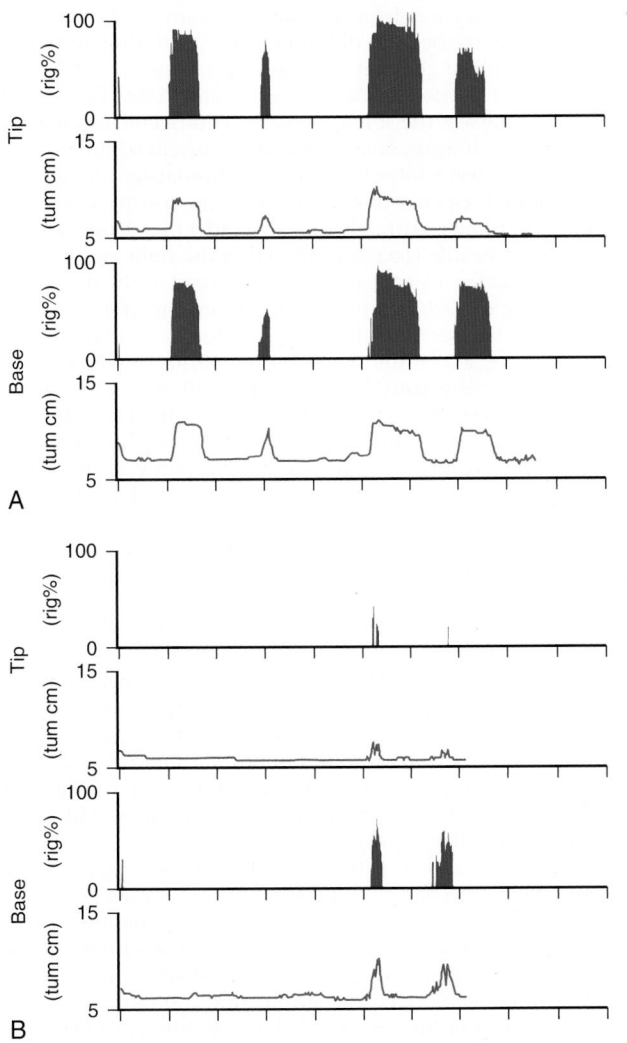

A

B

Figure 27-9. The RigiScan device has been designed to measure penile rigidity during home nocturnal monitoring. A, A study in a patient with at least two episodes of well-sustained, completely rigid nocturnal erections. B, A study with two episodes of poorly sustained, poorly rigid nocturnal erections. Such home studies fail to document sleep quality.

include four to five erectile episodes per night, mean duration longer than 30 minutes, an increase in circumference of more than 3 cm at the base and more than 2 cm at the tip, and maximal rigidity greater than 70% at both base and tip (Cilurzo et al, 1992). A computerized program has yielded standardized data measurements according to cumulative distribution of time-intensity measures, defined as tumescence activity units (TAU) and radial rigidity activity units (RAU) (Burris et al, 1989; Levine and Carroll, 1994). Potential limitations of Rigiscan include the fact that radial rigidity does not accurately predict axial rigidity (Allen et al, 1993; Licht et al, 1995) and considerable variability apparently exists even in normal subjects (Levine and Carroll, 1994). Further, the manner of testing does not allow verification of the presence of REM sleep.

NPT electrobioimpedance (NEVA, American Medical Systems, Inc., Minnetonka, MN) is a device introduced more recently that assesses volumetric changes in the penis during nocturnal erections (Knoll and Abrams, 1999). The device consists of three small electrode pads applied to the hip and the penile base and glans and a small recording device attached to the patient's thigh. In operation, an undetectable alternating current is transmitted from the glans electrode to the hip ground, and the penile base electrode measures impedance and changes in penile length. Impedance measures decrease in concert with increases in cross-sectional area of the penis during nocturnal tumescence. Further investigation is needed to establish the relationship of volumetric changes and the rigidity of the penis. Similar to Rigiscan, the technique also does not include REM sleep monitoring and correlations.

In summary, NPTR monitoring is an attractive approach for objectively evaluating the somatic basis of erectile ability, theoretically devoid of psychological interference. However, it has several apparent shortcomings, which limit its routine use for diagnostic purposes (Jannini et al, 2009). Central issues are that the testing does not indicate the cause and severity of ED and that the results may be poorly reproducible. Another fundamental issue is whether the testing appropriately evaluates wakeful, sexually relevant erections. Indeed, erections observed during NPTR monitoring do not unequivocally equate with erections sufficient for sexual performance, and false-positive results are possible for various clinical situations (e.g., multiple sclerosis). False-negative results may occur in aging patients and in patients with depression or anxiety, which may conditionally affect the physiology of sleep-related erectile phenomena. Nonetheless, NPTR monitoring may be considered in special circumstances such as when the cause of ED is obscure and noninvasive testing is desirable.

Audiovisual and Vibratory Stimulation

Alternative erectogenic methods can be used in conjunction with diagnostic testing of erectile function. **Erotic stimulation by explicit videotape material with monitoring has been used as a reliable as well as a time- and cost-effective alternative to NPTR for differentiating between organic and psychogenic ED presentations** (Sakheim et al, 1987; Bancroft et al, 1991). **It is also considered more physiologic, consistent with erectile behavior when awake.** The testing has potential limitations, with possible false-negative responses occurring in the presence of endocrine abnormalities (Carani et al, 1992; Greenstein et al, 1995) and false-positive responses occurring in psychological situations such as erotic excitement inhibition (Chung and Choi, 1990). As one may infer, these methods can be applied in conjunction with other stimulatory conditions (e.g., pharmacologic erection testing) as well as erectile function assessment approaches (e.g., Rigiscan monitoring) (Katlowitz et al, 1993; Martins and Reis, 1997).

Neuroimaging

Diagnostic techniques to evaluate central mechanisms of male sexual arousal have contributed to the psychophysiologic investigation of ED. Positron emission tomography (Miyagawa et al, 2007) and functional magnetic resonance imaging (Park et al, 2001;

Montorsi et al, 2003; Mouras et al, 2003; Ferretti et al, 2005) have been used in association with video sexual stimulation or an erectogenic pharmacologic stimulus (e.g., oral apomorphine). Studies have documented key brain regions associated with sexual arousal that induce penile erection (i.e., anterior cingulate, insula, amygdala, hypothalamus, and secondary somatosensory cortices). Interestingly, functional abnormalities in the brain have been shown in patients with psychogenic ED, suggesting that this diagnosis may be attributable to an actual biologic basis. More investigation in this area is necessary before determining its clinical role.

Psychological Evaluation

The psychological evaluation of ED addresses psychogenic contributions to clinical presentations, essentially psychological and interpersonal factors interfering with erectile function. These aspects should not be underestimated, and it is well documented in population studies that ED is associated with anxiety, depression, low degrees of self-esteem, negative outlook on life, self-reported emotional stress, and a history of sexual coercion (Feldman et al, 1994; Laumann et al, 2007). The urologist's role in initiating a psychological evaluation is not necessarily complicated, and a basic attempt to use queries about a patient's psychological health is helpful in assessing sexual health (Rowland et al, 2005).

The diagnostic interview is central to the psychological evaluation, and this process should be straightforwardly handled. Readily discernible causes of sexual dysfunction may be elicited, such as fear of failure, performance anxiety (for widowers, this may include complex interactions of dating, new partners, and unresolved mourning/guilt), insufficient sexual stimulation, loss of attraction for the partner, adjustment to a chronic illness or surgery, and relationship conflicts. In addition, causes that are less immediately discernible may be identified to include unresolved parental attachments, sexual identity issues, history of sexual trauma, occurrence of extramarital affairs, and cultural-religious taboos (Leach and Bethune, 1996; Laumann et al, 2007).

The interviewer should be mindful of the possibility of a primary psychogenic ED presentation (Turnbull and Weinberg, 1983). In the absence of organic risk factors, a primary psychogenic ED causation may be suspected. Further support for the diagnosis may follow the confirmation of noncoital erections (i.e., masturbatory, nocturnal, or when awakening). Clinical subtypes of psychogenic ED may be further identified: (1) generalized versus situational, and (2) lifelong (primary) versus acquired (secondary, including substance abuse or major psychiatric illness).

The interviewer should also inquire about relationship factors (Rosen, 2001). Relationship conflicts may be the source of psychogenic ED or otherwise may exacerbate organic ED. A couple's issues include intimacy and trust, status and dominance, loss of sexual attraction, ability to achieve sexual satisfaction without erection, and communication problems. Important information may derive not just from interviewing the patient alone, and interviews both with the couple together and of partners separately may provide insight.

Complex intrapsychic causes of sexual dysfunction are often relevant for the ED presentation and may become evident during the diagnostic interview. The clinical history may show a significant traumatic life experience, cultural or religious strife, compulsive sexual behavior, or neurotic process. It may suggest the presence of serious psychiatric comorbidities such as substance abuse, depressive symptoms, anxiety disorder, or personality disorder. It is recognized that the urologist may not have the professional background, comfort, or time to address these issues definitively, and a referral to a psychological expert for further attention would certainly be appropriate.

Neurologic Evaluation

The neurologic evaluation of ED is concerned with neurogenic associations with ED presentations. The importance of testing for deficits in the neurologic system relates to the principal regulatory role of this system for governing erectile function. Target sites for evaluation include peripheral, spinal, and supraspinal centers as well as both somatic and autonomic pathways involved in this biologic response. In line with this purpose, several diagnostic tests have been introduced. However, thus far they have had limited impact on routine clinical management decisions, and much of the available testing in this realm is reserved for research protocols and medicolegal investigations (Giuliano and Rowland, 2013). Additionally, fundamental problems surround the lack of sensitivity, reproducibility, reliability, and validity for many of these tests. This concern is particularly so for autonomic function tests, distinct from somatic function testing, which has been shown to be reproducible and valid. Otherwise, tests that could be most useful for evaluating penile erection, for example, neurotransmitter release, are altogether undeveloped.

Somatic Nervous System

Biothesiometry. This test represents a technique to assess afferent sensory function of the penis (Padma-Nathan, 1988). Testing involves a handheld electromagnetic device placed on the pulp of the index fingers, both sides of the penile shaft, and the glans penis. Measurements of sensory perception threshold are obtained in response to various amplitudes of vibratory stimulation. Investigators have questioned the usefulness of penile glans biothesiometry, which does not accurately portray neurophysiologic function of the dorsal penile nerve because of limitations in recording responses to vibratory stimuli of glanular skin (Bemelmans et al, 1995).

Sacral Evoked Response: Bulbocavernosus Reflex Latency. This test is used to assess the somatosensory reflexogenic mechanism of penile erection. Testing consists of a direct-current stimulator, which delivers square-wave impulses via two stimulating ring electrodes placed around the penis, one secured near the corona and the other secured 3 cm more proximally, and a recorder that gauges responses via concentric needle electrodes placed in the right and left bulbocavernous muscles. Latency period is measured as the interval from the beginning of each stimulus to the beginning of each response. An abnormal latency time, defined as a value more than three standard deviations above the mean (30 to 40 ms), indicates a high probability of neuropathology (Padma-Nathan, 1988). However, the use of this test has been questioned, and it has been shown that a full battery of electrophysiologic tests evaluating limb nerve function is more sensitive in diagnosing neuropathy than such tests specific to pudendal nerve function alone (Vodusek et al, 1993; Ho et al, 1996).

Dorsal Nerve Conduction Velocity. This test in concept extends from pudendal nerve function reflex testing and involves electrophysiologic stimulation with two stimulating electrodes placed at the glans and the base of the penis for obtaining two bulbocavernosus reflex latency measurements. Conduction velocity of the dorsal nerve is represented by dividing the distance between the two stimulating electrodes by the difference in latency times recorded from both sites. An average conduction velocity of 23.5 m/s with a range of 21.4 to 29.1 m/s is found in normal subjects (Gerstenberg and Bradley, 1983). Abnormal nerve conduction velocities were found to be diagnostic for neurogenic ED in patients with diabetes (Kaneko and Bradley, 1987).

Genitocerebral Evoked Potential. This test is designed to assess afferent sensory mechanisms and stimulus processing at spinal and supraspinal nervous system levels. The testing requires complex electronic equipment for recording the evoked potential waveforms overlying the sacral spinal cord and cerebral cortex in response to dorsal penile nerve electrical stimulation (Spudis et al, 1989). Central conduction time is recorded as the difference between the latency times after stimulation of the first replicated spinal response and the first replicated cerebral response (Padma-Nathan, 1988). The test has been questioned as having poor discriminatory value of response latencies (Pickard et al, 1994). However, it may still serve as an objective tool to define characteristics of afferent penile sensory dysfunction in patients with subtle abnormalities on neurologic examination.

Autonomic Nervous System

Heart Rate Variability and Sympathetic Skin Response. The test of heart rate control (mainly parasympathetic) consists of measuring heart rate variations during quiet breathing, deep breathing, and in response to raising the feet. Normative parameters have been documented. The test of sympathetic skin response involves producing an electrical shock stimulus at a certain location, for example, median or tibial nerve, and recording the evoked potential elsewhere, for example, contralateral hand or foot or penis. Recording from the penis is considered to be a potentially useful method of testing penile autonomic innervation (Daffertshofer et al, 1994). **Penile Thermal Sensory Testing.** This test serves to assess the conductance of small sensory nerve fibers, which are affected by autonomic disturbances consistent with neuropathy. The testing measures thermal threshold. In studies of the penis, it seems to correlate well with the clinical determination of neurogenic ED (Lefaucheur et al, 2001; Bleustein et al, 2003). **Corpus Cavernosum Electromyography and Single Potential Analysis of Cavernous Electrical Activity.** This test offers a direct recording of cavernous electrical activity, which varies between penile flaccidity and tumescence (Wagner et al, 1989; Leddy et al, 2012). In the normally flaccid penis, electrical activity is described as exhibiting a rhythmic slow wave with intermittent bursts of activity. As penile tumescence occurs (such as in response to visual sexual stimulation or after intracavernosal injection of a smooth muscle relaxant), this activity ceases. During detumescence, the baseline electrical activity returns. Patients with suspected autonomic neuropathy were demonstrated to display a discordant pattern, having continued electrical activity during erectogenic stimuli (Wagner et al, 1989). Recording techniques have been standardized, and normative values have been defined to include maximum peak-to-peak amplitudes between 120 and 500 mV and mean potential durations of 12 seconds (Stief et al, 1994). However, the clinical utility of this test remains in question (Kellner et al, 2000; Jiang et al, 2003).

Hormonal Evaluation

The hormonal evaluation for ED explores an endocrinologic basis for the sexual dysfunction and recognizes accumulating evidence that endocrinopathies potentially impact the physiology of penile erection (Traish and Guay, 2006; Mirone et al, 2009). **Several endocrine conditions are particularly relevant in this regard: hypogonadism (decrease or absence of hormonal secretion from the gonads), hyperthyroidism (excessive thyroid hormone release), and diabetes (altered modulation of androgen function** (Wang et al, 2011; Maggi et al, 2013). The diagnostic evaluation may be undertaken in view of their possible influences on erectile function. The clinical history may raise suspicion regarding the diagnosis, although the clinical presentation of an endocrinopathy may be variable. Several questionnaires have been proposed for use in screening, particularly with respect to hypogonadism (Morley et al, 2000; Daig et al, 2003; Heinemann, 2005). A new psychometrically validated hypogonadism screener has been developed to identify men with symptoms of hypogonadism (Rosen et al, 2011). However, their general lack of specificity for most presentations and the lack of sensitivity for some others has limited their widespread applications (Morales et al, 2007). The central feature of this evaluation involves biochemical testing for serum hormonal levels (Bhasin et al, 2010).

Serum Testosterone Measurements

Much focus in assessing the impact of endocrinopathies on male sexual function has centered on the role of androgens. Androgen deficiency or low testosterone levels are observed in as few as 2% and as many as 33% of men presenting clinically with ED (Korenman et al, 1990; Citron et al, 1996; Soran and Wu, 2005). Differences in patient populations under study likely account for the variation in statistics. In acknowledging that aging may represent

the primary cause of declining androgens, thought leaders have variously applied such terms as androgen deficiency of the aging male (ADAM), partial androgen deficiency of the aging male (PADAM), hypoandrogenism, symptomatic late-onset hypogonadism (SLOH), and andropause to designate this association.

It is important to understand the biology of testosterone production and function so as to proceed with its evaluation in laboratory. **Testosterone circulates in three fractions: free (0.5% to 3%), tightly bound to sex hormone–binding globulin (SHBG) (~30%), and loosely bound to albumin and other serum proteins (~67%)** (Basaria and Dobs, 2001; Freeman et al, 2001). **Free testosterone and albumin-bound portions comprise the bioavailable testosterone fraction. The relative concentrations of the carrier proteins (SHBG and albumin) serve to modulate androgen function.** Numerous conditions can alter the SHBG fraction and accordingly affect bioavailable testosterone to some extent even if the total testosterone measurement is unchanged (Bhasin et al, 2010). Decreased SHBG is associated with moderate obesity, nephrotic syndrome, hypothyroidism, and the use of glucocorticoids, progestins, and androgenic steroids, and it produces an elevation in bioavailable testosterone. Increased SHBG is associated with aging, hepatic cirrhosis, hyperthyroidism, human immunodeficiency virus infection, and the use of anticonvulsants and estrogens, and it produces a lowering in bioavailable testosterone. Despite the observation that lower levels of SHBG are associated with insulin resistance (Stellato et al, 2000), variable SHBG levels have been documented in diabetic men, possibly because of confounding obesity and aging factors, and the diagnosis of hypogonadism in this population should rely on the measurement of a low bioavailable testosterone level (see later) (Kapoor et al, 2007).

Theoretically, the unbound or free fraction measurement of testosterone offers the most relevant determination of testosterone bioavailability. However, commercial assays for free testosterone are known to be inconsistent and have been considered as invalid by some investigators (Vermeulen et al, 1999; Ly et al, 2010; Field and Wheeler, 2013). **The best indicator of androgen status is the calculated bioavailable testosterone (free testosterone and albumin-bound testosterone).** A formula for this calculation is found on the website of the International Society for the Study of the Aging Male at http://www.issam.ch/freetesto.htm, and this formula requires entries for the values of total testosterone and SHBG. In men with serious liver disease or hypoalbuminemia, entry of the serum albumin value may be useful for obtaining the best calculation.

For screening purposes, measurement of total serum testosterone level is generally sufficient. It is recommended that the blood draw be performed between 7:00 AM and 11:00 AM when there is a peak serum testosterone level, accounting for the fact that diurnal variation occurs in younger and middle-aged men (Wang et al, 2009). **The typical reference range for the total testosterone measurement is 280 to 1000 ng/dL. Because of individual variability, it is recognized that the normal range for testosterone beyond which replacement therapy should be initiated remains unresolved.** If the testosterone level is below or at the low limit of normal, blood draw should be repeated for confirmation. On the other hand, a mildly abnormal testosterone level might be found to be normal in 30% of patients on repeat testing (Bhasin et al, 2010). The clinical scenario, such as the presence of conditions that alter testosterone carrier proteins, may prompt further testing and assessment decisions.

Serum Gonadotropin Measurements

When proceeding with a second total testosterone determination, assessment of LH and prolactin should also be included. Measurement of serum gonadotropins will help to localize the source of the hypogonadism. It is understood that testosterone release involves the integrative activity of the hypothalamic-pituitary-gonadal axis and its regulatory feedback mechanisms, and disruption at any level of this axis may account for hypogonadism (Bhasin et al, 2010). A result of low testosterone is decreased negative feedback to the hypothalamus and pituitary, causing increased secretion of LH and follicle-stimulating hormone (FSH). Elevated serum LH and FSH releases are appropriate pituitary responses to low serum testosterone levels, which is consistent with testicular failure (primary hypogonadism). In contrast, normal or low serum LH and FSH releases in the setting of low serum testosterone levels indicate an inappropriate response and suggest a central disorder (secondary hypogonadism).

Serum Prolactin Measurement

Hyperprolactinemia causes hypogonadism by suppression of gonadotropin-releasing hormone from the hypothalamus, which impairs the pulsatile LH secretion required for serum testosterone production by the gonads (Morales et al, 2004). An additional possible mechanism for sexual dysfunction, specifically loss of sexual libido, in patients with hyperprolactinemia independent of the circulating level of testosterone relates to an interference of the peripheral conversion of testosterone to dihydrotestosterone (DHT) (Lobo and Kletzky, 1983). **Suspicion of hyperprolactinemia is raised in the patient with low serum testosterone and low or inappropriately normal LH.** However, controversy surrounds the consideration of routine determinations of prolactin in men with ED, with some indicating the low yield in doing so (Johnson and Jarow, 1992; Govier et al, 1996) and others finding that low serum testosterone or low sexual desire does not always coincide with the diagnosis (Buvat and Lemaire, 1997; Johri et al, 2001). Causes of the condition include various medications such as antipsychotic agents, tricyclic depressants and opiates, prolactin-secreting tumors, hypothyroidism, hypothalamic lesions, renal insufficiency, cirrhosis, and chest wall lesions (Zeitlin and Rajfer, 2000; Molitch, 2005).

Magnetic Resonance Imaging Scans

Cases of central (hypogonadotropic) hypogonadism as well as unexplained hyperprolactinemia prompt central imaging of the pituitary. This evaluation commonly involves magnetic resonance imaging, which can identify structural abnormalities (Citron et al, 1996; Petak et al, 2002; Rhoden et al, 2003). **Generally accepted guidelines provide indications for pituitary imaging: cases of severe central hypogonadism (testosterone <150 ng/dL) and suspicion of pituitary disease (i.e., panhypopituitarism, persistent hyperprolactinemia, or symptoms of tumor mass effect).**

Serum Thyroid Function Tests

Hyperthyroidism is associated with ED, possibly by increasing aromatization of testosterone into estrogen (which raises levels of SHBG) (Morales et al, 2004) **or by increasing adrenergic tone (which causes smooth muscle contractile effects or exerts psychobehavioral effects)** (Carani et al, 2005). Symptoms of hyperthyroidism, such as hyperactivity, irritability, heat intolerance, palpitations, fatigue, and weight loss, are often reported, and physical signs such as tachycardia, tremor, goiter, and eyelid retraction are often identified. The diagnosis is made biochemically by measurement of high levels of thyroid hormone (total or free thyroxine [T_4] or triiodothyronine [T_3]) with a low-serum thyroid-stimulating hormone level.

TREATMENT CONSIDERATIONS

The treatment of ED axiomatically follows an appropriate diagnostic workup. Although current interventions are both etiologically specific and nonspecific, an intervention that is specific for the cause of ED ideally offers the opportunity to treat ED with a corrective purpose in mind. **Current recommendations adhere to a patient goal-directed focus to therapy and specify that therapeutic options are presented according to a step-care clinical**

> ### KEY POINTS: DIAGNOSTIC EVALUATION
>
> - The basic evaluation of ED consists of a detailed case history, physical examination, and proper laboratory tests.
> - The sexual history should define the characteristics of the ED presentation according to such features as its onset, duration, conditions, severity, and etiology.
> - Cardiac risk assessment and risk reduction interventions are appropriate when necessary for all patients presenting for ED evaluations.
> - The hormonal evaluation for ED explores an endocrinologic basis for the disorder, with special consideration given to hypogonadism, hyperthyroidism, and diabetes as possible influences.
> - Questionnaires and other patient self-report measures offer practical help in documenting the presence, severity, and responsiveness to treatment of ED.
> - Specialized evaluation and testing may be required for individuals with complicated or atypical presentations of ED, and they potentially offer improved therapeutic outcomes for these presentations.

management approach (Fig. 27-10) (Montague et al, 2005; Hatzichristou et al, 2010).

Lifestyle Modification

The risk of developing ED is significantly associated with the presence of comorbid health conditions such as diabetes, cardiovascular disease, and metabolic syndromes that are either preventable or to a minimal extent treatable in endeavoring to optimize health status (Kostis et al, 2005). It stands to reason that optimization of these diseases offers opportunities to prevent the development of ED or to ameliorate its extent (Glina et al, 2013).

Epidemiologic studies have shown examinations of potentially modifiable risk factors and in some instances have provided support that risk modification may indeed improve erectile function. For instance, several reports have suggested that the discontinuation of cigarette smoking results in a recovery of functional erection status (Mannino et al, 1994; Feldman et al, 2000; Bacon et al, 2006). A beneficial role of increasing exercise for those with a sedentary lifestyle in men with ED was also evident (Feldman et al, 1994; Derby et al, 2000). In a prospective study, obese men with moderate ED and no overt symptoms of cardiovascular disease showed significant improvements in IIEF scores after exercise and weight control when compared with a control group that followed an educational program alone (Esposito et al, 2004). Significant changes in body mass index, C-reactive protein, and physical activity scores were observed in the intervention group compared with the control group. Mediterranean-style diets and a reduction in caloric intake have been found to improve erectile function in men with metabolic syndrome (Esposito et al, 2006). A change to a no-nose saddle from a conventional saddle was shown to recover erectile function, presumably by alleviating perineal trauma, in a short-term interventional study of men with ED associated with occupational bicycle riding (Schrader et al, 2008).

Reports indicating that ED is potentially ameliorated by lifestyle modifications of risk factors that predispose this sexual dysfunction are most illuminative. The role of lifestyle modifications to prevent or to treat ED has gained support by way of systematic reviews and meta-analysis (Kupelian et al, 2010; Gupta et al, 2011; Porst et al, 2013). The mechanisms of this effect may include reduced cardiovascular risk factors, increased serum testosterone levels, and overall improved mood and self-esteem (Gupta et al, 2011; Meldrum et al, 2012; Glina et al, 2013). **Ongoing clinical and basic science investigation may further affirm the benefits of lifestyle modification and clarify its mechanistic basis.**

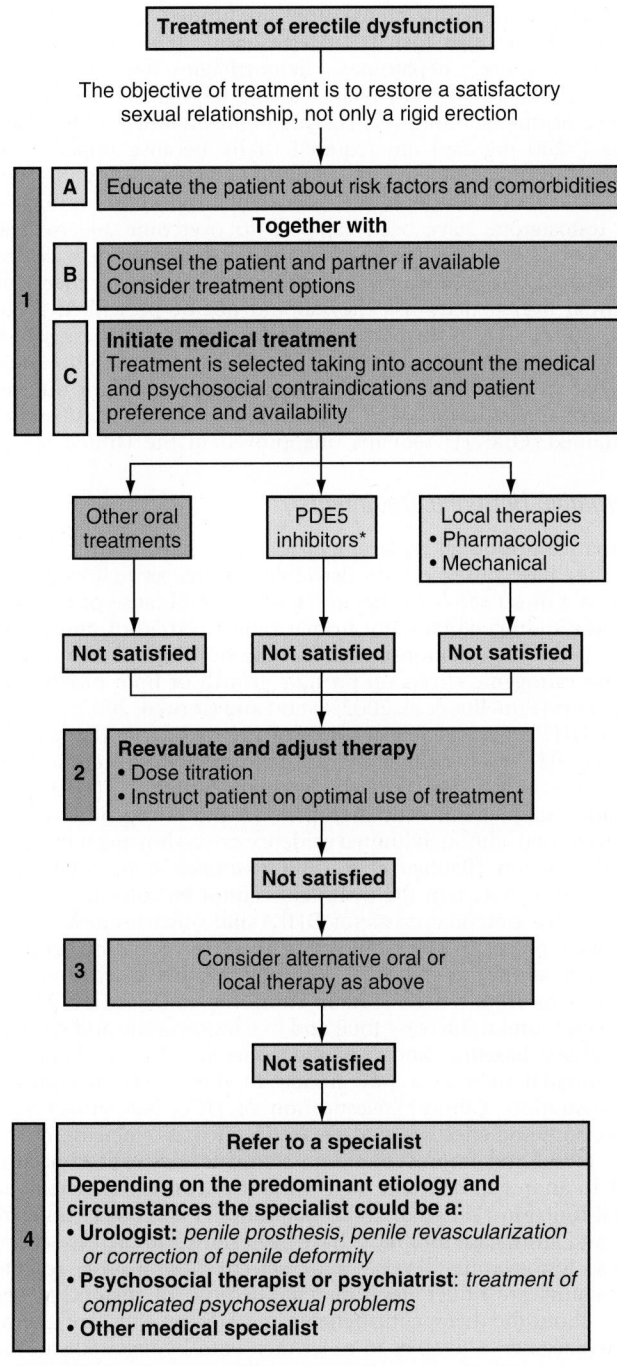

Similarly, in patients suffering adverse sexual dysfunction effects from the use of SSRIs (e.g., ED, retarded ejaculation), treatment strategies such as drug substitution (e.g., bupropion, nefazodone, buspirone, mirtazapine), drug holidays, SSRI dosage reduction, watchful waiting, and administration of PDE5 inhibitors have enabled sexual function recovery (Rosen et al, 1999b; Nurnberg et al, 2001).

Psychosexual Therapy

Because of the frequent interplay of psychological and interpersonal factors in clinical presentations of ED, it is hardly surprising to consider that psychosexual therapy should be included in the therapeutic armamentarium for this sexual dysfunction. A strong limitation in this area is that evidence-based investigation and well-controlled, large-scale outcome research that documents the efficacy of interventions are generally lacking. In practice, psychosexual therapy does represent an ill-defined combination of interventions and interpretations, based on behavioral, relational, psychoanalytic, and cognitive psychology concepts. **A variety of interventions are used: systematic anxiety reduction/ desensitization, sensate focus, interpersonal therapy, cognitive-behavior therapy, sex education, couples' communication and sexual skills training, and masturbation exercises (Althof et al, 2005). Integrated treatments, which combine psychosexual interventions with medical therapies such as oral therapy, intracavernosal injection, or vacuum device therapy, have also proved successful in managing ED presentations, particularly those associated with motivational obstacles (Hawton, 1998; Althof et al, 2005).** It is understandable that the common urologist may not feel comfortable or does not possess the necessary training to address complicated psychosocial concerns. However, for mild to moderate psychosocial matters, the urologist may be prepared to proceed with a "biopsychosocial" model that minimally involves awareness of psychosocial issues and preparedness to counsel a patient or couple about normal sexual function and acceptable sexual behaviors (Althof and Needle, 2011). Collaborative efforts with a mental health clinician who has expertise in psychosexual therapy may be necessary to implement intensive therapy techniques.

Hormonal Therapy

A prescription of hormonal therapy is considered so as to impact the clinical presentation of ED for the patient in whom a hormonal disturbance is identified. The urologist's role is fitting for the treatment of primary hypogonadism and hyperprolactinemia, whereas endocrinologists would be considered as the foremost consultants for other endocrinopathies.

Testosterone Replacement

Androgen replacement addresses straightforwardly the clinical complaint that is associated with hypogonadism. As a general principle of sex steroid replacement therapy, serum hormone levels to be achieved daily throughout 24 hours should ideally achieve normal reference values and resemble the normal diurnal pattern. **Evaluating serum testosterone levels both before and during treatment is imperative, although the efficacy of testosterone supplementation is best judged by clinical response rather than a precise testosterone determination. Current recommendations suggest that a short (e.g., 3-month) therapeutic trial is justified, and, in the absence of a response, testosterone administration should be discontinued** (Wang et al, 2009; Bhasin et al, 2010). Potential adverse effects of androgen therapy (i.e., erythrocytosis, sleep apnea, urinary symptoms, prostate cancer progression risk, gynecomastia, acne) should be recognized (Morales et al, 2004; Wald et al, 2006). **Monitoring of patients on therapy consists of a baseline assessment that includes digital rectal examination and serum PSA testing along with laboratory evaluation (i.e., hemoglobin/ hematocrit levels, liver function tests, cholesterol level, and lipid**

Figure 27-10. **Treatment algorithm for erectile dysfunction recommended by the International Consultations on Sexual Medicine.** PDE5, phosphodiesterase type 5.

Medication Change

It is possible that a certain medication is an offending factor resulting in the clinical presentation of ED. After this inference is made, an appropriate next step would be to change to a different dose or type of medication entirely, considering that this action may reverse ED in some patients (Ralph and McNicholas, 2000). For instance, switching antihypertensive therapies from thiazide diuretics and β-blockers to calcium channel blockers and renin-angiotensin system inhibitors (i.e., angiotensin-converting enzyme inhibitors and angiotensin receptor blockers) may recover erectile function in men developing ED in this clinical setting.

profile) followed by the assessment of treatment efficacy after 3 to 6 months and annually thereafter to ascertain symptom response and any adverse events (Morales et al, 2004; Bhasin et al, 2010). Short-acting preparations may be preferred in favor of long-acting depot preparations in the initial treatment of patients, so that therapy can be discontinued on the occasion of an adverse event (Wang et al, 2009).

For the treatment of hypogonadism, several testosterone preparations are offered and can be delivered by various routes: intramuscular, subcutaneous, transdermal (patch and gel), buccal, and oral (Edelstein et al, 2006; Morgentaler et al, 2008; Wang et al, 2009; Bhasin et al, 2010; Corona et al, 2011). A brief description of available therapies follows (see also Table 27-6).

Intramuscular. Testosterone enanthate or cypionate, an injectable depot preparation of testosterone, is delivered by deep intramuscular injection (200 to 250 mg every 2 to 3 weeks). The schedule of therapy results in supraphysiologic levels of testosterone for 72 hours with a steady exponential decline to subphysiologic levels by 10 to 12 days. Alternative dosing of 100 mg every 7 to 10 days can be considered in situations when patients experience symptomatic mood changes or sexual fluctuations associated with documented early hypogonadal troughs. Another parenteral preparation, testosterone propionate, is also delivered intramuscularly at a dosage of 200 mg every 2 to 3 days because of its shorter half-life, and it may also display serum testosterone fluctuations. Testosterone undecanoate (TU), as a depot formulation consisting of 750- or 1000-mg dosages administered at 10-week dosing intervals, has been used in Europe since 2003 although it is not yet available in the United States.

Subcutaneous. Pellets offer a subcutaneous, long-acting depot formulation of testosterone. Testopel is a pellet containing 75 mg of testosterone. Dosing usually requires 2 to 6 pellets (150 to 450 mg testosterone) implanted subcutaneously every 3 to 6 months.

Transdermal. Transdermal delivery options comprise patches and gels, with a delivery approach that intentionally simulates normal circadian levels of testosterone. When patients apply medication in the morning, higher initial absorption will mimic normal diurnal variation.

Testoderm was approved initially as a scrotal patch administered daily without adhesive (4 to 6 mg), but it came under disuse because of difficulties with its application, the requirement for scrotal shaving, and the finding that it significantly produced high levels of DHT by conversion by 5α-reductase activity that is plentifully present in the scrotal skin. Testoderm TTS represented an alternative formulation avoiding the inconveniences of the scrotal application. Its application is to the arm, back, or buttock as a 5-mg patch. Androderm, an alternative product, delivers 2.5 or 5 mg of testosterone daily. Both patches have been associated with itching, chronic skin irritation, and allergic contact dermatitis. The skin irritation is alleviated by the local application of cortisone cream. Patients are advised to alternate application sites and avoid sun-exposed areas.

AndroGel (testosterone 1% gel) is a topical gel pack that contains 50, 75, or 100 mg of testosterone, with only 10% of the drug being absorbed during a 24-hour period. Testim, also providing 1% testosterone, is an alternative product packaged as a 5-g tube containing 50 mg of testosterone. Both are similarly applied once daily in the morning to clean, dry skin on the shoulders, upper arms, or abdomen, and it is allowed to dry before dressing. Axiron (testosterone 2% solution) is another transdermal product approved by the U.S. Food and Drug Administration (FDA), consisting of 30 mg of testosterone applied to each axilla once daily using a metered applicator. Special considerations for axillary administration include the concealable location and high permeability of the axilla, which has a relatively high level of 5-α reductase activity.

Buccal. Striant refers to a tabletlike, mucoadhesive treatment system (30 mg of testosterone) that continuously delivers medication. It is applied twice daily to the gum tissue above the incisors allowing testosterone to be absorbed through the buccal mucosa.

Oral. Oral testosterone preparations are limited. Concern is associated with the liver toxicity of testosterone (i.e., hepatitis, cholestatic jaundice, hepatomas, hemorrhagic liver cysts, and hepatocellular carcinoma) related to the large doses necessary to achieve normal serum levels (Bagatell and Bremner, 1996). Large doses (>200 mg/day) are required orally because much of the administration is rendered metabolically inactive during the "first-pass" circulation through the liver. Chemical modifications of oral testosterone have been explored to overcome adverse reactions. Both 17α-methyltestosterone and fluoxymesterone have been formulated, but because of their patient variability of effect with potential liver toxicity risk they should not be prescribed (Wang et al, 2009). TU, as an oral formulation in oleic acid, is safe by partly escaping hepatic inactivation (Köhn and Schill, 2003). However, it has shown a large individual variability for the time of maximal responses as well as when maximal serum testosterone is attained. Oral TU remains unapproved in the United States.

Alternative Hormone Treatments

Alternative hormonal replacement therapies have been suggested, and they have posed certain desirable features as well as caveats. DHT as a direct mode of therapy is attractive because of its action as a pure androgen that is not aromatizable to estradiol, and accordingly it has been demonstrated that the hormone does not exert adverse estrogenic effects on prostate growth or lipid profile measurements (Kunelius et al, 2002; Sakhri and Gooren, 2007). A therapeutic DHT gel is available at a dose of 125 to 250 mg/day, yielding plasma DHT levels comparable to physiologic testosterone levels (Kunelius et al, 2002). Dehydroepiandrosterone (DHEA), a hormone supplement with androgen-like and estrogen-like effects, has been used, although limited evidence exists showing it improves sexual function (Baulieu et al, 2000; Morales et al, 2004). It is important to note that the treatment cannot be considered harmless, and the potential exists for DHEA and other nontestosterone androgen precursor preparations (e.g., DHEA-S, androstenediol, androstenedione) to stimulate hormone-sensitive diseases such as breast or prostate cancer. Human chorionic gonadotropin (HCG) has been found to increase total and free testosterone and estradiol 50% above baseline, and it would conceivably be of benefit to hypogonadal men in a way similar to the effects of androgen administration. Clinical investigation of HCG has shown some anthropometric effects (i.e., decrease in fat mass, increase in lean body mass) and improvements in serum testosterone concentrations in androgen-deficient men without documented benefits for sexual function (Liu et al, 2002; Tsujimura et al, 2005). Antiestrogens and aromatase inhibitors have been shown to increase endogenous testosterone levels, and selective androgen receptor modulators are under development. Because of insufficient evidence about the therapeutic benefits and adverse effects of alternative replacement therapies in older men with hypogonadism, they are not currently recommended for use (Wang et al, 2009).

Hyperprolactinemia Treatments

The treatment of hyperprolactinemia is undertaken with the acknowledgment that testosterone replacement therapy is neither corrective nor sufficient to improve sexual function. The therapeutic objective, rather, is to identify and address the underlying cause, which may then ameliorate ED. Offending drugs, such as estrogens, morphine, sedatives, and neuroleptics, should be discontinued (Molitch, 2008). A prolactin-secreting adenoma should be treated medically and if necessary surgically. Bromocriptine, a dopamine agonist that lowers prolactin level and restores testosterone to normal, serves to reduce the size of the tumor. Neurosurgical ablation becomes necessary if the therapeutic response to medication does not occur or visual effects are noted in association with optic-nerve compression (Gillam et al, 2006). Erection recovery is most evident after treatment of men with significant serum elevations of prolactin (higher than 40 ng/mL) (Netto Júnior and Claro, 1993).

TABLE 27-6 Testosterone Preparations

FORMULATION	CHEMICAL STRUCTURE	T½	STANDARD DOSAGE	ADVANTAGES	DISADVANTAGES
ORAL AGENTS					
Testosterone undecanoate	17-α-hydroxyl-ester	4 hr	120-240 mg 2-3 times daily	Oral convenience Modifiable dosage	Serum testosterone levels and clinical responses vary Must be taken with meals
Methyltestosterone	17-α-alkylated	3.5 hr	20-50 mg 2-3 times daily	Oral convenience Modifiable dosage	Potential hepatotoxicity Treatment considered obsolete
Mesterolone	1-alkylated	8 hr	100-150 mg 2-3 times daily	Oral convenience Modifiable dosage	Nonaromatizable to estrogen
INTRAMUSCULAR AGENTS					
Testosterone enanthate	17-α-hydroxyl-ester	4-5 days	250 mg every 2-3 wk	Low cost Modifiable dosage	Wide fluctuations in circulating T levels Multiple injections Relative higher risk of polycythemia
Testosterone cypionate	17-α-hydroxyl-ester	8 days	200 mg every 2-3 wk	Low cost Modifiable dosage	Wide fluctuations in circulating T levels Multiple injections
Testosterone propionate	17-α-hydroxyl-ester	20 hr	100 mg every 2 days	Low cost	Wide fluctuations in circulating T levels Multiple injections Relative higher risk of polycythemia
Testosterone undecanoate	17-α-hydroxyl-ester	34 days	1000 mg every 10-14 wk	Testosterone levels maintained within normal range Long lasting Less frequent administration	Pain at injection site
SUBCUTANEOUS AGENTS					
Surgical implants	Native testosterone	—	4-6 200-mg implants lasting ≤6 mo	Treatment only twice per yr	Placement is invasive Risk of extrusion and site infections
CONTROLLED-RELEASE T-BUCCAL FORMULATION AGENTS					
Testosterone buccal	Native testosterone	12 hr	30 mg 2 times daily	Testosterone levels within physiologic range	Possible oral irritation Twice-daily irritation Unpleasant taste
TRANSDERMAL AGENTS					
Testosterone patches	Native testosterone	10 hr	5-10 mg/day	Mimics circadian rhythm Simple administration	Skin irritation Daily administration
Testosterone gel 1%-2%	Native testosterone	6 hr	5-10 g/day	Testosterone levels maintained within normal range Flexible dose modification Skin irritation less common than with patches	Possible transfer during intimate contact Daily administration
Testosterone solution 2%	Native testosterone	NA	60-120 mg/day	Testosterone levels maintained within normal range	Possible transfer during intimate contact Daily administration

NA, not available; T, testosterone; T½, drug half-time.

Modified from Corona G, Rastrelli G, Forti G, et al. Update in testosterone therapy for men. J Sex Med 2011;8:639–54.

Pharmacologic Therapies

The premise of pharmacologic therapies is that they simulate the biochemical and molecular mechanisms of action naturally governing the erectile response. **Conceptually, erectogenic therapies serve strategically either to promote proerectile mechanisms or to oppose antierectile mechanisms, at both peripheral and central levels of the neurovascular axis responsible for penile erection** (Rowland and Burnett, 2000). At a peripheral level, these mechanisms influence corporeal smooth muscle tone. Promotion of proerectile mechanisms is achieved by either inducing corporeal smooth muscle activation through cell-receptor agonists or effectors of tissue relaxant pathways (e.g., stimulating second messenger cyclic nucleotide [cyclic guanosine monophosphate {cGMP} or cyclic adenosine monophosphate {cAMP}] synthesis) or inhibiting the deactivation of smooth muscle relaxation pathways (e.g., inhibiting phosphodiesterases), whereas opposition of antierectile mechanisms are achieved by decreasing smooth muscle contraction through receptor antagonists of tissue contractile pathways (e.g., alpha$_1$-adrenergic inhibitors). At a central nervous system level (i.e., brain or spinal cord), neuronal pathways are affected, and potential opportunities exist to promote proerectile pathways (e.g., agonists of dopaminergic D$_2$ receptors in the medial hypothalamus) or to oppose antierectile pathways (e.g., antagonists of 5-HT$_{1A/2}$ [serotonergic] receptors in the spinal cord).

Diverse therapies have been touted throughout time, although their efficacy and safety characteristics have not always been clearly defined. Current standards of regulatory agency approval have helped to clarify the qualifications of commercially developed and marketed therapies (Hirsch et al, 2004).

Oral Therapy

Orally administered medication for ED meets many of the attributes of "ideal therapy," which include convenience, simplicity, and noninvasiveness (Morales et al, 1995). Oral therapies are increasingly in demand to meet the therapeutic objective of clinical efficacy as well.

Phosphodiesterase Type 5 Inhibitors. This class of medication was famously inaugurated as an effective ED treatment in the United States following the FDA approval of sildenafil citrate (Viagra, Pfizer, Inc., New York, NY) in 1998, vardenafil hydrochloride (Levitra, Bayer Schering Pharma AG, Berlin, Germany), and tadalafil (Cialis, Lilly LLC, Indianapolis, IN) in 2003, and avanafil (Stendra, Vivus Inc., Mountain View, CA) in 2012 (Bruzziches et al, 2013; Porst et al, 2013). **PDE5 inhibitors similarly work to block the catalytic action of the enzyme that degrades cGMP, the downstream effector of the erection mediator nitric oxide, which** then facilitates the signal transductional mechanisms of corpus cavernosal smooth muscle relaxation required for penile erection. **It is important to recognize that the medications augment but do not induce the erectile response and the induction of penile erection requires the release of nitric oxide from penile nerve endings and vascular endothelium under the influence of sexual stimulation** (Burnett, 2005). The high concentration of PDE5 inhibitors in the smooth muscle of the penile corpora cavernosa accounts for the selectivity of their effect.

Despite their similar modes of actions, PDE5 inhibitors differ somewhat in their biochemical properties, pharmacokinetic profiles, and clinical performances (Table 27-7). The chemical structure of PDE5 inhibitors are similar, containing a guaninelike base, a riboselike or desoxyribose-like system, and a phosphate diester-like bond, which confers their ability to bind effectively to the catalytic site of the PDE5 enzyme. The chemical structures of sildenafil and vardenafil are similar, unlike that for tadalafil, and this difference serves to explain some phenomenologic distinctions observed between these agents (Corbin and Francis, 1999). The chemical structure of avanafil differs from the standard model of the other three agents, which may account for some of its selective actions (Kedia et al, 2013). **Distinct from the actions of tadalafil and avanafil, sildenafil and vardenafil cross-react to a greater extent with phosphodiesterase (PDE) type 6, which is expressed in the retina, and this difference may explain the complaint of visual disturbances observed with sildenafil and vardenafil use.** Tadalafil minimally cross-reacts with PDE type 11, unlike the other three PDE5 inhibitors, although the significance of this effect is unclear. The remaining side effects commonly observed with PDE5 inhibitor treatment are associated with inhibition of PDE5 localized in other target tissues, such as vascular and gastrointestinal smooth muscle. Tadalafil possesses a longer half-life of elimination than the other three PDE5 inhibitors. This feature suggests a longer therapeutic window uniquely afforded for tadalafil, which may translate into increased convenience for couples having sexual intercourse with this agent.

All four PDE5 inhibitors have demonstrated equivalent efficacy and tolerability in clinical trials for the treatment of ED of varying severity and cause (Carson and Lue, 2005; Hellstrom, 2007; Giuliano et al, 2010; Bruzziches et al, 2013; Porst et al, 2013; Yuan et al, 2013). Trial designs for these agents have differed, limiting useful comparisons among them, and superiority cannot be claimed for any particular agent in the absence of directly comparative studies (Carson and Lue, 2005; Khera and Goldstein, 2011). **In general, the agents effectively result in successful sexual intercourse rates of approximately 70%** (Carson and Lue, 2005; Khera and Goldstein, 2011). A somewhat reduced intercourse success rate of 40% to 50% has been reported in diabetic patients with ED (Fonseca et al, 2004;

TABLE 27-7 Comparison of Four Phosphodiesterase Type 5 Inhibitors Currently Available in the United States

	SILDENAFIL	VARDENAFIL	TADALAFIL	AVANAFIL
Cmax (ng/mL)	450	20.9	378	2153
Tmax (hr)	0.8	0.7-0.9	2	0.3-0.5
Onset of action (min)	15-60	15-60	15-120	15-60
Half-life (hr)	3-5	4-5	17.5	3-5
Bioavailability	40%	15%	Not tested	30%
Fatty food	Reduced absorption	Reduced absorption	No effect	Reduced absorption
Recommended dosage	25, 50, 100 mg	5, 10, 20 mg	5, 10, 20 mg	50, 100, 200 mg
Side effects:				
Headache, dyspepsia, facial flushing	Yes	Yes	Yes	Yes
Backache, myalgia	Rare	Rare	Yes	Rare
Blurred/blue vision	Yes	Rare	Rare	No
Precaution with antiarrhythmics	No	Yes	No	No
Contraindication with nitrates	Yes	Yes	Yes	Yes

Cmax, maximal plasma concentration; half-life, time required for elimination of one half of the medication from plasma; Tmax, time required to attain Cmax.

Safarinejad, 2004) and in patients with ED associated with radical prostatectomy in general (Hatzimouratidis et al, 2009). However, the intercourse success rate for patients after bilateral nerve-sparing radical prostatectomy specifically is somewhat better than for the entire group, and reports have commonly documented rates that approach 60% to 70% for functional erections with therapy.

According to standard dosing recommendations, patients are instructed to take the medications on demand between 30 and 60 minutes before intended sexual activity. This lead-time interval is specified to take advantage of the duration by which the medications achieve peak serum concentrations (i.e., approximately ½ hour for avanafil, 1 hour for sildenafil and vardenafil, and 2 hours for tadalafil). Although the onset of activity has been documented to occur possibly within 20 minutes for each agent, this characteristic is less important to patients than erection hardness and maintenance of erections with therapy (Claes et al, 2008). A daily dosing regimen has been approved for tadalafil as an alternative treatment schedule to afford patients greater convenience in having sexual intercourse while using this agent (Porst et al, 2006; Shabsigh et al, 2010). **Optimization of effect for all PDE5 inhibitors is also achieved by applying sexual stimulation properly as a prerequisite for nitric oxide release, by reducing food intake, which may delay drug absorption, by escalating drug dosing as needed, and by repeating attempts with the medications several times (up to nine or ten attempts affords maximal probability of success)** (McCullough et al, 2002; Barada, 2003; Shindel, 2009). **Correcting or improving adverse health conditions (e.g., glycemic control, hyperlipidemic control, androgen replacement), which affect drug efficacy, has also been demonstrated as potentially beneficial** (Guay, 2003; Sadovsky et al, 2009). As evidence of therapeutic efficacy, patient and partner satisfaction with therapy (as shown for sildenafil) has been well demonstrated (Montorsi and Althof, 2004). Suboptimal acceptance or lack of long-term adherence to therapy (up to 47% of patients) has been reported, which may indicate the influence of psychosocial factors or challenges of a treatment that requires repeated dosing (Seftel, 2002; Al-Shaiji and Brock, 2009).

BOX 27-1 Warnings and Drug Interactions

The package inserts of all four phosphodiesterase type 5 (PDE5) inhibitors warn against their use in patients with severe cardiovascular diseases and left ventricular outflow obstruction (e.g., aortic stenosis, idiopathic subaortic stenosis), those with severely impaired autonomic control of blood pressure, and patients not studied in clinical trials (U.S. prescribing information of Viagra, Cialis, and Levitra and Stendra, September 2013). These include patients with:

- Myocardial infarction, stroke, or life-threatening arrhythmia within the previous 6 mo
- New York Heart Association class II or greater heart failure or coronary artery disease causing unstable angina
- Resting hypotension (<90/50 mm Hg) or hypertension (>170/100 mm Hg)
- Known hereditary degenerative retinal disorders including retinitis pigmentosa
- Severe hepatic impairment (Child-Pugh C) or end-stage renal disease requiring dialysis

Certain drugs such as ketoconazole and itraconazole and protease inhibitors such as ritonavir can impair the metabolic breakdown of PDE5 inhibitors by blocking the CYP3A4 pathway. Such agents may increase blood levels of inhibitors, requiring a PDE5 dose reduction. On the other hand, agents such as rifampin may induce CYP3A4, enhancing the breakdown of inhibitors and requiring higher PDE5 doses. Kidney or hepatic dysfunction may require dose adjustments or warnings.

Patients using PDE5 inhibitors should be thoroughly counseled regarding precautions (Box 27-1). Cardiovascular safety using this class of compounds has been well demonstrated, although it should be emphasized that given the cardiovascular risks of sexual activity and potential for adverse drug interactions with this therapy, cardiovascular risk assessment and stabilization should be considered for all men before the institution of PDE5 inhibitor therapy. **Controlled and postmarketing studies involving these agents have shown that they do not cause an increase in myocardial infarction or death rates when compared with expected rates in study control populations** (Jackson et al, 2006a; Hellstrom, 2007; Nehra, 2009). In addition, patients with known coronary artery disease or heart failure receiving PDE5 inhibitors did not exhibit worsening ischemia, coronary vasoconstriction, or worsening hemodynamics on exercise testing or cardiac catheterization. Caution is advised for the use of PDE5 inhibitors in patients with certain conditions: aortic stenosis, left ventricular outflow obstruction, hypotension, and hypovolemia. The agents have a minimal effect on QTc interval (Morganroth et al, 2004). Vardenafil among PDE5 inhibitors is not recommended in patients who take type 1A antiarrhythmics (e.g., quinidine or procainamide) or type 3 antiarrhythmics (e.g., sotalol or amiodarone) or in patients with congenital prolonged QT syndrome.

Nitrate use in any form (e.g., sublingual nitroglycerin, isosorbide dinitrate, other nitrate preparations used to treat angina, amyl nitrite, and amyl nitrate "poppers") represents an absolute contraindication. Past use of nitrates, that is, more than 2 weeks before the use of PDE5 inhibitors, is not considered a contraindication. **If angina occurs during sexual activity when using a PDE5 inhibitor, patients should cease this activity and seek emergency care immediately.** They should inform medical personnel that a PDE5 inhibitor was taken and should avoid nitroglycerin use for a period of 24 hours for sildenafil and vardenafil and 48 hours for tadalafil (Cheitlin et al, 1999). If acute myocardial infarction occurs with the use of PDE5 inhibitors, usual therapies, with the exception of organic nitrates, may be administered. If hypotension results from PDE5 inhibitor use, patients should be placed in the Tredelenburg position and given intravenous fluids along with administration of α-adrenergic agonists (e.g., phenylephrine) as needed. Refractory hypotension warrants intra-aortic balloon counterpulsation, as specified by the American College of Cardiology/American Heart Association guidelines. **No pharmacologic antidote to the PDE5 inhibitor/nitrate interaction exists. Caution is advised when PDE5 inhibitors are coadministered with α-adrenergic blockers, because both agents are vasodilators with blood pressure lowering effects.**

Side effects observed with PDE5 inhibitor therapy include headache (7% to 16%), dyspepsia (4% to 10%), flushing (4% to 10%), myalgia/back pain (0% to 3%), nasal congestion (3% to 4%), and visual disturbances (e.g., photophobia, blue vision) (0% to 3%). Randomized, controlled trials have documented that flushing and visual side effects are more common in patients receiving sildenafil or vardenafil, whereas back pain/myalgia is more common in patients receiving tadalafil. These events have been found to be mild and to abate with time, and the side effects prompt discontinuation only in few patients (Hellstrom, 2007; Porst et al, 2013). **The concern has been posed with PDE5 inhibitor therapy regarding the development of nonarteritic anterior optic neuropathy (NAION), which can cause blindness, although several systematic reviews of the safety of this class of compounds have not shown an increased risk of NAION or other adverse ocular events associated with their use** (Laties, 2009; Porst et al, 2013). Affected patients in postmarketing reports possibly carried risk factors for blindness to include hypertension, diabetes, and hyperlipidemia. At this time, despite the absence of a proven link between PDE5 inhibitor use and serious ocular disorders, physicians should continue to advise patients to stop use of PDE5 inhibitors and to seek immediate medical attention as a safety measure in the event of a sudden loss of vision (Laties, 2009; Porst et al, 2013).

The interest in extending the use of PDE5 inhibitors beyond an on-demand erectogenic role and rather applying them to recovery or maintenance of the natural vitality of the penis in the face of an ED-associated disease state or condition has been investigated. This proposal has been considered particularly in the clinical context of radical prostatectomy and has been introduced as a therapeutic strategy à la "penile rehabilitation," by which the medications are taken in some regularly scheduled fashion to promote the recovery of spontaneous erectile function. Presently, this role remains unclear, owing to limited well-designed and conducted (i.e., randomized, controlled) clinical trials of PDE5 inhibitor use in this clinical setting (Mulhall et al, 2013). In one supportive trial involving sildenafil treatment of 36 weeks starting 4 weeks after the surgery, 27% of patients using the agent recovered erections defined as "good enough for sexual activity" compared with 4% of patients on placebo at about 1 year after surgery (Padma-Nathan et al, 2008). However, in another trial involving vardenafil treatment of 9 months either on-demand or daily starting 14 days after surgery, erection recovery was no different in patients using vardenafil by either form of administration or placebo at about 1 year after surgery (Montorsi et al, 2008). Another trial randomizing patients to the use of sildenafil nightly or on-demand for 12 months with a 1-month washout showed that erection recovery was not different between patient groups (Pavlovich et al, 2013). Randomized, controlled trials in other ED contexts have also failed to show sustained natural erectile function improvement after discontinuing continuous regimens of PDE5 inhibitor therapy (Zumbé et al, 2008; Burnett et al, 2009).

The notion of combining PDE5 inhibitors with other ED therapies such as vasoactive penile pharmacotherapies has been proposed (Lau et al, 2006; McMahon et al, 2006). This strategy is to be considered "off-label," and clinical precautions are advised.

α-Adrenoceptor Antagonists. Phentolamine mesylate is a nonspecific α-adrenergic receptor antagonist with equal affinity for blocking both α_1- and α_2-adrenoreceptors. Its mode of action presumably is to produce corporeal smooth muscle relaxation by blocking the (antierectile) postsynaptic α_1-adrenergic receptor (Juenemann et al, 1986). Clinical trials suggested an efficacy rate in men with minimal ED of approximately 40% (Goldstein, 2000). The drug was considered to be relatively safe, with less than 10% of patients using the 40-mg dosage experiencing headaches, facial flushing, or nasal congestion. However, further investigation is required before determining whether it will produce erectile responses of sufficient quality for reliable sexual intercourse, particularly in men with more severe ED.

Yohimbine hydrochloride (Yocon), an indolalkylamine alkaloid derived from the bark of the yohimbe tree, reportedly exerts central effects on the mediation of penile erection operating as an α_2-adrenoreceptor antagonist (Clark, 1991; Giuliano and Rampin, 2000). Originally proposed to be an erectogenic and aphrodisiac agent, the drug has been investigated as an authentic ED treatment. It is conventionally prescribed orally at a dosage of 5.4 mg three times daily with observation for improvement throughout at least a month. A meta-analysis of all randomized, placebo-controlled trials involving yohimbine suggested a superior effect for the medication compared to placebo (Ernst and Pittler, 1998). **However, the drug does not appear to enable successful sexual intercourse any better than placebo in men with confirmed organic ED** (Montague et al, 1996; Telöken et al, 1998). Adverse effects appear to be relatively infrequent but include hypertension, anxiety, tachycardia, and headache. Although yohimbine may be well tolerated, its modest results suggest that it may be best limited to men with psychogenic ED (Porst et al, 2013).

Dopaminergic Agonists. Apomorphine (Uprima, TAP Pharmaceutical Products Inc., Lake Forest, IL) is a dopaminergic agent activating D_1 and D_2 receptors at a central level within the paraventricular nucleus of the brain, indicating its particular relevance in the treatment of men with psychogenic ED (Lal et al, 1987). The medication is administered in sublingual form with a dosage range of 2, 4, and 6 mg, and it has no erectile efficacy if it is swallowed (Heaton, 2000). It has a rapid onset of action, with a mean time to erection of 12 minutes. Apomorphine achieves a maximal plasma concentration in 50 minutes, although its window of opportunity extends for approximately 2 hours from administration. In clinical trials involving men with ED of varying severities and etiologies, the drug achieved a successful sexual intercourse rate of 50.6% at the 4-mg dosage compared with the 33.8% placebo rate (Heaton, 2000). Side effects include nausea (16.9%), dizziness (8.3%), yawning (7.9%), somnolence (5.8%), sweating (5%), and emesis (3.7%). Syncope occurred in 0.6% of patients using the medication at the highest recommended dosage, and this was accompanied by a prodrome consisting of nausea, vomiting, sweating, dizziness, and light-headedness but no cardiac sequelae. Side effects were minimized when patients were titrated from higher to lower dosages. The drug achieved regulatory approval for commercialization by European authorities in early 2001, but it has not been so approved in the United States.

Melanocortin-Receptor Agonists. Melanocortin analogues (e.g., melanotan II, PT-141) have been studied showing efficacy in inducing erectile responses in early clinical trials (Wessells et al, 2000; Diamond et al, 2004). These drugs operate centrally at melanocortin-4 receptors, which have been implicated in controlling food intake and energy expenditure as well as modulating erectile function and sexual behavior. Flushing and nausea have been reported as side effects. The drugs have not achieved regulatory approval for the treatment of ED.

Serotonin-Receptor Effectors. Trazodone (Desyrel) is an antidepressant that has been associated with priapism, prompting its "off-label" investigation as a possible treatment for ED (Lal et al, 1990). It is purported to work through mechanisms at the spinal-cord level with multiple serotonergic effects (Allard and Giuliano, 2001). The active metabolite of trazodone acts as an agonist of the proerectile $5-HT_{2C}$ receptor through reuptake inhibition, with some affinity for the $5-HT_{2A}$ receptor, although it may also operate as an antagonist of antierectile $5-HT_{1A}$ receptors (Andersson and Wagner, 1995). Rigorous evaluations have not shown clinical efficacy that exceeds placebo responses in eliciting penile erection (Costabile and Spevak, 1999). Given its potential side effects (i.e., drowsiness, nausea, emesis, blood pressure changes, urinary retention, and priapism) and general lack of effect, this medication would appear to have a limited role for ED treatment.

Other Oral Therapies. Additional possibilities for the oral treatment of ED, including L-arginine (the amino acid precursor of nitric oxide), L-dopa (dopamine precursor), limaprost (prostaglandin E_1), and naltrexone (opioid antagonist), have been proposed (Burnett, 1999). Each of these agents has a plausible mechanism of action to induce erections. However, they remain insufficiently studied, and their clinical roles remain unclear (Porst et al, 2013).

Intracavernosal Injection

The discovery in 1982 that vasoactive agents, delivered by injection into the penis, induced erections is credited with launching the movement toward medical therapies for the treatment of ED (Virag, 1982; Zorgniotti, 1985). **Since that time, there has been an explosion of basic scientific and clinical research leading to the development and use of various locally administered vasoactive medications having mechanisms of action that result in corporeal smooth muscle relaxation.** Although a host of medications have been explored for this purpose, three medications are used regularly in clinical practice: alprostadil, papaverine, and phentolamine (Table 27-8). **These have been administered clinically as a single agent (i.e., monotherapy) or in various combinations (e.g., bimix, trimix). Combination therapy offers a synergistic mechanism of the vasoactive agents to elicit maximal erectile responses, particularly among patients who have failed monotherapy** (Zorgniotti and Lefleur, 1985; Bennett et al, 1991; Floth and Schramek, 1991; Khera and Goldstein, 2011; Porst et al, 2013). This alternative may also be used to circumvent side effects of a certain agent (e.g., penile pain associated with alprostadil).

A general rule of thumb is to start with a small dose of medication, especially in patients with nonvasculogenic forms of ED. In-office self-injection training and education are recommended before home injection, and this opportunity may also be used to

TABLE 27-8 Intracavernosal Pharmacotherapies

TRADE NAME	DRUG	DOSAGES	EFFICACY (INTERCOURSE)
Caverject	Alprostadil (Prostin VR)	5-40 µg/mL	≈70%
Viradal/Edex	Alprostadil (Prostin VR)	5-40 µg/mL	≈70%
Bimix	Alprostadil + phentolamine	20 µg/mL + 0.5 mg/mL	≈90%
Bimix Androskat (EU)	Papaverine + phentolamine	30 mg/mL + 0.5 mg/mL	≈90%
Trimix	Alprostadil + papaverine + phentolamine	10 µg/mL + 30 mg/mL + 1.0 mg/mL	≈90%
Invicorp	VIP + phentolamine	NA	≈80%

EU, European Union; NA, not available; VIP, vasoactive intestinal polypeptide.

titrate medication toward a dosage that safely yields an erection of sufficient rigidity for sexual intercourse yet lasts no more than an hour (Bénard and Lue, 1990; Fallon, 1995). **The therapy is contraindicated for men with psychological instability, a history or risk for priapism, histories of severe coagulopathy or unstable cardiovascular disease, reduced manual dexterity (although the partner can be trained in the injection technique), and use of monoamine oxidase inhibitors (because of the risk of precipitating a life-threatening hypertensive crisis in the event that an intracavernosal α-adrenergic agonist is used to reverse a priapic episode)** (Sharlip, 1998).

Alprostadil. Alprostadil (Prostin VR) is a synthetic form of a naturally occurring fatty acid, prostaglandin E_1, which binds with specific receptors on smooth muscle cells and activates intracellular adenylate cyclase to produce cAMP, which in turn induces tissue relaxation through a second messenger system (Palmer et al, 1994). It currently is the only FDA-approved injectable medication for ED, and it is marketed for this purpose under the trade names Caverject (Pfizer Inc., New York, NY) and Viradel/Edex (Schwarz Pharma, Milwaukee, WI) (Linet and Ogrinc, 1996; Porst, 1996; Buvat et al, 1998). After intracavernosal injection, the medication is locally metabolized by 96% within 60 minutes and does not appreciably enter the peripheral circulation (van Ahlen et al, 1994). **At dosages of 10 to 20 µg, alprostadil produces full erections in 70% to 80% of patients with ED** (Linet and Neff, 1994; Khera and Goldstein, 2011; Porst et al, 2013). The most common side effects of treatment are pain at the injection site or during erection (in 11% of patients), hematoma/ecchymosis (1.5%), prolonged erection/priapism (1% to 5%), and penile fibrotic lesions (2%) (Linet and Ogrinc, 1996). **Perceived advantages of alprostadil for intracavernosal pharmacotherapy relative to other agents are lower incidences of prolonged erection, systemic side effects, and penile fibrosis. Disadvantages include a higher incidence of painful erection and higher cost, and, after reconstitution into liquid from powder, alprostadil has a shortened half-life if not refrigerated.**

Papaverine. Papaverine, an alkaloid isolated from the opium poppy, is a nonspecific PDE inhibitor that prevents the degradation of cAMP and cGMP so that these cyclic nucleotides accumulate in smooth muscle cells and thereby increasingly promote tissue relaxation (Kukovetz et al, 1975). The compound also blocks voltage-dependent calcium channels along the membrane wall, thus impeding calcium influx to the cell, a process known to trigger smooth muscle contraction (Brading et al, 1983; Sunagane et al, 1985). Papaverine is metabolized in the liver, and the plasma half-life is 1 to 2 hours. Its general efficacy in promoting penile erection after intracavernosal administration is approximately 60% (Porst et al, 2013). The drug is inexpensive and stable at room temperature. However, disadvantages include commonly observed liver enzyme elevations, priapism risk (up to 35%), and penile fibrosis risk (1% to 33%), which have led to its abandonment as monotherapy (Lakin et al, 1990; Fallon, 1995; Porst, 1996; Moemen et al, 2004).

Phentolamine. In addition to its purported oral role for ED therapy, phentolamine mesylate is more familiarly applied as an intracavernosal agent (Regitine). Although its erectogenic effect is mediated by blocking the (antierectile) postsynaptic α_1-adrenergic

receptor (Sironi et al, 2000), because of its potential inhibition of the prejunctional α_2-adrenergic receptor, which interferes with norepinephrine reuptake, the drug's tissue relaxant effect for penile erection is believed to be antagonized (Juenemann et al, 1986). This dual effect of the drug probably accounts for its limited success when administered intracavernosally as a sole agent (Blum et al, 1985). It has a short plasma half-life (30 minutes). Common side effects associated with the drug include systemic hypotension, reflex tachycardia, nasal congestion, and gastrointestinal upset.

Vasoactive Intestinal Polypeptide. Vasoactive intestinal polypeptide (VIP), a hormone having 28 amino acids originally isolated from the small intestine, was proposed early on to be the elusive nonadrenergic noncholinergic (NANC) mediator of penile erection because of its potent vasodilatory effects in various tissues (Adaikan et al, 1986). Its mechanism of action in smooth muscle is achieved through specific protein receptor binding and activation of adenylate cyclase, thereby promoting synthesis of cAMP and subsequent tissue relaxation (Anderson and Wagner, 1995). The drug has had disappointing effects when administered alone, although when separately combined with other drugs such as papaverine and phentolamine, erection responses were elicited (Kiely et al, 1989; Dinsmore and Wyllie, 2008). VIP in combination with phentolamine (Invicorp) is currently being sought for regulatory approval in the United States.

Intraurethral Suppositories

The administration of vasoactive drugs via the urethral channel of the penis was introduced with the hope of affording a less invasive procedure than intracavernosal needle injections to induce penile erection. **This technique relies on the absorption of the medication through the mucosal lining into the surrounding corpus spongiosum, with passage via small vascular channels into the main erectile bodies, the corpora cavernosa.** The transfer of drug from the urethra to the cavernous tissue varies across men according to anatomic variability. Following an initial trial, which demonstrated that prostaglandin E_2 was effective in inducing full tumescence in 30% of patients and partial tumescence in 40% of patients (Wolfson et al, 1993), a synthetic formulation of prostaglandin E_1 was developed and the FDA approved it in November 1996 as MUSE (Medicated Urethral System for Erection, MEDA Pharmaceuticals, Inc., Somerset, NJ) (Hellstrom et al, 1996; Padma-Nathan et al, 1997). MUSE uses a suppository inserted into the urethral opening that dispenses a semisolid pellet (1×3 mm) of alprostadil (125, 250, 500, and 1000 µg dosages) into the distal urethra (3 cm from the external urethral meatus). Several technical procedures optimize the success of the treatment including properly depositing and manually distributing the medication into the penis and the patient's remaining in the upright position for several minutes after its application. In-office training and monitoring of initial response may afford advantages for optimizing technique and making dosage adjustments before performing the treatment at home.

A calculated final responder rate to MUSE is approximately 50%, and among responders approximately 70% of administrations result in sexual intercourse (Hellstrom et al, 1996;

Padma-Nathan et al, 1997; Guay et al, 2000; Khera and Goldstein, 2011; Porst et al, 2013). The combined use of an adjustable penile constriction band (ACTIS) was designed and was approved by the FDA to enhance the local retention and effect of the medication (Lewis, 2000). A transurethral bimix consisting of alprostadil and α_1-adrenergic antagonist prazosin (ALIBRA) was introduced and in a multicenter trial of nearly 400 patients was shown to increase the at-home responder rate for successful sexual intercourse from 47% with alprostadil alone to 70% with ALIBRA (Qureshi, 2001).

Intraurethral therapy is perceived to have a niche role, associated with its inferior efficacy both with regard to PDE5 inhibitors and intracavernosal self-injection therapy (Khera and Goldstein, 2011; Porst et al, 2013). The main indications for this therapy are patients who are nonresponsive to PDE5 inhibitors resulting from damage of the autonomic penile nerve supply (e.g., radical prostatectomy, cystectomy, and trauma) or those who wish to use the therapy in combination with PDE5 inhibitors. Another rare indication for intraurethral therapy is patients complaining about a soft (cold) glans syndrome, which may occur after penile prosthesis implantation or as a clinical entity itself (Porst et al, 2013).

The most common side effects of MUSE include local urogenital pain (approximately one third of patients) and minor urethral bleeding (5%) (Padma-Nathan et al, 1997; Guay et al, 2000). Other complications such as hypotension (3%), dizziness (4%), and priapism (0.1%) have been observed as well. MUSE is contraindicated in patients with known hypersensitivity to alprostadil, abnormal penile anatomy, and conditions that increase the risk of priapism. MUSE seems safe for female partners, producing only a 5.8% incidence of vaginal burning or itching, although it should not be used without a condom for intercourse with a pregnant woman.

Transdermal/Topical Pharmacotherapy

The notion to apply vasoactive drugs directly to the surface of the penis is consistent with the general appeal of many transdermal therapies (e.g., gels and creams) in medicine based on their delivery route: convenience, simplicity, and putatively limited systemic adverse effects. Several topical therapies have been explored for ED treatments, although certain obstacles have limited their widespread use. Nitroglycerin, a nitric oxide donor formulated as a 2% paste, was found to produce tumescence but rarely penile rigidity sufficient for sexual intercourse (Owen et al, 1989). This relative inefficacy combined with its headache side effects for both patient and partner following absorption and action of the drug as a potent systemic vasodilator have precluded its use in clinical practice. Papaverine, formulated as a gel, was investigated but then abandoned as a topical ED treatment when it was found that its large molecular size (molecular weight 376 Da) interfered with its transdermal absorption (Kim et al, 1995).

Alprostadil has been a more promising prospect, subjected to commercial development for penile glans administration in combination with transdermal delivery enhancers: alprostadil 0.3% in combination with a proprietary permeation enhancer, referred to as Vitaros (Apricus Biosciences, San Diego, CA), and alprostadil combined with NexACT, referred to as Alprox-TD (NexMed, Inc., Robbinsville, NJ). Applied intrameatally, such agents in clinical trials have shown efficacy with rates of vaginal penetration and intercourse success that were small but significantly greater than placebo rates and caused minor side effects of site-specific burning or warmth that were comparable to placebo rates (McVary et al, 1999; Goldstein et al, 2001; McMahon, 2002; Padma-Nathan and Yeager, 2006; Rooney et al, 2009; Porst et al, 2013). Prostaglandin E_1 ethyl ester, which is a prodrug of prostaglandin E_1, is believed to possess an improved transdermal permeation and less skin irritation than enhancing agents because of its esterification (Schanz et al, 2009). Applied to the shaft of the penis in early clinical trials, this drug achieved significantly higher rigidity scores than placebo. In general, transdermal therapy with alprostadil is likely to meet similar clinical roles as that assigned to transurethral pharmacotherapy. Further clinical trials will be useful to define and establish their place in the treatment of ED.

Medical Device

In patients who do not respond to or who decline oral or local vasoactive pharmacotherapeutic options, vacuum erection device therapy may be alternatively explored. **The principle of vacuum erection device therapy is to mechanically create negative pressure surrounding the penis to engorge it with blood and then restrain blood egress from the organ to maintain the erection-like effect** (Nadig et al, 1986; Broderick et al, 1992). Although the treatment does not produce a truly physiologic erection and the engorged blood predominantly consists of venous blood (Bosshardt et al, 1995), the effect resembles a normal erection and is sufficient for coitus. A particular feature is that the glans penis, and not solely the corpora cavernosa, is engorged with blood by the treatment, such that the treatment is further advantageous for patients experiencing glanular insufficiency (soft glans syndrome).

The standard vacuum erection device consists of a usually clear plastic suction cylinder and vacuum-generating source (manual or battery-operated pump) in one piece. It is placed directly over the flaccid penis and operated, and after the penis is erected an elastic constriction ring or band is positioned at the base of the penis; then the vacuum is released and the device is removed (Montague et al, 1996; McMahon, 1997). **The cylinder has a pressure-release valve designed to prevent penile injury from excessive negative pressure. Sexual intercourse may then ensue, although it is recommended that the ring should not be left in place for longer than 30 minutes. Prescription devices are advised, and metal or other inelastic rings are contraindicated.**

Efficacy rates as high as 90% have been reported for achieving satisfactory erections for ED associated with various severities and etiologies, but satisfaction rates with the device are lower, ranging commonly from 30% to 70% (Hellstrom et al, 2010; Porst et al, 2013). Attrition is reported to occur and may relate to lack of efficacy with more severe forms of ED, although long-term continuation rates have ranged up to 60% (Porst et al, 2013). Success is limited in patients with severe vascular abnormalities such as proximal venous leakage or arterial insufficiency or fibrosis secondary to priapism or prosthesis infection (Marmar et al, 1988). Patient preferences also dictate long-term success. The device is more acceptable to older men in a steady relationship compared to young, single men. Among basic expectations of the treatment, patients should be informed of possible local discomfort or pain associated with the constriction band, a pivoting effect of the penis because turgidity exists only distal to the band's location, a cyanotic discoloration and coolness of the penis resulting from extracorporeal congestion, and trapping of the ejaculation caused by urethral constriction (Witherington, 1989; Sidi et al, 1990; Cookson and Nadig, 1993). Common complications are minor and include penile pain and numbness, difficult ejaculation, ecchymosis, and petechiae, and major complications (e.g., penile skin necrosis, urethral varicosities, Fournier gangrene) are infrequent. Patients receiving anticoagulant therapy (e.g., aspirin, warfarin) and patients with bleeding disorders should use the device with caution (Limoge et al, 1996). Special uses for this therapy have been sought. It has been successfully combined with oral, intracavernosal, and intraurethral pharmacotherapies to produce erectile responses (Marmar et al, 1988; Chen et al, 1995; John et al, 1996; Chen et al, 2004; Canguven et al, 2009). The device has enhanced erectile effects in the presence of a malfunctioning penile prosthesis (Sidi et al, 1990; Korenman and Viosca, 1992). Further, it may offer a means to preserve the elasticity of penile tissues after priapism or penile prosthesis explantation (Moul and McLeod, 1989; Soderdahl et al, 1997) or after surgical correction of Peyronie disease (Yurkanin et al, 2001), and it has been suggested to facilitate erection recovery after treatments for prostate cancer (Raina et al, 2006; Köhler et al, 2007).

Surgery

Surgical interventions have always served an important role in the armamentarium of ED treatments. **They are often applied in the** face of penile injury resulting from genital or pelvic trauma, penile structural deformity occurring in association with Peyronie disease, or possibly cavernosal fibrosis secondary to prolonged ischemic priapism or infection. They are also considered when medical therapy for ED is contraindicated, unsuccessful, or undesirable.

Penile Prosthesis Surgery

Penile prosthesis or implant surgery is a mechanism for creating penile rigidity that differs from a physiologic or pharmacologically induced erection. Malleable (semirigid) and inflatable (hydraulic) devices are both currently available for this purpose. Details of this treatment option are presented elsewhere.

Penile Revascularization Surgery

Based on the requirements of inflow of blood and its retention in the penis for penile erection to occur, it is hardly a wonder to think that vascular surgeries have aggressively been pursued to facilitate or restore these biologic processes.

Arterial Revascularization. In concept, arterial revascularization surgery was designed to create arterial inflow to the corpora cavernosa, in turn addressing the presentation of arteriogenic ED. Several procedures have been described to meet this objective, similarly creating an anastomosis of the inferior epigastric artery either to the corpus cavenosum directly or to vascular conduits of the penis such as the dorsal artery (i.e., revascularization), the deep dorsal vein (i.e., arterialization), or the deep dorsal vein with venous ligation (i.e., arterialization with venous reconstruction) (Hellstrom et al, 2010). Success of these surgeries has been variable and depends on careful patient selection. Penile arteriography is required to establish a penile arterial anatomic defect, and other organic causes of ED (e.g., venous incompetence) that would limit surgical success should be excluded. **According to the current literature, the following inclusion criteria should be met when selecting patients for arterial surgery: age less than 55 years, nonsmoker, nondiabetic, absence of venous leakage, and radiographic confirmation of stenosis of the internal pudendal artery** (Hellstrom et al, 2010; Sohn et al, 2013). **The highest success rates are reported in young men (less than 30 years of age) with isolated arterial stenosis following perineal or pelvic trauma** (Babaei et al, 2009). Complications of arterial revascularization surgery include glans hyperemia (13%), shunt thrombosis (8%), and inguinal hernias (6.5%) (Manning et al, 1998; Kawanishi et al, 2004).

Venous Reconstruction. Venous reconstruction was proposed to prevent the pathologic blood egress from the penis, understandably serving to correct veno-occlusive ED. Most surgical procedures have centered on ligating or embolizing penile veins (e.g., superficial dorsal vein, deep dorsal vein, crural vein) or surgically compressing the penile crura (e.g., crural plication/ligation, pericavernoplasty) (Hellstrom et al, 2010). **Success with these surgeries has not been affirmed, owing primarily to inaccurate or deficient methods for diagnosing and correcting the relevant anatomic defect. The optimal surgical approach remains to be defined, and thus venous reconstructive surgery is presently considered investigational** (Montague et al, 2005; Hellstrom et al, 2010; Sohn et al, 2013). Reported complications of this surgery include glanular hypo/anesthesia, skin necrosis, wound infections, penile curvature/shortening, and glans hyperemia.

Combination Therapies

It is well recognized that many patients with ED will not respond acceptably to monotherapy, with nonresponder rates documented as high as 40% of patients (Porst et al, 2013). Some patients indeed may achieve optimal therapeutic responses by combining treatment options. In addition, it is possible that a dose-limiting adverse effect is associated with ED monotherapy such that combined treatments may then seem advantageous. Multiple combinations may

certainly be proposed for ED treatment. The extant literature describes several successful combinations: oral PDE5 inhibitors with psychosocial counseling (Althof et al, 2005), oral PDE5 inhibitors with testosterone replacement therapy (Shabsigh et al, 2004), oral PDE5 inhibitors with transurethral alprostadil (Mydlo et al, 2000; Nehra et al, 2002), oral PDE5 inhibitor and intracavernosal pharmacotherapy (McMahon et al, 1999), oral PDE5 inhibitor and vacuum erection device (Chen et al, 2004; Canguven et al, 2009), intracavernosal pharmacotherapy and vacuum erection device (Chen et al, 1995), transurethral pharmacotherapy and vacuum erection device (John et al, 1996), and transurethral pharmacotherapy and penile prosthesis surgery (Benevides and Carson, 2000). **Caution is advised when initiating combination therapy to observe for potential complications that may be compounded by combined treatments, and in-office evaluations before continuing treatments at home may be considered to offer an additional measure of safety.**

Alternative Therapies

Alternative therapies have long been considered for the treatment of ED, from herbs, ointments, and concoctions of antiquity to vitamins, nutraceuticals, and dietary supplements in commercial supply today. The movement toward alternative medicines in this field actually gained momentum during the past decade with the emergence of effective oral therapy in the form of PDE5 inhibitors, which created avenues for producing PDE5 inhibitor-like counterfeit and imitation substances and promoting regulatory agency unapproved products in general. Indeed, the true efficacies of proposed alternative therapies (e.g., ginkgo biloba, L-arginine, Korean red ginseng) remain uncertain in the absence of evidenced benefit in rigorously performed, randomized, controlled clinical trials (Moyad et al, 2004; Khera and Goldstein, 2011). The success of these products is ascribed in some measure to the known placebo effect of agents to treat ED, which has been observed to amount to as much as 25% to 50% in properly conducted clinical trials. **Before the use of alternative therapies can be advocated, further research that demonstrates their mechanisms of action and meaningful efficacies must be performed.**

KEY POINTS: TREATMENT CONSIDERATIONS

- An informed decision-making process that combines goals and preferences of the patient (and partner) and balanced and thorough guidance of the clinician should dictate the best therapeutic option.
- Although definitive evidence is necessary to affirm the benefits of risk modification for preserving erectile health, recommendations are offered to maintain a healthy and fit lifestyle for this purpose.
- Patient education and counseling and application of medical therapies as initial forms of ED management constitute basic management in common practice.
- Psychosexual therapy offers a role in the integrative management of ED.
- Several pharmacotherapies administered by various modalities including oral, intracavernosal, intraurethral, and transdermal/topical routes are successfully applied or are under study as ED treatments.
- Vacuum erection device therapy offers an alternative to oral or local vasoactive pharmacotherapeutic options for ED.
- Surgical intervention, principally penile prosthesis surgery, represents an important ED treatment and may be considered when medical (nonsurgical) therapy is contraindicated, unsuccessful, or undesirable.
- Arterial revascularization surgery is offered only to selected patients with ED who meet stringent clinical and radiographic criteria for surgical success.

FUTURE DIRECTIONS

Impressive progress has been made in the field of ED management, encompassing all areas of epidemiology, basic scientific research, clinical investigation, and health services research. Future directions will assuredly continue with particular interest directed to new therapeutics. In the near future, pharmacotherapies will likely remain center stage, further driven by research discoveries in the molecular and cellular mechanisms responsible for the erectile response. Technologic advances in the way of interventional devices have rapidly gained interest. Alternatives such as implanting zotarolimus-eluting peripheral stents in atherosclerotic lesions of the internal pudendal arteries (Rogers et al, 2012) and low-intensity extracorporeal shockwave therapy applied to the penis (Vardi et al, 2012) are currently under study, supporting the idea that these and other such interventions may achieve the goal of restoring erectile function or improving it effectively for the long term. Futuristic approaches such as gene therapy, stem-cell therapy, and tissue engineering have been mainly advanced at the preclinical stage of development with the same long-term purpose, although their eventual roles remain eagerly anticipated. The future of this field looks exciting and should foster the very best outcomes for patients experiencing ED.

REFERENCES

The complete reference list is available online at www.expertconsult.com.

SUGGESTED READINGS

Bhasin S, Cunningham GR, Hayes FJ, et al. Testosterone therapy in men with androgen deficiency syndromes: an Endocrine Society clinical practice guideline. J Clin Endocrinol Metab 2010;95:2536–59.

Khera M, Goldstein I. Erectile dysfunction. Clin Evid (Online) 2011;Jun 29:1803.

Lewis RW, Fugl-Meyer KS, Corona G, et al. Definitions/epidemiology/risk factors for sexual dysfunction. J Sex Med 2010;7:1598–607.

Montague DK, Jarow JP, Broderick GA, et al. Chapter 1: the management of erectile dysfunction: an AUA update. J Urol 2005;174:230–9.

Montorsi F, Adaikan G, Becher E, et al. Summary of the recommendations on sexual dysfunctions in men. J Sex Med 2010;7:3572–88.

Porst H, Burnett A, Brock G, et al. SOP conservative (medical and mechanical) treatment of erectile dysfunction. J Sex Med 2013;10:130–71.

28 Priapism

Gregory A. Broderick, MD

Priapism is a persistent erection arising from dysfunction of the mechanisms regulating penile tumescence, rigidity, and flaccidity. A correct diagnosis of priapism is a matter of urgency requiring identification of the underlying hemodynamics.

Scientific organizations have recommended guidelines for the management of priapism, including the American Urological Association (AUA) in 2003 (www.auanet.org) and the International Society for Sexual Medicine in 2006 (www.issm.info). Both groups have noted that the literature on priapism is composed mainly of small case series and individual case reports and includes inconsistent definitions and methodologies with few long-term erectile function outcome data. Recent case series have included detailed methodology including duration of priapism, cause of priapism, and erectile function outcomes. The basic science on the pathogenesis of priapism and clinical research supporting the most effective treatment strategies are summarized in this chapter. Recommendations for best clinical practice and suggestions for research are made.

DEFINING PRIAPISM

Priapism is a full or partial erection that continues more than 4 hours beyond sexual stimulation and orgasm or is unrelated to sexual stimulation.

Ischemic Priapism (Veno-Occlusive, Low-Flow)

Ischemic priapism is a persistent erection marked by rigidity of the corpora cavernosa (CC) and little or no cavernous arterial inflow. In ischemic priapism there are time-dependent changes in the corporal metabolic environment with progressive hypoxia, hypercarbia, and acidosis. The patient typically reports penile pain after 6 to 8 hours, and the examination reveals a rigid erection. The condition is analogous to a muscle compartment syndrome, with initial occlusion of venous outflow and subsequent cessation of arterial inflows. Well-documented histologic changes occur within the corporal smooth muscle as a consequence of prolonged ischemia. **Interventions beyond 48 to 72 hours of onset may help relieve erection and pain but have little benefit in preserving potency.** Histologically, by 12 hours corporal specimens show interstitial edema, progressing to destruction of sinusoidal endothelium, exposure of the basement membrane, and thrombocyte adherence at 24 hours. After 48 hours thrombus can be found in the sinusoidal spaces, and smooth muscle necrosis with fibroblast-like cell transformation is evident (Spycher and Hauri, 1986). **Ischemic priapism is an emergency. When left untreated, resolution may take days and erectile dysfunction (ED) invariably results** (Fig. 28-1A and B).

Stuttering Priapism (Intermittent)

Stuttering priapism is characterized by a pattern of recurrence. The term has historically described recurrent unwanted and painful erections in men with sickle cell disease (SCD) (Serjeant et al, 1985). Patients typically awaken with an erection that persists for several hours. Males with SCD may experience stuttering priapism from childhood; in these patients the pattern of stuttering may increase in frequency and duration, leading to a full episode of unrelenting ischemic priapism. Any patient who has experienced an episode of ischemic priapism is also at risk for stuttering priapism.

Nonischemic Priapism (Arterial, High-Flow)

Nonischemic priapism is a persistent erection caused by unregulated cavernous arterial inflow. Typically, the corpora are tumescent but not rigid and the penis is not painful. A history of blunt trauma to the penis or an iatrogenic needle injury is common. Whatever the mechanism of injury, the result is a disruption of the cavernous arterial anatomy creating an arteriolar-sinusoidal fistula. **The cavernous environment does not become ischemic and cavernous blood gases do not show hypoxia, hypercarbia, or acidosis. This type of priapism, once properly diagnosed, does not require emergent intervention.** Beyond the acute trauma, patients do not report pain. Normal erectile function has been reported after recovery from the initial event, despite persistence of nonsexual partial erection.

PRIAPISM: HISTORICAL PERSPECTIVES

The term *priapism* has its origin in reference to the Greek god Priapus, who was worshipped as a god of fertility and protector of horticulture. Priapus is memorialized in sculptures for his giant phallus. The first recorded account of priapism in English medical literature appears in the *Lancet* and is attributed to Tripe (1845). Historically, the most commonly cited observation on this condition in North American literature is Frank Hinman Sr.'s

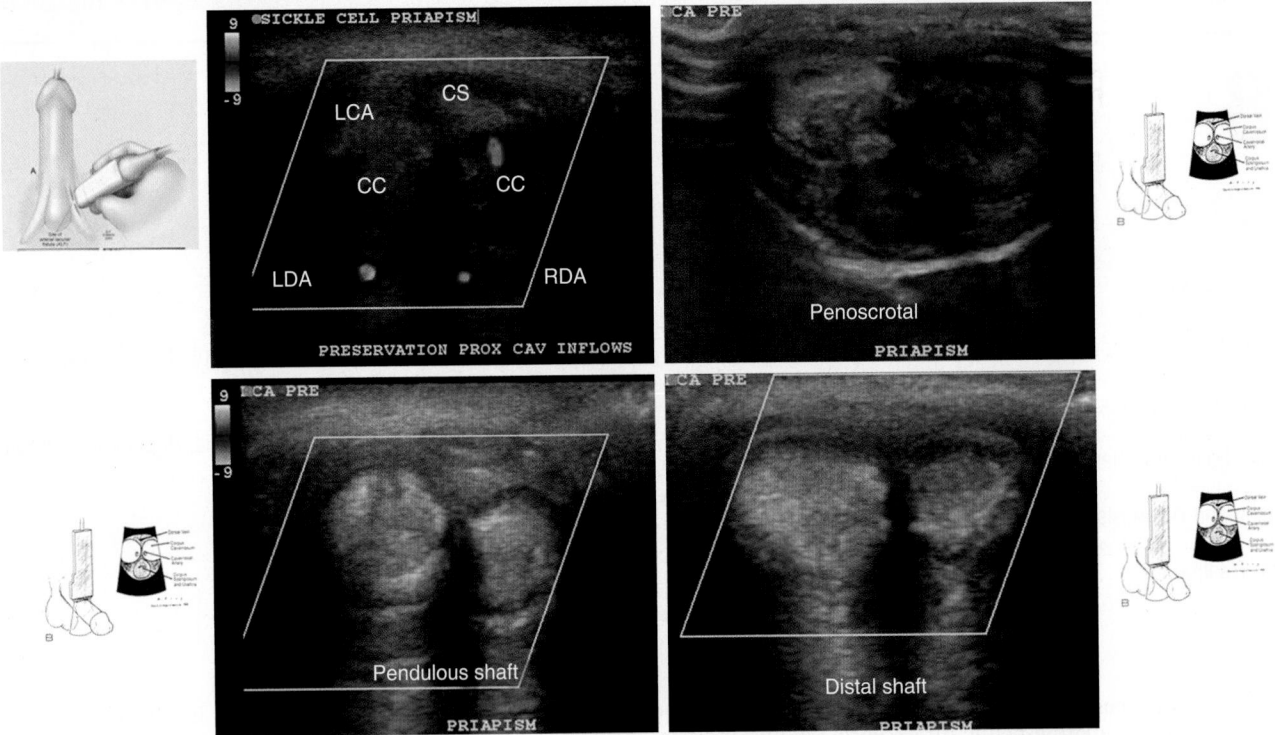

Figure 28-1. This 21-year-old Nigerian man had erectile dysfunction after recurrent episodes of sickle cell ischemic priapism. A, Transperineal imaging with color Doppler shows preservation of cavernous arterial inflow at the origin in the corpora cavernosa. B to D, Increasing echogenicity on gray-scale ultrasound of the penile shaft: penoscrotal, pendulous shaft, and distal shaft. These findings are the result of recurring ischemic priapism, which leaves the patient with distal corporal fibrosis. CC, corpora cavernosa; CS, corpus spongiosum; LCA, left cavernous artery; LDA, left dorsal artery; RDA, right dorsal artery.

landmark article describing the natural history of priapism (Hinman, 1914). Subsequently in 1960 his son, Frank Hinman Jr., proposed that venous stasis, increased blood viscosity, and ischemia were responsible for priapism and emphasized that failure to correct these abnormalities in the penile environment was essentially responsible for treatment nonresponse (Hinman, 1960). Advances in our understanding of the physiology of erection and the pathophysiology of ED substantiated early hypotheses that prolonged veno-occlusion within the corporal bodies is analogous to a compartment syndrome. Hauri and colleagues demonstrated the radiologic differences between veno-occlusive and arterial priapism (1983).

Frank Hinman (1914) first described "acute transitory attacks of priapism" as opposed to persistence or rapid recurrence of a single episode. The actual term *stuttering priapism* is attributed to Emond and colleagues (1980) in observations of patients with SCD in a Jamaican clinic. Stuttering priapism episodes were seen to increase in frequency and length, leading to major, unrelenting occurrence of ischemic priapism. Attempts to manage SCD patients with stuttering ischemic priapism resulted in the early recommendation for hormonal suppression of nocturnal erections and stuttering with estrogen (Serjeant et al, 1985).

Nonischemic priapism is described far less commonly than ischemic priapism in the urologic literature. **Nonischemic priapism is invariably associated with antecedent perineal or penile trauma.** It was first described in the English literature by Burt (Burt et al, 1960).

EPIDEMIOLOGY AND PATHOPHYSIOLOGY OF PRIAPISM

Etiology of Ischemic Priapism (Veno-Occlusive, Low-Flow)

Ischemic priapism accounts for the majority of cases described in the literature. The erection of ischemic priapism may begin with

---

KEY POINTS: PRIAPISM DEFINITIONS

- Priapism is a full or partial erection that continues more than 4 hours beyond sexual stimulation and orgasm or is unrelated to sexual stimulation.
- Ischemic (low-flow) priapism is a persistent erection marked by rigidity of the CC, with little or no cavernous arterial inflow.
- Nonischemic (arterial, high-flow) priapism is a persistent erection caused by unregulated cavernous arterial inflow. The corpora are tumescent but not rigid, and the erection is not painful.
- Stuttering priapism describes a pattern of recurrence. The term has traditionally described recurrent prolonged and painful erections in men with SCD.

---

sexual stimulation or the administration of pharmacologic agents. **Once an erection persists beyond 4 hours and is not relieved by orgasm or pharmacologic reversal, the pathophysiologic phenomena of ischemic priapism have begun.** Erections lasting up to 4 hours are by consensus defined as "prolonged"; manufacturers of erection-facilitating pharmacotherapies (oral, injectable, and intraurethral) recommend that the patient seek emergent medical consultation for prolonged erection.

Population-based studies estimate cases per 100,000 person-years (the number of patients with a first episode of priapism divided by the accumulated amount of person-time in the study population). Cases per 100,000 person-years have been calculated in several countries; these data depend on recording of presentations to clinics and hospitals where cases are registered. Kulmala and colleagues (1995) calculated the cases per 100,000 person-years to be 0.34 to 0.52 from 1975 to 1990 in Finland; Eland and colleagues (2001) calculated the cases in the Netherlands to be 1.5 per 100,000 person-years; Earle and colleagues (2003) calculated 0.84 per 100,000 person-years in Australia from 1985 to 2000. These reported incidence rates were statistically significantly affected by the introduction and proliferation of intracavernous vasoactive injections for the management of ED; in Finland during the last 3 years of the study the incidence of priapism doubled to 1.1 cases per 100,000 person-years. These and other reports on the epidemiology and etiology of priapism are also greatly influenced by the prevalence of SCD in the populations described. **The lifetime probability of a man with SCD developing ischemic priapism ranges from 29% to 42%** (Emond et al, 1980). Two retrospective analyses—the Nationwide Inpatient Sample (NIS) and the Nationwide Emergency Department Sample—provide estimates of the incidence of priapism in the United States. Chrouser and colleagues (2011) accessed data from the NIS (1998 to 2006); the NIS database extrapolation suggests that 1868 to 2960 patients with priapism are admitted annually to hospitals in the United States. In the actual sample (4237 hospitalizations), 30% of patients were white, 61.1% were black, and 6.3% were Hispanic; 41.9% of patients had a diagnosis of SCD; and 36.2% of patients required penile surgery. The mean age at time of hospital admission for priapism associated with SCD was 23.8 years and for non-SCD was 40.8 years. Roghmann and colleagues (2013) looked at the Nationwide Emergency Department Sample. They estimated that from 2006 to 2009 there were 32,462 emergency department visits for priapism. The number of emergency department visits for priapism in the United States was higher during summer, and 13.3% of patients were admitted to the hospital.

In 1986 Pohl and colleagues reported on 230 cases. The cause of priapism was identified as idiopathic in the majority; 21% of cases were associated with alcohol or drug use or abuse, 12% with perineal trauma, and 11% with SCD (Pohl et al, 1986). Although SCD is a predominant cause of veno-occlusive priapism in the literature, there is a wide variety of reported associations from urinary retention to insect bites (Hoover and Fortenberry, 2004). Priapism has even been reported after spider bites and envenomation from the Brazilian banana spider, *Phoneutria nigriventer* (Andrade et al, 2008; Villanova et al, 2009). The genus *Phoneutria* (from the Greek for "murderess") has eight species. *P. nigriventer* is known to hide in dark and moist places, wander the jungle floor, and stow away within banana shipments. *P. nigriventer* is blamed for most cases of envenomation in Brazil; the venom contains a neurotoxin that has calcium channel blocking properties, inhibits glutamate release, and inhibits calcium reuptake and glutamate reuptake. Bites can cause intense pain, loss of muscle control—paralysis, breathing problems—asphyxiation, and priapism. Two peptides isolated from the venom of *P. nigriventer* have been directly linked with the induction of persistent and painful erections in mammals (Tx2-5 and Tx2-6) (Leite et al, 2012). The protein has been named *eretina* and has been shown to have a highly specific interference at the molecular level with the nitric oxide pathway (NO). Penile erection has been induced in vivo with eretina by direct intraperitoneal injection with a minimum effective dose of 0.006 µg/kg (Andrade et al, 2008).

Hematologic dyscrasias are a major risk factor for ischemic priapism. Priapism has been described as a complication of SCD, thalassemia, hereditary spherocytosis, paroxysmal nocturnal hemoglobinuria, glucose-6-phosphate dehydrogenase deficiency, glucose-6-phosphate isomerase deficiency, and congenital dyserythropoietic anemia (Burnett, 2005; Kato, 2012). **Thrombotic disease states have also been cited as precipitants of ischemic priapism;** these conditions include asplenia, erythropoietin use, hemodialysis with heparin use, and cessation of Coumadin therapy. Intracavernous heparin given as a therapy for priapism caused by rebound hypercoagulable states has actually worsened the condition (Fassbinder et al, 1976; Bschleipfer et al, 2001). **Priapism may occur in patients with excessive white blood cell (WBC) counts.** The incidence of priapism in adult male patients with leukemia is 1% to 5% (Chang et al, 2003). Hyperleukocytosis causes priapism in these patients; it

is believed that mechanical pressure on abdominal veins secondary to splenomegaly causes congestion of cavernous outflow and sludging of leukemic cells within the CC. When priapism occurs in the oncology setting, evaluation and management of the predisposing condition must accompany interventions directed at the penis. In hematologic malignancies, leukapheresis and cytotoxic therapy (hydroxyurea, cytosine arabinoside) may reduce the numbers of circulating WBCs (Ponniah et al, 2004; Manuel et al, 2007). **Priapism secondary to metastatic infiltrating solid lesions rather than leukemoid reaction is extremely rare.** In most case reports of metastatic priapism, the primary malignancy is genitourinary (prostate and bladder). Metastatic infiltration of the penis may proceed with solid replacement or focal deposits within the CC, glans, and corpus spongiosum. Theoretically, metastatic deposits within the corpora could obstruct venous outflow, resulting in ischemic priapism. Depending on the status of the patient, metastatic lesions may be managed expectantly, with partial or total penectomy, chemotherapy, or irradiation. These cases are too rarely and poorly described to define best practice recommendations (Robey and Schellhammer, 1984; Chan et al, 1998; Guvel et al, 2003; Celma Doménech et al, 2008) (Box 28-1).

Sickle Cell Disease

Blood dyscrasias are a risk factor for ischemic priapism. SCD priapism has traditionally been ascribed to stagnation of blood within the sinusoids of the CC during physiologic erection, secondary to obstruction of venous outflow by sickled erythrocytes (Lue, 2002). Nelson and Winter (1977) described a series of cases in which SCD was the primary cause of ischemic priapism in 23% of adults and 63% of children. **Sickle cell hemoglobinopathy accounts for at least a third of all cases of priapism,** and, indeed, prevalence of ischemic priapism varies significantly within the population of males in a community with SCD. **From Emond and colleagues' 1980 observational study comes the most commonly quoted incidence: Among 104 men attending an outpatient sickle cell clinic in Kingston, Jamaica, the incidence of priapism in men with homozygous sickle cell (SS) disease was 42%** (Emond et al, 1980). In a U.S. clinical series, Tarry and associates (1987) found that 6.4% of male children in an outpatient sickle cell clinic had a history of priapism. Adeyoju and colleagues (2002), in an international multicenter observational study of SCD, mailed or interviewed 130 patients attending SCD clinics in the United Kingdom and Nigeria. Respondents ranged in age from 4 to 66 years old, with a mean age of 25. The authors cited mean age of onset of priapism as 15 years, with 75% of patients having their first episode before age 20 and rare first-time presentations by the third decade of life. In the questionnaires a clear distinction was made between acute severe prolonged priapism lasting longer than 24 hours requiring emergency attention and stuttering recurrent priapism of shorter and self-limiting duration. In this population the incidence of acute priapism was 35%; of these patients, 72% gave a history of stuttering priapism. The median frequency of occurrence of stuttering priapism was three times per month; the median duration of each episode was 1.2 hours, with the longest being 8 hours. Precipitating events reported from greatest to least were sexual arousal or intercourse, fever, sleep, cold weather, and dehydration. Self-administered regimens were analgesics, drinking water, and exercise. Twenty-one percent of patients reporting a history of priapism also reported ED. Only 7% of young men who had not experienced priapism were even aware that priapism was a potential complication of their SCD. On the basis of the World Health Organization global prevalence map of SCD, Aliyu and colleagues (2008) estimated that 20 to 25 million individuals worldwide have homozygous SCD: 12 to 15 million in sub-Saharan Africa, 5 to 10 million in India, and 3 million in other world regions. They also found that 70,000 patients with SCD live in the United States (Aliyu et al, 2008).

The sickle cell genetic mutation is the result of a single amino acid substitution in the β-globin subunit of hemoglobin S (HbS). The clinical features are seen in homozygous SCD patients: chronic hemolysis, vascular occlusion, tissue ischemia, and

BOX 28-1 Causes of Priapism

α-ADRENERGIC RECEPTOR ANTAGONISTS
Prazosin, terazosin, doxazosin, tamsulosin

ANTIANXIETY AGENT
Hydroxyzine

ANTICOAGULANTS
Heparin, warfarin

ANTIDEPRESSANTS AND ANTIPSYCHOTICS
Trazodone, bupropion, fluoxetine, sertraline, lithium, clozapine, risperidone, olanzapine, chlorpromazine, thioridazine, phenothiazines

ANTIHYPERTENSIVES
Hydralazine, guanethidine, propranolol

ATTENTION-DEFICIT/HYPERACTIVITY DISORDER AGENTS
Methylphenidates (Concerta, Daytrana, Focalin, Metadate, Methylin, Quillivant, Ritalin)
Atomoxetine (Strattera)

RECREATIONAL DRUGS
Alcohol, cocaine (intranasal and topical), crack cocaine, marijuana

GENITOURINARY CONDITIONS
Straddle injury, coital injury, pelvic trauma, kick to penis or perineum, arteriovenous or arteriocavernous bypass surgery, urinary retention

HEMATOLOGIC DYSCRASIAS
Sickle cell disease, thalassemia, granulocytic leukemia, myeloid leukemia, lymphocytic leukemia, multiple myeloma, hemoglobin Olmsted variant, fat emboli associated with hyperalimentation, hemodialysis, glucose-6-phosphate dehydrogenase deficiency

HORMONES
Gonadotropin-releasing hormone, testosterone

INFECTIOUS (TOXIN-MEDIATED) CAUSES
Scorpion sting, spider bite, rabies, malaria

METABOLIC CONDITIONS
Amyloidosis, Fabry disease, gout

NEOPLASTIC CAUSES (METASTATIC OR REGIONAL INFILTRATION)
Prostate, urethra, testis, bladder, rectum, lung, kidney

NEUROGENIC CONDITIONS
Syphilis, spinal cord injury, cauda equina compression, autonomic neuropathy, lumbar disk herniation, spinal stenosis, cerebral vascular accident, brain tumor, spinal anesthesia, cauda equina syndrome

VASOACTIVE ERECTILE AGENTS
Papaverine, phentolamine, prostaglandin E_1, oral phosphodiesterase type 5 inhibitors, combination intracavernous therapy

Modified from Lue TF. Physiology of penile erection and pathophysiology of erectile dysfunction and priapism. In: Walsh PC, Retik AB, Vaughan ED, et al, editors. Campbell's urology. Philadelphia: Saunders; 2002. p. 1610–96.

end-organ damage. HbS polymerizes when deoxygenated, injuring the sickle erythrocyte, activating a cascade of hemolysis and vaso-occlusion. Membrane damage results in dense sickling of red cells, causing adhesive interactions among sickle cells, endothelial cells, and leukocytes. Hemolysis releases hemoglobin into the plasma. Free hemoglobin reacts with NO to produce methemoglobin and nitrate. This is a scavenging reaction; the vasodilator NO is oxidized to inert nitrate. Sickled erythrocytes release arginase-I into blood plasma, which converts L-arginine into ornithine, effectively removing substrate for NO synthesis. Oxidant radicals further reduce NO bioavailability. The combined effects of NO scavenging and arginine catabolism result in a state of NO resistance and insufficiency termed *hemolysis-associated endothelial dysfunction* (Morris et al, 2005; Rother et al, 2005; Kato et al, 2007; Aliyu et al, 2008).

Contemporary science implicates hemolysis and reduced NO in the pathogenesis of pulmonary hypertension, leg ulcers, priapism, and stroke in SCD patients, whereas increased blood viscosity is believed to be responsible for painful crises, osteonecrosis, and acute chest syndrome (Kato, 2012; Kato et al, 2006). SCD patients with priapism have a fivefold greater risk of developing pulmonary hypertension. SCD priapism is also associated with reduced hemoglobin levels and increased hemolytic markers: reticulocyte count, bilirubin, lactate dehydrogenase, and aspartate aminotransferase. Cerebral vascular accidents are more frequent, close to episodes of full-blown priapism; the ASPEN syndrome (association of SCD, priapism, exchange transfusion, and neurologic events) describes cerebral vascular accidents in SCD patients who have received exchange transfusions (Siegel et al, 1993; Merritt et al, 2006). Sickle cell trait is considered a benign condition; a few complications have been associated with

extreme physical exertion. There have been case reports of sickle cell trait as the predisposing factor to ischemic priapism (Larocque and Cosgrove, 1974; Birnbaum and Pinzone, 2008).

Iatrogenic Priapism: Intracavernous Injections

Prolonged erection is more commonly reported than is priapism after therapeutic or diagnostic injection of intracavernous vasoactive medications (Broderick and Lue, 2002). Despite the introduction of effective oral medications for ED in 1998, intracavernous injection (ICI) remains an important therapeutic option for men with severe ED in whom a phosphodiesterase type 5 (PDE5) inhibitor fails or who cannot take PDE5 inhibitors because they require or include nitrates. In many communities patients receiving intracavernous medications for ED will outnumber patients with SCD. **Priapism after ICI is a problem all urologists will encounter and must be prepared to manage.** In a review of worldwide reports on ICI programs, Junemann and colleagues (1990) noted that diagnostic injection resulted in 5.3% of men getting ischemic priapism, and 0.4% of men reported priapism after injecting at home. In papaverine-based ICI programs, reports of prolonged erections and priapism are poorly distinguished and range from 0% to 35% (Broderick and Lue, 2002). In worldwide clinical trials of the Alprostadil Study Group, prolonged erection (defined as 4 to 6 hours) was described in 5% of patients, and priapism (longer than 6 hours) in 1% (Porst, 1996). In the United States the approved label and package insert for one product (alprostadil [Caverject]) cites the frequency of prolonged erection (4 to 6 hours) as 4% and frequency of priapism as 0.4%. The label recommends that "to minimize chances of prolonged erection or priapism Caverject should be titrated slowly to the lowest effective dosage." In papaverine/phentolamine/alprostadil ICI programs, prolonged erections have been reported in 5% to 35% of patients (Broderick and Lue, 2002).

Iatrogenic Priapism: Oral Phosphodiesterase Type 5 Inhibitors and Medications for Attention-Deficit/Hyperactivity Disorder

All PDE5 inhibitors have similar side effects related directly to their mode of action, tissue content of substrate, and pharmacologic selectivity for type 5 inhibition versus other phosphodiesterase enzymes. Side effects occurring in 2% or more of patients include headache, flushing, dyspepsia, rhinitis, light sensitivity, and myalgia. Morales and colleagues (1998) analyzed data from 4274 men who received double-blind treatment with sildenafil or placebo for up to 6 months and 2199 who received long-term open-label sildenafil for up to 1 year. No cases of priapism (erection lasting longer than 4 hours) were reported. No cases of priapism were reported by Montorsi and colleagues (2004) in a multicenter, open-label, 24-month extension of 8- or 12-week double-blind, placebo-controlled studies assessing the long-term efficacy, safety, and tolerability of tadalafil in 1173 men with ED. Nonetheless, the **indications and usage section of the U.S. Food and Drug Administration (FDA)–approved product labeling (U.S. prescribing information [USPI]) for PDE5 inhibitors** does contain this warning: "**There have been rare reports of prolonged erection greater than 4 hours and priapism (painful erections >6 hours duration) for this class of compounds.**" Both the USPI and European Summary of Product Characteristics label information contain warning or precautionary language about the use of these agents in men who have conditions predisposing them to priapism. The FDA approved Cialis (tadalafil) as an oral treatment for ED (2.5 mg, 5 mg, 10 mg, and 20 mg) in 2003. Once-daily tadalafil (2.5 mg and 5 mg) was approved for oral treatment of ED in 2008, and subsequently in 2011 tadalafil (2.5 mg and 5 mg) was approved for the signs and symptoms of benign prostatic hyperplasia (BPH) and treatment of ED. Tadalafil 5 mg daily caused no priapism in a phase 2 clinical study of 281 men with history of lower urinary tract symptoms secondary to BPH for 6 weeks, followed by dosage escalation to 20 mg once daily for 6 weeks (McVary et al, 2007). **The 2013 label for the most recently approved PDE5 inhibitor, Stendra (avanafil 50 mg, 100 mg, 200 mg), contains virtually identical precautionary wording as prior labels for as-needed (PRN) oral forms of sildenafil, vardenafil, and tadalafil: "There have been rare reports of prolonged erection greater than 4 hours and priapism (painful erections greater than 6 hours)."**

From 1999 to 2007 there were at least nine case-based reports of oral PDE5 inhibitor use and adult priapism and at least one pediatric patient (Aoyagi et al, 1999; Kassim et al, 2000; Sur and Kane, 2000; Goldmeier, 2002; McMahon, 2003; Wilt and Fink, 2004; Galatti et al, 2005; King et al, 2005; Kumar et al 2005; and Wills et al, 2007). **Most case reports detailing priapism after use of a PDE5 inhibitor reveal histories of increased risk for priapism: SCD, spinal cord injury, use of a PDE5 inhibitor recreationally, use of a PDE5 inhibitor in combination with ICI, history of penile trauma, use of psychotropic medications, or use of recreational drugs.** Wills and coworkers (2007) described a 19-month-old boy weighing 10 kg who accidentally ingested up to six tablets of sildenafil 50 mg. The child had persistent sinus tachycardia and partial erection for 24 hours; the authors presume this was a high-flow priapism (HFP) because the shaft was neither completely rigid nor painful. Erection in the child subsided spontaneously after overnight intravenous hydration and observation.

In 2013 the FDA issued a warning that methylphenidate medications used in the treatment of attention-deficit/hyperactivity disorder (ADHD) may result in prolonged erection or priapism. The FDA also warns that atomoxetine, another ADHD drug, has been linked to reports of priapism in children, teens, and adults. Drug therapy in ADHD is used in children, adolescents, and adults to increase the ability to pay attention and decrease impulsiveness and hyperactivity. The 2012 Summary Health Statistics for U.S. Children: National Health Interview Survey (Bloom et al, 2013) estimated that more than 6.4 million children ages 4 to 17 have been diagnosed with ADHD; this represents a 41% increase over a decade. The Centers for Disease Control and Prevention (CDC) further estimate that two thirds of these children are prescribed methylphenidate medications (Centers for Disease Control and Prevention, 2013).

Methylphenidate is a central nervous system stimulant; atomoxetine is a selective norepinephrine reuptake inhibitor. The FDA cautions that physicians may be tempted to switch patients from methylphenidate medications to atomoxetine but that priapism is actually more common in patients taking atomoxetine (U.S. Food and Drug Administration, 2013). **The median age of male patients taking methylphenidate who developed priapism (erection lasting longer than 4 hours) was 12.5 years.**

KEY POINTS: ISCHEMIC PRIAPISM AS A COMPLICATION OF ERECTILE DYSFUNCTION THERAPY

- Prolonged erection is more commonly reported than priapism after therapeutic or diagnostic injection of intracavernous vasoactive medications.
- In worldwide clinical trials of alprostadil, prolonged erection (defined as 4 to 6 hours) occurred in 5% of administrations, and priapism (longer than 6 hours) in 1%.
- In clinical practice, ICI of Trimix (papaverine, phentolamine, and alprostadil) results in prolonged erections in 5% to 35% of administrations.
- Few case reports have documented priapism after PDE5 inhibitor therapy. These reports suggest that men were at increased risk for priapism because of SCD, spinal cord injury, use of a PDE5 inhibitor recreationally, use of a PDE5 inhibitor in combination with ICI, history of penile trauma, use of psychotropic medications, or abuse of narcotics.
- Methylphenidate medications and atomoxetine used in the treatment of ADHD may result in prolonged erection or priapism.

Etiology of Stuttering (Intermittent) Priapism

Stuttering (intermittent) priapism describes a pattern of recurrent priapism. The term has traditionally been used to describe recurrent unwanted and painful erections in men with SCD. **Patients typically awaken with an erection that persists up to 4 hours and becomes progressively painful secondary to ischemia. SCD patients may experience stuttering priapism from childhood. Any patient who has experienced ischemic priapism is at risk for stuttering priapism. Patients with stuttering priapism will experience repeated painful intermittent attacks up to several hours before remission.** Affected young men suffer embarrassment, sleep deprivation, and performance anxiety with sexual partners (Chow and Payne, 2008). In a study of 130 patients with SCD, Adeyoju and colleagues (2002) reported that 46 (35%) had a history of priapism and, of these, 33 (72%) had a history of stuttering priapism. In 75% of patients the first episode of stuttering priapism occurred before the age of 20. Two thirds of males with SCD ischemic priapism at presentation will describe prior stuttering attacks (Jesus and Dekermacher, 2009). **Commonly reported precipitants of full-blown SCD priapism are stuttering nocturnal or early morning erections, dehydration, fever, and exposure to cold** (Broderick, 2012).

Etiology and Pathophysiology of Nonischemic (Arterial, High-Flow) Priapism

HFP is a persistent erection caused by unregulated cavernous arterial inflow. The epidemiologic data on nonischemic priapism is almost exclusively derived from small case series or individual case reports. Nonischemic priapism is much rarer than ischemic priapism, and the cause is largely attributed to trauma. Forces may be blunt or penetrating, resulting in laceration of the cavernous artery or one of its branches within the corpora. The cause most commonly reported is a straddle injury to the crura. Other mechanisms include coital trauma, kicks to the penis or perineum, pelvic fractures, birth canal trauma to the newborn male, needle lacerations, complications of penile diagnostics, and vascular erosions complicating metastatic infiltration of the corpora (Witt et al, 1990; Brock et al, 1993; Dubocq et al, 1998; Burgu et al, 2007; Jesus and Dekermacher, 2009). Although accidental blunt trauma is the most common cause, **HFP has been described after iatrogenic injury from cold-knife urethrotomy, Nesbitt corporoplasty, and deep dorsal vein arterialization** (Wolf and Lue, 1992; Liguori et al, 2005). Any mechanism that lacerates a cavernous artery or arteriole can produce unregulated pooling of blood in sinusoidal space with consequent erection. Nonischemic priapism is typically delayed in onset compared with the episode of blunt trauma (Ricciardi et al, 1993). **Sustained partial erection may develop 24 hours after perineal or penile blunt trauma.** It is believed that the hemodynamics of a nocturnal erection disrupts the clot and the damaged artery or arteriole ruptures; the unregulated arterial inflow creates a sinusoidal fistula. As healing progresses with clearing of clot and necrotic smooth muscle tissue, the fistula forms a pseudocapsule. **Formation of a pseudocapsule at the site of fistula may take several weeks to months.**

Contemporary reports suggest that HFP may have a unique subvariety. **Several authors have noted that after either aggressive medical management of ischemic priapism or surgical shunting, priapism may rapidly recur with conversion from ischemia to high flow.** HFP has been reported after aspiration and injection of α-adrenergics in the management of ischemic priapism (McMahon, 2002; Rodriguez et al, 2006; Bertolotto et al, 2009). Color Doppler ultrasonography (CDU) has shown formation of an arteriolar-sinusoidal fistula at the site of intervention (needle laceration or shunt site) (Fig. 28-2). On rare occasions after reversal of ischemic priapism, a new high-flow hemodynamic state of the cavernous arteries occurs with no evidence of fistula. **This presentation of HFP should be suspected in patients in whom rapid recurrence, persistence of erection with partial penile rigidity, or stuttering priapism not associated with pain is evident. Nonfistula type of arterial priapism is the result of dysregulation of cavernous inflows.** Nonfistula arterial priapism is a rare complication after management of ischemic priapism (Seftel et al, 1998; Cruz Guerra et al, 2004; Wallis et al, 2009). Penile tenderness to palpation is easily confused with the ongoing ache of persistent ischemia. Soft-tissue edema and ecchymosis render the physical examination findings equivocal after medical and surgical maneuvers to alleviate priapism. **Dysregulated arterial inflows with or without a fistula can best be distinguished from persistent ischemic priapism by CDU.**

> ### KEY POINTS: HIGH-FLOW PRIAPISM
>
> - Nonischemic priapism is much rarer than ischemic priapism.
> - HFP results from laceration or disruption of a cavernous artery or arteriole.
> - The most common cause is a straddle injury to the crura.
> - Other mechanisms include coital trauma, kicks to the penis or perineum, pelvic fractures, birth canal trauma to the male newborn, needle lacerations, complications of penile diagnostics, and vascular erosions complicating metastatic infiltration of the corpora.
> - HFP has been described after iatrogenic trauma from cold-knife urethrotomy, corporoplasty, and penile revascularization procedures.

Priapism in Children

Priapism in children and adolescents is most commonly related to SCD. The literature suggests that the incidence of priapism in pediatric sickle cell clinics is 2% to 6% (Tarry et al, 1987; Jesus and Dekermacher, 2009). The majority of SCD priapism is ischemic. In the newborn period, fetal hemoglobin predominates, not HbS (Burgu et al, 2007). SCD phenotypes related to ischemic or occlusive crises are unlikely to be evident while fetal hemoglobin persists. Newborn priapism is an extremely rare phenomenon with only limited case reports and rare application of contemporary diagnostic modalities. Erection is frequently elicited in males during the newborn period. In male newborns, simple tactile stimulation such as diaper changing, bathing, and urethral catheterization may result in erection; the erection quickly subsides after cessation of stimuli. Fewer than 20 cases of newborn priapism have been reported in the literature, and rarely has the cause been defined; causes have included polycythemia, blood transfusion, and birth canal trauma (Amlie et al, 1977; Leal et al, 1978; Shapiro, 1979; Walker and Casale, 1997). The majority of cases have been conservatively managed with spontaneous resolution reported from hours to days. Minimally invasive diagnostics (CDU) should be performed (Pietras et al, 1979; Meijer and Bakker, 2003). In children who develop priapism after straddle trauma, every effort should be made to localize the arteriolar-sinusoidal fistula. Hatzichristou and colleagues (2002) reported that identification of the fistula by Doppler ultrasound coupled with direct manual compression softens the high-flow erection and may speed spontaneous resolution. They suggested that this noninvasive therapy likely works in children and not adults because the perineum has considerably less subcutaneous fat and because crural bodies are more easily compressed.

MOLECULAR BASIS OF ISCHEMIC AND STUTTERING PRIAPISM

Advances in our understanding of the molecular basis of priapism have drawn significantly from both in vitro and in vivo experimental studies using animal models. Data on the true inciting mechanisms involved in ischemic priapism are emerging. **Ischemic priapism consists of an imbalance of vasoconstrictive and vasorelaxatory mechanisms predisposing the penis to hypoxia and acidosis. In vitro studies have demonstrated that when corporal smooth muscle strips and cultured corporal smooth muscle cells are exposed to hypoxic conditions, α-adrenergic stimulation fails to induce corporal smooth muscle contraction** (Broderick and Harkaway, 1994; Saenz de Tejada et al, 1997; Muneer et al, 2005). Extended periods of severe anoxia significantly impair corporal smooth muscle contractility and cause significant apoptosis of smooth muscle cells and, ultimately, fibrosis of the CC.

In experimental animal models of ischemic priapism, lipid peroxidation, an indicator of injury induced by reactive oxygen species (ROSs), and increased hemo-oxygenase expression occur in the penis during and after ischemic priapism (Munarriz et al, 2003; Jin et al, 2008). Additional pathophysiologic mechanisms involved in the progression of ischemia-induced fibrosis are the upregulation of hypoxia-induced growth factors. Transforming growth factor-β (TGF-β) is a cytokine that is vital to tissue repair. However, excess amounts may induce tissue damage and scarring. Upregulation of TGF-β occurs during hypoxia and in response to oxidative stress (Moreland et al, 1995; Jin et al, 2008). It is hypothesized that TGF-β may be involved in the progression of the corporal smooth muscle to fibrosis (Bivalacqua et al, 2000; Jeong et al, 2004).

Transgenic mouse models of SCD manifest priapism (Beuzard, 1996; Bivalacqua et al, 2009b). There have been two major discoveries in elucidation of the molecular mechanism of ischemic priapism. Mi and colleagues (2008) have shown that transgenic sickle cell mice CC have enhanced smooth muscle relaxation to electrical field stimulation. Transgenic sickle cell mice and mice lacking endothelial NO synthase (eNOS) gene expression display

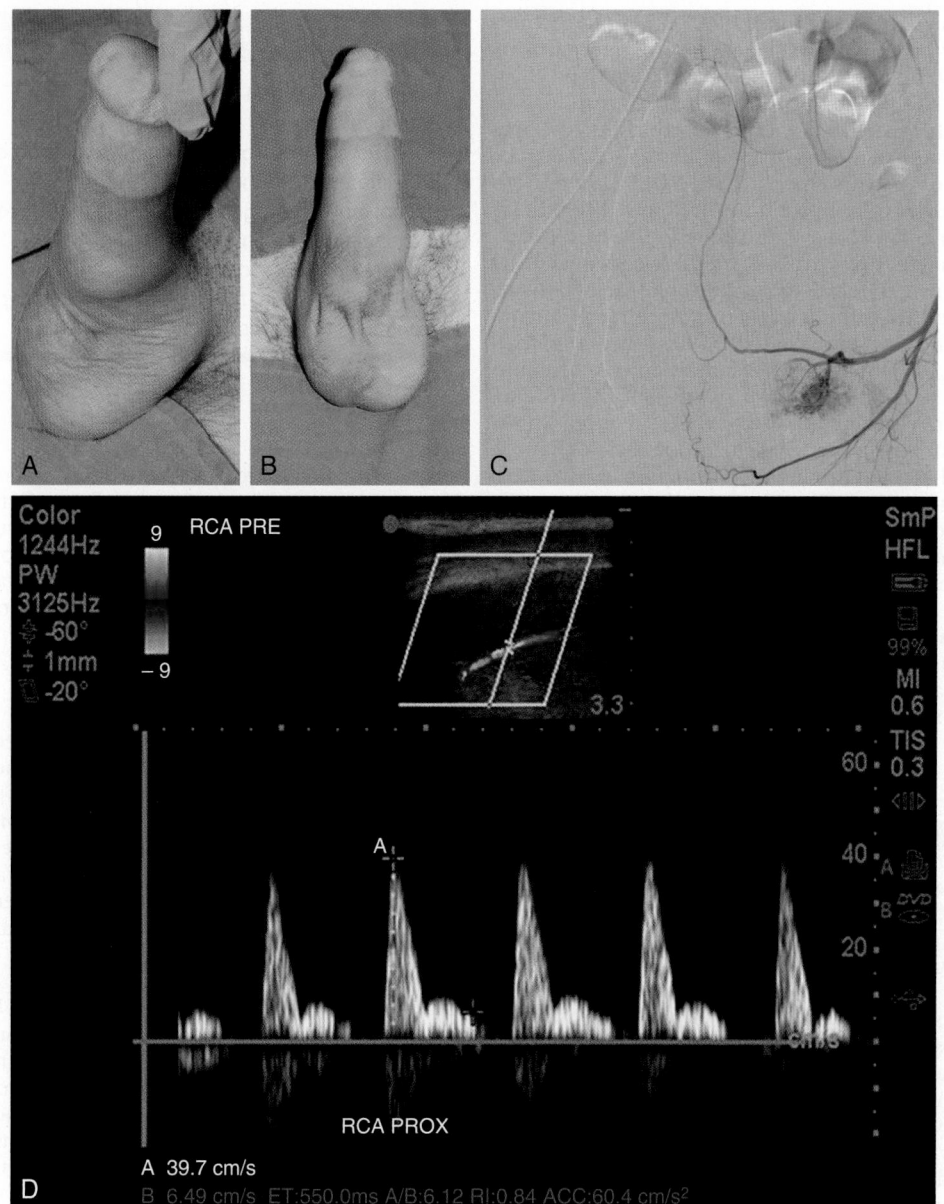

Figure 28-2. A, A 21-year-old white man with a history of ischemic priapism after binging with alcohol, marijuana, and energy drinks. Patient had a series of penile shunt procedures in attempts to reverse ischemic priapism: Winter, Al-Ghorab, bilateral corpora cavernosa to spongiosum. Six months later he sought evaluation for embarrassing persistent partial erection; consistent with converting from ischemic to high-flow priapism, he had no pain. **A,** Tumescent shaft with glans scar. **B,** Penoscrotal bulging at site of cavernospongiosal shunts. **C,** Angiogram of fistula originating at the bulbourethral artery. **D,** Doppler flows with peak systolic velocity of 39 cm/sec and 6 cm/sec; end diastolic flow and resistive index, 84.

supraphysiologic erections and spontaneously phasic priapic activity in vivo (Bivalacqua et al, 2006, 2007).

Endothelial cells actively regulate basal vascular tone and vascular reactivity by responding to mechanical forces and neurohumoral mediators with the release of a variety of relaxing and contracting factors. In the penis the vascular endothelium is a source of vasorelaxing factors such as NO and adenosine, as well as vasoconstrictor factors such as RhoA/Rho-kinase. Recent evidence suggests that in states of priapism there may be aberrant NO and adenosine signaling, thus identifying a potential role for NO/cyclic guanosine monophosphate (cGMP), as well as adenosine and RhoA/Rho-kinase signaling in the pathophysiology of ischemic priapism (Champion et al, 2005; Mi et al, 2008; Bivalacqua et al, 2009a).

eNOS−/− mutant mice have an exaggerated erectile response to cavernous nerve stimulation and have phenotypic changes in erectile function consistent with priapism (Champion et al, 2005; Bivalacqua et al, 2006). Mice lacking the *eNOS* gene manifest a priapism phenotype through mechanisms involving defective PDE5 regulatory function in the penis, resulting from altered endothelial NO/cGMP signaling in the organ (Lin et al, 2003; Bivalacqua et al, 2006). Supporting this hypothesis, PDE5 expression is significantly reduced in corpora cavernosa smooth muscle cells (CCSMCs) grown under anoxic and hypoxic cell culture conditions (Lin et al, 2003). **In the context of molecular dysregulation, the cyclic nucleotide cGMP is produced in low steady-state amounts under the influence of priapism-related destruction of the vascular endothelium and thus reduced endothelial NO activity; this** situation downregulates the set point of PDE5 function, secondary to altered cGMP-dependent feedback control mechanisms (Champion et al, 2005; Bivalacqua et al, 2006; Burnett and Bivalacqua, 2007). **When NO is neuronally produced in response to an erectogenic stimulus or with nocturnal erections, cGMP production surges in a manner that leads to excessive erectile tissue relaxation because of basally insufficient PDE5 enzyme to degrade the cyclic nucleotide. In addition, reduced Rho-kinase activity (contractile mediator) may contribute to the susceptibility of corporal tissue to excessive relaxation via two distinct molecular mechanisms. Two distinct molecular mechanisms appear to act in concert to promote stuttering ischemic priapism: enhanced vasorelaxation by uninhibited cGMP and diminished contractile effects of Rho-kinase.** Transgenic sickle cell mice also have significant reductions in penile NO/cGMP signaling leading to deficient PDE5 expression and activity, as well as reduced RhoA/Rho-kinase expression, which causes them to manifest enhanced erectile responses and recurrent priapism (Champion et al, 2005). Another potential cause of enhanced corporal smooth muscle relaxation in SCD-associated priapism is elevated penile adenosine levels, which cause the CC to be in a chronically vasodilated state (Mi et al, 2008). **Taken together, these data suggest that ischemic priapism and, most important, stuttering priapism are direct results of NO imbalance resulting in aberrant molecular signaling, PDE5 dysregulation, adenosine overproduction, and reductions in Rho-kinase activity, translating into enhanced corporal smooth muscle relaxation and inhibition of vasoconstriction in the penis.**

KEY POINTS: SICKLE CELL DISEASE AND PRIAPISM

- Sickle cell hemoglobinopathy accounts for at least a third of all cases of ischemic priapism.
- The sickle cell genetic mutation is the result of a single amino acid substitution in the β-globin subunit of hemoglobin.
- Clinical features are seen in homozygous SCD patients: chronic hemolysis, vascular occlusion, tissue ischemia, and end-organ damage.
- Hemolysis and reduced NO are central in the pathogenesis of pulmonary hypertension, leg ulcers, priapism, and stroke in SCD patients.
- Increased blood viscosity is responsible for painful crises, osteonecrosis, and acute chest syndrome.
- SCD patients may experience stuttering priapism from childhood.
- SCD patients with stuttering priapism will experience repeated painful intermittent attacks up to several hours before remission.
- Stuttering priapism in SCD is the result of molecular dysregulation with enhanced corporal smooth muscle vasorelaxing forces and inhibition of vasocontractile forces in the penis.

EVALUATION AND DIAGNOSIS OF PRIAPISM

History

In order to initiate appropriate management, the physician must determine whether the underlying priapism hemodynamics are ischemic or nonischemic. **Emergency management of ischemic priapism is recommended. Ischemia should be suspected when** the patient has progressive penile pain associated with the duration of erection; has used a known drug associated with priapism; has SCD or another blood dyscrasia; or has a known neurologic condition, especially those affecting the spinal cord. Stuttering priapism history is one of recurrent episodes of prolonged erections, usually nonresolving morning erections. **Nonischemic priapism should be**

BOX 28-2 Elements in Taking the History of Priapism

Duration of erection
Presence of pain
Previous episodes of priapism and method of treatment
Baseline erectile function
Use of any erectogenic therapies (both prescription and nutritional supplements)
Medications and recreational drugs
Sickle cell disease, hemoglobinopathies, hypercoagulable states
Trauma to the pelvis, perineum, or penis

---

suspected when there is no pain and the erection duration has not been accompanied by progressive discomfort. There is a history of straddle injury, coital trauma, blunt trauma to the penis or perineum, penile injection, penile surgery, or a diagnostic procedure of the pelvic and penile vessels. The onset of post-traumatic HFP in adults and children may be delayed by hours to several days after the initial injury (Box 28-2).

Physical Examination

Inspection and palpation of the penis are recommended to determine the extent and degree of tumescence and rigidity; the involvement of the cavernous bodies; the presence of pain; and the evidence of trauma to the perineum. **In ischemic priapism the corporal bodies will be completely rigid; the glans penis and corpus spongiosum are not.** Although malignancies rarely cause priapism, examination of the abdomen, testicles, perineum, rectum, and prostate may help identify a primary cancer. Malignant infiltration of the penis causes indurated nodules within or replacing corporal tissue. The subtle differences in the penile examination findings may be apparent to the experienced urologist but can be overlooked by emergency personnel on initial evaluation (Fig. 28-3A to F). If physical examination reveals the penis to be nontender, tumescent, or partially erect, nonischemic priapism should be suspected. **In nonischemic priapism the corpora will be tumescent but not completely rigid.** In children and adults with HFP, depending on the location of trauma and time since the traumatic event, there may be residual bruising at the perineum from straddle injury (Table 28-1).

Laboratory Testing

Evaluation should include a complete blood count (CBC), WBC count with blood cell differential, platelet count, and coagulation profile to assess anemia, rule out infection, detect hematologic abnormalities, and ensure that the patient can safely tolerate surgical interventions should initial medical management fail. **In African-Americans, a sickle cell preparation and hemoglobin electrophoresis should be requested.** Other hematologic abnormalities may cause priapism, including leukemia, platelet abnormalities, and thalassemia, and these should be sought if the cause is not evident. An elevated reticulocyte count is nonspecific and may be present in both priapism caused by SCD and thalassemia. Urine and serum toxicology panels should be done if recreational narcotic or prescription psychoactive drugs are suspected from the history. **A corporal blood gas by aspiration is recommended in the emergency evaluation of priapism. The corporal blood aspirate differentiates ischemic from nonischemic priapism. Aspiration may be both diagnostic and therapeutic. Visual inspection of the color and consistency of an initial penile aspirate will reveal dark deoxygenated blood with a "crankcase oil" appearance in ischemic priapism. The initial corporal aspirate may be sent for blood gas testing to document pH, PO_2, and PCO_2** (Table 28-2). CDU should be initiated if the history

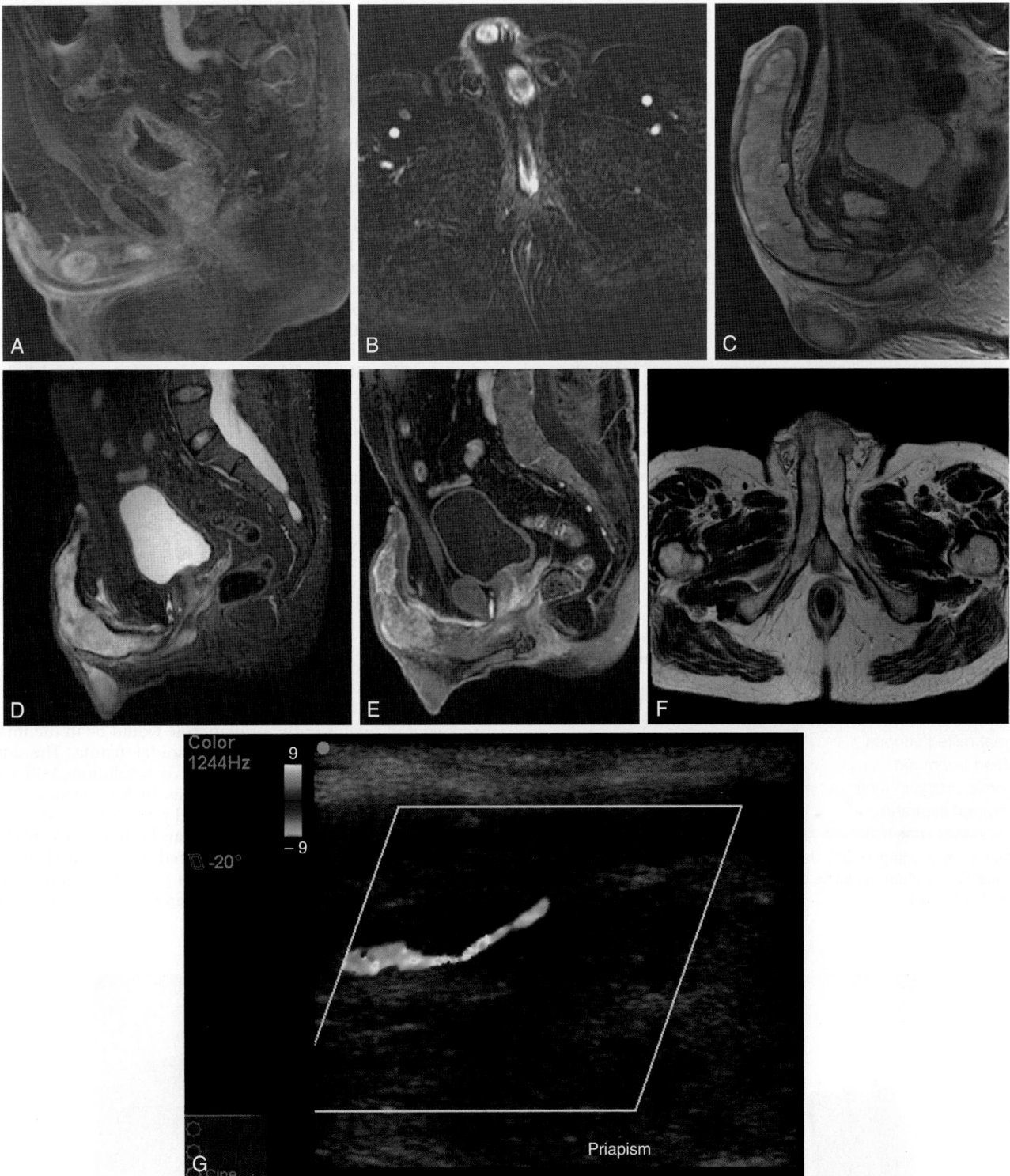

Figure 28-3. A, Sagittal magnetic resonance imaging (MRI) scan of the penis showing metastatic deposits of prostate cancer to the corpus cavernosum. **B,** Coronal MRI image from the same patient. Note the proximal and distal metastatic deposits of prostate cancer. **C,** T2-weighted MRI showing chondrosarcoma replacing corpus cavernosum. **D to F,** A 50-year-old white man with neurofibromatosis with a 6- to 12-month history of partial erection and progressive penile deformity. He was referred with a diagnosis of Peyronie disease. Penile biopsies showed malignant peripheral nerve sheath tumor or neurofibrosarcoma. T2- and T1-weighted MRI images show large irregular masses replacing corpora cavernosa. **G,** Color Doppler imaging shows irregular right cavernous artery with high flow. (C, Courtesy David Ralph.)

suggests penile or perineal trauma or if the corporal aspirate reveals well-oxygenated blood (Fig. 28-4).

Penile Imaging

CDU of the penis and perineum is recommended in the evaluation of priapism. CDU is an adjunct to the corporal aspirate

TABLE 28-1   Key Findings in Priapism

FINDINGS	ISCHEMIC PRIAPISM	NONISCHEMIC PRIAPISM
Perineal trauma	Seldom	Usually
Hematologic abnormalities	Usually	Seldom
Recent intracorporal injection	Sometimes	Sometimes
Corpora cavernosa fully rigid	Usually	Seldom
Penile pain	Usually	Seldom
Abnormal penile blood gas	Usually	Seldom
Cavernous inflow (on Doppler)	Seldom	Usually

Modified from Montague DK, Jarow J, Broderick GA, et al. American Urological Association guideline on the management of priapism. J Urol 2003;170:1318–24.

TABLE 28-2   Typical Blood Gas Values

SOURCE	Po_2 (mm Hg)	Pco_2 (mm Hg)	PH
Normal arterial blood (room air)	>90	<40	7.40
Normal mixed venous blood (room air)	40	50	7.35
Ischemic priapism (first corporal aspirate)	<30	>60	<7.25

Modified from Montague DK, Jarow J, Broderick GA, et al. American Urological Association guideline on the management of priapism. J Urol 2003;170: 1318–24.

in differentiating ischemic from nonischemic priapism. **Patients with prolonged ischemic priapism will have no blood flow in the cavernous arteries;** the return of the cavernous artery waveform will accompany successful detumescence. **Patients with nonischemic priapism have normal to high blood flow velocities** detectable in the cavernous arteries; an effort should be made to localize the characteristic blush of color emanating from the disrupted cavernous artery or arteriole (Broderick and Lue, 2002). Examination of the entire penile shaft and perineum is recommended; this can be done with the patient supine but frog-legged (Fig. 28-5). **Penile arteriography should be reserved for the management of HFP, when embolization is planned; arteriography is too invasive as a diagnostic procedure to differentiate ischemic from nonischemic priapism** (Burnett, 2004). **The data from penile blood gas assessments become confusing after interventions. CDU should always be considered in the evaluation of a full or partial erection after treatments for ischemic priapism. The differential diagnosis includes resolved ischemia with penile edema, persistent ischemia, and conversion to high-flow state.** Chiou and colleagues (2009a) have recommended that to accurately categorize presentations as nonischemic or ischemic, careful interpretation of CDU hemodynamics must be done in conjunction with the clinical assessment. They describe eight patients with priapism after ICI (duration ≤7 hours), all of whom showed presence of cavernous arterial inflows with varied peak systolic velocities and end-diastolic velocities. They concluded that most patients with priapism after ICI (and duration <7 hours) have a hemodynamic picture of mixed arteriogenic and veno-occlusive priapism. In their series, men with idiopathic ischemic priapism longer than 20 hours showed no detectable cavernous arterial inflows.

There have recently been reports on the use of magnetic resonance imaging (MRI) in priapism. Kirkham and colleagues (2008) noted that there are **three possible roles for MRI** to help in the assessment of priapism; the primary role would be in the **imaging of a well-established arteriolar-sinusoidal fistula.** The authors acknowledge that a limitation of MRI is resolution; MRI cannot demonstrate small vessels as clearly as high-frequency Doppler sonography or angiography. The second role would be in ischemic priapism to **demonstrate the presence and extent of tissue thrombus and corporal smooth muscle infarction.** Ralph and coworkers (2009) used MRI to assess 50 patients presenting with refractory ischemic priapism. All patients had priapism lasting from 24 to 72

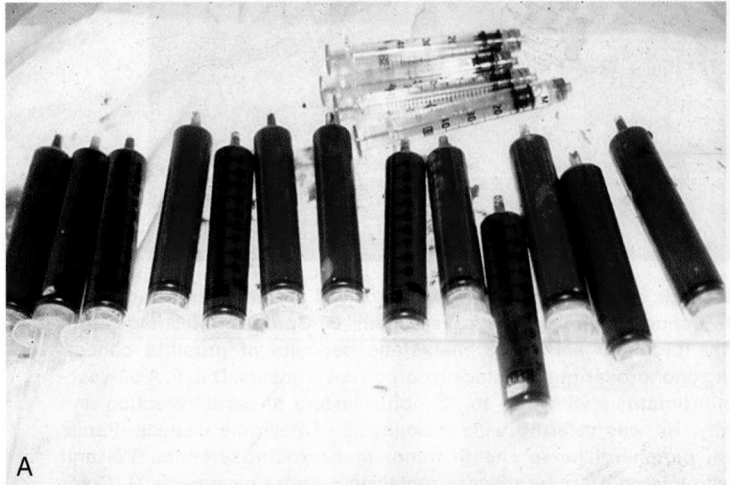
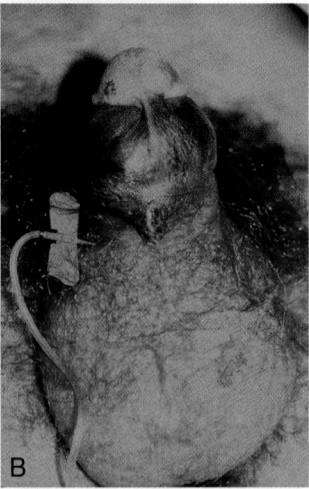

Figure 28-4. A, The initial corporal aspirate in ischemic priapism shows dark, deoxygenated blood. Subsequent aspirations will show brighter blood as corpus cavernosum is reoxygenated by inflow. Empty syringes are from successive injections of phenylephrine. **B,** A butterfly needle for aspiration and injection should be placed at the penoscrotal junction. Initial attempts in the emergency department failed to reverse priapism because of distal placement of the butterfly needle and failure to repeat aspiration and injections of an α-adrenergic agent.

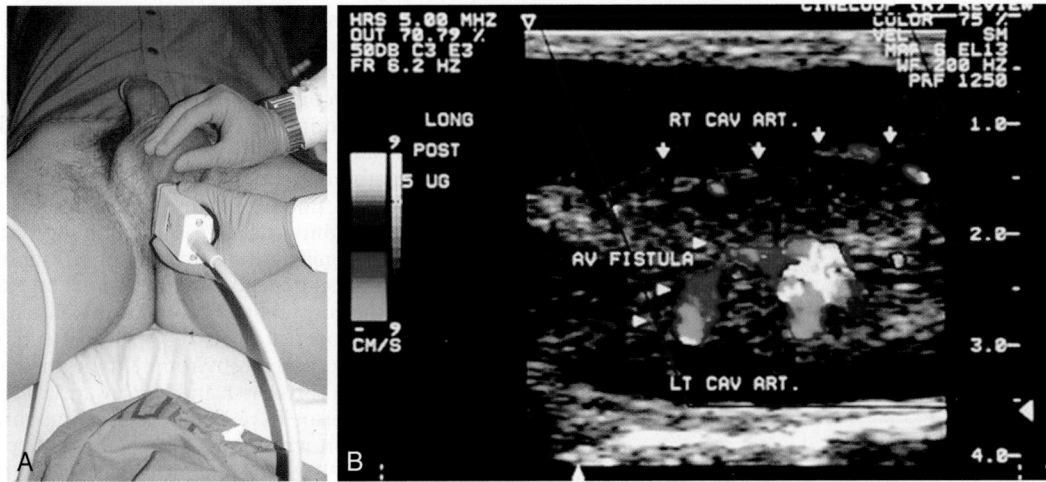

Figure 28-5. **A,** Examination of the crural bodies is required when searching for arterial sinusoidal fistula after straddle injury. **B,** Color Doppler image of arterial sinusoidal fistula of left cavernous artery.

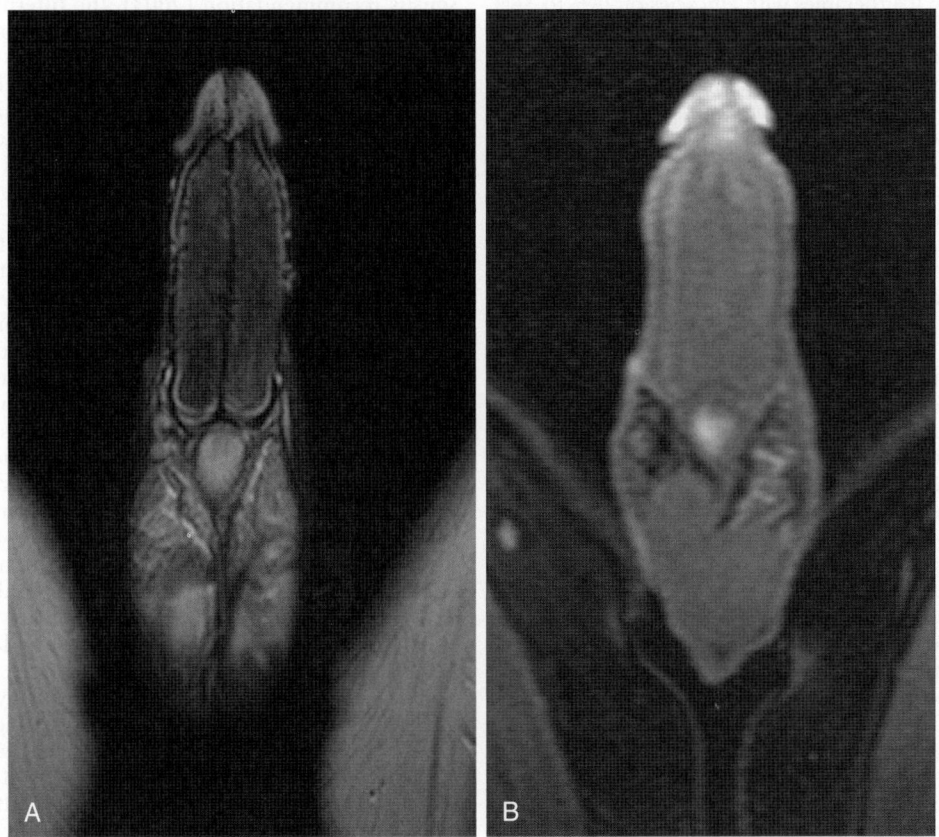

Figure 28-6. **A,** T2-weighted magnetic resonance image showing cavernous body thrombosis. **B,** Same patient. There is no enhancement after gadolinium infusion. At operation, extensive smooth muscle necrosis and thrombus were found. Patient had untreated ischemic priapism lasting several days. (Courtesy David Ralph.)

hours, and each had failed medical and surgical interventions. Patients underwent MRI to characterize the extent of smooth muscle necrosis before placement of penile prosthesis (Fig. 28-6). The third role for MRI would be in the **imaging of corporal malignancy or metastasis** with corporal smooth muscle replaced by malignant tissue or with true ischemic priapism caused by obstruction of venous outflow.

MEDICAL TREATMENTS

Ischemic Priapism

Historically, first aid was applied by the patient or recommended by a health practitioner unfamiliar with the hemodynamics of priapism; these interventions included ejaculation, ice packs, cold baths, and cold water enemas. Each of these remedies was thought to end erection by inducing vasoconstriction. Some historical reports advised voiding and exercise. Oral sympathomimetic drugs (etilefrine, pseudoephedrine, phenylpropanolamine, and terbutaline) have been reported to effectively reverse prolonged erection (<4 hours) initiated by ICI therapies with efficacies of 28% to 36% (Lowe and Jarow, 1993). Lowe and Jarow (1993) compared oral terbutaline with pseudoephedrine or placebo in 75 patients with prolonged erection induced by ICI of alprostadil; they reported detumescence in 38% of cases with terbutaline, 28% with pseudoephedrine, and 12% with placebo. In a follow-up study Priyadarshi (2004) specifically investigated the efficacy of oral terbutaline in the management of prolonged erection after ICI (papaverine/chlorpromazine); he administered oral terbutaline 5 mg or placebo to men with persisting erection for more than 2.5 hours. Detumescence was achieved in 42% and 15% of cases, respectively, treated with terbutaline or placebo. Terbutaline treatment was unsuccessful in 58% of cases; all of those patients responded to ICI of an α-adrenergic agent.

Every practice administering diagnostic ICI or teaching ICI must be prepared to manage priapism. In my experience, when a vasoactive injection results in a prolonged erection with duration longer than 1 hour but shorter than 4 hours, aspiration may not be necessary. Phenylephrine (200 μg) injected with an ultrafine needle and 1-mL syringe may reverse the erection. Reversing a prolonged erection will spare the patient and the office staff the complexity of treating full-blown ischemic priapism.

Oral agents are not recommended in the management of acute ischemic priapism (>4 hours). The recommended initial treatment of ischemic priapism is the decompression of the CC by aspiration. Aspiration will immediately soften the erection and relieve pain. Aspiration alone may relieve priapism in 36% of cases. The AUA Guidelines Panel (2003) advised that there were not sufficient data to conclude that aspiration followed by saline intracorporal irrigation was any more effective than aspiration alone (Montague et al, 2003). Subsequently, Ateyah and colleagues (2005) reported that a combination of corporal blood aspiration and cold saline irrigation effectively terminated priapism in 66% of cases compared with aspiration alone (24%). **Data to support the efficacy of cold saline are limited. Aspiration should be repeated until no more dark blood can be seen coming out from the corpora and fresh bright red blood is obtained. This process leads to a marked decrease in the intracavernous pressure, relieves pain, and resuscitates the corporal environment, removing anoxic, acidotic, and hypercarbic blood.** A single, large-bore, 19-gauge needle should be inserted at the penoscrotal junction at the 3 or 9 o'clock position to avoid piercing the dorsal neurovascular bundle. The surgeon should compress the penile shaft between the thumb and first digit, just below the 19-gauge needle, aspirating the shaft until it is soft. With the needle left in place, the shaft is permitted to refill. Compression is reapplied and aspiration repeated. These maneuvers may need to be serially

repeated. Several small, empty syringes should be available (3-mL to 12-mL syringes).

Corporal aspiration, if unsuccessful, should be followed by α-adrenergic injection or irrigation. Aspiration followed by the ICI of sympathomimetic drugs was recommended by the AUA Guidelines Panel in 2003 (Montague et al, 2003; Broderick et al, 2010). Sympathomimetic drugs (phenylephrine, etilefrine, ephedrine, epinephrine, norepinephrine, metaraminol) cause cavernous smooth muscle contraction. In the laboratory, normal cavernous smooth muscle preparations from humans, rabbits, and rodents show concentration-dependent contractions on exposure to phenylephrine, if the corporal environment is well oxygenated and has a normal pH (Broderick et al, 1994). In patients, time-dependent changes in the corporeal environment begin within 6 hours of persistent erection (Broderick and Harkaway, 1994). Animal models of ischemic priapism have demonstrated impairment in smooth muscle contraction with progressive acidosis, hypoxia, and glucopenia (Broderick, 1994; Saenz de Tejada et al, 1997; Munnarriz et al, 2006; Muneer et al, 2008). Corpus cavernosum specimens from patients with prolonged priapism show no contractions to high-dose phenylephrine in vitro.

Phenylephrine is a relatively selective α_1-adrenergic receptor agonist with minimal β-mediated ionotropic and chronotropic cardiac effects; it is the agent of choice according to AUA consensus recommendation (2003), the International Consultation on Sexual Medicine (2010), and the European Association of Urology guideline on priapism (2014) (Montague et al, 2003; Broderick et al, 2010; Salonia et al, 2014). There are no comparative trials of sympathomimetics in the management of priapism, nor are there studies of dosage tolerance to report. In terms of corporal physiology, α-adrenergic agonists are vasoconstrictors of cavernous artery and arterioles. Intracavernous administration of an α-adrenergic agent should contract cavernous smooth muscles, allowing sinusoidal blood to egress from subtunical veins. On the other hand, a β-adrenergic agonist, which would relax cavernous smooth muscle and dilate the cavernous artery and arterioles, could promote oxygenated arteriolar blood to enter the cavernous spaces and wash out deoxygenated blood. Metaraminol is a pure α-adrenergic agent; etilefrine, phenylephrine, and epinephrine are mixed α- and β-adrenergic agonists. Terbutaline is a pure β agonist. Case reports with these agents show varying efficacy from 43% to 81%. In addition to the specific reversal agent, there is clearly a time-dependent efficacy for pharmacologic reversal of priapism. For acute pharmacologic management of ischemic priapism, the intracavernous administration of dilute solutions of phenylephrine or epinephrine is most commonly described in the United States. In Europe etilefrine is commonly described. Etilefrine is a phenylephrine related β-adrenergic and α-adrenergic agonist. It is available in oral and parenteral formulations internationally (effortil, ethylandrianol, ethylphenylephrine, phetanol, ethyl noradrianol). Currently, pseudoephedrine, phenylpropanolamine, and ephedrine are the orally active adrenergic agents available in the United States. Pseudoephedrine (Sudafed) is regulated under the Combat Methamphetamine Epidemic Act of 2005, which banned over-the-counter sales of cold medicines containing pseudoephedrine. It is available "behind the counter" without a prescription. Neither Sudafed (pseudoephedrine) nor Sudafed PE (phenylephrine) have been evaluated as oral agents for the reversal or prevention of priapism in the United States. Phenylephrine is typically diluted in normal saline to a concentration of 100 to 200 μg/mL; it is administered intracavernously as a 1-mL injection every 3 to 5 minutes. Administration should be intermittent over the course of an hour. **In my experience, phenylephrine can be concentrated as 200 μg/mL in saline and administered intermittently as 0.5 mL to 1.0 mL every 5 to 10 minutes to a maximum dosage of 1 mg. This will permit up to 10 separate injections of 0.5 mL (100 μg each) or 5 separate injections of 1 mL (200 μg each). The penis is aspirated between successive injections by tightly pinching the shaft at the penoscrotal junction, just below the site of needle insertion. Aspiration should continue until the distal shaft is empty and collapses. This removes deoxygenated**

acidic blood. **Then phenylephrine is injected. Gradually the compression at the penoscrotal junction is released, allowing the shaft to refill with fresh blood.** Extremes of age and preexisting cardiovascular diseases should be taken into consideration before intracavernous sympathomimetic administration. **Serial monitoring of blood pressure and pulse should be performed during and immediately after ICI of sympathomimetic drugs. Potential side effects of intracavernous sympathomimetics include headache, dizziness, hypertension, reflex bradycardia, tachycardia, and irregular cardiac rhythms.** Davila and colleagues (2008) reported subarachnoid hemorrhage in a patient with SCD ischemic priapism. The patient was a 24-year-old African-American man who reported sudden and severe headache immediately after intracorporal administration of phenylephrine 500 μg/mL repeated every 3 minutes for a total of 4 mL (2000 μg = 2 mg). In 2005 the Pennsylvania Patient Safety Authority published an advisory, *Let's Stop This "Epi"demic! Preventing Errors with Epinephrine.* The report describes a case of a 16-year-old boy who received 4 mL of undiluted 1:1000 epinephrine solution intracavernously to treat priapism. The physician thought the 1:1000 ratio on the epinephrine 1 mg/mL label meant the solution had been prediluted with 1000 mL of fluid (Pennsylvania Patient Safety Authority, 2006). **Whichever intracavernous sympathomimetic agent is chosen for the management of ischemic priapism, urologists are well advised to consult their pharmacies and develop clear mixing and dosage protocols for safe administration** (Fig. 28-7).

SCD and hematologic malignancies are rare but important causes of ischemic priapism. Classically, treatment of SCD-induced ischemic priapism involved analgesics, hydration, oxygen, bicarbonate, and exchange transfusion. Unfortunately, acute neurologic complications may follow exchange transfusions. Hematologists have begun to question the emphasis on intravenous hydration, sodium bicarbonate for alkalinization, and exchange transfusion as first line therapy for SCD-associated priapism (Kato, 2012).

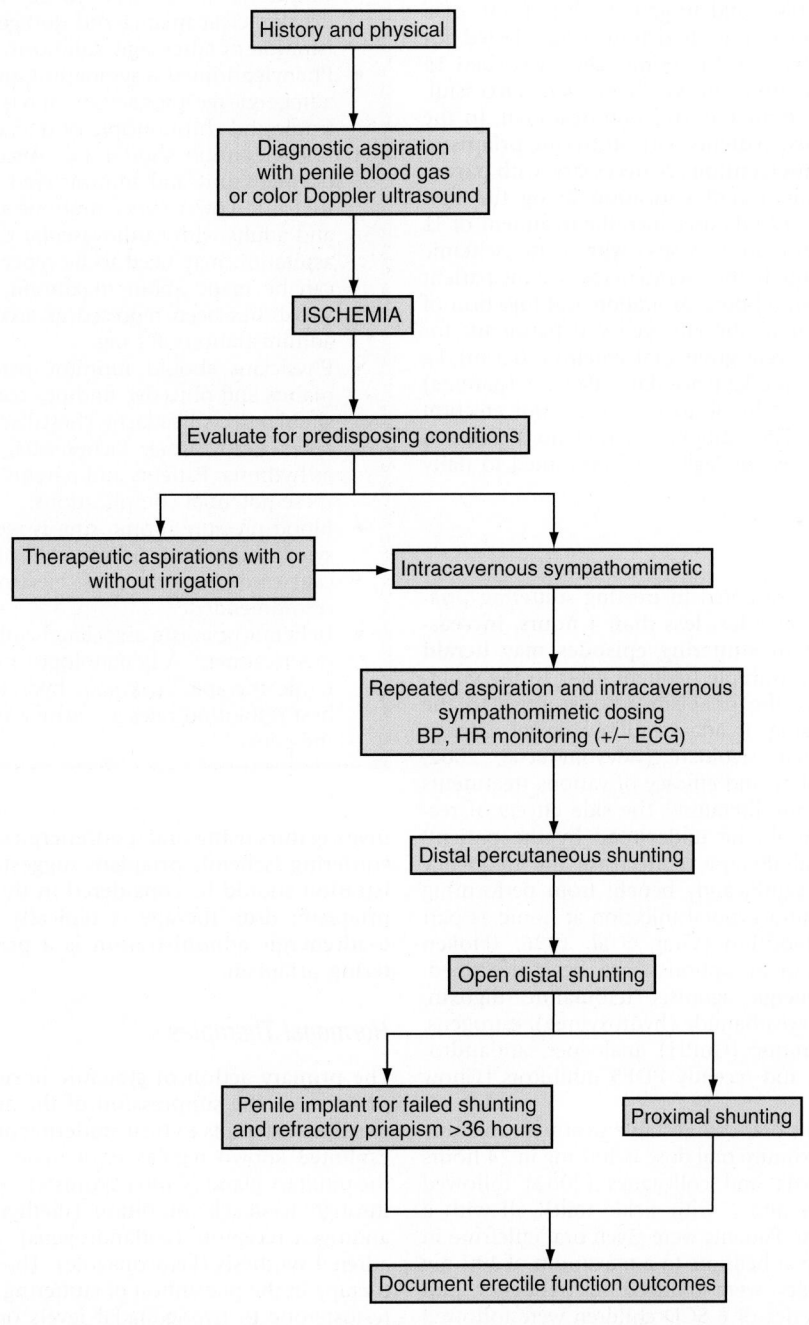

Figure 28-7. Algorithm for managing ischemic priapism. BP, blood pressure; ECG, electrocardiogram; HR, heart rate.

Hydroxycarbamide (hydroxyurea) is a hematologic agent used in the management of vaso-occlusive crises in sickle cell patients (Saad et al, 2004; Morrison and Burnett, 2012). The proposed mechanisms of action are increase in production of hemoglobin F; reduction of leukocytes, platelets, and reticulocytes; and promotion of release of NO. **In the best interests of the patient, the urologist should seek hematologic consultation in the management of boys and men with SCD priapism but remain assertive that hematologic therapy alone is not effective management of SCD priapism** (Rogers, 2005). A 2006 report suggested that blood transfusion may have no effective role in the treatment of sickle cell–induced priapism (Merritt et al, 2006). **Reports from hematology centers suggest high success rates with use of penile aspiration, injection, and irrigation with intracavernous sympathomimetics for SCD priapism** (Mantadakis et al, 2000). Mantadakis and colleagues (2000) conducted a prospective trial for the management of children with SCD with prolonged erection, ages 3 to 18 years (no placebo group). For erections lasting longer than 4 hours and less than 12 hours, emergency department interventions were local anesthetic, cavernous aspiration, and irrigation with 10 mL of a 1:1,000,000 solution of epinephrine. If detumescence lasted for 30 minutes, patients were discharged to home. They described 15 patients receiving 39 interventions, of which 37 were successful; 67% required only one aspiration and irrigation treatment. **In the management of SCD pediatric patients with stuttering priapism, several levels of escalating intervention are necessary, with parental and emergency department staff education being the first level.** Gbadoe and colleagues (2001) described the treatment of 11 SCD patients (ages 30 months to 15 years) with acute ischemic priapism or stuttering priapism. In their series of cases, if the patient had priapism lasting less than 6 hours, aspiration and injection of 5 mg of etilefrine was given in the emergency department; for stuttering priapism, patients were given oral etilefrine 0.5 mg/kg nightly for 1 month, or 0.25 mg/kg twice daily. Patients (parents) also administered injections at home to reverse painful erection lasting longer than 1 hour. The authors reported no significant hypertension and only one case of "agitation" attributed to daily administration.

Stuttering Priapism

Various factors need to be considered in treating stuttering priapism. **Although an episode may last less than 4 hours, increasing frequency or duration of stuttering episodes may herald a major ischemic priapism.** Multiple frequent visits to the emergency department to resolve the priapism are disruptive to the patient's life and embarrassing. If attacks follow sexual activity, patients may become sexually avoidant (Adeyoju et al, 2002; Chow and Payne, 2008). Safety and efficacy of various treatments are poorly characterized in the literature. The side effects of recommended medications should be understood by the patient. Patients on chronic medical therapy to decrease the frequency of stuttering episodes may significantly benefit from performing a single sympathomimetic intracorporal injection at home as part of a personal treatment algorithm (Virag et al, 1996; Teloken et al, 2005). Multiple treatment options have been described: oral and injectable α-adrenergic agonists, terbutaline, digoxin, the antisickling agent hydroxycarbamide (hydroxyurea), estrogens, gonadotropin-releasing hormone (GnRH) analogues, antiandrogens, baclofen, gabapentin, and recently PDE5 inhibitors (Chow and Payne, 2008).

Etilefrine is available as an oral or injectable treatment in some European countries. The maximum oral dose is 100 mg in 24 hours (Okpala et al, 2002). Okpala and colleagues (2002) followed 18 adults (17 SCD patients and 1 with sickle trait), all with a history of stuttering priapism. Patients were given oral etilefrine in escalating doses from 25 mg at bedtime to a maximum of 100 mg each day. Stuttering episodes were reduced in frequency and duration in 72%. A small series of 6 SCD children were followed with administration twice daily with 0.25 mg of etilefrine per kilogram (Gbadoe et al, 2002). **The experience of multiple**

KEY POINTS: MEDICAL MANAGEMENT OF ISCHEMIC PRIAPISM

- Oral therapy is not recommended for the treatment of acute ischemic priapism.
- The initial treatment of ischemic priapism is decompression by aspiration.
- Aspiration should be repeated until oxygenated blood is seen to refill the corpora.
- Aspiration should be followed by the ICI (or irrigation) of a diluted α-adrenergic drug.
- Worldwide availability of adrenergic agents varies; effective reversal of priapism has been documented with dilute injections of ephedrine, epinephrine, etilefrine, metaraminol, or phenylephrine. Phenylephrine is the agent of choice recommended by AUA, International Consultation on Sexual Medicine, and European Association of Urology guidelines.
- Clinicians are advised to consult their pharmacies and develop clear mixing and dosage protocols for safe administration of adrenergic solutions.
- Phenylephrine is a sympathomimetic drug with selective α_1 adrenergic receptor actions; it has minimal β-mediated ionotropic and chronotropic cardiac effects.
- Phenylephrine should be concentrated as 200 μg/mL in normal saline and administered intracavernously as 0.5 mL to 1 mL. Lower concentrations should be used in children and adults with cardiovascular disease. Administration and aspiration may need to be repeated. No recommendations can be made about maximum safe dosage. Hypertensive stroke has been reported as a complication of cumulative administration of 2 mg.
- Physicians should monitor patients for subjective complaints and objective findings consistent with known undesirable effects: headache, chest discomfort, acute hypertension, reflex bradycardia, tachycardia, palpitations, and cardiac arrhythmia. Patients and parents should be informed about these potential complications.
- Blood pressure monitoring is recommended with repeated sympathomimetic administration. In patients with significant cardiovascular risks, electrocardiogram monitoring is recommended.
- Ischemic priapism associated with SCD requires intracavernous treatment. A hematologist may provide concurrent systemic therapies (oxygen, hydration, transfusion), but the best resolution rates are achieved with therapies directed at the penis.

investigators using oral α-adrenergics in the management of SCD stuttering ischemic priapism suggests that limited daily administration should be considered in the management of stuttering priapism; drug therapy is typically initiated at bedtime. Oral α-adrenergic administration is a preventative strategy for stuttering priapism.

Hormonal Therapies

The primary action of systemic hormonal therapy in stuttering priapism is the suppression of the androgenic effects on penile erection. Attempts to treat stuttering priapism with hormones have exploited known regulators of male sexual function by targeting the pituitary gland (GnRH agonists), suppressing pituitary function through feedback inhibition (diethylstilbestrol [DES]), blocking androgen receptors (antiandrogens), and reducing testicular and adrenal synthesis (ketoconazole). The common goal of hormonal therapy in the prevention of stuttering priapism is to reduce serum testosterone to hypogonadal levels or block testosterone's effects on the penis. In the only randomized placebo-controlled trial, a synthetic estrogen, **DES,** caused termination of the stuttering episodes in all patients who received treatment (Chinegwundoh and Anie, 2004). However, in more than 50% of patients (5 of 9) priapism recurred after treatment cessation. Similar results have been described by others in case reports (Gbadoe et al, 2002; Shamloul and el Nashaar, 2005). Long-term estrogen therapy is not recommended because of the potential cardiovascular side effects. **GnRH analogues,** goserelin acetate and leuprolide acetate, have been described in case reports (Levine and Guss, 1993; Shamloul and el Nashaar, 2005). Chronic therapy with GnRH analogues in combination with penile injection of α-adrenergics as needed has been reported in the management of ischemic stuttering priapism (Steinberg and Eyre, 1995). Discontinuation of GnRH analogues typically leads to stuttering resumption. **Antiandrogens** including flutamide, bicalutamide, and chlormadinone have been used to interrupt stuttering priapism, and their use has been detailed in case reports. Antiandrogens may have benefit to patients over the GnRH analogues because they are orally administered and because some patients continue having sexually stimulated erections (Costabile, 1998; Dahm et al, 2002; Yamashita et al, 2004). Abern and Levine (2009) used nightly administration of the antifungal agent **oral ketoconazole and prednisone** to suppress nocturnal erections as a preventive strategy for recurrent ischemic priapism in 8 patients followed for 1.5 years. The protocol required titrating dosages and monitoring of nocturnal erections and serum testosterone levels; mean testosterone levels fell from a baseline of 475 ng/dL to 275 ng/dL. The fall in testosterone levels appeared to be a surrogate for efficacy in preventing significant episodes of priapism. Ketoconazole inhibits steroidogenesis in the adrenal and gonadal tissues; it has a half-life of 8 hours. Ketoconazole inhibits cortisol production, necessitating concomitant prednisone administration. In the Abern and Levine protocol, men with recurring ischemic priapism were treated with ketoconazole 200 mg given orally (PO) every 8 hours and prednisone 5 mg at bedtime for 2 weeks, followed by ketoconazole nightly without prednisone supplementation. Rachid-Filho and colleagues (2009) have described the efficacy of oral **5α-reductase inhibitors** (finasteride) in the management of sickle cell stuttering priapism. They administered finasteride to 35 patients over 120 days in doses that decreased monthly from 5 mg/day to 3 mg/day and then 1 mg/day in the final month. This was not a controlled trial, but careful observation of stuttering episodes was made. They found at the beginning of treatment that the mean number of episodes of stuttering priapism per patient was 22.7, and at the end of 4 months the mean number of episodes per patient was 2.1. The optimal effects were found at 5- and 3-mg daily doses. Six of 35 patients in this study developed painless gynecomastia. Finasteride is a 5α-reductase inhibitor approved in the United States for management of symptomatic BPH (Proscar 5 mg) and male pattern alopecia (Propecia 1 mg); finasteride and dutasteride are type II 5α-reductase inhibitors. This class of drugs reduces conversion of testosterone to dihydrotestosterone, which is believed to be many times more potent at the cellular level. Paradoxically, when measured during clinical trials, serum testosterone levels go up in healthy controls and patients administered finasteride or dutasteride. Neither drug is approved for use in patients with stuttering ischemic priapism.

Baclofen

Studies in both rats and humans suggest that baclofen inhibits penile erection and ejaculation, through γ-aminobutyric acid (GABA) receptor activity. In rats, stimulation of $GABA_B$ receptors in the lumbosacral spinal cord inhibits erection (Bitran et al, 1988; Paredes and Agmo, 1995; Vaidyanathan et al, 2004). Denys and colleagues (1998) reported on nine men with multiple sclerosis or spinal cord injuries who were treated for 44 months with intrathecal baclofen for muscle spasticity; eight of nine reported decreased erectile function, which reversed on cessation of baclofen. Rourke and colleagues (2002) first reported on the use of oral nightly baclofen 40 mg in the management of recurrent priapism in patients with neurologic lesions. D'Aleo and colleagues (2009) were the first to report on the use of an intrathecal pump to administer baclofen

180 μg daily for the management of skeletal muscle spasm and recurrent priapism in a patient with spinal cord injury; the patient was refractory to treatment with oral administration of 75 mg/day but responded to a test dose of 25 μg intrathecally. The neurologic literature generally fails to categorize these erectile events as ischemic or nonischemic. Triggering events may be tactile nonsexual stimulation causing repeated reflexogenic erections. Better characterization of these unwanted erections in men with upper motor neural lesions is necessary to appreciate hemodynamics, inciting events, duration, and impact on erectile function. There have been reports to the FDA that men with baclofen infusion pumps experience a withdrawal syndrome when those pumps fail. The withdrawal syndrome has been characterized by return of spasticity, agitation, sleeplessness, and priapism. Advanced symptoms resemble autonomic dysreflexia and may include rhabdomyolysis. The syndrome responds to oral baclofen dosing until intrathecal therapy can be resumed. In non-neurogenic patients, daily administration of baclofen is associated with drowsiness, nausea, complaints of fatigue, and ED. Recurrent reflexogenic erections are clearly an unwanted condition associated with muscle spasticity in men with spinal cord lesions and neurologic disease, but it remains to be demonstrated whether the duration and hemodynamics of such erectile events are similar to ischemic stuttering priapism typical in SCD.

Phosphodiesterase Type 5 Inhibitors in the Management of Stuttering Priapism: A Counterintuitive Treatment Strategy

Bialecki and Bridges (2002) first reported on sildenafil having a paradoxic effect in controlling stuttering priapism in three patients with SCD. Although this proposal would immediately seem illogical on the basis of the understanding that PDE5 inhibitors exert erectogenic effects, there is a scientific basis for using these agents to treat priapism.

In a small case series, Burnett and colleagues showed that daily sildenafil or tadalafil therapy reduces ischemic priapism episodes in men with stuttering priapism (Burnett et al, 2006a). **When used in long-term regimens unassociated with erection stimulatory conditions, PDE5 inhibitor therapy alleviates recurrent priapism episodes in men with SCD-associated priapism without affecting normal erectile capacity** (Burnett et al, 2006b; Bivalacqua et al, 2009a). The working theory is that surges of cGMP go unchecked because of downregulated levels of PDE5; this results in stimuli such as nocturnal erection, which causes unchecked corporal smooth muscle relaxation. In initial series, the short-acting PDE5 inhibitor sildenafil citrate was given at a dose of 25 mg oral daily, with escalation to 50 mg daily. Subsequently these investigators reported on tadalafil at a dose of 5 or 10 mg taken orally three times weekly. Multicenter, randomized, double-blind, placebo-controlled clinical trials are underway. PDE5 inhibitors should be started under conditions of complete penile flaccidity, not during a stuttering episode. Efficacy is seen after a week or more of administration.

SURGICAL MANAGEMENT OF ISCHEMIC PRIAPISM

Surgical management of ischemic priapism is indicated after repeated penile aspirations and injections of sympathomimetics have failed or if such an attempt has resulted in a significant cardiovascular side effect. At present there is a paucity of data regarding the timing of surgical intervention following initiation of medical treatment, although the 2004 International Consultation on Sexual Medicine in Paris recommended corporal aspiration and α-adrenergic agonists for at least 1 hour before consideration of shunting (Pryor et al, 2004). **Early surgical intervention may be preferable in patients with malignant or poorly controlled hypertension or for men who are using monoamine oxidase inhibitor medications contraindicating α-adrenergic therapies.** A comprehensive discussion and documentation that includes baseline erectile function, duration of priapism, risks and benefits of the surgery, and ED should be held with the patient or guardian and an informed consent form signed by the patient or guardian.

Shunting

It is generally accepted that the longer an episode of ischemic priapism lasts, the greater the likelihood of compromised erectile function in the future. Early reviews concluded that priapism lasting longer than 24 hours was associated with a 90% ED rate (Pryor and Hehir, 1982). Kulmala and colleagues (1996) reported 92% erectile function preservation among patients with ischemic priapism reversed in less than 24 hours, but only 22% preservation of erectile function among men with priapism lasting longer than 7 days. Recommendations based on well-documented erectile function outcomes are few. One recent study does document erectile function outcomes by contemporary standards (International Index of Erectile Function [IIEF]). Bennett and Mulhall (2008) carefully documented 39 patients with SCD priapism who came to their emergency department over 8 years; men were routinely interviewed for erectile function status within 4 weeks of priapism and interventions. Of the 39 African-American men followed, 73% acknowledged prior episodes of stuttering; 85% had previously been diagnosed with SCD; but only 5% had been counseled in SCD clinics or were aware that priapism was a complication of SCD. A standard protocol of aspiration and phenylephrine injection was performed; shunting for failure of medical management was performed in 28%. In patients in whom priapism was reversed, spontaneous erections (with or without use of sildenafil) were reported in 100% of men when priapism was reversed by 12 hours; 78% when reversed by 12 to 24 hours; and 44% when reversed by 24 to 36 hours. In this contemporary series of SCD patients, no men reported the return of spontaneous erections after priapism lasting 36 hours or more. **The International Society for Sexual Medicine**

Standards Committee (expert opinion) stated that shunting is to be considered for ischemic priapism events lasting 72 hours or less. Consideration should be given to foregoing a shunt in priapism events lasting longer, in particular when cavernous thrombosis is evident and no blood can be aspirated from the corporal bodies (Pryor et al, 2004; Mulhall, 2006).

The objective of shunt surgery is reoxygenation of the cavernous smooth muscle. The shared principle of shunt procedures is to reestablish corporal inflow by relieving venous outflow obstruction; this requires creation of a fistula between the CC and glans penis, CC and corpus spongiosum, or CC and dorsal or saphenous veins. Shunt procedures are subdivided on the basis of anatomic location on the penis (Lue and Pescatori, 2006) (Fig. 28-8).

- Percutaneous distal shunts—Ebbehoj (1974), Winter (1976), or T shunt (Brant et al, 2009)
- Open distal shunt—Al-Ghorab (Hanafy et al, 1976; Borrelli et al, 1983) or corporal snake (Burnett and Pierorazio, 2009)
- Combined T shunt and corporal snake maneuver—Zacharakis and colleagues (2014b)
- Open proximal shunt—Quackles (1964) or Sacher and colleagues (1972)
- Saphenous vein—Grayhack and colleagues (1964)
- Deep dorsal vein shunt—Barry (1976)

A distal cavernoglanular shunt should be the first choice of shunting procedures because it is technically easier to perform than proximal shunting. Percutaneous distal shunting is less invasive than open distal shunting and can be performed with local anesthetic in the emergency department. The most recently described distal shunt (Brant et al, 2009) creates a T-shaped shunt between the CC and glans penis. Brant and associates (2009) describes 13 men with priapism durations longer than 24 hours (in 6 of 13, other distal or proximal shunt procedures had failed). All T shunts were performed after penile anesthetic block; in 12 of 13 patients, the priapism was successfully reversed by initial intervention. In T shunting a No. 10 blade is placed vertically through the glans 4 mm away from the meatus; the blade pierces through the glans to the CC and is rotated 90 degrees away from the urethra and removed (Fig. 28-9). Deoxygenated blood is milked out of the wound. The glans is then sutured with absorbable suture. The authors recommend discharge home if the penis remains flaccid for 15 minutes (Brant et al, 2009). If erection returns or persists, a second T shunt is recommended on the opposite side of the meatus. When ischemic priapism has been present for more than 36 hours, immediate placement of bilateral T shunts is recommended, with passage of 20-Fr dilators into the fistula tract and well into the CC down to the crus. This technique is more traumatic and will require general anesthesia. Burnett and Pierorazio (2009) have described a similar technique to resolve ischemic priapism refractory to first-line interventions. Their procedure, known as the *corporal snake,* is a modification of the Al-Ghorab corporoglanular shunt (see Fig. 28-8B and Fig. 28-10). With the patient under general anesthesia, a 2-cm transverse incision is made on the glans; the distal tips of the rigid CC are incised and grasped with 2-0 stay sutures or Kocher clamps. Deoxygenated blood is milked out of the CC, but rather than excising a wedge of tunica and underlying CC muscle, a 7/8 Hegar dilator is advanced through each of the tunica windows proximally several centimeters to release blood and thrombus. The penis is made flaccid by repeated manual compression and release; the glans skin is then approximated with 4-0 chromic sutures; a urethral catheter is placed, and lightly compressive dressing is applied to the genitalia.

Segal and associates (2013) retrospectively reviewed the Johns Hopkins Hospital experience with the corporal snake maneuver. Ten patients with ischemic priapism with a mean duration of 75 hours (range 24 to 288 hours) refractory to medical intervention and simple distal shunting (Winter or Ebbehoj) were treated surgically with the corporal snake maneuver; in 8 the priapism resolved, and they had no postoperative recurrence during 6-month follow-up. In 2 patients the priapism did not respond; they were treated by insertion of inflatable penile implant at time of presentation. Complication rates were significant (20%); complications

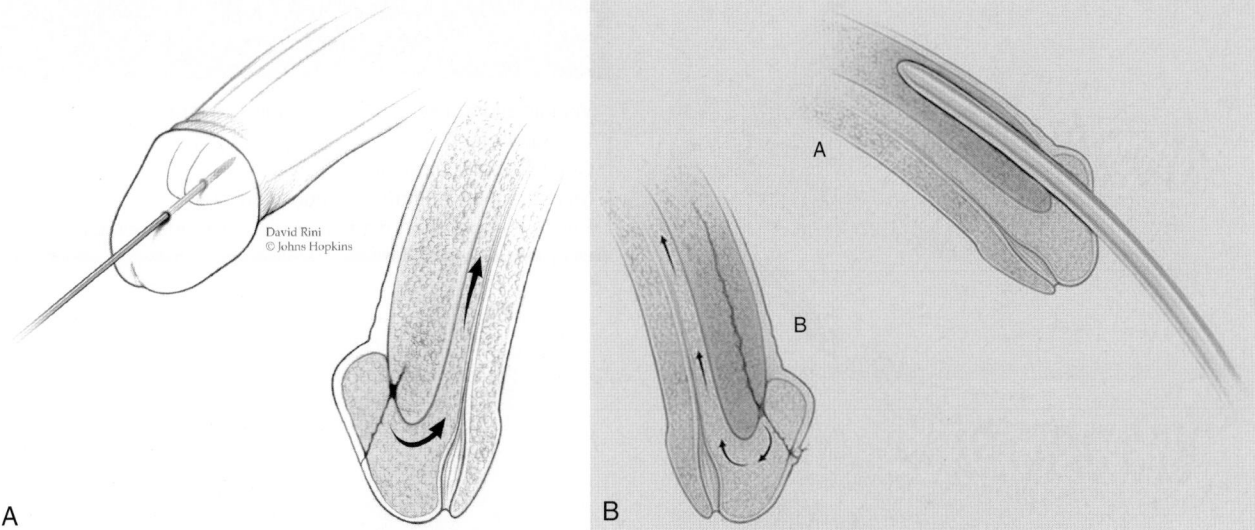

Figure 28-8. **A,** Winter shunt. The distal cavernoglanular shunt procedure is depicted by the transglanular placement of a large-bore needle or angiocatheter in the distal glans and corpus cavernosum. **B,** Corporal snake maneuver is a modification of the Al-Ghorab shunt. After excision of a 5-mm circular core of distal tunica albuginea, a 7/8 Hegar dilator is inserted down each corporal body through the tunica window. (A, © Brady Urological Institute; B, from Burnett AL, Pierorazio PM. Corporal "snake" maneuver: corporoglanular shunt surgical modification for ischemic priapism J Sex Med 2009;6:1171–76.)

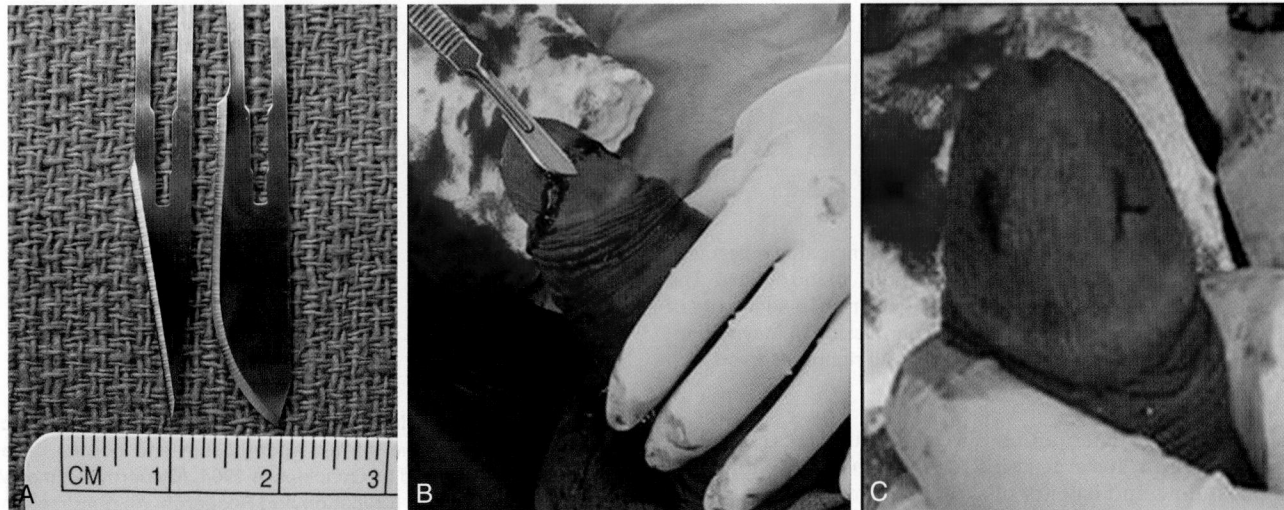

Figure 28-9. **A,** A No. 11 blade is used for an Ebbehoj percutaneous cavernoglanular shunt, and a No. 10 blade is used for a T shunt. **B and C,** Note the differences between the Ebbehoj and T shunts. In the Ebbehoj technique the No. 11 blade leaves a straight incision into the glans and corpus cavernosum. In the creation of a T shunt the No. 10 blade is rotated 90 degrees after insertion and is withdrawn. In both the percutaneous techniques deoxygenated blood is milked out of the open wounds; once bright red blood is seen, the skin is closed, leaving the deeper incision of the open fistula. In either procedure the maneuver may be repeated on the opposite corpus. (Courtesy Dr. Tom Lue.)

included wound infection, penile skin necrosis, and urethrocutaneous fistula. The authors documented sexual health function outcomes in these patients treated for refractory priapism lasting 24 to 288 hours; all had significant complaints of ED at 6 months, with 2 of 8 receiving subsequent penile implants (Segal et al, 2013). Zacharakis and colleagues (2014b) described the efficacy and outcomes of combining the T shunt (Brant et al, 2009) with the corporal snake maneuver in 45 patients. All were refractory to medical reversal of ischemic priapism. The combined distal surgical technique was successful in resolving the acute priapism if duration was less than 24 hours but had limited efficacy in cases of priapism exceeding 48 hours. Corporal needle biopsies were performed in

each patient and documented smooth muscle necrosis, worsening as a function of time and uniform in all men with more than 48 hours of ischemia. At 6 months, erectile function outcomes were assessed by the erectile function domain score from the IIEF-5. T shunt with corporal snake tunneling successfully reversed ischemic priapism in all patients with less than 24 hours' duration, but at 6 months ED was reported by 50% of men. The authors (Zacharakis et al, 2014b) conclude that the cutoff for reversing ischemic priapism in the hopes of preserving future erectile function is 48 hours. They advise that management of refractory ischemic priapism of longer than 48 hours' duration should include discussion of immediate insertion of a penile implant.

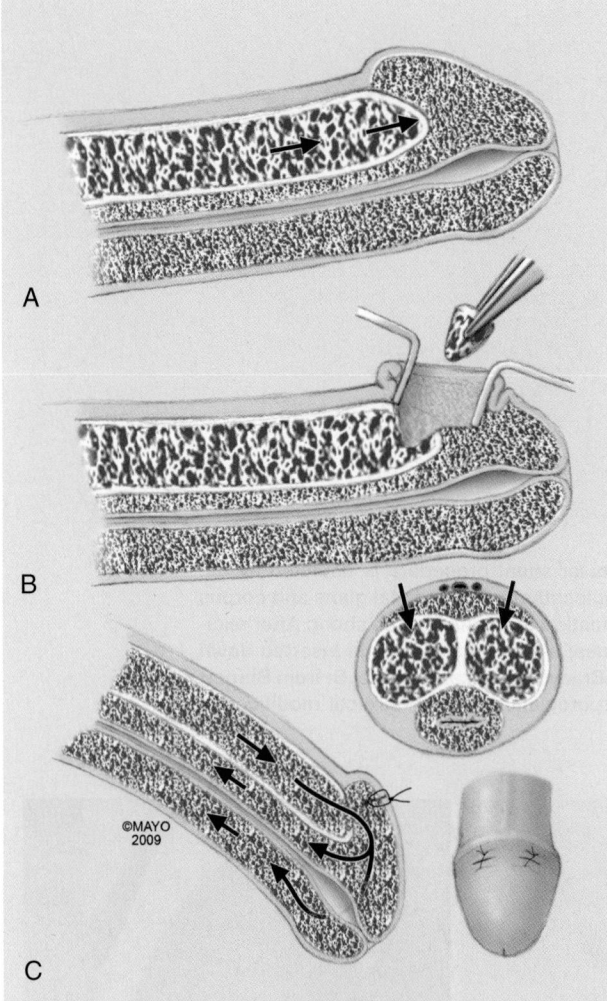

Figure 28-10. **An open corporoglanular shunt is indicated if percuta-neous shunting fails to reestablish cavernous blood inflow. The Al-Ghorab shunt requires the excision of circular cone segments of the distal tunica albuginea (5 × 5 mm). (By permission of Mayo Foundation for Medical Education and Research. All rights reserved.)**

BOX 28-3   Assessing Corpora Cavernosa Shunt Patency

Visualization of bright red blood in corporal aspirate
Corporal blood gas
Color Doppler ultrasonography
Measurement of intracavernous pressure
Penile compression maneuver (squeeze and release)

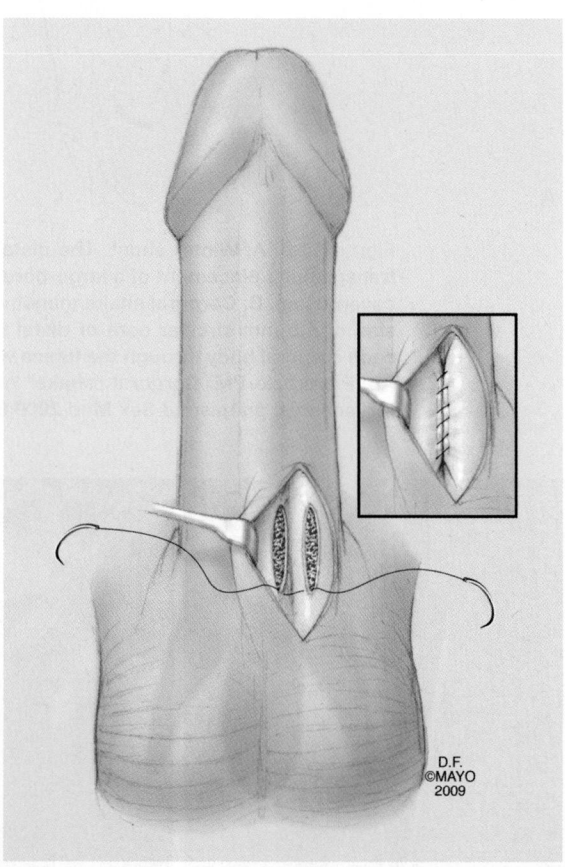

Figure 28-11. **The proximal open shunt technique to establish com-munication between the corpus spongiosum and corpus caverno-sum was first described by Quackles in 1964. (By permission of Mayo Foundation for Medical Education and Research. All rights reserved.)**

The key factors determining successful surgical reversal of ischemic priapism are evacuation of thrombus, reestablishing cavernous inflow, and patency of shunt. Theoretically, larger open shunt procedures are likely to result in higher shunt patency rates; there are no data comparing percutaneous and open distal shunts. The surgeon must be guided by familiarity with various techniques: percutaneous shunting, open distal shunting, proximal shunting, and vein shunting. Although distal shunting can be performed with penile block and sedation in the emergency department, open shunting, especially that requiring passage of dilators into the CC, will likely require general anesthesia and an operating room suite. At the completion of the shunt, patency can be verified in the oper-ating room and subsequently the recovery room in a number of ways: bright oxygenated blood should be seen emanating from the corporal bodies; intracavernous pressures should fall; the penis should detumesce and refill with sequential compression and release; and CDU should show resumption of cavernous artery inflow (Lue, 2002; Nixon et al, 2003; Chiou et al, 2009a) (Box 28-3). Complications of shunting include penile edema, hema-toma, infection, urethral fistula, penile necrosis, and pulmonary embolism. Distal shunt failures may be the consequence of inad-equate size and/or formation of a clot at the site. Distal shunt failure invariably leads to further surgical interventions. Shunts cut through the collagen-rich tunica albuginea; collagen-activated platelets and fibrin form as a reaction to surgical injury and will work to seal off

the shunt. Premature thrombosis of the site could lead to shunt failure. Three suggestions have been made to prevent shunt obstruc-tion and subsequent failure: (1) compressive penile dressings should be avoided; (2) the patient should periodically squeeze and release the distal penis to "milk" the shunt maintaining patency; and (3) anticoagulation should be considered with shunting. The literature contains only one such recommendation for perioperative anticoagulation for the prevention of premature shunt obstruction in ischemic priapism. That regimen includes preoperative aspirin 325 mg coupled with subcutaneous heparin 5000 units and post-operative aspirin 81 mg daily for 2 weeks (Lue and Garcia, 2013).

The most commonly described proximal shunt is the unilat-eral shunt, described by Quackles in 1964 (Fig. 28-11). Proximal corpus cavernosum to spongiosum (CC-CS) shunt procedures require a trans-scrotal or transperineal approach (Quackles, 1964). There are no data comparing bilateral (Sacher et al, 1972) and unilateral CC-CS shunts (Quackles, 1964). Typically, bilateral shunts are staggered; the right side and left side are separated by a distance of at least 1 cm in an effort to minimize the risk of urethral stricture at the point of CC-CS communication (Fig. 28-12). If

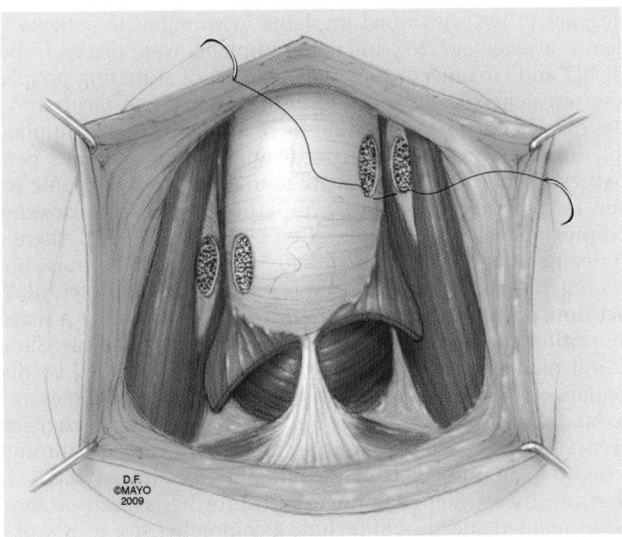

Figure 28-12. Bilateral shunts are staggered. The right and left sides are separated by a distance of at least 1 cm in an effort to minimize the risk of urethral stricture at the point of corpus cavernosum to spongiosum communication (Sacher et al, 1972). (By permission of Mayo Foundation for Medical Education and Research. All rights reserved.)

proximal shunting fails, some have advocated saphenous vein bypass or deep dorsal vein shunt (Fig. 28-13). A wedge of tunica albuginea is removed and the vein is anastomosed end to side of CC. There are no comparative trials of vein shunting for ischemic priapism. Authors have described a significant risk of saphenofemoral vein thrombus and pulmonary embolism with vein shunting (Kandel et al, 1968).

Immediate Implantation of Penile Prosthesis

Unfortunately, **the natural history of untreated ischemic priapism or priapism refractory to interventions is severe fibrosis, penile length loss, and complete ED** (see Fig. 28-1). Kelami (1985) described the implantation of the Small-Carrion penile prosthesis through an infrapubic incision in the management of postpriapic ED. Bertram and colleagues (1985) described six postpriapic cases of penile prosthesis; five of the six men had successful implantation of semirigid prostheses. Both groups described extensive corporal fibrosis and suggested that semirigid implants were preferable because inflatable implants would not overcome the corporal fibrosis sufficiently to erect the penis. Douglas and colleagues (1990) reported on penile prosthesis in five SCD postpriapic men; they described a surgical technique of tunneling and corporal excavation. Inadvertent damage to the tunica albuginea was common, as was subsequent migration of hardware; 11 additional procedures were required after the initial implants. The average time from priapism to implant in Douglas's series was 4 years. Monga and

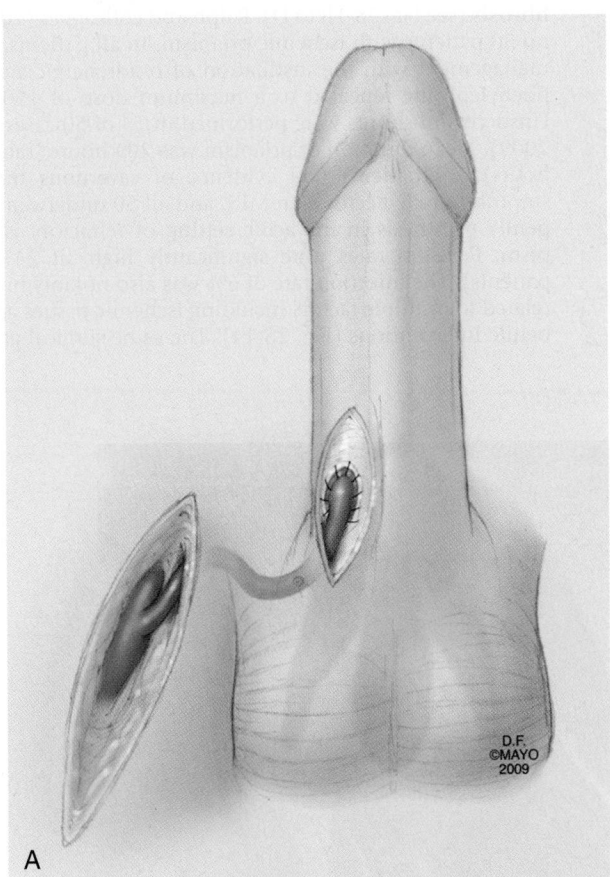

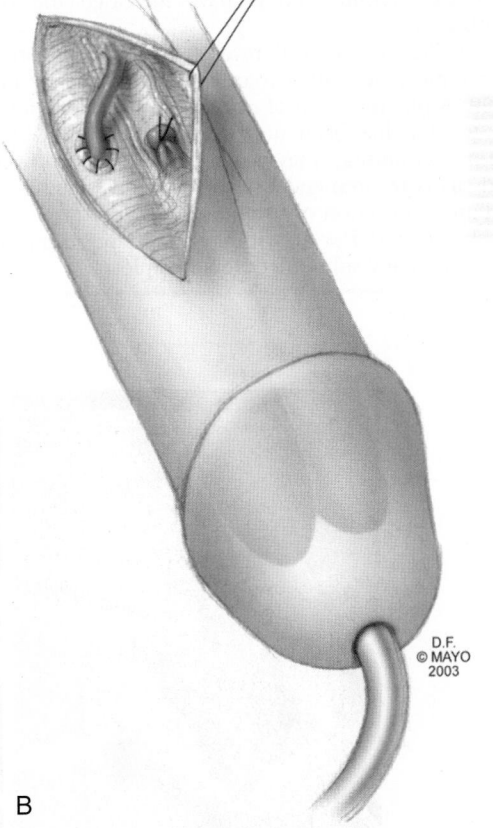

Figure 28-13. A, Venous bypass to control ischemic priapism was first described by Grayhack and colleagues in 1964. The Grayhack shunt mobilizes the saphenous vein below the junction of the femoral vein and anastomoses the vein end to side into the corpus cavernosum. **B,** Deep dorsal vein (DDV) shunt with distal ligation of DDV and anastomosis of proximal DDV to corpus cavernosum. A wedge of tunica albuginea is removed. (By permission of Mayo Foundation for Medical Education and Research. All rights reserved.)

colleagues (1996) described implants in young SCD patients (six patients, average age 26); inflatable implants were placed to both treat ED and circumvent ongoing episodes of stuttering priapism. These researchers suggested that both potency and recurrent episodes of ischemic priapism could be managed by "early" implantation. **Some have suggested performing an immediate penile prosthesis procedure in the acute management of ischemic priapism in patients in whom sympathomimetic intracavernous therapies and shunting have failed** (Rees et al, 2002). There are two distinct advantages to immediate implantation: corporal fibrosis is not yet established, and penile length may be preserved. **The exact time point at which prosthetic insertion becomes a reasonable option for managing ischemic priapism is unclear.** Should medical management of ischemic priapism be followed by distal percutaneous shunt, by open distal shunt, and subsequently by proximal shunting before penile implant? Should men with delayed presentation of ischemic priapism and evident corporal thrombus be triaged to an immediate penile implant procedure? What is clear is that any discussion pertaining to early prosthesis insertion should be documented and should include a comprehensive review of the theoretic advantages and actual risks. Compared with prosthesis insertion in a typical patient with ED, **there are significantly higher rates of complications noted in priapism cases: infection, urethral injury, device migration, device erosion, and revision surgeries.** The surgeon must be familiar with the additional technical concerns posed by weaknesses in the tunica albuginea in the region of prior shunts.

The advantages of early penile implantation in the acute management of ischemic priapism are preservation of penile length and technically easier implant insertion. Delayed placement of penile prosthesis is technically challenging because of corporal fibrosis (see Fig. 28-1B to D). Ralph and colleagues (2009) reported on 50 patients with ischemic priapism. In all patients, conservative management with the instillation of α-adrenergic agents (200 μg phenylephrine repeated to a maximum dose of 1500 μg) failed. Unsuccessful shunts were performed in 13 of 50 cases (Ralph et al, 2009). Mean duration of priapism was 209 hours (range 24 to 720 hours). All patients had evidence of cavernous thrombus and smooth muscle necrosis on MRI, and all 50 underwent insertion of penile prosthesis in the acute setting of refractory ischemic priapism. Revision rates were significantly high, at 24% (12 of 50 patients). The infection rate of 6% was also notably high and likely related to multiple factors including ischemic tissues and preceding penile interventions (Fig. 28-14). The same surgical group recently

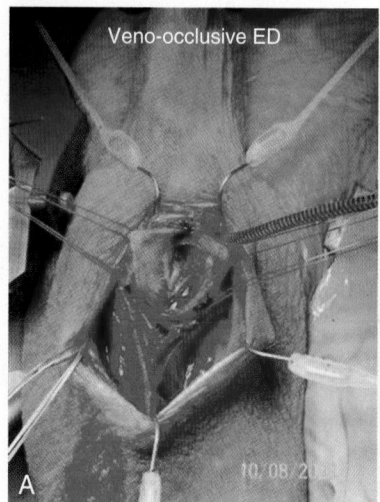
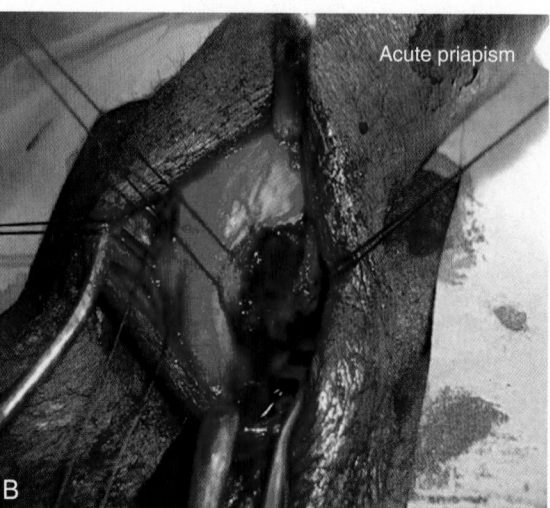

Figure 28-14. **A penoscrotal surgical approach for insertion of inflatable penile implant in a white male patient with severe veno-occlusive erectile dysfunction (ED) (A) and a sickle cell disease patient with acute ischemic priapism refractory to pharmacologic interventions and shunting for 48 hours (B). (A, Courtesy G. A. Broderick, MD; B, courtesy David J. Ralph, MD.)**

KEY POINTS: SURGICAL MANAGEMENT OF ISCHEMIC PRIAPISM WITH IMMEDIATE PENILE IMPLANT

- The natural history of untreated ischemic priapism or priapism refractory to interventions is severe fibrosis, penile length loss, and complete ED.
- The advantages of early penile implantation in the acute management of ischemic priapism are preservation of penile length and easier insertion.
- Document baseline erectile function, duration of priapism, history of stuttering, and prior interventions.
- Consider penile prosthesis in the following circumstances:
  - Aspiration and sympathomimetic ICI have failed.
  - Distal and proximal shunting procedures have failed.
  - Ischemia has been present for longer than 36 hours.
- Consider an MRI before surgery or corporal biopsy at the time of implant to document corporal smooth muscle necrosis.
- There are higher rates of revision surgery and complications noted in priapism cases resulting from infection, urethral injury, device migration, and device erosion.

compared two cohorts of patients undergoing penile implant for refractory ischemic priapism. An early insertion cohort was operated on at a mean of 7 days after onset of priapism, and the delayed cohort was operated on at a mean of 5 months after priapism. In the early insertion group, satisfaction and ability to have intercourse was 96%; in the delayed group, corporal fibrosis made surgery technically more difficult and overall patient satisfaction was 60% (Zacharakis et al, 2014a).

INTERVENTIONAL ANGIOGRAPHY IN THE MANAGEMENT OF ARTERIAL (NONISCHEMIC, HIGH-FLOW) PRIAPISM

Arterial priapism is not an emergency. Spontaneous resolution or response to conservative therapy has been reported in up to 62% of published series (Montague et al, 2003; Pryor et al, 2004). Persistent partial erection from HFP may be evident for months to years, without adverse impact on erectile function (Bastuba et al, 1995). Kumar and colleagues (2006) described a case of HFP in a 24-year-old patient 10 days after straddle injury on a bicycle. The patient had no erection for the first 4 days after injury. Examination revealed a tumescent penis that was compressible. Penile aspiration and blood gas analysis revealed oxygenated corporal blood. CDU of the cavernous artery revealed arteriosinusoidal fistula. Partial erection spontaneously resolved 4 days after diagnostic evaluation, with the patient reporting normal erections 2 weeks later. The authors hypothesized that in patients with blunt penile and perineal trauma, an arteriolacunar fistula forms; these fistulae, unlike arteriovenous communications, may spontaneously resolve because the less rigid walls of the lacunae are prone to spontaneous thrombosis. Onset of HFP is typically delayed for 72 hours after injury. The erection is partial, not rigid, and not painful. Although the site of perineal trauma may have hematoma, spreading of the hematoma to the shaft should raise suspicion of rupture of tunica albuginea; this would be highly unusual in blunt perineal (straddle) injury. The pathophysiology of HFP is unregulated arteriolacunar fistula from disruption or crush injury to terminal branches of the cavernous artery. Fistula is typically unilateral. Because there is no restriction of venous outflow, erection is partial and bendable. Patients do report additional engorgement with sexual stimulation, with return to partial erection after climax.

There are no comparative outcome studies of intervention versus conservative management in HFP; there are sufficient case descriptions, especially in children, to recommend initial watchful

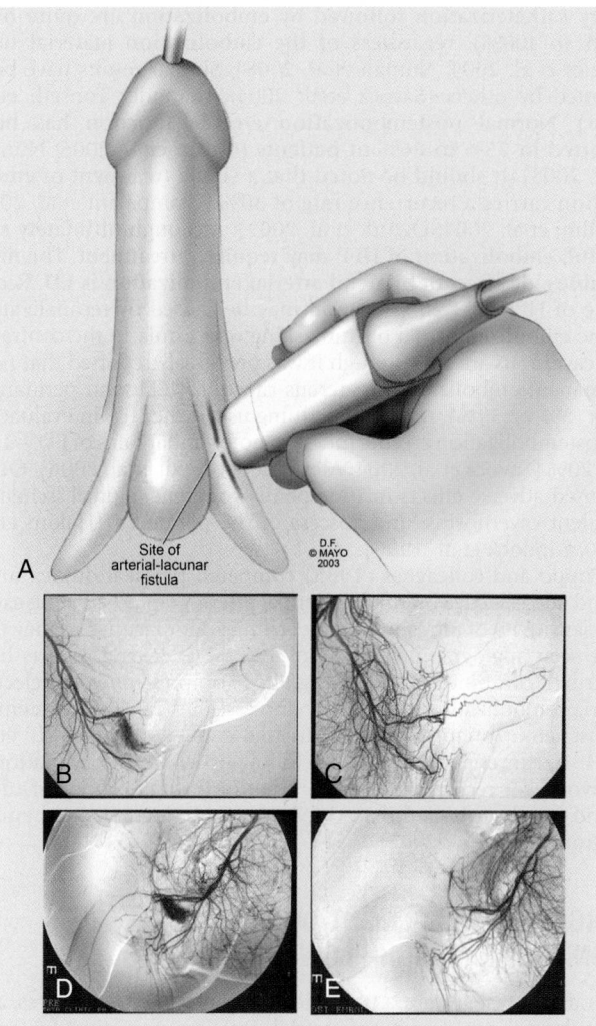

Figure 28-15. Color Doppler ultrasonography of the penis and perineum is recommended in the evaluation of priapism when the history or examination findings suggest penile trauma (A). Doppler sonography for localization of a fistula correlates well with selective pudendal angiography (B to E); a characteristic fistula blush is shown (B and D), along with normal arteriograms (C and E). (A, By permission of Mayo Foundation for Medical Education and Research. All rights reserved.)

waiting (Nehra, 2006). Initial observation is recommended for this type of priapism. Conservative measures include ice applied to the perineum and site-specific compression. **Cavernous aspiration has only a diagnostic role in HFP. Repeated aspirations, injection, and irrigation with intracavernous sympathomimetics have no role in the treatment of nonischemic priapism.**

Patients demanding immediate relief can be offered selective arterial embolization. The pathognomonic arteriographic finding is an arteriolacunar fistula; a characteristic intracavernosal cone-shaped blush of contrast is seen at the site of the cavernous artery or arteriole laceration (Fig. 28-15). Selective internal pudendal catheterization and subsequent embolization have been reported with various agents: microcoils, polyvinyl alcohol, *N*-butylcyanoacrylate, gel-foam, and autologous blood clot (Kuefer et al, 2005). Permanent materials pose a greater theoretic risk of ED; many authors recommend use of autologous blood clot and absorbable gels (Pryor et al, 2004; Kim et al, 2007). Autologous blood clot has a low risk of foreign body reaction, or antigenicity; it is a temporary occlusive agent and should permit recanalization of the cavernous artery (Park et al, 2001). **The success rates with selective pudendal**

artery catheterization followed by embolization are quite high (89% to 100%), regardless of the embolization material used (Kuefer et al, 2005; Numan et al, 2008). Similar results have been reported by others (Savoca et al, 2004; Alexander Tønseth et al, 2006). **Normal postembolization erectile function has been reported in 75% to 86% of patients** (Cakan et al, 2006; Numan et al, 2008). **It should be noted that a single treatment of embolization carries a recurrence rate of 30%** (Ciampalani et al, 2002; Gandini et al, 2004; Ozturk et al, 2009). **Although ultimately successful, embolization of HFP may require retreatment. The most notable side effect of bilateral arterial embolization is ED.** Recurrence of HPF after embolization may be caused by recanalization of the embolized fistula or unmasking of a fistula in the contralateral cavernous artery. Although it was previously reported that nonpermanent embolization materials cause less ED than permanent ones (5% vs. 39%), reports describing use of the IIEF in evaluation of postembolization erectile function note similar rates of ED—15% and 20% (Savoca et al, 2004; Alexander Tønseth et al, 2006). Other reported adverse effects include penile gangrene, gluteal ischemia, purulent cavernositis, and abscess of the perineum (Hakim et al, 1996; Sandock et al, 1996).

Puppo and colleagues (1985) compared perineal duplex ultrasound and selective internal pudendal arteriography, showing excellent sensitivity of ultrasound in detecting arteriolacunar fistulae that were seen angiographically (12 of 12 cases). Several reports have described combined ultrasound-guided compression with selective arterial embolization to increase success rates in the treatment of nonischemic priapism (Hatzichristou et al, 2002; Bartsch et al, 2004; Cakan et al, 2006). If the follow-up clinical examination is equivocal for recurrence of HFP, a perineal duplex Doppler ultrasound can determine the need for repeat arteriography and embolization (Kim et al, 2007).

SURGICAL MANAGEMENT OF ARTERIAL (NONISCHEMIC, HIGH-FLOW) PRIAPISM

Arterial priapism is not a urologic emergency. HFP is painless, and there have been reports of partial erection persisting for years (Nehra, 2006). Any intervention must follow a comprehensive discussion with the patient regarding risks and benefits of any of the procedures advocated by the clinician. **In cases of long-standing arterial priapism in which a pseudocapsule around the fistula has developed, surgical ligation has been reported to be successful. Formation of a pseudocapsule may take weeks to months after trauma. Corporal exploration before the formation of a pseudocapsule may result in ligation of the cavernous artery** rather than selective ligation of the fistula. Currently this intervention is reserved for patients who do not wish to pursue expectant management or who are poor candidates for angioembolization. It is also reserved for patients who refuse the procedure; for patients in places where technology is not available; and for patients in whom angioembolization has failed (Ji et al, 1994; Berger et al, 2001; Mulhall, 2006). The surgical approach is transcorporal. Intraoperative Doppler ultrasound guidance is recommended (Fig. 28-16).

SUMMARY

Priapism is a full or partial erection that persists more than 4 hours beyond sexual stimulation and orgasm or is unrelated to sexual stimulation. Prompt diagnosis and appropriate management are

---

KEY POINTS: EVALUATION AND MANAGEMENT OF HIGH-FLOW PRIAPISM

- Arterial priapism is not an emergency and may be managed expectantly.
- Diagnosis of HFP is best made by penile or perineal CDU.
- Penile aspiration and injection of α-adrenergic agents is not recommended for HFP.
- Angioembolization should be preceded by a thorough discussion of chances for spontaneous resolution, risks of treatment-related ED, and lack of significant consequences expected from delaying interventions.
- Overall success rates with embolization are high, although a single treatment carries a recurrence rate of 30% to 40%.
- When angioembolization fails or is contraindicated, surgical ligation is reasonable.
- Formation of a pseudocapsule at the site of a sinusoidal fistula may take weeks to months after trauma.
- CDU guidance is recommended during exploration to locate fistulae.

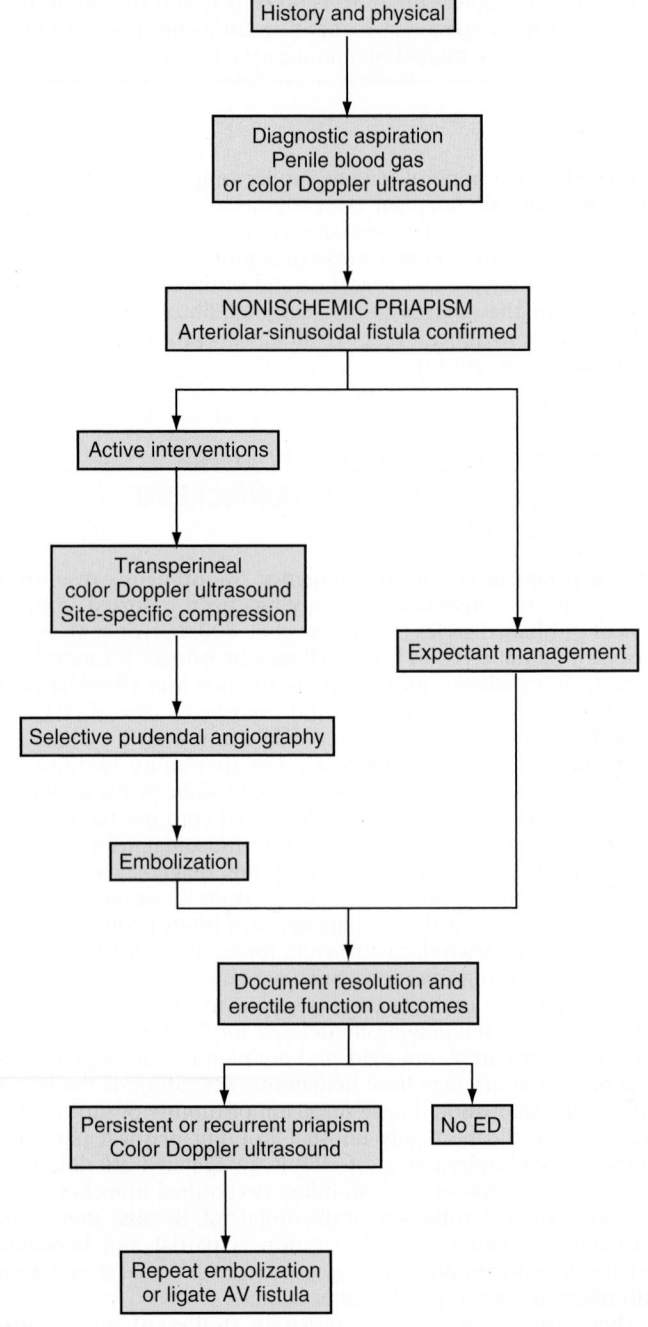

Figure 28-16. Algorithm for managing high-flow priapism. AV, arteriovenous; ED, erectile dysfunction.

necessary to spare patients ineffective interventions and optimize erectile function outcomes. Ischemic priapism (veno-occlusive, low-flow) is a persistent erection marked by rigidity of the CC. In ischemic priapism there are time-dependent changes in the corpora with progressive hypoxia, hypercarbia, and acidosis. Ischemic priapism is a urologic emergency. Treatment for ischemic priapism is administered in stepwise manner: decompression of the corpora by needle aspiration, injection and irrigation with a dilute sympathomimetic drug, surgical shunting, and consideration of immediate penile implant in refractory cases. Ischemic priapism is a common pathologic consequence of SCD. Stuttering ischemic priapism describes a pattern of prolonged morning erections that are unwanted and painful in boys and adolescents with SCD. Any patient who has experienced an episode of ischemic priapism is also at risk for stuttering priapism. HFP (nonischemic priapism, arterial priapism) is a persistent erection caused by unregulated cavernous arterial inflow. Typically, the corpora are tumescent but not rigid and the penis is not painful. A history of blunt trauma (a straddle injury) or an iatrogenic needle injury to the penis is common. The cavernous environment in HFP does not become ischemic, and cavernous blood gases do not show hypoxia, hypercarbia, or acidosis. HFP, once properly diagnosed, does not require emergent treatment. Urologists intervening to treat priapism should use standardized questionnaires to document the history of the prolonged erection: onset, trauma, medical history of blood dyscrasias, use of illicit substances, prior events, prepriapism erectile function, recurrence after each intervention, and recovery of erectile function. Documenting erectile function outcomes on the basis of duration of ischemic priapism, time to interventions, and types of interventions will establish evidence-based guidance on how and when to apply those interventions.

REFERENCES

The complete reference list is available online at www.expertconsult.com.

SUGGESTED READINGS

Bastuba MD, de Tejada IS, Dinlenc CZ, et al. Arterial priapism: diagnosis, treatment and long-term follow up. J Urol 1995;151:1231–7.

Bennett N, Mulhall J. Sickle cell disease status and outcomes of African American men presenting with priapism. J Sex Med 2008;5(5):1244–50.

Bivalacqua TJ, Champion HC, Mason W, et al. Long-term phosphodiesterase type 5 inhibitor therapy reduces priapic activity in transgenic sickle cell mice. J Urol 2006;175:387.

Brant WO, Garcia MM, Bella AJ, et al. T-shaped shunt and intracavernous tunneling for prolonged ischemic priapism. J Urol 2009;181:1699–705.

Broderick GA. Priapism and sickle-cell anemia: diagnosis and nonsurgical therapy. J Sex Med 2012;9:88–103.

Broderick GA, Kadioglu A, Bivalacqua TJ, et al. Priapism: pathogenesis, epidemiology, and management. J Sex Med 2010;7:476–500.

Burnett AL, Bivalacqua TJ, Champion HC, et al. Feasibility of the use of phosphodiesterase type 5 inhibitors in a pharmacologic prevention program for recurrent priapism. J Sex Med 2006;3:1077–84.

Chan PTK, Begin LR, Arnold D, et al. Priapism secondary to penile metastasis: a report of two cases and a review of the literature. J Surg Oncol 1998;68(1):51–9.

Chiou RK, Aggarwal H, Chiou C, et al. Colour Doppler ultrasound hemodynamic characteristics of patient with priapism before and after therapeutic interventions. Can Urol Assoc J 2009a;3(4):304–11.

Kato GJ. Priapism in sickle-cell disease: a hematologist's perspective. J Sex Med 2012;9:70–8.

Ozturk MH, Gumus M, Donme H, et al. Materials in embolotherapy of high-flow priapism: results and long-term follow-up. Diagn Interv Radiol 2009;15(3):215–20.

Ralph DJ, Garaffa G, Muneer A, et al. The immediate insertion of a penile prosthesis for acute ischaemic priapism. Eur Urol 2009;56:1033–8.

Salonia A, Eardley I, Giuliano F, et al. European Association of Urology guidelines on priapism. Eur Urol 2014;65:480–9.

Seftel A, Haas CA, Brown SL, et al. High flow priapism complicating veno-occlusive priapism: pathophysiology of recurrent idiopathic priapism? J Urol 1998;159:1300–1.

Zacharakis E, Raheem AA, Freman A, et al. The efficacy of the T-shunt procedure and intracavernous tunneling (snake maneuver) for refractory ischemic priapism. J Urol 2014b;191:164–8.

29 Disorders of Male Orgasm and Ejaculation

Chris G. McMahon, MBBS, FAChSHM

Ejaculatory dysfunction is one of the most common male sexual disorders. The spectrum of ejaculatory dysfunction **extends from premature ejaculation (PE), through delayed ejaculation, to a complete inability to ejaculate (known as anejaculation) and includes retrograde ejaculation, painful ejaculation, and the recently described postorgasmic illness syndrome (POIS).**

The sexual response cycle comprises the four interactive stages of **desire, arousal, orgasm, and resolution.** During sexual activity, increasing levels of sexual arousal reach a threshold that triggers the ejaculatory response, which then typically terminates the sexual episode for the male. The perception of the striated muscle contractions and resulting semen expelled during ejaculation, mediated through sensory neurons in the pelvic region, gives rise to the experience of orgasm, a distinct cortical event, experienced phenomenologically both cognitively and emotionally.

Ejaculatory latency, the time extending from the onset of penile stimulation to the moment of ejaculation, represents a continuum of time that shows variation across men and, within men, across situations. Although the great majority of men appear to reach ejaculation and orgasm after several minutes of penile vaginal stimulation and are, along with their partners, quite satisfied with the latency of their ejaculatory response, others report dissatisfaction. Specifically, some men ejaculate very rapidly after, or sometimes even before, penetration and do so with minimal stimulation. Others may ejaculate only with great difficulty or not at all, even after prolonged stimulation.

ANATOMY AND PHYSIOLOGY OF THE EJACULATORY RESPONSE

The ejaculatory reflex comprises sensory receptors and areas, afferent pathways, cerebral sensory areas, cerebral motor centers, spinal motor centers, and efferent pathways (Fig. 29-1). Neurochemically, this reflex involves a complex interplay between **central serotonergic and dopaminergic neurons, with secondary involvement of cholinergic, adrenergic, oxytocinergic, and γ-aminobutyric acid (GABA) neurons.**

Based on functional, central, and peripheral mediation, the ejaculatory process is typically subdivided into three phases: **emission, ejection (or penile expulsion), and orgasm.** Emission consists of contractions of seminal vesicles and the prostate, with expulsion of sperm and seminal fluid into the posterior urethra, and is mediated by sympathetic nerves (T10 to L2). Ejection is mediated by somatic nerves (S2 to S4), and involves pulsatile contractions of the bulbocavernosus and pelvic floor muscles together with relaxation of the external urinary sphincter. Ejection also involves a sympathetic spinal cord reflex, on which there is limited voluntary control. The bladder neck closes to prevent retrograde flow; the bulbocavernous, bulbospongiosus, and other pelvic floor muscles contract rhythmically, and the external urinary sphincter relaxes. Intermittent contraction of the urethral sphincter prevents retrograde flow into the proximal urethra (Yeates, 1987). Orgasm is the result of cerebral processing of pudendal nerve sensory stimuli resulting from increased pressure in the posterior urethra, sensory stimuli arising from the verumontanum, and contraction of the urethral bulb and accessory sexual organs.

Many neurotransmitters are involved in the control of ejaculation, including dopamine, norepinephrine, serotonin, acetylcholine, oxytocin, GABA, and nitric oxide (McMahon et al, 2004a). Of the many studies conducted to investigate the role of the brain in the development and mediation of sexual functioning, dopamine and serotonin have emerged as essential neurochemical factors. **Whereas dopamine promotes seminal emission/ejaculation via D_2 receptors, serotonin is inhibitory.** Serotonergic neurons are widely distributed in the brain and spinal cord and are predominantly found in the brainstem, raphe nuclei, and the reticular formation. Currently, multiple serotonin (5-HT) receptors have been characterized: 5-HT_{1A}, 5-HT_{1B}, 5-HT_{2A}, 5-HT_{2B}, etc. (Peroutka and Snyder, 1979). Stimulation of the 5-HT_{2C} receptor with 5-HT_{2C} agonists results in delay of ejaculation in male rats, whereas stimulation of postsynaptic 5-HT_{1A} receptors results in shortening of ejaculation latency (Ahlenius et al, 1981), leading to the hypothesis that men with PE may have hyposensitivity of 5-HT_{2C} and/or hypersensitivity of the 5-HT_{1A} receptor (Waldinger, 2002; Waldinger and Oliver, 2005).

PREMATURE EJACULATION

Classification of Premature Ejaculation

In 1943 Schapiro proposed classification of PE into two types, B and A (Schapiro, 1943). In 1989 Godpodinoff renamed both types as **lifelong (primary) and acquired (secondary) PE** (Godpodinoff, 1989). Over the years, other attempts to specify subtypes have occurred (e.g., global vs. situational, the effect of a substance, etc.).

Lifelong PE is a syndrome characterized by a cluster of core symptoms, including early ejaculation at nearly every intercourse within 30 to 60 seconds in the majority of cases (80%) or between 1 to 2 minutes (20%), with every or nearly every sexual partner and from the first sexual encounters onward (Waldinger, 1998; McMahon, 2002).

Acquired PE differs in that men develop early ejaculation at some point in their life, which is often situational, having previously had normal ejaculation experiences. The main distinguishing features between presentations of these two syndromes are the

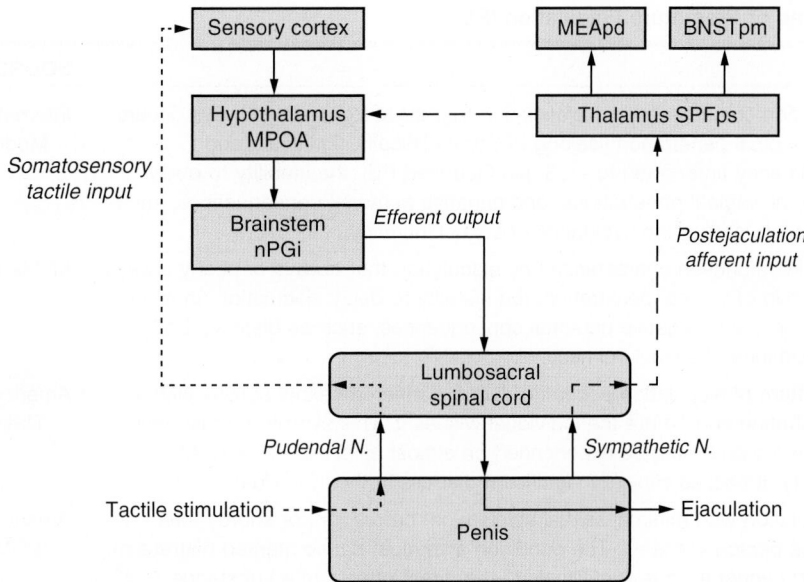

Figure 29-1. Central nervous system areas involved before, during, and after ejaculation. Somatosensory tactile input from the penis/genitals ascends to the cerebral cortex. Efferent pathways project from the hypothalamus to the sacral spinal cord and genitals. After ejaculation, information is returned from the genitals to several brain areas. BNSTpm, posteromedial bed nucleus of stria terminalis; MEApd, posterodorsal medial amygdala; MPOA, medial preoptic area; N, nerve; nPGi, nucleus paragigantocellularis; SPFps, medial parvicellular subparafasicular nucleus of thalamus. (From Waldinger MD. The neurobiological approach to premature ejaculation. J Urol 2002;168:2359–67.)

time of onset of symptoms and the reduction in previously normal ejaculatory latency of acquired PE.

Community-based normative intravaginal ejaculation latency time (IELT) research and observational studies of men with PE demonstrated that although **IELTs of less than 1 minute have a low prevalence of approximately 2.5% in the general population,** a substantially higher percentage of men with normal IELT report PE (Patrick et al, 2005; Waldinger et al, 2005a, 2009). To take account of this diversity, Waldinger and Schweitzer (2006b, 2008) proposed a new classification of PE in which **four PE subtypes are distinguished on the basis of the duration of the IELT, frequency of reports, and course in life. In addition to lifelong PE and acquired PE, this classification includes natural variable PE (or variable PE) and premature-like ejaculatory dysfunction (or subjective PE).** Men with variable PE occasionally experience an early ejaculation. It should not be regarded as a disorder, but as a natural variation of the ejaculation time in men (Waldinger, 2013). On the other hand, men with subjective PE report PE while actually having a normal or even extended ejaculation time (Waldinger, 2013). The report of PE in these men is probably related to psychological and/or cultural factors. In contrast, the consistent early ejaculations of lifelong PE suggest an underlying neurobiologic functional disturbance, whereas the early ejaculation of acquired PE is more related to underlying medical causes. Serefoglu and colleagues (2010, 2011) confirmed the existence of these four PE subtypes in a cohort of men in Turkey. Recently, Zhang and associates (2013) and Gao and colleagues (2013) using a similar methodology confirmed similar prevalence rates of the four PE subtypes in China to that reported by Serefoglu and associates (2010, 2011). This new classification and continued research into the diverse phenomenology, cause, and pathogenesis of PE are expected to provide a better understanding of the four PE subtypes (Waldinger and Schweitzer, 2008). Although the pathogenesis of lifelong and acquired PE differs, the presence of shared dimensions, such as a lack of ejaculatory control and the presence of negative personal consequences, suggests a potential for a single unifying definition of both lifelong and acquired PE. With

continued research into the two other PE subtypes, variable PE and subjective PE, it may be appropriate to expand this unifying definition in the future.

Definition of Premature Ejaculation

Research into the treatment and epidemiology of PE depends heavily on how PE is defined. The **medical literature contains several univariate and multivariate operational definitions of PE** (Masters and Johnson, 1970; American Psychiatric Association, 1994; World Health Organization, 1994; Metz and McCarthy, 2003; Colpi et al, 2004; McMahon et al, 2004b; Montague et al, 2004; Jannini et al, 2005; Waldinger et al, 2005b; McMahon et al, 2008b) (Table 29-1). Each of these definitions characterizes men with PE using all or most of the accepted dimensions of this condition: ejaculatory latency, perceived ability to control ejaculation, reduced sexual satisfaction, personal distress, partner distress, and interpersonal or relationship distress. **None of these definitions was supported by evidence-based clinical research.**

These authority-based definitions are discussed in detail on the Expert Consult website.

International Society for Sexual Medicine Definition of Premature Ejaculation

In the last decade, substantial progress has been made in the development of evidence-based methodology for PE epidemiologic and drug treatment research using the objective IELT and subjective validated patient-reported outcome (PRO) measures. In October 2007, **the International Society for Sexual Medicine (ISSM) convened an initial meeting of the first Ad Hoc ISSM Committee for the Definition of Premature Ejaculation to develop the first contemporary, evidence-based definition of lifelong PE.** Evidence-based definitions seek to limit errors of classification and thereby increase the likelihood that existing and newly developed therapeutic strategies are truly effective in carefully selected dysfunctional

TABLE 29-1 Definitions of Premature Ejaculation (PE)

DEFINITION	SOURCE
PE is a male sexual dysfunction characterized by ejaculation that always or nearly always occurs before or within 1 min of vaginal penetration (lifelong PE) or a clinically significant and bothersome reduction in latency time, often to ~≤ 3 min (acquired PE), the inability to delay ejaculation on all or nearly all vaginal penetrations, and negative personal consequences, such as distress, bother, frustration, and/or the avoidance of sexual intimacy.	International Society of Sexual Medicine, 2014
Lifelong PE is a male sexual dysfunction characterized by ejaculation that always or nearly always occurs before or within 1 min of vaginal penetration, the inability to delay ejaculation on all or nearly all vaginal penetrations, and negative personal consequences, such as distress, bother, frustration, and/or the avoidance of sexual intimacy.	McMahon et al (ISSM), 2008b
A persistent or recurrent pattern of ejaculation occurring during partnered sexual activity within ~1 min after vaginal penetration and before the individual wishes it. This symptom must have been present for at least 6 mo and must be experienced on almost all or all (~75%-100%) occasions of sexual activity. It causes clinically significant distress in the individual.	American Psychiatric Asociation (DSM-5), 2013
Persistent or recurrent ejaculation with minimal sexual stimulation, before, on, or shortly after penetration and before the person wishes it. The condition also must cause marked distress or interpersonal difficulty and cannot be due exclusively to the direct effects of a substance.	American Psychiatric Asociation (DSM-IV-TR), 2000
For individuals who meet the general criteria for sexual dysfunction, the inability to control ejaculation sufficiently for both partners to enjoy sexual interaction, manifest as either the occurrence of ejaculation before or very soon after the beginning of intercourse (if a time limit is required, before or within 15 secs) or the occurrence of ejaculation in the absence of sufficient erection to make intercourse possible. The problem is not the result of prolonged absence from sexual activity.	World Health Organization (ICD-10), 1994
The inability to control ejaculation for a "sufficient" length of time before vaginal penetration. It does not involve any impairment of fertility, when intravaginal ejaculation occurs.	Hatzimouratidis et al (EAU Guidelines on Disorders of Ejaculation), 2010
Persistent or recurrent ejaculation with minimal stimulation before, on, or shortly after penetration and before the person wishes it, over which the man has little or no voluntary control, which causes the man and/or his partner bother or distress.	McMahon et al (ICUD), 2004b
Ejaculation that occurs sooner than desired, either before or shortly after penetration, causing distress to one or both partners.	Montague et al (AUA Guideline on the Pharmacologic Management of PE), 2004
The man does not have voluntary, conscious control or the ability to choose in most encounters when to ejaculate.	Metz and McCarthy, 2003
The Foundation considers a man a premature ejaculator if he cannot control his ejaculatory process for a sufficient length of time during intravaginal containment to satisfy his partner in at least 50% of their coital connections.	Masters and Johnson, 1970
Men with an IELT <1 min (belonging to the 0.5th percentile) have "definite" PE, and men with IELTs between 1 and 1.5 min (0.5th to 2.5th percentile) have "probable" PE (see Fig. 29-2). In addition, a grading of severity of PE should be defined in terms of associated psychological problems. Thus both definite and probable PE need further psychological subclassification in asymptomatic, mild, moderate, and severe PE.	Waldinger et al, 2005c
PE is diagnosed on the basis of the pathologic IELT, as measured by the stopwatch method, with a feeling of loss of voluntary control and/or distress or relational disturbances, as measured by PRO.	Jannini et al, 2005

AUA, American Urological Association; DSM-IV-TR, *Diagnostic and Statistical Manual of Mental Disorders* (4th edition, Text Revision); DSM-5, *Diagnostic and Statistical Manual of Mental Disorders* (5th edition); EAU, European Association of Urology; ICUD, International Consultation on Urological Diseases; IELT, intravaginal ejaculation latency time; ISSM, International Society of Sexual Medicine; PRO, patient-reported outcome.

populations (Metz and McCarthy, 2003). After critical evaluation of the published data, the committee unanimously agreed that the constructs that are necessary to define lifelong PE are time from penetration to ejaculation, inability to delay ejaculation, and negative personal consequences from PE, and they recommended the following definition (McMahon et al, 2008a):

Lifelong PE is a male sexual dysfunction characterized by the presence of all of these criteria: 1) ejaculation that always or

nearly always occurs prior to or within about 1 minute of vaginal penetration; 2) the inability to delay ejaculation on all or nearly all vaginal penetrations; and 3) negative personal consequences such as distress, bother, frustration, and/or the avoidance of sexual intimacy.

However, the committee was unable to identify sufficient published objective data to craft an evidence-based definition of acquired PE. The committee anticipated that future studies would generate sufficient data to develop an evidence-based definition for acquired PE.

In April 2013 the ISSM convened a second Ad Hoc ISSM Committee for the Definition of Premature Ejaculation in Bangalore, India. The brief of the committee was to evaluate the current published data and attempt to develop a contemporary, evidence-based definition of acquired PE and/or a single unifying definition of both acquired and lifelong PE. Members unanimously agreed that although lifelong and acquired PE are distinct and different demographic and etiologic populations, they can be jointly defined, in part, by the constructs of time from penetration to ejaculation, inability to delay ejaculation, and negative personal consequences from PE. The committee agreed that the presence of these mutual constructs was sufficient justification for the development of a single unifying definition of both lifelong and acquired PE. Finally, the committee determined that the presence of a clinically significant and bothersome reduction in latency time, often to approximately 3 minutes or less, was an additional key defining dimension of acquired PE.

The second Ad Hoc ISSM Committee for the Definition of Premature Ejaculation (2013) defined PE (lifelong and acquired PE) as a male sexual dysfunction characterized by the following:
- **Ejaculation that always or nearly always occurs before or within approximately 1 minute of vaginal penetration (lifelong PE) or a clinically significant and bothersome reduction in latency time, often to approximately 3 minutes or less (acquired PE)**
- **The inability to delay ejaculation on all or nearly all vaginal penetrations**
- **Negative personal consequences, such as distress, bother, frustration, and/or the avoidance of sexual intimacy**

The unified ISSM definition of lifelong and acquired PE represents the first evidence-based definition for these conditions. **This definition should form the basis for the office diagnosis of lifelong PE and the design of PE observational and interventional clinical trials. It is limited to men engaging in vaginal intercourse because few studies are available on PE research in homosexual men or during other forms of sexual expression.** This definition intentionally includes a degree of diagnostic conservatism and flexibility. The 1-minute IELT cutoff point for lifelong PE should not be applied in the most absolute sense, because approximately 10% of men seeking treatment for lifelong PE have IELTs of 1 to 2 minutes. The phrase "within approximately 1 minute" must be interpreted as giving the clinician sufficient flexibility to diagnose PE also in men who report an IELT as long as 90 seconds. Similarly, a degree of flexible clinical judgment is key to recognition and interpretation of a bothersome change in ejaculatory latency with reduction of premorbid latency to 3 minutes or less in men with acquired PE. Men who report these ejaculatory latencies but describe adequate control and no personal negative consequences related to their rapid ejaculation do not merit the diagnosis of PE.

The rationale for the ISSM definition of lifelong and acquired PE is fully explored on the Expert Consult website.

Diagnostic and Statistical Manual of Mental Disorders (DSM-5) Definition of Premature Ejaculation

Based on the same data that supported the ISSM definition of lifelong PE, **the recently published DSM-5 definition of PE** (American Psychiatric Association, 2013) now includes an objective ejaculatory latency criterion. DSM-5 defines PE as follows:

A persistent or recurrent pattern of ejaculation occurring during partnered sexual activity within approximately 1 minute following vaginal penetration and before the individual wishes it. This symptom must have been present for at least 6 months and must be experienced on almost all or all (approximately 75%-100%) occasions of sexual activity. It causes clinically significant distress in the individual.

The DSM-5 definition of PE requires clinicians to specify PE as either lifelong or acquired and as generalized or situational. In addition, the DSM-5 definition of PE distinguishes between mild PE (ejaculation occurring within ~30 seconds to 1 minute of vaginal penetration), moderate PE (ejaculation occurring within ~15 to 30 seconds of vaginal penetration), and severe PE (ejaculation occurring before sexual activity, at the start of sexual activity, or within ~15 seconds of vaginal penetration).

Prevalence of Premature Ejaculation

Reliable information on the prevalence of lifelong and acquired PE in the general male population is lacking. PE has been estimated to occur in 4% to 39% of men in the general community (Reading and Wiest, 1984; Nathan, 1986; Spector and Boyle, 1986; Spector and Carey, 1990; Grenier and Byers, 1997; Laumann et al, 1999; Porst et al, 2007) and is often identified as the most common self-reported male sexual disorder (Jannini and Lenzi, 2005). However, **a substantial disparity exists between the incidence of PE in epidemiologic studies that rely on patient self-report of PE and/or inconsistent and poorly validated definitions of PE** (Laumann et al, 1999; Patrick et al, 2005; Giuliano et al, 2008) and, as suggested by community-based stopwatch studies of the IELT, the interval between penetration and ejaculation (Waldinger et al, 2005a). The latter demonstrates that the **distribution of the IELT is positively skewed, with a median of 5.4 minutes (range, 0.55 to 44.1 minutes), decreases with age, varies across countries,** and supports the notion that IELTs of less than 1 minute are statistically abnormal compared to those in men in the general Western population (Fig. 29-2) (Waldinger et al, 2005a).

Prevalence data derived from patient self-report will be appreciably higher than prevalence estimates based on clinician diagnosis using the more conservative ISSM definition of PE. The following studies demonstrate the varying prevalence estimates ranging from 30% down to 3%. Data from The Global Study of Sexual Attitudes and Behaviors (GSSAB), an international survey investigating the attitudes, behaviors, beliefs, and sexual satisfaction of 27,500 men and women 40 to 80 years of age, reported the global prevalence of PE (based on subject self-report) to be approximately 30% across all age groups (Nicolosi et al, 2004; Laumann et al, 2005). Perception of "normal" ejaculatory latency varied by country and differed when assessed by either the patient or the partner (Montorsi, 2005). A core limitation of the GSSAB survey stems from the fact that the youngest participants were 40 years of age, an age when the incidence of PE might be different from that of younger males (Jannini and Lenzi, 2005). Contrary to the GSSAB study, the Premature Ejaculation Prevalence and Attitude Survey found the prevalence of PE among men 18 to 70 years of age to be 22.7% (Porst et al, 2007). The real prevalence of PE is difficult to assess in clinical practice (Jannini and Lenzi, 2005).

Basile Fasalo and associates (2005) reported that 2658 of 12,558 men (21.2%) attending a free andrologic consultation self-diagnosed PE, the majority describing acquired PE (14.8%) and 4.5% describing lifelong PE. In contrast, Serefoglu and colleagues (2010) reported that the majority of PE treatment–seeking patients described lifelong PE (62.5%) compared to acquired PE (16.1%). Similar findings were reported by Zhang and coworkers (2013) who found that the majority of 1988 Chinese outpatients described lifelong PE (35.6%) or acquired PE (28.07%). These data provide evidence that patients with lifelong and acquired PE comprise the majority of the patients who seek treatment for PE. In addition, a disparity appears to exist between the incidence of the various PE subtypes in the general community and in men actively seeking treatment for PE.

Consistent with this notion, **Serefoglu and colleagues (2011) subsequently reported an overall PE prevalence of 19.8% comprising lifelong PE (2.3%), acquired PE (3.9%), variable PE (8.5%), and subjective PE (5.1%).** Using similar research methodology, Gao and associates (2013) reported that 25.80% of 3016 Chinese men reported PE, with similar prevalence of lifelong (3.18%), acquired (4.84%), variable PE (11.38%), and subjective

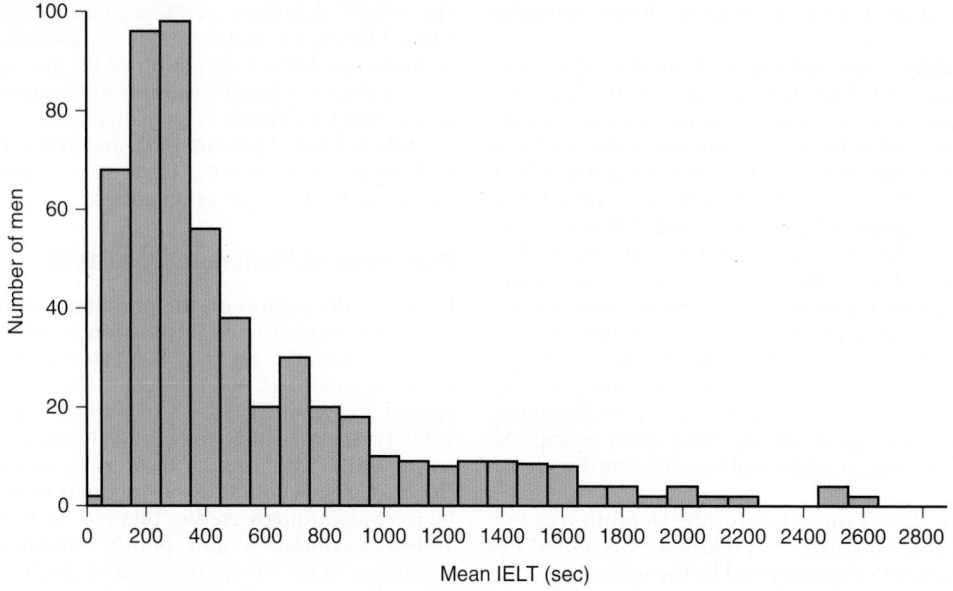

Figure 29-2. Distribution of intravaginal ejaculatory latency times (IELT) values in a random cohort of 491 men. (From Waldinger M, Quinn P, Dilleen M, et al. A multinational population survey of intravaginal ejaculation latency time. J Sex Med 2005;2:492–7.)

PE (6.4%). Of particular interest is the report of Serefoglu and colleagues (2011) that men with acquired PE are more likely to seek medical treatment than men with lifelong PE (26.53% vs. 12.77%). This finding was confirmed by Gao and coworkers (2013), who demonstrated that patients with acquired PE were more likely to seek (17.12% vs. 14.58%) and plan to seek (36.30% vs. 27.08%) treatment for their PE than men with lifelong PE. These data suggest that the prevalence of acquired PE in the community is approximately 4% among sexually active adults and that these patients are more likely to seek medical treatment.

Causes of Premature Ejaculation

Historically, attempts to explain the cause of PE have included a diverse range of biologic and psychological theories. Most of these proposed causes are not evidence based and are speculative at best. Although men with lifelong and acquired PE appear to share the dimensions of short ejaculatory latency, reduced or absent perceived ejaculatory control, and presence of negative personal consequences from PE, they remain distinct and different demographic and etiologic populations (Porst et al, 2010).

Lifelong Premature Ejaculation

Waldinger and colleagues (1998) hypothesized that lifelong early ejaculation in humans may be explained by either a hyposensitivity of the 5-HT_{2C} and/or hypersensitivity of the 5-HT_{1A} receptor. Recent studies suggest that **in some men, neurobiologic and genetic variations could contribute to the pathophysiology of lifelong PE**, as defined by the ISSM criteria and that the condition may be maintained and heightened by psychological/environmental factors (Janssen et al, 2009).

Acquired Premature Ejaculation

Acquired PE is commonly due to **sexual performance anxiety** (Hartmann et al, 2005), psychological or relationship problems (Hartmann et al, 2005), **ED** (Laumann et al, 2005), occasionally prostatitis (Screponi et al, 2001), or hyperthyroidism (Carani et al, 2005) or during withdrawal/detoxification from prescribed (Adson and Kotlyar, 2003) or recreational (Peugh and Belenko, 2001) drugs. Consistent with the predominant organic cause of acquired

PE, men with this problem are usually older, have a higher mean body mass index (BMI), and have a greater incidence of comorbid disease, including hypertension, sexual desire disorder, diabetes mellitus, chronic prostatitis, and ED, than men with lifelong, variable, and subjective PE (Basile Fasolo et al, 2005; Porst et al, 2010; Serefoglu et al, 2010; Serefoglu et al, 2011; Gao et al, 2013; McMahon et al, 2013; Zhang et al, 2013).

Premature Ejaculation and Sexual Performance Anxiety, Psychological Problems, and Relationship Problems

Anxiety has been reported as a cause of PE by multiple authors and is entrenched in the folklore of sexual medicine as the most likely cause of PE despite scant empirical research evidence to support any causal role (Jern et al, 2007; Janssen et al, 2009). Several authors suggest that **anxiety activates the sympathetic nervous system and reduces the ejaculatory threshold as a result of an earlier emission phase of ejaculation** (Janssen et al, 2009).

Hypoactive sexual desire may lead to PE, as a result of an unconscious desire to abbreviate unwanted penetration. Similarly, diminished sexual desire can be a consequence of chronic and frustrating PE.

Female sexual dysfunctions (such as anorgasmia, hypoactive sexual desire, sexual aversion, sexual arousal disorders, and sexual pain disorders, such as vaginismus (Dogan and Dogan, 2008) also may be related to acquired PE.

Premature Ejaculation and Comorbid Erectile Dysfunction

Recent data demonstrate that as many as half of subjects with ED also experience PE (Basile Fasolo et al, 2005; Laumann et al, 2005; Porst et al, 2007).

Premature Ejaculation and Prostate Disease

Acute and chronic lower urogenital infection, prostatodynia, or chronic pelvic pain syndrome (CPPS) is associated with ED, PE, and painful ejaculation (Waldinger et al, 2005c; Donatucci, 2006; Zohdy, 2009; Rowland et al, 2010). **Several studies report PE as the main sexual disorder symptom in men with chronic prostatitis or CPPS, with a prevalence of 26% to 77%** (Rowland et al,

2010). The exact pathophysiology of the links among chronic prostatitis, ED, and PE is unknown. It has been hypothesized that prostatic inflammation may result in altered sensation and modulation of the ejaculatory reflex, but evidence is lacking (Donatucci, 2006; Shamloul and El-Nashaar, 2006; Sharlip, 2006). It has been reported that antibiotic treatment of microbiologically confirmed bacterial prostatitis in men with acquired PE resulted in a 2.6-fold increase in IELT and improved ejaculatory control in 83.9% of subjects (El-Nashaar and Shamloul, 2007).

Premature Ejaculation and Hyperthyroidism

The majority of patients with thyroid hormone disorders experience sexual dysfunction. Studies suggest a significant correlation between PE and suppressed thyroid-stimulating hormone (TSH) values in a selected population of andrologic and sexologic patients. The 50% prevalence of PE in men with hyperthyroidism fell to 15% after treatment with thyroid hormone normalization (Carani et al, 2005). Although occult thyroid disease has been reported in the elderly hospitalized population, it is uncommon in the population who present for treatment of PE and routine **TSH screening is not necessary unless clinically indicated** (Atkinson et al, 1978).

Evaluation of Men Reporting Premature Ejaculation

Medical History

Men presenting with self-reported PE should be evaluated with a **full medical and sexual history, a focused physical examination, inventory assessment of erectile function, and any investigations suggested by these findings.** Inclusion of the partner in the management process is an important but not mandatory ingredient for treatment success. Some patients may not understand why the clinician wishes to include the partner, and some partners may be reluctant to join the patient in treatment. However, if partners are not involved in treatment, they may be resistant to changing the sexual interaction (Donahey and Miller, 2000). A cooperative partner can enhance the man's self-confidence, skills, self-esteem, and sense of masculinity and more generally assist the man to develop ejaculatory control (Perelman, 2003). This is in turn likely to lead to an improvement in the couple's sexual relationship, as well as the broader aspects of their relationship. No controlled studies have been done on the impact of involving partners in treating PE. However, a review of treatment studies for ED demonstrated the important role of including a focus on interpersonal factors on treatment success (Mohr and Bentler, 1990).

Patients expect clinicians to inquire about their sexual health (Schein et al, 1988). Often patients are too embarrassed, shy, and uncertain if sexual complaints belong in the health care professional's office (Humphrey and Nazareth, 2001). Inquiry into sexual health gives patients permission to discuss their sexual concerns and also screens for associated health risks (e.g., cardiovascular risk and ED). Box 29-1 lists recommended and optional questions that patients who report PE should be asked (McMahon et al, 2004b; Althof et al, 2010). The recommended questions establish the diagnosis and direct treatment considerations and the optional questions gather detail for implementing treatment. Finally, the committee recommends that the health care providers take a medical and psychosocial history.

Diagnosis of Premature Ejaculation

The ISSM definition of PE should form the basis for the diagnosis of PE. A significant population of men with self-reported PE fails to satisfy the criteria of the ISSM definition of PE. This parallels the substantial disparity between the self-reported incidence of PE in epidemiologic studies (Laumann et al, 1999) and that suggested by community-based normative stopwatch IELT studies (Waldinger et al, 2005a). This population has recently been categorized as having either variable PE or subjective PE (Waldinger et al, 2006b;

BOX 29-1 Recommended and Optional Questions to Establish the Diagnosis of Premature Ejaculation (PE) and Direct Treatment

RECOMMENDED QUESTIONS FOR DIAGNOSIS OF PE
What is the time between penetration and ejaculation (coming)?
Can you delay ejaculation?
Do you feel bothered, annoyed, and/or frustrated by your PE?

OPTIONAL QUESTIONS
Differentiate Lifelong and Acquired PE
When did you first experience PE?
Have you experienced PE since your first sexual experience on every/almost every attempt and with every partner?

Assess Erectile Function
Is your erection hard enough to penetrate?
Do you have difficulty in maintaining your erection until you ejaculate during intercourse?
Do you ever rush intercourse to prevent loss of your erection?

Assess Relationship Impact
How upset is your partner with your PE?
Does your partner avoid sexual intercourse?
Is your PE affecting your overall relationship?

Previous Treatment
Have you received any treatment for your PE previously?

Impact on Quality of Life
Do you avoid sexual intercourse because of embarrassment?
Do you feel anxious, depressed, or embarrassed because of your PE?

From Althof SE, Abdo CH, Dean J, et al. International Society for Sexual Medicine's guidelines for the diagnosis and treatment of premature ejaculation. J Sex Med 2010;7:2947–69.

Waldinger and Schweitzer, 2008). Men with subjective PE report PE but have a normal ejaculatory latency typically of 2 to 6 minutes but on some occasions as long as 25 minutes. It is characterized by a preoccupation with a subjective but false perception of PE with an ejaculation latency time (ELT) within the normal range but often with reduced ejaculatory control.

Determination of Intravaginal Ejaculation Latency Time

Self-estimation by the patient and partner of IELT should be used to determine IELT in clinical practice. Stopwatch measures of IELT are widely used in clinical trials and observational studies of PE, but have not been recommended for use in routine clinical management of PE. Despite the potential advantage of objective measurement, stopwatch measures have the disadvantage of being intrusive and potentially disruptive of sexual pleasure or spontaneity. More recently, studies have indicated that patient or partner self-report of ejaculatory latency correlate relatively well with objective stopwatch latency and might be useful as a proxy measure of IELT (Althof, 1998; Pryor et al, 2005; Rosen et al, 2007; McMahon, 2008a). Because patient self-report is the determining factor in treatment seeking and satisfaction, it is recommended that self-estimation by the patient and partner of ejaculatory latency be accepted as the method for determining IELT in clinical practice.

Patient-Reported Outcome Measures

Standardized assessment measures such as validated questionnaires and PRO measures can be used as an adjunct to a full medical and sexual history and self-estimation of ejaculatory latency in the evaluation of men presenting with self-reported PE. These measures are all relatively new and were developed primarily for use as research tools. Some have shown good psychometric properties and are potentially valuable adjuncts for clinical screening and assessment.

Several PE measures have been described in the literature (Yuan et al, 2004; Althof et al, 2006; Arafa and Shamloul, 2007; Symonds et al, 2007a, 2007b; Patrick et al, 2008; Serefoglu et al, 2009), although only a small number have undergone extensive psychometric testing and validation. Five validated questionnaires have been developed and published to date. Currently, two questionnaires have extensive databases and meet most of the criteria for test development and validation: the **Premature Ejaculation Profile (PEP)** and the **Index of Premature Ejaculation (IPE)** (Althof et al, 2006; Patrick et al, 2008). A third brief diagnostic measure, the **Premature Ejaculation Diagnostic Tool (PEDT)**, has a modest database and is available for clinical use (Symonds et al, 2007a). Two other measures, the Arabic and Chinese PE Questionnaires, have minimal validation or clinical trial data available and are not recommended for clinical use.

Further details of PRO measures are available on the Expert Consult website.

Assessment of Erectile Function

The presence of comorbid ED should be evaluated using a validated instrument such as the International Index of Erectile Function (IIEF) or the IIEF-5 (SHIM). Normal erectile function should be defined as an IIEF Erectile Function Domain of 26 or greater or IIEF-5 greater than 21 (Rosen et al, 1997; Cappelleri et al, 2001). Recent data demonstrate that as many as half of subjects with ED also experience PE (Jannini et al, 2005). In the European Premature Ejaculation Study (PEPA), ED was present in 31.9% of men with PE compared to 11.8% of men without PE (Porst et al, 2007). In the GSSAB, the odds ratio for ED in men with PE ranged from 6.0 in Europe and as high as 11.9 in South America (Laumann et al, 2005). Consistent with this, ED is more prevalent in men with acquired PE than lifelong PE (Basile Fasolo et al, 2005). PE is also more common with increasing severity of ED after adjustment for age (Corona et al, 2004: El-Sakka, 2006, 2008). Men with ED may either require higher levels of stimulation to achieve an erection or intentionally "rush" intercourse to prevent early detumescence of a partial erection, resulting in ejaculation with a brief latency (Jannini et al, 2005). This may be compounded by the presence of high levels of performance anxiety related to their ED, which serves to only worsen their prematurity. However, caution should be exercised in the diagnosis of comorbid ED in men with PE, because 33.3% of potent men with PE confuse the ability to maintain erections before and after ejaculation, record contradictory response/s to some/all questions of the SHIM, especially Q3 and Q4, and receive a false-positive SHIM diagnosis of ED (McMahon, 2009).

Physical Examination

Current literature suggests that the diagnosis of lifelong PE is based purely on the medical history because there are no predictive physical findings or confirmatory investigations (McMahon, 2005). As differentiation of lifelong PE and acquired PE may be difficult in either young men or men with no or few previous sexual partners and/or limited sexual experience, a physical examination is highly desirable and represents an opportunity for screening for cardiovascular or gender-specific diseases. However, **in men with acquired PE, a physical examination is mandatory in an effort to identify the cause of the PE** and to alleviate its possible cause (Jannini et al, 2006b). The presence of ED should be evaluated either by medical history or with the assistance of a validated instrument. Laboratory or imaging investigations are occasionally required based on the patient's medical history. A digital prostate examination, routine in an andrologic setting for all men over 40, is useful in identifying possible evidence of prostatic inflammation or infection (Jannini et al, 2006a).

Treatment of Premature Ejaculation

Figure 29-3 is a flow chart for the management of PE (Rowland et al, 2010). **Multiple psychosexual and pharmacologic treatments are available for PE.** Men with lifelong PE are best managed with PE pharmacotherapy alone or **in combination with graded levels of patient and couple psychosexual therapy.** Men with acquired PE should receive cause-specific treatment (e.g., psychosexual counseling or ED pharmacotherapy, alone or in combination with PE pharmacotherapy). Men with natural variable PE or PE-like ejaculatory dysfunction should be primarily treated with psychosexual education and graded patient and couple psychotherapy.

Psychosexual Therapy

All men seeking treatment for PE should receive basic psychosexual education or coaching (Althof, 2006c, 2007; Perelman, 2003, 2006). This may include providing information on the prevalence of PE and general population IELT to dispel myths about PE, information on enjoyable sexual activities to extend the man and his partner's sexual repertoire, as well as strategies to address avoidance of sexual activity or unwillingness to discuss sex with his partner. These educational strategies are designed to give the man the confidence to try the medical intervention, reduce performance anxiety, and modify his maladaptive sexual scripts.

Additional information on the role of psychosexual therapy in the *management of PE is available on the Expert Consult website.*

Pharmacologic Treatment

Several forms of pharmacotherapy have been used in the treatment of PE (Giuliano and Clement, 2012). These include the use of **topical local anesthetics, SSRIs, tramadol, phosphodiesterase type 5 (PDE5) inhibitors, and α-adrenergic blockers.** The use of topical local anesthetics, such as lidocaine, prilocaine, or benzocaine, alone or in association, to diminish the sensitivity of the glans penis is the oldest known pharmacologic treatment for PE (Schapiro, 1943). The introduction of the SSRIs paroxetine, sertraline, fluoxetine, and citalopram and the tricyclic antidepressant (TCA) clomipramine has revolutionized the treatment of PE. These drugs block axonal reuptake of serotonin from the synaptic cleft of central serotonergic neurons by 5-HT transporters, resulting in enhanced 5-HT neurotransmission and stimulation of postsynaptic membrane 5-HT receptors.

Treatment with Selective Serotonin Reuptake Inhibitors and Tricyclic Antidepressants. PE can be treated with **on-demand SSRIs such as dapoxetine or off-label clomipramine, paroxetine, sertraline, and fluoxetine or with daily dosing of off-label paroxetine, clomipramine, sertraline, fluoxetine, or citalopram.**

Dapoxetine. Dapoxetine has received approval for the treatment of PE in over 50 countries worldwide. Dapoxetine has not received marketing approval for the United States by the U.S. Food and Drug Administration. It is a **rapid-acting and short–half-life SSRI with a pharmacokinetic profile supporting a role as an on-demand treatment for PE** (Pryor et al, 2006). No drug-drug interactions associated with dapoxetine, including phosphodiesterase inhibitor drugs, have been reported. In randomized controlled trials (RCTs), dapoxetine 30 mg or 60 mg taken 1 to 2 hours before intercourse is more effective than placebo from the first dose, resulting in **2.5- and 3.0-fold increases in IELT, increased ejaculatory control, decreased distress, and increased satisfaction.** Dapoxetine was comparably effective in men with lifelong and acquired PE (Porst et al, 2010) and was similarly effective and well tolerated in men with PE and comorbid ED treated with PDE5 inhibitor drugs (McMahon et al, 2013). Treatment-related side effects were

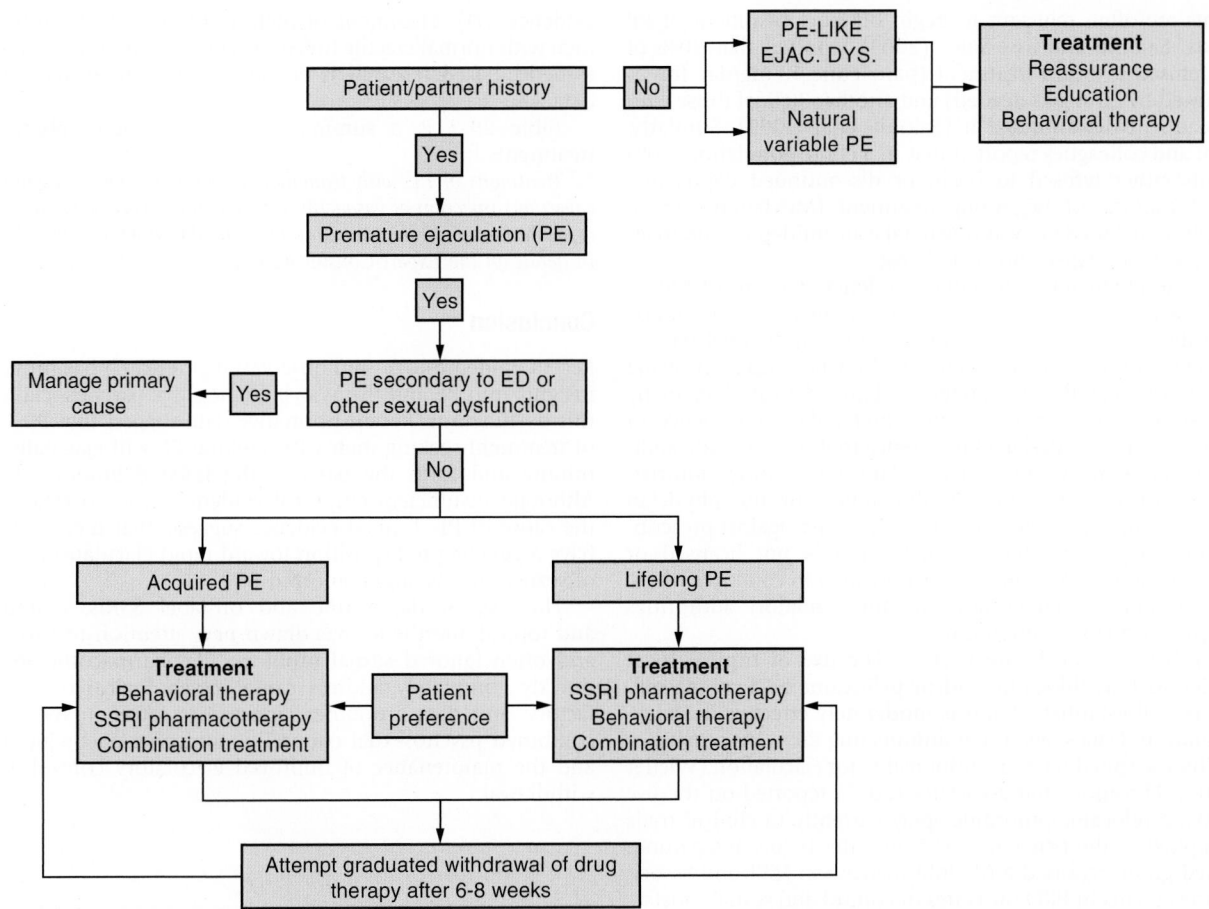

Figure 29-3. Algorithm for the office management of premature ejaculation (PE). ED, erectile dysfunction; EJAC. DYS., ejaculation dysfunction; SSRI, selective serotonin reuptake inhibitor.

uncommon and dose dependent and included nausea, diarrhea, headache, and dizziness (McMahon et al, 2011). They were responsible for study discontinuation in 4% (30 mg) and 10% (60 mg) of subjects. There was no indication of an increased risk for suicidal ideation or suicide attempts and little indication of withdrawal symptoms with abrupt dapoxetine cessation (Levine, 2006).

Off-Label Selective Serotonin Reuptake Inhibitors and Tricyclic Antidepressants. Daily treatment with off-label paroxetine 10 to 40 mg, clomipramine 12.5 to 50 mg, sertraline 50 to 200 mg, fluoxetine 20 to 40 mg, and citalopram 20 to 40 mg is usually effective in delaying ejaculation. A meta-analysis of published data suggests that **paroxetine exerts the strongest ejaculation delay, increasing IELT approximately 8.8-fold over baseline** (Waldinger et al, 2004b).

Ejaculation delay usually occurs within 5 to 10 days of starting treatment, but the full therapeutic effect may require 2 to 3 weeks of treatment and usually is sustained during long-term use (McMahon, 2002). Adverse effects are usually minor, start in the first week of treatment, and may gradually disappear within 2 to 3 weeks. They include **fatigue, yawning, mild nausea, diarrhea, or perspiration.** Anecdotal reports show that decreased libido and ED are less frequently seen in nondepressed men with PE treated by SSRIs compared to depressed men treated with SSRIs (Waldinger, 2007). Neurocognitive adverse effects include significant **agitation and hypomania in a small number of patients, and treatment with SSRIs should be avoided in men with a history of bipolar depression** (Marangell et al, 2008).

Platelet serotonin release has an important role in hemostasis (Li et al, 1997) and SSRIs, especially with concurrent use of aspirin and nonsteroidal anti-inflammatory drugs, may be associated with

increased risk for upper gastrointestinal bleeding. Priapism is a rare adverse effect of SSRIs and requires urgent medical treatment. Long-term SSRI use may be associated with **weight gain and an increased risk for type 2 diabetes mellitus** (Fava et al, 2000). In men with normal semen parameters, **paroxetine has been reported to induce abnormal sperm DNA fragmentation in a significant proportion of subjects, without a measurable effect on semen parameters.** The fertility potential of a substantial number of men on paroxetine may be adversely affected by these changes in sperm DNA integrity (Tanrikut et al, 2010).

Systematic analysis of RCTs of antidepressants (SSRIs and other drug classes) in patients with depressive and/or anxiety disorders indicates **a small increase in the risk for suicidal ideation or suicide attempts in youth but not adults.** In contrast, the risk for suicidal ideation has not been found in trials with SSRIs in nondepressed men with PE. Caution is suggested in prescribing SSRIs to young adolescents with PE aged 18 years or less, and to men with PE and a comorbid depressive disorder, particularly when associated with suicidal ideation (Khan et al, 2003). Patients should be advised to **avoid sudden cessation or rapid dose reduction of daily dosed SSRIs, which may be associated with an SSRI withdrawal syndrome** (Black et al, 2000).

On-demand administration of clomipramine, paroxetine, sertraline, and fluoxetine 3 to 6 hours before intercourse is modestly efficacious and well tolerated but is associated with substantially less ejaculatory delay than daily treatment in most studies (Kim and Paick, 1999; McMahon and Touma, 1999; Strassberg et al, 1999; Waldinger et al, 2004a). On-demand treatment may be combined with either an initial trial of daily treatment or concomitant low-dose daily treatment (McMahon and Touma, 1999).

Patients are often reluctant to begin off-label treatment of PE with SSRIs. Salonia and associates (2009) reported that 30% of patients refused to begin treatment (paroxetine 10 mg/day for 21 days followed by 20 mg as needed) and another 30% of those who began treatment discontinued it (Salonia et al, 2009). Similarly, Mondaini and colleagues reported that in a clinic population, 90% of patients either refused to begin or discontinued dapoxetine within 12 months of beginning treatment (McMahon, 2002). Reasons given included not wanting to take an antidepressant, treatment effects below expectations, and cost.

The decision to treat PE with either on-demand dosing of dapoxetine (where available) or daily dosing of off-label SSRIs should be based on the treating physician's assessment of individual patient requirements. Although many men with PE who engage in sexual intercourse infrequently may prefer on-demand treatment, many men in established relationships may prefer the convenience of daily medication. Well-designed preference trials will provide additional insight into the role of on-demand dosing. In some countries, off-label prescribing may present difficulties for the physician because the regulatory authorities strongly advise against prescribing for indications in which a medication is not licensed or approved. Obviously this complicates treatment in countries where there is no approved medication and the regulatory authorities advise against off-label prescription.

Off-Label Topical Local Anesthetics. The use of topical local anesthetics such as lidocaine and/or prilocaine as a cream, gel, or spray is well established and is moderately effective in delaying ejaculation. Data suggest that diminishing the glans sensitivity may inhibit the spinal reflex arc responsible for ejaculation (Wieder et al, 2000). Dinsmore and associates (2007) reported on the use of PSD502, a lidocaine-prilocaine spray currently in clinical trials that is applied to the penis at least 5 minutes before intercourse. The treated group reported a 6.3-fold increase in IELT and associated improvements in PRO measures of control and sexual satisfaction (Dinsmore et al, 2007; Henry et al, 2008). Minimal reports have been made of penile hypoanesthesia and transfer to the partner as a result of the unique formulation of the compound. Other topical anesthetics are associated with significant penile hypoanesthesia and possible transvaginal absorption, resulting in vaginal numbness and resultant female anorgasmia unless a condom is used (Busato and Galindo, 2004).

Phosphodiesterase Type 5 Inhibitors. Off-label on-demand or daily dosing of PDE5 inhibitors is not recommended for the treatment of lifelong PE in men with normal erectile function. ED pharmacotherapy alone or in combination with PE pharmacotherapy is recommended for the treatment of lifelong PE or acquired PE in men with comorbid ED. PDE5 inhibitors sildenafil, tadalafil, and vardenafil are effective treatments for ED. Several authors have reported experience with PDE-5 inhibitors alone or in combination with SSRIs as a treatment for PE (Abdel-Hamid et al, 2001; Chia, 2002; Erenpreiss and Zalkalns, 2002; Linn et al, 2002; Salonia et al, 2002; Chen et al, 2003; Li et al, 2003; Lozano, 2003; Tang et al, 2004; Mattos and Lucon, 2005; McMahon et al, 2005; Sommer et al, 2005; Zhang et al, 2005; Atan et al, 2006; Sun et al, 2007; Mattos et al, 2008; Aversa et al, 2009; Mathers et al, 2009; Jannini et al, 2011). The putative role of PDE5 inhibitors as a treatment for PE is speculative and based only on the role of the nitric oxide (NO)/cyclic guanosine monophosphate (cGMP) transduction system as a central and peripheral mediator of inhibitory nonadrenergic, noncholinergic nitrergic neurotransmission in the urogenital system (Mamas et al, 2003). Although systematic reviews of studies on the PDE5 inhibitor drug treatment of PE have failed to provide robust empirical evidence to support a role of PDE5 inhibitors in the treatment of PE, with the exception of men with PE and comorbid ED (McMahon et al, 2006a; Asimakopoulos et al, 2012), recent well-designed studies do support a potential role for these agents, suggesting a need for further evidence-based research (Aversa et al, 2009).

Some evidence supports the efficacy and safety of off-label, on-demand, or daily dosing of PDE5 inhibitors in the treatment of lifelong PE in men with normal erectile function (level of evidence 4D). Treatment of lifelong PE with PDE5 inhibitors in men with normal erectile function is not recommended, and further evidence-based research is encouraged to understand conflicting data.

Table 29-2 is a summary of recommended pharmacologic treatments for PE.

Treatment of PE with tramadol, α_1-adrenoceptor antagonists, intracavernous injection of vasoactive drugs, acupuncture, surgical neurotomy, cryoablation, and neuromodulation of the dorsal penile nerve is discussed in detail on the Expert Consult website.

Conclusion

Recent epidemiologic and observational research has provided new insights into PE and the associated negative psychosocial effects of this dysfunction. Recent normative data suggest that 80% to 90% of treatment-seeking men with lifelong PE will ejaculate within 1 minute and form the basis of the ISSM definition of lifelong. Although insufficient empirical evidence exists to clearly identify the cause of PE, limited evidence suggests that men with PE may have a genetic predisposition toward rapid ejaculation, high levels of sexual anxiety, and comorbid ED.

The use of dapoxetine and off-label SSRIs, clomipramine, and topical anesthetics has drawn new attention to this common and often ignored sexual problem. PE pharmacotherapy fails to directly completely address causal psychological or relationship factors, and data are either lacking or scarce on the efficacy of combined psychosexual counseling and pharmacologic treatment and the maintenance of improved ejaculatory control after drug withdrawal.

KEY POINTS: PREMATURE EJACULATION

- PE is a common sexual dysfunction.
- PE is associated with negative psychological consequences, including distress, bother, and frustration that may affect quality of life, partner relationships, self-esteem, and self-confidence and can act as an obstacle to single men forming new partner relationships.
- The evidence-based ISSM definition of lifelong and acquired PE should form the basis of the office diagnosis of lifelong PE.
- Limited evidence suggests lifelong PE has a genetic basis and acquired PE is most often the result of sexual performance anxiety, psychological or relationship problems, and/or ED.
- Oral SSRI drugs and topical anesthetic drugs are effective and safe treatments for PE.
- Psychosexual cognitive behavioral therapy has a limited role as a first-line treatment for PE but has an important role as an adjunct to pharmacotherapy, especially in men with acquired PE resulting from sexual performance anxiety.
- Men with acquired PE, most often secondary to comorbid ED, hyperthyroidism, chronic lower urogenital infection, prostatodynia, or CPPS, should receive appropriate cause-specific treatment alone or in combination with an SSRI.

DELAYED EJACULATION, ANEJACULATION, AND ANORGASMIA

Any psychological or medical disease or surgical procedure that interferes with either central control of ejaculation or the peripheral sympathetic nerve supply to the vas and bladder neck, the somatic efferent nerve supply to the pelvic floor, or the somatic afferent nerve supply to the penis can result in delayed ejaculation, anejaculation, retrograde ejaculation, and/or anorgasmia. Thus the

TABLE 29-2   Drug Therapy for Premature Ejaculation (PE)

DRUG	DOSE	DOSING INSTRUCTIONS	INDICATION	COMMENTS	LEVEL OF EVIDENCE
Dapoxetine	30-60 mg	On demand, 1-3 hr before intercourse	Lifelong PE Acquired PE	Approved in >50 countries	High
Paroxetine	10-40 mg	Once daily	Lifelong PE Acquired PE		High
Sertraline	50-200 mg	Once daily	Lifelong PE Acquired PE		High
Fluoxetine	20-40 mg	Once daily	Lifelong PE Acquired PE		High
Citalopram	20-40 mg	Once daily	Lifelong PE Acquired PE		High
Clomipramine	12.5-50 mg	Once daily	Lifelong PE Acquired PE		High
	12.5-50 mg	On demand, 3-4 hr before intercourse	Lifelong PE Acquired PE		High
Tramadol	25-50 mg	On demand, 3-4 hr before intercourse	Lifelong PE Acquired PE	Potential risk for opiate addiction	Low
Topical lignocaine/ prilocaine	Patient titrated	On demand, 20-30 min before intercourse	Lifelong PE Acquired PE		High
Alprostadil	5-20 μg	Patient administered intracavernous injection 5 min before intercourse	Lifelong PE Acquired PE	Risk for priapism and corporal fibrosis	Very low
PDE5 inhibitors	Sildenafil 25-100 mg Tadalafil 10-20 mg Vardenafil 10-20 mg	On demand, 30-50 min before intercourse	Lifelong and acquired PE in men with normal erectile function		Very low
			Lifelong and acquired PE in men with ED	? Improved efficacy if combined with SSRI	Moderate

ED, erectile dysfunction; PDE5, phosphodiesterase type 5; SSRI, selective serotonin reuptake inhibitor.

causes of delayed ejaculation, anejaculation, and anorgasmia are manifold.

Definition, Terminology, and Characteristics of Men with Delayed Ejaculation

Delayed ejaculation (DE), retarded ejaculation (RE), or inhibited ejaculation (IE) are probably the least common, least studied, and least understood of the male sexual dysfunctions. Yet their impact is significant in that it typically results in a lack of sexual fulfillment for both the man and his partner, an effect further compounded when procreation is among the couple's goals of sexual intercourse.

Problems with "difficulty" in ejaculating may range from varying delays in the latency to ejaculation to complete inability to ejaculate (anejaculation). Reductions in the volume, force, and sensation of ejaculation may occur as well. At the extremes are anejaculation (time) and retrograde ejaculation (direction), but more commonly encountered are IE, RE, and DE. A final disorder, anorgasmia, refers to a perceived absence of the orgasm experience, independent of whether any or all of the physiologic concomitants of ejaculation have taken place.

Terminology and Definition

RE, DE, IE, inadequate ejaculation, idiopathic anejaculation, primary impotentia ejaculations, and psychogenic anejaculation all have been used synonymously to describe a delay or absence of male orgasmic response. If a distinction is to be made, usually IE is characterized by the complete absence of ejaculation, although no clear consensus exists. Herein, the preferred terminology DE is meant to describe any and all of the ejaculatory disorders resulting in a delay or absence of ejaculation.

DSM-IV-TR defines DE as follows (American Psychiatric Association, 2000):

The persistent or recurrent delay in, or absence of, orgasm after a normal sexual excitement phase during sexual activity that the clinician, taking into account the person's age, judges to be adequate in focus, intensity, and duration. The disturbance causes marked distress or interpersonal difficulty; it should not be better accounted for by another Axis I (clinical) disorder or caused exclusively by the direct physiologic effects of a substance or a general medical condition.

Similarly, the Second International Consultation on Sexual Dysfunction defines DE as the persistent or recurrent difficulty, delay in, or absence of attaining orgasm after sufficient sexual stimulation, which causes personal distress (McMahon et al, 2004a).

No clear criteria exist as to when a man actually meets the conditions for DE, because operationalized criteria do not exist. Given that most sexually functional men ejaculate within approximately 4 to 10 minutes after intromission (Patrick et al, 2005), a clinician might assume that **men with latencies beyond 25 or 30 minutes (21 to 23 minutes represents approximately 2 standard** deviations above the mean) who report distress or men who simply cease sexual activity because exhaustion or irritation qualify for this diagnosis. Such symptoms, together with the fact that a man and/or his partner decide to seek help for the problem, are usually sufficient for a DE diagnosis.

Epidemiology of Delayed Ejaculation

The prevalence of ejaculatory disorders is unclear, partly because of the dearth of normative data for defining the duration of "normal" ejaculatory latency, particularly regarding the right "tail" of the distribution (i.e., beyond the mean latency to orgasm). Furthermore, larger epidemiologic studies have not subdivided various types of ejaculatory disorders (e.g., delayed vs. absent), further limiting our knowledge. In general, DE is reported at low rates in the literature, rarely exceeding 3% (Laumann et al, 1999; Simons and Carey, 2001; Perelman, 2004). The prevalence of DE appears to be moderately and positively related to age, which is not surprising in view of the fact that ejaculatory function as a whole tends to diminish as men age.

Failure of ejaculation can be a **lifelong problem or an acquired problem. It may be global and happen in every sexual encounter or be intermittent or situational.** Normative descriptive data from large samples of men with DE have not been available, but a recent analysis identified 25% of a clinical sample with lifelong DE, with the remainder reporting a secondary problem (Perelman, 2004). Although coital anejaculation is frequently the treatment driver (especially for extremely religious individuals referred for fertility problems), men also seek treatment when distressed by their inability to achieve orgasm in response to manual, oral, or vaginal stimulation by their partner. Many men with acquired DE can masturbate to orgasm, whereas others, for multiple reasons, will not or cannot. Loss of masturbatory capacity secondary to emotional or physical trauma also is seen. Approximately 75% of one clinical sample could reach orgasm through masturbation, whereas the remainder either would not or could not (Perelman, 2004).

Similar to men with other types of sexual dysfunction, **men with DE indicate high levels of relationship distress, sexual dissatisfaction, anxiety about their sexual performance, and general health issues**—significantly higher than sexually functional men. In addition, along with other sexually dysfunctional counterparts, men with DE typically report lower frequencies of coital activity (Rowland et al, 2005). A distinguishing characteristic of men with DE—and one that has implications for treatment—is that they usually have little or no difficulty attaining or keeping erections; in fact they are often able to maintain erections for prolonged periods. But despite their good erections, they report low levels of subjective sexual arousal, at least compared with sexually functional men (Rowland et al, 2004b).

Cause of Delayed Ejaculation and Anejaculation

DE and anejaculation may be lifelong or acquired, global, or situational. A number of pathophysiologic conditions have been associated with ejaculatory problems (Box 29-2). These include congenital disorders as well as ones caused by psychological factors, treatment of male pelvic cancers with surgery or radiotherapy, neurologic disease, endocrinopathy, infection, and treatment for other disorders. When a medical history or symptomatology so indicates, investigation of such possible causes may be necessary. **The most common causes of DE seen in clinical practice are psychogenic IE, degeneration of penile afferent nerves and pacinian corpuscles in the aging male, hypogonadism, diabetic autonomic neuropathy, treatment with SSRI antidepressants and major tranquilizers, radical prostatectomy or other major pelvic surgery, or radiotherapy.**

Psychological Delayed Ejaculation

Psychogenic DE, often described as **IE,** is usually related to **sexual performance anxiety,** which may draw the man's attention away

---

> **BOX 29-2**   Causes of Retrograde Ejaculation, Delayed Ejaculation, Anejaculation, and Anorgasmia
>
> **AGING MALE**
> Degeneration of penile afferent nerves
>
> **PSYCHOGENIC**
> Inhibited ejaculation
>
> **CONGENITAL**
> Müllerian duct cyst
> Wolffian duct abnormality
> Prune belly syndrome
>
> **ANATOMIC CAUSES**
> Transurethral resection of prostate
> Bladder neck incision
>
> **NEUROGENIC CAUSES**
> Diabetic autonomic neuropathy
> Multiple sclerosis
> Spinal cord injury
> Radical prostatectomy
> Proctocolectomy
> Bilateral sympathectomy
> Abdominal aortic aneurysmectomy
> Para-aortic lymphadenectomy
>
> **INFECTIVE**
> Urethritis
> Genitourinary tuberculosis
> Schistosomiasis
>
> **ENDOCRINE**
> Hypogonadism
> Hypothyroidism
>
> **MEDICATION**
> α-Methyldopa
> Thiazide diuretics
> Tricyclic and SSRI antidepressants
> Phenothiazine
> Alcohol abuse
> SSRI, selective serotonin reuptake inhibitor.

---

from erotic cues that normally serve to enhance arousal. Other psychodynamic explanations emphasize psychosexual development issues and have attributed lifelong DE to a wide range of conditions, including fear, anxiety, hostility, orthodoxy of religious belief, and relationship difficulties (Munjack and Kanno, 1979; Waldinger and Schweitzer, 2005). Although some of these factors may contribute to DE in individual men, no well-controlled studies provide broad support, at this point, for any of the various hypotheses mentioned previously (Waldinger and Schweitzer, 2005).

Masters and Johnson (1970) were the first to suggest that DE in some men might be associated with **orthodoxy of religious belief.** Such beliefs may limit the sexual experience necessary for learning to ejaculate or may result in an inhibition of normal function. Many devoutly religious men have masturbated only minimally or not at all, and, for some, guilt and anxiety about "spilling seed" may have led to idiosyncratic masturbatory patterns, which in turn resulted in DE. Such men often had little contact with women before marriage and, although they may have dated, were less likely than their secular counterparts to experience orgasm with a partner, especially through intercourse.

Idiosyncratic and vigorous masturbation styles that cannot be replicated during intercourse with a partner, or an "autosexual" orientation in which men derive greater arousal and enjoyment from masturbation than from intercourse, are risk factors for DE (Perelman, 2005; Perelman and Rowland, 2006). These men precondition themselves to possible difficulty attaining orgasm with a partner and, as a result, experience acquired DE. They appear able to achieve erections sufficient for intercourse despite a relative absence of subjective arousal (Apfelbaum, 1989), and their erections are taken as erroneous evidence by both the man and his partner that he was ready for sex and capable of achieving orgasm. Disparity between the reality of sex with the partner and the sexual fantasy used during masturbation may inhibit sexual arousal and thus represent another contributor to DE (Perelman, 2001).

Endocrinopathy

Hypothyroidism is commonly strongly associated with DE, whereas hyperthyroidism is rarely associated with PE (Carani et al, 2005; Corona et al, 2006). Similarly, **hypogonadism** and low testosterone are associated with DE or anejaculation (Corona et al, 2008, 2011, 2012). **Hyperprolactinemia,** via inhibition of hypothalamic gonadotropin-releasing hormone GnRH is associated with low testosterone, reduced sexual desire, ED, and DE. The effect of prolactin on ejaculation is possibly mediated via its action on the serotinergic system (Corona et al, 2006, 2009).

Iatrogenic Causes

Any prescribed or recreational drug that changes the levels of neurotransmitters such as serotonin, dopamine, or oxytocin that are involved in the central or peripheral neurocontrol of ejaculation may affect ejaculatory latency.

SSRIs are commonly used for the treatment of depression and are associated with a high incidence of sexual dysfunction, with up to 60% reporting some form of treatment-related sexual dysfunction, most commonly ejaculatory dysfunction (Montejo et al, 2001; Delgado et al, 2005; Madeo et al, 2008). Treatment with **antipsychotics,** probably resulting from either a direct and/or indirect dopamine antagonism (Hull et al, 2004) or increased prolactin levels (Roke et al, 2012), is also commonly associated with DE and retrograde ejaculation (Madhusoodanan and Brenner, 1996; Raja, 1999). Retrograde ejaculation associated with antipsychotics is thought to be due to antagonistic effects on the α-adrenergic system at the level of the bladder neck (Holtmann et al, 2003).

Treatment of Male Pelvic Cancers

Overall quality of life and sexual functioning have evolved as key issues in the management of patients with cancer. Because of modern surgical techniques, improved quality of drugs for chemotherapy, and modern radiation techniques, more patients can be successfully treated without largely compromising sexual functioning.

Prostate Cancer

Prostate cancer has become the most common nonskin malignancy in men in Western countries. External-beam radiotherapy (EBRT) and brachytherapy (BT) are, together with the open or robotic radical prostatectomy (RP/RALP), the most common and effective treatments for localized prostate cancer. Despite the introduction of very modern radiotherapy (RT) techniques, sexual functioning after prostate cancer treatment remains problematic for many patients. **After RP/RALP, men no longer ejaculate, but maintain a sense of orgasm** that can vary from less to more intense than preoperatively and may experience arousal urinary incontinence or climacturia— that is, urinary incontinence at orgasm.

Ejaculatory disturbances after RT of prostate cancer were reported as early as the 1980s (Van Heeringen et al, 1988). More recent studies have evaluated the impact of RT on sexual desire, ejaculation, and orgasm. **After EBRT, a decline in sexual desire was reported by 43% of 64 patients and a decreased frequency of orgasm by 57%; all men reported a decrease in ejaculate volume** (Helgason et al, 1995). Using a validated questionnaire, Borghede and Hedelin (1997) reported a decrease in the ability to ejaculate in 56% of the patients. Good prognostic factors for sexual functioning preservation after RT were low age and higher frequency of intercourse.

Early RT studies also assessed sexual functioning. Herr (1979) reported already in 1979 on 51 patients treated with retropubic iodium-125 seeds, with loss of ejaculate experienced by 6% of the patients. In a later study, dry ejaculation was reported by 16% of the patients after BT (Kwong et al, 1984). In both studies, all patients had previously undergone a transurethral resection of the prostate (TURP). For the first time a discomfort with ejaculation was mentioned in two studies (up to 25% of the patients) (Kleinberg et al, 1994; Arterbery et al, 1997). This result is quite common in clinical practice after BT, because of edema of the prostate possibly reducing the elasticity of the urethra and inducing discomfort with ejaculation. In some patients, discomfort with ejaculation did not disappear even 18 to 24 months after BT (Beckendorf et al, 1996). Also, decreased interest in sex, sexual desire, and libido was mentioned in up to 50% of the patients evaluated (Beckendorf et al, 1996; Arterbery et al, 1997; Borghede and Hedelin, 1997; Joly et al, 1998).

Several studies on the cause of post-RT decreased libido and ejaculatory disorders have been reported. Daniell and associates (2001) studied retrospectively levels of testosterone and other hormones after RT of prostate cancer. Testosterone was found to be low 3 to 8 years after EBRT, with lower levels found in older patients. Although testes are very sensitive to radiation, spermatogenesis is more easily affected than androgen productions. The radiation dose calculated in the testes of men irradiated for prostate cancer is only 3% to 8% of the dose that could possibly affect androgen production and could explain a decrease in testosterone. A TURP carries a high incidence of retrograde ejaculation because it is thought to disrupt the closure mechanism of the vesical neck; this could explain ejaculatory disturbances in most patients after previous TURP.

Rectal Carcinoma

Not much is known about sexual functioning after RT of rectal carcinoma. Preoperative RT for rectal cancer has been associated with a reduction in the rate of local relapse and possibly an advantage in survival. Preoperative RT with the total mesorectal excision in low-stage rectal cancer has become a common procedure in Europe. **A sharp dissection of the mesorectum associated with visualization and preservation of the pelvic autonomic nerve leads to excellent results regarding erectile and ejaculatory functioning.** Only one study has specifically studied the effects of preoperative RT for rectal carcinoma on male sexual functioning and concluded that it may impair male sexual functioning (Bonnel et al, 2002). However, numbers were too small to draw final conclusions.

Testicular Cancer

Germ cell tumors of the testis are relatively rare, accounting for approximately 1% of all male cancers. The long-term survival for early disease approaches 100%. Because testicular cancer affects mainly young men in their sexual and fertile life, sexual functioning and ejaculatory disorders are particularly important. The side effects of retroperitoneal lymph node dissection (RPLND) for residual mass after chemotherapy for nonseminomatous cancer are better documented than sexual sequelae of elective abdominal RT for seminoma. **Anejaculation occurs in the majority of the patients in non–nerve-sparing techniques.** As a result of careful anatomic studies, the technique of RPLND has been **modified with nerve sparing so that antegrade ejaculation is now maintained in 80%**

TABLE 29-3 Correlation of Erection, Ejaculation, and Intercourse with Level and Severity of Spinal Cord Injury

CORD LESION		REFLEXOGENIC ERECTIONS (%)	PSYCHOGENIC ERECTIONS (%)	SUCCESSFUL COITUS (%)	EJACULATION (%)
Upper motor neuron	Complete	92	9	66	1
	Incomplete	93	48	86	22
Lower motor neuron	Complete	0	24	33	15
	Incomplete	0	1	100	100

From Comarr AE. Sexual function among patients with spinal cord injury. Urol Int 1970;25:134–68.

to 100% of patients (van Basten et al, 1997). Libido and orgasm seem to be normal in these patients.

After RT, deterioration in sexual functioning has been reported in 1% to 25% of the patients (Schover et al, 1986; Tinkler et al, 1992; Jonker-Pool et al, 1997; Caffo and Amichetti, 1999; Incrocci et al, 2002). Tinkler and colleagues (1992) reported on 237 patients after orchiectomy and abdominal RT and compared these data to 402 age-matched controls. In almost all parameters studied, including erection, ejaculation, and libido, patients scored less than controls (reduction in orgasm, in libido, and interest in sex). Specifically, there was no difference in the ability to ejaculate during sexual activity, but the patients undergoing RT reported a noticeable reduction in the amount of semen compared to before treatment. Caffo and Amichetti (1999) evaluated toxicity and quality of life in 143 patients treated for early-stage testicular cancer. Of these, 23% reported a decreased libido, 27% problems with getting an orgasm, and 38% ejaculation disturbances, including PE. A decrease in sexual desire, orgasm, and volume or semen was negatively correlated with age (Schover et al, 1986). Jonker-Pool and associates (1997) reported on three groups of patients, after RT, wait and see, and chemotherapy. Patients undergoing RT reported decreased libido in 22% compared to 12% in the wait-and-see group and 30% in the chemotherapy group. Decrease or absence of ejaculate was reported in 15%, 7%, and 21% in the three groups, respectively; decreased orgasm was found in 15%, 12%, and 30%, respectively. Although the differences were not statistically significant, in the RT group, ejaculation and orgasm disturbances were higher than in the wait-and-see group. Similar results were reported by Arai and coworkers (1997). PE was reported in up to half of the patients (Arai et al, 1997; Incrocci et al, 2002), but it was the same as recalled before treatment (Incrocci et al, 2002).

The superior hypogastric plexus is responsible for ejaculation and is mediated by the sympathetic system; it is a fenestrated network of fibers anterior of the lower abdominal aorta. The hypogastric nerves exit bilaterally at the inferior pole of the superior hypogastric plexus and have connections with the S1 to S2 roots. Normal emission requires integrity of this system. During RPLND, these nerves are difficult to recognize and might be damaged, resulting in decreased semen volume or dry ejaculation. Pathways for ejaculation are included in the RT fields for rectal and prostate carcinomas. Damage of the sympathetic nerves could be caused by radiation, but the dose does not seem enough to completely explain the dysfunction. Orgasm is even more complex than ejaculation, because it is also affected by cortical input.

Neurologic Disorders

Degeneration of penile fast-conducting afferent nerves and pacinian corpuscles in the **aging male, diabetic autonomic neuropathy, multiple sclerosis, and spinal cord injury** are often associated with DE/anejaculation.

Spinal Cord Injury

The ability to ejaculate is severely impaired by spinal cord injury (SCI). Bors and Comarr highlighted the impact of the level and completeness of SCI on the postinjury erectile and ejaculatory

capacity (Bors and Comarr, 1960; Comarr, 1970) (Table 29-3). **Unlike erectile capacity, the ability to ejaculate increases with descending levels of spinal injury. Fewer than 5% of patients with complete upper motor neuron lesions retain the ability to ejaculate.** Ejaculation rates are higher (15%) in patients with both lower motor neuron lesions and an intact thoracolumbar sympathetic outflow. Approximately 22% of patients with an incomplete upper motor neuron lesion and almost all men with incomplete lower motor neuron lesions retain the ability to ejaculate. In patients capable of successful ejaculation, the sensation of orgasm may be absent and retrograde ejaculation often occurs.

Several techniques for obtaining semen in men with SCI with ejaculatory dysfunction have been reported. **Vibratory stimulation** is successful in obtaining semen in up to 70% of men with SCI (Brindley, 1984). The use **of electroejaculation** to obtain semen by electrical stimulation of efferent sympathetic fibers of the hypogastric plexus is an effective and safe method of obtaining semen. Brindley (1986) reported that 71% of men with SCI who underwent electroejaculation achieved ejaculation. However, both vibratory stimulation and electroejaculation are associated with **a significantly high risk for autonomic dysreflexia.** Pretreatment with a fast-acting vasodilator such as nifedipine minimizes the risk for severe hypertension, should autonomic dysreflexia occur with either form of treatment (Steinberger et al, 1990).

Semen collected from men with SCI is often initially senescent and of poor quality with a low sperm count and reduced sperm motility but may improve with subsequent ejaculations. This poor semen quality may be due to chronic urinary tract infection, dilution of sperm content with urine, chronic use of various medications, elevated scrotal temperature as a result of prolonged sitting, and stasis of prostatic fluid. Testicular biopsies in men with SCI demonstrate a wide range of testicular dysfunction including hypospermatogenesis, maturation arrest, atrophy of seminiferous tubules, germinal cell hypoplasia, interstitial fibrosis, and Leydig cell hyperplasia. In addition, prostatitis secondary to prolonged catheterization, epididymitis, and epididymo-orchitis can precipitate obstructive ductal lesions and testicular damage. Ohl and associates (1989) reported that sperm density and motility were higher in those with incomplete lesions. In a recent collective analysis of 40 paraplegic patients, 22 successfully produced pregnancies by natural insemination or assisted reproductive techniques (Dahlberg et al, 1995).

Congenital Disorders

Typical congenital problems include müllerian duct obstruction, caused by failure of complete absorption of müllerian duct remnants in males; wolffian duct abnormalities, which may compromise vas deferens, ejaculatory duct, and seminal vesicle functioning; and prune belly syndrome.

Infective Disorders

Sexually transmissible infections such as gonorrhea or nonspecific urethritis can produce cicatrization and obstruction anywhere in the male reproductive tract, especially if treatment is delayed. Urinary infection, especially if complicated by epididymitis, also can produce obstruction that may be situated at the ejaculatory duct level. Schistosomiasis is endemic in large parts of Africa and is seen with increasing frequency in tourists returning from Africa who have contracted the disease while enjoying water sports. The disease may manifest with hemospermia (McKenna et al, 1997), and fibrosis and calcification may lead to genital obstruction. Genitourinary tuberculosis can cause great damage to the male reproductive tract, and because healing occurs with calcification, the lesions may be irreparable.

Evaluation of Men with Delayed Ejaculation

Evaluation of men presenting with DE or anejaculation should include **a full medical and sexual history, a focused physical examination, determination of serum testosterone levels, and any additional investigations suggested by these findings.**

Assessment begins by determining whether DE is lifelong or acquired, global or situational (Box 29-3). Evaluation includes establishment of how often a man can ejaculate during intercourse and the time elapsed between penetration and ejaculation, the IELT. If ejaculation fails to occur, the duration of thrusting before suspension of intercourse, the reasons for suspension of intercourse (e.g., fatigue, loss of erection, a sense of ejaculatory futility, or partner request), and whether ejaculation can occur during postcoital self- or partner-assisted masturbation must be determined. The presence or absence of premonitory ejaculatory sensation during intercourse or masturbation suggests achievement of sufficient arousal to almost attain the ejaculation threshold. Variables that improve or worsen performance are noted. The man's ability to relax, sustain, and heighten arousal and the degree to which he can concentrate on sensations are noted.

The presence and extent of patient, partner, or interpersonal related negative psychological consequences such as bother, distress, frustration, or the avoidance of sexual contact should be established. The frequency of intercourse and the identity of the initiator of sexual contacts are useful surrogate measures for these negative psychological consequences. The quality of the nonsexual relationship also should be explored.

In men with acquired DE, previous illness, surgery, medications, or life events or circumstances should be reviewed. The events may include a variety of life stressors and other psychological factors (e.g., after his wife's mastectomy the man is afraid of hurting her and therefore is only partially aroused). Societal and religious attitudes that may interfere with excitement are noted, such as the "spilling of seed as a sin."

A focused physical and genital examination to determine whether the testes and epididymes are normal and whether the vasa are present or absent on each side, supported by a screening morning total testosterone level and any other hormonal or imaging investigations indicated by either history or physical examination, will identify or exclude organic disease. Digital rectal examination to determine prostate size, anal sphincter tone, and quality of the bulbocavernous reflex is indicated in most men, with the exception of young men with situational and clear psychogenic IE. The presence of a neuropathy may require electrophysiologic evaluation of neural pathways controlling ejaculation, pudendal somatosensory and motor evoked potentials, sacral reflex arc testing, and sympathetic skin responses.

The occurrence of orgasm in the absence of prograde ejaculation suggests retrograde ejaculation and can be confirmed by the presence of spermatozoa in postmasturbation first-void urine. If the cause of DE is unclear, culture of expressed prostatic secretion and urine, urine cytology, and serum prostate-specific antigen will exclude prostatitis and bladder and prostatic cancer. Ultrasound scan of the testicles and epididymes may define any local disease.

Patients with unilateral or bilateral ejaculatory duct obstruction or congenital absence of vasa usually present with thin/runny low-volume semen, aspermia, and infertility. Seminal analysis demonstrates azoospermia or oligospermia with low concentration of fructose and a low pH. Ultrasound scanning of the entire urinary system and referral to a urologist is indicated because coexisting renal anomalies may be present. Bilateral absence or malformation of the vasa may be associated with the cystic fibrosis gene (Mickle et al, 1995).

Treatment of Men with Delayed Ejaculation or Anejaculation

Figure 29-4 is a flow chart for the management of DE (Rowland et al, 2010). Treatment should be cause specific, address the issue of infertility in men of reproductive age, and may include **patient/couple psychoeducation and/or psychosexual therapy, pharmacotherapy, or integrated treatment.** Men/partners of reproductive age undergoing pelvic surgery should be informed of the risk for infertility as a result of anejaculation and the availability of sperm harvesting and assisted reproductive techniques.

Whether a clear pathophysiologic cause is present or absent, patients might be counseled to consider **lifestyle changes, including enjoying more time together to achieve greater intimacy, minimizing alcohol consumption, making love when not tired, and practicing techniques that maximize penile stimulation such as pelvic floor training** (Waldinger and Schweitzer, 2005). Neuropathic DE is usually irreversible, and therefore the patient might be counseled to seek alternative methods to achieve mutual sexual satisfaction with his partner.

BOX 29-3 Recommended and Optional Questions to Establish the Diagnosis of Delayed Ejaculation (DE) and Direct Treatment

RECOMMENDED QUESTIONS FOR DIAGNOSIS OF DE

For Diagnosis

How often can you ejaculate during sexual intercourse?

During intercourse, how long after penetration does it take for you to either ejaculate or stop intercourse?

When you cannot ejaculate during sexual intercourse, how often do you feel that you are close to ejaculation?

If you cannot ejaculate, why do you stop intercourse?

Do you ever feel that you have ejaculated but fail to release semen?

Do you feel bothered, annoyed, and/or frustrated by your DE?

How often can you ejaculate during masturbation by yourself or with your partner?

OPTIONAL QUESTIONS

Differentiate Lifelong and Acquired DE

When did you first experience DE?

Have you experienced DE since your first sexual experience on every/almost every attempt and with every partner?

Assess Erectile Function

Is your erection hard enough to penetrate?

Do you have difficulty in maintaining your erection during intercourse?

Assess Relationship Impact

How upset is your partner with your DE?

Do you or your partner avoid sexual intercourse?

Is your DE affecting your overall relationship?

Previous Treatment

Have you received any treatment for your DE previously?

Impact on Quality of Life

Do you feel anxious, depressed, or embarrassed because of your DE?

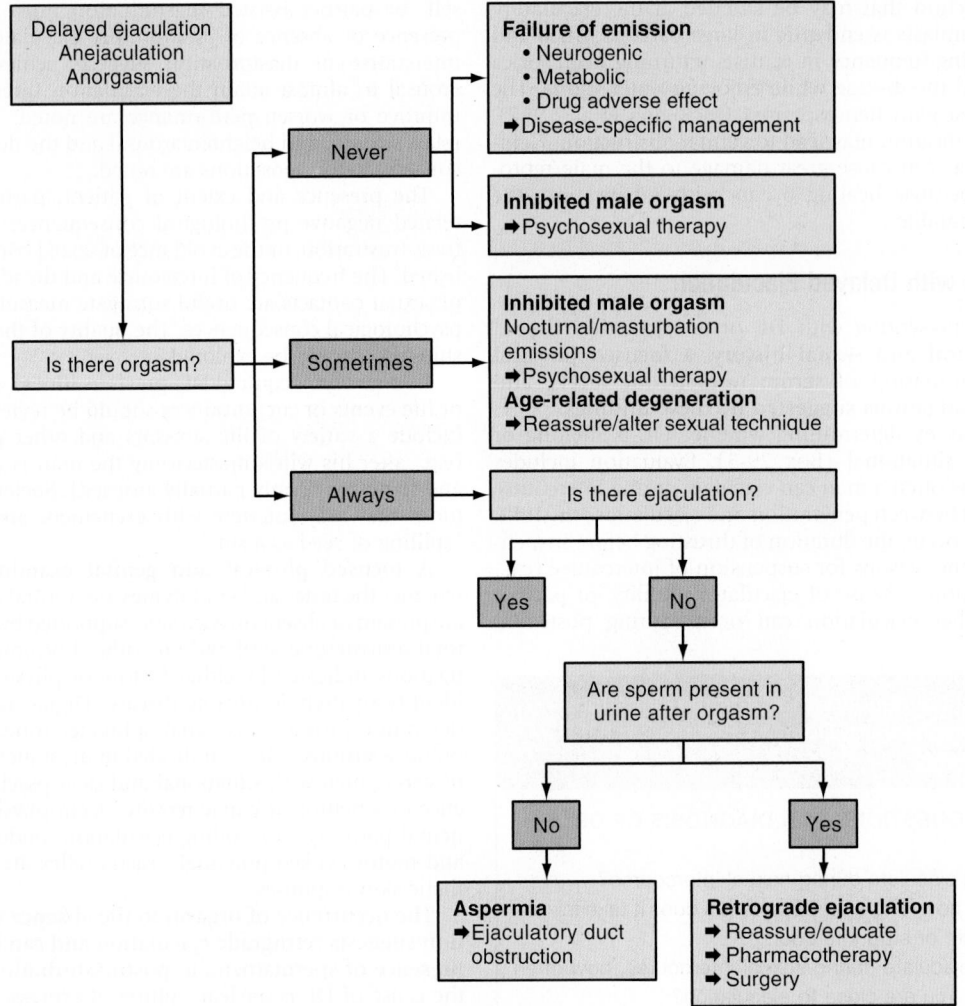

Figure 29-4. Algorithm for the office management of delayed ejaculation, anejaculation, and anorgasmia.

Psychological Strategies in the Treatment of Delayed Ejaculation

If organic and pharmacologic causes have been eliminated, **referral to an expert psychosexual therapist** is usually indicated to evaluate the causative psychological and behavioral issues. Beneficial effects through psychotherapy depend on the severity of the DE and the individual's receptiveness to engage in counseling and adhere to the counselor's recommendations.

Additional information on the role of psychosexual therapy in the management of DE is available on the Expert Consult website.

Pharmacotherapy in the Treatment of Delayed Ejaculation

Drug treatment of DE or IE ejaculation has met with **limited success** (Table 29-4). **These drugs facilitate ejaculation by either a central dopaminergic, antiserotonergic, or oxytocinergic mechanism of action or a peripheral adrenergic mechanism of action.** However, no drugs have been approved by regulatory agencies for this purpose and most drugs that have been identified for potential use have limited efficacy, impart significant side effects, or are as yet considered experimental in nature. **Results are relatively poor in men with psychogenic DE and neuropathic DE.**

α_1-Adrenergic receptor agonists such as on-demand **precoital pseudoephedrine** (60 to 120 mg 1 to 2 hours before intercourse) or the **selective norepinephrine reuptake inhibitor (SNRI) antidepressant reboxetine** (4 to 8 mg daily) which inhibits synaptic noradrenaline reuptake have limited efficacy. The antihistamine **cyproheptadine**, a central serotonin antagonist, is anecdotally

TABLE 29-4 Drug Therapy for Delayed Ejaculation and Anejaculation

	DOSAGE	
DRUG	**AS NEEDED**	**DAILY**
Cabergoline	—	0.5-2 mg every 3 days
Amantadine	100-400 mg (for 2 days before coitus)	100-200 mg twice daily
Pseudoephedrine	60-120 mg (1-2 hr before coitus)	—
Reboxetine	—	4-8 mg
Oxytocin	24 IU intranasal during coitus	—
Bupropion	—	150 mg/day or twice daily
Buspirone	—	5-15 mg twice daily
Cyproheptadine	4-12 mg (3-4 hr before coitus)	—

associated with the reversal of anorgasmia induced by the SSRI antidepressants, but no controlled studies have been reported (McCormick et al, 1990; Ashton et al, 1997). These studies suggest an effective dose range of 4 to 12 mg 3 to 4 hours before intercourse, with administration on a chronic or on-demand basis. However, significant dose-related sedative effects are likely to diminish its overall efficacy.

Amantadine, an indirect stimulant of dopaminergic nerves both centrally and peripherally, has been reported to stimulate sexual behavior and ejaculation in SSRI antidepressant–induced anorgasmia when administered on demand (100 to 400 mg 2 days before coitus) or chronically (100 to 200 mg twice daily) (Balogh et al, 1992).

A variety of other pharmacologic agents, including **cabergoline, bromocriptine, bupropion, and buspirone** have been anecdotally reported as potential DE pharmacotherapy, despite an absence of large-population RCTs. Of interest is the recent single case report of the **intracoital administration of intranasal oxytocin** in a case of treatment-resistant anorgasmia (Ishak et al, 2008). However, in the absence of robust RCT data, oxytocin cannot be recommended as a treatment for DE.

KEY POINTS: DELAYED EJACULATION

- The causes of DE and anejaculation are manifold.
- Failure of ejaculation can be a lifelong problem (25%) or an acquired problem (75%). It may be global and occur in every sexual encounter or be intermittent or situational.
- Treatment of men with DE should be cause specific and address the issue of infertility in men of reproductive age.
- Drug treatment of men with DE or anejaculation has had limited success.

RETROGRADE EJACULATION

Antegrade (normal) ejaculation requires a closed bladder neck (and proximal urethra). **Surgical procedures that compromise the bladder neck closure mechanism may result in retrograde ejaculation.** Transurethral incision of the prostate (TUIP) results in retrograde ejaculation in 5% (Hedlund and Ek, 1985) to 45% (Kelly et al, 1989) of patients and is probably related to whether one or two incisions are made and whether the incision includes primarily the bladder neck or extends to the level of the verumontanum. The importance of contraction of the urethral smooth muscle at the level of the verumontanum has been hypothesized to be important in preventing retrograde ejaculation (Reiser, 1961). TURP carries a higher incidence of retrograde ejaculation than does TUIP. The reported incidence of retrograde ejaculation after TURP ranges from 42% (Edwards and Powell, 1982) to 100% (Quinlan et al, 1991). Although these men may have some antegrade ejaculation and usually experience orgasmic sensation, both events may be reduced as part of the changes that occur in the male sexual response as a man ages. Retrograde ejaculation is more common in diabetes mellitus than in age-matched controls ($P < .01$), has been reported in 30% of men with diabetes mellitus, and is not statistically associated with duration of diabetes mellitus, BMI, waist circumference, or hemoglobin A1c or total testosterone levels (Waldinger et al, 2005a).

Retrograde ejaculation and failure of emission can be distinguished by examination of a postmasturbatory specimen of urine for the presence of spermatozoa and fructose. The finding of more than 5 to 10 sperm per high-power field in a postejaculation urine specimen confirms the presence of retrograde ejaculation. In patients with low-volume ejaculate, the finding of more sperm in the urine than in the antegrade ejaculate indicates a significant component of retrograde ejaculation (Sigman and Howards, 1998).

Treatment of Retrograde Ejaculation

Retrograde ejaculation can be surgically treated with bladder neck reconstruction but results remain consistently poor (Abrahams et al, 1975; Lipshultz et al, 1981). Drug treatment is the most promising approach. As mentioned earlier, α-adrenergic sympathetic nerves mediate both bladder neck closure and emission. Several sympathomimetic amine agents have been described as useful with mixed results (Kedia and Markland, 1975). These drugs include **pseudoephedrine, ephedrine, midocrine, and phenylpropanolamine.** These agents work by stimulating the release of noradrenaline from the nerve axon terminals but also may directly stimulate both α- and β-adrenergic receptors. The most useful is pseudoephedrine, which is administered at a dose of 120 mg 2 to 2.5 hours precoital. The TCA **imipramine,** which blocks the reuptake of noradrenaline by the axon from the synaptic cleft is also occasionally useful. The usual dose is 25 mg twice daily. The current feeling is that long-term treatment with imipramine is likely to be more effective. Although medical treatment may not always produce normal ejaculation, it may result in some prograde ejaculation. In patients who do not achieve antegrade ejaculation with either surgery or medication, sperm retrieval and artificial insemination is an alternative approach. The basic method of sperm retrieval involves recovery of urine by either catheter or voiding after masturbation and then centrifugation and isolation of the sperm.

KEY POINTS: RETROGRADE EJACULATION

- TURP and diabetic autonomic neuropathy are the most common causes of retrograde ejaculation.
- Retrograde ejaculation and failure of emission can be distinguished by examination of a postmasturbatory specimen of urine for the presence of spermatozoa and fructose.
- Pharmacotherapy is associated with variable degrees of success and includes agents such as pseudoephedrine, midodrine, and imipramine.

PAINFUL EJACULATION

Painful ejaculation, or odynorgasmia, is a poorly characterized syndrome. It may be associated with **urethritis, BPH, acute or chronic prostatitis, CPPS, seminal vesiculitis, seminal vesicular calculi, or ejaculatory duct obstruction** (Weintraub et al, 1993; Corriere, 1997; Kochakarn et al, 2001; Nickel et al, 2005). Often, no obvious etiologic factor can be found. **Painful ejaculation occurs in 17% to 23% of men with LUTS/BPH** (Frankel et al, 1998; Tubaro et al, 2001; Brookes et al, 2002; Vallancien et al, 2003). Men with BPH and painful ejaculation have more severe LUTS and report greater bother. In addition, they report a higher incidence of ED and a reduced ejaculation volume, compared to men with LUTS only (Rosen et al, 2003). Treatment of men with LUTS with α-blocking drugs may be associated with painful ejaculation. A lower incidence of pain has been reported with the uroselective $α_1$-blocking drug, alfuzosin (van Moorselaar et al, 2005). Management should focus on treatment of the underlying cause.

POSTORGASMIC ILLNESS SYNDROME

POIS is a recently described but poorly characterized "orphan" disease comprising a **collection of symptoms that include severe myalgia and fatigue associated with a flulike state that occurs within 30 minutes of orgasm.**

Additional information on POIS is available on the Expert Consult website.

CONCLUSION

Recent epidemiologic and observational research has provided new insights into PE and the associated negative psychosocial effects of this dysfunction. The recently developed multivariate evidence-based ISSM definition of lifelong and acquired PE provides the clinician a more discriminating diagnostic tool and should form the basis of the office diagnosis of lifelong PE.

Although insufficient empirical evidence exists to unequivocally identify the cause of PE, limited evidence suggests that lifelong PE may have a genetic basis and that acquired PE is most often due to sexual performance anxiety, psychological or relationship problems, and/or ED and to a lesser extent, chronic prostatitis, CPPS or hyperthyroidism.

Current evidence suggests that psychosexual cognitive behavioral therapy has a limited role in the contemporary management of PE and confirms the efficacy and safety of oral SSRI drugs and topical anesthetic drugs. It is likely that dapoxetine, despite its modest effect on ejaculatory latency, has a place in the management of PE, which will eventually be determined by market forces once the challenge of regulatory approval has been met. Treatment with tramadol, intracavernous injection therapy, or alternative methods of drug delivery cannot be recommended until the results of large, well-designed RCTs are published in major international peer-reviewed medical journals.

DE and anejaculation are more common as men age and have manifold organic and psychogenic causes. They have a significant impact on sexual fulfilment for both the man and his partner and may result in infertility. Treatment of men with DE represents one of the most significant challenges in sexual medicine and outcome results are often disappointing.

REFERENCES

The complete reference list is available online at www.expertconsult.com.

SUGGESTED READINGS

Althof SE, Abdo CH, et al. International Society for Sexual Medicine's guidelines for the diagnosis and treatment of premature ejaculation. J Sex Med 2010;7:2947–69.

Corona G, Mannucci E, et al. Psychobiological correlates of delayed ejaculation in male patients with sexual dysfunctions. J Androl 2006;27:453–8.

Janssen PK, Bakker SC, et al. Serotonin transporter promoter region (5-HTTLPR) polymorphism is associated with the intravaginal ejaculation latency time in Dutch men with lifelong premature ejaculation. J Sex Med 2009;6:276–84.

McMahon CG, Althof SE, et al. An evidence-based definition of lifelong premature ejaculation: report of the International Society for Sexual Medicine (ISSM) ad hoc committee for the definition of premature ejaculation. J Sex Med 2008;5:1590–606.

McMahon CG, Jannini E, et al. Standard operating procedures in the disorders of orgasm and ejaculation. J Sex Med 2013;10:204–29.

Rowland D, McMahon CG, et al. Disorders of orgasm and ejaculation in men. J Sex Med 2010;7(4 Pt 2):1668–86.

Waldinger MD, McIntosh J, Schweitzer DH. A five-nation survey to assess the distribution of the intravaginal ejaculatory latency time among the general male population. J Sex Med 2009;6:2888–95.

30 Surgery for Erectile Dysfunction

J. Francois Eid, MD

Penile prostheses have been used to treat erectile dysfunction (ED) since the mid 1970s (Scott et al, 1973; Small et al, 1975). In the United States, approximately 20,000 penile prosthetic devices are implanted annually, accounting for 75% of the global market (Mulcahy and Wilson, 2006; Garber, 2008). The primary goal of penile implant surgery is to restore erections that most closely resemble normal function in terms of rigidity, girth expansion, and length expansion. Because ED is often associated with feelings of inadequacy, disappointment, and loss of self-confidence, an additional goal of implant surgery is to improve a patient's quality of life and self-esteem. **Men who experience ED constantly think about their dysfunction. After prosthetic surgery for ED, they experience a sense of freedom that is very similar to being cured. This feeling is not reported by men who use other temporary treatment options for ED** (Rajpurkar and Dhabuwala, 2003).

Indications for a penile prosthetic device include failure or rejection of more conservative therapy for ED, Peyronie disease in which ED and erectile deformity coexist, irreversible organic etiology of ED, penile fibrosis, post priapism and unresponsive to more conservative treatment, phalloplasty following radical penile cancer surgery or gender change, and psychological impotence after failure of all other treatment (Anderson et al, 2007; Al-Enezi et al, 2011). Prosthetic implants are considered the most effective method for obtaining an artificial erection in patients with ED who are unresponsive to or cannot tolerate other treatment (Bettocchi et al, 2010).

TYPES OF PROSTHESES

There are two broad categories of penile implants, semirigid rods and inflatable devices, both of which were introduced almost 40 years ago and have undergone significant design improvements since that time (Scott et al, 1973; Small et al, 1975). The devices in both categories can be used to achieve penile rigidity, but there are differences in cosmetic appearance, and semirigid rods do not permit flaccidity. **The selection of a device may depend on a physician's surgical experience, insurance coverage, and patient preference and anatomy and/or history.**

Semirigid Rods

Semirigid rods are paired, solid cylinders that fill each corpus cavernosum. They can be further subdivided into malleable and positional devices (Figs. 30-1 and 30-2). A malleable device has a central core that allows a patient to position the penis upward for sexual intercourse and downward at other times. A positional device incorporates a series of articulating polyethylene discs with a central

metal cable support, which make it better able to maintain upward and downward positions. Semirigid rods are typically available in several diameters and lengths. Advantages of these prostheses are that they are relatively inexpensive, easy to implant (although a larger incision of the tunica albuginea is required), and easy to use. They also have a relatively low mechanical failure rate. Drawbacks are that they simulate a constant erection, may be difficult to conceal, and do not increase penile girth (Jain and Terry, 2006; Montague, 2011). Also, with semirigid rods, the capsule of scar tissue that forms around the device loosens up over time, decreasing the quality of the erection. Because the elastic tunica albuginea wants to retract when stretched to the erect length, the distal tip of the rigid device is more likely to atrophy or migrate toward the distal portion of the glans and potentially to erode through the meatus (see Figs. 30-1 and 30-2).

Inflatable Prostheses

Inflatable prostheses are designed to approximate normal function more closely by permitting girth and length expansion during erection and penile flaccidity when not in use. They consist of two hollow intracorporeal cylinders, each of which fills a corpus cavernosum. The cylinders are inflated with saline solution to produce penile rigidity during sexual activity and are deflated after intercourse. Inflatable prostheses can be subdivided further into two-piece and three-piece devices. The two-piece device consists of the two cylinders and a scrotal pump (Fig. 30-3). Reservoirs in the proximal portion of the cylinders are prefilled with saline and preconnected to the pump via silicone tubing. Pressing a valve mechanism in the pump transfers the solution from the reservoirs into the distal, inflatable portion of each cylinder. Bending the cylinders down for several seconds activates a release valve that deflates the device by allowing the fluid to flow back to the reservoirs. Cylinders are typically available in several widths and lengths to permit a more customized fit. Rear tip extensions allow the length of a two-piece prosthesis to be further tailored to each patient.

The three-piece device consists of the two hollow cylinders, a scrotal pump, and a saline-filled reservoir (Fig. 30-4). Silicone tubing connects the cylinders to the pump and the pump to the reservoir. Repeatedly squeezing the pump transfers saline from the reservoir to the cylinders until adequate rigidity is achieved, and pressing a valve mechanism in the pump causes the fluid to flow back to the reservoir. Similar to the two-piece devices, three-piece devices are also typically available in several widths and lengths and come with optional rear tip extensions. One-touch release models and other more recent innovations in pump design facilitate deflation.

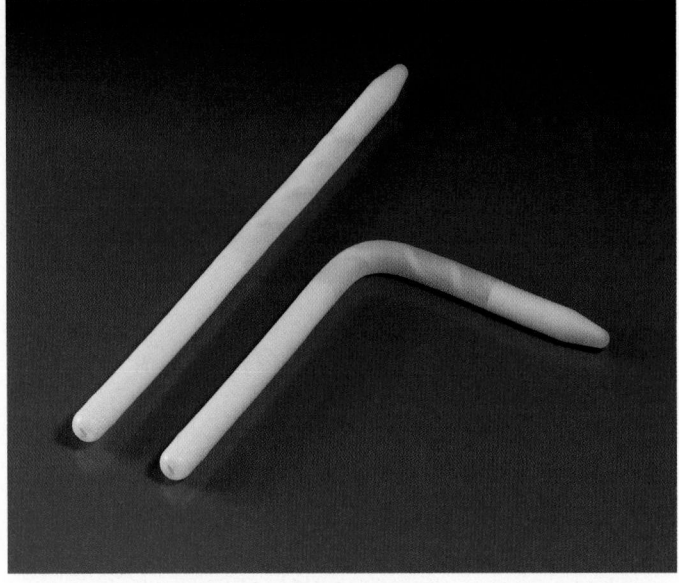

Figure 30-1. **Coloplast Genesis malleable prosthesis. (Courtesy Coloplast Corp., Minneapolis, MN.)**

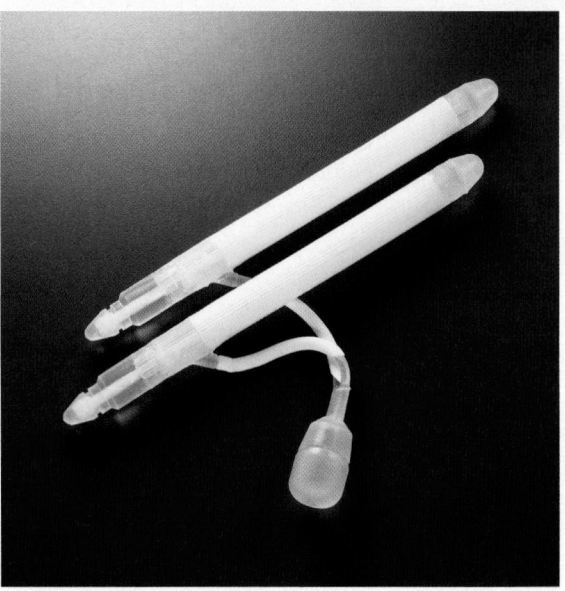

Figure 30-3. **Ambicor two-piece prosthesis. (Courtesy American Medical Systems, Minnetonka, MN.)**

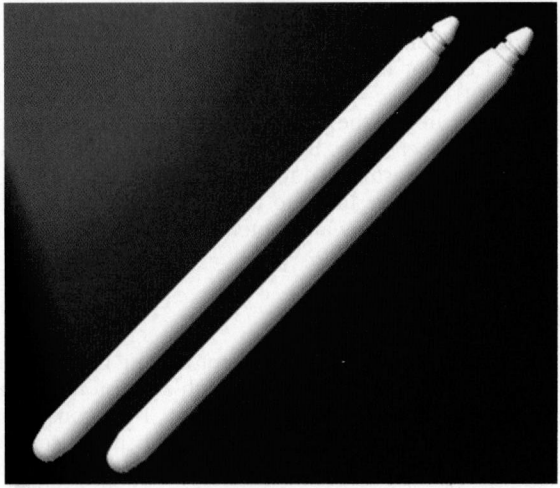

Figure 30-2. **Spectra positional prosthesis. (Courtesy American Medical Systems, Minnetonka, MN.)**

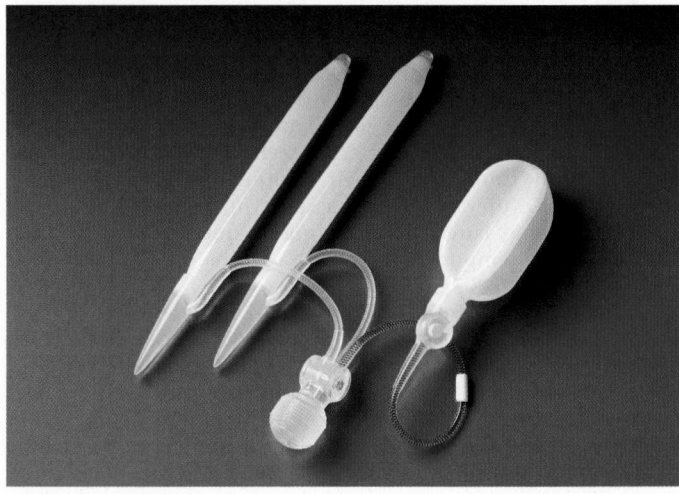

Figure 30-4. **Coloplast Titan Zero Degree angle cylinders with Touch pump and reservoir with lockout valve prosthesis. (Courtesy Coloplast Corp., Minneapolis, MN.)**

An advantage of a two-piece device over a three-piece device is that there is no need to implant a separate reservoir; this facilitates the surgery for the urologist and may be useful with patients in whom placement of the reservoir is extremely difficult because of colostomy, ileostomy, kidney transplant, or extensive pelvic surgery. A two-piece device also reaches full inflation with fewer squeezes of the pump. However, the pump is very small and hard, making it difficult for patients to manipulate. Also, implantation of a two-piece device requires a larger incision of the tunica albuginea. **In comparison, a three-piece device acts and feels more like a natural erection. It is more rigid when inflated and is more flaccid when deflated** (Fig. 30-5).

Initially, semirigid prostheses were more popular than inflatable devices, primarily because they were easier to implant and rarely required mechanical revision (Wilson and Mulcahy, 2006). However, this preference diminished as mechanical reliability improved. At the present time in the United States, 70% of patients are implanted with three-piece inflatable devices, 20% are implanted with two-piece devices, and 10% are implanted with semirigid rods. Elsewhere, approximately half of all patients are implanted with semirigid rods, and half are implanted with inflatable devices, primarily owing to cost considerations (Mulcahy and Wilson, 2006).

PREOPERATIVE PATIENT EVALUATION AND PREPARATION

Although penile prosthetic surgery is a highly effective treatment for ED, it is an irreversible procedure accompanied by numerous risks, which makes careful patient evaluation and preparation critical. Thorough preoperative assessment and education can help ensure that a patient is a good candidate for the procedure. It also helps identify the best type of prostheses for any specific circumstance. See Table 30-1 for more details about selection of a prosthesis.

The patient's first visit should be informational in nature; the focus should not be on decision making. It is important that the patient understand the efficacy of the various treatment options available for ED and potential contraindications for penile prosthetic surgery (Box 30-1). Giving a patient the opportunity to

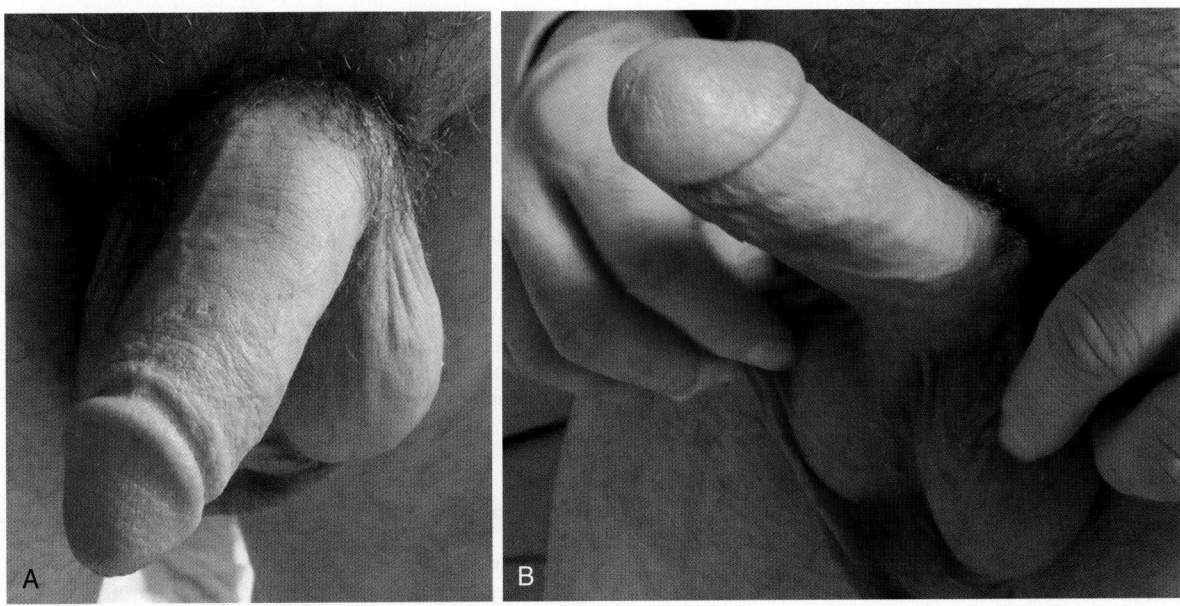

Figure 30-5. A and B, Patient with Coloplast Titan Zero Degree angle cylinders and Touch pump showing the flaccid and erect penis.

TABLE 30-1 Selection of a Prosthesis

CIRCUMSTANCE	RECOMMENDED PROSTHETIC	RATIONALE
Fibrosis (e.g., secondary to priapism)	Narrow-cylinder AMS CXR* or Coloplast Narrow†	Inadequate corporeal space
Peyronie disease/penile curvature	AMS CX*, Coloplast Titan†, or malleable	Allows girth expansion but no length expansion so will not exacerbate curvature
Limited manual dexterity or mentally disabled	Malleable or semirigid rods	Easier to manipulate
Penis length <20 cm	AMS CX*, AMS LGX*, or Coloplast Titan†	Allows for maximum amount of fluid transfer between cylinders and reservoir for best rigidity and flaccidity
Small narrower penis	AMS LGX*	Cylinder lengthens by 18% and narrow corporeal cavity prevents deformity of cylinders on inflation
Abdominoperineal resection Femora-femoral bypass Cystectomy with neobladder	Two-piece device—AMS Ambicor*	Avoids reservoir placement
Extensive abdominal/pelvic surgery Open and post-robotic prostatectomy	AMS Ambicor* or three-piece device—AMS CX or LGX with Conceal Reservoir*	Place reservoir in a submuscular location above the transversalis fascia
Neurologic impairment	AMS CX with soft cylinders	Lower risk of erosion
Atrophic tunica albuginea	AMS CX*	
Older patients with frail tissues and weak hands	AMS CX with Momentary Squeeze Pump*	AMS cylinders are softer, and Momentary Squeeze Pump is easier to deflate
Younger patients with larger, more robust penises	Coloplast Titan with Zero Degree Angle cylinders with Touch pump†	Rounder and wider shaft when cylinders are inflated Smaller, more discreet pump
Penis length >20 cm in length and >21 mm in girth	Coloplast Titan 20, 22 cm or XL 24-28 cm Zero Degree Angle cylinders†	Titan cylinders expand to 22 mm girth vs. 18 mm girth for AMS CX

*American Medical Systems (AMS), Minnetonka, MN.
†Coloplast Corp., Minneapolis, MN.

handle a sample prosthesis and see how it works facilitates actual use of the device after it is implanted (Bettocchi et al, 2010); however, seeing the entire three-piece device on the first visit can be intimidating and overwhelming. It is best for patients first to see a video and photos of implanted patients to appreciate the look and function of a prosthesis. Next, the patient can be given the opportunity to handle a model of the pump only, without having to handle the reservoir and cylinders. It is important to ensure patients understand that sensation, orgasm, and ejaculatory function are not altered by a penile prosthesis and that nothing is removed to insert the implant. On seeing the device, patients are often concerned about the size of the incision required to implant it, and they should be reassured that only a 1-inch incision is necessary.

A thorough review of the patient's medical, surgical, and sexual history is critical to evaluating the efficacy of previous nonsurgical treatment, selecting the most appropriate type of prosthesis, identifying contraindications, and mitigating risk factors for potential adverse events (Ulloa et al, 2008; Wilson and Mulcahy, 2006). For example, any detected infection should be eradicated before surgery, and glycemic control should be optimized in diabetic patients. Box 30-1 contains a list of potential contraindications for penile prosthetic surgery.

The appointment should also include a complete urologic examination, including a penile Doppler ultrasound study after intracorporeal injection of a vasodilating agent to assess severity of ED, vascular flow, tumescence, and penile anatomy. After a penile injection, the penis is more easily stretched, and abnormalities such as shortening, hourglass deformity, and curvature are revealed and can be evaluated. **This is also a good time to measure and record the length of the stretched penis and show the patient what size he should expect from the implant. These measurements can be recorded on a flow sheet and made available during the surgery to confirm that intraoperative measurements of the penis with the cylinders inflated match the measurements obtained in the office.**

Finally, informed consent should be obtained from the patient after a discussion that addresses the surgical procedure and postoperative recovery, potential complications (especially complications that may require surgical intervention), and expected outcome. Ensuring that the patient (and, ideally, his partner) has realistic expectations is essential to a positive outcome (Anderson et al, 2007). It is important for the patient to understand that the procedure is irreversible and that positioning the device permanently alters the corpora cavernosa, resulting in the loss of any preexisting erectile capability. **Patients should also be made aware that the preoperative length of the fully stretched flaccid penis is typically the maximal length that can be obtained after prosthetic surgery and that the procedure may result in a degree of penile shortening and glans softening** (Montague and Angermeier, 2003).

To help reduce the incidence of postoperative infection, patients are instructed to wash with chlorhexidine soap for 3 days before the surgery. The American Urological Association also recommends preoperative administration of prophylactic antibiotics for both gram-positive and gram-negative organisms for any open procedures involving prosthetic implantation (Wolf et al, 2008). Finally, patients should be instructed to avoid taking aspirin and nonsteroidal anti-inflammatory drugs for 7 days before surgery because such medication can increase the risk of postoperative bleeding. Patients with drug-eluting stents or a history of coronary artery disease are exceptions to this rule and should continue taking low-dose aspirin (81 mg) including on the day of the surgery.

KEY POINTS: PREOPERATIVE PATIENT PREPARATION

- Patients are often concerned about the size of the incision required to implant the device and should be reassured that only a 1-inch incision is necessary.
- It is important the patient understands that the procedure is irreversible and that positioning the device permanently results in the loss of any preexisting erectile capability.
- Patients should know that the preoperative length of the fully stretched flaccid penis is typically the maximal length that can be obtained after prosthetic surgery.
- Ensuring that the patient (and, ideally, his partner) has realistic expectations is essential to a positive outcome.

SURGICAL PREPARATION AND APPROACH

The surgical approach varies depending on the surgeon's preference and on the type of prosthetic device implanted. This section focuses on implantation of a three-piece inflatable device because this type is most commonly used in the United States. The three-piece device can be inserted through a scrotal or infrapubic incision. Each approach offers the surgeon and the patient advantages and disadvantages. Reservoir placement is easier when choosing the infrapubic approach. More precise pump positioning and better cylinder input pump tube concealment are achievable through the scrotal approach, which is described in this section. When planning to implant a standard three-piece device (i.e., 12 to 14 mm), it is recommended also to have a narrower or semirigid device (i.e., 9 to 11 mm) available at the time of surgery; this provides the flexibility to use the narrower option if implanting a multicomponent device becomes difficult because of unanticipated anatomic constraints. For example, it is better to implant a narrower device than attempt vigorous dilation of a fibrotic, scarred corpora and risk urethral *perforation*. Over time, the narrower device will dilate the corpora, and it may be possible to replace it with a three-piece device 3 to 6 months later.

To the extent possible, it is important to minimize the duration of the surgery, decreasing the risk of infection. This can be facilitated by using a dedicated surgical instrument set that, along with sutures and other necessary equipment, is kept close at hand. The specific instruments, sutures, needles, and cylinder sizes that should be available in the operating room have been described elsewhere (Eid, 2003). It is critical that all instruments are thoroughly scrubbed of all potential debris before undergoing final sterilization. Infection risk is reduced further by using as few instruments as possible and limiting the extent to which they must be passed back and forth with the scrub nurse. Ideally, operating room traffic should be minimized, and laminar flow ventilation should be used to reduce surgical site infection further.

General, local, spinal, or regional anesthesia is administered at the discretion of the anesthesiologist. A benefit of spinal anesthesia is that it blocks the parasympathetic and sympathetic nervous systems, causing penile dilation and facilitating the surgery. Blood flow to the legs is also increased, which decreases the risk of deep vein thrombosis. A disadvantage of spinal anesthesia is that it necessitates a longer stay in the recovery room and the placement of an indwelling urinary catheter, which needs to be removed within 24 to 48 hours. A risk with general anesthesia is that the typical cough reflex after extubation could potentially herniate the reservoir.

The patient is admitted for a penile implant on the day of surgery and discharged the same day. (Admission to an outpatient surgery center is preferable to hospital admission because the latter increases the risk of cross-contamination from sick patients.) The patient showers before surgery with an antiseptic chlorhexidine scrub and is placed in a supine position on the operating room table. The table should be flexed in a manner that elevates the pelvis and flattens the lower abdomen; this permits a more proximal exposure of the crura and stretches the lower abdominal muscles to provide countertraction for placement of the reservoir. The patient is shaved and undergoes a presurgical chlorhexidine soap scrub of the genital area. The skin is painted with a chlorhexidine/70% alcohol preparation, and intravenous antibiotics are administered to protect against gram-positive and gram-negative organisms, based on the profile of antibiotic-resistant bacteria most commonly found in the institution. An iodophor drape with a small fenestration is used to cover exposed skin while permitting access to the penis and scrotum. A Foley catheter is inserted, capped, and palpated to identify the urethra, which is then avoided for the remainder of the surgery. Finally, a Scott retractor is secured with tubing across the base of the penis. The use of large, blunt yellow hooks instead of the smaller, sharp blue hooks provides better exposure and minimizes the risk of damaging the device or surgical gloves.

From this point forward and depending on the surgeon's preference, it is possible to use a novel "no touch" surgical technique designed to reduce penile prosthesis infection (Eid et al, 2012). With this technique, all surgical instruments used to make the skin incision before cylinder placement are considered contaminated and removed from the surgical field, and everyone on the operating field who has touched skin replaces their surgical gloves (Fig. 30-6).

A study evaluating the no touch technique reported a 0.46% infection rate (Eid et al, 2012). However, regardless of the technique used, exposure of all of the components of the device to the patient's skin must be minimized because most penile prosthesis infections are caused by skin flora that attach to the device and are then introduced into the patient.

Cylinder Placement

A high scrotal approach on the median raphe, approximately 1 inch inferior to the junction with the penis, is preferable to the classic penoscrotal approach because it allows the incision to be limited to 1 inch, which permits quick closure without scarring and less postoperative bleeding, swelling, and pain. This approach also facilitates access to the penis in obese or thin men. The high scrotal approach is also preferable to an infrapubic approach because the latter increases the tendency of the pump to migrate to a high scrotal position, making it more visible in the anterolateral aspect of the scrotum and leaving the tubing easily palpable at the base of the penile shaft. Scrotal skin is mobilized over the shaft of the base of the penis, and surrounding tissue is pushed laterally by securing the Foley catheter and urethra between the thumb and index finger (see Fig. 30-6).

Dissection can be minimized by making the incision straight down toward the urethra. This incision reduces postoperative swelling and edema and results in a thick layer of subcutaneous tissue allowing for complete isolation of tubing from skin suture line and better incision closure. The scrotal location of the incision also allows for deeper placement and concealment of input tubing to the pump (see Fig. 30-6). A small fenestration is then made in the 3M Steri-Drape 1012 that is placed to cover the operative field and the Scott retractor loosely. Four additional blunt hooks are used to secure the opening in the drape to the edges of the scrotal incision, retracting the cut edges of the skin and drape by securing the hooks on the retractor frame (Fig. 30-7). The remainder of the procedure is performed through the opening, eliminating all direct and indirect contact between the implant and the skin.

The tunica albuginea of each corpus cavernosum is identified on either side of the urethra (Fig. 30-8), secured with 3-0 polydioxanone suture (PDS) RB-1, and incised 1 cm lateral to the urethra (Fig. 30-9). The incision should be limited to the tunica albuginea and avoid cavernosal muscle tissue. Positioning the corporotomy close to the urethra allows direct downward orientation of the tubing between the cylinder and the pump and makes it less likely that the patient will be able to palpate the tubing at the base of his penis.

Blunt scissors are used to develop a space between the tunica albuginea and cavernosal muscle (Fig. 30-10) in both directions to

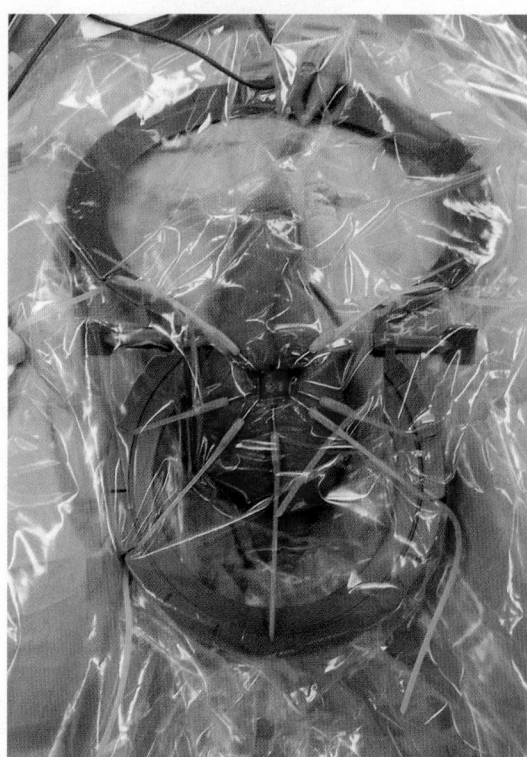

Figure 30-7. **The 3M Steri-Drape 1012 Fluoroscope Drape with opening secured to scrotal incision with yellow hooks.**

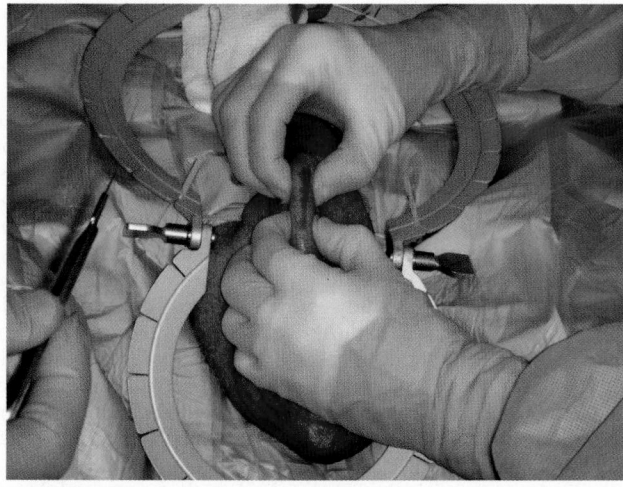

Figure 30-6. **Securing the Foley catheter and urethra.**

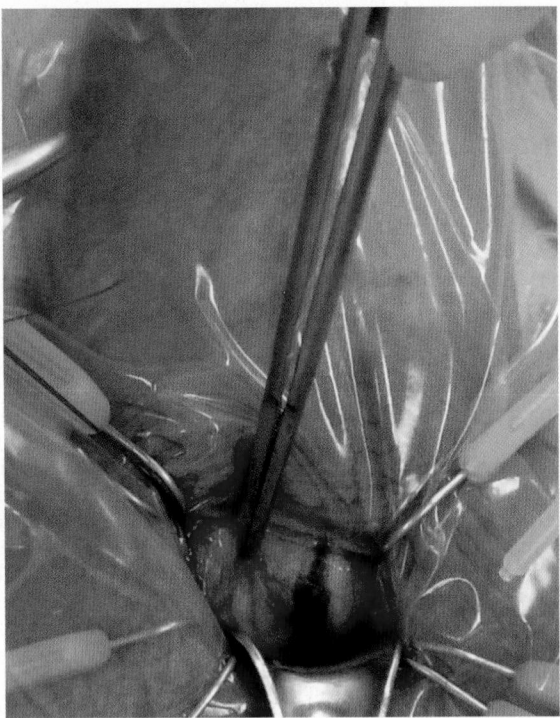

Figure 30-8. Left tunica albuginea is marked 1 cm lateral to the urethra.

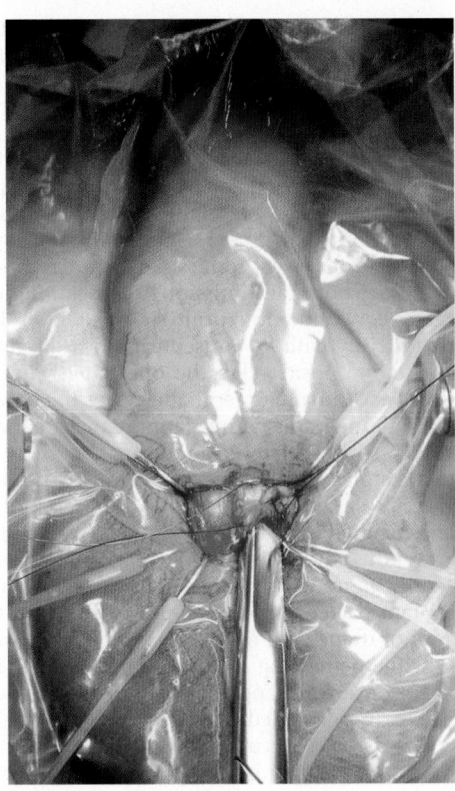

Figure 30-10. Initial dilation with blunt-tip Mayo curved scissors.

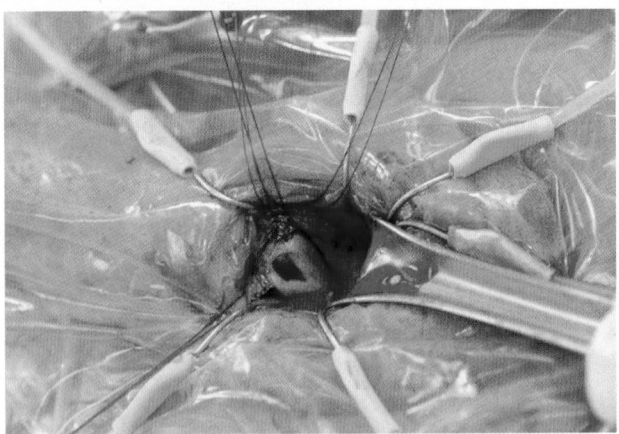

Figure 30-9. Position and size of corporotomy.

allow sequential dilation of the corpora using Dilamezinsert (Lone Star Medical Products, Stafford, TX) or Hegar dilators. More than half of surgery-related complications when implanting cylinders occur during this part of the procedure (Henry and Wilson, 2007). **The use of force is unnecessary and should be avoided to prevent perforation of the tunica albuginea and damage to the urethra at the meatus or the crus, which can occur during either distal or proximal dilation** (Sadeghi-Nejad, 2007). The use of special dilators (e.g., Rossello [Coloplast Corp., Minneapolis, MN] or Uramix [Uramix, Inc., Lansdowne, PA] double-blade cavernotome dilators or Otis urethrotome) can help decrease the risk of perforation in the presence of corporeal fibrosis (Bettocchi et al, 2008).

To prevent distal or proximal crossover into the contralateral corpus during initial dilation, constant traction should be applied to the shaft of the penis by pulling on the glans, and the curvature of the scissors should be maintained away from the midline of the penis, with the tips next to the tunica albuginea (see Fig. 30-10). It is preferable to dilate at the level of the venous plexus at

the periphery of cavernosal muscle tissue (vs. centrally through cavernosal muscle). **If crossover occurs, it is usually preferable to recognize it and correct it during this part of the procedure, rather than after further dilation or insertion of the cylinders.**

To correct a distal perforation, the damaged corpus apex should first be exposed through a transverse incision of the skin and tunica albuginea near the glans. A small hole can usually be located distally on the medial aspect of the cavernosal cavity and repaired using separate PDS stitches. The distal apex of the corpora needs to be closed with a second running suture, and a slightly shorter prosthetic cylinder is selected for the perforated side; this is necessary to prevent the distal tip of the cylinder from resting on the urethral suture repair. A more conservative approach would be to terminate the procedure and bring the patient back for implantation 3 months later. The disadvantage of this strategy is that the length of the shaft is foreshortened, and dilation of the scarred corpora is much more difficult. If the perforation occurs after both corpora are dilated, a semimalleable cylinder can be placed in the nonperforated side to preserve penile length. Use of a Dacron or Gore-Tex sleeve should be avoided because of the markedly increased risk of infection and ingrowth into the graft, which makes it impossible to remove. To evaluate proximal perforation during surgery, a dilator can be placed in each crura, and their heights can be compared to confirm that one has penetrated too deeply inside the perineum. Repair involves anchoring the cylinders to the surrounding corpora tissue by placing stitches above and below the input tubing, which prevents the cylinder from proximal migration and allows the perforation to heal. Alternatively, nonabsorbable sutures can be used to create a sling through the solid portion of the inflatable cylinder (Bettocchi et al, 2008). A study comparing prosthetic implantation with or without corpora dilation suggested that dilation is unnecessary in primary implantation cases. The investigators reported that patients receiving an implant without the use of dilation experienced less postoperative pain and increased penile length compared with patients in whom dilators were used to facilitate cylinder insertion (Moncada et al, 2010).

To select an optimally sized cylinder, the corporeal lengths should be measured distally and proximally with respect to a fixed

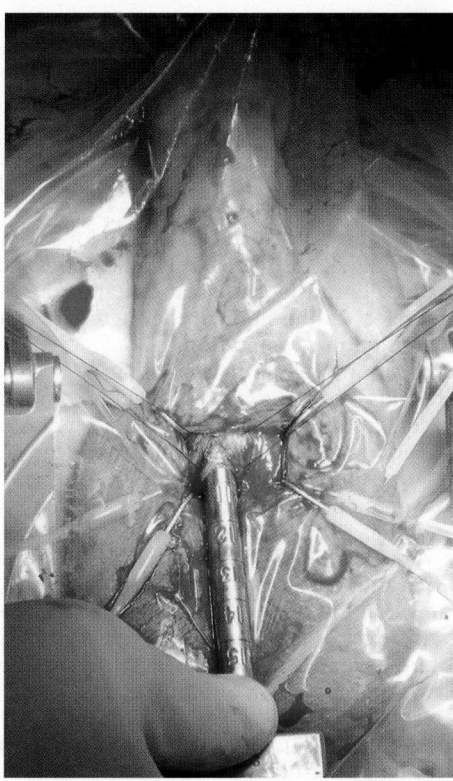

Figure 30-11. **Dilamezinsert is used to obtain distal measurement.**

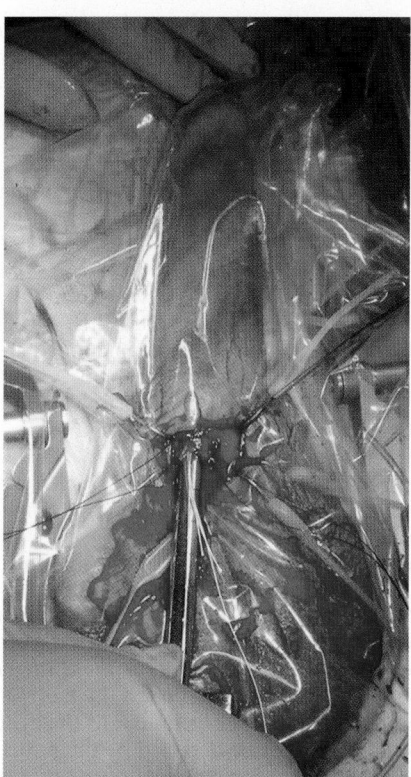

Figure 30-12. **Furlow introducer is used to pass right cylinder traction suture.**

point of reference, such as a traction suture (Fig. 30-11). Oversized cylinders can result in erosion and an S-shaped penile deformity, which can cause increased wear at the flexion point of the curve and lead to mechanical failure (Wilson et al, 1996; Montague, 2011). Conversely, an undersized cylinder may not adequately support the glans; this can be easily addressed by adding rear tip extenders. **It is important not to overstretch the penis over the measuring instrument, especially when measuring the proximal portion.** Creating an artificial erection by irrigating the corpora with saline can help assess if the penis is straight or curved. Noting the presence or absence of irrigant leakage from the meatus around the catheter can also help evaluate the possibility of urethral injury.

When a cylinder is selected, the device is opened on the surgical field and prepared for implantation by purging air from the cylinders and pump. The traction suture from the distal tip of each cylinder is secured to a Keith needle and passed into the distal aspect of the penile shaft and through the glans penis with the Furlow introducer (Fig. 30-12).

Damage to the device is avoided by passing both sutures and Keith needle before placing a cylinder into a corpora (Bettocchi et al, 2010). Because most cylinders are preconnected to the pump, it is important to orient the cylinders such that the two input tubes to the pump do not cross over each other. After each traction suture has been passed through the glans penis, the proximal portion of each cylinder is inserted first. The cylinder is folded on itself, and when the distal tip is placed in the corporeal orifice, the traction suture is pulled to insert the rest of the cylinder.

Each cylinder must lay flat in the corpora when traction is applied on the suture. Any folds observed in the cylinder indicate that it may be too long or that the rear tip is not properly positioned.

When both cylinders have been inserted, a 60-mL syringe filled with saline is used as a surrogate reservoir to inflate the cylinders to evaluate erection size and quality. The cylinders are then deflated, and the penis is reexamined to ascertain correct cylinder sizing. This test can also help identify cylinder malfunction or damage should it occur. If the cylinder length needs adjustment, the saline should

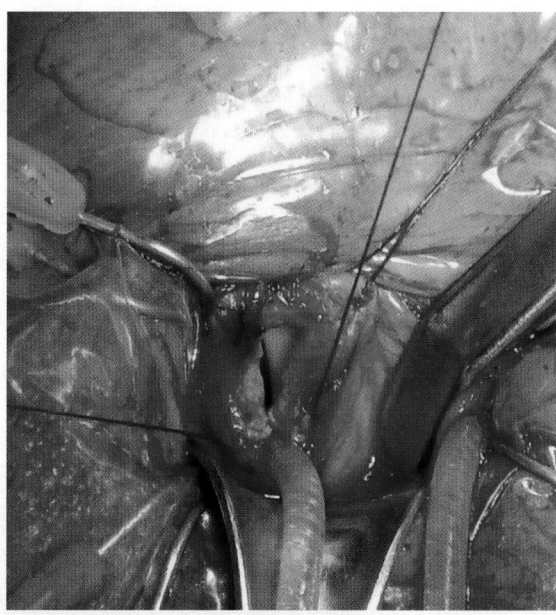

Figure 30-13. **Watertight closure of right corporotomy.**

be completely removed from the cylinder before removing the cylinder from the corpora and changing or removing the rear tip extender; this facilitates the adjustment and decreases the chance of damaging the cylinder. **Each time a cylinder is removed, adjusted, and repositioned into the corpora, it can become contaminated and its sterility can be compromised, especially if it comes into contact with skin.**

A watertight closure of the corporotomy can be achieved with a running 3-0 PDS using a hemostatic stitch or by approximating the previously placed tagging 3-0 PDS (Fig. 30-13). Although the former approach takes more time and can potentially cause needle injury to the cylinder, it is preferable because it creates a watertight closure. When the corporotomy is closed, the pump should be activated and deactivated several times while assessing cylinder size and integrity. **If the latter approach is used, and a watertight closure is not achievable, a drain should be placed at the end of the procedure to evacuate bleeding and prevent scrotal hematoma.**

Pump Placement

Placement of the pump before the reservoir minimizes skin contact time while the reservoir is being placed. Allis clamps are used to provide gentle traction to the scrotal fascia, and a flap is developed beneath the urethra for a distance of 2 to 3 cm. A long, closed nasal speculum is introduced into a 1-cm incision made in the scrotal fascia, approximately 1 to 2 cm from the urethra, and directed upward between both testicles and toward the bottom of the scrotum. The speculum is used to form a pocket in the scrotal sac, in the fatty layer between the testicular tunica vaginalis and slightly behind the testicles (Fig. 30-14).

It is important to keep the blades of the speculum closed until the tips reach the bottom of the scrotal sac to prevent excessive dilation of the pouch, which should fit snugly around the pump. This prevents posterior pump migration, which renders it less accessible to the patient. **The pump should be positioned such that the deflation footprint is easily accessible to the patient yet unobtrusive, and the tubing between the pump and the cylinders should be placed so that it cannot be detected by the patient and sexual partner.** After obtaining complete hemostasis, the opening in the scrotal fascia can be closed. Bleeding around the pump causes an inflammatory reaction and hematoma formation, and a thick capsule develops around the pump. Use of the implant is delayed, and it is difficult to activate the device.

Reservoir Placement

Before reservoir placement, it is important to ensure the bladder is empty to avoid bladder perforation. While applying upward traction to the penis, the base of the crus is palpated, and Scarpa fascia is bluntly divided. In this manner, a defect is created between the crus of the penis medially and the spermatic cord laterally. Next, the operator's finger is oriented toward the pubic ramus, and the external inguinal ring is identified. The tip of a large blunt Mayo curved scissors is placed over the pubic ramus by sliding it between the base of the penis and the operator's finger. After tilting the scissors at a 90-degree angle with the plane of the abdominal wall and positioning the tip of the scissors just over the pubic ramus, a small 0.5-cm defect is made in the floor of the inguinal canal with the

blunt Mayo scissors. **It is important to limit the excursion of the scissors to a 1-cm depth and to maintain the scissors on the pubic ramus.** Incomplete perforation of the floor of the inguinal canal should be avoided because it will cause separation of transversalis fascia from the undersurface of the internal oblique muscle. This will cause a decrease in the countertraction of the transversalis fascia, making it more difficult to puncture the floor of the inguinal canal and access the space of Retzius. When the defect of the floor is made, the scissor is removed and exchanged for a nasal speculum with 8-cm-long blades (Fig. 30-15). **It is unnecessary to dilate the space of Retzius vigorously, and great care must be taken not to make a large defect in the floor of the inguinal canal resulting in reservoir herniation or migration.**

This part of the procedure may be difficult in a patient after hernia repair and transversalis fascia thickening owing to mesh and previous surgery. In such cases, it may be necessary instead to make a separate incision for adequate reservoir placement or to implant the reservoir in a submuscular location. The latter approach may make the reservoir palpable and possibly visible (Henry and Wilson, 2007; Al-Enezi et al, 2011). Catastrophic outcomes, such as injury to bowel or a major blood vessel or placing the reservoir into the bladder, colon, and vena cava, have occurred in the past when attempting to place the reservoir in this manner in patients with previous pelvic surgery. **Placement of the reservoir in the space of Retzius should be performed only in patients who have not undergone surgery previously. Submuscular reservoir placement with a flat reservoir (AMS Conceal; American Medical Systems [AMS], Minnetonka, MN) or a separate incision (Fig. 30-16) should always be performed in all patients after robotic prostatectomy, radical cystectomy, and abdominoperineal resection and in patients with history of pelvic fracture with bladder rupture and pelvic surgery.** However, positioning the reservoir above the transversalis fascia in a submuscular position can lead to autoinflation of the device, which occurs when the fluid pressure within the reservoir is greater than the back-pressure limits of the pump (Levine and Hoeh, 2012).

When the space of Retzius is entered with the long nasal speculum, it is opened, and the surgeon's index finger is used to confirm

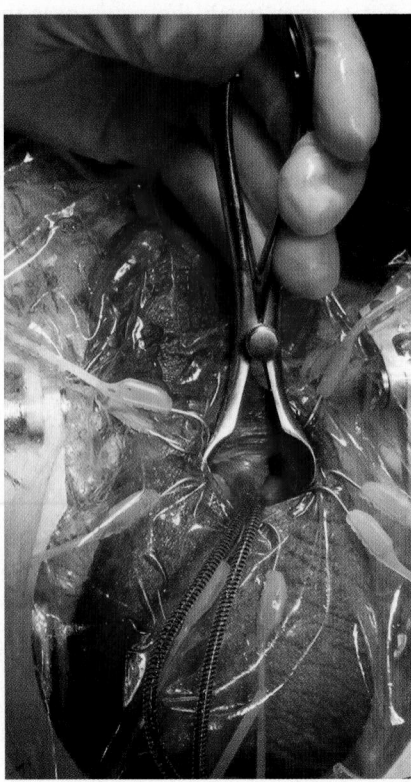

Figure 30-15. Placement of reservoir into space of Retzius.

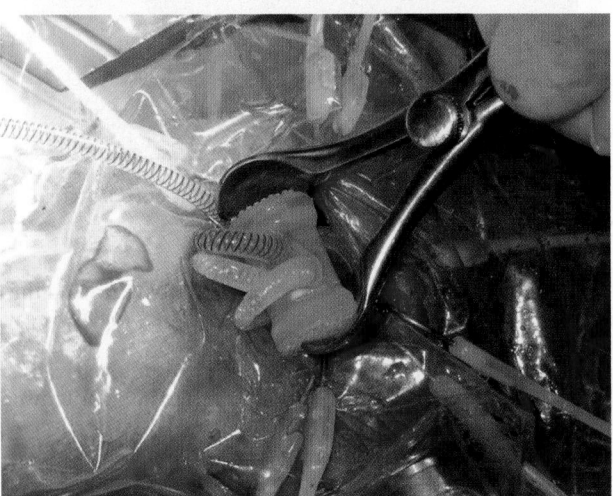

Figure 30-14. Placement of pump into scrotal sac.

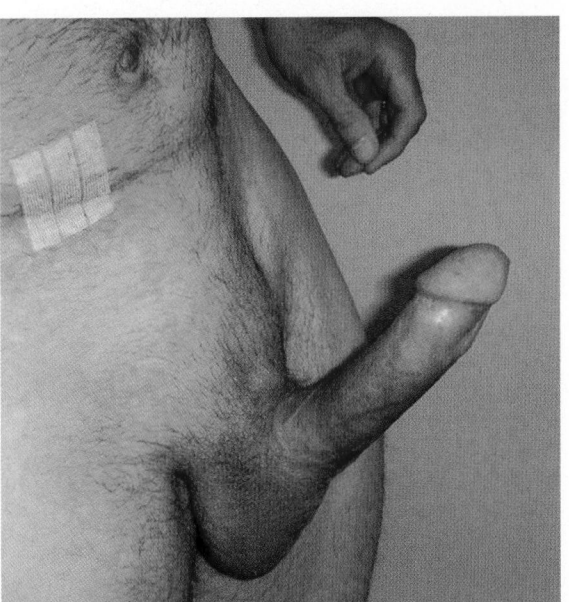

Figure 30-16. Right lower quadrant incision for submuscular placement of reservoir in a patient after robotic prostatectomy. Coloplast Titan 24-cm XL cylinders are shown inflated 2 weeks postoperatively.

its position. An empty reservoir is placed through the nasal speculum next to the bladder, the speculum is removed, and the reservoir is filled with the appropriate amount of saline. A back-pressure test performed by applying gentle pressure on the lower abdominal wall. A palpable reservoir or back-pressure of saline noted into the syringe is an indication that it has not been properly positioned. A surrogate test should then be performed, using a syringe as the reservoir, to confirm proper reservoir placement and check for back-pressure. It is important that the prosthesis is completely deflated before tubing from the pump is trimmed and connected to tubing from the filled reservoir. **Every effort must be made to maintain the reservoir full during the immediate postoperative period to prevent autoinflation of the device later on.** Allowing healing to occur over a partially filled reservoir limits its ability to store an adequate volume of saline. If hematuria if present at this point, it could potentially indicate injury to the bladder wall, which must be ruled out before closing.

Closure

At this point, the surgical site should be irrigated and reexamined for hemostasis. When hemostasis is confirmed, Buck fascia and the dartos muscle are closed, followed by closure of the skin. A benefit of using nonabsorbable sutures are the warm baths (lying flat, not sitting) started on postoperative day 3, which help relieve pain, decrease any swelling or edema, and keep the scrotum clean. The catheter can be removed the morning after the surgery by the patient at home, and the stitches are removed after 14 days.

The use of a closed-suction drain to reduce the risk of hematoma after inflatable penile implant surgery is controversial. Two retrospective studies investigating the use of drains did not produce conclusive results, and there have been no randomized controlled clinical trials evaluating the efficacy of using a drain after implant surgery (Wilson et al 1996; Sadeghi-Nejad et al, 2005; Kramer et al, 2011). Proponents posit that draining the scrotum can decrease edema, increase comfort, and decrease the time to initiation of device cycling. Opponents argue that draining increases the risk of infection, drain fracture, bleeding during placement, and damaging the device and inconveniences the patient, who then has to return to the clinic the following day to have the drain removed (Sadeghi-Nejad et al, 2005; Kramer et al, 2011). A review of articles addressing penile prosthetic infection published in Medline and EMBASE

databases from 2000 to 2012 concluded that no recommendation can be made about the use of surgical drains to reduce infection rates associated with penile prosthetic surgery (Elmussareh et al, 2013). **If the surgeon is not satisfied with hemostasis, the surgical area should be drained.**

KEY POINTS: SURGICAL PREPARATION AND APPROACH

- Minimizing surgery duration decreases the risk of infection.
- Exposure of all of the components of the device to the patient's skin should be minimized.
- During dilation, the use of force is unnecessary and should be avoided to prevent perforation of the tunica albuginea.
- Narrower inflatable and semirigid devices should be available for all cases in the event that implanting a three-piece device becomes difficult.
- Placement of the reservoir in the space of Retzius should not be performed in patients with prior pelvic surgery.
- A closed-suction drain should be used if the surgeon is not satisfied with hemostasis.

POSTOPERATIVE CARE

When implanting a penile prosthesis, the outcome is very dependent on the nature of postoperative care. Because the surgery is typically an outpatient procedure or involves a 23-hour stay, the Foley catheter and drain (if used) are removed the morning after surgery (Garber, 2008). The efficacy of postoperative prophylactic antibiotics has not been demonstrated in prospective studies and remains controversial. Although there is no consensus regarding the type or duration of antibiotic administration postoperatively, a survey of 216 urologists found that most prescribed antibiotics for 7 days after surgery and favored quinolones (Koves et al, 2011; Wosnitzer and Greenfield, 2011; Elmussareh et al, 2013).

During the first week, the patient should avoid sitting on the scrotum (this can push the pump upward) and lifting more than 15 pounds or any other activities that could cause displacement of the reservoir into the inguinal canal. **Brief-style underwear should be worn for the first month, with the penis placed on the lower abdomen and oriented toward the umbilicus until the device is first inflated. Such positioning promotes capsule formation around the cylinders and will orient the erection in an upward direction.** It also helps prevent downward curvature during the healing process (Wilson and Mulcahy, 2006; Montague, 2011).

If the type of device implanted does not include a lock-out valve on the reservoir, the patient should be warned about the potential for postoperative autoinflation, which typically occurs following intra-abdominal pressure increase. This autoinflation can be embarrassing and increases the risk of cylinder erosion (Abbosh et al, 2012). Should autoinflation occur, the patient may need to return to the clinic earlier than usual for instruction about how to deflate the device. At 3 months, the capsule that forms around the reservoir typically protects it from any pressure increase and decreases the incidence of autoinflation (Wilson and Mulcahy, 2006). **It is important for the patient to understand that capsule formation should occur when the reservoir is full, and the reservoir should not be left in a partially filled state for extended periods. If the capsule forms around a partially filled reservoir, the capsule will restrict future expansion of the reservoir, prohibit complete cylinder emptying, and potentially cause autoinflation, resulting in a need for surgical revision.** Abbosh and colleagues (2012) described the use of outpatient laparoscopic capsulotomy to treat this problem.

The extent to which a patient experiences postoperative pain varies depending on his tolerance and any preexisting conditions (e.g., neuropathy). Scrotal bruising and swelling are common, with scrotal hematoma typically receding without surgical intervention (Wilson and Mulcahy, 2006). An oral narcotic is often required the first week, followed by nonsteroidal anti-inflammatory medication as needed. Ice packs may be used intermittently.

The first postoperative visit typically occurs at 2 weeks to assess wound healing and manage any signs of autoinflation. During this visit, it is critical to identify early signs or symptoms of local infection. The patient again returns to the clinic at approximately 4 weeks after surgery for an appointment focusing on how to operate the device. Initial inflation of the prosthesis may be difficult, and the patient should be instructed to cycle the device (i.e., inflate and deflate it) during warm baths twice each day for the next month to facilitate its use. The patient can then attempt sexual intercourse as soon as he feels comfortable using the device. Additional postoperative instructional visits may be necessary, depending on each patient's experience. Subsequent follow-up at 3 months, 6 months, and then annually should be scheduled to assess healing, particularly cylinder tip position in the glans; device functioning; and patient satisfaction.

COMPLICATIONS

Complications can occur during surgery or postoperatively. Complications that can occur during surgery include organ injury/perforation, cylinder crossover, and damage to the device during implantation. These are addressed in Surgical Preparation and Approach. Complications that can occur postoperatively are addressed in the following sections.

Infection

Infection is a serious complication of prosthetic surgery and represents significant pain and suffering for an elective procedure. The incidence of infection is estimated to be approximately 4% for primary implants before the introduction of specially coated devices and 10% for revision implants (Henry et al, 2004); however, this may reflect underreporting because of discontinuity of care (Muench, 2013). **Research suggests that most infections are caused by bacteria on the skin that attach to the device and are then introduced into the patient.** Because infections are infrequent and evidence suggests that skin bacteria are relatively innocuous, physicians tend to assume that such contamination is inevitable and focus their efforts on managing the contamination by irrigating, using antibiotic-coated implants, and administering IV antibiotics (Henry et al, 2008; McKim and Carson, 2010), overlooking surgical technique (i.e., avoiding touching the skin) as an adjunct to decrease the potential source of infection further.

Knowing the time line of presentation of a suspected infected prosthesis can help guide early management and diagnosis. For example, at the 2-week postoperative interval, if the patient does not seem to improve and reports persistent or increased pain, one must resist the temptation to prescribe oral antibiotics. If the device is not infected, the patient should experience a clinical improvement within the next 7 to 14 days. If the device is infected, antibiotics are useless at this point and may delay diagnosis. Fever, erythema, swelling, elevated white blood cell count, and incision drainage are late signs and symptoms of infection and are usually not observed at this postoperative visit. The sooner an infection is diagnosed, the better the chance for successful salvage. Imaging studies such as scrotal sonography, computed tomography scan, and magnetic resonance imaging are not helpful in making an early diagnosis. Tethering of the pump may also be a sign of infection but can sometimes be caused by inflammation and capsule formation from a hematoma. Capsule formation improves over time, whereas inflammation persists or becomes more pronounced. **Close patient follow-up and weekly examinations with evaluation of white blood cell count are important when an infection is suspected. Clinical deterioration with persistence of pain and tethering at 3 to 4 weeks postoperatively signals an infection, and aggressive early salvage should be considered before systemic symptoms,**

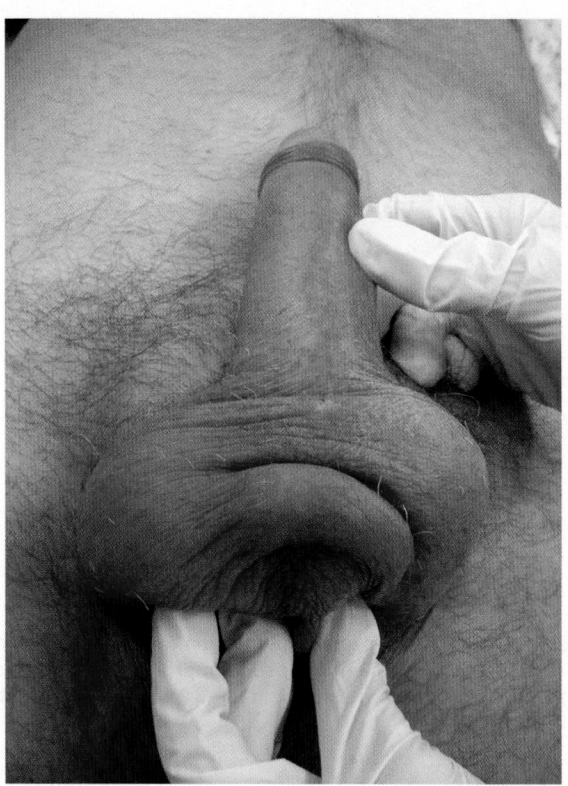

Figure 30-17. Tethering of pump consistent with early infection of prosthesis.

such as fever, elevated white blood count, erythema, and abscess formation of scrotum, occur (Fig. 30-17).

The bacterial contamination that causes infection most often occurs at the time of surgery and typically involves organisms that colonize the skin, such as *Staphylococcus epidermidis, Staphylococcus aureus,* and *Candida albicans.* These organisms can persist despite perioperative antibiotics. When they reach a critical mass, they excrete a biofilm in which they can live in a decreased metabolic state, causing no clinical symptoms until at least 4 to 6 weeks and sometimes years after implantation (Wilson and Mulcahy, 2006). **Because of the biofilm, the use of systemic antibiotics to treat symptomatic patients is typically insufficient, and infection necessitates the removal of all device components as well as any permanent sutures or graft material used during corporeal reconstruction. Attempts to remove only part of an infected device typically result in persistent infection** (Garber, 2008).

Traditionally, after removal of an infected implant, a surgeon waited several months before considering replacement. However, severe cavernosal fibrosis after explantation complicates replacement surgery, contributing to a 50% success rate even for experienced surgeons. The fibrosis also causes significant penile shortening and potential loss of sensation, which has a negative impact on patient satisfaction (Muench, 2013). Introduction of a "salvage" procedure involving removal of the infected prosthesis, wound washout, and immediate device replacement helped facilitate reimplantation and preserve penile length (Brant et al, 1996; Jain and Terry, 2006). When indicated (i.e., for chronic and nonpurulent infection), salvage success rates can exceed 84% if the procedure includes thorough wound irrigation with a series of antibiotic and antiseptic solutions, followed by a change of surgical gowns, gloves, drapes, and instruments; placement of a new device; wound closure without drains; and oral antibiotics for 1 month (Mulcahy, 2000; Henry et al, 2005; Garber, 2008). More recent research suggests that aggressive washout with normal saline combined with meticulous sterile technique may further improve postsalvage infection and reoperation rates (Masson, 2012). The salvage technique can also be used when a device requires replacement for reasons other than infection (Henry et al, 2005. **Salvage is contraindicated in patients presenting with enterococcus, tissue necrosis, sepsis, diabetic ketoacidosis, or cylinder erosion into the urethra** (Mulcahy 2003; Wilson and Mulcahy, 2006).

When malfunctioning penile prostheses are removed, they are often found to be colonized with pathogenic bacteria, even in the absence of clinical infection. For example, Silverstein and colleagues (2006) used scanning laser microscopy to determine that 80% of prostheses explanted because of mechanical malfunction were colonized with gram-positive rods, cocci, and fungal elements, and Henry and associates (2004) reported that culture-positive bacteria were found in 70% of patients with clinically uninfected penile prostheses. However, according to a study by Kava and colleagues (2011), less than 10% of devices removed because of malfunction or rerouted because of extrusion were colonized with pathogenic bacteria. The authors also found that there was no correlation between culture-positive patients and postoperative infection. They suggested that their findings may differ from findings of other investigators because of their use of a preoperative, adjuvant, alcohol-based skin preparation.

More recently, a novel surgical technique has been developed to facilitate delayed implantation of a replacement device. Swords and coworkers (2013) described the insertion of a temporary filler consisting of an antibiotic cast of synthetic high-purity calcium sulfate into the corpus cavernosum when an infected device is removed. This "spacer" provides constant delivery of local antibiotic to the infected area and reabsorbs within 30 to 60 days, at which time a new prosthetic device can be implanted.

Specially coated three-piece devices have been developed by both AMS (Minnetonka, MN) and Coloplast Corporation (Minneapolis, MN) to inhibit bacterial adhesion and proliferation. The AMS 700 devices are impregnated with InhibiZone, a coating on the external surface of the device that elutes rifampin and minocycline to inhibit bacterial growth. The Coloplast Titan prosthesis has a hydrophilic polyvinylpyrrolidone coating that absorbs and elutes any antibiotic solution in which it is soaked. The introduction of these coatings within the past decade has decreased the incidence of infection by 50% to 70%, even after 11 years of follow-up (Carson et al, 2011; Mandava et al, 2012; Serefoglu et al, 2012). **This decreased incidence confirms our hypothesis that infections are caused by contamination of the prosthesis at the time of implantation.** It appears that the antibiotics eluting from the devices and/or the slippery surfaces of the implant reduce the proliferation and attachment of the relatively milder, late-appearing types of bacteria noted earlier. However, although such coatings have significantly decreased overall infection rates, more aggressive and earlier-appearing bacteria, such as *Enterococcus, Escherichia coli,* and *Pseudomonas aeruginosa,* are now causing infection at increasing rates (Eid et al, 2012).

Risk factors for infection may be related to patient history, intraoperative conditions, or postoperative variables. Risk factors related to patient history include poor patient hygiene, spinal cord injury, urinary tract infection, distant sites of infection, and revision surgery performed for previous device infection; however, it is unclear whether revision surgery for mechanical failure is associated with higher rates of infection (Cakan et al, 2003; Kava et al, 2011; Selph and Carson, 2011; Elmussareh, 2013; Muench 2013) Diabetes mellitus may also be a risk factor, although studies report conflicting results. For example, a large retrospective study with a follow-up period of up to 7.7 years found a higher incidence of first revisions owing to infection in diabetic patients compared with nondiabetic patients; however, other studies have not found a difference in the incidence of infection between the two groups (Lotan et al, 2003; Mulcahy and Carson, 2011). It is also unclear whether poorly controlled diabetes and immunosuppression are associated with an increased infection risk (Bishop et al, 1992; Wilson et al, 1998; Elmussareh et al, 2013). **Intraoperative risk factors for infection may include inadequate skin preparation with alcohol/chlorhexidine; prolonged surgical time (i.e., >2 hours); prolonged and repeated exposure of components of the** prosthesis to patient's skin; frequent repositioning and resizing of the cylinder, pump, or reservoir; scrotal hematoma (particularly if liquefied); and not changing gloves before handling the device. A postoperative variable associated with infection risk is prolonged hospitalization.

A review of studies focusing on penile prosthetic infection between 2000 and 2012 suggested that the most important factors to minimize the risk of device infection include the use of antibiotic-coated prostheses and procedures that decrease inoculating bacteria into the surgical wound (i.e., alcohol skin preparation, a no touch surgical technique, and perioperative antibiotic use) (Elmussareh et al, 2013). Although the use of perioperative antibiotics reduces infection, there are no specific guidelines recommending antibiotic protocols, and a wide range of practice patterns exists among urologists performing prosthetic surgery (Wosnitzer and Greenfield, 2011).

KEY POINTS: INFECTION

- Knowing the time line of presentation of a suspected prosthetic infection can help guide early management and diagnosis.
- Infection necessitates the removal of all device components as well as any permanent sutures or graft material used during corporeal reconstruction.
- Factors that minimize the risk of device infection include the use of antibiotic-coated prostheses and procedures that decrease inoculating bacteria into the surgical wound (i.e., alcohol skin preparation, a no touch surgical technique, and perioperative antibiotic use).

Device Malfunction

Device malfunction is becoming less common as prosthesis design improves over time (Bettocchi et al, 2010). A historical prospective study estimating long-term survival rates of first-time implants (N = 2384) found that freedom from mechanical breakage was 79.4% at 10 years and 71.2% at 15 years (Wilson et al, 2007). **The most common types of malfunction in a three-piece prosthetic device depend on the manufacturer and include cracks in the silicone tubing, leaks at the site where the tubing connects to the pump, leaks within the cylinder, cylinder aneurysm, and pump disruption** (Garber, 2008). Autoinflation, which is discussed elsewhere in this chapter, has been observed to occur in 2.4% to 11% of devices overall, but this incidence decreased to 1.3% in devices with lockout valves (Carson et al 2000; Wilson et al, 2002). Reservoir-related mechanical malfunction is also rare, and it is unclear whether a functioning reservoir should be replaced during revision surgery to address other issues (Levine and Hoeh, 2012).

If malfunction occurs within a few months after implantation, replacement of only the defective component should be considered, especially if this avoids a repeat corporeal incision. **After the device has been in place for more than 2 years, complete replacement is indicated** (Jain and Terry, 2006). Other options following malfunction include no treatment or device removal without replacement. When choosing the latter, it is important for the patient to understand that because the cavernosal space is now empty, the tunica albuginea will retract, scar tissue will form inside the penis, and the penis will become permanently shorter.

Other Complications

Postoperative complications occurring less frequently than infection and device malfunction include erosion, S-shaped penile deformity, poor glans support, and scrotal hematoma. Erosion typically occurs months or years after implantation and can manifest in several different locations. For example, an oversized cylinder, especially the semimalleable type, is most likely to erode into the meatus at the level of the glans. The pump and input tubes to the cylinders can erode at the level of the scrotal skin if placed too superficially, although an indolent low-grade bacterial infection is most often the reason for this (Natali, 2010; Talib et al, 2013). Similarly, the reservoir can erode into the bowel or bladder if either is fixed in place by adhesions resulting from previous surgery or radiation; however, this is very uncommon (Levine and Hoeh, 2012). **Regardless of the location, erosion always necessitates complete removal of all the components of the device and possible salvage replacement.** If only one of the cylinder tips has eroded through the meatus, the entire device needs to be removed, including the pump and reservoir, and a malleable cylinder is placed in the noneroded side only, to prevent shortening of the penis. The perforation must be allowed to heal for 8 to 12 weeks before reimplantation is attempted (Natali, 2010).

An S-shaped penile deformity can occur after incomplete distal dilation of the corpora cavernosa and/or implantation of an oversized cylinder (Wilson et al, 1996; Bettocchi et al, 2008). This complication also necessitates device replacement. In contrast, implantation of an undersized cylinder can result in poor glans support; however, this can be treated by adding rear tip extenders or by replacing the cylinders with the correct size without disturbing the scrotal pump.

Because blood collects in dependent areas of the body, scrotal hematoma can follow implantation of a three-piece prosthesis, with reported incidence ranging from 0.7% to 3.6%. Attempts to decrease the development of scrotal hematoma include keeping corporotomies small, closing with a running watertight suture, and using hemostatic sealant (Cohen and Eid, 2014). Kramer and colleagues (2011) published an analysis of the risks and benefits related to the use of closed-suction drains. In the absence of a large, prospective, randomized trial, it is unclear which course of action is most beneficial, and the final decision is largely a matter of surgeon preference. **In my opinion, it is better to use a drain than to risk hematoma. Blood in the scrotal sac causes significant inflammation and formation of a thick fibrous capsule around the pump, which makes it very difficult for the patient to manipulate the pump when healed.** Additionally, a liquefying hematoma provides iron and nutrients, making it an ideal setting for bacterial growth and infection.

SPECIAL CASES

Several situations make implantation of a penile prosthesis particularly challenging. These include previous pelvic surgery (which is addressed in Surgical Preparation and Approach), Peyronie disease, priapism, scleroderma and lupus, and previous radical prostatectomy.

Peyronie disease is characterized by focal fibrotic replacement of healthy tunica albuginea; this most commonly causes curvature of the penis toward the location of the scar and results in ED (Mulcahy and Wilson, 2006). A prosthetic implantation procedure similar to that described in Surgical Preparation and Approach has been found to straighten the erection adequately in approximately 40% of patients (Chaudhary et al, 2005). Otherwise, penile straightening may be required and typically involves manual modeling during which the tunical plaque is fractured over an inflated cylinder at the time of implantation by forcibly bending the penis in a direction opposite the curvature. Plication or tunical incision/excision with or without grafting may rarely be necessary (Hudak et al, 2013; Segal and Burnett, 2013). Mulhall and associates (2005) developed an algorithm for the surgical treatment of Peyronie disease and ED that involves objective assessment of penile deformity using dynamic infusion cavernosometry and cavernosography, followed by administration of erectogenic therapy. The authors found that patients who did not respond to erectogenic therapy and underwent penile prosthetic surgery had excellent results. Other studies subsequently reported that surgical placement of an inflatable penile prosthesis is an effective treatment option for Peyronie disease (Levine et al, 2010; Chung et al, 2013). However,

another study suggested that Peyronie disease compromises inflatable prosthetic device durability and increases malfunction rates, possibly owing to stress on the device during surgery, use, or both (DiBlasio et al, 2010).

Priapism is defined as a full or partial erection that continues for more than 4 hours beyond intercourse or is unrelated to sexual stimulation (Tausch et al, 2013). If left untreated, the resulting fibrosis is usually distal, extensive, and dense, making it very difficult to dilate with conventional instruments (Wilson and Mulcahy, 2006; Martinez-Salamanca et al, 2011). A review of surgical procedures to facilitate prosthetic implantation and improve outcomes in such situations suggests that scar incision should include a combination of techniques (i.e., extensive wide excision, multiple incisions minimizing excision, corporeal counterincisions, corporeal excavation technique, or Shaeer technique) as well as cavernotomes and smaller prostheses (Shaeer and Shaeer, 2007; Martinez-Salamanca et al, 2011). A retrospective analysis of prosthetic implantation in 17 patients with postpriapism ED found that although all patients were successfully implanted without major postoperative complications, 2 patients experienced urethral injury secondary to extensive corporeal fibrosis (Durazi and Jalal, 2008).

The use of radical prostatectomy to treat prostate cancer often results in ED. Some clinicians assume that implantation of a three-piece prosthetic device is contraindicated in such situations because of a perceived increased risk of intraoperative injury. To address these concerns, two studies investigated the use of penile prostheses after radical prostatectomy. In the first, Lane and colleagues (2007) reported that of 115 consecutive patients receiving a three-piece inflatable penile prosthesis after prostatectomy, none experienced intraoperative complications, including injury to the bladder or iliac vessels, with successful blind entry into the retropubic space in all cases. In the second study, Menard and associates (2011) examined surgical complication and patient satisfaction rates in subjects receiving a penile implant after radical prostatectomy and found that the procedure was associated with low morbidity and high satisfaction, especially with respect to erectile function; however, they noted that fibrosis in the retropubic space may necessitate a second incision for reservoir placement or use of a two-piece device instead of a three-piece device. Nevertheless, there have been several catastrophic mishaps related to implantation of a penile prosthesis after prostatectomy, such as placing the reservoir in the bladder, sigmoid colon, or vena cava and injury to the bladder or bowel. **In my opinion, the reservoir should always be placed through a separate incision (if the implant is performed via a penoscrotal approach) and placed in a submuscular position.** Although robotic prostatectomy can be performed through an extraperitoneal approach, most prostatectomies are performed transabdominally, and the peritoneum is not closed after the prostate is removed. Under this circumstance, a second incision (preferably on the right side to avoid the sigmoid) or submuscular reservoir placement must always be performed.

PATIENT SATISFACTION

In general, patient satisfaction with penile prosthetic implantation for ED has increased over the past 40 years, seemingly at least partly as a result of mechanical and design enhancements (Trost et al, 2013). **Patient satisfaction with penile prosthetic implantation is currently the highest among all of the treatments for ED** (Mulcahy, 2010; Rajpurkar and Dhabuwala, 2003). Bernal and Henry (2012) reviewed all relevant research published over the past two decades and identified nine studies meeting their inclusion criteria (e.g., >30 subjects, three-piece device, written in English), all of which indicated that patients report high satisfaction rates. This seems to be the case regardless of device manufacturer or older age (Brinkman et al, 2005; Villarreal and Jones, 2012; Chung et al, 2013).

In a study designed to identify specific factors that affect overall satisfaction, 21 patients were surveyed preoperatively about their expectations and asked to rate their satisfaction 4 months postoperatively (Kramer and Schweber, 2010). **The investigators found an inverse correlation between patients' expectations and postoperative satisfaction, suggesting that helping patients have realistic expectations and providing them with an accurate description of the procedure result in higher satisfaction after implantation.**

Factors associated with postoperative dissatisfaction include a diagnosis of Peyronie disease, a history of radical prostatectomy, and a body mass index of 30 (Akin-Olugbade et al, 2006). The most common postoperative complaint associated with the reduction of overall satisfaction is loss of penile length (Lee and Brock, 2013). Strategies to preserve penile size after prosthetic implantation can be implemented before insertion, intraoperatively, or after insertion. Henry and colleagues (2012) conducted a prospective, multicenter study to assess patient satisfaction and axial rigidity of a cylinder that is longer in length than other available prostheses. The investigators concluded that the longer cylinders had great rigidity based on objective and subjective assessment. They also reported that patients had excellent satisfaction rates after implantation of the longer cylinders.

CONCLUSION

Penile prosthetic surgery is a highly effective treatment option for patients with ED who fail first-line and second-line therapy. Over the past 40 years, refinements in surgical technique have significantly reduced the rates of infection and other complications, and innovations in prosthetic design have had a positive impact on device malfunction rates. High levels of patient and partner satisfaction exceed that of many other, less invasive treatment options and reflect the fact that penile implants have become the "gold standard" for the treatment of advanced ED.

Please visit the accompanying website at www.expertconsult.com to view
videos associated with this chapter.

REFERENCES

The complete reference list is available online at www.expertconsult.com.

SUGGESTED READINGS

Al-Enezi A, Al-Khadhari S, Al-Shaiji TF. Three-piece inflatable penile prosthesis: surgical techniques and pitfalls. J Surg Tech Case Rep 2011;3(2): 76–83.

Eid JF, Wilson SK, Cleves M, et al. Coated implants and "no touch" surgical technique decreases risk of infection in inflatable penile prosthesis implantation to 0.46%. Urology 2012;79(6):1310–5.

Elmussareh M, Goddard JC, Summerton DJ, et al. Minimising the risk of device infection in penile prosthetic surgery: a UK perspective. J Clin Urol 2013;6(5):280–8.

Muench PJ. Infections versus penile implants: The war on bugs. J Urol 2013;189(5):1631–7.

Mulcahy JJ. Current approach to the treatment of penile implant infections. Ther Adv Urol 2010;2(2):69–75.

31 Diagnosis and Management of Peyronie Disease

Laurence A. Levine, MD, FACS, and Stephen Larsen, MD

GENERAL CONSIDERATIONS

Peyronie disease (PD) was first known as *induratio penis plastica*. It was subsequently named after Francois Gigot de la Peyronie because he was the first to describe and offer treatment for it in a paper published in 1743 (Peyronie, 1743). But Guilielmus de Saliceto in the 13th century and Gabriele Falloppio in the 15th century had previously reported on this abnormality of the penis (Musitelli et al, 2008).

PD is currently recognized as a wound-healing disorder of the tunica albuginea (Devine and Horton, 1988) **that results in the formation of an exuberant scar, occurring presumably after an injury to the penis activates an abnormal wound-healing response** (Van De Water, 1997; Greenfield and Levine, 2005; Ralph et al, 2010; Levine and Burnett, 2013). **The resulting scar or plaque is inelastic and therefore results in penile deformity including curvature, indentation, hinge effect, and shortening and is frequently accompanied by erectile dysfunction (ED). One of the most important characteristics of this particular wound-healing disorder is that once the scar has occurred, it does not undergo normal remodeling and therefore the scar and deformity persist** (Del Carlo et al, 2008). Progress with treatment of PD has been limited by an incomplete understanding of its pathophysiology, and this lack of understanding has resulted in an inability to prevent the disease from starting and to prevent progression once it has occurred. This, combined with the fact that there is no known reliable treatment to reverse the scarring process, makes PD a challenging disorder to treat.

Multiple misconceptions have been held for decades about PD. Many of these misconceptions have been carried forward and appear to have compromised the proper assessment and early treatment of men with PD (LaRochelle and Levine, 2007). These include that Peyronie is a rare disorder. **On the contrary, we now know that the prevalence of PD is somewhere between 3% and 20%, and in certain populations such as those with diabetes mellitus and ED the prevalence may be even higher** (Lindsay et al, 1991; La Pera et al, 2001; Rhoden et al, 2001; Schwarzer et al, 2001; Sommer et al, 2002; Mulhall et al, 2004b; El-Sakka, 2006; Arafa et al, 2007; DiBenedetti et al, 2011). Another misconception is that PD has a reasonable likelihood of resolving spontaneously. As a result, men are often told by their physicians that nothing can be done during the acute phase and they should wait 6 months to a year, because there is a "good chance" that the disease process will resolve. **We now know from multiple natural history studies that full spontaneous resolution is extremely rare and that it is more likely that within the first 12 to 18 months after presentation, if no treatment is offered, up to 50% of patients will experience worsening of their deformity** (Mulhall et al, 2006). Another misconception is that PD is a disorder that occurs only in middle-aged men. Multiple studies have demonstrated that it can occur in teenagers to men in their late 70s (Levine and Dimitriou, 2000; Kadioglu et al, 2002; Tal et al, 2012). Why this process occurs more commonly in middle-aged men is unclear, but theories include that the aging tunica is more apt to be injured in men who are susceptible to the disease, which activates the abnormal wound-healing process (Devine and Horton, 1988; Jarow and Lowe, 1997).

It is also a disorder that appears to go through an active phase during which the scar can grow, resulting in progressive deformity and pain. However, once it stabilizes, there is rarely further progression (Box 31-1).

NATURAL HISTORY

An understanding of the natural history of PD is critical to counseling patients and selection of treatment options. There are two phases. **The first is the active (acute) phase, which is commonly associated with painful erections and changing deformity of the penis. This is followed by a stable (chronic) phase, which is characterized by stabilization of the deformity and disappearance of painful erections** (Devine et al, 1997; Jalkut et al, 2003; Ralph et al, 2010; Kadioglu et al, 2011a). It would seem intuitive that once the scarring process has begun, there would be a progressive increase in deformity; but we have found that up to 20% of patients will experience a sudden onset of deformity that can be as great as 90 degrees.

It has been reported that PD can completely resolve in some patients, but this is probably a misconception. It is more likely that some men who traumatize their penises develop curvature secondary to the local inflammatory process. In some of these patients the inflammation resolves before scarring sets in. Thus the patient who has resolution of his deformity may not have had PD at all, but rather a slow-healing wound that simply takes longer to undergo the proper remodeling found with normal wound healing. **Spontaneous regression has been looked at in several contemporary natural history studies that have suggested that no more than 13% of patients will have some improvement of their deformity over the first 12 to 18 months after onset of the disease process**

BOX 31-1 Peyronie Disease Caveats

- Peyronie disease is not rare.
- It does not have a high likelihood of spontaneous resolution.
- It is not a disease of only middle-aged men.
- It is not a disease of only Caucasian men.
- Trauma to the flaccid and erect penis appears to activate the scarring process in susceptible men.
- Erectile dysfunction is frequently found in men with Peyronie disease.
- Plaque calcification is not an indication of mature, chronic-phase disease.

when not treated (Kadioglu et al, 2002; O'Brien et al, 2004; Mulhall et al, 2006; Hatzimouratidis et al, 2012). **The key point to remember is that complete spontaneous resolution of PD is a rare occurrence.** Recently, Berookhim and associates (2014) reported on a group of men who elected to have no treatment of their PD. In this study it appeared that the later the man sought evaluation in the first year after the onset of symptoms, the less likely that he would experience further deformity when left untreated (Berookhim et al, 2014).

EPIDEMIOLOGY

Incidence

The incidence of PD varies widely depending on the population being screened—from 0.39% to 20.3%, with most current estimates of the incidence of PD being between 3% and 9% and the peak age of onset of PD in the early 50s (Schwarzer et al, 2001; Mulhall et al, 2004a). It was previously held that this was a disorder primarily of Caucasian men of northern European descent. **It is now recognized that men of every race can develop PD.** The variation in recognition of and reporting on this disorder in certain populations may be a result of the interest and presence of physicians with expertise in PD, as well as cultural mores that may make it more or less comfortable for men to share information about changes in their sexual function with a health care provider (Lindsay et al, 1991; Arafa et al, 2007). A recent Japanese study looked at a total of 1090 men undergoing a routine health check and demonstrated the prevalence of PD in healthy men to be quite low at 0.6% (Shiraishi et al, 2012). In a large U.S. Web-based survey, 16,000 randomly selected men over the age of 18 years were asked to self-report the symptoms, diagnosis, or treatment of PD. In this study, 0.5% to 0.8% of respondents had received a diagnosis of or treatment for PD, whereas 13% of respondents admitted to having symptoms of PD such as penile deformity or palpable plaque (DiBenedetti et al, 2011). **The estimated number of unknown cases seems to be much greater than the number of symptomatic patients seeking treatment** because autopsy data demonstrate that 22 out of 100 men have at least a mild form of the disease (Smith, 1969). Therefore the prevalence of PD seems to be equivalent to if not greater than that of important public diseases such as diabetes and urolithiasis, both established to be present in 3% to 4% of the general population (Sommer et al, 2002). **It is worthwhile to note that the actual rates of PD may be higher than self-reported studies would suggest,** because men with PD may be reluctant to discuss the signs and symptoms of this embarrassing condition.

The incidence of symptomatic PD may be increasing, which is perhaps explained by an increasing tendency to obtain medical help, increasing awareness that may be secondary to people seeking information on the Internet, or increasing use of pharmacologic treatments for ED (e.g., phosphodiesterase inhibitors, intracavernosal injectable agents) (Hellstrom, 2003). **Phosphodiesterase inhibitors have not been suggested to directly contribute** to the development of PD; rather, their associated use in those with medical conditions such as diabetes that contribute to ED is the likely explanation, because these men now experience erections with deformities they would not have realized were present. At this time there is no suggestion that use of phosphodiesterase type 5 (PDE5) inhibitors should worsen or provoke PD. On the other hand, more recent in vitro and animal model studies have suggested that use of PDE5 inhibitors, as nitric oxide (NO) donors, has an antifibrotic effect that may be beneficial for the patients with PD (Valente et al, 2003; Ferrini et al, 2006; Gonzalez-Cadavid and Rajfer, 2009; Chung et al, 2011a). Treatments for ED, including intracorporeal injection therapy and vacuum devices, have also been implicated as a cause of PD (Carrieri et al, 1998; Jalkut et al, 2003; Bjekic et al, 2006). What seems more likely is that these treatments are designed to create a stronger erection, which can then be injured during a sexual encounter, activating the disease process in the susceptible individual. **To date there is no evidence that any medicines such as beta blockers or phenytoin cause PD.**

Associated Conditions

Aging

PD is most commonly diagnosed in the fifth decade of life. **A linear increase in prevalence can be seen from ages 30 to 49 with an exponential increase in prevalence at age 50 and up** (Sommer et al, 2002). Mulhall and associates (2004b) demonstrated an increased prevalence of 8.9% in a population being screened for prostate cancer in a study in which the mean patient age was 68 years (Mulhall et al, 2004b). PD may also occur in young men. PD patients under age 40 tend to be seen during the acute phase after rapid onset of disease with a penile deformity and pain on erection (Tefekli et al, 2001). Studies have shown that approximately 10% of men with PD are younger than 40 years (Levine and Dimitriou, 2000). In addition, Tal and associates (2012) reported on 32 teens diagnosed with PD over a 10-year period with a mean age of 18 (Tal et al, 2012). Sixteen percent reported antecedent trauma, and 37% reported subsequent ED. A high level of distress was reported by 94% of these young men, with 34% seeking treatment for an anxiety or mood disorder (Tal et al, 2012). **The increased prevalence of PD with age is likely a reflection of the increased likelihood of comorbid medical conditions contributing to the development of ED such as hypertension, hyperlipidemia, diabetes, and low testosterone, all of which have been suggested as possible causative factors associated with PD.** Hypothetically, it could also reflect the reduced tissue elasticity that naturally occurs with aging, predisposing this tissue to stretch-related injury.

Diabetes

One of the more interesting recently studied associations is that of diabetes mellitus and PD. **The prevalence of diabetes in men with PD has been reported to be as high as 33.2%, which is much higher than in the general population** (Kadioglu et al, 2002; Bjekic et al, 2006; Cowie et al, 2010). Conversely, the prevalence of PD among diabetics has been shown to be increased when compared with the general population, with a reported rate of 8.1% to 20.3% depending on the specific population being screened (El-Sakka and Tayeb, 2005; Tefekli et al, 2006; Arafa et al, 2007). This may reflect particular patient populations, ethnic groups, referral patterns, and expertise of the physicians treating the disorder. Longer duration of diabetes and poor glucose control have also been shown to significantly increase the severity of PD with respect to duration of PD, deformity, curvature, and erectile function (El-Sakka and Tayeb, 2005; Kendirci et al, 2007). A recent retrospective study suggested that plaque size and pain may decrease as underlying diabetes is treated (Cavallini and Paulis, 2013). This was a small retrospective study, and further prospective studies are necessary to confirm these results.

One theory for the apparent association between PD and diabetes is that men with diabetes are at a higher risk for ED, which may

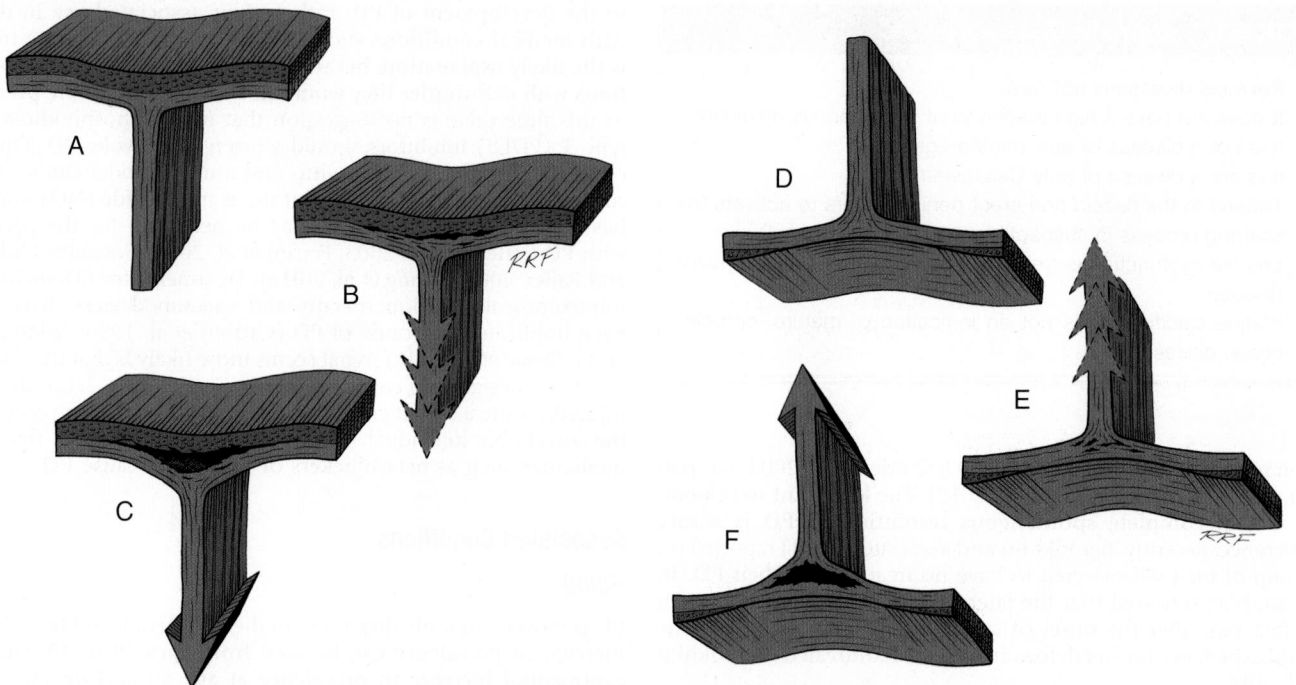

Figure 31-1. Demonstration of the mechanism of injury during buckling injuries to the penis. A, Fibers of the septal strands dorsally fan out and are interwoven with the inner circular lamina fibers of the tunica albuginea. The outer lamina consists of longitudinal fibers. B, In the chronic mechanism of Peyronie disease, less turgid erections allow flexion of the penis during intercourse, producing elastic tissue fatigue, further reducing elasticity of the tissue and leading to multiple smaller ruptures of the fibers of the tunica with smaller collections of blood, possibly producing multiple scars. C, In the acute mechanism of Peyronie disease, bending the erect penis out of column produces tension on the strands of the septum, delaminating the layers of the tunica albuginea. Bleeding occurs, and the space fills with clot. The scar generated by the response of the tissue to this process becomes the Peyronie disease plaque. D, Illustration of the situation on the ventrum of the penis, where the bilaminar arrangement of the tunica albuginea becomes thinned, with the midline being monolaminar. The fibers of the septal strands fan out and are interwoven with the inner circular layer. There is no outer circular layer. E, In the chronic mechanism of Peyronie disease, less turgid erections allow buckling of the penis as in B. F, In the acute mechanism of Peyronie disease, buckling of the erect penis out of column produces tension on the strands of the septum, causing the septal fibers to tear.

predispose to injury during intercourse because of the less rigid penis pivoting back and forth, potentially resulting in a tissue fatigue–type fracture, activating the scarring disorder (Devine and Horton, 1988) (Fig. 31-1). Another theory suggests that diabetes may lead to decreased compliance of tissues as a result of increased collagen cross-linking (Aronson, 2003). This may make minor injuries less prone to normal remodeling.

Erectile Dysfunction

ED appears to be more common in men with PD than in the general population (Ralph et al, 2010). **The prevalence of ED in men with PD has been reported to be 37% to 58%** (Kadioglu et al, 2002; Usta et al, 2004; Casabé et al, 2011; Chung et al, 2011b). In a duplex ultrasound study of 76 men with PD and ED, 36% had evidence of penile arterial insufficiency and 59% had veno-occlusive disease as the cause of their ED (Lopez and Jarow, 1993). In our review of their own clinical experience, approximately 80% of men with PD also have reported diminished rigidity. Half of these men had ED before the onset of PD, usually as a result of the typical vascular risk factors for ED (e.g., smoking, diabetes, hypertension, dyslipidemia), whereas the other half developed ED subsequent to the onset of the PD. **The prevalence of associated comorbidities is higher in patients with PD and ED than in patients with PD, which may indicate that hypertension, smoking,** hypercholesterolemia, diabetes mellitus, and hyperlipidemia are more likely related to ED than to the pathogenesis of PD (Usta et al, 2004). This later onset may be attributable to changes in penile geometry and/or psychological inhibition, which is difficult to determine even in studies in which duplex ultrasound and cavernosometry are used (Levine and Coogan, 1996; Kadioglu et al, 2002).

Psychological Aspects

PD is not only a physically deforming but also a psychologically devastating disorder. Multiple studies have now demonstrated the frequent association of psychological distress in men with PD including diminished self-esteem, shame, embarrassment, self-disgust, anxiety, loss of sexual confidence, and depression, all of which can compromise the man's relationships at home, at work, and in the bedroom (Gelbard et al, 1990; Jones, 1997; Rosen et al, 2008; Smith et al, 2008a). **Penile shortening and the inability to have intercourse are the two most common and consistent risk factors for emotional distress and relationship problems associated with PD** (Rosen et al, 2008; Smith et al, 2008a).

Psychosocial stress is reported by 77% to 94% of men with PD (Gelbard et al, 1990; Tal et al, 2012; Nelson and Mulhall, 2013). Contemporary studies using a validated measure of depression (Center for Epidemiologic Studies Depression Scale [CESD]) have demonstrated moderate to severe depression in 48% of PD patients, and these rates typically increase with the duration of PD (Nelson et al, 2008). PD also commonly affects the patient's sexual partner, causing feelings of helplessness as well as feelings of personal responsibility for the PD caused by trauma during intercourse, and sadness over loss of intimacy (Rosen et al, 2008).

In an effort to develop a valid outcome measure for assessing psychosocial and sexual consequences of PD, Rosen and associates (2008) conducted a study composed of a series of focus groups with 28 PD patients and identified common concerns. These concerns were grouped into four core domains: (1) physical appearance and self-image, (2) sexual function and performance, (3) PD-related pain and discomfort, and (4) social stigmatization and isolation (Rosen et al, 2008). With these data, a validated Peyronie's Disease Questionnaire (PDQ) was developed; patient-reported estimates of penile curvature severity correlated with PDQ domains, whereas objective measures of penile curvature did not. Thus for some patients even a lesser degree of curvature may be highly bothersome or provoke distress (Hellstrom et al, 2013). This is also evidenced by the fact that self-estimates of penile curvature in men with PD differ from objective measures by an average of 20 degrees, with 54% of patients overestimating their curvature (Bacal et al, 2009). It is important to remember that despite "successful treatment" that may allow the patient to be sexually functional again, there is often persistent psychological distress, presumably because of the residual changes to the patient's pre-PD penis (Gelbard et al, 1990; Jones 1997). It is critical that the physician recognize these psychological effects, not only to enhance the trust between the patient and physician, but also to identify more advanced indicators of depression, which should initiate referral to a sex therapist, psychologist, or psychiatrist (Levine, 2013).

Radical Prostatectomy

Both prostate cancer and PD are most prevalent in men after their fifth decade of life. The evidence to support or refute a link between radical prostatectomy and PD is limited. In a study of 1011 post–radical prostatectomy patients, Tal and associates (2010) demonstrated an incidence of PD of 15.9% with a mean time to development of disease of 13.9 months (Tal et al, 2010). Although postoperative erectile function was not a predictor of development of PD, younger age at time of prostatectomy and white race were reported risk factors for developing PD after radical prostatectomy. The authors concluded that prospective controlled studies are needed to elucidate the incidence of PD after radical prostatectomy and determine if radical prostatectomy has a causative role in the pathogenesis of PD (Tal et al, 2010).

Ciancio and Kim (2000) also examined the effects of prostatectomy on penile fibrosis and sexual dysfunction. Eleven percent of all patients undergoing prostatectomy developed fibrotic changes in the penis. This fibrosis led to penile curvature in 93%, "waistband" deformity in 24%, and palpable plaques in 69%. Therefore, it does appear that men undergoing radical prostatectomy by an open or robotic approach have a higher risk of developing PD than the general population. The mechanism responsible for this is not known but may include perioperative penile trauma, neurogenic consequences, or as we believe is local release of cytokines that activate the abnormal wound-healing process in men susceptible to PD.

Hypogonadism

The possibility that low serum testosterone may be associated with PD has also been investigated. Results of studies have varied on this topic. Moreno and Morgentaler (2009) demonstrated that severity of curvature was worse in men with low free and total testosterone. Rhoden and associates could demonstrate no such association and concluded in their study that androgen serum levels and sexual dysfunction had no association to PD (Rhoden et al, 2010).

The presence of hypogonadism in patients with PD has been suggested to exaggerate the severity of PD. Nam and associates (2011) showed in a study of 106 patients with PD that curvature, plaque size, ED, and response to medical therapy were worse in patients with testosterone deficiency and concluded that further studies are needed to confirm this relationship. Cavallini and associates (2012) investigated whether testosterone replacement in hypogonadal men with PD would affect treatment with intralesional verapamil injection. In these patients, supplementation with testosterone improved the efficacy of intralesional verapamil compared with those who did not receive testosterone replacement. Plaque area and penile curvature were also more severe in hypogonadal men with PD (Cavallini et al, 2012).

Collagen Disorders

There does appear to be an association of PD with other collagen disorders such as Dupuytren disease (DD). DD is believed to be transmitted in an autosomal dominant manner. The prevalence of DD in different geographic locations is extremely variable (0.2% to 56%), and it is not clear whether this is because of genetic or environmental factors. The literature concerning coexisting DD in patients with PD also demonstrates a very large range (0.01% to 58.8%) (Nugteren et al, 2011). As with PD, the prevalence of DD increases with age, from 7.2% among men in the age group of 45 to 49 years up to 39.5% in those 70 to 74 years old (Gudmundsson et al, 2000). Other studies have demonstrated DD in 21% to 22.1% of PD patients, as well as 6.7% who reported having a first-degree relative with DD (Carrieri et al, 1998; Nugteren et al, 2011). Other associated fibrotic conditions are contracture of the plantar fascia (Ledderhose disease) and tympanosclerosis, both of which are uncommon disorders (Box 31-2).

KEY POINTS: EPIDEMIOLOGY

- The incidence of PD varies widely depending on the population being screened and is likely much higher than once thought. Current estimates are between 3% and 9%, and the peak age of onset of PD is the early 50s.
- A linear increase in prevalence can be seen from ages 30 to 49, with an exponential increase in prevalence at age 50.
- PDE5 inhibitors have not been suggested to directly contribute to the development of PD; rather, their associated use in those with medical conditions that contribute to ED likely unmasks deformities that would have otherwise gone unrecognized.
- The prevalence of PD among diabetics has been shown to be 8.1% to 20.3% depending on the population screened, which is higher than in the general population. This may reflect particular patient populations, ethnic groups, referral patterns, and expertise of the physicians treating the disorder.
- The prevalence of ED in men with PD has been reported to be 37% to 58%.
- PD is not only a physically deforming but also a psychologically devastating disorder, with 48% of patients showing signs of moderate to severe depression; in general, these rates increase with the duration of PD. Penile shortening and inability to have intercourse are the two most common and consistent risk factors for emotional and relationship problems associated with PD.
- There appears to be an increased incidence of PD in men who have undergone radical prostatectomy, although further prospective studies are required to confirm this association.
- Although hypogonadism may be associated with PD, there is no clear evidence that it is a risk factor. Further study is indicated, and assessment of serum testosterone is recommended.

BOX 31-2   Associated Conditions

Aging
Diabetes
Erectile dysfunction
Psychological distress
Radical prostatectomy
Hypogonadism
Collagen disorders

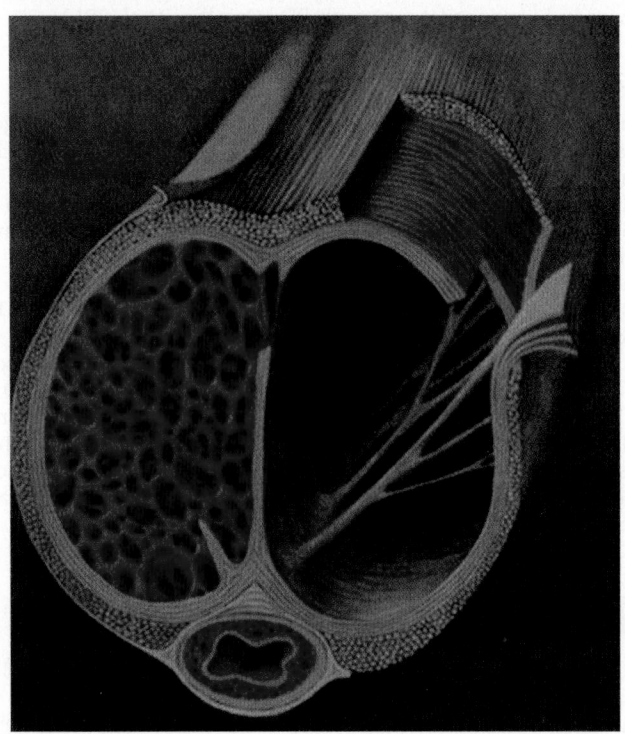

Figure 31-2. The outer layer bundles, which are coarser and directed in a longitudinal manner, often form an incomplete layer (regions 4 to 5 o'clock, 7 to 8 o'clock, and 11 to 1 o'clock) and condense to form ligament-like structures. Artist's drawing of penis depicts dorsal and ventral thickening and pillars. (Data from Brock G, Hsu GL, Nunes L, et al. The anatomy of the tunica albuginea in the normal penis and Peyronie's disease. J Urol 1997;157:276–81.)

PENILE ANATOMY AND PEYRONIE DISEASE

The exact cause of PD remains to be determined. Ongoing studies continue to clarify this disorder on the genetic, molecular, and anatomic level. The corpora cavernosa, the erectile bodies of the penis, surrounded by the tunica albuginea possess the ability to become rigid by becoming engorged with blood. **The tunica albuginea is a multilayered structure predominantly composed of type 1 collagen that is oriented with an inner circular and outer longitudinal layer interlaced with elastin fibers separated by an incomplete septum** (Gentile et al, 1996; Brock et al, 1997; Kelly, 2007). This septum is anchored into the inner circular layer and is key to the structural integrity of the tunica; without it, computer models have demonstrated that the stress generated by a full erection of one contiguous corporeal body would be sufficient to rupture the tunica albuginea (Mohamed et al, 2010). **These anchor sites are susceptible to microvascular trauma and tunical delamination, which may be one of the triggers leading to this disease** (Devine et al, 1997). The structure is further reinforced by intracavernous pillars, which anchor the tunica albuginea across the corpora cavernosa at the 2 to 6 o'clock and 10 to 6 o'clock positions, with finer pillars at the 5 and 7 o'clock positions (Fig. 31-2) (Brock et al, 1997). **It is**

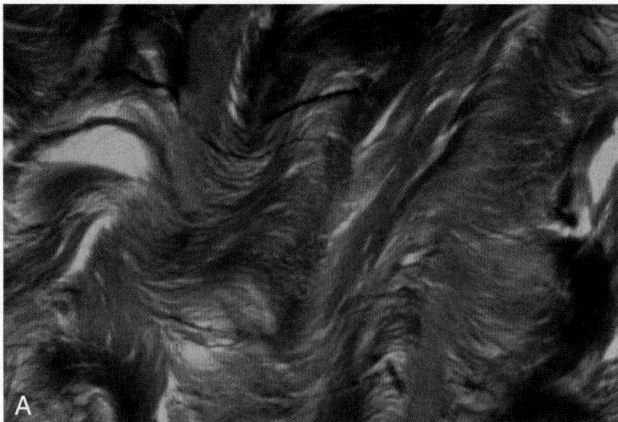

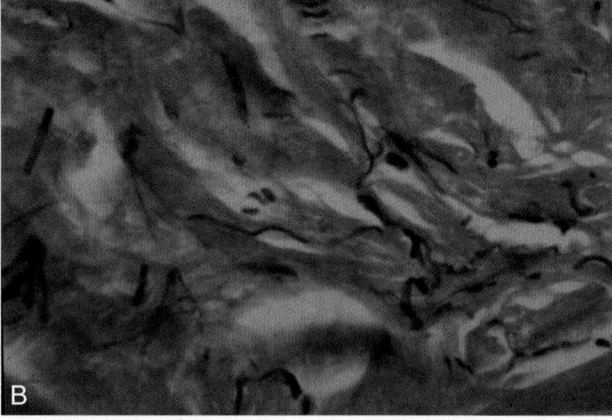

Figure 31-3. Photomicrographs of the tunica albuginea. A, Normal tunica albuginea demonstrating the polarized arrangement of collagen. **B,** Peyronie plaque demonstrating the nonpolarized arrangement of collagen and the haphazard arrangement of elastin. Collagen stains green; elastin stains black.

interesting to note that 60% to 70% of plaques are located on the dorsal aspect of the penis and are usually associated with the septum (Pryor and Ralph, 2002). It is possible that pressures on the penis during intercourse may cause a delamination between the two layers, activating the abnormal wound-healing process, which is trapped within the tunic, fostering the progressive scarring.

The longitudinal layer of the tunica albuginea is thinnest at the 3 and 9 o'clock positions of the corpora; it is completely absent between the 5 and 7 o'clock positions (Brock et al, 1997). This may contribute to greater ease of dorsal buckling and may explain why most PD patients exhibit dorsal curvature (Devine and Horton, 1988; Border and Ruoslahti, 1992; Brock et al, 1997; Devine et al, 1997; Jarow and Lowe, 1997). In normal tunical tissue, each layer appears to be distinct and is able to slide on the adjacent layer. The normal three-dimensional structure of the tunica affords great flexibility, rigidity, and tissue strength to the penis despite the fact that the tunica albuginea is quite thin—1.5 to 3.0 mm, depending on the position around the circumference. **Normal architecture is essentially lost consequent to this disease, resulting in what is known as a Peyronie "plaque," which when examined histologically demonstrates disorganization of collagen fibrils as well as a decrease in and disorganization of elastin resulting in penile deformity caused by asymmetrical expansion of the corpora** (Figs. 31-3 and 31-4) (Akkus et al, 1997; Brock et al, 1997; Devine et al, 1997; Costa et al, 2009). When expansion is limited at one point along the circumference of the corpora by the inelastic scar of the Peyronie plaque, deviation to that side occurs; a circumferential plaque may lead to an hourglass deformity (Akkus et al, 1997; Devine et al, 1997).

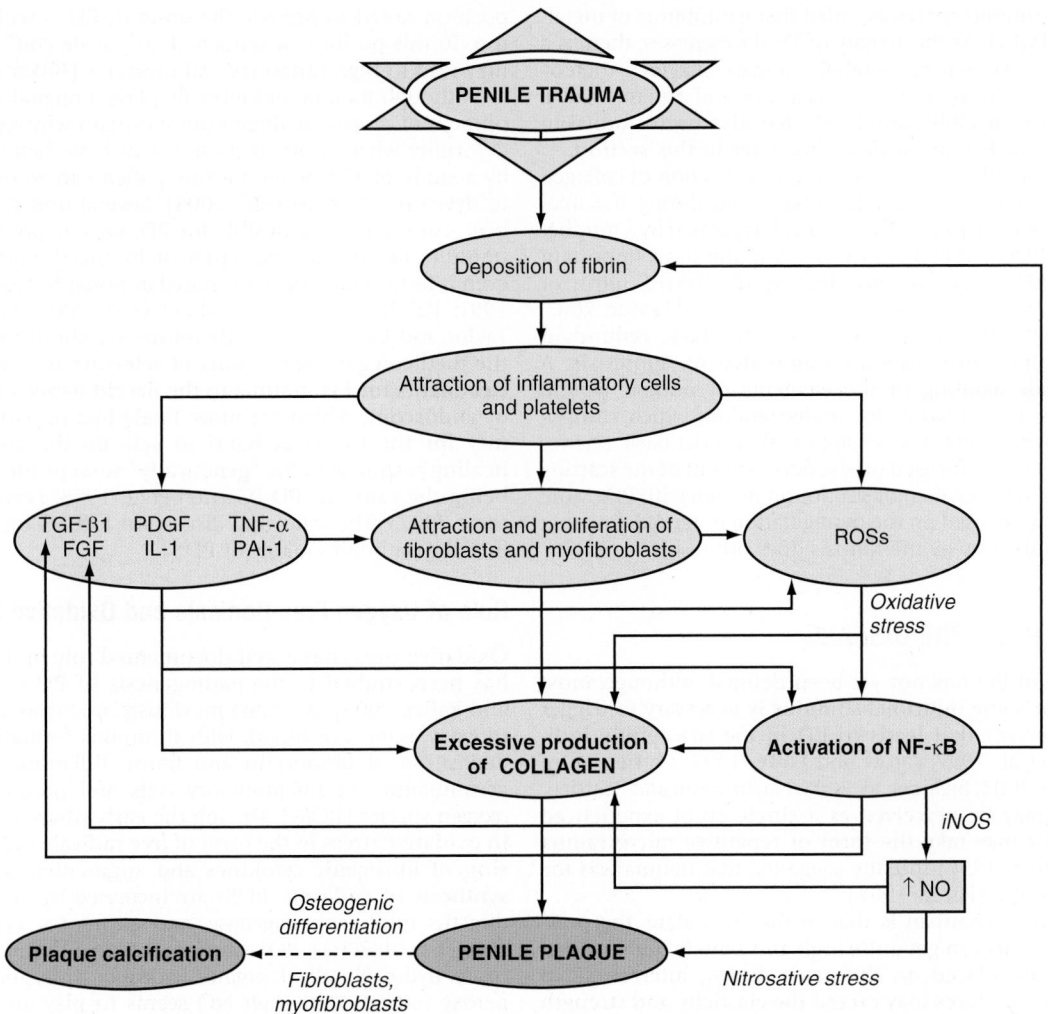

Figure 31-4. Pathogenetic mechanisms of Peyronie disease. FGF, fibroblast growth factor; IL-1, interleukin-1; iNOS, inducible nitric oxide synthase; NF-κB, nuclear factor-κB; NO, nitric oxide; PAI, plasminogen activator inhibitor; PDGF, platelet-derived growth factor; ROS, reactive oxygen species; TGF, transforming growth factor; TNF, tumor necrosis factor. (Data from Paulis G, Brancato T. Inflammatory mechanisms and oxidative stress in Peyronie's disease: therapeutic "rationale" and related emerging treatment strategies. Inflamm Allergy Drug Targets 2012;11:48–57.)

Impact of Wound Healing on the Development of Peyronie Disease

In general, PD has been described as a wound-healing disorder of the tunica albuginea. Recent investigations have focused on the mechanisms of wound healing, fibrosis, and scar formation and have correlated the findings with the PD population. Normal wound healing involves three phases: an acute phase, a proliferative phase, and a remodeling phase. These are not to be confused with the acute and chronic phases of PD previously described. By understanding the wound-healing process, one gains a better understanding of PD, targets for drugs used to treat PD, and the animal models that have been developed for the study of PD. In general, during the **acute phase,** blood vessel injury leads to extravasation of blood and aggregation and activation of platelets that release chemotactic agents that act as promoters in the wound-healing cascade by activating and attracting neutrophils during the first 24 hours after clot formation, macrophages after 48 hours, and finally lymphocytes after 72 hours (DiPietro, 1995). Macrophages phagocytose dead or potentially injurious material and destroy bacteria or other foreign cells via oxygen free radical reactions. In addition, macrophages activate keratinocytes, fibroblasts, and endothelial cells by releasing potent tissue growth factors, particularly transforming growth

factor-β (TGF-β), as well as other mediators such as TGF-α, heparin binding epidermal growth factor, fibroblast growth factor (FGF), and collagenase (DiPietro, 1995; Ravanti and Kahari, 2000).

The next phase of normal wound healing is the **proliferative phase,** which marks the shift toward tissue repair beginning at approximately 72 hours after injury and persisting for approximately 2 weeks. It is characterized by fibroblast and myofibroblast migration in response to TGF-β and platelet-derived growth factor (PDGF), as well as deposition of newly synthesized extracellular matrix (ECM) composed of type I and type III collagen, hyaluronan, fibronectin, and proteoglycans (Velnar et al, 2009). At this point, fibroblasts are stimulated by TGF-β to change into myofibroblasts, which contain thick actin bundles allowing for wound contraction. TGF-β also signals fibroblasts and myofibroblasts to synthesize types I and III collagen (Tomasek et al, 2002; Gelbard, 2008).

Finally, the **remodeling phase** begins and in the normal situation may last up to 1 or 2 years. The remodeling of an acute wound is tightly regulated by mechanisms that balance the simultaneous degradation and synthesis of collagen as well as other ECM macromolecules. Any alterations in this process may lead to abnormal wound healing with excessive scarring (Velnar et al, 2009). Matrix metalloproteinases (MMPs) (collagenases), produced by neutrophils, macrophages, and fibroblasts in the wound, are responsible for the degradation of collagen. They are subsequently held in check by inhibitory factors called tissue inhibitors of metalloproteinases (TIMPs). As the activity of TIMPs increases, there is a drop in matrix breakdown by metalloproteinase enzymes, thereby promoting new matrix accumulation (Ravanti and Kahari, 2000). **This balance between TIMPs and MMPs has also been studied in the pathogenesis of PD and is described later in this section.**

Over time the highly disorganized initial deposition of collagen matrix becomes more oriented and cross-linked during the final stages of the remodeling phase. The process is regulated by a number of factors, with PDGF, TGF-β, and FGF being the most important (Velnar et al, 2009), but also including MMPs, TIMPs, fibrin or plasminogen activator inhibitor-1 (PAI-1) (Taylor and Levine, 2007; Velnar et al, 2009). **Having accomplished this task, redundant fibroblasts and myofibroblasts are eliminated by apoptosis.** A fundamental understanding of the elements of normal wound healing provides a foundation for understanding which components may go awry in PD. It does appear that most basic science research in this field has focused on the development of the scarring process resulting in the exuberant scar found in men with PD. More recent research has focused on the dysregulation of remodeling that may be responsible for why the fibrosis does not resolve.

ETIOLOGY OF PEYRONIE DISEASE

The exact cause of PD has not yet been defined, although most would agree that some injurious stimulus is necessary to trigger the cascade of events that leads to PD in the susceptible individual (Devine et al, 1997; Jarow and Lowe, 1997; Carrieri et al, 1998; Jalkut et al, 2003; Bjekic et al, 2006; Nachtsheim and Rearden, 1996). **Trauma may be perceived as a single event experienced by the patient or may take the form of repetitive microtrauma to the penis.** Furey (1957) initially suggested that trauma was the primary cause of PD (Furey, 1957).

The proposed mechanism is that in the erect state, the pressures inside the penis can get quite high and acutely higher when external forces are placed on the penis during intercourse in particular. These pressures may exceed the elasticity and strength of the tunica tissues, resulting in a microfracture. A commonly held misconception is that the trauma to the penis must occur only when it is erect; however, in our experience we have noted that trauma to the flaccid penis may also trigger this process. In a recent review of our database of 228 patients who had recognized trauma to the penis shortly before the onset of PD, 16% reported a traumatic event to the flaccid penis (e.g., motor vehicle accident, sports-related injury). As the scar develops, there may also be an inflammatory response, resulting in the pain that can be present in the flaccid penis or when pressure is placed on the penis. Dorsal and ventral sheer stresses occurring during sexual activity may account for the more common dorsal location of plaques (Devine et al, 1997). Investigators have suggested that repetitive microtrauma to the penis leads to delamination of the tunica albuginea and vessels between the layers of the tunica (Somers and Dawson, 1997). This leads to microhemorrhage and initiates the woundhealing cascade described previously.

Carrieri and associates (1998) reported a 16-fold increase in PD in those who had undergone prior invasive procedures as well as a nearly 3-fold increase in PD in patients who had experienced genital and/or perineal trauma (Carrieri et al, 1998). It is also important to note that although trauma has been considered the most likely trigger activating PD, in our clinical experience no more than 30% of men recall a specific event involving injury to the penis close to the time when the scarring or pain began. Other investigators have reported 16% to 40% of patients having had antecedent trauma (Bjekic et al, 2006; Tal et al, 2012). An injury occurring during sexual activity appears to be the most common recognized event associated with the onset of PD. An association with trauma and position of intercourse has been proposed for some time, based on the assumption that certain positions may be more apt to cause injury. This has not been verified but it does appear from anecdotal experience that the most common sexual position noted to precede the onset of PD is with the partner on top. In this position, a sudden "faux pas de coit" or missed thrust may lead to high intracorporeal pressures (Bitker et al, 1988).

Although trauma undoubtedly plays a pivotal role in the development of disease, it alone cannot explain why some men develop deformity whereas others do not. This is no better illustrated than by a study of 193 penile fracture patients in whom none went on to develop PD (Zargooshi, 2004). Several underlying factors have been considered responsible for PD; genetic predisposition, autoimmune factors, an aberration of localized wound healing, and even infection have been proposed as possible causes (Devine et al, 1991; Ralph et al, 1996; Mulhall et al, 2002; Jalkut et al, 2003; Taylor and Levine, 2007). **Therefore, we should be careful about the medicolegal implications of referring to PD as the result of treatments for ED, trauma to the flaccid penis, or catheterization or endoscopy, which are more likely just providing an opportunity for the forces at hand to activate the abnormal woundhealing response in the "genetically" susceptible man rather than being the cause of PD** (Carrieri et al, 1998; Levine and Latchamsetty, 2002). The following discussion focuses on specific research into the pathophysiology of PD.

Role of Oxygen Free Radicals and Oxidative Stress

Oxidative stress has a well-documented role in tissue fibrosis and has been studied in the pathogenesis of PD (Gonzalez-Cadavid and Rajfer, 2005). As stated previously, microvascular trauma leads to extravasation of blood, with thrombus formation that leads to deposition of fibronectin and fibrin. Inflammation ensues with accumulation of inflammatory cells and production of reactive oxygen species (ROSs). **During the early phase of PD an increase in oxidative stress in the form of free radicals induces overexpression of fibrogenic cytokines and augmented transcription and synthesis of collagen.** ROSs are increased by TGF-β1, which also directly inhibits collagenase and promotes collagen synthesis (Magee et al, 2002). ROSs include superoxide anion, hydrogen peroxide, hydroxyl radical, organic hydroperoxide, alkoxy radicals, and peroxy radicals. Although NO seems to play an antifibrotic role, nitrosative stress as well as oxidative stress can lead to macromolecular damage, cytotoxic effects, lipid peroxidation, DNA fragmentation, collagen accumulation, and cellular dysfunction (Paulis and Brancato, 2012).

Role of Nitric Oxide in Peyronie Disease

NO is a small reactive free radical that acts as both an intracellular and an extracellular regulatory molecule. Wound cells, including monocytes, macrophages, and fibroblasts, have been shown to synthesize NO through a nuclear factor-κB (NF-κB)–activated inducible NO synthase (iNOS)–dependent mechanism after injury. The iNOS isoform produces NO; it is usually considered a defense mechanism against infection or cancer, is associated with inflammation, and is significantly increased in human and animal PD plaques (Gonzalez-Cadavid, 2009). NO synthesized by iNOS reacts with ROSs, thus reducing ROS levels and presumably inhibiting fibrosis. **The antifibrotic effects of NO may be mediated at least in part by the reduction of myofibroblast abundance and may lead to a reduction in collagen I synthesis** (Vernet et al, 2005). **NO may also play an antifibrotic role by activating guanylyl cyclase, thus producing cyclic guanosine monophosphate (cGMP), which has been suggested to inhibit plaque formation** (Ferrini et al, 2002; Valente et al, 2003).

Role of Myofibroblasts in Peyronie Disease

The excessive deposition of collagen and ECM accompanied by the loss of functional cells that characterizes tissue fibrosis is caused in some cases by the appearance and accumulation of myofibroblasts (Gonzalez-Cadavid, 2009). Twenty percent of cells cultured from PD tunica albuginea are in fact myofibroblasts, suggesting that they may be one of the primary factors leading to fibrosis in PD (Mulhall et al, 2002). Proposed mechanisms for the presence and persistence of myofibroblasts include a decrease in myofibroblast apoptosis, as well as stimulation of fibroblast transformation to myofibroblasts by TGF-β and mechanical stress, which has been associated with hypertrophic scarring (Darby and Hewitson, 2007; Gelbard, 2008). **Myofibroblast activation is a key event in the development of fibrosis. Trauma to the tunica albuginea secondary to microscopic delamination increases the adherence of fibroblasts to their surroundings, exposing them to changes in ECM tension, and in the presence of appropriate cytokines initiates their differentiation into myofibroblasts** (Gelbard, 2008). When tension diminishes, myofibroblasts tend to undergo apoptosis. Gelbard postulated that if myofibroblasts are continuously exposed to tension in the form of rigid corpora during erections, they may fail to undergo apoptosis and subsequently contribute to what appears to be a hallmark of PD—inappropriate and persistent stimulation of the wound-healing process (Gelbard, 2008).

Role of Transforming Growth Factor-β1 in the Etiology of Peyronie Disease

TGF-β1 has been shown to be significantly associated with PD (El-Sakka et al, 1997). **TGF-β is a strong activator of myofibroblasts and is known to be a potent fibrotic growth factor by stimulating the deposition of ECM.** TGF-β binds cell surface receptors and through a signal transduction cascade leads to the deposition and remodeling of ECM by stimulating cells to simultaneously **(1) increase the synthesis of most matrix proteins** (Ihn, 2002); **(2) decrease production of matrix-degrading proteases while increasing the production of inhibitors of these proteases** (Knittel et al, 1999); **and (3) modulate the expression of integrins** (Margadant and Sonnenberg, 2010). The action of TGF-β in tissue repair has been shown to involve an initiation of complex sequences of monocyte chemoattraction, induction of angiogenesis, and control of the production of cytokines and other inflammatory mediators (Border and Ruoslahti, 1992). Moreover, TGF-β stimulates the synthesis of individual matrix components including fibronectin, tenascin, collagens, and proteoglycans, while simultaneously blocking matrix degradation by decreasing the synthesis of proteases and increasing levels of protease inhibitors (Balza et al, 1988). All these events can be beneficial in tissue repair; however, the deposition of ECM at a site of tissue injury can lead to scarring and fibrosis. Furthermore, **the ability of TGF-β to induce its own production may be the key to the development of scarring and fibrosis** (Border and Ruoslahti, 1992). TGF-β1 is not the only member of the large TGF-β superfamily of growth and differentiation factors (GDFs) that have been implicated as fibrotic agents. Myostatin, also known as GDF-8, has been proposed not only as an inhibitor of myofiber formation but also as an inducer of fibrosis. Myostatin is expressed in the normal human tunica albuginea (TA) and overexpressed in PD plaque. Myostatin stimulates myofibroblast generation and collagen deposition in normal tunic and is upregulated by TGF-β1. Myostatin seems to potentiate the effects of TGF-β1 (Cantini et al, 2008).

Fibrotic Gene Expression in Peyronie Disease

A variety of profibrotic and antifibrotic factors contribute to the development of PD plaque that leads to deformity (Grazziotin et al, 2004). Qian and colleagues performed DNA microarray analysis of PD tissue obtained from patients undergoing surgery for PD. The most highly upregulated gene found in the PD plaque, *PTN* or *OSF1*, codes for a secreted heparin-binding protein thought to stimulate mitogenic growth of fibroblasts and osteoblast recruitment, and is possibly related to plaque ossification. Proteins responsible for cell proliferation, cell cycling, and apoptosis were found to be increased, whereas Id-2, an inhibitor of myofibroblast differentiation, was downregulated. The second most upregulated gene, *MCP-1*, is critical to the inflammatory response and ossification (Graves, 1999; Graves et al, 1999). Genes related to myogenic

conversion during wound healing and fibroblast differentiation into myofibroblasts were upregulated, whereas collagenase IV, which is critical for collagen degradation and is decreased in fibrosis, was downregulated (Magee et al, 2002). Qian and associates (2004) performed a study comparing gene expression profiles of PD patients with those of DD patients. A series of 15 genes were upregulated and none were downregulated in the PD plaque versus the normal TA. Of the genes upregulated, the ones most prominently increased were MMPs involved in collagen breakdown, specifically *MMP-2* or *MMP-9* in one half of the PD plaques, in addition to genes involved in actin-cytoskeleton interactions required for fibroblasts and myofibroblasts to generate the contractile forces (Qian et al, 2004). According to the findings of another study, the lower expression of apoptotic genes may cause the persistence of collagen-producing cells that are upregulated, consequently resulting in plaque formation. Similar expression levels of apoptotic genes in both tunica albuginea and Peyronie plaques may be caused by the generalized physiopathologic alterations in the tunica albuginea that lead to plaque formation at a vulnerable region subjected to recurrent trauma (Zorba et al, 2012).

Del Carlo and colleagues (2008) investigated the role of MMPs and TIMPs in the pathogenesis of PD by using harvested plaque from patients who had PD. PD tissue samples were found to have diminished or absent levels of MMP-1, MMP-8, and MMP-13 compared with matched perilesional tunica and non-PD controls. PD fibroblasts were cultured with soluble MMPs and TIMPs after treatment with TGF-β or interleukin-1β (IL-1β). They found that IL-1β stimulation increased the production of MMP-1, MMP-2, MMP-8, MMP-9, MMP-10, and MMP-13 in PD fibroblasts, whereas TGF-β increased the production of only MMP-10 and decreased the production of MMP-13, suggesting that PD fibroblasts can be induced to make MMPs (Del Carlo et al, 2008). Baseline aberrant expression of p53, a cell cycle–regulating protein, has been demonstrated in PD fibroblasts as well as an absent response to sublethal DNA damage. This suggests a role for an aberration in the p53 pathway in the pathogenesis of this condition (Mulhall et al, 2001a).

When all this information is taken together, it is not hard to understand why there are myriad clinical presentations and treatments for this very complex disease. A variety of alterations may be present in a given patient, which may manifest as fibrosis with penile deformity (see Box 31-2). This has been demonstrated by Qian and colleagues, who found **marked heterogeneity in gene expression profiles among men with PD** (Qian et al, 2004). As suggested by the ensuing section on medical therapy, different medical treatments that target different disease mechanisms may not work uniformly among the PD population (see Fig. 31-4).

KEY POINTS: ANATOMY AND ETIOLOGY

- The longitudinal layer of the tunica albuginea is thinnest at the 3 and 9 o'clock positions of the corpora; it is completely absent between the 5 and 7 o'clock positions. This absence of the longitudinal layer ventrally may contribute to greater ease of dorsal buckling and may explain why most PD patients exhibit dorsal curvature.
- Normal architecture is essentially lost consequent to this disease, resulting in what is known as a Peyronie plaque, which when examined histologically demonstrates disorganization of collagen fibrils as well as a decrease and disorganization of elastin, resulting in penile deformity caused by asymmetric expansion of the corpora.
- Antecedent trauma has been reported in 16% to 40%; most would agree that some injurious stimulus is necessary to trigger a cascade of events that lead to PD in the susceptible individual.
- Oxygen free radicals, oxidative stress, NO, myofibroblasts, TGF-β1, and fibrotic gene expression all play a key role in the development of PD and are key avenues for future research to further elucidate the exact mechanism behind the development of PD.

SYMPTOMS

The most frequent presenting symptoms of patients with PD include penile pain, erect deformity, and palpable plaque, as well as ED (Pryor and Ralph, 2002; Smith et al, 2008b; Chung et al, 2011a). Many men who have PD visit the doctor with a self-misdiagnosis of ED. Not all patients experience pain or are able to palpate a plaque, but the shortening, hinge effect, distal softening, and curvature, when present, are readily recognized. Pain, when present in the acute phase, can occur in the flaccid condition with palpation of the plaque, with erection, or during intercourse. Once the disease process is stable, most pain will resolve, but in some men the pain persists with what has been referred to as "torque" pain associated with a pulling sensation on the plaque when a strong erection occurs (Levine and Larsen, 2013). This should not be confused with the inflammatory pain of the acute phase.

Although curvature can be one of the most recognized and distressing deformities associated with PD, many men are capable of sexual activity with curvature up to 60 degrees, particularly if the curvature is dorsal and more gradual along the shaft. Men with ventral or lateral curvatures may have a more difficult time with intromission because of discomfort. Yet, it is not uncommon to hear that the partner does not complain of discomfort during coitus, regardless of the degree or direction of curvature. Patient estimates of curvature are unreliable. One study demonstrated that 50% of patients overestimated their degree of curvature by an average of 20 degrees (Bacal et al, 2009). Classification by degree of curvature was introduced by Kelami (1983). One center reported on the distribution of curvature by the Kelami classification and found that 39.5% of patients had 30 degrees (mild) or less, 35% had 31 to 60 degrees (moderate), and 13.5% had more than 60 degrees of curvature (severe); 12% had no curvature but did experience an hourglass deformity resulting in an unstable erection (Kadioglu et al, 2011b).

The PD plaque can manifest in a variety of configurations including cords; simple nodules; coinlike, irregular dumbbell shapes; or I-beam plaques. It appears that virtually all plaques have a septal component, which supports the concept of delamination of tunical fibers as a result of axial forces on the septum (Jordan, 2007). Pure septal plaques have also been reported and may result in narrowing, shortening, or no recognized deformity at all (Bella et al, 2007).

The orientation of the plaque usually defines the deformity. Therefore patients with a simple dorsal plaque are most apt to have dorsal curvature; but if there is transverse or spiraling scarring, which can be partial or circumferential, this could result in varying degrees of indentation including an hourglass deformity, which can result in an unstable penis, or a hinge effect as a result of the inability to tolerate axial forces in the erect condition (Pryor and Ralph, 2002). The distal softening of the shaft beyond the plaque is also difficult to understand, because dynamic infusion cavernosometry and cavernosography (DICC) studies have found that the pressures within the corpora cavernosa are equal, when measured, proximal and distal to the plaque (Jordan and Angermeier, 1993). The cause of distal flaccidity remains speculative and includes local cavernosal fibrosis extending from the involved tunic (Ralph et al, 1992) and site-specific venous leak.

EVALUATION OF THE PATIENT

As with all medical conditions, a detailed history is a critical part of the evaluation of the man with PD (Levine and Greenfield, 2003). The intake interview should focus on presenting signs and symptoms such as pain, deformity, and palpable plaque. The assessment should also include whether onset was gradual or sudden and the estimated time that symptoms began; it should be determined whether there was any inciting event that may have triggered the process, including direct external penile trauma to the

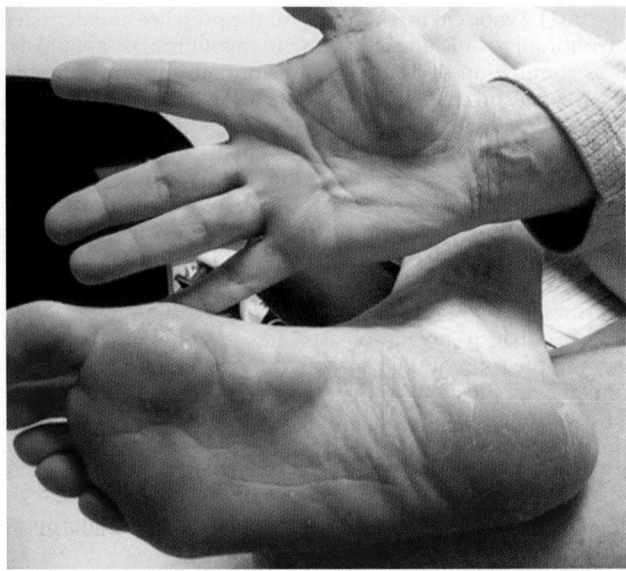

Figure 31-5. This patient had physical evidence of Dupuytren, Ledderhose, and Peyronie diseases.

flaccid or erect penis or instrumentation. The patient should be asked whether there is any personal or family history of other fibrotic disorders including DD and Ledderhose disease (Fig. 31-5). **Patients should be carefully queried as to their erectile capacity, but ultimately the question is whether the patient is capable of intromission or incapable because of deformity and/or diminished rigidity. A useful question that has been shown to be an effective predictor of postoperative erectile function is "If your penis was straight with the same quality of rigidity that you have now, do you think it would be adequate for penetrative sexual activity?"** (Levine and Greenfield, 2003; Taylor et al, 2012). Clearly if the patient does not feel his erections would be satisfactory with or without pharmacotherapy, this can help direct the patient to treatment with a penile prosthesis and straightening maneuvers; nonsurgical or other surgical approaches could result in improvement of deformity, but if there is persistent ED, such treatment would likely not give the patient a sexually functional erection.

Further information to be obtained from the sexual history will be whether there are any vascular risk factors for ED, including a history of diabetes, hypertension, elevated cholesterol, and smoking. This is also a useful time to determine if there are issues with premature or delayed ejaculation. A list of medications may also indicate underlying medical conditions that may predispose to ED.

The recently validated PD questionnaire (PDQ) (Rosen, 2008; Hellstrom et al, 2013) addresses not only the concerns of the patient regarding structural changes of the penis but also how PD affects his overall psychological condition. The current questionnaire has 15 questions assessing three domains, including (1) Peyronie psychological and physical symptoms (six items), (2) penile pain (three items), and (3) the effects of PD symptoms (six items). Each domain is intended to be an independent measure, and the scores are not summed for a total instrument score. Higher scores indicate a greater negative impact. With further experience, it may prove to be a useful assessment tool for patients making treatment decisions. The PDQ can be downloaded at www.auxilium.com/PDQ.

The value of a photograph taken at home of the erect penis has been controversial because of the inability to adequately represent and measure a three-dimensional deformity (Ohebshalom et al, 2007; Bacal et al, 2009). At the current time, with the prevalence of smartphones, a photograph can be taken by the patient from above and from the side in the erect state, which can be useful during the initial consultation to get a general impression of the direction and severity of the deformity.

The physical examination should include a general assessment of the femoral pulses, appearance of the flaccid penis, and whether it is circumcised. **To assess the Peyronie plaque, the penis should be examined on stretch, which allows easier identification of the plaque (Fig. 31-6). The location of the plaque may be useful to**

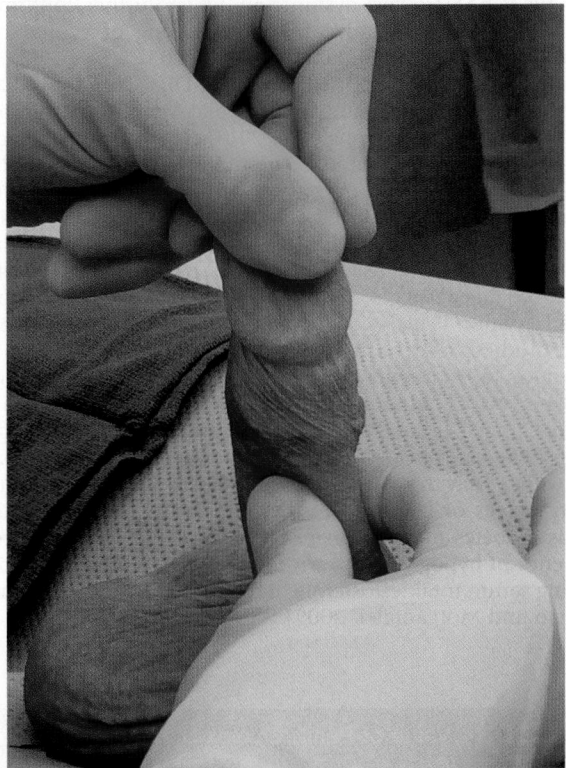

Figure 31-6. Palpation of penis on stretch facilitates identification of plaque.

record, but measurement of the size of the plaque with any modality has been found to be inaccurate because the plaque is rarely a discrete lesion (Bacal et al, 2009; Ralph et al, 2010; Hatzimouratidis et al, 2012; Levine and Burnett, 2013). It has irregular borders and often extends into a septal cord (Levine and Greenfield, 2003; Ralph et al, 2010). **Furthermore, there is no evidence that a reduction in plaque size as a result of treatment is at all associated with improvement of deformity** (Levine and Burnett, 2013). **The stretched penile length (SPL) is also a critical parameter to measure at the initial consultation. This is performed by placing the penis on stretch by grasping the glans and pulling at a 90-degree angle away from the body** (Wessells et al, 1996). It is our preference to measure from the pubis to the corona dorsally, as these are two fixed points and facilitate repeated measurement during the course of treatment and follow-up. The consistency of the plaque may be recorded. A "rock hard" plaque may be an indicator of calcification but will need to be confirmed with some form of imaging, preferably ultrasonography (Fig. 31-7). A calcified plaque is readily identified on ultrasonography because of the hyperdensity of the plaque with shadowing behind it. Computed tomography and magnetic resonance imaging have little value in the evaluation of the man with PD, but further investigation is ongoing to determine whether these modalities can provide prognostic information (Andresen et al, 1998; Hauck et al, 2003).

Only recently has it been recognized that calcification may occur early after the onset of the scarring process, and therefore the previously held notion that calcification is an indication of chronic, severe, and/or mature disease appears untrue (Levine et al, 2013). Calcification is most likely the result of a different genetic subtype of PD in which there is activation of genes involved in osteoblastic activity (Vernet et al, 2005). Why some plaques undergo mineralization and others do not remains unknown, but it does appear that the extent of mineralization may have a bearing on a successful response to nonsurgical therapy; men with more extensive calcification are less likely to benefit from nonsurgical treatment (Chung et al, 2011a). Several investigators have indicated that intralesional injection therapy with verapamil and interferon (IFN) is less likely to be successful in men with significant calcification (Levine et al, 2002; Hellstrom et al, 2006). This is because the drug will not be able to get into or effect change within this

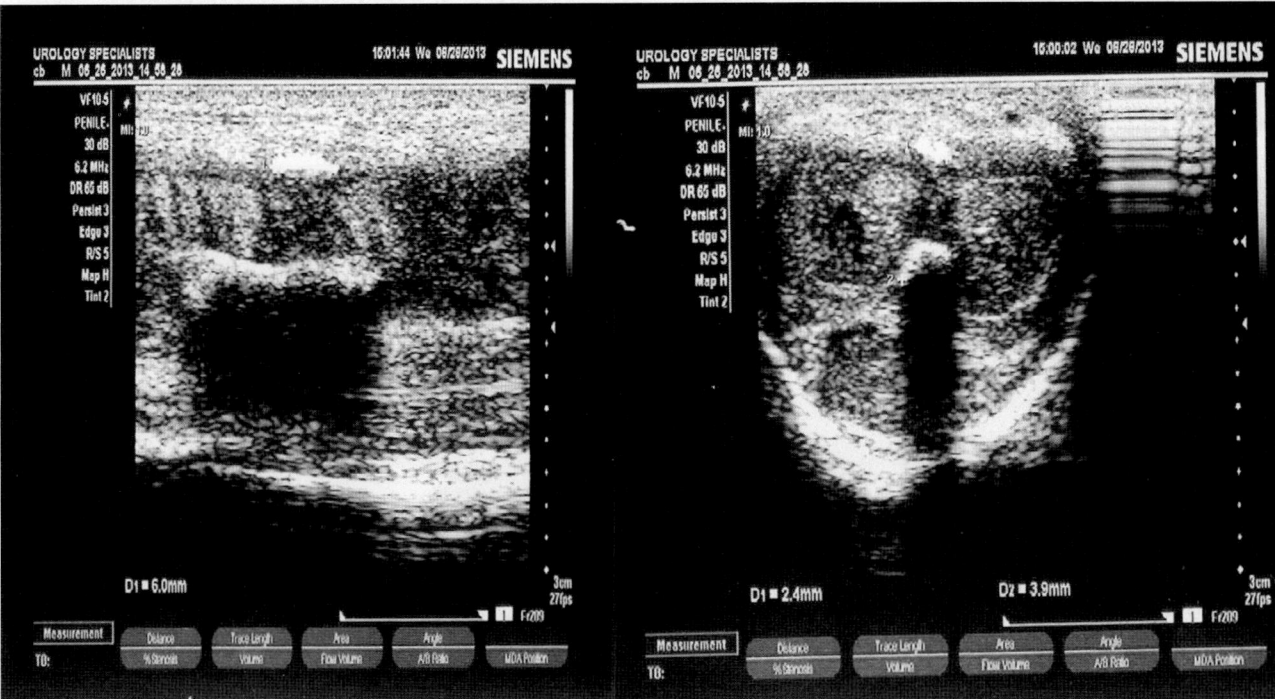

Figure 31-7. This ultrasound image demonstrates areas of dorsal and ventral calcification. Note shadowing behind calcified plaques.

mineralized tissue. Furthermore, investigators have also suggested that patients with extensive calcification are more apt to proceed to placement of a penile prosthesis (Breyer et al, 2007; Chung et al, 2012b). **Recently a calcification grading system was published. The investigators found that patients with grade 3, or the most extensive, calcification (>1.5 cm in any dimension or multiple plaques ≥1.0 cm) were more likely to undergo surgery when they also had satisfactory erectile function. This is in contradistinction to those who had less severe calcification of grade 1 (<0.3 mm) or grade 2 (0.3 to 1.5 cm) or no calcification in whom there was no evidence of an increased likelihood of proceeding to surgery** (Levine et al, 2013).

The role of vascular testing has not been clearly defined. In centers that see many men with this disorder, duplex ultrasound analysis is routinely performed as part of the initial evaluation, especially for those who are considered surgical candidates (Ralph et al, 2010; Hatzimouratidis et al, 2012; Levine and Burnett, 2013). Assessment of penile deformity in the erect state is critical to the evaluation. This has been shown to be most accurately measured after an office vasoactive injection as compared with a home photograph or vacuum-induced erection (Ohebshalom et al, 2007). **The benefits of a complete duplex ultrasound assessment include identification of calcification during initial surveillance in the flaccid state, assessment of penile vascular flow parameters after intracavernosal injection of vasoactive agent, observation of the erectile response to the vasoactive injection compared with the patient's sexually induced erection at home, and provision of the best opportunity to objectively assess deformity** (Figs. 31-8

and 31-9; Box 31-3). **These parameters are absolutely critical to the decision process for the patient who is considering surgery** (Fig. 31-10).

Several studies have demonstrated that preoperative erectile function correlates strongly with postoperative results (Jordan and Angermier, 1993; Levine and Greenfield, 2003; Taylor et al, 2012). In an analysis of the relationship of penile deformity to the vascular status of PD, patients with ventral curvature were most likely to have cavernous veno-occlusive dysfunction, which further confirms the concern about postoperative ED after grafting of ventral curves (Lowsley and Boyce, 1950; Kendirci et al, 2005).

Some authors have reported the use of DICC as a tool to assess penile vascular integrity and in particular venous leakage before surgery (Jordan, 2007; Alphs et al, 2010). This test appears to add unnecessary invasiveness and expense and provides little value to the diagnostic evaluation over a well-done dynamic penile duplex ultrasonography. Although no standard evaluation for assessment of penile sexual sensitivity has been established, light touch and biothesiometry can be used (Levine and Burnett, 2013). Biothesiometry has been suggested to be an indirect measure of penile sexual sensation. This is controversial because no definitive controlled studies have been reported (Padma-Nathan, 1988). The assumption is that the vibratory nerves travel with the unique sexual nerves of the penis. Therefore, vibratory appreciation with the index fingers used as the positive control and anterior thighs as the negative control can be a surrogate assessment of sexual sensation, which may be compromised by scar infiltration into the sensory nerves or because of other underlying systemic disorders such as diabetes mellitus. In response to the proposed increased prevalence of hypogonadism with PD, we recommend obtaining a morning serum total testosterone level during the initial evaluation (Moreno and Morgantaler, 2009).

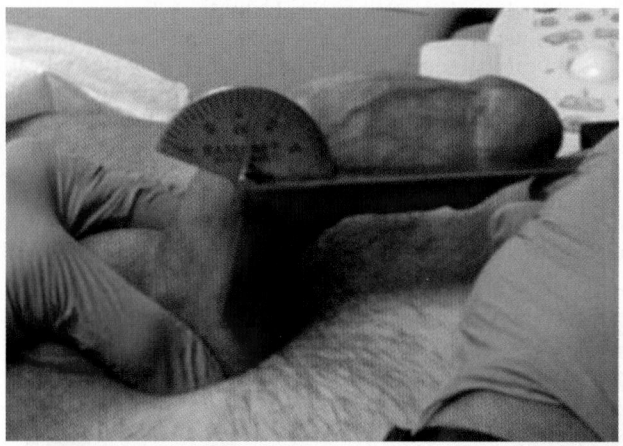

Figure 31-8. Measurement of curvature with goniometer.

> **BOX 31-3** Value of Penile Duplex Ultrasonography for Peyronie Disease
>
> - Identification and measurement of plaque calcification
> - Identification of corporeal fibrosis
> - Observation of erectile response to vasoactive intracavernosal injection
> - Measurement of penile vascular parameters (peak systolic velocity, end-diastolic velocity, and resistive index)
> - Optimum objective measurement of erect penile deformity (curvature, girth irregularities, hinge effect)

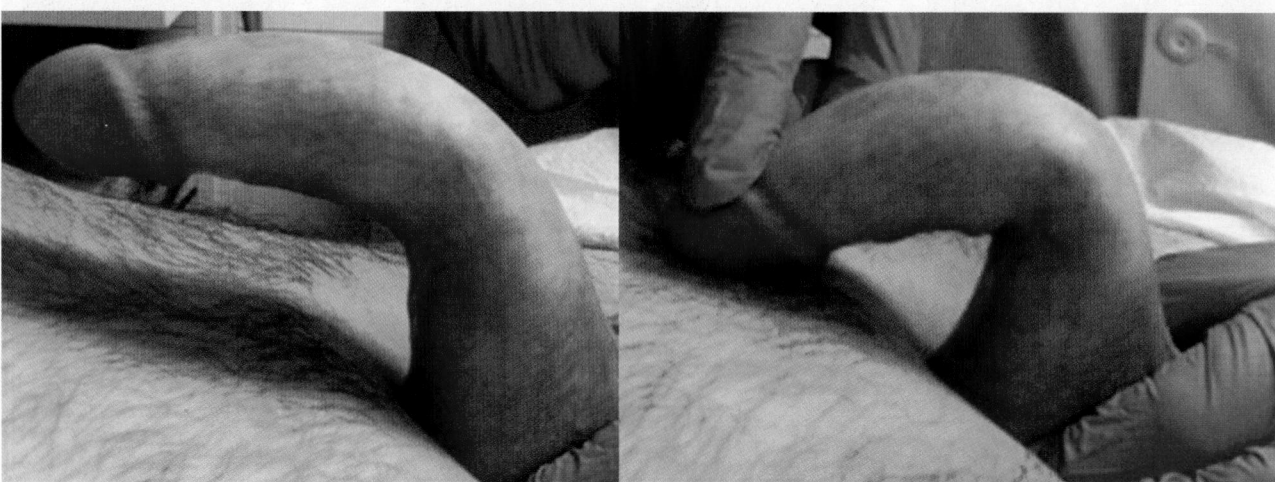

Figure 31-9. Instability or a hinge effect of the erect penis caused by indentation is demonstrated in this severely dorsally bent penis with application of axial pressure.

TREATMENT PROTOCOLS

Multiple treatment protocols have been developed and published. It should be recognized that these algorithms serve only as guidelines and that individualization is key to patient success, which depends on specific findings from the history, physical examination, duplex ultrasonography, and patient goals (Levine and Lenting, 1997; Levine and Greenfield, 2003; Bokarica et al, 2005; Ralph et al, 2010; Hatzimouratidis et al, 2012).

NONSURGICAL TREATMENT OF PEYRONIE DISEASE

Myriad nonsurgical treatments for PD have been offered since the time of de la Peyronie. Medical therapy until very recently has been compromised by suboptimal studies that failed to demonstrate meaningful results owing to small numbers of subjects, lack of a control group, lack of randomization, and limited objective measurements (Schaeffer and Burnett, 2012). **In addition, the variety of disease presentations and its poorly understood cause contribute to treatments that have not addressed the underlying pathophysiology of this wound-healing disorder.** In this section, we review the contemporary treatments and focus on placebo-controlled studies when possible.

Some patients require only reassurance, particularly if there is no difficulty or pain for the patient or his partner in accomplishing penetrative sex. Patients should also be reassured that this is not a disorder that will degenerate into a cancer and is therefore not life-threatening.

Oral Medications

Potaba

Potassium aminobenzoate (Potaba) is a member of the vitamin B complex. Its mechanism of action has not been studied since 1959, when Zarafonetis and Horrax **demonstrated in fibroblast cell cultures that potassium aminobenzoate can reduce the formation of collagen.** According to this in vitro study, it is believed that this drug decreases serotonin levels by increasing monoamine oxidase

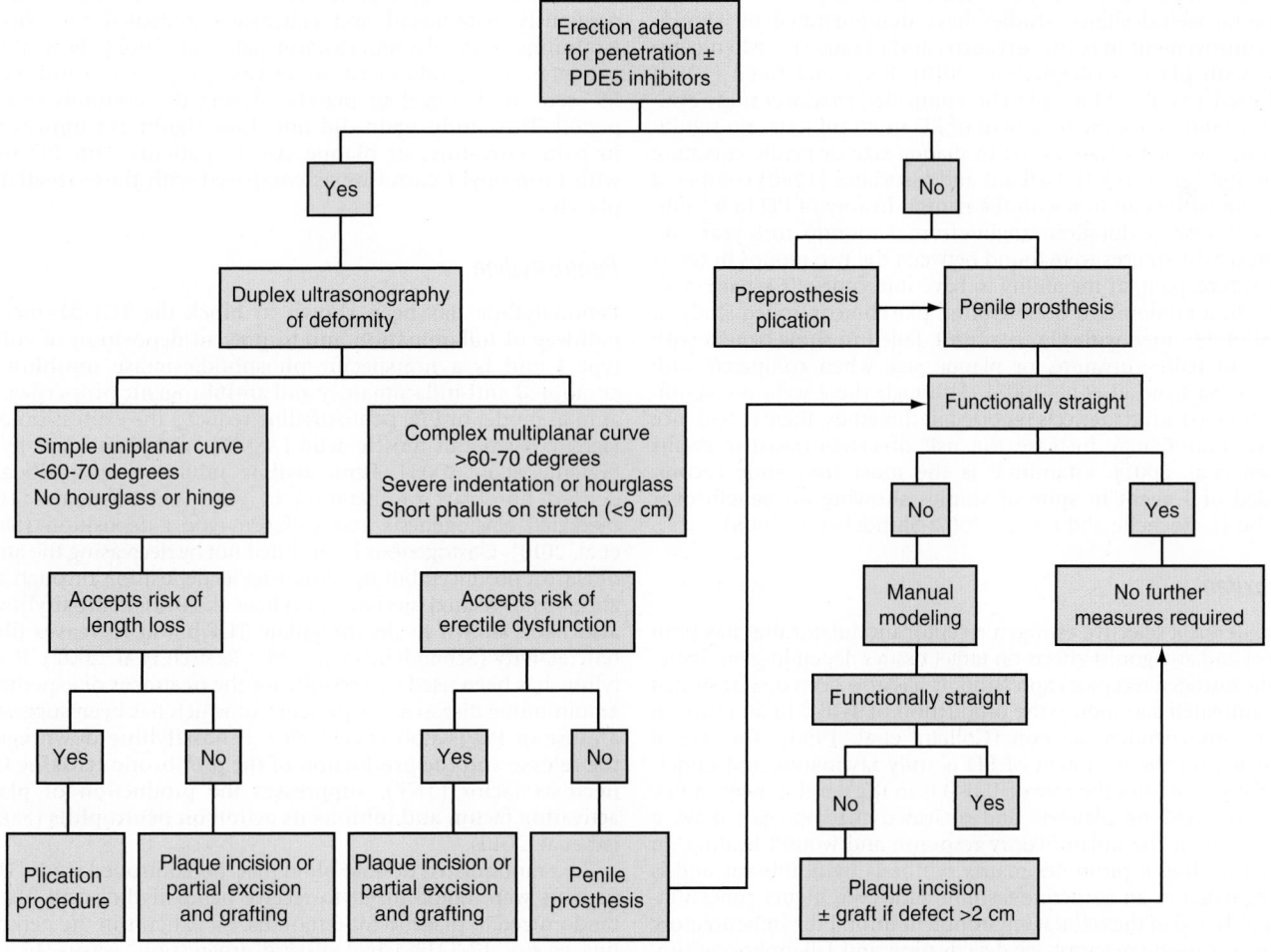

Figure 31-10. Algorithm for the surgical management of Peyronie disease. PDE5, phosphodiesterase type 5.

activity, resulting in enhancement of the endogenous antifibrotic properties of tissues (Zarafonetis and Horrax, 1959).

In a randomized double-blind placebo-controlled trial of 103 treatment-naive PD patients with noncalcified plaque, 51 patients were assigned to treatment with potassium *p*-aminobenzoate and 52 to placebo. Mean plaque size decreased in the treatment arm, whereas plaque size remained stable over 12 months of follow-up in the placebo arm. Penile deviation remained stable in those receiving active drug; penile curvature deteriorated significantly in 32.5% of those receiving placebo. No significant differences concerning decrease in pain could be observed between the two groups. The authors concluded, "Potassium paraaminobenzoate appears to be useful to stabilize the disorder and prevent progression of penile curvature" (Weidner et al, 2005). No severe adverse events occurred in the study; however, acute hepatitis associated with administration of potassium aminobenzoate for PD has been reported (Roy and Carrier, 2008). **Because there is little evidence of benefit with potassium amino benzoate in placebo-controlled trials and it is expensive and difficult to consume (24 tablets daily), we do not recommend its use.**

Vitamin E

Vitamin E is one of the oldest described oral treatments for the treatment of PD (Scardino and Scott, 1949). Vitamin E, a fat-soluble vitamin metabolized in the liver and excreted in bile, is an antioxidant that **is thought to limit oxidative stress of ROSs known to be increased during the acute and proliferative phases of wound healing.** Increased free-radical expression and a prolonged inflammatory phase of wound healing have been demonstrated in PD. **Treatment with vitamin E inactivates circulating free radicals that otherwise would inhibit NO from exerting its positive effects on vascular smooth muscle** (Safarinejad et al, 2007).

Several well-designed studies have demonstrated no significant improvement in pain, curvature, and plaque size when compared with placebo (Ralph et al, 2010). Pryor and Farell (1983) conducted a double-blind, placebo-controlled crossover study evaluating vitamin E for the treatment of PD in 40 subjects. No significant improvements were noted in plaque size or penile curvature (Pryor and Farell, 1983). Gelbard and associates (1990) compared treatment with vitamin E with the natural history of PD in 97 subjects with disease duration ranging from 3 months to 8 years; no significant differences were found between the two groups in terms of curvature, pain, or the ability to have intercourse (Gelbard et al, 1990). In a randomized double-blind placebo-controlled study of a total of 236 men with PD, vitamin E failed to show benefit with respect to pain, curvature, or plaque size when compared with placebo (Safarinejad et al, 2007). Although there were no significant observed adverse effects reported in this study, there is evidence that vitamin E may increase the risk of cerebrovascular events (Brown et al, 2001). **Vitamin E is the most frequently recommended oral agent in spite of studies showing no benefit over placebo** (LaRochelle and Levine, 2007; Shindel et al, 2008).

Tamoxifen

Tamoxifen is a selective estrogen receptor modulator that has both agonist and antagonist effects on target tissues depending on tissue-specific estrogen receptor expression. It has also been demonstrated that tamoxifen can induce the production of TGF-β in an estrogen receptor–independent fashion (Colletta et al, 1990). The use of tamoxifen for the treatment of PD is truly fascinating and underscores how complex the role of TGF-β is in the development of PD. TGF-β released by platelets and activated macrophages plays a central role in the inflammatory response and wound healing. In normal healing it promotes matrix synthesis by fibroblasts and is self-regulated in an autocrine fashion. However, higher concentrations of TGF-β in the cellular environment inhibit the inflammatory response, causing macrophage deactivation and T-lymphocyte suppression, thus preventing further fibrogenesis (Wahl et al, 1989). This was the initial reasoning for Ralph and associates (1992) to

report in a nonrandomized study on the initial use of tamoxifen for the treatment of PD (Ralph et al, 1992).

The initial beneficial effects previously reported were not confirmed in a randomized placebo-controlled trial of 25 patients with PD (Teloken et al, 1999). **The study demonstrated no significant improvement with respect to pain, penile deformity, or plaque size when compared with placebo** (Teloken et al, 1999).

Colchicine

Colchicine has been demonstrated to have several different potential mechanisms of action in the treatment of PD. **By binding to tubulin and causing it to depolymerize, colchicine inhibits cell mitosis, mobility, and adhesion of leukocytes; inhibits transcellular movement of collagen; and stimulates the production of collagenase** (Taylor, 1965; Ehrlich and Bornstein, 1972; El-Sakka et al, 1999).

In a randomized double-blind placebo-controlled study to determine the effectiveness and safety of colchicine, 84 PD patients with noncalcified plaque were randomized to colchicine or placebo. Objective measurements did not demonstrate any difference in plaque size or penile curvature. **There were no substantial differences in response to treatment based on duration of disease or within the three Kelami classification groups** (Kelami, 1983). **Significant drug-related adverse effects in the colchicine group included gastrointestinal upset with diarrhea** (Safarinejad, 2004).

Carnitine

Carnitine is a trimethylamine molecule that plays a unique role in cell energy metabolism (Reda et al, 2003). **L-Carnitine is hypothesized to act by increasing mitochondrial respiration and decreasing free radical formation** (Bremer, 1983).

In the same double-blind placebo-controlled study mentioned previously, Safarinejad and colleagues compared the effects of L-carnitine with placebo (Safarinejad et al, 2007). Fifty-nine PD patients were randomized to receive propionyl-L-carnitine and 59 were randomized to placebo during the 6-month treatment period. **This study again did not show significant improvement in pain, curvature, or plaque size in patients with PD treated with propionyl-L-carnitine as compared with those treated with placebo.**

Pentoxifylline

Pentoxifylline has been shown to block the TGF-β1–mediated pathway of inflammation and to prevent deposition of collagen type I and is a nonspecific phosphodiesterase inhibitor with combined anti-inflammatory and antifibrogenic properties. In an animal model of PD, pentoxifylline reduced the expression of collagen I, α-smooth muscle actin (ASMA), and plaque size by 95% (Valente et al, 2003). Pentoxifylline inhibits tunica albuginea–derived fibroblast proliferation in vitro and attenuates TGF-β–mediated elastogenesis and collagen type I deposition (Shindel et al, 2010). Elastogenesis is inhibited not by decreasing the amount of elastin produced but by inhibiting its deposition through an α_1-antitrypsin–related mechanism (Lin et al, 2010). **Pentoxifylline has also been shown to downregulate TGF-β and increases fibrinolytic activity** (Schandené et al, 1992; Raetsch et al, 2002). Pentoxifylline has been used successfully for the treatment of experimental autoimmune diseases, the presence of which has been suggested as a cause of PD (Ralph et al, 1996). **Pentoxifylline downregulates the release and the production of the profibrotic cytokine tumor necrosis factor (TNF), suppresses the production of platelet-activating factor, and inhibits its action on neutrophils** (Safarinejad et al, 2010).

In a randomized double-blind placebo-controlled study, 114 PD patients were randomized to receive pentoxifylline and 114 were randomized to placebo for 6 months. Of patients in the pentoxifylline group, 12 (11%) had disease progression, versus 46 (42%) in the placebo group. **Improvement in penile curvature and plaque volume was significantly greater in patients treated with** pentoxifylline than with placebo. The increase in International Index of Erectile Function (IIEF) total score was significantly higher in the pentoxifylline group. One patient discontinued the medication because of adverse effects. There were no adverse effects in any of the vital signs or in the laboratory data. Pentoxifylline is a peripheral vasodilator and could induce hypotension; consequently, blood pressure should be monitored during treatment with this drug. The most common side effects include nausea, vomiting, dyspepsia, malaise, flushing, dizziness, and headache (Safarinejad et al, 2010).

Phosphodiesterase Type 5 Inhibitors

PDE5 inhibitors have been shown to be safe and effective in treating ED in patients with PD (Levine and Latchamsetty, 2002). Recently tadalafil was shown to significantly improve IIEF and quality-of-life (QoL) scores when used in conjunction with extracorporeal shock-wave therapy (ESWT) as compared with ESWT alone (Palmieri et al, 2012). There was no advantage with respect to deformity.

PDE5 inhibitors have also been suggested as treatment for PD. By increasing the levels of cGMP, PDE5 inhibitors can inhibit collagen synthesis and induce fibroblast and myofibroblast apoptosis, thus acting as antifibrotic agents by inhibiting scar development (Valente et al, 2003; Gonzalez-Cadavid and Rajfer, 2010).

In a study by Chung and associates (2001), 35 men with an isolated septal scar received tadalafil 2.5 mg daily over a 6-month period, after which 24 patients (69%) had resolution of the septal scar. The authors concluded that low-dose daily tadalafil is a safe and effective treatment option in septal scar remodeling (Chung et al, 2011a).

Intralesional Injection

Verapamil

Calcium channel blockers were originally found to inhibit the incorporation of proline into ECM protein, thus leading to the conclusions that cellular calcium metabolism appears to regulate ECM production and that hypertrophic disorders of wound healing may respond to therapy with calcium channel antagonist drugs (Lee and Ping, 1990).

Verapamil is a calcium channel blocker that has been shown to significantly affect fibroblast function on several levels, including cell proliferation, ECM protein synthesis and secretion, and collagen degradation. In vitro Peyronie plaque fibroblast proliferation is inhibited by 65% by verapamil at a concentration of 100 to 1000 mg/mL (Anderson et al, 2000). These changes may allow intralesional verapamil to retard, prevent, or possibly reverse plaque formation and progression of PD (Levine and Estrada, 2002). Recently a study demonstrated the mechanism of action of intralesional verapamil injection versus normal saline in a rat model. After verapamil injection there were histologic changes as well as reduced plaque size and penile curvature. Verapamil injection also resulted in decreased collagen and elastin fibers, as well as reduced ASMA, an indicator of myofibroblast activity (Chung et al, 2013b).

The first reported use of verapamil for the treatment of PD was by Levine and associates and was the first new intralesional treatment since steroid injection was introduced in 1957 (Furey, 1957; Levine et al, 1994). This was a nonrandomized dose-escalating study in 14 men who received biweekly injections of verapamil for 6 months. Subjectively, there was significant improvement in plaque-associated penile narrowing (100%) and curvature (42%). Objectively, a decreased plaque volume of more than 50% was noted in 30% of the subjects. Plaque softening was noted in all patients, and 83% noticed that plaque-related changes in erectile function had arrested or improved. There was no toxicity, nor did symptoms recur when improvement was noted. This preliminary study suggested that intralesional verapamil may be an economical and sensible nonoperative approach to the treatment of PD warranting further study (Levine et al, 1994). In a larger noncontrolled study, verapamil injection resulted in a reduction of pain in 97%

of the patients, an improvement in sexual function in 72%, a subjective reduction of deformity in 86%, an improvement in distal rigidity in 93%, and an objective reduction of curvature in 54% (mean curve reduction of 25 degrees) (Levine, 1997).

Rehman and associates (1998) performed a single-blind study on 14 PD patients who were randomly assigned to injection with verapamil or saline. This study demonstrated a significant improvement in plaque size, plaque-associated penile narrowing, and quality of erection in the verapamil-treated men versus the control group. There was no significant difference with respect to penile curvature. There was no local or systemic toxicity except for an occasional ecchymosis or bruise at the injection site (Rehman et al, 1998). Bennett and colleagues showed in a shorter 3-month trial of 94 patients improvement in curvature in 18%, no change in 60%, and worsening in 22% and concluded that intralesional verapamil can at a minimum stabilize penile deformity (Bennett et al, 2007).

Currently, intralesional verapamil is one of the leading treatment options for the conservative management of PD despite the fact that some studies have not shown as favorable a response as described earlier (Shindel et al, 2008). In a recent randomized single-blind placebo-controlled trial, Shirazi and associates (2009) randomized 80 patients to receive intralesional verapamil and 40 patients to receive local saline injection. This study demonstrated no significant difference with respect to plaque size, pain, curvature, plaque softening, or improvement in sexual dysfunction in the active drug and control groups. This study concluded that although some trials have demonstrated intralesional verapamil to be an effective treatment for PD, further larger-scale studies are warranted given these negative findings to assess the effectiveness of intralesional verapamil for the treatment of PD (Shirazi et al, 2009). This study highlights the potential for inconsistent results for men with PD, which may vary because of patient selection, presence of calcification, plaque location, drug administration technique, and sample size. Drug concentration has also been evaluated, and although 10 mg/10 mL is the most commonly used dose and volume, Cavallini and associates (2007) showed a greater response to injection when 10 mg of verapamil was diluted with 20 mL of injectable saline (Cavallini et al, 2007). Poor candidates for this treatment include those with extensive calcification, curvature of greater than 90 degrees, or ventral curvature, in which it is difficult to adequately infiltrate the plaque (Levine et al, 2002). Predictors of success with intralesional verapamil include younger age (below age 40) and curvature greater than 30 degrees (Moskovic et al, 2011).

Nicardipine

Nicardipine is a dihydropyridine (DHP) type of calcium channel blocker. An in vitro study has suggested that it is more effective than a non-DHP type, verapamil, in reducing glycosaminoglycan biosynthesis and ECM production (Gürdal et al, 1992). Soh and associates (2010) performed the only study on the effectiveness of nicardipine for the treatment of PD. A total of 74 patients were assigned randomly to nicardipine versus saline. Nicardipine demonstrated a significant reduction of pain, improvement in IIEF-5 score, and reduction of plaque size when compared with placebo. Penile curvature was significantly improved in both the active drug and placebo groups without significant difference. There were no severe side effects, such as hypotension or other cardiovascular events (Soh et al, 2010).

Interferon Alfa-2b

IFN alfa-2b was first investigated as a treatment for PD in 1991 in the in vitro studies by Duncan and associates (1991). In fibroblasts derived from Peyronie plaques, the addition of IFN alfa-2b decreased their rate of proliferation in a dose-dependent fashion, decreased the production of extracellular collagen, and increased the production of collagenase (Duncan et al, 1991).

In a single-blind, multicenter, placebo-controlled, parallel study to assess the safety and efficacy of intralesional IFN alfa-2b,

Hellstrom and associates (2006) randomized a total of 117 consecutive PD patients to IFN alfa-2b or saline. Improvement in penile curvature, plaque size and density, and pain resolution was significantly greater in patients treated with IFN alfa-2b versus placebo. **The treatment group demonstrated a mean decrease in curvature of 27% or 13.5 degrees versus 9% or 4.5 degrees in the placebo group. Although these results were statistically significant, the question arises whether the small difference between the IFN and saline is clinically significant when taking into account the significant cost of the drug and its side effect profile, which frequently includes flulike symptoms** (fever, chills, and arthralgia) and minor penile swelling with ecchymosis. All these symptoms were effectively treated with over-the-counter nonsteroidal anti-inflammatory agents ingested before the injection procedure, and none lasted longer than 36 hours (Hellstrom et al, 2006). **This study was important because it was the first multicenter randomized placebo-controlled trial of intralesional injection for PD. It also was important because it showed that saline injection had little to no effect on penile deformity.**

Clostridial Collagenase

The first U.S. Food and Drug Administration (FDA)–approved drug for the treatment of PD, collagenase *Clostridium histolyticum* (CCH), is produced by the bacterium *C. histolyticum* and selectively degrades collagen types I and III in connective tissues despite the presence of TIMPs, which have been shown to be elevated in PD as well as to increase apoptosis of fibroblasts (Morales et al, 1983; Matsushita et al, 2001; Del Carlo et al, 2008; Syed et al, 2012). The recent flurry of investigation on this drug has come many years after the first time it was examined as a treatment for PD by Gelbard and associates (1982), who demonstrated that CCH significantly reduced the size of PD plaques, whereas elastic fibers, vascular smooth muscle, and axonal sheaths were not affected (Gelbard et al, 1982).

In the **first prospective, randomized, double-blind, placebo-controlled study of CCH, 49 men with PD were treated with CCH, resulting in significant improvements in plaque size and penile deformity** (Gelbard et al, 1993). All patients with a penile bend of 30 degrees or less and/or palpable plaque less than 2 cm responded (N = 3); 36% of patients with a penile bend of 30 to 60 degrees and/or 2 to 4 cm of palpable plaque responded; and 13% of patients with a penile bend of greater than 60 degrees and/or greater than 4 cm of palpable plaque responded. CCH was well tolerated, with no allergic reactions and no significant changes in laboratory parameters (Gelbard et al, 1993). Further investigation was encouraged but took years owing to absence of industry support.

In a phase 2 trial, **25 patients with PD received three intralesional injections of 10,000 units of CCH over 7 to 10 days, with a repeat of treatment at 3 months to assess change from baseline in penile deviation angle and plaque size** (Jordan, 2008). **A decrease in deviation angle of at least 25% was achieved in 58% of patients, and 95% of patients experienced a reduction in plaque size** (Jordan, 2008). More than 50% of patients in this series were considered "very much improved" or "much improved" at all time points in the study; approximately one third were considered to show minimal improvement or no change, resulting in an investigator's assessment of "worse."

In a **phase 2b trial, 147 patients with PD were enrolled in a randomized, double-blind, placebo-controlled trial of CCH or placebo, with a second randomization to modeling or nonmodeling** (Gelbard et al, 2012). **Patients receiving CCH and modeling had a significant change in curvature of the penis and decrease in the PD symptom effect score compared with placebo** (Gelbard et al, 2012).

The phase 3 IMPRESS (Investigation for Maximal Peyronie Reduction Efficacy and Safety Studies) I and II trials examined the clinical efficacy and safety of CCH intralesional injections in subjects with PD (Gelbard et al, 2013). A total of 417 and 415 subjects, respectively, went through a maximum of four treatment cycles, each separated by 6 weeks. Men received up to eight injections of 0.58 mg CCH, two injections per cycle separated by approximately 24 to 72 hours with the second injection of each followed 24 to 72 hours later by penile plaque modeling. Men were stratified by baseline penile curvature (30 to 60 degrees versus 61 to 90 degrees) and randomized to CCH or placebo 2 : 1 in favor of active drug. Post hoc meta-analysis of IMPRESS I and II data revealed that **men treated with CCH showed a mean 34% improvement in penile curvature, representing a mean change of −17.0 degrees ± 14.8 degrees per subject, compared with a mean 18.2% improvement in placebo-treated men, representing a mean change of −9.3 ± 13.6 degrees per subject ($P < .0001$). The mean change in PD symptom effect score was significantly improved in treated men versus men on placebo (−2.8 ± 3.8 vs. −1.8 ± 3.5, $P = .0037$). Patients with extensive calcification, ventral plaques, and disease duration less than 12 months were excluded.** Although serum antibodies to CCH developed in virtually all patients studied, no adverse events were noted as a result. The primary and frequently noted side effect was varying degree of ecchymosis and local penile bruising. Serious adverse events included corporeal rupture in three patients and penile hematoma in three patients. All three corporeal ruptures and one of the three penile hematomas were successfully repaired surgically; another hematoma was successfully drained percutaneously (Gelbard et al, 2013). **Further experience will help determine which patients may benefit most from CCH. This may depend on direction of curve, size of plaque, prevalence of calcification, and duration of disease, among other factors to be determined. A recent presentation did demonstrate that surgical correction with plication or grafting could be successfully performed after CCH injection without added technical difficulty** (Larsen and Levine, 2012). CCH received FDA approval for the treatment of PD in December 2013.

Topical Drug Application

Several studies have evaluated the effectiveness of topically applied agents for the treatment of PD. Topical application avoids the pain and trauma of intralesional injection therapy. The first study of topical application of a drug, β-aminopropionitrile, showed no benefit with respect to deformity change (Gelbard et al, 1983).

Topically applied liposomal recombinant human superoxide dismutase (lrhSOD) has also been studied in a randomized placebo-controlled trial (Riedl et al, 2005). This substance is proposed to act as an oxygen free radical scavenger, which might interrupt inflammatory cascades and thereby limit further disease progression. Penile curvature was improved by 5 to 30 degrees in 23% of patients and pain was significantly reduced as well ($P = .017$) compared with placebo after 4 weeks. The authors concluded that lrhSOD is an easily given, safe, and effective local therapeutic for the painful phase of PD (Riedl et al, 2005). No further studies have been performed regarding the use of lrhSOD. Therefore at this time the data are insufficient to recommend its use.

Fitch and associates (2007) reported on the use of topical verapamil for the treatment of PD (Fitch et al, 2007). Two simultaneous three-armed, double-blind, placebo-controlled studies were conducted in this pilot study. In this study topical verapamil improved curvature in 14 of 18 patients (77.8%) with mean curvature improvement of 43.6%. This study also boasted reduction in plaque size in 100% of participants, as well as improvement in erectile function in 72.7%. This study was originally aimed at comparing verapamil to topical trifluoperazine, **but because of the severity of side effects (anxiety, agitation, blurred vision, insomnia, and depression), topical trifluoperazine was discontinued before completion of randomization.** The results of this study have been called into question given the small sample size, lack of a true placebo, and absence of objective measures (Levine, 2007). In addition, simple topical administration of verapamil has been shown to be ineffective in achieving tissue levels within the tunica albuginea sufficient for therapeutic effect (Martin et al, 2002).

At this time, no topically applied agent has been shown to be effective in the treatment of PD.

Electromotive Drug Administration

Transdermal drug delivery was proposed to be superior to oral or injection therapy because it bypasses hepatic metabolism and minimizes the pain of injection. Unlike topical verapamil gel, electromotive drug administration (EMDA) with verapamil has been found to deliver detectable levels of the drug to the tunica albuginea (Martin et al, 2002; Levine et al, 2003).

A double-blind, placebo-controlled trial to determine the effectiveness of verapamil delivered through EMDA randomized a total of 42 PD patients to verapamil versus saline. Treatments were performed twice weekly for 3 months. **Both verapamil and saline groups demonstrated essentially equivalent reduction of curvature. The study concluded that further research is necessary to determine whether electric current alone may have a role in the treatment of PD** (Greenfield et al, 2007). Overall, EMDA was well tolerated in each group and it was noted by all patients to be easy and convenient to perform at home. The only adverse event reported by patients was temporary mild erythema at the treatment site (Greenfield et al, 2007).

In another prospective placebo-controlled study with transdermal EMDA, Di Stasi and associates (2004) randomized patients to receive verapamil and dexamethasone versus placebo. Those receiving active drug demonstrated significant decreases in plaque volume as well as penile curvature from 43 degrees to 21 degrees, which was significant when compared with placebo. Significant pain relief occurred in both groups, transient in the control group and permanent in the study group. All patients experienced temporary erythema at the electrode site. There were no other side effects (Di Stasi et al, 2004). **Although this approach has limited evidence of benefit, it has not been adopted in most centers.**

Extracorporeal Shockwave Therapy

The mechanism of action involved in ESWT for PD is unclear. However, there are two purported hypotheses: (1) Shock waves cause direct damage to the penile plaque, and (2) ESWT increases the vascularity of the targeted area by generating heat, which leads to the induction of an inflammatory reaction, resulting in lysis of the plaque and removal by macrophages (Gholami et al, 2003).

In the first prospective randomized double-blind placebo-controlled clinical trial evaluating ESWT for the treatment of PD, 100 treatment-naive PD patients with disease duration less than 12 months were randomly allocated to either ESWT (n = 50) or placebo (n = 50). For the placebo group, a nonfunctioning transducer was employed. Patients randomized to ESWT demonstrated improvements in pain, IIEF-5 score, and mean QoL score. **Plaque size and penile curvature were not significantly different in the treatment and placebo groups.** After 24 weeks, mean IIEF-5 score and mean QoL score were stable in the ESWT group, whereas mean visual analog scale (VAS) score was significantly lower when compared with baseline in both groups. It is interesting to note that after 24 weeks, mean plaque size and mean curvature degree were significantly worse in the placebo group when compared with both baseline and ESWT values. **This difference was less than 3 degrees, which, although statistically significant, is of no clinical significance** (Palmieri et al, 2012).

Recently a second placebo-controlled, prospective randomized single-blind study was performed in which 102 PD patients were randomly assigned (n=51) to ESWT or placebo (Hatzichristodoulou et al, 2013). Pain decreased in 17 of 20 (85.0%) patients in the ESWT group and in 12 of 25 (48.0%) patients in the placebo group. Penile deviation was not reduced by ESWT and worsened in 40% and 24.5% of patients in the ESWT and placebo groups, respectively ($P=.133$). Change in sexual function and plaque size reduction was not different between the two groups. In addition, plaque size increased in five patients (10.9%) receiving ESWT only. **The authors concluded that despite some potential benefit of ESWT with regard to pain reduction, it should be emphasized that pain usually resolves spontaneously with time. Given this and the fact** that deviation may worsen with ESWT, the treatment cannot be recommended.

Penile Traction

Controlled stretching of the penis, or "penile traction," by a device that holds the penis in a cradle and subjects it to **tension appears to meet a previously unmet need within the population of PD patients for a noninvasive, nonsurgical first-option treatment modality.**

Traction has been shown in nonpenile tissue models to induce cellular proliferation by several pathways (Ilizarov, 1989; Sun et al, 1996; Molea et al, 1999; Assoian and Klein, 2008; Bueno and Shah, 2008). It can also trigger scar remodeling; it has been shown that tension applied to tissues leads to a reorientation of collagen fibrils parallel to the axis of stress (Molea et al, 1999; Shapiro, 2008) These changes are the result of a process referred to as *mechanotransduction* whereby mechanical stimuli are converted into chemical responses within the cell (Alenghat and Ingber, 2002). Several signaling cascades are activated by tension on the cytoskeleton, which leads to a proliferative response as well as activation of various genes (Assoian and Klein, 2008). An **in vitro study to determine the cellular effects of traction on PD cells demonstrated a significant decrease in ASMA in the strained compared with nonstrained PD cell cultures, whereas an increase in MMPs involved in collagen degradation was observed.** In contrast, cytokines and proteins involved in fibroblast replication and inflammation such as ASMA, heat shock protein 47 (HSP47), and TGF-β1 receptor were not upregulated (Chung et al, 2013a). Several studies have been performed examining the clinical effects of traction for the treatment of PD, although none have been controlled trials.

Levine and associates (2008) first demonstrated the use of penile traction for the treatment of PD in a pilot study of 10 men. In nearly all (90%), prior medical therapy had failed. Traction was applied as the only treatment for 2 to 8 hr/day for 6 months. All subjects underwent pretreatment and post-treatment physical examination including measurement of stretched flaccid penile length and biothesiometry. Subjectively, all men noted reduced curvature estimated at 10 to 40 degrees, increased penile length (1 to 2.5 cm), and enhanced girth in areas of indentation or narrowing. **Objective measures demonstrated reduced curvature in all 10 men of up to 45 degrees; average reduction for the group was 33%, from 51 degrees to 34 degrees. SPL increased 0.5 to 2.0 cm, and erect girth increased 0.5 to 1.0 cm with correction of hinge effect in four out of four men.** It is important to note that results were maintained at 6 months after completion of therapy. The IIEF erectile function domain score increased from 18.3 to 23.6 for the group. There were no adverse events including skin changes, ulcerations, hypoesthesia, or diminished rigidity (Levine et al, 2008).

Gontero and associates (2009) performed a phase 2 prospective study on 15 PD patients with a curvature not exceeding 50 degrees with mild or no ED. Penile curvature decreased from an average of 31 degrees to 27 degrees at 6 months, which was not statistically significant. Mean stretched and flaccid penile length increased by 1.3 and 0.83 cm, respectively, at 6 months. Results were maintained at 12 months. Overall treatment results were subjectively scored as acceptable in spite of limited curvature improvements, which varied from "no change" to "mild improvement." **The investigators concluded that the use of a penile extender device provided only minimal improvements in penile curvature but a reasonable level of patient satisfaction, probably attributable to increased penile length. The selection of patients with stabilized disease, many with calcified plaques, and penile curvature not exceeding 50 degrees may have led to outcomes underestimating the potential efficacy of the treatment** (Gontero et al, 2009).

Recently a prospective nonrandomized study was conducted administering traction to PD patients in the acute phase, defined as progressive penile curvature exceeding 15 degrees and/or pain at rest or at erection in the last 12 months (Martínez-Salamanca et al, 2014). A total of 55 patients underwent traction for 6 months and were compared with 41 patients also in the acute phase who did not. Patients were advised to use the device at least 6 hours a day and no more than 9 hours, preventing its use during sleep. Mean duration of use was 4.6 hours per day (3.1 to 9.2 hours). Also, patients were taught to remove the device for at least 30 minutes every 2 hours to prevent glans ischemia. **The mean curvature decreased from 33 degrees at baseline to 15 degrees at 6 months and 13 degrees at 9 months with a mean decrease of 20 degrees in the traction group.** VAS score for **pain decreased from 5.5 to 2.5 after 6 months** ($P<.05$). The percentage of patients who were not able to achieve penetration decreased from 62% to 20% ($P<.03$). Without this intervention, deformity increased significantly, stretched flaccid penile length decreased, VAS score for pain increased, and erection hardness worsened. **Furthermore, the need for surgery was reduced in 40% of patients who would otherwise have been candidates for surgery and simplified the complexity of the surgical procedure (from grafting to plication) in one of every three patients.** Treatment-related adverse events included two cases of erythema in the balanopreputial sulcus, which resolved with stopping traction for 24 to 48 hours. Fourteen patients (25.5%) reported some degree of discomfort. Worsening of erectile function over the treatment period was not observed, **and the overall satisfaction rate was 85%** (range 60% to 90%) at 9 months. No case of sensory change after traction was reported (Martínez-Salamanca et al, 2014). **In our opinion, traction therapy has the potential to be the most effective nonsurgical treatment to recover lost length, reduce curvature, and enhance girth.** It is critical that the patient wear the device for 3 or more hours per day to get satisfactory results.

Vacuum Therapy

Application of a penile vacuum device to mechanically straighten the penis has been evaluated in one published noncontrolled study in which subjects wore the vacuum device for 10 minutes twice per day for 12 weeks. This study demonstrated a reduction in the angle of curvature by 5 degrees to 25 degrees in 21 of 31 patients. Three patients' curvature worsened, and in seven the curvature remained unchanged. Fifty-one percent were satisfied with this outcome; the other 49% went on to surgical correction (Raheem et al, 2010). Although vacuum erection devices are usually considered safe, it would seem that the short-term duration of stretching forces on the penis would not induce the desired physical changes known to occur with mechanotransduction with prolonged stretch therapy. Several complications such as the development of PD, urethral bleeding, skin necrosis, and penile ecchymosis have been reported with concomitant use of constriction rings and when inappropriately elevated pressures are applied to the penis for an extended period of time (Kim et al, 1993; Ganem et al, 1998).

Combination Therapy

One study investigated whether the combination of the mechanical effects of penile traction with the chemical effects of intralesional verapamil and oral medications (pentoxifylline and L-arginine) could have a synergistic effect on the tunica albuginea and Peyronie plaque (Abern et al, 2012). All patients were given oral pentoxifylline and L-arginine, with 39 electing to undergo traction and 35 choosing not to use traction. Both treatment groups had a statistically significant reduction in erect penile curvature. The traction group had a reduction from a mean of 44.4 degrees (standard deviation [SD] 27.5 degrees) at baseline to a mean of 33.4 degrees (SD 25.3 degrees) after the 24-week protocol ($P = .03$). Patients not using traction had a reduction from a mean of 36.6 degrees at baseline (SD 18.5 degrees) to a mean of 21.5 degrees (SD 19.3 degrees) after treatment ($P < .01$). There were no statistically significant differences in curvature outcomes between the two groups. In patients using traction, SPL increased overall by a mean 0.3 cm (SD 0.9 cm) after treatment, which trended toward statistical significance ($P = .06$), whereas the men not using traction lost an average of 0.7 cm (SD 1.1 cm) of length, which was not statistically different ($P = .46$) (Abern et al, 2012). Unfortunately, this study did not control for duration of traction therapy, and some men included in the traction group applied the device for only 1 to 2 hr/wk, whereas others wore it for over 50 hr/wk. An analysis of traction duration and deformity change demonstrated that wearing the device on average three or more hours per day allowed reliable measured deformity improvement, which occurred in a dose-response fashion.

Another combination study examined the effects of combining verapamil injection and verapamil iontophoresis with or without the use of a combination pill that contained vitamin E (36 mg), p-aminobenzoic acid (100 mg), propolis (as galangin 100 mg), blueberry anthocyanins (80 mg), soy isoflavones (50 mg), *Muira puama* (25 mg), damiana (25 mg), and *Persea americana* (50 mg). Intergroup analysis revealed greater plaque size reduction (−30.8% vs. −18.0%) and greater percentage with reduction of curvature (85% vs. 53.5%) with use of the combination pill (Paulis et al, 2013b).

Radiation Therapy

Radiation therapy has been proposed as a treatment for PD since 1964 (Duggan, 1964). **In vitro studies suggest that low-dose radiation therapy has a potent anti-inflammatory effect, inhibiting leukocyte-endothelium interactions** (Arenas et al, 2012). In recent years, radiation therapy has been proposed as a treatment for pain that was thought to be "abnormally persistent." In 1975 a retrospective study examined the use of radiation therapy and found it to be no more effective than no treatment (Incrocci et al, 2000). **It is the consensus of multiple experts in the field that radiation should be avoided because of potential risk of malignant change and increase in the risk of ED in aging patients** (Ralph et al, 2010; Hatzimouratidis et al, 2012; Mulhall et al, 2012).

Conclusion

At this time it is our opinion that combination therapy will offer **the best opportunity for improvement by creating a synergy between the chemical effects of the oral and/or injectable agents and the mechanical effects of external forces on the penis. The recent addition of an FDA-approved treatment (injectable CCH) provides what appears to be a sensible nonsurgical treatment option for PD.** Further experience will allow better discrimination as to the optimum candidates. Clearly, it appears that the goal of nonsurgical treatment at a minimum should be to prevent progression of deformity during the acute phase. Reducing deformity to improve sexual function and reduce the effects of the scarring is the ultimate goal of all treatment for PD (Tables 31-1, 31-2, and 31-3).

SURGICAL MANAGEMENT

Indications

Surgical reconstruction is indicated for men with deformity that precludes satisfactory sexual intercourse or causes pain for themselves or their partner during sexual relations or because of distress as a result of the appearance of the erect penis (Kadioglu et al, 2006).

Surgery remains the gold standard treatment to most rapidly and reliably correct the deformity associated with PD; and for men who also have ED, placement of a penile prosthesis can provide rigidity for penetrative sexual activity. The indications for surgical correction include stable disease, which is defined as disease that is at least 1 year from onset, and at least 6 months of stable deformity. These indications have not been formally studied but appear to be generally accepted by experts in the field (Jordan, 2007; Ralph et al, 2010; Levine and Burnett, 2013). Other indications include a deformity that compromises or makes impossible the patient's ability to engage in sexual intercourse because of the nature of the deformity and/or inadequate rigidity, and patients in whom conservative therapy has failed (Box 31-4). No single surgical approach is universally defined as the

KEY POINTS: NONSURGICAL TREATMENT OF PEYRONIE DISEASE

- Patients who have no pain or difficulty in accomplishing penetrative sex may require only reassurance, because this is not a disorder that will degenerate into a cancer and is not life-threatening.
- A poor understanding of the cause of this wound-healing disorder contributes to the fact that to date, conservative treatments often yield inconsistent and clinically insignificant improvements in deformity.
- Currently, no oral agent has been shown in placebo-controlled trials to result in clinically meaningful improvement in curvature.
- Topical therapy and ESWT have not been shown to reduce penile deformity.
- Intralesional verapamil and IFN alfa-2b have shown evidence of reduced curvature and improved sexual function. Yet most studies are not controlled trials. These agents at a minimum appear to result in deformity stabilization during the acute phase.
- The first FDA-approved drug for the treatment of PD, CCH is produced by the bacterium *C. histolyticum* and selectively degrades collagen types I and III. Mean curvature reduction in the phase 3 trials in the treatment arm was 34% (17 degrees) vs. 18.2% (9.3 degrees) for placebo. Further experience will help determine which patients may benefit most from CCH, which may depend on direction of curve, size of plaque, prevalence of calcification, and duration of disease. The volume of patients seeking treatment for PD may increase over the coming years as public awareness increases with the advent of use of this drug.
- Combination therapy, also known as a "three-armed approach" using daily pentoxifylline and L-arginine, biweekly verapamil injections, and daily traction likely provides the best opportunity for deformity improvement by creating a synergy between the chemical effects of the oral and/or injectable agents with the mechanical effects of external forces on the penis.

standard of care (Kendirci and Hellstrom, 2004; Gur et al, 2011) because there are multiple factors to consider, including severity of curvature, direction of curvature, presence of a hinge effect, erection quality, and patient goals. An algorithm for surgical decision making is presented in Figure 31-10 (Levine and Larsen, 2013).

Preoperative consent is critical because patients with PD are distressed and frequently emotionally devastated. It has been reported that men who have undergone treatment for PD are often not satisfied with their results because of their expectation for recovery of their pre-Peyronie penile appearance (Jones, 1997). **It is therefore important to have a frank discussion with the patient so that he understands the limitations of the operation, as well as to set appropriate expectations regarding outcomes to optimize patient satisfaction** (Jordan and McCammon, 2007; Ralph et al, 2010). **The patient should understand that there is a possibility of persistent or recurrent curvature, reduction of penile erect length, diminished rigidity, and decreased sexual sensation** (Box 31-5). Persistent or recurrent curvature is unusual but has been shown in up to 16% of men, the great majority of whom do not require another operation (Taylor and Levine, 2007; Ralph et al, 2010). **The patient should understand that the goal is to make the penis "functionally straight," which expert opinion defines as a residual deformity of 20 degrees or less** (Ralph et al, 2010; Levine and Burnett, 2013). The European Association of Urology (EAU) guidelines committee on PD defines successful curvature correction as 15 degrees or less of residual curvature (Hatzimouratidis et al, 2012). Change in penile erect length is more likely with plication than with grafting, although all surgical correction procedures have been associated with some length loss. This is extremely important for the patient to understand preoperatively because 70% to 80% of patients initially have loss of length as a result of the fibrotic disease process (Pryor and Ralph, 2002; Jordan and McCammon, 2007; Ralph et al, 2010). Thus, further loss of length can be a major concern. Having stretched flaccid penile length documented preoperatively permits comparison with postoperative length. Diminished rigidity has long been reported after surgery, and studies have demonstrated that up to 50% of men may have some degree of postoperative reduction in rigidity, which may respond to a PDE5 inhibitor. Rigidity will not likely be

TABLE 31-1 Oral Agents for Peyronie Disease (PD)

TREATMENT	MECHANISM OF ACTION	STUDY OUTCOMES	ADVERSE EFFECTS
Potaba	Decreases serotonin levels by increasing monoamine oxidase activity, resulting in enhancement of the antifibrotic properties of tissues	Decreased plaque size, no decrease in curvature	Anorexia, nausea, fever, skin rash, hypoglycemia, acute hepatitis
Vitamin E	Antioxidant, limits oxidative stress of reactive oxygen species shown to be increased in PD	No benefit	Possible cerebrovascular events, nausea, vomiting, diarrhea, headache, dizziness
Tamoxifen	Induces the production of TGF-β in an estrogen receptor–independent fashion, theoretically causing macrophage deactivation and T-lymphocyte suppression, thus preventing further fibrogenesis	No benefit	Alopecia, retinopathy, thromboembolism, pancytopenia
Colchicine	Microtubule depolymerization; inhibits cell mitosis, mobility, adhesion of leukocytes, and transcellular movement of collagen and stimulates the production of collagenase	No benefit	Myelosuppression, diarrhea, nausea, vomiting
Carnitine	Increases mitochondrial respiration; decreases free radical formation	No benefit	Seizures, diarrhea, nausea, stomach cramps, vomiting
Pentoxifylline	Blocks the TGF-β1–mediated pathway of inflammation; prevents deposition of collagen type I; is a nonspecific phosphodiesterase inhibitor; decreases platelet-activating factor	Decreased curvature in 33% of patients, mean 23 degrees	Nausea, vomiting, dyspepsia, malaise, flushing, dizziness, and headache

TGF, transforming growth factor.

TABLE 31-2 Intralesional Agents for Peyronie Disease (PD)

TREATMENT	MECHANISM OF ACTION	STUDY OUTCOMES	ADVERSE EFFECTS
Verapamil	Calcium channel blocker inhibits fibroblast proliferation, extracellular matrix protein synthesis and secretion; increases collagenase activity.	Reduction of curvature and plaque-associated penile narrowing, improvement in quality of erection	Nausea, lightheadedness, penile pain, ecchymoses
Nicardipine	DHP type of calcium channel blocker. In vitro study demonstrated that it is more effective than a non-DHP type, verapamil, in reducing glycosaminoglycan biosynthesis and production of extracellular matrix, such as collagen.	Reduction of pain, improvement in IIEF-5 score, and reduction of plaque size; no benefit in curvature	No severe side effects, such as hypotension or other cardiovascular events
Interferon alfa-2b	Decreases plaque fibroblast proliferation in dose-dependent fashion, decreases the production of extracellular collagen, and increases the production of collagenase.	Decrease in curvature of 27% (13.5 degrees) vs. 9% (4.5 degrees) in the placebo group	Sinusitis, flulike symptoms (fever, chills, and arthralgia), and minor penile swelling with ecchymosis
Clostridial collagenase	Selectively degrades collagen types I and III in connective tissues despite the presence of TIMPs, which have been shown to be elevated in PD and to increase apoptosis of fibroblasts.	Decrease in penile curvature by 34%, mean decrease of 17 degrees vs. 18%, mean decrease 9.3 degrees in placebo; PD symptom bothersomeness score significantly improved vs. placebo	Contusions, ecchymoses, corporeal rupture

DHP, dihydropyridine; IIEF, International Index of Erectile Function; TIMPs, tissue inhibitors of metalloproteinases.

TABLE 31-3 External Force Application for Peyronie Disease

TREATMENT	MECHANISM OF ACTION	STUDY OUTCOMES	ADVERSE EFFECTS
Electromotive drug administration	Bypasses hepatic metabolism, increases concentration of drug to target tissues compared with topical application alone	Verapamil alone: no benefit Verapamil + dexamethasone: decreases in plaque volume as well as penile curvature from 43 degrees to 21 degrees	Temporary erythema at the electrode site
Extracorporeal shockwave therapy	Direct damage to the penile plaque; increases vascularity of the targeted area inducing an inflammatory reaction, resulting in lysis of the plaque and removal by macrophages	Improvements in pain, IIEF-5 score, and mean QoL score; no curvature reduction	Local petechiae and ecchymoses
Penile traction	Decreases α-smooth muscle actin, increases matrix metalloproteinases involved in collagen degradation	Length increased 0.5-2.0 cm; girth increased 0.5-1.0 cm; curvature mean decrease of 20 degrees; pain decreased; softening or shrinking of plaque; overall satisfaction 85%	Erythema in the balanopreputial sulcus, discomfort
Vacuum therapy	Unknown; mechanical effects similar to traction have been suggested	Reduction in the angle of curvature by 5-25 degrees in 21 of 31 patients	Development of PD, urethral bleeding, skin necrosis, and penile ecchymosis
Radiation therapy	Anti-inflammatory effects via functional modulation of the adhesion of white blood cells to activated endothelial cells and modulation of the induction of nitric oxide synthase in activated macrophages	No clinical benefit	Possible malignant change, increased risk of ED in elderly

ED, erectile dysfunction; IIEF, International Index of Erectile Function; QoL, quality of life.

BOX 31-4 Indications for Surgery

- Stable deformity for at least 6 months from onset of symptoms
- Inability to engage in satisfactory penetrative sexual intercourse because of deformity and/or inadequate rigidity
- Failed conservative treatment
- Desire for most rapid and reliable result

BOX 31-5 Preoperative Consent

Set expectations regarding outcome.
- Persistent or recurrent curvature: The goal is "functionally straight" (curvature <20 degrees)
- Change in length: The result is more likely shorter with plication than with grafting.
- Diminished rigidity
  - ≥5% in all studies—grafting more than plication
  - ≥30% if suboptimal preoperative rigidity—dependent on preoperative erectile quality
- Decreased sexual sensation
  - Typically resolves in 1 to 6 months
  - Rarely compromises orgasm or ejaculation

improved by penile straightening, and therefore in patients who already have significant ED that does not respond to oral medication, placement of a penile prosthesis should be offered (Taylor and Levine, 2007; Ralph et al, 2010). Men who are considering penile straightening procedures without a penile prosthesis should be carefully evaluated for the quality of their preoperative erections, which does appear to be the most reliable predictor of postoperative ED (Flores et al, 2011; Taylor et al, 2012). In some men with PD and ED the correction of the penile geometry resulted in improved rigidity (Pescatori et al, 2003). **Regardless, it is of critical importance that the patient understand that any operation done on the penis to correct PD may result in diminished rigidity, and that this may subsequently be treated successfully with oral PDE5 inhibitors, injection therapy, or a vacuum device; and those in whom these approaches fail can have a penile prosthesis implanted with little to no additional difficulty** (Kendirci and Hellstrom, 2004; Levine et al, 2010; Chung et al, 2012c). Decreased sexual sensation has been examined and reported on infrequently, but it does appear that around 20% of men will describe some reduction in penile sensitivity, rarely interfering with orgasm or ejaculation. During the acute postoperative period there can be hyperesthesia or hypoesthesia, which tends to resolve and stabilize within 6 to 12 months postoperatively (Taylor and Levine, 2008; Ralph et al, 2010). **The primary determinants for the choice of surgical approach are based on two factors, including quality of the preoperative erection hardness and severity of deformity, including curvature and indentation. In men who have rigidity that is adequate for coital activity with or without pharmacotherapy, tunica plication techniques and plaque incision or partial excision with grafting may be used. Tunica plication techniques are recommended for those who have a simple curvature of less than 70 degrees, those with absence of an hourglass or hinge effect, and those in whom the anticipated loss of length would be less than 20% of the total erect length** (Levine and Lenting, 1997; Ralph and Minhas, 2004; Mulhall et al, 2005). **The estimated penile length loss can be determined during preoperative testing while the penis is erect by measuring the difference in length between the long and short sides of the penis. Grafting procedures are recommended for those with more complex curves of greater than 60 to 70 degrees and/or a destabilizing hourglass resulting in a hinge effect. This hinge effect results in**

a buckling or unstable penis, which makes penetrative sex difficult. **These men must have strong, sexually induced rigidity to reduce the likelihood of postoperative ED** (Flores et al, 2011; Taylor et al, 2012) (Table 31-4). **For the man who has PD and ED that is refractory to medical therapy, published algorithms have indicated that penile prosthesis placement is the procedure of choice** (Levine and Dimitriou, 2000; Mulhall et al, 2005; Ralph et al, 2010; Levine and Burnett, 2013). This procedure allows for correction of the deformity while also addressing the ED. If curvature is not satisfactorily corrected with the prosthesis inflated during surgery, additional straightening maneuvers may be performed. We recommend manual modeling as the first step as initially reported by Wilson and Delk (1994). If there is residual curvature in excess of 30 degrees after modeling, then a relaxing incision in the tunica albuginea overlying the area of maximum curvature can be made. It is recommended that if the incisional defect is greater than 2 cm, a biograft (i.e., pericardium or small intestine submucosa) should be placed over the defect to prevent cicatrix contracture of the incision or herniation of the prosthesis (Levine and Dimitriou, 2000; Ralph et al, 2010). Plication techniques have been recommended to be performed before placement of the prosthesis to correct curvature in lieu of manual modeling (Rahman et al, 2004; Dugi and Morey, 2010). In this circumstance, if the curvature is dorsal, the erectile deformity can be defined with injection of a vasoactive drug and infusion of saline, then sutures are placed in a Lembert fashion to cause ventral shortening and correction of the curve.

Tunical Shortening Procedures

Penile plication aims to shorten the longer (or convex) side of the tunica albuginea to match the length to the shorter side (Syed et al, 2003; Ralph, 2006). **Advantages to these approaches include shorter surgical time, good cosmetic outcomes, minimal effect on rigidity, simple and safe surgery, and effective straightening** (Hudak et al, 2013; Hatzimouratidis et al, 2012). **Disadvantages include shortening and failure to correct an hourglass or hinge.** A study of failures with the Nesbit procedure identified three factors associated with an unsatisfactory outcome, including impaired preoperative erectile function, penile shortening of greater than 2 cm, and penile deformity greater than 30 degrees (Andrews et al, 2001). Multiple surgical plication techniques have been offered for PD, beginning with the Nesbit procedure (Nesbit, 1965) (Fig. 31-11). This technique uses excision of an elliptical segment of the tunica on the contralateral side of the curvature. In the setting of a ventral curvature, once Buck's fascia has been elevated, small wedges of the dorsal tunica albuginea are excised and then the defect is closed, typically with permanent suture. Multiple variations on this approach have evolved, including the Yachia procedure, which uses the Heineke-Mikulicz technique (Yachia, 1990; Yachia, 1993). In the setting of a dorsal curvature, a short (0.5 to 1.5 cm), full-thickness vertical incision is made on the ventral shaft tunic, opposite the area of maximum curvature, which is then closed transversely to shorten the ventral aspect and correct the curvature (Fig. 31-12). This approach must be used carefully so that the length of the incision is not too long, such that transverse closure could result in further narrowing of the shaft, possibly resulting in an unstable erection. Several authors have suggested that this approach has a lower risk of perceived penile shortening (Klevmark et al, 1994; Nooter et al, 1994; Sulaiman and Gingell, 1994; Kümmerling and Schubert, 1995; Poulson and Kikeby, 1995; Ralph et al, 1995; Savoca et al, 2000; Savoca et al, 2004).

Imbrication procedures are used to avoid making a full-thickness tunical incision and fold the tunica to correct curvature. The techniques of tunical plication without incision were introduced in 1985 by Essed and Schroeder, who used nonabsorbable sutures placed in a figure-of-eight fashion to enable the knots to be buried (Essed and Schroeder, 1985). Two years later, Ebbehoj and Metz (1987) described their plication technique using multiple rows of sutures to shorten the longer side for congenital curvature (Ebbehoj and Metz, 1987). The 16-dot procedure has become a popular variation

TABLE 31-4 Outcomes for Plaque Excision or Incision and Grafting

GRAFT MATERIAL	AUTHOR AND DATE	PATIENTS (N)	MEAN FOLLOW-UP (MONTHS)	STRAIGHT AT LATEST FOLLOW-UP (%)	ED (%)	SATISFACTION RATES (%)
Dermal grafts	Wild et al, 1979	10	11	60	6	70
	Levine, 1997	15	11	73	12	70
	Chun et al, 2001	48	19.6	80	25	73
	Kovac and Brock, 2007	50	45	94	NR	NR
	Chung et al, 2011a	6	102	50	NR	35
Saphenous vein grafts	El-Sakka et al, 1998	113	9.72	96	12	92
	Kadioglu et al, 1999	20	13.2	75	5	NR
	Montorsi et al, 2000	50	12	80	6	96
	Akkus et al, 2001	58	16	86	7	92
	Adeniyi et al, 2002	51	32	82	8	88
	Hsu, 2003	24	31.2	96	4	100
	Kalsi et al, 2005	113	>60	80	23	60
	Kim et al, 2008	20	>12	85	35	NR
Buccal mucosa	Shioshvili et al, 2005	26	38	92	8	NR
	Cormio et al, 2009	15	13	100	0	93
Proximal crura	Teloken et al, 2000	7	6	86	0	86
	Schwarzer et al, 2003	31	NR	84	19	94
	Da Ros et al, 2012	27	NR	96	4	70
Tunica vaginalis	Das, 1980	15	4-16	87.5	0	100
	O'Donnell, 1992	25	42.2	88	68	NR
Dura mater	Fallon, 1990	40	12-72	95	25	NR
	Sampaio et al, 2002	40	12-24	95	15	NR
Temporalis fascia	Gelbard and Hayden, 1991	12	NR	100	0	100
Fascia lata	Kalsi et al, 2006	14	31	79	7	93
Small intestinal submucosa (SIS 4-layer)	Breyer et al, 2007	19	15	63	53	Score of 2.7/5.0
	Kovac and Brock, 2007	13	7.8	77	NR	85
	Lee et al, 2008	13	14	100	54	NR
	Staerman et al, 2010	33	14	67	11	79
	Chung et al, 2010	17	75	77	13	NR
Bovine pericardium	Egydio et al, 2002	33	19	88	0.0	NR
	Knoll, 2007	162	38	91	21	NR
Tutoplast pericardial graft	Hellstrom and Reddy, 2000	81	58	79	20	78
	Leungwattanakij et al, 2001	19	22	84	16	74
	Usta et al, 2003	11	14	91	NR	NR
	Levine et al, 2003	40	22	98	30	92
	Kovac and Brock, 2007	13	30	100	NR	NR
	Chung et al, 2011a	81	58	91	32	75
	Taylor and Levine, 2008	23	79	87	NR	NR
Acellular dermis	Adamakis et al, 2011	5	6	100	0	100
Synthetic materials	Faerber and Konnak, 1993	9	17.5	100	0	100
TachoSil	Licht et al, 1997	28	22	61	18	30
	Horstmann et al, 2011	43	63	41	9	20

ED, erectile dysfunction; NR, not reported.

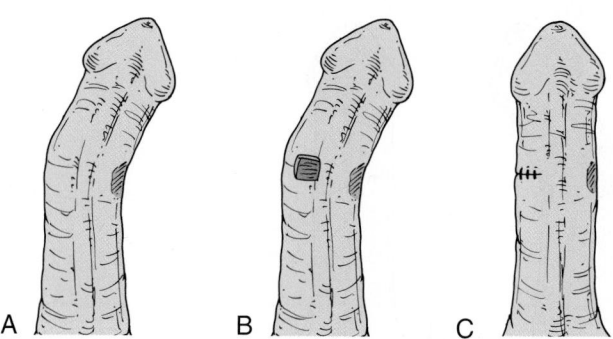

Figure 31-11. A, The Nesbit procedure employs a transverse elliptical incision of the tunica albuginea. **B,** This is done contralateral to the area of greatest curvature. **C,** The defect is closed transversely with permanent suture with or without the addition of absorbable suture.

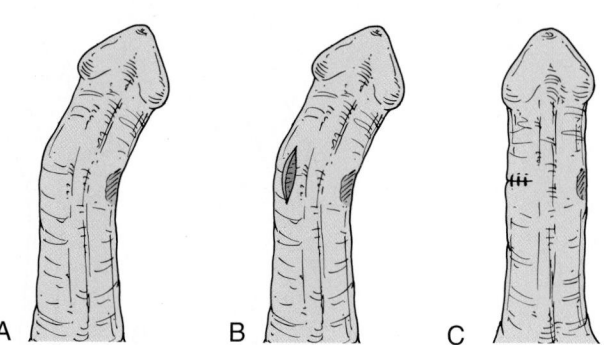

Figure 31-12. A, The Yachia procedure employs a full-thickness vertical incision **(B)** in the tunica albuginea contralateral to the area of greatest curvature and is closed transversely **(C)** without removal of tunica albuginea.

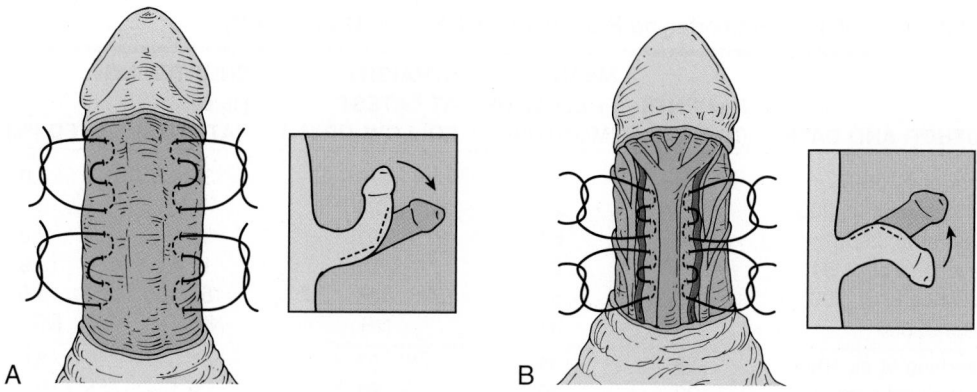

Figure 31-13. The dot procedure employs no incision. The tunica albuginea is plicated with permanent suture using an extended Lembert-type suture placement following four dots per plication. **A,** Suture placement for dorsal curve. **B,** Suture placement for ventral curve.

of tunical shortening in which there is no incision into the tunic but the tunica albuginea is plicated with permanent suture using an extended Lembert-type suture placement technique (Gholami and Lue, 2002; Brant et al, 2007; Rolle et al, 2005) (Fig. 31-13). Another plication variation is the Levine modification of the Duckett-Baskin tunica albuginea plication (TAP), which was originally used for children with congenital curvature. Here, a partial-thickness incision is made transversely on the contralateral side to the point of maximum curvature (Baskin and Duckett, 1994; Levine, 2006). A pair of transverse parallel incisions 1 to 1.5 cm in length are made through the longitudinal fibers but do not violate the inner circular fibers of the tunic. As a result, the underlying cavernosal tissue is not disturbed, which is thought to reduce the likelihood of postoperative ED. These incisions are separated by 0.5 to 1.0 cm depending on the desired amount of shortening. The longitudinal fibers between the two transverse incisions are excised so as to reduce the bulk of the plication. This procedure is now done with a single central permanent suture (2-0 Tevdek suture, Teleflex Medical, Research Triangle Park, NC, or TiCron suture, Medline, Mundelein, IL) placed in an inverting vertical mattress fashion to bury the knot and then supported with absorbable suture (3-0 polydioxanone [PDS], Ethicon, Somerville, NJ) placed in a Lembert fashion to reduce the palpable nature of the plication and knots (Fig. 31-14).

The key is that all plication procedures shorten the long side of the penis and therefore can result in loss of length on that aspect of the penis. Studies have examined the loss of penile length after use of the TAP technique. The expected factors that predicted loss of length included the direction of curvature and the degree of curvature (Greenfield et al, 2006). Greenfield and colleagues (2006) found that men who had a ventral curvature of

greater than 60 degrees tended to have the greatest potential loss of penile length. Preoperative penile length and degree and direction of curvature deformity appear to correlate with postoperative satisfaction (Mulhall et al, 2005; Greenfield et al, 2006).

The drawbacks of any tunica plication procedure for PD are that it does not correct shortening and it potentially may enhance loss of penile shaft length. It does not address hinge or hourglass effect and may exacerbate it, resulting in an unstable penis. The plaque is also left in situ. Penile narrowing or indentation has been reported in up to 17% with these techniques. In addition, there can be pain associated with the knots and suture granulomas (Tornehl and Carson, 2004; Taylor and Levine, 2008; Ralph et al, 2010). Surgical straightening with plication procedures can be expected in 79% to 100% of patients, with a reported satisfaction rate of 65% to 100% (Van der Horst et al, 2004; Ding et al, 2010; Larsen and Levine, 2013). Recurrence of penile curvature deformity (greater than 30 degrees) has been reported in up to 12% in a limited number of long-term studies (Taylor et al, 2008; Levine and Burnett, 2013). The reported risk of new ED ranges from 0% to 38%, and diminished sensation has been reported in 4% to 21% with follow-up of up to 89 months. Other, less common complications include hematoma in up to 9% of patients, urethral injury in less than 2%, and phimosis in up to 5% (Tornehl and Carson, 2004; Kadioglu et al, 2011b; Larsen and Levine, 2013). The most recent International Consultation on Sexual Medicine (ICSM) published recommendations regarding plication procedures in 2010 and reported that there was "no evidence that one surgical approach provides better outcomes over another, but curvature correction can be expected with less risk of new ED" when compared with grafting procedures (Ralph et al, 2010) (see

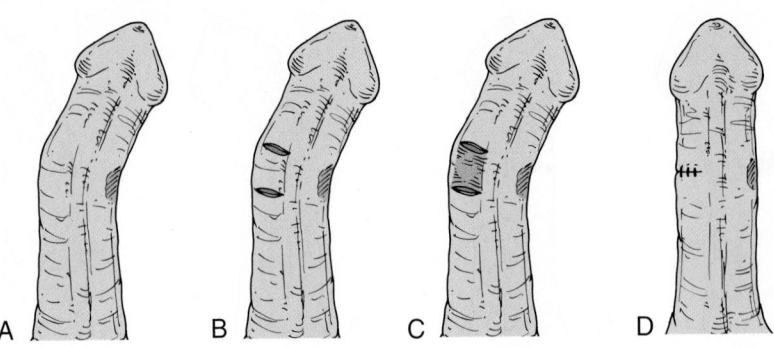

Figure 31-14. The tunica albuginea plication (TAP) procedure (A) employs a pair of transverse parallel incisions (B) separated by 0.5 to 1.0 cm. The incision is made through the longitudinal fibers but does not violate the inner circular fibers of the tunic. C, The longitudinal fibers between the two transverse incisions are removed to reduce the bulk of the plication. D, The defect is then brought together transversely.

TABLE 31-5 Outcomes of Tunical Shortening Procedure for Peyronie Disease (PD)

PROCEDURE	AUTHOR AND DATE	PATIENTS (N)	MEAN FOLLOW-UP (MONTHS)	STRAIGHT AT LATEST FOLLOW-UP (%)	SHORTENING (% OF PATIENTS)	ED (%)	SATISFACTION RATES (%)
Nesbit	Licht et al, 1997	28	22	79	37	4.0	79
	Schneider et al, 2003	48	25	23	44	0	75
	Syed et al, 2003	42	84	91	50	2.0	76
	Savoca et al, 2004	218	89	86.3	17.4	12.9	83.5
	Bokarica et al, 2005	40	81	88	15,* 100**	5.0	NR
	Ralph, 2006	9	31	NR	NR	NR	67
Plication	Geertsen et al, 1996	28	34	57	NR	3.5	82
	Levine and Lenting, 1997	22	20	91	9	9	NR
	Thiounn et al, 1998	29	34	79	NR	38	81,* 62**
	Schultheiss et al, 2000	61	39.8	70.5	45.9	3.3	NR
	Chahal et al, 2001	44	49	29	90	36	NR
	Gholami and Lue, 2002	124	31	85	41	6	96
	Van der Horst et al, 2004	28	30	83	NR	0	67.8
	Paez et al, 2007	76	70	42	NR	60	NR
	Kim et al, 2008	26	≥12	65	69	11	65
	Kadioglu et al, 2008	15	21	87	NR	NR	93
	Taylor and Levine, 2008	61	72	93	18	10	84
	Dugi and Morey, 2010	34	6	98	NR	2.9	93
Yachia	Licht et al, 1997	30	12	100	NR	NR	83
	Rehman et al, 1997	26	32	92	100	7.7	78
	Daitch et al, 1999	14	24.1	93	57	7	79

*Patient perceived shortening
**Objectively measured shortening
ED, erectile dysfunction; NR, not reported.

Table 31-5 for a summary of outcomes of tunical shortening procedures).

Tunical Lengthening Procedures (Plaque Incision or Partial Excision and Grafting)

Indications for plaque incision and grafting (PIG) or partial plaque excision and grafting (PEG) for surgical correction of PD includes greater complexity of disease with several (or all) of the following: curvature greater than 60 to 70 degrees, shaft narrowing, hinging, and extensive plaque calcification (Levine and Lenting, 1997; Kendirci and Hellstrom, 2004; Ralph et al, 2010; Kadioglu et al, 2011b; Levine and Burnett, 2013). Most important, for the patient to be a candidate for incision or PEG, he must have strong preoperative erections (Taylor et al, 2012). This can be determined during the patient interview, when he is asked directly, "If your penis was straight, would the quality of rigidity that you currently have allow penetrative sex?" Should the patient hesitate or note suboptimal-quality erections, a grafting procedure should not be performed unless the patient fully understands the risk of more advanced postoperative ED and the possible need for subsequent prosthesis placement to obtain optimal rigidity. Some men simply reject the idea that they need a prosthesis as a first-line surgical treatment. Others who might be considered candidates for tunica plication reject this approach because of fear of penile length loss. These men may be offered a grafting repair with the understanding that a penile prosthesis can be placed with minimal added difficulty at a later time. The advantage of performing the grafting procedure is that it would likely correct curvature and reestablish more normal shaft caliber while increasing the likelihood of some length recovery in the range of 0.5 to 3.0 cm.

Other factors have been reported in the literature as possible predictors of postoperative ED, including age older than 55 years, evidence of corporeal veno-occlusive dysfunction on duplex ultrasound analysis with a resistance index of less than 0.80, large tunica defect and graft size, ventral curvature, and curvature greater than 60 degrees (Leungwattanakij et al, 2001; Levine et al, 2005; Alphs et al, 2010; Flores et al, 2011). These predictors have been suggested as a result of single-center studies, with a limited number of patients in each cohort. Larger-scale studies indicate that the most critical criterion for any grafting procedure is the quality of preoperative erections (Flores et al, 2011; Taylor et al, 2012). **In fact, Jordan and Angermeier found that there was a linear association between preoperative and postoperative ED** (Jordan and Angermeier, 1993). **Expert opinion has been consistent that patients with ventral deformity do not do well with grafting procedures.** In fact, Hellstrom's analysis of the relationship of penile deformity to the vascular status of PD patients showed that men with ventral curvature had the greatest likelihood of having cavernous veno-occlusive dysfunction (Lowsley and Boyce 1950; Jordan and Angermeier, 1993).

Surgical grafting techniques include PIG and PEG. Historically, total excision of the plaque was practiced to "cut out the disease," resulting in onlays of large grafts with an unacceptably high rate of ED (Kendirci and Hellstrom, 2004; Kadioglu et al, 2006). Therefore, plaque incision was introduced in which a modified-H or double-Y incision is made in the area of maximum curvature (Gelbard, 1995). This allows the tunic to be expanded in this area, thereby correcting the curvature and shaft caliber but minimizing the underlying exposure of the cavernous tissue and thereby reducing the potential fibrosis of the cavernosal tissue and/or interrupting the delicate veno-occlusive mechanism, which has been considered the most likely contributor to postoperative ED with these grafting procedures (Dalton et al, 1991; Hatzimouratidis et al, 2012). Using the modified-H incision allows the correction of the curvature and shaft caliber. Gelbard (1995) has suggested that using multiple incisions and filling them with grafts would result in a smoother correction of curvature and potentially less injury to the underlying cavernosal tissue (Gelbard, 1995).

We favor PEG in which the area of maximum deformity is excised, particularly if it is associated with severe indentation. **An increasing number of patients with severe deformity have indentation that if not addressed may result in a straightened penis but with residual narrowing causing instability.** The corners of the defect are darted in a radial fashion to enhance correction of the narrowing in that area (Levine, 2011). Geometric principles have been applied to the grafting technique so as to obtain a properly sized graft with excellent correction of deformity (Egydio et al, 2004). This approach has been considered unnecessarily complex, and there have been reports of a higher rate of postoperative ED when this technique has been used (Flores et al, 2011). **It appears intuitive that to reduce the risk of postoperative ED, the key is to limit the trauma to the underlying cavernosal tissue to maintain the veno-occlusive relationship between the cavernosal tissue and the overlying tunica graft.**

Graft Materials

The ideal graft should approximate the strength and elastic characteristics of normal tunica albuginea; should have minimal morbidity and tissue reaction; should be readily available, not too thick, pliable, easy to size and suture, inexpensive, and resistant to infection; and should preserve erectile capacity (Gur et al, 2011; Kadioglu et al, 2007). Multiple autologous grafts have been used historically, including fat, dermis, tunica vaginalis, dura mater, temporalis fascia, saphenous vein, crura or albuginea, and buccal mucosa (Lowsley and Boyce, 1950; Devine and Horton, 1974; Das, 1980; Lue and El-Sakka, 1998; Teloken et al, 2000; Sampaio et al, 2002; Leungwattanakij et al, 2003; Kargi et al, 2004; Shioshvili et al, 2005; Kadioglu et al, 2007). These have fallen out of favor because of a need for extended surgery to harvest the graft as well as a second surgical site, which possesses its own potential complications of healing, scarring, and possible lymphedema. Crural and buccal grafts are compromised by the inability to get enough graft material for large defects (Hatzichristou and Hatzimouratidis, 2002; Schwarzer et al, 2003; Shioshvili et al, 2005). Synthetic polyethylene terephthalate (PETE, Dacron) and polytetrafluoroethylene (PTFE, Teflon) grafts have been used historically and are not recommended now because of the potential risk of infection, localized inflammatory response, and fibrosis (Devine et al, 1997; Brannigan et al, 1998). Finally, "off-the-shelf" allografts and xenografts have emerged, including processed pericardium from a bovine or human source, porcine intestinal submucosa, and porcine skin. The two most common grafts currently used are Tutoplast (Coloplast US, Minneapolis, MN), processed human and bovine pericardium, and porcine small intestinal submucosa (SIS) grafts (Surgisis ES, Cook Urological, Spencer, IN) (Hellstrom, 1994; Hellstrom and Reddy, 2000; Knoll, 2001; Levine and Estrada, 2003). These packaged processed grafts are being used with increased frequency because of their ease of use and reduction in operating times. The pericardial grafts are thin, are strong, do not contract, and have no reports of infection or rejection. Chun and associates (2001) performed a comparison of dermal and non-Tutoplast processed human cadaveric pericardial grafts in the modified Horton-Devine procedure. Overall, 92% of patients were able to achieve successful coitus with or without assistance. These researchers reported a 33% overall recurrence rate, with 26% of patients who received dermal grafts and 44% of patients who received pericardial grafts experiencing recurrence. However, this study did not report on the severity of recurrence, and all these patients were able to achieve erections suitable for coitus. Satisfaction rates were similar, and those who underwent pericardial grafting had shorter operative times as well as decreased morbidity associated with the absence of a graft donor site (Chun et al, 2001). The SIS grafts have similar advantages to pericardium, except there have been reports of graft contraction, particularly with one-ply grafts, with associated recurrent curvature in the 37% to 75% range (Santucci et al, 2005; John et al, 2006; Breyer et al, 2007; Kovac and Brock, 2007; Taylor and Levine, 2008). Other reported postoperative complications with SIS grafts include subgraft hematoma in 26% and an infection rate of 5% (Breyer et al, 2007).

Tissue-engineered graft materials have been considered more recently and potentially offer the advantage of having a graft seeded with cellular material, which may enhance the take of the graft and potentially reduce local tissue fibrosis with diminished postoperative ED. Adipose tissue–derived stem cell–seeded SIS, human acellular matrix tunica albuginea grafts, and autologous tissue-engineered endothelialized tunica albuginea grafts have been investigated for incision and excision procedures (Schultheiss et al, 2004; da Silva et al, 2011; Imbeault et al, 2011; Ferretti et al, 2012; Ma et al, 2012). Imbeault and associates (2011) demonstrated in vitro creation of artificial tunica albuginea using human dermal fibroblast and human endothelial cells. They concluded that this tissue-engineered endothelialized tubular graft was structurally similar to normal tunic with a high burst pressure and adequate mechanical resistance. Furthermore, the autologous property of this model could represent an advantage compared with other available grafts (Imbeault et al, 2011). Such studies may help elucidate future medical treatments for PD using tissue-engineered grafts for the reconstruction of the tunica albuginea. The biomechanical properties, compatibility with the tunica albuginea, and effective neovascularization of the tissue-engineered grafts need to be investigated further before such basic research can be applied in practice.

Grafting Surgical Technique

Once the patient has achieved satisfactory general anesthesia, it is advised that the patient receive a dose of intravenous antibiotics and that the deep venous thrombosis protection apparatus be applied. The dorsal SPL should be measured. An artificial erection is then created by injecting a vasoactive drug (papaverine, Trimix, prostaglandin E_1) via a 21-gauge butterfly needle placed through the glans into the corpus cavernosum. Saline can be infused to create a full rigid erection, which allows visualization and measurement of the deformity, including curvature and areas of indentation with or without hinge effect. The preferred approach for grafting procedures is a circumcising incision made approximately 1.5 to 2 cm proximal to the corona, or through a previous circumcision site. The penis is degloved down to the Buck fascia, at which point hemostasis is obtained with bipolar cautery. It is advisable for the surgeon to use loupe magnification to reduce the likelihood of injury to neurovascular structures. With the shaft exposed, the erection can again be re-created, demonstrating the area of maximum deformity. In the circumstance of a dorsal or dorsal-lateral curvature, the Buck fascia, with the enclosed neurovascular bundle, is elevated by making a pair of parallel incisions just lateral to the urethral ridge, through the Buck fascia to the tunica albuginea. The Buck fascia is carefully elevated off the tunic. Typically this can be done with delicate, sharp dissection, but occasionally, if there is significant adhesion between the Buck fascia and the tunic, bipolar cautery can be used to elevate this with minimal risk of permanent nerve injury. Once the Buck fascia is elevated off the area of maximum deformity, a full erection is re-created. The area of maximum deformity is marked for incision or partial plaque excision. This allows excision and expansion of areas of severe indentation. It should be noted that even with a pure lateral curvature, the tunic to be excised must traverse through the dorsal septum, because this is the anchor point of the scar and if it is not taken, substantial residual curvature will likely remain (Jordan, 2007). When extensive calcification extends beyond the area of partial plaque excision, the calcified component can be removed, leaving the outer lamina intact because the calcification involves the inner circular fibers. Once the rectangular defect is established, the corners are darted in a radial fashion so as to help to recover normal shaft caliber in the area of indentation. We have simplified the geometric principle technique by ensuring that the lateral sides of the defect are of equal length (Egydio et al, 2004; Levine, 2011). In doing this, we create a uniform-sized square or rectangle, which virtually always allows satisfactory correction of lateral and dorsal curvature. Often the proximal transverse length will be longer than the distal transverse length because of distal tapering of the shaft. The penis can now be measured on stretch again; typically there will be increased dorsal length from 0.5 to 3.0 cm. Stay sutures of 4-0 PDS (Ethicon, Somerville, NJ) are placed in the four corners of the defect and at the midpoint transversely, distally, and proximally. With these stay sutures on stretch, the defect can be measured longitudinally and transversely. Our preference is to use a Tutoplast processed pericardial graft (Coloplast, Minneapolis, MN), because there is usually little graft contraction. The graft should be sized no more than 10% larger than the measured defect on stretch. Porcine SIS grafts (Cook Urological, Spencer, IN) need to be oversized by 25%. Once the graft has been cut to size, it is secured in place with the previously placed stay sutures; then, with 4-0 PDS placed in a running fashion, the graft is secured to the defect. If a large defect is created, it may be advisable to place several interrupted 4-0 PDS sutures in the area of the septum to reduce the volume of blood that can accumulate under the graft. An artificial erection is again reestablished; if there is significant residual curvature, this can be addressed with tunica plication. We have found that this is necessary in up to 25% of patients. In patients who have a more prolonged curve or in those who have substantial indentation in one area as well as a more distal curvature, the grafting should be performed in the area of indentation, and plication is used to address any residual

dorsal or lateral curve once grafting has been completed. In this circumstance a single graft can be used, which has not been shown to have a higher rate of postoperative ED than when multiple grafts are used but does have the advantage of shorter operative time. Once satisfactory deformity correction has been accomplished, the Buck fascia is reapproximated with running 4-0 chromic, and the shaft skin is reapproximated to subcoronal skin with interrupted 4-0 chromic in a horizontal mattress fashion. Of note, for those patients who are uncircumcised and do not have any evidence of phimosis, a circumcision is not necessary (Garaffa et al, 2010); but if there is any question of excessive redundant foreskin and/or phimosis, then circumcision should be performed to reduce the likelihood of postoperative paraphimosis (Garaffa et al, 2010). The penis is dressed with Xeroform gauze (3M, St. Paul, MN) placed over the circumcising incision, and then a Coban wrap (3M, St. Paul, MN) is placed distal to proximal, providing gentle compression. Typically the dressing is left in place for 3 days and then removed, at which point the patient may shower. Submersion of the wound is not advised because this may encourage wound separation.

Postoperative Management

The postoperative rehabilitation period is critical to reduce the risk of postoperative ED and length loss as well as to optimize straight healing. We find it useful to liken the importance of postoperative rehabilitation after penile surgery to the importance of the rehabilitation needed for successful orthopedic joint replacement. Typically a patient is seen 2 weeks after surgery, at which point massage and stretch therapy are initiated (Horton et al, 1987). The patient is instructed to grasp the penis by the glans and gently stretch it away from the body and then with his other hand to massage the shaft of the penis for 5 minutes twice per day for 2 to 4 weeks. The massage and stretch can be performed by the patient's partner for the second 2 weeks if possible. This will reinitiate the sexual experience for the couple and hopefully diminish the fear of reinjuring the penis, for which the partner may feel responsible. Investigators have recommended the use of nocturnal PDE5 inhibitors to enhance postoperative vasodilation, which may help support graft take, reduce cicatrix contraction, and theoretically preserve cavernosal tissue, thereby reducing postoperative ED (Levine et al, 2005). Finally, external penile traction devices have been encouraged and have been recently shown to reduce length loss postoperatively and can even enhance length gain after both grafting and plication procedures (Levine et al, 2013). In a recent report, SPL in patients who used postoperative traction therapy was shown to increase after plication and PEG procedures by +0.85 cm and +1.48 cm, respectively, versus length changes of −0.53 cm and +0.24 cm in the plication and PEG groups in which postoperative traction was not used. In fact 50% of the plication and 89% of the PEG patients using postoperative traction had measured length gain. The reported average daily use was 2.5 hours for 4.5 days per week for an average duration of 3.8 months. There was no patient reported with postoperative length loss among those who used postoperative traction therapy, and although not statistically significant, there was a trend of higher satisfaction for erect length in the groups in which postoperative traction was used. Traction is recommended to be used for 3 or more hours per day, beginning 3 to 4 weeks after surgery, once the wound can tolerate the pressures of the stretching device for 3 months (Rybak et al, 2012).

In a review of the published reports on grafting for PD over the past 12 years, satisfactory straightening was found in 74% to 100% of patients, but postoperative ED, which does not have a uniform definition in the literature and may include reduced rigidity, compared with preoperative rigidity, to complete loss of rigidity, has been reported in 5% to 54% of patients. Diminished sensation after grafting has been reported in a few series with a follow-up of less than 5 years (Taylor and Levine, 2008). In the few single-center surgical outcome reviews with 5 or more years of follow-up, ED has been reported in up to 24%, with recurrent or persistent curvature in the 8% to 12% range (Montorsi et al, 2004; Kalsi et al, 2005; Chung et al, 2011a; Usta et al, 2003). See Table 31-4 for a summary of the outcomes for penile straightening with plaque incision or excision and grafting.

Penile Prosthesis for Men with Peyronie Disease

Indications

In men with PD and concurrent ED refractory to PDE5 inhibitors, penile prosthesis placement is the procedure of choice (Levine and Lenting, 1997; Levine and Dimitriou, 2000; Kendirci and Hellstrom, 2004; Ralph and Minhas, 2004; Mulhall et al, 2005). **Additional straightening maneuvers may be necessary, including manual modeling and incising of the tunica albuginea with or without grafting.** Recently, transcorporeal approaches have been used before modeling or relaxing incisions; the plaque is incised or stretched from within the corporeal body (Shaeer, 2011; Perito and Wilson, 2013).

Techniques for Straightening When Placing a Penile Prosthesis for Peyronie Disease

An inflatable penile prosthesis (IPP) appears to be the preferred surgical implant, as the pressure within the cylinders allows for superior correction of curvature with manual modeling, as well as improved girth enhancement. Malleable prostheses, when used for PD historically, were associated with narrow, cold, and less than natural erections (Montorsi et al, 1993; Ghanem et al, 1998; Marzi et al, 1997).

Manual modeling via the penoscrotal approach is recommended with a high-pressure inflatable cylinder, but all available three-piece and two-piece devices have been used successfully to correct deformity (Wilson and Delk, 1994; Montague et al, 1996; Montorsi et al, 1996; Levine et al, 2001; Chung et al, 2012c). Our approach is to place the prosthesis cylinders first, followed by closing of the corporotomies. With use of a surrogate reservoir attached to the pump tubing, the prosthesis can be filled to full rigidity, which will allow visualization of the deformity. To protect the pump from the high pressures that may occur during manual modeling, shodded hemostat clamps are applied to the tubing between the pump and the cylinders. The penis is then bent in the contralateral direction to the curvature. It is recommended to try to hold the penis in this position for 60 to 90 seconds, but experience has suggested that around 30 seconds may be all that is possible. Once the modeling has been performed, the penis can be reassessed by instilling more fluid, reapplying the hemostats, and then performing the modeling procedure repeatedly until satisfactory curvature correction has been attained. **The modeling technique should be a gradual bending rather than a violent maneuver, because this will reduce the likelihood of inadvertent tearing of the tunic or injury to the overlying neurovascular bundle.** Urethral injuries during performance of this technique as a result of distal extrusion of the prosthetic cylinders at the fossa navicularis have been reported (Wilson and Delk, 1994; Wilson et al, 2001). To reduce the likelihood of this occurring, the bending hand should be placed on the shaft of the penis rather than on the glans, to avoid downward pressure on the tips of the cylinders. The other hand should be grasping the base of the penis with pressure over the corporotomies, which will provide support to this area and reduce the likelihood of disruption of the suture line.

Published reports on the use of modeling have indicated that successful straightening can be expected in 86% to 100% with no higher incidence of device revision; sensory deficit after manual modeling is rare but remains a potential complication that should be discussed with the patient preoperatively (Wilson and Delk, 1994; Montague et al, 1996; Wilson et al, 2001; Levine et al, 2010; Chung et al, 2012c). Although it would appear that for more severe curvature more advanced techniques are necessary, published experience has suggested that manual modeling may be used as first-line therapy for correction of curvature after prosthesis implantation (Levine et al, 2010; Chung et al, 2012c). An alternative to this would be to perform a tunic plication contralateral to the curvature before

placement of the prosthesis to correct the curvature (Rahman et al, 2004; Dugi and Morey, 2010). When there is residual curvature of greater than 30 degrees or residual indentation causing the inflated cylinder to buckle, tunical incision is recommended after elevation of the Buck fascia in that area (Levine and Dimitriou, 2000).

The transverse penoscrotal skin incision will allow access to virtually the entire shaft, except when the curvature is distal and dorsal on the shaft, so degloving the penis is not always necessary. The tunical incision is made with the cylinders deflated, using the cautery to release the tunic with an effort to preserve cavernosal tissue over the implant. When Titan cylinders (Coloplast, Minneapolis, MN) are used, the energy should be less than 30 watts to reduce potential cylinder thermal injury (Hakim et al, 1996). Once the incision has been made, the cylinders are reinflated and further modeling can be performed to optimize deformity correction. **Although there is not a clearly accepted approach, grafting is recommended when the defect measures greater than 2 cm in any dimension to reduce cicatrix contracture and cylinder herniation** (Levine and Dimitriou, 2000; Carson and Levine, 2014). **Historically, synthetic grafts were used, but currently biografts of pericardium or porcine SIS are recommended. Use of locally harvested dermal grafts is not recommended, because there is risk of transferring bacteria to the prosthesis.**

There have been limited publications looking at the long-term results with regard to outcomes and satisfaction with inflatable penile prostheses in men with PD and ED. Levine and associates (2010) reported on 90 consecutive men undergoing placement of an IPP, with 4% having satisfactory straightening with prosthesis placement alone, 79% having satisfactory curvature correction with prosthesis and modeling, 4% requiring tunical incision, and 12% having incision and pericardial grafting for correction of curvature. There was no evidence that the additional maneuvers increased the rate of mechanical failure or infection with up to 8 years of follow-up. In the nonvalidated questionnaire used in this study, overall patient satisfaction was 84%, whereas only 73% were satisfied with curvature correction. This may indicate a flaw in the design of the questionnaire, but may also reflect the general disappointment and frustration of patients with PD (Levine et al, 2010). Thus, preoperative counseling and setting appropriate expectations as with any prosthesis placement are critical (Akin-Olugbade et al, 2006). It is recommended that preoperative discussion also be focused on the goal of obtaining "functional straightness," in which a residual curvature of 20 degrees or less in any direction would likely not compromise sexual activity and may correct in time as a result of tissue expansion caused by the cylinders. A comparison of outcomes between the two three-piece inflatable devices in North America found no significant advantage with respect to device reliability, infection, or patient satisfaction (Chung et al, 2012c).

By far the most common postoperative complaint heard from men who have undergone penile prosthesis placement is length loss (Montague, 2007). The first to objectively evaluate penile length change after prosthesis implantation were Wang and associates, who demonstrated decreases of 0.8, 0.75, and 0.74 cm at 6 weeks, 6 months, and 1 year after surgery, respectively (Wang et al, 2009). This is of particular concern in the PD population, who often already have loss of penile length. Any additional length loss as a result of the implant may be distressing to the patient and should be addressed preoperatively. For those men who cannot tolerate any further length loss, a recent small pilot study using traction therapy before penile prosthesis placement in men with PD as well as other disorders causing penile shortening (e.g., prosthesis explants, radical prostatectomy) did demonstrate that after 3 to 4 months of daily traction for an average of 3 hours or more per day, there was no further loss of length after prosthesis placement, and the majority had gained some length (0.5 to 2.0 cm) compared with the pretraction SPL (Levine and Rybak, 2011). Postoperative prolonged cylinder inflation has been recommended to maintain penile length and decrease residual curvature; the device is kept inflated for 10 to 30 minutes daily for 3 months starting 6 weeks after surgery. See Table 31-6 for a summary on the outcomes of penile straightening with penile prosthesis placement.

TABLE 31-6 Outcomes of Penile Prosthesis Implantation for Peyronie Disease

AUTHOR AND DATE	PROSTHESIS TYPE	PATIENTS (N)	MEAN FOLLOW-UP (MONTHS)	ADDITIONAL STRAIGHTENING MANEUVERS (%)	SATISFACTION RATES (%)
Garaffa et al, 2011	Inflatable	129	NR	37	86
	Malleable	80	NR	16	72
Levine et al, 2010	Inflatable	90	49	96	84
DiBlasio et al, 2010	Inflatable	79	20	11	NR
Wilson and Delk, 1994	Inflatable	138	NR	8	NR
Montague et al, 2007	Inflatable	72	NR	8	67
Chaudhary et al, 2005	Inflatable	46	12	61	93
Rahman et al, 2004	Inflatable	5	22	100	100
Levine and Dimitriou, 2000	Inflatable	46	39	NR	NR
Akin-Olugbade et al, 2006	Inflatable	18	≥6	22.2	60
Usta et al, 2003	Inflatable	42	21 (12-48)	30	84
Wilson et al, 2001	Inflatable	104	60	0	99
Carson et al, 2000	Inflatable	63	NR	NR	88
Morganstern et al, 1997	Inflatable	309	42	NR	NR
Montorsi et al, 1996	Inflatable	33	17	40	79

NR, Not reported.

KEY POINTS: SURGICAL MANAGEMENT

- Surgical correction of PD with or without penile prosthesis placement remains the gold standard to correct deformity and is indicated when deformity or rigidity compromises or prevents penetrative sexual activity.
- Surgical candidates need to undergo a detailed and comprehensive consent process so that the patient will understand the potential limitations of the surgery and will have appropriate personal expectations, thereby improving postoperative satisfaction.
- For the man with satisfactory preoperative rigidity with curvature less than 60 to 70 degrees without significant indentation, some form of tunica plication is indicated. There does not appear to be any one plication technique that has been demonstrated to be superior to others, as no head-to-head comparative trials have been published.
- Men who have more severe, complex deformity but who have strong preoperative erectile function and no evidence of venous insufficiency on duplex ultrasound analysis should be considered candidates for straightening with plaque incision or PEG.
- The complications associated with these operations include incomplete straightening, recurrent curvature, shaft shortening, diminished penile sexual sensation, and ED.
- It appears that the nature of the graft is less likely the determining factor with respect to postoperative ED. On the other hand, optimum outcomes are most likely a result of proper patient selection with respect to preoperative erectile status as well as operative technique.
- For men who have inadequate rigidity and PD, penile prosthesis placement with straightening maneuvers as necessary should be considered first-line surgery.

CONCLUSION

PD is far more common than previously thought and is a growth area in urology, not only for clinical practice but also for basic science research. The mysteries of this wound-healing disorder need to be clarified, and this will likely yield better treatment options as well as potential strategies to prevent progression. It should be recognized that there are acute and stable phases and that surgery should be offered only after the scarring process has been stable for 3 to 6 months. Patients with PD should be counseled that complete correction of the deformity, including curvature, indentation, and shortening, is not likely and that the goal is to allow the patient to function sexually again. The devastating psychological impact of this disease is important to recognize, and psychological counseling is occasionally indicated and should be offered. For patients in the acute phase, not offering any therapy does little for their emotional and physical distress and may allow progression of deformity. Offering nonsurgical treatment including oral, injection, and/or mechanical therapy may stop progression and possibly improve deformity and sexual function. When surgery is indicated, the goal is to correct the deformity and prevent worsening of ED so that penetrative sexual activity is possible. The patient must understand that recovery of his pre-PD penis is not likely and that surgery carries the risk of incomplete straightening and recurrent curvature, further shaft shortening, change in sexual sensitivity, and, most important, diminished postoperative rigidity. For men with drug-refractory ED and PD, placement of a penile prosthesis with straightening maneuvers is the best approach to address both problems with one operation.

Please visit the accompanying website at www.expertconsult.com to view videos associated with this chapter.

REFERENCES

The complete reference list is available online at www.expertconsult.com.

SUGGESTED READINGS

Gonzalez-Cadavid NF, Rajfer J. Mechanisms of disease: new insights into the cellular and molecular pathology of Peyronie's disease. Nat Clin Pract Urol 2005;2:291–7.

Gur S, Limin M, Hellstrom WJ. Current status and new developments in Peyronie's disease: medical, minimally invasive and surgical treatment options. Expert Opin Pharmacother 2011;12(6):931–44.

Hatzimouratidis K, Eardley I, Giuliano F, et al. European Association of Urology. EAU guidelines on penile curvature. Eur Urol 2012;62(3):543–52.

Jalkut M, Gonzalez-Cadavid N, Rajfer J. Peyronie's disease: a review. Rev Urol 2003;5(3):142–8.

Levine LA, Burnett AL. Standard operating procdures for Peyronie's disease. J Sex Med 2013;10:230–44.

Mulhall JP, Schiff J, Guhring P. An analysis of the natural history of Peyronie's disease. J Urol 2006;175(6):2115–8, discussion 2118.

Ralph D, Gonzalez-Cadavid N, Mirone V, et al. The management of Peyronie's disease: evidence-based 2010 guidelines. J Sex Med 2010;7(7):2359–74.

Taylor FL, Levine LA. Peyronie's disease. Urol Clin North Am 2007;34(4):517–34.

32

Sexual Function and Dysfunction in the Female

Alan W. Shindel, MD, MAS, and Irwin Goldstein, MD

SEXUAL WELLNESS

At a technical consultation on sexual health sponsored by the World Health Organization, sexual wellness was defined as (World Health Organization, 2006):

1. A state of physical, emotional, mental, and social well-being in relation to sexuality
2. Not merely the absence of disease, dysfunction, and/or infirmity
3. An important and integral aspect of human development and maturation
4. A human right

Diminished sexual function is associated with impaired quality of life and well-being (Laumann et al, 1999; Davison et al, 2009). Many urologists underestimate the prevalence of female sexual concerns and do not routinely make the assessment of sexual wellness a part of their practice (Bekker et al, 2009) despite evidence that many women in urologic clinics have sexual issues (Elsamra et al, 2010).

Relatively few women discuss sexual issues with their provider (Lindau et al, 2007). There are myriad reasons for this failure to address the issues; an important example is failure of the physician to broach the subject with the patient (MacLaren, 1995; Sadovsky et al, 2006; Sobecki et al, 2012). Despite a common perception that sexuality is not of importance to older women, studies have indicated that sex remains a concern even for a substantial number of elderly women.

Data referable to this may be found on the Expert Consult website.

A basic understanding of female sexual response is important, as urologic conditions and procedures have the capacity to markedly influence female sexual wellness. **The astute urologist will be aware of how sexual function may influence or be influenced by urologic conditions and will address these issues with patients.**

FEMALE SEXUAL RESPONSE

The Sexual Response Cycle

William Masters and Virginia Johnson were among the first to report on the physical aspects of sexual response (Masters and Johnson, 1966). According to their observations, sexual response begins with **the arousal phase. The arousal phase is characterized by vulvar and clitoral swelling, vaginal lubrication and lengthening, nipple erection, increased genital sensitivity, tachycardia,** tachypnea, and subjective pleasure and excitement (Masters and Johnson, 1966; Basson et al, 2010b). The sexual arousal phase is followed by the **plateau phase during which sexual excitement/ arousal continues** (Masters and Johnson, 1966).

Orgasm may follow a variable period of arousal and sexual stimulation. **Orgasm is a "variable, transient peak sensation of intense pleasure, creating an altered state of consciousness usually accompanied by involuntary, rhythmic contraction of the pelvic striated circumvaginal musculature, with concomitant uterine and anal contractions and myotonia, usually with an induction of well-being and contentment"** (Masters and Johnson, 1966; Meston et al, 2004).

Female orgasm has a long and controversial history; for centuries there was denial that such an entity even existed in healthy women. Female orgasm (and how it can and should be obtained) continues to be a highly controversial topic (Colson, 2010). Many women climax from direct or indirect stimulation of the clitoris; others may experience orgasm during vaginal penetration with or without stimulation of the clitoris or vulva. Some healthy women do not experience orgasm during vaginal penetration under any circumstances (Masters and Johnson, 1966; Wallen and Lloyd, 2011). Anal stimulation may also play a role in attaining orgasm for a minority of women (Herbenick et al, 2010b).

After orgasm(s) there is a **resolution phase** as sexual excitement declines back to baseline levels. In women this involves reduction in pelvic blood flow, relaxation of nipple erection, and restoration of heart rate to resting levels. Sexual excitement declines to resting levels; a sense of sexual satiety and lack of desire for additional sexual activity is typical of this phase (Masters and Johnson, 1966).

There is a wide range of normal sexual response in women (Bancroft and Graham, 2011). Some women may not experience orgasm during partnered sex; others may have one or several orgasms before a return to the resting state (Fig. 32-1) (Masters and Johnson, 1966). **This heterogeneity in sexual response is not** *necessarily* associated with differing levels of sexual satisfaction.

In the 1970s, Kaplan added the concept of sexual **desire** to the linear response model. **Sexual desire was postulated to precede the development of arousal** (Kaplan, 1977). In the early 2000s, Basson stated that a linear response may not be reflective of what women experience during sex. An alternative hypothesis is that intrinsic, active sexual desire is not an essential component of sexual health for all women. Some women may have a reactive desire that occurs in response to sexual initiation by a partner or by other external stimuli. **In such women, sexual response may**

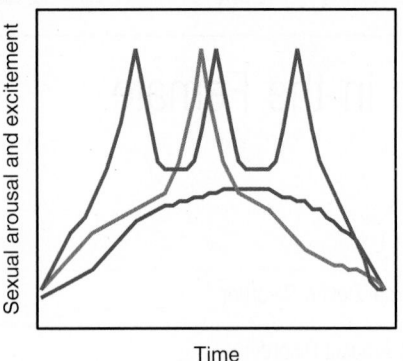

Figure 32-1. This linear sexual response cycle corresponds approximately to the models of Masters and Johnson (1966) and Kaplan (1977). Sexual arousal/excitement increases during sexual activity, reaching a peak with orgasm and eventually declining to baseline. Heterogeneity is present in female sexual response, with some women experiencing a single orgasm during a sexual encounter *(orange line)*. Other women may experience multiple orgasms *(red line)* or no orgasm *(blue line)*. Each of these patterns may be normal in a given woman.

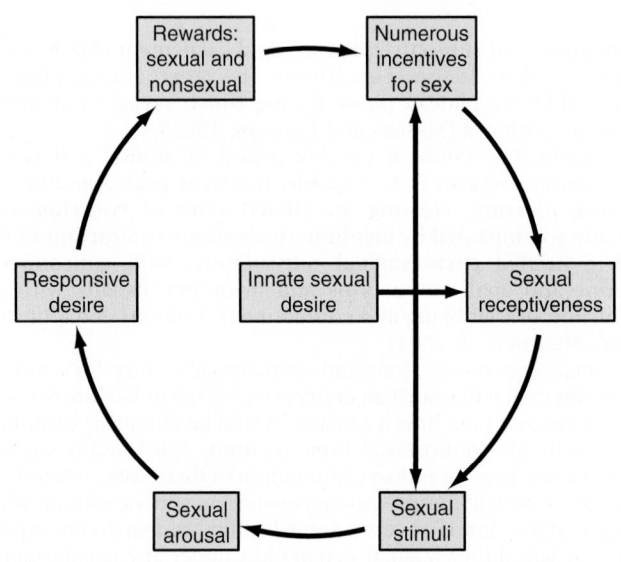

Figure 32-2. This circular sexual response cycle corresponds to the model of Basson (2002). In this model, sexual activity may occur in response to sexual desire or to previous rewards from sexual activity. With positive reward, sexual incentives are increased and sexual activity becomes more likely.

follow a circular model in which sexual activity leads to intra- and interpersonal rewards. This prompts sexual interest and receptiveness to additional sexual experiences (Fig. 32-2) (Basson, 2002). The various sexual response models are useful as a means of classification but should not be interpreted as a fixed pattern applicable to every woman and/or in every circumstance (Bancroft and Graham, 2011).

Studies on models of sexual response are discussed in more detail on the Expert Consult website.

Pelvic Anatomy and Genital Sexual Response

A detailed discussion of pelvic anatomy can be found on the Expert Consult website.

Pelvic anatomy relevant to female sexual response includes the clitoris (glans and crura), labia major and minora, the vulvar vestibule, the vagina, the vestibular bulbs, and the LA muscle (O'Connell et al, 2008). **Engorgement with blood of genital tissues is the**

unifying theme of the genital events underlying female sexual arousal (Suh et al, 2004; Yang et al, 2006). The clitoris (both glans and bulbs) is composed of erectile tissue with large dilated vascular spaces. The vascular spaces of the vagina, labia minora, and urethra are spongy but lack the large sinusoidal spaces of the clitoris; these structures may swell but do not become rigid with arousal (Yang et al, 2006).

Increased blood flow leads to attenuation of sodium reabsorption and increased oncotic pressure within the vaginal walls (Munarriz et al, 2002a). **Increased oncotic pressure produces a transudative ultrafiltrate that crosses into the vaginal lumen, producing vaginal lubrication** (Fig. 32-4 on the Expert Consult website) (Martin-Alguacil et al, 2006). Aquaporins are critical for the translocation of fluid across the vaginal mucosa. These soluble proteins translocate between the cytoplasm and the cell membrane, permitting efflux of transudate fluid through the vaginal epithelium (Kim et al, 2009). There are no glandular elements in the vagina itself. There may be some contribution to vaginal lubrication from small cervical glands and to external lubrication from vestibular (also known as Bartholin) glands around the vaginal introitus and/or the urethral Skene glands; these contributions are thought to be relatively minor (Woodard and Diamond, 2009).

Genital responses are controlled in large part by the autonomic nervous system. Generally, the parasympathetic nervous system enhances sexual response by vasodilation. The sympathetic nervous system opposes sexual responses by vasoconstriction but does play an important role in pelvic contractions with orgasm (O'Connell et al, 2008). The somatic nervous system plays a role in transmission of sensation and control of motor neurons to the pelvic floor (Schober and Pfaff, 2007).

Details on nongenital sites relevant to sexual arousal are included on the Expert Consult website.

Molecular Mechanisms

Molecular mechanisms and neuroanatomic information relevant to female sexual response are discussed on the Expert Consult website.

Neurophysiology

Serotonin

Serotonin is an important CNS neurotransmitter and is intimately linked to sexual response. Serotonergic receptors are present in the peripheral nervous system, vasculature, and vestibular glands (Fetissof et al, 1985; Frohlich and Meston, 2000). Serotonergic agonists induce vascular smooth muscle contraction by action on the 5-HT_{2A} receptor (Yang and Mehta, 1994). **Generally, serotonergic drugs (e.g., selective serotonin reuptake inhibitors [SSRIs]) have an inhibitory effect on sexual desire, arousal, and orgasm** (Balon, 2006).

More information is available on the Expert Consult website.

Dopamine and Oxytocin

Centrally, dopamine and oxytocin have been implicated as proorgasmic. Oxytocinergic and dopaminergic agonists increase sexual arousal and initiate sexual solicitation when released in the MPOA (Caldwell et al, 1989; Graham et al, 2012).

Oxytocin is synthesized in the PVN of the hypothalamus (Jenkins and Nussey, 1991) and has central and peripheral effects; it appears to mediate pair bonding in some species (Moscovice and Ziegler, 2012). In humans, oxytocin is released with orgasm and the intensity of sensation appears to correlate with the amount released (Blaicher et al, 1999; Meston and Frohlich, 2000).

Norepinephrine

Norepinephrine is the predominant sympathetic nervous system neurotransmitter in the peripheral nervous system. **Tonic** contraction of genital vasculature and suppression of arousal response are mediated by norepinephrine (Giuliano et al, 2002).

The administration of the adrenergic antagonist phentolamine has been shown to increase objective parameters of female sexual response (Rosen et al, 1999b); adrenergic agents have also been shown to reduce clitoral engorgement (Pescatori et al, 1993). Hence, there is indirect evidence of a role for the adrenergic neurotransmitter norepinephrine in opposing genital vasodilatory responses in humans as well. This effect is parsimonious with the known effects of adrenergic neurotransmitters in other vascular tissues, and this suggests that basal sympathetic tone to the female genital organs is mediated in large part by norepinephrine (Giuliano et al, 2002).

Other Neurotransmitters Relevant to Sexual Response

VIP plays a role in the CNS with respect to pair bonding during noncoital sexual intimacy (Eriksson and Uvnas-Moberg, 1990). This relationship is in addition to the important peripheral effects of VIP in the female genitalia. γ-Aminobutyric acid (GABA) and glutamate are neurotransmitters (inhibitory and excitatory, respectively) (Giuliano et al, 2002) that play a role in regulating interneuronal fibers at the level of the lumbar spinal cord. These interneurons integrate sexual stimuli (Schober and Pfaff, 2007). Acetylcholine plays a relatively minor excitatory role in female genital response. Anticholinergics have little effect on vaginal blood flow in humans (Wagner and Levin, 1980) and animals (Giuliano et al, 2001).

Hormonal Aspects of Sexual Response

Estrogens

Estrogens are the primary "female" sex steroids and estradiol (E) is the most significant of these. Estrogens act by binding to estrogen receptors (ERs). The alpha subtype (ER-α) is the most common isoform in the genitalia, although the beta subtype (ER-β) has also been detected (Hodgins et al, 1998; Saunders et al, 2000).

Estrogens have CNS effects relevant to sexual response (Rachman et al, 1998). **Estrogens maintain female genital tissue integrity and thickness** (Martin-Alguacil et al, 2006). Peak E levels occur at the midpoint of the menstrual cycle and are associated with maximal vaginal mucosal thickness and glycogen content; it is parsimonious to hypothesize that this is an evolutionary adaptation to facilitate sexual activity during the fertile window (Farage and Maibach, 2006). **With menopause there is a marked decline in genital sensitivity, vaginal thickness, collagen content, baseline moisture, and acidity** (Fig. 32-5 on the Expert Consult website). This may occur because of downregulation of VIP activity in the hypoestrogenic environment (Farage and Maibach, 2006; Martin-Alguacil et al, 2006).

Women with serum E levels less than 50 pg/mL have a markedly increased risk of vaginal dryness and pain during sexual activity (Sarrel, 2000). **Menopausal women who start E hormone replacement (vaginal or systemic) typically report increased sexual interest and enjoyment, less sexual pain, and greater orgasmic potential** (Nathorst-Boos et al, 1993; Dennerstein et al, 2005). Similar findings have been reported in women using selective estrogen receptor modulators (SERMs) and the novel synthetic hormone tibolone (Laan et al, 2001). The benefit of estrogenic therapies in nonselected menopausal women is less clear (Nastri et al, 2013). E replacement has been associated with increased risk of venous thromboembolism; some reports have also suggested that E replacement may predispose women to carcinogenesis (breast or endometrial) and cardiac disease. The issue of E replacement remains controversial (Utian et al, 2008).

E has been shown to enhance sensory fields, nerve density, and tissue mechanical properties that drive sensitivity in the genital tissues of experimental animals (Komisaruk et al, 1972; Kow and Pfaff, 1973; Pfaff et al, 1977). This effect may be mediated by E modulation of local sensory mediators important in genital sensation (Martin-Alguacil et al, 2006). E has also been shown to effect

recovery of pudendal nerves after trauma in animal models (Kane et al, 2004).

Although hypoestrogenism is associated with changes in sexual function and activity, many women with low serum estrogen report sexual interest and sexual activity that is satisfying (Cawood and Bancroft, 1996; Avis et al, 2009). Furthermore, postmenopausal women often maintain the capacity for vaginal lubrication; change in vaginal blood flow with sexual arousal is similar in healthy pre- and postmenopausal women (Laan and van Lunsen, 1997). With adequate sexual stimulation, vaginal lubrication may compensate for decreased baseline vaginal moisture (Berman et al, 1999). Postmenopausal sexual satisfaction is most strongly predicted by satisfactory sexual activity before menopause (Bachmann and Leiblum, 1991). **Ergo, estrogen status is important but not entirely predictive of sexual satisfaction in women** (van Lunsen and Laan, 2004). Sexual distress in older women may also be lower in some cases because of declines in sexual interest, which reduces the psychoemotional toll of declines in sexual functionality common in aging (Hayes and Dennerstein, 2005).

Testosterone

Testosterone (T) is the "male" sex hormone, but it is present in small quantities in women. Approximately 50% of circulating T in premenopausal women is produced by the adrenal glands with the remaining 50% produced by the ovaries (Judd et al, 1974). Activity of T is influenced by binding to sex hormone–binding globulin (SHBG) and weak binding to albumin. T bound to SHBG tends not to exert biologic effects (Bachmann and Oza, 2006).

Androgen receptors (ARs) are present in female genital tissues (Hodgins et al, 1998). The activity of the AR is of critical import in determining androgenic response to circulating T. Variations in AR activity result from a variety of factors; there has been intense interest on the trinucleotide (CAG) repeats on the AR primer (Chamberlain et al, 1994). Longer CAG repeats tend to reduce activity of the enzyme; this may influence the efficacy of serum T in producing clinically meaningful effects, although evidence to support this hypothesis in women is currently scant (Davison and Davis, 2011).

There is evidence that T plays a role in sexual appetitive behavior, maintenance of genital tissue integrity, and sexual arousal responses in women (Van Goozen et al, 1997; Riley and Riley, 2000; Traish et al, 2010). Low androgen levels are associated with a decline in sexual activity and desire (Bachmann and Leiblum, 1991). However, the relationship between T and sexuality in women is inconsistent (Davis et al, 2005; Brotto et al, 2010).

T levels decline with age in women although the rate of decrease slows after age 35. Because a substantial proportion of women's androgens are derived from adrenal sources, the decline in T production with menopause is gradual. The postmenopausal ovary produces T; women who are surgically menopausal after oophorectomy experience a more marked decline in T compared to women who are naturally menopausal (Davison et al, 2005). As SHBG levels rise with age, many postmenopausal women will experience a decline in bioavailable T, particularly if they use supplemental estrogen (another common cause of rising SHBG) (Bachmann and Oza, 2006).

Exogenous androgen increases sexual desire, arousal, and orgasmic response in women with low baseline serum androgen levels (Braunstein et al, 2005; Somboonporn et al, 2005; Shifren et al, 2006; Blumel et al, 2008; Davis et al, 2008b). A role for exogenous T in management of vulvovaginal atrophy has been demonstrated in some small studies (Witherby et al, 2011). Potential adverse effects of T treatment include application site reactions, hirsutism, acne, vaginal bleeding, and dyslipidemia (Braunstein et al, 2005; Braunstein, 2007). **There have also been substantial concerns about the risk of increased incidence of carcinogenesis, particularly hormone-sensitive tumors such as breast and endometrial** (Braunstein, 2007). The majority of long-term observation studies have not suggested a significant increase in cancer risk for women taking exogenous T for as long as 2 years (Braunstein, 2007; Davis et al, 2009; Jick et al, 2009).

An association has been reported between high serum androgen level and cardiovascular disease in women (Janssen et al, 2008). However, a 19-year longitudinal study in postmenopausal women did not detect any link between sex hormone levels and cardiovascular mortality (Barrett-Connor and Goodman-Gruen, 1995). Additionally, a long-term study in 365 female-to-male (FtM) transgender persons receiving supplemental androgen did not detect an increase in risk of cardiovascular disease (Asscheman et al, 2011). Additional data on long-term safety are needed (White et al, 2012).

T for women is off-label use in the United States. Careful discussion and documentation between patient and provider are essential if T supplementation is considered in women (Shifren et al, 2006; Wierman et al, 2010).

Dehydroepiandrosterone

Dehydroepiandrosterone (DHEA) is a weak androgen produced by the adrenal cortex. DHEA may be converted into androstenedione, a precursor to both T and E. Like T, DHEA levels tend to decline with increasing age (Davison et al, 2005).

In a study of more than 1000 Australian women, those with sulfated DHEA levels in the bottom 10th percentile experienced an increased risk for lower sexual desire, arousal, and responsiveness (Davis et al, 2005). **However, the role of supplemental DHEA in female sexual function is not established** (Arlt, 2004; Davis et al, 2011).

The Menstrual Cycle and Sexuality

Menstruation is under the regulation of several hormones, principally E (Bancroft and Graham, 2011). E gradually increases during the follicular phase and causes endometrial proliferation. Stability of the endometrium is maintained by the action of progesterone (P). E leads to a surge in LH production from the pituitary, triggering ovulation and initiating the luteal phase. T levels rise during the follicular phase to a peak around the time of ovulation (Roney and Simmons, 2013). In many women sexual desire peaks during the ovulatory phase (Burleson et al, 2002); these data are subject to several limitations (Brown et al, 2011) and there is substantial variability among women (Burleson et al, 2002; Sheldon et al, 2006; Wallen and Lloyd, 2011). After ovulation, E, P, and T gradually decline, leading to sloughing of the endometrium and the beginning of the menstrual phase (Wallach, 1970).

Hormonal contraceptives (oral, subcutaneous, injectable) modulate E to prevent ovulation. Hormonal contraceptives tend to reduce serum T (Coenen et al, 1996; Kovalevsky et al, 2010; Battaglia et al, 2012) and raise serum SHBG (Warnock et al, 2006). This synergistically lowers bioavailable T and may contribute to sexual side effects (Coenen et al, 1996). **Specific changes reported in some women using hormonal contraception include decreased sexual desire, atrophy and pain in the labia and genital tissues, decreased intercourse frequency, and decreased orgasmic function** (Fig. 32-6 on the Expert Consult website) (Battaglia et al, 2012). Some women tolerate hormonal contraception without discernible perturbation of their sexual life; several studies have reported no objective or subjective changes in sexual function in women using hormonal contraceptives (Shirtcliff et al, 2002; Greco et al, 2007; Flyckt et al, 2009; Kovalevsky et al, 2010; Lee et al, 2011). However, some women may be particularly sensitive to the androgen-lowering effects of hormonal contraception (Bancroft and Graham, 2011). The benefits of hormonal contraceptives for birth control and other concerns (e.g., dysmenorrhea, acne, etc.) should be balanced against these potential risks. Use of an agent with androgenic effects may be of benefit in women with sexual issues related to hormonal contraception (Davis et al, 2013).

Pelvic Floor Musculature

Contraction of the LA produces straightening and dilation of the vagina and elevation of the cervix (Shafik, 2000). The bulbospongiosus and ischiocavernosus muscles, located superficially and circumferential to the distal vagina, contract to increase distal vaginal tone and pressure during sexual arousal and orgasm (Shafik, 1993).

Kegel and Graber reported that the strength of the LA is directly related to sexual pleasure and orgasmic response in women (Kegel, 1952; Graber and Kline-Graber, 1979). Hypotonicity of these muscles may impair sexual response (Graziottin, 2005) and contribute to sexual problems resulting from pelvic organ prolapse and incontinence (Strohbehn, 1998). **Hypertonicity of the LA may predispose women to pain with vaginal penetration (**Rosenbaum and Owens, 2008).

MENTAL ASPECTS OF SEXUAL RESPONSE IN WOMEN

Mental and physical arousal may occur independently of one another in women. Women exposed to erotic imagery consistent with sexual orientation and preference typically experience subjective arousal and increased vaginal blood flow. Women may also have genital responses to sexual imagery that is mentally unappealing (e.g., images of the nonpreferred gender, images of nonpreferred sexual activities, etc.) despite the absence of subjective arousal (Laan et al, 1995; Chivers et al, 2007).

Additional information on sexual arousal in women is available on the Expert Consult website.

KEY POINTS: FEMALE SEXUAL RESPONSE

- Sexual response in women may be triggered by a number of intrinsic or extrinsic factors.
- NO, VIP, and a variety of other cellular messengers play important roles in female genital arousal responses.
- The CNS integrates erotic stimuli and exerts control of genital responses during arousal.
- E and T play important roles in maintaining genital tissues and modulating sexual response.
- Psychological, emotional, and mental factors play a substantial role in sexual response.

EVALUATION OF SEXUAL WELLNESS IN WOMEN

History

Sexuality and sexual health are sensitive topics and many patients (particularly older women) are hesitant to discuss these topics with their health care providers (Roos et al, 2012). Discomfort may stem from personal embarrassment or shame about sexuality, fear of embarrassing the provider, a sense that nothing can be done, a sense that sexual dysfunction is not a medical problem and/or not a significant problem to be addressed, or a simple lack of time during health care encounters (Nicolosi et al, 2006b). Unfortunately, many providers also have difficulty initiating conversations about sex for reasons similar to those given by patients (Merrill et al, 1990; Tsimtsiou et al, 2006). Many providers also report a lack of training in how to appropriately address sexuality with patients (Parish and Rubio-Aurioles, 2010; Shindel et al, 2010).

Sexual health inquiry can be incorporated into a general urologic clinic visit. Normalizing statements (e.g., "Many patients have questions or concerns about their sexual life") may help the patient to feel at ease discussing sex issues (Sadovsky et al, 2006). **A simple, open-ended question (e.g., "What concerns or questions do you have about sexuality?") is recommended as an initial screen** (Kingsberg and Althof, 2009). Yes/no questions (e.g., "Are there any problems with your sexual life that you wish to discuss with me?," "Are you satisfied with your sexual life?," "Are you having any bothersome sexual issues?") may be a more expedient and practical means to screen for sexual concerns in some contexts (Roos et al, 2012); if an affirmative response is provided to these screeners, follow-up with open-ended questions will likely produce more nuanced and informative responses (Kingsberg and Althof, 2009).

Allowing the woman to voice any concerns she has about her sexual life and satisfaction is one of the most basic but critical interventions that providers may make on behalf of sexual wellness. **The opportunity to discuss sexuality issues with a professional may substantially decrease sex-related distress** (Goldstein and Alexander, 2005).

Additional advice on taking a sexual history is available in the online supplement.

Surveys

Validated sexuality surveys are simple, unobtrusive, and reliable (Rosen, 2002; Kingsberg and Althof, 2009). In clinical practice, these instruments are useful as means to initiate a conversation about sexual issues (Clegg et al, 2012). **Survey instruments cannot replace a detailed history and physical examination** (Kingsberg and Althof, 2009). A 2010 study indicated that some female partners of men with ED had persistently low survey metric scores despite increases in sexual satisfaction (Conaglen et al, 2010).

Information on survey instruments is available on the Expert Consult website.

Evaluation of the Partner

Sexual distress is linked to incompatibility with the partner (Witting et al, 2008). **Hence involvement of the sexual partner is critical in the management of any sexual health concern.** Education of the partner may be of particular importance given the generally low knowledge of female sexual response in the community (Goldstein and Alexander, 2005).

Additional information on partner evaluation is available in the online supplement.

Physical Examination

A general physical examination including vital signs is required. The patient should be assessed for evidence of endocrinopathy, nerve injury, diabetes, or obesity (Goldstein and Alexander, 2005; Basson et al, 2010b). **Evaluation of the genitals should start with careful inspection of the external genitalia including mons pubis, labia majora, labia minora, clitoris, and vulvar vestibule. This superficial examination may show genital lesions, erythema that may predispose to sexual pain disorders, redundancy of the labia, or atrophy of the external genitalia** (Fig. 32-7 on the Expert Consult website) (Goldstein and Alexander, 2005; Basson et al, 2010b). Vulvar skin conditions are common and can lead to a variety of sexual concerns. Examples include eczema, psoriasis, contact dermatitis, fungal infections, apthous ulcers, and drug reactions.

Some dermatoses are specific to the vulva and are described on the Expert Consult website.

Testing for genital neuropathy may be accomplished by application of heat/cold stimuli, vibration, and/or application of a toothpick or small pin. A simple assessment for urinary incontinence (cough test, Q-tip test, etc.) is warranted. Urinary symptoms are associated with sexual problems and are within the scope of practice for urologists to manage.

Bimanual examination of the vagina is performed to assess for pelvic organ prolapse and ovarian pathology (Goldstein and Alexander, 2005). Assessment of the LA should be included as part of the bimanual examination (Rosenbaum and Owens, 2008). A speculum examination should be considered.

Assessment of vaginal pH is a simple, inexpensive test. High pH implies E deficiency and/or disruption of the normal vaginal microbiome; this may have relevance to recurrent infection, vulvovaginal atrophy, or other issues and should be performed routinely (Bachmann et al, 1999).

Serum and Other Laboratory Studies in the Evaluation of Sexual Wellness

The role of serum studies in evaluation of female sexual wellness is controversial (Goldstein and Alexander, 2005; Basson et al, 2010b). Serum chemistry, lipids, and glycosylated hemoglobin should be assayed, as these are low-risk tests for common problems potentially relevant to female sexual function. **Assessment of sex steroids, particularly serum E and T, should be considered if there is concern for significant endocrinopathy** (Utian et al, 2008; Kingsberg, 2009).

Serum T testing is controversial because of questions of relevance and precision of results; most widely available assays for T are not precise at the levels typical in women (Stanczyk et al, 2003; Bancroft and Graham, 2011). The timing of assay with respect to menstrual cycle should be clearly defined. T should be assayed in the morning between days 8 and 14 of a 28-day menstrual cycle (Davison and Davis, 2011). Mass spectroscopy is a preferred means for assessing T levels in women but is typically not available outside of research settings (Stanczyk, 2006). Radioimmune assay (RIA) has been shown to possess acceptable precision in quantifying androgen levels in women. The decision to measure serum T should only be made after consultation with the patient about the unknowns and with a clear sense of what will be done with the data if the test result is concerning for androgen insufficiency (Bachmann et al, 2002; Bachmann and Oza, 2006).

In the setting of very low sex steroid levels, prolactin may be assessed. Elevated prolactin is associated with decreased sexual desire and suppression of serum T levels (Atis et al, 2010). Assay of hormones such as DHEA (Munarriz et al, 2002b) and dihydrotestosterone (DHT) may be considered, but the usefulness of these tests is unclear (Davis et al, 2011).

Additional information on physiologic and sensory testing is available on the Expert Consult website.

KEY POINTS: EVALUATION OF SEXUAL WELLNESS IN WOMEN

- A complete history (medical, sexual, partner, etc.) and thorough physical examination (particularly of the genitals) is fundamental to evaluation of sexual wellness in women.
- Many patients are reticent to ask questions about sex; providers should initiate conversations about sexuality.
- Questionnaires and adjunctive testing are of benefit in some cases but do not replace history and physical examination.

SPECIAL POPULATIONS

Pregnancy

Pregnancy has biologic and psychological ramifications for a woman's sexuality (Farage and Maibach, 2006; Pauleta et al, 2010). **Sexual activity is generally safe in pregnancy.** Adaptation to the physical and emotional challenges of gravidity influence a woman's experience of her sexuality. Obstetrical involvement and advice are critical (Millheiser, 2012).

Sexual problems are generally most common in the third trimester (Leite et al, 2009). Women in the later stages of pregnancy may find some sexual positions uncomfortable; these may in some cases be resolved by use of alternative sexual positions or assistive cushions/furniture. Caution should be exercised when considering sexual activity in women with a history of cervical incompetence; repeated trauma to the cervix from vaginal penetration and prostanoids in semen may theoretically contribute to increased risk of preterm labor.

Delivery may be traumatic to the vulva and perineum. Vaginal tears, operative vaginal delivery, and episiotomy may be a source of persistent pain during intercourse with larger tears portending greater risk (Signorello et al, 2001; Leeman and Rogers, 2012). There is evidence of pelvic floor denervation and loss of pelvic floor strength in as many as 80% of women giving birth (Allen et al, 1990). **It does not appear that there is a significant difference in postpartum sexual function between women who deliver by Caesarean section and those who deliver vaginally** (Leeman and Rogers, 2012).

Although about 90% of women have resumed sexual activity by 3 months postpartum (Brubaker et al, 2008), several studies indicate that FSFI scores have not returned to baseline by that time point (Pauls et al, 2008). A major risk factor for this change may be dyspareunia, which has been reported in approximately half of postpartum women at 3 months (Barrett et al, 2000); the prevalence of dyspareunia after 3 months is generally lower (Lal et al, 2011), suggesting a decline in postdelivery dyspareunia with time.

Lactation involves robust production of the hormone prolactin, which tends to suppress estrogens and androgens; this may contribute to declines in sexual desire and dyspareunia from loss of hormone effect on genital tissues (Leeman and Rogers, 2012). The stressors of parenting a newborn and recovery from delivery are short-term barriers to sexual activity, which in some cases may lead to long-term sexuality issues (Pauleta et al, 2010).

Racial/Ethnic Minorities

Some differences in the prevalence of sexual concerns likely stem from cultural factors (Laumann et al, 2005). Perceptions of what is normal will dictate whether a woman believes the sexual issues she is experiencing are problematic (Anderson et al, 2011). Women from conservative or repressive environments tend to report lower levels of sexual satisfaction (Laumann et al, 2006). Awareness of cultural paradigms is useful; however, individual women may not conform to stereotypes of their culture.

A 2005 study reported on differences in sexual concerns of American women of Asian, European, and African ancestry. There was a high prevalence of concerns in women of all racial groups; however, the nature of those specific concerns differed. Compared to white women, African-American women were less likely to express concerns about vaginal lubrication and attractiveness but were more likely to be concerned about sexually transmitted diseases. Asian-American women were less likely than white women to report issues of sexual desire, arousal, orgasm, and dissatisfaction with sexual life although there was a slightly higher rate of concern about vaginal penetration (Nusbaum et al, 2005).

The Boston Area Community Health Study reported a lower odds ratio for sexual issues in women of black race compared to Latino and white women (Rosen et al, 2009a). A study of low-income breast cancer survivors indicated that Latino women had higher prevalence of a variety of sexual concerns (low desire, low arousal, lack of satisfaction, difficulty with orgasm) compared to Caucasian women even after controlling for covariables (Christie et al, 2010).

Physiologic differences may exist between racial/ethnic groups; these may be driven by genetics, cultural factors, and physical factors (Ravel et al, 2011). For example, serum T tends to be lower in women of African and Latino backgrounds relative to Caucasians and East Asians (Randolph et al, 2003). Whether these differences are clinically meaningful is fertile ground for future research.

Women Who Have Sex with Women and Transgender Persons

Between 1% and 2% and between 1% and 4% of women in the United States identity as lesbian or bisexual, respectively (Aaron et al, 2003; Conron et al, 2010; Herbenick et al, 2010b). Transgender persons account for 1% or less of the population but are increasingly visible in Western nations. Transgender persons include female to male (FtM or "transmen"), male to female (MtF or "transwomen"), and individuals who elect not to categorize themselves into a gender category. A person may identify as transgender without using cross-gender hormonal replacement or having gender reassignment surgery (Persson, 2009).

A provider who is not generally familiar with women who have sex with women (WSW) and transgender persons should take time to develop rapport and ask respectful questions to elucidate fully the precise nature of sexual concerns. Tactful questions and avoidance of assumptions about sexual proclivity are essential. The majority of patients will respond well to questions for clarification if such questions are asked in a respectful and nonjudgmental fashion (Stott, 2013). Care must be individualized to the patient's gender identify, sexual orientation, and sexual concerns (Wierckx et al, 2014).

Additional information on WSW and transgender persons is available on the Expert Consult website.

Disabled Women

Disabilities are mental and/or physical impairments (congenital or acquired) that limit an individual's capacity to function independently. Physical disabilities such as chronic pain, back injury, arthritis, spinal cord injury, multiple sclerosis (MS), cerebrovascular injury, amputations, and/or metabolic diseases may make sexual activity difficult or uncomfortable (Basson et al, 2010a). **However, many persons with even severe disabilities are able to adapt their sexual lives and practices to obtain a satisfying expression of their sexuality.** Providers should not assume that disabled persons cannot or should not enjoy a healthy sexual life (Tepper et al, 2001; Kreuter et al, 2011).

CNS injury or lesion can be particularly damaging to sexuality. Women with lesions of the spinal cord often report diminished genital sensation, loss of sexual self-esteem, difficulty with orgasm, and dissatisfaction with sexual responses (Tepper et al, 2001). Interestingly, genital sensation is preserved in some women with spinal cord injury. This appears to be mediated by vagus nerve fibers that bypass the spinal cord and project to the nucleus tractus solitarii region of the medulla oblongata (Komisaruk et al, 2004).

The issue of sexual activity in mentally disabled persons is an ethically and legally challenging issue (Appel, 2010). Respect for human rights warrants that a person with mental disability should not be denied the right to sexual pleasure (Greenspan, 2002); at the same time, issues of consent and coercion are difficult to resolve in persons with cognitive impairments (Spiecker and Steutel, 2002). Careful consideration and ethics consultation should be considered when such cases arise (Kennedy, 2003).

Victims of Sexual Violence

The lifetime prevalence of rape (forcible sexual penetration) or attempted rape in American women is estimated at 18% (Black et al, 2011). Data from other regions of the world suggest about 1 in 3 women globally will experience intimate partner violence or sexual violence perpetrated by a nonpartner (World Health Organization, 2013). **The prevalence of sexual abuse/violence against women underscores the importance of provider education on addressing sexuality in survivors.**

Sexual dysfunction is a common consequence of sexual violence and/or coercion (Nusbaum et al, 2005). Physical trauma to the genitals may predispose to pain from injury or muscle dysfunction (Postma et al, 2013). More relevant for the majority of cases is the psychological toll of having been forced into unwanted sexual contact. Multidisciplinary management is recommended; the primary goals of therapy are to empower the woman to feel in control of her sexuality and to dissociate consensual sexual activity from traumatic experiences (Basson et al, 2010b; Daglieri and Andelloux, 2013).

Female genital cutting is a special case of sexual violence that is addressed on the Expert Consult website.

Women with Urologic Concerns

Overactive bladder, stress urinary incontinence, and incontinence with sexual activity have been identified as independent risk factors for FSD in numerous studies (Rosen et al, 2009b; Wehbe et al, 2010). The prevalence of sexual dysfunction and/or decreased sexual activity in women with lower urinary tract symptoms varies between 19% and 50% depending on population and means of assessment. Women with urinary issues are twice as likely to report disruption of sexual life compared to their peers (Chen et al, 2013). Painful bladder syndromes and interstitial cystitis have also been linked to impairment of sexual response, sexual avoidance, and sexual pain in up to 88% of affected women (Bogart et al, 2011; Gardella et al, 2011).

Management of overactive bladder and/or stress incontinence has been clearly linked to positive changes in sexual response for women (Rogers et al, 2008; Wehbe et al, 2010). **However, placement of transvaginal mesh for pelvic organ prolapse or stress incontinence may contribute to dyspareunia, alteration of vaginal lubrication, and/or discomfort for sexual partners (**Helstrom and Nilsson, 2005; Boyles and McCrery, 2008). **Procedures that involve placement of slings may disrupt neurovascular innervations to the genital organs (**Benson and McClellan, 1993). While the risks of pelvic surgery for prolapse and/or incontinence are real several studies have reported improvements in sexual function after mesh placement; in many cases improvement is driven by resolution of incontinence and/or prolapse-related sexual dysfunction (Roovers et al, 2006; Altman et al, 2009).

Gynecologic Surgery Patients

The effects of hysterectomy on sexual function are mediated in large part by the indication for the procedure (Roovers et al, 2003); women who experience sexual dysfunction from gynecologic conditions (e.g., leiomyoma, endometriosis, etc.) (Helstrom, 1994; Grimes, 1999) are more likely to benefit from surgery whereas those without sexual issues at baseline may experience worsening of sexual function (Dennerstein et al, 1977; Carlson, 1997).

Cancer Patients

Sexual issues are common in women after pelvic cancer surgeries such as cystectomy/urethrectomy, vulvectomy, colectomy, abdominoperineal resection, and proctectomy (Raina et al, 2007; Donovan et al, 2010; Philip et al, 2013). Sexual dysfunction is also a risk of pelvic radiotherapy as a primary or adjuvant treatment (Incrocci and Jensen, 2013). Disruption of pelvic neurovasculature, side effects of treatment, and body image issues may predispose to impairment of sexual responses and pain (Raina et al, 2007).

In cystectomy and/or urethrectomy the anterior vaginal wall may be partially resected or otherwise compromised, leading to difficulty with vaginal penetration (Yang et al, 2006). Disruption of the nerve innervation to the external genitalia, vagina and clitoris is a common risk during cystectomy/urethrectomy (Stenzl et al, 1995). A 2004 study indicated that difficulty with orgasm, desire, and arousal are very common in women after radical cystectomy. **Slightly less than half of female cystectomy patients engage in coital intercourse after cystectomy and slightly over half report a decline in sexual life satisfaction** (Zippe et al, 2004).

 Issues in cancer survivorship are discussed in more detail on the Expert Consult website.

KEY POINTS: SPECIAL POPULATIONS

- A woman's sexuality may be affected by medical, sociocultural, and life factors.
- Sensitivity to the sexual wellness needs of minority populations and/or women who have suffered trauma is an essential component of professionalism.

FEMALE SEXUAL DYSFUNCTION
Semantics and Controversy

Female sexual dysfunction (FSD) is an umbrella term that encompasses distressing situations that interfere with a woman's ability to enjoy a satisfying sexual life. FSD is not truly a diagnosis but rather an umbrella term that may encompass one or more distressing situations that interfere with a woman's ability to enjoy a satisfying sexual life.

Controversies regarding FSD are addressed on the Expert Consult website.

Epidemiology

There is marked variability in the prevalence of sexual issues between regions (Laumann et al, 2006). Prevalence of sexual issues in the general female population is ambiguous due to selection bias, limited data collection, and variation/disagreement about what constitutes a sexual problem. Studies on the prevalence of FSD are presented in Table 32-1.

Disruption of sexual response and sexuality-related distress may occur independently. In a U.K. study of female twins only 37% of women with sexual dysfunction (assessed by Female Sexual Function Index [FSFI]) had concomitant sexual distress (assessed by the Female Sexual Distress Scale [FSDS]) (Burri et al, 2011). It is also important to note that not every sexually distressing situation is a sexual dysfunction; a woman may have distress about sexuality that is related to interpersonal issues rather than a disturbance in her own sexual response. The same twin study from the United Kingdom demonstrated that up to 16% of women who had "normal" sexual function per the FSFI still reported significant sexual distress. In cases of sexual distress without sexual dysfunction, interpersonal and/or psychological issues (Burri et al, 2011) were the principal bothersome issues. In a study of over 31,000 women in the United States, 43% of women had a sexual concern but just 22% endorsed sexual distress; just 12% had a sexual problem and distress (Shifren et al, 2008). A similar Finnish study reported a 34% prevalence of FSD, 36% prevalence of sexual distress, and a 20% prevalence of concomitant sexual dysfunction and distress (Witting et al, 2008).

Due to ambiguity in terminology, Raina et al (2007) have suggested a tripartite classification system:
1. *Sexual complaints* are expressions of discontent associated with sexual function. Women with sexual complaints are likely to have issues related to their partner and/or their personal experience of sexuality. Education on the anatomy and physiology of sexual response as well as communication and interpersonal skills may be sufficient to resolve many sexual complaints
2. *Sexual dysfunction* is a disturbance in one more or more phases of the sexual response cycle and/or pain during sexual activity. Women with sexual dysfunction may compensate for it in some fashion and thus preserve a sense of sexual satisfaction or at least contentment.
3. *Sexual disorder* is the combination of sexual dysfunction and personal distress relating to the sexual dysfunction. These women merit complete evaluation to assess for etiology and treatment options.

Whether one adheres to this classification scheme or not, it is always important when evaluating research or seeing a patient to gauge personal distress as this is a very important determinant of which treatments are indicated/desired.

Sexual dysfunction is more frequent in older women; *sexual complaints* may be more frequent in younger women (Roos et al, 2012). Similarly, distress related to sexual issues appears to be higher in premenopausal versus menopausal women (Berra et al, 2010); this may be due in part to adaptation on the part of some older women. The highest prevalence of sexual concerns with attendant distress is in women aged 45-64 (Shifren et al, 2008). It is reasonable to hypothesize that this is an age group in whom sexual activity remains a priority despite physical changes of menopause and advancing age, which may compromise sexual response. Distress is

TABLE 32-1 Epidemiology of Female Sexual Dysfunction (FSD) in General Populations

STUDY	REGION	POPULATION	FSD DEFINITION	FSD PREVALENCE	NOTES
Laumann et al, 1999	USA	1749 women aged 18-59	Yes on ≥1 PRO	43%	
Oksuz and Malhan, 2006	Turkey	518 women aged 18-55	FSFI ≦25	48%	
Nicolosi et al, 2005	Asia	3350 women aged 40-80	Sometimes or occasionally experiencing >1 PRO	32% to 82%	Lack of interest most common
Nicolosi et al, 2006b	Anglophone Countries	3006 women aged 40-80	Sometimes or occasionally experiencing >1 PRO	28% to 57%	Lack of interest most common
Nicolosi et al, 2006a	Europe	5023 women aged 40-80	Sometimes or occasionally experiencing >1 PRO	23% to 46%	Lack of interest most common
West et al, 2008	USA	1944 women aged 30-70	PFSF ≧ 40 = low desire PFSF* < 40 + PDS† ≧ 60 = HSDD	Low desire 36%; HSDD 8%	Assessment of sexual desire only
Valadares et al, 2008	Brazil	315 women aged 40-65 with 11+ years of school	PEQ score ≦7	36%	
Shifren et al, 2008	USA	31,581 women aged 18+	CSFQ response of "never" or "rarely"	43%	Sexual distress was 22% with combined distress and FSD in 12%
Witting et al, 2008	Finland	6601 women aged 18-33	FSFI <26.55	35%	
Chedraui et al, 2009	Ecuador	409 women aged 40-59	FSFI <26.55	56%	Lubrication and pain domains were lowest
Rosen et al, 2009b	USA	3202 women aged 30-79	FSFI <26.55	40%	Only 51% sexually active in past 4 wk
Blumel et al, 2009	Latin America	7243 women aged 40-59	FSFI <26.55	57%	74% sexually active
Ishak et al, 2010	Malaysia	163 women aged 18-65	Malaysian FSFI ≦55	26%	
Echeverry et al, 2010	Colombia	410 women aged 18-40	FSFI <26.5	30%	
Shindel et al, 2011	USA	1241 women aged 25 ± 3	FSFI <26.55	50%	
Mezones-Holguin et al, 2011	Peru	335 women aged 40-59	FSFI <26.5	35%	
Shindel et al, 2012	North America	1566 WSW aged 18-86	Modified FSFI <26.55	25%	
Moghassemi et al, 2011	Iran	149 women aged 43-64	FSFI <26.5	87%	
Zhang and Yip, 2012	Hong Kong	1410 women aged 19-49	Face-to-face interview using DSM-IV-TR criteria	38%	

*From Derogatis L, Rust J, Golombok S, et al. Validation of the profile of female sexual function (PFSF) in surgically and naturally menopausal women. J Sex Marital Ther 2004;30:25–36.
†From Derogatis L, Rust J, Golombok S, et al. A patient-generated multinational inventory to measure distress associated with low desire (PDS). International Society for the Study of Women's Sexual Health (ISSWSH) 2004 Annual Meeting, Atlanta, Georgia, October 28-31, 2004.
CSFQ, Changes in Sexual Functioning Questionnaire; DSM-IV-TR, *Diagnostic and statistical manual for mental disorders,* fourth edition, text revision; FSFI, female sexual function index; HSDD, hypoactive sexual desire disorder; PDS, personal distress scale; PEQ, personal experiences questionnaire; PFSF, profile of female sexual function; PRO, patient reported outcomes; WSW, women who have sex with women.

TABLE 32-2 Prevalence and Definition of Female Sexual Dysfunctions

	PREVALENCE*	DEFINITION†
Hypoactive sexual desire/low libido	9%-60%	Diminished feelings of sexual interest or desire, absence of sexual thoughts, and/or lack of receptivity to sexual activity‡
Sexual arousal disorder/sex not pleasurable	5%-51%	**Genital Female Sexual Arousal Disorder**: Disruption of clitoral erection, vaginal vasocongestion, vaginal lubrication
Difficulty with genital lubrication	8%-60%	**Psychological Female Sexual Arousal Disorder:** Absent or markedly diminished feelings of excitement or pleasure in response to sexual stimuli
		Mixed Female Sexual Arousal Disorder: GFSAD and PFSAD
Persistent genital arousal disorder	~1%	Persistent, recurrent, intrusive, and/or distressing sensations of genital arousal not related to sexual stimulation and that do not resolve after orgasm
Female orgasmic disorder	7%-65%	Lack of experience of orgasm or diminished orgasm intensity despite high sexual arousal after a period of sufficient sexual stimulation and arousal
Sexual pain disorders	4%-42%	**Dyspareunia:** Persistent/recurrent pain with attempted/complete vaginal entry with a penis, finger, or other object
		Vaginismus: as vaginal spasm or pain in response to penetration with a penis, finger, or other object despite a desire for penetration to occur‡
Anxiety about sexual performance	6%-16%	N/A

*Laumann et al, 1999; Nicolosi et al, 2005, 2006a, 2006b; Shifren et al, 2008; West et al, 2008; Witting et al, 2008; Garvey et al, 2009.
†Waldinger et al, 2009; Basson et al, 2010b.
‡The term *vaginismus* is no longer preferred, as it includes significant semantic baggage as a psychological disorder.

also more frequent in women who are partnered; a woman who is unpartnered may not be concerned with sexuality and will not have bother stemming from being unable to satisfy her partner.

FSD has been linked to increasing age (Hisasue et al, 2005; Ponholzer et al, 2005; Oksuz and Malhan, 2006; Valadares et al, 2008; Blumel et al, 2009; Chedraui et al, 2009), **menopausal symptoms** (Oksuz and Malhan, 2006; Valadares et al, 2008; West et al, 2008; Chedraui et al, 2009; Nappi and Lachowsky, 2009), **absence of partner** (Valadares et al, 2008), **age of partner** (Chedraui et al, 2009), **partner sexual dysfunction** (Hisasue et al, 2005; Blumel et al, 2009; Chevret-Measson et al, 2009; Zhang and Yip, 2012), **marital discord** (Zhang and Yip, 2012), urinary incontinence (Rosen et al, 2009b; Kim et al, 2011), **urinary symptoms** (Blumel et al, 2009; Rosen et al, 2009b; Mezones-Holguin et al, 2011; Shindel et al, 2012), **depression** (West et al, 2008; Rosen et al, 2009b; Echeverry et al, 2010), **tobacco use** (Oksuz and Malhan, 2006; Roos et al, 2012), **sedentary lifestyle** (Esposito et al, 2010), **infertility** (Millheiser et al, 2010), **HIV infection** (Wilson et al, 2010), **hypothyroidism** (Atis et al, 2010), **diabetes** (Giraldi and Kristensen, 2010), **sleep apnea** (Subramanian et al, 2010), **and poor general health** (Valadares et al, 2008; Blumel et al, 2009; Ishak et al, 2010; Navaneethan et al, 2010).

Several factors have conflicting data on association with FSD. **Estrogen replacement has been linked to both better** (Chedraui et al, 2009) **and worse** (Blumel et al, 2009) **sexual function in postmenopausal women.** Similarly, both **higher** (Chedraui et al, 2009) **and lower** (Blumel et al, 2009; Echeverry et al, 2010) **educational achievement have been linked to risk of FSD.** Conflicting data have been reported on the role of obesity in FSD. Some studies have reported **lower rates of sexual activity and sexual desire** (Smith et al, 2012) **in obese women and in women with metabolic syndrome** (Martelli et al, 2012); however other studies (Christensen et al, 2011) have suggested that **among women who are sexually active, obesity** (Christensen et al, 2011) **and metabolic syndrome** (Kim et al, 2011) **are not linked to sexual dysfunction.** Although data are ambiguous, concern for general health dictates that practitioners should encourage patients to maintain healthy body weight (Goldstein and Alexander, 2005).

Classification

Linear sexual response cycles have served as the foundation for most modern classification systems for FSD (Masters and Johnson, 1966).

While the linear model may not perfectly reflect sexual response in every woman it does represent a convenient means to organize diagnostic criteria. A summary of specific female sexual issues and their estimated prevalence is presented in Table 32-2. **There is substantial comorbidity between sexual issues in women** (Giles and McCabe, 2009).

The fifth edition of the *Diagnostic and Statistical Manual for Mental Disorders* (DSM-5) incorporated several changes to diagnostic criteria for FSD. DSM-5 emphasizes that FSD should be categorized as lifelong versus acquired and generalized versus situational. Duration of at least 6 months is required to apply a diagnosis except in the case of medication-induced sexual dysfunction.

In the DSM-5 sexual desire and arousal disorders in women have been combined into "female sexual interest/arousal disorder." This change was to address concerns that active sexual desire is not present in all sexually healthy women (Basson, 2002) and that some women do not differentiate sexual arousal from desire (Graham et al, 2004; Brotto et al, 2009). Similarly, **the DSM-IV terms "vaginismus" and "dyspareunia" have been combined into "genito-pelvic pain/penetration disorder" in DSM-5.** These recategorizations were controversial (Derogatis et al, 2010).

There has been scant research using these new diagnoses; in the interest of simplicity we will outline this chapter according to previous diagnostic categories (Basson et al, 2004).

KEY POINTS: FEMALE SEXUAL DYSFUNCTION

- FSD is a controversial topic but one of great importance to many women.
- A variety of medical and psychosocial issues have been clearly linked to risk of sexual concerns in women.
- Classification of female sexual disorders remains controversial; however, most classification schemes recognize disorders of sexual desire/interest, arousal, orgasm, and sexual pain.

HYPOACTIVE SEXUAL DESIRE DISORDER

Etiology

There are numerous causes for low sexual desire in women. Hubin and colleagues (2011) proposed five axes relevant to hypoactive

TABLE 32-3 Risk Factors for Hypoactive Sexual Desire Disorder

Cognitive	Lack of knowledge, negative anticipation, distractions, negative body image, depression
Physiologic	Neurologic, hormonal, surgical, iatrogenic, age
Behavioral	Avoidance, detachment linked to routine, habituation to infrequent sex
Emotional	Guilt, anxiety, insecurity, conflict
Environmental	Work/family obligations, poor communication, decreased attraction, societal influence

Modified from Hubin A, De Sutter P, Reynaert C. Etiological factors in female hypoactive sexual desire disorder sexologies. 2011;20:149–57.

BOX 32-1 Medications Associated with Female Sexual Dysfunction

Antiandrogens
  Spironolactone
  LHRH agonists
Anticonvulsants
Anticholinergics
Antidepressants
Antiestrogens
  Tamoxifen
  Raloxifene
  LHRH agonists
Antihistamines
Antihypertensives
  Diuretics
  β-blockers
  Calcium channel blockers
Chemotherapy
  Cyclophosphamide
Corticosteroids
Hormones
  Contraceptives
  GnRH agonists
Metoclopramide
Metronidazole
Recreational drugs
  Alcohol
  Amphetamines

GnRH, gonadotropin-releasing hormone; LHRH, luteinizing hormone–releasing hormone.

Modified from Jha S, Thakar R. Female sexual dysfunction. Eur J Obstet Gynecol Reprod Biol 2010;153:117–23.

sexual desire disorder (HSDD): cognitive, physiologic, behavioral, emotional, and environmental (Table 32-3). **Women who do not experience desire at baseline but who respond to sexual initiation and are not distressed do not meet criteria for HSDD** (Basson, 2002).

It is important to clarify that many early studies characterized sexual desire in terms of spontaneous sexual interest and desire. There is increasing evidence that for many women absence of sexual desire may be typical and not associated with distress. This relationship may be compounded by the self-attribution theory, which articulates that individuals may determine personal beliefs based on their personal behaviors rather than vice versa. For example, a woman who does not think about or initiate sex but who is receptive to sexual stimuli and enjoys sexual activity may (mistakenly) conclude that she is not interested in sex (Eccles and Wigfield, 2002).

Events or issues that occurred prior to onset of decreased sexual desire should be assessed. Common precipitating factors include hormonal changes, medication use, changes in relationship status, or life stressors (Brotto et al, 2010). It is very common for women to experience a reactive decline in sexual desire in the presence of other impediments to sexual activity. It may also be helpful to elucidate whether the decline in sexual interest is mental, emotional, or both. A subtle but important distinction may exist between absence of visceral desire for sex (nonspecific and colloquially referred to as "being horny") and absence of intellectual interest in sexual pleasure/intimacy (which may be related to psychosocial and partner issues). Patients may not be able to differentiate but this inquiry could provide valuable insights.

Hypoestrogenism has been clearly linked to decreased sexual desire in women, primarily in association with menopause. Women who are surgically menopausal report more severe perturbation of sexual desire relative to nonmenopausal women (de Almeida et al, 2011) and naturally menopausal women (West et al, 2008). Androgen deficiency has also been linked to decreased sexual interest in women (Warnock et al, 1997).

Psychosocial stressors have a marked effect on sexual interest in women. Depression is prevalent and includes a well-known association with HSDD. The HSDD Registry for women reported that up to one third of women with HSDD also report clinically significant depressive symptoms (Clayton et al, 2012). Sexual interest also declines with increasing relationship duration and/or with partner conflict (Segraves, 2002). Interestingly, although aging is associated with declines in sexual desire, associated distress may also decrease; this may account for the relatively lower rate of HSDD in older women compared to younger women (West et al, 2008).

The use of medications, particularly antidepressants of the SSRI class, is associated with HSDD (Montejo et al, 2001; Clayton et al, 2006). Other classes of medication commonly associated with HSDD in women are presented in Box 32-1; virtually every medicine has at least anecdotally been linked to a risk for sexual problems.

Treatment

At the time of this writing, there is no approved pharmacotherapy for HSDD in women. Attention to psychosocial issues and partner variables is of critical import. Stress reduction strategies, maintenance of general health, and addressing relationship issues are generally regarded as positive interventions, although empiric studies are scant.

Sexual interest can be an end unto itself and sexual desire can be positively perceived even in the absence of sexual activity (Wallen and Lloyd, 2011). This finding argues against the regulatory agency mandate that the end point of greatest interest in the treatment of HSDD is "satisfying sexual events" (Derogatis et al, 2011). Many women endorse satisfaction from sexual desire or a "desire to be desired"; this does not require a sexual encounter (satisfying or otherwise) to yield benefit (Meana, 2010; Bancroft and Graham, 2011). These topics remain controversial and speak to the need for more focused qualitative research on the fundamental underpinnings of women's sexual function.

Psychosexual Therapy

There are numerous mental health approaches to addressing HSDD in women. The general goals of therapy include education on sexual physiology and response, determination of type and frequency of sexual activity that is personally desired, and developing interpersonal communication skills (Kingsberg and Althof, 2009; Althof, 2010).

Cessation/Modulation of Medical Therapy

The ideal resolution of sexual problems related to a medication is cessation or substitution with a less side-effect–prone medication that produces similar effects. This is a preferred management strategy for SSRI-associated sexual dysfunction. Alternative strategies include "drug holidays," decreased dosages, and alternative agents acting as replacements or adjuncts (Ahrold and Meston, 2009; Fabre et al, 2011; Clayton et al, 2013; Taylor et al, 2013).

A meta-analysis of adjunctive treatments for SSRI-induced sexual dysfunction confirmed that twice-daily dosing with bupropion 150 mg improved sexual function outcomes; benefit was not realized with a single daily dose (Taylor et al, 2013). The 5-HT_{1A} partial agonist buspirone (20 to 60 mg/day) has also shown superior efficacy compared to placebo (50% remission for buspirone vs. 20% for placebo) for the management of sexual symptoms in women taking an SSRI for major depression (Landen et al, 1999). A randomized study of women taking SSRIs for depressive symptoms indicated that on-demand use of sildenafil (50 to 100 mg on demand) enhanced orgasmic function relative to placebo (Nurnberg et al, 2008).

Estrogens

E plays an important role in sexual desire for women (Nappi and Polatti, 2009). Correction of E deficiency has been associated with improvement in female sexual function, including desire (Gast et al, 2009; Nastri et al, 2013). This may occur by direct action on libido or by improvement in sexual arousal response and reduction in genital pain resulting from vulvovaginal atrophy.

Androgens

Supplementation with T increases sexual desire in women with low libido and low serum androgen levels (Lobo et al, 2003; North American Menopause Society, 2005). Studies on androgen for the management of HSDD in women are presented in Table 32-4. T has also been shown to improve other aspects of sexual function such as orgasm, pleasure concerns, responsiveness, and self-image (Davis et al, 2006; Shifren et al, 2006; Davis et al, 2008a, 2008b). Although most studies have investigated T as an adjunct to estrogen (in premenopausal women or in postmenopausal women already taking an estrogen supplement), a number have also investigated T monotherapy and have shown similar benefit with respect to sexual interest, desire, and sexual events (Davis et al, 2008b). T supplementation may work in part by increasing general markers for quality of life such as feelings of health, energy, and sense of well-being (Shifren et al, 2000). Mood and affect are crucially important in sexual response, and enhancement of these parameters may be of great benefit (Middleton et al, 2008).

A T patch was approved in Europe as a treatment for HSDD in women; the product was subsequently withdrawn (European Medicines Agency, 2012). The T-patch treatment did not achieve approval in the United States because of concerns about long-term safety and a perceived lack of clarity regarding the concept of female androgen insufficiency. Currently there is no approved androgen-based treatment for sexual-interest disorders in women in the United States (Wierman et al, 2006). Off-label T is used in women by some clinicians (Bachmann et al, 2002; Goldstein and Alexander, 2005).

Use of tibolone, flibanserin, bremelanotide, and other drugs for HSDD is detailed on the Expert Consult website.

FEMALE SEXUAL AROUSAL DISORDER

Female sexual arousal disorder (FSAD) may refer to the disruption of genital responses (GFSAD), to psychological arousal responses (PFSAD), or mixed FGSAD and PFSAD (Basson et al, 2010b).

Etiology

Atherosclerotic lesions reduce genital blood flow and responsiveness in animal models of FSD (Park et al, 2000; Traish et al, 2010). Vascular or neurologic disease may also contribute to GFSAD (Goldstein and Berman, 1998; Traish et al, 2010). Pelvic surgery (gynecologic, urologic, or colorectal) may also perturb genital innervations (particularly the autonomic innervation of the pelvic nerve) and vascular supply (Raina et al, 2007). Nicotine is associated with impairment of genital response (Harte and Meston, 2008). Diabetes represents a special risk factor for FSD, as it may be associated with neurologic, vascular, and/or hormonal defects (Kim et al, 2009; Giraldi and Kristensen, 2010) in addition to marked psychological morbidity (Bitzer and Alder, 2009).

In addition to their known effects on sexual desire, antidepressants may also impair genital arousal responses. Animal models have demonstrated inhibition of genital vasodilation from pelvic nerve stimulation after administration of antidepressant medications including SSRIs and serotonin/norepinephrine reuptake inhibitors (Angulo et al, 2004). In this same study there was some difference within class, suggesting that effects may be not be universal for all antidepressants or in all women. Furthermore, as depression itself is a risk factor for sexual dysfunction, some women may experience improvement in sexual satisfaction when treated with antidepressant drugs (Ishak et al, 2013).

The hormonal milieu may have a profound influence on genital tissues; hence endocrinopathy is an important cause of GFSAD. Perturbation of genital response (thinning of vagina, dryness, rise in pH) is often attributable to hypoestrogenism from menopause (Bachmann et al, 1999).

PFASD typically originates from psychological causes. Common examples include dissatisfaction with a sexual partner, nonsexual stressors that reduce mental energy required for fostering of sexual interest, and depression (Basson et al, 2010b).

Evaluation of Female Sexual Arousal Disorder

Appropriate characterization of FSAD is required to determine etiology and potential avenues for intervention. A precise history is critical to this process. Time of onset and associated factors should be assessed. Attention to the woman's feelings and relationship status is also of critical import (Brotto et al, 2010).

Treatment of Female Sexual Arousal Disorder

Psychosocial

Attention to psychosocial factors mediating FSAD is always an important component of treatment. These issues may or may not be primary in causing FSAD but they will be present to some extent in virtually every case. These issues should be addressed, or appropriate referral to a therapist should be made early in treatment.

Devices

The Eros Clitoral Therapy Device (Eros-CTD) is a battery-powered vacuum-driven suction device designed to be applied to the clitoris. In a validation study it was shown to enhance sensation, arousal, and orgasmic potential in women with and without sexual concerns (Billups et al, 2001).

Outside the realm of medical devices there exists a wide variety of sexual enhancement products. Examples include vibrators/massagers, dildos, and devices used for erotic/fantasy role-play (Queen, 2013). These devices may be of great usefulness in improving sexual response. Studies have indicated that many women use and have used vibrators for sexual stimulation; vibrator use has been associated with better scores on the FSFI (Herbenick et al, 2009, 2010a). Fantasy role-play and power exchange activities such as consensual bondage/domination/sadomasochism (BDSM) are used for sexual stimulation by small but significant numbers of women (Moser and Kleinplatz, 2006; Richters et al, 2008).

TABLE 32-4 Randomized Controlled Trials of Testosterone Therapy for Hypoactive Sexual Desire Disorder (HSDD)

STUDY	N	TREATMENT	DIFFERENCE VS. PLACEBO					
			SSE	PFSF-AROUSAL	PFSF-DESIRE	PDS	BISF-W	AE
Braunstein et al, 2005	447 women with HSDD, surgically menopausal, on estrogen	T transdermal patch (150-450 µg/day)	NR	8*	~5*	NS	NR	6%
Simon et al, 2005	562 women with HSDD, surgically menopausal, on estrogen	T transdermal patch (300 µg/day)	1.1†	5†	5†	−7.7†	NR	−2%
Davis et al, 2006	77 women with HSDD, surgically menopausal, on estrogen	T transdermal patch (300 µg/day)	0.5	19†	10†	−19.3†	NR	−1%
Shifren et al, 2006	238 women with HSDD, naturally menopausal on estrogen	T transdermal patch (300 µg/day)	1.6†	26%†	5.8†	−9†	NR	6%
El-Hage et al, 2007	36 women with HSDD, surgically menopausal, on estrogen	T transdermal cream (10 mg/day)	NR	NR	NR	NR	8.2†	NR
Davis et al, 2008a	261 women with decrease in satisfying sex, premenopausal	T transdermal spray (2.8-9 mg/day)	0.4-0.8†	NR	NR	NR	NR	11%-16%
Davis et al, 2008b	814 women with HSDD, menopausal, not on systemic estrogen‡	T transdermal patch (150 or 300 µg/day)	1.4*	~10†	~8†	~−11†	NR	0%
Panay et al, 2010	272 women with HSDD, naturally menopausal (26% on estrogen)	T transdermal patch (300 µg/day)	1.2†	~14†	7.6†	11.5†	NR	9%

AE, incidence of adverse events; BISF-W, Brief Index of Sexual Functioning for Women; NR, not reported; NS, not significant; PFSF, profile of female sexual function; PDS, personal distress scale; SSE, satisfying sexual event/mo; T, testosterone.
*Significant differences only with 300 µg/day patch.
†Statistically significant ($P < .05$).
‡Women taking vaginal estrogens continued on stable dosing regimens.

Some sexual enhancement products are marketed as "novelty items" not actually for use in sexual contexts to limit manufacturer liability for potential injuries. Urologists need not be experts in such devices but should advise patients to use reasonable cautions to prevent trauma (e.g., laceration, electric shock, numbness, loss inside a body cavity, etc.) (Aaronson and Shindel, 2010).

Oral Pharmacotherapy

PDE5I have been of great interest in treating FSAD because of the similarities in the mechanisms of vascular engorgement between men and women (Kim et al, 2003; Munarriz et al, 2003). Taken in aggregate, the data are conflicting on the efficacy of sildenafil (50 to 100 mg) for FSAD (Chivers and Rosen, 2010). The greatest efficacy of these drugs has been demonstrated in women with clearly defined etiologies for impairment of genital response, typically

neurologic lesions such as spinal cord injury, MS, or diabetes (Sipski et al, 2000; Dasgupta et al, 2004; Caruso et al, 2006). **PDE5 inhibitors are not approved for use in women and hence any use of these drugs in women is off label.**

Details on apomorphine, transdermal agents, lubricants, and hormones are detailed on the Expert Consult website.

PERSISTENT GENITAL AROUSAL DISORDER

Persistent genital arousal disorder (PGAD) is persistent, recurrent, intrusive, and/or distressing sensations of genital arousal that are not related to sexual stimulation and that do not resolve after orgasm (Basson et al, 2010b). Genital sensations associated with PGAD include throbbing, lubrication, pelvic congestion, sense of imminent hygasm without climax, and unprovoked orgasm (Waldinger and Schweitzer, 2009). The degree of distress is apparent from the fact that more than 20% of women presenting with PGAD in one series requested clitorectomy for management (Waldinger and Schweitzer, 2009). On the other hand, unprovoked sexual arousal may engender positive feelings in some women (Leiblum and Chivers, 2007).

Reliable data on the prevalence of PGAD are scant (Leiblum and Nathan, 2001; Waldinger et al, 2009). A survey of 96 women presenting to a sexual health clinic indicated that just one patient met the full five-point criteria for PGAD. Importantly, about one third reported at least one symptom of PGAD (Garvey et al, 2009). Whether this represents a continuum of PGAD severity or a difference in subjective perception of bother is unclear.

Etiology

PGAD has been associated with a dysfunction of sexual beliefs (Carvalho et al, 2013) and restless legs syndrome (Waldinger and Schweitzer, 2009). PGAD has also been associated with anxiety and obsessive-compulsive symptoms (Leiblum and Chivers, 2007), dietary soy intake (Amsterdam et al, 2005), sleep disturbances (Wylie et al, 2006), periclitoral masses (Bedell et al, 2014), spinal tumors, withdrawal of SSRI medications (Goldmeier et al, 2006; Leiblum and Goldmeier, 2008), and pelvic arteriovenous malformations (Goldstein et al, 1995).

The largest series of women with confirmed PGAD included 18 Dutch women. It was reported that two thirds of the women presenting with PGAD were menopausal. Also noted was a high (55%) prevalence of pelvic varices; it is unclear whether or not menopause and the prevalence of pelvic varices are related, as varices are common in older women (Waldinger et al, 2009). Additional evaluations (brain MRI, pelvic MRI, electroencephalogram, transvaginal ultrasound, and serum hormone levels) were not conclusively demonstrative of any abnormalities (Waldinger et al, 2009). However, clinical examination of these women demonstrated that two thirds of them had restless legs syndrome and/or overactive bladder (Waldinger and Schweitzer, 2009). Many women also reported exacerbation of PGAD symptoms with stress. The authors hypothesized that PGAD may be a manifestation of nonsexual "hyperexcitability" of the genitals.

Evaluation

A careful physical examination may show genital anomalies that predispose to recurrent and unwanted sexual stimulus. Hormonal evaluation is warranted. If there are other neurologic signs, spinal MRI may be of some use.

Treatment

Waldinger and colleagues (2009) reported durable efficacy of the benzodiazepine drug clonazepam (0.5 to 1.5 mg/day) in reducing PGAD symptoms in 56% of treated subjects; benefit was also reported in some women from treatment with tramadol 50 mg or oxazepam 10 mg (Waldinger and Schweitzer, 2009).

Cognitive/behavioral treatments have been proposed, including training to direct attention away from genital sensations and the reduction of overall anxiety (Leiblum and Chivers, 2007). Women with this poorly understood disorder have very positive responses to empathy and support from their providers (Waldinger and Schweitzer, 2009).

FEMALE ORGASMIC DISORDER

Etiology

For diagnosis of female orgasmic disorder (FOD), the term "sufficient sexual stimulation" must be kept in mind. A substantial number of healthy women do not climax from vaginal penetration; others may experience climax from penetration but only after prolonged stimulation. These are normal variants of female sexual response.

There is a widespread cultural belief (derived in large part by the theories of Sigmund Freud) that vaginal penetration should lead to orgasm and that an absence of orgasm from penetration is indicative of psychopathology (Freud, 1905). Some authors have reported superior sexual and life functioning in women who climax from vaginal penetration (Nicholas et al, 2008; Brody and Costa, 2011). Although coitus-associated orgasms may be physically possible but inhibited in some women, there is no reliable data indicating that women who rely on stimulation of the glans clitoris for sexual climax are abnormal (Colson, 2010). Such women should be encouraged to explore nonpenetrative sexual stimuli that lead to climax without being informed that they are frigid or otherwise dysfunctional.

The quality of the relationship influences a woman's capacity to experience orgasm during sex. Poor communication (Kelly et al, 2004) and relationship conflict (Dennerstein et al, 1999) are associated with a lower likelihood of orgasm in women. Psychosocial issues and depression also exert a substantial negative influence on orgasmic capacity in women (Laumann et al, 1999). Antidepressant drugs are associated with FOD (Rosen et al, 1999a).

There are conflicting data on whether orgasm problems are more frequent based on sociodemographic variables. No definite trends have been identified based on age, ethnicity, or menopausal status (Graham, 2010). Similarly, there has been investigation of genetic or hereditary factors; preliminary results have suggested that there may be some genetic component related to difficulty with orgasm but further studies are needed (Witting et al, 2009). Surgical therapy or disruption of the genitals has been linked to FOD in women; this is most likely a result of psychological distress and/or disruption of the earlier phases of sexual response (Graham, 2010).

Evaluation

The general evaluation of sexual health should be performed. It should be determined whether or not the woman is receiving the adequate sexual stimulation that leads to orgasm for her (Basson et al, 2000). Assessment of patient/partner perceptions is essential.

Treatment

Directed masturbation is one of few therapies that has been shown efficacious for FOD (Andersen, 1981; Heiman and Meston, 1997). Frank and honest discussion between partners on preferred erotic activity is essential. This may require education of the woman and her partner on the normalcy of variations in sexual preferences and responses. Incorporation of clitoral or other erotic stimulation may be a satisfactory means to resolve FOD in some women.

Other behavioral interventions are detailed on the Expert Consult *website.*

There are no approved pharmacotherapies for FOD. PDE5I enhance orgasmic response in women with decreased sexual desire related to the use of SSRI drugs (Nurnberg et al, 2008) and in postmenopausal women with orgasmic dysfunction (Cavalcanti et al, 2008). Use of these drugs in women is off label. Estrogens and androgens may be of benefit for women with FOD (Gast et al, 2009). These effects are likely driven by enhancement of earlier phases of sexual response and no study groups have investigated hormone manipulations with a primary end point of orgasm.

SEXUAL PAIN DISORDERS

Etiology

Genital and sexual pain disorders are often complex and multifactorial (Pauls and Berman, 2002). Regardless of initial etiology, pain with intercourse is likely to trigger a number of physical and psychological defense mechanisms that will further increase pain with sexual activity (Pauls and Berman, 2002). For instance, a woman with neuroproliferative vestibulodynia who experiences pain with

BOX 32-2   Conditions Commonly Associated with Sexual Pain

SUPERFICIAL
Neuroproliferative vestibulodynia
Vulvar dermatoses
Vulvovaginal atrophy
Condyloma

DEEP
Endometriosis
Interstitial cystitis
Pelvic floor muscle dysfunction
Uterine leiomyoma
Pelvic inflammatory disease
Pelvic fracture
Pelvic radiation
Vulvovaginal atrophy

Modified from Boardman LA, Stockdale CK. Sexual pain. Clin Obstet Gynecol 2009;52:682–90; and Vallier HA, Cureton BA, Schubeck D. Pelvic ring injury is associated with sexual dysfunction in women. J Orthop Trauma 2012;26:308–13.

intercourse will likely experience anxiety and impairment of genital arousal/lubrication with her next sexual encounter. Enhanced pelvic muscle tone may occur as a defense mechanism. This constellation of downstream effects will generally compound on one another. There is often a substantial delay between the onset of symptoms and the presentation for evaluation, and many presenting women have experienced genital pain as a result of numerous contributing factors (Pauls and Berman, 2002).

A list of conditions known to be associated with sexual pain disorders is presented in Box 32-2. **Studies in adolescent and young adult women (<25 years of age) indicated that between 20% and 57% report pain with intercourse** (Landry and Bergeron, 2009). **Sexual pain is also prevalent in older women, most commonly from vulvovaginal atrophy** (Farage and Maibach, 2006). The most common cause of vulvovaginal atrophy is estrogen deficiency related to menopause (surgical or natural) (North American Menopause Society, 2013). Pelvic radiation may also contribute to vaginal atrophy (Incrocci and Jensen, 2013).

Superficial dyspareunia may result from neuroproliferation of the vulvar vestibule. The vulvar vestibule is of endodermal origin and is hence embryologic and histologically distinct from the adjacent vaginal mucosa and vulvar squamous epithelium (O'Connell et al, 2008). This area may become hypersensitive, with tactile allodynia prohibitive of sexual contact (Zolnoun et al, 2006). Vulvar dermatoses are common and may be frequently missed as causes of superficial dyspareunia (Burrows et al, 2008). A retrospective review of patients seen in a tertiary referral center for vulvovaginal disorders reported that more than 60% of women had some form of vulvar dermatosis (Bowen et al, 2008). Deep dyspareunia has been associated with other gynecologic conditions such as uterine leiomyoma, ovarian cysts, and endometriosis (Vercellini et al, 2012).

The importance of mental, cognitive, and partner-related factors cannot be overlooked in any pain disorder. Anxiety and mood disorders are common in women with dyspareunia; attention to these factors is an essential part of treatment (Basson et al, 2010b). Women with high levels of relationship intimacy and partner support generally report less bother related to sexual pain disorders (Bois et al, 2013). Women from conservative, religious, and/or sexually repressive backgrounds are more likely to report sexual pain (Yasan and Gurgen, 2009). Pain that is prohibitive of sexual activity may also occur in victims of sexual abuse or trauma (Nusbaum et al, 2005; World Health Organization, 2013). Fear of pain, catastrophizing

thoughts (i.e., exaggerated negative thoughts about pain), and loss of self-efficacy (e.g., thoughts such as "I'll never be able to have good sex" or "there is nothing I can do to make it hurt less") have all been linked to worse pain with sexual activity. Loss of self-efficacy has been reported as the most influential mental variable in patients with genital pain during sex (Desrochers et al, 2009).

Evaluation

The onset of sexual pain is very relevant; a woman who experienced lifelong difficulty with sexual activity may have a congenital or psychological etiology for pain. A woman who previously enjoyed sexual activity but now finds it painful is likely to have a musculoskeletal, pelvic, genital, dermatologic, or psychological etiology.

Evaluation of sexual pain relies heavily on physical examination. Careful inspection of the entirety of the external genitalia is essential, as subtle pathology may be easily missed. Inspection of the vulva and labia majora may show dermatologic conditions such as lichen planus (LP), lichen simplex chronicus, lichen sclerosus, vulvar intraepithelial neoplasia (VIN), genital condyloma, contact dermatitis, or other lesions (Fig. 32-11 on the Expert Consult website). A biopsy may be warranted but should only be ordered to rule in or rule out a specific diagnosis.

After inspection of the vulva and labia majora, the labia minora, clitoris, and vulvar vestibule should be examined. Some degree of erythema is normal along the crease of the labia minora. Bartholin gland cysts, inflammation of Skene glands, clitoral phimosis, vulvar erythema, and labial fissures may be detected (Goldstein and Burrows, 2008). The endodermally derived vulvar vestibule is a site for superficial dyspareunia resulting from neuroproliferation (Fig. 32-12 on the Expert Consult website) (O'Connell et al, 2008). The line of demarcation between the endodermal vestibule, the ectodermal vulva, and the mesodermal vagina is subtle; precise examination is key to appropriate diagnosis. Regression/resorption of the labia minora is an important and often overlooked anomaly that is most commonly observed in women who are hormonally deficient (Goldstein and Burrows, 2008).

Assessment for vulvar sensation and tactile allodynia is recommended. This may be accomplished by application of a cotton swab, heat/cold, or a biothesiometer. Women with neuroproliferative vestibulodynia will have marked pain with even light contact against the vestibular tissue (Goldstein and Burrows, 2008).

Transvaginal palpation of the levator ani (LA) is essential. Transanal palpation may be an option in women unable to tolerate vaginal penetration. The patient should be asked to characterize palpation as pressure (normal) or pain (abnormal). Localization of pain permits more focal physical therapy and/or trigger-point injections. Palpation of the adnexa, uterus, and the pudendal nerves in the vicinity of the ischial tuberosity completes the examination (Goldstein and Burrows, 2008).

Treatment

The clitoris may not be involved in pain syndromes of the vestibule and vagina. Hence women with a sexual pain disorder may be able to experience sexual pleasure and bonding with a partner by means of clitoral stimulation. This may be a useful means to foster or maintain sexual intimacy while issues of vaginal and/or pelvic pain with intercourse are being addressed. A multimodal approach to the management of sexual pain is advisable. Psychobehavioral intervention to reduce anxiety surrounding sexual activity is crucial (Rosenbaum, 2011). Cognitive behavioral therapy, psychodynamic, and other therapeutic approaches have been used (Bergeron et al, 2001).

Treatment of Abdominopelvic Processes

Gynecologic conditions (uterine leiomyoma, cystic ovarian disease, endometriosis, labial fusion, vaginal septum, etc.) and other pelvic disorders (irritable bowel, Crohn disease, etc.) may predispose women to dyspareunia. Appropriate medical or surgical treatment may be of benefit in addressing sexual dysfunction although adjunctive therapies may be required (Basson et al, 2010b).

Empiric Medical Therapy

Empiric therapies advanced for sex-related pain include fluconazole, cromolyn sodium, botulinum toxin injection, capsaicin, local anesthetics, desipramine, tricyclic, and novel antidepressants, anticonvulsants, montelukast, enoxaparin, monoclonal antibodies to tumor necrosis factor-α, sacral nerve stimulation, and combination therapies. The level of evidence supporting these interventions as empiric therapy is generally sparse (Kamdar et al, 2007; Koninckx et al, 2008; Bertolasi et al, 2009; Ramsay et al, 2009; Basson et al, 2010b).

Vulvar Dermatoses

Vulvar dermatoses are best managed with reassurance and routine hygiene. Antihistamines may be beneficial to break the cycle of warranted itching that exacerbates the condition of lichen simplex and contributes to other entities. Steroids should not be used empirically for the management of any sexual pain disorder without a diagnosis. Steroid therapy may be indicated in some specific cases; before treatment with steroids is initiated it is prudent to consider biopsy, particularly because there is a small but finite risk of malignant transformation in lichen sclerosus and LP (Salim and Wojnarowska, 2005).

Vulvovaginal Atrophy

Vaginal moisturizers are agents designed to restore baseline lubriciousness of the vagina. Such agents may be of use in addressing uncomfortable vaginal dryness and have been shown to enhance sexual pleasure for many women. It is important to note that such agents are not designed for use as sexual lubricants; they tend to dry out from friction during intercourse. There are numerous commercially available lubricants intended for use during sexual contact (see Female Sexual Arousal Disorder) (Herbenick et al, 2011a).

Systemic or local administration of estrogens has been linked to improvements in vaginal atrophy related to hypoestrogenism (North American Menopause Society, 2007) Local estrogen therapies need not be combined with progestins for endometrial protection when used at low doses (North American Menopause Society, 2013). A variety of estrogen preparations are available for local use; these may be administered as vaginal creams, suppositories, rings, pessaries, or tablets. Systemic absorption of vaginal estrogen preparations is generally very low (Weisberg et al, 2005; Simon et al, 2010; North American Menopause Society, 2013) and hence local therapy may be preferable for patients and providers who are concerned primarily with genital effects. Systemic estrogens may be of use in some women (Bachmann, 1995) but their use must be carefully considered in light of some controversy about long-term health risks (Utian et al, 2008; Jick et al, 2009).

Local and systemic androgens have also been investigated for the management of vaginal symptoms in women. Pilot studies have suggested improvements in symptoms of dyspareunia and vaginal pH after administration of local androgens with no changes in systemic T or E levels (Witherby et al, 2011). A meta-analysis of T therapy has confirmed a generalized benefit with respect to sexual function (arousal, lubrication, and pain) in women who received T supplementation, although safety data are limited (Somboonporn et al, 2005).

Intravaginal DHEA has also been used for treatment of dyspareunia related to vulvovaginal atrophy and has been shown to be superior to placebo for improvement in vaginal histology, pH, and pain with intercourse (Labrie et al, 2011). Further research on the safety and efficacy profile of T and DHEA for vulvovaginal atrophy is warranted (Nappi and Davis, 2012).

Ospemifene is the first nonestrogen treatment approved by the FDA for the management of dyspareunia in postmenopausal women. Ospemifene is a SERM that includes estrogenic activity in bone and in the vaginal epithelium (Rutanen et al, 2003). Randomized controlled trials of oral ospemifene, 30 to 60 mg/day, have demonstrated superiority to placebo for improving vaginal histology, vaginal pH, and dyspareunia (Bachmann et al, 2010; Portman et al, 2013). The most common side effects of ospemifene are hot flashes, candidiasis, and urinary tract infection (Bachmann et al, 2010). In 1-year extension studies of ospemifene, continued benefits were noted with respect to dyspareunia. There was a low rate (0% to 1%) of endometrial proliferation; no carcinomas of the breast or endometrium were identified (Goldstein et al, 2013; Simon et al, 2013).

Musculoskeletal Dysfunction/Scarring

Pelvic floor physiotherapy is a treatment for pelvic/sexual pain related to musculoskeletal disorders. Directed massage, exercise, and pelvic floor biofeedback may durably ameliorate some forms of sexual pain (Rosenbaum, 2005; Bergeron et al, 2008). Progressive dilator therapy may be conducted in the office or at home for management of pain associated with penetration. The patient receives a set of progressively larger polymer dilators that can be inserted into the vagina. The size of the dilators inserted is increased gradually with the eventual goal of comfort with vaginal penetration. Compliance tends to be low without support and involvement from the provider (Rosenbaum, 2011).

Vaginal suppositories containing the benzodiazepine drug diazepam (10 mg) have been advocated by some experts for pelvic pain syndromes including dyspareunia. The FDA has not approved these medications for this indication, but several case reports have suggested efficacy as part of a multimodal treatment regimen (Rogalski et al, 2010). Muscle relaxants have also been used with the intent of decreasing somatic muscle contraction. These may be administered systemically or locally. Botulinum toxin may be effective as an injection for high-tone pelvic floor muscle dysfunction with vaginal spasm (Bertolasi et al, 2009; Goldstein et al, 2011; Nesbitt-Hawes et al, 2013).

Provoked/Neuroproliferative Vestibulodynia

Vulvar vestibulectomy is efficacious in the management of pain in the superficial external vulva related to neuroproliferation (Goldstein et al, 2006). A randomized study indicated superior results (based on intention to treat) of vestibulectomy compared to cognitive-behavioral therapy and biofeedback for dyspareunia (Bergeron et al, 2001). Benefits of treatment were maintained up to a follow-up of 2½ years post-treatment (Bergeron et al, 2008). Experienced and/or well-trained providers may offer vulvar vestibulectomy to patients who are carefully selected. **Patient selection is critical; this procedure should only be offered in the setting of neuroproliferative vestibulodynia affecting the vulvar vestibule** (Goldstein et al, 2006). Complete excision of all tissue between the Hart's line (junction between keratinized skin and mucosa) and the hymenal ring, with reapproximation of the vaginal mucosa to the vulvar skin, permits a satisfactory cosmetic result with removal of all affected tissue (Fig. 32-13 on the Expert Consult website) (Goldstein, 2006).

CONCLUSIONS

Female sexual function and dysfunction are important aspects of urologic practice. Urologists should be aware of the urologic ramifications of sexual issues and vice versa. Appropriate treatment (or referral) of women with sexual concerns will improve patient satisfaction and treatment compliance.

KEY POINTS: FEMALE SEXUAL CONCERNS

- The etiology of sexual concerns in women is often multifactorial.
- There is substantial overlap between sexual concerns in women.
- There are few approved pharmacotherapies for female sexual concerns; there are a number of treatments, but many of these are off label.
- A multidisciplinary approach to sexual concerns with sensitivity to the woman's unique situation is most likely to be effective.
- Psychosocial support is critical in the management of any sexual concern.

REFERENCES

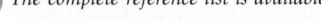

The complete reference list is available online at www.expertconsult.com.

SUGGESTED READINGS

Bachmann G, Oza D. Female androgen insufficiency. Obstet Gynecol Clin North Am 2006;33:589–98.

Basson R, Wierman ME, van Lankveld J, et al. Summary of the recommendations on sexual dysfunctions in women. J Sex Med 2010b;7:314–26.

Davis SR, Moreau M, Kroll R, et al. Testosterone for low libido in postmenopausal women not taking estrogen. N Engl J Med 2008;359:2005–17.

Giuliano F, Rampin O, Allard J. Neurophysiology and pharmacology of female genital sexual response. J Sex Marital Ther 2002;28(Suppl. 1):101–21.

Goldstein I, Alexander JL. Practical aspects in the management of vaginal atrophy and sexual dysfunction in perimenopausal and postmenopausal women. J Sex Med 2005;2(Suppl. 3):154–65.

Kingsberg S, Althof SE. Evaluation and treatment of female sexual disorders. Int Urogynecol J Pelvic Floor Dysfunct 2009;20(Suppl. 1):S33–43.

Laumann EO, Paik A, Rosen RC. Sexual dysfunction in the United States: prevalence and predictors. JAMA 1999;281:537–44.

Shifren JL, Monz BU, Russo PA, et al. Sexual problems and distress in United States women: prevalence and correlates. Obstet Gynecol 2008;112:970–8.

Wehbe SA, Whitmore K, Kellogg-Spadt S. Urogenital complaints and female sexual dysfunction (Pt. 1). J Sex Med 2010;7:1704–13, quiz 1703, 1714–15.

33

Surgical, Radiographic, and Endoscopic Anatomy of the Retroperitoneum

Drew A. Palmer, MD, and Alireza Moinzadeh, MD

Body Surface Landmarks

Posterior Abdominal Wall

Lumbodorsal Fascia

Retroperitoneal Fasciae and Spaces

Gastrointestinal Viscera

Vasculature

Lymphatic System

Nervous Structures

To the astute urologist, anatomic knowledge of the retroperitoneum is critical for success. This chapter provides a thorough description of retroperitoneal anatomy, including the genitourinary organs, musculature, bony structures, fasciae, vessels, lymphatics, neural structures, and gastrointestinal viscera. See Table 33-1 on the Expert Consult website for a review of the anatomic and surgical history of the retroperitoneum.

The retroperitoneum can be described as the entirety of the structures contained anteriorly by the posterior reflection of the peritoneum, posteriorly by the abdominal wall, cranially by the diaphragm, and caudally by the extraperitoneal pelvic structures (Fig. 33-1). The last term must be distinguished from *extraperitoneal space,* which includes the retroperitoneum and the space that circumferentially surrounds the abdominal cavity (Miralis and Skandalakis, 2009, 2010a, 2010b, 2010c, 2010d).

The contents of the retroperitoneum include the **kidneys, ureters, adrenals, pancreas, portions of the duodenum, ascending colon, descending colon, arterial structures including the aorta and its branches, venous structures including the inferior vena cava (IVC) and its tributaries, lymphatics, lymph nodes, sympathetic trunk, and lumbosacral plexus** (Fig. 33-2 on the Expert Consult website and Box 33-1; also see Fig. 33-1).

BODY SURFACE LANDMARKS

The ability to identify abdominal organs using physical examination has great utility for clinical diagnosis and operative planning. The location of the kidneys can be estimated based on their relationship to the bony structures of the posterior abdominal wall (Fig. 33-3). The upper pole of the left kidney is typically located at the level of the 11th rib. The right kidney lies lower than the left, with its upper pole at the level of the 12th rib. The lower poles of the kidneys are between the L3 and L4 vertebrae, and **the renal hila are approximately at the level of L1.**

POSTERIOR ABDOMINAL WALL

Flank Muscles (Figs. 33-4 to 33-7 and Table 33-2)

The most superficial of the flank muscles is the **external oblique,** which lies beneath the subcutaneous fascia. It originates from ribs

5 through 12, and its muscle fibers travel inferomedially inserting at the iliac crest and ending in the midline at the linea alba. **The inferior border of the aponeurosis of the external oblique forms the inguinal ligament.** Deep to the external oblique lies the **internal oblique,** which originates from the lumbodorsal fascia and the

---

BOX 33-1   Organs and Structures of the Retroperitoneum

ORGANS
Kidneys (PR)
Ureters (PR)
Adrenal glands (PR)
Portions of the duodenum (SR)
Ascending colon (SR)
Descending colon (SR)
Pancreas (SR)

VESSELS
Abdominal aorta (and its branches)
Inferior vena cava (and its tributaries)
Ascending lumbar veins
Portal vein
Lumbar lymph nodes
Lumbar lymphatic trunks
Cisterna chyli

NERVES
Branches of the lumbosacral plexus
Sympathetic trunk
Autonomic plexuses
Autonomic ganglia

PR, primarily retroperitoneal; SR, secondarily retroperitoneal.
Modified from Miralis P, Skandalakis JE. Surgical anatomy of the retroperitoneal spaces—part I: embryogenesis and anatomy. Am Surg 2009;75(11):1091–7.

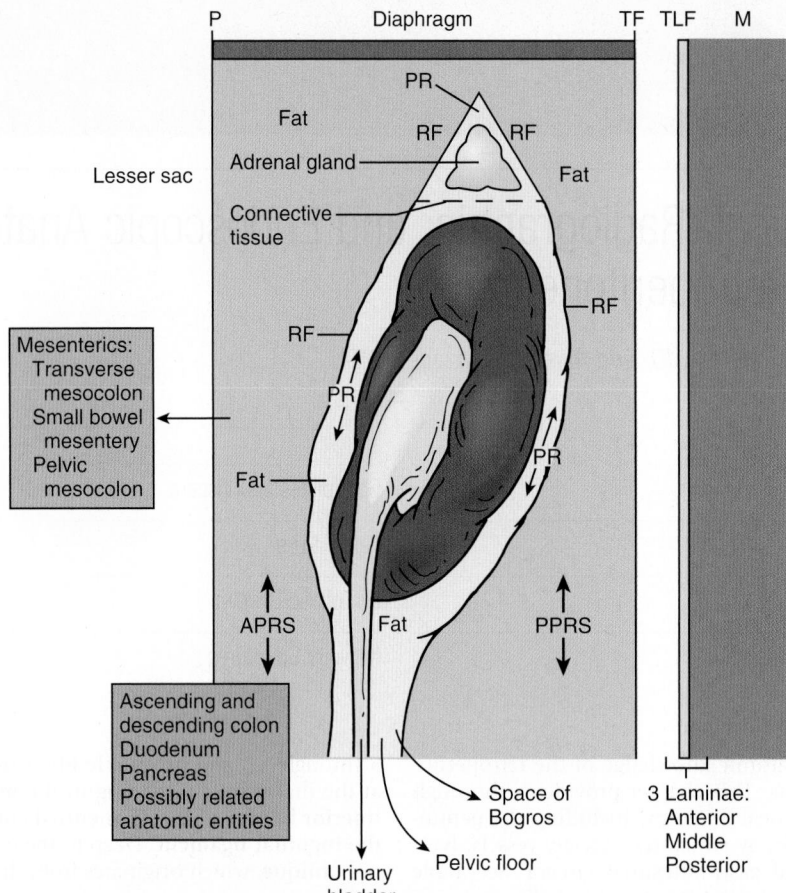

Figure 33-1. Diagram of retroperitoneal spaces. APRS, anterior pararenal space; M, muscles; P, peritoneum; PPRS, posterior pararenal space; PR, perirenal space; RF, renal fascia (Gerota fascia); TF, transversalis fascia; TLF, thoracolumbar fascia. (Modified from Skandalakis JE, Colborn GL. Skandalakis' surgical anatomy: the embryological and anatomic basis of modern surgery. Athens, Greece: Paschalides Medical Publications; 2004. p. 155.)

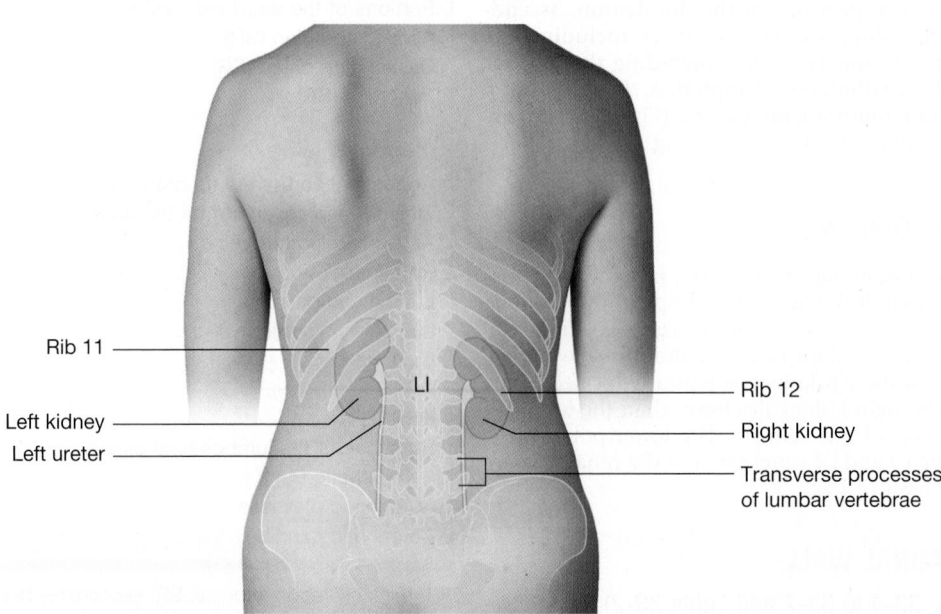

Figure 33-3. **Posterior view of the abdominal region of a woman with projections of the kidneys and ureters. (From Drake RL, Vogl AW, Mitchell AWM. Gray's anatomy for students. 2nd ed. Philadelphia: Churchill Livingstone; 2010.)**

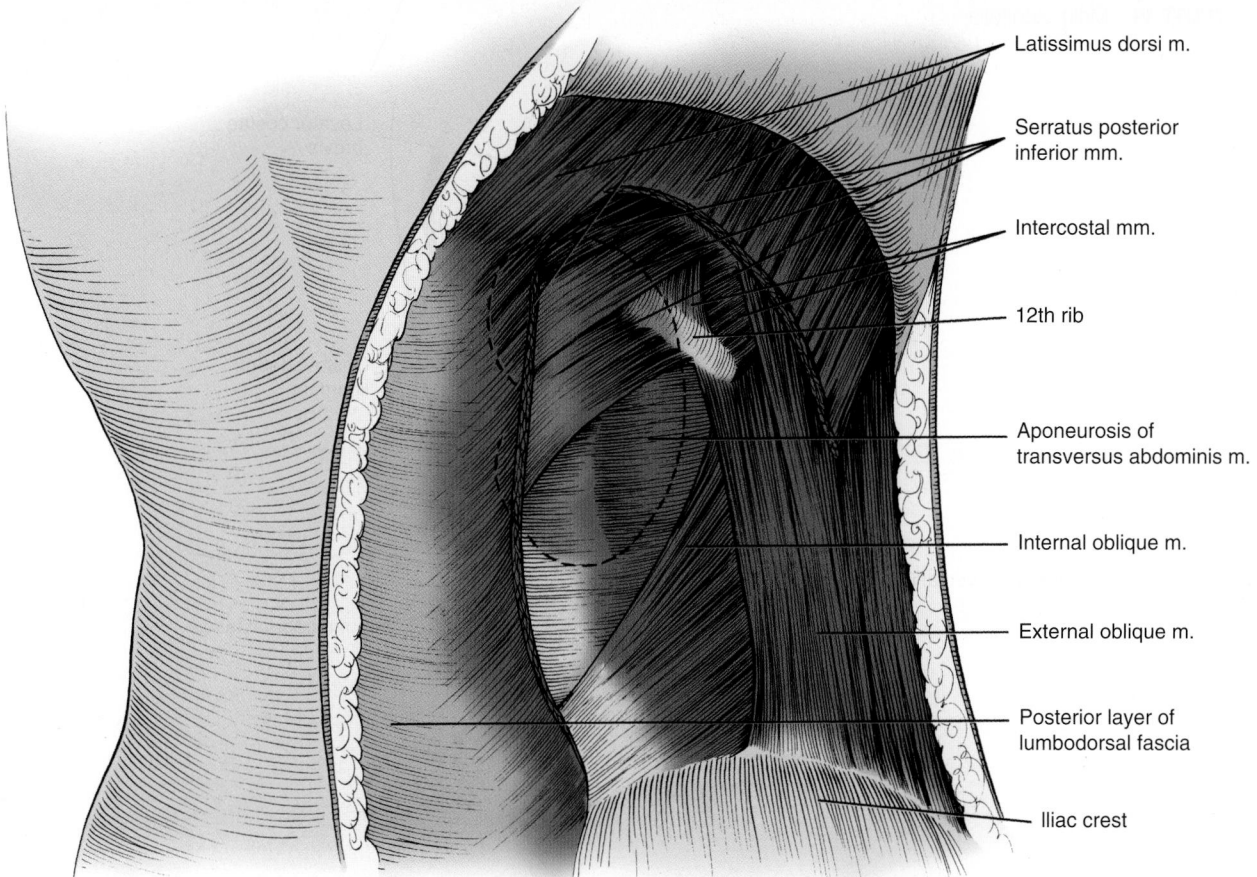

Latissimus dorsi m.

Serratus posterior inferior mm.

Intercostal mm.

12th rib

Aponeurosis of transversus abdominis m.

Internal oblique m.

External oblique m.

Posterior layer of lumbodorsal fascia

Iliac crest

Figure 33-4. Posterior abdominal wall musculature, superficial dissection. A section of the latissimus dorsi muscle has been removed. The location of the right kidney within the retroperitoneum is shown by the *dashed outline*.

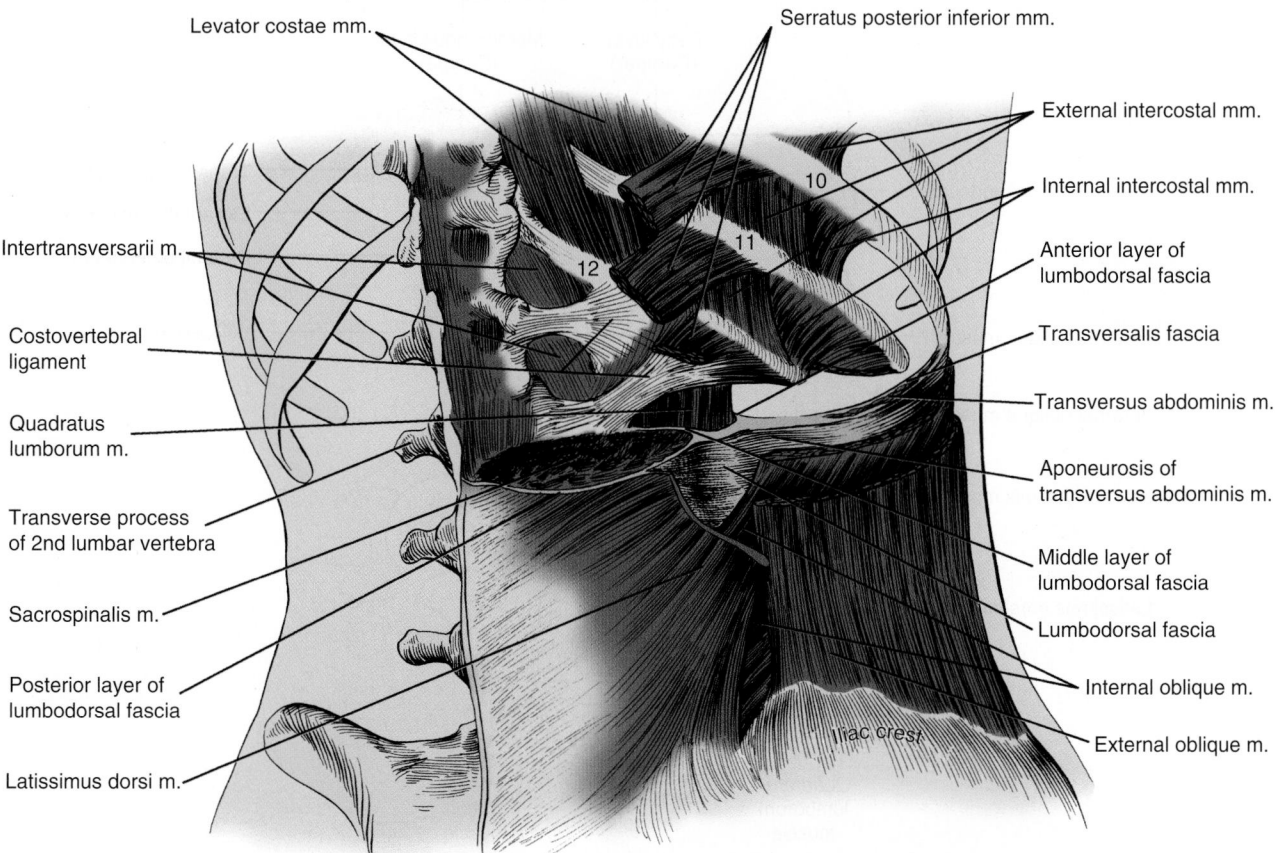

Levator costae mm.

Serratus posterior inferior mm.

External intercostal mm.

Internal intercostal mm.

Anterior layer of lumbodorsal fascia

Transversalis fascia

Transversus abdominis m.

Aponeurosis of transversus abdominis m.

Middle layer of lumbodorsal fascia

Lumbodorsal fascia

Internal oblique m.

External oblique m.

Intertransversarii m.

Costovertebral ligament

Quadratus lumborum m.

Transverse process of 2nd lumbar vertebra

Sacrospinalis m.

Posterior layer of lumbodorsal fascia

Latissimus dorsi m.

10

11

12

Iliac crest

Figure 33-5. Posterior abdominal wall musculature, intermediate dissection. The sacrospinalis muscle and three anterolateral flank muscle layers are seen in cut section, and the three layers of the lumbodorsal fascia posteriorly can be appreciated.

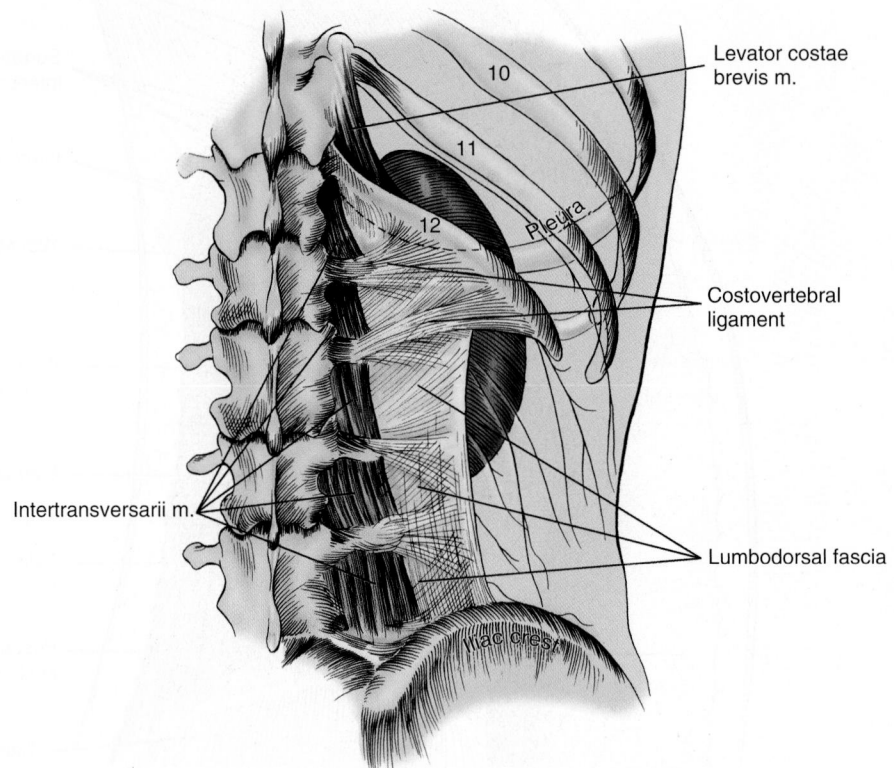

Figure 33-6. Posterior abdominal wall musculature, deep dissection. The lumbodorsal fascia and costovertebral ligament are visualized arising from the transverse processes of the lumbar vertebrae. The relationship of the kidney and pleura is also shown.

Labels on figure: Levator costae brevis m.; 10; 11; 12; Pleura; Costovertebral ligament; Lumbodorsal fascia; Intertransversarii m.; Iliac crest

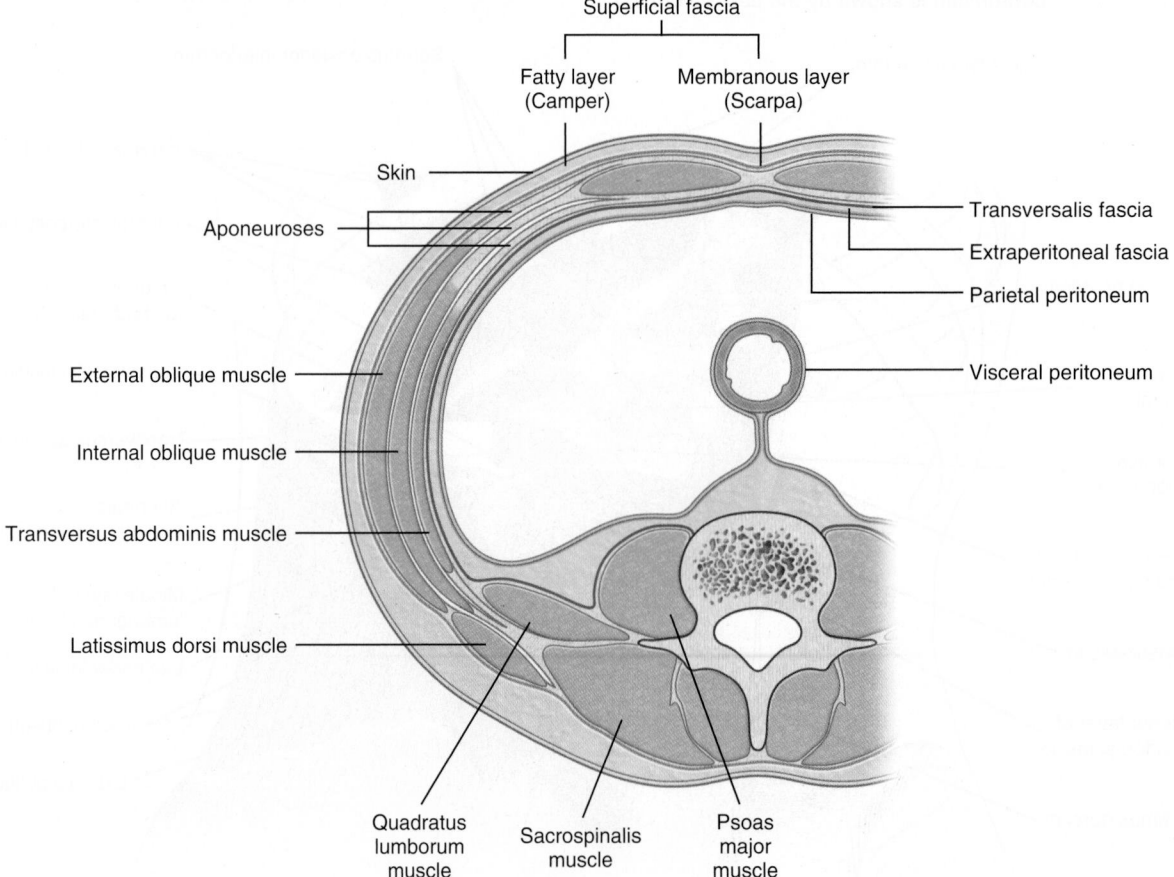

Figure 33-7. Transverse section showing layers of the lateral flank musculature. (From Drake RL, Vogl AW, Mitchell AWM. Gray's anatomy for students. 2nd ed. Philadelphia: Churchill Livingstone; 2010.)

Labels on figure: Superficial fascia; Fatty layer (Camper); Membranous layer (Scarpa); Skin; Aponeuroses; Transversalis fascia; Extraperitoneal fascia; Parietal peritoneum; Visceral peritoneum; External oblique muscle; Internal oblique muscle; Transversus abdominis muscle; Latissimus dorsi muscle; Quadratus lumborum muscle; Sacrospinalis muscle; Psoas major muscle

TABLE 33-2 Musculature of the Posterior and Lateral Abdominal Wall

MUSCLE	ORIGIN	INSERTION	FUNCTION
Erector spinae	Sacrum and vertebrae	Lower ribs and vertebrae	Extension of spine
External oblique	Ribs 5-12	Lateral lip of iliac crest, aponeurosis ending in linea alba	Compress abdominal contents, flexion of trunk
Internal oblique	Lumbodorsal fascia, iliac crest, inguinal ligament	Lower four ribs, aponeurosis ending in linea alba, pubic crest	Compress abdominal contents, flexion of trunk
Transversus abdominis	Lumbodorsal fascia, medial lip of iliac crest, ribs 7-12	Aponeurosis ending in linea alba, pubic crest	Compress abdominal contents
Psoas major	T12-L5 vertebrae	Lesser trochanter of femur	Flexion of hip
Psoas minor	T12 and L1 vertebrae	Pelvic brim, iliopubic eminence	Weak flexion of lumbar vertebral column
Iliacus	Iliac fossa, sacrum	Lesser trochanter of femur	Flexion of the hip
Quadratus lumborum	5th lumbar vertebra, iliac crest	L1-L4 vertebrae, 12th rib	Depress and stabilize 12th rib, lateral bending of trunk

Modified from Drake RL, Vogl AW, Mitchell AWM. Gray's anatomy for students. Philadelphia: Churchill Livingstone; 2005.

iliac crest. It travels superomedially inserting at the lower ribs and linea alba. Each of these muscle layers is invested in a layer of fascia. The **transversus abdominis** muscle, named because of the *transverse* direction of its muscle fibers, lies deep to the internal oblique. Deep to the transversus abdominis muscle lies the **transversalis fascia,** which crosses the midline anteriorly and fuses with the lumbodorsal fascia posteriorly. These flank muscles function to flex, extend, and rotate the trunk and provide compression of the abdominal contents.

Psoas, Iliacus, Quadratus Lumborum, and Erector Spinae
(Fig. 33-8; also see Figs. 33-4 to 33-7 and Table 33-2)

The **psoas major** muscle arises from the 12th thoracic vertebra to the 5th lumbar vertebra to attach to the lesser trochanter of the femur after traveling along the pelvic brim posterior to the inguinal ligament. The psoas minor muscle, which may be absent in some individuals, originates at T12 and L1 and inserts at the pelvic brim and iliopubic eminence. The psoas major functions in flexion of the thigh at the hip joint and is innervated by the anterior rami of L1, L2, and L3. The **iliacus** muscle originates at the caudal aspect of the iliac fossa and the lateral sacrum to insert at the lesser trochanter of the femur. It functions in flexion of the thigh at the hip joint along with the psoas major. The **quadratus lumborum** lies posterior and medial to the psoas muscle and assists with lateral bending of the trunk and stabilization of the 12th rib. Its origin is at L5 and the iliac fossa, and it attaches to the inferior border of the 12th rib and the transverse processes of L1-L4. The **erector spinae (sacrospinalis)** is a large group of back muscles that function to extend the spine.

Spine

The spine consists of 7 cervical vertebrae, 12 thoracic vertebrae, 5 lumbar vertebrae, the sacrum, and the coccyx. Each vertebra has a large weight-bearing area called the **vertebral body** and a posterior and lateral arch that forms the vertebral foramen (Fig. 33-9 on the Expert Consult website). The **spinous process** projects posteroinferiorly, and the **transverse processes** project posterolaterally. The lumbar vertebrae are the most clinically significant in regard to the retroperitoneum. They are larger than the other vertebrae with generally long, thin transverse processes.

The vertebral column levels have different relationships with the spinal cord segmental levels at different locations within the

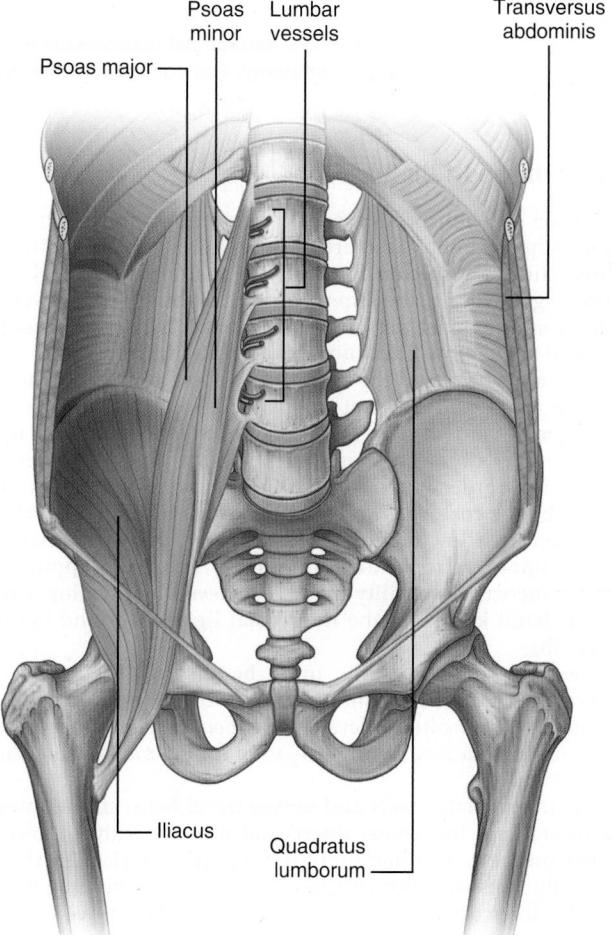

Figure 33-8. **Muscles of the posterior abdominal wall. (From Drake RL, Vogl AW, Mitchell AWM. Gray's anatomy for students. 2nd ed. Philadelphia: Churchill Livingstone; 2010.)**

spinal column. For example, the sacral spinal cord segmental levels typically begin between vertebral column level T12 and L1 in adults. When discussing spinal cord injury, one must be careful to specify vertebral column level versus spinal segmental level.

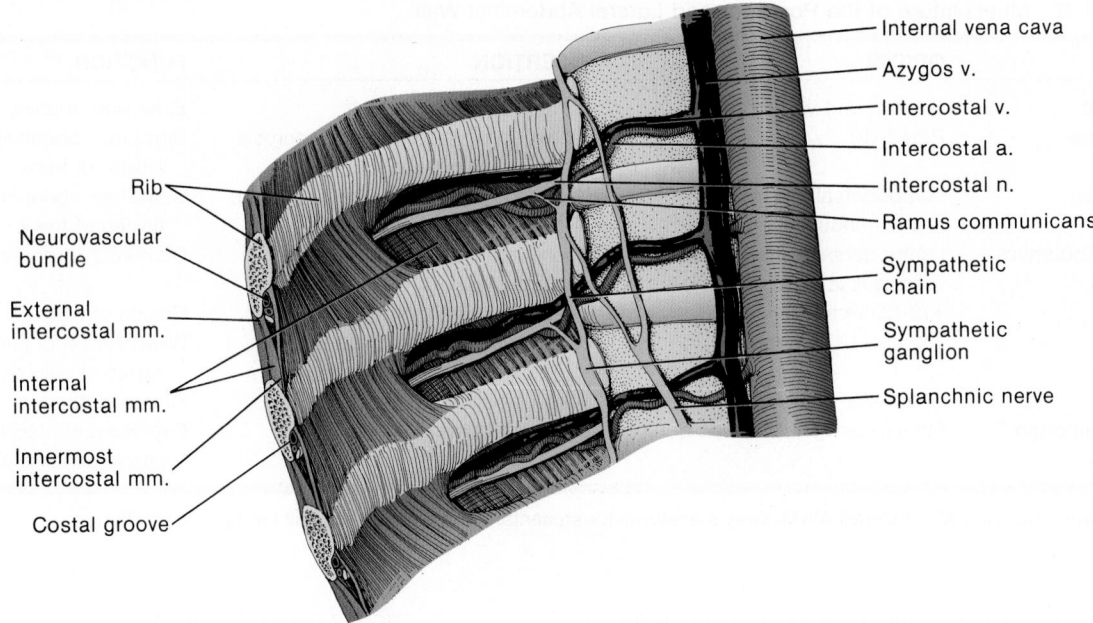

Figure 33-11. **Intercostal neurovascular bundle. (From MacLennan GT. Hinman's atlas of urosurgical anatomy. 2nd ed. Philadelphia: Saunders; 2012.)**

10th, 11th, and 12th Ribs

The lower ribs function to protect the retroperitoneal structures from traumatic injury. **Fracture of these lower ribs should lead to a high clinical suspicion for injury to the retroperitoneal structures** (Fig. 33-10 on the Expert Consult website). The lower ribs differ from the upper ribs given their shorter length with less pronounced angulation. The 10th rib articulates with the body of the vertebra at its head and the transverse process at its neck. The 11th rib lacks a neck and does not articulate with the transverse process. The angle of the 11th rib is less pronounced than that of the upper ribs. The 12th rib has no angle and is shorter than the other ribs. **Its inferior border is attached to the transverse processes of L1 and L2 by the costovertebral (lumbocostal) ligament, which can be incised to allow for increased mobility for greater exposure of the upper retroperitoneum during posterior approaches.** Similar increased mobility may be achieved by dividing a thick fibrous band known as the intercostal ligament found between other ribs.

The 11th and 12th ribs must be distinguished from the other ribs because they have no anterior connection with the sternum and are often referred to as *floating ribs*. These ribs are of clinical significance during palpation for the marking of a surgical incision.

The intercostal vessels and nerves travel between the internal intercostal and innermost intercostal muscles within the costal groove on the caudal margin of the superior rib (Fig. 33-11). The vein is the most superior structure with the artery running inferior to it. The intercostal nerve is the most inferior of the three structures and is often not protected by the costal groove.

LUMBODORSAL FASCIA

The **lumbodorsal (thoracolumbar) fascia** is composed of three distinct layers that invest the posterior abdominal wall musculature (Fig. 33-12). **These three layers merge into one as they travel laterally. A common access point to the retroperitoneum is near the tip of the 12th rib, where all layers have merged into one.** This single layer of lumbodorsal fascia merges with the aponeurosis of the transversus abdominis muscle anterolaterally. The **posterior lamella** originates medially from the spinous process of the lumbar vertebrae and covers the erector spinae muscles. The **middle lamella**

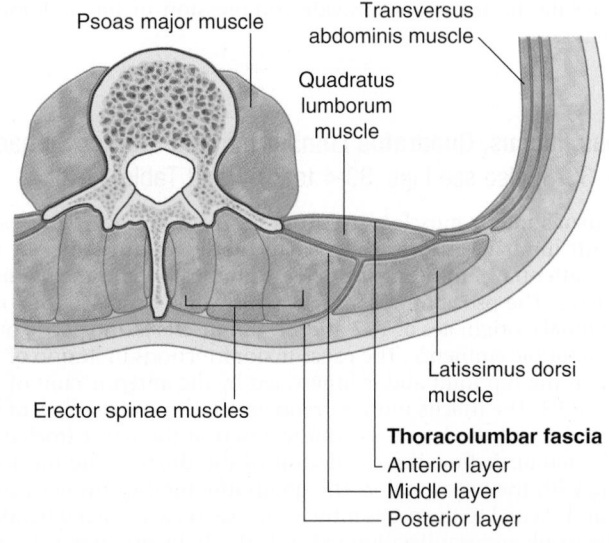

Figure 33-12. Lumbodorsal fascia and the deep back muscle. (From Drake RL, Vogl AW, Mitchell AWM. Gray's anatomy for students. 2nd ed. Philadelphia: Churchill Livingstone; 2010.)

separates these erector spinae muscles from quadratus lumborum. The anterior lamella covers the ventral surface of quadratus lumborum. Extending medially, the **anterior lamella** attaches to the vertebral transverse process and is continuous with the fascia that invests the psoas muscle.

The retroperitoneum can be entered without incising muscle using a dorsal lumbotomy incision (Fig. 33-13). This approach uses a vertical incision through the lumbodorsal fascia lateral to the erector spinae and quadratus lumborum muscles (Fig. 33-14 on the Expert Consult website).

RETROPERITONEAL FASCIAE AND SPACES

Derived from the mesoderm, the primitive mesenchyme differentiates to form a subcutaneous layer, body layer, and retroperitoneal

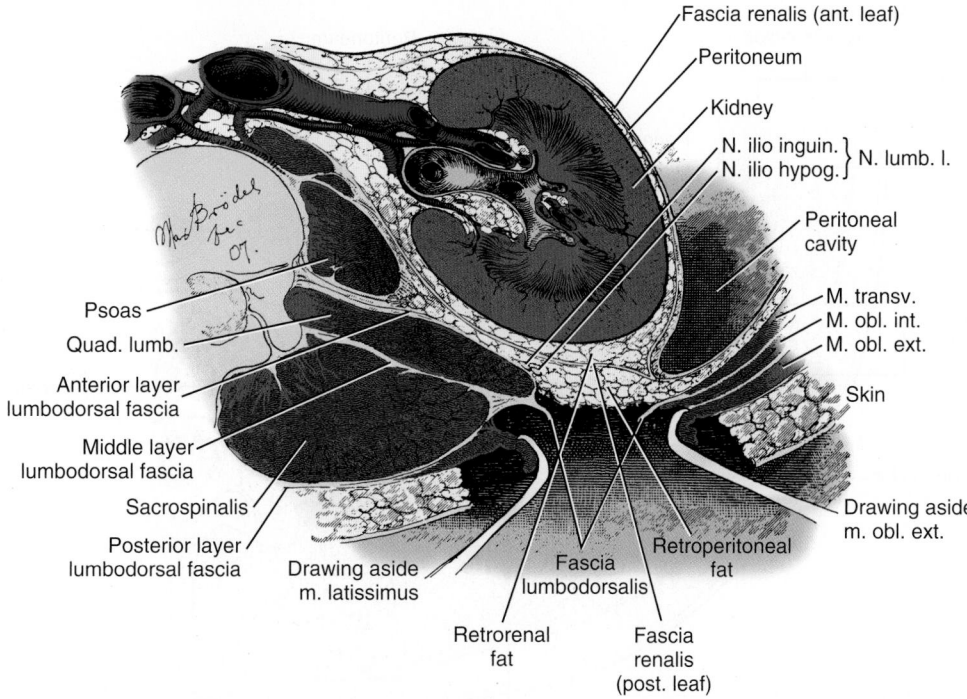

Figure 33-13. Transverse section through the kidney and posterior abdominal wall showing the lumbodorsal fascia incised. Through such a lumbodorsal incision, the kidney can be reached without incising muscle. (After Kelly and Burnam, from McVay C. Anson & McVay surgical anatomy. 6th ed. Philadelphia: Saunders; 1984.)

layer. The retroperitoneal layer forms three strata in late fetal development: the outer stratum, intermediate stratum, and inner stratum (Fig. 33-15 on the Expert Consult website). Historically, the retroperitoneum has been divided embryologically based on these three strata (Tobin, 1944). The **outer stratum** covers the epimysium of the abdominal wall muscles and becomes the transversalis fascia. The **intermediate stratum** is associated with the urinary organs, and the **inner stratum** is associated with the gastrointestinal organs (MacLennan, 2012). The aim is not to have the reader memorize what each embryologic stratum becomes during development. **Rather, these embryologic strata serve to categorize the retroperitoneal fasciae, which compartmentalize various spaces within the retroperitoneum.**

Transversalis Fascia and Posterior Pararenal Space

The outer stratum forms the **transversalis fascia,** which lies deep to the transversus abdominis muscle and superficial to the preperitoneal fat and peritoneum. Posterior to the kidney, the transversalis fascia remains anterior to the fascia surrounding the quadratus lumborum and psoas muscle (Fig. 33-16). **It may fuse medially with the posterior lamina of Gerota fascia, which is of clinical significance during retroperitoneal dissection because this fascia must be incised to allow access to the renal hilum.** This fusion creates the medial boundary of the **posterior pararenal space.** The anterior boundary is formed by the posterior lamina of Gerota fascia, and the posterior and lateral boundaries are formed by the transversalis fascia (Tobin, 1944).

Gerota Fascia (Renal Fascia) and Perirenal Space
(Figs. 33-17 and 33-18; also see Fig. 33-16)

The **anterior lamina** (fascia of Toldt or prerenal fascia) and the **posterior lamina** (fascia of Zuckerkandl or retrorenal fascia) of the renal fascia are derived from the intermediate stratum, which embeds the genitourinary organs. **They help to form the boundaries of the retroperitoneal spaces: the posterior pararenal space,** **perirenal space, and anterior pararenal space.** The two laminae together form the **renal fascia,** eponymously named *Gerota fascia,* after the Romanian anatomist Dimitrie D. Gerota (1867-1939). The **perirenal space** contains the adrenal, kidney, ureter, perirenal fat, renal vascular pedicle, and gonadal vessels. The perirenal fat is finer and lighter yellow in color compared with the coarser yellow-orange pararenal fat. The anatomy of the adrenal, kidney, and ureter is discussed in detail in their respective chapters.

The posterior lamina of Gerota fascia is thicker and more frequently visualized radiographically than the anterior lamina. These two layers merge laterally to form the **lateroconal fascia,** which separates the anterior and posterior pararenal spaces and continues anterolaterally deep to the transversalis fascia. There is some controversy regarding the medial and inferior extents of the perirenal space. Historically, it was assumed that there was no communication between the right and left perirenal spaces. However, based on in vivo cases and cadaveric injection studies, **there may be some communication across the midline below the level of the renal hilum** (Lim et al, 1998).

In addition, there has been no consensus on the patency and caudal extent of the perirenal space. Previously, it was suggested that the perirenal space is closed inferiorly by the fusion of Gerota fascia. However, in vivo cases and cadaveric injection studies demonstrated that the **perirenal space has a conelike shape that is open at its inferior extent in the extraperitoneal pelvis** (Lim et al, 1998). These boundaries are of tremendous clinical significance in the pathology of urologic disease because they function to contain perinephric fluid collections, which include urine (traumatic or iatrogenic urinary extravasation, obstructive uropathy with calyceal rupture), blood (traumatic or iatrogenic perinephric hematoma, ruptured aneurysm), or purulence (perinephric abscess or infected urinoma).

Anterior Pararenal Space and Inner Stratum

The **anterior pararenal space** is formed by the anterior lamina of the renal fascia posteriorly and the posterior layer of parietal peritoneum anteriorly (Fig. 33-19 on the Expert Consult website).

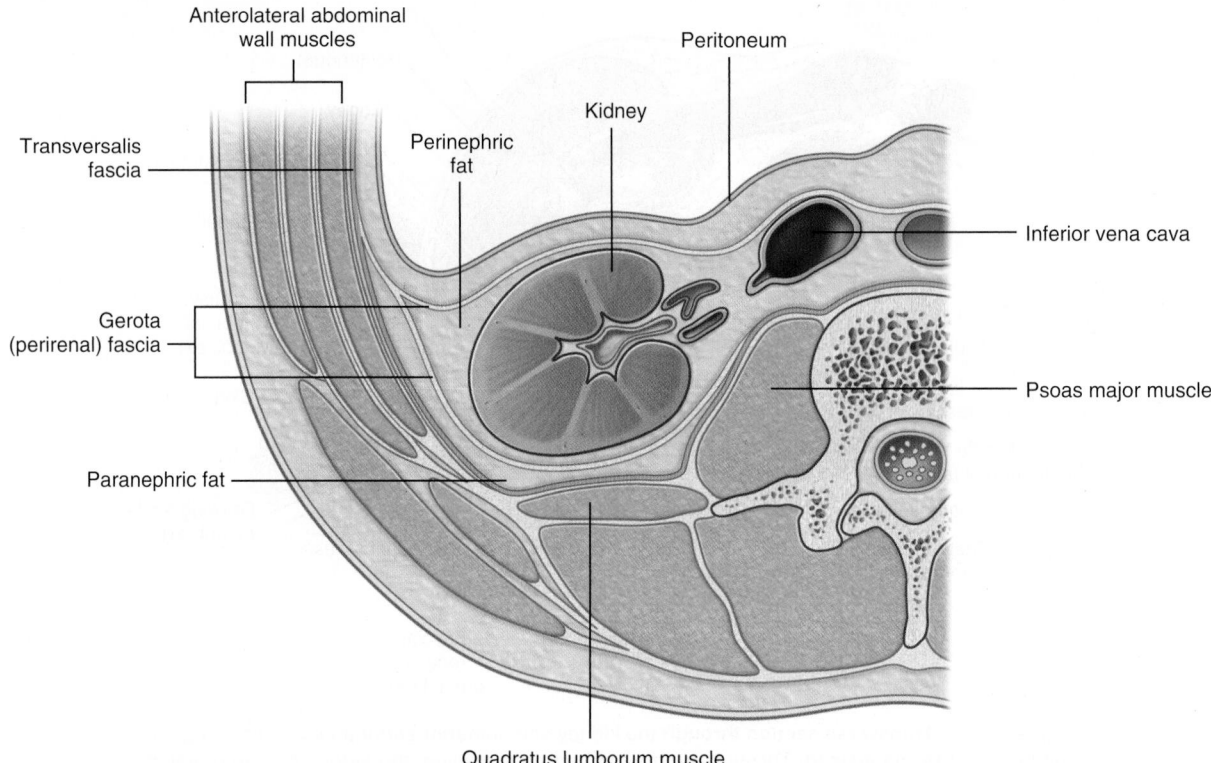

Figure 33-16. **Organization of the fasciae and fat surrounding the kidney. (From Drake RL, Vogl AW, Mitchell AWM. Gray's anatomy for students. 2nd ed. Philadelphia: Churchill Livingstone; 2010.)**

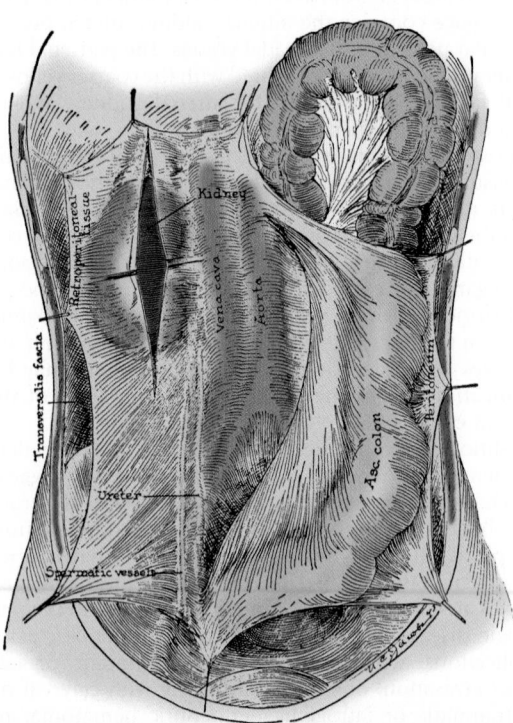

Figure 33-17. **Anterior view of Gerota fascia on the right side, split over the right kidney (which it contains) and showing inferior extension enveloping the ureter and gonadal vessels. The ascending colon and overlying peritoneum have been reflected medially. (From Tobin CE. The renal fascia and its relation to the transversalis fascia. Anat Rec 1944;89:295–311.)**

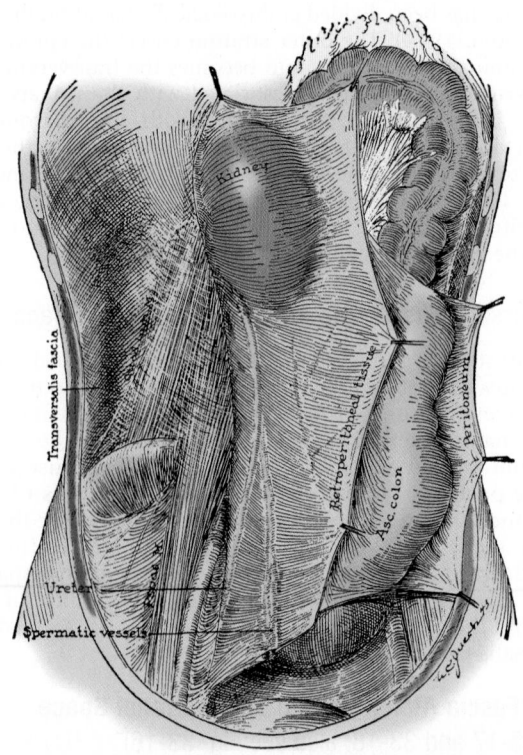

Figure 33-18. **Posterior view of Gerota fascia on the right side, rotated medially with the contained kidney, ureter, and gonadal vessels, exposing the muscular posterior body wall covered by the transversalis fascia. (From Tobin CE. The renal fascia and its relation to the transversalis fascia. Anat Rec 1944;89:295–311.)**

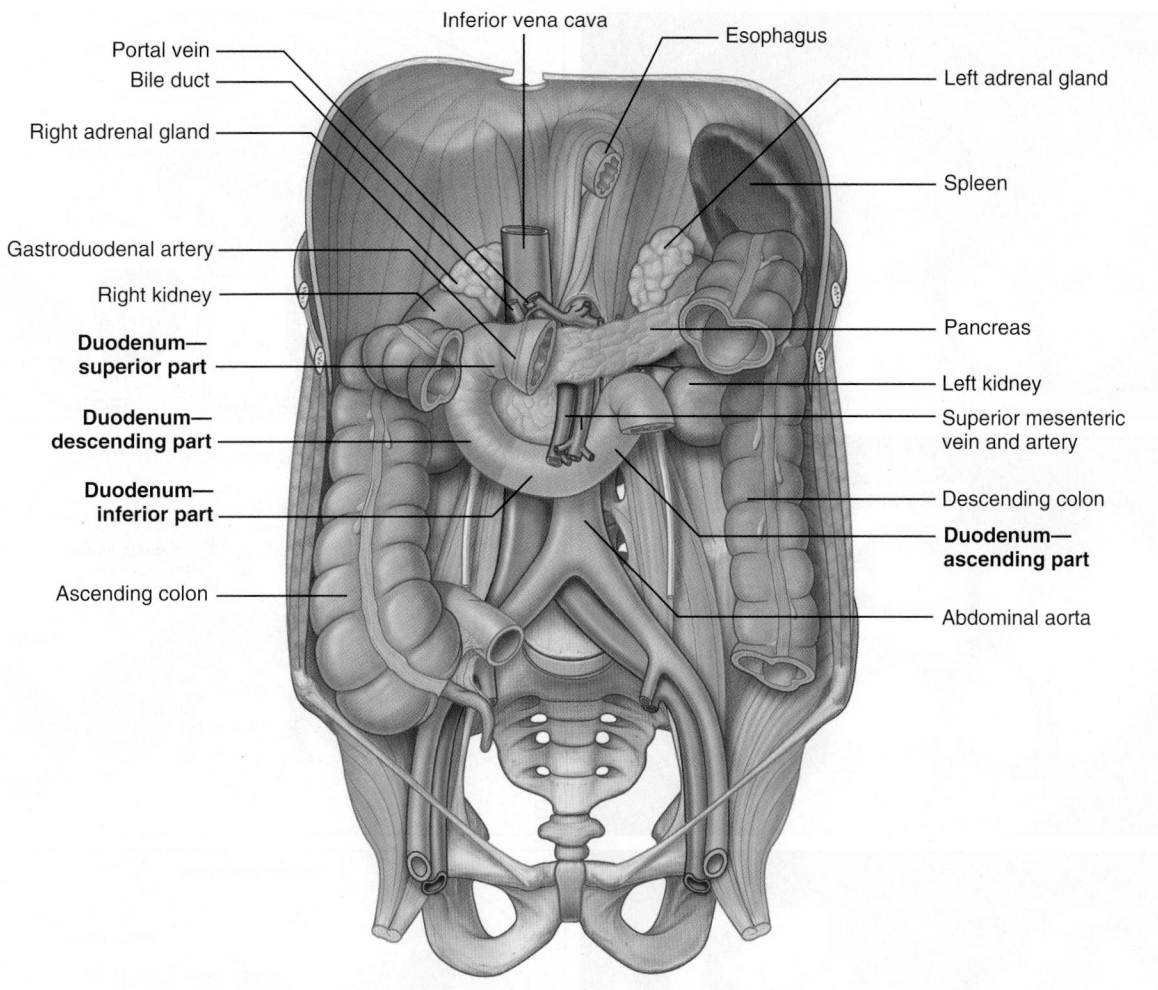

Figure 33-21. Colon, duodenum, and pancreas within the retroperitoneum. (From Drake RL, Vogl AW, Mitchell AWM. Gray's anatomy for students. 2nd ed. Philadelphia: Churchill Livingstone; 2010.)

Clinically, this space is significant because it can be developed to gain access to the kidney anteriorly when followed medially from the **white line of Toldt.** This classic landmark is created during embryogenesis when the inner stratum forms a multilayer fusion fascia with the primary dorsal peritoneum during the rotation and posterior attachment of the gastrointestinal viscera (Fig. 33-20 on the Expert Consult website). **During this event, the white line of Toldt is formed at the lateral border of the fusion of the colonic mesentery with the posterior peritoneum.**

The anterior pararenal space contains the secondarily retroperitoneal organs: the ascending and descending colon, pancreas, and second and third portions of the duodenum. These organs are intraperitoneal at one point during embryogenesis; however, they become retroperitoneal secondarily as they attach to the posterior abdominal wall when the inner stratum fuses with the primary dorsal peritoneum.

GASTROINTESTINAL VISCERA

The nonurologic viscera within the retroperitoneum includes the pancreas and parts of the duodenum and the colon (Figs. 33-21 and 33-22). The **pancreas** consists of four parts and has endocrine and exocrine functions. The head lies anterior to the IVC and is surrounded by the second portion of the duodenum. This portion is of concern for potential injury during right kidney procedures. The neck connects the head to the body, which crosses the abdomen anterior to the aorta and the origin of the superior mesenteric artery (SMA).

The tail of the pancreas is closely associated with the spleen and must be accounted for during left retroperitoneal surgery because of its proximity to the upper pole of the left kidney and left adrenal. In addition, the stomach is anterior to the upper pole of the left kidney and must be accounted for during transperitoneal left renal surgery (Fig. 33-23 on the Expert Consult website).

The **duodenum** is 20 cm to 25 cm in length and can be divided into four distinct parts. The first (superior) portion is intraperitoneal and extends from the pylorus to the neck of the gallbladder. The second (descending) and third (horizontal or inferior) portions of the duodenum are contained within the retroperitoneum. **The second, descending portion of the duodenum is of critical importance to the urologist because of its proximity to the right renal hilum. The duodenum may be mobilized medially using a *Kocher maneuver* to expose these right-sided retroperitoneal structures.** The common bile duct and the main pancreatic duct combine to enter the second portion of the duodenum at the ampulla of Vater (hepatopancreatic ampulla). The third portion of the duodenum crosses the body from right to left and lies posterior to the SMA and anterior to the aorta. The fourth and final portion ascends and becomes intraperitoneal as it transitions into the jejunum.

As with the duodenum, portions of the colon are secondarily retroperitoneal because they developed intraperitoneally but fused with the posterior abdominal wall during embryogenesis. The **ascending colon** and hepatic flexure overlie the right-sided retroperitoneal structures, and the splenic flexure and **descending colon** cover the left-sided retroperitoneal structures. To gain access

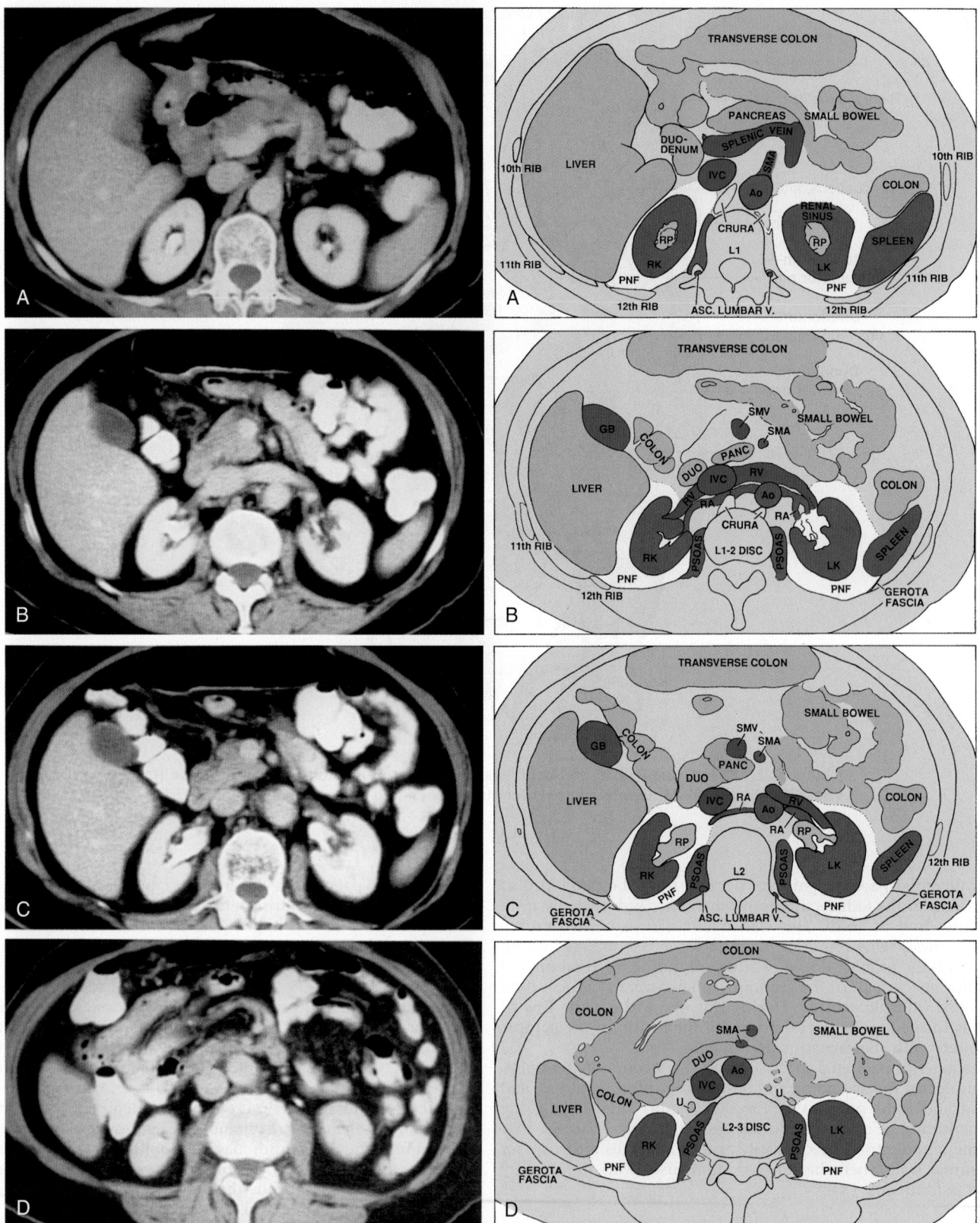

Figure 33-22. **Cross-sectional anatomy of the upper abdomen at the level of the kidneys demonstrated with transverse sections obtained by computed tomography. Sections are arranged from most cephalic to caudal. A, Section through the upper poles of the kidneys, superior to the renal vascular pedicles. B, Section through the level of the renal arteries and veins. C, Slightly more inferior section showing the renal pelves and relationship of the duodenum to the right renal hilum. D, Section through the lower poles of the kidneys showing the upper ureters. Ao, aorta; DUO, duodenum; GB, gallbladder; IVC, inferior vena cava; LK, left kidney; PANC, pancreas; PNF, perinephric fat; RA, renal artery; RK, right kidney; RP, renal pelvis; RV, renal vein; SMA, superior mesenteric artery; SMV, superior mesenteric vein; U, ureter.**

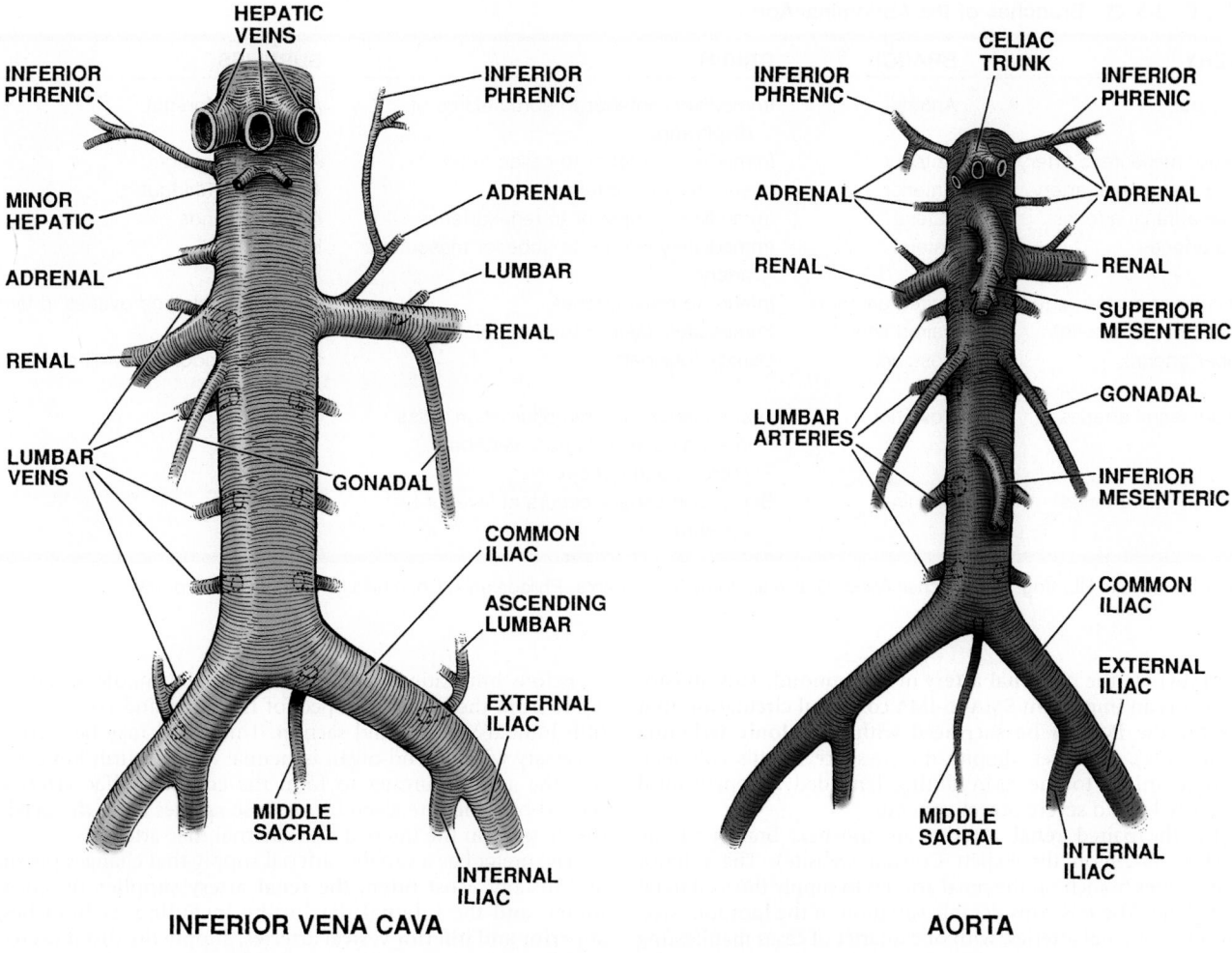

Figure 33-27. Inferior vena cava and its tributaries and abdominal aorta and its branches.

to the kidneys transperitoneally, the ipsilateral colon must be reflected medially in most instances. This can be performed by mobilizing the colon at the white line of Toldt, which visually represents the transition from the colonic visceral peritoneum to the posterior parietal peritoneum. **Care must be taken to divide the hepatocolic and splenocolic ligaments sharply when necessary to avoid iatrogenic injury to the liver and spleen, which is often due to excessive retraction during attempts to obtain adequate exposure.**

VASCULATURE

Arterial System

Arterial structures have three layers: the tunica intima (intima), tunica media (media), and tunica externa (tunica adventitia or adventitia) as shown in Figure 33-24 on the Expert Consult website. The **intima** consists of a layer of endothelial cells surrounded by subendothelial connective tissue. The **media** layer contains vascular smooth muscle cells and elastic connective tissue that control the caliber of the vessel. This layer is surrounded by the internal and external elastic laminae. The **adventitia** is the connective tissue sheath surrounding the vessel. It contains the nerves that control vasomotor tone and the vasa vasorum (Latin, "vessels of the vessels"), which are smaller vessels that supply the walls of larger vessels.

The major arterial structures of the retroperitoneum include the abdominal aorta (Figs. 33-25 and 33-26 on the Expert Consult website) and its branches (Fig. 33-27 and Table 33-3). Entering the abdomen through the aortic hiatus of the diaphragm at the level of

T12, the **abdominal aorta** courses centrally and to the left of the IVC. The first branches are the paired **inferior phrenic arteries,** which supply the inferior surface of the diaphragm (Fig. 33-28 on the Expert Consult website). The **superior adrenal artery** branches from the inferior phrenic artery and supplies the ipsilateral adrenal gland. **The superior arterial blood supply to the adrenal is constant; however, the middle and inferior arteries to the adrenal are variable. These arteries vary in number and location with the most common variant being the middle adrenal artery arising from the aorta and the inferior adrenal arising from the renal artery.**

The next branch of the abdominal aorta is the **celiac artery** (celiac trunk or truncus coeliacus) which is a short, unpaired artery that arises anteriorly at the midline at the level of T12. It gives origin to the left gastric, splenic, and common hepatic arteries, which supply the abdominal esophagus, stomach, duodenum, spleen, liver, and pancreas. Of surgical anatomic significance, the splenic vessels course on the cephalad aspect of the body and tail of the pancreas. When the inferior pancreatic edge is mobilized off the anterior renal fascia during adrenal or renal transperitoneal surgery, knowledge of the anatomic relationship between the splenic vessels and the pancreas is paramount to prevent vascular injury. The next branches are the paired middle adrenal arteries, which supply the ipsilateral adrenal gland as noted earlier.

The **SMA** branches next off the aorta, arising anteriorly in the midline at approximately the level of the middle adrenal arteries at L1-L2. It supplies the pancreas (inferior pancreaticoduodenal artery), small intestine, and most of the large intestine (ileocolic, right colic, and middle colic arteries). **The middle colic artery anastomoses with the left colic artery off the inferior mesenteric**

TABLE 33-3 Branches of the Abdominal Aorta

ARTERY	BRANCH	ORIGIN	SUPPLIES
Celiac trunk	Anterior	Immediately inferior to aortic hiatus of diaphragm	Abdominal foregut
Superior mesenteric artery	Anterior	Immediately inferior to celiac trunk	Abdominal midgut
Inferior mesenteric artery	Anterior	Inferior to renal arteries	Abdominal hindgut
Middle adrenal arteries	Lateral	Immediately superior to renal arteries	Adrenal glands
Renal arteries	Lateral	Immediately inferior to superior mesenteric artery	Kidneys
Testicular or ovarian arteries	Paired anterior	Inferior to renal arteries	Testes in male and ovaries in female
Inferior phrenic arteries	Paired lateral	Immediately inferior to aortic hiatus	Diaphragm
Lumbar arteries	Posterior	Usually four pairs	Posterior abdominal wall and spinal cord
Median sacral arteries	Posterior	Just superior to aortic bifurcation, pass inferiorly across lumbar vertebrae, sacrum, and coccyx	
Common iliac arteries	Terminal	Bifurcation usually occurs at level of L4 vertebra	

Modified from Drake RL, Vogl AW, Mitchell AWM. Gray's anatomy for students. Philadelphia: Churchill Livingstone; 2005. p. 331.

artery (IMA) via the marginal artery of Drummond. This anastomosis forms an important SMA-to-IMA collateral circulation that allows for the IMA to be sacrificed without colonic ischemia (Walker, 2009). However, despite the presence of this collateral circulation, injury to the SMA during left-sided retroperitoneal surgery may lead to severe bowel ischemia.

At L1, the paired **renal arteries** are the next branch of the aorta (Fig. 33-29 on the Expert Consult website). The inferior adrenal arteries branch off the renal arteries to supply the ipsilateral adrenal gland. There is considerable variation in the location, size, and number of renal arteries, with one quarter of cases manifesting with supernumerary renal arteries, which are more common on the right. The specific anatomic variations are discussed in depth in Chapter 42.

The **gonadal arteries** are the next paired branch of the aorta, typically arising anterolaterally from the aorta below the renal arteries. They may emerge from the renal artery in some variations, in which case they course with the gonadal vein. In males, the gonadal arteries are called the **testicular arteries,** and in females, they are called the **ovarian arteries.** The testicular arteries typically run anterior to the psoas, IVC, genitofemoral nerve, and ipsilateral ureter as they travel toward the internal inguinal ring.

The ovarian arteries arise from the anterolateral aspect of the aorta below the renal arteries. They travel anterior to the ureter and course medially as they pass through the infundibulopelvic ligament (suspensory ligament of the ovary) to the ovary. **There are extensive collaterals to the gonads in both sexes, allowing for ligation of the testicular and ovarian arteries without gonadal ischemia.**

The paired **lumbar arteries** arise posteriorly, adjacent to the bodies of the upper four lumbar vertebrae. They supply the posterior body wall and spine. In some instances, a fifth pair of lumbar arteries is present, arising from the middle sacral artery.

The **IMA** arises from the anterior aorta in the midline at the level of L3-L4 and supplies the colon from the splenic flexure to the upper rectum. The branches of the IMA are the left colic, sigmoid, and superior hemorrhoidal (rectal) arteries. The **sigmoid artery** branches into two to three inferior left colic arteries. As previously mentioned, the colonic branches of the IMA anastomose with the SMA via the marginal artery of Drummond and preclude colonic ischemia with IMA ligation. **The superior hemorrhoidal artery has collateral circulation with the inferior and middle hemorrhoidal arteries, which branch off the internal iliac arteries. These collaterals provide blood supply to the rectum and prevent ischemia during IMA ligation.**

Before bifurcation, the **median sacral** (middle sacral) artery arises from the posterior aspect of the aorta and courses over the fifth lumbar vertebra and sacrum. This vessel may be sacrificed if necessary without end-organ ischemia. At the fourth lumbar vertebra, the aorta bifurcates to form the **common iliac arteries.** No named branches are given off as these arteries enter the pelvis and divide to form the internal and external iliac arteries.

The ureter has a variable arterial supply that changes proximally and distally. **Most often, the renal artery supplies the proximal ureter, and the internal iliac artery including its branches, the superior and inferior vesical arteries, supply the distal ureter. The middle ureter is typically supplied by the aorta; however, it may also be supplied by the common iliac, gonadal, uterine, middle rectal, and vaginal arteries. In general, the abdominal (proximal) ureter receives its blood supply medially, and the pelvic (distal) ureter receives its blood supply from a lateral direction.**

Venous System

Although not as well defined, the layers of the venous system are similar to that of the arterial system. The layers from innermost to outermost are the intima, internal elastic lamina, media, external elastic lamina, and adventitia. As in the arterial system, the intima is composed of a layer of endothelial cells with subendothelial connective tissue. In the venous system, the internal and external elastic laminae are often poorly defined even in larger caliber vessels. The media layer of veins is significantly smaller than that of arteries and contains less vascular smooth muscle. Conversely, the venous adventitia is larger than the venous media and functions similar to the adventitia of the arterial system.

The venous system also differs from the arterial system with the presence of valves that prevent retrograde flow. These valves are typically bicuspid and they function to maintain the full venous blood flow toward the heart.

The major retroperitoneal venous structure is the IVC, formed from the confluence of the **common iliac veins,** inferior and to the right of the aortic bifurcation (see Fig. 33-27). The IVC ascends anterior to the vertebral bodies and to the right of the aorta through the retroperitoneum (Figs. 33-30 and 33-31 on the Expert Consult website). The infrarenal portion runs parallel and inferior to the aorta. On its ascent, the IVC becomes more anterior, and at the level of the diaphragm the great vessels are separated by the right crus of the diaphragm. **The IVC then enters the thorax through the central tendon of the diaphragm at the level of T8 and drains into the inferior aspect of the right atrium.**

The venous system is more variable than the arterial system; however, many venous structures run parallel with their arterial equivalent. The **median (middle) sacral vein** runs with its respective artery and typically drains into the left common iliac vein; however, it may enter into the angle created by convergence of the two common iliac veins. Avoiding these veins during fixation of the proximal limb of mesh during sacral colpopexy procedures is critical.

The **ascending lumbar veins** drain the posterior abdominal wall and run posterior to the psoas muscle and lateral to the spinal column (Fig. 33-32 on the Expert Consult website). They connect with the ipsilateral **lumbar veins,** which are variable in number and location compared with their arterial equivalents. These veins may assume a plexiform arrangement anterior to the vertebral bodies. **As the ascending lumbar veins enter the thorax, they become the hemiazygos vein on the left and the azygos vein on the right.**

In males, the **gonadal veins (testicular veins)** receive drainage from the pampiniform plexus, which is the venous complex that emerges from the testes. The testicular veins ascend through the retroperitoneum medially, running lateral to the respective artery and anterior to the ipsilateral ureter. The left testicular vein typically enters the inferior aspect of the left renal vein at a right angle; however, it may enter the IVC directly. The right testicular vein typically enters into the right anterolateral aspect of the IVC; however, it may enter into the right renal vein in 10% of cases. **These anatomic differences have clinical significance because the increased length and perpendicular entry of the left testicular vein into the left renal vein may account for the increased incidence of left-sided varicoceles.** This anatomic configuration may result in some element of increased back pressure in the left testicular vein compared with the right side. With the relative rarity of unilateral right-sided varicocele, a sudden-onset right varicocele should increase suspicion for a renal or retroperitoneal malignancy causing obstruction and poor venous outflow (e.g., right side renal cell cancer with venous thrombus). This clinical scenario should warrant retroperitoneal imaging to rule out malignancy.

The **ovarian veins** receive drainage from the pampiniform plexus adjacent to the ovarian hilum and travel through the infundibulopelvic ligament. As with the gonadal veins in males, the left ovarian vein enters the left renal vein, and the right ovarian vein empties into the anterolateral wall of the vena cava.

The **renal veins** course anteriorly to the renal arteries and empty into the lateral aspects of the vena cava at the level of L1. The right and left renal veins differ in length and tributaries with the right being shorter and typically having no tributaries. In rare cases, the right gonadal vein or a lumbar vein may empty into the right renal vein. In one sixth of cases, the renal vein is duplicated on the right side. The left renal vein is longer and typically receives the left gonadal vein at its caudal margin. At least one lumbar vein enters the left renal vein at or near the ostia of the gonadal vein. **The left adrenal vein is situated at the superior margin of the renal vein and in most patients inserts into the renal vein just medial to the gonadal vein.** The left adrenal vein occasionally is joined by the left inferior phrenic vein. The **right adrenal vein** is short, is single in number, has no tributaries, and drains directly into the posterolateral aspect of the vena cava. Although variable, the right inferior phrenic vein also typically drains into the superior portion of the IVC.

The gastrointestinal venous drainage does not mirror the arterial system as directly as the aforementioned venous structures. **The portal venous system receives venous blood from the bowel, spleen, pancreas, and gallbladder to be emptied into the liver** (Fig. 33-33 on the Expert Consult website). The **superior mesenteric vein (SMV)** receives venous drainage from the small intestine and the large intestine proximal to the splenic flexure. Tributaries of the SMV include the right gastro-omental, anterior and posterior inferior pancreaticoduodenal, jejunal, ileal, ileocolic, right colic, and middle colic veins. The SMV is joined by the splenic vein to form the **portal vein.** The tributaries of the **splenic vein** are the short gastric, left gastro-omental, pancreatic, and typically inferior mesenteric veins. The **inferior mesenteric vein** receives the venous

drainage from the colon distal to the splenic flexure. The portal vein splits into right and left branches, and the venous blood enters the endothelial lined hepatic sinusoids. After passing through these sinusoids, the venous blood leaves the liver through the hepatic veins, which enter the anterior aspect of the IVC before it crosses the diaphragm into the thorax. There are two groups of hepatic veins: the upper group, typically larger in caliber, and the lower group, which are typically smaller. **Occlusion of these hepatic veins can lead to Budd-Chiari syndrome, which is a form of progressive liver failure that often manifests rapidly with jaundice, ascites, abdominal pain, and hepatomegaly.**

LYMPHATIC SYSTEM

The lymphatic channels line tissue spaces and transport lymph to specialized areas of lymphoid tissue called lymph nodes. **The nodes typically have multiple afferent lymphatics and a single efferent lymphatic that drains into larger lymphatic vessels. Lymph generally flows cephalad from right to left until it returns to the venous circulation at the left innominate (brachiocephalic) vein.** Lymphatic fluid from the head, neck, right thorax, right arm, and right heart drains into the right innominate vein.

The lymphatic fluid from the pelvis and lower extremities drains into the internal iliac, external iliac, common iliac, obturator, and sacral nodes. These nodal regions then drain cephalad toward the lumbar nodes, whose efferent lymphatics form the lumbar trunks (Parker, 1935). The lumbar nodes are of considerable interest to the urologist because they provide the primary lymphatic drainage for structures supplied by lateral aortic arterial branches: the kidneys, adrenals, ureters, and gonads (Fig. 33-34). **For anatomic classification, three groups of lumbar nodes can be defined: left lumbar (aortic), interaortocaval (interaorticovenous), and right lumbar (caval) nodal groups.**

The left lumbar group includes the preaortic, left para-aortic (periaortic), and retroaortic nodes. The preaortic nodes are located anterior to the abdominal aorta, around the major anterior arterial branches that supply the gastrointestinal tract. The celiac, superior mesenteric, and inferior mesenteric nodes receive lymphatic drainage based on the anatomy of the similarly named arteries that supply the corresponding abdominal viscera. The efferents of these lymphatics coalesce to form the intestinal trunk. The left para-aortic region includes the nodes lateral to the midline of the aorta and medial to the left ureter. The retroaortic nodes are variably present and located between the aorta and vertebrae. The interaortocaval nodal group extends from the midline of the IVC to the midline of the aorta.

The right lumbar group includes the precaval, right paracaval, and retrocaval nodes. The precaval nodes are located on the anterior wall of the IVC. The right paracaval region includes the area lateral to the midline of the IVC, extending to the right ureter. The retrocaval nodes are present between the vena cava and the psoas muscle.

The testes are significant because they are embryologically retroperitoneal and have retroperitoneal blood supply and primary lymphatic drainage. When practically discussing testis malignancy, the three significant nodal regions are the left para-aortic, interaortocaval, and right paracaval. Elegant studies of early metastasis demonstrated the drainage pattern of the testes. **The left testis drains to the left para-aortic nodes with some drainage to the interaortocaval nodes.** There is no significant drainage to the right paracaval nodes, which is consistent with the general direction of lymphatic flow from right to left. **The right testis drains primarily to the interaortocaval nodes with some drainage to the right paracaval nodes. The left para-aortic region receives a small but appreciable amount of lymphatic drainage from the right testis, consistent with the aforementioned right-to-left flow.**

The efferent lymphatics of the lateral lumbar nodes coalesce to form the right and left lumbar trunks. Posterior to the right side of the abdominal aorta and anterior to the L1 and L2 vertebrae, these trunks come together at a saccular dilated structure known as the

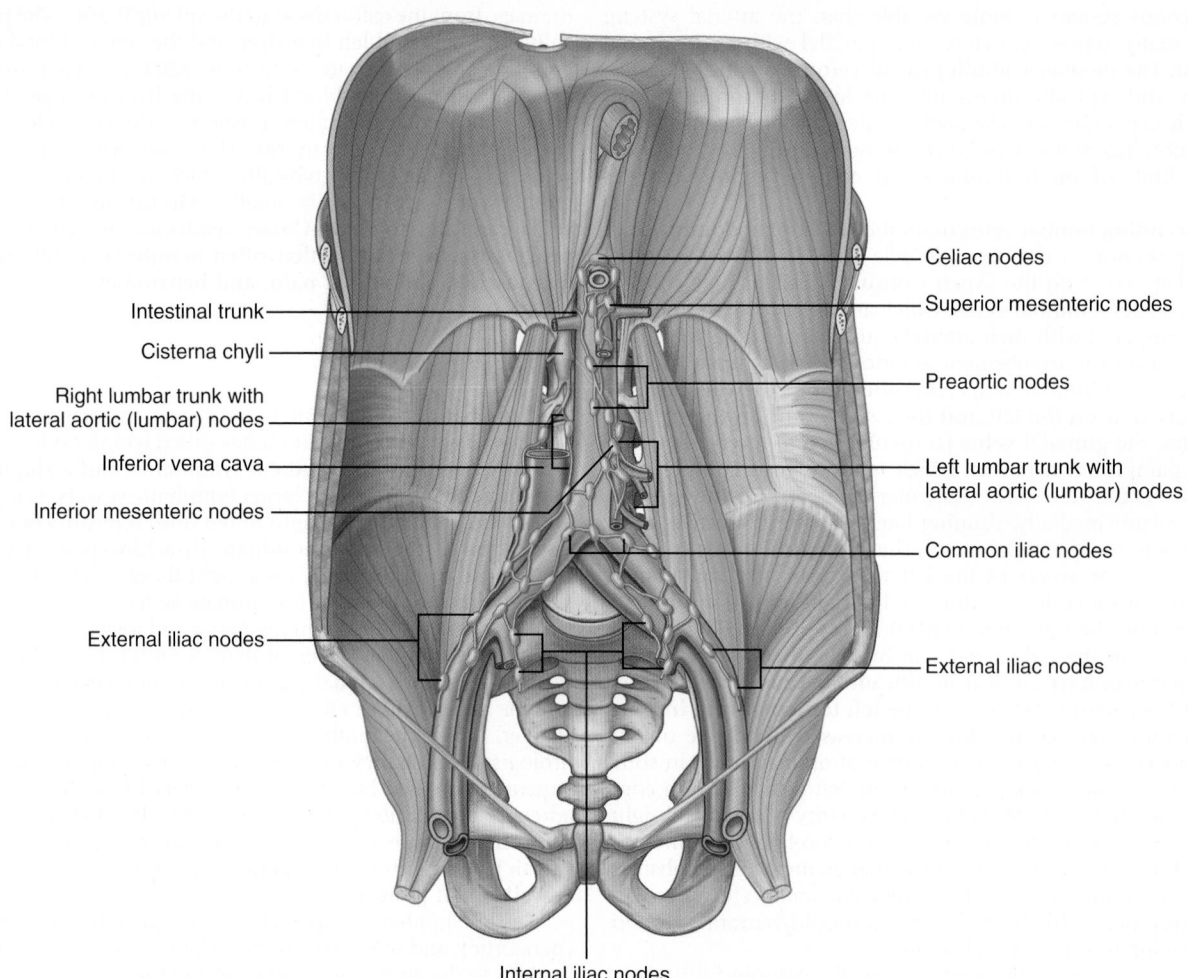

Intestinal trunk

Cisterna chyli

Right lumbar trunk with lateral aortic (lumbar) nodes

Inferior vena cava

Inferior mesenteric nodes

External iliac nodes

Celiac nodes

Superior mesenteric nodes

Preaortic nodes

Left lumbar trunk with lateral aortic (lumbar) nodes

Common iliac nodes

External iliac nodes

Internal iliac nodes

Figure 33-34. Retroperitoneal lymphatics. (From Drake RL, Vogl AW, Mitchell AWM. Gray's anatomy for students. 2nd ed. Philadelphia: Churchill Livingstone; 2010.)

cisterna chyli. This marks the beginning of the **thoracic duct,** which runs cephalad posterior to the aorta and empties into the left innominate vein.

NERVOUS STRUCTURES

The nervous structures of the retroperitoneum can be divided into the autonomic nervous system and the somatic nervous system. The autonomic system supplies efferent and afferent innervation to the abdominal viscera, blood vessels, and smooth muscle. The somatic system supplies efferent and afferent innervation to skeletal muscle, skin, and peritoneum.

Autonomic Nervous System

The general structure of the **autonomic nervous system** consists of two nerves with two cell bodies. The **preganglionic neuron** has a cell body within the central nervous system and an axon that extends into the peripheral nervous system, synapsing with another neuron within a ganglion. The second neuron is referred to as a **postganglionic neuron,** and its axon enters the structure in which it provides innervation. One caveat to this general structure is the neural anatomy of the adrenal gland. **The preganglionic fibers synapse directly with the cells of the adrenal medulla resulting in release of catecholamines. The adrenal can be considered a specialized ganglion of the autonomic nervous system.**

The autonomic system can be divided further into the parasympathetic and sympathetic nervous systems. The **parasympathetic nervous system** has craniosacral outflow because the preganglionic fibers originate from cranial nerves III, VII, IX, and X and from the ventral rami of the second, third, and fourth sacral nerves. The preganglionic fibers from S2-S4 form the pelvic splanchnic nerves, which provide parasympathetic innervation to the pelvic and abdominal viscera, which often contain the postganglionic parasympathetic fibers within their walls. The vagus nerve (cranial nerve X) also provides preganglionic parasympathetic fibers to the thoracic, abdominal, and pelvic viscera.

In contrast to the parasympathetic system, the preganglionic fibers of the **sympathetic nervous system** originate between the first thoracic and the second lumbar vertebral levels. These fibers exit the spinal cord from T1 to L2 through the ventral root and course through the corresponding spinal nerve and anterior rami into the ipsilateral sympathetic trunk (Fig. 33-35). The fibers then run medial to the psoas muscle along the anterolateral aspect of the spine. **The paired sympathetic trunks are in close proximity to the lumbar arteries and veins, which cross them perpendicularly.** The preganglionic fibers can synapse within the ganglia of the sympathetic trunk and send forth postganglionic fibers to the body wall and lower extremities. The preganglionic fibers also may leave the trunk as splanchnic nerves to synapse with the ganglia of the autonomic plexuses of the aorta (Fig. 33-36).

The first and largest of these plexuses is the celiac plexus, which contains paired ganglia that lie lateral to the celiac artery. Much of the autonomic innervation to the kidney, adrenal, renal

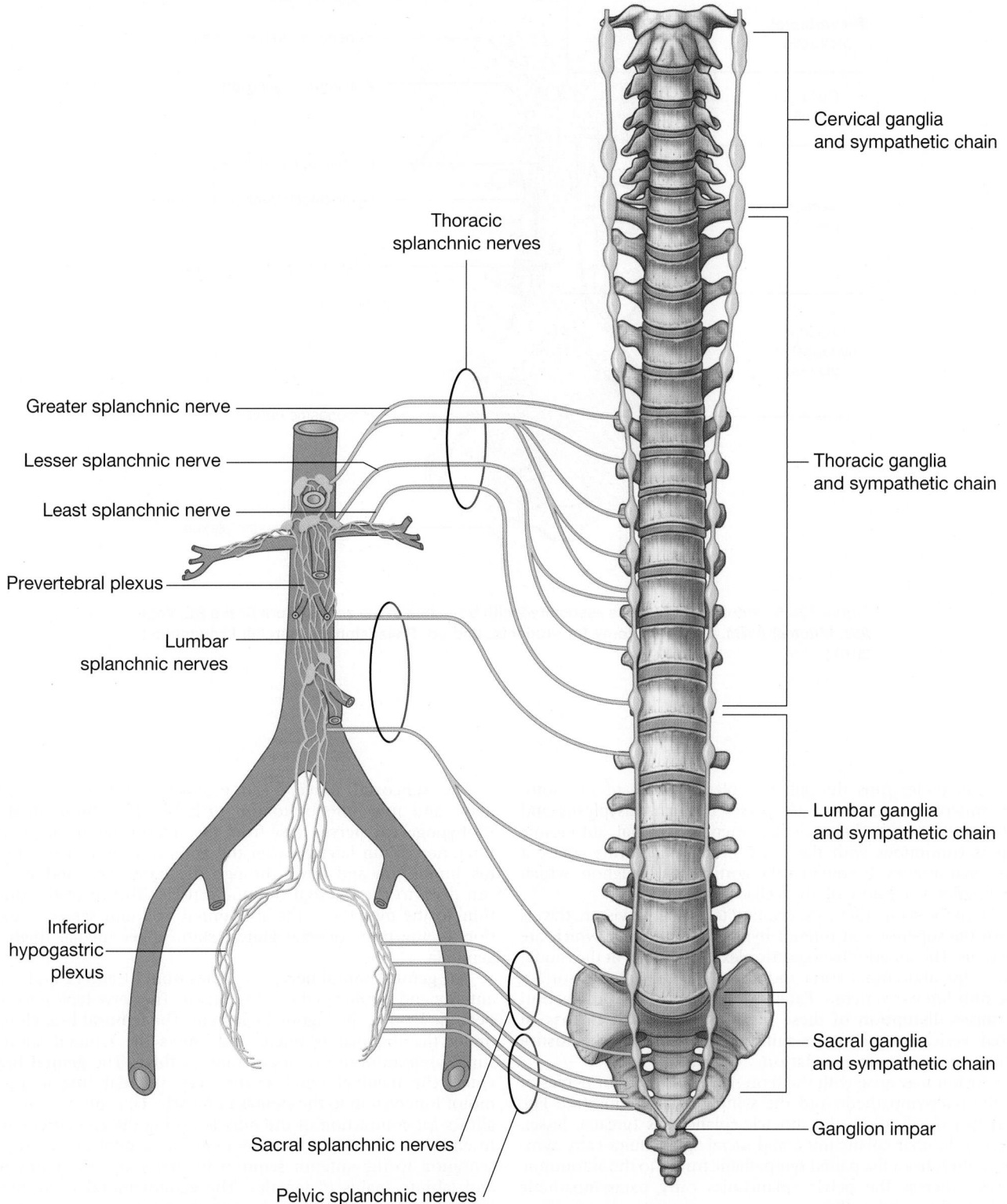

Figure 33-35. Sympathetic chain and splanchnic nerves. (From Drake RL, Vogl AW, Mitchell AWM. Gray's anatomy for students. 2nd ed. Philadelphia: Churchill Livingstone; 2010.)

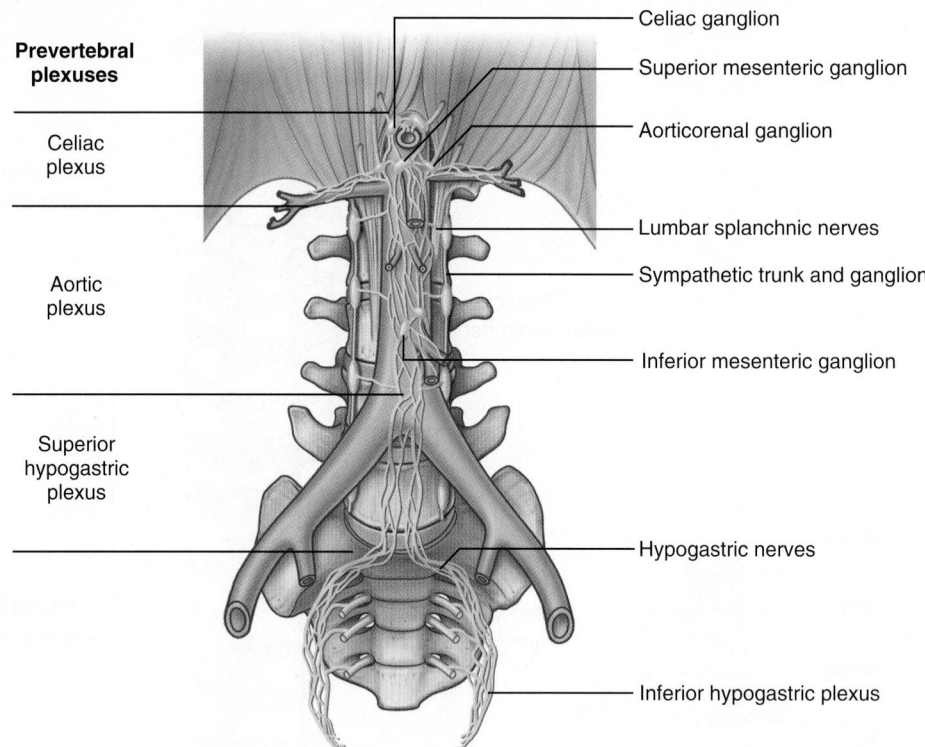

Prevertebral plexuses

Celiac plexus

Aortic plexus

Superior hypogastric plexus

Celiac ganglion

Superior mesenteric ganglion

Aorticorenal ganglion

Lumbar splanchnic nerves

Sympathetic trunk and ganglion

Inferior mesenteric ganglion

Hypogastric nerves

Inferior hypogastric plexus

Figure 33-36. **Autonomic plexuses associated with branches of the aorta. (From Drake RL, Vogl AW, Mitchell AWM. Gray's anatomy for students. 2nd ed. Philadelphia: Churchill Livingstone; 2010.)**

pelvis, and ureter runs through this plexus. Some of the autonomic innervation for the testes passes through this plexus and travels caudally with the testicular artery. The renal autonomic plexus is continuous with the celiac plexus and forms adjacent to the renal arteries. It contains the aorticorenal ganglion, which is an inferior extension of the celiac ganglion.

Much of the sympathetic innervation to the pelvic viscera travels through the superior and inferior hypogastric plexuses, which are contiguous. The superior hypogastric plexus originates at the caudal extent of the abdominal aorta and extends to the anterior surface of the fifth lumbar vertebra. **Extensive retroperitoneal dissection that causes disruption of these plexuses may result in loss of seminal vesicle emission or failure of bladder neck closure resulting in retrograde ejaculation.**

Confusion may arise with the term *splanchnic* used for nerves of both the parasympathetic and the sympathetic systems (see Fig. 33-35). For clarification, the thoracic splanchnics (greater, lesser, and least), lumbar splanchnics, and sacral splanchnics carry sympathetic fibers from the paired sympathetic trunks to the autonomic plexuses, whereas the pelvic splanchnics carry parasympathetic fibers from the sacral outflow.

Somatic Nervous System

The somatic sensory and motor nerves of the lower abdomen and lower extremities originate in the retroperitoneum. They form the lumbosacral plexus from the anterior rami of the lumbar and sacral nerves along with T12 (Fig. 33-37 on the Expert Consult website). The nerves arising from this plexus are in close proximity to the psoas muscle, with the superior nerves piercing the muscle, while the inferior nerves travel medial to the muscle body (Fig. 33-38). This plexus provides the cutaneous sensory innervation to the lower extremities (Fig. 33-39 and Table 33-4).

The **subcostal nerve** is an extension of the 12th thoracic nerve and runs inferior to the 12th rib. The **ilioinguinal and iliohypogastric nerves** arise from the anterior ramus of L1. These three nerves run laterally over the anterior aspect of the quadratus lumborum and travel through the transversus abdominis to run deep to the internal oblique muscle. They provide innervation to the muscles of the abdominal wall and sensory innervation to the posterolateral gluteal skin, upper medial thigh, and genitalia.

The **genitofemoral nerve** originates from L1 and L2 and courses anterior and parallel to the psoas muscle. The nerve typically divides near the level of the inguinal ligament. The **femoral branch** passes under the inguinal ligament and enters the femoral sheath to supply sensation to the upper anterior thigh. The **genital branch** enters the inguinal canal at the deep internal ring to provide motor innervation to the cremaster muscle. This motor component allows for contraction of the muscle during the cremasteric reflex. In addition to the motor component, the genital branch supplies sensation to the anterior scrotum in males and the mons pubis and labium majus in females. The genitofemoral nerve may be injured during a psoas hitch procedure (suture placement) and laparoscopic varicocelectomy (ligation). The **lateral cutaneous nerve of the thigh** (lateral femoral cutaneous nerve) arises from L2 and L3 and provides sensory innervation to the anterior and lateral thigh.

The **obturator nerve** originates from the anterior rami of L2-L4 posterior to the psoas muscle and courses inferiorly to the obturator canal. **The function of the obturator nerve includes hip adduction via motor innervation to the medial thigh compartment, which is of clinical significance during lateral transurethral resection and pelvic lymph node dissection.** Electrocautery employed during a transurethral resection of bladder tumor (TURBT) procedure may result in obturator nerve stimulation with

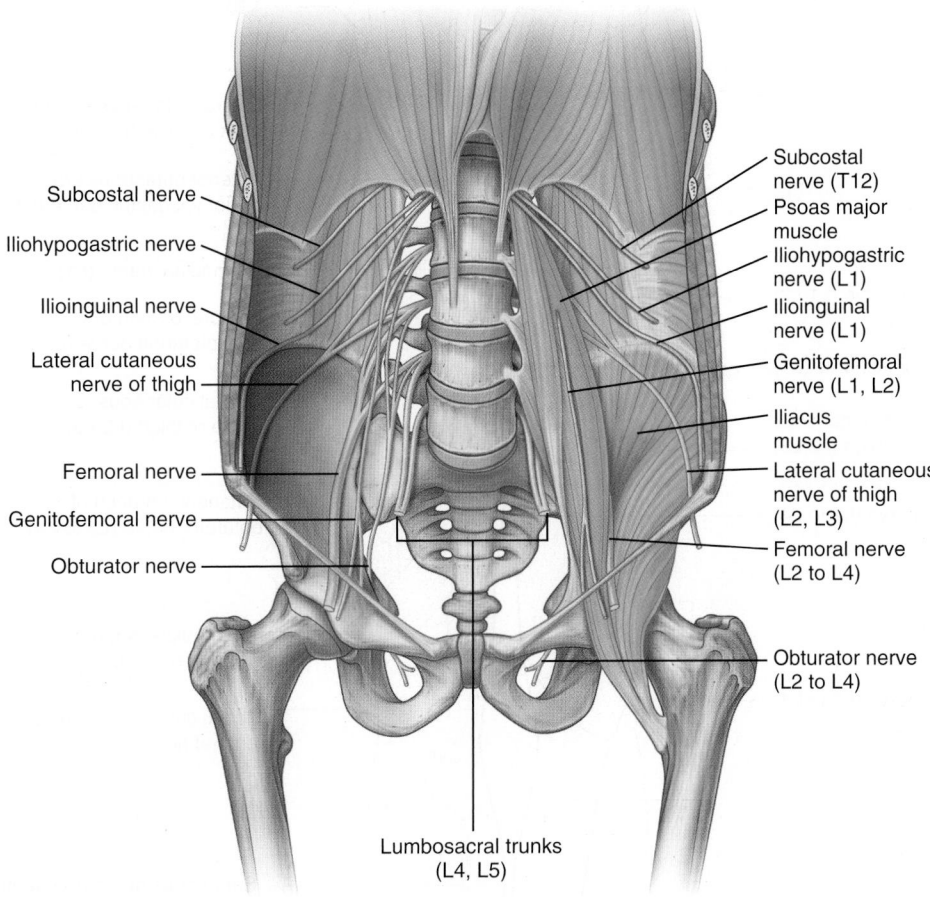

Figure 33-38. Lumbar plexus in the posterior abdominal region. (From Drake RL, Vogl AW, Mitchell AWM. Gray's anatomy for students. 2nd ed. Philadelphia: Churchill Livingstone; 2010.)

TABLE 33-4   Branches of the Lumbosacral Plexus

BRANCH	ORIGIN	SPINAL SEGMENTS	MOTOR FUNCTION	SENSORY FUNCTION
Subcostal	Anterior ramus T12	T12	Muscles of abdominal wall	Skin over hip
Iliohypogastric	Anterior ramus L1	L1	Internal oblique and transversus abdominis	Posterolateral gluteal skin and skin in pubic region
Ilioinguinal	Anterior ramus L1	L1	Internal oblique and transversus abdominis	Skin in upper medial thigh and the skin over either the root of the penis and anterior scrotum or the mons pubis and labium majus
Genitofemoral	Anterior rami L1 and L2	L1, L2	Genital branch: male cremasteric muscle	Genital branch: skin of anterior scrotum or skin of mons pubis and labium majus
				Femoral branch: skin of upper anterior thigh
Lateral cutaneous nerve of the thigh	Anterior rami L2 and L3	L2, L3	None	Skin on anterior and lateral thigh to the knee
Obturator	Anterior rami L2-L4	L2-L4	Obturator externus, pectineus, and muscles in medial compartment of thigh	Skin on medial aspect of thigh
Femoral	Anterior rami L2-L4	L2-L4	Iliacus, pectineus, and muscles in anterior compartment of thigh	Skin on anterior thigh and medial surface of leg

Modified from Drake RL, Vogl AW, Mitchell AWM. Gray's anatomy for students. Philadelphia: Churchill Livingstone; 2005.

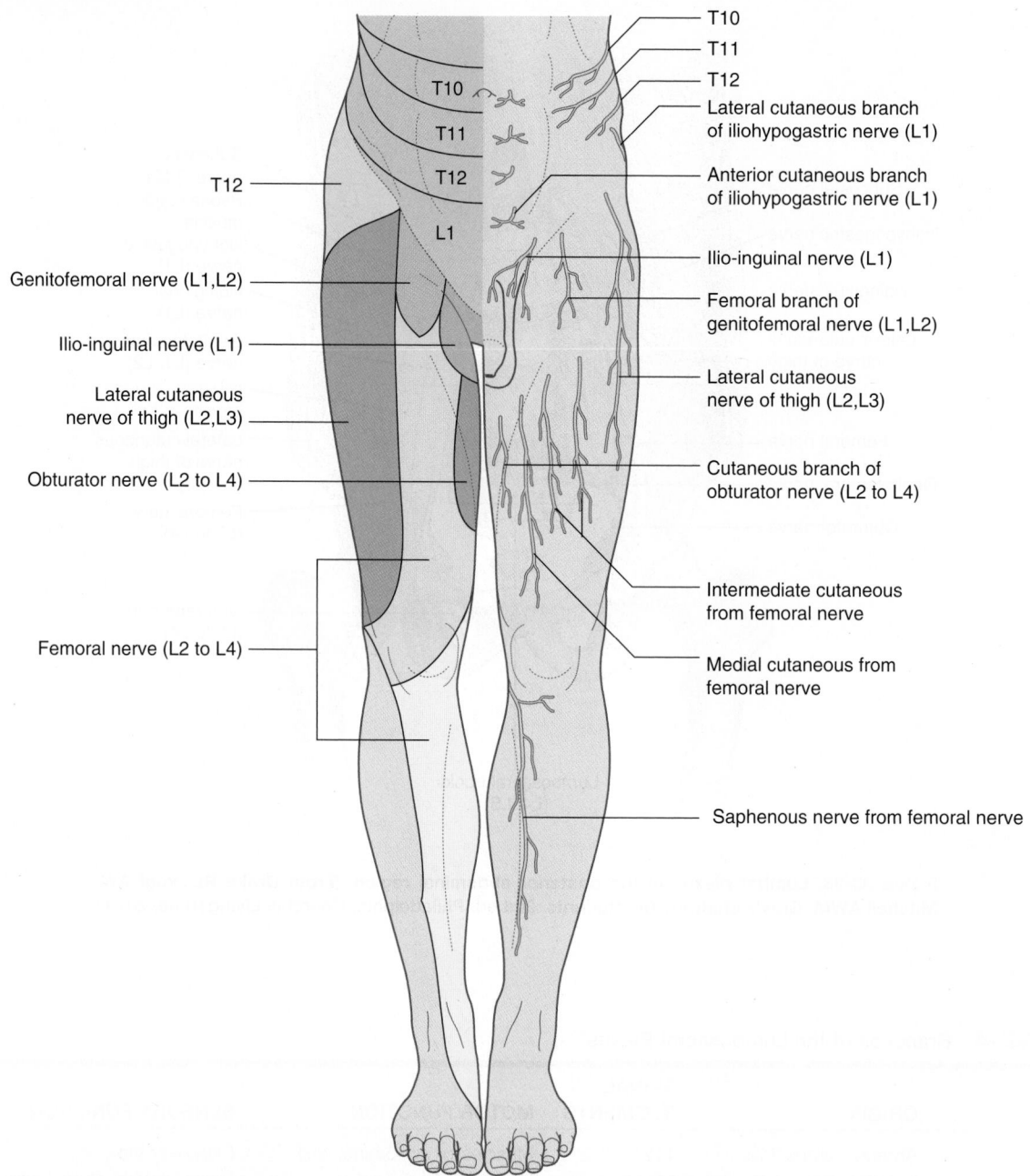

Figure 33-39. Cutaneous distribution of the nerves from the lumbar plexus. (From Drake RL, Vogl AW, Mitchell AWM. Gray's anatomy for students. 2nd ed. Philadelphia: Churchill Livingstone; 2010.)

subsequent rapid, forceful hip adduction. If this potential event is not anticipated and accounted for, severe bladder perforation may occur.

With its origin from the anterior rami of L2-L4, the **femoral nerve** provides efferent motor input to the muscles of the anterior thigh as well as the iliacus and pectineus, which are responsible for knee extension and hip flexion, respectively. The femoral nerve also gives sensory innervation to the skin over the anterior medial lower extremity. Compression of the femoral nerve may occur intraoperatively with placement of retractor blades inferolaterally against the inguinal ligament. Compression injury may result in a motor palsy to the quadriceps muscle, impairing extension at the knee.

Additionally, a stretch injury to the femoral nerve may occur with prolonged hip flexion in low lithotomy position used during minimally invasive pelvic surgery.

The **sciatic nerve** receives input from L4-S3 and provides the bulk of motor and sensory input to the lower extremities, including motor innervation to the posterior thigh compartment and all muscles in the leg and foot. Injury to this nerve may occur secondary to prolonged hip hyperflexion used during a high lithotomy position for vaginal and urethral procedures.

Please visit the accompanying website at www.expertconsult.com to view videos associated with this chapter.

KEY POINTS

- The retroperitoneum is contained anteriorly by the posterior reflection of the peritoneum, posteriorly by the abdominal wall, cranially by the diaphragm, and caudally by the extraperitoneal pelvic structures.
- The lumbodorsal fascia merges anterolaterally with the transversus abdominis muscle and is composed of three layers that cover the posterior abdominal wall musculature.
- The anterior and posterior laminae of Gerota fascia form the boundaries of the perirenal space, which has a conelike shape that is open caudally in the extraperitoneal pelvis.
- The retroperitoneal gastrointestinal structures are the pancreas, the second and third portions of the duodenum, the ascending colon, and the descending colon.
- The renal hila are at the level of L1, and the renal veins are anterior to the renal arteries.
- The lymph of the left testis drains to the left para-aortic nodes with some to the interaortocaval nodes, and the right testis drains primarily to the interaortocaval nodes with some to the right paracaval nodes and a small amount to the left para-aortic region. This drainage is consistent with global lymphatic flow from right to left.
- The parasympathetic autonomic nervous system has craniosacral outflow and the postganglionic fibers are often contained within the walls of the innervated viscera.
- The preganglionic sympathetic nervous system fibers exit from the spinal cord from T1 to L2 and may synapse within the sympathetic trunk or within the autonomic plexuses.
- The somatic nervous system provides sensory and motor innervation to the pelvis and lower extremities through the lumbosacral plexus.

REFERENCES

The complete reference list is available online at www.expertconsult.com.

SUGGESTED READINGS

Drake RL, Vogl AW, Mitchell AWM. Gray's anatomy for students. 2nd ed. Philadelphia: Churchill Livingstone; 2010.

MacLennan GT. Hinman's atlas of urosurgical anatomy. 2nd ed. Philadelphia: Saunders; 2012.

Smith JA, Howards SS, Preminger GM. Hinman's atlas of urologic surgery, 3rd ed. Philadelphia: Saunders; 2012.

34 Neoplasms of the Testis

Andrew J. Stephenson, MD, MBA, FACS, FRCS(C), and Timothy D. Gilligan, MD, MS

Germm Cell Tumors

Tumors of the Testicular Adnexa

Non–Germ Cell Tumors

N eoplasms of the testis constitute a morphologically and clinically diverse group of tumors, **of which more than 95% are germ cell tumors (GCTs). GCTs are broadly categorized as seminoma and nonseminoma germ cell tumor (NSGCT) because of differences in natural history and treatment. GCT is a relatively rare malignancy, accounting for 1% to 2% of cancers among men in the United States.** Approximately 95% of GCTs arise in the testis, and 5% are extragonadal in origin. With the development of cisplatin-based chemotherapy and the integration of surgery, GCTs have become a model of a curable neoplasm and serve as a paradigm for multidisciplinary treatment of cancer (Einhorn, 1981). In the era before cisplatin-based chemotherapy, the cure rate for patients with advanced GCT was 5% to 10%. At the present time, the long-term survival for men with metastatic GCT is 80% to 90%. With the successful cure of patients, an important treatment objective is minimizing treatment-related toxicity without compromising curability. Mortality from GCT is due to inherent resistance to cisplatin chemotherapy and the failure to eradicate fully residual disease elements in the early course of therapy.

Non-GCT tumors of the testis are rare and include sex cord–stromal tumors, lymphoid and hematopoietic tumors, tumors of the collecting duct and rete testis, and tumors of the testicular adnexa. A classification of testis neoplasms is presented in Box 34-1.

GERM CELL TUMORS

Epidemiology

In 2014, an estimated 8820 men were expected to develop testis cancer in the United States, and 380 were expected to die from this disease (Siegel et al, 2014). **In the United States, testis cancer is the most common malignancy among men 20 to 40 years old and the second most common cancer after leukemia among adolescent boys and young men 15 to 19 years old** (Horner et al, 2009). Testis tumors have three age peaks: infancy, age 30 to 34 years, and approximately age 60. **The incidence of bilateral GCT is approximately 2.5% (0.6% risk of synchronous and 1.9% risk of metachronous contralateral tumors)** (Fossa et al, 2005).

The incidence of testis cancer varies significantly according to geographic region. **Rates are highest in Scandinavia, Western Europe, and Australia–New Zealand; intermediate in the United States and United Kingdom; and lowest in Africa and Asia** (Weijl et al, 2000). **The incidence of testis cancer in the United States in non-Hispanic whites is five times higher than the incidence in blacks, four times higher than the incidence in Asians, and 78% higher than in Hispanics** (Horner et al, 2009).

The incidence of GCT appears to be increasing worldwide (McKiernan et al, 1999; McGlynn et al, 2005; Purdue et al, 2005). In the United States, the age-adjusted incidence rate for adolescent boys and men 15 to 49 years old increased from 2.9 per 100,000 in 1975 to 5.1 per 100,000 in 2004 (Holmes et al, 2008). Over this time period, incidence rates increased substantially more for seminoma than NSGCT (McGlynn et al, 2005; Powles et al, 2005). A stage migration of GCT has been observed in several countries partly secondary to increased awareness and earlier diagnosis. Between 1973 and 2001, the percentage of tumors diagnosed at a localized stage increased from 55% to 73% in the United States among white men. The stage distribution for African-American men remained stable during this time (McGlynn et al, 2005). **Only about 10% to 30% of men present with distant metastatic disease.** In the United Kingdom, the change in stage distribution over time is largely restricted to an increase in localized seminoma and a decrease in metastatic NSGCT; rates of localized NSGCT and metastatic seminoma are largely unchanged (McGlynn et al, 2005). **At the present time, localized seminoma is the most common presentation of GCT, representing approximately 50% of all men with GCT** (Powles et al, 2005).

Risk Factors

There are four well-established risk factors for testis cancer: cryptorchidism, family history of testis cancer, a personal history of testis cancer, and intratubular germ cell neoplasia (ITGCN). Infertile men also have a higher incidence of testis cancer. **Numerous studies have reported that more recent increases in testis cancer incidence can be largely attributed to birth-cohort effects, which implies that diet and/or other environmental factors play a major role in GCT carcinogenesis** (Liu et al, 1999; Huyghe et al, 2003; McGlynn et al, 2003; Richiardi et al, 2004; Bray et al, 2006; Verhoeven et al, 2008).

Men with cryptorchidism are four to six times more likely to have testis cancer diagnosed in the affected gonad, but the relative risk decreases to two to three times more likely if orchidopexy is performed before puberty (Dieckmann and Pichlmeier, 2004; Wood and Elder, 2009). A meta-analysis of cryptorchidism studies reported that the contralateral descended testis is also at **slightly increased risk** (relative risk 1.74 [95% confidence interval 1.01 to 2.98]) (Akre et al, 2009). Men with a first-degree relative with testis cancer have a substantially increased risk of testis cancer, and the median age at diagnosis in these men is 2 to 3 years younger than in the general population (Mai et al, 2009). A man's relative risk for testis cancer is 8 to 12 with an affected brother compared with 2 to 4 in men with an affected father (Westergaard et al, 1996; Sonneveld et al, 1999b; Hemminki and Chen, 2006). Men with a history of testis cancer have a 12-fold increased risk of developing GCT in the contralateral testis, but the 15-year cumulative incidence is only 2%.

Most GCTs arise from a precursor lesion, ITGCN (which is also referred to as carcinoma in situ). ITGCN is present in adjacent testicular parenchyma in 80% to 90% of cases of invasive GCT and is associated with a 50% risk of GCT within 5 years and 70% within 7 years (Skakkebaek et al, 1982; Dieckmann and Skakkebaek, 1999; Montironi, 2002). **Of patients with GCT, 5% to 9% have ITGCN within the unaffected contralateral testis, although the incidence of contralateral ITGCN increases to about 36% in men with testicular atrophy or cryptorchidism** (Dieckmann and

BOX 34-1 World Health Organization Classification of Testicular Tumors

Germ cell tumors
    Precursor lesions—intratubular malignant germ cells (carcinoma in situ)
    Tumors of one histologic type (pure forms)
        Seminoma
            Variant—seminoma with syncytiotrophoblastic cells
        Spermatocytic seminoma
            Variant—spermatocytic seminoma with sarcoma
        Embryonal carcinoma
        Yolk sac tumor
        Polyembryoma
        Trophoblastic tumors
            Choriocarcinoma
            Choriocarcinoma with other cell types
            Placental site trophoblastic tumor
        Teratoma
            Mature teratoma
            Dermoid cyst
            Immature teratoma
            Teratoma with malignant areas
    Tumors of more than one histologic type (mixed forms)—specify types and estimate percentage
Sex cord–gonadal stromal tumors
    Pure forms
        Leydig cell tumor
        Sertoli cell tumor
            Large-cell calcifying Sertoli cell tumor
            Lipid-rich Sertoli cell tumor
        Granulosa cell tumor
            Adult-type granulosa cell tumor
            Juvenile-type granulosa cell tumor
        Tumors of thecoma/fibroma group
        Incompletely differentiated sex cord–gonadal stromal tumors
        Mixed forms
    Unclassified forms
    Tumors containing germ cell and sex cord–gonadal stromal elements
        Gonadoblastoma
        Mixed germ cell and sex cord–gonadal stromal tumors, unclassified
Miscellaneous tumors
    Carcinoid tumor
    Tumors of ovarian epithelial types

Lymphoid and hematopoietic tumors
    Lymphoma
    Plasmacytoma
    Leukemia
Tumors of collecting ducts and rete
    Adenoma
    Carcinoma
Tumors of the tunica, epididymis, spermatic cord, supporting structures, and appendices
    Adenomatoid tumor
    Mesothelioma
        Benign
        Malignant
    Adenoma
    Carcinoma
    Melanotic neuroectodermal
    Desmoplastic small round cell tumor
Soft-tissue tumors
Unclassified tumors
Secondary tumors
Tumorlike lesions
    Nodules of immature tubules
    Testicular lesions of adrenogenital syndrome
    Testicular lesions of androgen-insensitivity syndrome
    Nodular precocious maturation
    Specific orchitis
    Nonspecific orchitis
    Granulomatous orchitis
    Malakoplakia
    Adrenal cortical rest
    Fibromatous peritonitis
    Funiculitis
    Residue of meconium peritonitis
    Sperm granuloma
    Vasitis nodosa
    Sclerosing lipogranuloma
    Gonadal splenic fusion
    Mesonephric remnants
    Endometriosis
    Epidermal cyst
    Cystic dysplasia
    Mesolithial cyst
    Others

Data from Vogelzang NJ, Scardino PT, Shipley WU, et al, editors. Genitourinary oncology. Philadelphia: Lippincott Williams & Wilkins; 1999.

Loy, 1996; Dieckmann and Skakkebaek, 1999). Gene expression profile analysis indicates that ITGCN develops before birth from an arrested gonocyte (Hussain et al, 2008; Sonne et al, 2009). In men with a history of GCT, the finding of testicular microlithiasis on ultrasound of the contralateral testis is associated with an increased risk of ITGCN (Karellas et al, 2007). **However, the significance of microlithiasis in the general population is unclear;** a study of 1500 Army volunteers found a 5.6% prevalence of microlithiasis, yet less than 2% of men with microlithiasis developed GCT within 5 years (DeCastro et al, 2008).

Pathogenesis and Biology

The carcinogenesis of GCTs is poorly understood (Looijenga et al, 2011; Turnbull and Rahman, 2011; Sheikine et al, 2012). As noted earlier, testicular GCTs develop from a precursor lesion,

ITGCN, which appears to develop from arrested primordial germ cells or gonocytes that failed to differentiate into presper-matogonia (Rajpert-de Meyts and Hoei-Hansen, 2007; Hussain et al, 2008; Looijenga et al, 2011). These cells are thought to lay dormant until after puberty, when they are stimulated by increased testosterone levels.

The increased incidence of testis cancer that started in the first half of the 20th century has been accompanied by an increased incidence of other male reproductive disorders, such as hypospadias, cryptorchidism, and subfertility (Rajpert-de Meyts and Hoei-Hansen, 2007; Sonne et al, 2008). These findings led to the hypothesis that testis cancer and these other disorders all resulted from a testicular dysgenesis syndrome, which resulted from environmental and/or lifestyle factors and genetic susceptibility. The specific environmental or lifestyle factors have not been defined. Increased prenatal estrogen exposure has been hypothesized as a risk factor, but this is controversial (Martin et al, 2008). There is stronger evidence that reduction in androgen activity can result in features of testicular dysgenesis syndrome, including cryptorchidism, hypospadias, and impaired spermatogenesis, but a direct link between reduced androgen signaling and ITGCN remains hypothetical (Sonne et al, 2008; Hu et al, 2009).

Evidence of environmental and lifestyle factors contributing to testis cancer includes the rapid increase in its incidence and findings that risk of second-generation immigrants is similar to their country of birth. In addition, mothers of children with testis cancer (but not the patients with testis cancer themselves) have been found to have higher blood levels of certain organic pollutants compared with other mothers (Sonne et al, 2008). Evidence for genetic factors includes the clustering of testis cancer in some families; the extreme difference in the rate of testis cancer in black and white Americans; and the finding of susceptibility loci on chromosomes 5, 6, and 12 in case-control studies (Mai et al, 2009). In addition, specific polymorphisms of certain genes, including the gene encoding c-KIT ligand, have been associated with an increased risk of testis cancer (Blomberg Jensen et al, 2008; Kanetsky et al, 2009; Turnbull and Rahman, 2011; Sheikine et al, 2012). Gonocytes depend on KIT ligand for survival, and the gene for this protein is located on the short arm of chromosome 12. **An increased number of copies of genetic material from the short arm of chromosome 12 is a universal finding in testicular and extragonadal germ cell tumors.** Of GCTs, 70% to 80% have an extra copy of chromosome 12 in the form of an isochromosome 12p (i[12p]), whereas the remainder show gain of 12p sequences detectable with fluorescence in situ hybridization (Looijenga et al, 2003). A connection between mutations or polymorphisms in c-KIT ligand and GCT has biologic plausibility.

One of the most striking features of GCTs is their sensitivity to cisplatin-based chemotherapy, which enables cure in most patients with widely metastatic disease. The specific biologic basis of this acute vulnerability to chemotherapy is incompletely understood but is thought to derive from the close relationship between GCTs and embryonal stem cells and gonocytes, which have a low threshold for undergoing apoptosis in response to DNA damage (Mayer et al, 2003; Schmelz et al, 2010). Gene expression analysis has found an upregulation of numerous genes that facilitate apoptosis, including *FasL*, *TRAIL*, and *Bax*, whereas *BCL-2* is downregulated (Schmelz et al, 2010). Expression patterns of genes controlling the G_1/S-phase checkpoint in GCTs appear to promote induction of apoptosis (Schmelz et al, 2010). In addition, GCTs lack transporters to export cisplatin from the cell and have a reduced ability to repair cisplatin-induced DNA damage (Mayer et al, 2003). GCTs have high intrinsic levels of wild-type p53 protein (which plays a role in mediating cell cycle arrest and apoptosis), and p53 mutations in GCTs are rare, yet differences have not been consistently found in p53 status when comparing chemosensitive and chemoresistant GCTs (Burger et al, 1998; Houldsworth et al, 1998). Similarly, expression of the antiapoptotic protein BCL-2 is low in GCTs, but BCL-2 levels do not distinguish chemosensitive and chemoresistant cell lines (Mayer et al, 2003). A small fraction of GCTs are resistant to chemotherapy, and the basis of that resistance remains obscure (Veenstra and Vaughn, 2011). Impaired DNA mismatch repair and activating *BRAF* mutations have been associated with treatment failure (Honecker et al, 2009; Looijenga et al, 2011; Veenstra and Vaughn, 2011; Sheikine et al, 2012).

Approximately 5% of GCTs are extragonadal in origin and develop in midline anatomic locations (retroperitoneum and mediastinum are most common). There are two main competing theories regarding the pathogenesis of extragonadal GCTs. The first hypothesizes that they originate from germ cells that mistakenly migrated along the genital ridge and were able to survive in an extragonadal environment. The second theory proposes a reverse migration from the testis to extragonadal locations (Chaganti and Houldsworth, 2000).

Primary mediastinal NSGCTs differ in several ways from NSGCTs originating in the testis or retroperitoneum (Moran and Suster, 1997a; Moran et al, 1997a, 1997b; Moran and Suster, 1998).

First, they are less sensitive to chemotherapy and have a poor prognosis with a 5-year overall survival of about 45% (Bokemeyer et al, 2002b). Mediastinal NSGCTs are more likely to have yolk sac tumor components and to be associated with elevations in serum α-fetoprotein (AFP) (Moran et al, 1997a; Bokemeyer et al, 2002b; Kesler et al, 2008). They are also associated with Kleinfelter syndrome and with hematologic malignancies that carry extra copies of the short arm of chromosome 12, as seen in adult GCT (Bokemeyer et al, 2002a; McKenney et al, 2007). **In contrast, mediastinal seminomas have a prognosis similar to testicular seminomas, and mature teratomas of the mediastinum have low metastatic potential and can generally be cured surgically** (Lewis et al, 1983; International Germ Cell Consensus Classification, 1997; Allen, 2002). **Primary retroperitoneal GCTs are indistinguishable biologically from testicular GCTs and carry the same prognosis.**

Histologic Classification

The histologic classification of GCTs is outlined in Box 34-2 (Sobin and Wittekind, 2002). **GCTs are broadly classified as seminoma and NSGCT, and the relative distribution is 52% to 56% and 44% to 48%, respectively** (McGlynn et al, 2005; Powles et al, 2005). **NSGCTs include embryonal carcinoma (EC), yolk sac tumor, teratoma, and choriocarcinoma subtypes, occurring either alone as pure forms or in combination as mixed GCT with or without seminoma** (Ulbright, 2005). Most NSGCTs are mixed tumors that are composed of two or more GCT subtypes. GCTs that contain both NSGCT subtypes and seminoma are classified as NSGCTs.

Intratubular Germ Cell Neoplasia

With the exception of spermatocytic seminoma, all adult invasive GCTs arise from ITGCN. ITGCN consists of undifferentiated germ cells that have the appearance of seminoma that are located basally within the seminiferous tubules. The tubule usually shows decreased or absent spermatogenesis, and normal constituents are replaced by ITGCN. The presence of ITGCN in an orchiectomy specimen in men with testis cancer does not have any prognostic implications with regard to the risk of relapse (von Eyben et al, 2004). ITGCN is much less frequent in GCTs in pediatric patients (Cheville, 1999).

BOX 34-2 World Health Organization Classification of Germ Cell Tumors

Intratubular germ cell neoplasia
Tumors of one histologic type (pure forms)
    Seminoma
        Seminoma with syncytiotrophoblastic cells
        Spermatocytic seminoma
    Embryonal carcinoma
    Yolk sac tumor
    Trophoblastic tumors
        Choriocarcinoma
        Trophoblastic neoplasms other than choriocarcinoma
        Monophasic choriocarcinoma
        Placental site trophoblastic tumor
    Teratoma
        Dermoid cyst
        Monodermal teratoma
        Teratoma with somatic type malignancy (malignant transformation)
Tumors of more than one histologic subtype (mixed forms)

From Sobin LH, Wittekind CH. UICC: TNM classification of malignant tumors. 6th ed. New York: Wiley-Liss; 2002.

Seminoma

Seminoma is the most common type of GCT. **On average, seminomas occur at an older average age than NSGCTs, with most cases diagnosed in the fourth or fifth decade of life** (Cheville, 1999). Grossly, seminoma is a soft tan-to-white diffuse or multinodular mass (Fig. 34-1A). Necrosis may be present but is usually focal and

not as prominent as in other GCTs. Seminomas consist of a sheet-like arrangement of cells with polygonal nuclei and clear cytoplasm, with the cells divided into nests by fibrovascular septa that contain lymphocytes (Fig. 34-1B) (Ulbright, 2005). Syncytiotrophoblasts, which stain positive for human chorionic gonadotropin (hCG), can be identified in about 15% of cases but are of no clear prognostic significance (Cheville, 1999). Lymphocytic infiltrates and

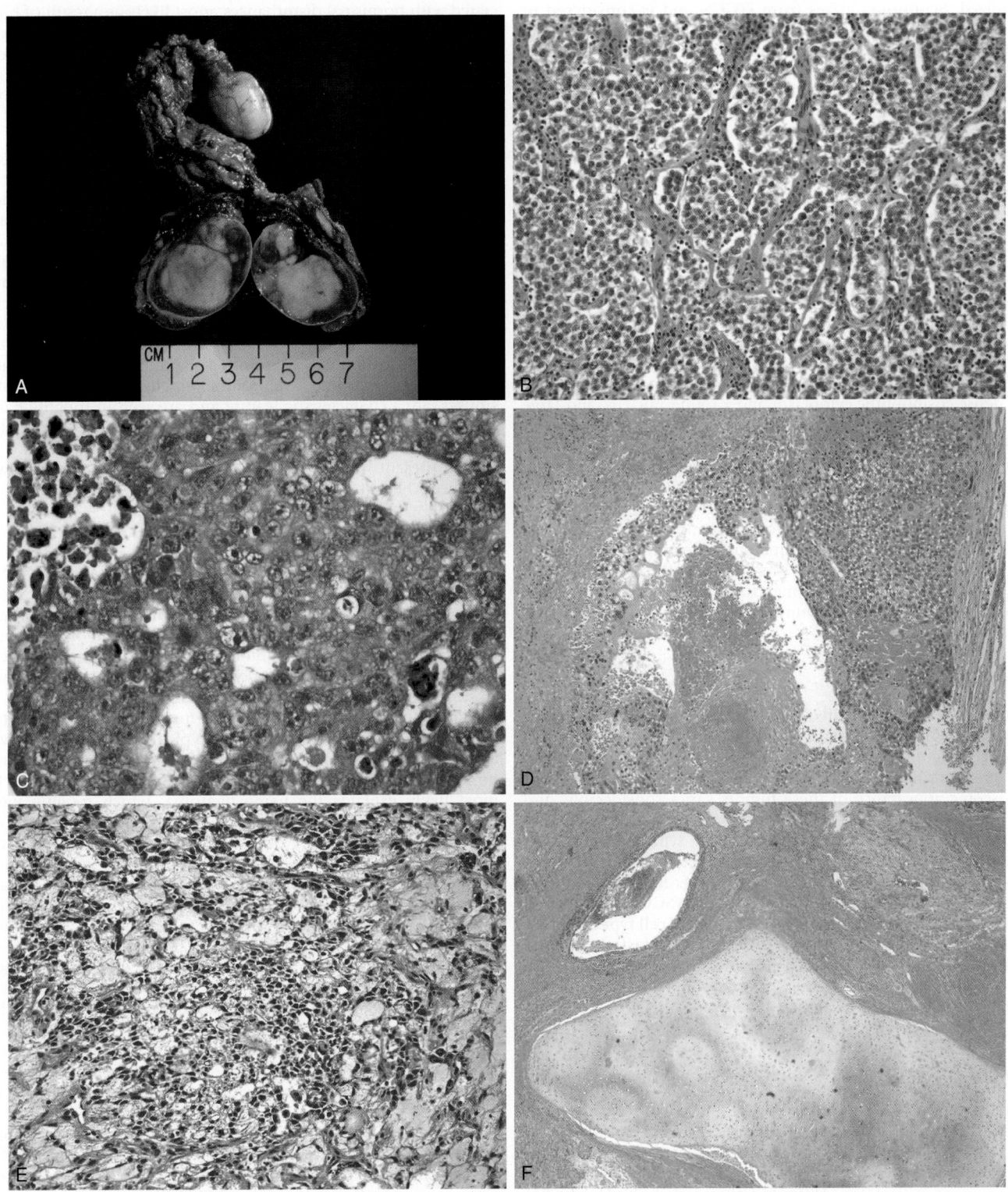

Figure 34-1. **A,** Gross section of testis containing seminoma. **B,** Seminoma (hematoxylin-eosin [H&E] stain). **C,** Embryonal carcinoma (H&E stain). **D,** Choriocarcinoma (H&E stain). **E,** Yolk sac tumor (H&E stain). **F,** Teratoma (H&E stain).

granulomatous reactions are often seen, and seminomas appear to be associated with an increased incidence of sarcoidosis (Rayson et al, 1998; Tjan-Heijnen et al, 1998). Seminomas may be confused with solid-pattern EC, yolk sac tumor, or Sertoli cell tumors (Ulbright and Young, 2008). Although immunohistochemical staining has a limited role in diagnosing GCTs, seminomas are typically negative for CD30, positive for CD117, and strongly positive for placental alkaline phosphatase (PLAP). Anaplastic seminoma was a previously recognized subtype of seminoma, but this distinction is of no clear biologic or clinical significance and is no longer recognized. **Seminoma arises from ITGCN and is considered to be the common precursor for the other NSGCT subtypes** (Ulbright, 2004). This ability of seminoma to transform into NSGCT elements has important therapeutic implications for the management of seminoma (discussed later) (Ulbright, 2004).

Spermatocytic Seminoma

Spermatocytic seminoma is rare and accounts for less than 1% of GCTs. Although classified as a variant of seminoma, these tumors represent a distinct clinicopathologic entity from other GCTs. **In contrast to other GCTs, spermatocytic seminomas do not arise from ITGCN, are not associated with a history of cryptorchidism or bilaterality, do not demonstrate i(12p), and do not occur as part of mixed GCTs** (Ulbright, 2005). Histopathologically, they differ from seminoma in that they do not stain for PLAP or glycogen (periodic acid–Schiff stain); nuclei are round; minimal lymphocytic infiltration is present; and three distinct cell types are present, including small lymphocyte-like cells, medium-size cells with dense eosinophilic cytoplasm and a round nucleus, and large mononucleated or multinucleated cells (Aggarwal and Parwani, 2009). The peak incidence is the sixth decade of life (Eble, 1994; Chung et al, 2004a). **It is a benign tumor (only three documented cases of metastases) and is almost always cured with orchiectomy** (Chung et al, 2004a; Horn et al, 2011). An exception to this rule are the rare cases of spermatocytic seminoma with sarcoma, which exhibit elements of sarcomatous differentiation, and anaplastic variant of spermatocytic seminoma; both of these entities are associated with widely metastatic chemotherapy-resistant disease and poor prognosis (Dundr et al, 2007; Narang et al, 2012; Wetherell et al, 2013).

Embryonal Carcinoma

EC consists of undifferentiated malignant cells resembling primitive epithelial cells from early-stage embryos with crowded pleomorphic nuclei (Ulbright, 2005). Grossly, EC is a tan-to-yellow neoplasm that often exhibits large areas of hemorrhage and necrosis. The microscopic appearance of these tumors varies considerably, and they may grow in solid sheets or in papillary, glandular-alveolar, or tubular patterns (Fig. 34-1C). In some cases, syncytiotrophoblasts are identified. EC is an aggressive tumor associated with a high rate of metastasis, often in the context of normal serum tumor markers. **EC is the most undifferentiated cell type of NSGCT, with totipotential capacity to differentiate to other NSGCT cell types (including teratoma) within the primary tumor or at metastatic sites.** As discussed subsequently, the presence and proportion of EC have been associated with an increased risk of occult metastasis in clinical stage (CS) I NSGCT. EC typically stains for AE1/AE3, PLAP, and OCT3/4 and does not stain for c-KIT.

Choriocarcinoma

Choriocarcinoma is a rare and aggressive tumor that typically manifests with extremely highly elevated serum hCG levels and disseminated disease. These tumors are typically deemed poor risk (stage IIIC) at diagnosis because of the serum hCG level and/or nonpulmonary organ metastases (Alvarado-Cabrero et al, 2014). **Choriocarcinoma commonly spreads by hematogenous routes,** and common sites of metastases include lungs, liver, and brain (Tinkle et al, 2001; Allen, 2002; Osada et al, 2004; Yokoi et al, 2008;

Alvarado-Cabrero et al, 2014). Microscopically, the tumor is composed of syncytiotrophoblasts and cytotrophoblasts, and the former stain positively for hCG (Fig. 34-1D) (Cheville, 1999). Seminoma and EC may also contain syncytiotrophoblasts. Areas of hemorrhage and necrosis are prominent. Similar to gestational trophoblastic disease, testicular choriocarcinoma is prone to hemorrhage, sometimes both spontaneously and immediately after chemotherapy is initiated, and such bleeding can be catastrophic, particularly when it occurs in the lungs or brain (Motzer et al, 1987; Yokoi et al, 2008; Kandori et al, 2010). In addition, choriocarcinomas are associated with hormonal disturbances, most likely as a result of highly elevated serum hCG. Stimulation of receptors for thyroid-stimulating hormone and luteinizing hormone by hCG (which shares an identical α subunit) can result in hyperthyroidism and elevated androgen production (Ulbright, 2005). Hyperprolactinemia also has been reported.

Yolk Sac Tumor

Pure yolk sac tumors (sometimes called endodermal sinus tumors) represent a very small fraction of adult gonadal and retroperitoneal GCTs but are more common in mediastinal and pediatric GCTs (Moran et al, 1997a; Moran and Suster, 1997b; Ross et al, 2002; Ulbright, 2005; Cao and Humphrey, 2011). Mixed GCTs often include elements of yolk sac tumor, which consists of a reticular network of medium-sized cuboidal cells with cytoplasmic and extracytoplasmic eosinophilic, hyaline-like globules (Epstein, 2010). Yolk sac tumors may grow in a glandular, papillary, or microcystic pattern. Schiller-Duval bodies, which resemble endodermal sinuses, are a characteristic feature and are seen in roughly half of cases (Fig. 34-1E). Cytoplasmic and extracellular eosinophilic hyaline globules are another characteristic histologic feature and can be present in 84% of cases. **Yolk sac tumors almost always produce AFP but not hCG.**

Teratoma

Teratomas are tumors that contain well-differentiated or incompletely differentiated elements of at least two of the three germ cell layers: endoderm, mesoderm, and ectoderm. Characteristically, all components are intermixed. Well-differentiated tumors are labeled mature teratomas, whereas tumors that are incompletely differentiated (i.e., similar to fetal or embryonal tissue) are labeled immature teratomas. **In adolescent boys and men, there is no clinical significance to the distinction between mature and immature teratomas, and histopathologists do not typically distinguish between the two entities.** Mature teratomas may include elements of mature bone, cartilage, teeth, hair, and squamous epithelium (a fact that most likely explains the name teratoma, which roughly means "monster tumor" in Greek) (Fig. 34-1F). The gross appearance of teratoma depends largely on the elements within it, with most tumors having solid and cystic areas. **Teratomas are generally associated with normal serum tumor markers, but they may cause mildly elevated serum AFP levels.** Approximately 47% of adult mixed GCTs contain teratoma; pure teratomas are uncommon (Leibovitch et al, 1995b; Simmonds et al, 1996).

In men, teratomas have a histologically benign appearance but are frequently found at metastatic sites in patients with advanced NSGCT. **Teratoma is resistant to chemotherapy.** Given its frequent presence at metastatic sites in advanced NSGCT, patients with residual masses after chemotherapy require consolidative surgical resection. The inherent chemoresistance of teratoma is a limitation to treatment strategies for NSGCT that use chemotherapy alone.

Despite their benign histologic appearance, teratomas contain many genetic abnormalities frequently found in malignant GCT elements, including aneuploidy, i(12p), and widely variable proliferative capacity (Castedo et al, 1989; Sella et al, 1991). Studies have also shown that cystic fluid from teratoma frequently contains hCG and AFP, confirming its malignant potential (Sella et al, 1991; Beck et al, 2004). The genetic instability of teratoma has important clinical implications. **Teratomas may grow uncontrollably, invade surrounding structures, and become unresectable (termed *growing teratoma syndrome*)** (Logothetis et al, 1982). **Rarely, teratoma may transform into a somatic malignancy, such as rhabdomyosarcoma, adenocarcinoma, or primitive neuroectodermal tumor** (Little et al, 1994; Comiter et al, 1998; Motzer et al, 1998). These tumors are called teratoma with somatic-type malignancy or teratoma with malignant transformation. These tumors frequently have abnormalities of i(12p), indicating their origin from GCT. Malignant transformation is highly aggressive, resistant to conventional chemotherapy, and associated with a poor prognosis (Comiter, 1998; El Mesbahi et al, 2007). Lastly, unresected teratoma in patients with advanced NSGCT may result in late relapse (Sheinfeld, 2003). All of these events may result in death.

KEY POINTS: GERM CELL TUMORS

- GCT is the most common solid malignancy among men 20 to 40 years old.
- Bilateral GCT occurs in 2% of men. A metachronous lesion is the most common presentation.
- The incidence of GCT is highest in whites and lowest in African-Americans.
- Cryptorchidism, personal or family history of GCT, and ITGCN are known risk factors for GCT.
- Orchidopexy for cryptorchidism performed before puberty is associated with a decreased risk of GCT.
- Approximately 70% of GCTs have an extra copy of chromosome 12 or i(12p), and this genetic marker may be used in the histopathologic diagnosis of GCT and non-GCT somatic malignancy arising from malignant transformation of teratoma.
- Approximately 5% of GCTs originate at extragonadal sites, most commonly mediastinum and retroperitoneum. Primary mediastinal NSGCTs are associated with a poor prognosis.
- Teratoma is histologically benign. Teratoma at metastatic sites arises from differentiation of metastatic embryonal carcinoma.
- Teratoma is resistant to chemotherapy.
- Teratoma is histologically benign but genetically unstable. It has unpredictable biology. Although uncommon, teratoma has the capacity to grow rapidly or undergo malignant transformation of ectodermal, mesodermal, or endodermal elements to form a non-GCT somatic malignancy.

Initial Presentation

Signs and Symptoms

The most common presentation of testis cancer is a painless testis mass. Acute testicular pain is less common and is caused by rapid expansion of the testis secondary to intratumor hemorrhage or infarction caused by rapid tumor growth. Pain is more commonly associated with NSGCT because these tumors tend to be more vascular and exhibit more rapid growth compared with seminomas. Patients frequently report a history of testicular trauma; incidental trauma is likely responsible for bringing the testis mass to the patient's attention for the first time. Patients may also complain of vague scrotal discomfort or heaviness. **Regional or distant metastasis at diagnosis is present in approximately one third of cases of NSGCT and 15% of cases of pure seminoma, and symptoms related to metastatic disease are the presenting complaint in 10% to 20% of patients** (Sonneveld et al, 1999a; Enewold et al, 2011). Bulky retroperitoneal metastasis may cause a palpable mass, abdominal pain, flank pain secondary to ureteral obstruction, back pain owing to involvement of the psoas muscle or nerve roots, lower extremity swelling secondary to compression of the inferior vena cava, or gastrointestinal symptoms. Pulmonary metastasis may manifest with dyspnea, chest pain, cough, or hemoptysis. Metastasis to supraclavicular lymph nodes may manifest as a neck mass. **Approximately 2% of men have gynecomastia,** resulting from elevated serum hCG levels, decreased androgen production, or increased estrogen levels (most commonly seen in men with Leydig cell tumors). **Although approximately two thirds of men with GCT have diminished fertility, it is an uncommon initial presentation.**

Physical Examination

The physician should carefully examine the affected and the normal contralateral testis, noting their relative size and consistency and palpating for any testicular or extratesticular masses. Atrophy of the affected or contralateral testis is common, particularly in patients with a history of cryptorchidism. Any firm area within the testis should be considered suspicious for malignancy and should prompt further investigations. A hydrocele may accompany a testis cancer and impair the examiner's ability to evaluate the testis. In this case, a scrotal ultrasound scan to evaluate the testis is warranted. The patient also should be examined for any evidence of palpable abdominal mass or pain, inguinal lymphadenopathy (particularly if he has had prior inguinal or scrotal surgery), gynecomastia, and supraclavicular lymphadenopathy. Auscultation of the chest for intrathoracic disease should be done.

Differential Diagnosis

The differential diagnosis of a testis mass includes epididymo-orchitis, torsion, hematoma, or paratesticular neoplasm (benign or malignant). Other diagnostic possibilities include hernia, varicocele, or spermatocele, although these usually can be distinguished from a testis mass by physical examination. **A firm intratesticular mass should be considered cancer until proved otherwise and should be evaluated further with a scrotal ultrasound scan. Patients with a presumptive diagnosis of epididymo-orchitis should be re-evaluated within 2 to 4 weeks of completion of an appropriate course of oral antibiotics.** A persistent mass or pain should be evaluated further with scrotal ultrasonography.

Diagnostic Delay

Diagnostic delay is a well-recognized phenomenon of this disease, with patients and physicians contributing to this delay. Patients with testis cancer are typically young and may be less inclined to seek medical evaluation for symptoms because of denial, ignorance, or limited access. **In prior studies, up to one third of testis tumors were initially misdiagnosed as epididymitis or hydrocele** (Bosl et al, 1981). For patients who present with signs or symptoms resulting from metastatic GCT, these may become the focus of the treating physician, who fails to diagnose GCT. These patients may be subjected to inappropriate treatment, diagnostic tests, and unnecessary surgery with subsequent delays in definitive therapy. Case reports describe patients undergoing exploratory laparotomy, neck dissection, or mastectomy for unsuspected metastatic GCT. The interval of delay is associated with advanced clinical stage, suboptimal response to chemotherapy, and diminished survival. Moul and colleagues (1990) reported a decrease in survival in patients with GCT treated during the period 1970 to 1987 with a diagnostic delay greater than 16 weeks, although a significant survival difference was not observed among patients treated in the cisplatin era. Stephenson and coworkers (2004) reported a higher proportion of men requiring intensive chemotherapy (multiple regimens, high-dose chemotherapy, and salvage chemotherapy) among men with a treatment delay greater than 30 days owing to unnecessary exploratory laparotomy.

Diagnostic delay can be avoided by efforts to improve patient and physician education. Physicians must consider the diagnosis of GCT in any adolescent boy or man from age 15 to 50 years with a firm testis mass, midline retroperitoneal mass, or mass in the left supraclavicular fossa.

Diagnostic Testing and Initial Management

Scrotal Ultrasonography

In men presenting with a testis mass, hydrocele, or unexplained scrotal symptoms or signs, **scrotal ultrasonography should be considered an extension of the physical examination because it is widely available, inexpensive, and noninvasive.** With high-frequency transducers (5 to 10 MHz), intratesticular lesions a few millimeters in size can be identified and readily distinguished from extratesticular pathology. On ultrasound scan, a typical GCT is hypoechoic, and two or more discrete lesions may be identified (Fig. 34-2). Heterogeneous echotexture within a lesion is more commonly associated with NSGCT because seminomas usually have a homogeneous echotexture. The presence of increased flow within the lesion on color Doppler sonography is suggestive of malignancy, although its absence does not exclude GCT. The association between testicular microlithiasis and GCT is not clearly defined, and this finding alone should not prompt further evaluation (DeCastro et al, 2008). **Given the 2% incidence of bilateral GCT, both testes should be evaluated with ultrasonography, although bilateral tumors at diagnosis are rare (0.5% of all GCTs), and metachronous presentation is more common** (Fossa et al, 2005).

In men with advanced GCT and a normal testicular examination, scrotal ultrasonography should be performed to rule out the presence of a small, impalpable scar or calcification, indicating a "burned-out" primary testis tumor. GCTs are among the most common neoplasms to undergo spontaneous regression, with seminoma being the most frequent subtype (Balzer and Ulbright, 2006). Radical orchiectomy should be performed in patients with sonographic evidence of intratesticular lesions (discrete nodule, stellate scar, coarse calcification) because ITGCN and residual teratoma are frequently encountered. Men with advanced GCT with normal testes on physical examination and ultrasound scan are considered to have primary extragonadal GCT.

The presence of small (<10 mm), impalpable intratesticular lesions in the absence of disseminated GCT or elevated serum tumor markers represents a diagnostic dilemma. Most of these lesions are benign (testicular cysts, small infarcts, Leydig cell nodules, or small Leydig cell or Sertoli cell tumors), although 20% to 50% may represent small GCTs (usually seminomas) (Hindley et al, 2003; Connolly et al, 2006; Muller et al, 2006; Shilo et al, 2012). The risk of malignancy increases with the size of the lesion, from 50% for lesions less than 1 cm to 80% or more for lesions 1 to 2 cm (Carmignani et al, 2005). Management options include inguinal orchiectomy, testis-sparing surgery involving inguinal exploration and excision (with frozen-section analysis to rule out GCT), and close observation with serial ultrasound scans (with exploration of growing lesions). Intraoperative ultrasonography is useful during surgical exploration of the testis to locate the lesion.

Serum Tumor Markers

Testis cancer is one of the few malignancies associated with serum tumor markers (lactate dehydrogenase [LDH], AFP, and hCG) that are essential in its diagnosis and management (Gilligan et al, 2010). Serum tumor marker levels should be obtained at diagnosis, after orchiectomy, to monitor for response to chemotherapy, and to monitor for relapse in patients on surveillance and after completion of therapy.

At diagnosis, AFP levels are elevated in 50% to 70% of low-stage (CS I, IIA, and IIB) NSGCT and 60% to 80% of advanced (CS IIC and III) NSGCT. EC and yolk sac tumors secrete AFP. Choriocarcinomas and seminomas do not produce AFP. Patients with pure seminoma in the primary tumor with an elevated serum AFP are considered to have NSGCT. The half-life of AFP is 5 to 7 days. AFP levels may also be increased in patients with hepatocellular carcinoma; cancers of the stomach, pancreas, biliary tract, and lung; nonmalignant liver disease (infectious, drug-induced, alcohol-induced, autoimmune); ataxic telangiectasia; and hereditary tyrosinemia.

hCG levels are elevated in 20% to 40% of low-stage NSGCT and 40% to 60% of advanced NSGCT. Approximately 15% of seminomas secrete hCG. hCG is also secreted by choriocarcinoma and EC. Levels greater than 5000 IU/L are usually associated with NSGCT. The half-life of hCG is 24 to 36 hours. hCG levels may be elevated in cancers of the liver, biliary tract, pancreas, stomach, lung, breast, kidney, and bladder. The α subunit of hCG is common to several pituitary tumors, and so **immunoassays for hCG are directed at the β subunit. Cross-reactivity of the hCG assay with luteinizing hormone may cause false-positive hCG elevations in patients with primary hypogonadism.** Elevated serum hCG results caused by hypogonadism normalize within 48 to 72 hours after administration of testosterone, and this can be done to distinguish between true-positive and false-positive hCG results. Marijuana use may also cause false-positive hCG results.

LDH levels are elevated in approximately 20% of low-stage GCT and 20% to 60% of advanced GCT. LDH is expressed in smooth, cardiac, and skeletal muscle. Lymphoma may also cause elevated LDH levels. Of the five isoenzymes of LDH, LDH-1 is the most frequently elevated isoenzyme in GCT. LDH-1 levels are correlated with the chromosome arm 12p copy number, which is frequently amplified in GCT. The magnitude of LDH elevation correlates with the bulk of disease. As a nonspecific marker for GCT, its main use is in the assessment of prognosis of GCT at diagnosis. The serum half-life of LDH is 24 hours.

Patients suspected to have a GCT should have blood drawn for serum AFP, hCG, and LDH before orchiectomy to aid in the diagnosis and to help interpret tumor marker levels after orchiectomy. For staging purposes, it is relevant to know whether serum tumor marker levels obtained before orchiectomy are declining after orchiectomy and, if so, how quickly. The results of serum tumor marker assays should not be used to guide decision making about whether or not to perform a radical orchiectomy because AFP or hCG levels in the normal range do not rule out GCT. A significantly elevated serum AFP can establish the diagnosis of NSGCT in a patient whose histopathologic diagnosis is pure seminoma because seminomas do not produce AFP. However, borderline-elevated values should be interpreted cautiously. **In rare patients who present with a testis, retroperitoneal, or mediastinal primary tumor and whose disease burden has resulted in a need to start treatment very urgently, substantially elevated serum AFP and/or hCG may be considered sufficient for diagnosis of GCT.** For such rare, medically unstable patients, treatment need not be delayed until histology results permit a tissue diagnosis. However, these patients should undergo radical orchiectomy after the completion of chemotherapy because the testis is a sanctuary site for

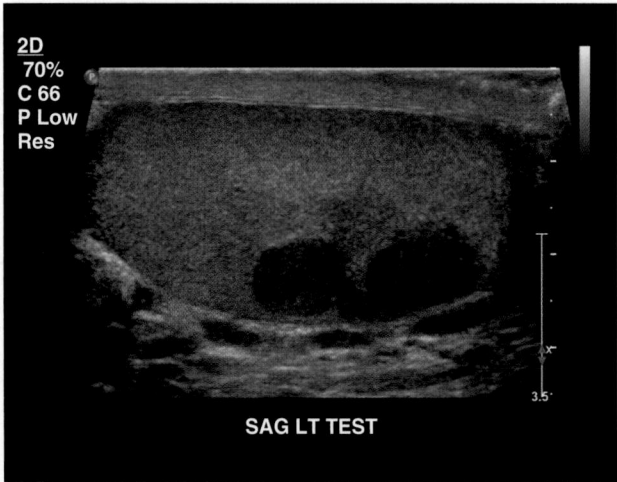

Figure 34-2. **Sagittal view of ultrasound of left testis showing multinodular hypoechoic intratesticular lesion confirmed to be pure seminoma at orchiectomy.**

Chapter 34 Neoplasms of the Testis **791**

malignant GCT owing to the blood-testis barrier, and the testis frequently contains residual invasive GCT, teratoma, or ITGCN (Geldart et al, 2002).

Radical Inguinal Orchiectomy

Patients suspected to have a testicular neoplasm should undergo a radical inguinal orchiectomy with removal of the tumor-bearing testicle and spermatic cord to the level of the internal inguinal ring. **A trans-scrotal orchiectomy or biopsy is contraindicated because it leaves the inguinal portion of the spermatic cord intact and may alter the lymphatic drainage of the testis, increasing the risk of local recurrence and pelvic or inguinal lymph node metastasis.** Because of the rapid growth of GCTs, orchiectomy should be performed in a timely manner; delays greater than 1 to 2 weeks should be avoided. Radical orchiectomy establishes the histologic diagnosis and primary T stage, provides important prognostic information from the tumor histology, and is curative in 80% to 85% of CS I seminoma and 70% to 80% of CS I NSGCT.

Histopathologic examination of the testis should identify the histologic type of the tumor (see Box 34-2) (Sobin and Wittekind, 2002), tumor size, multifocality, local tumor invasion (rete testis, tunica albuginea, tunica vaginalis, epididymis, spermatic cord, scrotum), primary T stage (Table 34-1) (Greene et al, 2002; Sobin and Wittekind, 2002), presence of ITGCN, invasion of blood or lymphatic vessels (termed *lymphovascular invasion*), and surgical margin status. For patients with mixed GCT, each individual tumor subtype should be identified including its relative proportion. Because of the relative rarity of GCT and the importance of primary tumor histology for treatment decision making, review of primary tumor specimens by experienced pathologists is recommended (Krege et al, 2008a, 2008b). In a randomized, multicenter clinical trial, 5 of 382 NSGCT specimens (1.3%) were reclassified as seminomas by centralized pathologic review (Albers et al, 2008).

Testis-Sparing Surgery

Testis-sparing surgery (or partial orchiectomy) is highly controversial and has no role in the treatment of a patient suspected to have a testicular neoplasm with a normal contralateral testis. However, it may be considered for organ-confined tumors less than 2 to 3 cm in size (30% of testicular volume) in patients with synchronous bilateral tumors or tumor in a solitary testis with sufficient testicular androgen production. It may also be considered for suspected benign tumor or indeterminate lesion less than 3 cm when serum AFP, hCG, and LDH are normal because the incidence of benign histology is 80% (Giannarini et al, 2010). Testis-sparing surgery is seldom feasible for larger tumors (>3 cm) because a complete excision frequently leaves insufficient residual testicular parenchyma for preservation. **When testis-sparing surgery is performed, intraoperative frozen-section analysis can distinguish between benign and malignant histology in most cases** (Tokuc et al, 1992; Elert et al, 2002). **Biopsy of the adjacent testicular parenchyma should be performed to rule out the presence of ITGCN. For patients with ITGCN, adjuvant radiotherapy to the residual testis using doses of 20 Gy or greater is usually sufficient to prevent the development of a GCT, while preserving Leydig cell function (and testicular androgen production).** Radiation at these doses causes permanent sterility of the treated testis. Leydig cell function may decline over time, and 40% of men who receive radiation therapy require supplemental testosterone (Petersen et al, 2002). The German Testicular Cancer Study Group reported no cases of local recurrence over a median follow-up of 91 months in 46 patients with small, organ-confined tumors who underwent testis-sparing surgery and received adjuvant radiotherapy for ITGCN (Heidenreich et al, 2001). In contrast, recurrent testis cancer developed in four of five men who did not receive adjuvant radiotherapy. Adjuvant radiotherapy may be delayed after testis-sparing surgery if fathering a child is desired, although close follow-up is mandatory (Giannarini et al, 2010).

Contralateral Testis Biopsy

Of patients with GCT, 5% to 9% have ITGCN in the normal contralateral testis (Dieckmann and Skakkebaek, 1999). In patients with an atrophic testis, history of cryptorchidism, or age younger than 40 years, the prevalence of ITGCN in the contralateral testis has been reported to be 36% (Dieckmann and Loy, 1996). An open inguinal biopsy of the contralateral testis may be considered in patients with risk factors for ITGCN or patients with suspicious lesions on preoperative ultrasound scan (Motzer et al, 2006).

TABLE 34-1 TNM Staging of Testicular Tumor: American Joint Committee on Cancer and Union Internationale Contre le Cancer

PRIMARY TUMOR (T)*

The extent of primary tumor is usually classified after radical orchiectomy and, for this reason, a *pathologic* stage is assigned.

pTx	Primary tumor cannot be assessed
pT0	No evidence of primary tumor (e.g., histologic scar in testis)
pTis	Intratubular germ cell neoplasia (carcinoma in situ)
pT1	Tumor limited to testis and epididymis without vascular/lymphatic invasion; tumor may invade into tunica albuginea but not tunica vaginalis
pT2	Tumor limited to testis and epididymis with vascular/lymphatic invasion or tumor extending through tunica albuginea with involvement of tunica vaginalis
pT3	Tumor invades spermatic cord with or without vascular/lymphatic invasion
pT4	Tumor invades scrotum with or without vascular/lymphatic invasion

REGIONAL LYMPH NODES (N)

Clinical (as Determined by Noninvasive Staging)

NX	Regional lymph nodes cannot be assessed
N0	No regional lymph node metastasis
N1	Metastasis with lymph node mass ≤2 cm in greatest dimension; or multiple lymph nodes, none more than 2 cm in greatest dimension
N2	Metastasis with lymph node mass, >2 cm, but not more than 5 cm in greatest dimension; or multiple lymph nodes, any one mass >2 cm but not more than 5 cm in greatest dimension
N3	Metastasis with lymph node mass >5 cm in greatest dimension

TABLE 34-1   TNM Staging of Testicular Tumor: American Joint Committee on Cancer and Union Internationale Contre le Cancer—cont'd

Pathologic (pN) (as Determined by Pathologic Findings of RPLND without Prior Chemotherapy or Radiotherapy)

pNX	Regional lymph nodes cannot be assessed
pN0	No regional lymph node metastasis
pN1	Metastasis with lymph node mass ≤2 cm in greatest dimension and ≤5 nodes positive, none more than 2 cm in greatest dimension
pN2	Metastasis with lymph node mass >2 cm but not more than 5 cm in greatest dimension; or >5 nodes positive, none more than 5 cm; or evidence of extranodal extension of tumor
pN3	Metastasis with lymph node mass >5 cm in greatest dimension

DISTANT METASTASIS (M)

MX	Distant metastasis cannot be assessed
M0	No distant metastasis
M1	Distant metastasis
M1a	Nonregional nodal or pulmonary metastasis
M1b	Distant metastasis at site other than nonregional lymph nodes or lung

SERUM TUMOR MARKERS (S)

SX	Marker studies unavailable or not performed
S0	Marker study levels within normal limits
S1	LDH <1.5 × N† *and* hCG (MIU/mL) <5000 *and* AFP (ng/mL) <1000
S2	LDH 1.5-10 × N *or* hCG (MIU/mL) 5000-50,000 *or* AFP (ng/mL) 1000-10,000
S3	LDH >10 × N *or* hCG (MIU/mL) >50,000 *or* AFP (ng/mL) >10,000

STAGE GROUPING

GROUP	T	N	M	S (SERUM TUMOR MARKERS)
Stage 0	pTis	N0	M0	S0
Stage I	pT1-4	N0	M0	SX
Stage IA	pT1	N0	M0	S0
Stage IB	pT2	N0	M0	S0
	pT3	N0	M0	S0
	pT4	N0	M0	S0
Stage IS	Any pT/Tx	N0	M0	S1-3
Stage II	Any pT/Tx	N1-3	M0	SX
Stage IIA	Any pT/Tx	N1	M0	S0
	Any pT/Tx	N1	M0	S1
Stage IIB	Any pT/Tx	N2	M0	S0
	Any pT/Tx	N2	M0	S1
Stage IIC	Any pT/Tx	N3	M0	S0
	Any pT/Tx	N3	M0	S1
Stage III	Any pT/Tx	Any N	M1	SX
Stage IIIA	Any pT/Tx	Any N	M1a	S0
	Any pT/Tx	Any N	M1a	S1
Stage IIIB	Any pT/Tx	N1-3	M0	S2
	Any pT/Tx	Any N	M1a	S2
Stage IIIC	Any pT/Tx	N1-3	M0	S3
	Any pT/Tx	Any N	M1a	S3
	Any pT/Tx	Any N	M1b	Any S

*Except for pTis and pT4, extent of primary tumor is classified by radical orchiectomy. Tx may be used for other categories in the absence of radical orchiectomy.
†N indicates the upper limit of normal for the LDH assay.
AFP, α-fetoprotein; hCG, human chorionic gonadotropin; LDH, lactate dehydrogenase; RPLND, retroperitoneal lymph node dissection.
From AJCC. Testis. In: Edge SE, Byrd DR, Compton CC, editors. AJCC cancer staging manual. 7th ed. New York: Springer; 2010. p. 469–73. Used with permission of the American Joint Committee on Cancer (AJCC), Chicago, Illinois. The original source for this material is the *AJCC Cancer Staging Manual,* Seventh Edition (2010), published by Springer Science and Business Media, LLC, www.springer.com.

Suspected Extragonadal Germ Cell Tumor

Approximately 5% of GCTs are of extragonadal origin (Bokemeyer et al, 2002b). Of patients with metastatic GCT without a testis mass, only one third definitively have a primary extragonadal GCT; one third have ITGCN in the testis, and one third have sonographic evidence of a "burned-out" primary tumor (Scholz et al, 2002). GCT should be considered in any male under 40 years with a midline mass. The presence of elevated serum AFP and/or hCG with a normal testicular evaluation is sufficient for the diagnosis of GCT, and histologic confirmation by biopsy is unnecessary before starting treatment. In cases of normal serum tumor markers, a biopsy of the mass should be performed to confirm the diagnosis of GCT before beginning treatment. A biopsy specimen showing poorly differentiated carcinoma represents a diagnostic dilemma if a primary tumor site cannot be confirmed. In this scenario, the diagnosis of extragonadal GCT with malignant transformation may be considered and supported by the expression of i(12p) in biopsy specimens. Patients with suspected extragonadal GCT should undergo inguinal orchiectomy at some point during their treatment course if the pattern of metastasis is consistent with a right-sided or left-sided testicular primary tumor or if there is sonographic evidence of a "burned-out" primary tumor.

KEY POINTS: DIAGNOSIS AND INITIAL MANAGEMENT OF GERM CELL TUMOR

- A solid intratesticular mass in a postpubertal male patient should be considered a GCT until proved otherwise.
- With rare exceptions, inguinal orchiectomy with high ligation of the spermatic cord should be performed in men suspected to have GCT. Trans-scrotal orchiectomy and biopsy should be avoided.
- Testis-sparing surgery for GCT is a consideration in highly selected patients who have a small tumor in either a solitary testis or synchronous bilateral testis masses, in whom preservation of the affected testis would provide sufficient testicular androgen production.
- Diagnostic delay is common in GCTs, and approximately one third of cases are initially misdiagnosed.
- If serum tumor marker levels were elevated before orchiectomy, they should be measured after orchiectomy to determine if levels are declining, stable, or rising. Serum tumor marker levels obtained before orchiectomy should not be used in management decisions.

Clinical Staging

The prognosis of GCT and initial management decisions are dictated by CS of the disease, which is based on the histopathologic findings and pathologic stage of the primary tumor, serum tumor marker levels measured after orchiectomy, and the presence and extent of metastatic disease as determined by physical examination and staging imaging studies. In 1997, an international consensus classification for GCT was developed by the American Joint Committee on Cancer (AJCC) and Union Internationale Contre le Cancer (UICC) (see Table 34-1). The AJCC and UICC staging systems for GCT are unique because, for the first time, a serum tumor marker category (S) based on postorchiectomy AFP, hCG, and LDH levels is used to supplement the prognostic stages as defined by anatomic extent of disease. **The AJCC and UICC staging systems were updated in 2002, and the new systems consider the presence of LVI in the primary as pT2 in an otherwise organ-confined tumor.** CS I is defined as disease clinically confined to the testis, **CS II** indicates the presence of regional (retroperitoneal) lymph node metastasis, and **CS III** represents nonregional lymph node and/or visceral metastasis.

Staging Imaging Studies

GCT follows a predictable pattern of metastatic spread, which has contributed to its successful management. **With the exception of choriocarcinoma, the most common route of disease dissemination is via lymphatic channels from the primary tumor to the retroperitoneal lymph nodes and subsequently to distant sites. Choriocarcinoma has a propensity for hematogenous dissemination. The retroperitoneum is the initial site of metastatic spread in 70% to 80% of patients with GCT.** Detailed mapping studies from retroperitoneal lymph node dissection (RPLND) series have increased understanding of the testicular lymphatic drainage and identified the most likely sites of metastatic spread (Sheinfeld, 1994). **For right testis tumors, the primary drainage site is the inter-aortocaval lymph nodes inferior to the renal vessels, followed by the paracaval and para-aortic nodes. The primary "landing zone" for left testis tumors is the para-aortic lymph nodes, followed by the inter-aortocaval nodes** (Donohue et al, 1982). **The pattern of lymph drainage in the retroperitoneum is from right to left.** Contralateral spread from the primary "landing zone" is common with right-sided tumors but is rarely seen with left-sided tumors and usually is associated with bulky disease. **More caudal deposits of metastatic disease usually reflect retrograde spread to distal iliac and inguinal lymph nodes secondary to large-volume disease and, more rarely, aberrant testicular lymphatic drainage. Retroperitoneal lymphatics drain into the cisterna chyli behind the right renal artery and right crus of the diaphragm.** Retrocrural lymph node metastasis may be visible in patients with retroperitoneal disease. From there, lymphatic spread occurs via the thoracic duct to the posterior mediastinum and left supraclavicular fossa.

Clinical Staging of the Abdomen and Pelvis. All patients with GCT should undergo staging imaging studies of the abdomen and pelvis. Computed tomography (CT) imaging with oral and intravenous contrast material is the most effective, noninvasive means of staging the retroperitoneum and pelvis. CT imaging also provides a detailed anatomic assessment of the retroperitoneum to identify anatomic anomalies that may complicate subsequent RPLND, such as a circumaortic or retroaortic left renal vein, lower pole renal artery, or retrocaval right ureter. Magnetic resonance imaging is an alternative to CT, although it is associated with longer examination times, higher cost, and less availability.

Enlarged retroperitoneal lymph nodes are found on CT in approximately 10% to 20% of seminomas and 60% to 70% of NSGCTs. The retroperitoneum is the most difficult area to assign CS accurately. **A consistent 25% to 35% rate of pathologically involved retroperitoneal lymph nodes has been reported for CS I NSGCT in the presence of a "normal" CT scan despite the improvements in CT imaging over the last four decades** (Fernandez et al, 1994). There is no consensus regarding size criteria for retroperitoneal lymph nodes that constitutes a "normal" CT scan. A size cutoff of 10 mm is frequently used to identify enlarged lymph nodes, but false-negative rates up to 63% have been reported when this size criterion is used. Among patients with CS IIA and IIB disease, clinical overstaging by CT (i.e., pathologically negative lymph nodes at RPLND despite enlarged lymph nodes on CT) is reported in 12% to 40% of patients.

An understanding of the primary drainage sites for left-sided and right-sided tumors has led to efforts to increase the sensitivity of abdominopelvic CT imaging by decreasing the size criteria for clinically positive lymph nodes in the primary landing zone. Leibovitch and colleagues (1995a) showed that using a size cutoff of 4 mm in the primary landing zone and 10 mm outside this region was associated with sensitivity and specificity for pathologic stage II disease of 91% and 50%, respectively. In a similar study, Hilton and associates (1997) reported sensitivity and specificity of 93% and 58%, respectively, using a cutoff of 4 mm for lymph nodes in the primary landing zone that were anterior to a horizontal line bisecting the aorta. **Based on this evidence, retroperitoneal lymph nodes 5 to 9 mm in size in the primary landing zone should be viewed with suspicion for regional lymph node metastasis, particularly if they**

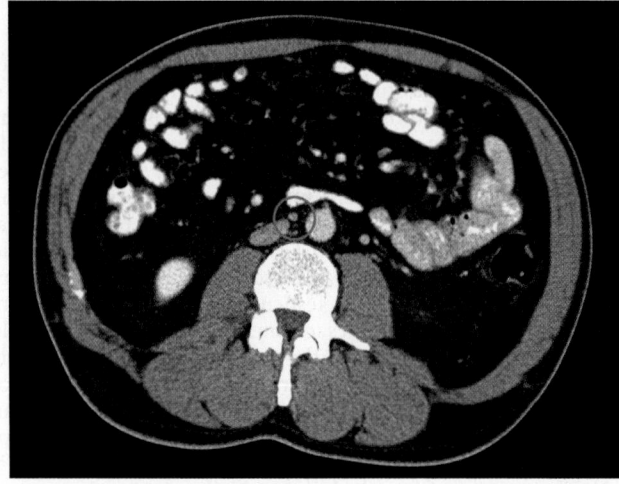

Figure 34-3. Postorchiectomy computed tomography image of the abdomen and pelvis in a patient with right testicular nonseminoma germ cell tumor showing a 7-mm lymph node in a primary landing zone. The lymph node was involved with teratoma at retroperitoneal lymph node dissection.

are anterior to the great vessels on transaxial images (Fig. 34-3). Because of the rapid growth of GCTs, it is advisable to base management decisions on CT imaging studies performed within 4 weeks of the initiation of treatment.

Malignant GCTs accumulate fluorodeoxyglucose (FDG), and several studies have investigated positron emission tomography with FDG (FDG-PET) in the staging of GCTs at diagnosis and assessing response after chemotherapy. Several small pilot studies suggested that FDG-PET can identify retroperitoneal metastasis in low-stage seminoma and NSGCT more precisely than CT (Albers et al, 1999). In a prospective trial of centrally reviewed FDG-PET studies in 111 contemporary patients with CS I NSGCT on surveillance, relapse was observed in 33 of 87 patients who were PET-negative with an estimated relapse-free rate of 63% (Huddart et al, 2007). The investigators concluded that FDG-PET is not sufficiently sensitive to stage CS I NSGCT accurately. de Wit and colleagues (2008) also reported that FDG-PET yielded only slightly better results than CT as a primary staging tool for low-stage NSGCT. **There is currently no role for FDG-PET in the routine evaluation of NSGCT and seminoma at the time of diagnosis.**

CS II disease is subclassified based on the size of regional lymph nodes as determined by abdominopelvic imaging into IIA (enlarged retroperitoneal lymph nodes ≤2 cm), IIB (enlarged retroperitoneal lymph nodes >2 cm but ≤5 cm), and IIC (enlarged lymph nodes >5 cm).

Pathologic Staging of the Abdomen and Pelvis. In selected European centers performing open RPLND and most laparoscopic RPLND series, RPLND is performed in patients with CS I or IIA NSGCT largely as a staging procedure without curative intent to identify the presence of regional lymph nodes and determine the need for subsequent chemotherapy (Nelson et al, 1999; Janetschek et al, 2000; Albers et al, 2003; Bhayani et al, 2003; Nielsen et al, 2007; Albers et al, 2008). Pathologic N stage differs from clinical N stage in that the former considers the number of lymph nodes involved: pN0, no regional lymph node metastasis; pN1, five or fewer lymph nodes involved, none larger than 2 cm; pN2, more than five lymph nodes involved and/or any lymph node 2 to 5 cm; pN3, any lymph node larger than 5 cm. In patients with pathologic stage II disease (pTany, pN1-3, M0), the risk of occult metastases (and relapse after RPLND) is closely related to the burden of regional lymph node metastasis (10% to 30% of pN1 vs. 50% to 80% for pN2-3). The pathologic N stage cannot be applied to RPLND specimens from patients who have received prior chemotherapy.

Chest Imaging

All patients with GCTs should undergo chest imaging before management decisions are made. Thoracic metastasis in the absence of retroperitoneal disease and/or elevated serum tumor markers is uncommon, particularly for seminomas. Routine chest CT imaging may be associated with a high rate of false-positive findings, which may complicate subsequent therapy (Horan et al, 2007). It is reasonable to obtain chest radiographs at the time of diagnosis as an initial staging study, and CT should be performed in patients with elevated serum tumor markers after orchiectomy, evidence of metastatic disease by physical examination or abdominopelvic CT imaging, or abnormal or equivocal findings on chest radiograph. It may be reasonable to order chest CT in patients with CS I NSGCT with evidence of LVI or EC predominance because some studies have reported a high rate of hematogenous metastasis to lung in the setting of a negative CT scan for retroperitoneal metastasis (Hermans et al, 2000; Sweeney et al, 2000). Mediastinal or hilar lymphadenopathy in the absence of retroperitoneal disease should raise the index of suspicion of non-GCT etiology such as lymphoma or sarcoidosis, and histologic confirmation of GCT by mediastinoscopy and biopsy should be performed before initiating systemic therapy (Hunt et al, 2009).

Visceral metastasis to bone and brain is uncommon in GCT in the absence of symptoms or other clinical indicators of disease. There is no role for routine bone scintigraphy or brain CT imaging at the time of diagnosis. A notable exception is brain CT imaging for patients with a highly elevated hCG (>10,000 mU/mL) because these levels are often associated with metastatic choriocarcinoma, which has a propensity for brain metastases.

Serum Tumor Markers

AFP, hCG, and LDH levels measured after orchiectomy are important for staging, prognosis, and treatment selection. All patients should have serum tumor markers drawn after orchiectomy to assess for appropriate decline according to half-life in patients with elevated levels before orchiectomy. Newly elevated and/or rising serum tumor marker levels after orchiectomy indicate the presence of metastatic disease, and these patients should receive induction chemotherapy. In the setting of a negative metastatic evaluation and slowly declining markers (i.e., not according to half-life), patients should be monitored closely and have levels checked periodically until the levels normalize or begin to rise. Stable AFP or hCG levels slightly above the normal range should be interpreted cautiously, and other causes for serum tumor marker elevation should be ruled out before management decisions are made. As with staging imaging studies, management decisions should be based on serum tumor marker levels measured within 4 weeks of the initiation of treatment.

Prognostic Classification of Advanced Germ Cell Tumors

An international, retrospective pooled analysis of 5202 patients with advanced NSGCT treated between 1975 and 1990 with platin-containing chemotherapy regimens (cisplatin or carboplatin) identified AFP, hCG, and LDH levels at the initiation of chemotherapy; the presence of nonpulmonary visceral metastasis; and primary mediastinal NSGCT as significant and independent prognostic factors for progression and survival (International Germ Cell Consensus Classification, 1997). In 660 patients with advanced seminoma, only the presence of nonpulmonary visceral metastasis was an important predictor of progression and survival (International Germ Cell Consensus Classification, 1997).

Based on these analyses, the International Germ Cell Cancer Collaborative Group (IGCCCG) risk classification for advanced GCT was developed (Table 34-2) (International Germ Cell Consensus Classification, 1997). **The IGCCCG risk group should be determined for each patient with metastatic GCT, and this should be used to guide treatment decision making on the choice of chemotherapy** (discussed later). This classification applies only to

TABLE 34-2 International Germ Cell Cancer Collaborative Group Risk Classification for Advanced Germ Cell Tumor

NONSEMINOMA	SEMINOMA
GOOD PROGNOSIS	
Testicular/retroperitoneal primary *and*	Any primary site *and*
No nonpulmonary visceral metastases *and*	No nonpulmonary visceral metastases *and*
Good markers—all of:	Normal AFP, any hCG, any LDH
AFP <1000 ng/mL *and* hCG <5000 IU/L (1000 ng/mL) *and* LDH <1.5 × *upper limit of normal (N)*	
56% of nonseminomas	90% of seminomas
5-year PFS 89%	5-year PFS 82%
5-year survival 92%	5-year survival 86%
INTERMEDIATE PROGNOSIS	
Testicular/retroperitoneal primary *and*	Any primary site *and*
No nonpulmonary visceral metastases *and*	Nonpulmonary visceral metastases *and*
Intermediate markers—any of:	Normal AFP, any hCG, any LDH
AFP ≥1000-10,000 ng/mL and ≤10,000 ng/mL *or* hCG ≥5000-50,000 IU/L and ≤50,000 IU/L *or* LDH ≥1.5 × N and ≤10 × N	
28% of nonseminomas	10% of seminomas
5-year PFS 75%	5-year PFS 67%
5-year survival 80%	5-year survival 72%
POOR PROGNOSIS	
Mediastinal primary *or*	No patients classified as poor prognosis
Nonpulmonary visceral metastases *or*	
Poor serum markers—any of: AFP >10,000 ng/mL *or* hCG >50,000 IU/L (10,000 ng/mL) *or* LDH >10 × *upper limit of normal*	
16% of nonseminomas	
5-year PFS 41%	
5-year survival 48%	

AFP, α-fetoprotein; hCG, human chorionic gonadotropin; LDH, lactate dehydrogenase; PFS, progression-free survival.
From International Germ Cell Consensus Classification: a prognostic factor-based staging system for metastatic germ cell cancers. International Germ Cell Cancer Collaborative Group. J Clin Oncol 1997;15: 594–603.

patients with advanced GCT at the time of diagnosis and is not applicable to patients with relapsed GCT. It is also based on the postorchiectomy serum tumor marker levels at the start of chemotherapy, not levels measured before orchiectomy.

According to IGCCCG criteria, approximately 56% of patients with advanced NSGCT are classified as good risk, 28% are classified as intermediate risk, and 16% are classified as poor risk, and the

5-year progression-free and overall survival rates for these patients are 89% and 92% (good risk), 75% and 80% (intermediate risk), and 41% and 48% (poor risk). There is no poor risk category for seminoma. Approximately 90% and 10% of patients with advanced seminoma are classified as good and intermediate risk by IGCCCG criteria, respectively, and the 5-year progression-free and overall survival rates for these patients are 82% and 86% (good risk) and 67% and 72% (intermediate risk). Van Dijk and colleagues (2006) published a meta-analysis of 10 studies of 1775 patients with NSGCT treated after 1989 and reported pooled 5-year survival estimates of 94%, 83%, and 71% for good-risk, intermediate-risk, and poor-risk patients by IGCCCG criteria. These results represent significantly improved survival compared with the original study (particularly for patients classified as poor risk) and are attributed to more effective therapy and more experience in treating patients with NSGCT.

The TNM system incorporates marker levels (S0-3) and nonpulmonary visceral metastasis in the staging of testis cancer. However, this system does not consider the differences in prognosis between seminomas and NSGCTs with nonpulmonary visceral metastasis. In the TNM system, both of these entities would be classified as stage IIIC, but IGCCCG would classify the former as intermediate risk and the latter as poor risk. The IGCCCG system is preferentially used for prognostic assessment and the selection of chemotherapy.

Sperm Cryopreservation

Although infertility is an uncommon presentation for GCT, up to 52% of men have oligospermia at diagnosis and 10% are azoospermic (Williams et al, 2009a). The limited data that exist suggest that roughly half of these men recover normospermia after orchiectomy (Carroll et al, 1987; Jacobsen et al, 2001). The germinal epithelium is exquisitely sensitive to platin-based chemotherapy and radiation therapy. **Virtually all patients become azoospermic after chemotherapy, and 50% and 80% of patients with normal semen parameters at diagnosis return to these levels within 2 and 5 years, respectively** (Bokemeyer et al, 1996a; Feldman et al, 2008). **Recovery of spermatogenesis after radiation therapy for seminoma may take to 2 to 3 years or longer** (Fossa et al, 1999b). RPLND may result in ejaculatory dysfunction in 80% or more of patients undergoing a full, bilateral template dissection without nerve sparing. Most men are able to father children after standard chemotherapy for GCTs; radiotherapy appears to have a more deleterious effect on fertility than chemotherapy (Huyghe et al, 2004). **Given the impact of treatments for testis cancer on fertility, men who are undecided or are planning future paternity are recommended to undergo sperm cryopreservation before treatment is initiated.** Sperm banking can be done before or after radical orchiectomy.

Treatment

Therapeutic Principles

The management of GCTs is governed by the potential for rapid growth and for cure in essentially all patients; **this translates into a need for rapid diagnosis and staging and expeditious application of appropriate treatment so as not to have patients die unnecessarily or experience side effects from treatment that would not have been required with earlier diagnosis and proper management.** After orchiectomy, staging imaging studies, serum tumor marker status should be performed and treatment plans should be developed as rapidly as can be reasonably accomplished.

The probability of cure even in the presence of metastatic disease has led to an aggressive approach with regard to the administration of chemotherapy and the performance of surgery after chemotherapy to resect residual masses. Chemotherapy is generally administered regardless of low white blood cell counts or thrombocytopenia, and nephrotoxic chemotherapy (cisplatin) is often administered even in the presence of moderate to severe renal insufficiency (Williams et al, 1987; Einhorn et al, 1989; Bajorin et al, 1993; Loehrer et al, 1995; Bokemeyer, et al, 1996b; Nichols et al, 1998; de Wit et al, 2001). Similarly, an aggressive surgical approach is taken to resect all sites of residual disease after chemotherapy for NSGCT even if this involves multiple anatomic sites. The young age and generally good health of patients with GCTs permits an aggressive treatment approach if needed.

Serum tumor markers strongly influence the management of GCTs, particularly NSGCTs. As discussed, **elevated serum AFP or hCG after orchiectomy indicates the presence of metastatic disease, and these patients are preferentially given chemotherapy.** For patients receiving chemotherapy, increasing serum tumor marker levels during or after therapy generally indicate refractory or relapsed disease, respectively. As discussed earlier, serum AFP, hCG, and LDH levels at the initiation of chemotherapy are important prognostic factors and influence the selection and duration of chemotherapy regimens (International Germ Cell Consensus Classification, 1997).

Testis cancer is a relatively rare disease, and general urologists and general oncologists do not typically treat a large volume of patients with GCTs. In addition, the treatment algorithms are complex and nuanced, and the data supporting certain treatments, such as RPLND, are based on data from a relatively small number of surgeons who have performed a large number of these operations (Donohue et al, 1993, 1995; Heidenreich et al, 2003; Stephenson, et al, 2005b; Williams et al, 2009b). Most urology residents in the United States complete their training having performed two or fewer RPLND procedures (Lowrance et al, 2007). Several studies reported improved survival when the treatment was provided at high-volume institutions (Aass et al, 1991; Harding et al, 1993; Feuer et al, 1994; Collette et al, 1999; Joudi and Konety, 2005; Suzumura et al, 2008). Whenever possible, patients with GCTs should be treated at high-volume centers, and RPLND should be performed by surgeons who are experienced with this operation.

Contrasting Seminoma and Nonseminoma Germ Cell Tumor

For treatment purposes, the distinction between seminoma and NSGCT is very important. Compared with NSGCT, seminoma has a more favorable natural history. In general, seminoma tends to be less aggressive, to be diagnosed at an earlier stage, and to spread predictably along lymphatic channels to the retroperitoneum before spreading hematogenously to the lungs or other organs. **At diagnosis, the proportion of patients with CS I, II, and III disease is 85%, 10%, and 5% for seminoma and approximately 33%, 33%, and 33% for NSGCT (Powles et al, 2005). Seminoma is also associated with a lower incidence of occult metastasis among patients with CS I (10% to 15% vs. 25% to 35% for NSGCT) and a lower risk of systemic relapse after treatment of the retroperitoneum (1% to 4% after radiotherapy for seminoma vs. 10% after RPLND for NSGCT),** which has important implications for the use of chemotherapy. Seminoma is less likely to have elevated serum tumor markers, and serum tumor markers do not range as high as in NSGCT. Also, serum tumor markers are not used in the IGCCCG risk classification of seminoma.

Compared with NSGCT, **seminoma is exquisitely sensitive to radiation therapy and platin-based chemotherapy.** Substantially lower radiation doses are required to eradicate seminoma compared with other solid tumors. **Radiation therapy is a standard treatment option for CS I, IIA, and IIB seminoma but has no role in NSGCT,** with the exception of treatment for brain metastases. Seminoma accounts for only 10% of advanced GCT cases despite the fact that it accounts for 52% to 56% of all GCTs. A poor prognosis IGCCCG risk category does not exist for advanced seminoma, and greater than 90% of metastatic cases are classified as good risk (compared with 56% for NSGCT) (International Germ Cell Consensus Classification, 1997). **The risk of teratoma at metastatic sites is generally not a consideration for advanced seminoma, which has important implications for the management of residual masses after chemotherapy. However, the potential for seminoma to transform into NSGCT elements is an important consideration in the management of patients who fail to respond to chemotherapy or who relapse after radiation therapy. Of patients with metastatic seminoma who relapse after treatment, approximately 10% to 15% have NSGCT elements at the site of relapse. An autopsy study showed that 30% of patients who die of seminoma have NSGCT elements at metastatic sites** (Bredael et al, 1982).

The risk of teratoma at metastatic sites has a substantial effect on treatment algorithms for NSGCT and necessitates the frequent use of postchemotherapy surgery (PCS) in patients with advanced disease. The risk of teratoma in the retroperitoneum in low-stage NSGCT has also influenced many clinicians to favor RPLND over chemotherapy in situations where the risk of occult distant metastases is low. As discussed earlier, teratoma is not sensitive to chemotherapy, and the outcome of patients with metastatic teratoma is related to the completeness of surgical resection.

Because GCTs are almost always cured, numerous clinical trials have been conducted in an attempt to minimize treatment and avoid unnecessary therapies in an effort to reduce short-term and particularly long-term side effects and toxicity. One approach has been to limit the number of patients who receive two interventions ("double therapy"): either surgery or chemotherapy and not both. **However, because NSGCTs are usually mixed tumors, and teratoma often exists at metastatic sites with other GCT elements, "cure" often requires chemotherapy to kill the chemosensitive components and surgery to remove teratomatous components.** It is widely accepted that the successful integration of systemic therapy and PCS is a major contributing factor to the improved cure rates for metastatic GCT seen over the past several decades. Although minimizing unnecessary treatment is an important goal, chemotherapy, radiation therapy, and CT imaging are associated with an increased lifetime risk of secondary malignant neoplasms (SMN) and/or cardiovascular disease (Meinardi et al, 2000; Zagars et al, 2004; Brenner and Hall, 2007; van den Belt-Dusebout et al, 2007; Tarin et al, 2009). In contrast, RPLND when performed by experienced surgeons is associated with a substantially more favorable long-term toxicity profile.

Intratubular Germ Cell Neoplasia

ITGCN is diagnosed by testicular biopsy performed for the investigation of infertility, contralateral testis biopsy in patients with GCT, or within the affected testis in a patient undergoing testis-sparing surgery. The rationale for treatment of ITGCN is based on the high risk of developing invasive GCT (Skakkebaek et al, 1982; Dieckmann and Skakkebaek, 1999). Treatment options include orchiectomy, low-dose radiotherapy, and close observation. The choice of therapy should be individualized based on the patient's desire for future paternity, the presence or absence of a normal contralateral testis, and the patient's desire to avoid testosterone replacement therapy. **Radical orchiectomy is the most definitive treatment, although low-dose radiotherapy (≥20 Gy) is associated with similar rates of local control with the prospect of preserving testicular endocrine function owing to the relative radioresistance of Leydig cells compared with germinal epithelium** (Heidenreich et al, 2001; Montironi, 2002; Dieckmann et al, 2003). **However, testosterone replacement therapy is ultimately required in up to 40% of patients, and patients should be monitored after radiotherapy for adequate testicular androgen production** (Heidenreich et al, 2001; Petersen et al, 2002). To preserve testicular endocrine function, dose reductions to less than 20 Gy have been investigated, but cases of recurrent ITGCN have been observed (Classen et al, 2003a; Dieckmann et al, 2003). For patients with a normal contralateral testis who desire future paternity, radical orchiectomy is preferred because scatter to the contralateral testis from radiotherapy may impair spermatogenesis. For patients with abnormal semen parameters but sufficient for assisted reproductive techniques, close surveillance with periodic ultrasound evaluation of the testis is a reasonable strategy with deferred therapy until successful pregnancy and/or development of GCT. Another option for these patients is testis exploration, sperm harvesting, and cryopreservation for assisted reproductive techniques and radical orchiectomy followed by testosterone replacement therapy.

Patients with ITGCN who are scheduled to receive cisplatin-based chemotherapy represent a unique circumstance because chemotherapy may reduce (but not eliminate) the risk of GCT. A study estimated the risk of testicular GCT after chemotherapy in a patient with ITGCN to be 21% at 5 years and 45% at 10 years (Christensen et al, 1998). These patients may be treated by low-dose radiotherapy after completion of chemotherapy, or they may undergo testis biopsy 2 years or more after chemotherapy with therapy reserved for patients with evidence of ITGCN (Krege et al, 2008a, 2008b).

Nonseminoma Germ Cell Tumor

Clinical Stage I Nonseminoma Germ Cell Tumor. Approximately one third of patients with NSGCT have CS I with normal serum tumor markers after orchiectomy. **The optimal management of these patients continues to generate controversy because the long-term survival associated with surveillance, RPLND, and primary chemotherapy approaches 100%.** Contributing to the controversy is the fact that occult metastases in the retroperitoneum or at distant sites are present in only 20% to 30% of patients overall. Any intervention after orchiectomy, with the potential for short-term and long-term morbidity, represents overtreatment for the 70% to 80% of patients with disease limited to the testis. Most centers employ a risk-adapted approach based on the probability of occult metastasis, although surveillance is the preferred approach at selected centers, regardless of a man's risk.

Risk Assessment. Numerous studies have attempted to identify histopathologic factors within the primary tumor that are predictive of the presence of occult metastasis. **The most commonly identified risk factors for occult metastasis are LVI and a predominant component of EC.** The definition of EC predominance in the literature varies from 45% to 90%. **The reported rate of occult metastasis (based on observed relapses on surveillance or lymph node metastasis at RPLND) with LVI and EC predominance varies from 45% to 90% and 30% to 80%, respectively** (Heidenreich et al, 1998; Sogani et al, 1998; Hermans et al, 2000; Sweeney et al, 2000; Alexandre et al, 2001; Roeleveld et al, 2001; Albers et al, 2003; Vergouwe et al, 2003; Nicolai et al, 2004; Stephenson et al, 2005a). **In the absence of these two risk factors, the risk of occult metastasis is less than 20%.** Other identified risk factors include advanced pT stage, absence of mature teratoma, absence of yolk sac tumor, presence of EC (regardless of the percent composition), percentage of MIB-1 staining, tumor size, and patient age. In a pooled analysis of 23 studies assessing predictors of occult metastasis in CS I NSGCT, Vergouwe and associates (2003) identified LVI (odds ratio 5.2), MIB-1 staining greater than 70% (odds ratio 4.7) and EC predominance (odds ratio 2.8) as the strongest predictors, and these factors were present in 36%, 55%, and 51% of patients.

As discussed previously, the results of abdominopelvic CT imaging should be considered when formulating treatment recommendations because a size cutoff of 1 cm is associated with a high false-negative rate. Retroperitoneal lymph nodes greater than 5 to 9 mm in the primary landing zone should be viewed with suspicion for regional lymph node metastasis.

Numerous risk groups and prognostic indices have been proposed based on the presence or absence of several of these risk factors, most commonly on the basis of LVI and EC predominance (Freedman et al, 1987; Read et al, 1992; Heidenreich et al, 1998; Sogani et al, 1998; Hermans et al, 2000; Alexandre et al, 2001; Albers et al, 2003; Nicolai et al, 2004; Stephenson et al, 2005a). **Classification of patients as low versus high risk based on LVI and EC predominance applies to the risk of occult metastatic disease in patients with CS I and should not be confused with the IGCCCG risk classification for metastatic NSGCT** (discussed previously). Only one of these prognostic models has been prospectively validated, and none have considered the results of staging CT imaging (Freedman et al, 1987; Read et al, 1992). Three prospective studies suggest that LVI and EC predominance may be associated with a risk of metastasis between 35% and 55%, not between 50% and 70% as has been reported in most older studies. A surveillance series from Princess Margaret Hospital reported a relapse rate of 52% among patients with LVI and/or pure EC (Sturgeon et al, 2011). Similarly, a series from British Columbia and Portland, Oregon, reported that LVI was associated with a relapse rate of 50%, whereas EC predominance was associated with a relapse rate of 33% (Kollmannsberger et al, 2010b). Likewise, a population-based surveillance study from Scandinavia reported a 42% relapse rate in patients with LVI (Tandstad et al, 2009). Lastly, only 18% of patients with CS I NSGCT treated by RPLND in a randomized trial had retroperitoneal lymph node metastasis despite the fact that 42% had evidence of LVI in the primary tumor (Albers et al, 2008). This lower than expected rate of occult metastasis may be due to greater scrutiny of staging CT imaging for abnormal lymph nodes and/or stage migration.

Surveillance. **The rationale for surveillance is based on the fact that 70% to 80% of patients with CS I NSGCT are cured by orchiectomy alone and the ability to salvage virtually all relapsing patients with chemotherapy based on the long-term cure rates achieved for chemotherapy for good-risk metastatic NSGCT** (International Germ Cell Consensus Classification, 1997). Surveillance offers the potential of reducing treatment-related toxicity by restricting treatment to patients with a proven need for it. Surveillance series have reported overall and disease-specific survival rates indistinguishable from rates seen with RPLND and primary chemotherapy. As a result, initial surveillance is regarded as a standard treatment option for CS I NSGCT. **The disadvantages of surveillance are that it is associated with the highest risk of relapse, the need for long-term (>5 years) surveillance, the potential for SMN owing to intensive surveillance CT imaging** (Brenner and Hall, 2007; Tarin et al, 2009), **and the more intensive therapy required to treat patients at the time of relapse than if they had received treatment at diagnosis.**

Published surveillance series have reported results on more than 3000 men, with a mean relapse risk of 28% and 1.2% cancer-specific mortality. The 11 largest series are summarized in Table 34-3 (Freedman et al, 1987; Read et al, 1992; Gels et al, 1995; Sogani et al, 1998; Colls et al, 1999; Sharir et al, 1999; Francis et al, 2000; Daugaard et al, 2003; Ernst et al, 2005; Tandstad et al, 2009; Kollmannsberger et al, 2010b; Tandstad et al, 2010; Sturgeon et al, 2011). **More than 90% of relapses occur within the first 2 years, but late relapses (>5 years) are seen in 1% of patients (5% in some reports)** (Daugaard et al, 2003; Sturgeon et al, 2011). In more contemporary series, 65% to 75% of relapses are contained in the retroperitoneum, with or without elevated serum tumor markers (Tandstad et al, 2009; Sturgeon et al, 2011). **Induction chemotherapy is the most common treatment used for patients with relapses because most have bulky (>3 cm) retroperitoneal lymphadenopathy, elevated serum tumor markers, or distant metastasis. However, patients with normal serum tumor markers and relapses limited to nonbulky (<3 cm)** retroperitoneal lymphadenopathy may be managed initially with RPLND (Stephenson et al, 2007).

The surveillance schedule employed in published series is highly variable, and no schedule has been demonstrated to be superior to another in terms of survival. Given that most relapses occur within the first 2 years, surveillance imaging and testing is intense in years 0 to 2, with less frequent testing in years 3 to 5. The risk of late relapse mandates surveillance beyond 5 years, but whether such surveillance should include CT scans is controversial. The frequency of abdominopelvic CT imaging varies across multiple series from 2 to 13 or more scans within the first 5 years of follow-up. A randomized trial of two versus five CT scans in years 1 to 2 reported no significant differences in survival, IGCCCG risk category at relapse, or CS at relapse (Rustin et al, 2007). Noncompliance with the prescribed surveillance schedule has been reported in 35% to 80% of patients in published series (Howard et al, 1995; Hao et al, 1998; Ernst et al, 2005).

Retroperitoneal Lymph Node Dissection. **The rationale for RPLND for CS I NSGCT is based on the following factors:** (1) retroperitoneum is the most common site of occult metastatic disease, with low risk of associated systemic disease; (2) 15% to 25% incidence of retroperitoneal teratoma (which is resistant to chemotherapy) in patients with occult metastasis; (3) low risk of abdominopelvic recurrence after full, bilateral template RPLND, obviating the need for routine surveillance CT imaging; (4) high cure rates after RPLND alone for patients with low-volume (pN1) retroperitoneal malignancy and teratoma (pN1-3); (5) avoidance of chemotherapy in greater than 75% or more of patients if adjuvant chemotherapy is restricted to patients with extensive retroperitoneal malignancy (pN2-3); (6) high salvage rate of relapses with good risk and induction chemotherapy; and (7) low short-term and long-term morbidity when nerve-sparing RPLND is performed by experienced surgeons. **In low-stage NSGCT, the therapeutic focus is the retroperitoneum, for which RPLND provides the most effective control with the lowest rates of serious long-term morbidity. The disadvantages of RPLND are that all patients undergo major abdominal surgery, it requires the availability of experienced surgeons and may not be deliverable to all patients, and it is associated with the highest rate of double therapy.**

The seven largest RPLND series for CS I NSGCT are summarized in Table 34-4 (Richie, 1990; Donohue et al, 1993; Hermans et al, 2000; Nicolai et al, 2004; Stephenson et al, 2005b; Albers et al, 2008; Williams et al, 2009b). The rate of pathologic stage II in these series ranges from 19% to 28%, and an estimated 66% to 81% of

TABLE 34-3 Surveillance Series for Clinical Stage I Nonseminoma Germ Cell Tumor

STUDY	NO. PATIENTS	RELAPSES (%)	MEDIAN FOLLOW-UP (mo)	MEDIAN TIME TO RELAPSE (mo)	SYSTEMIC RELAPSE*	GCT DEATHS (%)
Freedman et al, 1987	259	70 (32)	30	NR	61%	3 (1.2)
Read et al, 1992	373	100 (27)	60	3 (1.5-20)	39%	5 (1.3)
Gels et al,1995	154	42 (27)	72	4 (2-24)	71%	2 (1)
Sogani et al, 1998	105	27 (26)	136	5 (2-24)	37%	3 (3)
Sharir et al, 1999	170	48 (28)	76	7 (2-21)	79%	1 (0.5)
Colls et al, 1999	248	70 (28)	53	NR	73%	4 (1.6)
Francis et al, 2000	183	52 (28)	70	6 (1-12)	54%	2 (1)
Daugaard et al, 2003	301	86 (29)	60	5 (1-171)	66%	0
Ernst et al, 2005	197	58 (29)	54	6 (2-135)	22%	0
Kollmannsberger et al, 2010b	223	59 (26)	52	NR	NR	0
Sturgeon et al, 2011	371	104	76	7	33	3 (0.8)
Tandstad et al, 2009†	350	44 (13)	56	8	27%	1 (0.3)
Tandstad et al, 2010‡	129	19 (15)	123	8	37%	0

*Relapse with elevated serum tumor markers and/or relapse in tissue other than retroperitoneal lymph nodes.
†97% were lymphovascular invasion and low risk.
‡96% were lymphovascular invasion and low risk.
GCT, germ cell tumor; NR, not reported.

TABLE 34-4 Published Series of Retroperitoneal Lymph Node Dissection for Clinical Stage I Nonseminoma Germ Cell Tumor

STUDY	NO. PATIENTS	PS II (%)	TERATOMA IN RETROPERITONEUM	RELAPSE, PS I	RELAPSE, PS II	ADJUVANT CHEMOTHERAPY	GCT DEATHS (%)
Donohue et al, 1993	378	113 (30)	15%	12%	34%	13%	3 (0.8)
Hermans et al, 2000	292	67 (23)	NR	10%	22%	12%	1 (0.3)
Nicolai et al, 2004	322	61 (19)	NR	NR	27%	NR	4 (1.2)
Stephenson et al, 2005b	297	83 (28)	15%	6%	19%	15%	0
Williams et al, 2009b	76	37 (49)	NR	5%	11%	NR	0
Albers et al, 2008	173	31 (19)	NR	9%	NR	19%	0
Richie, 1990	99	35 (35)	NR	6%	15%	15%	0

GCT, germ cell tumor; NR, not reported; PS, pathologic stage.

these patients were cured after RPLND alone (Donohue et al, 1993; Hermans et al, 2000; Sweeney et al, 2000; Rabbani et al, 2001; Nicolai et al, 2004; Stephenson et al, 2005a, 2005b). The long-term cancer-specific survival with RPLND (with or without adjuvant chemotherapy) approaches 100%, and the risk of late relapse is negligible. Most RPLND series have reported retroperitoneal recurrences in less than 2% of patients, demonstrating its efficacy for control of disease of the retroperitoneum (Donohue et al, 1993; Hermans et al, 2000; Stephenson et al, 2005b).

A full, bilateral template dissection is associated with the lowest risk of abdominopelvic recurrence (<2%) and the highest rate of antegrade ejaculation (>90%) when nerve-sparing techniques are employed (Jewett, 1990; Donohue and Foster, 1998; Stephenson et al, 2005b; Eggener et al, 2007b; Subramanian et al, 2010). For this reason, it is now considered by many to be the standard of care for primary RPLND (Stephenson et al, 2011). A randomized trial of primary RPLND (plus adjuvant bleomycin-etoposide-cisplatin [BEP]×2 for pathologic stage II) versus BEP×1 chemotherapy for CS I NSGCT showed a significant improvement in 2-year progression-free survival with chemotherapy (99% vs. 92%), although no GCT deaths were observed in either arm (Albers et al, 2008). The local recurrence rate was 11% in patients with histologically negative retroperitoneal lymph nodes at RPLND, which was substantially higher than the local recurrence rate among all patients from experienced centers. The patients in this trial were treated at 61 different centers in Germany. The relative inexperience of surgeons and unilateral templates likely contributed to these poor results. **Patients who opt for RPLND should have this procedure performed by an experienced surgeon with a full, bilateral template dissection. Otherwise, patients should go on surveillance or receive primary chemotherapy.**

RPLND is a curative procedure in 60% to 90% of patients with pN1 disease and up to 100% of patients with teratoma only (regardless of the extent of lymph node involvement) (Pizzocaro and Monfardini, 1984; Williams et al, 1987; Richie and Kantoff, 1991; Rabbani et al, 2001; Sheinfeld et al, 2003; Stephenson et al, 2005b). The risk of relapse in patients with pN2-3 disease is greater than 50% (Vogelzang et al, 1983; Williams et al, 1987; Socinski et al, 1988; Stephenson et al, 2005b). With two cycles of adjuvant chemotherapy (most commonly BEP×2 or etoposide-cisplatin [EP]×2), relapses are reduced to 1% or less (Behnia et al, 2000; Albers et al, 2003; Kondagunta et al, 2004). **A randomized trial of adjuvant chemotherapy versus observation after RPLND for pathologic stage II showed a significant reduction in the risk of relapse (6% vs. 49%) but no difference in overall survival** (Williams et al, 1987). Adjuvant chemotherapy and observation are acceptable treatment options for patients with pathologic stage II disease, and patients should be informed of the risk of relapse after RPLND and the potential benefits and risks of these approaches.

Primary Chemotherapy. In contradistinction to adjuvant chemotherapy given for pathologic stage II disease after RPLND, primary chemotherapy refers to treatment administered to men with CS I NSGCT after orchiectomy. The goal of primary chemotherapy is to minimize the risk of relapse and to allow men to avoid RPLND and induction chemotherapy (for patients who relapse on surveillance). The rationale for primary chemotherapy is based on the efficacy of two cycles of chemotherapy to eradicate micrometastatic disease when given as adjuvant therapy after RPLND and the 20% to 25% need for chemotherapy despite RPLND (either as adjuvant therapy or for treatment of relapse) (Donohue et al, 1993; Hermans et al, 2000; Nicolai et al, 2004; Stephenson et al, 2005a). Primary chemotherapy offers patients the greatest chance of being relapse-free with any single treatment modality, and it can be delivered at community-based institutions (Tandstad et al, 2009, 2010). The disadvantages of primary chemotherapy are as follows: (1) it does not treat retroperitoneal teratoma and exposes patients to the potential for chemoresistant and/or late relapse (discussed later), (2) long-term surveillance CT imaging of the retroperitoneum is required, and (3) all patients are exposed to chemotherapy and the potential risk of late toxicity (e.g., cardiovascular disease and secondary malignancies). **The risk of late toxicity from two cycles of chemotherapy is poorly defined, although there appears to be no safe lower limit.**

Primary chemotherapy has been investigated in 12 published series, most of which have used BEP×2 (Table 34-5) (Abratt et al, 1994; Cullen et al, 1996; Pont et al, 1996; Ondrus et al, 1998; Bohlen et al, 1999; Amato et al, 2004; Chevreau et al, 2004; Oliver et al, 2004; Dearnaley et al, 2005; Albers et al, 2008; Tandstad et al, 2009, 2010). In men with LVI and/or EC predominance, it is possible to reduce the recurrence rate from 30% to 60% to about 2% to 3%. In 8 of the 12 series, no deaths from GCT were reported over an average median follow-up of 5 years. In the other four studies comprising 406 patients, 13 relapses (3%) were observed, and 6 (46%) of these relapsing patients died of GCT. **Although primary chemotherapy is associated with the lowest risk of relapse, these relapses are less amenable to salvage therapy because they are chemoresistant, particularly if they have received a regimen other than standard dose BEP. In contrast, patients who relapse after RPLND or on surveillance are chemotherapy-naive and are cured with chemotherapy in virtually all cases.** Although relapses are uncommon with primary chemotherapy, virtually all occur in the retroperitoneum; this mandates the use of surveillance abdominopelvis CT imaging in the follow-up of these patients. Many European institutions prefer BEP×2 to RPLND because the latter is primarily used as a staging procedure, performed without curative intent (Krege et al, 2008a, 2008b; Schmoll et al, 2009b).

A randomized trial and a population-based study investigated the use of BEP×1 as primary chemotherapy for CS I NSGCT (Albers et al, 2008; Tandstad et al, 2009). Over a median follow-up of less than 5 years in both studies, the risk of relapse after BEP×1 ranged from 1% to 3%, and cancer-specific survival approached 100% in

TABLE 34-5 Published Series of Primary Chemotherapy for Clinical Stage I Nonseminoma Germ Cell Tumor

STUDY	NO. PATIENTS	REGIMEN*	MEDIAN FOLLOW-UP (mo)	RELAPSES (%)	TIME TO RELAPSE (mo)	GCT DEATHS (%)
Abratt et al, 1994	20	BEP×2 (E: 360)†	31	0	NR	0
Cullen et al, 1996	114	BEP×2 (E: 360)	48	2 (1.8)	7, 18	2 (1.8)
Pont et al, 1996	29	BEP×2 (E: 500)	79	2 (2.7)	8, 27	1 (3.5)
Ondrus et al, 1998	18	BEP×2 (E: 360)	36	0	NR	0
Amato et al, 2004	68	CEB×2 (E: 360)	38	1 (1.5)	21	0
Bohlen et al, 1999	58	BEP×2 (E: 360); PVB×2 (20 pts)	93	2 (3.4)	22, 90	0
Chevreau, et al, 2004	40	BEP×2 (E: 360)	113	0	NR	0
Oliver et al, 2004	148	BEP×1 (n = 28); BEP×2 (n = 46); BOP×2 (n = 74) (E: 360)	33	6 (4.1)	NR	2 (1.4)
Dearnaley et al, 2005	115	BOP×2	70	3 (1.7)	3, 6, 26	1 (0.9)
Albers et al, 2008	191	BEP×1 (E: 500)	56	2 (1.0)	15, 60	0
Tandstad et al, 2009	382	BEP×1 (n = 312); BEP×2 (n = 70) (E: 500)	56	7 (1.8)	Range: 8-36	0
Tandstad et al, 2010	100	PVB×1 (n = 40) or PVB×2 (n = 60)	116	5	1, 9, 10, 27, 126	0

*Chemotherapy regimens: BEP, bleomycin-etoposide-cisplatin; BOP, bleomycin-vincristine-cisplatin; CEB, carboplatin-etoposide-bleomycin; PVB, cisplatin-vinblastine-bleomycin.
†E: 360 refers to an etoposide dose of 360 mg/m^2/cycle; E: 500 refers to an etoposide dose of 500 mg/m^2/cycle.
GCT, germ cell tumor; NR, not reported; pts, patients.

both studies. BEP×1 needs to be compared with BEP×2 in a randomized trial to verify its safety and efficacy.

Treatment Selection for Clinical Stage I Nonseminoma Germ Cell Tumor. There are no randomized trials that compare the standard treatment approaches for CS I NSGCT. A phase III, randomized trial compared BEP×1 versus unilateral, modified-template RPLND (with BEP×2 for patients with pathologic stage II disease) (Albers et al, 2008). Although a statistically significantly reduced risk of relapse was reported with BEP×1 (hazard ratio [HR] 0.13, 95% confidence interval 0.02 to 0.55), no cancer-specific deaths were reported in either arm. This trial has been criticized because it compared two nonstandard treatment approaches for CS I NSGCT (Sheinfeld and Motzer, 2008).

Given the excellent long-term survival with surveillance, RPLND, and primary chemotherapy, it is inappropriate to recommend any specific treatment option because there are relative advantages and disadvantages of each approach in terms of treatment-related toxicity, the need for subsequent treatment, and intensity of surveillance testing and imaging. Likewise, patient preferences may vary and should be considered. **Several clinical practice guidelines for CS I NSGCT have been published, and surveillance is generally recommended to low-risk patients, and surveillance, RPLND, or primary chemotherapy is recommended to high-risk patients** (Albers et al, 2005; Motzer et al, 2006; Hotte et al, 2008; Krege et al, 2008a, 2008b; Schmoll et al, 2009b; Stephenson et al, 2011). Nguyen and colleagues (2010) developed a decision-analysis model that considered cancer outcomes, treatment-related toxicity, and patient preferences for important post-treatment outcomes to define the optimal treatment for CS I NSGCT. Surveillance is associated with the highest quality-adjusted survival when the estimated risk of relapse is less than 33% to 37%, and active treatment (RPLND or primary chemotherapy) is favored when the risk of relapse is greater than 46% to 54%.

Clinical Stage IS Nonseminoma Germ Cell Tumor. CS IS is defined as the presence of elevated serum tumor markers after orchiectomy without clinical or radiographic evidence of metastatic disease. Studies of primary RPLND for CS IS NSGCT reported that 37% to 100% of patients subsequently required chemotherapy for retroperitoneal metastasis, persistently elevated serum tumor markers, or relapse (Davis et al, 1994; Saxman et al, 1996). **There is consensus that these patients should be treated similarly to patients with CS IIC and III and receive induction chemotherapy.** The cancer-specific survival after chemotherapy for CS IS is greater than 90% (Culine et al, 1996; International Germ Cell Consensus Classification, 1997). Slightly elevated and stable serum tumor marker levels after orchiectomy in patients without clinical evidence of disease should be interpreted cautiously because they may represent false-positive findings for disseminated NSGCT.

Clinical Stage IIA and IIB Nonseminoma Germ Cell Tumor. The optimal management of CS IIA and IIB NSGCT is controversial. **RPLND (with or without adjuvant chemotherapy) and induction chemotherapy (with or without postchemotherapy RPLND) are accepted treatment options with survival rates exceeding 95%.** No randomized trials have compared these treatment approaches. In a prospective, multicenter, nonrandomized trial of RPLND and two cycles of adjuvant chemotherapy versus induction chemotherapy, no significant differences in recurrence (7% for RPLND vs. 11% for chemotherapy) or overall survival were observed (Weissbach et al, 2000). A single-institution, nonrandomized, retrospective comparison of RPLND (and two cycles of adjuvant chemotherapy for pathologic stage II) and induction chemotherapy reported a significant reduction in the risk of recurrence with induction chemotherapy (98% vs. 79%), but cancer-specific survival approached 100% with both modalities (100% vs. 98%), patients undergoing RPLND received fewer cycles of chemotherapy (mean 4.2 vs. 1.4), and 51% of patients undergoing RPLND avoided chemotherapy (Stephenson et al, 2007).

The arguments in favor of RPLND for CS IIA and IIB are as follows: (1) 13% to 35% of patients have pathologically negative lymph nodes and avoid chemotherapy (Pizzocaro, 1987; Donohue et al, 1995; Weissbach et al, 2000; Stephenson et al, 2007); (2) approximately 30% have retroperitoneal teratoma, which is resistant to chemotherapy (Foster et al, 1996; Stephenson et al, 2007); (3) long-term cancer-specific survival is 98% to 100% with RPLND with or without adjuvant chemotherapy (Pizzocaro, 1987; Donohue et al, 1995; Weissbach et al, 2000; Stephenson et al, 2007); (4) 10% to 52% avoid any chemotherapy (Pizzocaro, 1987; Donohue et al, 1995; Weissbach et al, 2000; Stephenson et al, 2007); and (5) ejaculatory function is preserved in 70% to 90% of patients (Richie and Kantoff, 1991; Donohue et al, 1995; Weissbach et al, 2000). **The disadvantages of RPLND are as follows:** (1) additional therapy is required in 48% or more of patients, (2) 13% to 15% have persistence of disease after RPLND and require a full induction chemotherapy regimen, and (3) high-quality RPLND may not be deliverable at all institutions (Weissbach et al, 2000; Stephenson et al, 2007).

The arguments in favor of induction chemotherapy are the following: (1) a complete response is achieved and PCS is avoided in 60% to 78% of patients, (2) treatment can be delivered at community-based institutions, and (3) cancer-specific survival is 96% to 100% (Peckham and Hendry, 1985; Logothetis et al, 1987; Socinski et al, 1988; Ondrus et al, 1992; Horwich et al, 1994; Lerner et al, 1995; Culine et al, 1997; Debono et al, 1997; Weissbach et al, 2000; Stephenson et al, 2007). **The disadvantages of chemotherapy are the following:** (1) all patients are exposed to the risk of long-term toxicity of chemotherapy, and (2) patients who do not undergo postchemotherapy RPNLD are at risk of relapse with chemorefractory GCT.

Given that 13% to 35% of patients with CS IIA NSGCT have pathologically negative lymph nodes (a false-positive CT result), patients with indeterminate lesions on staging abdominopelvic CT imaging who are at otherwise low risk for metastatic disease may be observed closely initially to clarify subsequent treatment decisions. **Treatment considerations for CS IIA and IIB NSGCT include the risk of occult systemic disease, risk of retroperitoneal teratoma, short-term and long-term treatment-related morbidity, and need for double therapy.** The last consideration is of least importance but has strongly influenced opinion regarding the optimal treatment of these patients. As discussed earlier, because metastatic NSGCT frequently exists as chemosensitive malignant GCT and chemoresistant teratoma, "cure" often requires the combination of chemotherapy and surgery.

Experience with primary RPLND in low-stage NSGCT over the last two decades has identified parameters associated with systemic relapse. As with CS IS NSGCT, the presence of elevated AFP and hCG levels after orchiectomy is associated with an increased risk of systemic relapse after RPLND. Rabbani and colleagues (2001) reported relapses after RPLND in 4 of 5 patients (80%) with elevated postorchiectomy AFP or hCG levels compared with 7 of 45 patients (16%) with normal serum tumor markers. Stephenson and associates (2005b) identified the presence of elevated serum tumor markers (HR = 5.6, $P < .001$) and retroperitoneal lymphadenopathy greater than 3 cm (HR = 12.3, $P < .001$) as significant predictors of systemic relapse after RPLND. **There is consensus that patients with CS IIA and IIB NSGCT and elevated AFP or hCG levels or bulky lymph nodes (>3 cm) should receive induction chemotherapy.**

The presence of retroperitoneal teratoma is a limitation to any strategy for metastatic NSGCT that uses chemotherapy alone because it is resistant to chemotherapy. Overall, approximately 20% of patients with CS IIA and IIB have retroperitoneal teratoma, and this increases to 30% to 35% in patients with teratoma in the primary tumor (Donohue et al, 1995; Foster et al, 1996; Stephenson et al, 2005b). Residual microscopic teratoma may remain dormant and clinically silent throughout a patient's lifetime. It may also exhibit slow growth, which can be detected on surveillance CT imaging and is amenable to cure by surgical resection. However, growing teratoma syndrome, malignant transformation, and late relapse are the most serious (although rare) sequelae of unresected teratoma. **RPLND is preferred as initial therapy in patients at risk for retroperitoneal teratoma who are at otherwise low risk for systemic disease (normal serum tumor markers, lymphadenopathy <3 cm).**

Clinical Stage IIC and III Nonseminoma Germ Cell Tumor. Induction chemotherapy with cisplatin-based regimens is the initial approach used for the treatment of CS IIC and III NSGCT. As discussed previously, induction chemotherapy is also the preferred approach for CS IS and CS IIA and IIB with elevated AFP and hCG levels after orchiectomy. The specific regimen and

number of cycles are based on IGCCCG risk stratification (see Table 34-2) (International Germ Cell Consensus Classification, 1997).

The development of cisplatin-based chemotherapy represents the most important advancement in the treatment of GCT. Before the identification of cisplatin, complete responses to chemotherapy were achieved in 10% to 20% of patients, and the cure rate was only 5% to 10% (Einhorn, 1990). Long-term cure is now anticipated in 80% to 90% of patients with metastatic GCT. Randomized trials have evaluated the efficacy and safety of various drug combinations to determine the optimal regimen based on IGCCCG risk (Debono et al, 1997).

The initial landmark study was conducted at Indiana University using cisplatin-vinblastine-bleomycin (PVB)×4 in the 1970s and reported complete responses in 74% of patients and more than 70% long-term survivors (Beck et al, 2005). When it was demonstrated that etoposide could cure some patients with relapse after PVB chemotherapy, PVB×4 was compared with BEP×4 in a multicenter randomized trial. No significant difference in overall survival was seen between the two regimens (2-year survival 80%, $P = .11$), but BEP×4 was associated with less neuromuscular toxicity and was subsequently adopted as the standard regimen (Williams et al, 1987).

Chemotherapy for Good-Risk Nonseminoma Germ Cell Tumor

After BEP×4 became the standard regimen for advanced GCT, subsequent trials focused on reducing toxicity for patients with good-risk features and improving outcomes for patients with intermediate-risk and poor-risk disease. **For good-risk patients, two randomized trials showed that BEP×3 is not inferior to BEP×4** (Einhorn et al, 1989; Saxman et al, 1998; de Wit et al, 2001). With 184 patients enrolled in the U.S. study, 92% of patients in each arm were continuously disease-free with a minimum follow-up of 1 year, and four deaths in each arm at 10 years were reported in a later analysis (Einhorn et al, 1989; Saxman et al, 1998). An international European trial comparing BEP×3 versus BEP×4 in more than 800 IGCCCG good-risk patients reported similar outcomes with respect to 2-year progression-free survival (90% vs. 89%) and overall survival (97% in each arm) (de Wit et al, 2001). As a result of these studies, BEP×3 became the standard regimen for good-risk GCT.

To reduce toxicity, investigators have studied the effect of omitting bleomycin and substituting carboplatin for cisplatin. **All of the randomized trials in which a cisplatin regimen has been compared with a carboplatin regimen have reported superior outcomes with cisplatin** (Bajorin et al, 1993; Bokemeyer et al, 1996b; Horwich et al, 1997, 2000; Bokemeyer et al, 2004). **The issue of whether bleomycin can be safely omitted from cisplatin-based regimens in good-risk patients is much less clear and is one of the few remaining controversies in the management of advanced GCT.** The rationale for omitting bleomycin is based on the risk of pulmonary complications (including pulmonary fibrosis) and Raynaud phenomenon. All of these studies have shown a trend toward superiority for the bleomycin-containing regimen, although no significant survival advantage has been shown in any of the trials (Bosl et al, 1988; Levi et al, 1993). EP×3 is inferior to BEP×3 (Loehrer et al, 1995). A European randomized trial comparing BEP×4 with EP×4 (with reduced doses of etoposide) reported a significantly higher complete response rate (95% vs. 87%, $P = .008$) with BEP×3 but no difference in overall survival (de Wit et al, 1997). More recently, a French randomized trial comparing BEP×3 with EP×4 (using conventional doses of etoposide) failed to show a statistically significant difference in the risk of relapse or survival between the two regimens (Culine et al, 2007). **BEP×3 and EP×4 are both accepted regimens for patients with advanced GCT and good-risk features by IGCCCG criteria, and the 5-year overall survival is 91% to 94%** (International Germ Cell Consensus Classification, 1997; van Dijk et al, 2006).

Chemotherapy for Intermediate-Risk and Poor-Risk Nonseminoma Germ Cell Tumor

BEP×4 has been the standard regimen for advanced GCT with intermediate-risk and poor-risk features since 1987, and the corresponding 5-year survival rate is 79% for intermediate-risk patients and 48% for poor-risk patients (International Germ Cell Consensus Classification, 1997). Ifosfamide-based regimens using either etoposide-ifosfamide-cisplatin (VIP×4) or vinblastine-ifosfamide-cisplatin (VeIP×4) have been investigated in randomized trials and compared with BEP×4 (de Wit et al, 1998; Nichols et al, 1998; Hinton et al, 2003). The multicenter U.S. trial reported results on nearly 300 men with advanced GCT, with 13%, 23%, and 64% classified as good, intermediate, and poor risk by IGCCCG criteria (Nichols et al, 1998; Hinton et al, 2003). Comparing BEP×4 with VIP×4, the 2-year survival was 71% versus 74%, and the 5-year survival was 57% versus 62%; neither 2-year survival nor 5-year survival was significantly different (Nichols et al, 1998). The European study closed prematurely when the results of the U.S. study became available. Nevertheless, with 84 patients enrolled and more than 7 years' median follow-up, there were two deaths in the BEP×4 arm and one death in the VIP×4 arm, and overall survival at 5 years was greater than 80% (de Wit et al, 1998). In both BEP×4 versus VIP×4 trials, there were more deaths with BEP×4, but the differences were not significant. Because VIP×4 resulted in more high-grade hematologic and urologic toxicity, BEP×4 has remained the standard regimen for intermediate-risk and poor-risk GCT. However, these trials showed that comparable cancer outcomes could be achieved when ifosfamide is substituted for bleomycin. VIP×4 may be substituted for BEP×4 in patients with compromised pulmonary function and in patients in whom extensive chest surgery is likely to be performed to remove residual disease after chemotherapy (Kesler et al, 2008).

High-dose chemotherapy (HDCT) using carboplatin-etoposide–based regimens with autologous stem cell support (also termed *stem-cell rescue*) has been investigated as an alternative to BEP×4 in patients with GCT with a poor prognosis. The rationale for HDCT is the hypothesis that increasing dosage may overcome chemotherapy resistance. The most widely studied regimens have included carboplatin-etoposide alone or in combination with cyclophosphamide, ifosfamide, paclitaxel, or thiotepa (Beyer et al, 1996; Bokemeyer et al, 2002a; Einhorn et al, 2007; Kondagunta et al, 2007; Lorch et al, 2007; Kollmannsberger et al, 2009). Carboplatin is used in HDCT regimens because of dose-limiting nephrotoxicity and neuropathy with cisplatin. A randomized trial in 219 patients with intermediate-risk (21%) and poor-risk (79%) GCT randomly assigned to BEP×4 versus BEP×2 followed by two cycles of high-dose carboplatin-etoposide-cyclophosphamide and autologous stem cell support showed no significant difference in the 1-year durable complete response rate (48% vs. 52%, *P* = .5) or overall survival (Motzer et al, 2007). For patients in both arms, the 2-year survival was 83%, and the 5-year survival was 71%. However, toxicity was more severe for patients receiving HDCT. A smaller randomized trial also failed to demonstrate improved survival with HDCT compared with standard-dose regimens as first-line therapy for patients with metastatic GCT with poor prognosis (Droz et al, 2007). As a result, BEP×4 remains the standard first-line regimen in patients with intermediate-risk and poor-risk disease.

Although the standard chemotherapy for men with poor-risk disease has not changed in more than 20 years, the outcome of these men appears to have improved over time. In the original IGCCCG analysis, the 5-year overall survival for poor-risk patients was 48%, whereas survival rates of 60% or greater have been reported in subsequent multicenter randomized trials (Hinton et al, 2003; Droz et al, 2007; Motzer et al, 2007; Culine et al, 2008). A meta-analysis of 10 studies enrolling 1775 patients with disseminated NSGCT (including 456 poor-risk patients) reported that the pooled 5-year survival estimate for poor-risk patients was 71% (van Dijk et al, 2006).

Management of Residual Masses in Nonseminoma Germ Cell Tumor after Chemotherapy

To assess the response to first-line, cisplatin-based chemotherapy, patients are restaged with serum tumor markers and imaging studies of the chest, abdomen, and pelvis (including other sites of disease if present before chemotherapy). Patients are classified into the following categories based on their response to chemotherapy: (1) complete response, defined by normalization of serum tumor markers and resolution of radiographic disease (usually defined as residual masses ≤1 cm); (2) normalization of serum tumor markers with persistent radiographic tumor (partial remission–marker negative); (3) partial remission–marker positive; and (4) disease progression. Approximately 5% to 15% of patients fall into categories 3 and 4 and are typically managed with second-line (also termed *salvage*) chemotherapy (Einhorn et al, 1989; Mead et al, 1992; de Wit et al, 1997; Debono et al, 1997). There is clear consensus that patients with residual masses larger than 1 cm should undergo PCS (Albers et al, 2005; Motzer et al, 2006; Krege et al, 2008a, 2008b; Schmoll et al, 2009b). The management of patients with complete serologic and radiographic response is controversial, with some guidelines advocating close observation and others recommending PCS if the mass size before chemotherapy is greater than 3 cm (Albers et al, 2005; Motzer et al, 2006; Krege et al, 2008a, 2008b; Schmoll et al, 2009b).

The role of PCS for residual masses in patients with metastatic NSGCT is well established, and its rationale is based on several factors. Multiple large series of patients undergoing PCS for residual masses after first-line chemotherapy have consistently reported evidence of persistent GCT elements in the resected specimens in 50% or more. On average, histology of resected specimens demonstrates necrosis, teratoma, and viable malignancy (with or without teratoma) in 40%, 45%, and 15% of cases (Table 34-6) (Toner et al, 1990; Gerl et al, 1995; Steyerberg et al, 1995; de Wit et al, 1997; Debono et al, 1997; Hartmann et al, 1997b; Sonneveld et al, 1998; Stenning et al, 1998; Steyerberg et al, 1998; Hendry et al, 2002; Albers et al, 2004; Spiess et al, 2006b; Carver et al, 2007a). The 5-year overall survival of patients with complete resection of viable malignancy (with or without further chemotherapy) ranges from 45% to 77% (Toner et al, 1990; Fox et al, 1993; Gerl et al, 1995; Hartmann et al, 1997b; Donohue et al, 1998; Stenning et al, 1998; Fizazi et al, 2001; Spiess et al, 2006a; Carver et al, 2007a; Fizazi et al, 2008). In contrast, if left unresected, residual viable malignancy is destined to relapse, and only 25% to 35% of patients achieve durable remissions to second-line chemotherapy.

As discussed earlier, teratoma is resistant to chemotherapy and is present at metastatic sites in 15% or more of patients with disseminated NSGCT. The presence of metastatic teratoma is a limitation to any strategy for NSGCT that employs chemotherapy alone and necessitates the integration of chemotherapy and PCS in most patients with metastatic GCT. Unresected teratoma has the potential to exhibit rapid growth (growing teratoma syndrome), undergo malignant transformation, or cause late relapse, all of which may have lethal consequences. The outcome of metastatic teratoma is related to the completeness of surgical resection, and long-term survival is reported in 75% to 90% of patients who undergo PCS for residual teratoma (Toner et al, 1990; Hartmann et al, 1997b; Sonneveld et al, 1998; Stenning et al, 1998; Carver et al, 2007c). Lastly, in-field retroperitoneal relapse occurs in less than 2% of patients after a full, bilateral template RPLND, largely eliminating the need for radiographic surveillance of the abdomen and pelvis (Carver et al, 2007b).

Approximately 6% to 8% of PCS specimens contain evidence of non-GCT malignancy arising from malignant transformation of teratoma (Toner et al, 1990; Little et al, 1994; Carver et al, 2007c). The most common histology is rhabdomyosarcoma, and the presence of i(12p) or abnormalities of chromosome 12 in most specimens confirm its origin from GCT (Motzer et al, 1998). As with teratoma, the outcome of patients with malignant transformation is related to the completeness of surgical resection

TABLE 34-6 Histology of Postchemotherapy Residual Masses

STUDY	NO. PATIENTS	NECROSIS	VIABLE MALIGNANCY ± TERATOMA	TERATOMA ONLY
Steyerberg et al, 1995	556	45%	13%	42%
Carver et al, 2007a	504	49%	11%	39%
Hendry et al, 2002	330	25%	9%	66%
Debono et al, 1997	295	25%	7%	67%
Spiess et al, 2006b	236	41%	17%	42%
Albers et al, 2004	232	35%	31%	34%
Toner et al, 1990	185	47%	16%	37%
Steyerberg et al, 1998	172	45%	13%	42%
Stenning et al, 1998	153	29%	15%	55%
de Wit et al, 1997	127	35%	9%	56%
Oeschle et al, 2008	121	45%	21%	34%
Sonneveld et al, 1998	113	46%	9%	45%
Gerl et al, 1995	111	47%	12%	41%
Hartmann et al, 1997a	109	52%	21%	27%

TABLE 34-7 Histology of Postchemotherapy Residual Masses Less Than 20 mm in Size

STUDY	NO. PATIENTS	SIZE (mm)	NECROSIS	VIABLE MALIGNANCY ± TERATOMA	TERATOMA ONLY
Steyerberg et al, 1995	275	≤20	65%	5%	30%
Steyerberg et al, 1995	162	≤10	72%	4%	24%
Oldenburg et al, 2003	87	≤20	67%	7%	26%
Fossa et al, 1992	78	<20	68%	4%	29%
Fossa et al, 1989b	37	≤10	67%	3%	30%
Stephenson et al, 2007	36	≤5	69%	6%	25%
Toner et al, 1990	21	≤15	81%	7%	12%
Stomper et al, 1991	14	≤20	36%	14%	50%

because they are generally resistant to GCT-specific chemotherapy regimens. With complete resection, approximately 50% to 66% of patients survive, whereas most patients with incomplete resection experience rapid progression and death from GCT (Little et al, 1994; Comiter et al, 1998; Motzer et al, 1998; Lutke Holzik et al, 2003; Carver et al, 2007c). Chemotherapy specific to the transformed histology (e.g., sarcoma-specific regimen) has been investigated in two small series in selected patients with measurable disease limited to one histology. Partial responses were observed in 11 of 24 patients, 6 of whom are alive (Donadio et al, 2003; El Mesbahi et al, 2007).

Patients with necrosis only in the PCS specimens have a favorable prognosis, with relapse rates of 10% or less reported in most series (Toner et al, 1990; Hartmann et al, 1997b; Stenning et al, 1998; Carver et al, 2007a). Investigators have sought to identify factors that are reliably predictive of a high probability of necrosis to obviate the need for PCS in all patients with residual masses. In an early study, Donohue and coworkers (1987) reported that 0 of 15 patients without teratoma in the primary tumor and who achieved a 90% or greater reduction in the size of the residual mass with chemotherapy had no evidence of viable malignancy or teratoma at PCS. In contrast, seven of nine patients (78%) with teratoma in the primary tumor experiencing a similar reduction in the size of the metastasis with chemotherapy had evidence of viable malignancy and/or teratoma. **The absence of teratoma in the primary tumor, the percentage reduction in the retroperitoneal mass with chemotherapy, and the size of the residual mass have consistently been identified as predictors of necrosis in PCS specimens** (Toner et al, 1990; Stomper et al, 1991; Fossa et al, 1992; Steyerberg et al, 1995, 1998; Albers et al, 2004). However, despite statistical modeling using these and other factors, a consistent false-negative rate for necrosis of 20% has been reported (Steyerberg et al, 1995, 1998; Vergouwe et al, 2001). **The presence of** necrosis only in the retroperitoneum cannot be predicted with sufficient accuracy to obviate safely the need for PCS in patients with residual masses. An important concept is that the absence of teratoma in the primary tumor does not reliably exclude its presence in the retroperitoneum (Toner et al, 1990; Beck et al, 2002). Investigators have also studied the utility of FDG-PET in the prediction of the histology of residual masses after first-line chemotherapy. The utility of FDG-PET in the prediction of retroperitoneal histology for NSGCT is limited by the fact that teratoma is not FDG-avid. In a prospective study of 121 patients with residual masses after induction chemotherapy, the predictive accuracy of FDG-PET (56%) for viable malignancy or teratoma was no better than CT (55%) or postchemotherapy serum tumor markers (56%) (Oechsle et al, 2008). **FDG-PET has no role in the assessment of patients with NSGCT and residual masses after chemotherapy.**

Approximately 26% to 62% of patients experience a serologic and radiographic complete response to first-line chemotherapy (Einhorn et al, 1989; Dearnaley et al, 1991; Mead et al, 1992; Debono et al, 1997; Stenning et al, 1998; Ehrlich et al, 2010; Kollmannsberger et al, 2010a). **The optimal management of these patients is controversial.** Advocates of PCS for these patients argue that residual mass size (or percentage reduction with chemotherapy) cannot be used to exclude reliably the presence of residual disease within the retroperitoneum. **Numerous studies have demonstrated that, on average, patients with residual masses 20 mm or smaller have a 30% and 6% incidence of teratoma and viable malignancy, respectively** (Table 34-7) (Fossa et al, 1989b; Toner et al, 1990; Stomper et al, 1991; Fossa et al, 1992; Steyerberg et al, 1995; Beck et al, 2002; Oldenburg et al, 2003; Stephenson et al, 2007). In an analysis of 295 patients with GCT managed at Indiana University after induction chemotherapy, 77 (26%) experienced a complete serologic and radiographic response to chemotherapy; 92% were alive at 5 to 10 years with an observational strategy

(Debono et al, 1997). This result highlights the therapeutic benefit of PCS for patients with residual masses. **However, patients with complete serologic and radiographic response after induction chemotherapy represent a small minority of the overall population, indicating that observation is a reasonable option for only a select group of patients.** Two studies have confirmed the low risk of relapse (4% to 10%) and 97% to 100% cancer-specific survival in patients with residual masses less than 1 cm who were observed without PCS (Ehrlich et al, 2010; Kollmannsberger et al, 2010a). However, most of these patients were good risk by IGCCCG criteria and did not have teratoma in the primary tumor, highlighting their select nature.

Approximately one third of patients have residual masses at multiple anatomic sites (retroperitoneum, chest, and left supraclavicular fossa are the most common), and these patients should undergo resection of all sites of measurable residual disease (Toner et al, 1990; Gerl et al, 1994; Hartmann et al, 1997a; McGuire et al, 2003). Although some centers have described performing simultaneous RPLND, thoracotomy, or neck dissection, our practice is to perform infradiaphragmatic and supradiaphragmatic resections as separate procedures. **Discordant histology between anatomic sites is reported in 22% to 46% of cases** (Toner et al, 1990). In general, the histology of PCS specimens from nonretroperitoneal sites is more likely to show necrosis (60%) and less likely to show viable malignancy (10%) and teratoma (30%) (Toner et al, 1990; Gerl et al, 1994; Hartmann et al, 1997a; Steyerberg et al, 1997). In addition to the size of residual masses and the number of anatomic sites, the presence of necrosis in postchemotherapy RPLND specimens is highly predictive of necrosis at other sites (Steyerberg et al, 1997). Of patients undergoing PCS for residual masses at different sites, only 19 of 159 (12%) who had necrosis in the RPLND specimen had either viable malignancy or teratoma at other sites (Tiffany et al, 1986; Gerl et al, 1994; Brenner et al, 1996; Steyerberg et al, 1997; Tognoni et al, 1998; McGuire et al, 2003). **RPLND should be performed before PCS at other sites because the probability of residual disease in the retroperitoneum is highest, and RPLND histology is a strong predictor of histology at other sites. Observation of small residual masses at other sites is a reasonable option if the histology of the RPLND specimen is necrosis.**

As mentioned earlier, the 5-year survival for patients with viable malignancy in PCS specimens is 45% to 77%. The role of postoperative chemotherapy in this setting is controversial. Fox and colleagues (1993) reported that 14 of 27 patients (70%) undergoing PCS for viable malignancy were free of recurrence with adjuvant chemotherapy versus 0 of 7 patients who were observed. In an international pooled analysis of 238 patients with viable malignancy in PCS specimens, Fizazi and colleagues (2001) identified prechemotherapy IGCCCG intermediate-risk and poor-risk disease, incomplete resection, and greater than 10% viable malignancy in PCS specimens as important prognostic factors. Patients with zero, one, and two to three risk factors had a 5-year overall survival of 100%, 83%, and 51%. Overall, a significant improvement in 5-year relapse-free survival was observed with postoperative chemotherapy (73% vs. 64%, $P < .001$), but there was no difference in 5-year overall survival (74% vs. 70%, $P = .7$). In a subset analysis, patients with one risk factor had an improved 5-year survival with postoperative chemotherapy (88% vs. 56%, $P = .02$), but patients with zero (100% survival, with or without chemotherapy) and two to three risk factors (55% vs. 60%) did not. In a confirmatory study, this prognostic index was validated for relapse-free and overall survival, and no significant difference in these end points was observed among the patients who did and did not receive postoperative chemotherapy (Fizazi et al, 2008). **A complete resection of residual masses is the most critical determinant of outcome for patients with viable malignancy in PCS specimens after first-line chemotherapy. Immediate postoperative chemotherapy and surveillance may be reasonable options depending on the completeness of resection, IGCCCG risk group, and percent of viable cells.** There is no consensus on the appropriate chemotherapy regimen and the number of cycles that should be used in this setting.

The importance of PCS was highlighted in a randomized trial of BEP×3 versus EP×4 in 257 men with good-risk metastatic NSGCT (Culine et al, 2007). As part of this trial, PCS was not dictated by protocol, and only 52% underwent PCS, which frequently involved resection of residual mass only. Overall, 14 of 20 (70%) relapsing patients and 7 of 14 (50%) patients who died of GCT either did not undergo PCS or relapsed in the retroperitoneum after inadequate RPLND. **These results suggest a substantial proportion of deaths from GCT may be prevented by the appropriate integration of chemotherapy and surgery.**

Relapsing Nonseminoma Germ Cell Tumor

The treatment of relapsing NSGCTs depends on what treatment the patient previously received and, in certain cases, the location of the relapse. Patients who have never received chemotherapy have a much more favorable prognosis than patients who have already been treated with chemotherapy for disseminated disease.

Chemotherapy-Naive Nonseminoma Germ Cell Tumor Relapse. Chemotherapy-naive relapses occur in men with CS I NSGCT managed with either surveillance or RPLND and in men with CS IIA and IIB NSGCT treated with RPLND alone. Serum tumor markers are elevated 60% to 75% of the time in patients with CS I NSGCT who relapse on surveillance (Read et al, 1992; Gels et al, 1995; Sharir et al, 1999; Alexandre et al, 2001). **In general, these patients are treated with induction chemotherapy, with the specific regimen and duration of therapy determined by IGCCCG risk, and cure rates exceed 95%. Select CS I patients on surveillance who relapse in the retroperitoneum with nonbulky (<3 cm) tumor and normal serum tumor markers may be treated by induction chemotherapy or RPLND (particularly if teratoma was present in the primary tumor)** (Stephenson et al, 2007). The rationale for RPLND is to avoid or minimize the toxicity of chemotherapy, and long-term cure rates approach 100% with RPLND with or without adjuvant chemotherapy (Stephenson et al, 2007). CS I, IIA, and IIB patients who relapse after RPLND usually have involvement in the lungs or mediastinum. Virtually all of these patients are cured with first-line chemotherapy. Most relapses during surveillance or after RPLND occur within the first 2 years (Freedman et al, 1987; McLeod et al, 1991; Read et al, 1992; Albers et al, 1995; Gels et al, 1995; Sogani et al, 1998; Colls et al, 1999; Sharir et al, 1999; Francis et al, 2000; Daugaard et al, 2003; Stephenson et al, 2005b; Albers et al, 2008; Williams et al, 2009b; Zuniga et al, 2009; Kollmannsberger et al, 2010a). For the rare patient relapsing more than 2 years after orchiectomy or RPLND with normal tumor markers, biopsy or surgical resection should be strongly considered because of the likelihood of teratoma (Michael et al, 2000; Oldenburg et al, 2006). **Although the time to relapse is an important determinant of outcome in relapsing patients who have received prior chemotherapy, chemotherapy-naive patients who relapse more than 2 years after initial treatment have a prognosis similar to patients who relapse earlier.**

Nonseminoma Germ Cell Tumor Relapse Early after Chemotherapy. Men who relapse after previously receiving first-line chemotherapy are treated with second-line (salvage) chemotherapy. **Most relapses occur within 2 years of completing initial treatment, and these are classified as early relapse** (de Wit et al, 1998; Nichols et al, 1998; Michael et al, 2000; Culine et al, 2007; Motzer et al, 2007). **Relapses occurring more than 2 years after completion of initial therapy are classified as late relapse and differ substantially in terms of prognosis and therapy (discussed later).** Early relapsing patients who appear to have a particularly unfavorable prognosis are patients who fail to achieve a complete response to first-line therapy or who relapse within 6 months of achieving a complete response; these patients are frequently termed *incomplete responders* (Fossa et al, 1999c). **In an international pooled analysis of 1984 patients from 38 centers with relapse after first-line chemotherapy who received second-line chemotherapy, median progression-free survival was 10 months, and overall survival was 41 months** (Lorch et al, 2010). **Incomplete response to induction chemotherapy** (HR = 1.4 to 1.9), primary mediastinal NSGCT

(HR = 3.0), nonpulmonary visceral metastasis (HR = 1.3), and elevated AFP (HR = 1.3 to 2.0) and hCG (HR = 1.5) were associated with increased risk of progression with second-line chemotherapy.

As discussed earlier, etoposide and ifosfamide were demonstrated to have substantial activity in patients with relapse after first-line chemotherapy, and this led to investigation of VIP×4 as a second-line regimen for relapsed GCT after PVB×4 (Loehrer et al, 1986; Einhorn, 1990). VeIP×4 was also studied as a second-line regimen in men who had received prior etoposide from BEP regimens (Loehrer et al, 1998). Studies of VIP×4 and VeIP×4 reported long-term remission rates of 23% to 35% and overall survival rates of 32% to 53% (McCaffrey et al, 1997; Loehrer et al, 1998; Pico et al, 2005). Studies of paclitaxel in the early 1990s showed activity in relapsed GCT, which led to development of the paclitaxel, ifosfamide, and cisplatin (TIP) regimen, and relapse-free survival has been reported in 36% to 47% of patients (Kondagunta et al, 2005; Mardiak et al, 2005; Mead et al, 2005). **TIP×4, VIP×4, and VeIP×4 have never been compared in a randomized trial, and all are considered standard second-line regimens.**

HDCT has also been investigated as a second-line (and third-line) regimen in patients with GCT relapse, although its role as second-line therapy is controversial. Indiana University has amassed the largest, single-institution series comprising 184 consecutive patients with metastatic GCT that progressed after first-line (73%) or second-line (27%) chemotherapy; 94% of these patients received two or more courses of HDCT (Einhorn et al, 2007). Over a median follow-up of 4 years, 63% of patients were continuously disease-free, including 70% and 45% of patients who received HDCT as second-line and third-line therapy, respectively. An international matched-pair analysis comparing 74 patients treated at a single institution who received two to three cycles of VIP followed by one cycle of HDCT using carboplatin-etoposide-ifosfamide with 119 patients treated at multiple centers throughout Europe who received standard-dose, second-line chemotherapy using various regimens reported a 10% improvement in event-free and overall survival with HDCT (Beyer et al, 2002). HDCT was compared with standard-dose, second-line chemotherapy in a randomized controlled trial enrolling 280 patients from 43 institutions. Patients in the standard-dose arm received VIP×4 or VeIP×4, depending on whether they received prior etoposide during first-line therapy. Patients in the HDCT arm received VIP/VeIP×3 followed by one cycle of high-dose carboplatin-etoposide-cyclophosphamide (Pico et al, 2005). Over a median follow-up of 45 months, there were no significant differences in complete and partial response rates (56% in both arms) or 3-year event-free (35% vs. 42%, P = .16) and overall (53% in both arms) survival.

There are several potential explanations for the lack of benefit of HDCT in the randomized trial despite the favorable results reported in the two nonrandomized studies. First, the results from single-arm trials may be subject to selection bias from differences in case mix. In addition, the results achieved at high-volume institutions with unique experience with HDCT may not be reproducible at other institutions. Alternatively, the treatment strategy employed in the randomized trial may have been suboptimal in that three cycles of standard-dose chemotherapy and only one cycle of HDCT were given. The treatment philosophy at Indiana University is to take patients to HDCT as quickly as possible, limit the number of cycles of standard-dose chemotherapy so that patients are able to tolerate HDCT better, and to give two cycles of HDCT. In the randomized trial, only 73% of patients assigned HDCT were able to receive it, and deaths resulting from toxicity on the HDCT arm were twice as common as on the standard-dose arm (7% vs. 3%). In the Indiana University series, 94% of patients were able to receive two cycles of HDCT, and the treatment-related death rate was 2.7%. **Although HDCT as second-line therapy can cure a significant number of patients, the failure to demonstrate an improvement in survival compared with standard-dose regimens in three randomized trials (two as first-line therapy and one as second-line therapy) suggests it should not be considered a standard approach.** At the present time, HDCT

should be offered only at specialized centers with extensive experience.

Treatment options for high-risk patients with relapse (e.g., incomplete responders) include standard-dose, second-line chemotherapy or HDCT (if administered at a specialized, high-volume institution). Standard-dose, second-line chemotherapy is the preferred approach for patients who relapse more than 6 months after first-line chemotherapy. **Special mention is made of patients with declining or normalized serum tumor markers during first-line chemotherapy with enlarging (usually cystic) masses. These patients are considered to have growing teratoma syndrome. In these rare cases, chemotherapy is temporarily interrupted, and patients are taken for surgical resection. With complete surgical resection, the long-term prognosis for these patients is favorable** (Logothetis et al, 1982; Andre et al, 2000; Spiess et al, 2007).

For patients relapsing after second-line chemotherapy, subsequent options are HDCT (if not given previously) and regimens including various combinations of the following agents: gemcitabine, paclitaxel, oxaliplatin, and irinotecan (Pectasides et al, 2004; De Giorgi et al, 2006; Bokemeyer et al, 2008; Nicolai et al, 2009; Oechsle et al, 2011; Veenstra and Vaughn, 2011).

Management of Residual Masses after Salvage Chemotherapy. **Patients with serologic complete response to second-line chemotherapy with residual masses should undergo surgical resection after salvage chemotherapy.** Patients undergoing surgical resection after salvage chemotherapy differ from patients undergoing PCS of residual masses after first-line chemotherapy in several ways. A complete resection of residual masses is feasible in only 56% to 72% of patients (compared with ≥85% after first-line therapy) (Fox et al, 1993; Debono et al, 1997; Hartmann et al, 1997b; Stenning et al, 1998; Eggener et al, 2007a). The histology of post–salvage chemotherapy surgical specimens is characterized by higher rates of viable malignancy (53%) and lower rates of necrosis (26%) and teratoma (21%) compared with surgical specimens after first-line chemotherapy. The long-term survival of patients is also substantially poorer with 5-year survival rates of 44% to 61% in most series (Fox et al, 1993; Hartmann et al, 1997b; Donohue et al, 1998; Stenning et al, 1998). **Patients with viable malignancy in post–salvage chemotherapy surgical specimens have a particularly poor prognosis, and their survival is not improved with the use of postoperative chemotherapy.**

Desperation Surgery. Most patients with progressive disease despite first-line and second-line chemotherapy have a dismal prognosis. **However, a highly select group of patients with rising serum tumor markers who are deemed to have resectable disease limited to a single site (usually the retroperitoneum) may be candidates for salvage surgery, commonly referred to as desperation surgery.** Although published studies are limited to small, single-institution case series, 47% to 60% have normalization of serum tumor markers postoperatively, and long-term survival is reported in 33% to 57% of patients after desperation surgery with or without postoperative chemotherapy (Wood et al, 1992; Murphy et al, 1993; Eastham et al, 1994; Albers et al, 2000; Beck et al, 2005).

Nonseminoma Germ Cell Tumor Relapse Late after Chemotherapy. Late relapse after chemotherapy is defined as relapse occurring more than 2 years after treatment. Roughly 3% of patients with NSGCT experience a late relapse (Ronnen et al, 2005; Oldenburg et al, 2006). Because late relapse is rare, a biopsy should be performed to confirm the diagnosis, particularly when serum AFP and hCG are normal. **Late relapses can be divided into three histopathologic categories: viable malignancy (54% to 88%, yolk sac tumor most common), teratoma (12% to 28%), and malignant transformation (10% to 20%, adenocarcinoma most common)** (Baniel et al, 1995; Gerl et al, 1997; Michael et al, 2000; George et al, 2003; Sharp et al, 2008).

Risk factors for late relapse have not been definitively identified, but a history of prior relapse and the presence of teratoma in PCS specimens (potentially for incomplete resection) are associated with an increased risk (Gerl et al, 1997; Shahidi et al, 2002). Most men with a late relapse have only one site of disease.

Most late relapses occur in the retroperitoneum (50% to 72%), 17% occur in the lungs, 9% occur in the mediastinum, 7% occur in the neck, and 4% occur in the pelvis (Baniel et al, 1995; Gerl et al, 1997; George et al, 2003; Dieckmann et al, 2005; Oldenburg et al, 2006; Sharp et al, 2008). **Failure to control the retroperitoneum in the initial treatment phase is a major risk factor for late relapse. Serum AFP and hCG levels are elevated in about 50% and 25% of late relapses, respectively** (Oldenburg et al, 2006). Patients with elevated serum tumor markers as the only manifestation of late relapse should be monitored closely until there is measurable disease (George et al, 2003).

Until more recently, late relapse was associated with a worse prognosis than early relapses, although contemporary data suggest these patients may have a similar probability of cure. **In general, late relapse is resistant to chemotherapy, and the outcome is related to the ability to render patients disease-free by complete surgical resection** (Gerl et al, 1997; Shahidi et al, 2002; George et al, 2003; Dieckmann et al, 2005; Oldenburg et al, 2006; Sharp et al, 2008).

The importance of surgery is related to the fact that teratoma and malignant transformation are inherently chemoinsensitive, and viable malignancy is usually present in the setting of prior chemotherapy (platin-resistant). Of 32 patients with late relapse at Indiana University who received chemotherapy, only 6 (19%) achieved a complete response. Of the 49 patients treated initially with surgery, 45 (92%) were rendered disease-free (22 [45%] by surgery alone), and 29 (59%) are in complete remission. Overall, 69 (85%) patients achieved a disease-free state, and 58% were disease-free over a median follow-up of 25 months (George et al, 2003). In the Memorial Sloan-Kettering experience, the 5-year cancer-specific survival was 60%, and patients who had a complete surgical resection at the time of late relapse (60%) had significantly improved survival compared with patients without complete resection (40%) (79% vs. 36%, $P < .001$) (Sharp et al, 2008). The presence of symptoms and multifocal disease at late relapse were associated with inferior survival. In a German study of 72 patients with NSGCT and late relapse, 35 (49%) were in complete remission at last follow-up, most of whom were treated with a combination of chemotherapy and surgery (Dieckmann et al, 2005). The most favorable chemotherapy results for late relapse are with the TIP regimen (Kondagunta et al, 2005). **An aggressive surgical approach to resect all disease is appropriate either as the primary treatment or, in the setting of unresectable disease, after chemotherapy.**

Seminoma

Clinical Stage I Seminoma. Approximately 80% of patients with seminoma are CS I, and this is the most common presentation of testis cancer. **The management of these patients has undergone substantial changes over the past two decades, and surveillance, primary radiotherapy, and primary chemotherapy with single-agent carboplatin are now accepted treatment options.** More recent efforts have focused on reducing the therapeutic burden. **Platinum-based chemotherapy and infradiaphragmatic radiotherapy are associated with an increased risk of late cardiovascular toxicity and SMN** (Zagars et al, 2004; Travis et al, 2005; van den Belt-Dusebout et al, 2007; Beard et al, 2013). Minimizing target volume and dose has been investigated to reduce the toxicity of radiotherapy. Carboplatin is associated with less neurotoxicity, ototoxicity, and nephrotoxicity compared with cisplatin, but the risks of cardiovascular disease and SMN are largely unknown. In many instances, the short-term efficacy and safety of these approaches have been validated by randomized trials. **Long-term cancer control with each of these modalities approaches 100%.**

Primary Radiotherapy. The mainstay of treatment for CS I seminoma for the past four decades had been primary radiotherapy to the retroperitoneum and ipsilateral pelvis, termed *dog-leg configuration.* Published series of radiotherapy for CS I are listed in Table 34-8 (Fossa et al, 1989a; Warde et al, 1995; Fossa et al, 1999b; Classen et al, 2004; Jones et al, 2005; Oliver et al, 2005; Warde et al, 2005; Tandstad et al, 2011). **The optimal radiation dose has**

KEY POINTS: NONSEMINOMA GERM CELL TUMOR

- The optimal management of CS I NSGCT is controversial. Surveillance, primary RPLND, and primary chemotherapy with BEP×2 are accepted treatment options with long-term survival rates approaching 100% for each.
- A risk-adapted approach based on the presence of LVI and EC predominance is recommended. Surveillance is recommended for patients without these risk factors, and active treatment (RPLND or BEP×2) is recommended for patients with LVI and/or EC predominance. A non–risk-adapted approach, which includes surveillance as the recommended approach for all patients, is employed at some centers.
- Surveillance is not recommended for patients who are anticipated to be poorly compliant with follow-up imaging and clinical evaluation. The standard treatment approach for patients who relapse on surveillance is induction chemotherapy based on IGCCCG risk. However, selected patients with normal serum tumor marker levels and nonbulky (<3 cm) retroperitoneal adenopathy may also be managed with RPLND.
- BEP×2 is the standard regimen used for patients with CS I NSGCT who choose to receive chemotherapy. There is insufficient evidence at the present time to support BEP×1 as an acceptable alternative.
- A full, bilateral template with nerve sparing is the recommended approach for primary RPLND. Attempts to preserve ejaculatory function should not compromise oncologic efficacy. RPLND should be performed only by surgeons experienced with the procedure.
- Adjuvant chemotherapy after primary RPLND for pathologic stage II disease is associated with a substantial reduction in the risk of relapse but no difference in long-term survival compared with a strategy comprising observation with induction chemotherapy at the time of relapse. Adjuvant chemotherapy is usually recommended for patients with extensive retroperitoneal metastasis (pN2-3) and patients anticipated to be noncompliant with postoperative cancer surveillance imaging and testing.
- Induction chemotherapy and primary RPLND are accepted treatment options for patients with CS IIA and IIB NSGCT, with long-term cure in 95% or more. Induction chemotherapy is favored in patients with a high risk of occult metastatic disease on the basis of elevated serum tumor markers after orchiectomy and/or bulky (>3 cm) retroperitoneal lymphadenopathy.
- The management of patients with CS IS, IIC, and III NSGCT is induction cisplatin-based chemotherapy. The specific regimen and number of cycles is dictated by IGCCCG risk criteria. Patients with good-risk disease should receive BEP×3 or EP×4, and patients with intermediate-risk and poor-risk disease should receive BEP×4. With risk-appropriate chemotherapy and PCS, the survival of patients with good-risk disease is 89% to 94%, with intermediate-risk disease is 75% to 83%, and with poor-risk disease is 41% to 71%.
- Resection of all residual masses after chemotherapy is based on the incidence of residual cancer (either viable malignancy or teratoma) in 50% or more of patients.
- The use of adjuvant chemotherapy is controversial in patients with viable malignancy in residual masses after first-line chemotherapy.

not been defined; most centers use 20 to 30 Gy over 10 to 15 daily fractions (Fossa et al, 1989a; Warde et al, 1995; Fossa et al, 1999b). Long-term cancer-specific survival approaches 100%, and progression-free probability between 95% and 97% is reported (Fossa et al, 1989a; Warde et al, 1995; Fossa et al, 1999b; Warde et al, 2005; Kollmannsberger et al, 2010c; Tandstad et al, 2011). In-field recurrence after dog-leg radiotherapy is less than 1%,

TABLE 34-8 Radiation Therapy Series for Clinical Stage I Seminoma

STUDY	NO. PATIENTS	MEDIAN FOLLOW-UP (mo)	TARGET VOLUME	MEDIAN DOSE (Gy)	GCT DEATHS (%)	RELAPSE (%)	IN-FIELD RELAPSE (%)	PELVIC RELAPSE (%)
Fossa et al, 1989a	365	109	Dog-leg	40	4 (1)	13 (4)	1 (0.3)	0
Warde et al, 1995	194	97	Dog-leg	25	0	11 (6)	0	0
Warde et al, 2005	282	106	Dog-leg	25	0	14 (5)	—	—
Fossa et al, 1999b	242	54	Dog-leg	30	0	9 (4)	0	0
Fossa et al, 1999b	236	54	Para-aortic	30	1	9 (4)	2 (0.8)	4 (1.7)
Classen et al, 2004	721	61	Para-aortic	26	2 (0.3)	26 (4)	8 (1.1)	13 (1.8)
Jones et al, 2005	313	61	Para-aortic	30	1 (0.3)	10 (4)	3 (1)	6 (2)
Jones et al, 2005	312	61	Para-aortic	20	0	11 (4)	2 (0.6)	3 (1)
Oliver et al, 2005, 2011	904	78	Para-aortic	20-30	1 (0.1)	32 (4)	3 (0.3)	10 (1.6)
Tandstad et al, 2011	481	73	Dog-leg	25	0	4 (1)	2 (0.6)	—
Kollmannsberger et al, 2010c	159	65	Para-aortic	25	0	4 (2)	—	2(1)

GCT, germ cell tumor.

obviating the need for routine surveillance abdominopelvic CT imaging. Inguinal metastases are uncommon in patients without prior inguinal or scrotal surgery. **The most common sites of recurrence are the thorax and left supraclavicular fossa. Virtually all recurrences are cured with first-line chemotherapy.** Selected patients with isolated inguinal relapse may be salvaged with radiotherapy or surgical resection. **The surveillance of patients after dog-leg radiotherapy consists of regular clinical assessment, chest radiography, and serum tumor markers.**

Most patients experience some acute side effects with adjuvant radiotherapy, which typically include transient nausea, vomiting, and diarrhea, which are usually mild and self-limited. Acute grade II to IV hematologic toxicity occurs in 5% to 15% of patients (Fossa et al, 1999b). Moderate and severe late gastrointestinal toxicity (usually chronic dyspepsia or peptic ulcer disease) is reported in 5% and less than 2% of patients, respectively. The testicular germinal epithelium is exquisitely sensitive to ionizing radiation, and scatter dose to the contralateral testis may be significant despite protective shielding. After dog-leg radiotherapy, persistent oligospermia is reported in 8% (Fossa et al, 1999b). The issue of late cardiac toxicity and SMN is particularly germane for these patients given the long anticipated life expectancy. **The actuarial risk of developing SMN is estimated to be 18% at 25 years after radiotherapy for seminoma, and there is a 2.64% risk of dying of SMN at 15 years, representing an 89% increased risk of death from nontesticular cancer** (Travis et al, 2005; Beard et al, 2013). Secondary leukemia is linked with radiotherapy and chemotherapy, whereas an increased incidence of upper gastrointestinal tract, bladder, and possibly pancreas cancers is associated with radiotherapy.

To reduce the toxicity of radiotherapy, efforts to minimize the target volume and dose have been evaluated in randomized trials. The Medical Research Council (MRC) in the United Kingdom conducted a randomized trial of dog-leg versus para-aortic radiotherapy for CS I seminoma (Fossa et al, 1999b). The rationale for omitting radiotherapy to the ipsilateral pelvis is based on the low rate (1% to 3%) of pelvic lymph node involvement in patients without prior inguinal or scrotal surgery. Restricting radiotherapy to the para-aortic strip may reduce the risk of SMN and improve recovery of spermatogenesis. The 3-year relapse-free survival (96% vs. 97%) and overall survival (99% vs. 100%) in the para-aortic versus dog-leg

arms were similar, but patients receiving para-aortic radiotherapy had an improved short-term recovery of spermatogenesis (although no difference was seen at 3 years). However, the para-aortic arm experienced a significant increase in the rate of pelvic recurrence (2% vs. 0%, $P = .04$). The small but significant risk of pelvic recurrence necessitates the use of routine surveillance pelvic CT imaging with the associated increased cost and radiation exposure (Brenner and Hall, 2007).

The MRC and the European Organisation for the Research and Treatment of Cancer (EORTC) also conducted a randomized trial of 20 Gy versus 30 Gy para-aortic radiotherapy for CS I seminoma (Jones et al, 2005). The 5-year relapse-free survival (96% vs. 97%) and overall survival (99.6% vs. 100%) were similar, but patients receiving 20 Gy experienced less acute gastrointestinal toxicity, leukopenia, and lethargy (although results were similar at 12 weeks). Further follow-up is necessary to assess the durability of these results.

Surveillance. Given the potential for late toxicity with dog-leg radiotherapy, the 80% to 85% cure rate after orchiectomy, and the greater than 90% cure rates achieved with platin-based chemotherapy for advanced seminoma, surveillance has been evaluated at several centers. **Compared with NSGCT, surveillance for CS I seminoma is complicated by the limited utility of serum tumor markers to detect relapse and the need for long-term surveillance CT imaging because 10% to 20% of relapses occur 4 years or more after diagnosis** (Chung et al, 2002).

The largest surveillance series for CS I seminoma are listed in Table 34-9 (Horwich et al, 1992; von der Maase et al, 1993; Warde et al, 1995; Aparicio et al, 2003; Daugaard et al, 2003; Aparicio et al, 2005; Choo et al, 2005; Warde et al, 2005; Kollmannsberger et al, 2010c; Tandstad et al, 2011). **The 5-year relapse-free survival ranges from 80% to 86%, and cancer-specific survival approaches 100%. Of patients, 84% to 100% relapse in the retroperitoneum, and 18% to 24% have bulky retroperitoneal disease and/or distant metastases at the time of recurrence** (Horwich et al, 1992; von der Maase et al, 1993; Warde et al, 1995; Aparicio et al, 2003; Choo et al, 2005). Dog-leg radiotherapy is employed for treatment of relapse in 73% to 88% of patients, and cure rates of 70% to 90% are reported. Virtually all patients who relapse outside the retroperitoneum are cured with first-line chemotherapy.

TABLE 34-9   Surveillance Series for Clinical Stage I Seminoma

STUDY	NO. PATIENTS	MEDIAN FOLLOW-UP (mo)	GCT DEATHS (%)	RELAPSE (%)	RPN RELAPSE (%)	CS IIC-III RELAPSE (%)	SYSTEMIC RELAPSE (%)
Daugaard et al, 2003	394	—	0	69 (17)	—	—	—
Warde et al, 2005	348	106	1 (0.3)	55 (16)	—	—	—
Warde et al, 1995	172	50	1 (0.6)	27 (16)	24 (89)	5 (19)	1 (4)
von der Maase et al, 1993	261	48	1 (0.4)	49 (19)	46 (94)	12 (24)	1 (2)
Aparacio et al, 2003	143*	52	0	23 (16)	19 (84)	—	3 (13)
Horwich et al, 1992	103	62	0	17 (17)	17 (100)	3 (18)	1 (6)
Choo et al, 2005	88	145	0	17 (19)	15 (88)	3 (18)	2 (12)
Aparacio et al, 2005	100†	34	0	6 (7)	6 (100)	—	0
Tandstad et al, 2011	512	60	0	65 (14)	65 (100)	—	—
Kollmannsberger et al, 2010c	313	34	0	47 (19)	—	—	—

*Patients with lymphovascular invasion or clinical stage ≥T2 excluded.
†Patients with tumor size >4 cm or rete testis invasion excluded.
CS, clinical stage; GCT, germ cell tumor; RPN, retroperitoneal.

TABLE 34-10   Adjuvant Chemotherapy Series for Clinical Stage I Seminoma

STUDY	NO. PATIENTS	MEDIAN FOLLOW-UP (mo)	NO. CYCLES	GCT DEATHS (%)	RELAPSE (%)
Oliver et al, 2005, 2011	573	78	1	0	27 (5)
Steiner et al, 2002	108	60	2	0	2 (2)
Reiter et al, 2001	107	74	2	0	0
Dieckmann et al, 2000	93	48	1	0	8 (9)
Dieckmann et al, 2000	32	48	2	0	0
Oliver et al, 1994	78	51	2*	0	2 (2)
Aparacio et al, 2003	60	52	2	0	2 (3.3)
Aparacio et al, 2005	214	34	2	0	7 (4)
Tandstad et al, 2011	188	62	1	0	7 (4)
Kollmannsberger et al, 2010c	73	33	1-2	0	1 (2)

*33% of patients received 1 cycle of carboplatin.
GCT, germ cell tumor.

To detect and treat recurrences at an early stage, patients on surveillance should be followed with clinical assessment, chest radiography, serum tumor markers, and abdominopelvic CT imaging. Surveillance schedules employ assessments every 2 to 4 months in years 1 to 3, every 6 months in years 4 to 7, and annually thereafter. The necessary frequency of CT imaging is poorly defined; centers obtain CT imaging every 4 to 6 months in years 1 to 3, every 6 months in years 4 to 7, and annually thereafter. A trial from the MRC suggested that the frequency of surveillance CT imaging in low-risk CS I NSGCT in years 0 to 2 may be safely reduced from five times to two times without affecting survival or burden of therapy (Rustin et al, 2007). It is unclear whether these findings can be safely applied to surveillance for seminoma. Long-term follow-up is mandatory given the higher incidence of relapse after 5 years compared with NSGCT (Chung et al, 2002).

To select patients for active treatment better, investigators have endeavored to identify prognostic factors for occult metastasis. In a pooled analysis of three large surveillance series from the 1980s, tumor size larger than 4 cm and rete testis invasion were significant predictors of relapse in multivariable analysis (Warde et al, 2002). In contrast to NSGCT, LVI has not been identified as a significant predictor of relapse for CS I seminoma. The 5-year relapse rates for patients with zero, one, and two risk factors were 12%, 16%, and 32%. In this cohort, 21% of patients had both rete testis invasion and tumor size larger than 4 cm. Primary radiotherapy or carboplatin for all "high-risk" patients would still expose two thirds of patients with CS I seminoma (who are cured by orchiectomy) to unnecessary therapy. However, prospective validation of these risk factors is currently lacking.

Primary Chemotherapy with Single-Agent Carboplatin. **Primary chemotherapy with one to two cycles of single-agent carboplatin** has also been investigated as an alternative to primary radiotherapy with the potential for reduced late toxicity. The rationale for single-agent carboplatin is based on the 65% to 90% reported complete response rates observed among patients with advanced seminoma (Horwich et al, 2000) and its reduced toxicity compared with cisplatin. Oliver and colleagues (1994) first described the use of one to two cycles of carboplatin in 78 patients and reported only two relapses and no deaths. The published studies of carboplatin in CS I seminoma are listed in Table 34-10 (Dieckmann et al, 2000; Reiter et al, 2001; Steiner et al, 2002; Aparacio et al, 2003, 2005; Oliver et al, 2005; Kollmannsberger et al, 2010c; Aparacio et al, 2011; Tandstad et al, 2011). No deaths from seminoma have been observed, and 3- to 5-year relapse-free rates are 91% to 100%.

The MRC and EORTC conducted a randomized, phase III clinical trial of one cycle of carboplatin versus 20 to 30 Gy para-aortic radiotherapy in 1477 patients with CS I seminoma (Oliver et al, 2005, 2011). Over a median follow-up of 6.5 years, the 5-year relapse-free survival was similar (94.7% vs. 96%), and only one death was observed in the para-aortic radiotherapy arm. In this trial, patients receiving carboplatin experienced less lethargy and time away from work than patients receiving radiotherapy, and acute grade III to IV hematologic toxicity was observed in 4% of patients. Carboplatin was associated with a reduction in the rate of contralateral second-primary testis cancers (0.3% vs. 1.7%, $P = .03$).

A concern with one cycle of carboplatin is the potential for inadequate dosing leading to an increased risk of relapse. A higher relapse rate with one versus two cycles has been seen when comparing different studies, and a higher risk of relapse was reported among patients receiving an inadequate dose of carboplatin in the MRC/EORTC trial (Dieckmann et al, 2000; Oliver et al, 2008). The optimal dosing of carboplatin is calculated by the formula 7 × (glomerular filtration rate [mL/min] + 25) mg (Calvert and Egorin, 2002). **Carboplatin dosing should not be based on estimated glomerular filtration rate. It is recommended to base one cycle of carboplatin dosing on the results of radioisotope renal scans or administer two cycles of therapy.**

Given the low overall risk of relapse with CS I seminoma, the lack of prospectively validated markers to identify a high-risk population, and the potential for late toxicity with radiotherapy and carboplatin, many clinical practice guidelines now recommend surveillance as the preferred approach (Krege et al, 2008a, 2008b; Schmoll et al, 2009a). Surveillance enables 80% to 85% of patients to avoid treatment-related toxicity, and relapses are effectively salvaged with dog-leg radiotherapy in most cases. However, surveillance must be continued more than 5 years, and frequent CT imaging is required. For noncompliant patients or patients unwilling to accept surveillance, primary radiotherapy or primary chemotherapy with one to two cycles of carboplatin is recommended.

Clinical Stage IIA and IIB Seminoma. Approximately 15% to 20% of patients with seminoma have CS II disease; 70% of these patients have CS IIA and IIB. Dog-leg radiotherapy using 25 to 30 Gy (including a 5- to 10-Gy boost to involved areas) is employed at most centers. The higher radiation doses administered to CS IIA and IIB patients is generally well tolerated with acute grade III to IV gastrointestinal toxicity reported in 8% to 10% of patients (Classen et al, 2003b). Prophylactic radiation to the left supraclavicular fossa is no longer practiced because less than 3% of patients are likely to benefit(Zagars and Pollack, 2001; Chung et al, 2003). Long-term disease-free survival rates of 92% to 100% for CS IIA and 87% to 90% for CS IIB have been reported, with in-field recurrences reported in 0% to 2% and 0% to 7% of cases, respectively (Zagars and Pollack, 2001; Classen et al, 2003b; Chung et al, 2004b). Adding single-agent carboplatin to 30 Gy dog-leg radiotherapy reduced the relapse rate from 30% to 6% in one series, although further data are required to assess the utility of this approach (Patterson et al, 2001). **Relapses are cured in virtually all cases with first-line chemotherapy, and disease-specific survival approaches 100%. Routine surveillance CT imaging is unnecessary after complete resolution of disease.**

Induction chemotherapy using first-line regimens (BEP×3 or EP×4) is an accepted alternative to dog-leg radiotherapy. The Spanish Germ Cell Cancer Study Group reported on the use of BEP×3 or EP×4 in 72 patients with CS IIA and IIB seminoma (Garcia-del-Muro et al, 2008). Overall, 83% of patients achieved a serologic and radiographic complete response; only one patient (1.3%) had residual mass larger than 3 cm, and the two patients who underwent PCS for residual masses had necrosis only in the resected specimens. The 5-year relapse-free survival was 90%, and overall survival was 90% 95%. The SWENOTECA group similarly reported that there were no relapses among 73 CS IIA and IIB patients treated with cisplatin-based chemotherapy, whereas there were three relapses (10%) among 29 patients treated with radiotherapy. **Induction chemotherapy is preferentially given to** patients with bulky (>3 cm) and/or multiple retroperitoneal masses because the risk of relapse is lower than with dog-leg radiotherapy (Patterson et al, 2001; Chung et al, 2004b; Garcia-del-Muro et al, 2008).

Clinical Stage IIC and III Seminoma. As with NSGCT, patients with CS IIC and III seminoma are treated with induction chemotherapy, with the regimen and number of cycles determined by IGCCCG risk. Of patients with advanced seminoma, 90% are classified as good risk and should receive either BEP×3 or EP×4 chemotherapy. Complete radiographic responses are reported in 70% to 90% of patients, and the 5-year overall survival is 91% (Loehrer et al, 1987; Mencel et al, 1994; International Germ Cell Consensus Classification, 1997; Gholam et al, 2003). Only 10% of advanced seminomas have nonpulmonary visceral metastasis (classified as intermediate risk by IGCCCG criteria). With BEP×4 chemotherapy, the 5-year overall survival is 79% and progression-free survival is 75 (International Germ Cell Consensus Classification, 1997). Single-agent carboplatin in advanced seminoma is associated with inferior survival compared with cisplatin-based regimens (Bokemeyer et al, 2004).

Management of Residual Masses after Chemotherapy. **After first-line chemotherapy, 58% to 80% of patients have radiologically detectable residual masses** (Motzer et al, 1987; Puc et al, 1996; Duchesne et al, 1997; Fossa et al, 1997; Herr et al, 1997; Flechon et al, 2002; De Santis et al, 2004). **Spontaneous resolution of these masses is reported in 50% to 60% of cases, and the median time to resolution is 13 to 18 months** (Flechon et al, 2002; De Santis et al, 2004). **The histology of residual masses is necrosis and viable malignancy in 90% and 10% of cases, respectively** (Puc et al, 1996; Herr et al, 1997; Ravi et al, 1999; Flechon et al, 2002; De Santis et al, 2004). **PCS for seminoma is technically difficult (and frequently not feasible) because of the desmoplastic reaction that occurs after chemotherapy with resultant increased perioperative morbidity** (Mosharafa et al, 2003). Surgical complete resections in seminoma after chemotherapy are reported in only 58% to 74% of patients (compared with ≥85% after first-line chemotherapy for NSGCT) (Puc et al, 1996; Herr et al, 1997; Ravi et al, 1999; Flechon et al, 2002; De Santis et al, 2004). **Teratoma and malignant transformation are much less of a concern with advanced seminoma.** The management of postchemotherapy residual masses differs substantially for seminoma compared with NSGCT.

Investigators have endeavored to identify factors associated with a high risk of viable malignancy to justify PCS. **Postchemotherapy radiotherapy has no role in the management of residual masses** (Duchesne et al, 1997). **The size of residual masses is an important predictor of viable malignancy; 27% to 38% of discrete residual masses larger than 3 cm contain viable malignancy compared with 0% to 4% for masses smaller than 3 cm** (Puc et al, 1996; Herr et al, 1997; Flechon et al, 2002; De Santis et al, 2004). **FDG-PET has been found to be a useful adjunct to CT imaging to select patients for PCS** (De Santis et al, 2004). The specificity and sensitivity of a positive FDG-PET scan for masses larger than 3 cm were 100% and 80%, respectively. **Patients with discrete residual masses larger than 3 cm should be evaluated further with FDG-PET, and patients with positive PET scans should undergo PCS. PET-negative residual masses larger than 3 cm and masses less than 3 cm should be observed.** Inflammation and residual nonviable malignancy may cause a false-positive PET result if patients are scanned too soon after completing chemotherapy. FDG-PET should be delayed until at least 4 weeks after completion of chemotherapy.

Relapsed Seminoma

Chemotherapy-Naive Seminoma Relapse. Chemotherapy-naive relapse occurs in men with CS I seminoma on surveillance and in men with CS I and IIB seminoma treated with primary radiotherapy. **For the former patients, dog-leg radiotherapy is employed for treatment of relapse in 73% to 88% of patients, and cure rates of 70% to 90% are reported. Patients with bulky (>3 cm) retroperitoneal masses and systemic relapse should receive first-line chemotherapy, and salvage rates approach 100%.**

First-line chemotherapy cures virtually all patients who relapse outside the retroperitoneum after primary radiotherapy. Patients who relapse after single-agent carboplatin are considered to have chemotherapy-naive relapse and should receive first-line cisplatin-based chemotherapy.

Early Relapse of Seminoma after Chemotherapy. **An estimated 15% to 20% of patients with advanced seminoma relapse after induction chemotherapy, including 10% who achieve an initial complete response** (Loehrer et al, 1987; Mencel et al, 1994; International Germ Cell Consensus Classification, 1997). In general, patients with incomplete response to first-line chemotherapy or relapse after an initial major clinical response have a poor prognosis with long-term survival rates of 20% to 50% (Miller et al, 1997; Vuky et al, 2002; Gholam et al, 2003). The small number of patients with seminoma who require second-line chemotherapy has limited the evaluation of unique treatment strategies, and relapsing patients are treated on regimens that were largely developed for NSGCT relapse. In two small studies, the efficacy of VeIP×4 as second-line chemotherapy was evaluated in 36 patients with relapsed seminoma. Overall, 30 patients (83%) achieved a complete response to chemotherapy (with or without PCS), and 21 (53%) were continuously free of recurrence over a median follow-up of 72 to 84 months (Miller et al, 1997; Vuky et al, 2002). Vuky and coworkers (2002) also evaluated HDCT in 12 patients with advanced seminoma and an incomplete response to first-line chemotherapy, and 6 patients (50%) achieving a complete response remained free of recurrence. **An important consideration for patients with advanced seminoma who relapse after first-line chemotherapy is the potential for teratoma at the site of relapse. Patients with normal serum tumor markers should undergo biopsy before starting second-line chemotherapy.**

Late Relapse of Seminoma after Chemotherapy. In most published series, pure seminoma accounts for less than 8% of late relapse events (Baniel et al, 1995; George et al, 2003; Ronnen et al, 2005; Sharp et al, 2008). However, Dieckmann and colleagues (2005) reported a series of 122 patients with late relapse, of whom 50 (41%) had pure seminoma at diagnosis. Only 6 (12%) of these patients had received prior first-line chemotherapy, and most had received single-agent carboplatin or radiation therapy at diagnosis. Long-term control of cancer was achieved in 88% of patients. **Late relapse of seminoma may have a favorable prognosis, particularly in patients without prior exposure to cisplatin.**

Brain Metastases

About 1% of men with disseminated GCT have brain metastases detected before initiating chemotherapy, and between 0.4% and 3% develop brain metastases after first-line chemotherapy (Raina et al, 1993; International Germ Cell Consensus Classification, 1997; Fossa et al, 1999a). **Brain metastases are associated with choriocarcinoma and should be suspected in any patient with a very high serum hCG level** (Fossa et al, 1999a; Kollmannsberger et al, 2000; Salvati et al, 2006; Gremmer et al, 2008; Nonomura et al, 2009). **Choriocarcinomas are highly vascular and tend to hemorrhage during chemotherapy, and death rates of 4% to 10% secondary to intracranial hemorrhage have been reported** (Kollmannsberger et al, 2000; Nonomura et al, 2009). This risk must be considered in management of these patients, and neurologic changes need to be evaluated expeditiously.

The 5-year overall survival in patients with brain metastases is 33% for patients with disseminated NSGCT and 57% for patients with seminoma (International Germ Cell Consensus Classification, 1997). **Men who relapse in the brain after achieving a complete response to chemotherapy appear to have a worse prognosis than patients with brain involvement at diagnosis,** with overall survival rates of 39% to 44% for isolated brain metastases and 2% to 26% for brain metastases associated with other sites of disease (Fossa et al, 1999a; Kollmannsberger et al, 2000; Hartmann et al, 2003; Salvati et al, 2006; Gremmer et al, 2008; Nonomura et al, 2009). Case studies and pooled analyses of patients with GCT and brain metastases have reported outcomes with various

KEY POINTS: SEMINOMA

- The optimal management of CS I seminoma is controversial. Surveillance, primary radiotherapy (20 to 30 Gy to the paraaortic region with or without ipsilateral pelvis), and primary chemotherapy with carboplatin (one to two cycles) are accepted treatment options with long-term survival rates approaching 100% for each.
- Prognostic factors for occult metastases in CS I seminoma are not as well developed as for NSGCT. Given the overall low risk of occult metastases (15% to 20%), the inability to identify a high-risk population on the basis of histopathologic factors in the primary tumor, and the potential for late toxicity with primary radiotherapy, surveillance has become the recommended treatment approach for CS I seminoma.
- Surveillance is not recommended to patients who are anticipated to be poorly compliant with follow-up imaging and clinical evaluation. The standard treatment approach to patients who relapse on surveillance is dog-leg radiotherapy (25 to 35 Gy), although patients with bulky retroperitoneal lymphadenopathy or distant metastases should receive IGCCCG risk-appropriate first-line chemotherapy.
- Primary radiotherapy and primary chemotherapy with single-agent carboplatin are associated with similar rates of cure and survival. Patients who receive para-aortic radiotherapy and patients who receive carboplatin require periodic CT imaging in the surveillance of recurrent disease after treatment; this is not required for patients who receive dog-leg radiotherapy.
- Dog-leg radiotherapy (25 to 35 Gy) and first-line chemotherapy (BEP×3 or EP×4) are accepted treatment options for patients with CS IIA and IIB seminoma and nonbulky (<3 cm) retroperitoneal lymph node metastasis. First-line chemotherapy (BEP×3 or EP×4) is recommended for bulky (>3 cm) and/or multifocal retroperitoneal metastases.
- The first-line treatment of patients with CS IIC and III seminoma is cisplatin-based chemotherapy, and the specific regimen and number of cycles are dictated by IGCCCG risk criteria. Patients with good-risk disease should receive BEP×3 or EP×4, and patients with intermediate-risk disease should receive BEP×4.
- Patients with discrete, residual masses larger than 3 cm after first-line chemotherapy should undergo further evaluation with FDG-PET imaging. Patients with PET-positive residual masses should undergo PCS. Residual masses that are PET-negative or less than 3 cm can be safely observed after chemotherapy.

treatment strategies, but there are no randomized trials to define optimal management clearly (Spears et al, 1992; Fossa et al, 1999a; Kollmannsberger et al, 2000; Hartmann et al, 2003; Salvati et al, 2006; Gremmer et al, 2008; Nonomura et al, 2009). Treatment strategies include chemotherapy, surgical resection, whole-brain radiation therapy, and stereotactic radiosurgery, with most patients receiving multimodal therapy. **Patients with brain metastases at diagnosis should receive BEP×4 chemotherapy followed by resection of residual masses.** The benefit of radiation therapy in this setting is unclear (Fossa et al, 1999a; Kollmannsberger et al, 2000; Hartmann et al, 2003). At our institution, radiation therapy is considered only for patients with unresectable residual lesions not amenable to stereotactic radiosurgery because of concerns of radiation-induced neurotoxicity (Doyle and Einhorn, 2008). **Patients who relapse in the brain after first-line chemotherapy should be treated with second-line chemotherapy followed by resection and/or radiation therapy** (Fossa et al, 1999a; Hartmann et al, 2003). For men who relapse in the brain and at other anatomic sites, the prognosis is very poor, particularly if it is not the first relapse.

Treatment-Related Sequelae

Sequelae of treatment of testis cancer can be divided into late and early complications. Complications from orchiectomy and RPLND are discussed in Chapter 35 and are not reviewed here except to note that the main issues after RPLND are midline scar, ejaculatory dysfunction, small bowel obstruction, and perioperative complications. Also, there is an increased incidence of hypogonadism after orchiectomy for GCT.

Early Toxicity

Cisplatin-based chemotherapy is associated with numerous early complications and side effects, including fatigue, myelosuppression, infection, peripheral neuropathy, hearing loss, diminished renal function, and death. The death rate from toxicity has ranged from 0% to 2.4% during chemotherapy for good-risk disease and from 3% to 4.4% during standard first-line chemotherapy for intermediate-risk and poor-risk disease (de Wit et al, 1998; Nichols et al, 1998, 2001; Toner et al, 2001; Culine et al, 2007, 2008). The impact of chemotherapy and radiation therapy on spermatogenesis has been discussed previously. Most men are able to father children after treatment for GCT but paternity rates are lower for men treated with radiation therapy and/or chemotherapy (Huyghe et al, 2004; Brydoy et al, 2005). Early complications of radiation therapy include fatigue, nausea and vomiting, leukopenia, and dyspepsia (Fossa et al, 1999b; Jones et al, 2005; Oliver et al, 2005).

Late Toxicity

Numerous long-term sequelae have been reported in GCT survivors, including peripheral neuropathy, Raynaud phenomenon, hearing loss, hypogonadism, infertility, SMN, and cardiovascular disease (Brydoy et al, 2009; Fossa et al, 2009; Rossen et al, 2009; Gilligan, 2011). Symptoms of Raynaud phenomenon and peripheral neuropathy have been reported in 20% to 45% and 14% to 43%, respectively, of GCT survivors (Brydoy et al, 2009; Rossen et al, 2009). Significant hearing loss and/or tinnitus after cisplatin-based chemotherapy is reported in 20% to 40% of patients and can be documented via audiometry in 30% to 75%. Hypogonadism has been documented in about 10% to 20% of patients treated with orchiectomy alone, 15% to 40% of patients treated with radiation therapy, and 20% to 25% of patients treated with first-line chemotherapy regimens (Nord et al, 2003; Lackner et al, 2009).

Large population-based studies of GCT survivors have reported an increased risk of death from gastrointestinal and cardiovascular diseases after radiation therapy and an increased risk of death from infections, cardiovascular diseases, and pulmonary diseases after chemotherapy (Fossa et al, 2007). Patients treated with both radiation and chemotherapy have the highest risk of death from nonmalignant causes. The increased cardiovascular disease incidence and mortality in GCT survivors is particularly well documented (Meinardi et al, 2000; Huddart et al, 2003; Fossa et al, 2007; van den Belt-Dusebout et al, 2007; Fossa et al, 2009). The etiologies of these cardiovascular complications are not well understood, but putative contributing factors are radiation-induced or chemotherapy-induced vascular injury and chemotherapy-induced cardiac injury and metabolic syndrome (Nuver et al, 2005; Altena et al, 2009).

The risk of SMN is a particular concern. The incidence of non–germ cell malignancies is 60% to 100% higher in GCT survivors treated with cisplatin-based chemotherapy or radiation therapy compared with the general population and 200% higher in patients who received both radiation and chemotherapy (Travis et al, 2005; Richiardi et al, 2007). The risk of death from non–germ cell malignancies in GCT survivors treated with radiation or chemotherapy is less well defined but appears to be doubled compared with the general population (Fossa et al, 2004). The frequent use of body CT imaging in the surveillance of patients after therapy is another source of radiation that may increase the risk of SMN (Brenner and Hall, 2007; Chamie et al, 2008; Tarin et al, 2009).

NON–GERM CELL TUMORS

Sex Cord–Stromal Tumors

Sex cord–stromal tumors are rare, comprising approximately 4% of testis neoplasms. The term *sex cord–stromal tumor* refers to neoplasms containing Leydig cells, Sertoli cells, granulosa cells, or thecal cells. **Approximately 90% of these tumors are benign, and 10% are malignant.** Histologic criteria have been developed to help distinguish between benign and malignant histology and include tumor size larger than 5 cm, necrosis, vascular invasion, nuclear atypia, high mitotic index, increased MIB-1 expression, infiltrative margins, extension beyond the testicular parenchyma, and DNA ploidy (Kim et al, 1985; Cheville et al, 1998). Most malignant cases are associated with two or more of these features. **However, the presence of metastatic disease is the only reliable criterion for making this distinction.**

Leydig Cell Tumors

Leydig cell tumors account for 75% to 80% of sex cord–stromal tumors. There is no association with cryptorchidism. Most of these tumors occur in men 30 to 60 years old, although approximately one fourth occur in children. Adults may present with painless testis mass, testicular pain, gynecomastia (as a result of androgen excess and peripheral estrogen conversion), impotence, decreased libido, and infertility. Boys usually present with a testis mass and isosexual precocious puberty (prominent external genitalia, pubic hair growth, and masculine voice).

Diagnostic workup should include serum tumor markers and testicular ultrasound examination. The ultrasound appearance of these tumors is variable and is indistinguishable from GCT. In the presence of gynecomastia, infertility, depressed libido, or precocious puberty, luteinizing hormone, FSH, testosterone, estrogen, and estradiol should also be drawn (these should be measured after orchiectomy if the diagnosis is not suspected preoperatively). When the diagnosis is confirmed, patients should undergo chest-abdomen-pelvis CT imaging for staging purposes.

In the past, radical inguinal orchiectomy was the initial treatment of choice. If the diagnosis is suspected preoperatively, given the 90% incidence of benign histology, testis-sparing surgery may be considered for lesions less than 3 cm with intraoperative frozen-section histologic confirmation (Carmignani et al, 2006, 2007). **Completion orchiectomy should be performed if GCT histology is seen (either on intraoperative frozen section or on final pathology) or if malignant features (listed earlier) are present on final pathologic examination of the resected tumor.**

Given the rarity of these tumors, they are often not suspected preoperatively, and most patients undergo radical orchiectomy. Benign lesions are usually small, yellow to brown, and well circumscribed, without areas of necrosis or hemorrhage. Histologically, the tumors consist of uniform, polygonal cells with round nuclei. Reinke crystals are present in 25% to 40% of cases and appear as densely eosinophilic, needlelike or rhomboid structures within the cytoplasm. These tumors must be distinguished from Leydig cell hyperplasia that occur in atrophic testes and adjacent to GCTs, in which Leydig cells infiltrate between seminiferous tubules without displacing or obliterating them. Malignant behavior has not been reported in a prepubertal patient. Older patients are more likely to have malignant tumors.

The most frequent metastatic sites are the retroperitoneum and lung. RPLND is reasonable in selected cases with adverse features, although high rates of progression are observed in cases with pathologically involved nodes, suggesting a staging role only for RPLND (Mosharafa et al, 2003). **Metastatic Leydig cell tumors are resistant to chemotherapy and radiation therapy, and survival is poor** (Mosharafa et al, 2003). Ortho,para-DDD, a potent inhibitor of steroidogenesis, may produce partial responses in patients with metastasis and excess androgen production, but cure is impossible (Schwarzman et al, 1989). Surveillance is recommended for patients without clinical or pathologic features suggestive of malignancy. There are no widely accepted criteria for follow-up, but patients should be monitored at regular intervals with clinical assessment, hormonal profile (including luteinizing hormone, FSH, testosterone, estrogen, and estradiol), and CT imaging of the chest, abdomen, and pelvis for 2 years. **Persistent Leydig cell dysfunction and hypogonadism may occur after excision of the primary tumor, and 40% of men may require testosterone supplementation postoperatively** (Conkey et al, 2005).

Sertoli Cell Tumor

Sertoli cell tumors constitute less than 1% of testis neoplasms. The median age at diagnosis is 45 years, but rare cases in boys have been reported. Rarely, these tumors are associated with Peutz-Jeghers syndrome and androgen insensitivity syndrome and are frequently bilateral (either synchronous or metachronous). There is no association with cryptorchidism. Gynecomastia is evident in one third of patients. **As for Leydig cell tumors, testis-sparing surgery can be considered for tumors less than 3 cm given the high incidence of benign histology (90%). For tumors larger than 3 cm or if intraoperative frozen-section or final pathologic analysis reveals GCT or malignant features, radical inguinal orchiectomy should be performed.** The tumors are well circumscribed, yellow-white or tan, with uniform consistency. Microscopically, the tumors contain epithelial elements resembling Sertoli cells with varying amounts of stroma organized into tubules. These tumors may be misinterpreted as seminomas leading to errors in the selection of treatment. **Diagnostic workup; staging studies; and criteria for treatment, surveillance, and follow-up are similar to Leydig cell tumors.**

Granulosa Cell Tumors

Granulosa cell tumors of the testis are exceedingly rare. The juvenile type is benign and is the most frequent congenital testis tumor (most frequently occurring in infants <6 months old), accounting for 7% of all prepubertal testicular neoplasms. The adult type resembles granulosa cell tumors of the ovary. Gynecomastia and increased estrogen secretion are common. Testis-sparing surgery may be considered for tumors less than 3 cm if the diagnosis is suspected preoperatively. Otherwise, radical inguinal orchiectomy is recommended. Treatment of the primary tumor is curative because these tumors appear to have limited metastatic potential.

Gonadoblastoma

Gonadoblastoma is a mixed germ cell–sex cord–stromal tumor composed of seminoma-like germ cells and sex cord cells showing Sertoli differentiation. They occur almost exclusively in patients with gonadal dysgenesis and intersex syndromes. Of affected individuals, 80% are phenotypic females, usually presenting with primary amenorrhea. The remaining patients are phenotypic males, almost always presenting with cryptorchidism (with the dysgenic gonad in the inguinal or abdominal location), hypospadias, and some form of female internal genitalia. **These tumors should be considered an in situ form of malignant GCT because approximately 50% of patients develop an invasive GCT (usually seminoma, although yolk sac tumor and EC can occur)** (Ulbright, 2004). Gonadoblastomas do not metastasize, but metastasis of the malignant GCT elements may occur. **Bilateral orchiectomy is required because of the risk of bilateral tumors (40%)** (Scully, 1970). For patients with malignant GCT, subsequent workup for metastatic disease with or without treatment should be initiated.

Miscellaneous Testis Neoplasms

Dermoid and Epidermoid Cyst

Dermoid and epidermoid cysts are rare benign neoplasms that are thought to arise from benign germ cells with retained embryonic properties or from displaced metaplastic mesothelial cells (Ye and Ulbright, 2012). Grossly, they are well-circumscribed, unilocular cystic masses filled with keratinized debris that may have a laminated appearance, which gives them the characteristic "onion peel" appearance on ultrasound scan. Dermoid cysts are differentiated from epidermoid cysts by the presence of adnexal structures such as glandular elements, adipose tissue, and cartilage. Dermoid and epidermoid cysts are distinguished from teratoma by the absence of ITGCN in the adjacent testis. **Enucleation or partial orchiectomy may be performed, although the lesion should be thoroughly sampled by a pathologist to rule out GCT or ITGCN.**

Adenocarcinoma of the Rete Testis

Adenocarcinoma of the rete testis is a rare but highly malignant neoplasm arising from the collecting system of the testis. The usual presentation is a painless testis mass with hydrocele. More than 50% of patients present with metastatic disease, and the overall median survival is 1 year. RPLND may be curative in patients with limited retroperitoneal lymph node metastasis. Chemotherapy and radiation therapy are ineffective.

Secondary Tumors of the Testis

Lymphoma

Primary testicular non-Hodgkin lymphoma is a rare tumor representing only 1% to 2% of all cases of lymphoma. Most commonly, lymphoma involves the testis through dissemination from extratesticular sites (Ulbright, 2004). Of cases, 85% occur in men older than 60 years. **Non-Hodgkin lymphoma is the most common testicular neoplasm in men older than age 50. Bilateral testicular involvement occurs in 35% of cases.** It usually manifests as a painless testicular mass in an older man. Approximately 25% of men have systemic symptoms (fever, night sweats, weight loss). Central nervous system involvement at diagnosis is reported in 10% of men. The initial treatment is radical inguinal orchiectomy. Men with testicular non-Hodgkin lymphoma should be referred to a hematologist-oncologist for staging investigations and subsequent therapy. Most cases are associated with systemic disease, and the overall prognosis is poor.

Leukemic Infiltration

The testis is a frequent site of relapse in boys with acute lymphocytic leukemia. Most boys are in complete remission at the time of testicular enlargement. **The diagnosis can usually be made by biopsy, and orchiectomy is unnecessary. Local control can be achieved with low-dose radiotherapy (20 Gy), and treatment**

should include the contralateral testis because of the frequent risk of bilateral involvement. Overall, the prognosis is poor because most patients have associated systemic disease.

Metastases

Metastases to the testis are rare. Bilateral involvement occurs in 15% of patients. The most common primary tumors are prostate, lung, melanoma, colon, and kidney. Although treatment is largely dictated by the primary tumor, orchiectomy may be considered for palliative reasons.

TUMORS OF THE TESTICULAR ADNEXA

Paratesticular tumors are rare and account for approximately 5% of intrascrotal neoplasms, roughly 75% of which arise from the spermatic cord.

Adenomatoid Tumor

Adenomatoid tumor is the most common paratesticular tumor, most commonly involving the epididymis (although these tumors may also arise within the testicular tunicae or the spermatic cord). The most common presentation is a small (0.5 to 5 cm), painless paratesticular mass detected on routine examination in a man in his third or fourth decade. **These tumors are benign and managed by inguinal exploration and surgical excision.** On microscopic examination, tumors are composed of epithelial-like cells that contain vacuoles and fibrous stroma.

Cystadenoma

Cystadenoma of the epididymis corresponds to benign epithelial hyperplasia. The lesions are usually multicystic, and the walls are studded with nodules of epithelial cells arranged in a glandular or papillary configuration. **Approximately one third of cases occur in patients with von Hippel-Lindau disease, which are usually bilateral.** The lesions are usually small and painless and are detected on routine examination in a young man.

Mesothelioma

Paratesticular mesothelioma arises from the tunica vaginalis and usually manifests as a painless scrotal mass in association with a hydrocele. These tumors most commonly occur in older adults but may be encountered in any age group. **Benign and malignant cases have been described, with the distinction based on atypia, mitotic activity, and invasion** (Ulbright, 2004). Malignant cases may be associated with asbestos exposure. **Treatment is radical inguinal orchiectomy.** RPLND may be considered in patients with malignant tumors without widespread metastatic disease. The role of chemotherapy for these tumors is poorly defined.

Sarcoma

Sarcomas of the spermatic cord, epididymis, and testis are the most common genitourinary sarcomas in adults. **Liposarcoma is the most common histologic subtype in adults,** followed by leiomyosarcoma, malignant fibrous histiocytoma, rhabdomyosarcoma, and fibrosarcoma (Coleman et al, 2003; Ulbright, 2004; Dotan et al, 2006; Rodriguez et al, 2014). **Embryonal rhabdomyosarcoma is the most common histologic subtype in men younger than age 30.** Sarcomas most commonly arise from the spermatic cord and are located in the intrascrotal region; primary mesenchymal tumors of the testis are exceedingly rare. These tumors usually manifest as a painless, palpable mass, and most are large (>5 cm in size) (Dotan et al, 2006). Ultrasonography demonstrates a solid mass, although it cannot distinguish between benign and malignant pathology. **Any solid mass in the scrotum external to the tunica albuginea should be explored through an inguinal approach, and a biopsy should**

be performed. Liposarcomas of the spermatic cord in the inguinal canal may be mistaken for inguinal hernia or lipoma, and CT or magnetic resonance imaging is helpful to distinguish between these entities.

Most patients have localized disease at diagnosis. **Sarcomas should be managed initially through an inguinal approach with wide excision of the spermatic cord and testis with high ligation. Patients with an initial incomplete resection should undergo repeat wide excision** (Coleman et al, 2003). **The primary pattern of failure is local, particularly for liposarcoma** (Ballo et al, 2001; Montgomery and Fisher, 2003; Khandekar et al, 2013). **Some authors have advocated for postoperative radiation therapy for all paratesticular sarcomas, particularly for liposarcomas and for tumors for which the adequacy of local control is in doubt** (Ballo et al, 2001; Hazariwala et al, 2013). **However, the efficacy of this approach is debated** (Fagundes et al, 1996; Coleman et al, 2003; Khandekar et al, 2013). Systemic chemotherapy should be given to patients with evidence of retroperitoneal or distant metastases. **In the presence of a normal metastatic evaluation, patients with sarcomas other than liposarcoma should undergo RPLND, and postoperative chemotherapy should be given to patients with retroperitoneal lymph node metastasis** (Dang et al, 2013). Given that the lymphatic drainage of the spermatic cord includes the ipsilateral pelvis, inguinal, and retroperitoneal lymph nodes, treating these areas with lymphadenectomy or radiation therapy should be considered. The long-term survival of men with paratesticular sarcoma is approximately 50%, with liposarcoma having the most favorable prognosis and malignant fibrous histiocytoma and leiomyosarcoma having the least favorable prognosis (Coleman et al, 2003; Rodriguez et al, 2014).

REFERENCES

The complete reference list is available online at www.expertconsult.com.

SUGGESTED READINGS

Albers P, Siener R, Krege S, et al. Randomized phase III trial comparing retroperitoneal lymph node dissection with one course of bleomycin and etoposide plus cisplatin chemotherapy in the adjuvant treatment of clinical stage I nonseminomatous testicular germ cell tumors: AUO trial AH 01/94 by the German Testicular Cancer Study Group. J Clin Oncol 2008; 26:2966–72.

De Santis M, Becherer A, Bokemeyer C, et al. (2-18)Fluoro-deoxy-D-glucose positron emission tomography is a reliable predictor for viable tumor in postchemotherapy seminoma: an update of the prospective multicentric SEMPET trial. J Clin Oncol 2004;22:1034–9.

Debono DJ, Heilman DK, Einhorn LH, et al. Decision analysis for avoiding postchemotherapy surgery in patients with disseminated nonseminomatous germ cell tumors. J Clin Oncol 1997;15:1455–64.

Dieckmann KP, Skakkebaek NE. Carcinoma in situ of the testis: review of biological and clinical features. Int J Cancer 1999;83:815–22.

Dotan ZA, Tal R, Golijanin D, et al. Adult genitourinary sarcoma: the 25-year Memorial Sloan-Kettering experience. J Urol 2006;176:2033–8, discussion 2038–9.

Einhorn LH. Treatment of testicular cancer: a new and improved model. J Clin Oncol 1990;8:1777–81.

Feldman DR, Bosl GJ, Sheinfeld J, et al. Medical treatment of advanced testicular cancer. JAMA 2008;299:672–84.

Fossa SD, Gilbert E, Dores GM, et al. Noncancer causes of death in survivors of testicular cancer. J Natl Cancer Inst 2007;99:533–44.

Fossa SD, Oldenburg J, Dahl AA. Short- and long-term morbidity after treatment for testicular cancer. BJU Int 2009;104:1418–22.

George DW, Foster RS, Hromas RA, et al. Update on late relapse of germ cell tumor: a clinical and molecular analysis. J Clin Oncol 2003;21:113–22.

International Germ Cell Consensus Classification: a prognostic factor-based staging system for metastatic germ cell cancers. International Germ Cell Cancer Collaborative Group. J Clin Oncol 1997;15:594–603.

Kollmannsberger C, Moore C, Chi KN, et al. Non-risk-adapted surveillance for patients with stage I nonseminomatous testicular germ-cell tumors: diminishing treatment-related morbidity while maintaining efficacy. Ann Oncol 2010;21:1296–301.

Motzer RJ, Amsterdam A, Prieto V, et al. Teratoma with malignant transformation: diverse malignant histologies arising in men with germ cell tumors. J Urol 1998;159:133–8.

Motzer RJ, Nichols CJ, Margolin KA, et al. Phase III randomized trial of conventional-dose chemotherapy with or without high-dose chemotherapy and autologous hematopoietic stem-cell rescue as first-line treatment for patients with poor-prognosis metastatic germ cell tumors. J Clin Oncol 2007;25:247–56.

Oliver RT, Mead GM, Rustin GJ, et al. Randomized trial of carboplatin versus radiotherapy for stage I seminoma: mature results on relapse and contralateral testis cancer rates in MRC TE19/EORTC 30982 study (ISRCTN27163214). J Clin Oncol 2011;29:957–62.

Stephenson AJ, Bosl GJ, Motzer RJ, et al. Retroperitoneal lymph node dissection for nonseminomatous germ cell testicular cancer: impact of patient selection factors on outcome. J Clin Oncol 2005;23:2781–8.

Stephenson AJ, Bosl GJ, Motzer RJ, et al. Nonrandomized comparison of primary chemotherapy and retroperitoneal lymph node dissection for clinical stage IIA and IIB nonseminomatous germ cell testicular cancer. J Clin Oncol 2007;25:5597–602.

Steyerberg EW, Keizer HJ, Fossa SD, et al. Prediction of residual retroperitoneal mass histology after chemotherapy for metastatic nonseminomatous germ cell tumor: multivariate analysis of individual patient data from six study groups. J Clin Oncol 1995;13:1177–87.

Travis LB, Fossa SD, Schonfeld SJ, et al. Second cancers among 40,576 testicular cancer patients: focus on long-term survivors. J Natl Cancer Inst 2005;97:1354–65.

Vergouwe Y, Steyerberg EW, Eijkemans MJ, et al. Predictors of occult metastasis in clinical stage I nonseminoma: a systematic review. J Clin Oncol 2003;21:4092–9.

35

Surgery of Testicular Tumors

Kevin R. Rice, MD, Clint K. Cary, MD, MPH, Timothy A. Masterson, MD, and Richard S. Foster, MD

In addition to its remarkable chemosensitivity, testicular germ cell tumor (GCT) is among the most surgically curable malignancies. Before the development of effective chemotherapeutic regimens for testicular GCT, investigators at Walter Reed Army Hospital were able to achieve a nearly 50% durable cure rate for patients demonstrating node-positive disease at primary retroperitoneal lymph node dissection (RPLND) (Patton et al, 1959). At the present time, nearly 80% of patients presenting with clinical stage I (CS I) testicular nonseminomatous germ cell tumor (NSGCT) are cured with orchiectomy alone (Warde et al, 2002; Hotte et al, 2010), whereas 60% to 80% of patients with pathologic stage II (PS II) NSGCT can be cured with primary RPLND (Donohue et al, 1993a; Stephenson et al, 2005). In the setting of larger volume metastatic disease requiring induction chemotherapy, approximately 90% of patients with residual retroperitoneal masses are cured by postchemotherapy retroperitoneal lymph node dissection (PC-RPLND) (Donohue et al, 1990). This chapter describes the management decision-making processes, operative techniques, and outcomes for testicular cancer surgery. This chapter provides the urologist with the foundation necessary to manage surgically the primary tumor as well as regional retroperitoneal metastases for all stages of testicular cancer.

MANAGEMENT OF TESTIS MASS

History and Physical Examination, Ultrasonography, and Preorchiectomy Evaluation

The presentation of a testicular mass warrants a prompt and thorough investigation. **Principal to this evaluation is understanding the temporal development of any associated symptoms, characterizing the scrotal contents with careful physical and ultrasound examination, and obtaining appropriate serologic tests** (Robson et al, 1965; Sandeman, 1979; Bosl et al, 1981; Thornhill et al, 1987; Richie, 1993; Honig et al, 1994; Petersen et al, 1999; Jacobsen et al, 2000; Simon et al, 2001). Timely recognition and diagnosis are paramount in the treatment of a given cancer at its earliest and most curable stage (Post and Belis, 1980; Oliver, 1985; Gascoigne et al, 1999; Chapple et al, 2004; Moul, 2007). Physical examination is the most crucial part of the evaluation of the testis mass. Although not mandatory, ultrasound examination can provide important details of tumor characteristics and document radiographically the laterality of the lesion (Horstman et al, 1992; Shah et al, 2010; Goddi et al, 2012). Additionally, documentation

of the characteristics of the contralateral testicle is essential because synchronous testicular masses have been reported in approximately 1% of patients (Bokemeyer et al, 1993; Coogan et al, 1998; Che et al, 2002; Holzbeierlein et al, 2003; Pamenter et al, 2003; Fossa et al, 2005; Hentrich et al, 2005). Obtaining serum tumor marker (STM) values, including α-fetoprotein, human chorionic gonadotropin, and lactate dehydrogenase, aids in solidifying a diagnosis of GCT and serves as a baseline to compare serologic trends after orchiectomy. Placement of a testicular prosthesis at the time of radical orchiectomy should be discussed before surgery.

Radical Orchiectomy

In patients in whom a testicular malignancy is suspected, radical orchiectomy is the diagnostic and therapeutic treatment of choice. The approach is via an inguinal incision, allowing for complete removal of the ipsilateral testis, epididymis, and spermatic cord to the level of the internal inguinal ring.

Technique

The patient is positioned supine on the operating room table. Proper preparation of the skin should encompass the abdomen above the umbilicus cranially, the bilateral mid-to-lower thigh caudally, and the external genitalia through to the perineum posteriorly. After sterile draping of the surgical field, exposure of the ipsilateral anterior superior iliac spine, pubic tubercle, and scrotum is required. Palpation and marking the overlying skin of the external inguinal ring can facilitate orientation of the medial extent of the inguinal canal.

The incision, typically 3 to 5 cm in length, is made with a transverse orientation overlying the inguinal canal following the lines of Langer. In circumstances in which a mass is too large to be delivered through the standard incision, the incision can be extended down along the anterior scrotum in a hockey-stick fashion. When the external oblique fascia is exposed and the external ring is identified, the inguinal canal should be opened along its course laterally for approximately 4 cm. In an obese patient, self-retaining instruments such as a Weitlaner or Gelpi retractor often prove helpful or necessary to provide exposure. With the external oblique fascia open, care should be taken to identify the ilioinguinal nerve for prospective preservation. This structure courses parallel to spermatic cord, typically along the cephalad aspect of its anterior surface. When the nerve is safely displaced, the spermatic cord is mobilized within the canal at the level of the pubic tubercle, where it can be encircled with a Penrose drain. After division of the external spermatic fascia and cremasteric fibers that surround the spermatic cord, gentle traction can be placed in the cephalad direction to draw the testicle toward the incision. Delivery of the testicle can be facilitated by applying external pressure to the ipsilateral hemiscrotum. After division of the gubernaculum, the spermatic cord is mobilized to the level of the internal inguinal ring until the peritoneal reflection is visualized. At this level, the vas deferens and gonadal vessels are dissected out, ligated, and divided separately. Ligation and division are typically performed with nonabsorbable suture, leaving a 1- to 2-cm suture tail on the stump of the gonadal vessels to facilitate identification at RPLND. Individually ligating the vas deferens from the remainder of the spermatic cord facilitates retrieval of the distal spermatic cord stump during subsequent RPLND because the vas deferens is not taken as part of this specimen.

After irrigation of the wound and close inspection for hemostasis, the ilioinguinal nerve is positioned safely in the floor of the inguinal canal, and closure of the external oblique aponeurosis is performed. A two- or three-layer closure of the subcutaneous and skin layers is completed, and sterile dressings are applied. In general, scrotal support and fluff dressings are helpful to avoid unnecessary scrotal swelling and hematoma formation for the first 48 to 72 hours.

Partial Orchiectomy

Because of the high rate of long-term survivors after testis cancer therapy, functional issues pertaining to treatment-related side effects and preservation of quality of life have emerged (Skakkebaek, 1975; Jacobsen et al, 1981; Klein et al, 1985; Haas et al, 1986; Kressel et al, 1988; Robertson, 1995; Carmignani et al, 2004). **Partial orchiectomy should be considered in patients with a polar tumor measuring 2 cm or less and an abnormal or absent contralateral testicle.** In circumstances in which the malignant nature of the tumor is uncertain, inguinal exploration and excisional biopsy can be done. In general, these operations should be performed in very select patients in whom the benefits of organ preservation are thought to outweigh the risks of local tumor recurrence. In patients with a normal contralateral testis, elective testis-sparing surgery is not advised.

Technique

The approach to partial orchiectomy is identical to the approach of a radical inguinal orchiectomy. The use of ischemia with or without hypothermia has been questioned by some authors and can be omitted if the resection time is limited to less than 30 minutes (Giannarini et al, 2010). With sterile towels draping the field to avoid contamination, intraoperative ultrasonography can be used to facilitate localization of the mass. When the mass is identified, a scalpel can be used to incise the tunica albuginea overlying the mass. When the approach is from the ventral midline, a vertical incision along the long axis of the testis is preferred. Otherwise, incisions localized medial or lateral to the ventral midline should be oriented horizontally to follow the course of the segmental arteries beneath the tunica albuginea.

Once identified, the tumor is enucleated preferably with a small rim of surrounding seminiferous tubules insulating the mass. In the presence of a confirmed GCT, the association of concomitant intratubular germ cell neoplasia in the surrounding parenchyma of the ipsilateral testis warrants consideration for completion radical orchiectomy or adjuvant radiotherapy to the remnant testis to reduce the risk of recurrent disease. Because of this risk, some clinicians choose to omit parenchymal biopsies in the setting of confirmed GCT and recommend treatment of all remnants with radical orchiectomy or adjuvant therapy. If radical orchiectomy is not performed, the tunica is closed with absorbable suture, and the testis is placed back into the dependent portion of the scrotal compartment and secured at three points of internal fixation to the gubernaculum or medial septum of the scrotum.

Adjuvant radiotherapy with a dosage of 18 to 20 Gy is recommended to prevent local tumor recurrence in all patients treated with partial orchiectomy for the management of GCT in a functionally solitary testis (Heidenreich et al, 2001; Krege et al, 2008; Giannarini et al, 2010). In these patients, the only benefit of partial orchiectomy is preservation of Leydig cell function. **Any local recurrence within the ipsilateral testis occurring with or without adjuvant therapy should be managed with completion radical orchiectomy.**

Delayed Orchiectomy

Most testicular cancers are initially diagnosed at the time of orchiectomy. However, in a small subset of patients with widespread and/or symptomatic GCT, the diagnosis is made based on biopsy of a metastatic lesion or empirically based on clinical and serologic features. In these unique settings, initiation of systemic chemotherapy supersedes diagnostic orchiectomy (Ondrus et al, 2001). **Because of high discordance of pathologic response rates within the testis, a delayed orchiectomy is recommended for all patients with NSGCT after induction chemotherapy, even in the setting of a complete response in the retroperitoneum** (Snow et al, 1983; Simmonds et al, 1995; Leibovitch et al, 1996; Ondrus et al, 2001).

The role of delayed orchiectomy is more controversial in patients with presumed primary retroperitoneal/extragonadal GCT. In studies in which biopsy of the testis was performed in these cases, intratubular germ cell neoplasia was seen in 42% of patients (Daugaard et al, 1992). Among such patients who are observed after chemotherapy, approximately 5% develop a metachronous testicular cancer (Hartmann et al, 2001). **Radical orchiectomy has been advocated when the metastatic pattern of retroperitoneal disease lateralizes to the expected distribution of a testicular primary.** In a small cohort series at Indiana University, 71% of patients with presumed extragonadal GCT undergoing a postchemotherapy delayed orchiectomy had histologic evidence of teratoma or necrosis within the testis, the latter suggesting a burned-out primary or complete response to chemotherapy (Brown et al, 2008). If observation of the testis is elected, monthly self-examinations and periodic physician assessment are warranted.

Postorchiectomy Evaluation

After orchiectomy, review of the pathologic findings along with incorporation of appropriate radiographic and serologic studies is necessary to determine clinical stage. Contrast-enhanced computed tomography (CT) with intravenous and oral contrast agents is the most effective means to accomplish this; however, magnetic resonance imaging may serve as a suitable alternative. Fluorodeoxyglucose-labeled positron emission tomography (PET) and lymphoangiography serve little to no role in the staging of GCTs after initial diagnosis. Similar to the evaluation before orchiectomy, assessment of STM (α-fetoprotein, human chorionic gonadotropin, lactate dehydrogenase) values and trends after orchiectomy completes the initial evaluation before patient counseling regarding management options.

KEY POINTS: MANAGEMENT OF THE TESTIS MASS

- Radical inguinal orchiectomy with high ligation of the spermatic cord is the definitive diagnostic and initial therapeutic step for management of testicular cancer in most cases.
- Partial orchiectomy should be considered only in selected patients with a polar mass measuring 2 cm or less and an abnormal or absent contralateral testicle.
- In the rare patient whose disease is sufficiently advanced/symptomatic to warrant immediate initiation of systemic chemotherapy, delayed orchiectomy should be performed given the potential for residual disease.

RETROPERITONEAL LYMPH NODE DISSECTION

All GCT subtypes demonstrate a propensity for predictable lymphatic spread to the retroperitoneum. Choriocarcinoma has also demonstrated a predilection for hematogenous spread. Depending on the presence and bulk of retroperitoneal disease and STM status, RPLND may be incorporated into management of the testicular GCT in the primary or postchemotherapy setting. **Although the approaches and techniques of primary RPLND and PC-RPLND are similar, these are fundamentally distinct surgeries. The rationale for primary RPLND is that, in contrast to most malignancies, testicular GCT is surgically curable in most patients with low-volume regional (retroperitoneal) lymphatic metastases. Conversely, the rationale for performing PC-RPLND in patients with residual retroperitoneal masses is that unresected teratoma and/or viable malignancy predispose the patient to disease progression and death.** In this section, we discuss similar technical considerations and exposure for primary RPLND and PC-RPLND. However, the surgeon must be aware of the aforementioned basic philosophical distinctions between these two surgeries. The retroperitoneal lymph node regions are illustrated in Figure 35-1.

The following list provides definitions of the different subtypes of RPLND that are discussed throughout this chapter:

- **Primary RPLND**—RPLND performed after orchiectomy for CS I or low-volume CS II NSGCT with normal postorchiectomy STMs.
- **PC-RPLND**—RPLND performed after completion of induction systemic chemotherapy. This procedure is generally performed when there is a residual retroperitoneal mass and normal postchemotherapy STMs. At some centers, PC-RPLND is performed even when there is a clinical complete remission (CR) to chemotherapy (discussed later).
- **Salvage PC-RPLND**—PC-RPLND performed after completion of induction and salvage (standard or high-dose) chemotherapy.

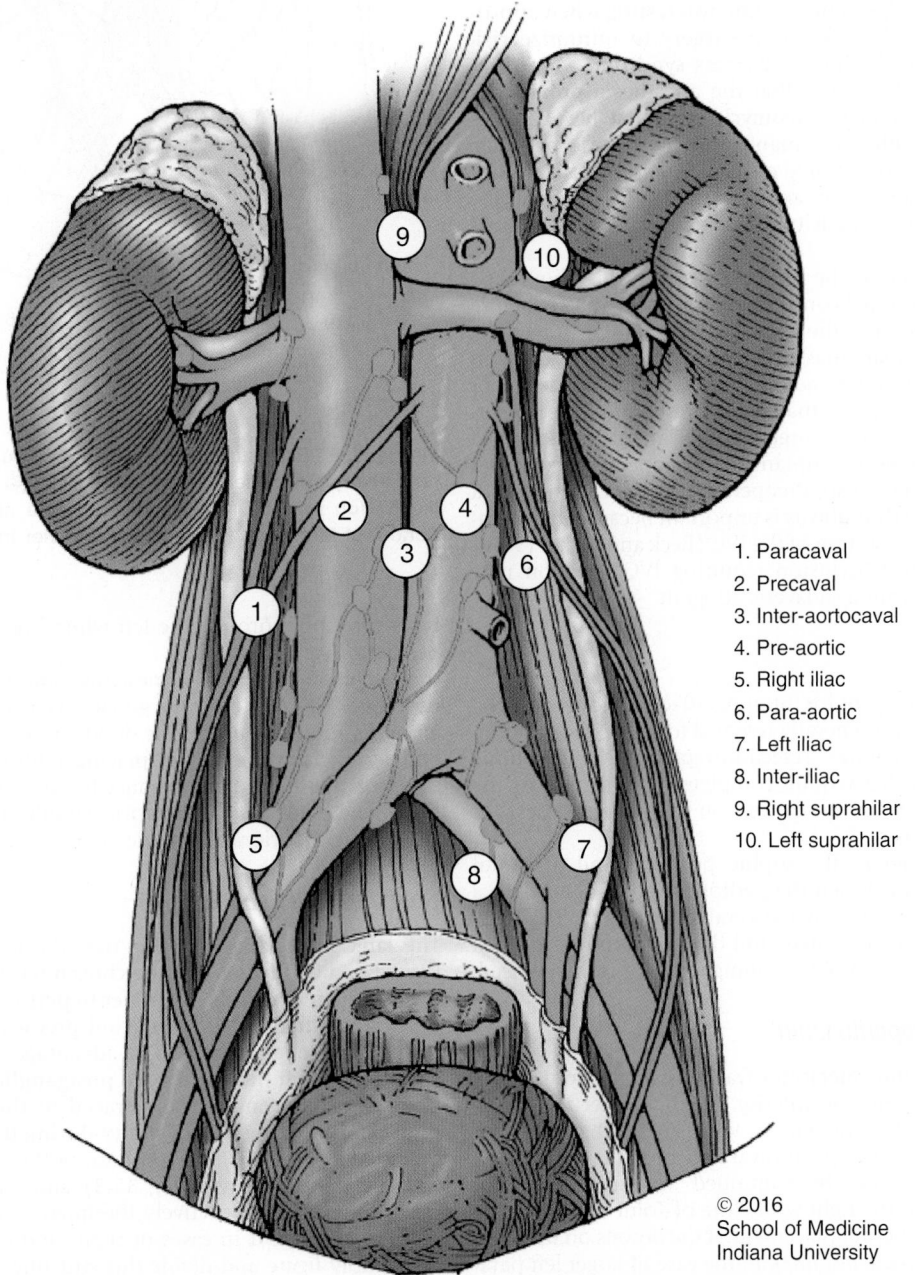

1. Paracaval
2. Precaval
3. Inter-aortocaval
4. Pre-aortic
5. Right iliac
6. Para-aortic
7. Left iliac
8. Inter-iliac
9. Right suprahilar
10. Left suprahilar

© 2016
School of Medicine
Indiana University

Figure 35-1. Retroperitoneal lymph node regions. (© 2016 Section of Medical Illustration in the Office of Visual Media at the Indiana University School of Medicine. Published by Elsevier Inc. All rights reserved.)

- **Desperation PC-RPLND**—PC-RPLND performed despite STM elevation.
- **Reoperative RPLND**—PC-RPLND performed in a patient who has undergone prior primary RPLND or PC-RPLND.
- **Resection of late relapse**—PC-RPLND performed for retroperitoneal recurrence 24 months or later after CR to primary therapy (which may or may not have included RPLND).

Preoperative Planning

We do not recommend bowel preparation or dietary modifications before RPLND. STMs should be checked within 7 to 10 days of surgery. Increased quantities of blood products should be considered for patients requiring more complex resections. Preoperative sperm banking should be offered to patients who desire future paternity if retroperitoneal masses are in the path of the postganglionic sympathetic nerve fibers. **It is important for the urologist to have a medical oncology partner who possesses the clinical ability to assess bleomycin toxicity, to limit the dose when necessary and to obtain pulmonary function testing when appropriate before sending the patient to surgery to minimize risk of postoperative acute respiratory distress syndrome. Additionally, the surgeon should ensure that the anesthesia provider is aware of any prior receipt of bleomycin and that he or she is familiar and comfortable with management of these patients.** Specifically, low fraction of inspired oxygen (FIO_2) and conservative intraoperative fluid resuscitation are important in minimizing the risk of postoperative lung toxicity (Goldiner et al, 1978; Donat and Levy, 1998).

Preoperative CT scan of the abdomen and pelvis should be thoroughly reviewed at initial consultation and immediately before surgery. A current CT scan of the chest is also required in patients with a history of pulmonary masses, planned concurrent resection of thoracic disease, or other radiographic/serologic evidence of disease progression. We prefer that preoperative imaging be performed within 6 weeks of that surgery date. Careful inspection of imaging can usually prevent unplanned intraoperative consultations of other surgical specialists. Preoperative identification of total inferior vena cava (IVC) thrombosis is important because the operation is made simpler by resection of the IVC (Beck and Lalka, 1998). Patients with incomplete occlusion requiring IVC resection may require reconstruction with a cadaveric allograft.

Surgical Technique

An orogastric tube is sufficient for intraoperative gastric decompression. Nasogastric tubes are generally reserved for patients with duodenal invasion that requires resection/repair or high-volume retroperitoneal masses that require complete mobilization of the mesentery and placement of the bowels on the patient's chest for the duration of the surgery.

The patient is placed in the supine position, and a ventral midline incision is made. When the peritoneal cavity is entered, a thorough inspection of abdominal viscera is performed. The falciform ligament is identified, ligated, and divided to minimize risk of hepatic retraction injury. A self-retaining retractor is then placed.

Exposure of the Retroperitoneum

For smaller paracaval and interaortocaval masses, the root of the mesentery is opened from the inferior tip of the cecum to the medial aspect of the inferior mesenteric vein (Fig. 35-2, *green dotted line*). In the case of large interaortocaval and/or paracaval masses, the mesenteric incision can be continued around the inferior portion of the cecum to the right white line of Toldt and up to the foramen of Winslow to permit placement of the bowels on the chest (see Fig. 35-2, *right purple dotted line*). In the case of larger left paraaortic masses, the inferior mesenteric vein is often ligated and divided to improve exposure of the left retroperitoneum (see Fig. 35-2, *left purple dotted line*). Alternatively, in the case of a modified left template dissection for CS I disease, the para-aortic packet can

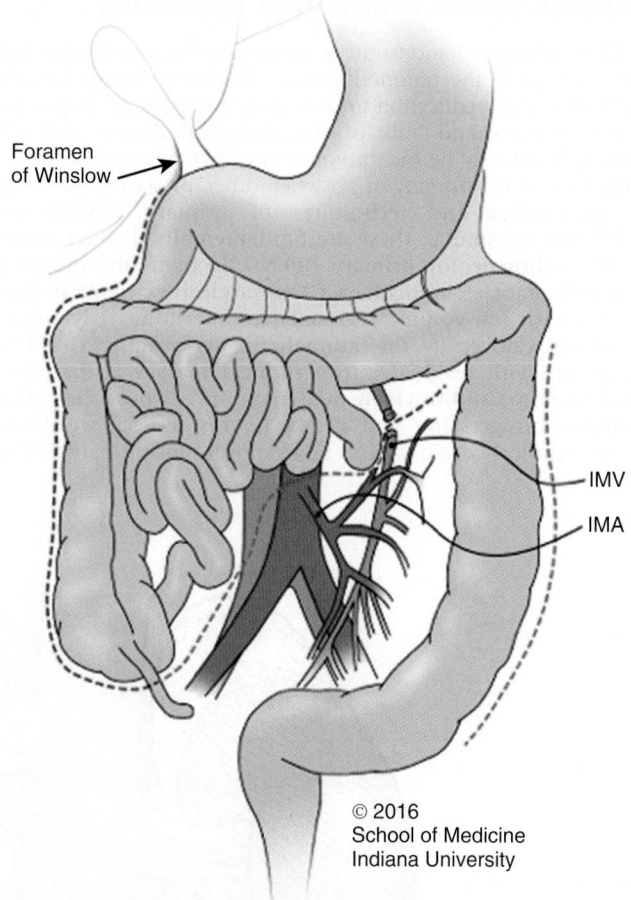

Foramen of Winslow

IMV

IMA

© 2016
School of Medicine
Indiana University

Figure 35-2. Exposure of the retroperitoneum. IMA, inferior mesenteric artery; IMV, inferior mesenteric vein. (© 2016 Section of Medical Illustration in the Office of Visual Media at the Indiana University School of Medicine. Published by Elsevier Inc. All rights reserved.)

be approached through the left white line of Toldt (see Fig. 35-2, *red dotted line*).

The plane between the mesentery and the retroperitoneal fat is developed by identifying the gonadal vein and developing the plane along its anterior surface. The duodenum is dissected off of the IVC and left renal vein. Before placing retractors in this region, the superior mesenteric artery must be identified (usually by palpation). The blades of the retractors should then be placed on either side of the superior mesenteric artery.

Split and Roll Technique

The large lymphatics coursing over the left renal vein should be ligated and divided. **When the chosen template includes splitting over both great vessels, we prefer to perform the split on the aorta first rather than the IVC to avoid precaval right-sided accessory lower pole renal arteries. The advantage of performing the IVC split first is that the right-sided postganglionic sympathetic nerve fibers can be identified and traced to the superior hypogastric plexus minimizing risk of injury during the aortic split.** The split is started at the 12 o'clock position of the aorta, immediately inferior to the left renal vein (Fig. 35-3), and continued caudally taking care to identify prospectively the inferior mesenteric artery (IMA) and (1) preserve it in cases of right modified template RPLND or (2) doubly ligate and divide this structure to expose the left paraaortic region in cases of full bilateral dissection. If a nerve-sparing technique is to be performed, the split should be stopped at the IMA, and postganglionic sympathetic fibers should be identified before proceeding caudally.

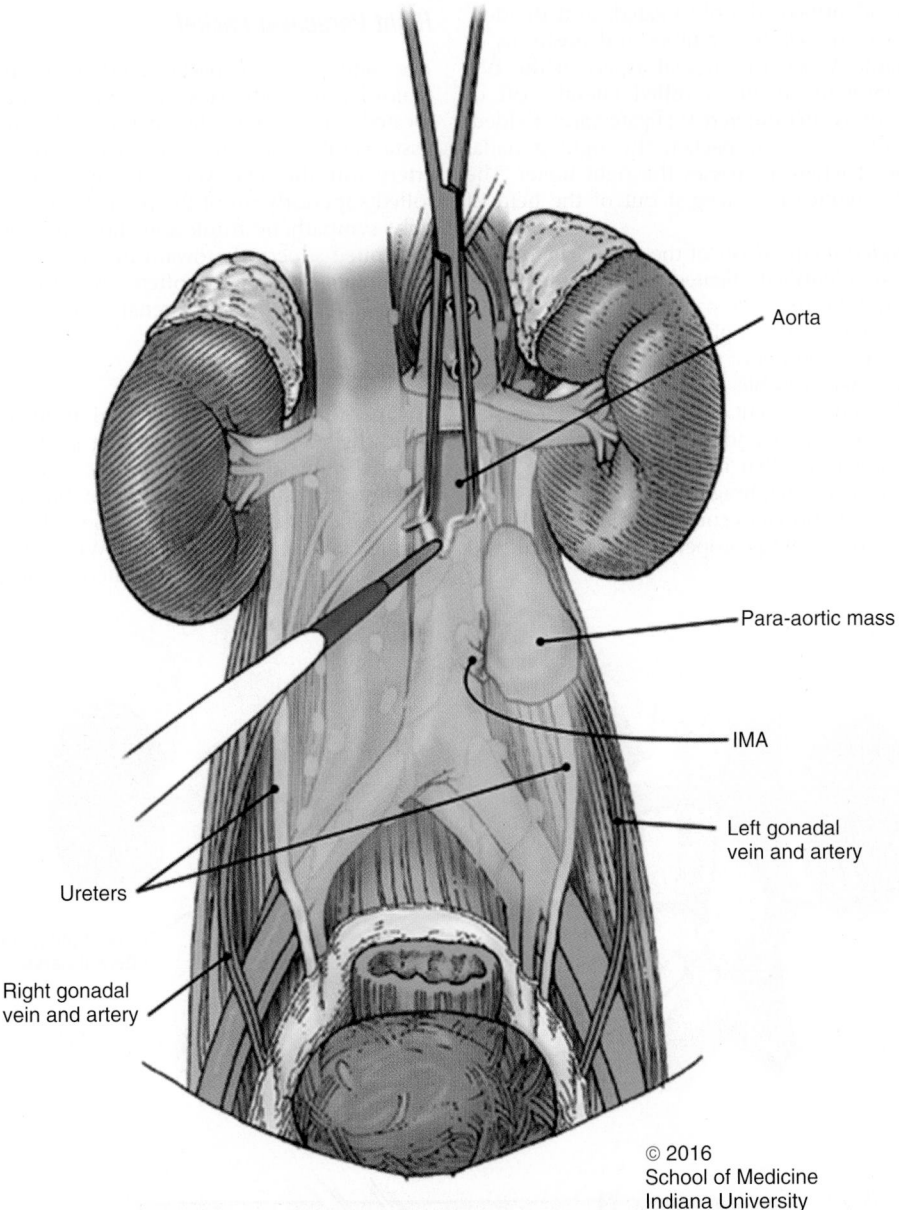

Aorta

Para-aortic mass

IMA

Left gonadal
vein and artery

Ureters

Right gonadal
vein and artery

© 2016
School of Medicine
Indiana University

Figure 35-3. The split-and-roll technique. IMA, inferior mesenteric artery. (© 2016 Section of Medical Illustration in the Office of Visual Media at the Indiana University School of Medicine. Published by Elsevier Inc. All rights reserved.)

Left Para-aortic Packet

As mentioned previously, the left para-aortic packet can be approached laterally through the left white line of Toldt or medially through the mesenteric root depending on which template is used. The left gonadal vein is doubly ligated and divided where it crosses the left ureter. The ureter is swept laterally and placed behind a retractor to minimize risk of subsequent injury. The split is continued down the 12 o'clock position of the aorta and left common iliac artery until the left ureter is reached. The lymphatic tissue is rolled laterally off of the aorta and left common iliac artery. The three left-sided lumbar arteries located between the renal hilum and aortic bifurcation are identified, doubly ligated, and divided.

The packet is rolled inferiorly off of the left renal vein. The left gonadal and lumbar vein (when present) are doubly ligated and divided where they drain into the left renal vein. The lateral aspect of the packet is dissected off of the lower pole of the kidney and ureter.

The caudal extent of the packet is rolled superiorly off of the posterior body wall. The left genitofemoral nerve and sympathetic

trunk should be identified and preserved when possible. The lumbar veins and body wall ends of the divided lumbar arteries should be identified and controlled. The packet is rolled up to the crus of the diaphragm. Lymphatics should be ligated as they course through the crus and into the retrocrural region. When the para-aortic resection is complete, tension on the ureteral retractor should be released to prevent prolonged ischemia.

Interaortocaval Packet

If a right-sided nerve-sparing technique is to be performed, the IVC split and roll is performed next. Otherwise, the medial side of the aorta can be controlled first. The IVC split is performed from the renal hilum to the crossover of the right common iliac artery where it is continued inferolaterally until the right ureter is reached. The right gonadal vein is doubly ligated and divided at the IVC. The lymphatic tissue is rolled medially off of the IVC. The nerves are visible running obliquely along the lateral edge of the packet as it is peeled off the medial border of the IVC. The lumbar veins located between the renal hilum and the common iliac veins are identified, doubly ligated, and divided. In contrast to the lumbar arteries, the number and positions of the veins are unpredictable. When the medial aspect of the IVC has been controlled, lymphatic tissue is rolled laterally off of the IVC, and any lumbar veins encountered are ligated and divided. Before harvesting the interaortocaval packet, the right gonadal vein is ligated and divided where it crosses the right ureter. The ureter is placed behind a retractor to keep it out of the field of dissection.

Lymphatic tissue is rolled medially off of the aorta. The medial three lumbar arteries are identified, ligated, and divided (Fig. 35-4C). The interaortocaval lymph node packet is harvested off of the anterior spinous ligament. The right sympathetic trunk is encountered at the right lateral border of the interaortocaval packet and should be preserved when possible. As the packet is rolled off of the anterior spinous ligament, the cut ends of the lumbar vessels should be controlled as they enter and exit the body wall. The superior aspect of the packet is rolled inferiorly off of the renal vessels exposing the crus of the diaphragm. Taking care to avoid injury to the renal artery, the lymphatics coursing into the retrocrural region must be ligated to prevent postoperative lymph leak and chylous ascites.

Right Paracaval Packet

The right paracaval packet tends to be the smallest of the three major lymph node packets because the right kidney and ureter are located very close to the lateral border of the IVC. The lymphatic tissue is rolled laterally and superiorly off of the right common iliac artery until the crossover of the right ureter is reached. The tissue is rolled superiorly off of the psoas fascia, taking care to preserve the right sympathetic trunk and the genitofemoral nerve. This roll is continued superiorly toward the right renal hilum and crus of the diaphragm. This packet often tapers to nothing and crosses under the IVC before the actual renal hilum is reached.

Gonadal Vein

The peritoneal lining is opened immediately over the gonadal vein. The ureter should be swept posteriorly off of the vein. The gonadal vein is placed on gentle traction and bluntly dissected down to the internal ring. If the orchiectomy was performed properly, the distal cut end of the gonadal vein and suture ligature should be easily retrievable. When the left gonadal vein is approached through the mesenteric root, it must be passed under

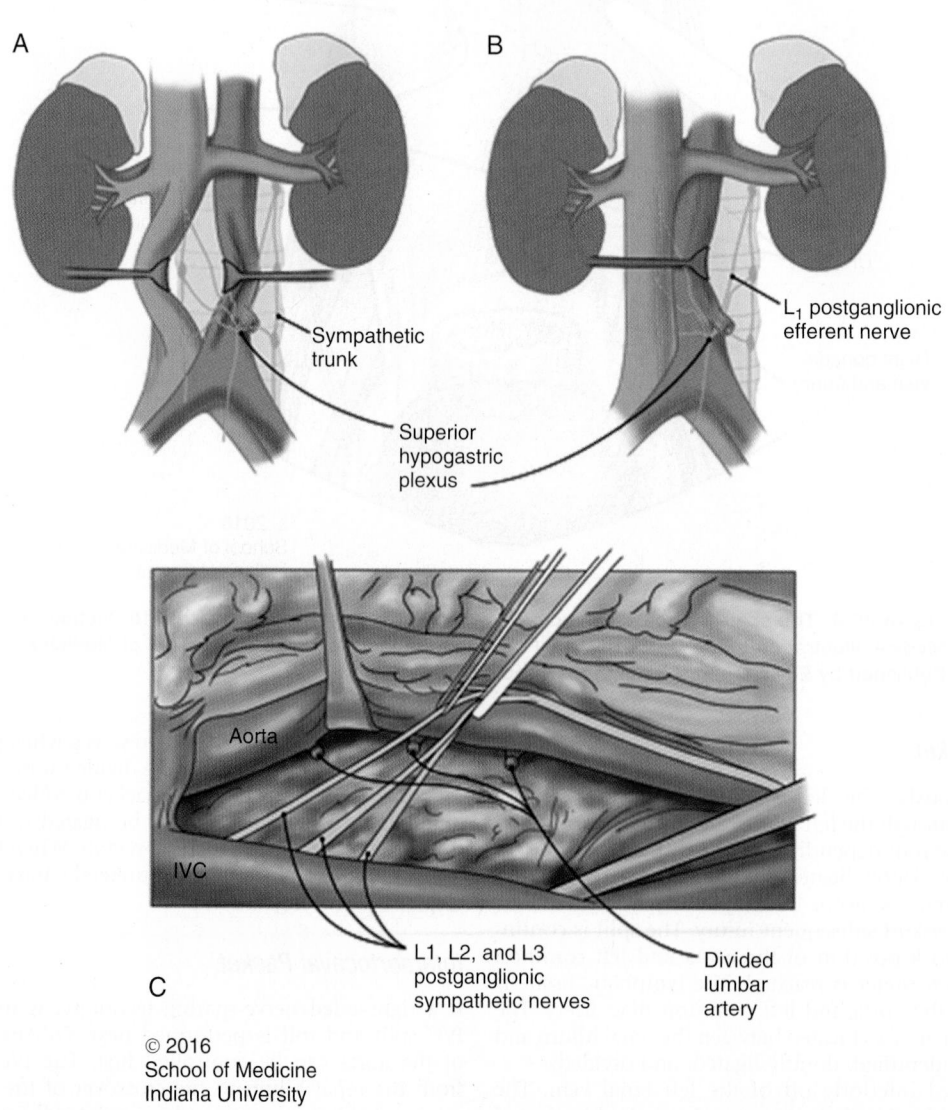

© 2016
School of Medicine
Indiana University

Figure 35-4. Nerve-sparing technique. A, Location of right-sided postganglionic sympathetic nerves. **B,** Location of left-sided postganglionic sympathetic nerves. **C,** Right-sided nerve-sparing technique with ligated lumbar arteries. IVC, inferior vena cava. (© 2016 Section of Medical Illustration in the Office of Visual Media at the Indiana University School of Medicine. Published by Elsevier Inc. All rights reserved.)

the mesentery of the sigmoid colon before it is resected down to the left internal inguinal ring.

Nerve-Sparing Technique

The anatomy of the four postganglionic efferent sympathetic fibers (L1 through L4) involved in antegrade ejaculation demonstrates significant variability from patient to patient. The L2 and L3 fibers are usually fused. Although the L2 through L4 fibers tend to take a more anterior course along the aorta and common iliac vessels, the L1 fiber takes a more shallow, caudal, and oblique course, exiting the sympathetic trunk near the level of the ipsilateral renal hilum. An intraoperative photograph of the bilateral nerve-sparing technique is shown in Figure 35-5.

The left-sided postganglionic sympathetic nerves are first identified as they course along the lateral border of the aorta and left common iliac artery and onto the anterior surface of these vessels immediately caudal to the IMA (see Fig. 35-4B). A Kittner sponge can be used to sweep the fatty connective tissue gently away revealing the shiny off-white nerve fibers running obliquely over the aorta and joining the contralateral postganglionic fibers in the superior hypogastric plexus. Fibers can be tagged with vessel loops to provide continued gentle traction as they are dissected to their origins at the sympathetic trunk. Alternatively, the left sympathetic trunk can be identified first distal to the level of the IMA and traced cranially until the postganglionic fibers are sequentially encountered.

The right-sided postganglionic nerve fibers are best identified as the precaval and interaortocaval lymphatic tissue is rolled medially off of the IVC. The postganglionic fibers can be seen coursing obliquely in an anterior and inferior direction toward the superior hypogastric plexus (see Figs. 35-4A and 35-5). These can be cleared of overlying tissue using a Kittner sponge. As described previously, the individual fibers should be encircled with vessel loops to place them on traction as they are traced down to their origins in the right sympathetic trunk.

When the nerve fibers have been dissected free for the entirety of their courses through the RPLND template, the lymphatic packets

around the fibers should be dissected. The specimen must be sequentially passed through the web of postganglionic fibers as it is released from the body wall. Care must be taken to avoid injuring the fibers during specimen harvest and obtaining hemostasis. The nerve fibers often exit the sympathetic trunks in close proximity to the lumbar vessels, which puts them at particular risk of collateral injury if lumbar bleeding is encountered.

Closure and Postoperative Care

When the RPLND is complete, the resection bed should be carefully inspected for any residual lymphatic tissue, lymph leaks, and hemostasis. Lymph leaks can be controlled with placement of metal clips. The abdomen should be copiously irrigated with warm sterile water in an attempt to discover any bleeding vessels in spasm. The posterior parietal peritoneum should be reapproximated with a simple running 2-0 chromic suture. This maneuver is designed to prevent the small bowel from scarring to the great vessels and retroperitoneum. Additionally, in the setting of full mobilization of the root and ascending colon, reapproximation of the mesentery is thought to decrease the risk of volvulus. When the retroperitoneum is closed, the small bowel should be run for its entire length to rule out unrecognized retractor injuries. Additionally, the liver, colon, and stomach should be inspected. Surgical drains are not routinely placed. However, large-volume retroperitoneal, retrocrural, or duodenal resections may require a drain. We leave a Penrose drain for large-volume resections, given the propensity of postoperative abdominal third spacing. This drain is typically removed after the patient has resumed a regular diet and drainage remains serous and less than 100 mL for 24 hours.

In the absence of bowel repair/anastomoses, patients are given sips of ice chips on the evening of surgery. On postoperative day 1, patients are advanced to unlimited clear liquids, and they are encouraged to spend most of the day in a chair and ambulating. If patients tolerate clear liquids, they are advanced to a regular diet and transitioned off of intravenous pain medications on postoperative day 2. Patients are typically discharged between postoperative days 3 and 5 depending on how quickly they are able to tolerate a

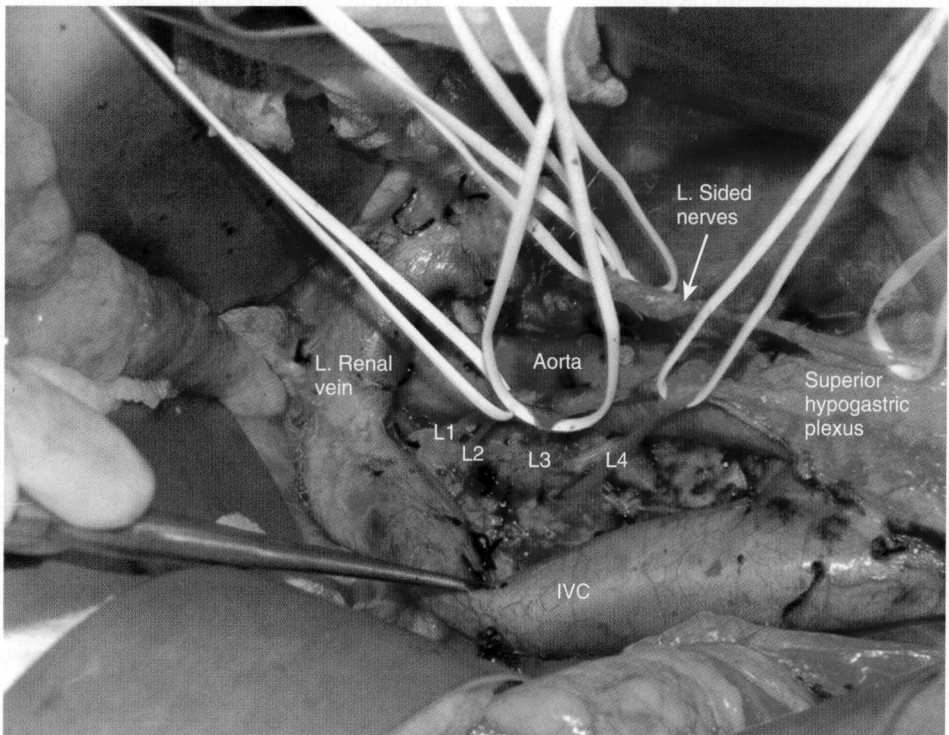

Figure 35-5. Bilateral nerve-sparing technique. IVC, inferior vena cava; **L.,** left; **L1 through L4, right-sided postganglionic sympathetic nerves.**

regular diet. Patients undergoing larger resections tend to have longer inpatient stays.

AUXILIARY PROCEDURES

The following discussion of auxiliary procedures applies to PC-RPLND because these procedures are rarely, if ever, required during primary RPLND. The incidence of auxiliary procedures at the time of PC-RPLND ranges from 24% to 45% in the literature (Beck et al, 2009; Heidenreich et al, 2009; Winter et al, 2012). The most common auxiliary procedure is a nephrectomy, followed by vascular reconstruction or resection. As the volume of retroperitoneal disease increases, so does the likelihood of requiring resection of adjacent organs and/or structures.

Nephrectomy

Nephrectomy at the time of PC-RPLND is the most commonly performed auxiliary procedure. The incidence of nephrectomy at PC-RPLND ranges from 5% to 31% (Base and Navratil, 1984; Beck and Lalka, 1998; Nash et al, 1998; Stephenson et al, 2006; Djaladat et al, 2012; Cary et al, 2013). Table 35-1 summarizes studies reporting on simultaneous nephrectomy and associated risk factors.

Recognition of preoperative risk factors associated with nephrectomy at PC-RPLND is vital for surgical planning and patient counseling. **Nephrectomy is usually needed in high-risk settings such as salvage RPLND, desperation RPLND, resection of late relapse, or reoperative RPLND. Additional risk factors include retroperitoneal mass size and location of primary tumor** (i.e., left vs. right testicle). In the Indiana University study, men with retroperitoneal mass size greater than 10 cm had a ninefold increase in odds of nephrectomy compared with men with retroperitoneal mass less than 2 cm. Left-sided primary tumors with left paraaortic retroperitoneal masses had significantly increased odds of nephrectomy compared with right-sided tumors (odds ratio 5.44, $P < .0001$) (Cary et al, 2013). Other reports supported this finding (Heidenreich et al, 2009; Djaladat et al, 2012). This finding is due to the fact that left-sided primary tumors metastasize to the paraaortic region near the renal hilum compared with metastasis of right-sided primary tumors to the interaortocaval landing zone.

It is important to consider postoperative renal function after nephrectomy because these patients may require postoperative adjuvant chemotherapy. Studies from Indiana University and Memorial Sloan-Kettering Cancer Center (MSKCC) reported a decline in renal function after nephrectomy (Nash et al, 1998; Stephenson et al; 2006). However, this decreased renal function neither resulted in the need for renal replacement therapy nor compromised subsequent adjuvant or salvage chemotherapy when necessary. Despite changes in renal function, most patients are able to tolerate subsequent chemotherapy if needed and avoid renal replacement therapy.

Major Vascular Reconstruction

Inferior Vena Cava Resection

Most cases requiring IVC resection have bulky stage disease (stage IIb or higher). **The incidence of IVC resection reported in the literature ranges from 5% to 10%** (Beck and Lalka, 1998; Nash et al, 1998; Winter et al, 2012). In 1991, Donohue and colleagues reported 40 patients who underwent IVC resection without reconstruction. In this study, the three indications for caval resection were necessity for tumor clearance (38%), vena caval scar occlusion (14%), and vena caval tumor thrombus (48%). The decision for en bloc caval resection was justified by the adverse nodal pathology, which included active cancer in 63% and teratoma in 31% of the specimens. For patients with lower extremity edema and imaging concerning for IVC compression/occlusion, venacavography, ultrasonography, or magnetic resonance imaging is helpful to assess for flow through the IVC and guide intraoperative decision making.

A German study reported on 34 patients with IVC interventions during PC-RPLND (Winter et al, 2012). There were 23 complete IVC resections performed with four patients having an IVC reconstruction using a polytetrafluoroethylene graft. The authors found that retroperitoneal mass size ($P < .0001$) and International Germ Cell Cancer Collaborative Group (IGCCCG) intermediate/poor risk ($P = .005$) were associated with the need for an IVC intervention on univariate analysis. The probability for an IVC intervention was 20.4% for patients with retroperitoneal mass size 5 cm or larger and IGCCCG intermediate/poor risk. Conversely, patients with retroperitoneal mass size smaller than 5 cm and good-risk disease had only a 2.7% probability for an IVC intervention.

Routine reconstruction of the vena cava after resection is not required. Data on 65 infrarenal IVC resections without reconstruction by Beck and Lalka (1998) support this approach. This study

TABLE 35-1 Risk Factors and Indications for Nephrectomy at Postchemotherapy Retroperitoneal Lymph Node Dissection*

STUDY	PATIENTS UNDERGOING Nx, N (INCIDENCE %)	TIME PERIOD	INDICATIONS/RISK FACTORS
Cary et al, 2013	265 (14.8)	1980-1997	RP mass size Year of surgery Primary tumor site Salvage chemotherapy Elevated markers
Djaladat et al, 2012	12 (14.1)	2004-2010	Left-sided hilar mass
Heidenreich et al, 2009	7 (4.6)	1999-2007	Encasement of renal vessels/ureter
Stephenson et al, 2006	32 (5)	1989-2002	Salvage RPLND Desperation RPLND Redo RPLND Late relapse
Nash et al, 1998	162 (19)	1974-1994	Involvement of renal structures Venous thrombus Poor renal function Combination of above

*Not all studies performed formal statistical analyses for predictive risk factors because of small sample size.
Nx, nephrectomy; RP, retroperitoneal; RPLND, retroperitoneal lymph node dissection.

evaluated the long-term sequelae of IVC resection using a survey developed by an international consensus conference on chronic venous disease held by the American Venous Forum (Beebe et al, 1996). The median follow-up for these patients was 89 months. Of patients, 75% had a disability score of 0 to 1 (none or mild disability). Only one patient had the highest possible disability score. Although these patients are at higher risk for chylous ascites and other periprocedural complications (Baniel et al, 1993), long-term venous congestion seems to be less of an issue; this is particularly true if there is complete occlusion with development of collateral circulation present preoperatively. Slow progressive retroperitoneal tumor growth with accompanying desmoplastic reaction to chemotherapy likely results in a gradual occlusion of caval blood flow allowing for adequate development of venous collateral circulation. The development of this collateral venous return likely results in less morbidity from caval resection in patients with testis cancer compared to patients with acute IVC occlusion.

Aortic Resection and Reconstruction

In some cases, retroperitoneal tumor encasement of the aorta requires en bloc aortic resection with reconstruction to remove the retroperitoneal mass adequately. **When this clinical situation occurs, it is crucial to alert additional surgical teams (i.e., vascular surgery) preoperatively to ensure successful clinical outcomes.** It is ideal to anticipate the need for aortic replacement preoperatively to allow proper patient counseling and time to coordinate between surgical services. An aortic tube graft is most commonly used for reconstruction; however, an aortobi-iliac graft may be used depending on the extent of tumor involvement.

Several studies evaluated the indications for aortic resection and its morbidity. In 2001, Beck and colleagues reported 15 patients who underwent aortic replacement during PC-RPLND. **Over a 30-year span involving more than 1200 patients, approximately 1% required this procedure.** Two thirds of these patients had received at least one course of salvage chemotherapy and/or had elevated STMs at the time of surgery. The indication for aortic replacement in these patients was tumor fixation to the aorta, with en bloc resection of the aorta deemed necessary for complete tumor removal. The retroperitoneal pathology in this group revealed active cancer in 80% and teratoma in 20%. At a median follow-up of 34 months, 33% of these patients were disease-free. Given the chemoresistant nature of the disease and bulky tumor burden surrounding the aorta in most of these patients with advanced GCT, aortic resection is a worthwhile undertaking and may provide a therapeutic benefit in a significant proportion of patients. In a multi-institutional German study of 402 patients who underwent PC-RPLND, 6 patients required aortic resection with graft placement (Winter et al, 2012). Although not statistically significant, there was a trend toward aortic replacement occurring more commonly in patients with residual mass size 5 cm or larger and having IGCCCG intermediate/poor risk.

When the decision for aortic resection has been made, the principles of the operation do not change substantially. The IVC should be dissected away from the mass and aorta using the split-and-roll technique with division of lumbar veins. The left ureter should be freed from the retroperitoneal mass. If the tumor does not encroach on the left renal hilum, this is also dissected free. The vascular surgery team assists with this dissection to ensure adequate length of the aorta cranial and caudal to the tumor, which allows for proximal and distal vascular control and ease of graft anastomoses. The aorta is cross-clamped and resected en bloc with the retroperitoneal mass. Lumbar arteries are divided during this process. Before cross clamping, the patient is usually administered intravenous heparin to minimize the risk of arterial thrombosis. The graft is sewn into place using standard vascular surgery principles.

Hepatic Resections

Patients with hepatic involvement at initial presentation fall into the IGCCCG poor-risk classification. Based on the initial 1997

publication of the IGCCCG risk stratification scheme, patients in this risk category have a 5-year overall survival (OS) of 48%. Patients with liver metastasis represent approximately 6% of patients with advanced GCTs (International Germ Cell Consensus Classification, 1997).

Jacobsen and colleagues (2010) evaluated the concordance between retroperitoneal and liver histology in patients who largely underwent simultaneous resections. The authors identified 59 patients with advanced GCT who underwent a liver resection. Of all hepatic specimens, 73% contained necrosis only, and the histologic concordance between retroperitoneal and liver necrosis was 94%. The authors concluded that management of hepatic lesions must be individualized, but that observation may be warranted for liver lesions requiring complicated hepatic surgery. Conversely, other groups found the histologic concordance between the retroperitoneum and liver less reliable (Hartmann et al, 2005; You et al, 2009). Nevertheless, necrosis is the most common histology found in the liver after chemotherapy in these studies. **Observation of liver lesions is warranted in some cases, particularly when hepatic involvement may require extensive resection.** Use of intraoperative frozen-section analysis of core biopsy specimens of liver lesions may provide additional information when deciding whether or not to resect hepatic lesions.

Pelvic Resections

Pelvic lymph node dissection is rarely needed during PC-RPLND. The largest series to date on pelvic metastases among patients undergoing RPLND was presented as an abstract on 137 (5%) of 2722 patients treated from 1990 to 2009. Mean pelvic mass size was 6.5 cm. The pelvic mass was managed by pelvic excision alone in 28%, pelvic excision with primary RPLND in 3%, and pelvic excision with PC-RPLND in 69%. Pelvic pathology revealed necrosis, sarcoma, teratoma, and active cancer in 16%, 5%, 55%, and 24%. **Factors associated with pelvic metastases were initial clinical stage, extragonadal primary, and prior groin surgery** (e.g., inguinal hernia repair) (all $P < .001$) (Mehan et al, 2011).

MSKCC reported their findings on 44 (2%) patients who underwent pelvic lymph node dissection during the course of management (Alanee et al, 2013). Mean pelvic mass size was 4 cm. Pelvic histology in this series revealed active cancer in 19 (43%) and teratoma in 17 (39%). No patient reported a history of prior scrotal or inguinal surgery. Overall, the need for pelvic lymph node dissection is rare; approximately 80% of patients with a pelvic mass had either teratoma or active cancer on final histology warranting resection in patients with pelvic disease.

Management of Supradiaphragmatic Disease

Approximately 10% to 20% of patients with a diagnosis of testicular cancer have evidence of supradiaphragmatic disease at presentation or go on to manifest intrathoracic spread at some point in the course of their illness (Kesler et al, 2011). Pulmonary metastases of testicular GCT represent disease spread via the hematogenous route, whereas mediastinal and cervical metastases represent lymphatic spread. Approximately 80% of mediastinal metastases are confined to the lower (retrocrural) and middle visceral mediastinum (Kesler et al, 2011). GCT found in the anterior mediastinum usually indicates a mediastinal primary GCT.

Studies evaluating comparative histology of retroperitoneal and thoracic disease have demonstrated pathologic discordance ranging from 25% to 50%. Most of these patients harbor the more aggressive pathology in the retroperitoneum (Gerl et al, 1994; Gels et al, 1997; Steyerberg et al, 1997; Besse et al, 2009). Steyerberg and colleagues (1997) reported on a multi-institutional study of 215 patients undergoing thoracotomy after cisplatin-based induction chemotherapy in an attempt to predict thoracic histology. RPLND histology was a strong predictor of histology at thoracotomy with 89% of patients with necrosis at RPLND having necrosis only in the chest. **It is generally recommended that if these resections are to be staged, RPLND should be performed first because the finding** of retroperitoneal necrosis/fibrosis may spare select patients unnecessary thoracic resection. Determining if and when to proceed with resection of thoracic disease in the setting of retroperitoneal necrosis is a decision that needs to be based on the expertise of a multidisciplinary testicular cancer team that has extensive experience in dealing with this disease. Kesler and colleagues (2011) recommended resection of any residual postchemotherapy thoracic mass larger than 1 cm. The exception to this rule would be a patient with extensive residual masses requiring a potentially morbid resection in the setting of necrosis only at RPLND.

Resection of Retrocrural Disease

Description of the surgical approach to most supradiaphragmatic disease is beyond the scope of this chapter. However, the surgical approach to and timing of resection of retrocrural disease is often intimately related to RPLND. The retrocrural space presents a surgical challenge given its anatomic location, and surgical approaches to retrocrural disease have evolved over time. Most of these cases are performed in combination with the thoracic surgery team. At Indiana University, early efforts employed a thoracoabdominal incision or a separate midline laparotomy and posterior thoracotomy. A more recent technique used for residual lower retrocrural disease is a midline laparotomy employing a transabdominal transdiaphragmatic approach that can be performed at the same time as RPLND (Fig. 35-6). This approach was first described by Fadel and associates (2000) in 18 patients who had simultaneous resection of masses located in the retroperitoneum and lower mediastinum. The rationale for this approach was to minimize the morbidity of a thoracotomy when feasible. Kesler and colleagues (2003) published results on 268 patients with mediastinal metastases who underwent mediastinal dissection for NSGCT. A transabdominal transdiaphragmatic approach was used in 60 (13.2%) of these patients. Operative morbidity was low with three (1.1%) operative deaths in the entire cohort, which represented patients with extensive/bulky residual disease.

The timing of retrocrural resection depends in part on whether there is contiguous disease in the retroperitoneum. Generally, if small-volume retrocrural disease exists concurrently with a retroperitoneal mass, this is approached through a single transabdominal and transdiaphragmatic incision simultaneously. If large-volume retroperitoneal teratomatous disease exists requiring a prolonged surgical time for RPLND, the retrocrural and mediastinal resection can be staged. If the mediastinal disease is not contiguous, the timing of mediastinal dissection is guided in part by the pathology of the retroperitoneum. This rationale is based on studies evaluating concordance between retroperitoneal and thoracic pathology discussed earlier.

KEY POINTS: AUXILIARY PROCEDURES

- Nephrectomy is the most commonly required auxiliary procedure. It is more common with large left-sided masses and when PC-RPLND is performed in high-risk settings.
- Routine IVC reconstruction is unnecessary when en bloc resection is performed in the setting of complete or near-complete IVC occlusion.
- Given the complex vascular reconstruction required, every effort must be made preoperatively to identify patients who require en bloc aortic resection.
- Given the high incidence of necrosis, the decision to proceed with hepatic resection needs to be based on retroperitoneal pathology (when available) and predicted morbidity of hepatic resection as determined by hepatic surgical specialists.
- Pathologic discordance between retroperitoneal and thoracic disease is common, with more aggressive histology being found more commonly in the retroperitoneum. If procedures are to be staged, RPLND should be performed first.
- When patients harbor residual masses in the retroperitoneum and the retrocrural region, consideration should be given to simultaneous PC-RPLND and retrocrural resection using a transabdominal, transdiaphragmatic approach to the latter.

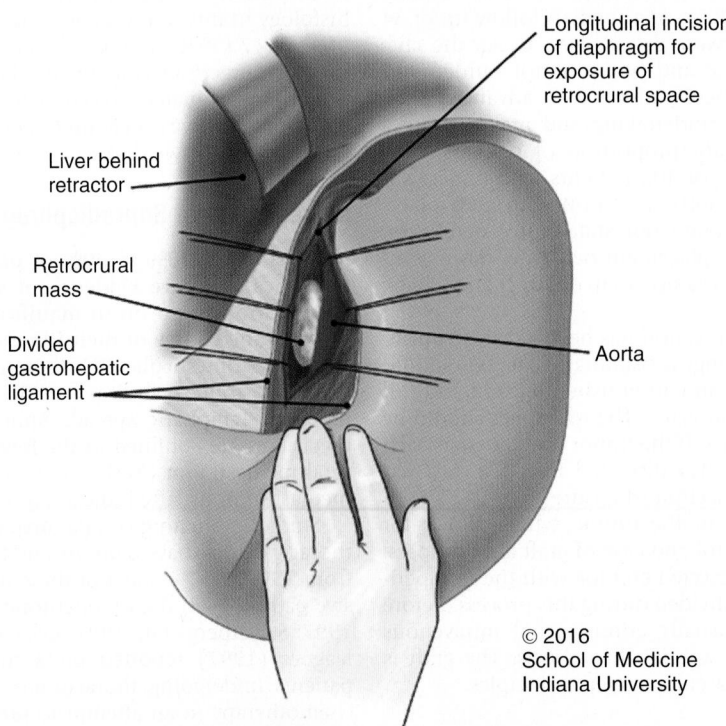

Longitudinal incision of diaphragm for exposure of retrocrural space

Liver behind retractor

Retrocrural mass

Divided gastrohepatic ligament

Aorta

© 2016
School of Medicine
Indiana University

Figure 35-6. Transabdominal, transdiaphragmatic approach to retrocrural mass. (© 2016 Section of Medical Illustration in the Office of Visual Media at the Indiana University School of Medicine. Published by Elsevier Inc. All rights reserved.)

SURGICAL DECISION MAKING

This section discusses the decision-making process involved in determining when to perform RPLND, the extent of dissection, and when to administer postoperative chemotherapy. The indications for, advantages of, and disadvantages of primary RPLND are discussed in Chapter 34 and are not repeated here.

Management of Clinical Complete Remission to Induction Chemotherapy

There is little debate that patients with disseminated testicular cancer who achieve a complete serologic remission but harbor a residual retroperitoneal mass after induction chemotherapy require PC-RPLND. However, the management of patients who achieve complete radiographic (no residual mass >1 cm) and serologic remission of metastatic GCT is controversial. Approximately 70% of men who receive cisplatin-based chemotherapy for stage II or higher testicular cancer can be expected to demonstrate complete resolution of measurable disease. Management options for these patients include observation or PC-RPLND.

Proponents of observation cite the excellent long-term survival demonstrated by patients managed nonoperatively. In a study of 141 men observed after demonstrating clinical CR to induction chemotherapy alone, Ehrlich and associates (2010) reported 15-year recurrence-free survival (RFS) of 90% and cancer-specific survival (CSS) of 97%. In a similar study of 161 patients with median 4.5-year follow-up, Kollmansberger and colleagues (2010) reported RFS of 93.8% and CSS of 100%.

Investigators at MSKCC recommended performing PC-RPLND on all patients with a history of retroperitoneal metastases even in the setting of a clinical CR because of the potential for residual microscopic disease. In 2006, Carver and coworkers reported on 532 patients undergoing PC-RPLND at MSKCC. Of 154 patients demonstrating a residual mass 1 cm or smaller on cross-sectional imaging performed after chemotherapy, 22%, 1%, and 5% demonstrated teratoma, teratoma/GCT, and GCT at PC-RPLND.

The main issue at the center of this debate is the natural history of microscopic residual teratoma. The concerns expressed by proponents of PC-RPLND in patients with clinical CR is that microscopic teratoma left in the retroperitoneum may lead to growing teratoma syndrome, late relapse, or malignant transformation to somatic-type malignancy. Proponents of observation propose that microscopic teratoma is biologically inert in most cases. Table 35-2 lists the results of three retrospective studies evaluating these two management strategies for patients with clinical CR to chemotherapy alone. Survival outcomes were excellent using either approach (Karellas et al, 2007; Ehrlich et al, 2010; Kollmannsberger et al, 2010). The two questions that remain to be answered are: (1) Does performing PC-RPLND in these patients prevent cancer-specific deaths? (2) Would the number needed to treat to prevent one death be low enough to justify this approach?

Use of Modified Templates in Primary Retroperitoneal Lymph Node Dissection

As the patterns of lymphatic spread of GCT have been defined, various RPLND templates have been proposed with the goal of balancing therapeutic efficacy with potential morbidity. Historically, RPLND involved removal of all lymphatic tissue contained in a contemporary bilateral infrahilar template in addition to resection in the interiliac region down to the bifurcation of the common iliac vessels (Ray et al, 1974). Full bilateral suprahilar dissections were performed routinely at some centers as well (Donohue et al, 1982a). Sometimes performed through a large thoracoabdominal incision, these resections were necessary to provide the best chance for durable cure because of the absence of curative chemotherapy for GCT and were associated with significant perioperative morbidity as well as rendering most patients anejaculatory (Donohue and Rowland, 1981).

In the 1970s and 1980s, the development of curative cisplatin-based chemotherapeutic regimens (Einhorn and Donohue, 1977), elucidation of distinct lymphatic spread for right-sided versus left-sided testicular tumors (Ray et al, 1974; Donohue et al, 1982b; Weissbach and Boedefeld, 1987), and description of surgical techniques to preserve the postganglionic sympathetic nerve fibers involved in seminal emission and antegrade ejaculation (Jewett et al, 1988; Colleselli et al, 1990; Donohue et al, 1990) significantly altered management of the retroperitoneum in patients with testicular GCT. In 1974, Ray and colleagues presented a series of 283 patients undergoing RPLND at MSKCC from 1944 to 1971. Dissections were predominantly infrahilar and evolved from a full bilateral dissection to a "modified bilateral" dissection as the primary landing zones of right-sided versus left-sided primaries became apparent. These modified bilateral templates were very similar to modified unilateral templates with the exception that lymphatic tissue below the IMA was routinely resected. The detailed description of distinct templates based on the laterality of the testicular primary was the first of its kind and set the stage for further refinement.

Donohue and colleagues (1982b) published a pathologic lymph node mapping study performed at Indiana University on 104 patients found to have pathologically positive nodes (pN+) at primary RPLND. Full bilateral dissections to include bilateral suprahilar dissections were performed on every patient. Investigators found that left-sided tumors were most likely to metastasize to the left para-aortic lymph nodes, whereas right-sided tumors were most likely to metastasize to interaortocaval and precaval regions. Spread to contralateral retroperitoneum and suprahilar regions was rare but increased with tumor bulk. Metastasis to the interiliac region was rare. This study confirmed the relatively predictable pattern of the lymphatic spread of testicular GCTs and provided strong pathologic evidence for the use of "modified bilateral" templates proposed by Ray and colleagues (1974) in patients with low-stage retroperitoneal disease. Omission of the contralateral retroperitoneum and interiliac regions resulted in the preservation of antegrade ejaculation in most patients. Omission of suprahilar regions decreased the risk of

---

TABLE 35-2 Management of Patients Experiencing a Clinical Complete Remission to Induction Chemotherapy

	EHRLICH ET AL, 2010	KOLLMANNSBERGER ET AL, 2010	KARELLAS ET AL, 2007
Management	Observation	Observation	PC-RPLND
No. patients	141	161	147
Follow-up (yr)	15.5	4.3	3
Good risk (%)	77	94	98
DFS (%)	91	94	97
CSS (%)	97	100	NR

CSS, cancer-specific survival; DFS, disease-free survival; NR, not reported; PC-RPLND, postchemotherapy retroperitoneal lymph node dissection.

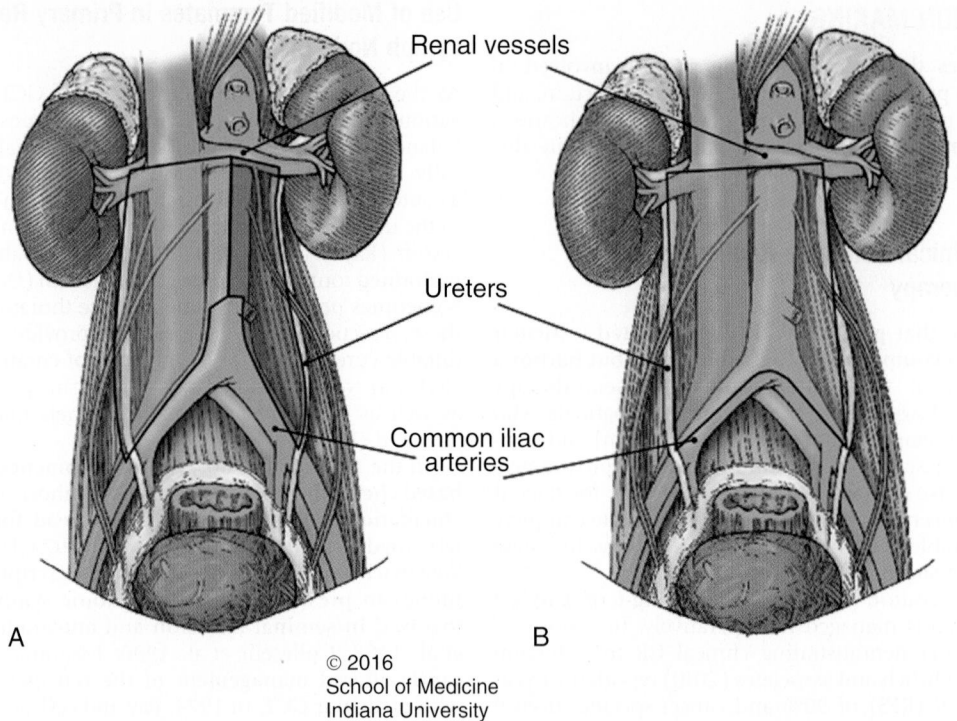

Renal vessels

Ureters

Common iliac arteries

A

B

© 2016
School of Medicine
Indiana University

Figure 35-7. Retroperitoneal lymph node dissection templates. A, Modified unilateral templates—right-sided shaded in yellow, left-sided shaded in purple. B, Modified bilateral template—shaded area. (© 2016 Section of Medical Illustration in the Office of Visual Media at the Indiana University School of Medicine. Published by Elsevier Inc. All rights reserved.)

postoperative chylous ascites, renovascular injuries, and pancreatic complications.

In 1987, Weissbach and Boedefeld reported a multi-institutional retrospective review of 214 patients with nonbulky PS II disease. The authors recommended a more reduced left-sided template including the para-aortic and upper preaortic nodes. The authors also proposed that a frozen section be sent from the primary landing zone; if the section was positive, a full bilateral infrahilar RPLND should be performed.

The end result of these template studies has been a more efficient, less morbid, and maximally effective RPLND. There is still significant debate among experts regarding the ideal extent of surgical templates. **Most experts agree that suprahilar/retrocrural and interiliac resections can safely be omitted from the standard RPLND template. However, controversy exists regarding the need to resect the contralateral retroperitoneal lymphatic tissue. The** boundaries of the modified unilateral templates and a full bilateral template are demonstrated in Figure 35-7.

Eggener and colleagues (2007b) reviewed a series of 500 patients undergoing primary RPLND for CS I or IIA testicular cancer at MSKCC. Bilateral infrahilar dissection was usually performed. The authors analyzed the 191 patients (38%) with PS II disease for the anatomic distribution of positive-node packets and applied five modified templates to these results. They reported that 3% to 23% of patients with pathologically positive nodes were found to have disease outside of the modified unilateral template depending on which one was applied. Extratemplate disease was seen more commonly with right-sided than left-sided tumors. **Given these results, the authors recommended full bilateral infrahilar nerve-sparing RPLND for patients with CS I or IIA testicular cancer.**

To date, no prospective or retrospective studies have compared the modified unilateral templates with the full bilateral templates. As discussed earlier, CSS and OS approach 100% in all series. Expanding the templates cannot be expected to improve either of these outcomes. The question is whether performance of a full bilateral infrahilar RPLND would prevent

retroperitoneal relapses that would occur after a properly performed modified unilateral template. When comparing series from centers that use the modified unilateral templates with series from centers that use the bilateral infrahilar templates, outcomes are very similar (Table 35-3) (Donohue et al, 1993a; Hermans et al, 2000; Nicolai et al, 2004; Stephenson et al, 2005). Although the MSKCC series reported an increased proportion of patients being cured by surgery alone, patients with pN2 disease routinely receive adjuvant postoperative chemotherapy at that center (Stephenson et al, 2005). In the first Indiana study, most of the node-positive patients were randomly assigned to observation versus adjuvant chemotherapy on protocol (Donohue et al, 1993a). In the more recent Indiana study, pN1 patients and most pN2 patients were observed with chemotherapy reserved for patients who experienced recurrence and pN3 patients (Hermans et al, 2000).

The appropriate boundaries of the primary RPLND template are controversial. Use of the templates recommended in the studies by Ray, Donohue, Weissbach, and Eggener and their colleagues will undoubtedly result in excellent survival outcomes. The question of which template offers greatest balance of oncologic control and minimization of morbidity remains unanswered.

Use of Modified Templates in Retroperitoneal Lymph Node Dissection after Chemotherapy

Donohue and colleagues first reported their experience performing consolidative RPLND after cisplatin-based chemotherapy in 1982. Most tumors containing teratoma and/or viable malignancy were located in their respective primary landing zones. However, given the frequent contralateral crossover in the setting of bulky disease and the inability to obtain reliable confirmation of histology intraoperatively, the authors stressed the importance of the PC-RPLND being "as complete as possible" (Donohue et al, 1982a). **The standard PC-RPLND became resection of all macroscopic disease**

TABLE 35-3 Selected Primary RPLND Series

STUDY	NO. PATIENTS	NO. pN+ (%)	RECURRENCE RATE FOR PN0 (%)	RECURRENCE RATE FOR pN+ MANAGED WITH RPLND ALONE (%)	FOLLOW-UP (yr)	CSS (%)
Donohue et al, 1993a	378	112 (29.6)	31 (12)	22 (34)	6.2	99.2
Stephenson et al, 2005	308	91 (29.5)	NR (7)	NR (34)	4.9	99.7
Hermans et al, 2000	292	66 (22.4)	23 (10.2)	7 (22.6)	3.8	100.0
Nicolai et al, 2004	322	60 (20)	NR	NR	7.2	98.8

CSS, cancer specific survival; NR, not reported; pN+, histologically postive lymph nodes; pN0, histologically negative lymph nodes; RPLND, retroperitoneal lymph node dissection.

along with a full bilateral infrahilar dissection. This approach provides excellent local control of the retroperitoneum, but is associated with significant morbidity including anejaculation in patients in whom a nerve-sparing technique is not possible.

Several groups investigated whether modified unilateral templates can safely be applied to appropriately selected patients in the postchemotherapy setting (Wood et al, 1992; Herr, 1997; Rabbani et al, 1998; Ehrlich et al, 2006; Beck et al, 2007; Carver et al, 2007a; Steiner et al, 2008; Heidenreich et al, 2009). Table 35-4 lists the results from several studies examining distribution of positive lymph nodes (teratoma and/or viable malignancy) and/or reporting outcomes after selective use of the modified unilateral templates in the postchemotherapy setting. When bilateral dissections were performed, rates of disease outside the unilateral template ranged from 18% to 32% (Carver et al, 2007a). However, rates of disease outside of the unilateral template and outside of macroscopic disease ranged from 2% to 18.6%. Variability in these percentages is likely a function of patient selection and the specific template used. Safe use of the unilateral modified templates in the postchemotherapy setting relies on selection of the correct template as well as appropriate patient selection. **Patients meeting the following criteria may be considered for modified unilateral template PC-RPLND according to data emerging from centers performing these surgeries:**

1. Well-defined lesion measuring 5 cm or less confined to the primary landing zone of the primary tumor on imaging before and after chemotherapy
2. Normal postchemotherapy STMs
3. IGCCCG good/intermediate risk

Figure 35-8 shows representative CT images for candidates for modified unilateral versus bilateral template PC-RPLND. Use of these selection criteria has resulted in in-field retroperitoneal recurrence rates of 0% to 1%, antegrade ejaculation rates of 85% to 94%, and CSS of 98% to 100% at postoperative follow-up times of 2.6 to 7.8 years (Beck et al, 2007; Steiner et al, 2008; Heidenreich et al, 2009). **Although these data are encouraging with regard to the use of the modified unilateral templates in PC-RPLND, the standard of care for patients requiring postchemotherapy resection remains resection of all macroscopic disease and a full bilateral infrahilar template RPLND. To date, there have been no prospective studies comparing outcomes in patients undergoing bilateral versus modified unilateral template PC-RPLND. If unilateral modified templates are to be used at PC-RPLND, strict adherence to the above-listed selection criteria is important.**

Adjuvant Chemotherapy for Pathologic Stage II Disease at Primary Retroperitoneal Lymph Node Dissection

Primary RPLND alone is curative in approximately 70% of patients with pN1-2 disease, and nearly all patients who experience recurrence are successfully salvaged at the time of recurrence (Donohue et al, 1993a, 1995; Nicolai et al, 2004; Stephenson et al, 2005). Evaluation of two cycles of adjuvant cisplatin-based

chemotherapeutic regimens has consistently demonstrated near-complete elimination of post-RPLND recurrences (Williams et al, 1987; Behnia et al, 2000; Kondagunta et al, 2004). **However, pro forma use of adjuvant chemotherapy for pN+ patients would result in overtreatment of approximately 70% of patients without any change in OS. Conversely, treating patients with pN1 and pN2 disease in the adjuvant rather than salvage setting spares patients with recurrent disease full-induction chemotherapy (in most cases one additional cycle of bleomycin, etoposide, Platinol or two additional cycles of etoposide, Platinol).** Investigators have attempted to determine which PS II patients are most likely to experience recurrence after primary RPLND.

Although the bulk of retroperitoneal disease encountered at primary RPLND has traditionally been viewed as a predictor of disease recurrence in the absence of adjuvant chemotherapy, this predictive value has not been consistently demonstrated when examining outcomes in patients with PS IIA and IIB disease. Most data demonstrating a direct relationship between retroperitoneal tumor burden and relapse come from early reports in which microscopic disease was separated out from low-volume macroscopic disease (both of which are now grouped together in PS IIA) (Vugrin et al, 1981; Fraley et al, 1985). When evaluating recurrences in the observation arm of a prospective randomized multi-institutional trial evaluating adjuvant cisplatin-based chemotherapy, Williams and coworkers (1987) reported recurrence rates of 40% for patients with microscopically positive nodes, 53% for patients with macroscopic nodal disease smaller than 2 cm, and 60% for patients with disease larger than 2 cm. However, this numeric trend did not reach statistical significance. Several retrospective studies reported no difference in recurrence rates when comparing PS IIA and IIB patients managed with postoperative observation (Pizzocaro and Monfardini, 1984; Donohue et al, 1993b; Nicolai et al, 2010; Al-Ahmadie et al, 2013). In two reports on patients with CS II NSGCT managed with primary RPLND, larger retroperitoneal tumor bulk was associated with increased recurrence rates (Donohue et al, 1995; Weissbach et al, 2000). It is unclear from these retrospective series what selection factors were used to determine which PS II patients were given adjuvant chemotherapy.

Additional histologic characteristics such as number and proportion of positive lymph nodes removed (Beck et al, 2005a; Al-Ahmadie et al, 2013), histology of viable GCT (Beck et al, 2005a; Al-Ahmadie et al, 2013), and extranodal extension (Beck et al, 2007; Al-Ahmadie et al, 2013) have failed to predict reliably patients who are more likely to experience recurrence when managed on post-RPLND surveillance. Patients with PS II disease demonstrating teratoma only in the retroperitoneal specimen demonstrate very low recurrence rates. Given this finding and the chemoresistance of teratoma, adjuvant chemotherapy is not recommended in these patients.

There is general agreement that compliant patients with pN1 disease can be safely observed after RPLND. The management of patients with pN2 disease is controversial. Some investigators recommend two cycles of adjuvant chemotherapy in these patients (Kondagunta and Motzer, 2007). The practice at Indiana University

TABLE 35-4 Studies Evaluating the Use of Modified Unilateral Templates in Postchemotherapy Retroperitoneal Lymph Node Dissection

STUDY	NO. PATIENTS	N+ OUTSIDE TEMPLATE (%)	N+ OUTSIDE TEMPLATE AND MACROSCOPIC DISEASE (%)	IN-FIELD RP RECURRENCE AFTER B/L RPLND (%)	IN-FIELD RP RECURRENCE AFTER U/L RPLND (%)	PRESERVATION OF EJACULATION IN TEMPLATES	FOLLOW-UP (yr)	CSS
Wood et al, 1992	113	14 (21.4)	9 (8)	NA	NA	NA	NA	NA
Herr, 1997	62	NR	NR	1 (4)	1 (2.7)	NR	6	89%
Rabbani et al, 1998	50	12 (24)	1 (2.6)	1 (2.6)	1* (9.1)	50%	4-5	96%-100%
Ehrlich et al, 2006	50	9 (18)	1 (2)	0	0	NA	4.4	NR
Beck et al, 2007	100	NA	NA	NA	0	NR	2.6	100%
Steiner et al, 2008	102	NA	NA	NA	1 (1)	94%	7.8	99%
Carver et al, 2007a	269	20-86 (7-32)	50 (18.6)	NR	NR	NR	3.75	NR
Heidenreich et al, 2009	152	NA	NA	1 (1.9)	0	85%	3.25	98%

*Occurred in patient who underwent tumorectomy only.
B/L, bilateral; CSS, cancer-specific survival; NA, not applicable; N+, histologically positive lymph nodes; NR, not reported; RP, retroperitoneal; RPLND, retroperitoneal lymph node dissection; U/L, unilateral.

KEY POINTS: SURGICAL DECISION MAKING

- Patients experiencing a clinical CR to induction chemotherapy generally should be observed. There is some debate regarding the benefit of PC-RPLND in these patients because of the potential for microscopic residual disease.
- The predictable lymphatic spread of testicular GCT has allowed for the establishment of the modified templates for use in patients with low-stage disease.
- The standard of care for PC-RPLND in patients with residual masses includes resection of all macroscopic residual disease and a full bilateral infrahilar template dissection. When modified unilateral templates are used in this setting, strict adherence to the above-outlined criteria is necessary to ensure proper patient selection.
- Administering two cycles of adjuvant cisplatin-based chemotherapy to patients with PS II disease demonstrating viable GCT nearly eliminates postoperative recurrences without affecting OS.

is to offer postoperative surveillance to patients with pN2 disease at primary RPLND.

HISTOLOGIC FINDINGS AT POSTCHEMOTHERAPY RETROPERITONEAL LYMPH NODE DISSECTION AND SURVIVAL OUTCOMES

The report from Indiana in 1982 on postcisplatin cytoreductive surgery was important in that it established the three major histologic categories encountered at PC-RPLND (Donohue et al, 1982a). In that report, teratoma, fibrosis, and viable GCT were encountered in roughly equal proportions. Since that time, refinement in primary chemotherapeutic regimens and clearer indications for resection have resulted in a decreasing number of patients demonstrating viable malignancy at PC-RPLND. **The relative frequencies of fibrosis, teratoma, and viable GCT reported in more contemporary series have generally been 40%, 45%, and 15%** (Steyerberg et al, 1995; Donohue et al, 1998; Hendry et al, 2002; Albers et al, 2004; Carver et al, 2006; Spiess et al, 2007).

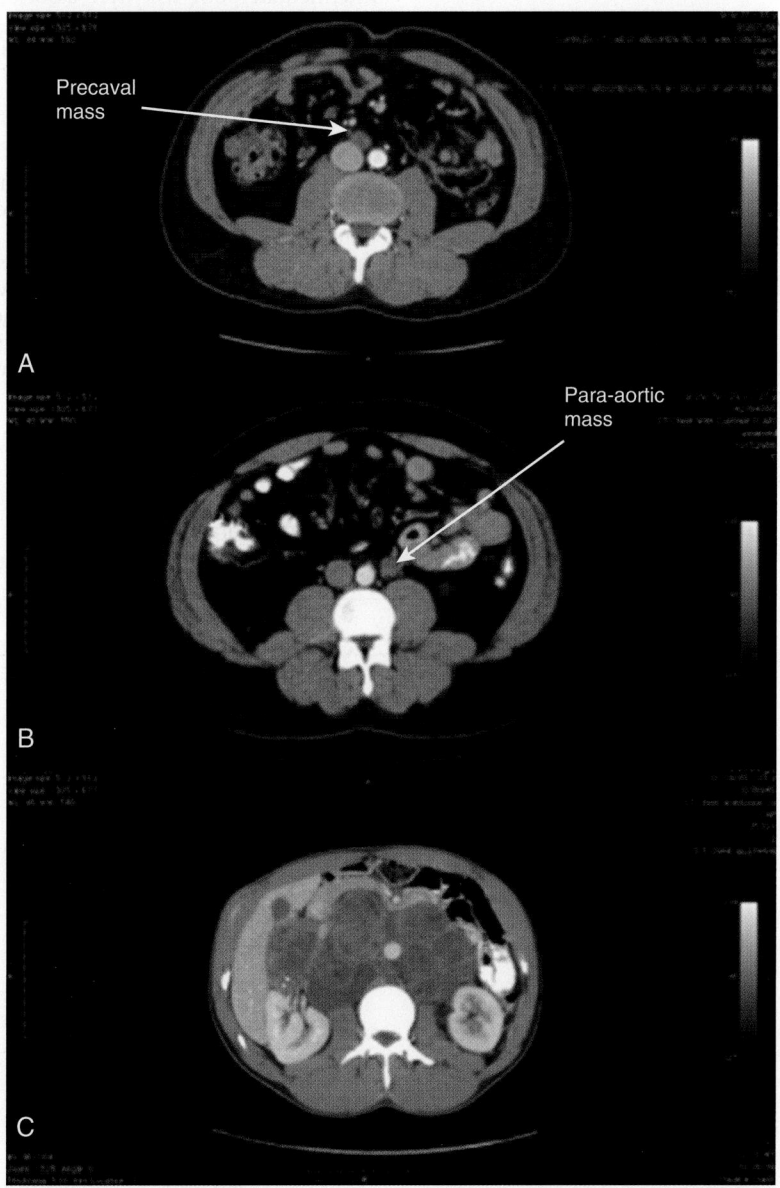

Figure 35-8. Computed tomography images of postchemotherapy residual retroperitoneal masses. A, This patient could be considered a candidate for modified right template postchemotherapy retroperitoneal lymph node dissection (PC-RPLND). B, This patient could be considered a candidate for modified left template PC-RPLND. C, This patient would require an extensive bilateral PC-RPLND.

Outcomes by Histology

Fibrosis, teratoma, and viable malignancy are associated with distinct survival outcomes when encountered at PC-RPLND. Survival outcomes as reported in the literature can be found in Table 35-5. The variability of figures within each histologic group is a function of era of treatment, level of pretreatment, study inclusion criteria, and length of follow-up.

Fibrosis/Necrosis

The finding of fibrosis/necrosis only at postchemotherapy resection is associated with favorable RFS and CSS because it indicates a total malignant cell kill in most patients. It can be inferred that the retroperitoneal metastatic deposits harbored no chemoresistant germ cell elements and that any other subclinical metastatic deposits were likely cleared by chemotherapy. CSS and RFS can be expected to approach 95% in these patients (Donohue and Foster, 1994; Carver et al, 2007c; Maroni et al, 2008).

Teratoma

In 1986, Loehrer and colleagues published the first report dedicated to examining outcomes in patients found to have teratoma only at PC-RPLND. With RFS of 61% and CSS of 82.3%, this series reported poorer outcomes than would be seen in later studies. **According to more contemporary outcomes, patients demonstrating teratoma only at PC-RPLND can be expected to demonstrate 80% to 90% RFS and 85% to 95% CSS** (Jansen et al, 1991; Donohue and Foster, 1994; Carver et al, 2006). Investigators found larger mass size after chemotherapy, presence of somatic-type malignancy, and mediastinal primaries to be associated with increased risk of recurrence (Loehrer et al, 1986; Jansen et al, 1991; Carver et al, 2007b). However, even in the setting of massive retroperitoneal teratoma (>10 cm), 98% CSS has been reported (Beck et al, 2009).

Viable Malignancy

Persistent viable malignancy encountered at PC-RPLND is associated with a poorer prognosis than teratoma or fibrosis. **Reported long-term survival in this group typically ranges from 50% to 70%** (Jansen et al, 1991; Donohue et al, 1998; Fizazi et al, 2001; Spiess et al, 2007; Kundu et al, 2010).

In a multi-institutional review of 238 patients with viable malignancy at PC-RPLND, Fizazi and associates (2001) determined three factors associated with poorer prognosis: (1) incomplete resection, (2) 10% or greater viable malignancy, and (3) IGCCCG intermediate/poor risk stratification at initial diagnosis. Patients with none of these risk factors were classified as "favorable" and demonstrated a 90% 5-year progression-free survival (PFS) and 100% 5-year OS. Patients with one risk factor were classified as "intermediate risk" (5-year PFS 76%, 5-year OS 83%), and patients with two or more risk factors were classified as "poor risk" (5-year PFS 38%, 5-year OS 51%). In a review of 41 patients treated at M.D. Anderson Cancer Center who were found to have viable GCT at PC-RPLND, larger tumor dimension and IGCCCG intermediate/poor risk were associated with increased recurrence rate, whereas persistently elevated α-fetoprotein and prior receipt of salvage chemotherapy were associated with poorer CSS (Spiess et al, 2007).

Adjuvant Chemotherapy

Adjuvant chemotherapy for viable malignancy at PC-RPLND has never been evaluated in a prospective randomized controlled trial. However, early experience revealed a very poor prognosis when these patients were observed postoperatively (Einhorn et al, 1981). **It was recommended that patients demonstrating viable GCT at PC-RPLND receive postoperative adjuvant cisplatin-based chemotherapy. Although the specific regimen has varied, the number of courses administered in the adjuvant setting after PC-RPLND has generally been two.**

TABLE 35-5 Survival Outcomes by Histologic Findings at Postchemotherapy Retroperitoneal Lymph Node Dissection

STUDY	NO. PATIENTS	FOLLOW-UP (yr)	RFS	CSS
FIBROSIS				
Donohue and Foster, 1994	150	>2	NR	93
Eggener et al, 2007a*	36	4.3	NR	85
Carver et al, 2007c	113	NR	95	NR
Maroni et al, 2008	184	4	92.1	NR
TERATOMA				
Loehrer et al, 1986	51	NR	61	82.3
Jansen et al, 1991	26	7.7	88.5	88.5
Donohue and Foster, 1994	273	>2	NR	93.4
Eggener et al, 2007a*	15	4.3	NR	77
Carver et al, 2006	210	3	85.4	94
Beck et al, 2009	99	3.5	76.8	98
VIABLE MALIGNANCY				
Jansen et al, 1991	23	7.9	54.5	64
Fox et al, 1993	133	3	30.8	42.8
Donohue et al, 1998	122	9	39	51.5
Fizazi et al, 2001	238	7.2	64	73
Eggener et al, 2007a*	10	4.3	NR	56
Spiess et al, 2007	41	3.9	50	71
Kundu et al, 2010	90	NR	62	71

*All patients received salvage chemotherapy before postchemotherapy retroperitoneal lymph node dissection.
CSS, cancer-specific survival; NR, not reported; RFS, recurrence-free survival.

Fizazi and colleagues (2001) found that adjuvant chemotherapy was associated with statistically superior PFS without statistical improvement in OS. When dividing patients into the aforementioned viable GCT risk categories, only patients in the intermediate-risk group demonstrated statistically significant improvements in 5-year PFS and OS. **Adjuvant chemotherapy seemed to be unnecessary in favorable-risk patients and ineffective in poor-risk patients.** In the absence of randomization, these outcomes were likely heavily influenced by selection bias. Similarly, when evaluating patients with viable GCT after salvage RPLND, patients did not appear to benefit from two postoperative cycles of cisplatin-based chemotherapy (Fox et al, 1993; Kundu et al, 2010). Adjuvant chemotherapy is generally not recommended in this setting.

KEY POINTS: HISTOLOGIC FINDINGS AT POSTCHEMOTHERAPY RETROPERITONEAL LYMPH NODE DISSECTION AND OUTCOMES

- Approximately 90% long-term survival can be expected among patients with fibrosis and/or teratoma only at PC-RPLND. This number decreases to 50% to 70% for patients demonstrating viable GCT at PC-RPLND.
- Two cycles of adjuvant chemotherapy are generally recommended in patients with viable GCT at PC-RPLND after induction chemotherapy.

POSTCHEMOTHERAPY RETROPERITONEAL LYMPH NODE DISSECTION IN HIGH-RISK POPULATIONS

Salvage Retroperitoneal Lymph Node Dissection

Patients undergoing PC-RPLND after salvage chemotherapy demonstrated higher rates of persistent viable malignancy and worsened survival outcomes compared with patients who received first-line chemotherapy only (see Table 35-5). Typically, OS and CSS ranged from 60% to 75% in this group (Fox et al, 1993; Donohue et al, 1998; Eggener et al, 2007a). When comparing only patients found to have viable malignancy at PC-RPLND, Fox and associates (1993) reported CSS of 58.5% in patients having received induction chemotherapy only versus 36.7% in patients having received salvage chemotherapy.

Reported experience with RPLND after high-dose chemotherapy (HDCT) is limited (Table 35-6). In 2004, Rick and colleagues reported results in 57 patients undergoing PC-RPLND after HDCT. They observed 59% RFS and 65% CSS at a median follow-up of 7.3 years. Similarly, Cary et al (2011) reported 71% OS at a median follow-up of 4.2 years in 77 patients undergoing RPLND after HDCT.

Desperation Retroperitoneal Lymph Node Dissection

In general, patients with elevated STMs after chemotherapy are not considered candidates for RPLND and are given standard or high-dose salvage chemotherapy. However, a surgical cure remains

---

TABLE 35-6 Postchemotherapy Retroperitoneal Lymph Node Dissection in High-Risk Populations

STUDY	NO. PATIENTS	TERATOMA (%)	FIBROSIS (%)	VIABLE MALIGNANCY (%)	FOLLOW-UP (yr)	CSS OR OS
SALVAGE						
Fox et al, 1993	163	NR	NR	55	5	36.7*
Donohue et al, 1998	166	NR	NR	NR	9.7	61.4
Eggener et al, 2007a	71	21	51	28	5	74
HDCT						
Rick et al, 2004	57	16	38	46	7.3	65
Cary et al, 2011	77	33.8	27.3	39	4.2	71
DESPERATION						
Donohue et al, 1998	150	NR	NR	NR	9.7	66
Ravi et al, 1998	30	26.7	27.6	46.7	4.8	57
Albers et al, 2000	30	11	25	64	11	57
Beck et al, 2005c	114	34.2	12.3	53.5	6	53.9
Ong et al, 2008	48	25	17	58	4.3	69
REDO						
McKiernen et al, 2003	56	37.5	28.6	33.9	4.1† 2.4‡	56
Sexton et al, 2003	21	67	24	24	4.7	63
Heidenreich et al, 2005	18	33.3	44.4	22.2	1.9	89
Willis et al, 2007	54	35	9	56	5	94.2
Pedrosa et al, 2014	203	34	14.8	51.2	5	61.2
LATE RELAPSE						
Baniel et al, 1995a	81	19	0	81	4.8	56.8
George et al, 2003	83	17	0	78	2.4	74.7
Dieckmann et al, 2005	72	NR	NR	NR	NR	58.3
Sharp et al, 2008	75	19	3	78	4.5	61

*Includes only patients with viable malignancy in the survival analysis.
†Follow-up for postchemotherapy retroperitoneal lymph node dissection.
‡Follow-up for primary retroperitoneal lymph node dissection.
CSS, cancer-specific survival; HDCT, high-dose chemotherapy; NR, not reported; OS, overall survival.

possible in selected cases in which chemotherapy has failed to normalize STMs. **Desperation RPLND is resection performed in the setting of elevated STMs.** Pathologic findings at desperation RPLND are listed in Table 35-6. In a review of 114 selected patients undergoing desperation RPLND, Beck and colleagues (2005c) reported a 5-year OS of 53.9% at a median follow-up of 6 years. OS was poorest in patients with viable malignancy demonstrated in the resection specimen, patients who had previously received salvage chemotherapy, patients with increased human chorionic gonadotropin before surgery, or patients who underwent repeat RPLND. Patients who received first-line chemotherapy only and demonstrated declining (but not normalizing) STMs were most likely (>75%) to demonstrate fibrosis and/or teratoma at RPLND. Further chemotherapy would not likely have benefited most of these patients. **The authors recommended use of the following selection criteria for desperation RPLND: declining or plateauing STMs after chemotherapy, slowly rising STMs after initial clinical CR to chemotherapy, resectable disease at one or two sites, and as a last resort in a patient with resectable disease and rising STMs after exhausting all reasonable chemotherapeutic options.** In a subsequent report on 48 patients by Ong and colleagues (2008), patients with fibrosis at PC-RPLND demonstrated poorer OS than patients with viable malignancy or teratoma likely indicating systemic metastases outside of the retroperitoneum. Patients with postoperative normalization of STMs demonstrated significantly improved OS. This finding was the only prognostic factor that remained robust to multivariable analysis. Outcomes reported in several retrospective desperation series are listed in Table 35-6 (Donohue et al, 1998; Ravi et al, 1998; Albers et al, 2000).

Reoperative Retroperitoneal Lymph Node Dissection

Repeat resection of retroperitoneal recurrence after primary or PC-RPLND has been termed *reoperative* or *redo RPLND*. CSS has been reported to range from 55% to 65% (Donohue et al, 1998; McKiernan et al, 2003; Sexton et al, 2003; Heidenreich et al, 2005; Willis et al, 2007). The reported histologic findings and survival outcomes in reoperative series are listed in Table 35-6. There appears to be a high incidence of GCT with somatic-type malignancy in this population, with a reported incidence of 15% to 20%. Given the technical difficulty of reoperative resections, complications have been reported to occur in approximately one third of patients (McKiernan et al, 2003; Pedrosa et al, 2014). Poorer survival outcomes have been reported in patients demonstrating viable GCT at reoperative RPLND and patients with prior receipt of salvage chemotherapy (McKiernan et al, 2003; Pedrosa et al, 2014).

In most cases, the need for reoperative RPLND likely represents an inadequate primary resection. Several reported findings support this idea. Most patients experience recurrence within the primary landing zone (McKiernan et al, 2003; Heidenreich et al, 2005). Pedrosa and colleagues (2014) reported that ipsilateral recurrence was associated with incomplete ipsilateral lumbar vessel ligation and an unresected ipsilateral gonadal vein. Similarly, Willis and colleagues (2007) reported that 46% of reoperative cases demonstrated retroaortic and/or retrocaval disease, indicating that these regions were omitted from prior RPLND. Using good technique at initial RPLND decreases the likelihood of having to perform a reoperative RPLND.

Late Relapse

Late relapse is defined as recurrence of GCT 24 or more months after CR to primary treatment modalities. This is a rare phenomenon that occurs in 2% to 4% of patients with GCT (Baniel et al, 1995a; Gerl et al, 1997). The retroperitoneum is the most common site of late relapse (Baniel et al, 1995a). Approximately 80% of cases of late relapse contain viable GCT with yolk sac tumor predominating (Baniel et al, 1995a; Michael et al, 2000; George et al, 2003; Sharp et al, 2008). Additionally, there appears to be a disproportionately high incidence of GCT with somatic-type malignancy. When late relapse occurs in patients who previously received chemotherapy, it is rarely cured by chemotherapy. **Surgical extirpation should be the initial management of all patients with resectable disease at late relapse. Patients with widespread and/or unresectable disease should be offered chemotherapy in an effort to downsize the tumor burden and render the disease resectable.** Reported OS is usually around 60%. Predictors of poorer survival outcomes include viable malignancy or somatic-type malignancy at late relapse, prior chemotherapy, and incomplete resection (Baniel et al, 1995a; George et al, 2003; Sharp et al, 2008).

> ### KEY POINTS: POSTCHEMOTHERAPY RETROPERITONEAL LYMPH NODE DISSECTION IN HIGH-RISK POPULATIONS
>
> - PC-RPLND performed as a salvage, desperation, or reoperative procedure or in the setting of late relapse is associated with significantly poorer survival outcomes than PC-RPLND performed after complete serologic response to induction chemotherapy.
> - Viable GCT is encountered in an increased proportion of patients within all of these subpopulations. Additionally, somatic-type malignancy is seen with increased frequency in patients undergoing reoperative RPLND and patients undergoing resection of late relapse disease.
> - In general, patients with elevated STMs after induction chemotherapy should receive salvage chemotherapy. Only patients satisfying the above-outlined selection criteria should be considered for desperation RPLND.
> - Reoperative RPLND generally indicates an inadequate prior RPLND. Increased complication rates and poorer survival outcomes in this setting highlight the importance of proper surgical technique at initial RPLND.
> - Late relapse in patients who previously received chemotherapy is generally chemoresistant. First-line management of late relapse in all patients with resectable disease should be surgical extirpation.

SURGICAL OUTCOMES, FUNCTIONAL CONSIDERATIONS, AND COMPLICATIONS OF RETROPERITONEAL LYMPH NODE DISSECTION

Lymph Node Counts

Higher lymph node counts have been associated with improved oncologic outcomes in various malignancies (Herr et al, 2002; Le Voyer et al, 2003; Schwarz and Smith, 2006, 2007). Given these findings, some investigators have proposed that node counts be used as surrogates for adequacy of lymphadenectomy. In recent years, several groups have investigated lymph node counts in primary and PC-RPLND (Carver et al, 2010; Risk et al, 2010; Thompson et al, 2010, 2011). Although investigators at MSKCC reported a direct correlation between node count and node positivity when evaluating patients with primary RPLND (Thompson et al, 2010), no such association was appreciated in two other studies (Liberman et al, 2010; Risk et al, 2010). Significant variability in lymph node counts, demonstrated by wide interquartile range and large standard deviation, indicates that node counts are not useful when assessing adequacy of an individual surgery (Risk et al, 2010; Thompson et al, 2010). However, surgeons and treatment centers may consider reviewing their own mean or median lymph node counts to determine if their numbers reflect those reported in the literature for the templates used. If lymph node counts are consistently lower than published standards, there may be a problem related to thoroughness of surgery and/or pathologic processing of specimens obtained.

Retroperitoneal Lymph Node Dissection and Fertility

Fertility in Patients Undergoing Retroperitoneal Lymph Node Dissection

Preserving fertility in men undergoing RPLND is more complex than simply sparing their postganglionic sympathetic nerves. Subfertility in a significant proportion of patients presenting with newly diagnosed testicular cancer is well documented. **When including all stages of disease, approximately 40% to 60% of patients presenting with testicular GCT have been reported to demonstrate abnormal parameters on semen analysis** (Fossa et al, 1985; Lange et al, 1987; Hansen et al, 1991; Foster et al, 1994). Baseline subfertility needs to be taken into account when evaluating paternity rates after RPLND.

Ejaculatory Dysfunction and Retroperitoneal Lymph Node Dissection

For successful antegrade ejaculation of sperm-containing semen to occur, several processes need to occur in coordinated fashion, as follows: (1) smooth muscle contraction in the vasa deferentia, seminal vesicles, and prostate resulting in seminal emission and prostate glandular secretion along with (2) closure of the bladder neck to prevent retrograde ejaculation and (3) rhythmic contractions of the ischiocavernosus, bulbospongiosus, and levator ani muscles expelling semen from the urethra. Processes 1 and 2 require efferent neurologic input from the L1 through L4 postganglionic sympathetic fibers, which coalesce with their contralateral counterparts in the superior hypogastric plexus. From the hypogastric plexus, these nerve fibers continue caudally to the seminal vesicles, ampulla of the vasa deferentia, vasa deferentia proper, bladder neck, and prostate (Donohue et al, 1990).

Before the development of unilateral modified RPLND templates and nerve-sparing techniques, most patients undergoing bilateral RPLND were rendered anejaculatory (Donohue and Rowland, 1981). In light of the successful nerve preservation techniques established for radical retropubic prostatectomy by Walsh and Donker (1982), testicular cancer surgeons sought to refine the surgical technique of RPLND with the goal of preserving antegrade ejaculation without compromising diagnostic and therapeutic efficacy. **Techniques were altered in two ways: (1) changing the boundaries of dissection** (Pizzocaro et al, 1985; Weissbach et al, 1985) **and (2) prospectively identifying postganglionic sympathetic fibers and the superior hypogastric plexus so that these structures could be preserved during subsequent lymphadenectomy** (Jewett et al, 1988).

Early studies on ejaculatory outcomes after modified unilateral template RPLND without nerve-sparing technique reported postoperative antegrade ejaculation in 75% to 87% of patients (Fossa et al, 1985; Pizzocaro et al, 1985; Weissbach et al, 1985). **However, in a more recent series, Beck and colleagues (2010) reported preservation of antegrade ejaculation in 97% of men undergoing modified unilateral template dissection without ipsilateral nerve-sparing technique.** These superior outcomes likely reflect improved understanding of the anatomy of postganglionic sympathetic nerve fibers allowing for the avoidance of damage to contralateral fibers caudal to the IMA.

Nerve-sparing RPLND results in preservation of antegrade ejaculation in 90% to 100% of patients (Jewett and Torbey, 1988; Donohue et al, 1990; Heidenreich et al, 2003; Beck et al, 2010). Although Jewett and Torbey (1988) reported temporary postoperative anejaculation in most patients, Donohue (1993) observed no such anejaculatory period. In the study by Jewett and Torbey (1988), bilateral template RPLND was performed in all patients, whereas ipsilateral nerve-sparing and modified unilateral template dissections were performed in most patients in the study by Donohue (1993). Neurapraxia likely accounted for the temporary anejaculation reported by Jewett and Torbey (1988).

In addition to demonstrating the efficacy of unilateral template dissection and nerve-sparing techniques in preserving antegrade ejaculation, these studies provided evidence that these new techniques did not compromise oncologic outcomes. With follow-up ranging from 10 months to nearly 5 years, only one retroperitoneal recurrence was reported in the aforementioned series. However, heterogeneous indications for use of post-RPLND adjuvant chemotherapy almost certainly affected recurrence rates.

Over the last 30 years, refinements in the technique of primary RPLND and PC-RPLND have resulted in a significant decrease in the incidence of postoperative ejaculatory dysfunction. Through the use of modified unilateral dissection templates and/or nerve-sparing techniques, preservation of antegrade ejaculation can be expected in greater than 90% of patients in whom at least one of these modalities can be employed. **Postoperative paternity can be expected in approximately 75% of men undergoing primary nerve-sparing RPLND** (Beck et al, 2010). Fertility after PC-RPLND has not been established because chemotherapy-induced disruption of spermatogenesis can persist for several years after completion of therapy (Lampe et al, 1997).

Complications of Retroperitoneal Lymph Node Dissection

The overall complication rate for primary RPLND has been reported to range from 10.6% to 24% (Baniel et al, 1994; Heidenreich et al, 2003; Subramanian et al, 2010). **Reported complication rates for PC-RPLND range from 20% to 30%** (Baniel et al, 1995b; Subramanian et al, 2010). Given the paucity of studies on this topic, predictors of complications after RPLND have been inconsistent. When evaluating primary RPLND, investigators at Indiana University reported lower complication rates associated with unilateral dissection and more recent era of surgery. The German Testicular Cancer Study Group found no such correlation between RPLND template and complications. However, investigators reported increased complication rates when RPLND was performed by surgeons with a lower volume of cases and/or at lower volume centers, leading to a recommendation to centralize RPLND to high-volume centers and to minimize the number of surgeons performing these surgeries at each center.

Table 35-7 summarizes reported complications in primary RPLND and PC-RPLND. A review of the incidence, prevention, and management of select complications follows.

Pulmonary Complications

Major pulmonary complications are extremely rare after primary RPLND but have been reported to occur in approximately 3% to 5% of patients after PC-RPLND (Baniel et al, 1994, 1995b; Heidenreich et al, 2003; Subramanian et al, 2010). Because most patients who undergo PC-RPLND have received bleomycin-containing induction chemotherapy, acute respiratory distress syndrome and prolonged postoperative ventilation account for most of these major complications. **The incidence of bleomycin-related perioperative pulmonary complications can be minimized by avoiding aggressive intraoperative and postoperative intravenous fluid resuscitation and keeping FIO_2 as low as is safely possible** (Goldiner et al, 1978; Donat and Levy, 1998). The importance of working with an anesthesiologist who has experience in managing patients who previously received bleomycin cannot be overstated. Pulmonary complications are most likely to be encountered in patients with large-volume pulmonary disease, particularly if simultaneous retroperitoneal and thoracic resections are to be performed (Baniel et al, 1995b).

Ileus

The reported rates of postoperative paralytic ileus range widely in the primary RPLND (0% to 18%) and PC-RPLND (2.2% to 21%) settings. This variation likely stems from differences in the definitions of ileus. In relatively low-volume PC-RPLND, an orogastric tube is used and removed at the conclusion of the procedure. In

TABLE 35-7   Complications of Retroperitoneal Lymph Node Dissection

	PRIMARY RPLND			PC-RPLND	
	BANIEL ET AL, 1994	**HEIDENREICH ET AL, 2003**	**SUBRAMANIAN ET AL, 2010**	**BANIEL ET AL, 1995b**	**SUBRAMANIAN ET AL, 2010**
No. patients	478	239	112	603	96
Overall complications (%)	10.6	19.7	24	20.7	32
Major complications (%)	8.2	5.4	3	NS	8
Mortality (%)	0	0	0	0.8	1
Major pulmonary (%)	1.9	0.8	0.9	5.1	3.1
Minor pulmonary (%)	0.2	0.4	3.6	5.1	3.1
Chylous ascites (%)	0.2	2.1	2	2	2
Symptomatic lymphocele (%)	0.2	1.7	0	1.7	1
Ileus (%)	NR	2.1	17.9	2.2	20.8
Wound infection (%)	4.8	5.4	0.9	4.8	4
Pulmonary embolism (%)	0	0.8	0.9	0.1	3.1
Ureteral injury (%)	0.2	0.4	0.9	0.9	0
Small bowel obstruction (%)	2.3	0.4	2.7	2.3	1.8
Postoperative hemorrhage (%)	0	0.8	0	0.3	1

NR, not reported; NS, not studied; PC-RPLND, postchemotherapy retroperitoneal lymph node dissection; RPLND, retroperitoneal lymph node dissection.

higher volume disease, the probability of significant ileus is greater, and a nasogastric tube should be used.

Lymphocele

The incidence of subclinical lymphocele after RPLND is unknown. However, it is thought that lymphoceles are relatively common and clinically insignificant in most cases. Symptomatic retroperitoneal lymphoceles are extremely rare with reported rates ranging from 0% to 1.7% (Baniel et al, 1994, 1995b; Heidenreich et al, 2003; Subramanian et al, 2010). Symptoms can be related to ureteral compression, displacement of abdominal viscera (if very large), or secondary infection. CT scan demonstrates a thin-walled cystic lesion in the resection bed. Air within the lymphocele and/or rim enhancement should raise concern for an infection. **Meticulous attention to ligation of large-caliber lymphatics during resection likely decreases the risk of developing a symptomatic lymphocele.** Treatment of symptomatic and/or infected lymphoceles includes percutaneous drainage with systemic antibiotics reserved for infected lymphoceles. Additionally, in the setting of infected lymphocele, one should consider leaving an indwelling drain rather than simple percutaneous aspiration.

Chylous Ascites

Chylous ascites refers to the accumulation of chylomicron-containing lymphatic fluid in the peritoneal cavity. **Chylous ascites has been reported to occur in 0.2% to 2.1% of patients undergoing primary RPLND and 2% to 7% of patients undergoing PC-RPLND** (Baniel et al, 1994, 1995b; Heidenreich et al, 2003; Evans et al, 2006; Subramanian et al, 2010). Patients typically present with complaints of increasing abdominal fullness, anorexia, nausea, vomiting, abdominal pain, and dyspnea. Patients often have a fluid wave on abdominal examination, which can help distinguish ascites from an ileus. Additionally, accumulated peritoneal fluid results in significant weight gain. Fluid has a milky color if paracentesis is performed. Chylous ascites is alkaline, stains positive for Sudan black, and demonstrates a triglyceride concentration greater than that of serum. However, these tests are usually unnecessary because clinical examination and/or gross inspection of aspirating fluid should be enough to confirm the diagnosis.

Suprahilar resections are thought to carry a higher risk for chylous ascites because of disruption of the cisterna chyli and its contributing lymphatics. The cisterna chyli is located at the level of the L1-2 vertebral bodies, medial to the posterior surface of the aorta in the retrocrural space. The association of IVC resection and chylous ascites is thought to be related to increased venous pressure below the level of the IVC producing increased capillary leak and ultimately third spacing of lymphatic fluid into the retroperitoneum (Baniel et al, 1993). In a review of the M.D. Anderson Cancer Center experience, Evans and colleagues (2006) found increased number of preoperative cycles of chemotherapy, increased estimated blood loss, and longer operative time to be associated with development of chylous ascites.

We recommend a graduated approach to the management of chylous ascites. In general, patients with symptomatic chylous ascites should first be managed with paracentesis. Although an indwelling drain can be left, we recommend simple paracentesis with consideration of low-fat/medium-chain triglyceride diet and intramuscular octreotide. If ascites reaccumulates, an indwelling drain should be placed. If these dietary modifications have already been instituted, patients should be given nothing by mouth, and total parenteral nutrition should be initiated. Although the use of octreotide in the setting of chylous ascites has not been studied in the urologic literature, it has demonstrated efficacy in minimizing chylous leaks after hepaticopancreaticobiliary surgery (Shapiro et al, 1996; Kuboki et al, 2013). Persistent high-volume chylous drainage (>100 mL/24 hr) despite these modifications is exceedingly rare. When it does occur, options include continued observation with conservative management, placement of a peritoneovenous (LeVeen) shunt, or surgical exploration with attempted ligation of the lymphatic leak. The latter two options should be reserved as last resorts. Peritoneovenous shunts have been reported to be associated with a significant incidence of occlusion and/or malfunction often requiring revision after placement, sepsis, and potentially fat embolization (Evans et al, 2006). Regardless of treatment modality that ultimately results in resolution of chylous ascites, consideration should be given to a continued low-fat diet with medium-chain triglycerides for 1 to 3 months after resolution of lymph leak.

Venous Thromboembolism

Venous thromboembolism (VTE) rates reported after primary RPLND and PC-RPLND are consistently low; this is likely the result of a young, otherwise healthy patient population. The rate of pulmonary embolism after primary RPLND has been reported to be less than 1% (Baniel et al, 1994; Heidenreich et al, 2003; Subramanian et al, 2010). After PC-RPLND, the rates range from 0.1% to 3.1% (Baniel et al, 1995b; Subramanian et al, 2010). The incidence of deep venous thrombosis is more difficult to determine because these cases are not consistently reported in the literature and are likely most often asymptomatic. Reported rates range from 0% to 1% in primary RPLND and PC-RPLND (Heidenreich et al, 2003; Subramanian et al, 2010).

All patients undergoing RPLND should have sequential compression devices placed before induction, which should be maintained throughout the hospital course. Ambulation should be resumed on postoperative day 1 in virtually all cases. The use of pharmacologic prophylaxis has never been evaluated in patients undergoing RPLND. Prophylactic subcutaneous low-dose unfractionated heparin or low-molecular-weight heparin has demonstrated efficacy in decreasing VTE rates in postoperative patients (Collins et al, 1988; Kakkar et al, 1993). The potential disadvantages are an increased risk for postoperative hemorrhage and anecdotal reports of increased risk for lymphocele. Retrospective studies on patients undergoing radical prostatectomy reported conflicting results with regard to the effect of postoperative pharmacologic thromboprophylaxis on pelvic lymphocele formation (Bigg and Catalona, 1992; Koch and Jr, 1997; Schmitges et al, 2012). The decision to use pharmacologic thromboprophylaxis needs to be made based on the low incidence of VTE in patients undergoing RPLND and extrapolation of data based on risk/benefit data from other surgeries and specialties. **Pharmacologic thromboprophylaxis is likely most important in patients who are at an increased risk for postoperative VTE, such as patients with a personal history of VTE, obesity, known hypercoagulable condition, or older age.**

Neurologic Complications

In the Indiana PC-RPLND review, no cases of paraplegia were noted. Seven cases of peripheral nerve injury were reported (Baniel et al, 1995b). All of these cases were secondary to patient positioning and potentially retractor placement (femoral neurapraxia). Careful attention to appropriate patient positioning by the surgical and anesthesia teams is important in minimizing peripheral nerve damage. In a review of 268 patients undergoing postchemotherapy resection of mediastinal disease for testicular or primary retroperitoneal GCT, Kesler and colleagues (2003) reported 6 patients (2.2%) with paraplegia. **Patients with bulky mediastinal and retroperitoneal disease are at an increased risk of developing paraplegia. The likelihood of neurologic complications increases with the scale of para-aortic resection.**

Mortality

Reported mortality after primary RPLND is essentially zero (Baniel et al, 1994; Heidenreich et al, 2003; Capitanio et al, 2009; Subramanian et al, 2010). Mortality after PC-RPLND is extremely rare and generally reported to be less than 1% (Baniel et al, 1995b; Capitanio et al, 2009; Subramanian et al, 2010). In a review of the Indiana University experience, 5 of 603 patients (0.8%) died after PC-RPLND (Baniel et al, 1995b). Causes of death were severe respiratory distress in two patients, multiple organ failure in one patient, fungal sepsis in one patient, and myocardial infarction after aorticoduodenal fistula in one patient. In a population-based study of 882 patients having undergone RPLND, Capitanio and colleagues (2009) used the Surveillance, Epidemiology, and End Results (SEER) database to determine if mortality rates previously reported by centers of excellence were applicable to the community. Although receipt of chemotherapy was not reported, there were no mortalities among patients with localized disease, whereas mortality rates of 0.8% and 6% were reported among patients with retroperitoneal disease and distant metastases, respectively.

RETROPERITONEAL LYMPH NODE DISSECTION IN UNIQUE SITUATIONS

Postchemotherapy Retroperitoneal Lymph Node Dissection for Seminoma

Pure seminoma is a particularly chemosensitive tumor with CR rates of 70% to 90% being reported in patients with disseminated disease treated with cisplatin-based chemotherapy (Loehrer et al, 1987; International Germ Cell Consensus Classification, 1997; Gholam et al, 2003). **Residual masses are relatively common after treatment of seminoma owing to the intense desmoplastic reaction occurring in response to chemotherapy. In most series of PC-RPLND performed for pure seminoma, viable malignancy is encountered in approximately 10% of cases,** with remaining patients demonstrating only fibrosis (Herr et al, 1997; Ravi et al, 1999; Flechon et al, 2002). **Additionally, PC-RPLND for seminoma has been associated with increased perioperative morbidity compared with PC-RPLND for NSGCT** (Friedman et al, 1985; Fossa et al, 1987; Mosharafa et al, 2003b). **Various thresholds for operative intervention have been derived with the common goal of avoiding an often unnecessary and potentially morbid surgery.**

In a review of 55 patients treated at MSKCC with pure testicular seminoma and available postchemotherapy retroperitoneal pathology (RPLND or biopsy), 30% of patients with masses 3 cm or larger had viable retroperitoneal seminoma or teratoma at resection, whereas none of the patients with smaller masses harbored residual disease (Herr et al, 1997). Investigators recommended RPLND in patients with pure seminoma with residual masses 3 cm or larger. Conversely, investigators at Indiana University reported no association between residual mass size and disease recurrence/progression on observation in their experience with 21 patients. The authors recommended observing all residual masses with resection reserved for patients demonstrating serologic or radiographic evidence of progression (Schultz et al, 1989).

More recently, PET has been used to assess for the presence of viable seminoma in residual masses. In this capacity, PET scans have a negative predictive value approaching 100%. However, false-positive PET scans have resulted in inconsistent positive predictive values ranging from 67% to 100% in two studies (De Santis et al,

2004; Lewis et al, 2006). **In light of these findings, some guidelines propose that patients without residual masses or a residual mass less than 3 cm be observed and patients with larger masses be evaluated with a PET scan 6 weeks after completing chemotherapy.** Patients with PET-avid masses are managed with RPLND, standard-dose salvage chemotherapy, or HDCT. Of these three modalities, HDCT has demonstrated the best survival outcomes with 92% OS when it is used in the second-line setting (Agarwala et al, 2011). In a review of 36 patients with pure seminoma demonstrating viable seminoma at PC-RPLND, Rice and colleagues (2012) reported a 54% CSS with only 9 patients (25%) remaining continuously disease-free after resection. **Given the superior survival outcomes associated with HDCT, this modality is preferred for most patients with pure seminoma who relapse after induction chemotherapy. However, PC-RPLND may continue to have a role for management of patients who relapse with focal, easily resectable masses to avoid the potential morbidity of HDCT. Ultimately, the decision needs to be made based on predicted morbidity of resection versus HDCT.**

Retroperitoneal Lymph Node Dissection for Sex Cord–Stromal Tumors

Sex cord–stromal tumors (SCSTs) account for 4% to 5% of all testicular neoplasms and include Leydig, Sertoli, and granulosa cell tumors as well as various combinations of these histologies. **It is estimated that 10% to 20% of adult SCSTs are malignant** (Kim et al, 1985; Grem et al, 1986; Kratzer et al, 1997). Although the presence of metastatic disease is the only reliable indicator of malignant phenotype, various primary tumor characteristics have been evaluated for their ability to predict aggressive behavior. **Features seeming to correlate with aggressive behavior have been fairly similar when examining the distinct subtypes of SCSTs. These characteristics include older age, primary tumor size larger than 4 to 5 cm, necrosis, mitotic rate greater than three to five per 10 high-power fields, moderate-to-severe nuclear atypia, infiltrative tumor margins/invasion of adjuvant structures, and lymphovascular invasion** (Kim et al, 1985; Dilworth et al, 1991; Kratzer et al, 1997; Young et al, 1998). Multiple features predictive of malignant phenotype frequently occur in the same patients, with patients demonstrating a malignant disease course often possessing two or three malignant characteristics (Kim et al, 1985; Young et al, 1998). Some experts recommended that tumors possessing two or more such features be categorized as malignant (Kratzer et al, 1997; Silberstein et al, 2013). However, prediction of malignant behavior based on histology is not as accurate as in GCT.

The role of RPLND in the treatment of SCST is unclear. **Arguments for use of RPLND in treatment of this disease are as follows: (1) Retroperitoneal nodes are consistently the most common (and likely the first) site of metastases in reported series** (Kim et al, 1985; Kratzer et al, 1997; Young et al, 1998); **(2) CS I patients can go on to develop retroperitoneal metastases at widely ranging time intervals indicating that early primary RPLND could perhaps prevent these recurrences** (Mosharafa et al, 2003a); **(3) there have been isolated reported cases of surgically cured patients with microscopic deposits of SCST in RPLND specimens** (Lockhart et al, 1976; Gohji et al, 1994; Mosharafa et al, 2003a; Silberstein et al, 2013); **and (4) although these tumors have been reported to demonstrate partial responses to chemotherapy, cures have not been documented.**

Arguments against performing RPLND are as follows: (1) Primary tumor histologic predictors of malignant behavior have demonstrated inconsistent performance making patient selection difficult (Mosharafa et al, 2003a; Silberstein et al, 2013), and (2) although there have been some surgical cures reported in the literature, follow-up is often too short to confirm cure, and most patients with positive retroperitoneal nodes die of their disease. **At the present time, no conclusive recommendation can be made regarding the use of RPLND in managing patients with SCST. The aforementioned advantages and disadvantages should be discussed with** the patient to allow him to make an informed decision regarding management.

KEY POINTS: RETROPERITONEAL LYMPH NODE DISSECTION IN UNIQUE SITUATIONS

- PC-RPLND is rarely performed in the setting of seminoma given the chemosensitivity of this histology, the technical difficulty of these resections, and the excellent response to HDCT.
- The role of RPLND in the treatment of SCST has not been definitively demonstrated given the rarity of malignant forms of these tumors.

CONCLUSION

Over the last 50 years, the field of testicular cancer has undergone a striking evolution through the parallel development and integration of more effective and less toxic chemotherapeutic regimens and the continued refinement of techniques for surgical resection. These advances have resulted in delivery of durable cures to more than 90% of patients with testicular cancer, while minimizing acute and long-term morbidity. These excellent outcomes can be achieved only through strict adherence to established therapeutic principles. Although treatment of patients with testicular cancer often requires an experienced multidisciplinary team, the successful management of nearly every patient with testicular cancer begins with his urologist. All urologists should have a thorough and nuanced understanding of the appropriate treatment of testicular cancer. This understanding helps to ensure expeditious delivery of appropriate medical and surgical treatment with early referral to high-volume centers when necessary. The success of surgical management of testicular tumors is measured not only by survival outcomes but also by minimizing morbidity through avoidance of unnecessary surgeries and functional preservation whenever possible.

Please visit the accompanying website at www.expertconsult.com to view videos associated with this chapter.

REFERENCES

The complete reference list is available online at www.expertconsult.com.

SUGGESTED READINGS

Baniel J, Foster RS, Gonin R, et al. Late relapse of testicular cancer. J Clin Oncol 1995;13:1170–6.

Carver BS, Bianco FJ Jr, Shayegan B, et al. Predicting teratoma in the retroperitoneum in men undergoing post-chemotherapy retroperitoneal lymph node dissection. J Urol 2006;176:100–3, discussion 103-4.

Carver BS, Shayegan B, Eggener S, et al. Incidence of metastatic nonseminomatous germ cell tumor outside the boundaries of a modified post-chemotherapy retroperitoneal lymph node dissection. J Clin Oncol 2007;25:4365–9.

Donohue JP, Leviovitch I, Foster RS, et al. Integration of surgery and systemic therapy: results and principles of integration. Semin Urol Oncol 1998;16:65–71.

Donohue JP, Thornhill JA, Foster RS, et al. Primary retroperitoneal lymph node dissection in clinical stage A non-seminomatous germ cell testis cancer. Review of the Indiana University experience 1965-1989. Br J Urol 1993;71:326–35.

Donohue JP, Zachary JM, Maynard BR. Distribution of nodal metastases in nonseminomatous testis cancer. J Urol 1982;128:315–20.

Eggener SE, Carver BS, Sharp DS, et al. Incidence of disease outside modified retroperitoneal lymph node dissection templates in clinical stage I or IIA nonseminomatous germ cell testicular cancer. J Urol 2007;177:937–42, discussion 942-3.

Ehrlich Y, Brames MJ, Beck SD, et al. Long-term follow-up of cisplatin combination chemotherapy in patients with disseminated nonseminomatous germ cell tumors: is a postchemotherapy retroperitoneal lymph node dissection needed after complete remission? J Clin Oncol 2010;28: 531–6.

Fizazi K, Tjulandin S, Salvioni R, et al. Viable malignant cells after primary chemotherapy for disseminated nonseminomatous germ cell tumors: prognostic factors and role of postsurgery chemotherapy—results from an international study group. J Clin Oncol 2001;19:2647–57.

Jewett MA, Kong YS, Goldberg SD, et al. Retroperitoneal lymphadenectomy for testis tumor with nerve sparing for ejaculation. J Urol 1988;139: 1220–4.

Stephenson AJ, Bosl GJ, Motzer RJ, et al. Retroperitoneal lymph node dissection for nonseminomatous germ cell testicular cancer: impact of patient selection factors on outcome. J Clin Oncol 2005;23:2781–8.

Williams SD, Stablein DM, Einhorn LH, et al. Immediate adjuvant chemotherapy versus observation with treatment at relapse in pathological stage II testicular cancer. N Engl J Med 1987;317:1433–8.

36 Laparoscopic and Robotic-Assisted Retroperitoneal Lymphadenectomy for Testicular Tumors

Mohamad E. Allaf, MD, and Louis R. Kavoussi, MD, MBA

Germ cell tumors (GCTs) are the most common malignancy in men between the ages of 15 and 35 (Carver and Sheinfeld, 2005). Testicular cancer is also one of the most curable solid-organ neoplasms, owing in large part to an excellent multimodal treatment paradigm that includes effective platinum-based chemotherapy and surgery (Einhorn, 1981). **Although contemporary survival rates for GCTs are more than 90%, cure rates and patient morbidity depend on selection of the management options.** Retroperitoneal lymph node dissection (RPLND) plays a major role in the management of patients with GCTs. The role of surgery continues to evolve owing to advances in chemotherapy regimens, clinical staging modalities, and continued surgical innovation (Sheinfeld and Herr, 1998; Allaf et al, 2005; Albers et al, 2008).

Primary chemotherapy is favored in Europe, whereas RPLND traditionally has been the management strategy of choice in the United States for high-risk patients with clinical stage I nonseminomatous germ cell tumor (NSGCT). RPLND can accurately stage the retroperitoneum and positively identify patients harboring metastases. In addition, patients with pathologic stage I disease are spared the toxicity and morbidity of any additional therapy because 90% or more experience long-term disease-free survival with surgery alone. Patients with pathologic stage II disease can learn more about the extent of their disease and make informed decisions regarding further therapy after RPLND. For patients in this group who harbor small-volume retroperitoneal disease (pN1), a properly performed RPLND can be curative in approximately 70% of men, so chemotherapy also can be avoided in this setting (Richie and Kantoff, 1991; Donohue et al, 1993; Rabbani et al, 2001). Because the retroperitoneum is the most frequent site of chemoresistant malignant GCT and teratoma, both of these processes are minimized with RPLND (Baniel et al, 1995). Some groups advocate RPLND as the treatment of choice for all men with clinical stage I NSGCT with teratoma in the orchiectomy specimen given the increased propensity of harboring teratoma in the retroperitoneum (Sheinfeld et al, 2003). RPLND eliminates these chemoresistant elements and maximizes therapeutic efficacy.

Traditionally, RPLND for GCTs has been performed via an open transabdominal or thoracoabdominal approach. Over the past two decades, minimally invasive approaches for the treatment of various malignancies have emerged and become popular. Since the early 1990s, retroperitoneal laparoscopic surgery has been used with proven benefits related to reducing perioperative morbidity, improving cosmesis, and shortening convalescence without compromising oncologic efficacy (Cadeddu et al, 1998; Allaf et al, 2004; Permpongkosol et al, 2005). Laparoscopic RPLND (L-RPLND) and more recently robotic-assisted RPLND (RA-RPLND) are technically demanding procedures that are increasingly being performed by experienced surgeons aiming to minimize morbidity while duplicating the open technique. **Given that untreated retroperitoneal disease and late relapses in the retroperitoneum are fatal and can be chemorefractory, it is of paramount importance that, as in open RPLND, a complete "cleanout" of lymph nodes is performed** (Whitmore, 1979; Borge et al, 1988; Baniel et al, 1995; Carver et al, 2005).

In this chapter, the evolution of L-RPLND and RA-RPLND is summarized. Controversies surrounding their use, surgical techniques, outcomes, and associated complications are discussed. The focus is on the management of low-stage NSGCTs and the role of these minimally invasive approaches after chemotherapy.

RATIONALE AND EVOLUTION

In an effort to decrease the morbidity associated with open RPLND, shortly after the introduction of laparoscopic renal surgery in 1991, several reports emerged documenting the feasibility of L-RPLND in the management of clinical stage I NSGCT (Rukstalis and Chodak, 1992; Stone et al, 1993; Klotz, 1994). Larger retrospective series followed suggesting decreased blood loss, shorter hospital stays, and faster return to normal activity compared with open RPLND, with preservation of antegrade ejaculation in more than 95% of patients (Gerber et al, 1994; Janetschek et al, 1994, 1996). An early multi-institutional retrospective analysis demonstrated preservation of antegrade ejaculation in all patients, short hospital stays (<3 days), and return to normal activity at 2 to 3 weeks postoperatively (Gerber et al, 1994). **The abbreviated convalescence allows patients who are candidates to receive chemotherapy with minimal delay.** These attractive early results encouraged others to investigate L-RPLND as a viable treatment option for low-stage NSGCT.

STAGING LAPAROSCOPIC RETROPERITONEAL LYMPH NODE DISSECTION AND CONTROVERSY

Of all laparoscopic applications to surgical urology, L-RPLND has raised the most controversy. This controversy is due to the technical difficulty of RPLND in general, the limited number of cases, and lack of interest at traditional centers of excellence. Laparoscopy is an access technique with the internal procedure being performed the same as with an open incision. Experience drives an equivalent dissection. In all early series and some contemporary studies, L-RPLND was used as a staging procedure (Bianchi et al, 1998; Janetschek et al, 2000). Patients not harboring occult metastases were identified and spared exposure to chemotherapy without undergoing open RPLND. In this form, L-RPLND was performed without retrocaval or retroaortic dissection, and chemotherapy was given to all patients harboring metastatic disease (including patients with pN1 disease). The decision to omit dissection behind the great vessels was based on the belief of a lack of isolated positive lymph nodes in this area (Holtl et al, 2002). Within this paradigm, the procedure was routinely aborted if positive lymph nodes were encountered, and chemotherapy was instituted in these cases (Bianchi et al, 1998; Nelson et al, 1999). **In contemporary series, this approach has been abandoned, and L-RPLND has evolved into a therapeutic procedure duplicating the open approach in its intent** (Allaf et al, 2005; Steiner et al, 2008; Hyams et al, 2012).

The use of restrictive template boundaries coupled with the universal use of chemotherapy in men harboring pathologic stage II disease generated criticism of published L-RPLND series. The controversy regarding the use of "staging" L-RPLND hinges on mapping studies demonstrating increased multifocality and contralateral disease in the presence of positive retroperitoneal nodes (Ray et al, 1974; Donohue et al, 1982; Weissbach and Boedefeld, 1987; Eggener et al, 2007). Critics argue that the liberal use of chemotherapy would not prevent relapses and compensate for incomplete resection.

DUPLICATION OF OPEN RETROPERITONEAL LYMPH NODE DISSECTION

At experienced centers at the present time, an exact replication of the open template is performed on all patients with NSGCT undergoing L-RPLND with wide templates and complete excision of retroaortic and retrocaval tissue, rendering the procedure both a staging and a therapeutic operation. Some groups perform a bilateral dissection on all patients, whereas others reserve bilateral dissection for patients with lymph node involvement (Allaf et al, 2005; Steiner et al, 2008).

DEVELOPMENT OF ROBOTIC-ASSISTED RETROPERITONEAL LYMPH NODE DISSECTION

Robotic technology has become ubiquitous within the urologic oncology community, and it is believed to have facilitated a minimally invasive approach to complex urologic operations such as radical prostatectomy and partial nephrectomy. Robotic technology has been shown to increase use of partial nephrectomy, likely owing to perceived ease in facility of this complex laparoscopic procedure (Patel et al, 2013). Given the wide range of robotic procedures performed by urologists and given that L-RPLND requires a complex laparoscopic skill set, small case series of RA-RPLND have emerged demonstrating safety and feasibility (Davol et al, 2006; Williams et al, 2011).

SURGICAL TECHNIQUE

L-RPLND is a technically challenging procedure associated with a steep learning curve and should be undertaken by experienced laparoscopic surgeons who are comfortable and adept with advanced

vascular techniques and open surgery in case of conversion. The indications for primary L-RPLND are identical to the indications for open RPLND and include clinical stage I or IIA disease, negative serum tumor markers, and the absence of comorbidities that would preclude safe surgery. In the postchemotherapeutic setting, L-RPLND has been limited mainly to small-volume residual disease; however, experienced surgeons have excised bulky tumors. **The surgical template for the procedure is dictated by laterality and intraoperative findings. Surgical margins should not be compromised to minimize morbidity, to preserve ejaculation, or because of technical constraints. The extent of the node dissection can be expanded based on intraoperative findings.**

Preoperative Patient Preparation and Technical Considerations

All patients considered candidates for L-RPLND must be fully informed of all treatment options, including open RPLND, chemotherapy, and surveillance. All potential complications including bleeding requiring blood transfusion; injury to adjacent organs (liver, bowel, gallbladder, kidney, ureter, pancreas, major vascular structures); and orthopedic, neurologic, or pulmonary complications as well as conversion to open surgery because of complications or incomplete resection should be discussed (Allaf et al, 2005; Winfield, 1998). Patients interested in future fertility are educated regarding preoperative sperm banking. Some surgeons advocate a low-fat diet 1 to 2 weeks before surgery to reduce the risk of chylous ascites, but data regarding this practice are not definitive. Patients undergo a mechanical bowel preparation the afternoon before surgery and take only clear liquids until midnight to decompress the bowels. Preoperative antibiotics are given before surgery, and antiembolism devices are placed on the lower extremities to minimize deep vein thrombosis.

Standard laparoscopic instruments are used throughout this procedure (e.g., atraumatic graspers, scissors, clip appliers, irrigation/suction device, and laparoscopic paddle retractor). Radiolucent polypropylene clips (Hem-o-lok; Weck Closure Systems, Triangle Park, NC) may minimize artifact on postoperative imaging of the retroperitoneum. In addition, a needle driver loaded with suture and adjunct hemostatic agents such as gelatin matrix (FloSeal Matrix Hemostatic Sealant; Fusion Medical Technologies, Fremont, CA) or oxidized cellulose (Surgicel; Ethicon, Piscataway, NJ) should be readily available in case of vascular injury. Sealing devices such as ultrasonic shears and bipolar devices should be used with caution and can be unreliable in sealing large lymphatic channels. A laparoscopic retractor is particularly useful for medial retraction of the bowel and alleviates the need to position the patient in a modified flank position. A gauze sponge placed in the abdomen can be helpful in tamponading bleeding.

Approach

Although some surgeons use an extraperitoneal approach (Hsu et al, 2003; Hara et al, 2004), most prefer a transperitoneal approach owing to the larger and more familiar working space. **Additionally, a transperitoneal approach facilitates bilateral dissection when warranted by allowing access to all four quadrants.**

Patient Positioning and Port Placement for Laparoscopic Retroperitoneal Lymph Node Dissection

After general anesthesia is induced, an orogastric tube and Foley catheter are inserted. The patient may be placed in the modified flank position (45 degrees) with the side of dissection elevated, but we prefer the supine position because it makes transitioning to a bilateral dissection less cumbersome and does not require patient repositioning (Fig. 36-1). Great care is taken to pad all pressure points to minimize the risk of nerve injury or rhabdomyolysis because these surgeries may require a longer time than their open

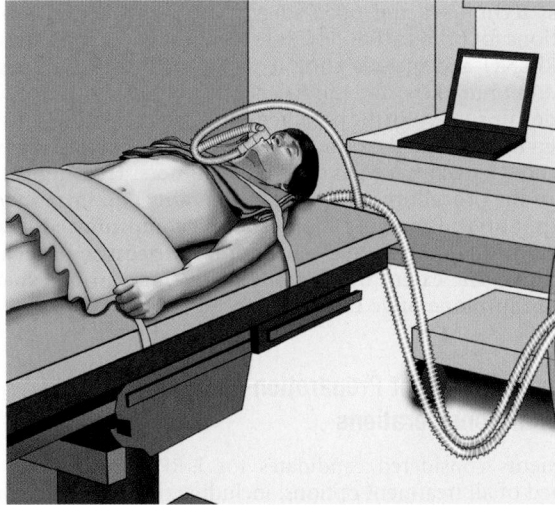

Figure 36-1. Patient positioning during laparoscopic retroperitoneal lymph node dissection. The arms are tucked, and the patient is padded and secured in a relatively supine position.

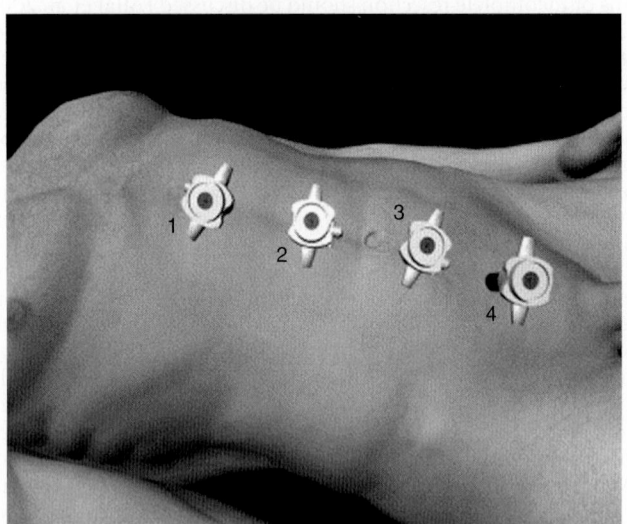

Figure 36-2. Port placement for laparoscopic retroperitoneal lymph node dissection. Four 10/12-mm, equally spaced trocars are placed in the midline.

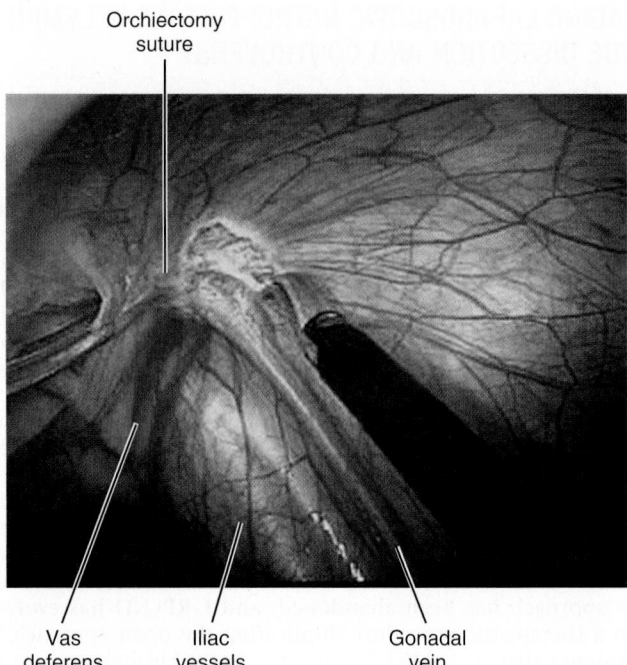

Figure 36-3. Incision of posterior peritoneum circumferentially around the inguinal ring.

counterpart. The patient must be secured to the operating table because tilt is needed to use gravity to help shift the bowel out of the operative field.

After intraperitoneal access is achieved (via a Veress needle or Hasson technique), four equally spaced, 10/12-mm laparoscopic ports are placed in the midline beginning 1 cm below the xiphoid process (Fig. 36-2). The umbilicus may not be incorporated as a port site. The large port size is essential to allow for the convenient introduction of larger (10/12-mm) instruments from varying angles. An additional 5-mm port may be placed in the midaxillary line midway between the iliac crest and ribs for additional retraction if needed. The bed is rotated maximally to allow optimal medialization of the bowel away from the operative field.

Right-Sided Dissection

The ascending colon is mobilized by incising the white line of Toldt from the pelvis and around the hepatic flexure. The second portion of the duodenum is identified and kocherized, providing exposure of the retroperitoneum including the medial para-aortic space on the left.

Spermatic Cord Dissection

The camera is moved to the second to the bottom trocar (trocar 3 in Fig. 36-2) to facilitate visualization during dissection of the spermatic cord stump. The peritoneum medial to the spermatic cord is incised, and the vas deferens is transected. The peritoneum is incised circumferentially around the inguinal ring (Fig. 36-3). With gentle traction on the cord, fibrous attachments and scar are incised until the suture on the spermatic cord is identified. The attachments are cut, and the cord is followed proximally along with surrounding nodal and fibroadipose tissue to the inferior vena cava (IVC). The ureter must be identified at all times to prevent inadvertent thermal injury. The spermatic vein and artery are ligated proximally and transected. The specimen is placed in an endobag and dropped on the contralateral side of the abdomen.

Lymphadenectomy

Although templates should be individualized to each case, we advocate removal of the right common iliac, paracaval, interaortocaval, preaortic, and medial para-aortic nodes (Fig. 36-4). Occasionally in obese patients (or when performing a full bilateral dissection), the left-most border of the dissection must be performed after rotating the table contralaterally to optimize exposure. The camera should be moved to the port second from the top. A paddle retractor is placed in the lowest trocar to protect and sweep the bowel medially.

The testicular vein stump is identified and minimally manipulated to prevent pseudoaneurysm formation with subsequent rupture. The tissues overlying the IVC are gently lifted and carefully incised longitudinally (Fig. 36-5). It is swept off the IVC in a "split and roll" fashion. Blunt dissection aids in further separating these lymphatic tissues toward and overlying the common iliac vessels inferiorly and renal hilum superiorly. Care must be taken to avoid injury of lower pole renal arteries, which are present in approximately 20% of cases, and accessory vessels crossing anterior to the IVC. The renal hilum is dissected to separate all fibroadipose tissue from the renal vein and artery as far under the IVC as possible. Next, the ureter is traced to its crossing over the common iliac vessels, and the lymphatic packet is separated from both of these structures.

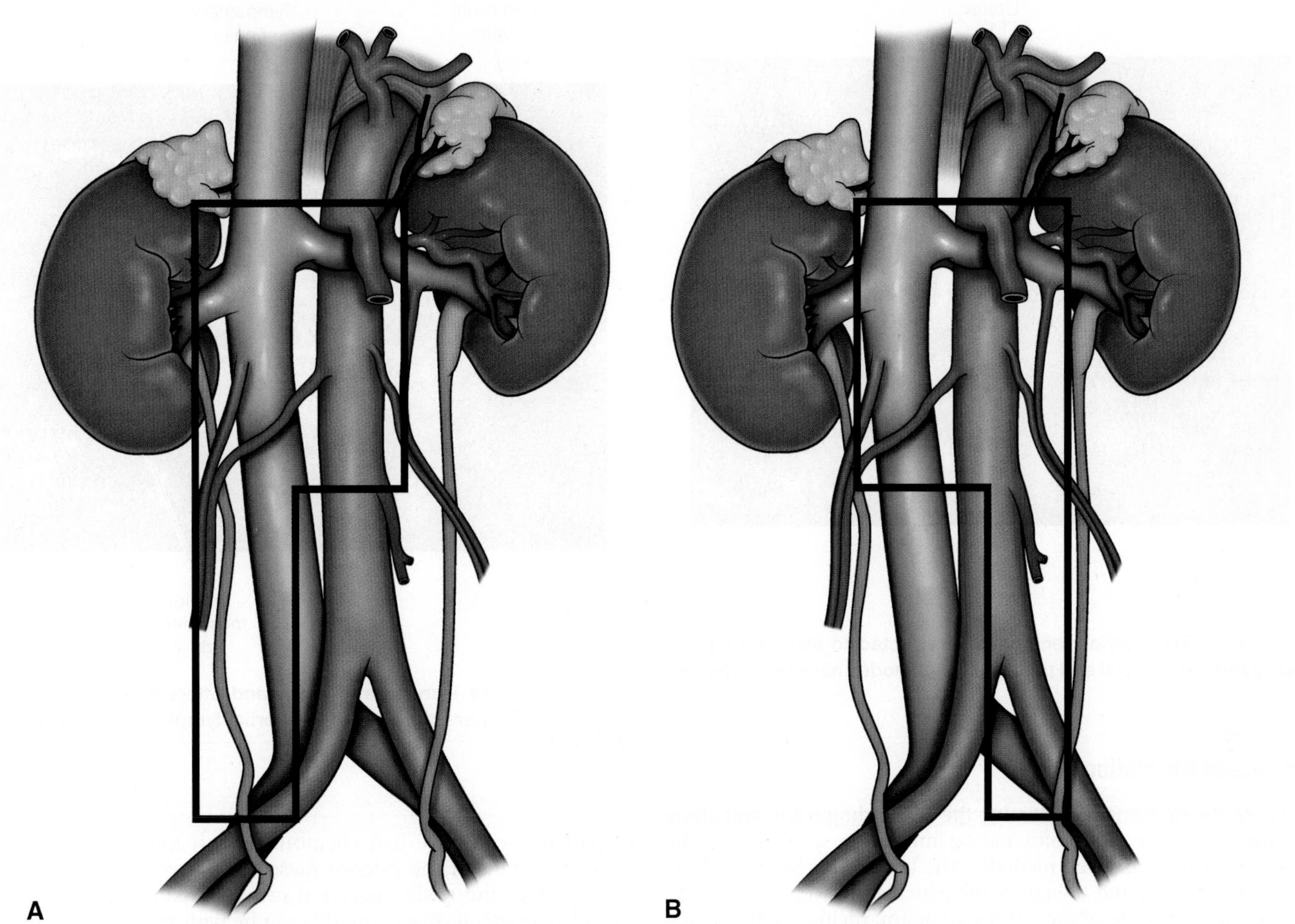

A

B

Figure 36-4. Suggested templates for right (A) and left (B) therapeutic laparoscopic retroperitoneal lymph node dissection. These templates can be expanded or contracted based on each patient's tumor.

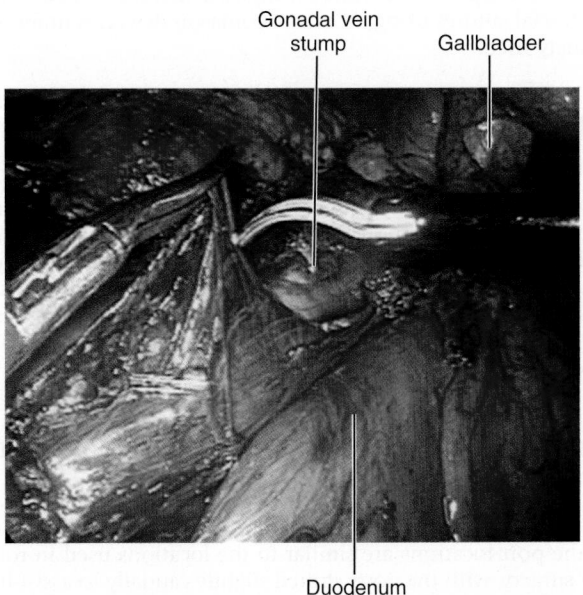

Gonadal vein stump

Gallbladder

Duodenum

Figure 36-5. Fibrofatty tissue overlying the inferior vena cava being incised to initiate the "split and roll" technique. The duodenum has been reflected medially, and the spermatic vein stump has been clipped and divided.

The "split" tissue along the IVC is "rolled" medially to expose the retrocaval space. Lumbar vessels are identified, clipped, and divided to allow splitting of the posterior lymphatic tissues (Fig. 36-6). After this splitting is accomplished, the tissues are released from their attachment to the spine and delivered laterally. Great care is taken to separate the lymph nodes from the sympathetic chain and postganglionic nerve fibers. The aorta is identified next, and the tissues overlying it are similarly split to the level of the inferior mesenteric artery and rolled medially to enter the retroaortic space. The lumbar arteries may be controlled if additional mobility is needed to mobilize the interaortocaval packet posteriorly. The aorta can be medially retracted, facilitating para-aortic node excision with careful preservation of the sympathetic chain laterally. The interaortocaval nodes finally are removed to complete the dissection.

An important technical point is to leave a long stump on the aorta/vena cava side when ligating lumbar vessels such that they can be grasped and controlled in the event a clip dislodges. Lumbar vessels that retract into the iliopsoas uncontrolled usually can be managed with pressure or a figure-of-eight suture placed deep into the muscle. Lacerations of the IVC and aorta may occur during this operation but in most cases do not mandate open conversion. Direct pressure usually prevents excessive hemorrhage and can achieve hemostasis without the need for additional maneuvers. Adjunct hemostatic agents also can be used successfully in this circumstance. If the bleeding persists, or in the case of arterial bleeding, direct pressure can be used temporarily before definitive repair is undertaken with intracorporeal suturing.

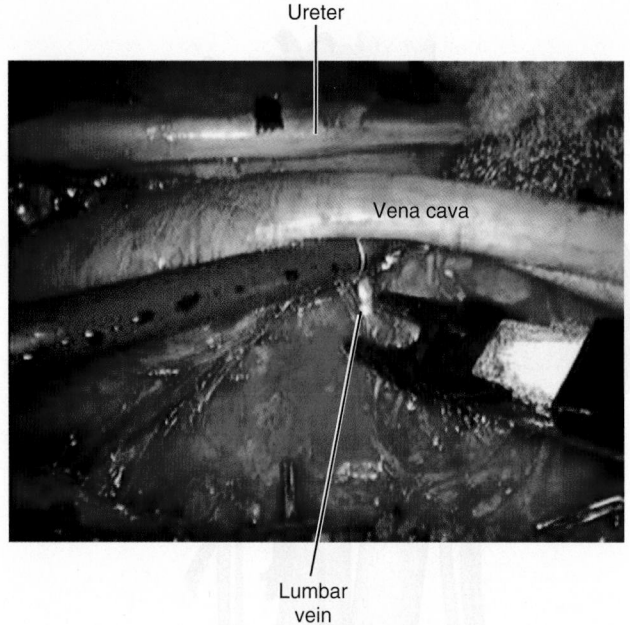

Figure 36-6. The inferior vena cava is retracted to allow for lumbar vein ligation. Paracaval and precaval lymph nodes have been cleared.

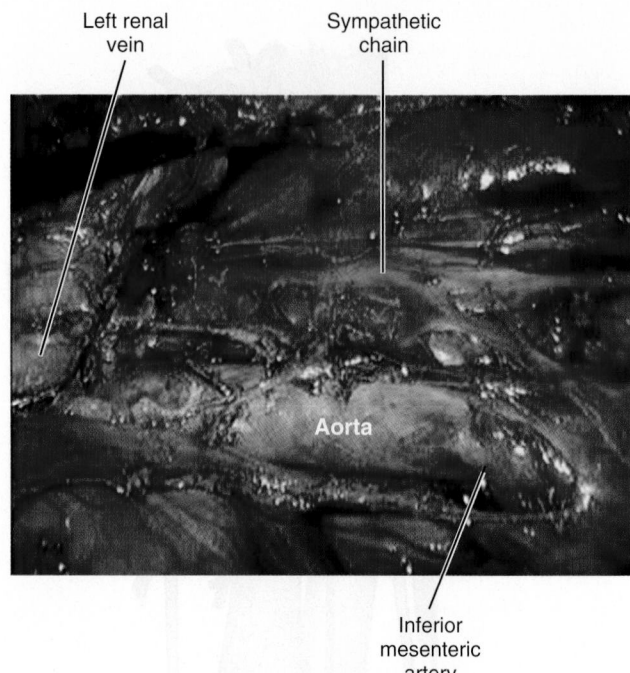

Figure 36-7. The sympathetic chain and efferent nerves are seen spared, while para-aortic and preaortic lymph nodes have been removed.

Left-Sided Dissection

The peritoneum is incised lateral to the descending colon and along the splenic flexure. The colorenal ligaments are severed, and the bowel is bluntly dissected medially. The lateral attachments of the spleen are incised, and the tail of the pancreas is swept medially to ensure wide exposure of the retroperitoneum, including the medial paracaval space.

Spermatic Cord Dissection

Analogous to what is done on the right side, the spermatic cord stump suture is identified after circumscribing the peritoneum at the inguinal ring. The spermatic vein along with adjacent lymph nodes is traced proximally to the renal vein and the artery to the aorta where they are ligated and cut. The cord is placed in an endobag for removal at the conclusion of the procedure.

Lymphadenectomy

We advocate removal of the left common iliac, para-aortic, preaortic, interaortocaval, and medial paracaval lymph nodes (see Fig. 36-4). The dissection can be expanded as needed. Lumbar veins draining into the renal vein are clipped and divided to allow full dissection of the renal hilum. The vein is cleaned off medially to the junction of the vena cava. A paddle retractor in the lowest trocar aids in dissection. The renal artery is completely freed of all lymphatic tissues. Clips are generously used to avoid postoperative leakage of lymph. The tissues overlying the aorta are split from the renal hilum to the level of the inferior mesenteric artery. Care should be taken to identify the right spermatic artery to avoid avulsion. In contrast to the tissues overlying the vena cava, the preaortic space may include postganglionic sympathetic nerves; care must be taken to separate the nodal tissue while preserving these nerves (Fig. 36-7). The ureter and common iliac vessels are separated from all fibroadipose tissue. The preaortic tissues are rolled medially down to the lumbar arteries. The lumbar vessels are controlled and cut, allowing excision of the retroaortic lymph nodes. The vena cava is identified, and using a "split and roll" approach, the paracaval, precaval, and interaortocaval lymph nodes are removed in the same manner as for a right-sided dissection. Care should be taken to identify any right-sided renal arteries to avoid inadvertent ligation.

In patients who have had chemotherapy, it may be necessary to ligate and transect the inferior mesenteric artery. If suspect nodes are detected, the node dissection can be expanded to perform a complete bilateral dissection; this can be performed from the same side using retraction.

At the conclusion of the operation, the lymph nodes are placed in an endobag and extracted. Each packet should be placed in a separate sac during dissection to help increase yield of nodal evaluation and count. The retroperitoneum is irrigated with warm water, and lymphostasis and hemostasis are ensured. The bowel and adjacent organs (liver, gallbladder, kidneys, ureters, pancreas, and spleen) are inspected carefully for injury. The trocar sites are closed with fascial sutures using a Carter-Thomason device. A drain is not routinely used.

Bilateral Laparoscopic Retroperitoneal Lymph Node Dissection

Bilateral dissections may be performed when necessary and usually can be undertaken without a change in patient positioning. When the side of primary tumor is completed with the templates described, a small amount of tissue is left just medial to the contralateral ureter and inferiorly toward the common iliac vessels. These tissues are dissected free, and a bilateral dissection is completed. It is easier to approach a bilateral dissection from the right side.

Robotic-Assisted Retroperitoneal Lymph Node Dissection
Port Placement and Technique

For RA-RPLND, we place the patient in a modified flank position, and the port locations are similar to the locations used in robotic renal surgery, with the ports shifted slightly caudally to assist in the iliac nodal dissection (Fig. 36-8). Use of the robotic fourth arm is preferred for improved retraction leaving the surgeon two working instruments. One or two 12-mm assistant ports may be used depending on surgeon preference. The general steps of the operation mirror the open and laparoscopic techniques. The robotic clip

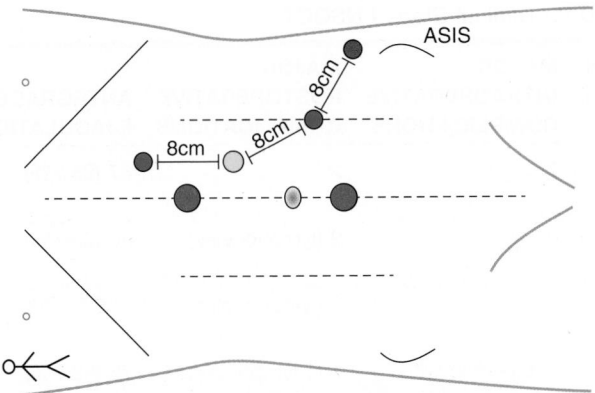

Figure 36-8. Port placement for robotic-assisted retroperitoneal lymph node dissection. *Yellow* **indicates camera port,** *green* **indicates 8-mm robotic ports, and** *red* **indicates 12-mm assistant ports. ASIS, anterior superior iliac spine.**

applier allows the surgeon to articulate the instrument while placing clips and can be particularly helpful in securing lumbar vessels. Depending on body habitus, dissection of the spermatic cord to the orchiectomy suture may require re-docking of the robotic arms and triangulating them toward the inguinal ring for a more direct approach to this area. An alternative technique has been described and entails placement of the patient in a steep Trendelenburg supine position with the robot docking from the patient's head (de Cobelli et al, 2013). The ports are placed in positions similar to robotic-assisted radical prostatectomy, but the field of dissection is reversed (toward the head).

POSTOPERATIVE CARE

Patients are extubated and transferred to the recovery area without nasogastric tube drainage. The patient may ambulate and resume a liquid diet the night of surgery. **Postoperative tachycardia may occur secondary to sympathetic stimulation** (Bahnson et al, 1989). Most patients can be discharged on postoperative day 1. Some surgeons advocate consumption of a low-fat diet for 1 to 2 weeks postoperatively.

PROSPECTIVE NERVE-SPARING TECHNIQUES

As in open RPLND, nerve-sparing techniques involve prospectively identifying, dissecting, and preserving the sympathetic chains, hypogastric plexus, and postganglionic fibers. With experience, these tissues can be readily identified as more fibrous compared with lymphatic tissue. On the right side, the postganglionic sympathetic fibers are most easily identified behind the IVC as they cross anterior to the aorta to insert in the hypogastric plexus. Their takeoff from the sympathetic chains is always near lumbar veins, so great care should be taken in clipping lumbar vessels. On the left side, it is easiest to identify the postganglionic sympathetic nerves at the ganglia as they leave the sympathetic chain and dissect them prospectively as they course anterior to the aorta before joining the hypogastric plexus. Care should be taken to avoid energy sources such as electrocautery when dissecting nerve fibers (Peschel et al, 2002; Bhayani et al, 2003; Abdel-Aziz et al, 2006; Steiner et al, 2008).

COMPLICATIONS

The most common reason for conversion to an open procedure is uncontrollable bleeding, and vascular injury is cited as the most common intraoperative complication (Bhayani et al, 2003;

Abdel-Aziz et al, 2006; Neyer et al, 2007; Kenney and Tuerk, 2008). Although bleeding and open conversion occurred frequently in older series, it is less common in more recent series. **In most contemporary series, the open conversion rate is less than 5%, but it has been reported as high as 11.8%** (Rassweiler et al, 2000; Neyer et al, 2007; Nielsen et al, 2007; Cresswell et al, 2008; Skolarus et al, 2008). **Conversion to an open procedure should never be viewed as a failure, and surgeons should be familiar with open RPLND should it be required.** Injury to major abdominal viscera also has been reported but appears to be a rare event (Neyer et al, 2007; Kenney and Tuerk, 2008).

Postoperative complication rates of 9% to 25% have been reported in contemporary series (Albqami and Janetschek, 2005; Neyer et al, 2007; Nielsen et al, 2007; Cresswell et al, 2008; Skolarus et al, 2008). Reported complications include chylous ascites, ileus, lymphocele, nerve injury, pulmonary embolus, *Clostridium difficile* colitis, retroperitoneal hematoma, and ureteral injury (Kenney and Tuerk, 2008). Retrograde ejaculation is a potential long-term source of morbidity for patients undergoing open RPLND and L-RPLND. **The rates of retrograde ejaculation have been consistently low with the laparoscopic approach and range from 0% to 14%** (Albqami and Janetschek, 2005; Neyer et al, 2007; Nielsen et al, 2007; Cresswell et al, 2008; Skolarus et al, 2008; Steiner et al, 2008). **With meticulous ligation of lymphatic channels, the incidence of chylous ascites should be less than 2%.** A summary of the morbidity of L-RPLND in the management of clinical stage I NSGCT is provided in Table 36-1. Although it is difficult to compare these data retrospectively with published open RPLND series, they appear to compare favorably. In one study of open primary RPLND, a 6% transfusion rate with a mean length of stay of 6 days was reported (Subramanian et al, 2010). Similar to L-RPLND, vascular injury was the most common intraoperative complication (4.5% of cases); 2 patients developed chylous ascites (1.8%) and 14 (12.5%) had an ileus. Antegrade ejaculation in this group of patients was 80%, and seven patients (6.3%) required reoperation (for small bowel obstruction [two patients], incisional hernia repair [four patients], and ureteral reconstruction [one patient]). Two patients required nephrectomy, one for a dysplastic kidney and the other for oncologic reasons.

The morbidity and open conversion rate of L-RPLND after chemotherapy is higher and seems to be experience dependent as well. Early series cited major complication rates of more than 50% (Palese et al, 2002) and high conversion rates (Rassweiler et al, 1996). However, similar to primary L-RPLND, more recent series from experienced centers show improvement in these parameters (Steiner et al, 2004; Permpongkosol et al, 2007). Steiner and colleagues (2004) reported on 68 L-RPLND procedures performed after chemotherapy and reported no open conversions. In another more limited report including 17 patients who underwent L-RPLND after chemotherapy, the authors reported no complications, transfusions, or open conversions (Maldonado-Valadez et al, 2007). Studies report preservation of antegrade ejaculation with experience (LeBlanc et al, 2001; Albqami and Janetschek, 2005; Corvin et al, 2005).

RESULTS AND CURRENT STATUS

There are no randomized trials comparing open RPLND and L-RPLND. Retrospective assessments suggest that patients undergoing L-RPLND have a significantly shorter hospital stay, decreased blood loss, greater quality-of-life scores, and faster return to normal activities (Janetschek et al, 1996; Abdel-Aziz et al, 2006; Poulakis et al, 2006). Results of RA-RPLND are limited to early reports demonstrating safety and feasibility.

Laparoscopic Retroperitoneal Lymph Node Dissection for Clinical Stage I Disease

Published reports of L-RPLND with long-term follow-up suggest that it is an effective treatment option for patients with low-stage

TABLE 36-1 Perioperative and Morbidity Outcomes of L-RPLND for Clinical Stage I NSGCT

STUDY	NO. PATIENTS	OR TIME (MEAN, MIN)	OPEN CONVERSION	EBL (mL)	LENGTH OF STAY (DAYS)	MAJOR INTRAOPERATIVE COMPLICATIONS	MAJOR POSTOPERATIVE COMPLICATIONS	ANTEGRADE EJACULATION
Hyams et al, 2012	91	NA	4	200	2.1	7	2	87 (95.7%)
Steiner et al, 2008	42*	323	0	125	4.8	0	2 (lymphoceles)	36 (85.7%)
Skolarus et al, 2008	19	250	0	145	1.5	0	4 (lymphoceles)	23/26† (88.5%)
Cresswell et al, 2008	79	177	1	NR	6	1 (bleeding with open conversion)	7 (1 lymphocele, 5 ureteral stenosis/injury, 1 pulmonary embolus)	78 (98.7%)
Albqami and Janetschek, 2005	103	217	3	144	3.6	3 (bleeding with open conversion)	0	217 (100%)
Bhayani et al, 2003	29	258	2	389	2.6	2 (bleeding with open conversion)	2 (1 lymphocele, 1 compartment syndrome)	28 (96.6%)
LeBlanc et al, 2001	20	230	0	<50	1.2	0	0	20 (100%)

*Data include 21 patients with clinical stage II disease.
†Ejaculation data given only as percentage of all patients (included are 7 patients with nonclinical stage I disease).
EBL, estimated blood loss; L-RPLND, laparoscopic retroperitoneal lymph node dissection; NA, not available; NR, not reported; NSGCT, nonseminomatous germ cell tumor; OR, operating room.

NSGCTs (Table 36-2). The staging accuracy of L-RPLND has been documented and consistent with open series in that 25% to 30% of men with clinical stage I NSGCT are found to harbor occult nodal disease. **A study with a mean follow-up of 7 years included 87 patients with clinical stage I disease and revealed a 9% and 0% relapse rate for patients with pN0 and pN+ disease, respectively, with all patients alive and free of disease at last follow-up** (Cresswell et al, 2008). The two retroperitoneal recurrences (2.5%) in this series occurred outside the dissection template, and all patients with pN+ disease were administered adjuvant chemotherapy. Examination of other large L-RPLND series confirms these findings, and recurrence rates and their patterns in this patient population are comparable to those of open RPLND series. The recurrence rate of patients found to have negative lymph nodes at L-RPLND is reported between 0% and 10%, which compares favorably with open RPLND series (Donohue et al, 1993; Hermans et al, 2000).

Despite the favorable long-term outcomes, the practice of universal chemotherapy in the adjuvant setting in patients with clinical stage I disease who are also harboring metastatic disease at L-RPLND has been the focus of critics who question the therapeutic efficacy of the technique. Approximately 70% of men found to have pN1 disease and who undergo a properly performed RPLND are cured and can avoid chemotherapy (Richie and Kantoff, 1991; Donohue et al, 1993; Rabbani et al, 2001). However, patients found to have pN1 disease can opt to receive two cycles of chemotherapy in the adjuvant setting with excellent long-term results rather than risk receiving three or four cycles of chemotherapy should they experience relapse. The decision to administer chemotherapy to patients with pN1 disease is a matter of preference and factors in the philosophy of the urologist and medical oncologist as well as the patient.

A report of 120 patients undergoing L-RPLND at one of four institutions in the United States included 10 patients with pathologic stage II disease who underwent surveillance (Nielsen

et al, 2007). At a mean follow-up of 34.8 months, none of the patients had experienced a retroperitoneal recurrence. **Additional reports omitting chemotherapy for patients with pN1 disease who underwent L-RPLND support its therapeutic efficacy, but further studies and follow-up are required** (Skolarus et al, 2008; Steiner et al, 2008).

The adequacy of L-RPLND also can be evaluated by examining patients found to have pathologic stage I disease. If L-RPLND was inadequate, certain patients with pathologic stage II disease would be mislabeled as having pathologic stage I disease, and a retroperitoneal recurrence would result. This supposition has not occurred because no retroperitoneal recurrence has resulted in a series of therapeutic L-RPLND where a full dissection has been performed (Bhayani et al, 2003; Porter and Lange, 2003; Nielsen et al, 2007; Skolarus et al, 2008; Steiner et al, 2008). The therapeutic efficacy of L-RPLND will continue to be tested as more patients found to have pathologic stage II disease are choosing observation after this technique with good results.

Laparoscopic Retroperitoneal Lymph Node Dissection for Clinical Stage II

Fewer reports exist examining the role of L-RPLND for patients with clinical stage II NSGCTs as a primary modality or in the postchemotherapeutic setting. Data regarding the use of primary L-RPLND in patients with clinical stage IIA disease are limited. Several authors have reported on the use of L-RPLND in the postchemotherapeutic setting (see Table 36-2). Albqami and Janetschek (2005) reported their experience with 59 patients with stage IIB or IIC disease who underwent L-RPLND after chemotherapy: Of the 43 patients with preoperative stage IIB disease with a mean follow-up of 53 months, 1 experienced a recurrence 24 months postoperatively along the external iliac nodes, outside the original template. Another group

TABLE 36-2 Oncologic Outcomes of Published L-RPLND Series for Patients with Clinical Stage I NSGCT

STUDY	NO. PATIENTS	FOLLOW-UP (MEAN, MONTHS)	NODE YIELD	N0/N+	NO. pN+ RECEIVING ADJUVANT CHEMOTHERAPY	NO. RECURRENCES*	DISEASE-FREE SURVIVAL
Hyams et al, 2012	91	38	26.1	N0: 63 N1: 21 N2: 7	21 (75%)	N0: (2 PU, 1 BC, 2 distant) N+: 0	100%
Steiner et al, 2008	21	17	22	N0: 16 N+: 5	0 (0%)	N0: 1 (PU) N+: 0	100%
Skolarus et al, 2008	19	23.7	23.8	N0: 13 N1: 6	5 (83.3%)	N0: 0 N+: 0	100%
Cresswell et al, 2008	79	84	14	N0: 60 N+: 19	19 (100%)	N0: 8 (3 PU, 2 RP, 1 PS, 1 BC) N+: 0	100%
Albqami and Janetschek, 2005	103	62	NR	N0: 77 N+: 26	26 (100%)	N0: 5 (3 PU, 1 RP, 1 BC) N+: 0	100%
Bhayani et al, 2003	29	72	20	N0: 17 N+: 12	10 (83.3%)	N0: 2 (PU, BC) N+: 1 (M)	100%
LeBlanc et al, 2001	20	15	9.8 (Rt) 17.7 (Lt)	N0: 14 N+: 6	6 (100%)	N0: 0 N+: 0	100%

*Recurrences: PU, pulmonary; RP, retroperitoneal, outside of template; BC, isolated biochemical; PS, port site.
L-RPLND, laparoscopic retroperitoneal lymph node dissection; Lt, left; NSGCT, nonseminomatous germ cell tumor; pN+, histologically positive lymph nodes; Rt, right.

(Maldonado-Valadez et al, 2007) reported on 17 patients and demonstrated the feasibility of L-RPLND after chemotherapy: Viable tumor was found in 3 patients, 2 of whom experienced retroperitoneal recurrences. Full bilateral RPLND, which is typically recommended in this setting, was not performed in these series (Stephenson and Sheinfeld, 2004).

Keeping in line with the goals of open RPLND performed after chemotherapy, Steiner and associates (2008) performed bilateral nerve-sparing L-RPLND on 19 postchemotherapy patients with stage IIB disease. The authors found teratoma in 4 patients, necrosis/fibrosis in 14 patients, and active tumor in 1 patient. This study included two patients with clinical stage IIA disease who underwent L-RPLND without adjuvant chemotherapy. No retroperitoneal recurrences were noted in either group at 17 months of follow-up. Longer follow-up and larger series are required to evaluate the efficacy of L-RPLND in the postchemotherapeutic setting.

SUMMARY

L-RPLND has been demonstrated to be a feasible, safe, and effective treatment option for men with clinical stage I NSGCT when performed at large-volume institutions by experienced laparoscopic surgeons. L-RPLND has evolved into a therapeutic operation duplicating the open procedure, with reports demonstrating efficacy and minimal morbidity. Data regarding L-RPLND for clinical stage II disease and for patients who have received chemotherapy are limited and associated with a longer learning curve. Early reports suggest that robotic-assisted surgery is emerging as yet another minimally invasive alternative to RPLND.

Please visit the accompanying website at www.expertconsult.com to view videos associated with this chapter.

> ### KEY POINTS
>
> - L-RPLND aims to decrease operative morbidity while duplicating the open approach.
> - The most common reason for conversion to an open procedure is bleeding, although this is a rare complication (<5%).
> - L-RPLND is an effective treatment option for patients with low-stage NSGCTs.
> - Reports omitting chemotherapy for patients with N1 disease who underwent L-RPLND support its therapeutic efficacy, but more studies and follow-up are required.
> - RA-RPLND is emerging as another minimally invasive alternative to open RPLND.

REFERENCES

The complete reference list is available online at www.expertconsult.com.

SUGGESTED READINGS

Allaf ME, Bhayani SB, Link RE, et al. Laparoscopic retroperitoneal lymph node dissection: duplication of open technique. Urology 2005;65:575–7.

Cresswell J, Scheitlin W, Gozen A, et al. Laparoscopic retroperitoneal lymph node dissection combined with adjuvant chemotherapy for pathological stage II disease in nonseminomatous germ cell tumours: a 15-year experience. BJU Int 2008;102:844–8.

Nielsen ME, Lima G, Schaeffer EM, et al. Oncologic efficacy of laparoscopic RPLND in treatment of clinical stage I nonseminomatous germ cell testicular cancer. Urology 2007;70:1168–72.

Steiner H, Zangerl F, Stohr B, et al. Results of bilateral nerve sparing laparoscopic retroperitoneal lymph node dissection for testicular cancer. J Urol 2008;180:1348–52, discussion 1352–3.

37 Tumors of the Penis

Curtis A. Pettaway, MD, Juanita M. Crook, MD, FRCPC, and Lance C. Pagliaro, MD

Cancers of the penis are uncommon tumors that are often devastating for the patient and frequently diagnostically and therapeutically challenging for the urologist. Although rare in North America and Europe, penile malignant neoplasms constitute a substantial health concern in many African, South American, and Asian countries.

Any discussion of penile cancers must begin by addressing both premalignant and malignant tumors of the penis. A description of these lesions serves to establish their anatomic, etiologic, and histologic relationship to squamous cell carcinoma, which is the most common malignant tumor of the penis, as well as to other malignant neoplasms that involve the penis. Developments in the etiologies of various premalignant and malignant penile tumors are reviewed in this chapter.

In this chapter, we review the epidemiology, etiology, and natural history of squamous carcinoma and its contemporary management. **Reports have confirmed the importance of pathologic stage and histologic features of the primary tumor as well as the presence and extent of lymph node metastasis in determining prognosis and treatment planning for penile squamous carcinoma** (Ravi, 1993a; McDougal, 1995; Theodorescu et al, 1996; Pizzocaro et al, 1997; Slaton et al, 2001). In addition, developments in staging of the disease, including novel imaging modalities and the use of dynamic sentinel node biopsy (DSNB), and modified surgical approaches to improve staging accuracy and reduce potential morbidities are presented. The selection of patients for organ-preserving surgical strategies is discussed.

The role of radiation therapy as both a primary treatment and a palliative measure is reviewed. Contemporary developments in chemotherapy as well as in combination therapy with multiple therapeutic modalities are also discussed. A contemporary scheme for the management of the inguinal region, based on histologic and clinical features, is presented.

Finally, the various nonsquamous malignant neoplasms that may involve the penis are reviewed and discussed.

PREMALIGNANT CUTANEOUS LESIONS

Please see the Expert Consult website for a discussion of premalignant cutaneous lesions (including Fig. 37-1), and virus-related dermatologic lesions.

SQUAMOUS CELL CARCINOMA

Carcinoma in Situ

Carcinoma in situ (Tis) of the penis is called *erythroplasia of Queyrat* by urologists and dermatologists if it involves the glans penis and prepuce or Bowen disease if it involves the penile shaft or the remainder of the genitalia or perineal region. This nomenclature has served to separate carcinoma in situ from the mainstream of thinking and reporting of penile carcinoma. However, the epidemiology and natural history of this lesion parallel those of early carcinoma of the penis, and carcinoma in situ can progress to invasive carcinoma.

The erythroplasia originally described by Queyrat in 1911 consists of a red, velvety, well-marginated lesion of the glans penis or, less frequently, the prepuce of the uncircumcised man (Aragona et al, 1985). It may ulcerate and may be associated with discharge and pain. On histologic examination the normal mucosa is replaced by atypical hyperplastic cells characterized by disorientation, vacuolation, multiple hyperchromatic nuclei, and mitotic figures at all levels. The epithelial rete extends into the submucosa and appears elongated, broadened, and bulbous. The submucosa shows capillary proliferation and ectasia with a surrounding inflammatory infiltrate that is usually rich in plasma cells. These microscopic features distinguish erythroplasia of Queyrat from chronic localized balanitis. HPV has been identified in penile carcinoma in situ (Pfister and Haneke, 1984). Progression to invasive carcinoma can occur in 10% to 33% of patients (Buechner, 2002; Bleeker et al, 2009).

In 1912 Bowen described an intraepithelial neoplasm of the skin associated with a high occurrence of subsequent internal malignant disease as a distinct entity. Bowen disease and erythroplasia of Queyrat are histologically similar (Graham and Helwig, 1973) (see Fig. 37-1C on the Expert Consult website). Both tumors are characterized by the noninvasive changes of carcinoma in situ. **Visceral malignant disease is not associated with erythroplasia of Queyrat, and subsequent case-control studies have shown no association of Bowen disease with internal malignant tumors** (Anderson et al, 1973). Thus penile carcinoma in situ does not in itself warrant a specific search for internal malignant tumors. **Bowen disease is characterized by sharply defined plaques of scaly erythema on the penile shaft. Crusted or ulcerated variants can occur. The appearance can be confused with bowenoid papulosis, nummular eczema, psoriasis, and superficial basal cell carcinoma. If it is not treated, then invasive carcinoma may arise in about 5% of patients** (Buechner, 2002). **When all cases of carcinoma in situ** are considered, metastasis is extremely rare but has been reported (Eng et al, 1995).

Treatment is based on proper histopathologic confirmation of malignancy with multiple biopsies of adequate depth to rule out invasion. When lesions are located on the foreskin, circumcision or excision with a 5-mm margin is adequate for local control (Bissada, 1992). In this regard, lesions on the glans penis are more difficult to treat by excisional strategies while maintaining normal penile anatomy. Recently several groups have described the technique of glans resurfacing for penile squamous carcinoma of the glans penis. In this technique the epithelium and subepithelial tissue of the glans penis are completely dissected off the underlying spongiosal tissue. The resulting defect is then closed with a skin graft. Early follow-up reveals very low rates of local recurrence (Hadway et al, 2006; Shabbir et al, 2011b). Alternative strategies include topical 5-fluorouracil cream (Lewis and Bendl, 1971; Graham and Helwig, 1973; Goette, 1974), 5% imiquimod cream (Danielson et al, 2003), and ablation with Nd:YAG (Landthaler et al, 1986; Frimberger et al, 2002a), potassium titanyl phosphate (KTP) 532-nm, or carbon dioxide lasers (Rosemberg and Fuller, 1980; Tietjen and Malek, 1998; van Bezooijen et al, 2001). Such strategies have been shown to produce excellent cosmetic and functional results. Radiation therapy can be used to treat tumors that are resistant to topical treatment, especially among patients who are not surgical candidates (Kelley et al, 1974; Grabstald and Kelley, 1980; Mazeron et al, 1984; McLean et al, 1993).

KEY POINTS: CARCINOMA IN SITU

- Carcinoma in situ (Tis) is an intraepithelial malignant process.
- Progression to invasive carcinoma may occur in 5% to 33% of patients if it is not treated.
- Metastasis has rarely occurred.
- Cancer eradication with organ-preserving strategies is the goal of therapy.

Invasive Carcinoma

Penile carcinoma accounts for 0.4% to 0.6% of all malignant neoplasms among men in the United States and Europe; it may represent up to 10% of malignant neoplasms in men in some Asian, African, and South American countries (Gloeckler-Ries et al, 1990; Vatanasapt et al, 1995). **However, reports suggest that the incidence of penile cancer is decreasing in many countries, including Finland, the United States, India, and other Asian countries** (Maiche, 1992; Frisch et al, 1995; Vatanasapt et al, 1995; Yeole and Jussawalla, 1997). The reasons are unclear but may be related in part to increased attention to personal hygiene.

Penile cancer is a disease of older men, with an abrupt increase in incidence in the sixth decade of life (Persky, 1977). In two studies the mean ages were 58 years (Gursel et al, 1973) and 55 years (Derrick et al, 1973). The tumor is not unusual in younger men; in one large series, 22% of patients were younger than 40 years and 7% were younger than 30 years (Dean, 1935); the disease has also been reported in children (Kini, 1944; Narasimharao et al, 1985). The Surveillance, Epidemiology, and End Results (SEER) database reveals no racial difference in incidence of penile cancer between black and white men in the United States (incidence for white men, 0.8 per 100,000; for black men, 0.7 per 100,000) (Vatanasapt et al, 1995).

However, a study using SEER data suggested that race is associated with outcome. Rippentrop and colleagues (2004) noted there were 1605 patients diagnosed with penile cancer from 1973 to 1998, with 22.4% (360) dying of the disease. They found factors independently predictive of worsened survival to be higher stage at diagnosis, age older than 65 years, African-American ethnicity, and disease within lymph nodes. These researchers demonstrated a statistically significant disease-specific risk of death that was 2.2-fold higher in African-American patients than in white patients. Although the reason for this disparity is likely to be multifactorial, possibilities include differences in cancer biology, in health care access, or in treatment. These provocative findings clearly deserve further study.

Etiology

The incidence of carcinoma of the penis varies according to circumcision practice, hygienic standard, phimosis, number of sexual partners, HPV infection, exposure to tobacco products, and other factors (Barrasso et al, 1987; Maiche, 1992; Maden et al, 1993; Misra et al, 2004).

Neonatal circumcision has been well established as a prophylactic measure that virtually eliminates the occurrence of penile carcinoma because it eliminates the closed preputial environment where penile carcinoma develops. The chronic irritative effects of smegma, a byproduct of bacterial action on desquamated cells that are within the preputial sac, have been proposed as a causative agent. Although definitive evidence that human smegma itself is a carcinogen has not been established (Reddy and Baruah, 1963), its relationship to the development of penile carcinoma has been widely observed. Improper hygiene can lead to buildup of smegma beneath the preputial foreskin, with resulting inflammation. Healing by fibrosis leads to phimosis of the preputial skin, which tends to perpetuate the cycle. Phimosis is found in 25% to 75% of patients described in most large series. Reddy and associates (1984) studied the foreskins of 26 men undergoing circumcision because of phimosis and found epithelial atypia in one third of the specimens.

Carcinoma of the penis is rare among the Jewish population, for whom neonatal circumcision is a universal practice (Licklider, 1961). Similarly, in the United States, where neonatal circumcision is widely practiced, penile cancer represents less than 1% of male malignant neoplasms. Among noncircumcising tribes of Africa and within Asian cultures in which circumcision is not practiced, penile cancer may amount to 10% to 20% of all male malignant neoplasms (Dodge, 1965; Narayana et al, 1982). Data from most large series show that penile cancer is rare among neonatally circumcised individuals but more frequent when circumcision is delayed until puberty (Frew et al, 1967; Gursel et al, 1973; Johnson et al, 1973). Adult circumcision appears to offer little or no protection from subsequent development of the disease (Maden et al, 1993). **These data suggest that the critical period of exposure to certain causative agents may have already occurred at puberty and certainly by adulthood, rendering later circumcision relatively ineffective as a prophylactic tool for penile cancer.**

Population-based data reveal that although neonatal circumcision is highly protective for invasive penile cancer, it does not afford the same level of protection for carcinoma in situ. Schoen and colleagues (2000) evaluated the incidence of invasive penile cancer or carcinoma in situ during a 10-year period and found only 2 cases of 89 (2.3%) occurring among neonatally circumcised men, whereas of 118 men with carcinoma in situ, 16 cases were noted among 102 men who were circumcised at birth for an incidence of 15.7%. Considering that the protective effects of circumcision on invasive penile cancer are likely to be mediated by avoidance of phimosis, it is noteworthy that another study associated phimosis with the development of invasive penile cancer but not carcinoma in situ (Hung-fu et al, 2001).

Male circumcision has also been shown to be effective against HIV type 1 (HIV-1) infection. This effect was shown to be specific by Reynolds and colleagues (2004). There was no protective effect of circumcision for other sexually transmitted diseases, such as herpes simplex virus type 2 infection, syphilis, or gonorrhea.

HPV infection and exposure to tobacco products appear to be associated with development of penile cancer. Epidemiologic data provided the first clues to a relationship between a sexually transmitted agent and cancer by demonstrating that the wives or ex-wives of men with penile cancer had a threefold higher risk of cervical carcinoma (Graham et al, 1979). Further investigation revealed that the male partners of women with cervical intraepithelial neoplasia had a significantly higher incidence of penile intraepithelial neoplasia (Barrasso et al, 1987). These same male patients were also found to have a greater incidence of HPV infection.

Polymerase chain reaction and in situ hybridization have provided increased evidence for a causative role of HPV by identifying specific DNA sequences from different HPV types in primary penile lesions (malignant and benign) but not in normal foreskins (Varma et al, 1991; Iwasawa et al, 1993). More than 25 types of HPV infect genital sites. HPV types 6 and 11 are most commonly associated with nondysplastic lesions such as genital warts, but these are also noted in nonmetastatic verrucous carcinomas. In contrast, HPV types 16, 18, 31, and 33 are associated with in situ and invasive carcinomas (Wiener and Walther, 1995). **HPV-16 appears to be the most frequently detected type in primary carcinomas and has also been detected in metastatic lesions** (Varma et al, 1991; Iwasawa et al, 1993; Wiener and Walther, 1995). As noted previously, the HPV genome encodes oncoprotein E6, which complexes with the tumor suppressor protein TP53, and oncoprotein E7, which binds the retinoblastoma (RB) protein, thus affecting cell cycle regulation (Munger et al, 1989; zur Hausen, 1996; Levi et al, 1998; Griffiths and Mellon, 1999) via the p14ARF/MDM2/p53 and p15INK4a/cyclin D/Rb pathways (Bleeker et al, 2009). Maden and colleagues (1993) **found that the incidence of HPV infection directly correlated with the number of lifetime sexual partners, which was also related to risk of penile cancer.** Furthermore, Castellsague and colleagues (1997) noted a direct correlation between the number of sexual partners, HPV-infected men, and incidence of cervical neoplasia among their female partners. Thus, for both cervical and penile cancer, HPV infection represents a preventable cause.

Poblet and coworkers (1999) reported on two patients with coexisting HIV-1 and HPV infection and postulated that HIV-1 could synergize with HPV to increase the progression of HPV lesions into penile carcinoma. Although there is evidence supporting this effect in cervical and anal neoplasia, definitive proof for penile cancer awaits further study (Northfelt, 1994).

Although HPV infection is probably an important factor in the development of penile cancer, its presence is not invariable (31% to 63% of patients with penile carcinoma test positive) (Wiener and Walther, 1995), **indicating that additional factors may be involved in the development of the disease or its subtypes.** Additional evidence includes a study by Rubin and associates (2001), who performed a sensitive polymerase chain reaction assay on penile cancer specimens from the United States and Paraguay and wrote their hypothesis-based essay. Overall, 42% of penile carcinomas were HPV positive. However, only 34.9% and 33.3% of keratinizing and verrucous carcinomas, respectively, were positive, whereas 80% and 100% of basaloid and warty tumor subtypes, respectively, exhibited HPV DNA. Other non–HPV-dependent molecular events leading to penile carcinogenesis have been described, including silencing of the CDK2NA locus via promoter hypermethylation, the expression of genes that target the INK4a/ARF locus, other gene mutations affecting TP53, and p14ARF, and MDM2 overexpression (reviewed in Ferreux et al, 2003; Bleeker et al, 2009).

Four studies have shown a significant association between exposure to cigarette smoke and development of penile cancer (Hellberg et al, 1987; Daling et al, 1992; Maden et al, 1993; Harish and Ravi, 1995). Hellberg and colleagues (1987) studied the smoking history of 244 men with penile cancer and matched controls. They found a significantly increased odds ratio for penile cancer based on whether an individual had smoked, and the risk increased with the number of cigarettes smoked. This observation held even when the presence of phimosis was controlled. **Harish and Ravi** (1995) **extended these observations by showing that all forms of tobacco products, including cigarettes, chewing tobacco, and snuff, were significantly and independently related to the incidence of penile cancer subsequent to multivariate regression analysis.** It has been hypothesized that tobacco products can act in the presence of HPV infection or bacteria associated with chronic inflammation to promote malignant transformation. These same risk factors are also common to other anogenital carcinomas (Daling et al, 1992; Maden et al, 1993).

Penile trauma may be another risk factor for penile cancer. The development of carcinoma in the scarred penile shaft after mutilating circumcision has been reported as a distinct entity (Bissada et al, 1986). Furthermore, Maden and colleagues (1993) found a greater than threefold risk of penile cancer in men with penile tears and rashes. A case-control study also revealed an odds ratio of 18:1 for the development of penile cancer for those men reporting a penile injury 2 years before the onset of the disease (Hung-fu et al, 2001).

Genital ultraviolet radiation, alone and combined with 8-methoxypsoralen, increases the risk of squamous carcinoma at genital sites. A 12-year follow-up study reported that the risk of penile and scrotal cancer was increased 286 times that of the general population for those exposed to ultraviolet A photochemotherapy and 8-methoxypsoralen (PUVA) (Stern, 1990). The risk was dose related. For those treated with ultraviolet B exposure, the risk was 4.6-fold enhanced. Another long-term follow-up study of PUVA-associated malignant neoplasia from Sweden revealed a 30-fold increased risk for skin cancer (but not for penile cancer) among males. In this study, PUVA was also associated with respiratory and pancreatic cancers (Lindelof et al, 1991). Lichen sclerosus (also known as balanitis xerotica obliterans) is a risk factor for the development of penile cancer. **Studies have shown the incidence of subsequent cancer with long-term follow-up to be between 2.3% and 9% of men with LS** (Depasquale et al, 2000; Micali et al, 2001). Velazquez and Cubilla (2003) studied LS occurring in association with penile cancer and noted its presence distinctly among the subset of penile carcinomas that were not associated with HPV.

Larger studies performed in areas where the disease is endemic, incorporating the many risk factors for penile cancer into a multivariate analysis, are clearly needed to define which factors independently confer risk. Thus far, no convincing evidence has been found linking penile cancer to other factors such as occupation, other venereal diseases (gonorrhea, syphilis, and herpes), marijuana use, or alcohol intake (Maden et al, 1993).

Prevention

The role of routine neonatal circumcision as a preventive strategy for penile cancer has been, to say the least, a controversial topic. The position of the American Academy of Pediatrics has changed over time with accumulating evidence from one of denial of any medical benefits (Schoen et al, 1989) to the more moderate position stating, **"There are potential medical benefits of newborn circumcision"** (Shapiro, 1999) to the most recent statement published in August 2012, which states, "Evaluation of current evidence indicates that the health benefits of newborn male circumcision outweigh the risks and that the procedure's benefits justify access to this procedure for families who choose it." Specific benefits in their data review included prevention of urinary tract infections, penile cancer, and transmission of sexually transmitted infections including HIV (American Academy of Pediatrics Task Force on Circumcision, 2012)

Any argument against circumcision must consider that penile carcinoma represents the only neoplasm for which there exists a predictable and simple means of prophylaxis to spare the organ at risk (Dagher et al, 1973). Although circumcision can obviate the disease, especially where facilities for daily hygiene may be lacking, it may not be as important in countries where good hygiene is practiced. Frisch and colleagues (1995) reported a falling incidence of penile cancer (from 1.15 per 100,000 men to 0.82 per 100,000 men) in the Danish population, which has a circumcision rate of only 1.6%. They attributed this trend to improved hygiene because the incidence of dwellings having a bath facility increased from 35% in the 1940s to 90% in the 1990s. Thus, considering the benefits of circumcision (including the prevention of infections, HIV infection and its transmission, and penile and cervical cancer), enhanced education about the potential benefits of circumcision, especially in developing countries, seems rational (Schoen et al, 1989; Reynolds et al, 2004; Kinkade et al, 2005).

Although neonatal circumcision and good hygiene to prevent the occurrence of phimosis represent important prevention strategies, additional efforts to prevent malignant transformation include avoidance of HPV infection potentially through condom use, of ultraviolet light exposure, and of tobacco products. Thus, modifiable behaviors can potentially prevent penile cancer (Munger et al, 1989; Maden et al, 1993; Harish and Ravi, 1995; Levi et al, 1998; Griffiths and Mellon, 1999; Bleeker et al, 2009).

As mentioned previously, HPV vaccination could play an emerging role in the future with respect to preventing transmission of HPV between males and females and potentially penile cancer. To date two prophylactic HPV vaccines are available (HPV 16/18 vaccine Cervarix [GlaxoSmithKline] and the quadrivalent HPV 16/18/6/11 vaccine Gardasil [Merck Sharp & Dohme]), and the efficacy of preventing HPV infection among HPV-negative young women and men has been demonstrated (Harper et al, 2004; Villa et al, 2005, Block et al, 2006; Bleeker et al, 2009; Giuliano et al, 2011).

KEY POINTS: EPIDEMIOLOGY, ETIOLOGY, AND PREVENTION

- Penile cancer is rare in developed countries and varies worldwide with age, circumcision, and hygiene practices.
- Recent epidemiologic data from the United States suggest a disparity in outcome, with African-Americans exhibiting poorer survival.
- Risk factors for development of penile cancer include lack of neonatal circumcision, phimosis, HPV infection, exposure to tobacco products, penile LS, and potentially penile trauma and exposure to PUVA.
- Histologic subtypes of penile cancer are correlated with HPV infection.
- Penile cancer represents a preventable disease in most cases via neonatal circumcision and/or behavior modification.

Natural History

Carcinoma of the penis usually begins with a small lesion that gradually extends to involve the entire glans, shaft, and corpora. The lesion may be papillary and exophytic or flat and ulcerative; if it is untreated, penile autoamputation may occur as a late result. The rates of growth of the papillary and ulcerative lesions are similar, but the flat, ulcerative tumor has a tendency toward earlier nodal metastasis and is associated with poorer 5-year survival rates (Dean, 1935; Marcial et al, 1962; Ornellas et al, 1994). Lesions larger than 5 cm (Beggs and Spratt, 1964) and those extending over 75% of the shaft (Staubitz et al, 1955) are also associated with an increased incidence of metastases and a decreased survival rate. However, others have not found a consistent relationship among lesion sizes, presence of metastases, and decreased survival (Ekstrom and Edsmyr, 1958; Puras et al, 1978).

Buck fascia acts as a temporary natural barrier to local extension of the tumor, protecting the corporeal bodies from invasion. Penetration of Buck fascia and the tunica albuginea permits invasion of the vascular corpora and establishes the potential for vascular dissemination. Urethral or bladder involvement is rare (Riveros and Gorostiaga, 1962; Thomas and Small, 1968).

The earliest route of dissemination from penile carcinoma is metastasis to the regional femoral and iliac nodes. A detailed description of lymphatic drainage of the penis is found elsewhere in this text and is well documented in the literature (Dewire and Lepor, 1992). Briefly, the lymphatics of the prepuce form a connecting network that joins with the lymphatics from the skin of the shaft. These tributaries drain into the superficial inguinal nodes (the nodes external to the fascia lata). The lymphatics of the glans join the lymphatics draining the corporeal bodies, and they form a collar of connecting channels at the base of the penis that drain by way of the superficial nodes. The superficial nodes drain to the deep inguinal nodes (those deep to the fascia lata). From there, drainage is to the pelvic nodes (external iliac, internal iliac, and obturator). Penile lymphangiographic studies demonstrate a consistent pattern of drainage that proceeds from superficial inguinal to deep inguinal to pelvic node sites without evidence of ipsilateral drainage (Cabanas, 1977, 1992). Multiple cross-connections exist at all levels of drainage, so that penile lymphatic drainage is bilateral to both inguinal areas.

Metastatic enlargement of the regional nodes eventually leads to skin necrosis, chronic infection, and death from inanition, sepsis, or hemorrhage secondary to erosion into the femoral vessels. Clinically detectable distant metastatic lesions to the lung, liver, bone, or brain are uncommon and are reported to occur in 1% to 10% of patients in most large series (Staubitz et al, 1955; Riveros and Gorostiaga, 1962; Beggs and Spratt, 1964; Derrick et al, 1973; Johnson et al, 1973; Kossow et al, 1973; Puras et al, 1978, reviewed in Pettaway et al, 2010). Such metastases usually occur late in the course of the disease after the local lesion has been treated. Distant metastases in the absence of regional node metastases are unusual.

Carcinoma of the penis is characterized by a relentless progressive course, causing death for the majority of untreated patients within 2 years (Beggs and Spratt, 1964; Skinner et al, 1972; Derrick et al, 1973). Rarely, long-term survival occurs, even with advanced local disease and regional node metastases (Furlong and Uhle, 1953; Beggs and Spratt, 1964). No report of spontaneous remission of carcinoma of the penis is known. Five percent to 15% of patients have been reported to develop a second primary neoplasm (Buddington et al, 1963; Beggs and Spratt, 1964; Gursel et al, 1973), and one series reported secondary carcinoma in 17% of patients (Hubbell et al, 1988).

Modes of Presentation

Signs

It is the penile lesion itself that usually alerts the patient to the presence of penile cancer. The presentation ranges from a relatively subtle induration or small excrescence to a small papule, pustule, warty growth, or more luxuriant exophytic lesion. It may appear as a shallow erosion or as a deeply excavated ulcer with elevated or rolled-in edges. Phimosis may obscure a lesion and allow a tumor to progress silently. Eventually, erosion through the prepuce, foul preputial odor, and discharge with or without bleeding call attention to the disease.

Penile tumors may arise anywhere on the penis but occur most commonly on the glans (48%) and prepuce (21%). Other tumors involve the glans and prepuce (9%), the coronal sulcus (6%), or the shaft (<2%) (Sufrin and Huben, 1991). This distribution of lesions may be the result of constant exposure of the glans, coronal sulcus, and interior prepuce to irritants (e.g., smegma, HPV infection) within the preputial sac, whereas the shaft is relatively spared.

Rarely, a mass, ulceration, suppuration, or hemorrhage in the inguinal area may be caused by nodal metastases from a lesion concealed within a phimotic foreskin. Urinary retention or urethral fistula from local corporeal involvement is a rare presenting sign.

Symptoms

Pain does not develop in proportion to the extent of the local destructive process and usually is not a presenting complaint. Weakness, weight loss, fatigue, and systemic malaise occur secondary to chronic suppuration. On occasion, significant blood loss from the penile lesion, the nodal lesion, or both may occur. Because local disease and regional disease are usually far advanced by the time distant metastases occur, presenting symptoms referable to such metastases are rare.

Diagnosis

Delay

Patients with cancer of the penis, more than patients with other types of cancer, seem to delay seeking medical attention (Lynch and Krush, 1969). In large series, 15% to 50% of patients delayed medical care for more than a year (Dean, 1935; Buddington et al, 1963; Hardner et al, 1972; Gursel et al, 1973). Explanations include embarrassment, guilt, fear, ignorance, and personal neglect. This level of denial is substantial, given that the penis is observed and handled on a daily basis.

Delay on the part of the physician in initiating both diagnosis and treatment may also be considerable. In some instances patients have been given prolonged courses of antibiotics or topical antifungal preparations before being referred for biopsy. Although some studies show that the difference in survival rates between patients with early presentation and those with later presentation is negligible (Ekstrom and Edsmyr, 1958; Johnson et al, 1973), other series show decreased survival with longer delay (Hardner et al, 1972). It appears logical that earlier diagnosis and treatment should improve outcome.

Examination

At presentation most lesions are confined to the penis (Skinner et al, 1972; Derrick et al, 1973; Johnson et al, 1973). The penile lesion is assessed with regard to size, location, fixation, and involvement of the corporeal bodies. Inspection of the base of the penis and scrotum is necessary to rule out extension into these areas. Rectal and bimanual examination provides information about perineal body involvement and presence of a pelvic mass. Careful bilateral palpation of the inguinal area for adenopathy is extremely important.

> ### KEY POINTS: NATURAL HISTORY AND PRESENTATION
>
> - Penile cancer often begins on the surface of the glans penis or in the preputial area, where it progressively enlarges.
> - Delay both in seeking medical attention and then in subsequent definitive biopsy is common.
> - Examination of both the penile primary tumor and the inguinal region is critical to treatment planning.
> - Metastasis occurs by embolization of tumor deposits from the penile tumor through penile lymphatics to the inguinal lymph nodes.
> - Distant metastases occur late in the history of the disease.

Biopsy

Confirmation of the diagnosis of carcinoma of the penis and assessment of the depth of invasion, the presence of vascular invasion, and the histologic grade of the lesion by microscopic examination of a biopsy specimen are mandatory before the initiation of any therapy. This provides insight into the therapeutic options for treatment of the primary lesion as well as the likelihood of nodal metastases in patients with no palpable adenopathy (McDougal, 1995; Lopes et al, 1996; Theodorescu et al, 1996).

Biopsy may be a separate procedure from definitive surgical treatment. A dorsal slit is frequently necessary to gain adequate exposure of the lesion for satisfactory biopsy. An alternative approach to treatment is biopsy with frozen-section confirmation followed by partial or total penectomy. Full informed consent must be obtained before the procedure. Velazquez and colleagues (2004) demonstrated the shortcomings of superficial diagnostic biopsies in a study evaluating specimens from 57 patients. There was difficulty in delineating the extent of depth in 91% of patients, discordance with the histologic grade in 30% of patients (specifically with

verrucous and mixed histologic patterns), and failure to detect any cancer in 3.5% of patients with well-differentiated cancers. The importance of obtaining an adequate biopsy specimen cannot be overemphasized.

Histologic Features

Most tumors of the penis are squamous cell carcinomas demonstrating keratinization, epithelial pearl formation, and various degrees of mitotic activity. The normal rete pegs are disrupted. Invasive lesions penetrate the basement membrane and the surrounding structures. Cubilla and associates (1993) originally divided penile cancers by growth pattern into superficially spreading squamous carcinoma, vertical growth carcinoma, verrucous carcinoma, and multicentric carcinoma. The superficially spreading carcinoma occurred most frequently, and inguinal lymph node metastases were found in 42% of patients. However, lymph node metastases were noted in 82% of patients with a vertical growth pattern, in none of those with a verrucous pattern, and in 33% of those with multicentric carcinomas. Subsequent to review of 61 cases from Memorial Sloan Kettering Cancer Center, Cubilla and colleagues (2001) classified the histologic types as follows: usual type, 59% of cases; papillary, 15%; basaloid, 10%; warty (condylomatous), 10%; verrucous, 3%; and sarcomatoid, 3%. Of note, both the basaloid and sarcomatous types were associated with aggressive behavior; 5 of 7 patients with these histologic patterns exhibited metastasis, and 5 of 8 (63%) died. In contrast, the verruciform histologic patterns were more favorable (1 patient with metastasis and no deaths). The typical squamous histologic type was intermediate in biologic potential; 14 of 26 patients exhibited metastases, and 13 of 36 (36%) died.

The basaloid variant, in addition to its aggressive behavior as noted previously, is associated with HPV expression in approximately 80% of cases (Gregoire et al, 1995; Cubilla et al, 1998, 2001; Rubin et al, 2001).

Squamous cell carcinomas have classically been graded using the Broders classification to define the level of differentiation on the basis of keratinization, nuclear pleomorphism, number of mitoses, and several other features (Broders, 1921; Lucia and Miller, 1992). This grading system was originally designed for squamous carcinoma of the skin and has been adapted by pathologists for penile squamous carcinoma. Four grades were originally described, but it is common for authors to modify this to a three-grade system by combining grades (Maiche et al, 1991). Low-grade lesions (grade 1 and grade 2) constitute 70% to 80% of the reported cases at diagnosis, whether a three- or four-grade system is used (Maiche et al, 1991). These well-differentiated lesions show cords of atypical squamous cells projecting downward from a hyperkeratotic epidermis. The lower-grade carcinomas typically demonstrate keratin, prominent intercellular bridges, and keratin pearls, characteristics that are absent in high-grade tumors. Almost half the tumors originating in the shaft are poorly differentiated (grade 3 and grade 4, depending on scale), whereas only 10% of tumors located in the prepuce are high-grade tumors (Maiche et al, 1991). Thus, grade and stage are often correlated.

Several studies have emphasized the association of high-grade disease with regional nodal metastases (Fraley et al, 1989; Ravi, 1993a; McDougal, 1995; Theodorescu et al, 1996; Heyns et al, 1997). Overall, there is a significant body of agreement as to the histologic features that characterize high tumor grade (grade 3 and grade 4) and its correlation with nodal metastasis. However, as noted previously, most tumors are of lower grades. Histologic features that would better stratify the prognosis for patients with invasive, low- to intermediate-grade penile cancers would be of value for management of patients.

Slaton and colleagues (2001) found that describing the percentage of poorly differentiated cancer in the primary penile tumor specimen correlated with lymph node metastasis. In this study, a semiquantitative system that estimated the amount of high-grade cancer (i.e., ≤50% vs. >50%) was significantly associated with nodal metastases and was more predictive than the Broders three-grade system in stratifying those with or without nodal metastasis.

However, Chaux and colleagues (2009) questioned these findings as they examined 117 specimens among patients undergoing primary tumor therapy and lymph node dissection. Over 50% of the tumors were actually heterogeneous with respect to grade, and among these tumors any proportion of grade 3 cancer was associated with lymph node metastasis. These disparate findings point to at least three problems with respect to grading and prognosis, including (1) lack of a uniform system, (2) reproducibility of interpretation, and (3) intratumoral heterogeneity of tumor components.

Vascular invasion by tumor cells has significant prognostic importance but may not be specifically mentioned in pathology reports. When vascular invasion is present, it provides valuable information. Four studies have assessed its presence or absence, and it was an important predictor of nodal metastasis in all the reports (Fraley et al, 1989; Lopes et al, 1996; Heyns et al, 1997; Slaton et al, 2001). **Thus the pathologist should specifically comment on the presence or absence of vascular invasion in the surgical specimen.**

Perineural invasion was recently found to be present in 36% of cases analyzed in a multi-institutional data set of 134 patients and was a strong predictor of lymph node metastasis (Velazquez et al, 2008).

KEY POINTS: BIOPSY AND HISTOLOGIC FEATURES

- Adequate tumor biopsy is essential to diagnosis and treatment planning.
- Squamous carcinoma histologic subtypes include usual type, papillary, basaloid, warty, verrucous, and sarcomatoid. They vary with respect to metastatic potential.
- Pathologic description of anatomic structures invaded (i.e., stage), the grade, and the status of vascular and perineural invasion provide important information to assess the risk of metastasis.

Laboratory Studies

The results of laboratory tests in patients with penile cancer are often normal. Anemia, leukocytosis, and hypoalbuminemia may be present in patients with chronic illness, malnutrition, and extensive suppuration at the area of the primary and inguinal metastatic sites. Azotemia may develop secondary to urethral or ureteral obstruction.

Hypercalcemia without detectable osseous metastases has been associated with penile cancer (Anderson and Glenn, 1965; Rudd et al, 1972). In a review from Memorial Sloan Kettering Cancer Center (Sklaroff and Yagoda, 1982), 17 of 81 patients (20.9%) were hypercalcemic. Hypercalcemia seems to be largely a function of the bulk of the disease. It is often associated with inguinal metastases and may resolve after excision of involved inguinal nodes (Block et al, 1973). **Parathyroid hormone and related substances may be produced by both tumor and metastases that activate osteoclastic bone resorption** (Malakoff and Schmidt, 1975). Medical treatment of hypercalcemia includes aggressive saline hydration to restore the extracellular fluid volume and to promote both sodium and calcium excretion. The administration of diuretics is performed if volume overload is suspected. Bisphosphonates (e.g., pamidronate, etidronate, and zoledronic acid) have become first-line therapy because they possess demonstrated efficacy as antiresorptive agents and are relatively safer than mithramycin, an older agent (Videtic et al, 1997; Morton and Lipton, 2000). For severe hypercalcemia associated with neurologic manifestations, the antiresorptive bisphosphonates can be combined with an agent that produces calciuria, such as calcitonin, to rapidly lower serum calcium levels.

Radiologic Studies

Primary Penile Tumor. **In patients with penile cancer both the primary tumor and the inguinal lymph nodes are readily assessed by palpation.** However, Horenblas and associates (1991) found that physical examination incorrectly established the actual pathologic stage in 26% of cases, with understaging in 10% and overstaging in 16%. It is clear that more accurate means of staging for penile tumors is needed.

Penile ultrasonography was performed on 16 patients referred for primary therapy by Horenblas and colleagues (1994). With use of a 7.5-MHz linear array small parts transducer they found that the ultrasound appearance of cancer was invariably hypoechoic. However, ultrasound examination often underestimated the thickness of tumors and could not delineate invasion into the subepithelial connective tissue of the glans penis from corpus spongiosum involvement (i.e., glanular stage T1 vs. glanular stage T2). However, the tunica albuginea separating the corpus cavernosum from the glans was easily identified in all patients, and the sensitivity for detecting corpus cavernosum invasion was 100%. This study confirmed the value of ultrasonography in assessing the primary tumor, as reported by others (Yamashita and Ogawa, 1989; Dorak et al, 1992).

Several studies have assessed the role of magnetic resonance imaging (MRI) in evaluating both the normal penis and its involvement by cancer. Vapnek and associates (1992) described the MRI appearance of the normal corpus cavernosum, corpus spongiosum, tunica albuginea, and Buck fascia. Of six patients with urethral cancer, the disease was accurately staged in five (83%). De Kerviler and colleagues (1995) used gadolinium contrast-enhanced MRI to compare both clinical and MRI findings with tumor pathologic stage. Clinical examination correctly staged six of nine tumors: MRI was correct in seven of nine cases but was not useful for clinical T1 lesions. Compared with MRI and ultrasonography, computed tomography (CT) has poor soft-tissue resolution and has not been useful for imaging the extent of the primary tumor (Vapnek et al, 1992).

Lont and associates (2003) directly compared physical examination with ultrasonography and MRI to assess their ability to determine the tumor stage. They evaluated 33 patients with penile squamous cell carcinoma, all of whom underwent ultrasound examination, MRI, and physical examination of the primary tumor. Findings were correlated with histologic evaluation of the specimens obtained at surgery with a focus on determining the invasion of the corpus cavernosum. The respective positive predictive value, sensitivity, and specificity for the study were as follows—physical examination: 100%, 86%, 100%; ultrasound examination: 67%, 57%, 91%; and MRI: 75%, 100%, 91%. This comparative study concluded that physical examination is reliable in determining corporeal invasion and that additional tests are mainly of value when physical examination cannot be properly performed.

The technique of artificial erection (by intracorporeal injection of prostaglandin E_1) may augment the use of contrast-enhanced MRI in staging of the primary tumor. A study by the European Institute of Oncology evaluated nine patients to compare clinical, pathologic, and MRI staging (Scardino et al, 2004). MRI aided by artificial erection and contrast enhancement was shown to be of value because it correlated with pathologic stage in eight of nine cases, whereas physical examination correlated with only five of nine cases. These data suggest that this novel MRI approach could be beneficial in staging of glanular tumors, specifically when physical examination findings are equivocal. **Thus, for small-volume glanular lesions, imaging studies add virtually no additional information to palpation in most patients. However, for lesions thought to invade the corpus cavernosum, contrast-enhanced MRI (perhaps augmented with artificial erection) may provide unique information, especially when physical examination** findings are equivocal and organ-sparing techniques are being considered.

Inguinal and Pelvic Region

Current Imaging Strategies among Clinical Node-Negative Patients. The ability to noninvasively determine the presence or absence of inguinal and pelvic metastases in patients with penile cancer remains problematic because physical examination exhibits varying reliability based on the grade and stage of the primary tumor as well as body habitus of the patient. Both CT and MRI techniques have depended on lymph node enlargement for detection of metastases but are unable to define the internal architecture of normal-sized nodes. Because CT and MRI have similar accuracy in determining lymphadenopathy in other cancers, CT has often been the imaging modality chosen in penile cancer to examine the inguinal and pelvic areas as well as to rule out more distant metastases.

Horenblas and associates (1991) compared the ability of physical examination, CT, and lymphangiography to assess the inguinal region in patients who were surgically staged or had prolonged follow-up. In 102 patients with a 39% prevalence of positive nodes, the sensitivity and specificity of physical examination were 82% and 79%, respectively. Of note, both CT and lymphangiography were performed in patients who were thought to have metastases. The sensitivity of lymphangiography was only 31%, but there were no false-positive results. Similarly, the sensitivity and specificity of CT were 36% and 100%, respectively. The combination of CT and lymphangiography performed simultaneously demonstrated equally poor sensitivity. Only one fifth of patients had positive nodes detected with either test. **On the basis of these data the authors concluded that CT and lymphangiography offer no useful additional information over physical examination, especially in patients with no palpable adenopathy.** An important caveat is that CT may have a role in examination of the inguinal region in obese patients or in those who have had prior inguinal surgery, in whom the physical examination may be unreliable.

Insights in the field of nanoparticle technology have been applied to imaging of genitourinary malignant neoplasms to enhance detection of microscopic metastases. Ferumoxtran-10 particles (size, 35 nm), administered at a dose of 2.6 mg of iron per kilogram of body weight intravenously combined with MRI, were capable of imaging microscopic metastasis in lymph nodes that were by size criteria normal (1 cm). Tabatabaei and colleagues (2005) evaluated lymphotropic nanoparticle-enhanced MRI (LNMRI) in seven patients with penile cancer who subsequently underwent groin dissection. Five of seven patients had no palpable adenopathy. LNMRI was highly sensitive and detected positive nodes in all five of these patients. Of note, the size range of the metastases was less than 1 cm in four patients. Unfortunately, no confirmatory studies were performed using this agent, and the compound is not currently available for routine use.

Squamous carcinoma was shown to take up the radiopharmaceutical fluorodeoxyglucose (FDG) and to be amenable to detection using combination positron emission tomography (PET) and CT. Scher and associates (2005) evaluated PET/CT among 13 patients with penile cancer who received injections of FDG. Five of the 13 patients had metastatic disease, and FDG-PET/CT detected it in 4 of them (80% sensitivity). However, in a follow-up study from the Netherlands, PET/CT was used in patients who were clinically node negative to determine the sensitivity among patients scheduled to undergo inguinal staging procedures. Among 5 patients with proven nodal metastasis, PET/CT was positive in only 1 (i.e., sensitivity of 20%) (Leijte et al, 2009a).

Among a similar cohort reported from this same group, ultrasound-guided needle aspiration was also shown to have limited sensitivity as well, detecting only 9 of 23 patients with proven metastases (sensitivity of 39%; Kroon et al, 2005a). Thus, among clinically node-negative patients, no current imaging modality has been shown to be sufficiently sensitive to detect microscopic metastases.

Current Imaging Strategies among Clinical Node-Positive Patients. Recent data among patients with proven inguinal metastases suggest that additional imaging may be of value in determining those patients with advanced disease who might do poorly when treated with surgery alone or could in fact exhibit occult distant metastases.

Graafland and colleagues (2011) evaluated the CT scan findings among a cohort of biopsy-proven patients with metastatic inguinal adenopathy to define if scan parameters could determine those with poor prognostic features subsequent to lymphadenectomy. They found that central necrosis or an irregular nodal border was highly sensitive and specific for any of the poor prognostic features including three or more positive nodes, extranodal extension (ENE) of cancer, or positive pelvic nodes.

In contrast to the clinically node-negative disease setting, one study has shown the potential value of PET/CT among patients with proven inguinal metastases. Graafland and coworkers (2009) studied PET/CT among 18 patients with biopsy-proven inguinal metastases and found PET/CT to have a sensitivity and specificity of 91% and 100%, respectively, for detecting pelvic lymph node metastases. In that study, PET/CT also identified several patients with distant metastases that were unsuspected. Thus, if confirmed, PET/CT may become an important study for detecting pelvic and distant metastasis.

In general, distant metastases occur late in the course of the disease, usually in patients with recognized significant inguinal and pelvic adenopathy. The most common metastatic sites are the lung, bone, and liver. Currently, in addition to chest, abdominal, and pelvic CT, radionuclide bone scintigraphy may be indicated to stage the extent of disease in patients thought to have widespread metastases (Vapnek et al, 1992).

KEY POINTS: RADIOLOGIC STUDIES

- Soft-tissue detail of penile tumors is best imaged by MRI.
- Physical examination provides the most reliable staging information for small distal lesions.
- Penile MRI performed in combination with artificial erection may provide unique staging information when physical examination findings are equivocal.
- Physical examination of the inguinal region remains the clinical gold standard for evaluating the presence of metastasis in the nonobese patient.
- CT or MRI can be useful in evaluating the inguinal region of obese patients and in those who have had prior inguinal surgery.
- Among patients with proven inguinal metastases, CT scan of the abdomen and pelvis may help to determine those patients with poor prognostic features for cure with surgery alone.
- PET/CT may be useful among patients with clinically detected inguinal metastases to define the presence of pelvic or distant metastasis.

Penile Cancer Staging

Seventh Edition TNM Penile Staging System. The seventh edition of the American Joint Committee on Cancer (AJCC) and Union for International Cancer Control (UICC) TNM staging system was published in 2010 and has become the consensus method for staging penile cancer (Table 37-1, Fig. 37-2) (Edge et al, 2010). With respect to the primary tumor, because grade and the presence of vascular invasion are established prognostic markers in predicting the risk of subsequent inguinal metastasis, the seventh edition TNM stratifies pT1 stage by their presence (i.e., high-grade tumors, vascular invasion present is pT1b) or absence (pT1b) (Slaton et al, 2001; Solsona et al, 2004; Ficarra et al, 2005). In addition, prostatic invasion (a rare finding) is now included in the pT4 designation.

Of considerable importance is that the seventh edition has both clinical and pathologic nodal staging descriptors to facilitate both

TABLE 37-1 American Joint Committee on Cancer (AJCC) Staging for Penile Cancer

PRIMARY TUMOR (T)	
TX	Primary tumor cannot be assessed
T0	No evidence of primary tumor
Tis	Carcinoma in situ
Ta	Noninvasive verrucous carcinoma*
T1a	Tumor invades subepithelial connective tissue without lymphovascular invasion and is not poorly differentiated (i.e., grade 3-4)
T1b	Tumor invades subepithelial connective tissue with lymphovascular invasion or is poorly differentiated
T2	Tumor invades corpus spongiosum or cavernosum
T3	Tumor invades urethra
T4	Tumor invades other adjacent structures

LYMPH NODES (N)	
NX	Regional nodes cannot be assessed†
pNX	Regional nodes cannot be assessed‡
N0	No palpable or visibly enlarged inguinal lymph nodes†
pN0	No regional lymph node metastasis‡
N1	Palpable mobile unilateral inguinal lymph node†
pN1	Metastasis in a single inguinal lymph node‡
N2	Palpable mobile multiple or bilateral inguinal lymph nodes†
pN2	Metastasis in multiple or bilateral inguinal lymph nodes‡
N3	Palpable fixed inguinal nodal mass or pelvic lymphadenopathy, unilateral or bilateral†
pN3	Extranodal extension of lymph node metastasis or pelvic lymph node(s), unilateral or bilateral‡

DISTANT METASTASIS (M)	
M0	No distant metastasis (no pathologic M0; use clinical M to complete stage group)
M1	Distant metastasis§

STAGE GROUPING			
Stage 0	Tis	N0	M0
	Ta	N0	M0
Stage I	T1a	N0	M0
Stage II	T1b	N0	M0
	T2	N0	M0
	T3	N0	M0
Stage IIIa	T1-3	N1	M0
Stage IIIb	T1-3	N2	M0
Stage IV	T4	Any N	M0
	Any T	N3	M0
	Any T	Any N	M1

*Broad pushing penetration (invasion) is permitted; destructive invasion is against the diagnosis.
†Based on palpation and imaging.
‡Based on biopsy or surgical excision.
§Lymph node metastasis outside the true pelvis in addition to visceral or bone sites.
From Edge SB, Byrd DR, Compton CC, et al. AJCC cancer staging manual. 7th ed. New York: Springer; 2010.

clinical and pathologic staging to better predict prognosis before definitive therapy. As pointed out by Leijte and colleagues (2008), the prognosis worsens for patients exhibiting greater degrees of palpable adenopathy (i.e., unilateral vs. bilateral vs. a fixed mass) or positive nodes on imaging versus those with clinically negative inguinal lymph nodes. Considering pathologic nodal factors further, the seventh edition stratifies patients with a single positive node from those with multiple or bilateral nodes and further recognizes the ominous prognosis (5% to 18% 5-year survival) associated with ENE of cancer (Srinivas et al, 1987; Ravi, 1993a; Lont et al, 2007).

Considering that the pathologic status of inguinal nodes is the driving factor determining survival, stage groupings (i.e., stage 0 to

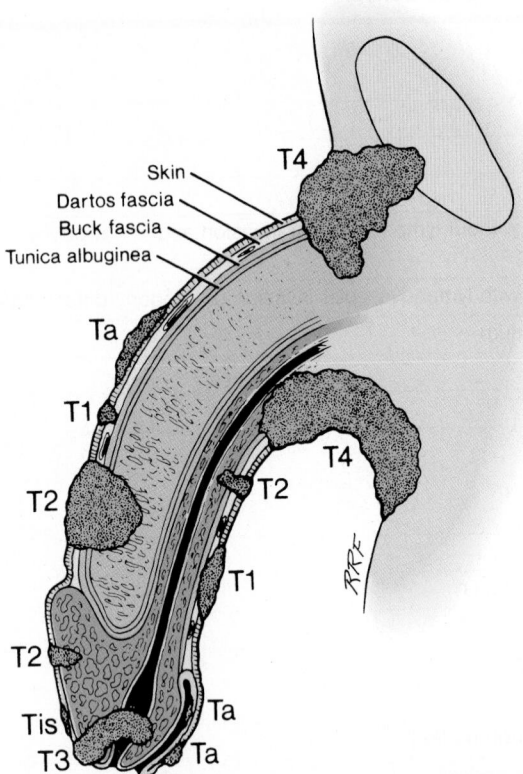

Skin
Dartos fascia
Buck fascia
Tunica albuginea

T4

Ta

T1

T2

Tis

T3

T4

T2

T1

Ta

Ta

T2

Figure 37-2. Because treatment decisions for inguinal node dissections are based on the characteristics of the primary lesion (see section on treatment of inguinal nodes), a careful assessment of the depth of invasion of the primary tumor is required. This diagram illustrates the importance of depth of invasion in assigning tumor (T) stage.

stage IV [see Table 37-1]) in the seventh edition TNM use the extent of nodal involvement as the major consideration. Thus the strength of the unified AJCC-UICC seventh edition TNM system (2010) is that it provides not only an accurate assessment of the primary tumor based on clinical staging (examination, biopsy) but also clinical and improved pathologic descriptors of lymph node status to predict outcome. Furthermore, the nodal status of the new TNM version has been externally validated among node-positive patients in a recent study from Shanghai (Zhu et al, 2011). In that study, stratification of recurrence-free survival among N1 to N3 categories was significantly better when comparing the seventh edition TNM to the prior sixth edition system.

Another recent important prognostic variable, lymph node density (LND), has been described. This variable describes the number of positive inguinal or pelvic nodes removed at surgery as a function of the total number of nodes removed. Thus, in addition to describing the number of positive lymph nodes, it also includes a potential quality variable in incorporating the total lymph node yield. Svatek and colleagues (2009) described this initially in a small series of 45 patients with proven inguinal metastasis, finding that LND was the strongest predictor of disease-specific survival, even when considering TNM stage and extracapsular extension. Zhu and colleagues (2011) confirmed this finding subsequently and also showed that LND retained its independent prognostic ability even when considering the improved seventh edition TNM staging system. Larger series of node-positive patients will be required to more precisely determine clinically useful cutoff values for LND as well as what constitutes an adequate lymph node yield at lymphadenectomy.

In the TNM staging system the primary tumor stage is assigned by biopsy (or even more reliably by complete resection) and

additional prognostic factors within the primary tumor now included in the TNM system (i.e., tumor grade and the presence of vascular invasion). In most cases the presence of palpable adenopathy, along with the histologic features of the primary tumor, determines the need for additional imaging studies. Positive fine-needle aspiration of palpably enlarged inguinal nodes or fine-needle biopsy of pelvic adenopathy identified by CT can assist in assigning nodal stage before therapy. In patients requiring surgical staging (palpable lymph nodes or those with adverse primary tumor histologic features), pathologic nodal status assigned according to seventh edition TNM stage provides valuable prognostic information. The suggested diagnostic criteria for current TNM staging are listed in Box 37-1.

KEY POINTS: STAGING

- Both clinical and pathologic factors related to the presence and extent of lymph node involvement determine survival and should be recorded.
- The current, seventh edition unified TNM staging system represents a consensus document that includes both clinical and pathologic descriptors that provide important prognostic information.

Differential Diagnosis

A number of penile lesions must be considered in the differential diagnosis of penile carcinoma. They include condyloma acuminatum, Buschke-Löwenstein tumor, and balanitis xerotica obliterans, as well as a number of infectious lesions (e.g., chancre, chancroid, herpes, lymphopathia venereum, granuloma inguinale, and tuberculosis). These diseases can be identified by appropriate skin tests, tissue studies, serologic examinations, cultures, or specialized staining techniques.

SURGICAL MANAGEMENT OF THE PRIMARY TUMOR

Organ Preservation

Surgical amputation of the primary tumor remains the oncologic gold standard for rapid definitive treatment of the penile primary tumor; local recurrence rates range from 0% to 8% (de Kernion et al, 1973; McDougal et al, 1986; Horenblas et al, 1992). Whereas amputation is often necessary for bulky stage T2 to T4 tumors, it has been shown to decrease sexual quality of life (Opjordsmoen and Fossa, 1994). This is relevant because approximately 55% of penile cancer patients are 60 years of age or younger and 30% are 55 years of age or younger (Narayana et al, 1982).

It is generally accepted that patients with penile primary tumors exhibiting favorable histologic features (stages Tis, Ta, T1; grade 1 and grade 2 tumors) are at a lower risk for metastases. These patients are also best suited for organ-sparing or glans-sparing procedures (Solsona et al, 2004). The goal of treatment is to preserve glans sensation where possible or at least to maximize penile shaft length. Such approaches include topical treatments (5-fluorouracil or imiquimod cream for Tis only), radiation therapy, Mohs surgery, limited excision strategies, and laser ablation (Sanchez-Ortiz and Pettaway, 2003; Solsona et al, 2004; Minhas et al, 2005; Crook et al, 2009, Alnajjar et al, 2012). This section focuses on novel insights into surgical strategies to achieve organ preservation. Radiation-based strategies are discussed later in the section on radiation therapy for the primary lesion.

Circumcision and Limited Excision Strategies

Circumcision, limited excisions of the glans, and glans removal with sparing of the penile shaft represent surgical strategies to maintain function and penile length. Historically, data on circumcision and limited excision of glanular lesions have been associated with recurrence rates from 11% to 50% (Hanash et al, 1970; Skinner et al, 1972; McDougal et al, 1986). However, the grade, size, and exact location of the lesion and the status of surgical margins were often unavailable in such reports.

Recent reports have suggested that conservative surgery may be performed safely in well-selected patients with discrete tumors by intraoperative frozen-section analysis (Davis et al, 1999; Bissada et al, 2003; Pietrzak et al, 2004; Minhas et al, 2005). **In addition, several studies have challenged the dictum establishing that a 2-cm surgical margin is required for all patients undergoing partial penectomy** (Hoffman et al, 1999; Agrawal et al, 2000). After performing a prospective histologic analysis of 64 penectomy specimens, Agrawal and associates (2000) concluded that tumor grade highly correlated with microscopic tumor spread. The maximum proximal histologic extent was 5 mm for grade 1 and grade 2 tumors and 10 mm for grade 3 tumors. Furthermore, "skip" lesions were not encountered. After performing a retrospective pathologic review of 12 penectomy specimens, Hoffman and colleagues (1999) also found 7 patients with disease of pathologic stage T1 or greater with microscopic margins measuring less than 10 mm. None of these patients had disease recurrence at a mean follow-up of 32.4 months. Pietrzak and colleagues (2004) documented the use of various techniques in a series of 39 patients to excise the tumor and to reconstruct or graft the glans and distal penis. With a mean follow-up of 16 months, only 1 patient (2.5%) who underwent a partial glans resection had a local recurrence. There were two early complications with grafts and two late complications with graft overgrowth intruding on the urethral meatus. Minhas and associates (2005) similarly performed either wide local excision or glans penis removal in 51 patients with margins of 0 to 10 mm in 48% and less than 2 cm in 98% of patients. With a median follow-up of 26 months, a local recurrence rate of 4% to 6% was noted. Limitations of this approach include proximal and distal deeply invasive tumors, high-grade tumors, and patients with poor health status who would not be candidates for salvage procedures if they experienced recurrence. A follow-up series from this same group that included 179 patients having undergone a variety of organ-sparing procedures including glansectomy, excisions, and distal corporectomy was recently reported (Philippou et al, 2012). With a mean follow-up of 43 months, the incidence of recurrence was 8.9% (16 patients). It is important to note that local relapse did not affect disease-specific survival. These results seem to suggest that a 2-cm margin may not be necessary for small tumors of lower grade in the presence of a negative frozen section. However, patients managed with limited excision techniques should be considered to be at a higher risk for local recurrence until longer-term follow-up and additional surgical series are available.

Another recent technique used in the surgical management of carcinoma in situ of the glans penis is *glans resurfacing*, also known as *glans stripping*. In this technique, subdermal dissection of the skin and subepithelial connective tissue off the underlying corpora spongiosa is performed. Shabbir and colleagues (2011a) described this procedure in 25 patients with clinical carcinoma in situ of the glans; they performed either a total or partial removal of all the glans surface tissue. Positive surgical margins were noted in 48% of patients overall but in only 20% of those having total removal. At a mean of 29 months, 5 patients underwent re-excision for unexpected invasive disease at the margin. One of 25 patients exhibited a clinical recurrence. Topical therapy was used for isolated positive margins with carcinoma in situ. Important considerations for this procedure are to document the absence of invasive cancer, to use topical therapy as an adjunct in the case of residual carcinoma in situ at a margin, and to perform careful follow-up.

Mohs Micrographic Surgery

Mohs microsurgery has historically had a positive impact on the management of penile carcinoma in situ and small superficially invasive tumors. As originally described by Mohs and colleagues (1985), it involves layer-by-layer complete excision of the penile lesion in multiple sessions (fixed tissue technique), with microscopic examination of the undersurface of each layer. Its sequential microscopic guidance offers improved precision and control of the negative margin while maximizing organ preservation. In a series of 29 consecutive cases of penile squamous cell carcinoma, the primary tumor was eradicated in 23 (92%) of 25 patients available for follow-up. Local recurrences were highly associated with tumor size (3 cm), advanced stage, and failure of previous definitive therapy (Mohs et al, 1992). These excellent results using a fixed tissue technique have not been reproduced with the currently used frozen-section methodology. Shindel and associates (2007) treated 33 patients with stage Tis (26 patients), T1 (4 patients), T2 (7 patients), and T3 (4 patients) penile cancer. Five procedures were terminated with positive margins. Of 25 patients with mean follow-up of 58 months, 8 (32%) developed recurrence. However, 7 of 8 were re-treated successfully with Mohs surgery. One patient who had progression of his disease died from it. **Thus Mohs microsurgery, as currently performed, may offer no additional benefit over surgical excision with intraoperative frozen-section assessment of margin status.**

Laser Ablation

The four most widely used laser energy sources are the CO_2, argon, Nd:YAG, and KTP lasers (Carpiniello et al, 1987; Malloy et al, 1988; von Eschenbach et al, 1991). Although the CO_2 laser has been widely used previously, the superficial depth of penetration (limited to 0.1 mm) makes it less than optimal for the treatment of penile carcinoma in situ or small T1 tumors. When the CO_2 laser is used, local recurrence rates have been shown to be as high as 50% (Bandieramonte et al, 1988; van Bezooijen et al, 2001). Conversely, the Nd:YAG laser results in protein denaturation at a depth of up to 6 mm by emitting at a wavelength of 1060 nm. Overall recurrence rates after laser ablation have been reported to be 7.7% for penile carcinoma in situ and have ranged from 10% to 25% for T1 lesions (Malloy et al, 1988; Windahl and Hellsten, 1995; Tietjen and Malek, 1998), but results from more contemporary series using the Nd:YAG laser exclusively have been more encouraging. **Frimberger** and colleagues (2002a) treated 29 men with carcinoma in situ and stage T1 tumors, combining Nd:YAG laser ablation with tumor base biopsies to ensure negative surgical margins. Only two recurrences (6.9%) were reported at a mean follow-up of 46.7 months, which is comparable to recurrence rates after partial penectomy. In an effort to reduce the incidence of positive surgical margins, Frimberger and associates (2002b) have proposed the use of autofluorescence and 5-aminolevulinic acid–induced fluorescence for targeting of frozen-section biopsy specimens.

Laser ablation is feasible and may achieve results equivalent to those of extirpative surgery, especially when it is performed in well-selected patients in conjunction with frozen-section biopsies. In addition, laser ablation has been associated with high rates of resumption of sexual activity (75%) and overall satisfaction (78%) (Windahl et al, 2004). However, until additional long-term studies become available, laser ablation should be performed with the understanding that local recurrences may develop and that close surveillance and patient self-examination are necessary for early detection. Although well-selected patients who develop small recurrent lesions may be candidates for repeated laser ablation, recurrences are best treated with wide local excision or partial amputation.

Contemporary Penile Amputation

Penile amputation remains the standard therapy for patients with deeply invasive or high-grade cancers. **Partial or total penectomy should be considered in patients exhibiting adverse features for cure by organ preservation strategies. These are consistently associated with tumors of size 4 cm or more, grade 3 lesions, and those invading deeply into the glans urethra or corpora cavernosa** (Mohs et al, 1992; Gotsadze et al, 2000; Kiltie et al, 2000). Because recurrence rates are higher with organ-preserving strategies, compliance with follow-up is also a consideration in recommending organ preservation versus amputation. Fortunately, most patients with recurrences that are detected and treated early are not adversely affected with respect to survival (Lont et al, 2006).

On the basis of contemporary results, organ preservation strategies should be discussed with patients exhibiting optimal tumor characteristics (stages Tis, Ta, T1; grade 1 and grade 2 tumors) to assist them in making informed decisions about therapy. (See Table 37-2 for treatment modalities for the primary penile tumor.)

KEY POINTS: SURGICAL TREATMENT OF THE PRIMARY TUMOR

- Patients with small lesions of low grade and stage (Tis, Ta, T1; grade 1 and grade 2) are the optimal candidates for organ preservation to maintain sexual quality of life.
- The goals of organ preservation are to maintain glanular tissue for sensory purposes when possible and/or to maintain penile length when glans penis preservation is not possible.
- Surgical modalities include limited excision strategies, Mohs surgery, and laser ablation.
- Local recurrence rates overall after organ preservation are higher than with traditional amputation; however, when local recurrences are detected and treated, early survival does not appear be adversely affected.
- Amputation remains the standard for large or deeply invasive lesions, to gain rapid tumor control.

TREATMENT OF THE INGUINAL NODES

The presence and the extent of metastasis to the inguinal region are the most important prognostic factors for survival in patients with squamous penile cancer. These findings affect the prognosis

TABLE 37-2 Treatment of the Primary Penile Tumor

STAGE	TREATMENT
Tis (glans)	Laser therapy, glans resurfacing; alternative: topical therapy
Ta, Tis (foreskin, shaft skin)	Surgical excision to achieve negative margin; alternatives: laser therapy, topical therapy (Tis only)
Ta, T1 grade 1-3 (glans)	Therapy based on size and position of lesion as well as potential side effects, excision, glans resurfacing procedures, glansectomy, radiotherapy (not indicated for Ta)
Ta, Tl grade 1-3 (foreskin, shaft)	Complete surgical excision to achieve negative margin
T2 (glans) without gross cavernosum involvement	Total glansectomy with or without corpora cavernosa transection to achieve negative surgical margins, partial penectomy, radiotherapy
T2 (corporeal invasion), T3	Partial or total penectomy
T4 (adjacent structures)	Consider neoadjuvant chemotherapy with surgical consolidation for responding patients if baseline resectability is a concern
Local disease recurrence after conservative therapy	Complete surgical excision to achieve negative surgical margins; may require partial or total penectomy; select patients with superficial low-grade recurrences may be candidates for repeat penile-conserving procedure
Radiotherapy	Select patients with T1-T2 tumors involving glans, coronal sulcus <4 cm

of the disease more than do tumor grade, gross appearance, and morphologic or microscopic patterns of the primary tumor.

Unlike with many other genitourinary tumors, which mandate systemic therapeutic strategies once metastasis has occurred, lymphadenectomy alone can be curative and should be performed. The biology of squamous penile cancer is such that it exhibits a prolonged locoregional phase before distant dissemination, providing a rationale for the therapeutic value of lymphadenectomy.

However, owing to the morbidity of traditional lymphadenectomy especially among patients with clinically negative groins, contemporary controversial issues include (1) the selection of patients for lymphadenectomy versus careful observation; (2) the types of procedures to correctly stage the inguinal region with low morbidity; and (3) multimodal strategies to improve survival among patients with bulky inguinal metastases.

In this rare disease, prospective randomized trials have not been performed to answer many of these questions. However, with the use of retrospective and prospective clinicopathologic data from several centers, treatment strategies are presented using the available data.

Contemporary Indications for Inguinal Lymphadenectomy

Prognostic Significance of the Presence and Extent of Metastatic Disease

Table 37-3 reveals data collected from 24 surgical series during a 37-year period. Patients proved to have no evidence of inguinal

TABLE 37-3 Carcinoma of the Penis: Prognostic Indicators for Survival

SERIES	NO. OF PATIENTS	CLINICAL AND PATHOLOGIC CHARACTERISTICS OF INGUINAL ADENOPATHY			5-YEAR SURVIVAL RATES (%)	
		PERCENTAGE WITH PALPABLE NODES	PERCENTAGE CLINICALLY FALSE POSITIVE (NODES PALPABLE, HISTOLOGIC FINDINGS NORMAL)	PERCENTAGE CLINICALLY FALSE NEGATIVE (NODES NONPALPABLE, HISTOLOGIC FINDINGS ABNORMAL)	INGUINAL NODES NEGATIVE*	INGUINAL NODES RESECTED AND POSITIVE†
Ekstrom and Edsmyer, 1958	229	33	48	—	80[a]	42
Beggs and Spratt, 1964	88	35	36	20	72.5	45
Thomas and Small, 1968	190	—	64	20	—	26
Edwards and Sawyers, 1968	77	—	—	0	68	25
Hanash et al, 1970	169	—	58[b]	2[b]	77[c]	—
Kuruvilla et al, 1971	153	39	63	10	69	33
Hardner et al, 1972	100	42	41[b]	16[b]	—	—
Gursel et al, 1973	64	53	60[b]	—	58	—
Skinner et al, 1972	34	29	40	—	75	20
					87[d]	50[d]
de Kernion et al, 1973	48	54	38[b]	—	84[e]	55[e]
Derrick et al, 1973	87	29	52	—	53	22
					76[d]	55[d]
Johnson et al, 1973	153	—	—	—	64.4	21.8
Kossow et al, 1973	100	51	49	25	—	—[f]
Puras et al, 1978	576	82	47	38[b]	89	67[g]
						29[h]
Cabanas, 1977	80	96	65	100	90	70[i]
						50[j]
						20[k]
Fossa et al, 1987	79	—	—	13	90	80[l]
						20[m]
Srinivas et al, 1987	199	63	14[n]	18	74	82[o]
						54[p]
						40[q]
						12[r]

Continued

TABLE 37-3   Carcinoma of the Penis: Prognostic Indicators for Survival—cont'd

| SERIES | NO. OF PATIENTS | CLINICAL AND PATHOLOGIC CHARACTERISTICS OF INGUINAL ADENOPATHY | | | 5-YEAR SURVIVAL RATES (%) | |
		PERCENTAGE WITH PALPABLE NODES	PERCENTAGE CLINICALLY FALSE POSITIVE (NODES PALPABLE, HISTOLOGIC FINDINGS NORMAL)	PERCENTAGE CLINICALLY FALSE NEGATIVE (NODES NONPALPABLE, HISTOLOGIC FINDINGS ABNORMAL)	INGUINAL NODES NEGATIVE*	INGUINAL NODES RESECTED AND POSITIVE†
McDougal et al, 1986	65	—	—	66	100	83[s] 66[t] 38[u]
Young et al, 1991	34	24	27	42	77	0
Horenblas et al, 1993	110	36	26	40	100	38
Ravi, 1993a	201	53	8	16	95	81[v] 50[w] 86[x] 60[y]
Ornellas et al, 1994	414	50	51[y]	39	87	29
Theodorescu et al, 1996	40	70	35	—	46	45
Puras-Baez et al, 1995	272	—	—	—	89	38

*On histologic or repeated physical examination.
†On histologic examination of adenectomy specimen.
[a]Majority of patients received prophylactic or preoperative radiation therapy to inguinal area.
[b]Histologic classification based on node biopsy, not node dissection.
[c]Corrected 5-year survival (i.e., patients dying before 5 years without evidence of disease are excluded).
[d]Patients dying free of cancer before 5 years are considered surgical cures.
[e]Three-year survival.
[f]Omitted.
[g]Positive findings in inguinofemoral nodes.
[h]Positive findings in inguinofemoral and pelvic nodes.
[i]Single inguinal node with positive findings.
[j]More than one inguinal node with positive findings.

[k]Three-year survival with positive findings in inguinal and pelvic nodes.
[l]N1-2.
[m]N3.
[n]After antibiotic therapy.
[o]One node positive.
[p]One to six nodes positive.
[q]More than six nodes positive.
[r]Bilateral nodes positive.
[s]Adjunctive adenectomy.
[t]Immediate therapeutic adenectomy.
[u]Delayed therapeutic adenectomy.
[v]One to three positive nodes.
[w]More than three positive nodes.
[x]Unilateral.
[y]Some lymph node dissection done without antibiotic pretreatment.

metastases on the basis of histologic examination of the inguinal nodes or repeated normal examination findings over time; the average 5-year survival rate was 73% (46% to 100%). In patients with resected inguinal metastases the 5-year survival averaged 60% (0% to 86%), but this varied widely and was directly attributable to the extent of nodal metastasis (see Table 37-3). This point is illustrated in several series shown in Tables 37-3 and 37-4. Patients with minimal nodal metastases (usually two or less) exhibited 5-year survivals that ranged from 72% to 88% compared with 0% to 50% when a greater degree of nodal involvement was present (see Table 37-4).

The extent of cancer in a lymph node was also of prognostic significance. Ravi (1993a) noted ENE of cancer in lymph nodes 4 cm in size, and only 1 of 17 patients (6%) undergoing lymphadenectomy survived 5 years. Finally, pelvic lymph node involvement has been a particularly ominous finding with respect to long-term survival; the combined results of several small series reveal an average 5-year survival of 14% when pelvic nodal

metastases are present (Table 37-5). **Taken together, these data suggest that the pathologic criteria associated with long-term survival after attempted curative surgical resection of inguinal metastases (i.e., 80% 5-year survival) include minimal nodal disease (up to two involved nodes in most series), unilateral involvement, no evidence of ENE of cancer, and absence of pelvic nodal metastases.**

Presence of Palpable Adenopathy as a Selection Factor for Inguinal Dissection

One can conclude from these data that it is advantageous to find and to treat nodal metastasis at the earliest possible opportunity. Data in Table 37-3 suggest that the presence of palpable adenopathy is associated with proven nodal metastasis in about 43% of cases on average (range 8% to 64%). In the remainder, lymph node enlargement is secondary to inflammation. Persistent adenopathy

TABLE 37-4 Five-Year Survival (%) Related to Extent of Nodal Metastasis

SERIES	NO. OF PATIENTS	NO. OF POSITIVE NODES	
		≤2	>2
Fraley et al, 1989	31	88%	7%
Johnson and Lo, 1984a	22	85%[a]	13%
Srinivas et al, 1987	119	82%	20% 54%[b]
Graafland et al, 2010	152	73%	27%
Ravi, 1993b	21	81%[c]	50%[d]
Pandey et al, 2006	102	76%[c]	8%[e] 0%[f]

[a]Approximate.
[b]A subset with one to six positive nodes.
[c]One to three positive nodes.
[d]More than three positive nodes.
[e]Four to five positive lymph nodes.
[f]More than five positive lymph nodes.

TABLE 37-5 Five-Year Survival Related to Pelvic Node Metastases

AUTHOR	NO. OF PATIENTS WITH POSITIVE NODES	5-YEAR SURVIVAL NO. (%)
de Kernion et al, 1973	2	1 (50)
Horenblas et al, 1993	2	0 (0)
Srinivas et al, 1987	11	0 (0)
Pow-Sang et al, 1990	3	2 (66)
Kamat et al, 1993	6	2 (33)
Ravi, 1993a	30	0 (0)
Lopes et al, 2000	13	5 (38)
Lont et al, 2007	25	4 (16)
Zhu et al, 2008	16	1 (6)
TOTAL	108	15 (14)

after treatment of the primary lesion and 4 to 6 weeks of antibiotic therapy is most often the consequence of metastatic disease. Similarly, the development of new adenopathy during follow-up is much more likely to be caused by tumor than inflammatory response. Thus historically a course of antibiotics was recommended for patients with suspicious nodes to potentially discern metastasis from cancer (Srinivas et al, 1987). However, several authors have raised the issue that this causes a significant delay and could affect survival, especially among patients who are likely to be truly positive by virtue of the stage or grade of the primary tumor (Kroon et al, 2005b; Pettaway et al, 2007). An alternative approach for such patients is to perform fine-needle aspiration cytology of palpable nodes either at the time of or immediately after treatment of the primary tumor. In the case of a positive result, definite therapy can be planned without a 4- to 6-week delay. Saisorn and associates (2006) reported a 93% sensitivity and a 91% specificity in 16 patients with palpable adenopathy (mean size 1.47 cm) undergoing fine-needle aspiration before lymphadenectomy. The recommendation for this procedure among patients with palpable nodes

was also incorporated in the European Association of Urology (EAU) Penile Cancer Guidelines. **Thus, although treatment of the primary tumor and a period of antibiotics are useful to help sterilize the inguinal region, this practice is no longer advocated as a tool to select patients who either should or should not undergo lymphadenectomy.** Should the fine-needle aspiration result be negative, depending on clinical suspicion, close observation, repeat aspiration, or excisional biopsy is performed because the false-negative rate of fine-needle aspiration cytology was 20% to 30% in two other older series (Scappini et al, 1986; Horenblas et al, 1991).

Evolving Indications for Lymphadenectomy in Patients without Palpable Adenopathy

Immediate versus Delayed Surgery

Considering the value of early detection and treatment of metastasis, **should inguinal lymphadenectomy (ILND) be routinely performed in patients with clinically normal groin examination findings at the time of presentation of the primary lesion?** This was the most controversial issue in the management of patients with squamous penile cancer previously; however, the pendulum has moved toward earlier lymphadenectomy in selected patients with penile cancer. As noted, the cure rate with ILND when nodes are positive for malignancy may be as high as 80%. A cure rate of this magnitude with surgery in the face of regional nodal metastases parallels the urologist's experience with testicular cancer, in which retroperitoneal lymphadenectomy provides cure in many patients with minimal nodal metastasis. In contrast, for other common genitourinary malignant neoplasms—bladder, prostate, and kidney—surgical cure in the presence of regional nodal metastases is rare. Given that node dissection can cure metastatic penile cancer, why is there debate about whether the procedure should be performed, especially given that regional node dissections are often advocated in other malignant neoplasms when evidence of their efficacy is marginal at best?

Morbidity versus Benefit

The reluctance to advocate automatic ilioinguinal lymphadenectomy (IILND) in all patients with penile cancer stems from the substantial morbidity the procedure can produce, as opposed to the relatively limited postoperative morbidity of pelvic or retroperitoneal lymphadenectomies. Early complications of phlebitis, pulmonary embolism, wound infection, flap necrosis, and permanent and disabling lymphedema of the scrotum and lower limbs were frequent after both inguinal and ilioinguinal node dissections (Skinner et al, 1972; Johnson and Lo, 1984a; McDougal et al, 1986; Fraley et al, 1989). **Postoperative complications have been reduced by improved preoperative and postoperative care; advances in surgical technique; plastic surgical consultation for myocutaneous flap coverage; and preservation of the dermis, Scarpa fascia, and saphenous vein, as well as modification of the extent of the dissection** (Catalona, 1988; Colberg et al, 1997; Bevan-Thomas et al, 2002; Coblentz and Theodorescu, 2002; Nelson et al, 2004). In the University of Texas MD Anderson Cancer Center experience, both the incidence and severity of lymphedema and skin edge necrosis were significantly decreased (Table 37-6, Fig. 37-3) (Bevan-Thomas et al, 2002).

Furthermore, experience has suggested that lymphadenectomy in the setting of microscopic disease may be less likely to produce complications than node dissection in the presence of bulky nodal metastases (Fraley et al, 1989; Ornellas et al, 1994; Coblentz and Theodorescu, 2002). This is presumably because of the reduced amount of lymphatic tissue removed, preservation of venous drainage, and less blood supply compromised. Together these factors affect the viability of skin flaps and lymphatic flow.

Mortality after ILND has been reported in association with surgery performed concomitantly with penectomy and after

TABLE 37-6   Lymphadenectomy Complications in Four Surgical Series

	JOHNSON AND LO (1984b)	RAVI (1993b)	ORNELLAS ET AL (1994)	BEVAN-THOMAS ET AL (2002)
No. of dissections	101	405	200	106
Period	1948-1983	1962-1990	1972-1987	1989-1998
COMPLICATIONS (%)				
Skin edge necrosis	50	62	45	8*
Lymphedema	50	27	23	23†
Wound infection	14	17	15‡	10
Seroma formation	16	7	6	10
Death	0	1.3	Not stated	1.8

*Significantly lower than in the three other reported series (all P = .0001).
†Significantly lower than in the series of Johnson and Lo (P = .0001).
‡Incidence among 85 lymphadenectomies performed by Gibson-type incision.
From Bevan-Thomas R, Slaton JW, Pettaway CA. Contemporary morbidity from lymphadenectomy for penile squamous cell carcinoma: the MD Anderson Cancer Center experience. J Urol 2002;167:1638–42.

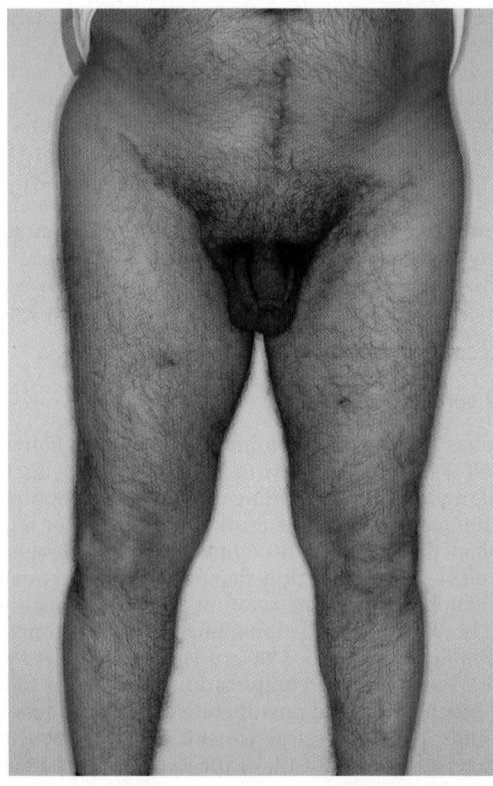

Figure 37-3. Postoperative appearance after contemporary lymphadenectomy. The patient's status is post right ilioinguinal lymphadenectomy and left superficial inguinal dissection for stage T2N1M0 squamous penile cancer. Mild edema is visible on the left 10 months after surgery. Patient remains without disease at 9 years.

palliative inguinal dissection. In both scenarios it was related to sepsis (Bevan-Thomas et al, 2002). An operative mortality of 3.3% was reported in earlier series (Beggs and Spratt, 1964). However, Johnson and Lo (1984a) and others (Ravi, 1993b; Ornellas et al, 1994; Coblentz and Theodorescu, 2002; Nelson et al, 2004) have reported no mortality in more recent series. Appropriate selection of patients along with routine preoperative antibiotic therapy and wound care to avoid septic complications has minimized this event.

Clearly, lymphadenectomy is not a trivial concern, even though morbidity appears to be decreasing. If a policy of routine lymphadenectomy were adopted in all patients with clinically negative lymph nodes, the average risk of false-negative examination findings (metastasis is actually present) would be approximately 29%, with wide-ranging variation (see Table 37-3). Stated another way, an average of 70% of patients could be subjected to the morbidity of ILND with no benefit. Potential reasons for false-negative examination findings include obesity, preexisting edema, and changes from prior therapy (radiation, inguinal surgery).

One alternative to immediate lymphadenectomy for all patients has been to observe patients with normal findings on inguinal examination. Lymphadenectomy is subsequently reserved for those patients who develop palpable lymph nodes. **The relevant question then becomes, can a delayed therapeutic dissection effectively salvage patients who have inguinal recurrence?**

Several studies have analyzed the survival of men undergoing early versus delayed lymphadenectomy according to pathologic evaluation of nodal status. McDougal and coworkers (1986) reported a series of 23 patients with invasive primary lesions and nonpalpable nodes; 9 patients were treated with immediate adjunctive lymph node dissection (6 had positive findings), and 14 were treated with surveillance and delayed lymph node dissection. The 5-year survival in the node-positive immediate adjunctive lymphadenectomy group was 83% (5 of 6 patients), whereas in the surveillance group the 5-year survival was 36% (5 of 14 patients). However, only 1 patient in the surveillance group had a node dissection. Presumably, the other 9 patients had progressed to inoperable local tumor or distant disease before presentation, emphasizing the role of careful, frequent follow-up and the difficulty of enforcing it. A third subset in this series had palpable nodes at presentation and had immediate therapeutic lymph node dissection, with 10 of 15 patients (66%) surviving 5 years (McDougal et al, 1986). The best results were from immediate adjunctive lymph node dissection (83%), with the next best from immediate therapeutic lymphadenectomy (66%). The worst results were from the surveillance and delayed lymphadenectomy group (36%), in whom dissection was delayed until palpable nodes developed. The interval of opportunity for cure in this third group appears to have been lost.

Similarly, Fraley and associates (1989) reported that immediate adjunctive lymphadenectomy resulted in a 5-year disease-free survival in 6 of 8 node-positive patients (75%) compared with 1 of 12 patients (8%) who had been observed and then treated with delayed lymphadenectomy when nodal enlargement occurred. Six other patients in that series also had unresectable adenopathy after initial surveillance, and all died of their disease. Although only 2 of 6 patients who had immediate lymphadenectomy had more than two positive nodes, all the patients treated by delayed lymph node dissection had three or more positive nodes.

Three other series suggest that early lymphadenectomy for varying degrees of "suspicious" or clinically positive nodes improves survival compared with the "surveillance" or delayed intervention approach in patients with clinically negative nodes (Johnson and Lo, 1984b; Ornellas et al, 1994; Kroon et al, 2005b). A series from the University of Texas MD Anderson Cancer Center compared 5-year disease-free survival of 14 patients undergoing early lymphadenectomy for clinically suspicious and histologically node-positive disease with that of 8 patients who were observed and later underwent lymphadenectomy when clinical nodal enlargement was undisputed (Johnson and Lo, 1984b). The primary tumors were of similar stage. The 5-year disease-free survival was 57% for early lymphadenectomy compared with 13% for delayed node dissection. Of note, the number of involved nodes in the immediate lymphadenectomy group (median, two) was half that of the delayed lymphadenectomy group (median, four), and no patient with more than two positive nodes survived more than 5 years.

Kroon and associates (2005b) from the Netherlands Cancer Institute compared survival of 20 patients found to have positive lymph nodes subsequent to prophylactic DSNB with that of 20 patients who underwent delayed inguinal dissection after proven nodal metastasis. The 3-year survival for patients detected during close surveillance was only 35% compared with 84% (P = .0017) for those undergoing early dissection. Pathologic evaluation of involved lymph nodes revealed ENE of cancer among 19 of 20 patients in the delayed group versus only 4 of 20 patients (P = .001) in the early group. Thus, despite careful follow-up, survival was adversely affected by the extent of cancer in involved lymph nodes.

A single large study from India disputes the magnitude of the value of early prophylactic dissection. Ravi (1993b) performed early prophylactic dissection in 113 patients with invasive penile cancer and compared the 5-year survival with that of 258 similarly staged patients who were initially observed. In the "early" group, 20 patients (18%) were found to have metastases, and all patients survived 5 years. The recurrence rate in the observed group was only 8% (21 patients). However, the 5-year survival in the patients who experienced recurrence was only 76% (compared with 100% in the early lymphadenectomy group). The enhanced survival of patients undergoing surveillance in India compared with other countries is probably attributable to patient selection factors, strict adherence to follow-up schedules, and aggressive treatment approach for recurrent disease (a combination of radiation and surgical resection) (Ravi, 1993a).

Thus, six series reveal an improvement in survival for patients undergoing early therapeutic versus delayed therapeutic dissection. Furthermore, five of the six series show that delayed therapeutic dissection can rarely salvage patients who experience recurrence. Taken together, these data suggest that a policy of immediate adjunctive or early lymphadenectomy gives greater assurance that surgical intervention will occur when tumor volume is small (see Table 37-4) (Johnson and Lo, 1984a; Fossa et al, 1987; Srinivas et al, 1987; Fraley et al, 1989; Ravi, 1993b; Kroon et al, 2005b).

Impact of Primary Tumor Histologic Features on Predicting Occult Nodal Metastasis

Although early lymphadenectomy improves survival in patients with inguinal metastases, the challenge remains to identify those patients who are truly lymph node negative to avoid the morbidity of traditional lymphadenectomy. **Data gained from analysis of a variety of histopathologic variables within the primary penile tumor allow the classification of patients into higher and lower risk groups for lymph node metastasis** (McDougal, 1995; Lopes et al, 1996; Theodorescu et al, 1996; Solsona et al, 2001; Ficarra et al, 2006).

Patients with primary tumors exhibiting carcinoma in situ or verrucous carcinoma have little or no risk for metastasis. Only two cases of metastasis in association with carcinoma in situ have been

TABLE 37-7 Penile Carcinoma: Corporeal Invasion and Incidence of Lymph Node Metastasis

STUDY	NO. OF PATIENTS	NO. OF POSITIVE NODES (%)	CLINICAL N STAGE
McDougal et al, 1986	23	11 (48)	N0
Fraley et al, 1989	29	26 (90)	N0
Theodorescu et al, 1996	18	12 (67)	N0
Villavicencio et al, 1997	37	14 (38)	N0
Lopes et al, 1996	44	28 (64)	NS
Heyns et al, 1997	32	15 (47)	NS
Solsona et al, 1992	42	27 (64)	NS

N, node; NS, not specified.

reported, and none of 47 cases of penile verrucous carcinoma has been shown to metastasize (Avrach and Christensen, 1976; Johnson et al, 1985; Seixas et al, 1994; Eng et al, 1995). Thus, patients with both Tis and Ta penile cancer are included in the low-risk group for inguinal metastases (Solsona et al, 2001, 2004).

In contrast, patients with corporeal invasion (stage pT2) in the penile tumor exhibit a high risk for metastasis. The average risk for inguinal metastasis among 225 patients in seven different series was 59% (Table 37-7). **The risk for metastasis among patients exhibiting corporeal invasion was similar irrespective of whether palpable adenopathy was present.**

Stage T1 penile cancers exhibit involvement of the subepithelial connective tissue only and lack involvement of the corpus spongiosum, corpora cavernosa, or urethra (Edge et al, 2010). Similarly staged tumors historically have been associated with a 4% to 14% incidence of nodal metastasis (Solsona et al, 1992; Villavicencio et al, 1997; Hall et al, 1998). Theodorescu and colleagues (1996) noted one exception to this relatively low rate of metastatic disease; 58% of patients (14 of 24) with pT1 primary tumors and initially negative nodes on clinical assessment subsequently developed inguinal nodal metastases. These data suggest that other variables present within the penile cancers of the cohort of patients studied (i.e., tumor grade and presence of vascular invasion) may have modified the effect of tumor stage on metastasis.

Several authors have evaluated the risk of nodal metastasis for stage T1 lesions according to tumor grade (Table 37-8). Among 73 patients with T1 grade 1 or grade 2 primary tumors, metastasis occurred in only 5 patients (7%). Recent data from Naumann and coworkers (2008), however, suggested that among T1 grade 2 tumors specifically, the risk of metastases could be higher than previously described. Among four series reporting specifically on the T1 grade 2 subset, in 129 initially node-negative patients, metastases occurred in 18 (14%) (see Table 37-8). However, 5 patients in this subset also exhibited either lymphatic or venous invasion (an adverse prognostic feature, see later). Ficarra and colleagues (2006) developed the first penile cancer nomogram using data from 175 patients. Based on tumor thickness and growth pattern, patients with T1 grade 2 tumors exhibited metastatic rates of 5% to 20%. Thus grade 2 tumors represent a heterogeneous group in which the histologic criteria used to describe grade 2 and the presence or absence of other poor prognostic features ultimately determine prognosis (Cubilla, 2009). In this regard the EAU guidelines assigned patients with T1 grade 2 tumors to the intermediate-risk category in which the risk of lymph node metastasis is greater than 16% (low risk) and less than 68% (high risk) (Solsona et al, 2004; Pizzocaro et al, 2010).

The presence of vascular invasion as a prognostic indicator of inguinal lymph node metastasis in squamous penile cancer is

now evident (Fraley et al, 1989; Lopes et al, 1996; Heyns et al, 1997; Slaton et al, 2001; Ficarra et al, 2005). Lopes and colleagues (1996) studied the prognostic value of lymphatic invasion in 146 patients with penile cancer. In a univariate analysis, clinical nodal stage, tumor thickness, lymphatic and venous embolization, and urethral infiltration were all associated with lymph node metastasis. However, subsequent to multivariate analysis, only venous and lym-

phatic invasion remained significant predictors for positive lymph nodes. Data from the University of Texas MD Anderson Cancer Center revealed that vascular invasion was absent in all patients with T1 tumors (Slaton et al, 2001). These patients were also lymph node negative at surgery. In contrast, patients with stage pT2 primary tumors exhibited nodal metastasis in 75% of cases (15 of 20) when vascular invasion was present but in only 25% of cases (3 of 12) when it was absent.

Ficarra and colleagues (2005) described prognostic factors for lymph node metastasis in 175 patients undergoing surgery for penile cancer in a multicenter study from the Northeast Uro-Oncological Group from Italy. Subsequent to multivariate statistical analysis, the presence of venous or lymphatic invasion and pathologic invasion of the corpus spongiosum or urethra were the only independent risk factors for lymph node metastasis among patients who were clinically lymph node negative. Taking this a step further and including the variables of tumor thickness, growth pattern, grade, venous or lymphatic invasion, corpus spongiosum or cavernosum involvement, urethral involvement, and palpable lymph nodes, Ficarra and colleagues (2006) developed a nomogram predicting inguinal lymph node involvement. The most important variables were venous or lymphatic invasion and the presence of palpable nodes in multivariate analysis. The concordance index of the nomogram was very good at 0.876. However, because of the complexity of the nomogram variables included, external validation of the nomogram has to date not been accomplished.

The presence of perineural invasion (Velazquez et al, 2008) and the microscopic front pattern of invasion (Guimares et al, 2006) have also been shown in recent studies to provide independent information with which to stratify a patient's risk of lymph node metastasis.

Molecular Prognostic Markers

Analysis of gene expression in penile cancer may have future implications with respect to the prediction of lymph node metastasis or survival. A review by Muneer and colleagues (2009) describes the status of several genes evaluated in tissue or serum that could have future prognostic implications with respect to predicting lymph node status or survival (Table 37-9). Zhu et al (2010) incorporated p53 expression into a nomogram that included T stage, grade, and the presence or absence of lymphovascular invasion. When compared with the EAU risk classification, the nomogram incorporating p53 would have resulted in 13 fewer lymph node dissections per

TABLE 37-8 Penile Carcinoma: Incidence of Nodal Metastasis for Stage T1, Grade 1 and Grade 2 Primary Tumors

AUTHOR	STAGE AND GRADE	NO. OF PATIENTS	NO. OF PATIENTS WITH METASTASIS (%)
Theodorescu et al, 1996	T1, G1	8	2 (25)
Solsona et al, 1992	T1, G1	19	0 (0)
McDougal, 1995	T1, G1-2	24	1 (4)
Heyns et al, 1997	T1, G1-2	9	1 (11)
Hungerhuber et al, 2006	T1, G1-2	13	1 (8)
TOTAL		73	5 (7)
Solsona et al, 1992	T1, G2	4	1 (25)
Solsona et al, 2001	T1, G2	4	1 (25)
Naumann et al, 2008*	T1, G2	16	7 (44)
Hughes et al, 2010	T1, G2	105	9 (9)
TOTAL		129	18 (14)

*Five tumors in node-positive group had lymphatic or venous invasion.

TABLE 37-9 Prognostic Molecular Markers of Lymph Node Status and Survival in Penile Cancer: Current Status

MARKER	ROLE	LYMPH NODE STATUS	SURVIVAL
Human papillomavirus (HPV)	High-risk types affect TP53 and RB function	Contradictory studies	Most studies show no correlation
TP53	Altered or mutated expression, increased proliferation, altered apoptosis, dedifferentiation	Preliminary data correlated with increased metastasis	Correlated with survival in T1 penile cancers only
CDKN2A	Inhibits RB function, enhancing proliferation	Not established	Not established
Squamous cell carcinoma antigen (TA-4)	Serum marker function unknown	Correlates with grossly evident metastases	No role
Ki-67	Nuclear protein associated with cycling cells	Predicts increased risk	No role
E-cadherin	Epithelial cell adhesion molecule lost in progression	Low expression associated with nodal metastasis	Low expression predicts worse survival
MMP-9	Matrix metalloproteinase family facilities invasion	No role	High expression predicts recurrence

RB, retinoblastoma protein.
Modified from Muneer A, Kayes O, Ahmed HU, et al. Molecular prognostic factors in penile cancer. World J Urol 2009;27:161–7.

100 patients, thus decreasing morbidity. These data suggest the potential value of incorporating molecular features into models to enhance prognostication. Presently, however, standardization of methodologies for assessment of gene expression and the lack of large tissue banks with well-annotated clinical data for validation studies hamper efforts to rigorously evaluate the potential usefulness of such biomarkers. Prospective multi-institutional studies analyzing both pathologic and molecular features are needed to further validate which pathologic and molecular variables best stratify a patient's risk for metastasis and survival.

Contemporary Evolving Indications for Expectant Management of the Inguinal Region

Data reviewed in the preceding paragraphs along with consensus guidelines demonstrate that patients with primary tumors exhibiting carcinoma in situ (Tis), verrucous carcinoma (Ta), and stage T1, grade 1 tumors exhibit a relatively low incidence of positive lymph nodes overall (0% to 16%) and are optimal candidates for watchful waiting strategies (Pompeo et al, 2009; Pizzocaro et al, 2010). Recommendations for the management of T1 grade 2 tumors vary based on quoted rates of subsequent metastases. The former EAU guideline (Solsona et al, 2004), although classifying such cases in the intermediate-risk group, recommended observation for T1 grade 2 tumors that lacked vascular invasion and exhibited a superficial growth pattern (i.e., absence of any other adverse features). This guideline was recently modified to recommend an inguinal staging procedure for this group of patients (Pizzocaro et al, 2010). Given the low rate of metastases of 9% overall in a recent study, we agree with the Société Internationale d'Urologie/ International Consultation on Urological Diseases (ICUD) recommendation that these patients may also be considered for observation (Pompeo et al, 2009; Hughes et al, 2010; see Table 37-9).This grouping of T1 grade 2 patients corresponds to the current AJCC TNM T1a classification (Edge et al, 2010). All other cases should be considered for surgical staging.

Patients with AJCC stage T1b or greater (see Table 37-1) as a group exhibit at least a 50% incidence of inguinal metastasis, so an inguinal staging procedure appears warranted. In addition, noncompliant patients with invasive primary tumors should be offered an inguinal staging procedure versus observation. Table 37-10 provides a guideline for more intensive follow-up of high-risk patients, especially within the first 2 years. **It is imperative for both the patient and the physician to adhere to such follow-up agreements and to be willing to intervene immediately if initial inguinal parameters change. Leijte and colleagues (2008) have documented that only a third of patients who were initially node negative but who subsequently develop an inguinal recurrence survive 5 years.**

TABLE 37-10 Penile Carcinoma: Suggested Follow-up for Patients with No Evidence of Inguinal Adenopathy Who Do Not Undergo Initial Lymphadenectomy

	INTERVAL	
YEAR	LOW-RISK GROUP*	HIGH-RISK GROUP†
1-2	3 months	2 months
3	4 months	3 months
4	6 months	6 months
5+	Annually	Annually

*Primary tumor stage Tis, Ta, and T1a.
†Primary tumor stage T1b or greater.

Indications for Modified and Traditional Inguinal Procedures

Modified Procedures

In patients with no evidence of palpable adenopathy who are selected to undergo inguinal procedures by virtue of adverse prognostic factors within the primary tumor, the goal is to define whether metastases exist with minimal morbidity for the patient. A variety of treatment options for this purpose have been reported and include fine-needle aspiration cytology, node biopsy, sentinel lymph node biopsy, extended sentinel lymph node dissection, dynamic sentinel lymph node biopsy, superficial dissection, and modified complete dissection. The technical aspects of many of these procedures are beyond the scope of this chapter but may be found in Chapter 39 and in the references by Horenblas and colleagues (2000) and Spiess and coworkers (2009).

Fine-Needle Aspiration Cytology. The experience with aspiration of clinically negative inguinal nodes guided by either lymphangiography or ultrasonography is limited. Scappini and associates (1986) performed fine-needle aspiration cytology under pedal or penile lymphangiography for nodal localization in 29 patients. Of 20 patients who had lymphadenectomy for histologic confirmation, there was complete agreement between aspiration cytology and histologic results. However, 2 of 9 patients whose cytologic analysis was negative subsequently died of metastatic disease, a presumptive 20% false-negative result. A series from Horenblas and colleagues (1991) also found that the sensitivity of fine-needle aspiration cytology was approximately 71% in 18 patients with clinically negative lymph nodes. This finding and the technical difficulty with lymphangiography make aspiration less practical as a staging technique for patients with no palpable lymph nodes. Kroon et al (2005a) described fine-needle aspiration cytology guided by ultrasonography as a preliminary study to surgical staging with DSNB. Thirty-four groins in 27 patients with clinically negative groins were found to have suspicious nodes by ultrasound examination and were aspirated. However, the sensitivity of the technique was only 39% subsequent to surgical staging. **Thus, at present, fine-needle aspiration cytology of clinically negative groins does not exhibit the sensitivity for it to be relied on as a staging modality.** However, direct aspiration of palpable inguinal nodes is easily performed, exhibited a sensitivity of 93% in a recent study, and, if positive, provides immediate information with which to advise patients about further treatment (Saisorn et al, 2006).

Sentinel Lymph Node Biopsy, Extended Sentinel Lymph Node Dissection, and Node Biopsy. The concept of sentinel lymph node biopsy as described by Cabanas (1977) is predicated on detailed penile lymphangiographic studies that have demonstrated consistent drainage of the penile lymphatics into a sentinel node or group of nodes located superomedial to the junction of the saphenous and femoral veins in the area of the superficial epigastric vein. In this series, when this sentinel node was negative for tumor, metastases to other ilioinguinal lymph nodes did not occur. Metastases to this node indicated the need for a complete superficial and deep inguinal dissection.

The accuracy of the sentinel node histology to identify inguinal node metastases was, however, questioned by a number of reports (Perinetti et al, 1980; Fowler, 1984; Wespes et al, 1986). Because nodal metastases became palpable within 1 year of sentinel node biopsy with normal findings in some patients in these series, a false-negative biopsy result must be presumed. In one large series, 5 of 41 patients (12%) with normal findings on sentinel node biopsy subsequently developed inguinal node metastases (Fossa et al, 1987). In Cabanas's series (1992), 3 of 31 patients with negative sentinel nodes died of disease, suggesting a false-negative rate for identifying metastases of 10%. McDougal and associates (1986) reported a 50% false-negative rate with inguinal node biopsy. A report by Pettaway and colleagues (1995), in which additional nodes around the sentinel node area were also removed, revealed that even this extended dissection was associated with a false-negative rate of 25%. The authors hypothesized that false-negative inguinal node biopsies were the result of anatomic variation in the position of the sentinel node within the inguinal field. **Thus, biopsies directed to a specific anatomic area can be unreliable in identifying microscopic metastasis and are no longer recommended.**

Dynamic Sentinel Node Biopsy. DSNB offers the potential for precise localization of the sentinel node with the lowest morbidity of any surgical staging technique (Kroon et al, 2005c). The goal of DSNB is to define where in the inguinal lymph node field the sentinel lymph node resides through use of a combination of visual (vital blue dyes) or gamma emission (hand-held gamma probe) techniques at the time of surgery.

The technique has been studied in patients with malignant melanoma and breast and vulvar carcinomas who required evaluation of the regional lymph nodes (Morton et al, 1992; Levenback et al, 1994; Albertini et al, 1996; Gershenwald et al, 1999). The technique involves intradermal injection of a vital blue dye (isosulfan blue or patent blue dyes) or technetium-labeled colloid adjacent to the lesion. The dye (or radioactive tracer) is transported by the afferent lymphatics to a specific node in the regional nodal basin. This node is designated the sentinel lymph node. In Morton's series of 237 patients with melanoma, the sentinel lymph node was identified in 194 patients. These patients then underwent full regional lymphadenectomy, with a false-negative sentinel node in only 1% of cases.

Several studies evaluating the results of DSNB as a staging tool in penile cancer are now available. Kroon and associates (2004) updated the Netherlands Cancer Institute experience, describing their experience using the combination of preoperative lymphoscintigraphy and intraoperative intradermally injected blue dye in 123 patients with penile cancer. They identified a sentinel node in 98% of patients, for a sensitivity rate of 82% and a false-negative rate of 18% (6 patients). Four of the 6 patients subsequently died of disease progression. Spiess and associates (2007) also noted a false-negative rate of 25% among 31 patients undergoing DSNB. The Netherlands Cancer Institute group subsequently instituted several changes, including (1) routine serial sectioning of the involved lymph nodes along with cytokeratin immunohistochemistry, (2) routine exploration of groins with low or no signal subsequent to preoperative or intraoperative studies, and (3) inguinal ultrasonography with fine-needle aspiration to detect subtle architectural changes (nonpalpable) in positive lymph nodes that could result in the redistribution of lymphatic flow (Kroon et al, 2005a).

In a multicenter update that included patients assessed with the modified DSNB protocol from two high-volume centers (the Netherlands Cancer Institute and St. George's Hospital in London) the false-negative rate was 7% (6 patients) among 323 patients (Leijte et al, 2009b). Three of 6 patients with recurrence (50%) either died or developed distant metastases. **Thus DSNB, when performed at high-volume centers using a standardized protocol, has an acceptable sensitivity, but deaths from penile cancer among initially node-negative patients still occurred.** This limits the applicability of this strategy to larger centers with experienced surgeons and nuclear medicine specialists.

Superficial and Modified Complete Inguinal Dissection. Both superficial inguinal and modified complete dissections have been proposed as staging tools for the patient without palpable inguinal lymphadenopathy. Superficial node dissection involves removal of those nodes superficial to the fascia lata. A complete IILND (removal of those nodes deep to the fascia lata contained within the femoral triangle as well as the pelvic nodes) is then performed if the superficial nodes are positive at surgery by frozen-section analysis. The rationale for superficial dissection is that two series have shown no positive nodes deep to the fascia lata unless superficial nodes were also positive (Pompeo et al, 1995; Puras-Baez et al, 1995). Furthermore, Spiess and colleagues (2007) showed that among the lymph node–negative cohort of patients undergoing DSNB followed by completion superficial dissection, no patient with a negative superficial dissection experienced recurrence, with more than 3 years of follow-up. A complete modified inguinal dissection was originally proposed by Catalona (1988) and involves smaller skin incision, limited field of inguinal dissection, preservation of the saphenous vein, and thicker skin flaps. This technique also avoids having to transpose the sartorius muscle to cover exposed femoral vessels. Unlike in superficial dissection, deep nodes within the fossa ovalis are also removed. Two reports involving 21 patients have confirmed the value of this technique, when it is properly performed, for identifying microscopic metastases with minimal morbidity (Parra, 1996; Colberg et al, 1997).

Thus, either superficial or complete modified inguinal dissection should adequately identify microscopic metastases in patients with clinically normal inguinal examination findings, without the need for a pelvic dissection if the inguinal nodes are negative. The disadvantage of the modified dissections is the higher overall complication rate (12% to 35%) when compared with DSNB (5% to 7%) (Kroon et al, 2005c; Spiess et al, 2009).

Limited dissections have the following advantages: More information is provided than by biopsy of a single node or group of nodes; the possibility of not identifying the sentinel node is limited by removal of all potential first-echelon nodes; and the dissection is readily performed by any surgeon experienced in inguinal surgery without the need for specialized equipment.

Minimally Invasive Inguinal Lymphadenectomy Using Laparoscopy or Robotic Techniques. Both the laparoscopic and robotic approaches to the inguinal region offer the potential for removing all of the inguinal lymph nodes at risk for disease while minimizing complications. The technical details of the contemporary procedure and early results have been described (Sotelo et al, 2007; Tobias-Machado et al, 2007; Matin et al, 2013). To date, the results of laparoscopic and robotic ILND have been comparable to those of open inguinal lymph dissection with comparable node counts achieved in both. A single case of inguinal recurrence reported at 12 to 33 months of follow-up and minor complications in about 20% of patients have been reported (Sotelo et al, 2009). However, in one study using a laparoscopic approach with over 600 days of follow-up, Master and colleagues (2012) noted minor complications in 27% of patients, with major complications noted in 14.6%. These were mainly infectious in nature and were managed with intravenous antibiotics or incision and drainage. Of note, among 41 dissections there was only a single case of skin edge necrosis. Matin and colleagues (2013), using a robotic-assisted approach, noted in a phase 1 pilot study that inguinal dissection appeared equivalent to an open approach in 18 of 19 (94.7%) patients when verified by a second surgeon using an open incision to inspect the same groin. Minimally invasive approaches, although promising as an inguinal staging tool, will require further validation with larger patient numbers and longer follow-up to better determine efficacy and complication rates compared with traditional approaches or DSNB.

Traditional Inguinal and Ilioinguinal Lymphadenectomy

In patients with resectable metastatic adenopathy, the potential therapeutic value of lymphadenectomy justifies the morbidity of treatment. The goals are to eradicate all obvious cancer, to provide coverage for exposed vasculature, and to provide rapid wound healing (primary closure or myocutaneous flap coverage). Several issues remain with respect to surgical decision making.

Should ILND be bilateral rather than unilateral for patients with unilateral adenopathy at initial presentation of the primary tumor? The answer to this question is yes. The anatomic crossover of penile lymphatics is well established, and bilateral drainage is the rule. In 43 of 54 patients (79%) undergoing intraoperative lymph node mapping at the Netherlands Cancer Institute, lymphatic drainage from the penis was bilateral (Horenblas et al, 2000). The contralateral node dissection may be limited to the area superficial to the fascia lata if no histologic evidence of positive superficial nodes is found at surgery by frozen-section analysis. Clinical support for a bilateral procedure is based on the finding of contralateral metastases in more than 50% of patients so treated, even if the contralateral nodal region was normal on palpation (Ekstrom and Edsmyr, 1958).

Should bilateral ILND be performed in patients with unilateral lymphadenopathy some time after the initial presentation and treatment of the primary tumor? It is generally believed that bilateral node dissection in this setting is not necessary. The recommendation of unilateral rather than bilateral node dissection with delayed presentation of unilateral lymphadenopathy is supported by the elapsed disease-free interval of observation on the normal side. If one assumes that nodal metastases will enlarge at the same rate, the clinical palpation of nodal metastases, if present in both groins, should appear at approximately the same time. The absence of clinical adenopathy on one side despite prolonged observation suggests freedom from disease on that side (Ekstrom and Edsmyr, 1958). However, this concept may not apply to all patients with delayed recurrence. Horenblas and colleagues (2000) noted that in patients with two or more unilateral metastases, contralateral occult metastases were noted in 30% of cases. Thus, in patients with a bulky unilateral recurrence, a contralateral inguinal staging procedure should be considered. Considering the current treatment recommendations for bilateral inguinal staging procedures in men at high risk for metastasis and the definition of low-risk groups for metastasis by use of available prognostic markers, this scenario should rarely occur.

Should pelvic lymphadenectomy (PLND) be performed in all patients with inguinal metastases, considering its potential for added morbidity and relatively low therapeutic value? This issue remains controversial, but recent data suggest that PLND may be omitted in select patients with limited inguinal metastases (Lont et al, 2007; Zhu et al, 2008; Pizzocaro et al, 2010). Patients with inguinal nodal metastases are at increased risk for spread to the pelvic nodes. Ravi (1993b) found no pelvic nodal metastases when inguinal nodes were negative but found positive pelvic nodes in 17 of 75 patients (22%) with one to three positive inguinal nodes and in 13 of 23 patients (57%) with more than three positive inguinal nodes. Srinivas and associates (1987) also found a similar correlation. Horenblas and colleagues (1993) showed that among patients with a single inguinal lymph node involved without extracapsular extension, the incidence of pelvic metastases was rare; they recommended avoiding pelvic dissection in such patients. Zhu and coworkers (2008) found that the sensitivity of CT for pelvic lymph node metastasis was only 37.5%. Use of the Cloquet node in predicting a positive pelvic node was only about 30% sensitive, as well. Important predictors were the number of positive nodes and lymph node size. Two contemporary studies addressing this issue have found a 0% to 12% incidence of pelvic lymph node metastasis when patients exhibited only one or two positive inguinal nodes, especially when extracapsular extension was absent and/or size was less than 3.5 cm (Lont et al, 2007; Zhu et al, 2008). Additional factors noted in these studies included the grade of the nodal metastasis and its TP53 status. Thus, patients with only a single small lymph node metastasis discovered at the time of inguinal dissection (i.e., no extracapsular extension, not high grade) may be at very low risk for pelvic metastasis and are potentially the optimal candidates in whom PLND can be avoided.

With respect to efficacy, the 5-year survival for patients with positive pelvic nodes averages around 14% (see Table 37-4). However, data from some of the smaller series suggest that in selected instances 5-year survival can occur in patients treated with surgery alone. In the series reported by Ravi (1993b), however, patients with even a single positive pelvic node did not survive 5 years (0 of 8 patients). The difficulty in determining the potential independent value of PLND as a therapeutic procedure is related to the small numbers of patients reported, the coexisting extensive inguinal adenopathy in patients with resectable pelvic nodes, and the failure to specify sites of relapse in patients undergoing IILND (i.e., inguinal versus pelvic versus distant site).

Thus, for patients undergoing ILND for curative intent (i.e., in whom preoperative studies reveal no pelvic adenopathy), PLND should routinely be considered in patients with two or more positive inguinal lymph nodes or when extracapsular nodal

extension is present. PLND in this setting serves as an effective staging tool for identifying those patients at increased risk for pelvic metastases in whom adjunctive therapy should be considered (Lont et al, 2007; Pizzocaro et al, 2010). Given the aforementioned indications, PLND can be performed simultaneously with ILND in the setting of higher volume inguinal metastases or as a secondary procedure after inguinal pathology is available. Alternatively, if pelvic nodal metastases are proven before lymphadenectomy (based on clinical findings), consideration should be given to neoadjuvant chemotherapeutic strategies followed by surgery (Leijte et al, 2007; Pagliaro et al, 2010; National Comprehensive Cancer Network [NCCN], 2012).

KEY POINTS: TREATMENT OF THE INGUINAL NODES

- The presence and extent of inguinal metastases determine survival in penile cancer.
- Patients with persistent palpable inguinal adenopathy should undergo an inguinal staging procedure.
- On the basis of the histologic features of the primary tumor, risk of lymph node metastases can be assessed in patients with no palpable adenopathy. DSNB, superficial ILND, or close follow-up can be recommended.
- Factors associated with a high cure in surgically treated patients include no more than two inguinal metastases, unilateral involvement, no ENE of cancer, and the absence of pelvic metastases. Patients with higher volumes of disease should be considered for adjuvant or neoadjuvant therapy.
- Morbidity of lymphadenectomy is decreasing in contemporary series.
- Superficial ILND reliably determines the presence of microscopic inguinal metastases without the need for specialized facilities but can have significant morbidity.
- Modified DSNB techniques to determine microscopic inguinal disease exhibit low morbidity, have been validated externally in higher-volume centers, and are now a recommended procedure in such centers.
- Laparoscopic and robotic ILND obtains lymph node yields that are comparable to those of open techniques when used in selected patients. Additional studies with larger patient numbers and longer follow-up are required before routine adoption into clinical practice.
- PLND is now recommended when more than one inguinal lymph node exhibits metastasis or when ENE of cancer is present.

Risk-Based Management of the Inguinal Region

A contemporary schema for management of the inguinal region is presented in Figure 37-4. Assumptions for these guidelines are that the primary tumor has been adequately controlled, that the pathologic stage of the primary tumor is available, and that an inguinal examination has been performed. CT of the abdomen and pelvis as well as chest radiography or other imaging studies should also be performed as clinically indicated.

Very Low-Risk Patients

Because the incidence of inguinal metastasis is anecdotal at best for patients with stage Tis or Ta primary tumors, observation is reasonable for those patients with normal inguinal examination findings (see Fig. 37-4A, *left*). For patients with palpable adenopathy, a course of antibiotics should reveal those whose adenopathy is related to infection versus metastasis. A persistently palpable node should undergo fine-needle aspiration cytology; if the result is negative, an excisional biopsy is recommended. If the biopsy finding is abnormal, ipsilateral inguinal dissection with contralateral superficial or modified complete dissection is performed. DSNB is an option in experienced centers.

Low- to Intermediate-Risk Patients (American Joint Committee on Cancer Stage T1a)

Several series have combined patients with stage T1 grade 1 and grade 2 tumors and have found them to exhibit less than a 10% incidence of inguinal metastasis (see Fig. 37-4A, *right*; see also Table 37-7). However, the incidence of metastasis among strictly T1 grade 2 tumors (25% to 44%) may be higher, and variable recommendations have been made. The recent EAU guidelines recommend inguinal staging for T1 grade 2 tumors (also stage T1a) among patients with clinically negative lymph nodes (Pizzocaro et al, 2010). However, observation is also an option for compliant patients in this setting (ICUD penile cancer guidelines found in Pompeo et al, 2009; NCCN penile cancer guidelines, 2012). Similar patients with palpable nodes on initial presentation should undergo fine-needle aspiration cytology. If the nodes are positive, the patients then undergo lymphadenectomy, as in Figure 37-4A. If they are negative, then a 4-week period of antibiotic therapy is reasonable. If adenopathy does not resolve, then either excisional biopsy and/or planned lymphadenectomy are reasonable options. Close

follow-up is indicated for patients whose nodes resolve after antibiotic therapy, although the overall risk in this group remains low.

High-Risk Patients (American Joint Committee on Cancer Stage T1b or Higher)

For the high-risk cohort, the incidence of inguinal metastasis ranges from 50% to 70% (see Fig. 37-4B). According to the recent guidelines, there is consensus that patients with poorly differentiated tumors, lymphovascular invasion, or pT2 or greater tumors should undergo an inguinal staging procedure (Pompeo et al, 2009; Pizzocaro et al, 2010; NCCN penile cancer guidelines, 2012). The surgical approach depicted in Figure 37-4B is designed to maximize detection and treatment for those with proven nodal metastasis while limiting the morbidity of those with negative lymph nodes at surgery. Thus surgical staging is indicated even in those patients with clinically normal inguinal examination findings. **In this setting, antibiotic use minimizes the risk of inguinal wound infections or septic complications after control of an infected primary tumor, rather than influencing the decision for surgical staging.**

Patients with normal inguinal examination findings are offered bilateral superficial dissection, complete modified dissection, or

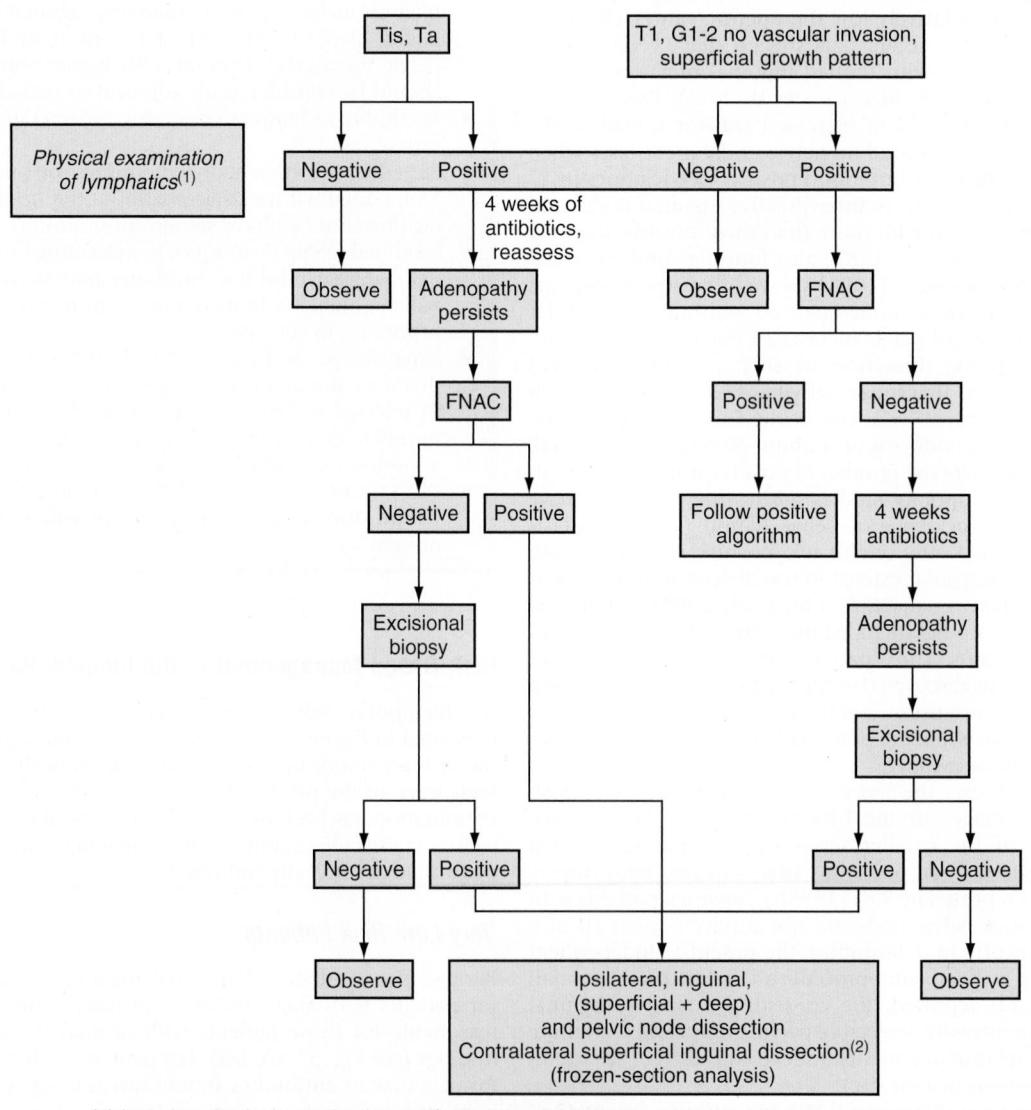

(1) Includes physical examination and/or imaging studies.

A (2) Complete modified dissection and dynamic sentinel node biopsy (experienced centers) acceptable.

Figure 37-4. **Management of regional disease. A, Low-risk patients.**

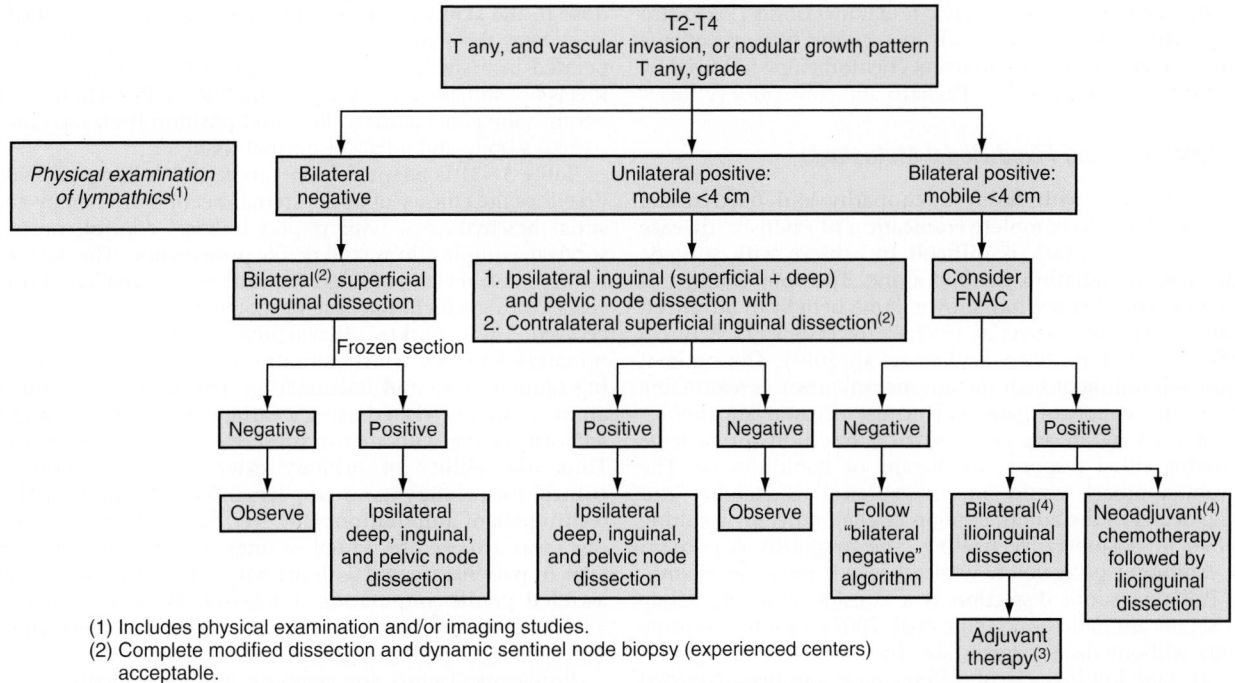

(1) Includes physical examination and/or imaging studies.
(2) Complete modified dissection and dynamic sentinel node biopsy (experienced centers) acceptable.
(3) Consider if >2 positive lymph nodes, or bilateral metastases, extranodal extension of cancer, or positive pelvic lymph nodes.
B (4) Either approach is acceptable.

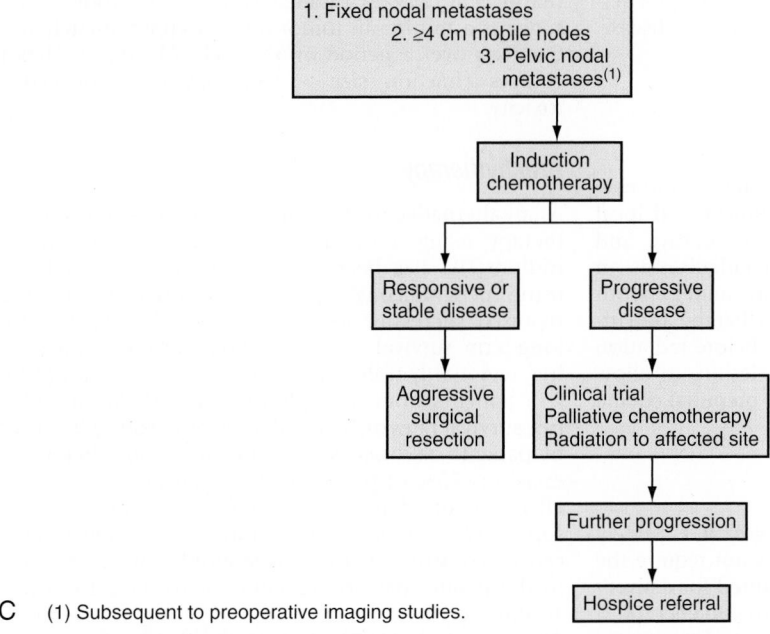

C (1) Subsequent to preoperative imaging studies.

Figure 37-4, cont'd **B, High-risk patients. C, Metastatic disease. FNAC, fine-needle aspiration cytology.**

DSNB (with the last offered in experienced centers). If frozen-section results reveal no metastasis, the procedure is concluded. For DSNB the results are based on permanent sections; thus further therapy is planned at a second setting if needed. If either side is positive, an ipsilateral inguinal dissection is performed. Pelvic dissection in the setting of a patient with no palpable adenopathy who is discovered to have positive inguinal metastasis at frozen section is optional and based on pathologic findings (Lont et al, 2007; Zhu et al, 2008). Patients with unilateral resectable adenopathy that is strongly suggestive of metastasis should undergo an ipsilateral ilio-inguinal dissection and a contralateral superficial or complete modified dissection. Frozen-section analysis then determines if deep inguinal or pelvic nodes should be excised. DSNB is another option

in managing the contralateral node-negative side. Palpable adenopathy of less than 4 cm was arbitrarily selected as a cutoff point for surgery as monotherapy because nodal metastases larger than 4 cm are associated with ENE of cancer (Ravi, 1993a).

For patients with bilateral palpable nodes that are strongly suggestive of metastasis, preoperative fine-needle aspiration cytology can be helpful for counseling of the patient as to the likelihood of the extent of surgery. For patients with negative results of fine-needle aspiration cytology, a staged surgical approach starting with superficial dissection is performed. Subsequent procedures in this setting depend on the results of frozen-section analysis. For patients requiring IILND because of metastases, adjuvant chemotherapy should be considered for those exhibiting more than two positive lymph nodes, ENE of cancer, or pelvic nodal metastasis (Pizzocaro et al, 2010). An alternative approach to consider among patients with bilateral metastases is neoadjuvant chemotherapy followed by surgical resection as described by Pagliaro and colleagues (2010).

Bulky Adenopathy and Fixed Nodal Metastasis

Survival in patients with bulky adenopathy and fixed nodal metastasis is related to complete eradication of extensive disease (see Fig. 37-4C). **This task is difficult to achieve with surgery, chemotherapy, or radiation therapy alone. The combination of surgery and chemotherapy has shown some benefit in advanced penile carcinoma** (Pizzocaro et al, 1997; Corral et al, 1998; Bermejo et al, 2007; Leijte et al, 2007; Pagliaro et al, 2010). The optimal integration and timing of such therapy are unknown. A reasonable approach in this cohort of patients is to use neoadjuvant chemotherapy followed by an aggressive surgical resection for patients demonstrating either response to therapy or stable disease. The neoadjuvant approach could improve surgical resectability and avoid long delays in the administration of chemotherapy resulting from delays in postoperative healing. The prognosis is poor in patients exhibiting progression while they are receiving chemotherapy. Palliative groin dissection is a consideration but rarely provides significant palliation (Leijte et al, 2007). Hemipelvectomy in patients without distant metastases has been reported (Block et al, 1973). Endoluminal vascular stents have also been reported to have transient success in preventing vascular erosion by tumor (Link et al, 2004). Clinical trials of novel systemic strategies and radiation therapy to affected areas provide the next level of care. With further progression, supportive care provided by hospice services can provide valuable support to patients with end-stage disease.

RADIATION THERAPY

Radiation Therapy for the Primary Lesion

Primary radiation therapy has significant curative potential and may permit relative preservation of penile form and function. If local control is not achieved, salvage surgery may still be curative, and therefore in a subset of men with penile cancer radiation as an initial strategy represents a reasonable treatment strategy. Both external-beam radiotherapy and interstitial brachytherapy are currently used in treating the primary penile tumor. Before radiation therapy, circumcision is necessary to expose the lesion, to allow resolution of any surface infection, and to prevent preputial edema and subsequent phimosis.

External-Beam Radiotherapy

External-beam radiotherapy has several advantages: It is widely available, delivers a homogeneous dose, and does not require the same expertise with respect to technical skills required for delivery of effective brachytherapy. In a review, Crook and coworkers (2009) described contemporary doses and fractions as ranging from 60 Gy in 25 fractions delivered over 5 weeks to 74 Gy in 37 fractions over 7.5 weeks. This contrasts with lower doses of 50 to 55 Gy cited in older series (McLean et al, 1993; Neave et al, 1993). One of the challenges of external-beam radiotherapy is to consistently position the penis in such a way as to be accessible by the radiation beam while not implicating adjacent normal tissues and structures. This is achieved by positioning the patient supine on the treatment couch and encasing the penis in a vertical position in a block of wax or Perspex with a central cylindric chamber. The block is bivalved for ease of application, which admittedly becomes more difficult as the course of radiotherapy progresses. The second consideration involves the physical nature of megavoltage radiation beams, which spare the skin surface and deliver the radiation dose at a depth in tissue. Penile cancer is of cutaneous origin and requires full treatment of the skin surface. Wax and Perspex are both tissue-equivalent materials, so the choice of these in fabricating an immobilization device effectively boluses the penis and brings the full

dose to the skin surface. An alternative has been described, which is to treat the patient in the prone position with the penis suspended in a small waterbath container (Vujovic et al, 2001), but this is not suitable for obese patients and can be technically difficult because the penis tends to float and position itself too close to the patient's body and adjacent normal tissue.

Table 37-11 is adapted from Crook and colleagues (2009), and describes the efficacy of both external-beam radiotherapy and interstitial brachytherapy with respect to local control, cause-specific survival, complications, and penile preservation. The data represent retrospective reviews of single institution series collected over many years, during which time staging systems and treatment techniques evolved. The data thus often represent a range of doses and fractionation schemes, which permits only limited conclusions regarding optimal dose and fractionation. **Five-year local control rates among patients treated using a variety of techniques ranged from 44% to 69.7% with penile preservation rates of 50% to 65%. Thus, the ability of primary external-beam radiotherapy to control the primary tumor appears inferior to traditional surgical techniques of amputation.** However, further local control in most cases was achieved by partial or total amputation and, **more than 50% of patients treated with primary external-beam radiotherapy avoided penile amputation.** Cause-specific survival ranged from 58% to 86% depending on primary tumor stage and lymph node status.

Prognostic factors for response among patients treated with external-beam radiotherapy include dose below 60 Gy, protracted treatment time exceeding 45 days or daily fraction less than 2 Gy in addition to stage T3, size exceeding 4 cm, and high-grade tumors (Sarin et al, 1997; Gotsadze, et al, 2000; Crook et al, 2009). This suggests a minimum tumor dose of approximately 66 Gy in 2-Gy fractions over a period of $6\frac{1}{2}$ weeks (45 days). Hypofractionated courses (fraction size >2 Gy) may be associated with worse toxicity.

Brachytherapy

As an alternative to external-beam radiotherapy, interstitial brachytherapy using a variety of radioisotopes but most commonly iridium-192 has been reported. Gerbaulet and Lambin (1992), using percutaneously placed interstitial iridium-192 implants, reported successful local control in 82% of 109 patients, with long-term survival rates of 75% to 80% in patients with tumor-free regional lymph nodes. Rozan and associates (1995) reviewed 259 patients from multiple centers, with 5- and 10-year disease-free survival rates of 78% and 67%, respectively. Twenty-two percent of patients also had surgery ranging from circumcision or local excision (75% of procedures) to total penectomy (4%). Late side effects occurred in 53% of the group. For noninvasive or very superficial tumors, a surface mold containing iridium-192 wires can be constructed. The plastic mold is worn in close apposition to the penile shaft for 12 hours or so daily for a period of 7 to 10 days for a total tumor dose of 60 Gy (El-Demiry et al, 1984; Akimoto et al, 1997). Because the depth of tumor invasion can be difficult to ascertain by clinical examination or imaging, and because a margin of full dose (comparable to the required surgical margin) is required beyond the macroscopic disease, the mold technique is rarely appropriate. Such superficial disease may now be treated more appropriately with laser or organ-sparing surgical techniques.

Crook and associates (2009) initially reported a cohort (1989-2000) of 30 men with cT1 to cT3 squamous cell carcinoma treated with iridium-192 delivered by 17- to 19.5-gauge steel needles held in a three-dimensional parallel array by predrilled acrylic plastic templates. With a median six needles (range 2 to 9), a prescribed dose of 60 Gy (range 55 to 65 Gy) was delivered during an average of 93 hours. With a median 34 months of follow-up, there were four local failures and four regional failures, and 1 patient required partial penectomy for radionecrosis. The 2-year actuarial local failure-free rate was 85%, and successful penile conservation was 83%. Obviously, tumors could only be clinically staged, and the

TABLE 37-11 Selected Series of Studies Reporting Local Control (LC) of Disease, Cancer-Specific Survival (CSS), Complications, and Penile Preservation for Men Treated with External-Beam Radiation Therapy (XRT) or Brachytherapy (BT) as Primary Treatment for Penile Cancer

STUDY	NO. OF PATIENTS	TYPE OF RT	DOSE (Gy)	F/U (mo) MEDIAN (RANGE)	LC BY RT AT 5 YEARS	CSS AT 5 YEARS	COMPLICATIONS	PENILE PRESERVATION
EXTERNAL BEAM								
McLean et al, 1993	26	XRT	35/10-60/25	116 (84-168)	61.5%	69%	7/26 unspecified	66% crude
Neave et al, 1993	20	XRT	50-55	36 mo minimum	69.7%	58%	10% stenosis	60%
Sarin et al, 1997	59	XRT	60/30	62 (2-264)	55%	66%	3% necrosis 15% stenosis	50% crude
Gotsadze et al, 2000	155	XRT	40-60	40	65%	86%	1 necrosis 5 stenoses	65%
Munro et al, 2001	13	XRT						
Zouhair et al, 2001	23	XRT						43%
Ozsahin et al, 2006	33	XRT/BT	52	62 (2-454)	44%	—	10% stenosis	52%
Mistry et al, 2007	18	XRT	55/16-50/20	62	63%	75%	2 necroses 1 stenosis	66% crude
BRACHYTHERAPY								
Mazeron et al, 1984	50	BT	60-70	(36-96)	78% crude		3 necroses 19% stenosis	74%
Delannes et al, 1992	51	BT	50-65	65 (12-144)	86% crude	85%	23% necrosis 45% stenosis	75%
Rozan et al, 1995	184	BT	63	139	86%	88%	21% necrosis 45% stenosis	78%
Soria et al, 1997	102	BT	61-70	111	77%	72%		72% (6 years)
Chaudhary et al, 1999	23	BT	50	21 (4-117)	70% (8 years)		0 necrosis 9% stenosis	70% (8 years)
Kiltie et al, 2000	31	BT	63.5	61.5	81%	85%	8 necroses 44% stenosis	75%
Crook et al, 2009	67	BT	60	48 (4-194)	87.5%	83.6%	12% necrosis 9% stenosis	88% 5 years 67% 10 years

F/U, follow-up; RT, radiation therapy.

authors stated that clinical distinction between cT1 and cT2 is subjective. Nodal failure related to tumor grade, but not tumor size. Kiltie and associates (2000), however, found local failures in 60% of tumors larger than 4 cm compared with 14% of tumors smaller than 4 cm. Mazeron and colleagues (1984) and Soria and coworkers (1997) both demonstrated more local failure as the tumor invaded the corpora and with tumor size larger than 4 cm. In the initial Crook series, prophylactic lymph node dissections were not routinely performed, and as one would expect, 50% of moderately or poorly differentiated tumors recurred regionally or distally (Crook et al, 2002). Therefore, selection of patients for prophylactic lymph node dissection is recommended to be the same as selection of patients undergoing surgical removal of the primary tumor.

The Crook series was updated in 2009 to 67 patients with a median follow-up of 4 years (range 0.2 to 16.2). At 10 years the actuarial cause-specific survival was 83.6%., and three late failures were observed (42, 64, 90 months). Penectomy was performed for 8 recurrences and 2 necroses for 5- and 10-year penile preservation rates of 88% and 67%, respectively. Inguinal lymph nodes in the most recent patients were managed with the same indications as for patients undergoing primary surgery, but with use of only biopsy information for determining high-grade disease and the presence of lymphovascular invasion. One predictor of local failure in this series was needle spacing—an increase in spacing (range 12 to 18 mm) decreased recurrences because of the wider lateral margin achieved. **Overall, local control** (see Table 37-11) **provided by interstitial brachytherapy appeared superior to that provided by external-beam radiotherapy, with 5-year local control rates of 70% to 87%. Penile preservation rates are highest at 5 years (74% to 88%), with some decrease at 8 to 10 years (67% to 70%)** (Crook et al, 2009).

Adverse Effects Associated with Radiotherapy

Acutely, after radiotherapy or brachytherapy one can expect moist desquamation at the treated site. This will be more extensive after external-beam radiotherapy because of the larger treatment volume. Re-epithelialization occurs in 4 to 8 weeks. Saline soaks and hygiene are important. Intercourse can be resumed when the patient is comfortable, but the use of additional water-based lubrication is recommended.

The two most common late side effects associated with radiotherapy are meatal stenosis and soft-tissue ulceration. Earlier series (from the 1960s to early 1970s) reported urethral fistula, stricture, or stenosis, with or without penile necrosis, pain, and edema (Kelley et al, 1974), in some instances necessitating secondary penectomy (Duncan and Jackson, 1972). Soft-tissue ulceration overall is reported in 0% to 23% of patients treated with external-beam or interstitial radiotherapy, with the higher rates associated with brachytherapy (see Table 37-11). In the case of persistent ulceration, a diagnostic dilemma exists in determining whether recurrent cancer is present; biopsy may be indicated. In general, ulceration is flat and superficial, with no raised or exophytic component. Close follow-up and treatment with antibiotics, vitamin E, and steroid creams are recommended. For cases resistant to these measures, a course of hyperbaric oxygen is often effective (Crook et al, 2009; Gomez-Iturriaga et al, 2011). The majority will heal with conservative management, but healing may take several weeks, and longer in diabetic patients. The more deeply invasive the original tumor, the longer healing can take. Meatal stenosis is reported in 10% to 45% of patients and may be related to increased dose per fraction in those treated with external-beam radiotherapy or needle spacing among those treated with brachytherapy. Meatal stenosis occurs later in follow-up (18 to 24 months) and may often be preceded by report of a weak, deviated or divided urinary stream. Intervention at this time using a meatal dilator will help to prevent subsequent unyielding fibrotic stenosis. Patients can be taught to do this themselves as required. If not appropriately managed, urethral strictures may occur late and may require a more formal dilation or, in very rare cases, urethroplasty.

The benefits of avoiding a mutilating surgical procedure are obvious, and although sexual function is typically reported to be preserved, the side effects of radiation on sexual quality of life have not been studied with validated instruments (Crook et al, 2009). Because brachytherapy irradiates much less of the penile shaft and erectile tissue, erectile function is more likely to be preserved than after external-beam radiotherapy. Patients and physicians must carefully consider the unique acute and long-term side effects of radiation therapy. For the elderly in whom sexual function is not an issue, partial penectomy may be quite acceptable, offering a prompt and effective treatment with relatively few side effects limiting activity in the postoperative period.

The organ-sparing benefits of radiation now must be compared with surgical choices such as laser therapy, Mohs micrographic surgery, and reconstructive surgery, all of which can provide organ sparing while minimizing functional loss. This emphasizes the need for multidisciplinary assessment and tertiary referral to centers where all options are available. Radiation may be the only solution for a patient with significant comorbidities who is not a surgical candidate.

Finally, as with any organ-sparing approach, extended follow up is essential. This must be emphasized to the patient at the time of the original treatment decision. Teaching self-examination and prompt reporting of concerns is also important. Local recurrence can be salvaged surgically without jeopardizing survival. Careful long-term follow-up is essential to detect recurrence promptly, and it must be recognized that recurrence may develop relatively late. In one series, 7 of 11 recurrences were detected after 2 years (63%) and 2 (18%) after 5 years (Mazeron et al, 1984). In terms of salvage surgery, Crook et al (2009) noted that external-beam radiotherapy typically treats much more of the penile shaft, whereas brachytherapy is more focal, leading to salvage options that are more likely to result in a partial penectomy than a total penectomy.

In summary, T1 and T2 tumors smaller than 4 cm with no or minimal extension beyond the coronal sulcus respond well to radiotherapy, and with careful planning, complications can be minimized (de Crevoisier et al, 2009). Brachytherapy can provide good local control and penile preservation with faster dose delivery (4 to 5 days rather than 6 to 7 weeks) compared with external-beam radiotherapy. For the patient who is an appropriate candidate for a radiation-based approach, the selection of external-beam radiotherapy versus brachytherapy may depend on the skill and experience of the radiation oncologist involved; external-beam radiotherapy may be more widely available. Crook and colleagues' series and review (2009) would suggest that the brachytherapy technique should be expanded and studied further in a multi-institutional fashion.

The treatment of locally advanced disease is clearly associated with a higher failure rate (local, regional, and distant), and the treatment approach must take into consideration regional nodes. For these patients, brachytherapy is not an option. Combined chemoradiotherapy radio sensitizers like cisplatin weekly—standard management in squamous carcinoma of the cervix—is well tolerated, is associated with excellent response rates, and may convert a patient with inoperable disease into a surgical candidate or alternatively may be used as definitive management (Rose, 2002). This approach will be studied in a cooperative international trial run through the International Rare Cancers Initiative (Nicholson et al, 2014).

Radiation Therapy for the Inguinal Areas

The presence and extent of lymph node involvement is such a key prognostic factor in the management of penile cancer that surgical evaluation of the inguinal regions is widely accepted. Surgical evaluation of high-risk, clinically node-negative patients is recommended so that additional treatment can be tailored to the actual pathology, rather than just offering "prophylactic" radiation to the inguinal nodes. A surgical approach to resectable adenopathy is also preferable because a dose that is sufficient to sterilize macroscopic disease in the groins is poorly tolerated (Murrell and Williams, 1965; Jensen, 1977; Kulkarni and Kamat, 1994). Furthermore, assessment of the treatment of the inguinal area by primary radiation therapy is hampered by the uncertainty arising from the inaccuracy of clinical staging and the frequent lack of histologic confirmation of nodal metastases. Table 37-3 summarizes the incidence of node positivity in clinically negative groins and suggests that radiation can be avoided in the majority of cases.

One of the largest series demonstrating a benefit of radiation therapy for lymph node metastases and/or distant metastases from penile cancer was published by Ravi and associates in 1994. One hundred and twenty patients with lymph node metastases and 9 with distant metastases were managed by radiation therapy alone (palliative) or in the preoperative or postoperative setting. Pertinent to the advanced disease presentation setting, 33 patients were treated with preoperative radiation therapy at 40 Gy over 4 weeks and subsequently had ILND. Of note, after radiation therapy and surgery, only 8% had evidence of ENE, and 3% recurred within the groin. This is relevant because in a prior report within a contemporary time frame (Ravi, 1993a), the incidence of ENE was 33% among patients treated with surgery alone, and groin recurrence was noted in 19%. The differences for both ENE and local recurrence were statistically lower ($P < .01$ and $P < .03$, respectively). The data are suggestive but not definitive that preoperative radiation therapy for nodes 4 cm or larger without skin fixation improved local control. The 5-year survival among the latter group was 70% (Ravi et al, 1994). These data are consistent with the beneficial effects seen when radiotherapy is used together with surgery or chemotherapy in other squamous malignancies such as vulvar, cervical, or anal carcinomas (Epidermoid anal cancer, 1996; Montana et al, 2000; Green et al, 2001). Such approaches should be further explored in the treatment of locally advanced penile cancer.

In the series by Ravi and colleagues (1994), palliative radiation therapy ameliorated symptoms in 56% of patients with fixed groin nodes, in 5 of 5 patients with painful bony metastases, and in 1 of /2 patients with spinal cord compression and paraplegia. However, pelvic and/or para-aortic radiation therapy was ineffective in patients with pelvic node metastases. Thus radiation therapy may be considered in patients with inoperable fixed and ulcerative inguinal lymph nodes who are not candidates for chemotherapy. On occasion, radiation to these areas is well tolerated, may result in significant palliation, and may postpone local complications for prolonged periods (Furlong and Uhle, 1953; Staubitz et al, 1955; Vaeth et al, 1970). Combined chemoradiotherapy is a promising approach, as previously mentioned, using weekly cisplatin as is successful in squamous carcinoma of the cervix (Rose, 2002).

Radiation has an important role to play as adjuvant therapy for surgically treated, pN+ patients. In a small retrospective study from Taiwan, Chen and colleagues (2004) reported regional failure rates after positive inguinal lymph node dissections in 11% (1 of 9) versus 60% (3 of 5) with and without adjuvant inguinal radiotherapy. Extrapolating from the published literature on vulvar cancer (Hyde et al, 2007), adjuvant radiotherapy 4500 cGy in 25 fractions over 5 weeks to the ipsilateral groin should be considered for patients with more than two positive nodes and for those with ENE. If the pelvic nodes are known to be clear, then the pelvis need not be included; but if pelvic node dissection has not been performed, then the radiation volume should extend to include the pelvis.

In summary, radiation therapy to the inguinal area is not recommended as prophylaxis for patients at high risk for inguinal node metastases. It is less effective therapeutically than a lymph node dissection for clinically involved nodes but should be considered as adjuvant treatment for those with more than two nodes positive or ENE. It may be useful for palliation in the situation of inoperable nodes and in a chemoradiotherapy approach may render inoperable disease resectable. Based on studies in other squamous malignancies, radiation as a part of a multimodal approach with chemotherapy and surgery among patients with advanced penile cancer should be further evaluated.

KEY POINTS: RADIATION THERAPY

- Primary radiation therapy for penile cancer may be successfully applied to select patients with T1 and T2 squamous cell carcinomas smaller than 4 cm with either external-beam radiotherapy or brachytherapy techniques.
- Salvage penectomy may be required after external-beam radiation or brachytherapy for persistent or recurrent disease or radiation necrosis. Lifelong careful follow-up is required.
- For patients selected for radiation therapy for the primary tumor, surgical management of inguinal lymph nodes should be recommended by the same criteria as for patients selected for surgical management of the primary tumor.
- Radiation to the inguinal area is not as effective as surgery for treatment of the inguinal nodes.
- Prophylactic radiotherapy has not been shown to alter the natural history of inguinal metastases and is not recommended.
- Integration of radiotherapy with surgery and chemotherapy in advanced disease requires further study.
- Palliative radiotherapy among patients with inoperable inguinal nodes may provide some benefit.

CHEMOTHERAPY

Advanced penile cancer manifesting as either bulky or unresectable regional disease or visceral metastases at initial presentation or disease recurrence is highly lethal because it is incurable in most cases with either surgery or radiotherapy alone (Ornellas et al, 1994; Ravi et al, 1994; Hegarty et al, 2006). Experience with single-agent or multiagent chemotherapy in this setting is limited because there are few phase 2 clinical trials and no randomized clinical trials. Several regimens have produced clinically meaningful

responses that have occasionally resulted in clearance of disease or facilitated surgical resection.

Single-Agent Chemotherapy

Gagliano and associates (1989) from the Southwest Oncology Group treated 26 patients, 12 of whom had received prior radiation, with low-dose (50 mg/m^2) cisplatin, and observed a 15% response rate of 1 to 3 months' duration and a median overall survival of 4.7 months. In a study from Memorial Sloan Kettering Cancer Center, 13 patients with extensive disease and either prior radiotherapy or chemotherapy were treated with cisplatin 70 to 120 mg/m^2 every 21 days. Three of 12 evaluable patients (25%) demonstrated responses (1 complete and 2 partial; duration 2 to 8 months; Ahmed et al, 1984).

Initial favorable reports from Japan suggested that bleomycin appeared to be effective in the treatment of penile and scrotal cancer. Ichikawa and associates reported a 50% response in 24 previously untreated patients with squamous carcinoma of the penis (Ichikawa et al, 1969; Ichikawa, 1977). A similar report from Uganda documented partial or complete tumor regression in 45% of treated patients (Kyalwazi et al, 1974). A review of 90 patients from the world literature demonstrated similar responses (Eisenberger, 1992). In a study by Ahmed and colleagues (1984), 14 patients were evaluable for response to single-agent bleomycin. There was one complete response, but the patient died from bleomycin pulmonary toxicity. There were also two partial responses, for an objective response rate of 21%. The median response duration was only 3 months (range 2 to 4).

Methotrexate produced responses in 8 of 13 patients (61%) treated at Memorial Sloan Kettering Cancer Center (Ahmed et al, 1984) with one complete response. However, median response duration even with the high response rate was 3 months (2 to 31 months), and one patient died from treatment-related sepsis. Methotrexate had been shown to be active in other reports (Mills, 1972; Garnick et al, 1979). Based on the Ahmed study, in which cisplatin, bleomycin, and methotrexate were given sequentially, there did not appear to be any obvious cross-resistance to the three agents. Subsequently a three-drug trial using cisplatin, bleomycin, and methotrexate was developed.

Combination Chemotherapy

The Southwest Oncology Group reported a phase 2 study using a modified regimen that reduced the total dose of cisplatin, bleomycin, and methotrexate. Haas and associates (1999) employed combination cisplatin, methotrexate, and bleomycin in 45 patients with locally advanced or metastatic penile cancer accrued from 31 different institutions. There were five complete and eight partial responses among 40 evaluable patients (32.5% response rate). The median duration of response was 16 weeks with an overall survival of 28 weeks (Haas et al, 1999). Although the response rate appeared encouraging, it was still within the 95% confidence interval (CI) for single-agent cisplatin, and there were five treatment-related deaths in the study (one from infection and four from pulmonary complications) (Ahmed et al, 1984; Gagliano et al, 1989; Haas et al, 1999). Thus this study failed to confirm the initial high response rate of single-agent methotrexate; the response rate was not significantly higher than that of single-agent cisplatin, and bleomycin pulmonary toxicity was significant (Haas et al, 1999).

Three additional contemporary trials, all including cisplatin, revealed significant activity while omitting the bleomycin and methotrexate. Theodore and colleagues (2008) reported the results of a European Organisation for Research and Treatment of Cancer (EORTC) phase 2 study in which 28 patients with locally advanced or metastatic disease (T3, T4, N1 to N3, or M1) received combination cisplatin and irinotecan. Patients were treated in either the neoadjuvant setting for four cycles before surgery (T3, N1 or N2) or up to eight cycles (T4, N3, M1 disease). Toxicity was acceptable, with no treatment-related deaths. Eight responses were noted (two complete, six partial) for an objective response rate of 30.8% (80%

CI 18.8% to 45%). Of note, three patients taken to surgery in the neoadjuvant setting were found to have no evidence of residual disease. The authors reported the trial as negative, however, because it was powered to show an objective response rate not less than 30% by CI.

A phase 2 clinical trial of neoadjuvant paclitaxel, ifosfamide, and cisplatin chemotherapy (TIP) was conducted at the University of Texas MD Anderson Cancer Center (Pagliaro et al, 2010). Eligible patients had stage Tx, N2 or N3 lymph node metastases, no evidence of distant metastases (M0), and no prior chemotherapy. Treatment consisted of four courses of TIP followed by bilateral inguinal lymph node dissections, unilateral or bilateral pelvic lymph node dissections, and surgical control of the primary tumor when appropriate. The objective response rate was 50% (15 of 30 patients), and the pathologic complete response rate was 10% (3 patients). Twenty-three patients completed four courses of TIP, and 22 of those underwent surgery. Nine patients (30% for the trial, 40.9% of those completing treatment) were alive and disease free at a median follow-up of 34 months. Nineteen deaths occurred as a result of progressive disease, and 2 from unrelated causes. Toxicity was acceptable and no treatment-related deaths occurred (Pagliaro et al, 2010). Thus the data for use of the TIP regimen suggest a response rate that may be significantly higher than that of single-agent cisplatin and better tolerance than with prior bleomycin- or methotrexate-containing regimens. Table 37-12 provides safety and efficacy data for cisplatin-containing chemotherapy regimens reported thus far. Treatment-related pulmonary toxicity and death were avoided with the absence of bleomycin.

A third prospective trial evaluated the combination of docetaxel, cisplatin, and 5-fluorouracil (TPF) in patients with locally advanced or metastatic penile cancer (Nicholson et al, 2013). The objective response rate was 38.5% (10 of 26 evaluable patients), and 65.5% of patients experienced at least one grade 3 or grade 4 event. The predetermined target response rate of 60% was not reached, and the authors concluded that similar results could be achieved with 5-fluorouracil and cisplatin and that the addition of docetaxel resulted in toxicity. The objective response rate to 5-fluorouracil and cisplatin in one retrospective series was 32% (8 of 25 patients) (Di Lorenzo et al, 2012)

Data from the aforementioned three prospective trials and one retrospective series suggest that patients with advanced, unresectable primary tumors or metastatic disease can benefit from cisplatin-based chemotherapy, and selected patients with bulky regional lymph node metastases appeared to benefit from post-chemotherapy lymphadenectomy. Negative pathology in lymph nodes was seen after neoadjuvant treatment with TIP (3 of 30 patients) and irinotecan and cisplatin (3 of 7 patients). For patients with unresectable primary tumors or bulky regional lymph node metastases, neoadjuvant treatment with a cisplatin-containing regimen may be effective and may allow curative resection. The optimal chemotherapy regimen has yet to be determined.

Adjuvant Chemotherapy

Historically, combination vincristine, bleomycin, and methotrexate therapy was administered in 12 weekly courses to 17 patients in the postoperative setting (12) or neoadjuvant setting (5) at the Milan National Tumor Institute. The patients treated were at high risk for recurrence with surgery alone; 9 showed extranodal tumor growth, 5 had pelvic nodal involvement, and 5 had bilateral metastases. At follow-up ranging from 18 and 102 months, only 1 relapse had occurred (Pizzocaro and Piva, 1988). Later, reports from this center further confirmed the value of adjuvant chemotherapy. Of 56 node-positive patients, 82% of the 25 patients receiving adjuvant vincristine, bleomycin, and methotrexate therapy survived 5 years, compared with 37% of 31 patients treated with surgery alone (Pizzocaro et al, 1995, 1997). In the neoadjuvant treatment group, partial responses were noted in 3 of 5 patients with extremely large (6 to 11 cm) nodal metastases. These three patients subsequently were completely resected and were free of tumor at intervals ranging from 20 to 72 months. These data have yet to be confirmed and will probably not be further studied, given the potential toxicities of bleomycin and methotrexate.

Postchemotherapy Surgical Consolidation

Shammas and colleagues (1992) reported on eight patients treated with the combination of cisplatin and 5-fluorouracil. Seven of the eight patients had Jackson stage III or IV disease, and two in this group had either pleural or lung metastases. One of 7 (14%) had a partial response with disappearance of lung metastases and post-surgical consolidation and lived for longer than 32 months. He received five cycles of therapy. Three patients with stable disease received only one or two cycles and survived for 2 or more to 11 months. Of note, two of three patients who ultimately had disease progression received three or four cycles of therapy and underwent surgical consolidation with survival times of 12 and 28 months from chemotherapy.

Thus, 2 of 7 patients (28%) who survived 28 and more than 32 months received significant palliation or cure from the combination. Corral and coworkers (1998) reported on the long-term follow-up of a prospective group of patients treated with bleomycin, methotrexate, and cisplatin. Among the cohort, 21 patients had penile carcinoma, with 10 of 21 (48%) having either N3 or M1

TABLE 37-12 Safety and Efficacy of Multidrug Penile Cancer Regimens without Bleomycin

	CHEMOTHERAPY	RESPONSE RATE	TREATMENT-RELATED DEATH	MEDIAN OVERALL SURVIVAL (mo)
Di Lorenzo et al, 2012*	Fluorouracil, 800-1000 mg/m^2/day, days 1-4 Continuous infusion cisplatin, 70-80 mg/m^2, day 1; cycle q3wk	32%	0/25	8
Pagliaro et al, 2010	Paclitaxel, 175 mg/m^2, day 1 Ifosfamide, 1200 mg/m^2, days 1-3 Cisplatin, 25 mg/m^2, days 1-3; cycle q3wk	50%	0/30	17.1†
Theodore et al, 2008	Irinotecan, 60 mg/m^2, days 1, 8, 15 Cisplatin, 80 mg/m^2, day 1; cycle q4wk	30.8%	0/28	4.7
Nicholson et al, 2013	Docetaxel, 75 mg/m^2, day 1 Cisplatin, 60 mg/m^2, day 1 Fluorouracil, 750 mg/m^2/day, days 1-5; cycle q3wk	38.5%	0/28	13.9

*Retrospective study.
†Neoadjuvant setting (N2-3, M0).

disease. The remainder had either N1 or N2 nodal metastases. Objective responses were noted in 12 (57%), including 2 of 5 with distant metastases. Six patients in the group (28.5%) achieved disease-free status with either chemotherapy alone (2) or surgery (3) or radiation therapy (1) with a median survival of 27.8 months. This was significantly longer than in those not achieving disease-free status (6.7 months, *P* = .004). Thus, this prospective study showed that a multidisciplinary approach to achieve disease-free status could prolong survival. Subsequently Leijte et al (2007) from the Netherlands Cancer Institute reviewed their experience with neoadjuvant chemotherapy in patients with initially "unresectable" penile cancer. The series included 20 patients treated with five different regimens including (1) single-agent bleomycin; (2) bleomycin, vincristine, and methotrexate; (3) cisplatin and 5-fluorouracil; (4) bleomycin, cisplatin, and methotrexate; and (5) cisplatin and irinotecan. The objective responses were evaluable in 19 (1 patient died because of bleomycin toxicity after 2 weeks), with 12 responses (63%, 2 complete, 10 partial). Surgical procedures included treatment of the primary tumor as well as inguinal and pelvic dissections. Additional soft-tissue resection including bone was sometimes required. Vascularized tissue flaps were used for inguinal reconstruction. Among 12 responders, only 9 went to surgery because 2 died of bleomycin-related complications and a third was deemed unfit for surgery. Eight of 9 responding patients taken to surgery (2 were pT0) were free of disease with a median follow-up of 20.4 months. This is in contrast to 3 nonresponders who went to surgery for palliative intent. All 3 died within 4 to 8 months as a result of locoregional recurrence. The implications of this study are that response to chemotherapy together with an aggressive surgical procedure provides the optimal scenario for significant palliation or potentially cure.

In a separate study Bermejo et al (2007) described the surgical considerations and complications among 10 patients who had either a response or stable disease after combination chemotherapy. The regimens included (1) bleomycin, methotrexate, and cisplatin; and (2) paclitaxel, ifosfamide, and cisplatin (TIP), or (3) paclitaxel and carboplatin. This cohort of patients exhibited bulky inguinal or pelvic metastases, with the only exclusions being patients with fixed pelvic masses or complete encasement of the femoral vessels. In addition to IILND, resection of the inguinal ligament, the inferior aspect of the rectus abdominis or external and internal oblique muscles, the spermatic cord and ipsilateral testicle, and segments of the femoral artery and vein (with subsequent patch or bypass grafting) was performed to achieve negative margins. Plastic surgery consultation was obtained for wound coverage, including the insertion of monofilament polypropylene mesh for abdominal wall defects and myocutaneous flaps of the sartorius, rectus abdominis, serratus anterior, and latissimus dorsi muscles. Among 5 patients exhibiting an objective response, 3 were alive and disease free at 48, 50, and 73 months. Two other patients died (1 of disease at 30 months, another of unknown causes at 21 months). Among the 5 remaining patients with stable disease, 3 were dead of disease within 7 months and 1 patient treated with bleomycin died of "failure to thrive" at 8 months. However, another patient treated with paclitaxel and carboplatin who achieved only stable disease was alive and disease free at 84 months. These data appear to reinforce the concept that response to systemic chemotherapy before surgery enhances the chance for long-term survival among those undergoing surgical resection. Related to systemic therapy, the authors reported that the TIP regimen was well tolerated and all three pT0 responses at surgery were among patients treated with TIP. This provided the rationale for the prospective phase 2 study discussed previously (Pagliaro et al, 2010). In that study, the patients with response to neoadjuvant TIP had significantly better overall survival (*P* = .001) and time to progression (*P* < .001) compared with those who did not.

Taken together, these data provide evidence that response to chemotherapy improves resectability and survival. Surgery among patients who do not respond to therapy may occasionally be associated with long-term survival but is more often associated with death because of either rapidly occurring locoregional recurrence or

distant metastases (Bermejo et al, 2007; Leijte et al, 2007; Pagliaro et al, 2010).

> ### KEY POINTS: CHEMOTHERAPY
>
> - Treatment with a cisplatin-containing regimen in advanced metastatic penile cancer should be considered because responses do occur and this may facilitate curative resection. The optimal chemotherapy regimen has yet to be determined.
> - The use of bleomycin in the treatment of men with penile cancer was associated with an unacceptable level of toxicity and is discouraged as first-line therapy.
> - Surgical consolidation to achieve disease-free status or palliation should be considered in fit patients with a proven objective response to systemic chemotherapy.
> - Among patients whose tumor progresses through chemotherapy, surgery is not recommended.

NONSQUAMOUS PENILE MALIGNANT NEOPLASMS

Nonsquamous penile malignant neoplasms are extremely rare. Pathologic descriptions and local and regional treatment options are available; however, outcomes and comparisons are limited to case reports and small retrospective series. Most reports establish the following features: (1) incidence of disease, (2) distinguishing pathologic features, (3) treatment recommendations, and (4) parallels (or lack thereof) to the same carcinoma in nongenital locations.

Basal Cell Carcinoma

Although basal cell carcinoma is frequently encountered on other sun-exposed cutaneous surfaces, it is rare on the penis (Fig. 37-5A). Fewer than 30 cases have been well documented (Goldminz et al, 1989; Ladocsi et al, 1998; Nguyen et al, 2006). The lesion can be seen anywhere on the penis but is commonly on the penile shaft. It is slow growing, and delay in diagnosis in one series ranged from 2 months to 50 years (Kim et al, 1994). **Treatment is by local excision, which is virtually always curative** (Hall et al, 1968; Goldminz et al, 1989). Only one case report describes what the authors believe to be the only reported case of metastatic penile basal cell carcinoma (Jones et al, 2000). Nguyen and colleagues (2006) reported two cases of basal cell carcinoma treated by Mohs surgery.

A benign variant of basal cell carcinoma, the premalignant fibroepithelioma of Pinkus, has been reported to occur on the penile shaft (Heymann et al, 1983). Diagnosis is made at excisional biopsy. Excision has been uniformly curative.

Melanoma and basal cell carcinoma rarely occur on the penis, presumably because the organ's skin is protected from exposure to the sun. Malignant neoplasms arising from the supporting structures of the penis are also rare and include any combination of tumors of smooth or striated muscle or of fibrous, fatty, or vascular tissue. Information about appropriate treatment of these malignant neoplasms is derived from the review of single case reports and small series (Belville and Cohen, 1992).

Melanoma

More than 150 cases of melanoma of the penis have been reported (Fig. 37-5B). Of 1200 melanomas treated at Memorial Sloan Kettering Cancer Center, only 2 were of penile origin (Das Gupta and Grabstald, 1965). At the University of Texas MD Anderson Cancer Center, less than 1% of all primary penile cancers were malignant melanomas (Johnson and Ayala, 1973; de Bree et al, 1997). **Melanoma manifests as a blue-black or reddish brown pigmented papule, plaque, or ulceration on the glans penis. It occurs on the prepuce less frequently.** Diagnosis is made by

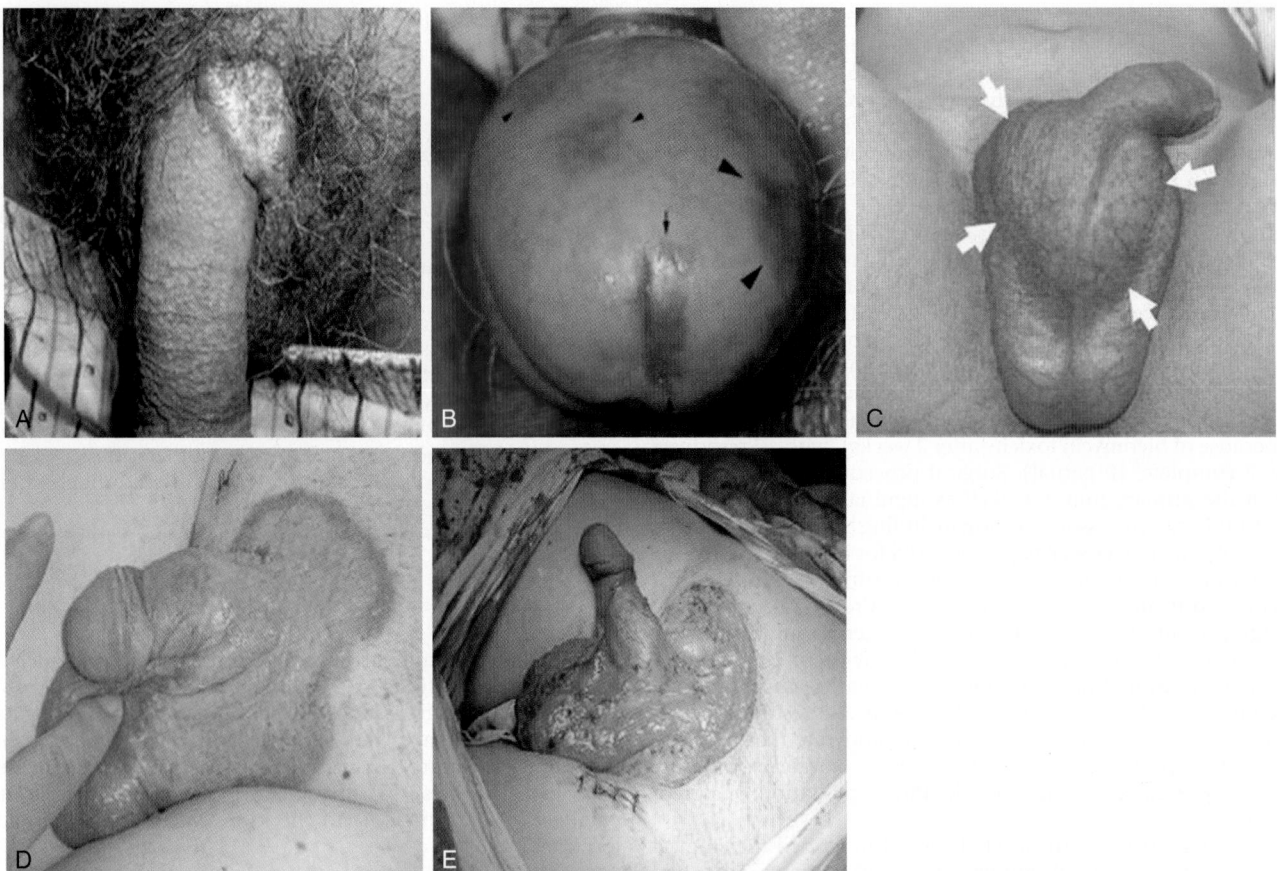

Figure 37-5. Clinical examination findings from non–squamous cell carcinomas involving the penis. A, Basel cell carcinoma. B, Melanoma. Note superficial spreading melanoma *(large arrowheads)*, melanoma in situ *(arrow)*, and two areas of possible melanosis *(small arrowheads)*. C, Leiomyosarcoma *(arrows)*. D, Paget disease. E, Paget disease after resection.

histologic examination of biopsy specimens, which demonstrate atypical junctional cell activity with displacement of pigmented cells into the dermis.

Prognostic characteristics that have been found significant for melanoma in other sites, such as depth of invasion (Clark staging) and thickness of the tumor (Breslow classification), have not been prospectively applied to penile lesions because experience with these lesions is limited. Sanchez-Ortiz and colleagues (2005) used the AJCC system for classifying cutaneous melanomas (Fleming, 1997) in the largest report to date on melanoma of the penis. This system incorporates elements of the Clark and Breslow staging systems. When this information is favorable, local excision is feasible. Distant metastatic spread has been found in 60% of patients studied (Abeshouse, 1958; Johnson et al, 1973; de Bree et al, 1997) in older series. However, Sanchez-Ortiz found that patients with early-stage melanomas had excellent outcomes if primary tumors were of low stage and regional lymph nodes were negative. Hematogenous metastases occur by means of the vascular structures of the corporeal bodies; lymphatic spread to the regional inguinal and pelvic nodes occurs by lymphatic permeation.

Surgery is the primary mode of treatment; radiation therapy and chemotherapy are of only adjunctive or palliative benefit. For stage I melanoma (localized lesion without metastases) and stage II melanoma (metastases confined to one regional area), adequate excision of the primary tumor by partial or total penile amputation together with en bloc bilateral ilioinguinal node dissection has historically been advocated (Johnson et al, 1973; Bracken and Diokno, 1974; Manivel and Fraley, 1988). In reviewing the University of Texas MD Anderson Cancer Center experience plus the literature to date, Sanchez-Ortiz and colleagues (2005) proposed a treatment algorithm for management of the primary tumor and

inguinal lymph nodes. For tumors of the foreskin, circumcision may be adequate. For glans tumors, a partial penectomy was recommended; and for glans-shaft tumors, a partial or total penectomy can be performed. The authors recommend bilateral modified inguinal lymph node dissections in all patients with lesions that are Breslow depth 1 mm or greater, with ulceration, or with Clark level IV or V involvement. Although dynamic sentinel lymph node biopsy techniques are increasingly used in more common sites of melanoma, their use in penile melanoma is unproven as yet. This is likely because of the rarity of the disease (Sanchez-Ortiz et al, 2006).

The prognosis for patients with penile melanoma is clearly dependent on stage of the primary tumor and the presence or absence of inguinal metastases. Contemporary staging and prognostic factors were reviewed by Sanchez-Ortiz and coworkers (2005). A report from the Netherlands (van Geel et al, 2007) focused on the concept of mucosal site penile melanomas—glans, meatus, fossa navicularis, and distal urethral. These lesions may appear more aggressive than cutaneous lesions, but greater delay in diagnosis may be a factor. In a pooled, retrospective analysis of 66 cases, the recurrence outcomes were similar for cutaneous melanomas of comparable tumor thickness.

Sarcomas

Primary mesenchymal tumors of the penis are rare. A thorough review of 46 such tumors from the Armed Forces Institute of Pathology revealed an equal number of benign and malignant lesions (Dehner and Smith, 1970). The patients ranged in age from newborn to the eighth decade of life. The presenting signs and symptoms of subcutaneous mass, penile pain and enlargement, priapism, and urinary obstruction were the same for both benign and malignant lesions. A sarcoma has been reported to masquerade as a Peyronie plaque (Moore et al, 1975).

Malignant lesions were found more frequently on the proximal shaft (Fig. 37-5C); benign lesions were more often located distally. The most common malignant lesions were those of vascular origin (hemangioepithelioma), followed in frequency by those of neural, myogenic, and fibrous origin (Ashley and Edwards, 1957). Single case reports of sarcomatous lesions have been published—for example, malignant fibrous histiocytoma (Parsons and Fox, 1988), angiosarcoma (Rasbridge and Parry, 1989), leiomyosarcoma (Planz et al, 1998), epithelioid sarcoma (Leviav et al, 1988), hemangioendothelioma (Kamat et al, 2004), and osteosarcoma (Sacker et al, 1994).

Sarcomas have been classified as superficial when they arise from the integumentary supporting structures and as deep when they develop from the corporeal body supporting structures (Pratt and Ross, 1969). Wide, local surface excision and partial penile amputation for the superficial tumors have been suggested and used successfully in isolated case reports (Pak et al, 1986; Dalkin and Zaontz, 1989). Total penile amputation has been reserved for tumors of deep corporeal origin. However, local recurrences are characteristic of sarcomas (Dehner and Smith, 1970). Fetsch and colleagues (2004), from the Armed Forces Institute of Pathology, have updated their series of 14 cases of leiomyosarcoma with review of the literature. They concluded that small lesions (smaller than 2 cm) were best managed with local resection, whereas deeper-seated tumor often necessitates partial or total amputation. Deep lesions at the base of the penis have the worst prognosis.

Regional metastases are rare. Unless adenopathy is palpable, node dissections are not recommended (Hutcheson et al, 1969). Distant metastases have also been unusual (Dehner and Smith, 1970). This supports aggressive local treatment in anticipation of cure. Radiation therapy and chemotherapy have not been used extensively enough for comment on their efficacy (Fetsch et al, 2004).

Kaposi sarcoma, which is usually a cutaneous manifestation of a generalized lymphoreticular disorder, may produce genital lesions but is now most frequently associated with HIV infection.

Extramammary Paget Disease

Extramammary Paget disease (EMPD) of the penis is rare, with fewer than 30 cases reported (Mitsudo et al, 1981; Macedo et al, 1997) up to the late 1990s. However, more recently several larger series have been reported from China and Korea (Yang et al, 2005; Wang et al, 2008). It appears grossly as an erythematous, eczematoid, well-demarcated area that cannot be clinically distinguished from erythroplasia of Queyrat, Bowen disease, or carcinoma in situ of the penis. Clinical presentation includes local discomfort, pruritus, and occasionally a serosanguineous discharge involving the penis, the scrotum, or even the perianal area (Fig. 37-5D and E). On microscopic examination, identification is clearly made by the presence of large, round or oval, clear-staining hydropic cells with hypochromatic nuclei (i.e., Paget cells). The cells often stain positively for cytokeratin 7 in addition to carcinoembryonic antigen and show gross cystic fluid protein but are S-100 protein negative (O'Connor et al, 2003). The tumor behaves as a slow-growing intraepithelial adenocarcinoma with cells derived from apocrine glands. With time the cells may become invasive with dermal tumor deposits metastasizing to regional lymph nodes via dermal lymphatics (Park et al, 2001 Hegarty et al, 2011). Of note, penoscrotal EMPD may be associated with other malignancies of the genitourinary tract, such as prostate, bladder, and renal malignancies (Chanda, 1985; Ojeda et al, 1987; Koh, 1995; Allan et al, 1998), and should be evaluated for their presence. In a recent series from MD Anderson Cancer Center among 20 reported patients, 9 (45%) had at least one other malignancy including prostate, bladder, renal, skin, esophageal, and rectal sites. Of note, 8 of the 9 patients were diagnosed with the other cancer before their diagnosis of EMPD.

Two reports from the Far East have added to the case series in the literature: 130 cases of penoscrotal Paget disease from China (Wang et al, 2008) and 36 from South Korea (Yang et al, 2005). In most cases only the skin and dermis must be resected with a gross margin of up to 3 cm. Positive margins may still occur, and frozen sections are recommended to guide the extent of resection. Local skin or scrotal flaps (Wang et al, 2008) can be used to cover the defects. Patients with a positive surgical margin are at a higher risk for recurrence, and additional resection is advised. In the series from Hegarty et al (2011), no recurrences were noted among patients with intraepidermal EMPD with negative surgical margins.

In a minority of cases the tumor may invade deeper structures, necessitating more extensive resection and reconstruction, as reported in case series (Hatoko et al, 2002; Fujisawa et al, 2008). If inguinal adenopathy is present, radical node dissection is advised (Hagan et al, 1975) but prognosis is poor (Yang et al, 2005). Hegarty and colleagues (2011) described the use of neoadjuvant docetaxel and carboplatin chemotherapy and surgical resection in two patients. One patient was alive with disease at 40 months, and the other had no evidence of disease at 13 months.

Adenosquamous Carcinoma

Adenosquamous carcinoma is a rare tumor characterized by both glandular and squamous histologic elements that are independent of the urethral glands. It manifests as a large (5 to 9 cm), firm, and grayish white granular exophytic mass involving the distal shaft or glans. On microscopic examination the glands contain mucin and are positive for carcinoembryonic antigen. In one reported case, the tumor was metastatic to a single inguinal node. This patient was managed with local excision of the primary tumor and a limited inguinal node dissection and lived 9 years after treatment. Other tumors were managed with local excision and surveillance (Cubilla et al, 1996). In only the seventh reported case (Romero et al, 2006), a patient with a bulky primary mass and inguinal lymph nodes underwent total penectomy and delayed ILND and PLND with a final pathologic stage of pT2N3M0 and was free of disease at 5-year follow-up.

Lymphoreticular Malignant Neoplasm

Primary lymphoreticular malignant neoplasm rarely occurs on the penis (Dehner and Smith, 1970). Leukemia may infiltrate the corpora, resulting in priapism (Pochedly et al, 1974). A thorough search for systemic disease is necessary when lymphomatous infiltration of the penis is diagnosed. If the penile lesion is indeed a primary tumor, systemic chemotherapy may be administered. It is the most effective therapy for local disease, for potential occult deposits that may exist elsewhere, and for preservation of form and function (Marks et al, 1988). Local low-dose radiation therapy has also been reported to be successful (Stewart et al, 1985).

Metastases

Metastatic lesions to the penis are unusual, with fewer than 300 cases reported in the literature (Belville and Cohen, 1992) until the early 1990s. Their infrequency is somewhat puzzling when one considers the rich blood and lymphatic supply to the organ and its proximity to the bladder, prostate, and rectal areas frequently involved with neoplasm. It is from these three organs that the majority of metastatic penile lesions originate (Abeshouse and Abeshouse, 1961). The most likely routes of spread are by direct extension, retrograde venous and lymphatic transport, and arterial embolism. Other sources of penile metastases emanate from the gastrointestinal tract, testis, and kidney (Belville and Cohen, 1992).

The most frequent sign of penile metastasis is priapism; penile swelling, nodularity, and ulceration have also been reported (McCrea and Tobias, 1958; Abeshouse and Abeshouse, 1961; Weitzner, 1971). Urinary obstruction and hematuria may occur. The most common histologic feature of penile invasion by metastatic lesions is the replacement of one or both corpora cavernosa, which explains the frequent occurrence of priapism. Solitary cutaneous, preputial, and glandular deposits are less common.

The differential diagnosis includes idiopathic priapism; venereal or other infectious ulcerations; tuberculosis; Peyronie plaque; and primary, benign, or malignant tumors.

Penile metastases represent an advanced form of virulent disease and usually appear rather rapidly after recognition and treatment of the primary lesion (Abeshouse and Abeshouse, 1961; Hayes and Young, 1967; Mukamel et al, 1987). On rare occasions a long period may elapse between the treatment of the primary lesion and the appearance of penile metastases (Abeshouse and Abeshouse, 1961) or the penile lesion may occur as the initial and only site of metastasis. In one report of 17 patients with penile metastases, 14 patients died of disseminated disease, with a median survival of 5 months after the diagnosis of penile metastases (Chaux et al, 2011).

Because of the association of a penile metastatic lesion with advanced disease, survival after its presentation is limited, and the majority of patients die within 1 year (Robey and Schellhammer, 1984; Mukamel et al, 1987; Fischer and Patrick, 1999). Successful palliative treatment may occasionally be possible in the case of solitary nodules or localized distal penile involvement if complete excision by partial amputation succeeds in removing the entire area of malignant infiltration (Spaulding and Whitmore, 1978). The prospect for surgical cure is minimal if proximal corporeal invasion is present. Penectomy is occasionally indicated after failure of other modalities to palliate intractable pain (Mukamel et al, 1987). Pain can also be managed by dorsal nerve section (Hill and Khalid, 1988). In general, radiation therapy has been unsuccessful, and chemotherapy has not been employed in a sufficient number of cases to warrant definitive recommendations.

KEY POINTS: NONSQUAMOUS MALIGNANT NEOPLASMS

- Basal cell carcinoma represents a highly curable variant with a relatively low metastatic potential.
- Sarcomas are prone to local recurrence; regional and distant metastases are rare. Superficial lesions can be treated with less radical procedures.
- Melanoma is an aggressive form of cancer but can be cured if diagnosed and treated with the appropriate surgical procedure at an early stage.
- EMPD disseminates by intraepidermal spread initially. Wide local excision to achieve negative margins is the therapy of choice. Invasive EMPD can be lethal.
- Penile metastases most often represent spread from a clinically obvious existing primary tumor. Prognosis is poor, and therapy should be directed toward the primary tumor site histology and local palliation.

REFERENCES

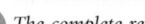 *The complete reference list is available online at www.expertconsult.com.*

SUGGESTED READINGS

Agrawal A, Pai D, Ananthakrishnan N, et al. The histological extent of the local spread of carcinoma of the penis and its therapeutic implications. BJU Int 2000;85:299–301.

Alani RM, Munger K. Human papillomaviruses and associated malignancies. J Clin Oncol 1998;16:330–7.

Alnajjar HM, Lam W, Bolgeri M, et al. Treatment of carcinoma in situ of the glans penis with topical chemotherapy agents. Eur Urol 2012;62(5):923–8.

Aragona F, Serretta V, Marconi A, et al. Queyrat's erythroplasia of the prepuce: a case-report. Acta Chir Belg 1985;85:303–4.

Bermejo C, Busby JE, Spiess PE, et al. Neoadjuvant chemotherapy followed by aggressive surgical consolidation for metastatic penile squamous cell carcinoma. J Urol 2007;177(4):1335–8.

Bevan-Thomas R, Slaton JW, Pettaway CA. Contemporary morbidity from lymphadenectomy for penile squamous cell carcinoma: the MD Anderson Cancer Center experience. J Urol 2002;167:1638–42.

Bhojwani A, Biyani CS, Nicol A, et al. Bowenoid papulosis of the penis. Br J Urol 1997;80:508.

Bleeker MC, Heideman DA, Snijders PJ, et al. Penile cancer: epidemiology, pathogenesis, and prevention. World J Urol 2009;27:141–50.

Buechner SA. Common skin disorders of the penis. BJU Int 2002;90:498–506.

Cabanas RM. Anatomy and biopsy of the sentinel lymph nodes. Urol Clin North Am 1992;19:267–76.

Castellsague X, Ghaffari A, Daniel RW, et al. Prevalence of penile human papillomavirus DNA in husbands of women with and without cervical neoplasia: a study in Spain and Colombia. J Infect Dis 1997;176:353–61.

Chaux A, Amin M, Cubilla AL, et al. Metastatic tumors to the penis: a report of 17 cases and review of the literature. Int J Surg Pathol 2011;19(5):597–606.

Chaux A, Torres J, Pfannl R, et al. Histologic grade in penile squamous cell carcinoma: visual estimation versus digital measurement of proportions grades, adverse prognosis with any proportion of grade 3 and correlation of a Gleason-like system with nodal metastasis. Am J Surg Pathol 2009;33(7):1042–8.

Coblentz TR, Theodorescu D. Morbidity of modified prophylactic inguinal lymphadenectomy for squamous cell carcinoma of the penis. J Urol 2002;168(Pt 1):1386–9.

Colberg JW, Andriole GL, Catalona WJ. Long-term follow-up of men undergoing modified inguinal lymphadenectomy for carcinoma of the penis. Br J Urol 1997;79:54–7.

Crook J, Grimard L, Tsihlias J, et al. Interstitial brachytherapy for penile cancer: an alternative to amputation. J Urol 2002;167:506–11.

Crook J, Ma C, Grimard L. Radiation therapy in the management of the primary penile tumor: an update. World J Urol 2009;27:189–96.

Cubilla A, Reuter V, Gregoire L, et al. Basaloid squamous cell carcinoma: a distinctive human papilloma virus–related penile neoplasm: a report of 20 cases. Am J Surg Pathol 1998;22:755–61.

Cubilla AL, Reuter V, Velazquez E, et al. Histologic classification of penile carcinoma and its relation to outcome in 61 patients with primary resection. Int J Surg Pathol 2001;9:111–20.

Danielson AG, Sand C, Weisman K. Treatment of Bowen's disease of the penis with 5% imiquimod cream. Clin Exp Dermatol 2003;28(Suppl. 1):7–9.

Di Lorenzo G, Buonerba C, Federico P, et al. Cisplatin and 5-fluorouracil in inoperable, stage IV squamous cell carcinoma of the penis. BJU Int 2012;110(11 Pt B):E661–6.

Dianzani C, Calvieri S, Pierangeli A, et al. Identification of human papilloma viruses in male dysplastic genital lesions. New Microbiol 2004;27:65–9.

Edge SB, Byrd DR, Compton CC, et al. Penis. AJCC Cancer Staging Manual. 7th ed. New York: Springer; 2010.

Eng TY, Petersen JP, Stack RS, et al. Lymph node metastasis from carcinoma in situ of the penis: a case report. J Urol 1995;153:432–4.

Ficarra V, Zattoni F, Artibani W, et al. Nomogram predictive of pathological inguinal lymph node involvement in patients with squamous cell carcinoma of the penis. J Urol 2006;175:1700–5.

Ficarra V, Zattoni F, Cunico SC, et al. Lymphatic and vascular embolizations are independent predictive variables of inguinal lymph node involvement in patients with squamous cell carcinoma of the penis. Gruppo Uro-Oncologico del Nord Est (Northeast Uro-Oncological Group) Penile Cancer data base. Cancer 2005;103:2507–16.

Frimberger D, Hungerhuber E, Zaak D, et al. Penile carcinoma: is Nd:YAG laser therapy radical enough? J Urol 2002;168:2418–21, discussion 2421.

Frisch M, Friis S, Kjaer SK, et al. Falling incidence of penis cancer in an uncircumcised population (Denmark, 1943–90). BMJ 1995;311:1471.

Giuliano AR, Lazcano E, Lina Villa L, et al. Circumcision and sexual behavior: factors independently associated with human papillomavirus detection among men in the HIM study. Int J Cancer 2009;124:1251–7.

Giuliano AR, Palefsky JM, Goldstone S, et al. Efficacy of quadrivalent HPV vaccine against HPV infection and disease in males. N Engl J Med 2011;364(5):401–11.

Graafland NM, Teertstra HJ, Besnard PE, et al. Identification of high risk pathological node positive penile carcinoma: value of preoperative computerized tomography imaging. J Urol 2011;185(3):881–7.

Graham JH, Helwig EB. Erythroplasia of Queyrat [review]. Cancer 1973;32:1396–414.

Greene FL, Compton CC, Fritz AG, et al. The penis. In: American Joint Committee on Cancer: staging atlas. New York: Springer; 2006. p. 287–92.

Gross G, Pfister H. Role of human papillomavirus in penile cancer, penile intraepithelial squamous cell neoplasias and in genital warts. Med Microbiol Immunol (Berl) 2004;193:35–44.

Grussendorf-Conen EI. Anogenital premalignant and malignant tumors (including Buschke-Löwenstein tumors). Clin Dermatol 1997;15: 377–88.

Haas GP, Blumenstein BA, Gagliano RG, et al. Cisplatin, methotrexate, and bleomycin for the treatment of carcinoma of the penis: a Southwest Oncology Group Study. J Urol 1999;161:1823–5.

Harish K, Ravi R. The role of tobacco in penile carcinoma. Br J Urol 1995;75:375–7.

Harmer MH. Penis (ICD-0187). TNM classification of malignant tumours. 3rd ed. Geneva: International Union Against Cancer; 1978. p. 126–8.

Hegarty PK, Suh J, Fisher M, et al. Penoscrotal extramammary Paget's disease: the University of Texas MD Anderson Cancer Center contemporary experience. J Urol 2011;186:97–102.

Horenblas S, Jansen L, Meinhardt W, et al. Detection of occult metastasis in squamous cell carcinoma of the penis using a dynamic sentinel node procedure. J Urol 2000;163:100–4.

Horenblas S, van Tinteren H, Delemarre JF, et al. Squamous cell carcinoma of the penis: accuracy of tumor, nodes and metastases classification system and role of lymphangiography, computerized tomography scan, and fine needle aspiration cytology. J Urol 1991;146:1279–83.

Horenblas S, van Tinteren H, Delemarre JF, et al. Squamous cell carcinoma of the penis. III. Treatment of regional lymph nodes. J Urol 1993;149: 492–7.

Hung-fu T, Morganstern H, Mack T, et al. Risk factors for penile cancer: results of a population-based case-control study in Los Angeles County. Cancer Causes Control 2001;12:267–77.

Johnson DE, Lo RK. Management of regional lymph nodes in penile carcinoma: five-year results following therapeutic groin dissections. Urology 1984;24:308–11.

Kroon BK, Horenblas S, Deurloo EE, et al. Ultrasonography-guided fine-needle aspiration cytology before sentinel node biopsy in patients with penile carcinoma. BJU Int 2005a;95:517–21.

Kroon BK, Horenblas S, Estourgie SH, et al. How to avoid false-negative dynamic sentinel node procedures in penile carcinoma. J Urol 2004;171(Pt 1):2191–4.

Kroon BK, Horenblas S, Lont AP, et al. Patients with penile carcinoma benefit from immediate resection of clinically occult lymph node metastases. J Urol 2005b;173:816–9.

Kroon BK, Lont AP, Valdes Olmos RA, et al. Morbidity of dynamic sentinel node biopsy in penile carcinoma [see comment]. J Urol 2005c;173: 813–5.

Kulkarni JN, Kamat MR. Prophylactic bilateral groin node dissection versus prophylactic radiotherapy and surveillance in patients with N0 and N1–2a carcinoma of the penis. Eur Urol 1994;26:123–8.

Leijte JA, Hughes B, Graafland NM, et al. Two-center evaluation of dynamic sentinel node biopsy for squamous cell carcinoma of the penis. J Clin Oncol 2009;27(20):3325–9.

Leijte JA, Kerst JM, Bais E, et al. Neoadjuvant chemotherapy in advanced penile carcinoma. Eur Urol 2007;52(2):448–94.

Leijte JA, Kirrander P, Antonini N, et al. Recurrence patterns of squamous cell carcinoma of the penis: recommendations for follow-up based on a two-centre analysis of 700 patients. Eur Urol 2008;54:161–9.

Lont AP, Besnard AP, Gallee MP, et al. A comparison of physical examination and imaging in determining the extent of primary penile carcinoma. BJU Int 2003;91:493–5.

Lont AP, Gallee MP, Meinhardt W, et al. Penis conserving treatment for T1 and T2 penile carcinoma: clinical implications of a local recurrence. J Urol 2006;176:575–80.

Lont AP, Kroon BK, Gallee MP, et al. Pelvic lymph node dissection for penile carcinoma: extent of inguinal lymph node involvement as an indicator for pelvic lymph node involvement and survival. J Urol 2007;177:947.

Lopes A, Hidalgo GS, Kowalski LP, et al. Prognostic factors in carcinoma of the penis: multivariate analysis of 145 patients treated with amputation and lymphadenectomy. J Urol 1996;156:1637–42.

Lucia MS, Miller GJ. Histopathology of malignant lesions of the penis. Urol Clin North Am 1992;19:227–46.

Maden C, Sherman KJ, Beckman AM, et al. History of circumcision, medical conditions, and sexual activity and risk of penile cancer. J Natl Cancer Inst 1993;85:19–24.

Master VA, Jafri SM, Moses KA, et al. Minimally invasive inguinal lymphadenectomy via endoscopic groin dissection: comprehensive assessment of immediate and long-term complications. J Urol 2012;188:1176–80.

Matin SF, Cormier JN, Ward JF, et al. Phase 1 prospective evaluation of the oncological adequacy of robotic assisted video-endoscopic inguinal lymphadenectomy in patients with penile carcinoma. BJU Int 2013; 111(7):1068–74.

McDougal WS. Carcinoma of the penis: improved survival by early regional lymphadenectomy based on the histological grade and depth of invasion of the primary lesion. J Urol 1995;154:1364–6.

Micali G, Nasca MR, Innocenzi D. Lichen sclerosus of the glans is significantly associated with penile carcinoma. Sex Transm Infect 2001;77: 226.

Minhas S, Kayes O, Hegarty P, et al. What surgical resection margins are required to achieve oncological control in men with primary penile cancer? BJU Int 2005;96:1040–3.

Misra S, Chaturvedi A, Misra NC. Penile carcinoma: a challenge for the developing world. Lancet Oncol 2004;5:240–7.

Mohs FE, Snow SN, Larson PO. Mohs micrographic surgery for penile tumors. Urol Clin North Am 1992;19:291–304.

Muneer A, Kayes O, Ahmed HU, et al. Molecular prognostic factors in penile cancer. World J Urol 2009;27:161–7.

Nelson BA, Cookson MS, Smith JA Jr, et al. Complications of inguinal and pelvic lymphadenectomy for squamous cell carcinoma of the penis: a contemporary series. J Urol 2004;172:494–7.

Nielson CM, Flores R, Harris RB, et al. Human papillomavirus prevalence and type distribution in male anogenital sites and semen. Cancer Epidemiol Biomarkers Prev 2007;16(6):1107–14.

Opjordsmoen S, Fossa SD. Quality of life in patients treated for penile cancer: a follow-up study. Br J Urol 1994;74:652–7.

Pagliaro LC, Crook J. Multimodality therapy in penile cancer: when and which treatments? World J Urol 2009;27:221–5.

Pagliaro LC, Williams DL, Daliani D, et al. Neoadjuvant paclitaxel, ifosfamide, and cisplatin chemotherapy for metastatic penile cancer: a phase II study. J Clin Oncol 2010;28(24):3851–7.

Park S, Grossfeld GD, McAninch JW, et al. Extramammary Paget's disease of the penis and scrotum: excision, reconstruction and evaluation of occult malignancy. J Urol 2001;166:2112–7.

Pettaway CA, Pagliaro LC, Theodore C, et al. Treatment of visceral, unresectable, or bulky/unresectable regional metastases of penile cancer. Urology 2010;76(2):S58–65.

Pettaway CA, Pisters LL, Dinney CP, et al. Sentinel lymph node biopsy for penile squamous carcinoma: the MD Anderson Cancer Center experience. J Urol 1995;154:1999–2003.

Philippou P, Shabbir M, Malone P, et al. Conservative surgery for squamous cell carcinoma of the penis: resection margins and long-term oncological control. J Urol 2012;188(3):803–8.

Pietrzak P, Corbishley C, Watkin N. Organ-sparing surgery for invasive penile cancer: early follow-up data. BJU Int 2004;94:1253–7.

Pietrzak P, Hadway P, Corbishley CM, et al. Is the association between balanitis xerotica obliterans and penile carcinoma under-estimated? BJU Int 2006;98(1):74–6.

Pizzocaro G, Algaba F, Horenblas S, et al. EAU penile cancer guidelines, 2009. Eur Urol 2010;57:1002–12.

Pizzocaro G, Piva L, Bandieramonte G, et al. Up-to-date management of carcinoma of the penis. Eur Urol 1997;32:5–15.

Poblet E, Alfaro L, Fernander-Segoviano P, et al. Human papillomavirus–associated penile squamous cell carcinoma in HIV positive patients. Am J Surg Pathol 1999;23:1119–26.

Pugliese JM, Morey AF, Peterson AC. Lichen sclerosus: review of the literature and current recommendations for management. J Urol 2007;178: 2268–76.

Ravi R. Correlation between the extent of nodal involvement and survival following groin dissection for carcinoma of the penis. Br J Urol 1993;72: 817–9.

Ravi R, Chaturvedi HK, Sastry DV. Role of radiation therapy in the treatment of carcinoma of the penis. Br J Urol 1994;74:646–51.

Reynolds SJ, Shepherd ME, Risbud AR, et al. Male circumcision and risk of HIV-1 and other sexually transmitted infections in India. Lancet 2004; 363(9414):1039–40.

Rippentrop JM, Joslyn SA, Konety BR. Squamous cell carcinoma of the penis: evaluation of data from the Surveillance, Epidemiology, and End Results Program. Cancer 2004;101:1357–63.

Rubin MA, Kleter B, Zhou M, et al. Detection and typing of human papillomavirus DNA in penile carcinoma. Am J Pathol 2001;159:1211–8.

Saisorn I, Lawrentschuk N, Leewansangtong S, et al. Fine-needle aspiration cytology predicts inguinal lymph node metastasis without antibiotic pretreatment in penile carcinoma. BJU Int 2006;97:1225–8.

Sanchez-Ortiz R, Huang SF, Tamboli P, et al. Melanoma of the penis, scrotum and male urethra: a 40-year single institution experience. J Urol 2005;173: 1958–65.

Scappini P, Piscioli F, Pusiol T, et al. Penile cancer: aspiration biopsy cytology for staging. Cancer 1986;58:1526–33.

Scardino E, Villa G, Bonomo G, et al. Magnetic resonance imaging combined with artificial erection for local staging of penile cancer. Urology 2004;63:1158–62.

Scher M, Seitz M, Reiser M, et al. ¹⁸F-FDG PET/CT for staging of penile cancer. J Nucl Med 2005;46:1460.

Seixas AL, Ornellas AA, Marota A, et al. Verrucous carcinoma of the penis: retrospective analysis of 32 cases. J Urol 1994;152:1476–9.

Shabbir M, Muneer A, Kalsi J, et al. Glans resurfacing for the treatment of carcinoma in situ of the penis: surgical technique and outcomes. Eur Urol 2011b;59(1):142–7.

Shapiro E. American Academy of Pediatrics policy statements on circumcision and urinary tract infection. Rev Urol 1999;1:154–6.

Shindel AW, Mann MW, Lev RY, et al. Mohs micrographic surgery for penile cancer: management and long-term follow-up. J Urol 2007;178:1980–5.

Slaton JW, Morgenstern N, Levy DA, et al. Tumor stage, vascular invasion and the percentage of poorly differentiated cancer: independent prognosticators for inguinal lymph node metastasis in penile squamous cancer. J Urol 2001;165:1138–42.

Solsona E, Algaba F, Horenblas S, et al. EAU guidelines on penile cancer. Eur Urol 2004;46:1–8.

Solsona E, Iborra I, Ricos JV, et al. Corpus cavernosum invasion and tumor grade in the prediction of lymph node condition in penile carcinoma. Eur Urol 1992;22:115–8.

Soria JC, Fizazi K, Kramar A, et al. Squamous cell carcinoma of the penis: multivariate analysis of prognostic factors and natural history in a monocentric study with a conservative policy. Ann Oncol 1997;8:1089.

Sotelo R, Sanchez-Salas R, Clavijo R. Endoscopic inguinal lymph node dissection for penile carcinoma: the development of a novel technique. World J Urol 2009;27:213–9.

Spiess PE, Izawa JI, Bassett R, et al. Pre-operative lymphoscintigraphy and dynamic sentinel node biopsy in staging penile cancer: results with pathologic correlation. J Urol 2007;177(6):2157–61.

Srinivas V, Morse MJ, Herr HW, et al. Penile cancer: relation of extent of nodal metastasis to survival. J Urol 1987;137:880–2.

Su CK, Shipley WU. Bowenoid papulosis: a benign lesion of the shaft of the penis misdiagnosed as squamous carcinoma. J Urol 1997;157:1361–2.

Svatek RS, Munsell M, Kincaid JM, et al. Association between lymph node density and disease specific survival in patients with penile cancer. J Urol 2009;182:2721.

Tabatabaei S, Harisinghani M, McDougal WS. Regional lymph node staging using lymphotropic nanoparticle enhanced magnetic resonance imaging with ferumoxtran-10 in patients with penile cancer. J Urol 2005;174:925.

Theodore C, Skoneczna I, Bodrogi I, et al. A phase II multicentre study of irinotecan (CPT 11) in combination with cisplatin (CDDP) in metastatic or locally advanced penile carcinoma (EORTC Protocol 30992). Ann Oncol 2008;19:1304.

Theodorescu D, Russo P, Zhang ZF, et al. Outcomes of initial surveillance of invasive squamous cell carcinoma of the penis and negative nodes. J Urol 1996;155:1626–31.

Tietjen DN, Malek RS. Laser therapy of squamous cell dysplasia and carcinoma of the penis. Urology 1998;52:559–65.

Tobias-Machado M, Tavares A, Ornellas AA, et al. Video endoscopic inguinal lymphadenectomy: a new minimally invasive procedure for radical management of inguinal nodes in patients with penile squamous cell carcinoma. J Urol 2007;177:953–7.

Vatanasapt V, Martin N, Sriplung MH, et al. Cancer incidence in Thailand, 1988–1991. Cancer Epidemiol Biomarkers Prev 1995;4:475–83.

Velazquez EF, Ayala G, Liu H, et al. Histologic grade and perineural invasion are more important than tumor thickness as predictor of nodal metastasis in penile squamous cell carcinoma invading 5 to 10 mm. Am J Pathol 2008;32:974–9.

Velazquez EF, Barreto JE, Rodriguez I, et al. Limitations in the interpretation of biopsies in patients with penile squamous cell carcinoma. Int J Surg Pathol 2004;12:139–46.

Velazquez EF, Cubilla A. Lichen sclerosus in 68 patients with squamous cell carcinoma of the penis: frequent atypias and correlation with special carcinoma variants suggests a precancerous role. Am J Surg Pathol 2003;27:1448–53.

Wang Z, Lu M, Dong GQ, et al. Penile and scrotal Paget's disease: 130 Chinese patients with long-term follow-up. BJU Int 2008;102:485–8.

Wiener JS, Walther PJ. The association of oncogenic human papillomaviruses with urologic malignancy. Surg Oncol Clin N Am 1995;4:257–76.

Windahl T, Skeppner E, Andersson SO, et al. Sexual function and satisfaction in men after LASER treatment for penile carcinoma. J Urol 2004;172:648–51.

Zhu Y, Ye D, Yao XD, et al. New N staging system of penile cancer provides a better reflection of prognosis. J Urol 2011;186(2):518–52.

Zhu Y, Zhang SH, Ye DW, et al. Predicting pelvic lymph node metastasis in penile cancer patients: a comparison of computed tomography, Cloquet's node, and disease burden of the inguinal lymph nodes. Onkologie 2008;31:37–41.

Zouhair A, Coucke PA, Jeanneret W, et al. Radiation therapy alone or combined surgery and radiation therapy in squamous-cell carcinoma of the penis? Eur J Cancer 2001;37:198–203.

38

Tumors of the Urethra

David S. Sharp, MD, and Kenneth W. Angermeier, MD

Benign Urethral Tumors

Male Urethral Cancer

Female Urethral Cancer

BENIGN URETHRAL TUMORS

Benign tumors of the urethra are quite rare, with only a few small series and case reports available in the literature. Leiomyoma, hemangioma, and fibroepithelial polyp are most frequently reported.

Leiomyoma

Leiomyomas of the urethra occur primarily in women, most commonly in the third and fourth decade of life. As of 1995, 36 cases had been reported in the English language literature (Leidinger and Das, 1995). Leiomyomas may be urethral or paraurethral in location, and tumor may protrude from the urethral meatus (Lee et al, 1995; Goldman et al, 2007). The most common clinical presentations include palpable anterior vaginal mass, irritative voiding symptoms, urinary tract infection, and hematuria. Obstructive urinary symptoms occur less frequently (Fry et al, 1988; Leidinger and Das, 1995). Leiomyomas also may be discovered incidentally during routine pelvic examination or an unrelated surgical procedure (Cornella et al, 1997). A percentage of these tumors have been reported to be hormonally sensitive based on changes in size during pregnancy and after delivery (Fry et al, 1988; Leidinger and Das, 1995). In many cases, diagnosis is aided by ultrasonography or magnetic resonance imaging (MRI). Paraurethral leiomyoma may be excised via a transvaginal approach, whereas intraurethral lesions are treated with transurethral resection (Cornella et al, 1997). Tumor recurrence is rare, and all reported urethral leiomyomas to date have followed a benign course (Goldman et al, 2007).

Hemangioma

Urethral hemangiomas are more common in males, and the majority of tumors initially described in the literature were located within the anterior urethra (Manuel et al, 1977). Most patients present within the second or third decade of life, although it is not uncommon for symptoms to have been present for years (Roberts and Devine, 1983). Urinary tract hemangiomas may be associated with the presence of cutaneous hemangiomas or congenital disorders such as Klippel-Trenaunay syndrome (Klein and Kaplan, 1975; Jahn and Nissen, 1991). The most common symptom of a urethral hemangioma is intermittent hematuria, which can be massive at times (Parshad et al, 2001). Bloody urethral discharge or hematospermia also may be noted. Diagnosis is made by cystoscopy, but this modality may underestimate the overall extent of the hemangioma (Manuel et al, 1977; Hayashi et al, 1997). MRI may be helpful in select cases to better delineate the extent of the lesion as with other tumors of the penis (Stewart et al, 2010). Smaller hemangiomas are generally treated with transurethral fulguration or laser; however, recurrent bleeding as a result of inadequate ablation may occur. In this setting, or when the hemangioma is more extensive, open excision with one- or two-stage urethral reconstruction may be required for cure (Roberts and Devine, 1983; Parshad et al, 2001).

Posterior urethral hemangioma has more recently been recognized as a cause of hematospermia and/or hematuria after ejaculation or erection in older men (Hayashi et al, 1997; Saito, 2008). The lesions typically occur between the verumontanum and the external urethral sphincter. The most common appearance is that of a small sessile lesion with associated varicosities, with pathology demonstrating cavernous hemangioma in most cases. Symptomatic posterior urethral hemangiomas respond well to transurethral resection and fulguration (Saito, 2008).

Fibroepithelial Polyp

Fibroepithelial polyps (FEPs) are benign tumors of mesodermal origin that can occur in the upper or lower urinary tract (Kumar et al, 2008). Urethral FEPs are rare and usually are diagnosed in males during the first decade of life (Aita et al, 2005). The most common clinical presentation in adults is restriction of the urinary stream, frequency, and dysuria (Kumar et al, 2008). Urinary retention is less common but has been reported (Salehi et al, 2009). Diagnosis is made by a combination of cystoscopy, retrograde urethrography, and voiding cystourethrography. FEPs are most commonly located in the posterior urethra in males (Tsuzuki and Epstein, 2005), but have been reported in the bulbar urethra (Kumar et al, 2008). They may arise from the urethra and protrude from the meatus in women (Yamashita et al, 2004; Aita et al, 2005). Transurethral resection is the treatment of choice and is usually curative. Pathologic examination is required to confirm the diagnosis and rule out a more aggressive lesion such as urothelial papilloma or inverted papilloma (Tsuzuki and Epstein, 2005).

MALE URETHRAL CANCER

General Considerations

Carcinoma of the male urethra is rare and usually manifests in the fifth decade of life (Dalbagni et al, 1999). A recent analysis of the National Cancer Institute Surveillance, Epidemiology, and End Results (SEER) database identified 2065 men diagnosed with primary urethral cancer in the United States between 1988 and 2006. Approximately 88% of the patients were white, and 8% African-American (Rabbani, 2011). **Etiologic factors include chronic inflammation resulting from a history of frequent sexually transmitted diseases, urethritis, and urethral stricture, and there is likely to be a causal role for human papillomavirus 16 in squamous cell carcinoma of the urethra** (Weiner et al, 1992; Cupp et al, 1996). The onset of malignant change in a patient with chronic urethral stricture disease may be insidious, and a high index of clinical suspicion is required to diagnose these tumors expediently. More than 50% of patients have a history of urethral stricture disease, almost 25% have a history of sexually transmitted disease, and 96% are symptomatic at presentation (Dalbagni et al, 1999). The most common manifesting symptoms are urethral bleeding, a palpable urethral mass, and obstructive voiding symptoms.

Pathology

Tumors of the male urethra are categorized according to location and histologic features of the cells lining the urethra (Mostofi et al, 1992) (Fig. 38-1). The bulbomembranous urethra is involved most frequently, accounting for 60% of tumors, followed by the penile urethra (30%) and prostatic urethra (10%). Although traditionally it has been held that the majority of primary urethral cancers were squamous cell carcinomas, the SEER study by Rabbani revealed transitional cell carcinoma in 77.6%, squamous cell carcinoma in 11.9%, adenocarcinoma in 5%, and other histologies in 5.5% (Rabbani, 2011). The histologic subtype of urethral cancer varies by anatomic location. Carcinomas of the prostatic urethra are of transitional cell origin in 90% and of squamous cell origin in 10%; carcinomas of the penile urethra are of squamous cell origin in 90% and of transitional cell origin in 10%; and carcinomas of the bulbomembranous urethra are of squamous cell origin in 80%, transitional cell origin in 10%, and adenocarcinoma or undifferentiated in 10% (Grigsby and Herr, 2000).

Urethral carcinoma in males can spread by direct extension to adjacent structures, usually involving the vascular spaces of the corpus spongiosum and the periurethral tissues, or it can metastasize through lymphatic embolization to regional lymph nodes. The lymphatics from the anterior urethra drain into the superficial and deep inguinal lymph nodes and occasionally into the external iliac lymph nodes. Tumors of the posterior urethra most commonly spread to the pelvic lymph nodes. Palpable inguinal lymph nodes occur in approximately 20% of cases and almost always represent metastatic disease, in contrast to penile cancer, in which a large percentage of palpable nodes may be inflammatory. Hematogenous dissemination is uncommon except in advanced disease.

Evaluation and Staging

The tumor, node, metastasis (TNM) staging classification is based on depth of invasion of the primary tumor and presence or absence of regional lymph node involvement and distant metastasis (Table 38-1). Examination under anesthesia, consisting of cystoscopy and bimanual palpation of the external genitalia, urethra, rectum, and perineum, aids in evaluating the extent of local involvement by tumor. Transurethral or needle biopsy of the lesion is also performed. Cytologic studies of voided urine do not seem to be a reliable method for diagnosis of primary urethral carcinoma. In one study, sensitivity was greatest in men with transitional cell carcinoma (80%) and in those with tumors involving the pendulous urethra (73%) (Touijer and Dalbagni, 2004). If rectal involvement is suspected on bimanual examination or by the patient's symptoms, an evaluation of the lower colon by barium enema study and flexible sigmoidoscopy is recommended to assist with surgical planning. Local soft tissue involvement, lymph node involvement, bone extension, and the presence of distant metastatic disease are best evaluated by a computed tomography (CT) scan of the chest, abdomen, and pelvis or in some cases by MRI. MRI may be particularly helpful for detecting invasion of the corpora cavernosa and is the most sensitive staging modality for the assessment of local tumor extent (Fig. 38-2) (Vapnek et al, 1992; Stewart et al, 2010).

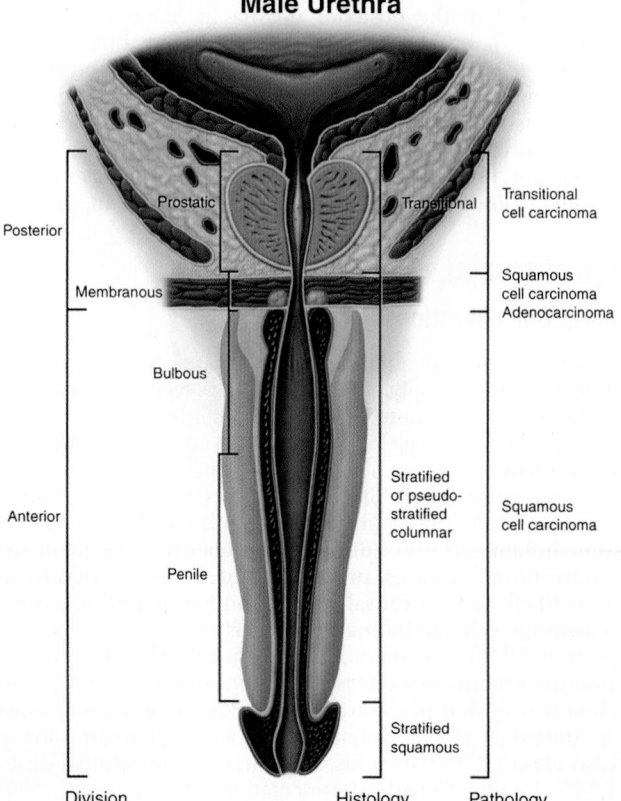

Figure 38-1. Anatomic regions of the male urethra and corresponding histology and histopathology.

TABLE 38-1 Urethral Cancer Tumor, Node, Metastasis Staging System

PRIMARY TUMOR (T) (MALE AND FEMALE)	
TX	Primary tumor cannot be assessed
T0	No evidence of primary tumor
Ta	Noninvasive papillary, polypoid, or verrucous carcinoma
Tis	Carcinoma in situ
T1	Tumor invades subepithelial connective tissue
T2	Tumor invades any of the following: corpus spongiosum, prostate, periurethral muscle
T3	Tumor invades any of the following: corpus cavernosum, beyond prostatic capsule, anterior vagina, bladder neck
T4	Tumor invades other adjacent organs
TRANSITIONAL CELL CARCINOMA OF THE PROSTATE	
Tis-pd	Carcinoma in situ, involvement of the prostatic ducts
T1	Tumor invades subepithelial connective tissue
T2	Tumor invades any of the following: prostatic stroma, corpus spongiosum, periurethral muscle
T3	Tumor invades any of the following: corpus cavernosum, beyond prostatic capsule, bladder neck (extraprostatic extension)
T4	Tumor invades other adjacent organs (invasion of the bladder)
REGIONAL LYMPH NODES (N)	
NX	Regional lymph nodes cannot be assessed
N0	No regional lymph node metastasis
N1	Metastasis in a single lymph node, 2 cm or less in greatest dimension
N2	Metastasis in a single lymph node, more than 2 cm but less than 5 cm in greatest dimension; or in multiple nodes, none greater than 5 cm
N3	Metastasis in a lymph node greater than 5 cm in greatest dimension
DISTANT METASTASIS (M)	
MX	Presence of distant metastasis cannot be assessed
M0	No distant metastasis
M1	Distant metastasis

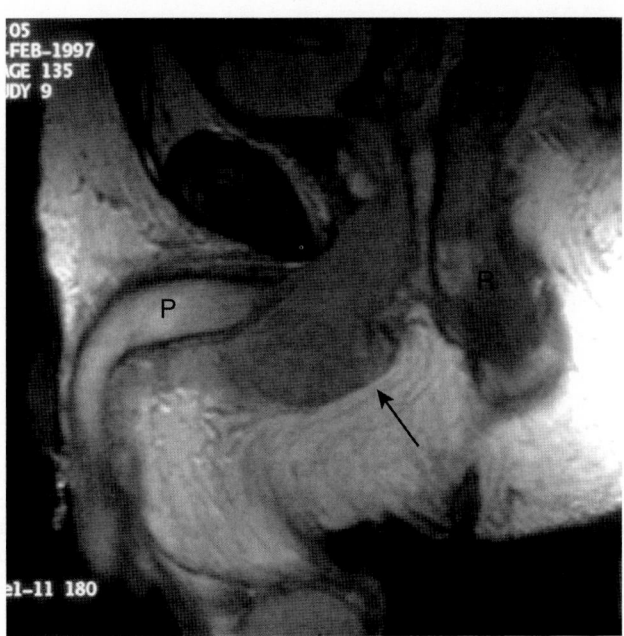

Figure 38-2. **Magnetic resonance image demonstrating large bulbo-membranous urethral cancer** *(arrow).* **P, penis; R, rectum.**

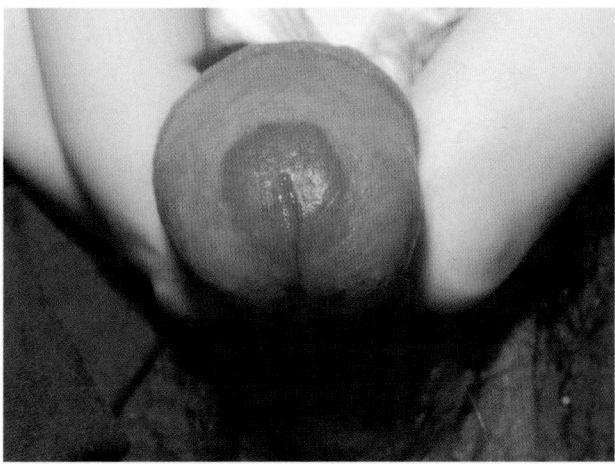

Figure 38-3. **Squamous cell carcinoma in situ (erythroplasia of Queyrat) of the glans penis surrounding the urethral meatus. The patient also had significant extension of disease into the distal urethra.**

Treatment

As in penile carcinoma, the primary form of treatment for men with urethral carcinoma is surgical excision. **In general, anterior urethral carcinoma is more amenable to surgical control, and the prognosis is better than that of posterior urethral carcinoma, which is often associated with extensive local invasion and distant metastasis** (Zeidman et al, 1992). A large series reported overall survival rates of 83% for low-stage tumors, 36% for high-stage tumors, 69% for anterior tumors, and 26% for those in the posterior urethra (Dalbagni et al, 1999). Similarly, a more recent study of 29 patients, 26 of whom underwent initial surgical excision, demonstrated 5-year overall survival rates of 67% for low-stage disease, 33% for high stage, 72% for anterior tumors, and 36% for posterior tumors. The majority of patients received some form of adjuvant radiation therapy or chemotherapy (Thyavihally et al, 2006).

Carcinoma of the Penile Urethra

Transurethral resection, local excision, or distal urethrectomy and perineal urethrostomy may be acceptable treatment in selected patients with superficial, papillary, or low-grade tumors. Long-term disease-free survival has been reported in this setting (Mandler and Pool, 1966; Konnak, 1980; Gheiler et al, 1998; Hakenberg et al, 2001; Karnes et al, 2010). Squamous cell carcinoma in situ of the perimeatal glans may extend into the distal urethra (Fig. 38-3) and has been successfully treated with partial glansectomy and distal urethrectomy with simultaneous urethral reconstruction (Nash et al, 1996) or penile urethrostomy (Fig. 38-4). In 2007, Smith and colleagues (2007) published results following penile-preserving surgery in 18 patients with squamous cell carcinoma of the penile urethra, 11 of whom had T2 and T3 disease. All underwent surgical excision with reconstruction and penile preservation, with no local recurrences. The authors therefore concluded that this was a feasible approach, and overall survival was not affected by the surgical procedure.

Partial penectomy with a 2-cm negative margin remains the traditional treatment for tumors infiltrating the corpus spongiosum and localized to the distal half of the penis. Excellent local control after this procedure has been documented (Kaplan et al, 1967; Ray et al, 1977; Anderson and McAninch, 1984; Hopkins et al, 1984; Dinney et al, 1994; Gheiler et al, 1998). If invasive

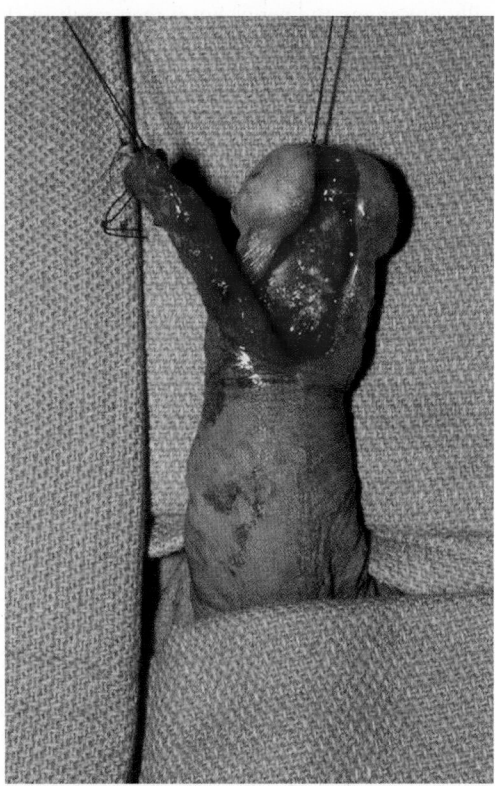

Figure 38-4. **Partial glansectomy and distal urethrectomy (same patient as in Figure 38-3). After negative margins were ensured, penile urethrostomy completed the procedure.**

disease extends to or involves the proximal penile urethra, total penectomy is required to obtain an adequate margin of excision (Fig. 38-5). A local recurrence rate of 13% has been reported after this procedure (Kaplan et al, 1967). It is important to emphasize that accurate staging is critical to avoid underestimation of the proximal extent of the tumor. Review of previous data would suggest that radical penectomy is an insufficient operation for bulbous urethral tumors (Zeidman et al, 1992).

Although some instances of tumor control by irradiation have been reported, in general, primary radiation therapy has been reserved for patients with early-stage lesions of the anterior urethra

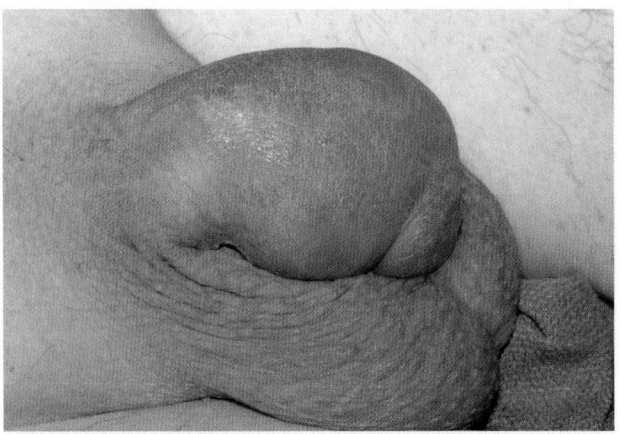

Figure 38-5. Large penile mass in a patient with transitional cell carcinoma of the penile urethra.

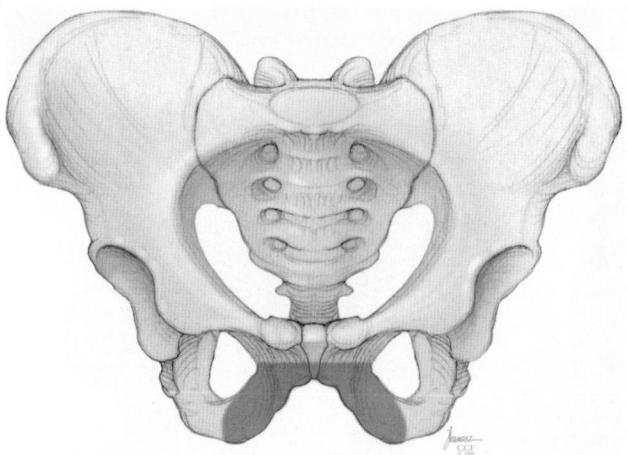

Figure 38-6. Shaded area outlines the portions of the ischiopubic rami excised at the time of inferior pubectomy during radical excision of bulbomembranous urethral cancer. (Reprinted with permission, Cleveland Clinic Center for Medical Art & Photography © 2003-2010. All Rights Reserved.)

who refuse surgery. A commonly used technique consists of parallel opposed fields with the penis suspended vertically by a urethral catheter (Heysek et al, 1985). Radiation therapy has the advantage of potentially preserving the penis, but it may result in skin ulceration or necrosis, urethral stricture, or chronic edema. The long-term results of radiotherapy are difficult to evaluate because few reports are available of male patients treated with this modality (Raghavaiah, 1978; Forman and Lichter, 1992; Koontz and Lee, 2010).

Chemoradiation has been reported as a treatment modality for patients with invasive anterior urethral cancer with the intent of genital preservation (Cohen et al, 2008). The study group included nine patients with disease in the penile urethra who received a defined protocol of mitomycin-C (MMC) and 5-fluorouracil (5-FU) along with concurrent external beam radiation therapy. Five patients demonstrated a durable complete response and required no further therapy except for treatment of urethral stricture. One patient underwent subsequent salvage surgery for local recurrence and remained with no evidence of disease at last follow-up examination. Although the number of patients is limited, this may represent a reasonable consideration for effective tumor treatment with the potential for genital preservation; further study is needed. The outcome of the entire patient cohort is discussed further in the following section.

As opposed to patients with penile cancer, survival benefit from prophylactic inguinal lymph node dissection in patients without palpable inguinal nodes has not been demonstrated with urethral cancer. However, cases of cure with limited nodal disease have been reported and therefore inguinal lymphadenectomy should be considered in the presence of palpable inguinal lymph nodes. This also serves to prevent local problems such as skin breakdown, wound drainage, and vascular erosion.

Carcinoma of the Bulbomembranous Urethra

Early lesions of the bulbomembranous urethra have been treated successfully by transurethral resection or by segmental excision of the involved urethral segment with an end-to-end anastomosis. Unfortunately, cases appropriate for limited resection are rare. **Poor survival figures have been recorded for all forms of treatment, but radical excision continues to be an important component of treatment in some patients.** Radical cystoprostatectomy, pelvic lymphadenectomy, and total penectomy often are required. Extending the operation to include in-continuity resection of the pubic rami and the adjacent urogenital diaphragm may improve the margin of resection and local control (Mackenzie and Whitmore, 1968; Shuttleworth and Lloyd-Davies, 1969; Bracken, 1982; Klein et al, 1983; Dinney et al, 1994). Limited cases of urethrectomy alone with perineal urethrostomy for infiltrating tumors confined to the corpus spongiosum have been reported (Hakenberg et al,

2001). Total urethrectomy with bladder preservation, bladder neck closure, and creation of a continent catheterizable stoma may be an alternative in select cases (Grivas et al, 2012). The benefit of these more conservative approaches needs to be weighed against the probability of local relapse or dissemination of disease.

Radical extirpation is performed with the patient in the low lithotomy position to allow perineal access. Standard abdominal mobilization of the bladder is completed, except for preservation of the endopelvic fascia and the anterior pubic attachments. A modified λ or inverted U-shaped perineal incision is performed, based just medial to the ischial tuberosities, with the apex in the mid-perineum. The ischiorectal fossae are developed as in perineal prostatectomy, and a tunnel is bluntly dissected just anterior to the rectum, extending from one fossa to the other. The inferior skin flap is mobilized by sharply dividing the intervening subcutaneous tissue and rectourethral muscle. The superior flap is mobilized by sharply incising the subcutaneous tissue to the superficial Colles fascia and then continuing bilaterally to the adductor musculature at the inferior pubic rami. Circumferential incision of the skin and dartos fascia at the penoscrotal junction is performed, and the corporeal bodies are mobilized for a short distance proximally from the superior aspect of the symphysis pubis to allow subsequent inferior pubectomy. Care must be taken not to carry this dissection too far proximally to avoid breaching the anterior aspect of a locally advanced tumor. The penis is passed downward through the perineal incision. Wider exposure may be gained by dividing the scrotum in the midline if necessary. The scrotum usually can be preserved; however, bulky tumors may necessitate sacrifice of portions of the scrotum or perineal skin. In this setting, the testicles may be preserved in thigh pouches.

To complete the pubic arch resection, the adductor musculature is sharply divided bilaterally from the length of the inferior pubic ramus along the medial margin of the obturator foramen. A Gigli saw is passed along the inferior ramus just posterior to the origins of the transverse perineal musculature. An inferiorly beveled transection is made bilaterally to simplify perineal delivery of the specimen. Alternatively, an osteotome may be used for this purpose. The entire symphysis may be resected for bulky urethral lesions involving the presymphyseal tissues. This is accomplished by division of the superior rami at their junction with the symphysis. For most lesions, however, the bulk of the symphysis can be preserved with resection of the subsymphyseal arch. This procedure is preferred, when possible, to preserve stability of the pelvic girdle, and it results in a much smaller pelvic floor defect. A Gigli saw passed through the obturator foramina, or an osteotome is used to incise the symphysis transversely, joining the foramina (Fig. 38-6). The specimen

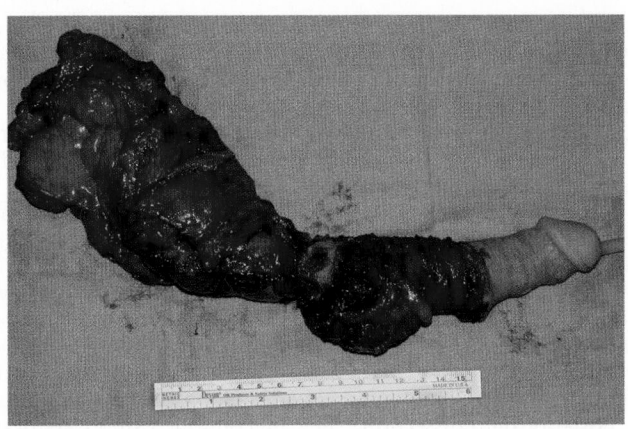

Figure 38-7. Surgical specimen after radical cystoprostatectomy, urethrectomy, penectomy, and inferior pubectomy for a large bulbomembranous squamous cell carcinoma.

is delivered en bloc (Fig. 38-7). After hemostasis is secure, the omentum is mobilized to cover the bowel. Large pelvic floor defects, such as occurring after total pubectomy, may be managed with a rectus abdominis muscle flap placed as a pelvic sling. Myocutaneous flaps can be fashioned to close large full-thickness perineal defects (Larson and Bracken, 1982).

Because of the relatively poor outcomes after surgery alone for advanced tumors of the posterior urethra, interest in multimodal therapy in this setting is increasing. Previous studies have evaluated the role of neoadjuvant chemotherapy in patients with advanced stage or metastatic disease. A regimen including methotrexate, vinblastine, doxorubicin, and cisplatin (M-VAC) has been noted to have activity against transitional cell carcinoma but was ineffective against other tumor histologic types (Scher et al, 1988). Dinney and colleagues (1994) reported long-term survival in four of eight patients who presented with metastatic urethral carcinoma and were treated with cisplatin-based chemotherapy and surgical excision. On the basis of this experience, their favored regimen consisted of cisplatin, bleomycin, and methotrexate for squamous cell carcinoma and M-VAC for transitional cell carcinoma.

In 2012 the group from MD Anderson conducted a retrospective study of 44 patients with urethral carcinoma to evaluate the role of cisplatin-based chemotherapy (Dayyani et al, 2013). The study included 28 females and 16 males, and all patients but one had T3 or T4 disease. Forty-three percent had N1 and 16% M1 disease. Histologic subtypes were mixed, with the majority being squamous cell carcinoma, adenocarcinoma, and urothelial carcinoma. Thirty-six patients received one of four platinum-based chemotherapy regimens. Five were complete responders (14%), and 72% of patients achieved a complete response or a partial response. The presented results were not stratified as to gender or histology. Surgical consolidation was then performed in 21 patients, and their mean overall survival was 25.6 months. Of the 9 patients, 4 (44%) with lymph node–positive disease at diagnosis were alive, with a minimum follow-up of more than 3 years. Based on this experience, the authors concluded that it is reasonable to consider neoadjuvant chemotherapy for T3b and T4 tumors, as well as high-risk T2 and T3a lesions.

The combination of chemotherapy and radiation therapy has shown some success in a small number of patients with localized and metastatic urethral cancer (Licht et al, 1995; Oberfield et al, 1996). More commonly, these forms of treatment are combined with surgery in a multimodal approach in patients with advanced stage or metastatic disease (Johnson et al, 1989; Gheiler et al, 1998; Grigsby and Herr, 2000). A more recent study reported 18 patients with invasive urethral carcinoma who were treated initially with chemoradiation consisting of MMC and 5-FU and concurrent external beam radiation therapy to the genitalia, perineum, and inguinal and iliac lymph nodes (Cohen et al, 2008). The number of anterior

and posterior cancers was equal, and 33% were N1 or N2. Fifteen patients demonstrated a complete response. Three nonresponders underwent salvage surgery and eventually died of their disease. Of the 15 patients who experienced complete response, 10 remained with no evidence of disease at last follow-up. In the other 5 patients, local recurrence only developed in 4, who underwent salvage surgery, and 2 remained with no evidence of disease. Mean 5-year disease-free survival after chemoradiation and salvage surgery was 72%. It is interesting to note that the previously identified risk factors of tumor grade, T stage, and presence of nodal metastasis were not predictive in this series (Rabbani, 2011). Although instrumentation or surgery for urethral stricture was required in all complete response patients without local disease recurrence, 11 of 18 overall were spared radical surgery after treatment. Although this report is one of the few with a consistent patient population and treatment regimen, further study of this approach is needed to confirm the findings of this single-institution series.

Management of the Urethra after Cystectomy

General Considerations

Contemporary series have demonstrated the incidence of urethral cancer recurrence that follows cystoprostatectomy to range from 2.1% to 11.1% after cutaneous diversion (Freeman et al, 1996; Hassan et al, 2004; Nieder et al, 2004) and 0.5% to 4% after construction of an orthotopic neobladder (Freeman et al, 1996; Hassan et al, 2004; Nieder et al, 2004; Varol et al, 2004). Early studies indicated that transitional cell carcinoma involving the prostatic urethra, particularly with stromal invasion, significantly increased the probability of postoperative urethral recurrence (Hardeman and Soloway, 1990; Freeman et al, 1996). A large number of patients undergoing radical cystectomy with urinary diversion was more recently analyzed, and demonstrated urethral tumor recurrence in 5% and 7% after 5 and 10 years, respectively (Stein et al, 2005). Involvement of the prostate with tumor (either superficial or invasive) and the form of urinary diversion were independent risk factors. Estimated 10-year incidence of urethral recurrence ranged from 4% in patients with no prostatic involvement and orthotopic diversion (lowest risk group) to 24% in those with invasive prostate disease and cutaneous diversion (highest risk group). **The low incidence of urethral recurrence after orthotopic bladder replacement has led most surgeons to feel comfortable proceeding with this form of diversion, as long as the findings on frozen-section biopsy of the distal prostatic urethral margin are normal at the time of cystoprostatectomy** (Freeman et al, 1996; Hassan et al, 2004; Nieder et al, 2004; Stein et al, 2005). Preoperative transurethral biopsy of the prostate to assess suitability for continent diversion does not correlate with final urethral margin when the preoperative biopsy is positive and has largely been abandoned in favor of intraoperative frozen section (Kassouf et al, 2008).

Approximately 40% of urethral recurrences are diagnosed within 1 year after cystoprostatectomy, with a median time to diagnosis of 18 months (Clark et al, 2004). However, cases of late urethral recurrence have been reported, indicating the need for prolonged surveillance in these patients (Schellhammer and Whitmore, 1976; Freeman et al, 1996). Urethral wash cytology has traditionally been recommended for urethral monitoring after cutaneous diversion and leads to earlier diagnosis of urethral recurrence than when evaluation is delayed until symptoms occur. However, the presumed survival benefit afforded by surveillance with urethral wash cytology over symptomatic presentation has been called into question (Lin et al, 2003). Voided urine cytology is part of standard surveillance in patients who have undergone orthotopic diversion. Patients with positive results for urine or urethral wash cytology or symptoms of urethral bleeding, discharge, or palpable mass are evaluated with cystoscopy and biopsy. Pelvic CT or MRI may be necessary to aid in assessment of the local extent of larger invasive tumors and to assess for metastatic disease. Patients who develop urethral carcinoma in situ after orthotopic diversion may respond to urethral perfusion with bacillus Calmette-Guérin, but this treatment is ineffective for those with papillary or invasive disease (Varol et al, 2004).

Total Urethrectomy after Cutaneous Diversion

The high or exaggerated lithotomy position provides optimal exposure for total urethrectomy, with the hips and knees gently flexed and the lower limbs abducted in boot-type stirrups. A modified λ or midline perineal incision (Fig. 38-8) is made, and the subcutaneous tissue and bulbospongiosus muscle are then divided in the midline and retracted to expose the corpus spongiosum. The corpus spongiosum is mobilized circumferentially near the level of the mid-bulbous urethra, and traction is applied to facilitate sharp dissection of the urethra distally, thus separating the corpus spongiosum from the adjacent corpora cavernosa. As dissection proceeds distally, the penis becomes inverted, the corpora cavernosa become bowed, and the glans recedes into the phallus. The penis is essentially turned inside out onto the perineum, and the dissection is completed to the base of the glans. To excise the meatus and glandular urethra, the penis is replaced in its anatomic position, and an

incision is made around the meatus and extended on each side down the ventral aspect of the glans. The distal urethra is then freed from its investments within the glans, and the isolated pendulous urethra is delivered onto the perineum. The deep spongiosum of the glans penis is reapproximated with 4-0 polydioxanone sutures in a horizontal mattress fashion; the surface layer is closed with interrupted 4-0 chromic sutures.

Proximal sharp dissection of the urethral bulb is carried out posteriorly and laterally, staying close to the bulb but avoiding entry, if possible, because bothersome bleeding will result. The urethra is detached from the corporeal bodies anteriorly to the level of the departure of the urethra from the bulb, leaving the specimen attached only by the membranous urethra itself. The bulbar arteries are usually identified at the 4-o'clock and 8-o'clock positions just inferior to the perineal membrane after they are transected during the posterior bulb dissection. They are controlled with electrocautery or suture ligature, or they can be ligated if they are identified before transection. **Care must be exercised in completing the proximal dissection, in view of the possible postcystectomy adherence of intestine to the superior surface of the urogenital**

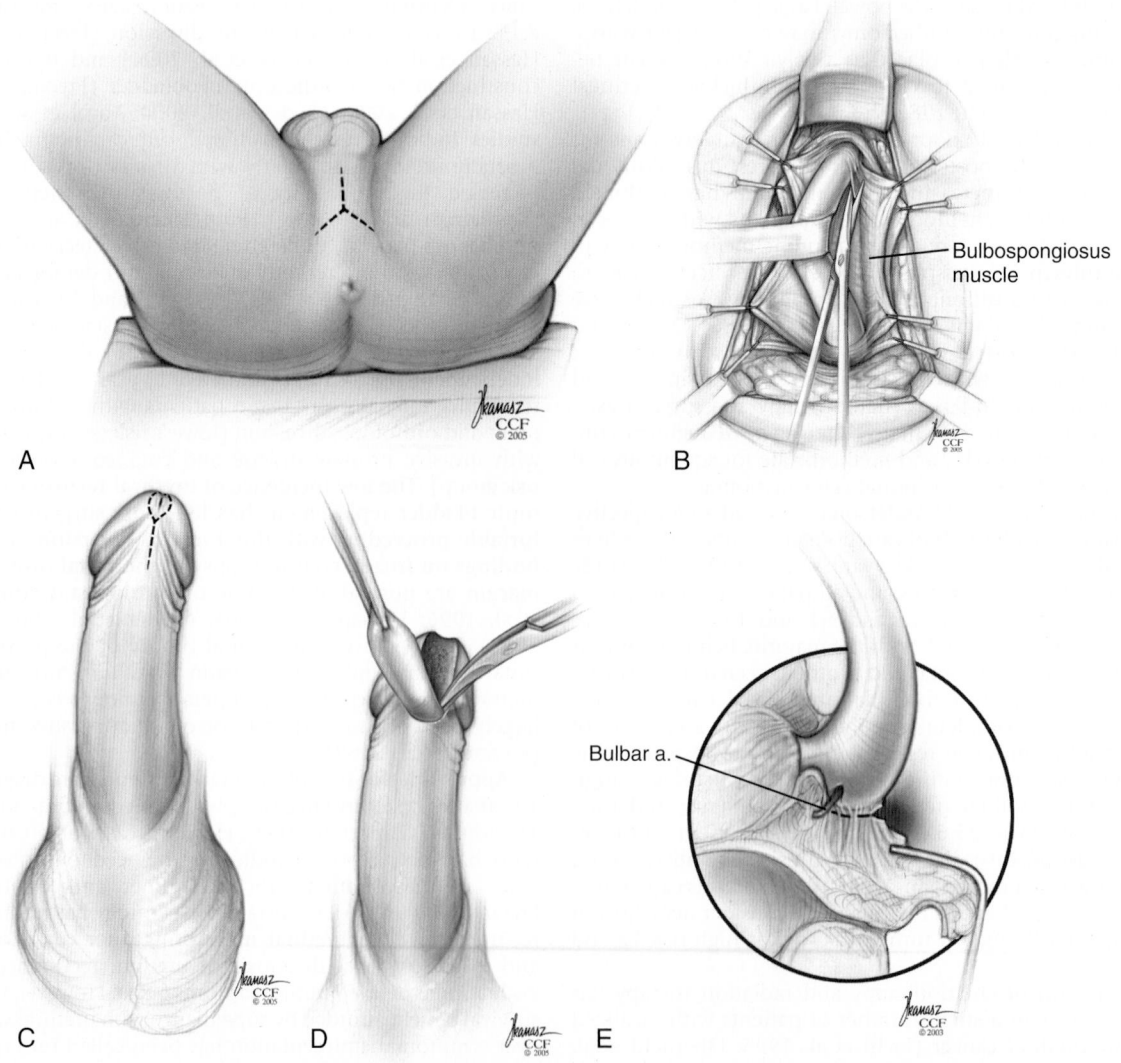

Figure 38-8. Secondary urethrectomy after previous cystoprostatectomy. A, Perineal incision. B, Division of bulbospongiosus muscle to expose the bulb of the corpus spongiosum and initial dissection of the urethra off of the corporeal bodies. C, Distal incision circumscribing the urethral meatus. D, Distal urethral dissection, which then connects to the proximal dissection at the level of the distal shaft. E, Sagittal view demonstrating posterior bulb dissection and location of the bulbar artery. (Reprinted with permission, Cleveland Clinic Center for Medical Art & Photography © 2003-2010. All Rights Reserved.)

diaphragm. This should be done under direct vision, and exposure can be aided by separating the crura of the corporeal bodies in the midline to open the intracrural space. All that remains of the membranous urethra proximally is an ill-defined fibrotic band, and it should be completely excised. Frozen-section analysis of this region adds some assurance that a negative proximal margin has been attained. A small suction drain is placed in the urethral bed and brought out through the perineum. Closure of the bulbospongiosus muscle, subcutaneous tissue, and skin with interrupted absorbable sutures completes the procedure, and a light pressure dressing is applied. Superficial hematoma, edema along the penile shaft, and infection are uncommon complications.

Total Urethrectomy after Orthotopic Diversion

Total urethrectomy after orthotopic urinary diversion is performed through an abdominoperineal approach. The patient is placed in lithotomy position with boot-type stirrups that can be adjusted during the procedure. Urethrectomy is carried out to the level of the membranous urethra. Abdominal exploration with lysis of adhesions and mobilization of the orthotopic neobladder is done to the level of the urethral anastomosis. Working with careful palpation from above and below, the area of the membranous urethra and the anastomosis are dissected free in their entirety. A circular area of the pouch adjacent to the anastomosis is excised to ensure an adequate surgical margin, and the specimen is delivered through the perineum. Bleeding from the musculature within the tunnel developed during excision of the membranous urethra can be bothersome and is best controlled with suture ligatures.

In most situations, urinary diversion is accomplished with an ileal conduit. **This often can be carried out with use of bowel from the orthotopic neobladder, which may be reconfigured when necessary, with care taken to incise the bowel along visible lines of previous closure with preservation of the mesenteric blood supply.** The remaining portions of the pouch are excised. If the existing diversion has an afferent limb (e.g., Studer pouch), this segment can be used to construct the conduit without the need for manipulation of the ureters (Bissada et al, 2004). Conversion to a continent cutaneous diversion also may be possible in selected patients, depending on intra-abdominal anatomy and the motivation of the patient (Bartoletti et al, 1999; Taylor et al, 2009).

KEY POINTS: MALE URETHRAL CANCER

- In general, anterior urethral carcinoma is more amenable to surgical control, and the prognosis is better than that of posterior urethral carcinoma, which is often associated with extensive local invasion and distant metastasis.
- As opposed to penile carcinoma, benefit from prophylactic inguinal lymph node dissection has not been demonstrated in urethral cancer.
- Because of the relatively poor outcomes after surgery alone for advanced tumors of the posterior urethra, multimodal therapy should be considered
- The low incidence of urethral recurrence after orthotopic bladder replacement has led most authors to feel comfortable proceeding with this form of diversion, as long as the findings on frozen-section biopsy of the distal prostatic urethral margin are normal at the time of cystoprostatectomy.
- In converting a patient to cutaneous conduit urinary diversion, bowel from the existing orthotopic neobladder often can be reconfigured with its blood supply intact and used for this purpose.

FEMALE URETHRAL CANCER

Epidemiology, Etiology, and Clinical Presentation

A primary malignant neoplasm arising from the female urethra is rare. The literature has reported that despite the female urethra being much shorter than its male counterpart, primary cancers of the urethra were more common in women than men (Narayan and Konety, 1992). However, more recent study has called this into question. Swartz and colleagues (2006) studied the incidence of primary urethral carcinoma in the United States and found that based on data from the SEER database, between 1973 and 2002, 1615 cases were identified, including 1075 men and 540 women. The ratio of female-to-male predominance had previously been reported as 4:1 (Narayan and Konety, 1992), but based on SEER data there is a 2:1 male-to-female predominance.

Female urethral carcinoma accounts for approximately 0.02% of female cancers (Fagan and Hertig, 1955) and less than 1% of cancers in the female genitourinary tract (Srinivas and Khan, 1987). More than 1200 cases are reported in the literature, most diagnosed in the fifth and sixth decades of life (Srinivas and Khan, 1987). Previously it was noted that approximately 85% of urethral carcinoma cases occur in white women (Terry et al, 1997); however, Swartz and colleagues (2006) reported a greater incidence of primary urethral cancers in African-American women than in white women. They found an overall annual incidence of 1.5 cases per million women, including 4.3 cases per million African-American women and 1.3 per million white women. In the Netherlands, overall crude annual incidence was 0.7 per million women, with peak incidence in the 80- to 84-year-old age group (Derksen et al, 2013).

Incidence appears to increase with age regardless of histologic subtype. The suggestion has been made that the disease is becoming even rarer, because the incidence appears to be decreasing over the time of the SEER study. Although it is likely that misclassification of the site of origin of tumors within the SEER database has led to some inaccuracy in the findings as reported by Swartz, other previous reports are likely biased by the tertiary referral center populations from which these reports originate.

Although the cause of urethral carcinoma in women has not been identified, several factors have been implicated. **Etiologic factors associated with the development of urethral carcinoma include leukoplakia, chronic irritation, caruncles, polyps, parturition, and human papillomavirus infection or other viral infections** (Mevorach et al, 1990; Grigsby and Herr, 2000). Female urethral diverticula also may predispose the patient to malignant change, with perhaps 5% of female urethral carcinomas arising within a diverticulum (Rajan et al, 1993). In a series of 90 women undergoing diverticulectomy, 5 (6%) were found to have invasive adenocarcinoma. Additionally, there was evidence of intestinal metaplasia and dysplasia in some patients (Thomas et al, 2008). Based on immunohistochemical analysis, adenocarcinomas appear to originate from different tissue origins, including (1) Skene glands as a prostatic homologue with resultant prostate-specific antigen positivity in some cases, (2) glandular metaplasia leading to columnar/mucinous adenocarcinoma, and (3) other sources leading to clear cell adenocarcinoma (Dodson et al, 1994; Murphy et al, 1999; Pongtippan et al, 2004; Reis et al, 2011; Papes and Altarac, 2013).

Anatomy and Pathology

Knowledge of urethral anatomy is essential for surgical excision and reconstruction. The female urethra has been divided into an anterior segment (distal third) and a posterior segment (proximal two thirds). **The distal third may be excised while urinary continence is maintained.** The proximal third of the urethra is lined by typical transitional urothelium and the distal two thirds by stratified squamous epithelium (Fig. 38-9). Along its length are submucosal glands composed of columnar epithelium. Lymphatic drainage differs along the course of the female urethra, as in men. Although crossover and communications are possible, lymphatics from the posterior urethra drain to the external and internal iliac and obturator lymph node chains. The anterior urethra and labia drain to the superficial and then to the deep inguinal lymph nodes (Carroll and Dixon, 1992).

The histology of the malignant neoplasm depends primarily on the site of origin within the urethra (see Fig. 38-9). Because of low numbers and varying patient populations, the most predominant

Female Urethra

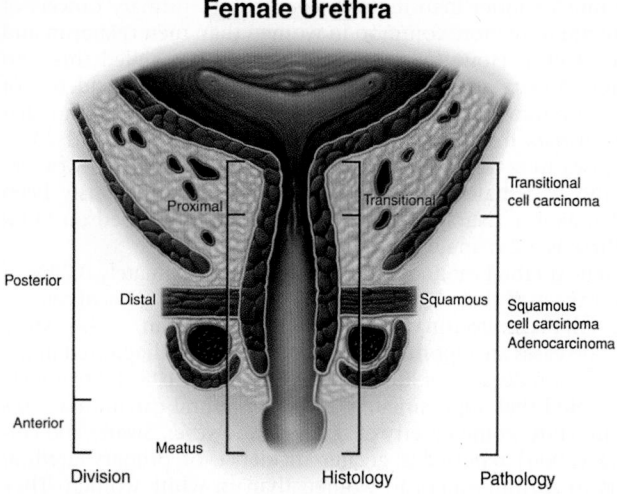

Figure 38-9. Anatomic regions of the female urethra and corresponding histology and histopathology.

cell type varies in different reported series. It is commonly believed that squamous cell carcinoma appears to be the most common histologic type, accounting for 30% to 70% of all cases. Urothelial carcinoma and adenocarcinomas are thought to be the next most common cell types (10% to 25% each). Swartz's review of SEER data found a small majority of cases were urothelial carcinomas and that among women, urothelial carcinoma, squamous cell carcinoma, and adenocarcinoma were noted in 30%, 28%, and 29% of cases, respectfully.

A study from Netherlands National Cancer Registry corroborated the SEER data and revealed that even in women, urothelial carcinoma remains the predominant cell type (Derksen et al, 2013). This study of 91 females with primary urethral carcinoma revealed urothelial carcinoma in 45%, squamous cell carcinoma in 19%, and adenocarcinoma in 29% of cases.

Other rarer cell types include lymphoma, neuroendocrine carcinoma, sarcomas, paragangliomas, melanoma, and metastasis (Johnson and O'Connell, 1983; Grabstald et al, 1966; Foens et al, 1991; Forman and Lichter, 1992; Grigsby and Herr, 2000; Swartz et al, 2006). Within urethral diverticula, an increased incidence of adenocarcinomas seems to exist, substantiating the theory that urethral diverticula in some women may arise from a glandular origin, such as the Skene glands (Spencer et al, 1990; Rajan et al, 1993; Gheiler et al, 1998; Thomas et al, 2008; Reis et al, 2011).

Diagnosis and Staging

The evaluation of women with suspected urethral carcinoma includes a thorough pelvic examination, evaluating for a palpable anterior vaginal mass for which the differential should include urethral diverticulum, urethral cancer, urethral polyp, or other benign neoplasm, such as a leiomyoma. Speculum examination should visualize the urethral meatus directly and evaluate for potential involvement of the vaginal wall and vulva. Diagnostic studies include cystourethroscopy and examination under anesthesia. MRI has been used to evaluate pelvic lesions because soft tissue contrast is superior to that with CT and it gives the best anatomic detail in this area. Additionally, MRI can assess local extension and lymph node involvement. Additional staging studies with chest radiograph or chest CT are appropriate. Bone scan may be performed if clinical suspicion exists of bony involvement as a result of bony symptoms or laboratory abnormalities such as elevated alkaline phosphatase or serum calcium. CT with positron emission tomography (CT/PET) may be useful in patients with metastatic disease although its utility is not accurately defined in urethral carcinoma. Serum prostate-specific antigen has been found to be elevated in a small number of case reports of females with adenocarcinoma, and it appears only

a minority of female patients with primary adenocarcinoma of the urethra have this elevated tumor marker (Dodson et al, 1994; Pongtippan et al, 2004). TNM staging for female urethral cancer is identical to that for male urethral cancer (see Table 38-1). Clinically palpable inguinal nodes are found in up to 30% of patients overall, and these are confirmed to be malignant in approximately 90% of cases. Up to 50% of patients with proximal or advanced urethral cancers may have palpable nodes. Pelvic nodal metastases are not uncommon, affecting 20% of cases. Metastasis outside of the pelvis at presentation is rare, however. During follow-up, another 15% of patients will develop metastatic nodal disease (Grigsby and Herr, 2000).

Treatment and Prognosis

Because of the rarity of this tumor and heterogeneity of disease, insufficient experience at any single institution within a reasonable period has precluded attempts to effectively define the natural history of the disease, recommendations for therapy, and follow-up of these patients (Grigsby and Herr, 2000). **Although it is conceivable that different histologic subtypes may affect prognosis and the propensity for route of disease spread, most studies have failed to detect any differences in survival based on histologic subtype** (Foens et al, 1991; Dimarco et al, 2004). Consequently, lesions of varying histologic type are often treated in a similar fashion. A recent survival analysis of SEER data in 359 women found that squamous cell carcinoma had a longer cancer-specific survival than urothelial or adenocarcinoma histologies (hazard ratio of 2.03 and 1.90, respectively) (Champ et al, 2012).

Treatment recommendations depend primarily on tumor location and clinical stage. Local excision, which should lead to excellent functional results, may be sufficient for the relatively uncommon small, superficial, distal urethral tumors. For more proximal and advanced urethral tumors, a more aggressive approach is warranted. **Compared with proximal urethral cancers, distal lesions are associated with improved survival.** Five-year disease-specific survival is reported at 71% for distal lesions, 48% for proximal lesions, and 24% for lesions that involve the majority of the urethra (Dalbagni et al, 1998). Surgical and radiotherapy series reflect overall 5-year survival rates of 30% to 40%. Unfortunately, little improvement has been made in treatment of this disease and survival rates have remained statistically unchanged for the last 50 years (Bracken et al, 1976; Prempree et al, 1984; Foens et al, 1991; Dalbagni et al, 1998; Dimarco et al, 2004).

In a study of SEER data encompassing 722 women with primary urethral cancer between 1983 and 2008, 359 women with non-metastatic disease were found to have enough data for cancer survival outcomes to be evaluated (Champ et al, 2012). They found that 5-year and 10-year overall survival was 43% and 32%, respectively. Cancer-specific survival at 5 and 10 years was estimated at 53% and 46%, respectively. Multivariate analysis revealed race (African-American), advanced stage, node-positive disease at time of surgery; nonsquamous histology; and advanced age as being associated with worse cancer-specific survival. Surgery was associated with improved survival, which was not seen for radiation therapy. These data do not indicate that radiation therapy lacks benefit, because selection bias and other confounding factors significantly affect interpretation of this result.

Data from the National Cancer Registry of the Netherlands evaluating 91 females with primary urethral carcinoma reported 46% of patients presenting with advanced disease (stage III or IV). Five-year survival rates of stage 0 to II, stage III, and stage IV were 67%, 53%, and 17%, respectively (Derksen et al, 2013).

Options for treatment of female urethral carcinoma include surgery, radiation therapy, and chemotherapy, alone or in combination. Treatment has trended toward a multimodality approach in recent years based on previously reported outcomes. Use of radiation therapy has increased compared to men treated for urethral carcinoma. In the study of SEER data by Champ and associates (2012), 72% had undergone some cancer-directed surgical procedure and 42% had undergone radiation. Data from the National

Cancer Registry of the Netherlands detailed treatment of 43% of patients with surgery, 16% with radiation, or radiation plus surgery in 22% (Derksen et al, 2013). Although representative of a heterogeneous group of studies, with varying treatment techniques and follow-up, reported results in case series with more than two patients based on primary treatment modalities are summarized in Tables 38-2 and 38-3 for early and advanced disease, respectively.

Distal Female Urethral Carcinoma

Small, exophytic, superficial tumors arising from the urethral meatus or distal third of the urethra may be surgically treated with circumferential excision of the distal urethra and inclusion of a portion of the anterior vaginal wall via a transvaginal approach. Frozen-section specimens of the proximal urethra should be obtained to ensure an adequate margin (Narayan and Konety, 1992). Laser coagulation of small distal tumors has been described (Staehler et al, 1985; Dann et al, 1989). In select patients with T2 or T3 cancer, bladder-sparing strategies also have been employed, if the tumor is more anterior, while an attempt is made to maintain a thorough resection. Dimarco and colleagues (2004) describe radical urethrectomy in the female patient, including excision up to the level of the bladder neck with wide resection of periurethral tissues and anterior vaginal wall. Urinary diversion is then accomplished with a catheterizable stoma (ileovesicostomy or appendicovesicostomy) to the native bladder. **Tumors in the distal (anterior) urethra tend to be low stage, and cure rates of 70% to 90% have been achieved with local excision alone.** However, in a study by Dimarco and colleagues (2004), 21% of patients with stage T2 or less tumors treated with partial urethrectomy had local recurrence. Other studies of partial urethrectomy, with or without

TABLE 38-2 Results of Various Treatment Modalities for Early Urethral Carcinoma in Women

TREATMENT	STUDY	NO. OF PATIENTS	SURVIVAL* NO. (%)
Radiotherapy	Weghaupt et al, 1984	42	30 (71)
	Pointon and Poole-Wilson, 1968	26	20 (77)†
	Taggart et al, 1972	15	8 (53)‡
	Grabstald et al, 1966	11	3 (27)
	Delclos et al, 1980	11	6 (55)
	Chu, 1973	11	7 (64)
	Antoniades, 1969	8	8 (100)§
	Prempree et al, 1984	6	6 (100)
	Johnson and O'Connell, 1983	5	3 (60)‖
	Klein et al, 1987	3	2 (66)¶
	TOTAL	**138**	**93 (67)**
Surgery	Grabstald et al, 1966	14	10 (71)
	Bracken et al, 1976	3	1 (33)
	Eng et al, 2003	4	4 (100)
	TOTAL	**21**	**15 (71)**
Radiotherapy plus surgery	Grabstald et al, 1966	3	2 (67)
	TOTAL	**3**	**2 (67)**

*Survival 5 to 6 years unless otherwise noted.
†Three-year survival.
‡Two-year survival with no evidence of disease.
§One patient dead of disease at 64 months.
‖Patients had no evidence of disease at 4 years.
¶Patients alive at 27 and 37 months.

radiation therapy, for lower stage lesions have recurrence rates of 0% to 50% (Hahn et al, 1991; Gheiler et al, 1998). Meatal stenosis is a common complication, and incidence may be decreased by spatulation of the urethra. Approximation of the anterior vaginal wall and labia may help prevent urinary incontinence, although a sling procedure or other procedure to treat urinary incontinence may need to be subsequently performed. Many authors report minimal complications and rare incontinence from partial urethrectomy, but one series noted de novo or worsening stress urinary incontinence in 42% of patients (Dimarco et al, 2004).

Radiation therapy, as well as surgery, has proved effective for the treatment of low-stage distal urethral carcinomas. An overall 5-year actuarial survival rate of 41% was reported in a series of 84 patients by Garden and colleagues (1993). This was subdivided into 5-year survival of 74% if only part of the urethra was involved and 55% if the entire urethra was involved. Survival appeared to be associated with clinical stage of the tumor (Garden et al, 1993). Radiation may be delivered as external beam, brachytherapy, or combined therapy. In a series of 42 patients treated at the University of Iowa, radiotherapy delivered with combined interstitial and external beam radiation provided fewer local failures (14%) than all radiation-treated patients (36%) or those treated by surgery alone (60%). However, 5-year survival rates for irradiated and surgically treated groups are similar (Foens et al, 1991). Although doses may vary widely, a dose between 55 and 70 Gy is reported in most series. Complication rates, now decreasing, have ranged from 20% to 40%, including urinary incontinence, urethral strictures, necrosis, fistula formation, cystitis, vulvar abscess, and cellulitis (Forman and Lichter, 1992). **Radiation may represent an alternative in women when surgical resection would negatively affect functional outcomes.** Significant morbidity has been noted with ilioinguinal lymphadenectomy. In addition, female urethral carcinoma often spreads systemically without regional lymph node involvement. Although studies are small, no evidence for improved survival after pelvic or inguinal lymphadenectomy has been found (Grabstald et al, 1966; Levine, 1980; Dimarco et al, 2004). These findings, as well as the inability to prognosticate likelihood for micrometastatic lymph node involvement, led to the recommendation against prophylactic or diagnostic lymphadenectomy. **Acknowledging that few objective data exist for making definitive decisions, recommendations for performing groin dissection have been made only for patients who present with positive inguinal or pelvic lymphadenopathy without distant metastasis or patients who develop regional adenopathy during surveillance.** Late inguinal lymph node recurrences up to 7 years have been noted. The technique of ilioinguinal lymphadenectomy is identical to the dissection performed in men for penile cancer (Narayan and Konety, 1992; Grigsby and Herr, 2000).

In patients with recurrent or radioresistant tumors, neoadjuvant irradiation followed by local excision resulted in a survival advantage over radiotherapy alone (Grabstald et al, 1966; Peterson et al, 1973; Allen and Nelson, 1978). Despite early and aggressive therapy for anterior lesions, local recurrence rates and mortality remain high. Further studies are necessary to evaluate the potential role of multimodality therapy in these patients.

Proximal Female Urethral Carcinoma

Proximal female urethral carcinomas are more likely to be high stage and may extend into the bladder and vagina. Results with anterior exenteration alone resulted in a 10% to 17% 5-year survival rate and a local recurrence rate of 67% (Bracken et al, 1976; Klein et al, 1983). The poor disease-specific survival and high local recurrence rates observed with single-modality treatment of advanced female urethral carcinoma have led to the recommendation of combination therapy (Dalbagni et al, 1998, 2001; Gheiler et al, 1998). Advanced female urethral carcinoma includes tumors in a proximal location, a lesion that encompasses the entire urethra, or a locally invasive lesion that involves external genitalia, vagina, or bladder. Anterior exenteration (cystourethrectomy), pelvic lymph node dissection, and wide vaginal or complete vaginal excision are often

TABLE 38-3 Results of Various Treatment Modalities for Advanced-Stage Urethral Carcinoma in Women

TREATMENT	STUDY	NO. OF PATIENTS	SURVIVAL* NO. (%)
Radiotherapy	Pointon and Poole-Wilson, 1968	52	21 (40)†
	Delclos et al, 1980	25	7 (28)
	Weghaupt et al, 1984	20	10 (50)
	Grabstald et al, 1966	19	1 (5)
	Antoniades, 1969	11	4 (36)‡
	Prempree et al, 1984	7	4 (57)
	Hahn et al, 1991	8	3 (38)
	Chu, 1973	8	0 (0)
	Johnson and O'Connell, 1983	7	4 (57)§
	TOTAL	**157**	**54 (34)**
Surgery	Grabstald et al, 1966	13	2 (15)
	Bracken et al, 1976	7	3 (43)‖
	Moinuddin Ali et al, 1988	3	0 (0)
	TOTAL	**23**	**5 (22)**
Radiotherapy + surgery	Grabstald et al, 1966	20	5 (25)
	Johnson and O'Connell, 1983	7	3 (43)
	Hahn et al, 1991	3	9 (0)
	Moinuddin Ali et al, 1988	4	2 (50)¶
	TOTAL	**34**	**19 (55)**
Radiotherapy + chemotherapy ± surgery	Gheiler et al, 1998	6	3 (50)**
	Dalbagni et al, 2001	4	2 (50)††
	TOTAL	**10**	**5 (50)**

*Survival 5 to 6 years unless otherwise noted.
†Three-year survival.
‡Two patients dead of disease at 8 and 21 years.
§No evidence of disease at 1, 1, 3, and 6 years.
‖No evidence of disease at 2 months and 3, 8, and 12 years.
¶Alive at 48 months.
**No evidence of disease at 6 months and 4 years.
††No evidence of disease at 1.5 and 4 years.

required to obtain negative surgical margins. If the lesion extends into the external genitalia, partial vulvectomy or labial excision may be necessary. Anterior exenteration is performed as for bladder cancer in a female patient, with a more extensive perineal portion of the procedure to provide wide margins around the urethra. The margins of the lymphadenectomy should include the Cloquet node distally and otherwise retain limits identical to the dissection encouraged for lymphadenectomy in bladder cancer. Anterior exenteration includes the en bloc removal of the entire urethra and bladder, the uterus and adnexa, and the anterior and lateral vaginal walls. On occasion, the entire vagina may need to be resected. The perineal portion is initiated by completing an inverted U-shaped incision to encircle widely around the urethral meatus. It has been suggested that this incision be extended onto the posterior vaginal wall to the labia minora and continued anteriorly to beyond and including the clitoris (Narayan and Konety, 1992). En bloc resection of the pubic symphysis and inferior pubic rami may be necessary if the lesion encroaches anteriorly at the pubis, although the necessity of bone resection has been questioned in ensuring durable local control when intraoperative irradiation is added in suspect cases (Dalbagni et al, 2001).

Radiotherapy alone for proximal invasive urethral carcinoma has yielded poor local control, and 5-year survival rates of 0% to 57% are reported (Grabstald et al, 1966; Johnson and O'Connell, 1983; Prempree et al, 1984; Narayan and Konety, 1992). An improved mean survival rate of 54% at 5 years resulted from the combination of radiation therapy and surgery for high-stage disease (Moinuddin Ali et al, 1988; Terry et al, 1997).

A combination of chemotherapy, radiation therapy, and surgery has been recommended for optimal local and distant disease control in advanced female urethral cancer. Patients whose treatment fails are thought likely to harbor micrometastatic disease at the time of primary treatment. For patients with squamous cell carcinoma, 5-FU plus MMC has been the most common empirically chosen regimen, in part because of its effectiveness against anal cancers (Kalra et al, 1985). For transitional cell cancers, either M-VAC or a gemcitabine regimen is recommended (Grigsby and Herr, 2000). Chemotherapy given concomitantly with radiation therapy has been shown to interfere with cell repair and thus act as a radiosensitizer. It is hoped that therapy based on this rationale may decrease local recurrence and improve survival by eliminating micrometastatic disease and preventing progression of local failures to systemic failures. The group at Memorial Sloan-Kettering has shown early results based on six patients with advanced proximal urethral tumors treated with a multimodality approach. The authors suggest that anterior exenteration with high-dose intraoperative brachytherapy followed by external beam radiation seems to improve local control. Studies must evaluate whether combined modality therapy proves to decrease distant metastasis and improve survival (Dalbagni et al, 1998, 2001).

For advanced female urethral cancer, we recommend primary chemotherapy and/or radiation therapy for locally advanced tumors. If a radiographic and endoscopic response is realized, consolidative surgery can be considered. Systemic chemotherapy should be considered for metastatic disease.

Urethral Recurrence after Cystectomy in Women

Orthotopic neobladder construction in women is now an established form of urinary diversion after radical cystectomy for transitional cell carcinoma. **The incidence of carcinoma involving the urethra in female patients undergoing cystectomy for bladder cancer ranges from 1% to 13%** (Coloby et al, 1994; Stein et al, 1995, 1998; Stenzl et al, 1995). Debate still exists as to whether involvement of the bladder neck is a contraindication to orthotopic diversion; a prospective study revealed that although all patients with urethral transitional cell carcinoma on final pathologic analysis of the cystectomy specimen had involvement of the bladder neck, more than 60% of women with bladder neck involvement had no evidence of urethral transitional cell carcinoma (Stein et al, 1998). Intraoperative frozen-section analysis of the urethral stump has been subsequently espoused by some authors to determine the feasibility of urethra-sparing cystectomy and orthotopic diversion (Stein et al, 1998).

Despite the reported incidence of urethral involvement in patients who have undergone cystectomy and the increased use of orthotopic diversion in women, few cases have been reported of subsequent urethral malignant neoplasms in patients who have undergone this procedure. A review of 1054 patients undergoing radical cystectomy at a single center with a median follow-up of 10 years included 211 women, 44 of whom had an orthotopic urinary diversion. None of the 44 women developed a urethral recurrence (Clark et al, 2004). Subsequently, this group from the University of Southern California reported their first case of primary urethral recurrence in female patients selected for orthotopic urinary diversion. The patient remained without evidence of disease at 4 years of follow-up after total urethrectomy, resection of neobladder neck, and conversion of the orthotopic reservoir to a continent cutaneous urinary diversion (Stein et al, 2008). A report by Taylor and colleagues from MD Anderson (2009) reported on 260 patients after radical cystectomy and orthotopic neobladder, 10 of whom were women. There were six urethral recurrences, all in male patients. In a study by Ali-el-Dein and colleagues (2004), 145 women underwent orthotopic urinary diversion, 61% for squamous cell carcinoma, and 21% for transitional cell carcinoma. At a median follow-up of 56 months, 2 patients (1.4%) developed an isolated urethral recurrence. One patient was reportedly not a surgical candidate, and the other patient underwent urethrectomy and conversion to a continent cutaneous reservoir but died 8 months later (Ali-el-Dein et al, 2004). One additional report described urethral transitional cell carcinoma in a woman after orthotopic diversion. This patient had a high-grade lesion of the bladder base with evidence of nodal metastasis. The patient was treated initially with chemotherapy, followed by urethral resection and conversion to a continent cutaneous diversion. The patient died 5 months later with visceral metastases (Jones et al, 2000). Limited experience to date precludes the ability to make definitive treatment recommendations for women with urethral cancer recurrence after orthotopic diversion. Urethrectomy and surgical resection of the area of the urethra-pouch anastomosis with conversion to a continent cutaneous urinary diversion seem feasible and reasonable in the absence of metastatic disease. Conversion to a cutaneous urinary conduit with use of reconfigured bowel from the existing orthotopic diversion is another option (Bissada et al, 2004).

KEY POINTS: FEMALE URETHRAL CANCER

- The three most common histologies for cancer of the female urethra are urothelial carcinoma, squamous cell carcinoma, and adenocarcinoma—each accounting for approximately 30% of cases.
- Compared with proximal urethral cancers, distal (anterior) lesions are associated with improved survival.
- Tumors in the distal urethra may be low stage, and cure rates of 70% to 90% have been achieved with local excision alone via a transvaginal approach. Radiation may represent an alternative when surgical resection would negatively affect functional outcome.
- Proximal female urethral carcinomas are more likely to be high stage and may extend into the bladder and vagina.
- Optimal treatment for advanced female urethral cancer is not well defined. Multimodal therapy is advocated. A combination of chemotherapy, radiation therapy, and surgery has been recommended for local and distant disease control.
- In appropriately selected women undergoing radical cystectomy and orthotopic diversion for bladder cancer, recurrence of cancer in the retained urethra is a rare event.

Please visit the accompanying website at www.expertconsult.com to view videos associated with this chapter.

REFERENCES

The complete reference list is available online at www.expertconsult.com.

SUGGESTED READINGS

Clark PE, Stein JP, Groshen SG, et al. The management of urethral transitional cell carcinoma after radical cystectomy for invasive bladder cancer. J Urol 2004;172:1342–7.

Cohen MS, Triaca V, Billmeyer B, et al. Coordinated chemoradiation therapy with genital preservation for the treatment of primary invasive carcinoma of the male urethra. J Urol 2008;179:536–41.

Dalbagni G, Donat SM, Eschwege P, et al. Results of high-dose rate brachytherapy, anterior pelvic exenteration and external beam radiotherapy for carcinoma of the female urethra. J Urol 2001;166:1759–61.

Dayyani F, Pettaway CA, Kamat AM, et al. Retrospective analysis of survival outcomes and the role of cisplatin-based chemotherapy in patients with urethral carcinomas referred to medical oncologists. Urol Oncol 2013;31:1171–7.

Dimarco DS, Dimarco CS, Zincke H, et al. Surgical treatment for local control of female urethral carcinoma. Urol Oncol 2004;22:404–9.

Grivas PD, Davenport M, Montie JE, et al. Urethral cancer. Hematol Oncol Clin North Am 2012;26:1291–314.

Karnes RJ, Breau RH, Lightner DJ. Surgery for urethral cancer. Urol Clin N Am 2010;37:445–57.

Rabbani F. Prognostic factors in male urethral cancer. Cancer 2011;117:2426–34.

39 Inguinal Node Dissection

Kenneth W. Angermeier, MD, Rene Sotelo, MD, and David S. Sharp, MD

Anatomic Considerations | Penile Cancer: Surgical Management of Regional Lymph Nodes

Despite ongoing clinical experience, treatment of squamous cell carcinoma of the penis remains primarily surgical. Early meticulous surgical management with close follow-up typically provides the best opportunity for cure. The most important factor determining survival in patients with penile cancer is the extent of lymph node metastases (Johnson and Lo, 1984; Srinivas et al, 1987; Ravi, 1993; Horenblas and van Tinteren 1994). The management of the inguinal lymph nodes therefore is a major component of the overall treatment strategy, and appropriate decision making with regard to lymph node assessment and excision is critical.

ANATOMIC CONSIDERATIONS
Penile Lymphatics

Squamous cell carcinoma of the penis spreads initially to regional lymph nodes before the occurrence of distant metastatic disease. Lymphatic spread occurs in a systematic fashion along the normal route of penile lymphatic drainage. The superficial lymphatic system consists of vessels draining the prepuce and skin of the penile shaft that converge dorsally and then divide at the base of the penis to drain into the right and left superficial inguinal nodes. The deep lymphatic system consists of drainage from the glans penis toward the frenulum, where large trunks are formed and encircle the corona to unite with those from the other side on the dorsum. They traverse the penis to the base within the Buck fascia, draining through presymphyseal lymphatics into the superficial inguinal nodes and the deep inguinal nodes of the femoral triangle. It is not uncommon for penile cancer to metastasize to the contralateral inguinal nodes because of crossover in the symphyseal region, and this needs to be taken into account in developing a treatment strategy. Drainage subsequently proceeds from the inguinal nodes to the ipsilateral pelvic lymph nodes. It is generally accepted that penile lymphatics drain to the inguinal nodes before proceeding into the iliac nodes (Riveros et al, 1967), although some anecdotal observations have suggested that penile lymphatics may at times drain directly to the external iliac nodes (Lopes et al, 2000). This observation is most likely related to undersampling of the inguinal nodes at the time of lymphadenectomy or at the time of pathologic review. **Although penile carcinoma metastatic to the inguinal lymph nodes confers a poorer prognosis overall, aggressive lymphadenectomy is associated with improved long-term survival and potential cure** (McDougal et al, 1986; Horenblas and van Tinteren, 1994). In addition, immediate resection of clinically occult lymph node metastases is associated with improved survival when compared with delayed resection of involved nodes at the time of clinical detection (Kroon et al, 2005). If the tumor has spread to the pelvic nodes, long-term survival is less than 10%.

Urethral Lymphatics

Urethral lymphatic drainage runs parallel to the urethra and is located within the mucous membrane and submucosa (Spirin, 1963). **This network is most dense in the area of the fossa** navicularis, and these branches join the lymphatics of the glans at the prepuce. The lymphatics of the penile urethra course laterally around the corpora cavernosa to join the vessels proceeding from the glans penis. Bulbar urethral drainage is more variable and may occur along the bulbar artery toward the medial retrofemoral node or may course under the pubis toward the anterior bladder wall, terminating in the retrofemoral and medial external iliac nodes (Wood and Angermeier, 2010).

Inguinal Anatomy

The inguinal lymph nodes are divided into superficial and deep groups, which are anatomically separated by the fascia lata of the thigh. The superficial group is composed of 4 to 25 lymph nodes that are situated in the deep membranous layer of the superficial fascia of the thigh (Camper fascia). The superficial inguinal nodes have been divided into five anatomic groups (Daseler et al, 1948): (1) central nodes around the saphenofemoral junction, (2) superolateral nodes around the superficial circumflex vein, (3) inferolateral nodes around the lateral femoral cutaneous and superficial circumflex veins, (4) superomedial nodes around the superficial external pudendal and superficial epigastric veins, and (5) inferomedial nodes around the greater saphenous vein (Fig. 39-1). The deep inguinal nodes are fewer and lie primarily medial to the femoral vein in the femoral canal. The node of Cloquet is the most cephalad of this deep group and is situated between the femoral vein and the lacunar ligament (Fig. 39-2). The external iliac lymph nodes receive drainage from the deep inguinal, obturator, and hypogastric groups. In turn, drainage progresses to the common iliac and para-aortic nodes.

The blood supply to the skin of the inguinal region derives from branches of the common femoral artery—the superficial external pudendal, superficial circumflex iliac, and superficial epigastric arteries. Complete inguinal dissection necessitates ligation of these branches. Viability of the skin flaps raised during the dissection depends on anastomotic vessels in the superficial fatty layer of the Camper fascia that course lateral to medial along the natural skin lines. Because lymphatic drainage of the penis to the groin runs beneath the Camper fascia, this layer can be preserved and left attached to the overlying skin when the superior and inferior skin flaps are fashioned. On the basis of this anatomy, a transverse skin incision least compromises this blood supply. In this fashion, serious skin slough is prevented in the majority of patients. The femoral nerve lies deep to the iliacus fascia and supplies motor function to the pectineus, quadriceps femoris, and sartorius muscles. In addition, this nerve provides cutaneous sensation to the anterior thigh and should be preserved. Some of the sensory branches, however, are commonly sacrificed in the regional node dissection.

The femoral triangle is bounded by the inguinal ligament superiorly, the sartorius muscle laterally, and the adductor longus medially. The floor of the triangle is composed of the pectineus muscle medially and the iliopsoas laterally. The location of the saphenofemoral junction is estimated to be at a point two fingerbreadths lateral and two fingerbreadths inferior to the pubic tubercle.

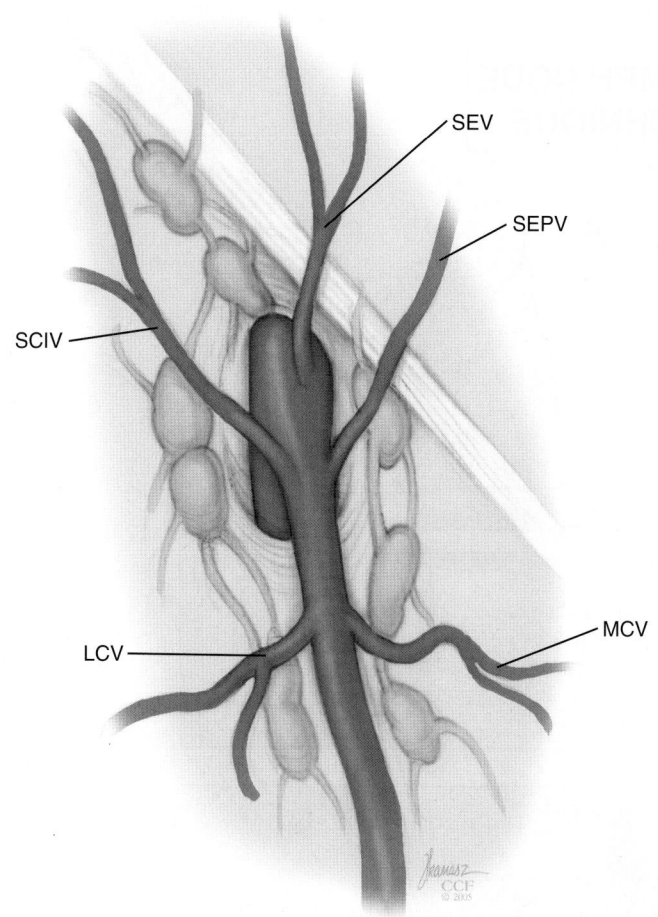

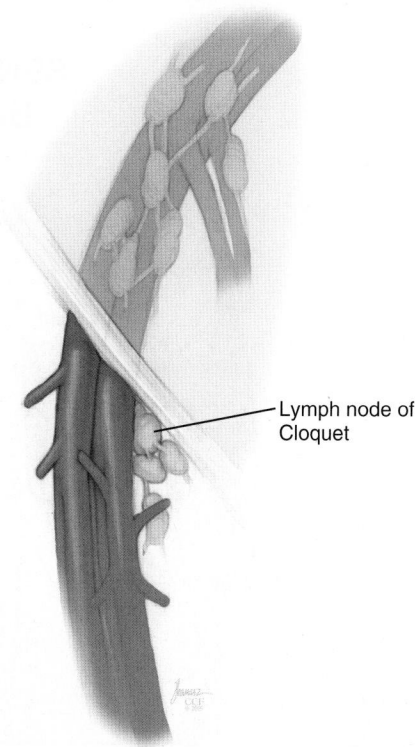

Figure 39-2. **Deep inguinal lymph nodes. (Reprinted with permission, Cleveland Clinic Center for Medical Art & Photography © 2003-2010. All rights reserved.)**

Figure 39-1. **Superficial inguinal lymph nodes and the branches of the saphenous vein. LCV, lateral cutaneous; MCV, medial cutaneous; SCIV, superficial circumflex iliac; SEPV, superficial external pudendal; SEV, superficial epigastric. (Reprinted with permission, Cleveland Clinic Center for Medical Art & Photography © 2003-2010. All rights reserved.)**

PENILE CANCER: SURGICAL MANAGEMENT OF REGIONAL LYMPH NODES

Clinically Negative Groins

Approximately 20% of patients with clinically nonpalpable inguinal nodes harbor occult metastases (Hegarty et al, 2006). Routine bilateral inguinofemoral lymph node dissection (IFLND) in these patients would overtreat 80% of them, subjecting them to potential increased morbidity. The optimal form of management would provide the ability to identify patients with metastatic penile cancer in this cohort who are potentially curable with surgical lymphadenectomy while at the same time avoiding unnecessary surgery in patients with pathologically negative inguinal nodes. Strategies to accomplish this include (1) improved prognostic algorithms and risk assessment based on the primary tumor's pathologic and clinical characteristics, (2) improved radiographic techniques, and (3) pathologic sampling of first-echelon nodes.

The indications for surgical assessment of inguinal lymph nodes when there is no palpable adenopathy are covered in Chapter 37. This section will focus on the techniques used for this purpose. The primary goal of these procedures is to accurately determine whether inguinal nodal metastases are present while minimizing patient morbidity.

Sentinel Node Biopsy

Sentinel lymph node biopsy is the technique to remove nodes that are first affected by the spread of metastatic disease. The theory is that certain cancers typically do not spread to other lymph nodes without the necessary and stepwise involvement of the sentinel node first. Based on anatomic studies, the concept of orderly lymphatic progression of metastatic cells from the primary tumor to the sentinel node does seem to be likely with regard to squamous cell carcinoma of the penis. This approach has gained acceptance as this concept has become more widely accepted, and has also proven effective for both breast cancer and melanoma.

The technique of sentinel node biopsy in patients with invasive squamous cell carcinoma of the penis and clinically negative inguinal regions was proposed by Cabanas (1977) after extensive study of lymphangiograms and anatomic dissections. A 5-cm incision is made parallel to the inguinal crease and centered two fingerbreadths lateral and inferior to the pubic tubercle. By insertion of the finger under the upper flap toward the pubic tubercle, the sentinel lymph node is encountered and excised (Fig. 39-3). Cabanas demonstrated that the sentinel node was always positive in patients with positive metastatic inguinal nodes at time of IFLND. In the absence of tumor in the sentinel node, no metastases were found in the other inguinal lymph nodes in 31 patients. In addition, he reported that this node (subsequently termed the *Cabanas node*) was positive in 4% of patients in whom the lymph nodes were not deemed clinically suspicious. It was concluded that routine excision of this sentinel node could identify patients with micrometastatic disease earlier than waiting for clinically palpable nodes, which was standard at the time.

Although Cabanas reported 90% survival in patients with normal findings on sentinel node biopsy, subsequent authors found the results to be less satisfactory, with false-negative rates of 18% to 25% (Perinetti et al, 1980; Wespes et al, 1986;

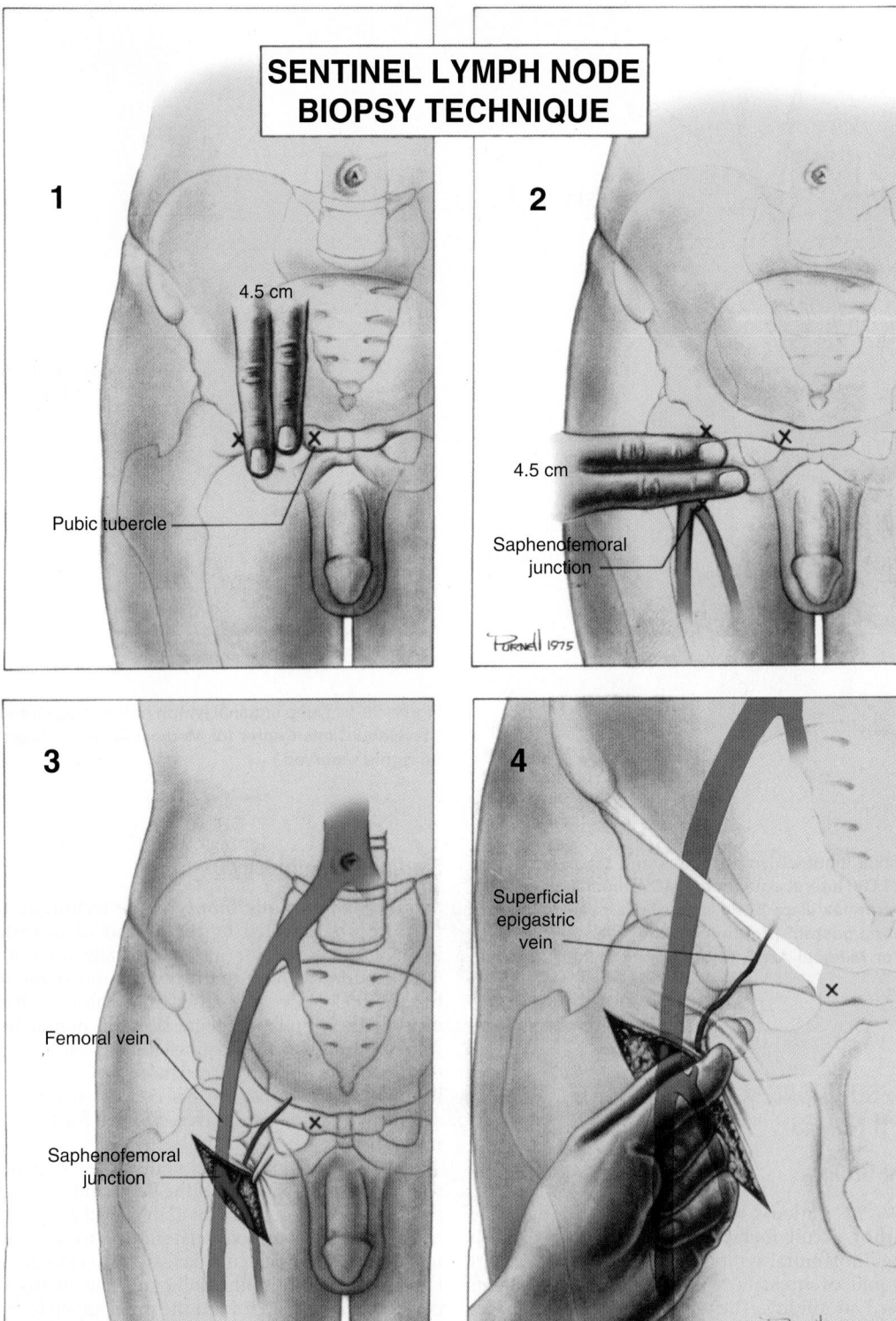

SENTINEL LYMPH NODE BIOPSY TECHNIQUE

1

4.5 cm

Pubic tubercle

2

4.5 cm

Saphenofemoral junction

Purnell 1975

3

Femoral vein

Saphenofemoral junction

4

Superficial epigastric vein

Purnell 1975

Figure 39-3. Sentinel lymph node biopsy technique as described by Cabanas in 1977. A 5-cm incision is made parallel to the inguinal crease and centered two fingerbreadths lateral and inferior to the pubic tubercle. By insertion of the finger under the upper flap toward the pubic tubercle, the sentinel lymph node is encountered and excised. (From Cabanas RM. An approach for the treatment of penile carcinoma. Cancer 1977;39:456–66.)

Srinivas et al, 1991). In large part, this is likely because this initial concept is based on a static location of the sentinel lymph node. As a result, this procedure is no longer recommended. In an attempt to improve sampling of the superficial nodal basin, Pettaway and colleagues (1995) evaluated extended sentinel node biopsy, during which all of the lymph nodes between the inguinal ligament and the superficial external pudendal vein were removed. This approach has also been abandoned because it resulted in a false-negative rate of 15% to 25% (Ravi, 1993; Pettaway et al, 1995).

Dynamic Sentinel Node Biopsy

Background

Renewed interest in sentinel lymph node biopsy for penile cancer returned as breast and melanoma treatments incorporated this approach successfully. Sentinel lymph node biopsy is now the preferred method of lymph node staging in breast cancer and melanoma (Warycha et al, 2009). The group at the Netherlands Cancer Institute (NKI) pioneered dynamic sentinel lymph node biopsy (DSNB) for staging in penile cancer beginning in 1994. **Since then, several groups have reported on the accuracy of DSNB in penile cancer as an alternative or adjunct to IFLND, and this procedure was included in the 2009 European Association of Urology (EAU) guidelines on penile cancer** (Pizzocaro et al, 2010). This method includes preoperative lymphoscintigraphy using technetium-99m nanocolloid, preoperative patent blue dye injection, and intraoperative guidance with a gamma ray detection probe to visualize the individual drainage pattern and accurately identify the sentinel node.

DSNB has undergone modifications to reduce false-negative rates. Initial reports out of the NKI revealed a relatively high false-negative rate of 22% (Tanis et al, 2002). Leijte and colleagues reported having found that patients staged by DSNB between 1994 and 2001 had an unsatisfactory false-negative rate of 19%. Further experience and refinement in their technique resulted in a reduction to a reported 5% in patients treated between 2001 and 2004 (Leijte et al, 2007). By combining the data from the NKI in Amsterdam (297 patients) and St. George's Hospital (SGH) in London (134 patients), a false-negative rate of 7% was subsequently achieved (Leijte et al, 2009). They reported a complication rate of 4.7% (28 of 592 explored groins), primarily infection, seroma or lymphocele, or delayed bleeding. A DSNB was classified as a false-negative procedure if a regional nodal recurrence was noted on follow-up after a negative DSNB. Of 323 patients in this study with 611 clinically negative groins, six such recurrences were noted, all within 15 months. The median follow-up for the paper was 17.9 months (range, 1 to 69 months) (Leijte et al, 2009). Subsequent data out of SGH reported on 500 inguinal basins in 264 consecutive men over a 6-year period (2004 to 2010). All patients had T1G2 or higher-stage disease of the primary tumor and nonpalpable nodes in one or both inguinal basins. Minimum follow-up was 21 months (median 57 months). Seventy-three positive inguinal basins (14.6%) in 59 patients (22.3%) were identified. The authors reported a false-negative DSNB rate of 5%. Twenty patients (7.6%) were identified with postoperative complications, half of which were lymphoceles.

Further outcomes of patients treated at NKI were reported based on time period of presentation. Of 1000 patients treated since 1956, 5-year cancer-specific survival increased for each cohort subsequently treated. In patients with cN0 disease, 5-year cancer-specific survival was 91% for patients treated between 1994 and 2012 versus 82% for patients treated between 1956 and 1993. Cancer-specific survival was better in patients treated during the DSNB era than those treated during the prophylactic bilateral IFLND era (Djajadiningrat et al, 2014).

Although the goal of treatment is to find all patients with potentially curable disease, false-negative rates of 5% to 10% are believed by many to be reasonably acceptable given the substantial reduction in morbidity. The ability of other centers to obtain results seen at NKI and SGH and generalize this method has been explored. A retrospective review of DSNB in a tertiary center in Sweden between 1999 and 2011 has been reported (Kirrander et al, 2012). Of 58 patients, 115 cN0 groins were analyzed with DSNB protocol. Two patients with a negative DSNB were noted to have a clinical recurrence, consistent with a false-negative rate of 15%. This study reported an evolving procedure at this institution; for instance, ultrasound was not used preoperatively in 45% of patients in the early time period. Nonetheless, the study confirms that this methodology and technique necessitate dedicated experience to gain optimal results. The false-negative rate of 15% is comparable with

early reports from other series and is expected to fall with increased use and overall experience. In comparison, in the breast cancer literature, recommendations exist that DSNB should be performed by surgeons with at least 20 procedures per year, with the first 20 including assistance from an experienced surgeon. Before routine adoption of the procedure, a false-negative rate below 5% is suggested (Kuehn et al, 2005). The learning curve has not been well established in penile cancer, although in the study of pooled data from NKI and SGH, none of the six recurrences consistent with false negatives occurred in the initial 30 procedures (Leijte et al, 2009). Because of the rarity of penile cancer, these expectations are challenging and provide support for a referral network approach to specialized centers.

Based on the aforementioned information, DSNB should be performed with the goal of a false-negative rate at 5% or lower. Reasons postulated for the false-negative rates seen in penile cancer include (1) selection or identification of the wrong node, (2) poor pathologic sectioning or sampling such that small cancer foci are missed, and (3) tumor occupying and obstructing lymphatic channels that allows for new lymphatics or arborization to occur, leading to unorthodox drainage (Srinivas et al, 1991; Kroon et al, 2004).

Technique

Figure 39-4 outlines the technique and methodology for DSNB as espoused by groups at SGH in London and NKI in Amsterdam (Hadway, et al, 2007; Leijte et al, 2007; Lam et al, 2013). Variations in the initial technique have been used to reduce false-negative rates (Kroon et al, 2004). Currently, inguinal ultrasound and fine-needle aspiration (FNA) cytology of suspect lymph nodes has been added as a preliminary step before lymphoscintigraphy. Patients with abnormal nodes on ultrasound undergo FNA, and only patients with negative FNA findings proceed to scintigraphy and DSNB. Patients with positive FNA findings undergo IFLND. The abnormal ultrasound findings used by the group at SGH to direct patients to FNA are outlined in Box 39-1. Ultrasound-guided FNA was added to the DSNB procedure in an attempt to circumvent false-negative results caused by tumor blocking and rerouting of lymphatics. Combined use of a radiotracer and blue dye is then performed to improve the identification of the sentinel node (Fig. 39-5). A meta-analysis performed by Sadeghi and colleagues revealed a pooled detection rate of 88.3%, which was improved to 90.1% if both blue dye and radiotracer were used (Sadeghi et al, 2012). Another change made to the initial DSNB protocol is that an inguinal exploration is performed after removal of the sentinel node. The groin is carefully palpated for suspicious nodes that failed to pick up any radioactive or dye tracer. Finally, a more accurate pathologic analysis of the resected node has also proven essential. A single section through a center of a node may miss micrometastatic disease. All nodes are submitted whole and embedded in paraffin. They are then serially sectioned in 2-mm increments and are evaluated with immunohistochemistry in addition to standard staining to avoid pathologic false negatives.

DSNB can be performed at the time of initial definitive primary tumor resection (after a biopsy of the penile lesion only), or after the primary tumor has been treated (with glans-preserving resection, partial or total penectomy). The group from Amsterdam has reported that postresection DSNB can be done with the technetium-99m nanocolloid injected around the resection wound or scar instead of around the tumor. They found comparable rates of sentinel node visualization (93%), sentinel node identification (100%), and detection of occult metastases (12%) when done after referral following primary tumor resection as when performed synchronously with the penile surgery (Graafland et al, 2010).

Follow-up

Strict follow-up is necessary to identify recurrences that can be managed surgically and potentially salvaged. For patients with a negative ultrasound and negative DSNB, clinical evaluation of the inguinal nodes is recommended. Examination in the office every 3

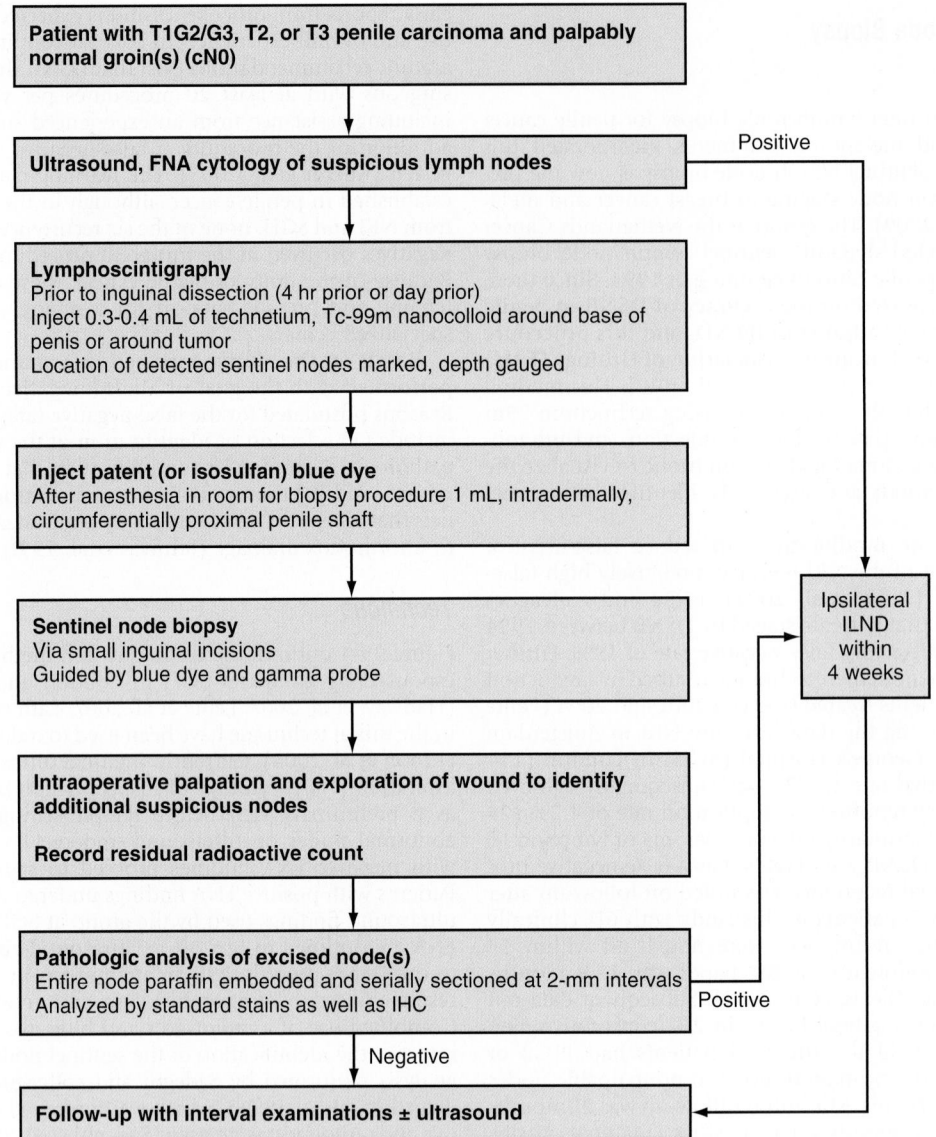

Patient with T1G2/G3, T2, or T3 penile carcinoma and palpably normal groin(s) (cN0)

Ultrasound, FNA cytology of suspicious lymph nodes

Lymphoscintigraphy
Prior to inguinal dissection (4 hr prior or day prior)
Inject 0.3-0.4 mL of technetium, Tc-99m nanocolloid around base of penis or around tumor
Location of detected sentinel nodes marked, depth gauged

Inject patent (or isosulfan) blue dye
After anesthesia in room for biopsy procedure 1 mL, intradermally, circumferentially proximal penile shaft

Sentinel node biopsy
Via small inguinal incisions
Guided by blue dye and gamma probe

Intraoperative palpation and exploration of wound to identify additional suspicious nodes

Record residual radioactive count

Pathologic analysis of excised node(s)
Entire node paraffin embedded and serially sectioned at 2-mm intervals
Analyzed by standard stains as well as IHC

Positive

Ipsilateral ILND within 4 weeks

Positive

Negative

Follow-up with interval examinations ± ultrasound

Figure 39-4. Flow diagram of technique and protocol for dynamic sentinel node biopsy. FNA, fine-needle aspiration; IHC, immunohistochemical markers; ILND, inguinal lymph node dissection. (Modified from Lam W, Alnajjar HM, La-Touche S, et al. Dynamic sentinel lymph node biopsy in patients with invasive squamous cell carcinoma of the penis: a prospective study of the long-term outcome of 500 inguinal basins assessed at a single institution. Eur Urol 2013; 63:657–63; and Leijte JA, Kroon BK, Olmos RA, et al. Reliability and safety of current dynamic sentinel node biopsy for penile carcinoma. Eur Urol 2007; 52:170–7.)

months for the first year, every 4 months for the second year, and every 6 months thereafter is recommended. Some patients may have a challenging inguinal nodal examination because of body habitus or lymphedema from prior procedures. In these patients ultrasound can be used. The role of computed tomography (CT), positron emission tomography (PET)-CT, or magnetic resonance imaging (MRI) is not well defined and sensitivity is suboptimal for low-volume metastatic disease. Finally, patients should be instructed on self-examination to be done at regular intervals (i.e., monthly) as an adjunct to their follow-up.

It is important to stress that DSNB remains a diagnostic procedure, allowing some men to avoid a therapeutic IFLND. Those with a positive DSNB should proceed to a full therapeutic lymphadenectomy. It is not appropriate for palpable lymphadenopathy and applies only to clinically negative nodes. In patients with palpable lymphadenopathy, inguinal lymphadenectomy is still recommended, as approximately one half of these patients will harbor pathologically positive lymph node metastases. Finally,

those centers employing DSNB need the experience and dedication of a multidisciplinary team of surgeons, nuclear medicine physicians, radiologists, and pathologists. The occurrence of a false negative is very serious, and salvage is usually difficult. The EAU and the International Consultation on Penile Cancer agree that DSNB is an acceptable staging procedure in the hands of experienced centers. Selection of patients is also dependent on acceptance and commitment of patients for regular follow-ups, as well as self-examination because of the possibility of false-negative findings (Hegarty et al, 2010). Whether the outcomes achieved by experienced centers can be reproduced at other small- or large-volume centers remains to be seen.

Superficial Inguinal Node Dissection

Superficial inguinal node dissection has been proposed as another method to surgically stage penile cancer patients without palpable lymphadenopathy. The procedure consists of removal of the nodal

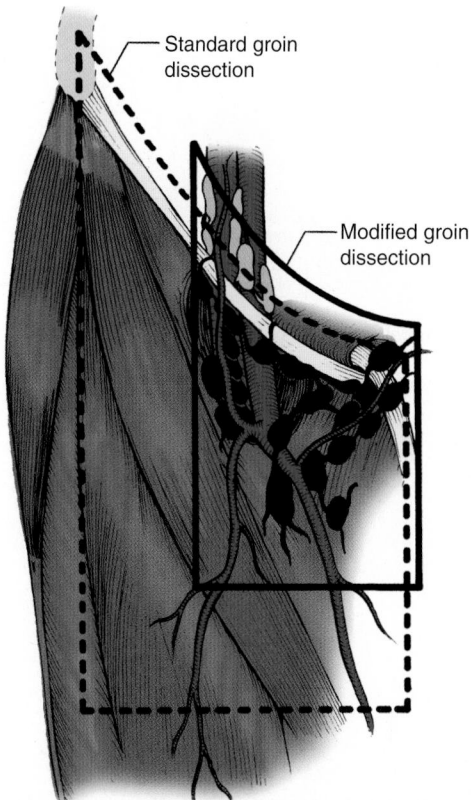

Figure 39-6. **Limits of standard and modified groin dissection. (From Colberg JW, Andriole GL, Catalona WJ. Long-term follow-up of men undergoing modified inguinal lymphadenectomy for carcinoma of the penis. Br J Urol 1997;79:54–7.)**

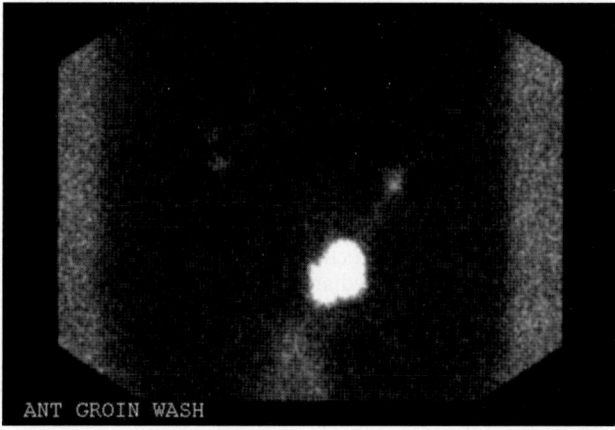

ANT GROIN WASH

Figure 39-5. **Lymphoscintigraphy: Dynamic images are obtained in multiple projections to provide location of the nodes with radiotracer uptake and their depth. Permanent marker is used to mark the location of each "hot" node. Here, there are two identified right sentinel inguinal lymph nodes and one left sentinel inguinal lymph node.**

packet superficial to the fascia lata and centered about the fossa ovalis and saphenofemoral junction. The peripheral boundaries of the dissection are similar to those described later for modified complete inguinal node dissection; however, the fascia lata is not opened. Previous studies have demonstrated no positive nodes deep to the fascia lata unless superficial nodes were also positive (Pompeo et al, 1995; Puras-Baez et al, 1995), which supports the efficacy of this procedure in surgical staging. In addition, a previous study of DSNB included a cohort of patients who underwent complete superficial node dissection. If the superficial nodes were negative, there were no recurrences with follow-up longer than 3 years (Spiess et al, 2007).

Modified Complete Inguinal Lymphadenectomy

In 1988, Catalona proposed a technique of modified inguinofemoral lymphadenectomy designed to provide staging information and therapeutic benefit similar to standard extended lymphadenectomy with less morbidity (Catalona, 1988) (Fig. 39-6). **Key aspects of the procedure are (1) shorter skin incision, (2) limitation of the dissection by excluding the area lateral to the femoral artery and caudal to the fossa ovalis, (3) preservation of the saphenous vein, and (4) elimination of the need to transpose the sartorius muscle.**

All of the superficial lymph nodes within the described area are removed, as are the deep inguinal nodes that are located primarily medial to the femoral vein to the level of the inguinal ligament.

The procedure begins by placing the patient into a frog-leg position. A 10-cm skin incision is made approximately 1.5 to 2 cm below the inguinal crease. Skin flaps are developed in the plane just beneath the Scarpa fascia for a distance of 8 cm superiorly and 6 cm inferiorly. The superior dissection is carried to the level of the external oblique fascia with exposure of the spermatic cord. A funiculus of lymphofatty tissue, extending from the base of the penis to the superomedial portion of the lymph node packet, is ligated and divided. Dissection commences in a caudad direction with removal of the superficial and deep inguinal nodes, with the boundaries consisting of the adductor longus muscle medially and the femoral artery laterally. The saphenous vein is identified and preserved, although a number of branches draining into it will need to be sacrificed. The nodal packet is dissected caudad to the level of the skin flap dissection (Fig. 39-7), at which point the lymphatics are carefully ligated and the specimen is delivered from the operative field (Fig. 39-8). A closed-suction drain is placed, and the incision is closed in standard fashion.

The false-negative rate for this procedure, in terms of detecting inguinal metastatic disease, ranges from 0% to 5.5% in the majority of published reports (Parra, 1996; Colberg et al, 1997; Coblentz and Theodorescu, 2002; Bouchot et al, 2004; d'Ancona et al, 2004).

Morbidity after modified complete inguinal lymphadenectomy consists primarily of minor complications including seroma or lymphocele (0% to 26%), lymphorrhea (9% to 10%), and wound infection or skin necrosis (0% to 15%). These have been self-limited in the majority of patients (Parra, 1996; Coblentz and Theodorescu, 2002; Jacobellis, 2003; Bouchot et al, 2004; d'Ancona et al, 2004; Spiess et al, 2009). Lower extremity edema has been reported in 0%

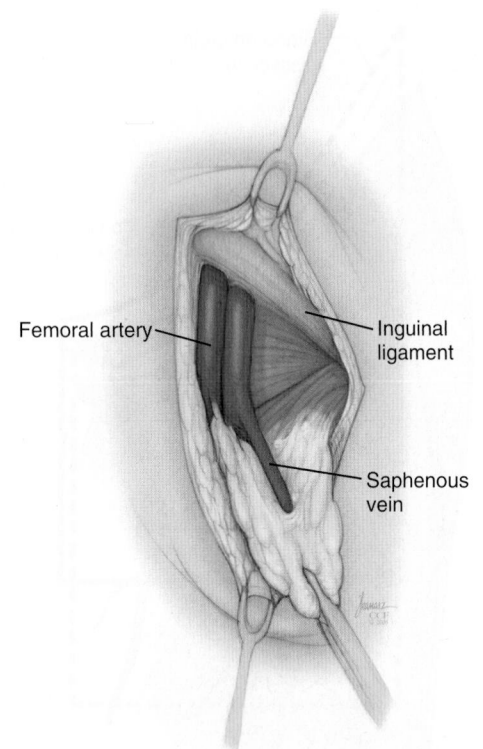

Figure 39-7. Modified inguinal lymphadenectomy. Lymph node packet is medial to the femoral artery and includes superficial and deep inguinal nodes. (Reprinted with permission, Cleveland Clinic Center for Medical Art & Photography © 2003-2010. All rights reserved.)

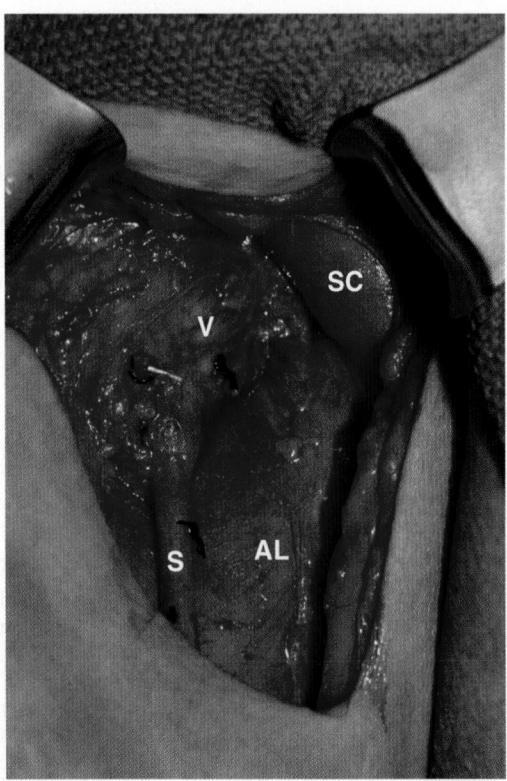

Figure 39-8. Intraoperative photograph of right inguinal region after modified lymphadenectomy. AL, adductor longus; S, saphenous vein; SC, spermatic cord; V, femoral vein.

to 36% of patients, and persistent clinically significant edema is uncommon.

The primary use of both superficial and modified complete inguinal lymphadenectomy currently is in patients with a primary tumor that places them at increased risk for inguinal metastasis and clinically negative groins on examination (stage T2 or greater, presence of vascular or lymphatic invasion, or high grade). These procedures allow for a more thorough assessment of the superficial inguinal nodal basin, do not require specialized equipment, and are associated with less morbidity than standard inguinal lymphadenectomy. If nodal metastasis is detected on frozen-section examination of the specimen, the procedure is converted to a standard radical IFLND.

Endoscopic and Robotic Inguinal Lymphadenectomy

Background

Endoscopic inguinal lymphadenectomy is a more recent technique with the potential for thorough excision of inguinal nodes with decreased morbidity. Bishoff and colleagues were first to report the use of endoscopic inguinal node dissection, in two cadavers and one patient with penile cancer (Bishoff et al, 2003). The patient required conversion to an open procedure because of inability to adequately mobilize the nodal mass superiorly. In 2006 Tobias-Machado and coworkers reported 10 patients who underwent bilateral lymphadenectomy for nonpalpable inguinal nodes. Standard open lymphadenectomy was performed on one side, and endoscopic on the other. Nodal counts were similar, with 20% complications on the endoscopic side, compared with 70% with open surgery (Tobias-Machado et al, 2006). Sotelo and colleagues reported the outcomes after 14 inguinal endoscopic lymphadenectomies in eight patients with clinical stage T2 squamous cell carcinoma of the penis, with a median operative time of 91 minutes and an average node yield of nine. No wound-related complications occurred (Sotelo et al, 2007). A detailed analysis of immediate and long-term complications using the Clavien classification system in 29 patients undergoing 41 endoscopic inguinal lymphadenectomy procedures revealed minor complications in 27%, and major complications in 14.6% (Master et al, 2012). There were no perioperative deaths. Similar experience has been reported in two recent smaller studies, demonstrating a yield of approximately 7 to 15 lymph nodes per groin and a 20% rate of seroma or lymphocele managed conservatively (Pahwa et al, 2013; Zhou et al, 2013).

In 2009, the first staged bilateral endoscopic operation performed robotically was reported (Josephson et al, 2009). Pathologic examination revealed no metastatic involvement in six superficial and four deep lymph nodes. The contralateral dissection occurred weeks later, and pathologic examination revealed five superficial and four deep negative nodes. There were no wound problems or lower extremity edema. Sotelo and colleagues reported performance of a bilateral procedure without repositioning the robot. Metastatic nodes were present bilaterally, with a yield of 19 lymph nodes on the right and 14 on the left (Sotelo et al, 2013). Matin and colleagues performed a thorough evaluation of the adequacy of a robotic inguinal lymph node dissection by subsequently opening the incision and having a second surgical oncologist look for unretrieved residual nodal tissue in 10 patients. The verifying surgeon's role was to inspect the surgical field to ensure that no additional superficial inguinal lymph nodes (e.g., above the fascia lata of the thigh) remained within the operative field. If additional tissue was removed at that time, it was sent for pathologic analysis to define whether it was nodal in origin and whether it contained metastasis. In one of these groins, two residual lymph nodes were recovered from below the Scarpa fascia along the superficial aspect of the inguinal field near the spermatic cord. No metastases were detected in these additional nodes. Among all patients undergoing robotic dissection, 18 of 19 fields (94.7%) were adequately dissected (Matin et al, 2013).

In summary, there is evidence to suggest that the morbidity of an endoscopic inguinal lymph node dissection is lower than

previously reported for open contemporary series with a similar number of nodes being harvested. The applicability of the robot is a more recent development and will need continued prospective evaluation in comparison with standard laparoscopic endoscopic procedures.

Surgical Technique

The patient is positioned on a split-leg table or in low lithotomy position to allow bilateral groin dissection without repositioning the robot. The assistant stands lateral to the right leg for a right-sided dissection and between the legs for the left side (Figs. 39-9 and 39-10). A Foley catheter is inserted in sterile fashion, after the inguinal and groin areas have been prepared and draped. Bony and soft tissue landmarks are marked on the skin surface, creating an inverted triangle in which the base is a line connecting the anterior superior iliac spine to the pubic tubercle, along the course of the inguinal ligament. The lateral boundary is the sartorius muscle angling toward the apex. The medial boundary is the adductor longus muscle, again extending toward the apex. These marks aid in correct trocar placement as well as in delineating the extent of dissection (Figs. 39-11 and 39-12).

A 2-cm incision is made 3 cm below the inferior aspect of the femoral triangle, approximately 25 cm below the inguinal ligament. A white subcutaneous layer is identified, which corresponds to the Scarpa fascia. Sweeping finger dissection is used to dissect the potential space beneath the Scarpa fascia to develop the skin flaps at the apex of the triangle out in both directions to two additional 8-mm ports (Fig. 39-13). These two primary robotic 8-mm ports are placed with finger-guided techniques laterally and medially. A

subcutaneous workspace is extended with the endoscope by sweeping with the lens itself (Fig. 39-14). The aim of this step is to create a superficial subcutaneous flap under the Scarpa fascia (Fig. 39-15). Alternatively, after the initial finger dissection, a 12-mm Origin balloon port trocar may be used (Origin Medsystems, Menlo Park, CA), set at 25 mm Hg for 10 minutes to create the space (Master et al, 2009). The workspace is then expanded with CO_2 insufflation at a pressure of 15 mm Hg. A 0-degree 10-mm lens is inserted, and one additional intervening 10-mm assistant port is placed between the camera and primary 8-mm working port on the assistant side. The robotic docking is performed as shown in Figures 39-9 and 39-10. The robot is located at 45 degrees contralateral to the first procedure (right side) and lateral to the patient in the second procedure (left side).

Our instrument preference is bipolar Maryland, or PK forceps in the left robotic arm, and monopolar scissors in the right arm to dissect the membranous and lymphatic tissue just deep to the Camper fascia. Every effort is made to completely develop the anterior working space to the inguinal ligament. The inguinal ligament is usually identified at the end of this dissection as being a transverse structure with white fibers, marking the superior limit of the dissection (Fig. 39-16). The boundaries of the dissection extend from the inguinal ligament superiorly, the sartorius muscle laterally, and the adductor longus muscle medially. One will be able to spare the saphenous vein in most patients, and the small branches of the femoral artery and vein may be clipped and divided (see Fig. 39-16). Identification of the adductor longus and sartorius muscles is facilitated by identifying the fascia of the respective muscles and correlating this to the previously made skin markings. The medial spermatic cord is seen medially. Inadvertent dissection

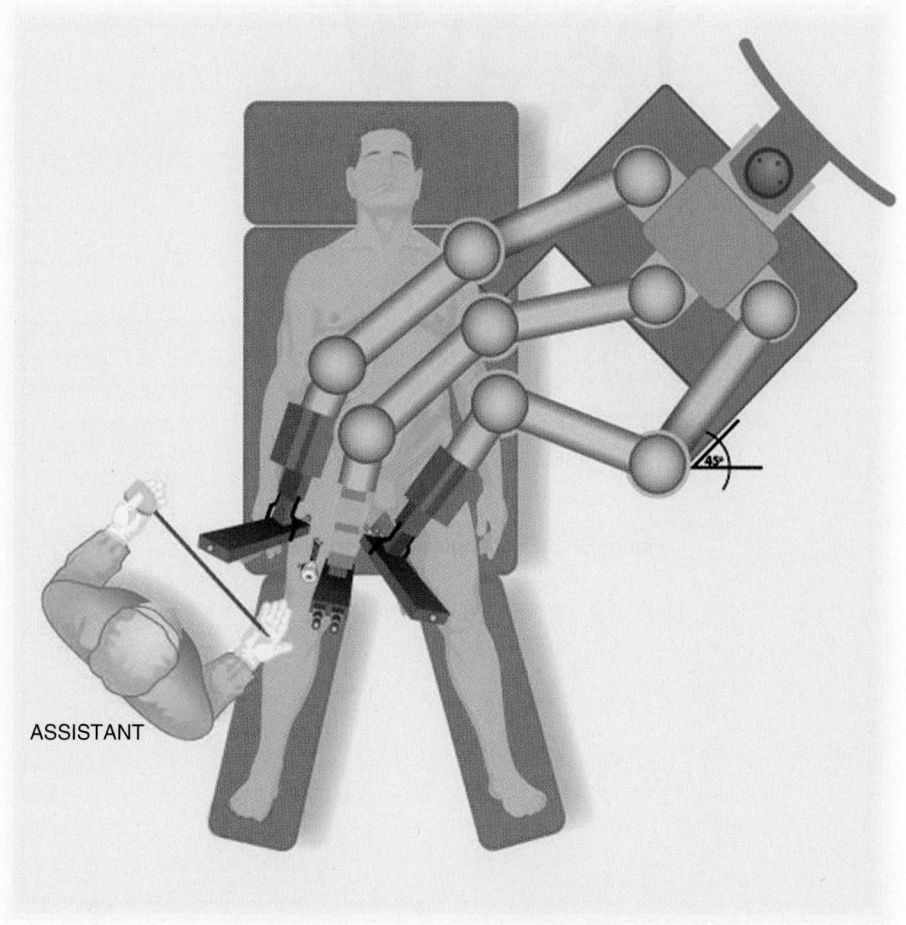

ASSISTANT

Figure 39-9. **Assistant position and robotic docking for right inguinal node dissection.**

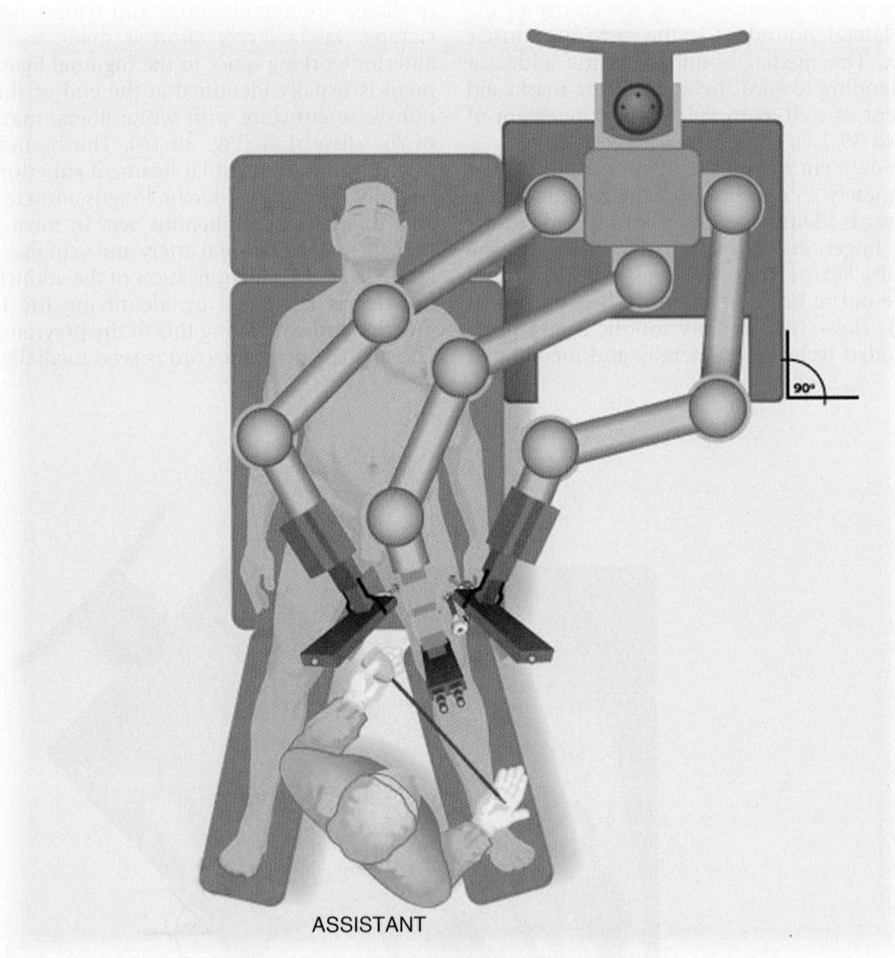

90°

ASSISTANT

Figure 39-10. **Left inguinal node dissection.**

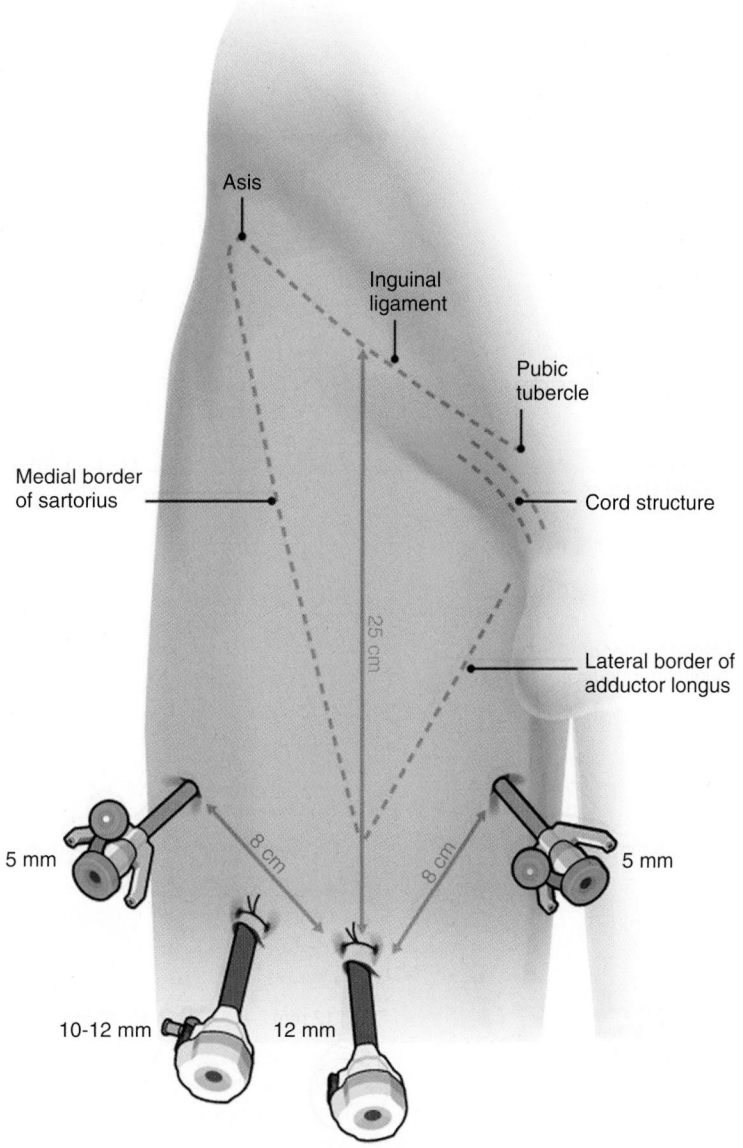

Figure 39-11. Landmarks and trocar placement for right inguinal node dissection.

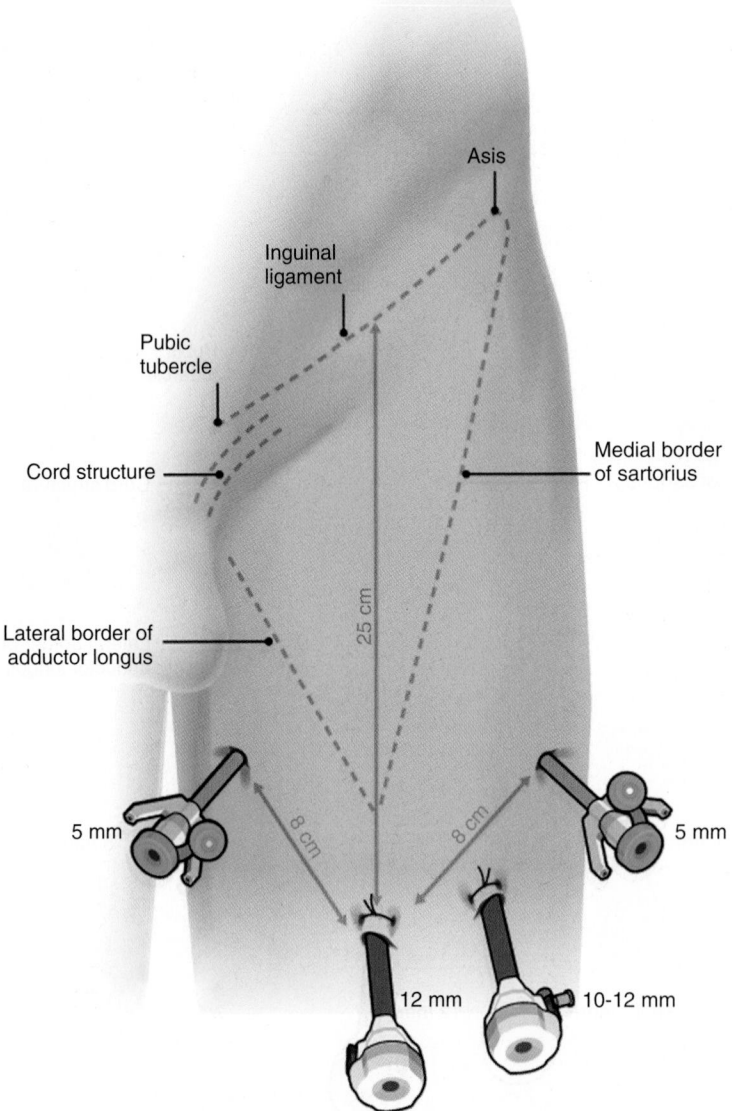

Figure 39-12. **Left inguinal node dissection.**

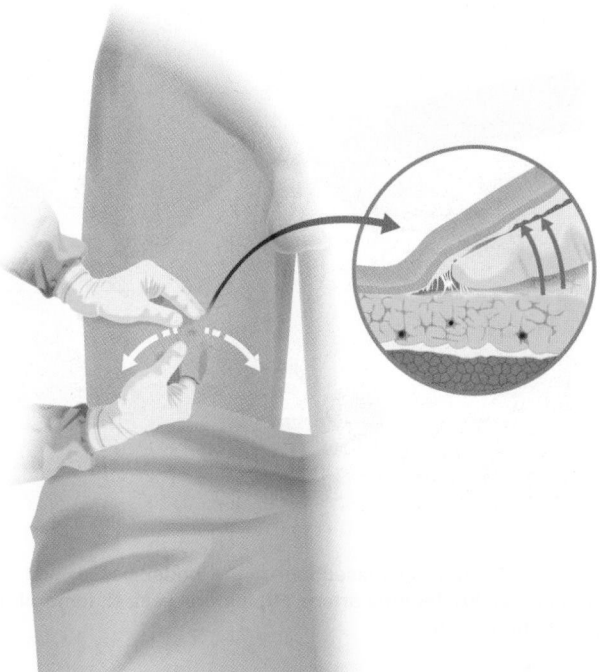

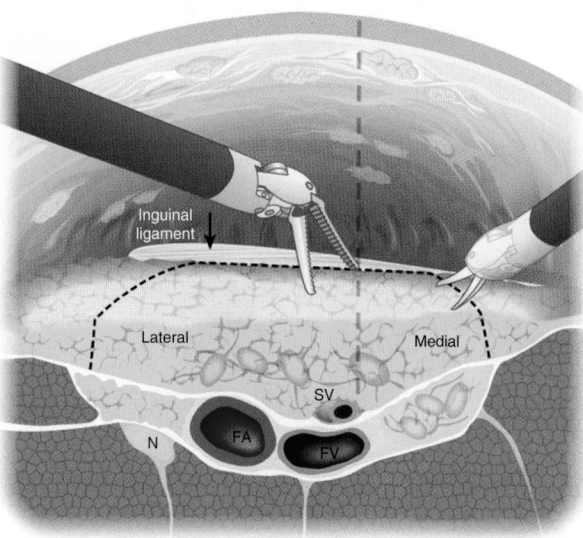

Figure 39-15. A superficial subcutaneous space is created under Scarpa fascia. FA, femoral artery; FV, femoral vein; N, femoral nerve; SV, saphenous vein.

Figure 39-13. Sweeping finger dissection dissects the potential space beneath Scarpa fascia to develop the skin flaps at the apex of the triangle.

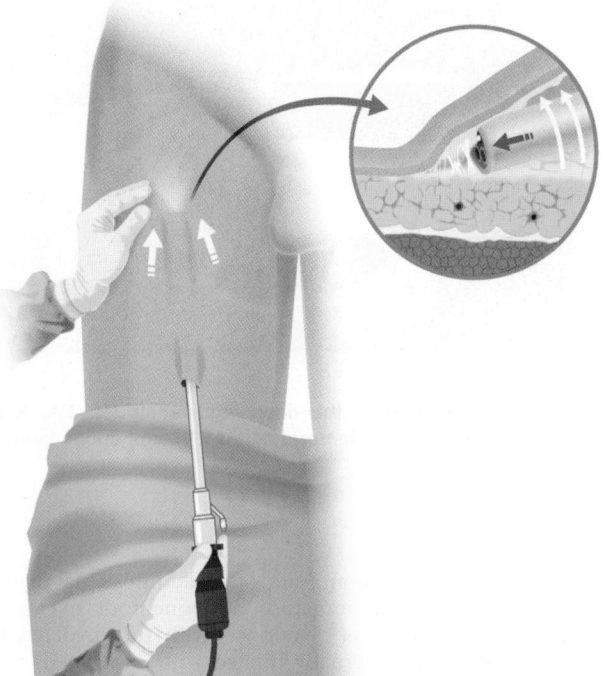

Figure 39-14. The subcutaneous workspace is extended with the endoscope by sweeping with the lens.

deep to the fascia lata is apparent when reddish muscular fibers are seen.

With blunt dissection, the nodal tissue can be rolled inward on both sides. This maneuver is continued inferiorly as much as possible from both sides to define the inferior apex of the nodal packet. The saphenous vein will be identified as it crosses the internal border of the dissection near the apex of the femoral triangle, and

following the vein leads the surgeon to the saphenous arch until its junction with the superficial femoral vein at the fossa ovalis. The dissection continues superiorly, where the packet is dissected off the fascia lata with a combination of sharp and blunt dissection. Typically the nondominant hand lifts the packet, and the monopolar scissors in the dominant hand advance the dissection. After the fossa ovalis is encountered, the packet is dissected away at its superolateral and superomedial limits, thereby narrowing the packet and pulling it away from the inguinal ligament. At this point the superficial and deep plane of dissection join and separate the package from the inguinal ligament (Fig. 39-17).

With the nodal packet circumferentially dissected except for its attachments to the saphenous arch, venous tributaries are clipped. Characteristic pulsations of the femoral artery serve as a nearby landmark. If possible, the packet will be released from the saphenous vein. If not, the vein can be ligated in the saphenous arch with Weck clips or an endovascular stapler. One must always attempt to preserve the saphenous vein whenever possible, however, to reduce the risk of postoperative lymphedema (Zhang et al, 2007).

The specimen is removed in an Endo Catch bag after extension of the camera trocar incision. Frozen section results determine whether a deep ipsilateral dissection will be required. We typically begin to create the working space in the other leg while waiting for results.

For the deep inguinal node dissection, the pneumoperitoneum is reestablished. The fascia lata medial to the saphenous arch is opened to expose the saphenofemoral junction. Inferomedial dissection around the femoral vein enables resection of the deep inguinal nodes (Master et al, 2009). This should be continued to the level of the femoral canal until the pectineus muscle is seen to ensure complete nodal retrieval (Fig. 39-18).

Insufflation pressure is then decreased to 5 mm Hg to confirm hemostasis. It is of great importance that meticulous control of lymphatics and excellent hemostasis be established to further reduce the risk of formation of lymphocele and/or hematoma, which could potentially become infected. A closed suction drain is positioned in the most dependent (caudal) portion of the lymphadenectomy field such that fluid tends to find the drain when the patient is upright. Trocar incisions are closed in standard fashion. The patient is allowed to ambulate the day of surgery and given a regular diet. Discharge is planned for the first postoperative day. A compressive elastic girdle, used for liposuction patients, is used to provide bilateral compression of the groins. In addition, elastic compression stockings are worn simultaneously and are used for 3

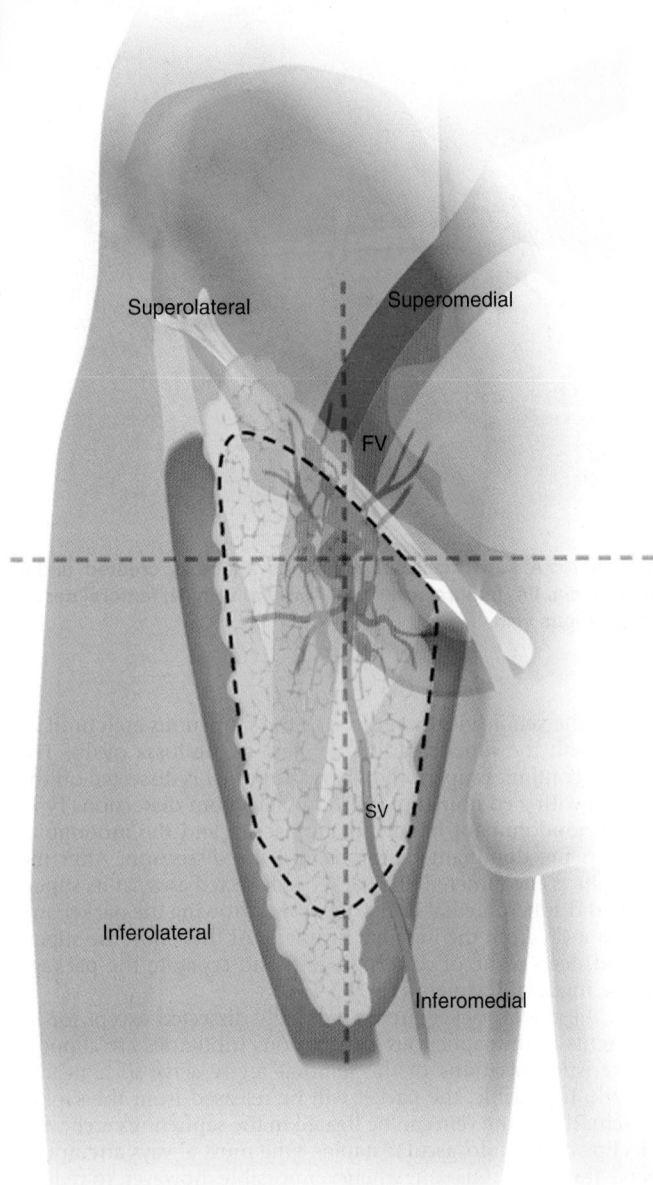

Figure 39-16. Boundaries of the inguinal node dissection. FV, femoral vein; SV, saphenous vein.

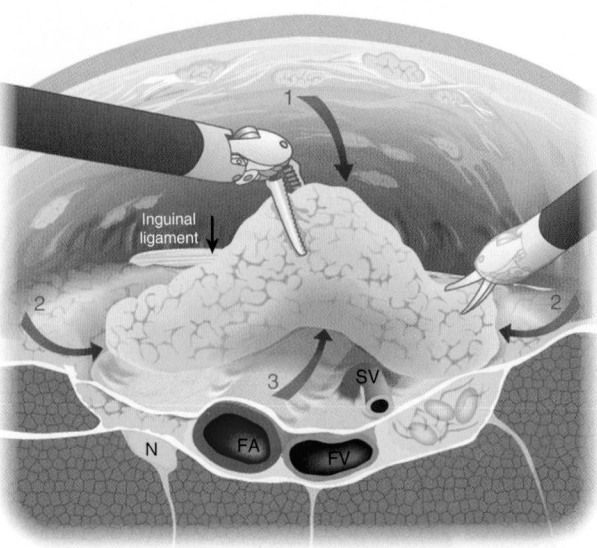

Figure 39-17. Steps in dissection of the nodal tissue; see corresponding text. FA, femoral artery; FV, femoral vein; N, femoral nerve; SV, saphenous vein.

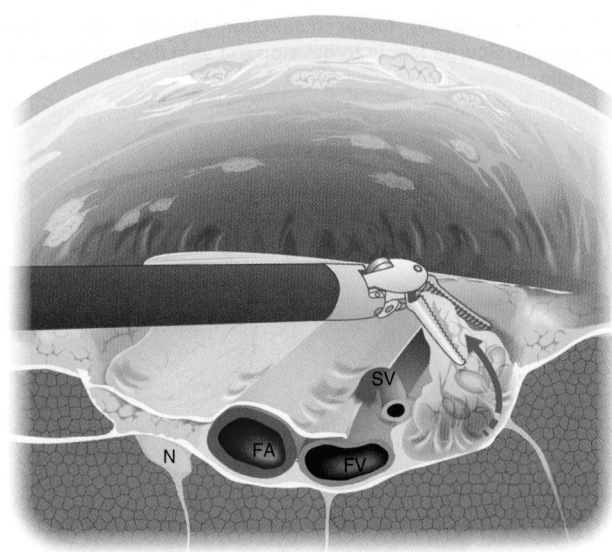

Figure 39-18. Resection of the deep inguinal nodes. FA, femoral artery; FV, femoral vein; N, femoral nerve; SV, saphenous vein.

months after surgery (Fig. 39-19). Broad-spectrum antibiotics are continued until after drains have been removed. Drains typically stay in place until the output is less than 50 mL per 24-hour period. All patients receive venous thromboembolism prophylaxis using fractionated or low-molecular-weight heparin.

Palpable Inguinal Adenopathy or Positive Inguinal Nodes

Radical Inguinofemoral Lymph Node Dissection

Radical IFLND is indicated in patients with resectable metastatic adenopathy and may be curative when the disease is limited to the inguinal nodes. We have also favored its use as a palliative procedure in patients with documented inguinal metastasis who are fit for surgery. If left unchecked, cancer-bearing inguinal nodes may lead to significant complications, such as infection or abscess with chronic foul-smelling drainage or life-threatening femoral hemor-

rhage (Fig. 39-20). Antibiotics are often administered preoperatively to reduce the inflammatory component of the regional adenopathy. The patient is positioned with the involved thigh slightly abducted and externally rotated with cushioned support under the flexed knee.

The inguinofemoral dissection is designed to cover an area outlined superiorly by a line drawn from the superior margin of the external ring to the anterior superior iliac spine, laterally by a line drawn from the anterior superior iliac spine extending 20 cm inferiorly, and medially by a line drawn from the pubic tubercle 15 cm down the medial thigh. In most situations the procedure is carried out through an oblique incision approximately 3 cm below and parallel to the inguinal ligament and extending from the lateral to the medial limit of the dissection (Fig. 39-21). If an area of the skin overlying the cancer-bearing nodes is invaded or adherent and requires excision, an elliptical incision is made around the involved skin and then extended medially and laterally. In this setting, the

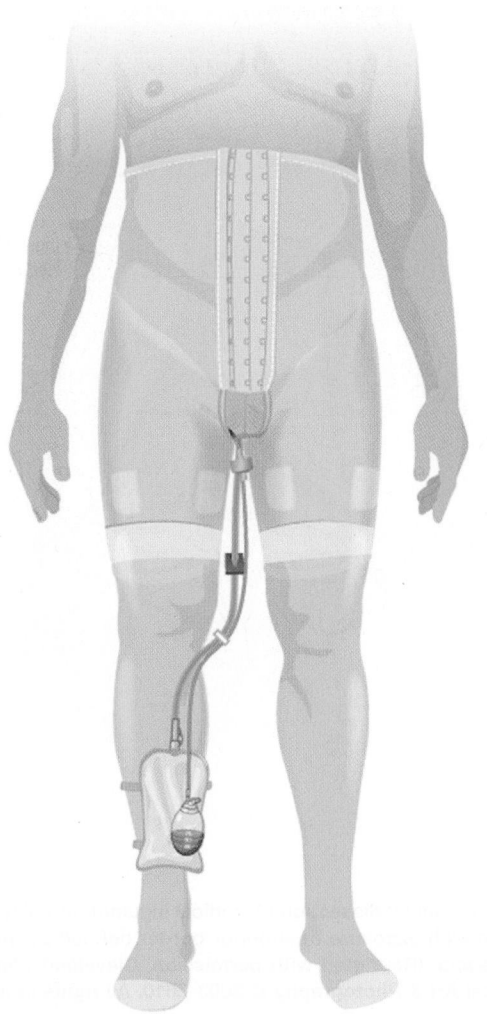

Figure 39-19. A compressive elastic girdle and elastic compression stockings are placed postoperatively.

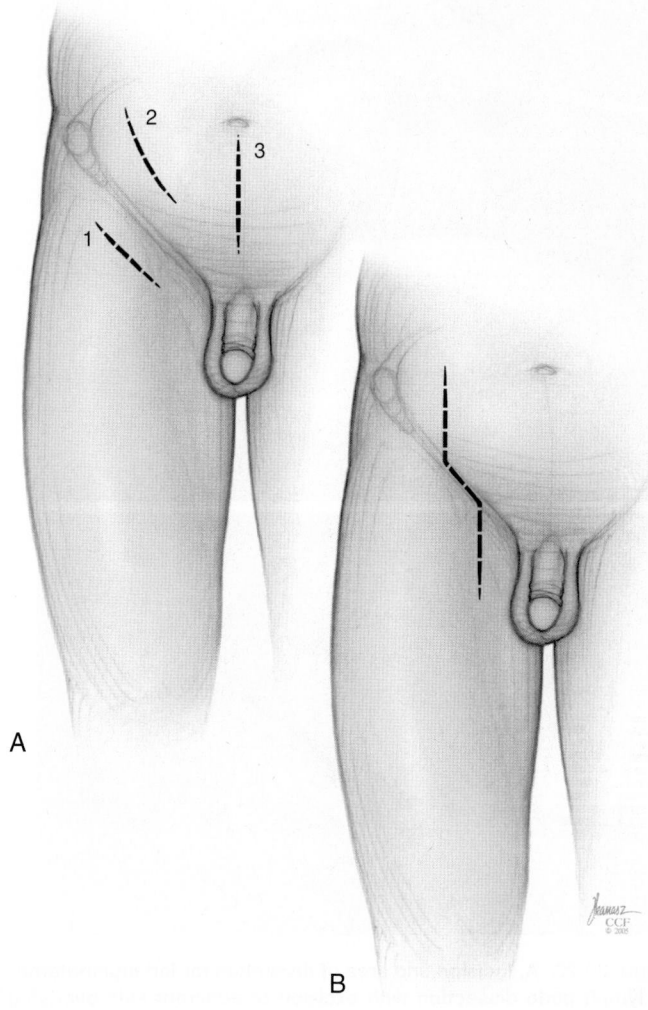

Figure 39-21. Ilioinguinal lymph node dissection. A, Incisions for inguinofemoral lymph node dissection (1), unilateral pelvic lymph node dissection (2), and bilateral pelvic lymph node dissection (3). B, Single-incision approach for ilioinguinal lymph node dissection. (Reprinted with permission, Cleveland Clinic Center for Medical Art & Photography © 2003-2010. All rights reserved.)

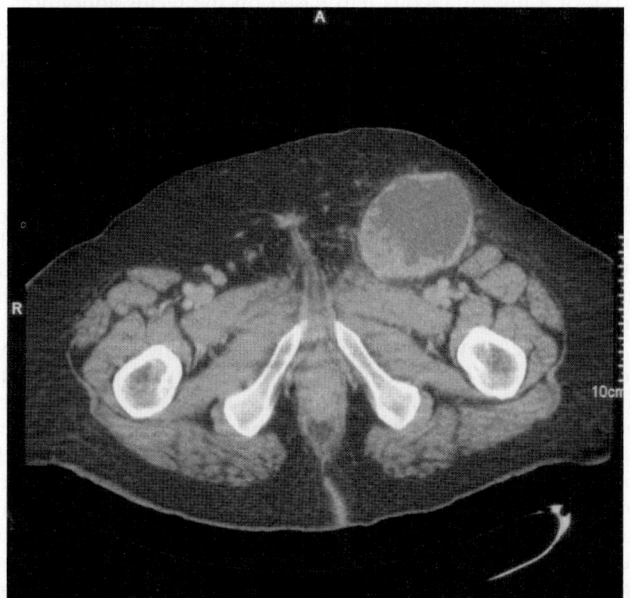

Figure 39-20. Pelvic computed tomographic scan of patient with penile carcinoma demonstrating large left inguinal metastasis overlying the femoral vessels.

incision may alternatively be extended superiorly from the lateral border of the ellipse and inferiorly from the medial border to make a single S-shaped incision for the iliac and inguinofemoral dissections (Fig. 39-22).

Superior and inferior skin flaps are developed in the plane just below the Scarpa fascia. The superior flap is elevated cephalad to a point 4 cm above the inguinal ligament, and the inferior flap to the limit of the dissection. The fat and areolar tissues are dissected from the external oblique aponeurosis and the spermatic cord to the inferior border of the inguinal ligament, forming the superior boundary of the lymph node packet (Fig. 39-23). The inferior angle of the inguinofemoral exposure is at the apex of the femoral triangle, where the long saphenous vein is identified and divided. In patients with minimal metastatic disease, it may be feasible and beneficial to spare the saphenous vein, and this should be considered (Fig. 39-24). Dissection is deepened through the fascia lata overlying the sartorius muscle laterally and the thinner fascia covering the adductor longus muscle medially. At the apex of the femoral triangle, the femoral artery and vein are identified, and dissection is continued superiorly along the femoral vessels. Superficial cutaneous perforating arteries are ligated as they are encountered on the

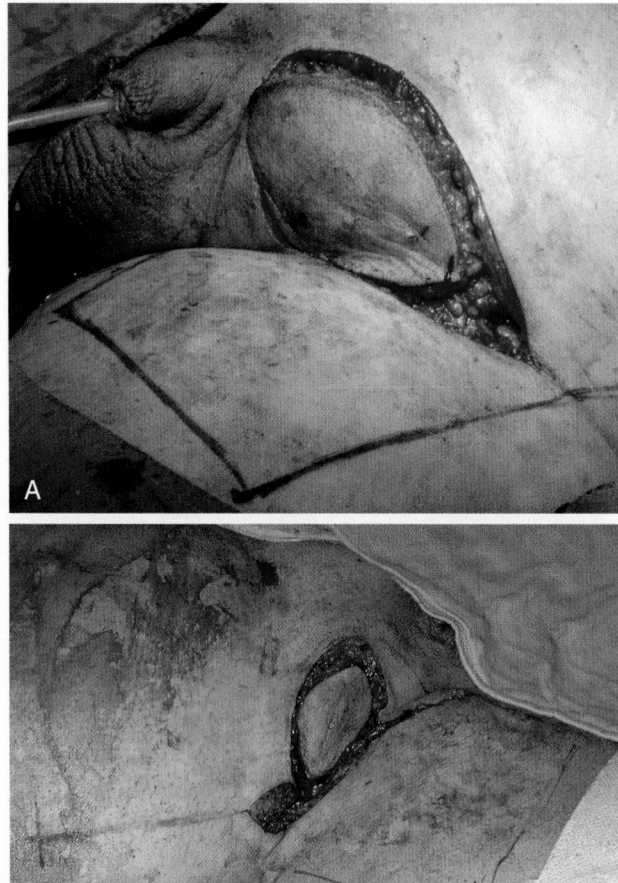

Figure 39-22. A, Incision and area of dissection for left inguinofemoral lymph node dissection with excision of adherent skin overlying nodal mass. **B,** Single-incision approach and area of dissection for right ilioinguinal lymph node dissection with excision of overlying skin.

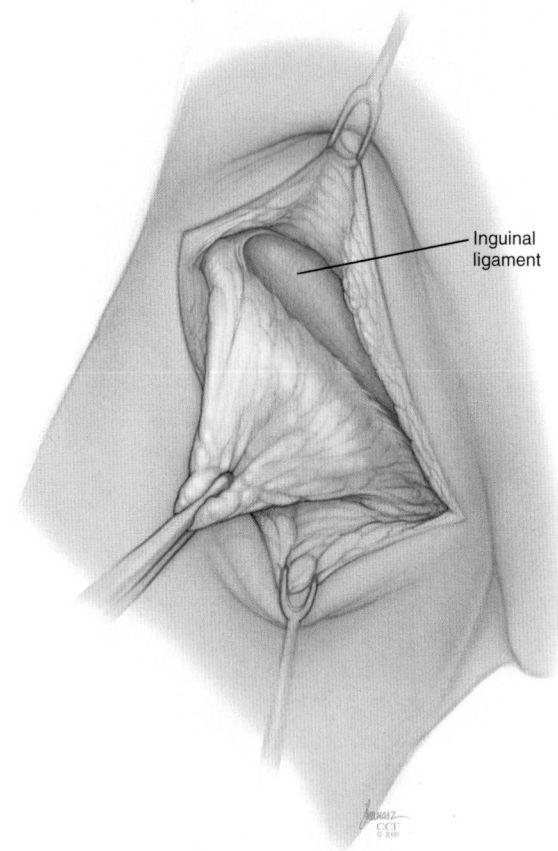

Inguinal ligament

Figure 39-23. Initial dissection for radical inguinofemoral lymph node dissection with exposure of superior border defined by the external oblique fascia. (Reprinted with permission, Cleveland Clinic Center for Medical Art & Photography © 2003-2010. All rights reserved.)

surface of the femoral artery. The saphenous vein is divided at the saphenofemoral junction, and the dissection is continued superiorly to include the deep inguinal nodes medial and lateral to the femoral vein until continuity with the pelvic dissection is attained at the femoral canal (Fig. 39-25). The anterior aspects of the femoral vessels are dissected, but the femoral vessels are not skeletonized, and the lateral surface of the femoral artery is not exposed. This avoids injury to the femoral nerve and the profunda femoris artery, and the femoral nerve is usually not visible as it runs beneath the iliacus fascia.

After the femoral triangle is dissected (Fig. 39-26), the sartorius muscle is mobilized from its origin at the anterior superior iliac spine and either transposed or rolled 180 degrees medially to cover the femoral vessels. The muscle is sutured to the inguinal ligament superiorly, and its margins are sutured to the muscles of the thigh immediately adjacent to the femoral vessels (Fig. 39-27). The femoral canal is closed, if necessary, by suturing the shelving edge of the Poupart ligament to the Cooper ligament, being careful not to compromise the lumen of the external iliac vein or to injure the inferior epigastric vessels in the process. Primary closure of the inguinofemoral dissection is usually possible with minimal or no further mobilization of the excision margins. When circumstances demand a large area of inguinal soft tissue sacrifice, primary closure may be obtained by scrotal skin rotation flaps (Skinner, 1974), an abdominal wall advancement flap (Tabatabaei and McDougal,

2003), or a myocutaneous flap based on the rectus abdominis or tensor fasciae latae (Airhart et al, 1982) for more extensive defects.

Closed-suction drains are placed under the subcutaneous tissue and brought out inferiorly. During closure, the skin flaps are sutured to the surface of the exposed musculature to decrease dead space. The skin is closed with absorbable subcutaneous sutures and staples. The patient is maintained on bed rest for 2 or 3 days, and pneumatic compression stockings are used. The drains are removed after 5 to 7 days, when drainage is less than 30 to 40 mL/day. Compression stockings are recommended postoperatively. We maintain the patient on a suppressive dose of a cephalosporin for 1 to 2 months until healed to decrease the incidence of erythema and cellulitis, and this seems to improve overall wound healing.

In the past, complications related to radical ilioinguinal lymphadenectomy have been significant. In contemporary series, early minor complications have been reported in 40% to 56% of dissections (Bevan-Thomas et al, 2002; Bouchot et al, 2004; Nelson et al, 2004; Spiess et al, 2009). These consist primarily of lymphocele, wound infection or necrosis, and lymphedema. Major complications, such as debilitating lymphedema, flap necrosis, and lymphocele requiring intervention, occur in 5% to 21% of patients (Bevan-Thomas et al, 2002; Nelson et al, 2004). Deep venous thrombosis (DVT) or pulmonary embolism (PE) has been reported in 4% to 7% of patients (Johnson and Lo, 1984; Ravi, 1993; Spiess et al, 2009). Efforts to minimize lower extremity lymphedema include early use of compression stockings and saphenous vein preservation when feasible. With regard to DVT and PE, sequential

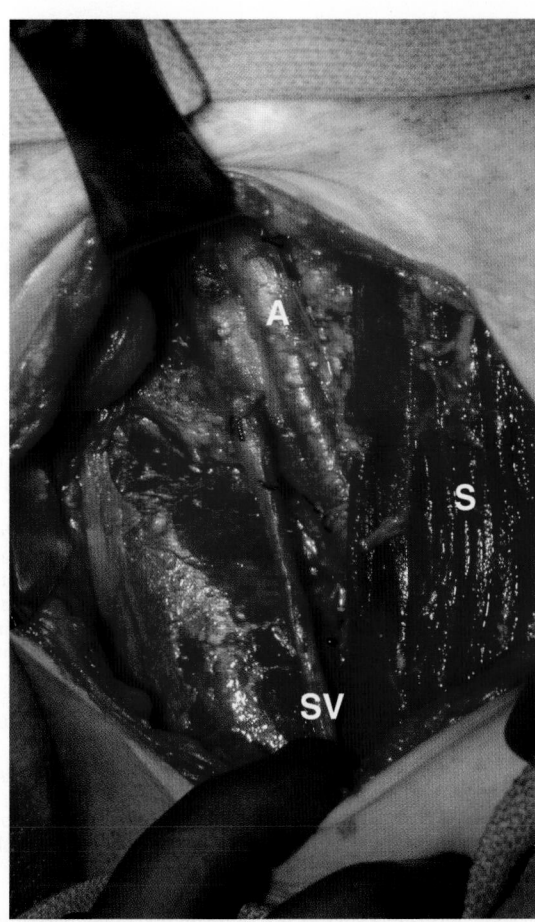

Figure 39-24. Intraoperative photograph after saphenous-sparing, radical, left inguinofemoral lymph node dissection. A, femoral artery; S, sartorius muscle; SV, saphenous vein.

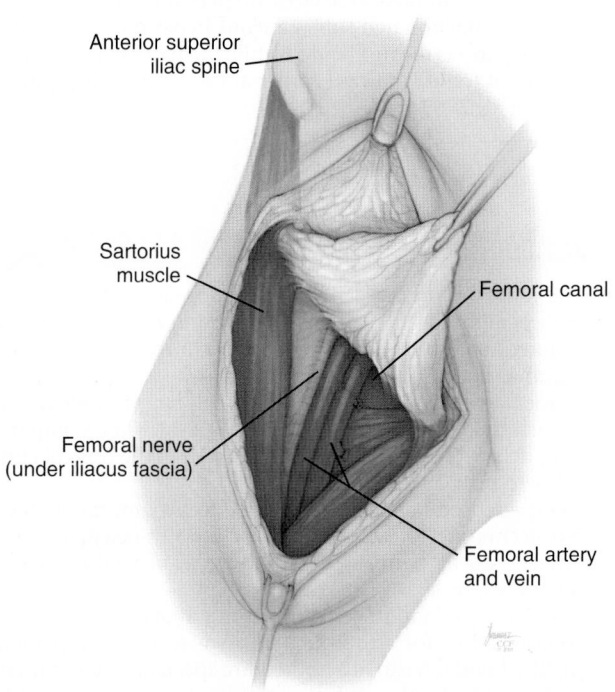

Figure 39-25. Inferior dissection during radical inguinofemoral lymph node dissection with removal of lymph node packet from the inferior border of the femoral triangle. After further lateral and medial dissection, the packet will remain in continuity with the pelvic dissection in the area of the femoral canal. (Reprinted with permission, Cleveland Clinic Center for Medical Art & Photography © 2003-2010. All rights reserved.)

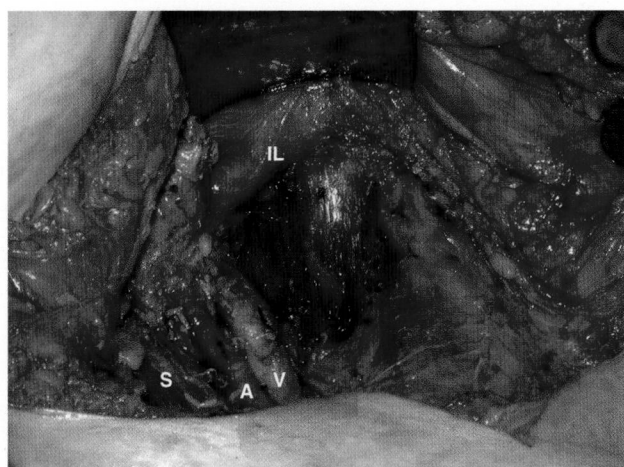

Figure 39-26. Intraoperative photograph after right radical inguinofemoral lymph node dissection in an obese patient. A, femoral artery; IL, inguinal ligament; S, sartorius muscle; V, femoral vein.

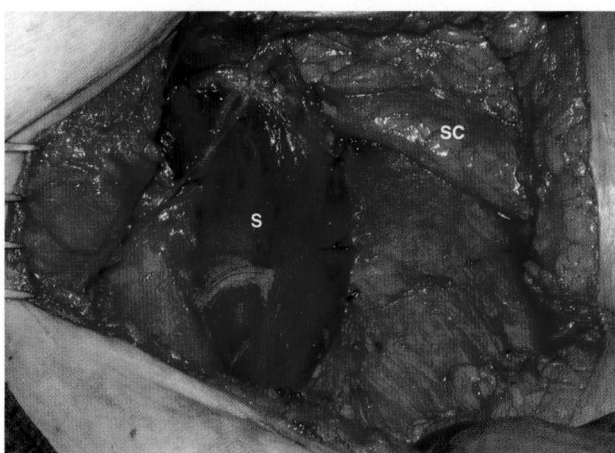

Figure 39-27. Sartorius muscle after detachment from the anterior superior iliac spine and 180-degree rotation medially, with suture fixation to the fascia of the inguinal ligament and the adductor longus. S, sartorius muscle; SC, spermatic cord.

lower extremity compression devices are placed before surgery. Use of prophylactic fractionated subcutaneous heparin or low-molecular-weight heparin is recommended while the patient is on bed rest, and the current trend is toward earlier ambulation when appropriate (Spiess et al, 2009).

KEY POINTS

- The most important factor determining survival in patients with penile cancer is the extent of lymph node metastases.
- Approximately 20% of patients with clinically nonpalpable inguinal nodes harbor occult metastases.
- Immediate resection of clinically occult lymph node metastases is associated with improved survival when compared with delayed resection of involved nodes at the time of clinical detection.
- In experienced hands, DSNB is an effective minimally invasive technique for assessment of clinically negative groins and should be performed with the goal of a false-negative rate of 5% or less.
- Superficial and modified complete inguinal lymph node dissections allow for a thorough assessment of the superficial inguinal nodal basin, do not require specialized equipment, and are associated with less morbidity than radical inguinal lymphadenectomy.
- There is early evidence to suggest that the morbidity of an endoscopic inguinal lymph node dissection may be lower than previously reported for open contemporary series with a similar number of nodes being harvested.
- Radical IFLND is indicated in patients with resectable metastatic adenopathy and may be curative when the disease is limited to the inguinal nodes.
- Penile cancer metastases to the pelvic lymph nodes do not occur in the setting of negative ipsilateral inguinal nodes.

REFERENCES

The complete reference list is available online at www.expertconsult.com.

SUGGESTED READINGS

Catalona WJ. Modified inguinal lymphadenectomy for carcinoma of the penis with preservation of saphenous veins: technique and preliminary results. J Urol 1988;140:306–10.

Djajadiningrat RS, Graafland NM, van Werkhoven E, et al. Contemporary management of regional nodes in penile cancer—improvement in survival? J Urol 2014;191:68–73.

Hagarty PK, Dinney CP, Pettaway CA. Controversies in ilioinguinal lymphadenectomy. Urol Clin North Am 2010;37:421–34.

Kroon BK, Horenblas S, Lont AP, et al. Patients with penile carcinoma benefit from immediate resection of clinically occult lymph node metastases. J Urol 2005;173:816–9.

Lam W, Alnajjar HM, La-Touche S, et al. Dynamic sentinel lymph node biopsy in patients with invasive squamous cell carcinoma of the penis: a prospective study of the long-term outcome of 500 inguinal basins assessed at a single institution. Eur Urol 2013;63:657–63.

Master VA, Jafri SM, Moses KA, et al. Minimally invasive inguinal lymphadenectomy via endoscopic groin dissection: comprehensive assessment of immediate and long-term complications. J Urol 2012;188:1176–80.

Matin SF, Cormier JN, Ward JF, et al. Phase 1 prospective evaluation of the oncological adequacy of robotic assisted video-endoscopic inguinal lymphadenectomy in patients with penile carcinoma. BJU Int 2013;111:1068–74.

McDougal WS, Kirchner FK, Edwards RH, et al. Treatment of carcinoma of the penis: the case for primary lymphadenectomy. J Urol 1986;136:38–41.

Pizzocaro G, Algaba F, Horenblas S, et al. EAU penile cancer guidelines 2009. Eur Urol 2010;57:1002–12.

Sadeghi R, Gholami H, Zakavi SR, et al. Accuracy of sentinel lymph node biopsy for inguinal lymph node staging of penile squamous cell carcinoma: systematic review and meta-analysis of the literature. J Urol 2012;187:23–31.

Spiess PE, Hernandez MS, Pettaway CA. Contemporary inguinal lymph node dissection: minimizing complications. World J Urol 2009;27:205–12.

Wood HM, Angermeier KW. Anatomic considerations of the penis, lymphatic drainage, and biopsy of the sentinel node. Urol Clin North Am 2010;37:327–34.

40 Surgery of the Penis and Urethra

Kurt A. McCammon, MD, FACS, Jack M. Zuckerman, MD,
and Gerald H. Jordan, MD, FACS, FAAP (Hon), FRCS (Hon)

Improvements in microsurgery, tissue transfer techniques, and tissue handling have expanded the repertoire of the urologic surgeon and the genitourinary reconstructive surgeon in particular. Urologists are now able to reconstruct congenital and acquired genitourinary abnormalities with greater facility. Microvascular and microneurosurgical techniques have made it possible to construct a phallus that allows a patient to void while standing and to enjoy erotic sensibility. Because the phallus has erotic sensibility and protective sensation, the patient can eventually have a prosthetic implantation that allows an acceptable sexual life. This chapter discusses the general principles of male genital reconstructive surgery; specifics include male urethral surgery, surgery for congenital and traumatic penile lesions, and complex fistula and obliterative issues associated with the posterior urethra.

PRINCIPLES OF RECONSTRUCTIVE SURGERY

Many techniques in reconstructive surgery require the transfer of tissue. Skin is one of those tissues, and **its properties vary from individual to individual and from place to place on the same individual.** Variable characteristics such as color, texture, thickness, extensibility, innate skin tension, and blood supply can be useful in various situations.

The term *tissue transfer* implies the movement of tissue for purposes of reconstruction. In contrast to extirpative surgery, **the transfer of tissue for reconstruction requires an intimate knowledge of the anatomy of the donor and the recipient sites as well as of the principles that allow the tissue to survive after it is transferred.**

The skin can be used as a model. The superficial layer of the skin is termed the *epidermis* (thickness, 0.8 to 1 mm). The deep layer of the skin is termed the *dermis*. The dermis has two layers: a superficial layer, the adventitial dermis (also called the papillary or periadnexal dermis, depending on the anatomy), and a deep layer, the reticular dermis. For genitourinary reconstruction, skin without adnexal structures is often used; the papillary dermis is synonymous with the adventitial dermis. Other tissues commonly transferred for genitourinary reconstruction include bladder and oral mucosa. The bladder epithelium is the superficial layer of the bladder; the deep layer of the bladder is termed the *lamina propria*, with superficial and deep layers. The oral mucosa is the superficial layer of much of the oral cavity, which also has a deeper layer termed the *lamina propria*, again with superficial and deep layers.

All tissue has physical characteristics: extensibility, inherent tension, and the viscoelastic properties of stress relaxation and creep. The physical characteristics of a transferred unit are primarily a function of the helical arrangement of collagen along with the elastin cross-linkages. The collagen-elastin structure is suspended in a mucopolysaccharide matrix that influences the viscoelastic properties.

Tissue can be transferred as a graft (Fig. 40-1). **The term *graft* implies that tissue has been excised and transferred to a graft host bed, where a new blood supply develops by a process termed *take*. Take requires approximately 96 hours and occurs in two phases. The initial phase, imbibition, requires about 48 hours.** During that phase, the graft survives by "drinking" nutrients from the adjacent graft host bed, and the temperature of the graft is less than the core body temperature. **The second phase, inosculation, also requires about 48 hours and is the phase in which true microcirculation is reestablished in the graft.** During that phase, the temperature of the graft increases to core body temperature. The process of take is influenced by the nature of the grafted tissue and the conditions of the graft host bed. Processes that interfere with the vascularity of the graft host bed interfere with graft take.

The epidermal, or epithelial layer, is a covering, the barrier to the "outside," and is adjacent to the superficial dermis, or superficial lamina. At approximately this interface is the superficial plexus. In the case of skin, the plexus is the intradermal plexus. There are some lymphatics in the superficial dermal or tunica layer. On the undersurface of the deep dermal layer or deep lamina is the deep plexus. In the case of skin, this is the subdermal plexus. The deep dermis contains most of the lymphatics and greater collagen content than found in the superficial dermal layer. The deep or reticular dermis is generally thought to account for the physical characteristics of the tissue.

If a graft is a split-thickness unit, it carries the epidermis or the covering. The graft also exposes the superficial dermal (intradermal or intralaminar) plexus. In most grafts, the superficial plexus comprises small but numerous vessels, which **conveys favorable vascular characteristics to a split-thickness unit.** The unit has few lymphatics, and **the physical characteristics are not carried, which accounts for the tendency of split-thickness units to be brittle and less durable.** The reticular dermis is not carried with the split-thickness unit (Jordan, 1993).

A mesh graft is usually an application of the split-thickness graft. After the harvest of a sheet graft, the sheet is placed on a carrier that cuts systematically placed slits in the graft. These slits can expand the graft by various ratios (i.e., 1.5:1, 2:1, 3:1). For

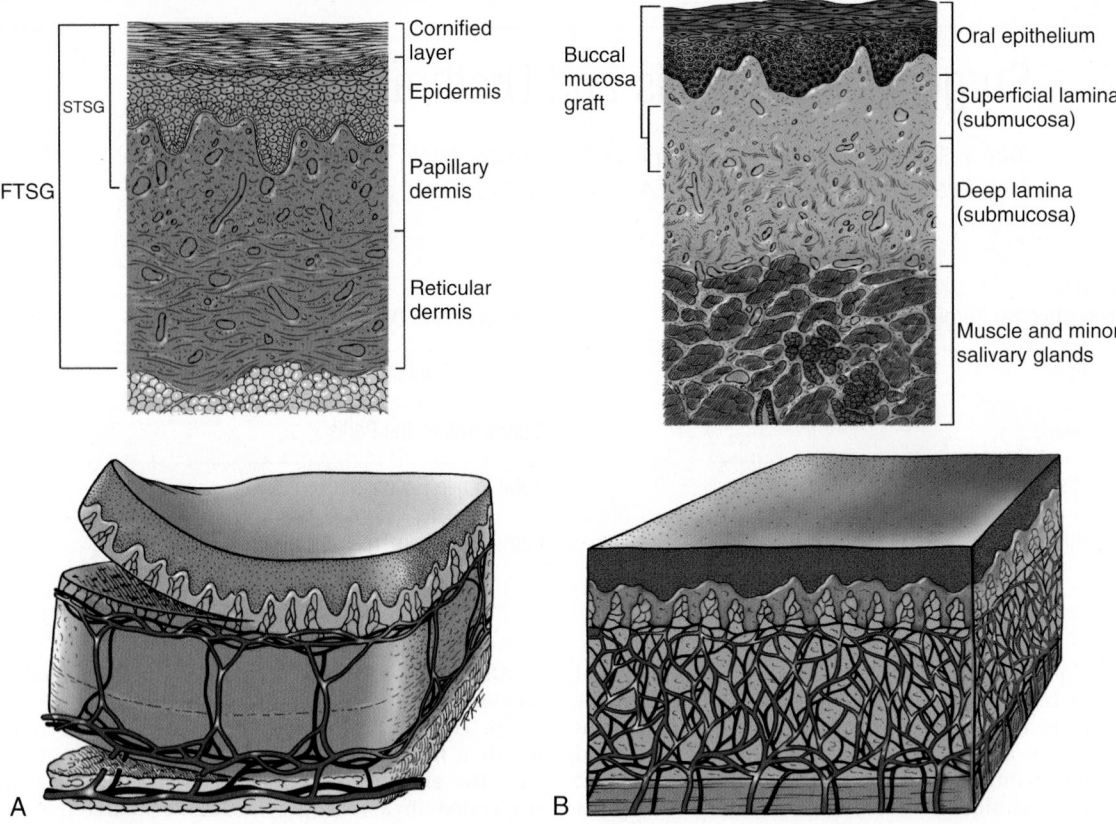

Figure 40-1. Cross-sectional diagrams (histologic appearance above, microvasculature below) of the skin. A, Cross-sectional diagrams of skin. B, Cross-sectional diagrams of oral mucosa. FTSG, full-thickness skin graft; STSG, split-thickness skin graft. (From Jordan GH, Schlossberg SM. Using tissue transfer for urethral reconstruction. Contemp Urol 1993;13:23.)

most genital reconstructive surgery, the slits are not for expansion but rather to allow subgraft collections to escape; in some cases, the slits allow the graft to conform better to irregular graft host beds (e.g., the testes in split-thickness skin graft scrotal construction). It has also been proposed that mesh grafts take readily because of increased levels of growth factors, possibly as a function of the slits. In general, full-thickness skin grafts are not meshed (Schreiter and Koncz, 1983; Jordan, 1993).

If a graft is a full-thickness unit, it carries the covering and the superficial dermis or lamina with all the characteristics attributable to that layer. However, it also carries the deep dermis or deep lamina. In skin, the subdermal plexus is exposed. In most cases, **the plexus is composed of larger vessels that are more sparsely distributed. The graft is fastidious in its vascular characteristics.** A full-thickness unit carries most of the lymphatics, and the physical characteristics are likewise carried with the transferred tissue (Devine et al, 1976; Jordan, 1993; Wessels and McAninch, 1996). Comparing the grafts that are most commonly used in genitourinary reconstructive surgery, **the split-thickness skin graft has favorable vascular characteristics but tends to contract** and be brittle when mature. **The full-thickness skin graft tends to have more fastidious vascular characteristics, but it does not contract as much and is more durable when mature** (see Fig. 40-1A). There is a difference between genital full-thickness skin (penile and preputial skin grafts) and extragenital full-thickness skin. This is probably a reflection of the increased mass of the graft in extragenital skin grafts. This increased mass makes the graft more fastidious, and the poor results reported with urethral reconstruction with extragenital full-thickness skin grafts are probably due to poor or ischemic take (Webster et al, 1984; Webster, 1987; Jordan, 1993). The posterior auricular graft (Wolfe graft) is an exception to the rule concerning extragenital skin. The postauricular skin is thin and

overlies the temporalis fascia and is thought to be carried on numerous perforators. The subdermal plexus of this graft mimics the characteristics of the intradermal plexus, and the total mass of the graft is more like that of the split-thickness unit. In the bladder epithelial graft, there is a superficial and a deep plexus; however, the plexuses are connected by many more perforators. **Bladder epithelial grafts tend to have more favorable vascular characteristics.** In the case of **oral mucosal grafts, there is a panlaminar plexus. The oral mucosal graft can be thinned, provided that a sufficient amount of deep lamina is carried to preserve the physical characteristics** (see Fig. 40-1B). **Oral mucosal grafts are thought to have optimal vascular characteristics** (Humby, 1941; Memmelaar, 1947). The thinned graft diminishes the total graft mass, while preserving the physical characteristics and not adversely affecting the vascular characteristics. The enthusiasm for the buccal mucosal graft seems well founded. The fact that the graft has a "wet epithelial" surface is likewise thought to be a favorable characteristic for many cases of urethral reconstructive surgery. The lingual, labial, and buccal grafts all vary in thickness and in substance. Because the labial mucosal grafts are thin, many surgeons prefer that donor site for reconstruction of the fossa navicularis (Jordan, 1993).

A series by Fichtner and colleagues (2004) reporting the use of "buccal mucosal" onlay grafts with mid-term and long-term results seems to suggest durability for these grafts. In that series, 67 patients were described, all with follow-up exceeding 5 years and some with 10 years of follow-up. All failures occurred within 12 months of the original procedure. More recent studies showed equal results with buccal and lingular grafts (Sharma et al, 2013). **The dermal graft has been used for years to augment the tunica albuginea of the corpora cavernosa.** When it is harvested, the graft exposes the intradermal plexus and the deep dermal plexus. The dermal graft takes readily (is not fastidious) and has the physical characteristics normal to skin. When it is properly prepared, the tunica vaginalis graft is essentially peritoneum. The tendency of peritoneum to take readily is well documented in the literature that examines adhesion formation and in the urology literature concerning the application of peritoneal grafts for reconstruction of the urinary tract. The literature fails to define accurately what the surgeon can expect regarding physical characteristics (Jordan, 1993). **Tunica vaginalis grafts have proved useful for small defects of the tunica albuginea of the corpora cavernosa, but aneurysmal dilation tends to develop when they are used for larger defects. Tunica vaginalis grafts have been tried for urethral reconstruction with uniformly poor results.**

As described in the urologic literature, vein grafts are perhaps not true grafts according to the terminology used in this chapter. Vein patches are widely used in vascular surgery. The premise is that the vein survives by endothelial direct perfusion and reestablishment of vein wall blood flow by perfusion of the vasa vasorum. The vascular literature is at odds with this concept. The intima is the endothelial layer; it is thin and easily injured during the process of vein harvest and preparation, with areas of endothelial sloughing noted. Inflammatory cells and fibrin adhere to the exposed basement membrane. However, the endothelium regenerates in the first 6 weeks. The media is a combination of smooth muscle and interlaced collagen. After graft harvest, smooth muscle injury is prominently noted and is thought to be related to warm ischemia. In more mature grafts, much of the smooth muscle is replaced by a process of fibrous transformation with collagen deposition. The adventitia is a loose collagenous network interspersed with vasa vasorum. Mature vein grafts show evidence of take to the vasa vasorum. However, the adventitia becomes incorporated by periadventitial connective tissues. Thrombosis in the vasa vasorum, early in the process of take, is not an unusual phenomenon. When vein grafts are exposed to arterial pressure and shear stress forces, the process colloquially described as "arterialization" occurs and is associated with changes of the vessel wall elastic properties, and the graft becomes rigid with low compliance. When these changes are noted, at least when veins are used for vessel replacement, the graft remains noncompliant throughout the remaining life of the graft (Szilagyi et al, 1973; Fuchs et al, 1978; Tolhurst and Haeseker, 1982). At the present time, vein "grafts" are being widely used for replacement of defects of the tunica albuginea of the corpora cavernosa. The pertinent points with regard to the transfer of vein patches to the corpora cavernosa and their long-term behavior have been inferred from the current vascular literature. Dermal grafts have been tried for urethral reconstruction, also with generally poor results. **Rectal mucosal grafts also have been proposed for urethral reconstruction, but little is known about their graft take.** In general, the vascularity of the bowel mucosa is based on the vascularity of the underlying muscle, with the mucosa carried on perforators. Little is found in the literature regarding the process of take of these grafts.

Tissue can be transferred as a flap. The term *flap* implies that the tissue is excised and transferred with the blood supply either preserved or surgically reestablished at the recipient site. Flaps can be classified by numerous criteria. Flaps can be classified on the basis of their vascularity and characterized as either random flaps (Fig. 40-2) or axial flaps (Fig. 40-3). A *random flap* is a flap without a defined cuticular vascular territory. The flap is carried on the dermal or laminar plexuses; the dimensions of random flaps can vary widely from individual to individual and from body site to body site. **The term *axial flap* means that there is a defined vessel in the base of the flap. There are three types of axial flaps. The direct cuticular axial flap is a flap based on a vessel superficial to the superficial layer of the deep body wall fascia (see Fig. 40-3A).** The classic example of a direct cuticular flap is the groin flap. A musculocutaneous flap (Fig. 40-4A) is based on the vascularity to the muscle. **The overlying skin paddle is carried on perforators.** If the muscle alone is carried as a flap, the overlying skin survives as a random unit. **The fasciocutaneous system of vascularity (Fig. 40-4B) is similar to the musculocutaneous system.**

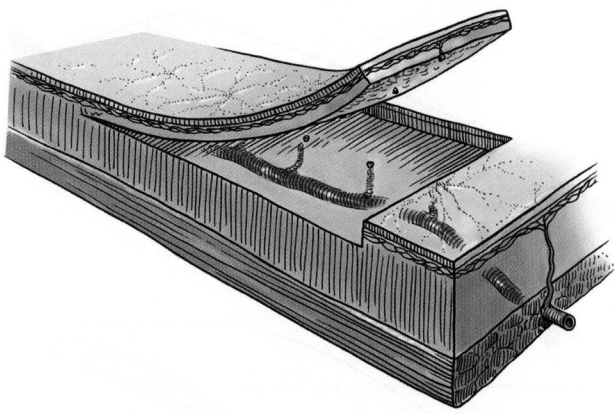

Figure 40-2. Random flap. The arterial perforators have been interrupted, and flap survival depends on the intradermal and subdermal plexuses.

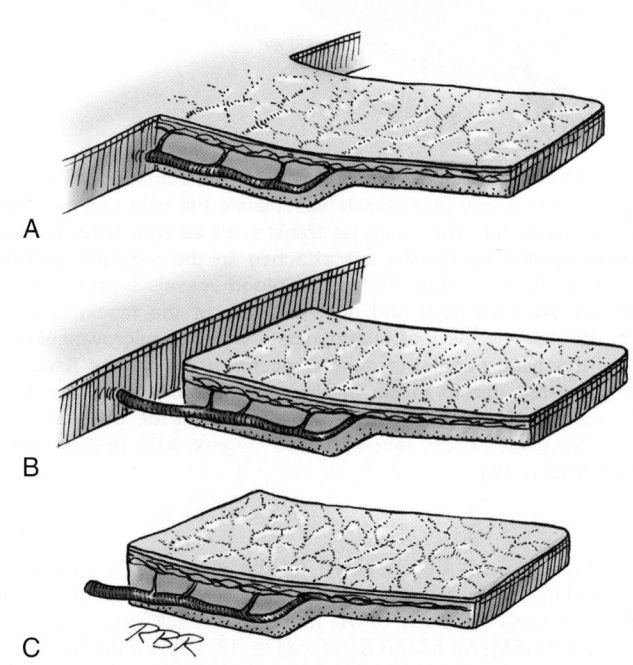

Figure 40-3. Axial flaps. Large vessels enter the base of the flaps. Survival depends on these vessels and on the random distal vascularity. **A,** Peninsula flap. The vascular continuity and the cutaneous continuity in the flap base are intact. **B,** Island flap. The vascular pedicle is intact; the cuticular continuity has been divided. These axial vessels are unsupported (dangling). **C,** Microvascular free-transfer flap. The free-flap cuticular and vascular connections are interrupted at the base of the flap. Vascular continuity is reconstituted in the recipient area by a microsurgical anastomosis. (From Jordan GH, McCraw JB. Tissue transfer techniques for genitourinary reconstructive surgery. AUA Update Series 1988;7:lesson 10.)

However, the deep blood supply is carried on the fascia (deep and superficial layers), and the overlying skin paddle is based again on perforators. One can transfer a fascial flap based on the deep blood supply associated with the flap; the overlying skin, if it is not carried with the flap, remains as a random unit (Ponten, 1981; Tolhurst and Haeseker, 1982; Cormack and Lamberty, 1984). It has been argued that fascia is relatively avascular and cannot serve as the "blood supply" to the fasciocutaneous unit. Actually, the fascial layer acts as a trellis—the vessels are carried much like the limbs of a vine (Jordan, 1993).

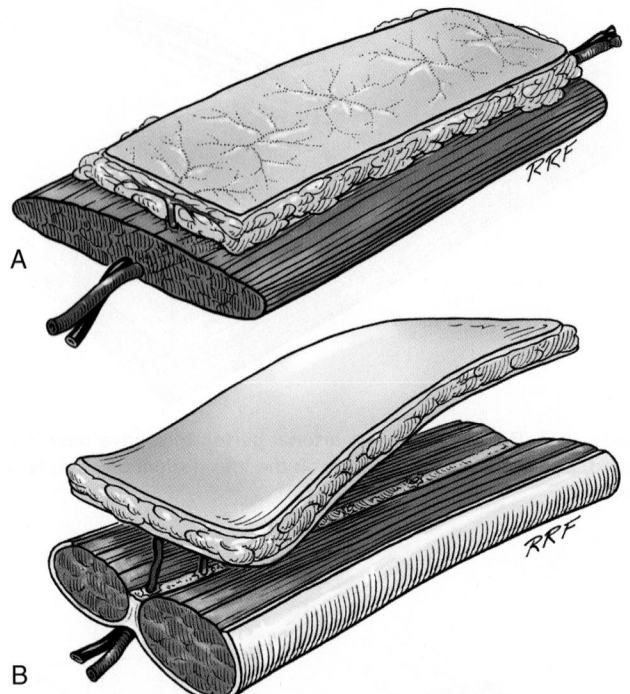

Figure 40-4. **A,** Musculocutaneous flap. Musculocutaneous perforators from the artery to a muscle vascularize the skin and overlying subcutaneous fat. They may be transferred as free flaps but are usually transferred locally, left attached to the vascular pedicle. **B,** Fasciocutaneous flap. Perforating blood vessels from rich plexuses on the superficial and deep aspects of the fascia connect to perforator vessels that communicate with the microvasculature of the overlying paddle. In genital reconstruction, these flaps are based on the dartos fascia of the penis or are free flaps from the forearm. (From Jordan GH, McCraw JB. Tissue transfer techniques for genitourinary reconstructive surgery. AUA Update Series 1988;7:lesson 10.)

A flap also can be classified by the elevation technique. A peninsular flap is a flap in which the vascular continuity and the cutaneous continuity of the flap base are left intact (see Figs. 40-2 and 40-3A). **An island flap (see Fig. 40-3B) is a flap in which the vascular continuity is maintained; however, the cuticular continuity is divided. A true island flap is elevated on dangling vessels. The microvascular free-transfer flap (free flap) (see Fig. 40-3C) has the vascular continuity and the cuticular continuity interrupted. The vascular continuity is then reestablished at the recipient site.**

The terminology is confusing. In genitourinary reconstructive surgical procedures, we tend to use the term *island flap.* As already mentioned, a true island flap is elevated on dangling vessels. However, the usual case is that a skin island or paddle is elevated either on the muscle, as in the gracilis musculocutaneous flap, or on the fascia, as in local genital skin flaps. The term *island flap* is not synonymous with the terms *skin island* and *skin paddle.* The usefulness of these flaps and grafts is illustrated in the discussion of surgical techniques later in this chapter. There is continued interest in the use of tissue-cultured grafts or "manufactured" grafts. The likelihood of someday being able to use off-the-shelf grafts or sheets of cultured material successfully is not far in the future (Chen et al, 1999; Atala, 2002; Rotariu et al, 2002; El-Kassaby et al, 2003; Bhargava et al, 2004).

Anatomy of the Penis and Male Perineum

 Please see the Expert Consult website for this section, including Figures 40-5 to 40-13.

Generalities of Reconstructive Surgical Techniques

With any surgical procedure, including reconstructive procedures of the external genitalia, there are basic rules and surgeons' biases regarding the best way to perform a certain operation. In this section, the differences are highlighted.

Reconstructive surgery is performed with all efforts aimed at minimizing tissue injury and promoting healing. Adequate visualization is essential. Surgical loupes are used by almost all surgeons performing adult and pediatric reconstructive genital surgery. A headlight or suction with attached light often adds to visualization, especially in deep perineal surgery. **In penile cases, such as reconstruction of the fossa navicularis or correction of penile curvature, bipolar cautery is used exclusively.** With cautery, the electrical charge is grounded either to a pad (monopolar) or to the opposite tong of the forceps (bipolar). In most instances, the field effects of the electricity are more confined with bipolar cautery. Because electricity is dissipated by conductors (in the case of human tissue, vessels, and nerves), there is a possibility of damage to these delicate structures. In other cases, monopolar cautery can be used in the superficial structures, but bipolar cautery is better during dissection around the corpus spongiosum, elevation of penile and scrotal flaps, division of the perineal intracorporeal space, and dissection of the dorsal neurovascular structures.

Appropriate instruments for genitourinary reconstructive surgery can commonly be found in a plastic surgery tray or on the peripheral vascular tray in the typical operating room. Some examples are fine tenotomy scissors, fine forceps, various skin hooks, and delicate needle holders. Sharp scissors that cut with minimal collateral trauma are essential. These instruments minimize tissue injury from manipulation and permit more precise dissection. For urethral surgery, a set of bougie à boule sizers is essential to check the caliber of the urethral lumen. McCrea urethral sounds are a good addition to the typical van Buren sounds available in the usual operating room. For calibration, sounds do not replace the need for bougie à boule calibrators. For posterior urethral reconstruction, a sound to pass through the cystostomy tract and prostate to find the proximal end for the reconstruction is often helpful. We find that a Haygrove staff serves this role nicely. Some centers use the cystoscope for this purpose, and often it suffices well, whereas at other times it is not as effective as the Haygrove-style sound.

The choice of suture material evolves on the basis of the surgeon's experience and bias. However, there are some common principles with which most surgeons would agree. First, in urethral surgery, absorbable suture is the rule. Typical choices for most surgeons are braided absorbable sutures or the family of monofilament absorbable sutures. Chromic suture is rarely used now because the choices of other absorbable sutures seem superior in virtually all cases. In the case of tension-free closures, very small sutures can be used. In some cases, tying the suture can be awkward, and a larger suture may be warranted, even though the anastomosis is tension free. The caliber of suture should be the smallest possible to line up the tissue, which is typically not under tension. There is no reason to use suture that is stronger than the tissues that are being sutured. Fine suture such as 5-0 and 6-0 chromic or polyglactin can be used to suture the epithelium to the adventitia of the corpus spongiosum to control bleeding. For a flap or graft repair, 4-0 to 6-0 suture is usually adequate. For primary anastomosis of the corpus spongiosum or for a posterior urethral reconstruction, 3-0 suture may be appropriate because of tying concerns. The needle should be tapered if possible except when, as in urethroplasty, for example, severe spongiofibrosis or scarring is present. Some typical choices are taper needles, such as RB-1, TF, and SH-1, and cutting needles, such as P-3 and PC-3. The UR-6 half-circle taper needle that is often used in radical prostatectomy can be helpful for deep perineal anastomosis of the urethra.

Surgical position and retraction are critical to attaining good results. If possible, procedures are done with the patient supine or prone. Many procedures that previously were done with the patient in the lithotomy position can be done with the patient in the frog-leg or split-leg position. For penile surgery, a Scott retractor with stay hooks (Lone Star Medical Products, Houston, TX, the Jordan-Bookwalter perineal retractor set (C. S. Surgical, Slidell, LA; J. Hugh Knight Instrument Company, New Orleans, LA), or the Omni-Tract perineal retractor (Omni-Tract Surgical, Division of Minnesota Scientific, St. Paul, MN) is helpful. Lithotomy or exaggerated lithotomy positions are used only for the minimal time necessary. With appropriate padding for the foot and positioning without pressure on the back of the leg, complications in the low-lithotomy position are minimal. When the patient is in the supine, split-leg, and low-lithotomy positions, venous compression stockings can be used. The controversy in positioning revolves around the use of the exaggerated lithotomy position. We prefer to use this position for all bulbar and posterior urethral reconstructions. Other surgeons use a lower lithotomy position. We find the more exaggerated position to be safe and believe that it provides unequaled access to the deep perineal structures (Angermeier and Jordan, 1994). Details of positioning, as we do it, are described later. To minimize the patient's time in the exaggerated position, all graft harvesting or flap elevation is done with the patient in the flat supine position.

In addition to proper diagnosis and planning, the surgical technique is important for the overall success of reconstructive surgery. In contrast to the results of extirpative surgery, the results of reconstructive surgery depend on methods that minimize tissue damage and maximize wound healing. The key ingredients are adequate visualization, appropriate choice of suture, delicate tissue handling, appropriate positioning, and adequate retraction.

> ## KEY POINTS: RECONSTRUCTIVE SURGICAL TECHNIQUES
>
> - Reconstructive surgery is performed with all efforts aimed at minimizing tissue injury and promoting healing. Loupe magnification is used by almost all surgeons performing adult and pediatric reconstructive surgery. For deep exposure, a headlight or lighted suction is advantageous. Instruments must be delicate because reconstructive surgery employs small sutures and small needles.
> - The choice of suture material evolves on the basis of the surgeon's experience. However, the caliber of sutures should be the smallest possible to align the tissue, which is not typically under tension. There is no reason to use suture that is stronger than the tissues being sutured.
> - The choice of surgical positioning is left to the surgeon's preference.
> - Proper diagnosis and planning of the surgical technique are important for the success of reconstructive surgery.

SELECTED PROCESSES

Urethral Hemangioma

Although **urethral hemangioma is a rare condition, it is usually persistent** and offers a challenge to the surgeon when excision is deemed necessary. Patients typically present with hematuria or a bloody urethral discharge and occasionally with obstructive symptoms. The lesions may be single or multiple, and the urethral meatus is a common location. Although the diagnosis is often made with cystoscopy, which readily visualizes the dilated blood vessels, the lesion often extends beyond the point at which it is seen with cystoscopy.

Because all reported cases of urethral hemangioma have been benign, management depends on the size and location of the lesion. Asymptomatic lesions do not require treatment and should be observed because hemangiomas can regress spontaneously. Symptomatic lesions that require treatment must be completely excised to prevent recurrence.

Although electrofulguration has been reported as a possible treatment of urethral hemangioma, it should be used only to control an acute episode. For smaller lesions, laser treatment has been successful and produces less scarring. Lasers that are used for this purpose include argon, potassium titanyl phosphate (KTP) (532 nm), and neodymium:yttrium-aluminum-garnet (Nd:YAG). The preferred treatment of larger lesions is open excision and urethral reconstruction; in some cases, this means circumferential reconstruction. Tubed graft reconstruction should be avoided; tubed flap reconstruction or tubed construction with mixed tissue transfer could be considered, although staged reconstruction is probably preferable. In addition, good initial success has been reported with polidocanol as a sclerosing agent for extensive urethral hemangiomas.

Reactive Arthritis

Reactive arthritis is characterized by a classic triad of arthritis, conjunctivitis, and urethritis. In addition, **some patients have had an episode of diarrhea that preceded the development of arthritis.** However, the classic triad is not present in most cases, and patients present with only arthritis affecting the knees, ankles, and feet in an asymmetrical distribution. The history of urethritis is obtained on detailed questioning.

Urethral involvement is usually mild and self-limited and constitutes a minor portion of the disease. In approximately 10% to 20% of patients, a glanular lesion is present. Referred to as **circinate balanitis,** this lesion **is diagnostic of reactive arthritis** and typically appears as a shallow, painless ulcer with gray borders. Occasionally, the lesion appears as small, red macules, 1 to 2 mm in diameter. When the urethritis is mild and self-limited, no treatment is necessary.

In rare cases, urethritis causes severe inflammation with necrosis of the mucosa, producing uncompromising stricture disease. We have been unsuccessful in excision and replacement of the urethra in these cases. Alternatively, we perform a perineal urethrostomy and excise the entire distal urethra. This approach may decrease the rheumatic manifestations associated with reactive arthritis.

Lichen Sclerosus

Lichen sclerosus (LS) was previously known as balanitis xerotica obliterans. LS is a chronic inflammatory hypomelanotic, lymphocyte-mediated skin disorder that in men involves the prepuce and glans and frequently leads to meatal stenosis and possible urethral involvement.

The reported incidence of LS in the Western population is 1 per 300 persons; however, the worldwide prevalence may be substantially different (Wallace, 1971; Dogliotti et al, 1974; Jacyk and Isaac, 1979; Datta et al, 1993). The peak ages of recognition in women are bimodal, with many cases noted before puberty and with another peak occurring in postmenopausal women (Tasker and Wojnarowska, 2003). In men, LS seems to peak between ages 30 and 50; however, LS has been described in people of all ages, from infants to elderly adults (Tasker and Wojnarowska, 2003). LS is commonly found at the time of circumcision when performed after the neonatal period (McKay et al, 1975; Rickwood et al, 1980; Garat et al, 1986; Ledwig and Weigland, 1989; Meuli et al, 1994). **LS is the most common cause of meatal stenosis and appears as a whitish plaque that may involve the prepuce, glans penis, urethral meatus, and fossa navicularis. If only the foreskin is involved, circumcision may be curative** (Akporiaye et al, 1997). In our experience, LS usually begins as a meatal or perimeatal process in a circumcised patient, but it may involve other areas of the preputial space in uncircumcised patients. In uncircumcised men, the prepuce becomes edematous and thickened and often may be adherent to the glans (Bainbridge et al, 1971). Diagnosis is made with biopsy. Several reports have suggested an association with chronic infection by a spirochete, *Borrelia burgdorferi* (Tuffanelli, 1987; Dillon and Ghassan, 1995; Shelley et al, 1999).

The first report of what was probably LS was published by Weir in 1875. He described a case of vulvar and oral "ichthyosis" (Weir, 1875). The term *balanitis xerotica obliterans* was first applied by Stühmer in 1928. Freeman and Laymon showed that balanitis xerotica obliterans and LS were probably the same process (Freeman and Laymon, 1941; Laymon and Freeman, 1944). In 1976, the International Society for the Study of Vulvar Disease devised a new classification system unifying the nomenclature and proposed the term *lichen sclerosus* (Friedrich, 1976).

The cause of LS has not been defined. Many mechanisms have been proposed. Koebner phenomenon relates the development of LS to trauma to an affected area (Lee and Phillips, 1994). A proposed mechanism is an autoimmune event. Autoantibodies to extracellular matrix protein 1 (ECM1) were detected in the serum of 67% of patients with LS and only 7% of control subjects, which would imply an autoimmune process (Oyama et al, 2003). Reports of LS associated with vitiligo, alopecia areata, thyroid disease, and diabetes mellitus also suggest a possible autoimmune basis. Reported oxidative damage of lipids, DNA, and protein in patients with LS may explain the mechanism of sclerosus, autoimmunity and carcinogenesis of LS (Sander et al, 2004).

An infectious cause was previously implicated (Tuffanelli, 1987; Ross et al, 1990), but a more recent case-control series found no association (Edmonds and Bunker, 2010). It has also been proposed that LS has a genetic origin, based on the observation of a familial distribution of cases (Marren et al, 1995). There have been reports of concomitant existence of the disease in identical twins (Thomas and Kennedy, 1986; Fallic et al, 1997) and nonidentical twins (Cox et al, 1986), with coexistence of dermatosis. The disease also has been seen in mothers and daughters (Shirer and Ray, 1987). Studies

on the human leukocyte antigen (HLA) have suggested a genetic component in patients with LS (Marren et al, 1995).

The combination of topical steroids and antibiotics may help stabilize the inflammatory process. Conservative therapy may be warranted in patients whose meatus can easily be maintained at 14 to 16 French (Staff, 1970). In these cases, intermittent catheterization with lubrication of the catheter and meatal dilator with 0.05% clobetasol (Temovate) may be adequate treatment. Long-term antibiotic therapy may also be helpful to improve inflammation because secondary infection of the inflamed tissue may occur. We have typically used tetracycline, but a trial of long-term penicillin or advanced-generation erythromycin therapy may be warranted (Shelley et al, 1999). This nonsurgical approach to treatment is used in patients who are not good surgical candidates for other medical reasons or in older patients and in younger patients who demonstrate stable disease. Secrest and colleagues (2008) proposed a link between hypogonadism and LS in male patients. These authors consistently showed diminished testosterone levels in patients with LS and analyzed whether replacement androgen therapy would be helpful.

Surgery is indicated in young patients with severe meatal stenosis. Because patients with long-standing meatal stenosis often have severe proximal urethral stricture disease, retrograde urethrography should be performed before therapy is initiated. A simple meatotomy is generally ineffective in patients with LS. Morey and colleagues (2007) showed that an extended meatotomy in patients with refractory stenosis was successful in 14 of 16 patients (87%). Malone (2004) described a ventral/dorsal meatotomy with an inverted V-shaped relaxing incision with the apex of the V close to the proximal limit of the dorsal meatotomy.

The etiology of stricture disease associated with LS is unclear. Possible causes include iatrogenic stricture resulting from repeated instrumentation and pressure voiding associated with meatal stenosis causing secondary intravasation of urine into the glans Littre (Fig. 40-14). In cases of early LS with only meatal involvement resulting in stenosis of the fossa navicularis, prompt reconstruction seems to be successful in the long-term and seems to avoid the sequelae of panurethral stricture disease. Most surgeons believe that because LS is a disease of genital skin, better tissue for reconstruction is the oral mucosa; techniques are discussed later (Mundy, 1994; Bracka, 1999). Long-standing cases with a long length of urethral stricture are amenable to techniques of reconstruction but are very challenging. It seems that except in the case of urethral stricture disease confined only to the meatus and fossa navicularis, staged oral graft reconstruction, at least in the short-term to midterm, seems to provide superior durable results. This may also be true in cases confined to the meatus and fossa navicularis because an analysis of patients reconstructed with the ventral transverse skin island technique showed a 50% recurrence rate even in those patients; the weakness of this analysis is that the data did not include biopsy proof that all patients had LS (Virasoro et al, 2007). We also see patients who present with a buried penis. This phenomenon occurs when the skin of the penile shaft has been lost because of severe inflammation, and the penis is trapped in the penopubic and scrotal area. These patients are often profoundly overweight, and many are diabetic; they have often had prior surgical procedures. Management of these patients is complex and ultimately determined by their desire and need for functional reconstruction. In some patients with severe urethral stricture disease, we have completely reconstructed the urethra; in others, we have simply performed a perineal urethrostomy. Perineal urethrostomy is usually technically straightforward because the rule in most patients with LS is to spare the proximal anterior urethra. We have proposed that, in many cases, the sparing of the proximal anterior urethra demonstrates the distribution of the glands of Littre for a given patient. Younger patients have requested mobilization and release of the penis with placement of a split-thickness skin graft. However, because the inflammation involves the glans penis (which is not removed), the secondary inflammation may also involve the skin graft. Lifelong monitoring of these patients for the secondary effects of inflammation is necessary.

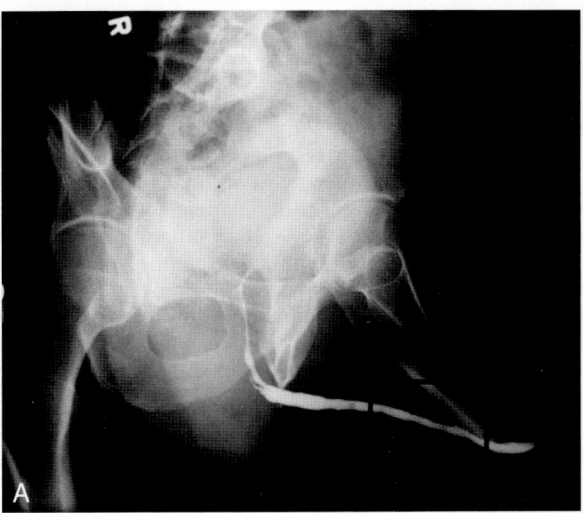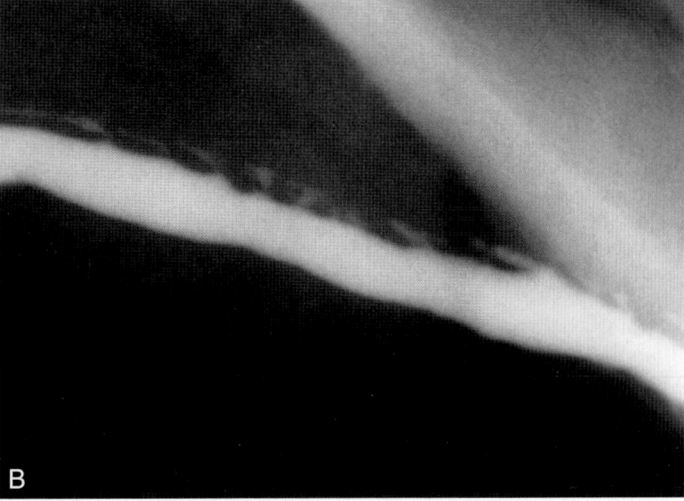

Figure 40-14. **A and B, Urethrography in a patient with urethral stricture disease associated with lichen sclerosus. The intravasation of contrast material into the dilated glands of Littre during voiding is illustrated. (From Jordan GH. Management of membranous urethral strictures via the perineal approach. In: McAninch J, Carroll P, Jordan GH, editors. Traumatic and reconstructive urology. Philadelphia: Saunders; 1996.)**

Finally, **several reports have suggested the development of squamous cell carcinoma in patients with a long history of LS** (Doré et al, 1990; Pride et al, 1993).

Amyloidosis

Amyloidosis of the urethra, although a rare disease, should be considered in the evaluation of any patient with a urethral mass. Patients may present with hematuria, dysuria, or urethral obstruction. Because the differential diagnosis includes urethral neoplasm, cystoscopy with transurethral biopsy is indicated. When the diagnosis is made, treatment should be based only on symptoms. Most patients can be observed expectantly and do not require aggressive treatment. Some patients require treatment for urethral stricture. Progression and recurrence are rare (Walzer et al, 1983; Dounis et al, 1985; Crook et al, 2002).

Urethrocutaneous Fistula

A urethrocutaneous fistula is a tract lined with epithelium that leads from the urethra to the skin. The size of a fistula can vary from pinpoint to large. **Urethral fistulae may be a complication of urethral surgery or develop secondary to periurethral infection associated with inflammatory strictures or treatment of a urethral growth** (condyloma or papillary tumor). **Treatment of a urethral fistula must be directed not only to the defect but also to the underlying process that led to its development.** Treatment varies according to the cause of the fistula. In cases of urethral reconstruction, especially reconstruction for hypospadias, fistula often occurs or recurs because of distal obstruction and high-pressure voiding. Additionally, in some cases in which multiple attempts at fistula closure have been attempted and failed, the tissues adjacent to the fistula are so scarred that staged reconstruction is needed to import "better tissue."

After urethral surgery, fistulae can develop immediately or as delayed complications. An early fistula is the result of poor local healing, possibly secondary to hematoma, infection, or tension with closure. In addition, breakdown of the urethra or overlying skin closure, or both, could occur. Very occasionally, with aggressive local care and continued urinary diversion, the fistula closes spontaneously.

Several techniques are used for fistula closure. Endoscopic and radiographic evaluation of the urethra must be performed before the repair in all cases. If the fistula is small and closure of the hole does not decrease the lumen of the urethra, a button of skin is removed from around the fistula, and its edges are cut flush with the urethral wall. The urethra is closed with small (6-0 or 7-0) absorbable sutures, inverting the epithelial edge, and the repair is tested to ensure that it is watertight. We prefer either polyglycolic acid (Vicryl) or polydioxanone suture. Subsequent layers are designed and closed to avoid superimposed suture lines. Without question, the safest diversion is a suprapubic catheter. However, in many cases, a silicone stent that reduces pressure during voiding for 7 to 14 days suffices. The operating microscope can be useful for the closure of small fistulae, allowing the use of 8-0 polyglycolic acid suture and limiting the size of the associated skin incision.

If the fistula is so large that simple closure would compromise the lumen of the urethra, local flaps often are required. However, if the adjacent tissues are thin and poorly visualized, closure of the fistula may become a staged urethral reconstruction as mentioned earlier. For larger fistulae, a suprapubic tube for diversion is probably prudent. Mobilization of flaps, such as the tunica dartos flap, may be necessary to secure adequate tissue interposition and avoidance of superimposed suture lines.

Fistulae associated with inflammatory strictures occur as periurethral tracts and develop secondary to high-pressure voiding of infected urine. As multiple tracts develop, this problem becomes what is known as a "watering pot perineum." Repair requires suprapubic drainage, and treatment of the infection requires incision and drainage of any abscesses present. We widely excise the fistula tracts and associated inflammatory tissue and wait 4 to 6 months before repairing the underlying stricture. Flap reconstruction, if donor tissues are available, may be used. However, a staged graft procedure (discussed later) is also an excellent choice. One must be cautious in a patient with urethral fistulae but without a history of chronic obstructive voiding symptoms. In many cases, fistula or periurethral abscess may be the hallmark symptom of urethral carcinoma.

Urethral Diverticulum

A congenital diverticulum is a transitional cell epithelium–lined pouch that is the result of either a distention of a segment of the urethra or the attachment of a structure to the urethra by a narrow neck (i.e., a müllerian remnant). In male patients, a congenital anterior urethral diverticulum may result from incomplete development of the urethra, with a defect in only the ventral wall and subsequent distention of this segment by the hydraulic force of the voiding stream (Valdivia et al, 1986; Bedos and Cibert, 1989; Ozgok et al, 1994). The downstream lip of the defect may serve as a valvular obstruction, increasing the pressure in the lumen, and subsequently the diverticulum enlarges. **Another possible etiology is injury of the urethra, which may cause an intraspongiosal hematoma.** This hematoma could create a paraurethral space and subsequent diverticulum or fistula. These defects can also be associated with urethral strictures (Bryden and Gough, 1999). It has also been suggested that congenital diverticula may represent giant cystic dilation of Cowper ducts (Gil-Vernet, 1977; Jiminez Cruz and Rioja Sanz, 1993). We do not favor this proposed suggested etiology because the diverticula seem to be slightly more distal than the expected location of Cowper ducts, and in our experience with reconstruction of a considerable number of these diverticula, no proximal limb of the ducts seems to exist in them. In many cases, endoscopic unroofing of the diverticulum remedies the voiding symptoms; although after unroofing, the patient commonly may note postvoid dribbling. Open repair essentially excises the redundancy of the urethra associated with the diverticulum. If the lumen is compromised, dorsal onlay by either graft or flap can be useful.

A congenital diverticulum in the prostatic urethra may be a large remnant of the müllerian duct associated with defects of diminished virilization. However, it often occurs in proximal hypospadias and represents an enlarged utricle (Devine et al, 1980). **These diverticula may not be demonstrated with voiding urethrography but are demonstrated with cystoscopy or retrograde urethrography.** The tip of a urethral catheter tends to catch in this opening, necessitating the use of something to direct the catheter tip toward the true lumen. Other than necessitating caution during evaluation, these diverticula do not usually cause problems or require treatment unless they are very large.

Large utricles can accumulate urine with voiding and then decompress after voiding. If they are large enough, the stasis of urine can be associated with recurrent urinary tract infection or difficult-to-manage "incontinence." A surgical approach to small lesions can be through a suprapubic incision, possibly opening the bladder to go through the center of the trigone. However, large diverticula can be approached trans-sacrally (Peña and Devries, 1982). Although this is a complex procedure, it seems to be associated with much less morbidity than an abdominal or a perineal approach and provides superior exposure. We excise the diverticulum after exposing and dissecting its communication with the urethra. After ensuring that there is no distal obstruction to interfere with healing, we close the urethra.

Diverticula of the female urethra are covered in Chapter 90.

Paraphimosis, Balanitis, and Phimosis

Paraphimosis, or painful swelling of the foreskin distal to a phimotic ring, occurs if the foreskin remains retracted for a prolonged time. Swelling is sufficient to make reduction of the foreskin over the glans difficult. **In a very young child, paraphimosis is often seen after the foreskin has been traumatically reduced during an examination or sometimes by overzealous parental attempts at hygiene.** Traumatic, sudden reduction of a tight foreskin should be avoided in all ages and circumstances. To reduce a paraphimosis, gentle steady pressure must be applied to the foreskin to decrease the swelling; with a child, this is best accomplished in a quiet room by a parent squeezing it in the hand. Elastic wrap may be helpful in some cases. Putting an ice pack on the area for a short time before gentle compression is helpful as an analgesic. When the swelling has been reduced, the surgeon can push against the glans with the thumbs, pulling on the foreskin with the fingers. Because paraphimosis tends to recur, a dorsal slit at a minimum or a circumcision should be carried out as an elective procedure at a later date. An occasional patient presents with acute paraphimosis that has been present for many hours to days; this is typically seen in an adolescent who is reluctant to reveal the problem to his parents. In these cases, reduction may be impossible, and paraphi-

mosis should be dealt with by emergency dorsal slit or circumcision. Considerable postoperative edema is the rule in these cases.

Balanitis, or inflammation of the glans, can occur as a result of poor hygiene, from failure to retract and clean under the foreskin. The subsequent swelling makes cleaning more difficult, but the inflammation usually responds to local care and antibiotic ointment. Oral antibiotic therapy occasionally may be necessary. Balanoposthitis is a severe form of balanitis and occurs when the phimotic band is tight enough to retain inflammatory secretions, creating what amounts to a preputial cavity abscess. Occasionally, an emergent dorsal slit is required.

Phimosis, or the inability to retract the foreskin, can result from repeated episodes of balanitis. In older patients, balanitis may be a presenting sign of diabetes. In these cases, circumcision may be warranted.

Urethral Meatal Stenosis

A small urethral meatus in a newborn probably would not be called to a urologist's attention unless the stenosis is associated with other congenital deformities (e.g., hypospadias) or causes voiding difficulties or urinary tract infection (Allen and Summers, 1974). If the urethral meatus of a boy appears exceptionally narrow and there are associated symptoms, a meatotomy should be considered. For this decision to be made, voiding should be observed to note that the meatus opens as a full, forceful stream is passed. If the stream is narrow and excessively forceful, stenosis is probably present. The occluding skin is generally a thin layer that sometimes can be seen to pouch out, with the meatus opening at the dorsal lip as the child voids. **Meatal stenosis in a boy appears to be a consequence of circumcision that then allows subsequent ammoniacal meatitis.** If the child is seen with ammoniacal meatitis, we usually start meatal dilation with 0.05% clobetasol cream. Within a week, the process seems to abate. Anecdotally, the fusion of the ventral-meatal skin that causes meatal stenosis can be avoided. Parents must be counseled about the cause—that is, a wet diaper pressing for prolonged periods against the tip of the glans.

A ventral urethral meatotomy sometimes can be accomplished with the use of local anesthesia. In a young child, general anesthesia is the preferred approach, avoiding trauma to the child, the parents, and the urologist. It is important to insert the anesthetic needle into the skin fold from the underside so that the tip of the needle can be observed and controlled. If insertion is done from the outside, the needle passes through both layers of the fold, and a wheal cannot be raised because of leakage of the anesthetic solution. After the meatotomy, the edges of the cut seal together unless they are kept open. The tip of a meatal dilator is the best instrument for this purpose. The child's parents are instructed to separate the edges gently with the tip of the dilator three times a day for 7 to 10 days. The surgeon should observe the parents carry out this procedure. Pediatric meatal dilators (see later product reference) are available; however, the tip of an ophthalmic antibiotic tube also works well, and the antibiotic ointment can be used as the lubricant.

Meatal stenosis occurs in adults after inflammation, specific or nonspecific urethral infection, and trauma (especially in association with indwelling catheters, urethral instrumentation, or radical prostatectomy in some cases). It also may be the result of the failure of a previous hypospadias repair. To perform a ventral meatotomy in a normally developed penis in adolescents and adults, it is often necessary to place sutures to approximate the urethral mucosal edge to control bleeding. This step usually requires three sutures: one at the apex and one on either side. We have found a dilator made by Cook Urological (Spencer, IN; Catalog No. 073406, adult 6 to 34 French; No. 073403, pediatric 6 to 10 French) to be helpful in keeping the meatus open. In some cases, it may be necessary to perform a dorsal rather than a ventral meatotomy. This procedure can be accomplished as a Y-V-plasty after the excision of any scarred ridge of neourethra. Dorsal meatotomy, although effective in opening the meatus, often creates a cosmetically suboptimal shape of the meatus. In an adult, it is unusual for the meatal stenosis to be an isolated finding. The stricture process usually involves the fossa navicularis to some extent as well.

Circumcision

Controversy continues regarding whether neonatal circumcision should or should not be performed (Poland, 1990; Schoen, 1990). Much attention has been focused on this issue, but despite this, many boys in the United States are circumcised. Ritual circumcision will continue; however, in ritual circumcision, it is not necessary to remove the skin but only to draw blood. **It is important not to circumcise any boy with a penile abnormality (e.g., hypospadias, chordee) that may require the foreskin during repair. Circumcision is indicated in a young boy who has had recurrent urinary tract infections thought to be associated with the redundant preputial skin.**

Most circumcisions performed just after birth are done with the Gomco clamp or one of the plastic disposable devices made for this purpose. Care should be taken to free the foreskin from the glans completely and to apply appropriate tension when the foreskin is pulled into the clamp. To prevent either a too generous or an inadequate circumcision, we find it useful to mark the foreskin carefully so that the correct level is ascertained. At our center, we perform neonatal circumcision with a penile block for anesthesia.

The most common complication is bleeding as a result of inadequate control with vascular compression. Application of an epinephrine-soaked sponge may help in controlling minimal venous bleeding. Infection can also occur and responds to local care. Any resulting skin separation should be repaired after the inflammation resolves. Minimal separation may be amenable to healing by secondary intention. Sometimes too much skin is removed, or the urethra is included in the clamp, resulting in a fistula. In many, if not most, cases in which excess skin is removed, closure can still be accomplished with aggressive frenuloplasty along with remaining skin closure by transposition of the remaining skin. If the entire penis is "scalped," it may be best managed with a split-thickness skin graft or with reapplication of the excised foreskin, after it is prepared properly as a graft. In complicated cases, burying the penis in the scrotum and repairing it at a later date may be prudent. **Monopolar electrocautery should be avoided in a neonatal circumcision because penile loss from the field distribution of the current can occur. The use of monopolar cautery with a Gomco or similar clamping device must be avoided because devastating loss of tissue can occur.**

A newborn who lost his penis because of a circumcision mishap should not be gender reassigned. Our experience with phallic construction includes many children and youths who had been converted to a female after a circumcision accident. As they passed through puberty, they realized that this sexual assignment was wrong. Most of these boys could undergo reconstruction in such a manner as to preserve reproductive function.

In adults, circumcision can be done with local anesthesia, by blocking the dorsal nerves at the base of the penis and circumferentially infiltrating the superficial layers of the penile base. In men and older boys, we favor a sleeve circumcision. With the foreskin in its retracted position, a marking pen outlines an incision, leaving a small preputial cuff. This mark should go straight across the base of the frenulum. This incision is made and carried through the dartos fascia to the superficial lamina of the Buck fascia. The foreskin is reduced, and a second incision is marked, following the outlines of the coronal margin and the V of the frenulum on the ventral side. The frenulum usually retracts into a V. In some cases, the frenulum can be lengthened by closing the edges of the V in a longitudinal orientation for a short length (frenuloplasty). If frenuloplasty is done, the proximal incision does not need to follow the V of the retracted frenulum because the ventral skin is straight. We make the skin incision and fulgurate bleeding vessels with bipolar cautery as the incision is deepened and the skin edge is mobilized. In older boys and men, the vessels are more substantial and not easily sealed by compression, no matter how vigorous. Circumcision clamps can be ineffective and are not recommended even

though larger sizes are available. After the sleeve of preputial skin has been removed, hemostasis is obtained, and the skin edges are reapproximated.

In younger boys, some surgeons may consider this sleeve procedure to be tedious and difficult. If this is the case, after the skin is marked, a dorsal slit is made through both layers of the prepuce back to the level of the corona. Following the marks, the two layers of the preputial skin are incised. Bleeders are controlled, and the skin edges are reapproximated.

Complications should be uncommon. Most patients develop some hyperesthesia of the glans, which resolves. A hematoma is probably the most common immediate complication. Some patients notice minor cosmetic imperfections that are functionally insignificant. One of the most distressing problems we see is a patient who complains that the surgeon has removed too much skin. To avoid this occurrence, a circumcision should be done precisely, and, whatever the procedure to be carried out, the incisions should first be marked with the skin lying undistorted on the shaft. Adults requesting circumcision must be carefully evaluated from a psychosexual standpoint because many of these patients who are the most persistent in requesting circumcision become the most dissatisfied after the surgery.

Circumcision has been shown in numerous studies to provide protection for men in areas where human immunodeficiency virus (HIV) is very prevalent (Auvert et al, 2005; Bailey et al, 2007; Gray et al, 2007). Circumcision has consistently been shown in well-conducted randomized controlled trials to reduce the risk of HIV acquisition in heterosexual African men by 50% to 60%. Similar prospective trials have not been performed in developed countries; however, retrospective data among heterosexual men in the United States showed a similar approximately 50% reduction in HIV prevalence among men with known exposure, suggesting the data may be extrapolated to this population. Additionally, male circumcision has been shown to reduce the risk for acquisition of herpes simplex virus type 2, human papillomavirus, genital ulcer disease, and some sexually transmitted bacterial infections (Tobian et al, 2014).

There is a biologic rationale for reduction in the spread of sexually transmitted infections, particularly HIV, with circumcision. Superficial Langerhans cells, $CD4^+$ T cells, and $CD8^+$ T cells are rich and less well protected by keratin on the inner aspect of the male foreskin and frenulum. When the foreskin is retracted during intercourse, this large and susceptible surface area is exposed allowing contact with HIV-infected secretions and subsequent risk for infection. Uncircumcised men have also been shown to have an increased frequency of genital ulcers and increased frequency of microtears during intercourse, both of which increase HIV transmission.

Despite the well-demonstrated benefit of circumcision in heterosexual men, the same benefit has not been shown for men who have sex with men (MSM). A large meta-analysis of more than 53,000 MSM did not demonstrate a statistically significant protection against HIV (Millett et al, 2008). Subgroup analysis demonstrated a trend toward reduced prevalence of HIV among MSM performing predominantly insertive rather than receptive anal intercourse, and others have corroborated these findings.

Failed Hypospadias Repair

In treating a patient in whom hypospadias repair has failed, it is important to obtain all available records to help determine what may have contributed to his complications. **A hypospadias repair may fail because of an inadequate correction of chordee or an inadequate urethra, with a stricture, fistula, or diverticulum** (Winslow et al, 1986). **It is often readily apparent from the records that not all aspects of the hypospadias deformity** (i.e., ventrally displaced meatus, ventral chordee, and some expression of inadequacy of ventral tissue fusion) **were addressed in the previous repairs.** Adults with urethral strictures are often seen who have had hypospadias surgery as children. Depending on the age of the patient and the preference of the treating urologist, a variety of different techniques may have been used to repair the original hypospadias. Many of these patients have persistent chordee and a subcoronal meatus. Adults also have been seen who have had long-standing evidence of urethral fistula. In addition, some patients may have clinical findings not related to hypospadias that should have been recognized previously, especially when hypospadias is part of an overlying intersex problem. In the past, problems associated with previous failures were caused by errors in design, technique, or postoperative care (Devine et al, 1978). **With more modern techniques available and with most hypospadias treated by surgeons with considerable experience, failures seem to be associated with perioperative infections or other factors that adversely affect wound healing.** At the present time, complex hypospadias repair failures are encountered with much less frequency, and most that are encountered are in patients who had previous procedures more than 15 to 20 years ago. Complications in these patients resulted not from poorly designed surgery at the time but rather from the "state of the art" at the time.

Evaluation of a failed hypospadias repair includes retrograde urethrography, voiding cystourethrography, and cystoscopy. In an older patient, a reliable preoperative assessment of residual chordee can be made on the basis of the history and photographs taken at home. In younger patients, complete evaluation of more complex situations with use of anesthesia may be necessary.

In an adult patient, a detailed discussion must occur regarding the positive and negative aspects of the various approaches. Patients who were initially operated on before the late 1970s probably underwent either a graft or some form of repair using almost exclusively ventral tissue. Some of these patients still have the remnants of a dorsal hood or enough dorsal skin for a dorsal transverse penile skin island type of reconstruction to be performed.

We believe that surgical correction of complex cases requires an aggressive approach by the surgeon (Secrest et al, 1993). However, with the advent and very common usage of the tubed incised plate repair, initially described by Snodgrass (1999), the nature of failures is different, and the approaches also are remarkably different. Based on our observations, the number of failed surgeries is less, the nature of graft salvage techniques is remarkably different, and the method of addressing residual curvature is different. It is possible to reincise the "urethral plate" and tubularize it if the plate is not scarred and possible to graft the plate dorsally if it is; if the tissues are badly scarred, many surgeons revert to staged reconstruction (Snodgrass et al, 2009). The use of flaps has a place in corrective procedures, and the excision of scarred tissues causing residual curvature likewise has its place. However, plication or corporoplasty techniques for correction of residual curvature have, for the most part, become the standard of care. Graft techniques for correction of curvature are used but with far less frequency than in years past.

Residual Genital Abnormality in Patients with Closed or Diverted Exstrophy

Residual genital defects in men who have had exstrophy repaired as children can cause functional, aesthetic, and psychologic problems. The effects of these problems are compounded in men who have undergone urinary diversion and who must wear stomal appliances, although with the improvement of continent diversions, this is less of a factor. Successful reconstruction is possible except in the most severe forms of bladder exstrophy or cloacal exstrophy—when the penis or the halves of the bifid penis are truly inadequate. Even then, if normal testes are present, the success of newer techniques of phallic construction (see subsequent discussion) should lend support to considering the option of raising such a child as a boy, possibly preserving his reproductive potential through puberty. In these very difficult cases, we think that the parents must be presented with both options, gender reassignment versus eventual phalloplasty. Remarkable progress has been made in the treatment of difficult cases (Johnston, 1975; Hendren, 1979; Jeffs, 1979; Snyder, 1990; Perovic et al, 1992; Gearhart et al, 1994; Mitchell and Bagli, 1996) and in techniques of primary closure. However, many patients need further genital surgery because they experience the hypertrophic growth spurt of the penis associated with puberty.

The goals of reconstructive surgery in male patients with exstrophy or epispadias are to produce a dangling penis with erectile bodies of satisfactory length and shape to allow sexual function and to construct a urethra that serves as a conduit for the passage of urine and ejaculate. However, experience has shown that in a patient with a diverted exstrophy and only a bladder remnant, construction of a urethra that is essentially defunctionalized is difficult. These urethras all eventually seem to fibrose and stenose. The bladder neck remnant becomes a cyst that is often colonized. Bouts of virulent epididymitis or the formation of what is really a bladder neck remnant abscess begin to occur. We have seen two patients who developed carcinoma of the prostate in a bladder neck remnant. The diagnosis in these patients was difficult, and the resultant surgery was even more difficult. Neither patient did well from the standpoint of treatment of the carcinoma. Both were seen before the aggressive use and better understanding of prostate-specific antigen.

Many patients who have undergone surgery as children do not present for correction of inadequacies of the external genitalia until after they have completed puberty and realize that their situation has not improved and is not likely to improve. Some have been in sexual situations and have encountered problems. We employ a systematic approach to accomplishing the reconstruction necessary to correct the anatomic defects in these patients (Devine et al, 1980; Winslow et al, 1988). Surgery is undertaken in a sequential fashion beginning with the simplest procedure that would achieve the desired functional result.

Lower abdominal wall scarring can be corrected or defects can be closed by fashioning peripenile flaps that are shaped like a W. In many patients, there may be wide diastasis recti that is really a ventral hernia. Anchoring of meshes or Gore-Tex can be difficult, and we have resorted to a fibular bone microvascular free transfer in several cases to reconstruct the continuity of the pubis, allowing effective closure of the abdominal hernia.

With more effective contemporary primary closure techniques, the adult reconstructive surgeon's place is primarily in the correction of hernia, or in the patient who has an inadequate penis either due to deformity, scarring, or improper gender reassignment.

TRAUMA TO THE GENITALIA

This topic is primarily covered in Chapter 101, but an additional description is included in the electronic version of this chapter. Please see the Expert Consult website for this section and Figure 40-15.

URETHRAL STRICTURE DISEASE

The term *urethral stricture* refers to anterior urethral disease, or a scarring process involving the urethral epithelium or spongy erectile tissue of the corpus spongiosum (spongiofibrosis) (Fig. 40-16). The spongy erectile tissue of the corpus spongiosum underlies the urethral epithelium, and the scarring process extends through the tissues of the corpus spongiosum in some cases and into adjacent tissues. **Contraction of this scar reduces the urethral lumen.** For example, if a normal urethra measures 30 Fr, its diameter is 10 mm, and the area of the lumen is approximately 78 mm^2. If scarring has resulted in a urethra that measures 15 Fr, the lumen is only 55 mm^2, or 29% reduced. It is evident that scar contraction caused by anterior urethral stricture disease can be asymptomatic for a while, but because the lumen is further reduced, it can be associated with marked voiding symptoms.

In contrast, posterior urethral "strictures" are not included in the common definition of urethral stricture. Posterior urethral stricture is an obliterative process in the posterior urethra that has resulted in fibrosis and is generally the effect of distraction in that area caused by either trauma or radical prostatectomy. Although the distraction defect can be lengthy in some cases, the

KEY POINTS: SELECTED PROCESSES

- Urethral hemangioma is a rare condition that is usually persistent. It can present a significant challenge to the surgeon. All reported cases of urethral hemangioma have been benign, and management depends on the size and location of the lesion.
- Reactive arthritis is characterized by a classic triad of arthritis, conjunctivitis, and urethritis. Urethral involvement is usually mild, self-limited, and a minor portion of the disease.
- LS previously was referred to as balanitis xerotica obliterans. Diagnosis is made through biopsy. LS is thought to be possibly premalignant for the development of squamous cell carcinoma of the glans. It is the most common cause of meatal stenosis. Management of patients with LS-related stricture is complex, and results to date are suboptimal. The management is determined by the desire of the patient and the need for functional reconstruction.
- Amyloidosis is a rare disease of the urethra and should be considered in the evaluation of any patient with a urethral mass. Patients present with hematuria, dysuria, or urethral obstruction.
- A urethrocutaneous fistula is a tract lined with epithelium that leads from the urethra to the skin. It may be a complication of urethral surgery or develop secondary to periurethral infection associated with inflammatory strictures or treatment of a urethral growth. Treatment of the urethral fistula must be directed not only to the defect but also to the underlying process that led to its development.
- A congenital urethral diverticulum is a transitional cell epithelium–lined pouch that is the result of either a distention of a segment of the urethra or the attachment of a structure to the urethra by a narrow neck. In male patients, "congenital" anterior urethral diverticulum may result from incomplete development of the urethra or possibly may be the result of straddle trauma that led to an intracorporeal spongiosal hematoma. Congenital diverticulum in the prostatic urethra is a remnant of the müllerian duct.
- Paraphimosis is a painful swelling of the foreskin distal to a phimotic ring. It occurs when the foreskin has been retracted and not reduced. Edema forms in the distal skin.
- Urethral meatal stenosis in a young boy appears to be a consequence of circumcision. The circumcision allows the development of ammoniacal meatitis, which can heal with a membrane across the ventral portion of the meatus. Controversy continues regarding whether neonatal circumcision should or should not be performed. If it is going to be performed, the circumcision needs to be adequate. The most common complication of neonatal circumcision, in our opinion, is when it is inadequately done.
- A patient with failed hypospadias repair can be complex. Many are victims of the technology of the time when they had their initial reconstruction. All patients with urethral involvement should be evaluated as if they have urethral stricture disease.
- Advanced techniques for the reconstruction of the exstrophy-epispadias complex have led to much better functional results and less need for secondary exstrophy reconstruction. Secondary exstrophy reconstruction is aimed at the area of the escutcheon, the dorsal base of the penis, the penile shaft, the urethra, and the penoscrotal junction.

actual process involving the tissues of the urethra is usually confined. By consensus of the World Health Organization conference, the term *stricture* is limited to the anterior urethra. Distraction defects are processes of the membranous urethra associated with pelvic fracture. Other narrowings of the posterior urethra are termed *urethral contractures* or *stenoses* (Bhargava et al, 2004).

Urethral Anatomy

Although urethral anatomy is described in the earlier section on anatomy, it is useful to re-emphasize key anatomic points. **The bulbous urethra is eccentrically placed in relation to the corpus spongiosum and is much closer to the dorsum of the penile structures** (see Fig. 40-6). As one moves distally, the pendulous or penile urethra becomes more centrally placed within the corpus spongiosum.

The genital skin has a dual (proximal and distal) and bilateral blood supply, forming a fasciocutaneous system (see Fig. 40-10). **The corpus spongiosum receives blood from the common penile artery, the terminal branch of the internal pudendal artery** (see Fig. 40-12). **The corpus spongiosum also has a dual blood supply—a proximal blood supply and a retrograde blood supply through the dorsal arteries as they arborize in the glans penis.**

Etiology

Any process that injures the urethral epithelium or the underlying corpus spongiosum to the point that healing results in a scar can cause an anterior urethral stricture. Most urethral strictures are the result of trauma (usually straddle trauma). This trauma to the urethra often goes unrecognized until the patient presents with voiding symptoms resulting from the obstruction of the stricture or scar. In most cases of straddle trauma, reconstruction of the bulbar urethral injury is possible (Park and McAninch, 2004). Iatrogenic trauma to the urethra still exists, but with the development of small endoscopes and the limitation of indications for cystoscopy in boys, we see fewer iatrogenic strictures today than in the past. The place of idiopathic urethrorrhagia with regard to strictures in children is unclear; some question whether it may be a cause of strictures in young boys regardless of whether the child underwent an endoscopic procedure (Rourke et al, 2003). No specific inciting factor has been identified as causing idiopathic urethrorrhagia. Histologic results from a patient of ours with resolving urethrorrhagia showed portions of tissues covered in part by squamous epithelium; other parts were covered by transitional epithelium; there were several areas of denuded epithelium with acute hemorrhage and neutrophilic infiltration; a few foci of microcalcification were shown; several mucus glands were found within the submucosal connective tissue as well as a few collections of amorphous material, likely mucin. These areas stained negatively with a special stain for amyloid. There was no evidence of viral cytopathic effect or malignancy. We did not see evidence of bacterial infection or viral inclusions. However, we have seen an increase in strictures associated with LS, and those strictures clearly behave much more like inflammatory strictures than traumatically induced isolated scars. Finally, posterior urethral injuries, traumatic by definition, result in obliterative or near-obliterative defects that are associated with extensive fibrosis interposed between the distracted ends of the urethra.

Inflammatory strictures associated with gonorrhea were the most commonly seen in the past and are less common now. With the advent of prompt and effective antibiotic treatment, gonococcal urethritis progresses less often to gonococcal urethral strictures. The place of *Chlamydia* and *Ureaplasma urealyticum* (i.e., nonspecific urethritis) in the development of anterior urethral strictures is unclear. No clear association between nonspecific urethritis and the development of anterior urethral stricture has been established.

As mentioned earlier, there is a definite association between the development of an inflammatory stricture and LS. LS usually begins with inflammation of the glans and inevitably causes meatal stenosis, if not a true stricture of the fossa navicularis. The cause of this distal penile skin and urethral inflammation is unknown. Some evidence suggests that the progression of the stricture eventually to involve the anterior urethra extensively may be due to high-pressure voiding that causes intravasation of urine into the glands of Littre, inflammation of these glands, and, perhaps, microabscesses and deep spongiofibrosis. Whether the urethral changes and eventual fibrosis are also related to bacterial injury has not been well defined. Although the use of antibiotics seems to limit obstructive voiding

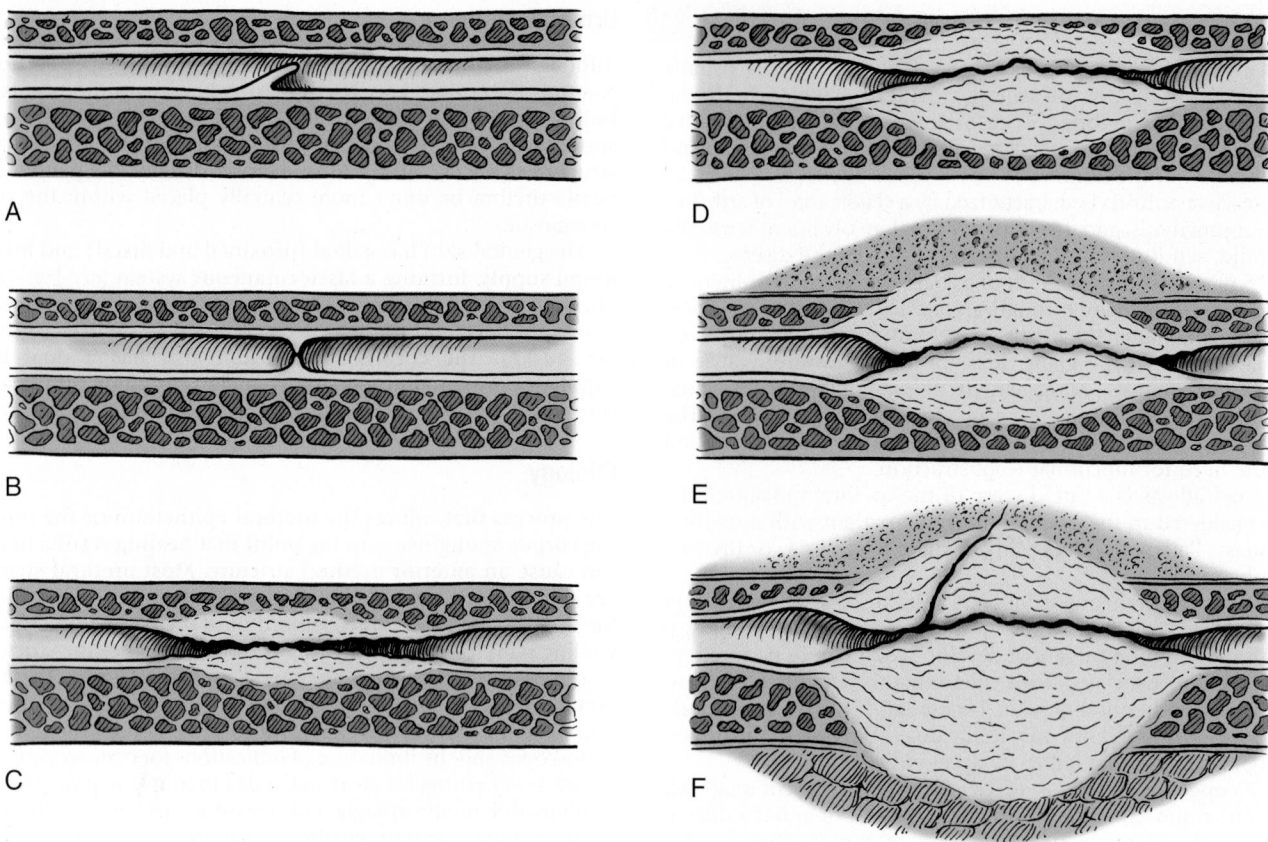

Figure 40-16. The anatomy of anterior urethral strictures includes, in most cases, underlying spongiofibrosis. A, Mucosal fold. B, Iris constriction. C, Full-thickness involvement with minimal fibrosis in the spongy tissue. D, Full-thickness spongiofibrosis. E, Inflammation and fibrosis involving tissues outside the corpus spongiosum. F, Complex stricture complicated by a fistula. This can proceed to the formation of an abscess, or the fistula may open to the skin or the rectum. (From Jordan GH. Management of anterior urethral stricture disease. Probl Urol 1987;1:199–225.)

symptoms in these patients, to our knowledge the literature does not show resolution of the stricture process with the use of antibiotics.

The entity known as a congenital stricture is difficult to understand. In embryologic development, if a stricture is found at a natural place where a fusion of structures occurs (i.e., the posterior and anterior urethra), a congenital stricture might be a reasonable assumption. However, the term *congenital stricture* is used by some authors to define a stricture for which there is no identifiable cause. We propose that it is reasonable to define a stricture as congenital only if it is not an inflammatory stricture, it is a short-length stricture, and it is not associated with a history of or potential for urethral trauma. These criteria limit the term *congenital stricture* to strictures of the anterior urethra found in infants before they attempt erect ambulation. So defined, congenital strictures are the rarest encountered.

Diagnosis and Evaluation

Patients who have urethral strictures most often present with obstructive voiding symptoms or urinary tract infections such as prostatitis and epididymitis. Some patients also present with urinary retention. However, on close inquiry, most of these patients are found to have tolerated notable voiding obstructive symptoms for a long time before progressing to complete obstruction.

When a patient cannot void, an attempt commonly is made to pass a urethral catheter. If the catheter does not pass, the nature of the obstruction is determined by dynamic retrograde urethrography. Most cases are managed with acute dilation, and there are many instances in which this is not the best course for the patient. When there is doubt, we determine the nature of the stricture when possible, and selectively place a suprapubic cystostomy catheter to treat the acute situation and allow time for a more appropriate treatment plan to be devised. The practice of blind passage of filiforms and blind dilation without knowledge of the anatomy of the urethral stricture is condemned. Although detailed imaging is not always available, flexible endoscopy is almost universally available in the United States. The stricture can be visualized, and guidewire placement under direct vision can be attempted.

For an appropriate treatment plan to be devised, it is important to determine the location, length, depth, and density of the stricture (spongiofibrosis). The length and location of the stricture can be determined with radiography, urethroscopy, and ultrasonography. The depth and density of the scar in the spongy tissue can be deduced from the physical examination, the appearance of the urethra in contrast-enhanced studies, and the amount of elasticity noted on urethroscopy. The depth and density of fibrosis are difficult to determine objectively. The absolute length of spongiofibrosis may not be evident on ultrasound evaluation. **Ultrasound examination can augment contrast-enhanced studies and is accurate in determining the length of narrow-caliber annularity** (Morey and McAninch, 1996b). Contrast studies of the urethra are best carried out by or under the direct supervision of the surgeon responsible for treatment of the patient.

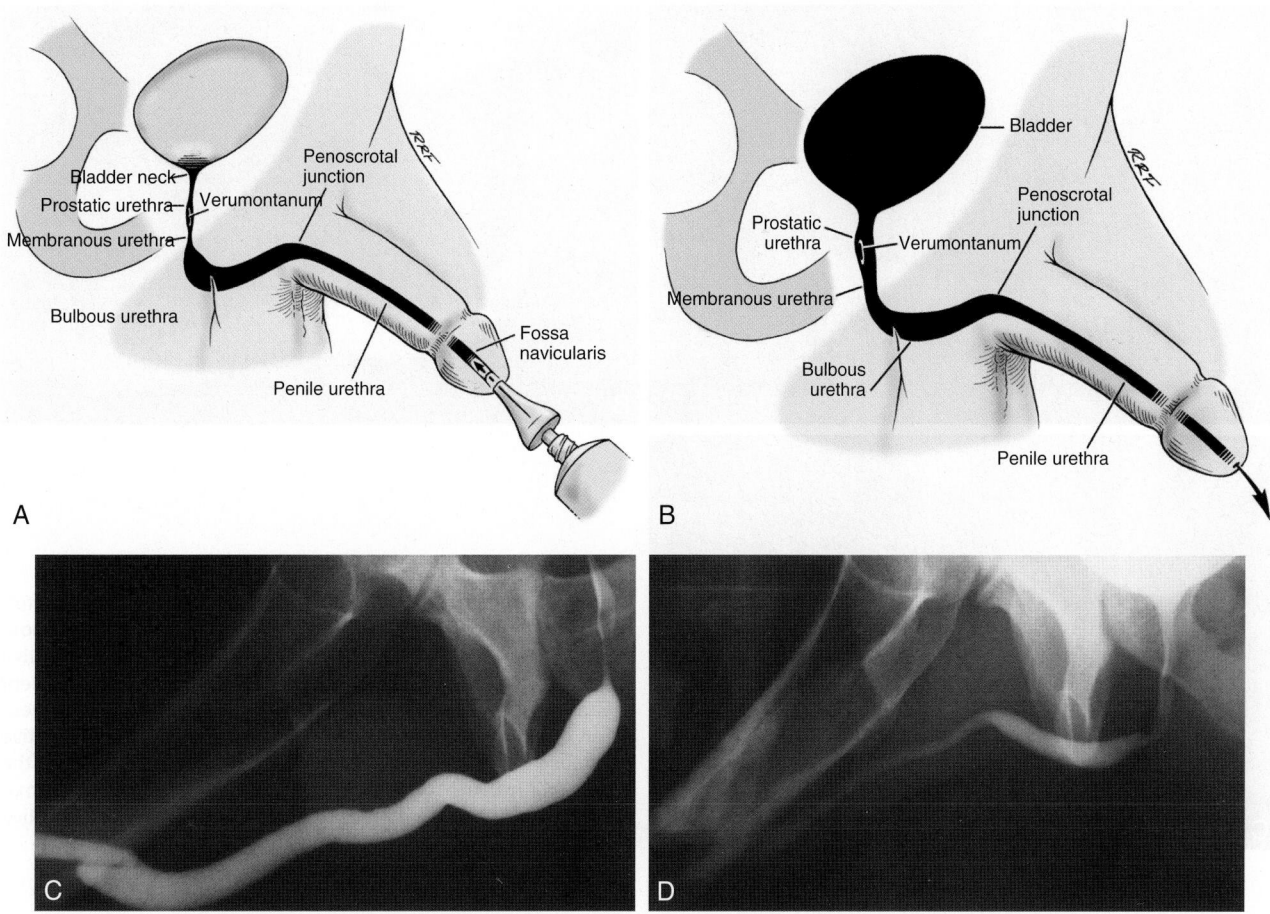

Figure 40-17. A, Representation of a dynamic retrograde urethrogram with the criteria of McCallum illustrated. **B,** Representation of a dynamic voiding urethrogram with the criteria of McCallum illustrated. **C,** Normal retrograde urethrogram. **D,** Normal voiding urethrogram. **(A and B,** Modified from McCallum RW. The adult male urethra. Radiol Clin North Am 1979;17:227–44.)

McCallum and Colapinto (1979a, 1979b) described the use of dynamic radiographic studies and emphasized the need for these studies to be dynamic as opposed to static (Fig. 40-17). At our center, imaging includes dynamic studies that are performed during retrograde injection of contrast material and while the patient is voiding. Even with gentle technique, extravasation during retrograde urethrography is possible in patients in whom the urethra is markedly inflamed. For this reason, contrast studies should be carried out with contrast material that is suitable for intravenous injection and used either directly from the bottle or diluted according to the manufacturer's guidelines. Contrast materials that have been thickened with lubricating jelly or anesthetic gels can be a source of problems and offer little with regard to enhancement of radiographic studies, and they do not make the studies more comfortable. Real-time ultrasound evaluation of the urethra after it has been filled with a lubricating jelly or saline has been described by Morey and McAninch (1996a, 1996b). However, it is a misconception that ultrasonography always directly visualizes the spongiofibrosis. Morey and McAninch (1996a, 1996b) believed that ultrasonography of the bulbous urethra possibly more accurately determines the length of the stricture, which could be important in considering an anastomotic repair. If the patient is not in steep lateral oblique position for retrograde urethrography, the length of the stricture will be underestimated. Finally, during contrast-enhanced urethrography, more than one projection may be necessary to visualize the stricture. Magnetic resonance imaging (MRI) is also being explored as an adjunct to the evaluation of urethral stricture and pelvic fracture urethral injuries (PFUIs). In

our experience, the use of MRI for routine strictures or pelvic fracture urethral distraction defects is not routinely beneficial. In the case of urethral tumors, we have found MRI to be invaluable. The experience of others is commensurate with ours (Pavlica et al, 2003). In a pelvic fracture urethral distraction defect, the alignment of the two urethral ends can be defined clearly.

Endoscopic examination may be necessary after contrast studies. The flexible cystoscope has simplified this evaluation, and when local anesthesia is used, there is little discomfort associated with it. The scope can be passed to the stricture, and it often is unnecessary to pass it beyond that level. In addition, it is not always necessary, and usually not beneficial, to dilate the stricture at the time of the initial endoscopic evaluation. Pediatric endoscopic equipment has proved to be extremely valuable for examination of the urethra proximal to a narrow-caliber area without the need to dilate the narrowest area. In a patient who cannot void and has a suprapubic tube, combined contrast studies with endoscopy are helpful in defining the stricture anatomy (Fig. 40-18).

It is imperative to evaluate the urethra completely proximal and distal to the stricture with endoscopy and bougienage during surgery to ensure that all the involved urethra is included in the reconstruction. Although hydraulic pressure generated by voiding may keep segments proximal to the stricture patent, unless these segments are included in the repair, they are at risk for contraction after obstruction of the narrow-caliber segment is relieved with reconstruction. For this reason, any abnormal areas of the urethra that are proximal to a narrow-caliber segment of the stricture must be treated with suspicion. If the lumen does not appear to

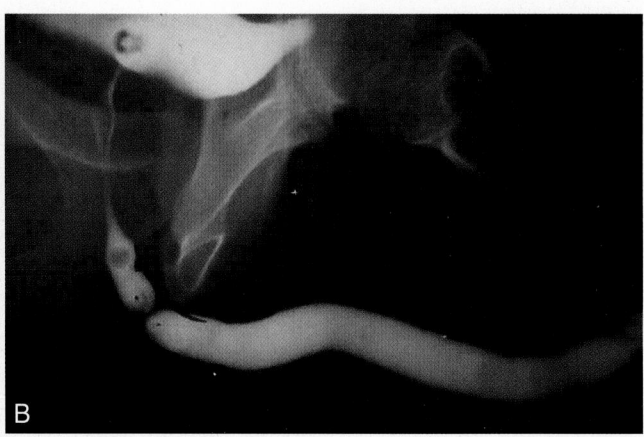

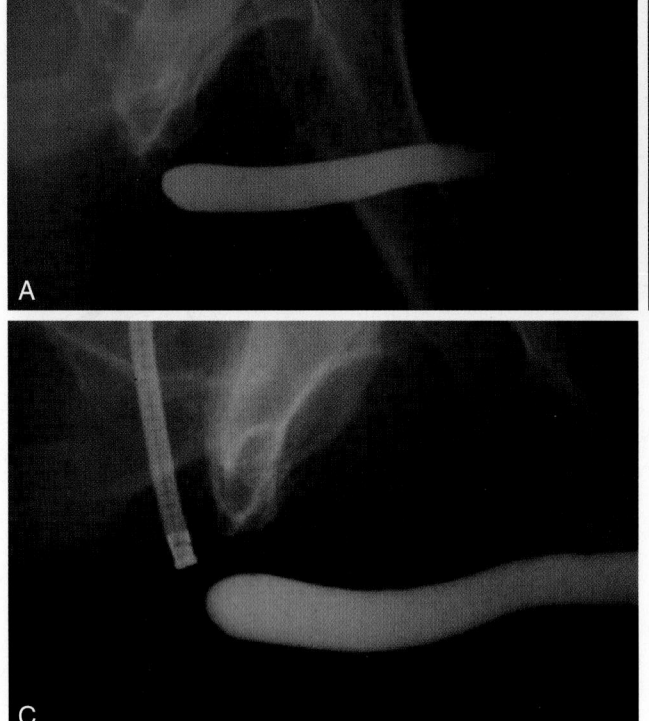

Figure 40-18. **Series of radiographs demonstrating the useful-ness of the combination of contrast enhancement with endos-copy. A, A retrograde urethrogram shows a totally obliterative process involving the proximal bulbous urethra. B, The patient was successful in relaxing to void; however, there is sugges-tion of a wide-caliber annular area proximal to the obliterative process of the bulbous urethra. C, Endoscopy through the suprapubic cystostomy tube clarifies the anatomy of the proxi-mal urethra and demonstrates the length of the obliterative process.**

demonstrate evidence of diminished compliance, we presume that area to be uninvolved in active stricture disease. However, coning down of the urethra suggests its involvement in the scar.

In some patients, the urethra proximal to a narrow area may remain confusing with regard to its potential for continued con-striction after reconstruction. In select patients, we have found it useful to place a suprapubic tube to defunctionalize the urethra. After 6 to 8 weeks, if there is to be constriction of an area that was hydrodilated with voiding, the tendency for that constriction to occur should become apparent.

Treatment

Although the treatment of urethral stricture disease dates to the foundations of urology, significant progress made during the last 50 years allows many of the most complex strictures to be reli-ably reconstructed in one stage. In the past, a concept known as the reconstructive ladder was used as a treatment guideline for urethral strictures. That concept was based on the principle that the simplest procedure should always be attempted first, and sometimes repeated after failure, before moving on to more complex approaches. This approach is considered archaic in modern urethral reconstruction.

The patient and the physician must have a good understand-ing of the goal of treatment before the treatment choice is made. Treatment options should be discussed with the patient, with care taken to emphasize the anticipated outcome with regard to potential cure. Some patients may prefer stricture management and choose to have periodic dilations in the office, at home, or in the hospital rather than undergo technically detailed open surgery. Others may have cure as a goal and choose surgical management. Many surgical procedures today have short-term and mid-term results approaching long-term success rates of more than 90% to 95% for many strictures.

KEY POINTS: URETHRAL STRICTURE

- The term *urethral stricture* refers to anterior urethral disease and is a scarring process that involves the epithelium and the spongy erectile tissue of the corpus spongiosum. Con-traction of the scar reduces the urethral lumen. Posterior urethral strictures are more correctly referred to as PFUIs; strictures of the prostatic urethra or bladder neck are prop-erly referred to as contractures or stenoses.
- The anterior urethra is invested by the corpus spongiosum, and as it proceeds proximally it is eccentrically placed in relation to the corpus spongiosum. The genital skin has a dual and bilateral blood supply, forming a fasciocutaneous vascular system. The vascularity of the corpus spongiosum is based on the common penile artery.
- In general, most anterior urethral strictures are the result of trauma. Inflammatory strictures associated with gonorrhea are rarely seen; however, strictures associated with LS have behavior similar to inflammatory strictures.
- Patients who have urethral strictures most often present with obstructive voiding symptoms or urinary tract infec-tions such as prostatitis and epididymitis. Patients who present with urinary retention, on close inquiry, have tol-erated notable voiding obstructive symptoms for a long time.
- For an appropriate treatment plan to be devised, it is important to determine the length, location, depth, and density of the spongiofibrosis. This determination can be done with a combination of contrast-enhanced studies, endoscopy, and selective ultrasonography. It is imperative to evaluate the urethra completely proximal and distal to the stricture with endoscopy. A pediatric cystoscope is useful.

Dilation

Urethral dilation is the oldest and simplest treatment of urethral stricture disease, and for a patient with an epithelial stricture without spongiofibrosis, it may be curative. **The goal of this treatment, a concept that is frequently forgotten, is to stretch the scar without producing more scarring.** If bleeding occurs during dilation, the stricture has been torn rather than stretched, possibly further injuring the involved area.

The least traumatic method to stretch the urethra is to use soft techniques over multiple treatment sessions. We believe that the safest method of urethral dilation currently available involves the use of urethral balloon-dilating catheters. These catheters may be attached to a filiform tip or passed over a guidewire or may come with an integral coudé tip. For initial dilation, we favor the use of balloons placed over wires that have been passed through the stricture under endoscopic control.

Dilation can be curative and, in the literature, in correctly selected patients, has short-term and mid-term efficacy rates equal to internal urethrotomy. Selection criteria are discussed in the following section on internal urethrotomy. The literature does not compare internal urethrotomy and dilation in randomized selection, and we do not have a true comparison but rather comparison by retrospective analysis (Steenkamp et al, 1997).

Internal Urethrotomy

Internal urethrotomy refers to any procedure that opens the stricture by incising it transurethrally. The urethrotomy procedure involves incision through the scar to healthy tissue to allow the scar to expand (release of scar contracture) and the lumen to heal enlarged. The goal is for the resultant larger luminal caliber to be maintained after healing.

With epithelial apposition, wound healing occurs by primary intention. Internal urethrotomy does not provide an epithelial approximation but rather aims to separate the scarred epithelium so that healing occurs by secondary intention. In healing by secondary intention, epithelialization progresses from the wound edges. As it progresses from the wound edge, epithelialization slows. In an effort to aid epithelialization, nature invokes the forces of wound contraction, not to be confused with scar contraction. Wound contraction closes the wound defect and limits the size of the area that requires epithelialization, hastening the healing of the surface defect. However, in the case of internal urethrotomy, wound contraction merely tries to reapproximate the edges of the scar, putting a race into effect. If epithelialization progresses completely before wound contraction significantly narrows the lumen, the internal urethrotomy may be a success. If wound contraction significantly narrows the lumen before completion of epithelialization, the stricture has recurred. Dubey and colleagues (2005) showed the extent of luminal narrowing to be a predictor of success with internal urethrotomy: The narrower the percent of narrowing, the worse the outcome, with a cutoff of 74% narrowing.

Many surgeons have learned to perform internal urethrotomy by making a single incision at the 12 o'clock position. However, this location might be questioned on the basis of the location of the urethra within the corpus spongiosum. On examination of a cross section of the corpus spongiosum, it can be seen that the thinnest portion of the anterior aspect is from 10 o'clock to 2 o'clock. The distance between the anterior wall of the urethra and the corpora cavernosa is likewise short in the bulbous urethra, and a single incision at 12 o'clock could rapidly penetrate the corpus spongiosum and extend into the triangular ligament; although it might not enter the corpora cavernosa, a deep cut could enter the intracrural space. Distally, although the anterior aspect of the corpus spongiosum is thicker, a deep incision in the more distal aspects of the anterior urethra would enter the corpora cavernosa, and these incisions have been associated with erectile dysfunction thought to be due to local cavernosal veno-occlusive dysfunction. Vigorous incisions at 10 o'clock and 2 o'clock in the bulbous urethra risk the same problem. If deep spongiofibrosis is present, stricture cure is

impossible by internal urethrotomy, and these deep incisions are unnecessary.

The most common complication of internal urethrotomy is recurrence of stricture. Less commonly noted complications of internal urethrotomy include bleeding (almost always associated with erections immediately after the procedure) and extravasation of irrigation fluid into the perispongiosal tissues. These complications are rare today because of the less frequent use of aggressive internal urethrotomy as a treatment modality for urethral strictures. Normal saline should be used as the irrigant when direct visual internal urethrotomy is performed. Additionally, with the use of deep urethrotomy incisions, another complication can be creation of a fistula between the corpus spongiosum and the corpora cavernosa and cavernosal veno-occlusive dysfunction.

A major problem with assessing the success rates of internal urethrotomy is that the nature of the strictures that have been treated with internal urethrotomy has been poorly reported. In addition, the literature is unclear regarding the goal of internal urethrotomy. For many, an internal urethrotomy is successful if it offers temporary relief. In many cases, internal urethrotomy has been reported as successful despite the fact that it has been associated with eventual stricture recurrence. A report by Santucci and McAninch (2001) using actuarial techniques showed the curative success rate of internal urethrotomy to be approximately 20% (Rosen et al, 1994). Evaluations by Pansadoro and Emiliozzi (1996) and others showed the curative success rate of direct visual internal urethrotomy to be approximately 30% to 35%. Their analysis also showed that there is virtually no increase in success rate with a second internal urethrotomy. **The data show that strictures at the bulbous urethra that are less than 1.5 cm in length and not associated with dense, deep spongiofibrosis (i.e., straddle injuries) can be managed with internal urethrotomy, with a 74% moderately long-term success rate.** The study by Pansadoro and Emiliozzi (1996) did not have any long-term successes for treated strictures outside the bulbous urethra. The variables associated with success of internal urethrotomy have been verified by other studies (Heyns et al, 1998). Many studies have shown that the success of reconstruction is diminished by multiple prior urethral dilations and internal urethrotomy (Stone et al, 1983; Albers et al, 1996; Heyns et al, 1998) (Boccon-Gibod, personal communication, 2005). Success rates with internal urethrotomy are not equal to success rates of open urethral reconstruction (Mandhani et al, 2005). Numerous analyses have sought to compare the cost-effectiveness of the practice of internal urethrotomy initially before consideration of open reconstruction. The analyses all differ in method and differ in findings (Rourke and Jordan, 2005; Wright et al, 2006; Wessells, 2009).

Several techniques have been employed to oppose the process of wound contraction and to prevent stricture recurrence. One method is to leave an indwelling Foley catheter for 6 weeks after urethrotomy, in the hope that the urethra will mold around the catheter as it heals. However, studies have shown that the failure rate of long-term catheterization after internal urethrotomy is similar to that seen with 3 to 7 days of catheterization, and even 6 weeks is insufficient time to oppose the forces of wound contraction.

Another technique used to oppose the forces of wound contraction after internal urethrotomy is home self-catheterization or home urethral obturation. After internal urethrotomy, patients generally have an indwelling catheter placed for 3 to 5 days. When the catheter is removed, the patient is started on a urethral obturation regimen. Most regimens require more frequent catheterizations early in the recovery period, with a tapering schedule during the next 3 to 6 months. Anecdotally, many surgeons have reported an improved cure rate with self-catheterization combined with internal urethrotomy. However, it has been our experience that the stricture inevitably recurs when the patient stops self-obturation, regardless of how long it has been used. That being understood, this approach can effectively manage the problems when it is combined with a urethral dilating regimen in a properly motivated patient. Colchicine, because it binds tubulin, has been used along with internal urethrotomy (Carney et al, 2007). Initial findings in a nonrandomized study also suggest that, perhaps by pharmacologically blocking tubulin and possibly wound contracture, the results of internal urethrotomy may be better. Mitomycin C with its antifibroblast and anticollagen activity when injected submucosally has been shown to decrease the risk of recurrence after a urethrotomy (Mazdak et al, 2007).

Urethral stents (removable or permanently implantable) are another modality used in opposing the forces of wound contraction after internal urethrotomy or dilation. Removable urethral stents are designed to prevent the process of epithelialization from incorporating the stent into the urethral wall and are left in place for 6 months to 1 year before they are removed. The greatest experience with these removable stents comes from Israel (Yachia and Beyar, 1991), and centers there report good success in small series. The Memokath stent is not currently available in the United States. It is a removable stent made of nitinol with varying success rates.

Most experience with permanently implantable stents comes from Europe and the United Kingdom. Milroy (1993) reported a success rate of 84% at 4.5 years with use of the permanently implantable UroLume (Rousseau et al, 1987; Sigwart et al, 1987; Milroy et al, 1988, 1989; Sarramon et al, 1990; Ashken et al, 1991; Krah et al, 1992; Sneller and Bosch, 1992; Verhamme et al, 1993; Badlani et al, 1995; Milroy and Allen, 1996; Jordan, 1997; Tillem et al, 1997; Brandes and McAninch, 1998; Shah et al, 2003). The UroLume, made of an alloy, is designed to be incorporated into the wall of the urethra and corpus spongiosum. Available data show that the stent is best employed for relatively short strictures of the bulbous urethra associated with minimal spongiofibrosis. However, these are the strictures that are most successfully reconstructed with open techniques that offer better long-term success rates. The North American Study Group 11-year data showed that of 179 patients originally enrolled in the North American Study, 24 patients completed 11 years of follow-up. The overall success rate for all patients enrolled at 11 years is less than 30% (Shah et al, 2003). A 10-year follow-up study from The Netherlands (De Vocht et al, 2003) reported results thought to "weaken the optimistic early results"; of 15 patients implanted, only 2 were satisfied with their stent at 10 years.

Permanently implantable stents are associated with unique complications. The stents must be **placed only in the bulbous urethra,** and when placed beyond the area of the scrotal urethra, placement has been associated with pain on sitting and intercourse. Some patients (particularly young patients) **complain of perineal pain,** often with vigorous activity, even after implantation of the stent in the deep bulbous urethra. In addition, **longer bulbous strictures require two stents that are overlapped.** These **stents can migrate** away from each other, leaving a gap between them where recurrence of stricture is inevitable. When this occurs, the stricture recurrence is excised, and a third stent is placed to span the gap.

There are also **specific contraindications to the use of the UroLume.** Patients who have undergone **prior substitution urethral reconstruction,** particularly where skin has been incorporated into the urethra, have been shown to be poor candidates for implantation with the UroLume stent because contact of the stent with the skin is associated with a virulent hypertrophic reaction. These patients experience postvoid dribbling, and the hypertrophic reaction can be so severe in some cases that functional recurrence of the stricture results. Another subset of patients shown to be **poor candidates for the UroLume includes patients with strictures associated with deep spongiofibrosis.** Patients who fall into this category **have had urethral distraction injuries and straddle injuries associated with deep fibrosis.** UroLume has been taken off the market and is currently not available for implantation. However, there are still many patients who will present with UroLume stents, and many will need treatment.

Lasers

Please see the Expert Consult website for this section.

To date, the results of laser urethrotomy are mixed. However, with the advent of new lasers and experience with them, future data may show better results.

Open Reconstruction: Excision and Reanastomosis

It has been demonstrated with certainty that the most dependable technique of anterior urethral reconstruction is the complete excision of the area of fibrosis, with a primary reanastomosis of the normal ends of the anterior urethra (Fig. 40-19) (Russell, 1914). The best results are achieved when **the following technical points are observed: The area of fibrosis is totally excised; the urethral anastomosis is widely spatulated, creating a large ovoid anastomosis; and the anastomosis is tension free.**

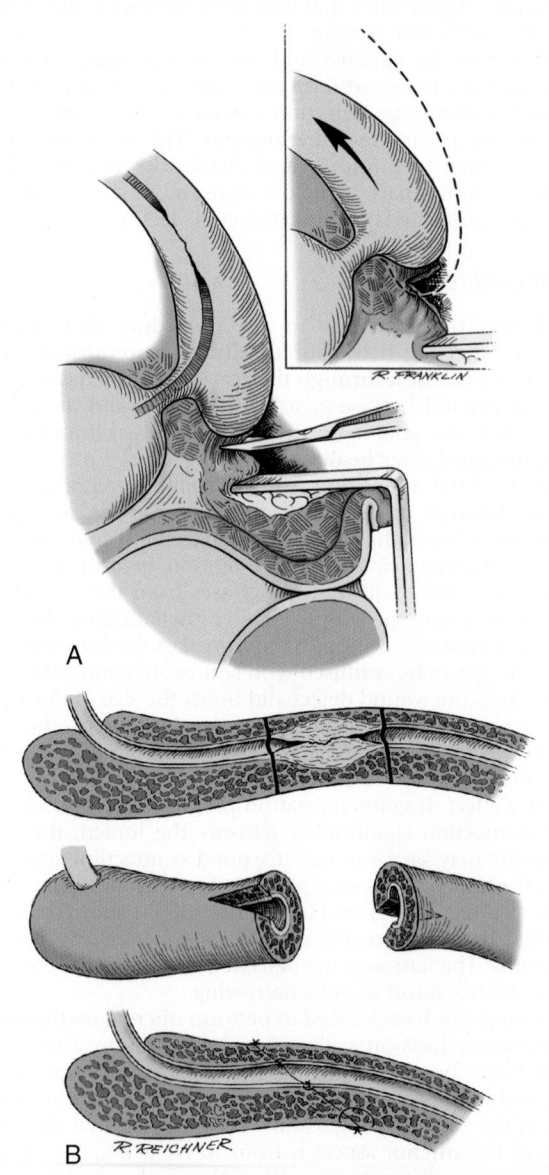

Figure 40-19. **Techniques for excision and primary reanastomosis of anterior urethral stricture. A, The bulbospongiosus is released from its attachment to the perineal body. The arteries to the bulb are not divided. This technique allows the urethra to be mobilized distally. This technique combined with development of the intracrural space can shorten the path of the urethra by approximately 1 to 1.5 cm. B, Technique of a primary spatulated anastomosis after excision of an anterior urethral stricture. (From Jordan GH. Principles of plastic surgery. In: Droller MJ, editor. Surgical management of urologic disease: an anatomic approach. Philadelphia: Mosby; 1992. p. 1218–37.)**

The success of this procedure relies on vigorous mobilization of the corpus spongiosum. With vigorous mobilization, dissection of Buck fascia to improve compliance, development of the intracrural space, and detachment of the bulbospongiosus from the perineal body, significant lengths of stricture can be excised and reanastomosed. Strictures of 1 to 2 cm are generally easily excised with reanastomosis. In some cases, strictures 3 to 5 cm can be totally excised, and a primary reanastomosis of the anterior urethra can be performed. For very proximal short-length bulbous strictures, tension-free anastomosis can be facilitated by the dissection of the membranous urethra (Fig. 40-20). As a rule, the closer the stricture is to the membranous urethra, the longer it can be and still be reconstructed with anastomotic techniques. For many proximal strictures, a single-layer anastomosis is preferable. When the length of stricture precludes total excision of fibrosis with primary anastomosis, tissue transfer is required. Morey and Kizer (2006) published a series of patients who had stricture excision with anastomosis for strictures up to 5 cm and pointed out that younger patients have more compliant tissue, allowing the limits to be stretched.

DeCastro and associates (2002) reported an interesting variant of excision with anastomosis for anterior stricture. In that case report, a patient had two independent areas of stricture apparently separated by totally normal urethra and corpus spongiosum. The authors excised both areas of stricture independently with respective anastomosis of each site. Although this case was successful, we think that the authors' considerable experience allowed them to achieve a successful result, and a safer reconstruction with use of onlay or augmented onlay might have been better.

Jordan and colleagues (2007) first reported the use of a vessel-sparing excision and reanastomosis of the bulbar urethra. The dissection is similar to the standard excision and reanastomosis (Fig. 40-21): The triangular ligament is divided, and the intracrural space is developed, the space between the membranous urethra and the proximal vasculature is developed, and these vessels are preserved (Fig. 40-22). The urethra is divided with the stenotic segment excised, the ends are spatulated, and the reanastomosis is performed. Andrich and Mundy (2012) described an alternative vessel-sparing technique for proximal strictures in which a longitudinal dorsal stricturotomy is performed and the stricture is excised from within the urethra without disrupting the spongiosum. After stricture excision, the ventral urethra is reapproximated primarily, and the longitudinal dorsal stricturotomy is closed horizontally, preserving the vasculature. Preserving the proximal blood supply to the bulbar urethra is advantageous in patients whose distal blood supply is compromised by trauma, previous surgery, or hypospadias. Another theoretical advantage would be a decrease in the risk of erectile dysfunction and potential decreased risk for erosion if subsequent artificial sphincter implantation were probable. Further studies need to be done to confirm the initial excellent results with the vessel-sparing technique and prove the theoretical advantages (Jordan, et al 2007; Gur and Jordan, 2008; Andrich and Mundy, 2012).

Four grafts that have been successfully used for primary urethral reconstruction are the full-thickness skin graft, bladder epithelial graft, oral mucosal graft, and rectal mucosal graft. Oral mucosal grafts, as mentioned earlier, can be taken from the cheek (buccal), the lip (labial), and the undersurface of the tongue (lingual). Split-thickness skin grafts have been used for staged anterior urethral reconstruction (Humby, 1941; Memmelaar, 1947; Pressman and Greenfield, 1953; Devine et al, 1976; Hendren and Crooks, 1980; Schreiter and Koncz, 1983; Webster et al, 1984; Hendren and Reda, 1986; Ransley et al, 1987; Burger et al, 1992; Jordan, 1993; El-Kassaby et al, 1996; Wessels and McAninch, 1996). The characteristics and microvascularity of some

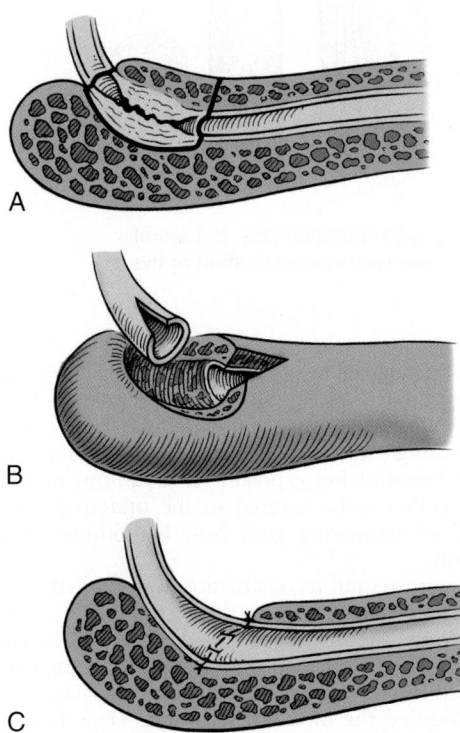

Figure 40-20. Technique of excision of very proximal bulbous urethral stricture with reanastomosis. This technique is facilitated by dissection of the membranous urethra. A, The area of the stricture is defined for excision. B, The stricture is excised, and both ends of the urethra are spatulated on the dorsal aspect. C, The anastomosis is complete.

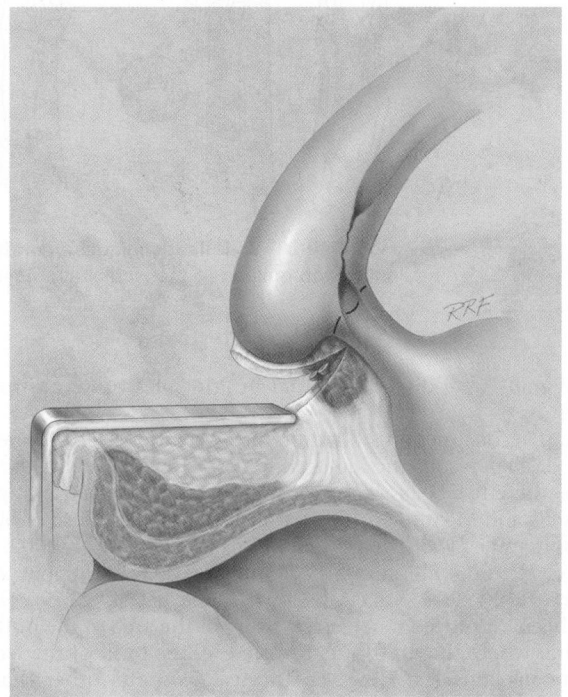

Figure 40-21. Diagrammatic representation of the dissection of the proximal corpus spongiosum, bulbospongiosum, and membranous urethra. The customary technique for dividing the urethra through the juncture of the membranous urethra with the proximal bulbous urethra—to perform an excision of stricture with a primary anastomosis. In this illustration, the proximal vasculature has been ligated and divided. The urethra can then be divided at the distal-most limits of the membranous urethra.

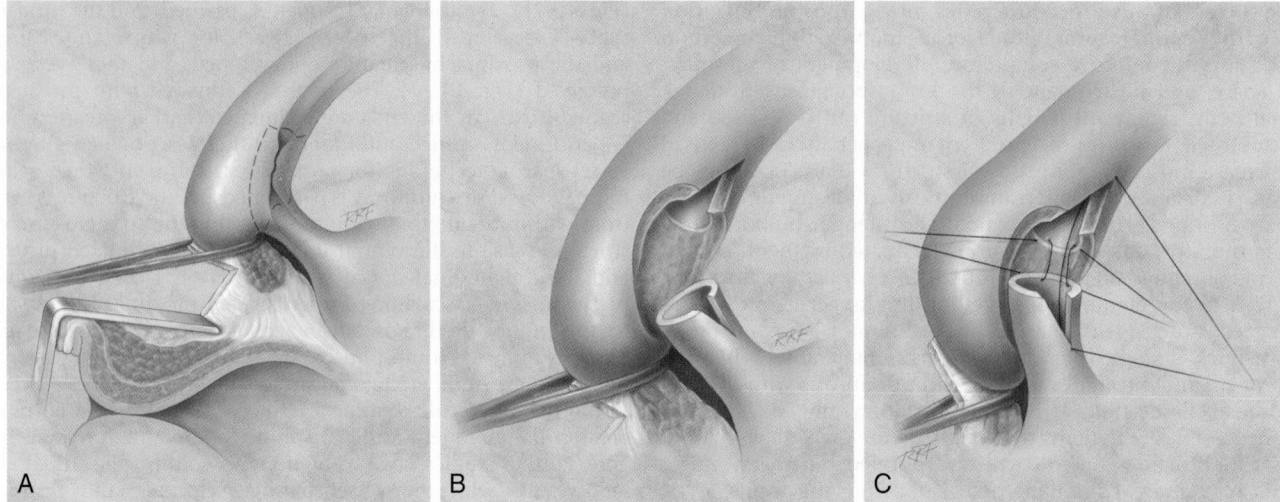

Figure 40-22. **Technique of vessel-sparing excision with primary anastomosis. The proximal corpus spongiosum, bulbospongiosum, and area of the proximal vessels and membranous urethra have been dissected. A, Dissection of the space between the proximal vasculature and the membranous urethra is illustrated. In this technique, the arteries to the bulb can be preserved, and the membranous urethra can be divided at its juncture with the bulbous urethra. The area of proximal stricture can be excised. B, The stricture has been excised before placement of the anastomotic sutures. C, Anastomotic sutures are placed to effect the spatulated anastomosis. At this center, customarily we alternate polydioxanone sutures with Monocryl; however, any acceptable absorbable suture can be used. The membranous urethra is spatulated on the dorsum as is the proximal bulbous urethra.**

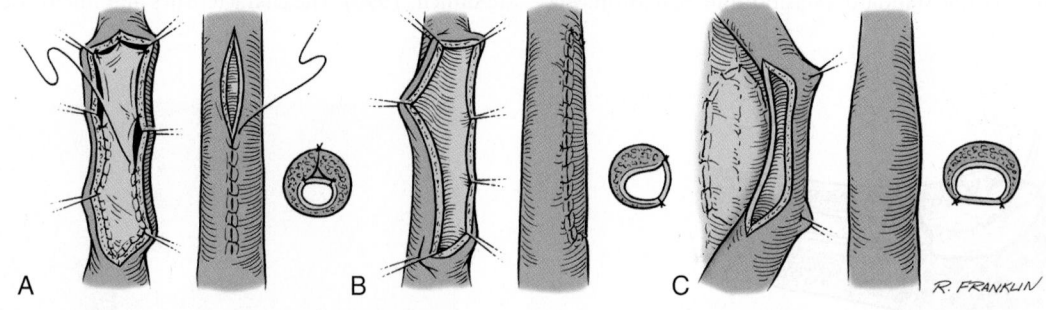

Figure 40-23. **Various techniques of graft onlay. A, Ventral onlay with spongioplasty. B, Lateral onlay with quilting to the ischiocavernosus muscle. C, Dorsal onlay with spread fixation of the graft.**

of the grafts were discussed earlier in Principles of Reconstructive Surgery.

Graft reconstruction of the urethra was almost abandoned in favor of flap reconstruction techniques. However, since the late 1990s, there has been a resurgence of interest in the use of grafts (Wessells and McAninch, 1996) and, specifically, the use of buccal mucosal grafts (Hellstrom et al, 1996; Weinberg et al, 2002; Barbagli et al, 2003; Elliott et al, 2003; Bhargava and Chapple, 2004; Kellner et al, 2004; Xu et al, 2004; Dubey et al, 2005). **Grafts have been employed most successfully in the area of the bulbous urethra, where the urethra is invested by the bulk of the ischiocavernosus muscles. However, the use of grafts other than in the area of the bulbous urethra and, in some cases, the use of tubed reconstruction are reported in increasing numbers.** The grafts can be applied to the ventrum of the urethra; however, a ventral urethrotomy seems to be advantageous only if use of the spongioplasty maneuver is contemplated (Fig. 40-23). The spongioplasty procedure requires that the corpus spongiosum adjacent to the area of the stricture be relatively normal and free of fibrosis. There are data to support the superiority of results with the dorsal onlay technique and other reports showing no difference in success.

In the past, we preferred to use lateral graft onlay (see Fig. 40-23B) or dorsal graft onlay (see Fig. 40-23C). Placement of the urethrostomy laterally allows exposure of the urethra while cutting through the corpus spongiosum, where it is relatively thinner, limiting bleeding and maximizing exposure. In addition, in the bulbous urethra, the graft can be sutured to the underlying muscle bed in the hope of improving graft–host bed immobilization and approximation.

The Monseur urethral reconstruction was applied in only a few select centers (Monseur, 1980). In this technique, the urethrostomy was made through the stricture on the dorsal wall. The edges of the stricture were sutured open to the underlying triangular ligament or corpora cavernosa, or both. Barbagli and associates (1995) subsequently modified the Monseur technique (Fig. 40-24). In their modification, the urethrostomy is performed through the stricture on the dorsal wall. In the area of the urethrostomy, a graft is applied and spread fixed to the triangular ligament or corpora cavernosa, or to both. The edges of the stricturotomy are sutured to the edges of the graft and to the adjacent structures. The results of this technique are excellent. The ventral and dorsal graft onlay techniques can be used with stricture excision and strip anastomosis (augmented

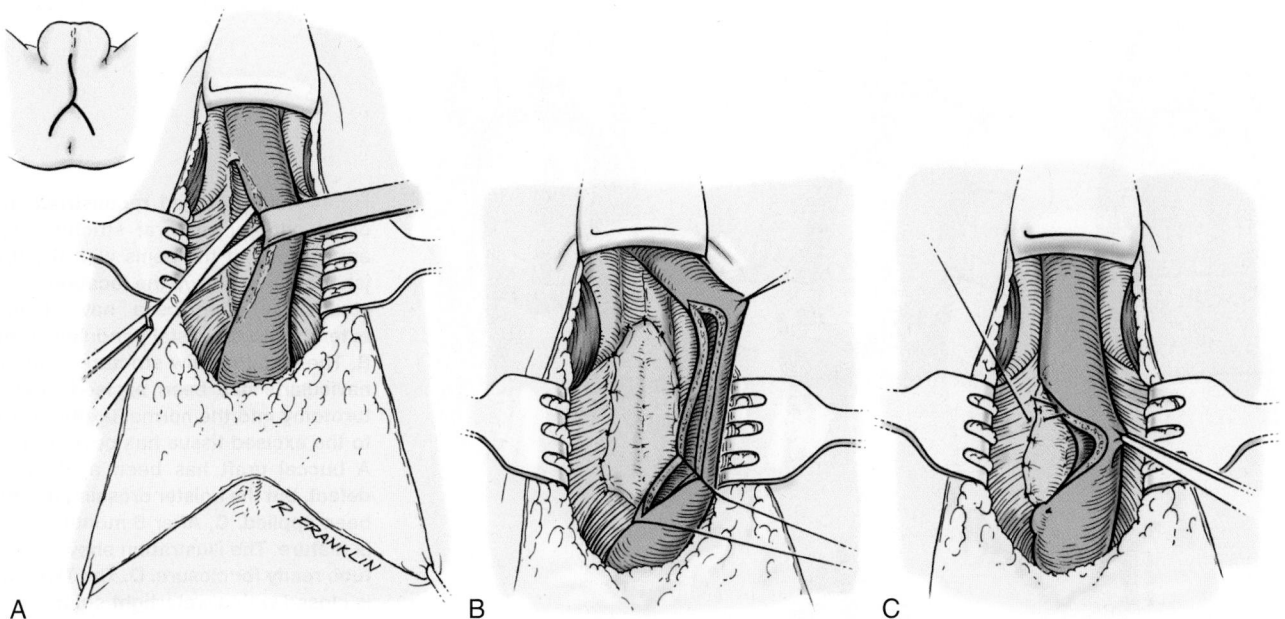

Figure 40-24. Technique of dorsal graft onlay popularized by Barbagli. A, The corpus spongiosum is detached from the triangular ligament and corpora cavernosa. B, A dorsal urethrostomy is performed. The graft is spread fixed to the corpora cavernosa. Note the pie-crusting incision. C, The edges of the stricturotomy are sutured to the graft and to the corpora cavernosa.

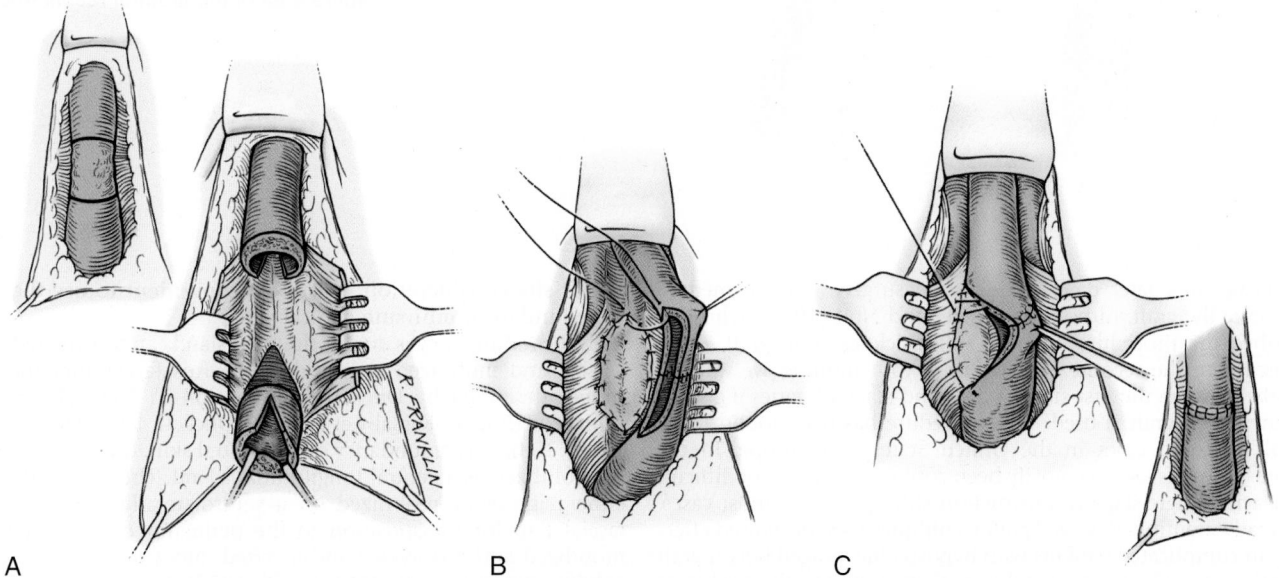

Figure 40-25. Technique of augmented anastomosis with graft onlay. A, The corpus spongiosum is detached from the triangular ligament and the corpora cavernosa. The area of spongiofibrosis is identified and marked, and the area of the narrowest caliber stricture is excised. The urethral ends are spatulated on the dorsum. B, A two-layer floor strip anastomosis is performed, and the graft is spread fixed to the corpora cavernosa. Note the pie-crusting incisions and the mattress sutures. C, The edges of the stricturotomy are sutured to the graft and to the corpora cavernosa.

anastomotic procedure) (Fig. 40-25). For proximal strictures, the vessel-sparing technique of augmented anastomosis depends on the surgeon's ability to excise the scarred epithelium and underlying corpus spongiosum tissue without the need to divide the corpus spongiosum completely.

Another option is the two-staged application of a mesh split-thickness skin graft, buccal mucosal graft, or posterior auricular full-thickness skin graft. In the first stage of the staged graft procedure, a medium-thickness split-thickness skin graft, a buccal mucosal graft, or a Wolfe graft is placed over the dartos fascia. If the graft is placed immediately onto the tunica albuginea or corpora cavernosa, the inability to mobilize the graft makes second-stage tubularization difficult. However, there is an advantage to having at least a midline strip of the graft adherent to the corpora

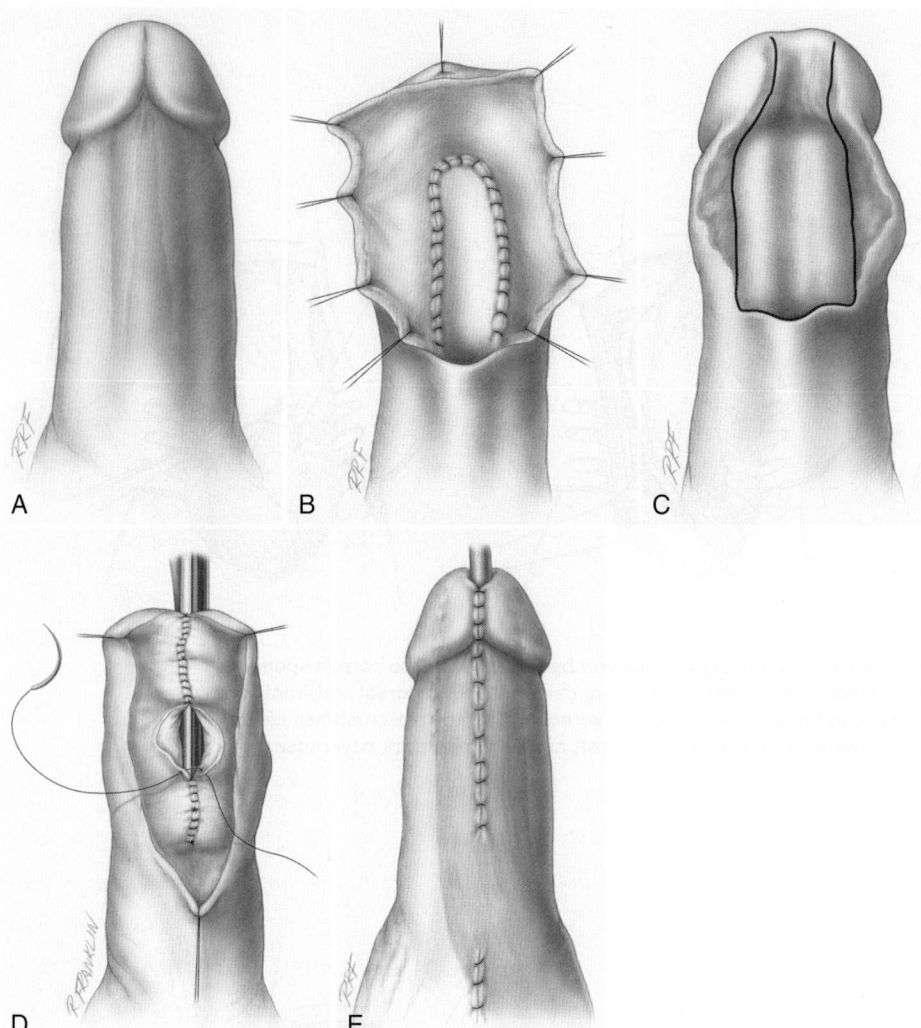

A

B

C

D

E

Figure 40-26. Staged reconstruction of a distal anterior urethral stricture. **A,** The appearance of the penis with the urethra (shaded area shows the location of a tight stenosis of the fossa navicularis that extends into the distal pendulous urethra). **B,** The distal narrow stricture of the fossa navicularis has been excised, and stricturotomy into the normal urethra proximal to the excised tissue has been performed. A buccal graft has been applied to the defect, but the bolster dressing has not yet been applied. **C,** After 6 months, the graft is mature. The illustration shows a Tiersch tube ready for closure. **D,** The Tiersch tube is closed with a watertight suture line. The distal urethra is usually calibrated to create a urethral lumen of approximately 28 Fr. **E,** Glans reconstruction and closure of the distal shaft has been performed (shaded area shows the tunica dartos flap that carries a parietal tunica vaginalis island). The flap is mobilized in this case from left hemiscrotum and transposed to cover the entire area of the urethral reconstruction.

cavernosa. At a later date, second-stage surgery is performed to tubularize the graft. Although Schreiter and Noll (1989), who first described the procedure of mesh split-thickness skin graft, often proceeded to the second stage within 3 to 4 months, we wait 12 months between the first-stage and second-stage surgeries if a split-thickness skin graft is used. This procedure has been found to be useful for select cases in the United States and Europe. In the United States, its use has mostly been confined to the most difficult cases, with single-stage reconstruction still applied to most cases. As already mentioned, staged graft techniques have been used effectively in complicated patients with hypospadias. Staged buccal graft operations have been successful in patients with LS with mid-term follow-up. In addition, in complicated patients with hypospadias, staged buccal grafts and posterior auricular skin grafts have been successfully employed (Fig. 40-26).

Numerous applications of genital skin islands, mobilized on either the dartos fascia of the penis or the tunica dartos of the scrotum, have been proposed for the repair of urethral stricture disease. In the past, these "flap operations" were considered separate procedures. We suggest that all these procedures are different applications of a single concept, as proposed by the microinjection studies of Quartey (1983). Skin islands can be viewed as passengers on fascial flaps, and the design of flaps for urethral reconstruction can be paralleled to the design of flaps for reconstruction in general.

There are **three important considerations for the use of flaps in urethral reconstruction: the nature of the flap tissue, the vasculature of the flap, and the mechanics of flap transfer.** The skin must be nonhirsute for urethral reconstruction. **In addition, for**

donor site consideration, it is most convenient to use the areas of redundant nonhirsute genital skin.**

If the redundancy is dorsal, the skin island can be oriented transversely and mobilized on the dorsal dartos fascia after the techniques described by Duckett and Standoli in 1984 (Fig. 40-27) (Duckett, 1986; El-Kassaby et al, 1986; Duckett, 1992; Duckett et al, 1993). If there is redundancy of the ventral skin, the skin island can be mobilized as a ventral longitudinal island. These islands can be either vigorously mobilized on a ventrolaterally oriented dartos fascial flap for transposition to the perineum or less vigorously mobilized and transposed and inverted into a pendulous urethral stricture defect (Fig. 40-28) (Orandi, 1972). Ventral islands can be oriented transversely (Fig. 40-29) and longitudinally. Longer skin islands can be mobilized by orienting the island ventrally and transversely at the distal extent. This "hockey stick" orientation allows islands 7 to 9 cm (Fig. 40-30). For distal strictures of the anterior urethra, including the fossa and meatus and the pendulous urethra, the islands can be advanced to reconstruct to the level of the meatus by either developing glans wings or elevating the ventral glans.

Where there is general redundancy to the penile skin, the islands can be oriented circumferentially. These "circular skin islands" are mobilized on the entire penile dartos fascia, and the mechanics of transposition suggest that they are most efficient when they are ventrally based, with the pedicle split dorsally. In some cases, circular skin islands 15 cm can be obtained (El-Kassaby et al, 1986; McAninch, 1993; Miller and McAninch, 1993). The so-called Q flap circular island design can provide even longer islands, sometimes necessary for complex long-length anterior urethral reconstruction (Morey et al, 2000).

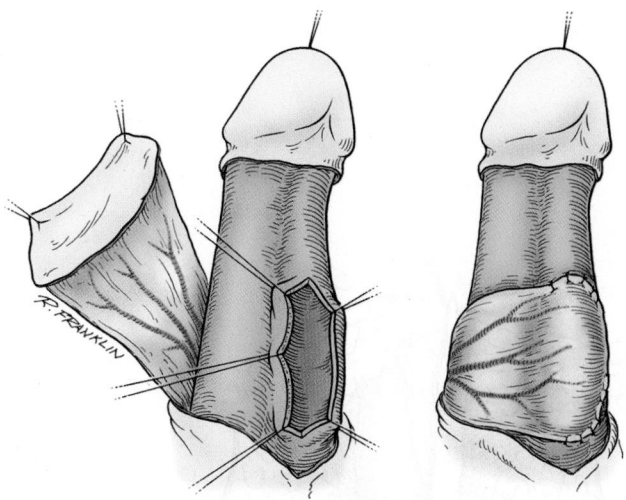

Figure 40-27. **A dorsal transverse island of penile skin applied to a stricture of the urethra. The flap has been elevated on the dartos fascia, and a lateral incision into the urethra has been made. The flap is secured in place *(right)*. (From Jordan GH. Management of anterior urethral stricture disease. In: Webster GD, editor. Problems in urology. Philadelphia: Lippincott; 1987. p. 217.)**

It is often beneficial to combine the excision of the stricture with a skin island onlay (Fig. 40-31) **or a graft onlay in an augmented anastomosis** (see Fig. 40-25). We have found that **segments of very narrow caliber (nearly or totally obliterating) are difficult.** These segments can often be completely excised; a roof or floor strip anastomosis of the urethra is performed, and the remaining urethrotomy defect is filled with either a graft or a skin island onlay. In some patients, there are relatively large nonhirsute areas of the scrotal skin that can be elevated on the tunica dartos of the scrotum. This flap has been maligned in the literature in the past. However, we and others have extensive experience with these flaps and, in select cases, have had very good results. The fascial flap must be based laterally, and so oriented, these flaps have been shown to be extremely reliable. Because the tunica dartos has a significant muscle component, the skin island must be carefully tailored. If these skin islands are correctly tailored at the outset, they are not attended with diverticular development as some have believed they were in the past. Scrotal skin islands are not our first choice; however, for difficult cases, they remain a reasonable option.

These procedures using skin islands oriented on the penile dartos fascia have also been useful for reconstruction of the fossa navicularis (Cohney, 1963; Blandy and Tresidder, 1967; Brannen, 1976; De Sy, 1984; Jordan, 1987; Armenakas et al, 1998). In the past, meatal strictures and strictures of the fossa navicularis were managed with repeated dilations or sequential meatotomies. Because these meatotomies were seldom successful in the long-term, techniques were developed that allowed the spatulation of random penile skin flaps into the meatotomy defects. These procedures functionally improved the results; however, the cosmetic appearance of the penis was suboptimal. With the use of skin islands elevated on the dartos fascia, excellent functional and cosmetic results became the norm. The design of these islands must take into consideration the location of hair on the shaft of the penis and the mechanics of flap transfer (i.e., transposition vs. advancement) (Figs. 40-32 and 40-33). In addition, full-thickness skin has been used to reconstruct the fossa navicularis, but when they can be avoided, skin grafts are not considered appropriate for reconstruction in cases of LS. As already mentioned, there is question about the use of skin islands in general in patients with LS.

The literature is clear that onlay procedures (graft or flap) are associated with a higher success rate than tubularized grafts or tubularized skin islands (Hendren and Crooks, 1980). **Tubularized grafts and skin islands should be avoided, if possible. When**

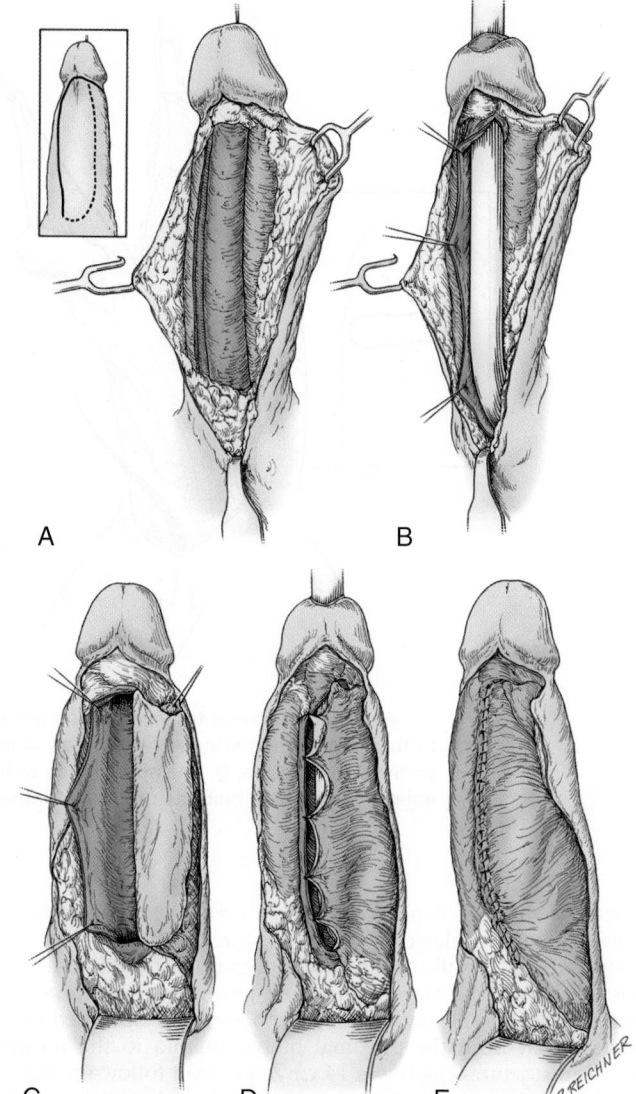

Figure 40-28. **Penile longitudinal skin island. The incisions to be made to mobilize the flap are demonstrated in the *inset*. The heavy line is the primary incision made full thickness through the dartos fascia and superficial Buck fascia lateral to the corpus spongiosum. A, Dissection elevates the dartos fascial flap well past the corpus spongiosum in the midline. B, A lateral urethrostomy placed to face the flap has opened the entire length of the stricture. C, The skin paddle of the flap has been developed by making the incision outlined by the dotted line *(inset)* and undermining the skin lateral to it. The medial edge of the flap has been fixed to the edge of the stricturotomy. D, The flap is inverted into the defect. E, A watertight subepithelial suture line has been completed with a running absorbable monofilament suture. The skin will be closed with subcutaneous sutures and interrupted cutaneous sutures. (From Jordan GH. Management of anterior urethral stricture disease. In: Webster GD, editor. Problems in urology. Philadelphia: Lippincott; 1987. p. 214.)**

tubularized segments cannot be avoided, the length of these segments can be limited by combining aggressive mobilization and excision. Without question, tubularized flaps provide better results than tubularized grafts. Where extremely long segments of the anterior urethra require reconstruction, a flap can be used distally and augmented by graft onlay proximally (Wessells et al, 1997). Where tubed reconstruction is required, in a small series with only short follow-up, the combination of a graft spread fixed to reestablish the "urethral plate" with flap onlay seems perhaps to

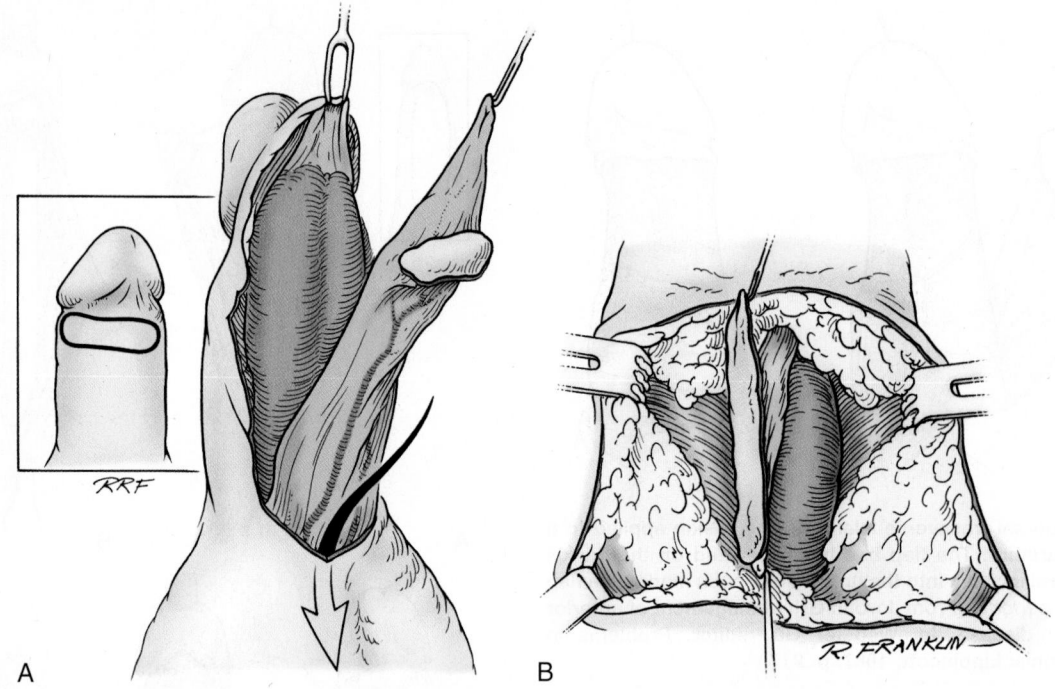

Figure 40-29. **A ventral transverse skin island is elevated on the penile dartos fascia, inverted to the area of the perineum where flap onlay is accomplished. A, The skin island is elevated on the dartos fascia. B, The appearance of the flap transposed to the area of the perineum for onlay in a proximal bulbous urethral stricture.**

be better than tubed flap reconstruction, even when it is employed in the onlay-tube-onlay configuration (Morey, 2001).

More recently, Kulkarni and colleagues (2012) published their approach to a single-stage panurethral reconstruction. Through a perineal incision and invaginating the penis, they described using a dorsal graft from the proximal bulbar urethra to the meatus. The mean stricture length was 14 cm, and mean follow-up was 59 months. The overall success rate was 83.7%; for primary repairs, the success rate was 86.5% compared with 61.5% in patients who failed a previous urethroplasty. Most of the recurrences the authors described were proximal.

A flap procedure that can be used as an alternative to split-thickness skin grafts when nonhirsute skin is unavailable is the epilated midline genital skin island. Similar to a split-thickness skin graft, this procedure must be viewed as a staged procedure, with the epilations being the initial stage or stages. Epilation can be accomplished with either a narrow-gauge needle and monopolar cautery or epilation needles and machines. The interval between the epilations must be 6 to 8 weeks, and urethral reconstruction cannot be accomplished until 10 to 12 weeks after the last epilation. The actual stricture repair involves elevation of the midline skin island, based on the dartos fascia of the penis and the tunica dartos of the scrotum. As with nonhirsute scrotal skin islands in general, the importance of meticulous tailoring of the scrotal portion of the island cannot be overemphasized.

Mundy (1994) analyzed a large series of urethral reconstructions. His data showed that when follow-up is limited to 1 year, the success rate with tissue transfer clusters is about 95%. However, with longer follow-up, there is deterioration over time. With excision and primary anastomosis, the success seen at 1 year seems to be more durable and does not appear to deteriorate at the same rate with time. We have reported our long-term data for excision and primary anastomosis with anterior urethral stenosis in 220 patients with a mean follow-up of 44 months; three recurrences were noted, two within the first 6 months and a third at 4 years. The rate of postoperative erectile dysfunction is 2%, with patients with severe straddle injuries being at

increased risk. **In a meta-analysis of graft onlay procedures compared with flap procedures, Wessells and McAninch (1998) showed equivalent results for graft operations and flap procedures,** and graft onlay procedures are technically far easier to perform. There are some cases where flap reconstruction would be expected to provide superior results (i.e., radiation strictures, patients with multiple operations, pendulous strictures). However, with the increased knowledge gained by the enthusiastic application of graft reconstruction, a paradigm for anterior reconstruction has been redefined. Although grafts have been used successfully for all segments of the anterior urethra, many authors think that, all other variables being equivalent, flaps are best suited for distal reconstruction, and grafts are best for proximal reconstruction (Greenwell et al, 1999).

Postoperative erectile dysfunction is an important issue. Our rates for anterior urethral anastomotic reconstruction were quoted earlier. **In an analysis by Coursey and colleagues (2001), 200 patients who underwent urethroplasty were studied. Overall, the rate of erectile dysfunction after urethroplasty was approximately equal to the rate after circumcision. Longer-segment reconstructions were associated with a higher risk of postoperative erectile dysfunction, although the patient's erectile function improved over time in many cases.**

Special mention is needed regarding reconstruction for strictures associated with LS. With the advent of flap techniques, many centers embraced these techniques for these strictures. However, analysis of results from patients with LS treated at several large centers showed a very high recurrence rate. Consequently, these centers adjusted the techniques by applying staged graft techniques (see Fig. 40-26). Staged graft techniques using skin grafts also had a very high recurrence rate in many analyses. **Theoretically, because LS is a skin condition, the use of skin as a flap, single-stage graft, or staged graft does not preclude involvement of the skin with the inflammatory process (Lee and Phillips, 1994; Akporiaye et al, 1997). Surgeons at numerous centers believe that staged oral graft techniques should be employed for reconstruction of strictures associated with LS.** Short-term follow-up results suggest better success

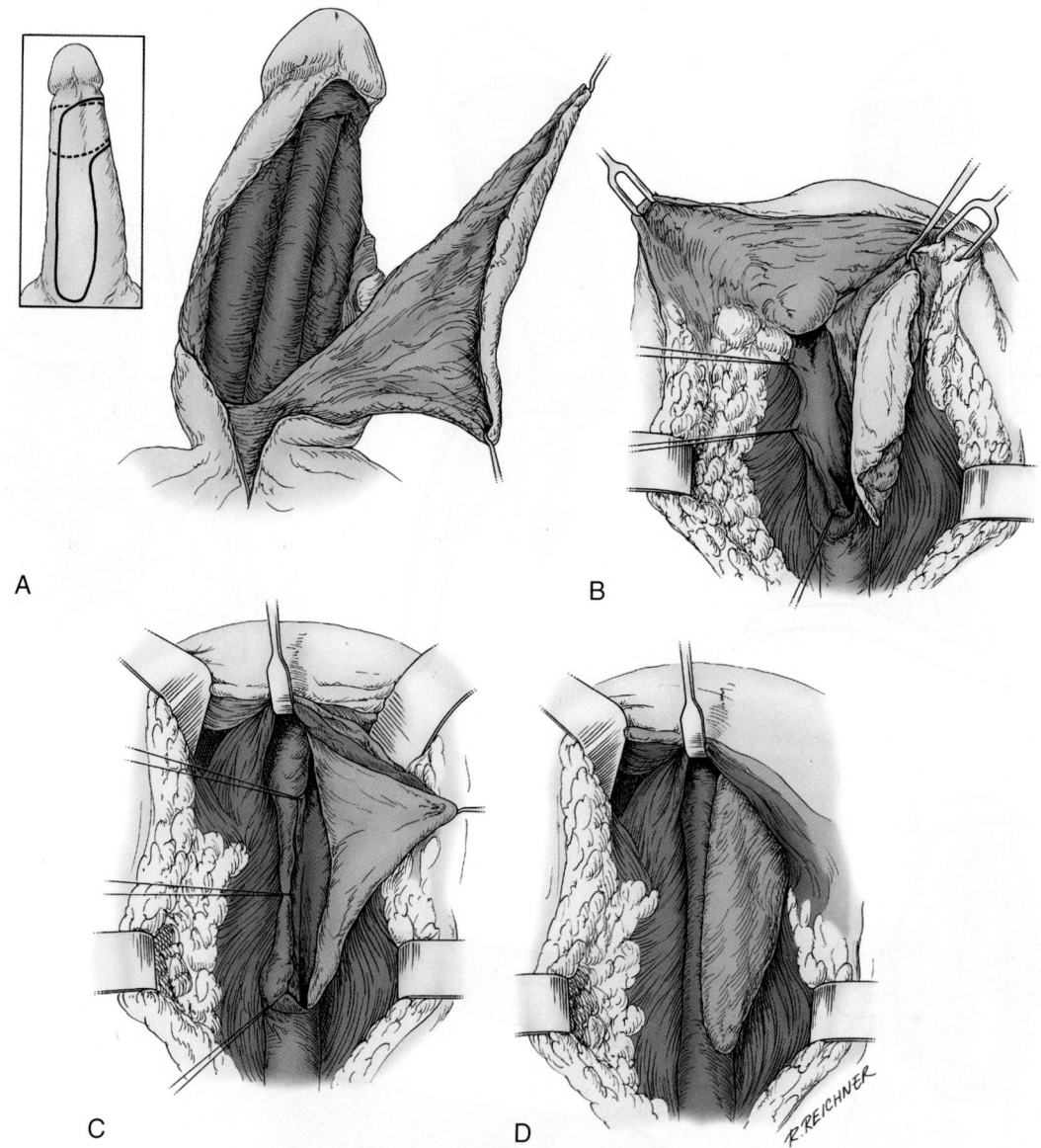

Figure 40-30. **Ventral skin island for long bulbous stricture.** The skin paddle of the flap is developed on the ventral midline of the penis and can be extended around the penile shaft at its distal end. **A,** The paddle of the flap has been incised, and its pedicle has been elevated. This pedicle includes Buck fascia and dartos fascia, denuding the tunica of the corpus spongiosum and the corpora cavernosa. The pedicle (the dartos fascia bilaterally) is based on the superficial external pudendal vessels and the internal pudendal vessels in the scrotum. Development of this pedicle allows the flap to be moved to any area of the urethra. **B,** The flap has been passed through a tunnel beneath the scrotum developed by dissection along the corpus spongiosum. A laterally placed urethrostomy has opened the urethral stricture. **C,** The deep edge of the flap is secured by the suture techniques previously described. **D,** Anastomosis of the flap has been completed. The pedicle can be seen extending beneath the scrotum. (From Jordan GH, McCraw JB. Tissue transfer techniques for genitourinary surgery, part III. AUA Update Series 1988;7:lesson 11.)

with this approach. Long-term follow-up results are unavailable. In a review of our experience in patients with a fossa navicularis stricture and LS, we noted a 50% recurrence in the stricture with a ventral transverse skin island (Virasoro et al, 2007).

PELVIC FRACTURE URETHRAL INJURIES

PFUIs are the result of blunt pelvic trauma and accompany about 10% of pelvic fracture injuries. Although total disruption of the urethra is possible with a straddle injury, these injuries most

commonly involve only the bulbous urethra. However, the ensuing spongiofibrosis can be associated with complete obliteration of the urethra. **Distraction injuries are unique to the membranous urethra.** Pelvic fracture distraction injuries of the membranous urethra have been compared with plucking an apple (prostate) off its stem (the membranous urethra). This analogy implies that the injury most frequently occurs at the apex of the prostate. However, experience shows that this is not the case, and the most frequent point of distraction is at the departure of the bulbous urethra from the membranous urethra (Andrich and Mundy, 2001; Mouraviev and Santucci, 2005). The distraction can

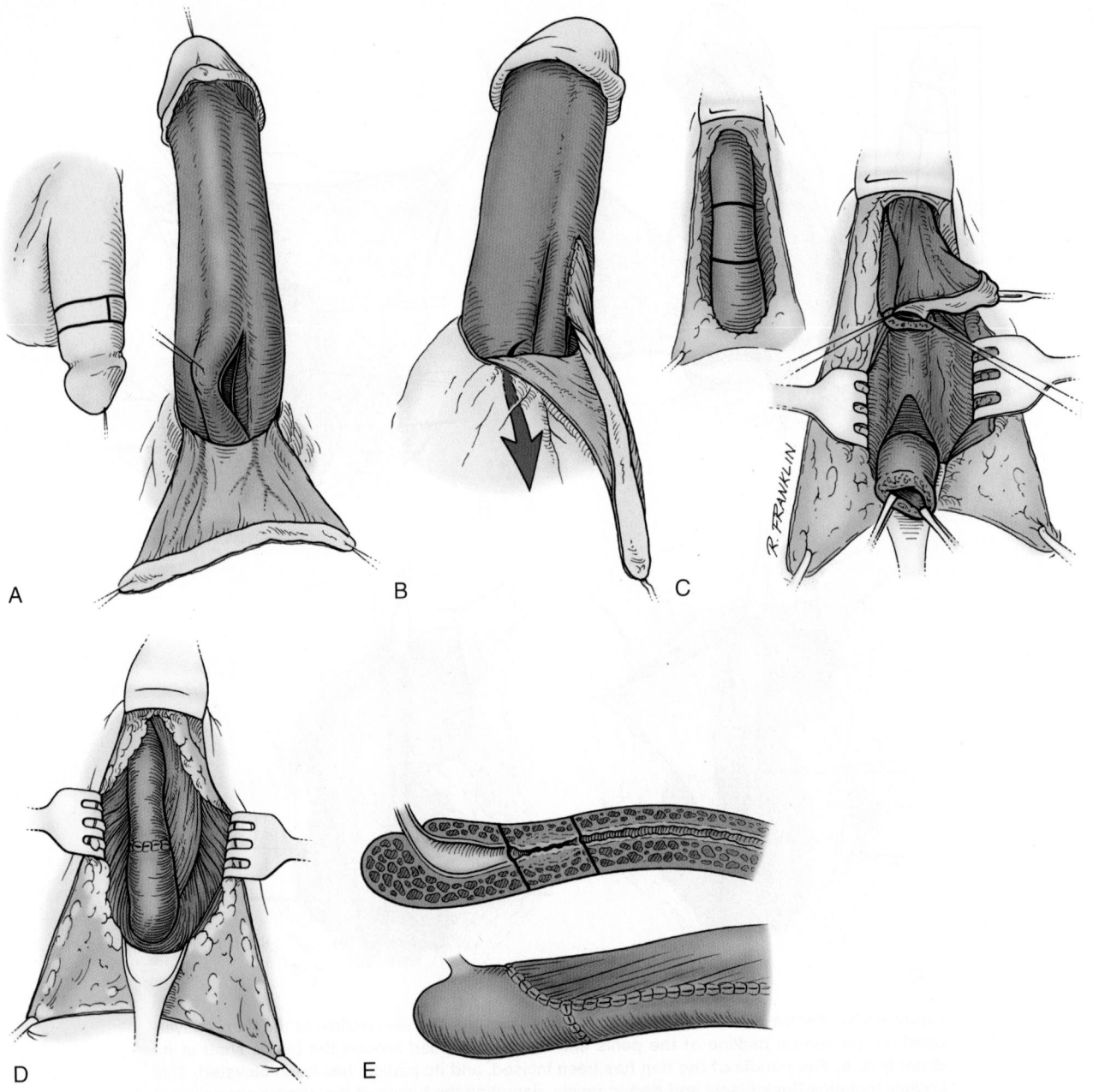

Figure 40-31. Reconstruction in a patient with a long anterior urethral stricture with a relatively short narrow-caliber section (technique of augmented anastomosis with circular skin island). A, A circular skin island is elevated on the dartos fascia. The patient is positioned flat on the table. **B,** The skin island onlay is begun, the rest of the flap is placed into the perineal dissection, and the penis is closed; the patient is then repositioned in the lithotomy position. **C,** The flap is retrieved through the perineal dissection. The narrow-caliber section is excised, and the urethra is spatulated on the dorsum. **D,** The onlay is completed, and the floor strip anastomosis is closed. **E,** Schematic of the surgery. (From Stack RS, Schlossberg SM, Jordan GH. Reconstruction of anterior urethral strictures by the technique of excision and primary anastomosis. Atlas Urol Clin North Am 1997;5:11–21.)

involve all or any portion of the membranous urethra between the departure of the bulbous urethra and the apex of the prostate. In postpubescent male patients, the injury seldom involves the prostatic urethra. In prepubescent male patients, in whom the prostatic urethra is more fragile, the injury can extend into that area.

Total distraction of the entire circumference of the urethra appears not to occur with many injuries. Instead, a strip of epithelium is left intact. In these patients, the placement of an aligning catheter may allow the urethra to heal virtually unscarred or with an easily managed stenosis. Because of flexible endoscopy equipment, the placement of an aligning catheter is straightforward. If distraction is complete, the catheter serves to align the obliterated urethral ends, and reconstruction is facilitated. Because of the ready availability of flexible cystoscopes, some centers acutely evaluate these injuries only with endoscopy. Clinicians who are enthusiastic for this approach believe that not only can the injury be completely evaluated, but also the entire process, including the placement of an aligning catheter, is expedited (Kielb et al, 2001). Aligning catheters are just what the name implies—a guide, not a mechanism for placing traction on the bladder and

KEY POINTS: TREATMENT OF URETHRAL STRICTURE

- In the treatment of urethral stricture disease, the patient and the physician must have a good understanding of the goals of treatment before the treatment choice is made.
- Urethral dilation is the oldest and simplest treatment of urethral stricture disease. However, the goal of dilation is to stretch the scar atraumatically. Dilation is seldom used curatively.
- Internal urethrotomy refers to any procedure that opens the stricture by incising it transurethrally. The factors that contribute to success of internal urethrotomy have been defined as follows: internal urethrotomy should be reserved for strictures of the bulbous urethra; the stricture should be less than 1.5 cm in length; and the stricture should not be associated with dense deep spongiofibrosis. Many studies have shown that repeated dilation and internal urethrotomies diminish the success rate of eventual open urethral reconstruction.
- Numerous lasers have been used for anterior urethral strictures. To date, the results of laser urethrotomy are mixed.
- Excision with primary anastomosis has proved to be the gold standard for repair of anterior urethral strictures. Previously, excision with primary anastomosis was thought to be a relatively limited procedure and applicable only for strictures less than 1.5 to 2 cm. However, with better understanding of the anatomy, longer strictures have been successfully addressed with excision and primary anastomosis.
- Some strictures require tissue transfer, and grafts and flaps have been successfully employed. A meta-analysis by Wessells and McAninch (1998) showed that the results of graft reconstruction and flap reconstruction are equivalent. The complexity of flap procedures is greater than that of graft procedures. The concept of augmented anastomosis can be used with graft and flap onlay and is thought to provide better results than just pure onlay in many cases. When flaps are employed for urethral reconstruction, conceptually all become one operation with multidimensional application.

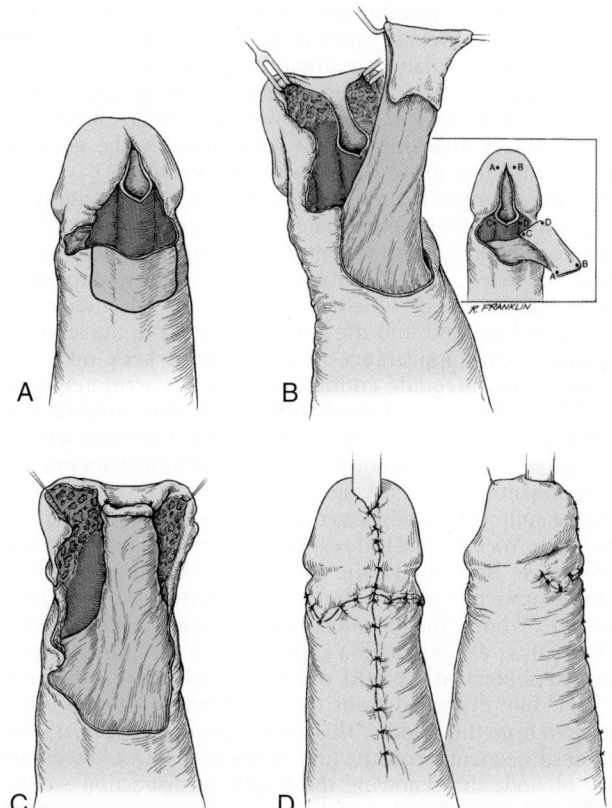

Figure 40-32. **Technique of reconstruction of the fossa navicularis after Jordan. A,** The ventral corpus spongiosum is exposed, and the urethra is opened ventrally through the area of stenosis. A transverse ventral skin island is outlined on the distal penile skin. **B,** The skin island is elevated on the ventral dartos fascia. **C,** The skin island is transposed and inverted into the meatotomy defect *(inset, B).* **D,** Appearance of the penis closed after the procedure. (A to C, From Jordan GH. Reconstruction of the fossa navicularis. J Urol 1987;138:1210; D, from Jordan GH. Reconstruction of the meatus–fossa navicularis using flap techniques. In: Schreiter F, editor. Plastic-reconstructive surgery in urology. Stuttgart: Georg Thieme; 1999. p. 338–44.)

prostate. Aligning catheters also seem to act as a drain as the pelvic hematoma liquefies, and perhaps the presence of the catheter may allow more rapid and complete resolution of the process (Cohen et al, 1991; Herschorn et al, 1992; Rehman et al, 1998; Mouraviev et al, 2005). Close follow-up after a voiding trial is essential because many of these patients experience stricture formation after removal of the aligning catheter and require definitive repair (Leddy et al, 2012).

Evaluation

As with the repair of any stricture or stenosis, it is important to define the precise anatomy of the pelvic fracture injury before treatment is undertaken (McCallum and Colapinto, 1979a, 1979b); this includes the depth, density, length, and location. In pelvic fracture urethral distraction defects, the depth and density of fibrosis are predictable. Although the location of the distraction injury has been shown to be an important factor in continence after reconstruction, this information should be a factor only in counseling of patients before the reconstruction and not in the treatment approach. The length of the defect is an important consideration and must be determined as precisely as possible.

Contrast studies are a first-line tool for the evaluation of PFUI. A cystogram outlines the bladder and provides information about rostral displacement of the proximal urethra. A lack of contrast material in the posterior urethra gives some information, albeit inconclusive, about the integrity of the bladder neck.

When the patient is successful in relaxing to void and the cystogram outlines the posterior urethra, a simultaneous retrograde urethrogram outlines the length of the injury defect.

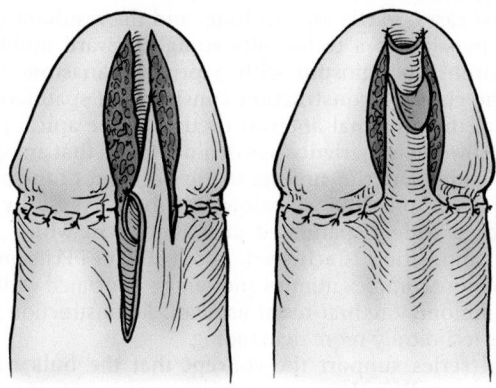

Figure 40-33. **Technique after De Sy, in which a ventral longitudinal skin island is advanced into the meatotomy defect. The skin island is developed by de-epithelialization of a portion of the longitudinal flap.** (From Jordan GH. Management of anterior urethral stricture disease. Probl Urol 1987;1:199–225.)

However, this situation is the exception rather than the rule, and retrograde urethrography is most useful for determining whether the anterior urethra is normal. If the anterior urethra is normal, **it has been our experience and the experience of others that a successful anastomotic repair is ensured.** A primary anastomosis has been shown to be possible even with some involvement of the anterior urethra. Even in cases of prior failed posterior urethral reconstruction, primary anastomotic repair is often feasible, although the failure rate is slightly higher in these cases (Chapple and Pang, 1999; Flynn et al, 2003; Koraitim, 2003; Shenfeld et al, 2004). **Primary anastomosis is unquestionably the goal in all patients until it is proved impossible to perform.**

When the proximal urethra is not visualized on a simultaneous cystogram with urethrogram, endoscopy through the suprapubic tract in combination with retrograde urethrography can be used to outline the defect. After the endoscopic appearance of the bladder neck is assessed, the flexible endoscope can be advanced through the bladder neck and into the posterior urethra to the level of the obstruction. **The appearance of the bladder neck on contrast studies or on antegrade endoscopy does not accurately predict the ultimate function of the bladder neck after urethral reconstruction** (Iselin and Webster, 1999). A simultaneous retrograde urethrogram outlines the anterior urethra, with the space not visualized representing the injury defect.

Some authors have advocated MRI for the evaluation of patients with PFUIs. We have had little experience with MRI for that purpose; however, we have found the information obtained on the few studies that we have done to be useful. In these cases, there was the question of bone interposition into the injury defect, and MRI outlined this. We evaluated a case in which the prostatic urethra appeared obliterated. On MRI, one could easily see that the prostate was not only distracted from the membranous urethra but also distracted from the bladder. This information was essential to planning of subsequent reconstruction in this case. It would seem intuitively obvious that knowing the length of distraction would be helpful in determining the precise approach and steps necessary for reconstruction. However, the literature is unclear on this matter (Andrich et al, 2003; Koraitim, 2004), and it is our experience that the surgeon must be prepared to exercise all options of reconstruction in virtually all such cases (McCallum and Colapinto, 1979a, 1979b).

Repair

The timetable for the reconstruction of PFUIs is determined by the type and extent of associated injuries. If possible, it is desirable to proceed within 4 to 6 months after trauma. However, orthopedic injuries of the lower extremities often necessitate a delay in proceeding with urethral reconstruction (Mundy, 1991; Follis et al, 1992; Brandes and Borrelli, 2001).

In most cases, PFUIs are not long, and the resultant obliteration is amenable to a technically straightforward mobilization of the corpus spongiosum with a primary anastomotic technique. The classic reconstruction consists of a spatulated anastomosis of the proximal anterior urethra to the apical prostatic urethra. However, experience has demonstrated that anastomosis of the proximal anterior urethra to any segment of the posterior urethra (apical, prostatic, or below) **can be successfully accomplished by a widely spatulated anastomosis in which optimal epithelial apposition is achieved.** About 10% of PFUIs are associated with more complex injuries and can be associated with fistulae (most commonly urethral rectal fistulae). Reconstruction of these injuries is technically more demanding.

Several series support the concept that the bulk of PFUIs, even the most difficult cases, can be managed by the perineal approach (Webster et al, 1983; Koraitim, 1985; Webster and Sihelnik, 1985; Webster et al, 1990; Morey et al, 1996; Koraitim, 1997; Flynn et al, 2003). A transpubic or an abdominal-perineal approach, as pioneered by Waterhouse and colleagues (1973), in our experience, is unnecessary for the reconstruction of distraction injuries. In addition, pubectomy can be associated with long-term sequelae, including shortening of the penis, destabilization of erection, and destabilization of the pelvis, resulting in a chronic pain syndrome with exercise. However, some surgeons continue to rely heavily on the transpubic approach (Koraitim, 1997; Das et al, 2004).

Alternatively, the above-and-below approach has merit when concomitant surgery is planned in the region of the bladder neck. We have found and Iselin and Webster (1999) reported that the competence of the bladder neck is difficult to assess accurately before the reestablishment of urethral continuity. In the past, great reliance was placed on whether the bladder neck was closed or open on cystography. However, contrast material may opacify the prostatic urethra when the bladder neck is more than adequately competent for continence. Similarly, confidence has been placed in the appearance of the bladder neck on endoscopic examination through the suprapubic tube. Again, even when an obvious scar is noted to involve the bladder neck, follow-up of these patients after urethral reconstruction establishes continuity of the urethra and finds many patients with more than adequate continence. Other patients are believed to have incontinence secondary to scar incarceration of the bladder neck, caused by the extensive fibrosis left behind by resolution of the hematoma. However, in our experience, this is an infrequent occurrence, and the appearance of the bladder neck by any modality available is not predictive of continence. It is currently our practice to reestablish the continuity of the urethra and, when there are concerns about continence, to forewarn the patient before the urethral reconstruction. If these patients find that they experience inadequate continence postoperatively, the problem is addressed in a subsequent procedure (Bhargava et al, 2004).

At the time of reconstruction, before the patient is placed in the lithotomy position, endoscopy is performed through the meatus and again through the suprapubic tube sinus. Endoscopy on the table is designed to ensure that there is no concomitant vesicolithiasis. The endoscopy is performed with a rigid endoscope, which is manipulated through the suprapubic tube sinus and the bladder neck and positioned against the area of total obliteration. On gentle manipulation of the endoscope, if the impulse of the endoscope tip is felt on the patient's perineum, the impulse is palpable when the perineum is opened, and an instrument is manipulated through the bladder neck during reconstruction. If the impulse is not palpable perineally at this time, it may not be palpable during dissection. We create a temporary vesicostomy in these cases, which allows us to position an instrument reliably through the bladder neck because the vesicostomy allows the surgeon to identify the bladder neck palpably before instrumentation of the posterior urethra. This maneuver has eliminated the occurrence of false passages with use of a sound such as the Haygrove staff through the suprapubic site and has eliminated the occurrence of misanastomosis of the anterior urethra to sites other than the apical proximal urethra.

We prefer the use of the exaggerated lithotomy position for the perineal approach (Fig. 40-34). This position is safe and provides optimal exposure to the area of the membranous and apical prostatic urethra (Angermeier and Jordan, 1994). A custom Skytron table, modified to allow the exaggerated lithotomy position, and a Stille-Scandia table, designed to place patients in the lithotomy position, are our preferences. The legs are carefully positioned in Allen-style or Guardian-style stirrups. Care is taken to avoid pressure on the lateral aspects of the lower extremities and calf muscles. The patient's hips are elevated into position by raising the buttocks portion of the operating table. The boots are positioned to avoid stretch injuries of the common peroneal nerves (see Fig. 40-34).

After the patient is correctly positioned, the perineal approach to reconstruction begins with an incision and dissection anterior to the transverse perinei musculature (anterior perineal triangle). This is in contrast to the approach posterior to the transverse perinei musculature (posterior anal triangle), which is useful for perineal prostatectomy. We use a λ-shaped incision (Fig. 40-35) that is carried sharply down to the midline fusion of the ischiocavernosus musculature (see Fig. 40-35A), then beneath the scrotum, to expose the uninvested portion of the corpus spongiosum. We then place a self-retaining ring retractor.

The fusion of the ischiocavernosus musculature is divided, and the musculature is cleanly dissected from the corpus spongiosum and bulbospongiosum (see Fig. 40-35B to D). The corpus spongiosum is detached from the triangular ligament and corpora cavernosa (see Fig. 40-35E), the bulbospongiosum is detached from the

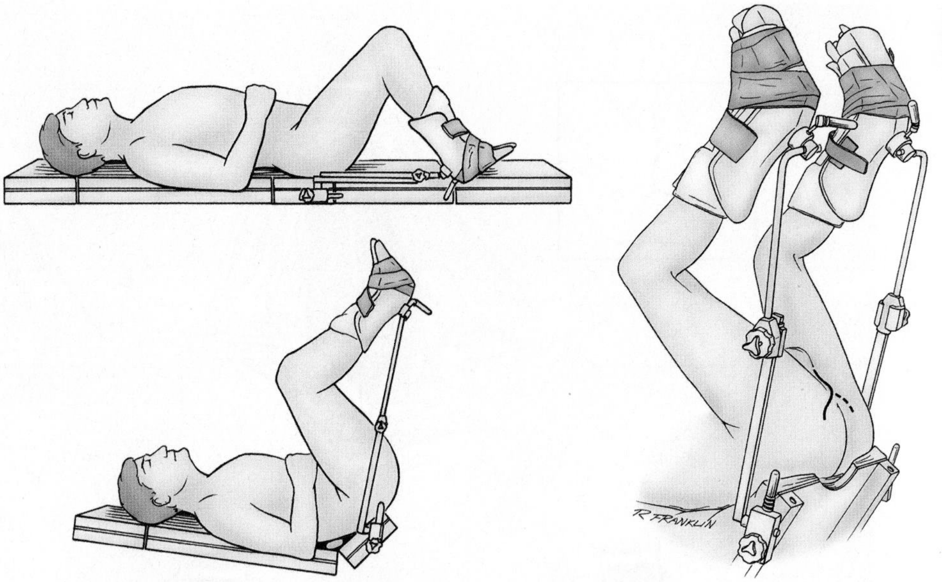

Figure 40-34. **Patient placed in an exaggerated lithotomy position. The hips have been rotated into position by elevation of the buttocks portion of a specially modified table. The legs are suspended from boot-style stirrups with as little flexion of the hips and knees as allowed by the design of the stirrups. (From Angermeier KW, Jordan GH. Complications of the exaggerated lithotomy position: a review of 177 cases. J Urol 1994;151:866–8.)**

perineal body, and the dissection is carried farther down to the infrapubic space. Posterior detachment of the bulbospongiosum is carried anteriorly, and the dissection is eventually carried through the area of fibrosis (see Fig. 40-35F).

In some cases, the proximal blood supply is encountered and must be controlled. We have found that these arteries are easily controlled with a sharp-tipped hemostat and monopolar cautery. Suture ligature should be avoided in the arteries to the bulbospongiosum because of their proximity to the nerves as they are coursing into the corpora cavernosa.

We divide the triangular ligament and vigorously develop the intracrural space down to the pubis (Fig. 40-36). If the dorsal vein is encountered, it is ligated and divided. It is important to ensure that the arteries were not rolled into the intracrural space if the tissues were dislocated during trauma. The penetration of the cavernosal arteries or the dorsal arteries, or both, into this space is commonly seen. If there is doubt about the nature of the vessels encountered, Doppler sonography should be performed. When the pubis is exposed, the periosteal elevator can be gently introduced onto the retropubic surface, releasing and allowing the descent of the tissues from beneath the pubis.

We introduce a Haygrove staff into the suprapubic sinus and through the bladder neck to the distal limits of the posterior urethra (see Fig. 40-35G and H). The impulse is palpated, and the fibrosis is resected until normal tissue planes are encountered. The tissue is submitted for histologic examination. The tip of the Haygrove staff is eventually concealed only by the normal urethral epithelium, at which point we open the epithelium and control it with either a skin hook or a stitch. We perform endoscopy to ensure that the urethrotomy is at the distal limits of the posterior urethra. If a tension-free anastomosis is thought to be impossible, we mobilize the corpus spongiosum beneath the scrotum from its attachment to the corpora cavernosa. Aggressive mobilization of the corpus spongiosum is the last maneuver undertaken because it is thought to have possible ill effects on the retrograde blood supply, which in a patient with pelvic fracture may be tenuous. Meticulous detachment of the investment of Buck fascia from the corpus spongiosum increases the compliance of the corpus and limits the need for aggressive mobilization.

It is important to try to avoid the creation of chordee during the repair of a distraction injury. To prevent chordee, the attachment cannot be carried beyond the area of the penoscrotal attachment. However, it is warranted in some cases to counsel patients preoperatively that they may have some chordee after aggressive mobilization that results in a primary anastomotic repair. Primary anastomotic repairs have success rates in the high 90% range. If a

technique of tissue transfer is needed, the long-term cure rates may eventually be only in the mid-80% range. Most of these patients are young. Successful, durable reconstruction is of paramount importance. If chordee results, it is most often mild and not disabling sexually; in our and other surgeons' minds, it is probably a fair trade for optimizing the urethral reconstruction. Development of the intracrural space—mobilization of the corpus spongiosum, infrapubectomy, and, if needed, rerouting of the corpus spongiosum—shortens the course that the corpus spongiosum must traverse and allows reconstruction without attendant chordee.

The proximal urethrotomy is spatulated so that it accepts at least a 32-Fr bougie à boule, and 10 to 12 anastomotic sutures are placed and tagged to allow identification of their position in the proximal anastomosis. We have used a combination of 3-0 Monocryl and 3-0 polydioxanone sutures for this purpose. No special needles are required for the placement of these sutures. However, a Heaney needle driver and a Ravitch needle driver can be useful in difficult cases. After spatulation of the proximal urethrotomy and placement of the sutures, we spatulate the proximal portion of the anterior urethra. The spatulation is continued until the urethrotomy accepts a 30-Fr to 32-Fr bougie à boule, and the anastomotic sutures are placed in their respective locations. Before seating the anastomosis, we introduce a soft silicone (Silastic) ribbed urethral stenting catheter through the anastomosis under direct vision. The wound is copiously irrigated to reduce the clot around the area of the anastomosis, and the anastomosis is seated.

Next, we reattach the corpus spongiosum to the corpora cavernosa and the bulbospongiosum to the perineal body. We place a small suction drain deep to the closure of the ischiocavernosus musculature and Colles fascia and a second one superficial to that closure and beneath the subcutaneous closure.

In cases in which the proximal urethra is significantly distracted in a rostral direction, the surgeon must be prepared to perform infrapubectomy (Fig. 40-37) or corporeal rerouting, or both (Fig. 40-38). Performance of the infrapubectomy, along with the development of the intercrural space, allows exposure of the apical prostatic urethra. When the prostatic urethra remains rostrally displaced, the impulse of the sound or instrument placed through the cystostomy tract into the bladder neck is often not readily apparent. In these situations, it is comforting to be able to palpate the bladder neck and the properly placed sound before embarking on a dissection beneath the pubis. In addition, if the rostral distraction is significant, the path of the anterior urethra over the hilum of the penis into the infrapubectomy often does not allow a tension-free anastomosis, and the infrapubectomy can be continued beneath

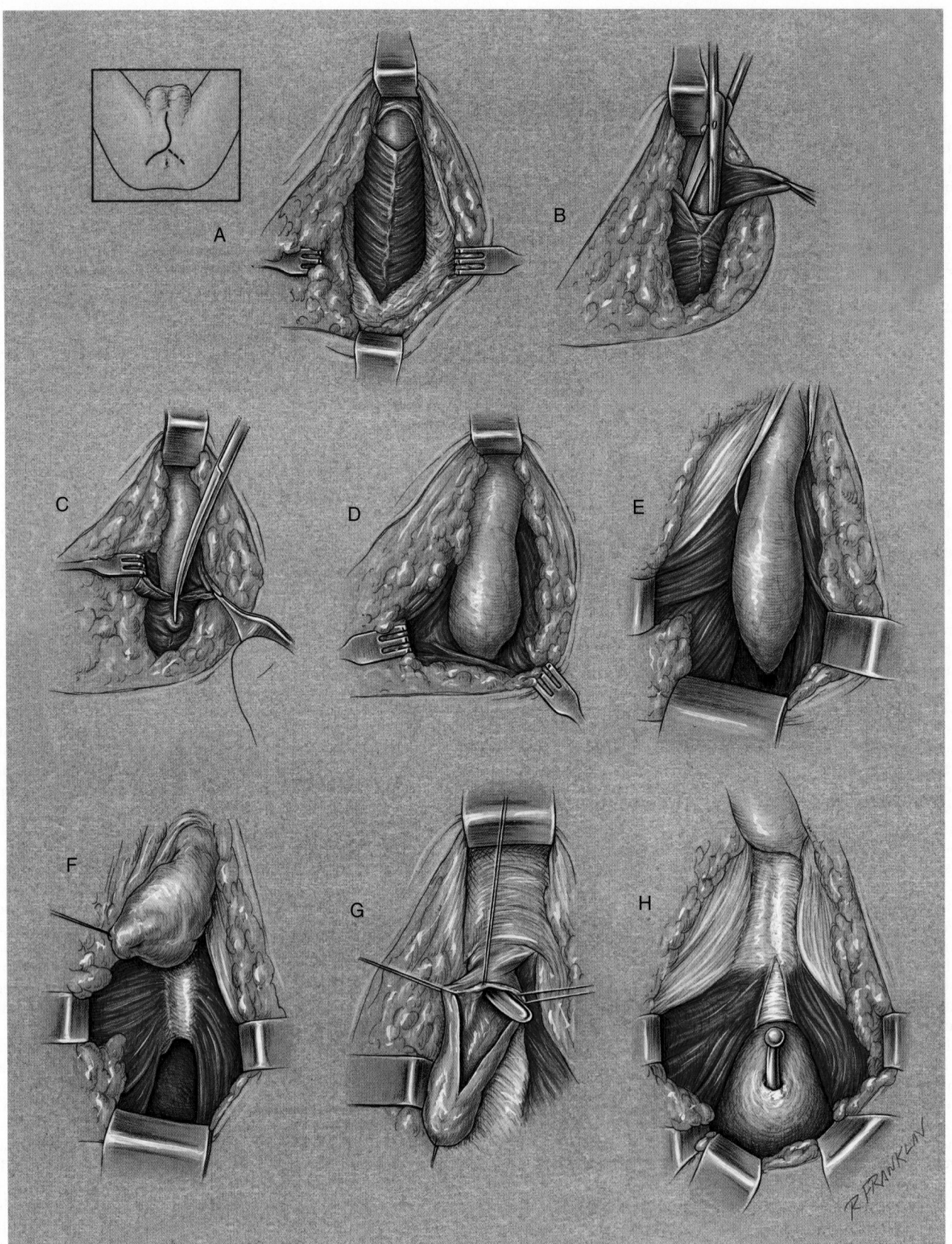

one side of the corpora cavernosa, allowing rerouting of the corpus spongiosum (see Fig. 40-38).

Postoperative Management

We use a small soft silicone (Silastic) stenting catheter. Urine is diverted via the suprapubic cystostomy, and the urethral catheter is plugged and serves as a stent only. After the reconstruction, patients are initially kept at bed rest for 24 to 48 hours and then ambulated and discharged with the suprapubic catheter and stenting urethral catheter in place. Patients are discharged on a regimen of oxybutynin and a suppressive antibiotic only if the preoperative urine culture was positive. The drains are removed as drainage allows.

A voiding trial with contrast material is performed between 21 and 28 days postoperatively. Patients are directed to stop taking oxybutynin 24 hours before the voiding trial. In anastomoses that are technically straightforward, the trial is performed at 21 days, and

in cases with more rostral distraction of the proximal urethra, the trial is delayed for 3 to 5 days longer. The trial involves removing the urethral catheter, filling the patient's bladder with contrast material, and instructing him to void. We do not use pericatheter retrograde urethrography to evaluate patients who have undergone urethral reconstruction. The voiding film is examined to ensure that there is no extravasation and that the reanastomosis appears widely patent. A urine culture specimen is also obtained, and the suprapubic catheter is plugged. The patient is allowed to void through the urethra for 5 to 7 days, and the suprapubic catheter is then removed. Approximately 6 months postoperatively and again 1 year later, patients are evaluated with flexible endoscopy. At that time, we consider the reconstruction to be mature, and it should be widely patent. If no symptoms have reappeared, we refer further follow-up examinations to the referring urologist.

We have almost completely replaced postoperative retrograde studies with flexible endoscopy. We have not found flow studies

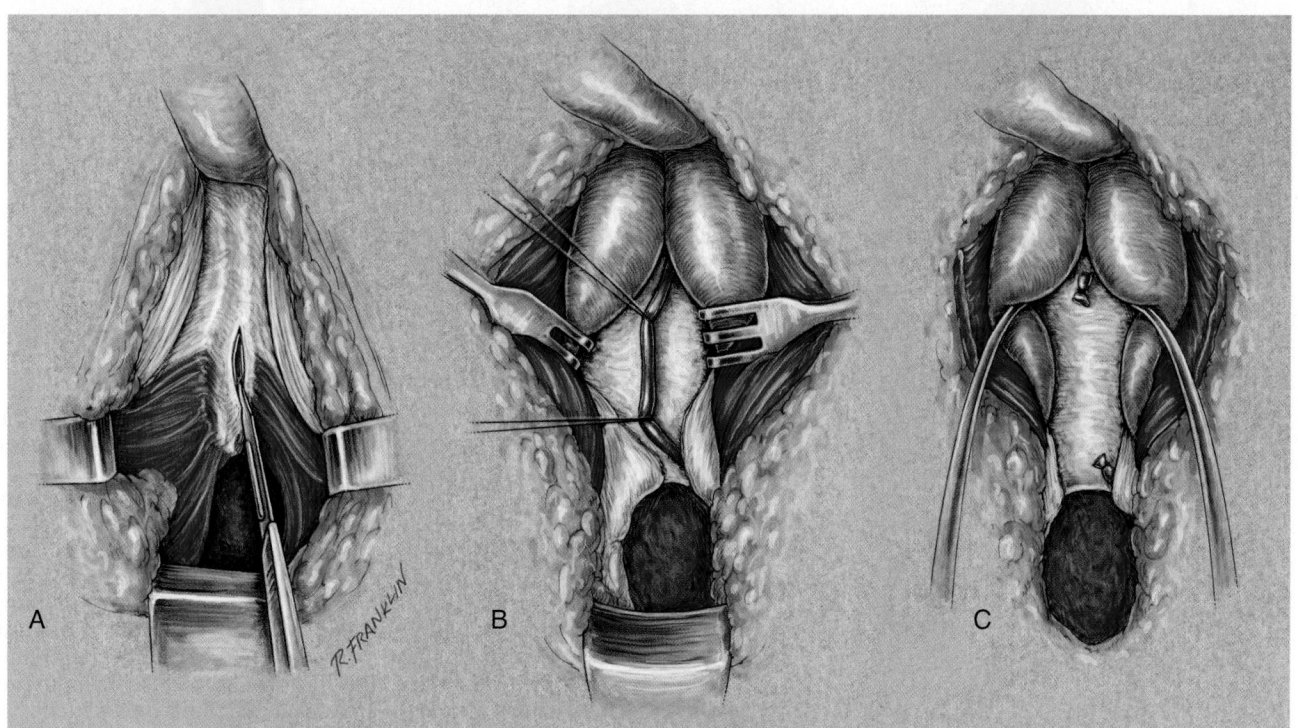

Figure 40-36. Division of the triangular ligament and development of the intracrural space. A, When the prostatic urethra is displaced, and the arc that the urethra must traverse needs to be shortened, that length can be shortened by incision of the triangular ligament. **B,** Incision and mobilization of the perichondrium and periosteum of the symphysis pubis to allow placement of retractors without trauma to the erectile bodies. Lateral displacement of the crura exposes the dorsal vein of the penis; after careful identification, the vein can be ligated and divided. **C,** Completion of the dissection affords additional exposure for resection of the fibrosis that surrounds the apex of the prostate and the proximal end of the disrupted urethra. (From Jordan GH. Reconstruction of the meatus–fossa navicularis using flap techniques. In: Schreiter F, editor. Plastic-reconstructive surgery in urology. Stuttgart: Georg Thieme; 1999. p. 338–44.)

Figure 40-35. Perineal repair of a membranous urethral stricture. A λ-shaped incision extends from the midline of the scrotum to the ischial tuberosities. **A,** Colles fascia has been opened to expose the midline fusion of the ischiocavernosus muscles and the tunica of the corpus spongiosum distal to the edge of the muscles. **B,** The scissors are introduced to develop the space between the muscle and the bulb of the urethra. **C,** An incision is made in the midline with the scissors, exposing the length of the bulb. **D,** The ischiocavernosus muscle is retracted to expose the full length of the bulb. **E,** The self-retaining retractor is placed to expose the inferior fascia of the genitourinary diaphragm. The bulb of the corpus spongiosum (bulbospongiosum) can be mobilized to gain access to the fibrosed area of the urethra. **F,** The fibrosed urethra is incised, freeing the bulb. **G,** The anterior urethra is opened to make an adequate lumen. **H,** The Haygrove staff has been passed through the suprapubic cystostomy. Resection of the fibrotic distraction defect has allowed it to pass into the perineum.

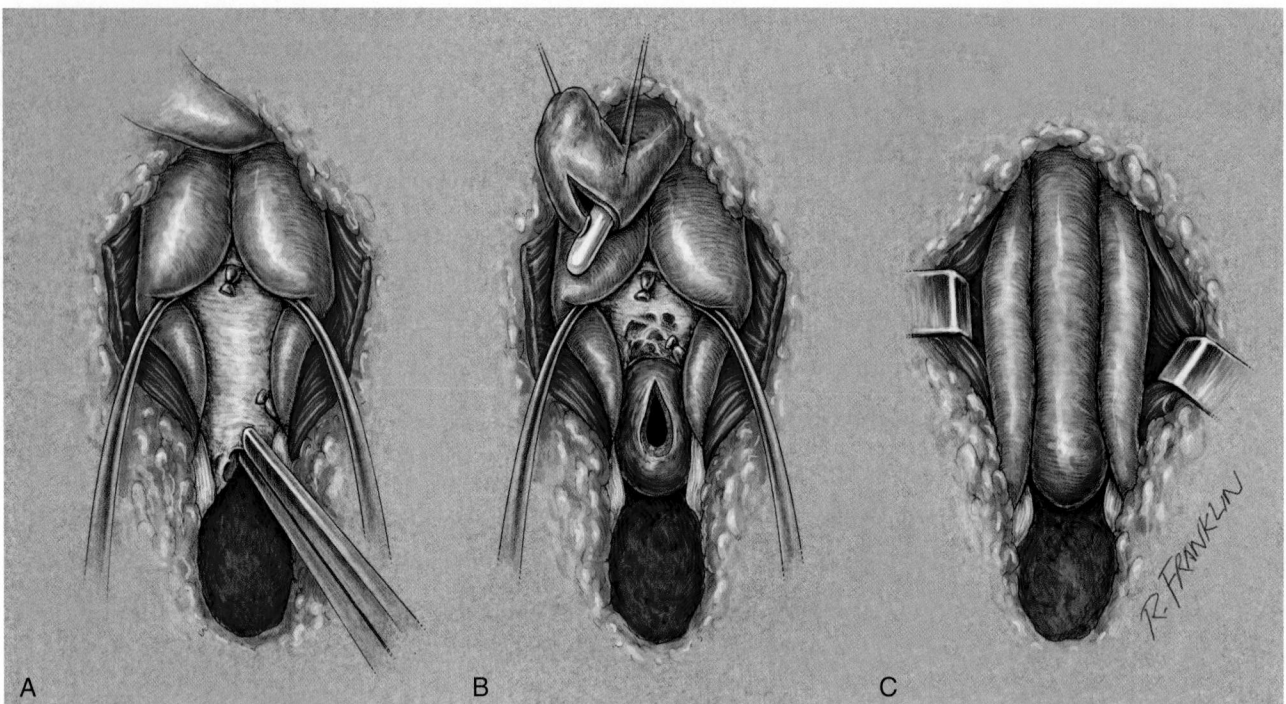

Figure 40-37. Infrapubectomy. If the prostate is elevated behind the symphysis pubis (A), the inferior aspect of the symphysis is resected with a Kerrison rongeur. As much of the bone can be removed as necessary (B) to afford a simple approximation of the ends of the urethra (C).

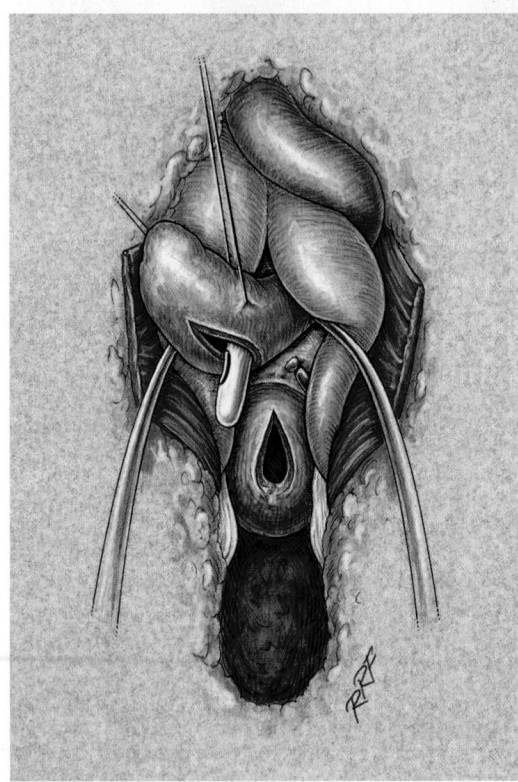

Figure 40-38. Resection of the pubis and rerouting of the urethra around the crus. When the prostate is markedly displaced, it may be necessary to expand the infrapubectomy. Sometimes, despite separation of the crura to the full extent possible, the two ends of the urethra do not meet when they are brought directly through the crus. It is necessary to bring the urethra lateral to one of the crura to make up this length.

to be valuable in observing these patients. In many cases (anterior urethral reconstruction), we have found that retrograde urethrography is more confusing than helpful.

With the use of the techniques discussed or similar techniques, curative rates for reconstruction of posterior PFUIs are in the high 90% range. In large centers, failures are not due to technical problems (i.e., anastomotic restenosis). In general, failures are indicative of ischemia of the proximal corpus spongiosum with ensuing stenosis of the mobilized corpus spongiosum. This occurs because, with mobilization, the corpus spongiosum, in essence, becomes a flap with the vascular pedicle being the retrograde vascularity from the arborization of the dorsal arteries through the glans (Fig. 40-39).

We have studied this phenomenon in trauma patients and have arrived at conclusions that we believe allow us to predict the patients at risk for this ischemic atrophy phenomenon. Initially, we used pudendal angiography to study all trauma patients who seemed to be at risk for bilateral deep internal pudendal artery injury at the time of trauma. These were patients who had evidence of injury to the dorsal penile nerves, patients in whom reconstruction had failed at other centers, patients with lateral impact pelvic fractures, and patients whose pelvic fractures were of the "windswept" variety (Brandes and Borrelli, 2001). We found that many patients had evidence of either unilateral or bilateral pudendal artery lesions, but that most had evidence of vascular reconstitution. **Patients with an intact pudendal artery on one side often were potent and were reliably cured with reconstruction. Patients with only reconstituted vessels, either unilateral or bilateral, never were potent but were reliably reconstructed.** We found that these patients were optimal candidates for penile arterial revascularization to improve potency. Because we noted this relationship to potency, we began evaluating patients with duplex ultrasonography. We found that patients with normal unilateral or bilateral pudendal arteries demonstrated normal arterial parameters on duplex evaluation. Patients with only reconstituted bilateral or unilateral arteries never had normal arterial parameters on duplex ultrasonography.

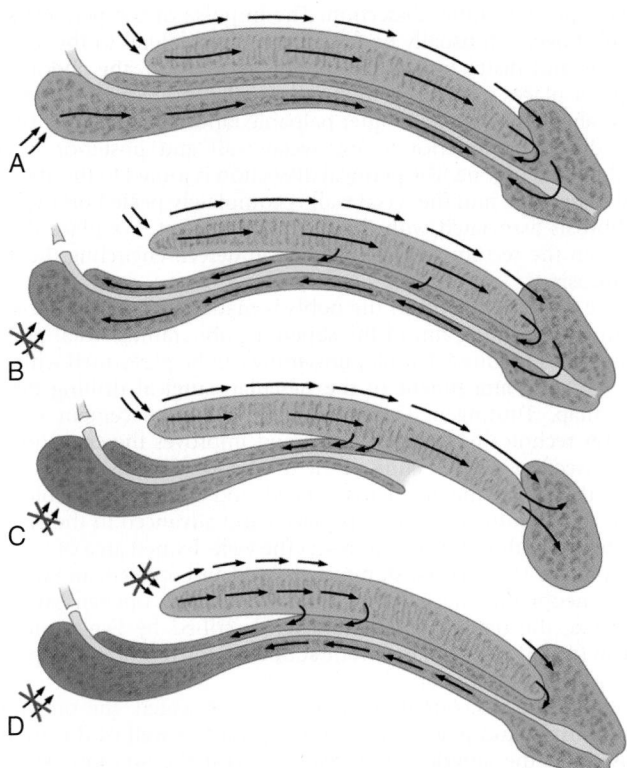

Figure 40-39. Diagrammatic representation of the deep vasculature of the penis. **A,** In the normal situation, through the common penile artery, flow is directed to the tip of the penis with arborization into the spongy erectile tissue of the glans penis. This provides retrograde flow into the corpus spongiosum. If the arteries of the bulb are intact, there is also antegrade arterial flow to the corpus spongiosum. **B,** With interruption of the arteries to the bulb and mobilization of the corpus spongiosum, all flow to the corpus spongiosum is retrograde through the common penile arterial system. **C,** In hypospadias, the distal corpus spongiosum may have been interrupted, with proximal mobilization of the corpus spongiosum and division of the arteries to the bulb. Even if the common penile circulation is intact to the tip of the penis, it may not adequately provide retrograde vascularity to the corpus spongiosum; ischemic stenosis can ensue. **D,** In the case of injury to the common penile artery, with elevation of the proximal corpus spongiosum and division of the arteries to the bulb, blood flow to the proximal corpus spongiosum may be inadequate, leading to ischemic necrosis or ischemic stenosis.

This information allows us to proceed to pudendal angiography only in patients with abnormal arterial parameters on duplex ultrasonography; patients with normal findings on ultrasonography predictably do well with reconstruction. Our data also show that patients do well with reconstruction if they have at least one side that is reconstituted, and the only patients at risk for ischemic stenosis are patients with bilateral complete obstruction of the internal pudendal vessels. In such patients, we perform penile arterial revascularization to augment the vascularity and, with that accomplished, proceed to urethral reconstruction (Jordan, 2005; Davies et al, 2009; Zuckerman et al, 2012). In many cases of pelvic fracture urethral distraction defects, erectile dysfunction is a consequence of the injury, although erectile dysfunction clearly results from the reconstructive surgery in some patients. We think that the incidence of injury to the pudendal arteries is drastically underreported and under-recognized. We and others believe that in many of these cases, the cause of erectile dysfunction is vascular (Brandes and Borrelli, 2001). However, there are at least a portion of patients

with neurogenic erectile dysfunction following PFUI, as some men experiencing ED following PFUI will have normal arterial inflow (Shenfeld et al, 2003; Metze et al, 2007).

Summary

Using the maneuvers outlined, we have found that virtually all distraction injuries can be reconstructed through a perineal approach with an anastomotic technique. Although the above-and-below approach is used when concomitant bladder neck surgery is performed, the inability to identify these patients accurately has led us to perform bladder neck surgery at a second setting. We have abandoned a transpubic approach as applied to posterior urethral distraction injuries.

Although we favor primary reconstruction of posterior urethral distraction injuries, other authors choose to manage these injuries endoscopically (Barry, 1989). We have found that the endoscopic management of PFUIs is not a simple procedure and must be undertaken only by a skilled and experienced surgeon. Many of these procedures can be categorized as a "cut-for-light" procedure. Although some surgeons report success, most cut-for-light procedures are not done with sufficient precision to allow adequate realignment of the urethra. We have seen many disasters that have resulted from these procedures and in most cases condemn the use of these modalities. In addition, no cut-for-light series compares favorably, with regard to long-term success rates, with series from large centers that use primary anastomotic techniques (Levine and Wessells, 2001).

In 1989, Marshall described his method of using stereotactic techniques for endoscopic alignment of the ends of the urethra. He emphasized the length of time it takes to obtain precise alignment before undertaking the endoscopic portion of the procedure. In his procedure, he passed a wire through the aligned ends of the urethra, minimally dilating the channel and widening it with transurethral resection. The scar is stabilized by a period of self-catheterization. While technically feasible, this approach has limited applicability for most patients. Patients whose medical condition, age, or concomitant orthopedic injury prevents them from being placed in the exaggerated lithotomy position or reconstructed using a transpubic approach may be managed with this technique.

In children, the goals of surgery are the same as in adults. In our experience, most children can undergo reconstruction by the same perineal exposure as used in adults. Exposure is more difficult, but nonetheless perineal anastomosis can be done (Hafez et al, 2005). However, the posterior, sagittal transsphincteric approach has been proposed as a better approach in children (Mathews et al, 1998; Peña and Hong, 2004). We agree that the posterior approach is an elegant method of exposure; however, with this approach, we have observed that surgeons tend to resort to techniques of substitution reconstruction where primary anastomosis could be done and, in our opinion, is superior. With our experience accumulating using the vessel-sparing approach to anterior urethral reconstruction—primary anastomosis and augmented anastomosis—we have extended the technique to select patients with pelvic fracture urethral reconstruction and have found the approach feasible with good results in a small number of patients. However, the advantage has not been proven.

VESICOURETHRAL DISTRACTION DEFECTS

Enthusiastic use of radical prostatectomy has led to increasing experience with patients who have had total obliteration of vesicourethral anastomosis. In some patients, there is distraction of the vesicourethral anastomosis with either a totally obliterating distraction defect or severe anastomotic stenosis. With increased use of robotic-assisted laparoscopic techniques we have seen a decrease in the number of significant anastomotic stenoses, and other authors have shown this as well (Breyer et al, 2010). This improvement may be secondary to reduction in anastomotic urine leaks, better mucosal apposition, and the running anastomosis allowed with the magnification and dexterity using the robotic approach.

As with other defects, it is important to determine the length of the defect accurately. This can be accomplished by simultaneous cystography with retrograde urethrography, simultaneous retrograde urethrography and antegrade endoscopy through the suprapubic tube, or both.

Numerous options are available for the management of these complex patients. Many of these patients have other medical problems, and it has been our observation that many have thick and small bladders, possibly contributing to the difficulty with the initial surgery. The ever-present issue of body habitus also must be considered and, in our opinion, contributes to problems with the initial anastomosis. An indwelling suprapubic tube must always be considered an option. In a patient who is significantly overweight, the results of aggressive reconstruction have not been good. The place for endoscopic techniques is covered later in this section; however, in the case of short-length distractions, we have had good success with aggressive incisions at the 3 o'clock and 9 o'clock positions followed in approximately 3 weeks with repeated incisions. Whether the holmium laser is better than the cold knife can be debated; the hot knife is unnecessary. If one must "core through" to establish continuity, endoscopic procedures have no place in our opinion except as discussed later. Vanni and colleagues (2011) published their experience with radial urethrotomy and intralesional injection of mitomycin C. They had an initial success rate of 72% in patients with recalcitrant strictures.

In some cases, a continent catheterizable bladder augmentation may be a better operation than aggressive functional reconstruction; in an obese patient, construction of a functional catheter channel can be difficult. Diversion must also be entertained, and in patients in whom functional reconstruction is not an obvious choice, it becomes a primary option.

If functional reconstruction is deemed possible, we think it is a reasonable choice, and our technique is as follows. We place the patient in a low-lithotomy position and use an abdominal-perineal combined approach. We make a lower midline incision, exposing the bladder and dissecting it from the lateral sidewall and further mobilizing the anterior bladder from beneath the pubis as aggressively as can be safely undertaken from above. We then open the peritoneum and develop the retrovesical space, again taking care to complete the dissection as safely as can be accomplished from above.

A second surgeon begins the perineal dissection by a curvilinear perineal incision similar to that used for a radical perineal prostatectomy. The dissection is posterior to the transverse perinei musculature (posterior anal triangle) and carried along the anterior rectal wall to the area where fibrosis is encountered from the prior

radical prostatectomy dissection. The impulse of the perineal surgeon's finger can usually be felt adjacent and lateral to the area of fibrosis and distraction at this point. In addition, the abdominal surgeon places a finger at the limits of the retrovesical dissection from above to provide another palpable landmark and to ensure a safe dissection anterior to the rectal wall and posterior to the bladder and trigone. The perineal dissection is joined to the abdominal dissection, and the rectal wall is completely peeled off the area of fibrosis associated with the distraction defect. We place drains between the rectum and the distraction defect, encircling the area of fibrosis.

The dissection beneath the pubis is made easier by the excision of an ellipse of the rim of the superior pubic ramus. Total pubectomy is not required. Partial pubectomy can be performed with the reciprocating attachment of the Aesculap surgical drilling device (Aesculap, Tuttlingen, Germany); this makes placement of the sutures technically straightforward and improves the exposure for the dissection and resection of the distraction fibrosis.

At this point, the bladder is opened, and the area of the bladder neck is determined. A sound is placed and advanced to the area of obliteration; this allows us to resect the well-defined area of fibrosis completely. The urethral stump is exposed and opened, and the site of the neobladder neck, having been identified, is opened. We marsupialize the bladder epithelium as described by Eggleston and Walsh (1985), place anastomotic sutures in the urethral stump, and pass a stenting catheter.

Before the vesicourethral anastomosis is seated, the omentum is mobilized and placed between the posterior wall of the anastomosis and the anterior rectal wall. We seat the anastomosis and wrap the omentum around the area of anastomosis, tagging it into place. The lateral vesical spaces are drained with closed suction drains, and a suprapubic tube is left in place when the vesicostomy is closed. We have been doing this procedure perineally with similar outcomes.

Postoperative care is the same as for a radical prostatectomy. Patients are discharged when their drainage and ambulation allow and their diet has been resumed. We evaluate patients 4 to 6 weeks postoperatively, with the stenting urethral catheter removed and the bladder filled by way of the suprapubic tube.

Because one attempt has failed in these patients, we generally are conservative with the timing of a voiding trial. In some cases, voiding trials are done at 2 to 3 weeks.

Our series continues to grow, and we continue to have excellent success in reconstruction. We have some patients who deem their continence adequate for their lifestyle; in the others, we have been successful with the placement of an artificial sphincter.

Other authors have proposed a different approach to these very difficult cases. In patients for whom multiple attempts at dilation or incision of these vesicourethral anastomotic stenoses have failed, Elliott and Boone (2001) proposed making an incision with placement of the UroLume endoprosthesis, followed at an interval by the placement of an artificial sphincter. They initially described nine men treated with this approach; seven of the men were satisfied with the results of their treatment at a mean follow-up of 17.5 months. Other authors (Mark et al, 1993; Kaplan, 2004; Anger et al, 2005) have proposed slight modifications of this approach and also report adequate patency and continence in these patients. With the removal of UroLume from the market, this approach is impossible.

COMPLEX FISTULAE OF THE POSTERIOR URETHRA

The increase in the performance of radical prostatectomy has also led to an increased incidence of vesicorectal or vesicourethrorectal fistulae. In most cases, these are small and managed by a transperineal, transanal-transsphincteric, or posterior approach. However, some cases are complex, with the fistulae associated with large granulated cavities. The problem is magnified when radiation (brachytherapy, external beam therapy, or both) is part of the equation. With radiation fistulae, many centers have gone to diversion with ileal conduit or bowel pouch as opposed to functional reconstruction. These cases have also been managed with the approach described earlier for vesicourethral distraction problems. However, the omentum serves an even more important purpose in these cases. In addition, with the increasing application of "minimally invasive" modalities for carcinoma of the prostate (i.e., brachytherapy, combined brachytherapy with external beam irradiation, higher dose external beam irradiation, and cryotherapy), the magnitude of complexity of these problems of prostatic urethral fistulae, granulated cavities, and severe rectal injury continues to increase. We have tried to approach these problems aggressively, with preservation of function where possible.

In many of these cases, salvage prostatectomy can be combined with rectosigmoid resection. In some cases, we have successfully reanastomosed the bladder to the membranous urethra. Preservation of continence has been mixed. In cases in which vesicourethral anastomosis is impossible, a urachal-peritoneal flap combined with a rectus abdominis muscle flap is used to bolster the closed bladder neck and to keep the closed bladder neck from sticking to the back of the pubis. The bladder is augmented, and a continent catheterizable channel is developed. In some cases, the continuity of the colon cannot be reestablished, and a colostomy is performed as distally on the descending portion of the colon as possible. Whenever continuity of the colon can be reestablished, a J-pouch colo-anal anastomosis is done. Omentum is used to envelop the rectal closure or to separate the rectal closure from the vesicourethral anastomosis. The combined abdominal-perineal approach that was previously described provides excellent safe exposure for management of these complex situations. The morbidity of this approach has been acceptable.

One must be careful in addressing the irradiated bowel. We had a patient who did well with his surgery for continent catheterizable augmentation and bowel closure, but when his colostomy was reversed, he developed an overwhelming colitis and a re-fistula, with an eventual septic death. Another patient had a breakdown of his bladder neck closure and to date remains with a large vesicoabdominal fistula. These cases must be individualized. When they go well, they go wonderfully well; when they do not, they become a disaster for the patient, the patient's family, and the surgeons involved.

Zinman reported a 10-year experience with the management of rectourethral fistulae (Vanni et al, 2009). The series comprised 33 patients who had fistulae and who had not undergone irradiation and 33 patients who had undergone irradiation. Mean follow-up for the entire series was about 20 months. The review was a retrospective review taken from office records and hospital records. All fistulae were repaired by an anterior transperineal approach using gracilis muscle interposition flaps and in some cases with a buccal graft. In this series, 100% of the nonirradiated fistulae were successfully closed with a mean follow-up of 20 months, 85% of the irradiated fistulae were closed in a single stage, and 12% required an additional procedure, with an ultimate closure rate of about 97%. In the nonirradiated group, there were no urethral strictures noted with long-term follow-up; five recurrent strictures were noted in the irradiated group. In the nonirradiated group, 91% of the patients had their bowel undiverted. In the irradiated group, 39% had long-term bowel diversion. Zinman believes that the use of muscle interposition flaps are integral to achieving good results, and the use of buccal mucosal grafts, where needed to augment the closure of the urinary tract, was also believed to be invaluable (Vanni et al, 2009). An estimation of ultimate urinary and bowel function is integral to the determination of the plan for reconstruction or diversion, or both. Also, the surgical approach chosen facilitates and limits options (i.e., of the bowel, the urethra, or tissue interposition) (Lane et al, 2006).

CURVATURES OF THE PENIS

Normal elasticity and compliance of all tissue layers of the penis are critical for erectile function, tumescence, and rigidity. Tissues

---

> ### KEY POINTS: VESICOURETHRAL DISTRACTION DEFECTS AND COMPLEX FISTULAE OF THE POSTERIOR URETHRA
>
> - Vesicourethral distraction defects are a complication of radical prostatectomy.
> - There are many options for management of these complex patients. An indwelling suprapubic tube must always be considered a long-term option. Likewise, in some cases, a continent catheterizable bladder augmentation may be a better operation than aggressive functional reconstruction. If functional reconstruction is deemed reasonable, we have employed an above-and-below technique, in which laparotomy is combined with a posterior perineal triangle dissection.
> - The interposition of omentum has been used for distraction defects and for complex fistulae. This approach allows safe mobilization of the rectum from the area of the distraction scar or from the fistula site.
> - When radiation is added, the complexity of reconstruction is magnified. The effects of radiation must be allowed to settle; tissue interposition is the rule, and functional reconstruction is impossible in many cases. Some think that diversion, in the case of patients who have received radiation, is the safest and best option.
> - Careful consideration of ultimate urinary and bowel function is integral to proper planning of surgery.

must expand in all dimensions as the penis engorges with blood; eventually, the tissues of the tunica albuginea and the septal fibers of the corpora cavernosa are stretched to the limits of their compliance, and tumescence is converted to rigidity. In the normal penis, the tissues are symmetrically elastic, and the erection is straight. In curvature of the penis, there is relative asymmetry of one aspect of the erect penis. In some cases, this condition arises from diminished compliance of one aspect of the tunica albuginea or outright foreshortening of one aspect of the erectile bodies.

The term *chordee* **means curvature,** but it is commonly used as if it refers to the tissues causing the curvature. This misuse of the term is seen in the statement "the chordee was resected"; properly phrased, the statement should be "the chordee can be corrected by resecting the inelastic tissues that are causing the chordee."

Curvatures of the penis can be congenital or acquired. Some confusion also exists in common usage of the term *congenital curvature of the penis.* **The terms** *congenital curvature of the penis* **and** *chordee without hypospadias* **have often been used interchangeably. We prefer to reserve the term** *chordee without hypospadias* **for patients in whom the meatus is properly located on the tip of the glans penis; a ventral curvature is associated with abnormalities of the ventral fascial tissues or corpus spongiosum, or both.** It has long been recognized that hypospadias is a condition that is associated in some patients with either a diminutive penis or a micropenis. Although a small penis is not diagnostic of hypospadias, it is highly unusual for a patient with hypospadias to have an exceptionally large erect penis. In contrast, other congenital curvatures of the penis (ventral, lateral, or dorsal) are inevitably associated with the finding of a large erect penis. Because **the trauma that results in acquired curvature is virtually always associated with intercourse, the occurrence of acquired curvature is nil before the onset of puberty.** We have seen some patients in whom there was a history of trauma during vigorous masturbation, but these patients are the exception. Similar to congenital curvatures of the penis, acquired curvatures may be dorsal, lateral, ventral, or complex.

Types of Congenital Curvature of the Penis

Please see the Expert Consult website for this section.

Chordee without Hypospadias in Young Men

Please see the Expert Consult website for this section.

Congenital Curvatures of the Penis

Patients with congenital curvature of the penis can have ventral, lateral (which is most often to the left), or, unusually, dorsal curvature. Photographs of the erect penis demonstrate a smooth curvature that generally involves the entire pendulous portion of the penile shaft.

Patients are usually otherwise healthy young men between the ages of 18 and 30 years. Many of these patients have noticed curvature before passing through puberty but have presumed it to be normal. However, with puberty, they discover that the curvature is not normal; or they become sexually active and discover that the curvature impedes their efforts; or they notice increasing curvature as they pass through puberty, and this, in their minds, clearly would preclude sexual intercourse. Occasionally, a patient waits until he is older than 30 years to deal with the anomaly; even less often, a younger adolescent may discuss his genitalia with his parents.

In circumcised patients, we make an incision through the circumcision scar, which in many cases is displaced well down on the penile shaft. However, even with relatively significant displacement of the circumcision scar on the shaft of the penis, the reincision should be through the circumcision scar. The penis is degloved by dissection of the layer immediately superficial to the superficial lamina of Buck fascia.

An artificial erection is obtained with normal saline infusion or pharmacologic agents. We do not routinely recommend a tourniquet device because constricting devices can conceal the proximal limits of the curvature; this is of most significance in cases of ventral curvatures, which frequently extend proximally. Occasionally, some element of perineal pressure is initially required, but these are patients with normal erectile function, and venous occlusive function is normal. The artificial erection demonstrates the character of the curvature and the location of maximal curvature. In patients with ventral curvature, there may be some illusion of thickening of the dartos and Buck fascia, and in these patients, the fibrous tissue is mobilized and completely excised. The corpus spongiosum is detached from the corpora cavernosa and mobilized from the glans to the penoscrotal junction.

After these tissues are excised, the artificial erection is repeated, and an occasional patient is found to have complete straightening. However, most patients experience a differential elasticity between the dorsal and the ventral aspects of the corporeal bodies, and although the curvature may have been lessened, it persists unless further procedures are done to straighten the penis.

In an adult patient with persistent curvature, there are two options for surgical correction: (1) to lengthen the ventral aspect of the penis by making transverse incisions in the ventral tunica and placing an autologous tissue graft (we currently use the small intestinal submucosal graft at our institution), and (2) to shorten the dorsal aspect of the penis by elevating the neurovascular bundle, excising an ellipse or ellipses from the dorsum of the tunica albuginea, and closing the defects in watertight fashion (Nesbit procedure [Nesbit, 1965]). **Because the size of the erect penis is usually not a problem in these cases of congenital curvature, we have chosen the second option and strenuously discourage ventral grafting in these patients.** The recovery period after this procedure is much shorter, and the variabilities of graft take do not have to be considered. In addition, when a graft is used, there is always the possibility, although uncommon, of the development of graft-induced veno-occlusive dysfunction. **In a 2000 consensus conference sanctioned by the World Health Organization, the committee on Peyronie disease and congenital curvature of the penis agreed that most, if not all, cases in men with the classic finding of congenital curvature of the penis were best managed with plication or corporoplasty techniques but not grafting techniques** (Jardin et al, 2000; Lue, 2004). This consensus was reiterated at the next World Health Organization conference. It is preferable to shorten the longer aspect of the penis in patients with congenital curvature. However, **if the patient falls into the category of chordee without hypospadias and shortness of the penis is an issue, we selectively use incisions with grafts to correct the curvature** (Devine and Horton, 1975).

After the decision has been made to proceed with excisions of ellipses of dorsal tunica, Buck fascia can be elevated, in concert with the dorsal neurovascular structures, by beginning just lateral to the corpus spongiosum and carrying the dissection dorsally across the midline. Alternatively, the tunica can be exposed by excising the deep dorsal vein of the penis and opening the inner lamina of Buck fascia. Elevation of the neurovascular structures is done by dissecting from the dorsal midline laterally around to the corpus spongiosum and from the coronal margin to the penopubic junction, limiting the effects of stretching the dorsal structures with exposure of the dorsum of the penis.

An artificial erection is obtained to plan the proposed ellipse excisions. We prefer to use several small ellipses rather than try to correct the curvature with one large ellipse. The first ellipse is usually positioned at the point of maximal concavity. The edges of the planned ellipse are apposed with a Prolene suture. The artificial erection is repeated to assess the effects of that excision. If there is good straightening in that area of the shaft, the incisions are again well marked, the plicating sutures are removed, and the ellipses of tunica are made with a sharp scalpel blade. By dissection in the space of Smith and removal of only an ellipse of tunica, the ellipses are carefully excised to avoid damage to the underlying erectile tissue or can be merely closed under the reapproximated edge of the defect in the tunica albuginea. The edge of the ellipse is reapproximated with a combination of interrupted 4-0 polydioxanone sutures and a watertight running 4-0 polydioxanone suture.

After closure, we repeat the artificial erection to assess the results of the first ellipse with the others. A final artificial erection should demonstrate the penis to be perfectly straight. In cases of ventral curvature or when complex curvatures are associated with an element of ventral curvature, a minimal degree of dorsal curvature after correction is acceptable. In most cases, as the sutures dissolve, the penis either remains minimally dorsiflexed or becomes perfectly straight.

The Buck fascia is closed. Two small suction drains are placed superficial to the Buck fascia but deep to the dartos fascia. We replace the skin sleeve, with its edges apposed with interrupted small Vicryl or Monocryl sutures. In all patients, we place a small Foley catheter and a small suction drain, and both are removed on the first postoperative day. Depending on the amount of edema and drainage, patients are discharged from the hospital on the evening of the first postoperative day or early the second postoperative day.

A congenital lateral curvature of the penis is often associated with some complexity of curvature; patients frequently notice lateral curvature in association with a ventral or, less commonly, a dorsal curvature. However, some patients present with only lateral curvature, with the right side larger than the left, and curvature to the left.

In some cases, a repair of the lateral curvature can be approached through a small incision at the point of maximal curvature. Laterally placed incisions on the penile shaft are not cosmetically optimal. We prefer a degloving incision after exposure of the deep penile structures; the point of maximal concavity is then marked. Prolene sutures are placed, and an artificial erection is performed again. The size of the ellipse is assessed, and the ellipse is excised and closed as discussed earlier.

As mentioned, most cases of lateral curvature are associated with complex curvatures. In these patients, the correction of the curvature is similar to that described for patients with ventral curvature, with incision through the circumcision scar with the skin reflected. In contrast to a ventral curvature, with a lateral curvature, the entire dorsal neurovascular bundle does not need to be reflected; it is seldom required and it is not considered beneficial to excise the deep dorsal vein in approaching the dorsum of the penis. The postoperative care is the same as described for a ventral curvature. For the uncommon patient with a congenital dorsal curvature of the penis, the repair is best accomplished by mobilizing the lateral aspect of the corpus spongiosum to allow small ellipses lateral to the midline to be positioned on the ventrum of the penis, by the technique described before.

Although described as a method for plication for curvature associated with Peyronie disease, corporoplasty, a procedure described by Yachia (1993), is also useful for the correction of congenital curvatures. The procedure consists of longitudinal incisions in the tunica albuginea with transverse closure. The "long side" is plicated without the need for excision; however, the plication is durable in that the tunica is opened and closed with a resulting scar, rather than reliance only on the strength of sutures as originally described by Nesbit (1965). With this technique, closure is done with absorbable monofilament suture.

Acquired Curvatures of the Penis

Acquired curvatures of the penis inevitably follow trauma to the penis. Many of these cases are associated with Peyronie disease, also believed to be associated with trauma to the penis during intercourse (Bella et al, 2007). Patients occasionally present who have had vigorous internal urethrotomy, with the incision extended outside the urethra and corpus spongiosum and involving the tunica of the corporeal bodies, causing scarring that is significant enough to be associated with curvature.

Acquired Curvatures of the Penis That Are Not Peyronie Disease

When a young man presents with an acquired curvature of the penis, one must always consider Peyronie disease. However, many men do not have true Peyronie disease. These patients, on close questioning, reveal a history of minimal lateral curvature of the penis and a clear memory of a lateral buckling injury that occurred during intercourse. In some cases, the patient remembers hearing a "snap" and notices immediate detumescence and significant ecchymosis of the penis. These patients are often referred with a diagnosis of Peyronie disease, but a diagnosis of curvature secondary to penile fracture is more accurate. Because of the noticeable events associated with fracture of the penis, many patients present acutely, and reconstruction can be accomplished at that time.

Occasionally, a patient or his primary care physician ignores the stigmata of the trauma (often described as "minimal" by patients), and the patient presents with a noticeable lateral scar that causes indentation of the lateral aspect of the penis and, in some cases, curvature. Patients who had preexisting lateral curvature may notice that their penis has been straightened by the trauma, but they are disturbed by the concavity caused by the scar. In others, the small linear scar causes a significant lateral curvature.

Another group of patients presents after a similar buckling trauma to the penis but without associated detumescence or ecchymosis. These patients report noticing that their erections were painful for a period after the trauma, and then a nodule developed in the lateral aspect of the penis. Eventually, they present with a lateral linear scar that has led to curvature and indentation at the site. We refer to this injury as a subclinical fracture of the penis. **The lesion of a subclinical fracture of the penis is believed to be due to the disruption of the outer longitudinal layer of the tunica albuginea during the buckling trauma. The inner, circular layer is not disrupted and maintains the blood-tight continuity of the corpus spongiosum. Another possible scenario is that both layers of the tunica albuginea are disrupted, but the overlying Buck fascia maintains its integrity. Some patients notice a pop with intercourse and a period of pain with erections, followed by curvature of the penis—usually dorsal. These patients probably tear the septal insertion completely. These patients have a similar presentation to patients with Peyronie disease.**

Patients usually have normal erectile function after subclinical or clinical fracture of the penis; there does not appear to be an association with concomitant global cavernosal veno-occlusive dysfunction. However, the association of cavernosal veno-occlusive dysfunction and trauma of the penis continues to be seen, and some patients have significant problems with erectile dysfunction after fracture-type injuries of the penis. These injuries are not associated with shortening of the penis. In most cases, the lack of erectile dysfunction and penile shortening help distinguish these patients from patients with Peyronie disease. If a detailed history leads one to suspect blighted erectile function, erectile function should be evaluated before proceeding with surgery. At our institution, we evaluate these patients with duplex ultrasonography and selectively with dynamic infusion cavernosometry and cavernosography.

Although foreshortening of the penis is not a characteristic of either the injury itself or the resulting scar in either of these injuries, these patients are not ideal candidates for contralateral plication procedures. This treatment would result in bilateral scars, which would cause bilateral indentations of the penis, and although the penis would have been straightened by the correction, most patients are upset by the cosmetic and functional result of a near-circumferential indentation of the penis. Instead, we excise the scar and place a graft to replace the corporotomy defect caused by the scar excision. Because these scars are on the lateral aspect of the penis, minimal mobilization of Buck fascia, associated dorsal neurovascular structures, and corpus spongiosum is required at the site.

The results of the surgical correction described have been extremely effective. Successful correction with a single operation has been achieved in all patients treated at our institution.

KEY POINTS: CURVATURES OF THE PENIS

- Curvatures of the penis can be acquired or congenital. Congenital curvatures of the penis can be categorized as chordee without hypospadias or congenital curvature of the penis.
- In general, chordee without hypospadias is a forme fruste of hypospadias. Although the meatus may not be abnormally placed, these patients usually have findings suggestive of hypospadias (i.e., malformation of the ventral structures of the penis). These patients are not characterized by large erect penises. In contrast, patients with congenital curvature of the penis seem to have exceptionally large erect penises.
- The entity of congenital curvature of the penis seems to be related to nonsymmetrical expansion of the erectile bodies, which must expand significantly during tumescence. Reconstruction in these patients generally is best accomplished by excision with plicating closure or pure plication techniques. The use of grafts is not recommended because of the unusual but real occurrence of graft-induced veno-occlusive dysfunction in certain patients.

TOTAL PENILE RECONSTRUCTION
General

The principal techniques of penile reconstruction were originally developed for treatment of trauma patients, and these patients were victims of war injuries in many injuries. In 1936, Bogaraz described a technique for phallic construction in a series of war-injured patients, and in 1944, Frumkin followed with a series from the Soviet Union. Aware of the work in the Soviet Union, Gillies and Harrison (1948) reported on a series of patients in whom they had accomplished penile reconstruction while stationed at a major hospital in the outskirts of London during World War II. In this series, numerous patients had a complete absence of the penis.

Initially, all procedures for phallic construction involved delayed formation and transfer of tubed abdominal flaps. These tubes were produced from random flaps of skin and because of their size were based on a tenuous blood supply. To allow new vascular patterns to become established in the transferred tissue, they were formed in stages, with a "delay" between the stages. In the "tube-within-a-tube" design, the inner tube allowed the placement of a baculum during intercourse, and the outer tube provided skin coverage. Patients voided through a proximal urethrostomy. This approach continued to be the "state-of-the-art" phallic construction and penile reconstruction until 1972, when Orticochea described total reconstruction of the penis using the gracilis musculocutaneous flap. In 1978, Puckett and Montie reported a series in which they constructed the penis with a tubed groin flap. In the early cases in this series, the flap was transferred in delayed fashion to the area of the penile stump. Later in the series, a microvascular free-transfer technique was employed.

In 1984, Chang and Hwang popularized the forearm flap, based on the radial artery, for phallic construction. Biemer (1988) reported a modification of the forearm flap, which was also based on the radial artery; in 1990, Farrow and colleagues reported their "cricket bat" modification of the radial forearm flap. **At the present time, forearm flaps are the most commonly employed method for total phallic construction and penile reconstruction.**

The forearm flap is usually harvested from the nondominant forearm. Preoperatively, the Allen test is used to screen patients carefully for arterial insufficiency. This test involves palpation of the radial and ulnar arteries in the wrist, with the patient making a tight fist to express blood from his hand. As he opens his hand, the fingers are pale, but if palmar circulation is normal and both arteries are patent, the fingers turn pink when one of the arteries is released. On the basis of either the Allen test or the patient's history, if there is any doubt about the integrity of the radial and ulnar arteries or the palmar arch, upper extremity angiography is performed.

As described, the forearm flap is a fasciocutaneous flap vascularized by the radial artery; however, the ulnar artery also vascularizes the forearm fascia and most of the forearm skin. The radial artery arises as a continuation of the brachial artery and proximally lies beneath the belly of the brachioradialis muscle, becoming more superficial at the wrist. The ulnar artery is also a continuation of the brachial artery and vascularizes a similar area of skin and underlying adipose tissue. The vascularity of the overlying skin is achieved by way of the underlying (antebrachial) fascia, which is the superficial fascia investing the musculature of the forearm.

The forearm flap can be elevated and transferred on the superficial fascia. The lateral and medial antebrachial cutaneous nerves appear proximally beneath the fascia. The cephalic, basilic, and medial antebrachial veins are also included in the flap and constitute a portion of the venous drainage. In some patients, the vena comitans is the dominant venous drainage system. At the time of flap transfer, it is imperative to assess the vena comitans and the superficial veins to determine which is the dominant system in the individual patient.

The various modifications of the forearm flap do not represent changes in the technique of flap elevation; rather, they are modifications in the design of the skin island and the relative position of the urethral paddle in relation to the skin that eventually becomes shaft coverage. Each of these modifications has advantages in different situations.

In the forearm flap as described by Chang and Hwang (1984), the shaft is covered with the radial aspect of the skin paddle. A de-epithelialized strip is made, and a second skin island, on the ulnar aspect of the skin paddle, is tubed to form the urethra. The urethral tube is rolled within the tube of skin to form a tube-within-a-tube design. In the white population, this flap has demonstrated a tendency to lead to ischemic stenosis of the lateral paddle, where the urethra is constructed.

In the cricket bat modification, the urethral tube extends distally, closely overlying either the radial or the ulnar artery. We have experience with elevation of the cricket bat modification on both arteries. Proximal to the urethral strip, a broader portion of the skin paddle provides coverage of the shaft. The urethral portion is tubed and transposed by inverting it into the center of the shaft portion of the skin paddle. The advantage of this modification lies in centering the urethral portion over the respective artery, in contrast to the Chinese design, in which the ulnar aspect is far distal from the radial artery,

with the potential for ischemic stenosis or loss of that portion. The cricket bat modification has been useful in trauma patients, particularly in patients who have a significant stump of erectile bodies and urethra left after the injury.

The modification by Biemer (1988) also centers the urethral portion of the flap over the artery. As described by Biemer, the flap is elevated on the radial artery and includes a vascularized piece of the radial bone intended to provide rigidity to the new penis. However, the inclusion of cartilage and bone has not been universally successful, and rigidity in these flaps is obtainable by the use of either an externally applied or an internally implanted prosthesis. If the bone is not elevated, the Biemer flap design can be elevated on either the radial or the ulnar artery. At our center, we most often elevate the flap on the ulnar artery, in a modification of the Biemer design.

Modifications of the Biemer design also include the glans construction technique that was originally described by Puckett and Montie (1978). In the original Biemer design, a central strip becomes the urethra, and lateral to that strip, two de-epithelialized portions and two lateral islands (lateral aspects of that skin paddle) are fused dorsally and ventrally to cover the shaft. With the modification of Puckett and colleagues (1982), a large island is left distally and flared back over the tip of the tubed flaps, creating the illusion of a glans penis. The Biemer design, especially when it is combined with Puckett's design for glanular construction, offers the best cosmetic results (Fig. 40-40).

There are several disadvantages to the use of a forearm flap for phallic construction. The major disadvantage of forearm flaps is the obvious donor site deformity. We have reconstructed the donor site with full-thickness skin grafts taken from the area of the inguinal crease or buttock, and the cosmetic result is far superior to that obtained when the donor site is reconstructed with split-thickness skin graft (even thick split-thickness skin). Additionally, morbidity can be reduced with mobilization of the intact forearm skin to reduce the grafting requirement and attempts to minimize the step between the skin and muscle bed. A second disadvantage lies in the **possibility of the development of cold intolerance in the hand of the donor side.** Early in our experience with the forearm flap, we reconstructed the radial artery with an interposition vein graft. We have since abandoned this procedure in most of our series and have not seen cold intolerance in our patients. Another disadvantage occurs in male and virilized transgender patients **when the forearm skin is hirsute because the hair can be problematic** if it is included in the portion of the flap used for urethral construction. In such patients, we try to identify the potential for the problem and refer them for epilation before surgery.

McRoberts and Sadove (2002) proposed the use of the fibular osteocutaneous flap for phallic construction. The fibula is elevated on the periosteal vessel along with the overlying skin paddle. As they described, urethral reconstruction is by tubed graft techniques, and their procedure had a 100% urethral complication rate. Kim and colleagues (2009) used a radial forearm osteocutaneous flap in 40 patients with reasonable results, although for many patients the incorporation of bone did not provide sufficient rigidity for sexual function over time. For patients who need vascularized tissue only to cover the shaft of the penis, we have used the upper lateral arm flap. This is a fasciocutaneous flap, and its cutaneous vascular territory is centered on the radial collateral artery. The skin of the lateral upper arm is thin, with little subcutaneous adiposity. To mark the location of the lateral intramuscular septum and the course of the superior radial collateral artery, we draw a line joining the insertion of the deltoid with the lateral epicondyle. We begin the dissection posteriorly, elevating the superficial fascia until the posterior lateral portion of the intramuscular septum has been identified. A potential disadvantage of this flap lies in the fact that the entire venous drainage depends on the vena comitans, and although superficial veins do traverse the flap, none of them seems to provide significant venous drainage. We have found the flap to be completely reliable so far, with no losses secondary to venous insufficiency.

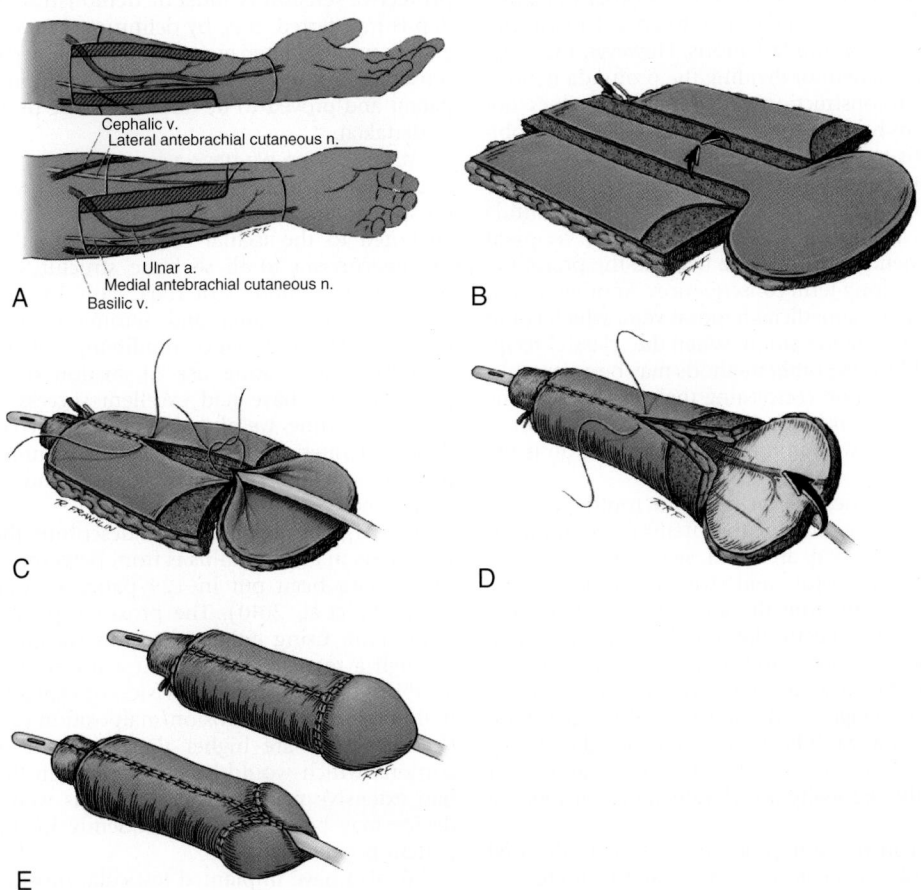

Cephalic v.
Lateral antebrachial cutaneous n.

Ulnar a.
Medial antebrachial cutaneous n.
Basilic v.

A

B

C

D

E

Figure 40-40. A, Schematic diagram of an ulnar forearm flap, modified Biemer design, on the patient's left (usually nondominant) forearm. **B,** Schematic of the elevated flap. The flap has been divided into skin islands by de-epithelializing the strips. Laterally are the shaft skin islands, medially is the urethral skin island, and distally is the integral glans, after the design of Puckett. **C,** Schematic of the configuration of the flap. Notice the urethral skin island has been tubularized to the level of the neomeatus. The lateral shaft skin islands are now in the process of being tubularized over the tubularized urethra. **D,** Schematic of the phallic flap as it is further configured. This view is of the dorsum. The ventral skin island has been closed over the urethra, and the dorsal skin islands are being collected. The integral glans will then be reflected over the dorsum of the flap. **E,** The appearance of the phallus after it is totally configured and transposed to the area of the "penis."

This flap has also been used for total phallic construction. For this purpose, the flap is expanded by tissue expander and elevated across the elbow, and the distal flap is elevated on the recurrent radial artery. As with the forearm flap, the donor site of an upper lateral arm flap can be disfiguring. However, because the scar is on the upper arm, it is more easily concealed beneath a shirtsleeve than a scar in the forearm. All the flaps described allow microneurosurgical coaptation of the flap cutaneous nerves with recipient nerves. With total phallic construction, the cutaneous nerves can be attached either to the dorsal nerves of the penis or to the dorsal nerves of the clitoris in a transsexual patient. When these nerves are unavailable, the nerves can be coapted to the pudendal nerve, which in most patients requires an interposition graft. These nerves are thought to provide the best restoration of erogenous cutaneous sensibility. We have also coapted the flap's cutaneous nerves to the ilioinguinal nerves, which provides sensation to the inner aspect of the thigh and the lateral aspect of the scrotum, and have achieved a reasonable degree of erogenous sensibility. The ilioinguinal nerve is also thought to provide a better degree of protective sensation (albeit less erogenous sensation) compared with the dorsal nerves (Monstrey et al, 2009).

In most patients, the deep inferior epigastric vessels are the recipient vasculature for flap transfer. These vessels are medial branches of the iliac system and lie on the dorsal (deep) aspect of the rectus abdominis muscle. The artery usually remains deep to the muscle, although an early penetration of the artery into the muscle can be observed in some patients. The artery classically bifurcates at the level of the umbilicus and is generally accompanied by two or more venae comitantes. These vessels have been elevated by several methods, and Lund and colleagues (1995) described their elevation for penile revascularization with laparoscopic techniques. When the deep inferior epigastric vessels are used, it is often necessary to include a saphenous vein for further venous runoff.

In some patients, these vessels are unavailable, and we have used a saphenous interposition graft to the superficial femoral artery. With use of this technique, we mobilize the saphenous vein well down the upper aspect of the thigh and then attach the vein to the femoral artery, making a temporary arteriovenous fistula. The fistula is divided, with the saphenous vein becoming the venous runoff and the interposition graft providing the arterial inflow. This system of recipient vessels is greatly inferior to a direct arterial anastomosis; because of this, in a few patients we have divided the profunda femoris vessel and vigorously dissected it from its other branches. We have then performed an end-to-end (artery-to-artery) anastomosis of the ulnar artery to the profunda femoris. However, the long-term consequences to the patient of dividing the profunda femoris are unclear. Immediate reconstruction of the profunda does not appear to be advantageous because the dissection required to mobilize the profunda femoris to become a recipient vessel requires the division of numerous proximal branches, and these would not be reconstructed with an immediate reconstruction of the profunda femoris. Mention of this as a potential means of "creating" recipient vessels is not to recommend the procedure because the procedure may yet have unacceptable long-term consequences. Another option in extreme cases is to use the superficial femoral vein, which could be reconstructed with a vein interposition. When the "classic" recipient vessels are unavailable, these other methods may be acceptable. However, we strenuously caution concerning their use because the long-term consequences are unknown. We believe that division of the superficial femoral artery with immediate reconstruction is the preferable choice.

In the latter part of our series, we included the routine transfer of gracilis muscle to cover the area of the urethral anastomosis, increasing the vascularity to that area and significantly altering the incidence of anastomotic fistula and stricture formation. We also elevated a bipedicled flap from the area of the penile shaft base, which is transposed beneath the phallic flap. This flap provides increased bulk and some modicum of scrotal construction, and when it is combined with the gracilis muscle, its thickness provides excellent coverage for the juncture of the flap with the base of the neoscrotum. Mobilization of a tunica dartos flap with tunica vaginalis pedicle, or a Martius flap in a transgender patient, may obviate the necessity to elevate and transpose a gracilis muscle flap.

During the phallic construction procedure, urine is diverted by means of a suprapubic cystostomy tube, and the urethra is stented with a No. 14 soft silicone (Silastic) catheter. A voiding study is usually performed between the third and fourth postoperative week.

Outcomes after forearm free-flap phalloplasty have now been reported from several centers. Even in centers of excellence for phallic construction, complications and reoperations seem to be the rule rather than the exception. Monstrey and colleagues (2009) reported the largest single-stage radial forearm phalloplasty series with 289 patients over 15 years. Urologic complications were seen in 41% of patients, the most common being fistula in 25%, stricture in 8.7%, and both in 9% of patients. Stricture treatment in this series required a multitude of procedures to achieve a patent urethra; however, fistulae healed spontaneously in most cases. Tactile sensation was achieved in all patients, and many were sexually active.

Similarly, Garaffa and coworkers (2010) published a series from the United Kingdom on 112 patients undergoing total phallic construction with a radial forearm free flap. Reconstructions at this center are performed in stages rather than a single stage. The urethral anastomosis is deferred until several months after the flap has demonstrated stability. At a median 26 months of follow-up, 99% of patients who had achieved urethral continuity were voiding anatomically through the phallus. Despite staging the procedure, strictures still developed in 10% and fistulae in 24% of patients. Most patients (71.5%) developed phallus sensation.

Vascular complications and graft loss are the most feared morbidities associated with free-flap phalloplasty. These are rare events with rates of total flap loss ranging from 0.6% to 5% and higher rate of partial loss or limited skin necrosis (Leriche et al, 2008; Monstrey et al, 2009; Garaffa et al, 2010). Occasionally, minimal loss of the phallus is amenable to local wound care, but more often these cases require debridement and split-thickness skin grafting for coverage.

Rigidity for intercourse in a patient with phallic construction is usually achieved by either an externally applied or a permanently implanted prosthesis. Prosthetic implantation is never undertaken until 1 year after phallic construction because protective sensibility must be demonstrated in the flap. When the flap is transferred, it is, by definition, rendered insensate. At about 3 to 4 months after reconstruction, as nerve regeneration occurs, sensation becomes noticeable. In addition, the urethra must be patent and proved to be durable before prosthetic implantation is undertaken.

At our center, we have a large series of patients with internally implanted devices. We have implanted hydraulic and articulated prostheses encased in Gore-Tex neocorpora. These devices are anchored to the ischial tuberosity and the pubis by anchoring the neocorpora to these bone structures. In most patients, we implant two cylinders or rods. Early in our series, we had problems with hematoma and seroma formation and subsequent infection. However, since modifying our antibiotic regimen and including the routine use of suction drains with the implant procedure, we have had excellent success with implantation. At the present time, we place the antibiotic-coated (Inhibizone) AMS 700CXR (American Medical Systems, Minnetonka, MN). The Titan prosthesis with hydrophilic coating and narrow base has also been used.

The largest published series describing the use of a mechanical prosthesis in a neophallus is from Belgium where a variety of prostheses have been put in 129 patients from 1996 through 2007 (Hoebeke et al, 2010). The proximal prosthesis was fixed to the pubic rami using either a Dacron sheath or permanent stitches through a rear tip extender. At a mean 30 months of follow-up, 41.1% of patients needed revision or explant for infection (11.9%), malfunction (13%), erosion/malposition (22.7%), or leak (9.2%). Complications are higher than seen for implants into normal corpora, which would be expected given that the neophallus has had extensive prior surgery, is not as well vascularized, and the device may be used more frequently in this traditionally young patient population.

We also have implanted testicular prostheses in many patients. In patients in whom we have used a hydraulic device, we have implanted the pump in one neohemiscrotum and a testicular prosthesis in the opposite one.

Reconstruction after Trauma

In many ways, the problems of trauma patients are more challenging to solve than the problems of patients who require total phallic construction. We have treated a large number of patients who have had devastating injuries to the penis after complicated prosthetic surgery or surgery to correct penile curvatures of Peyronie disease. The goal in these patients is to preserve the penile structures and function as much as possible and correct the deficiencies that are imposed on the patient by the trauma.

Acutely, urine must be diverted, necrotic tissue must be carefully debrided, and any foreign bodies that may have been implanted must be removed. Vigorous acute wound management stabilizes the wounds and allows active granulation to progress. In all trauma patients, an attempt should be made to save as many of the penile structures as possible.

Approximately 3 to 6 weeks after trauma, primary reconstruction can be undertaken, although we have elected to wait 4 to 6 months in some patients, depending on the situation. When significant adjacent tissue loss has occurred, the adjacent areas must be well reconstructed before proceeding with either phallic construction or penile reconstruction.

In a trauma patient, it is imperative that well-vascularized tissues be eventually transposed to the adjacent area, and reconstruction of these areas can be accomplished with numerous flaps. For groin reconstruction, the tensor fascia lata flap has been useful. The rectus femoris flap, characteristically long and large, can be transposed to the area of the lower abdomen and has been an extremely useful flap for inguinal and lower abdominal reconstruction. The gracilis muscle is an excellent flap for reconstruction of the perineum and the groin. Alternatively, the posterior thigh flap can be used for reconstruction of the groin and perineum and, in some cases, transposed to the lowermost portion of the lower abdomen. The rectus abdominis flap is a useful flap and can be elevated with a vertical or transverse skin paddle. In addition, the flap can be transposed to either the ipsilateral or the contralateral side. Care must be taken in a patient who has had lower abdominal external beam irradiation.

Variations of the flap designs described for complete phallic construction have been successfully applied in select patients for penile reconstruction. An example is one patient who sustained an injury to his penis from a shotgun blast. The blast injured a large portion of the patient's right corpus cavernosum, and most of the penile skin was either destroyed or used for urethral reconstruction. In this patient, a flap based on the Chinese design was elevated. However, because the urethral reconstruction was accomplished with a penile skin island, the ulnar portion of the flap was not needed for that purpose. The ulnar portion was de-epithelialized and tubularized to form bulk and a new right corporeal body. This patient is now sexually active, and the bulk of the tube's dermal section gives adequate support to his penis for intercourse.

Another patient required only distal urethral construction and glans reconstruction. For this patient, we based a flap on the Biemer design to construct a glans. The proximal portions of the flap were de-epithelialized, allowing fixation of the neoglans on the tips of the corporeal bodies, and an excellent functional and cosmetic result was achieved for this patient. The versatility of free-flap technology allows the solution of complex issues with reasonably acceptable functional and cosmetic results.

FEMALE-TO-MALE TRANSSEXUALISM

Female-to-male transsexual patients present a unique challenge, and no patient should be considered for definitive reassignment surgery without having undergone complex screening and evaluation by a team consisting of mental health professionals as well as surgeons who are skilled in undertaking transgender surgery. It is imperative that an ongoing, stable, therapeutic relationship be established between the patient and a mental health professional at the time of definitive gender reassignment surgery. At our institution, the Harry Benjamin criteria (Ramsey, 1996) are strictly adhered to, and surgery is accomplished by a team of urologists, plastic surgeons, and gynecologists.

In most patients, the first stage of female-to-male transsexual surgery consists of bilateral salpingo-oophorectomy, hysterectomy, vaginectomy, and urethral lengthening with colpocleisis. Even in virginal patients, our surgeons have become skilled at accomplishing a hysterectomy and bilateral salpingo-oophorectomy by way of transvaginal surgery. We perform a vaginectomy at the same operation, leaving the anterior vaginal wall to be transposed as a random flap to lengthen the female urethra and allow colpocleisis. Lengthening of the female urethra brings the base of the native urethra up to what will be the base of the phallic flap; along with the transfer of gracilis muscle, it has significantly altered our surgical results with regard to urethral anastomotic fistula and stricture. Urine is diverted with a suprapubic tube, and a voiding trial is performed in approximately 21 days. Patients are generally in the hospital for 2 to 3 days and return 3 to 4 months later for phallic construction.

For phallic construction in a transsexual patient, we elevate a bipedicled flap of skin, as already described, from the area where the phallic structure will be implanted and transpose it to the undersurface of the neopenis. The patient is generally in the hospital for 10 to 14 days after total phallic construction, and a voiding trial with contrast material is done at about 28 days postoperatively. After 1 year, when erogenous sensibility is demonstrated and the urethra is proved to be durable, prosthetic implantation is considered.

REFERENCES

The complete reference list is available online at www.expertconsult.com.

SUGGESTED READINGS

Aboseif SR, Breza J, Lue TF, et al. Penile venous drainage in erectile dysfunction: anatomical, radiological and functional considerations. Br J Urol 1989;64:183–90.

Akporiaye LE, Jordan GH, Devine CJ Jr. Balanitis xerotica obliterans (BXO). AUA Update Series 1997;16:166–7.

Chapple C, Barbagli G, Jordan G, et al. Consensus statement on urethral trauma. BJU Int 2004;93:1195–202.

Chapple CR, Pang D. Contemporary management of urethral trauma and the post-traumatic stricture. Curr Opin Urol 1999;9:253–60.

Coursey JW, Morey AF, McAninch JW, et al. Erectile function after anterior urethroplasty. J Urol 2001;166:2273–6.

Devine CJ Jr, Blackley SK, Horton CE, et al. The surgical treatment of chordee without hypospadias in men. J Urol 1991;146:325–9.

Fichtner J, Filipas D, Fisch M, et al. Long-term outcome of ventral buccal mucosa onlay graft urethroplasty for urethral stricture repair. Urology 2004;64:648–50.

Heyns CF, Steenkamp JW, de Kock ML, et al. Treatment of male urethral strictures: is repeated dilation or internal urethrotomy useful? J Urol 1998;160:356–8.

Iselin CE, Webster GD. The significance of the open bladder neck associated with pelvic fracture urethral distraction defects. J Urol 1999;162:34–51.

Jordan GH. The application of tissue transfer techniques in urologic surgery. In: Webster G, Kirby R, King L, et al, editors. Reconstructive urology. Oxford (UK): Blackwell Scientific; 1993. p. 143–69.

Levine J, Wessells H. Comparison of open and endoscopic treatment of posttraumatic posterior urethral strictures. World J Surg 2001;25:1597–601.

McCallum RW, Colapinto V. The role of urethrography in urethral disease. Part I. Accurate radiological localization of the membranous urethra and distal sphincters in normal male subjects. J Urol 1979a;122:607–11.

McCallum RW, Colapinto V. The role of urethrography in urethral disease. Part II. Indications for transsphincter urethroplasty in patients with primary bulbous strictures. J Urol 1979b;122:612–8.

McRoberts JW, Chapman WH, Answell JS. Primary anastomosis of the traumatically amputated penis: case report and summary of literature. J Urol 1968;100:751–4.

Morey AF, Metro MJ, Carney KJ, et al. Consensus on genitourinary trauma: external genitalia. BJU Int 2004;94:507–15.

Pansadoro V, Emiliozzi P. Internal urethrotomy in the management of anterior urethral strictures: long-term followup. J Urol 1996;156:73–5.

Quartey JK. One stage penile/preputial cutaneous island flap urethroplasty for urethral stricture: a preliminary report. J Urol 1983;129:284–7.

Rourke KF, McCammon KA, Sumfest JM, et al. Open reconstruction of pediatric and adolescent urethral strictures: long-term follow-up. J Urol 2003;169:1818–21, discussion 1821.

Webster GD, Mathes GL, Selli C. Prostatomembranous urethral injuries: a review of the literature and a rational approach to their management. J Urol 1983;130:898–902.

41 Surgery of the Scrotum and Seminal Vesicles

Frank A. Celigoj, MD, and Raymond A. Costabile, MD

The scrotum and its contents are unique body components because of their superficial anatomic location, which facilitates physical examination, imaging, and surgical access. Clinically, the external genitalia are one of the few organ systems in medicine that can have a significant psychosocial impact on a patient's well-being as well as their fertility potential. A significant reason that urologists must be thoroughly competent in dealing with conditions of the scrotum and scrotal contents is that physicians in other medical specialties are limited in their knowledge of scrotal anatomy, examination, disease entities, and treatment options. This unfamiliarity may seem perfunctory to most physicians, but it is of the utmost importance that urologists have a strong understanding of the anatomy, pathology, and surgical treatment of diseases that affect the external genitalia because of their significance in fertility potential and male endocrine function and impact on patient self-image.

SURGICAL ANATOMY OF THE SCROTUM

It is crucial to understand the blood supply to the organs within the scrotum when surgical intervention is indicated (Box 41-1). **The availability of multiple blood supplies to the testis allows continued testicular viability when one or two of the arteries are compromised by injury or ligation.** An understanding of scrotal anatomy readily permits accessibility for surgical procedures, including surgery of the scrotal wall, vasectomy, spermatocelectomy, surgery of the epididymis, hydrocelectomy, and surgical treatment of orchitis and orchialgia.

Spread of Scrotal Infections and Postoperative Fluids Based on Scrotal Anatomy

There is a predictable pathway for the spread of scrotal infections including Fournier gangrene and necrotizing fasciitis of the scrotum and postoperative fluids based on scrotal anatomy. **Anatomic barriers to the spread of necrotizing fasciitis include the dartos fascia of the penis and scrotum, Colles fascia of the perineum, and Scarpa fascia of the anterior abdominal wall. The testicles and epididymes are frequently spared in cases of necrotizing fasciitis of the scrotum** (Figs. 41-1 and 41-2) (Gupta et al, 2007).

PREOPERATIVE PREPARATION

Anesthetic Technique for Scrotal Surgery

Effective anesthetic techniques for scrotal surgery range from local injection with or without sedation to spinal to general anesthesia. The use of a spermatic cord block with local infiltration of 0.5% lidocaine without epinephrine is a simple, cost-effective anesthetic technique that can be implemented by the surgeon for outpatient scrotal surgical procedures. Regional cord block typically can be performed without premedication with satisfactory patient analgesia (Wakefield and Elewa, 1994; Magoha, 1998). Spermatic cord block can be used in patients with large hydroceles for anesthesia by initially percutaneously draining the hydrocele, performing the block, and then performing hydrocelectomy (Reale et al, 1998). Outpatient scrotal surgery performed with midazolam sedation and a local block with sedation reversal at the end of the procedure has a very high patient satisfaction rate (Birch and Miller, 1994).

Preoperative Preparation and the Use of Antibiotics in Scrotal Surgery

The overall infection rate with scrotal surgery is relatively low, ranging from zero to 10%. There is no difference in the incidence of postoperative wound infections or complications in patients undergoing hydrocelectomy or spermatocelectomy when comparing iodine-based versus chlorhexidine antiseptic preparations. Scrotal cases are considered as class II (clean-contaminated surgeries), which makes it reasonable to use preoperative antibiotics (Kiddoo et al, 2004). The American Urological Association (AUA) best practice policy statement on urologic surgery antimicrobial prophylaxis recommends a single dose of preoperative antibiotics if the patient has risk factors for infection, including advanced age, anatomic anomalies of the urinary tract, poor nutritional status, smoking, long-term corticosteroid use, immunodeficiency, externalized catheters, colonized endogenous or exogenous material, a distant coexistent infection, or prolonged hospitalization. The recommended antibiotic prophylaxis is a dose of a first-generation cephalosporin or clindamycin as an alternative antimicrobial (Wolf et al, 2008). **Patients who underwent preoperative clipping for hair removal the morning of surgery had a significantly lower**

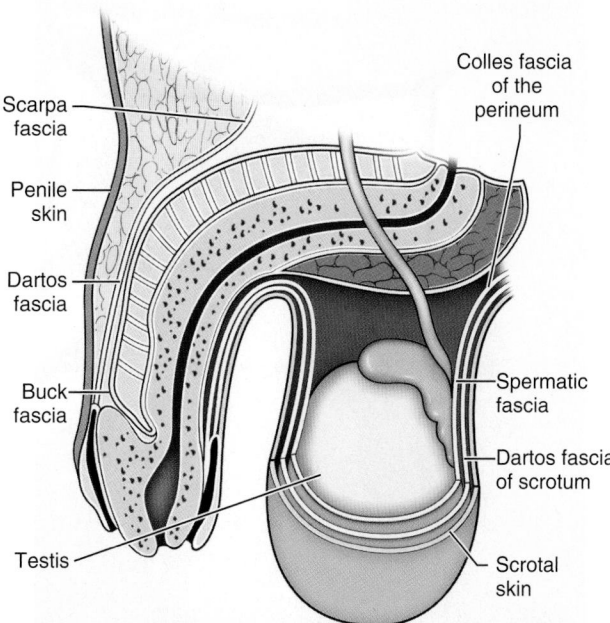

Figure 41-2. Sagittal view of anatomic barriers to the spread of infection. (Modified from Kavoussi PK, Costabile RA. Disorders of scrotal contents: orchitis, epididymitis, testicular torsion, torsion of the appendages, and Fournier's gangrene. In: Chapple CR, Steers WD, editors. Practical urology: essential principles and practice. London: Springer-Verlag; 2011.)

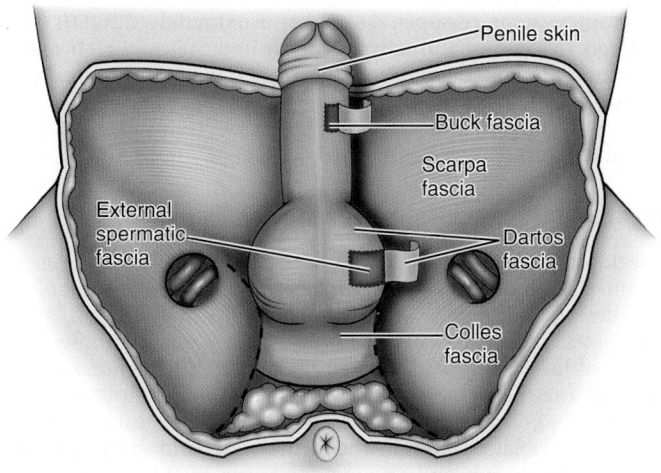

Figure 41-1. Anatomic barriers to the spread of infection. (Modified from Kavoussi PK, Costabile RA. Disorders of scrotal contents: orchitis, epididymitis, testicular torsion, torsion of the appendages, and Fournier's gangrene. In: Chapple CR, Steers WD, editors. Practical urology: essential principles and practice. London: Springer-Verlag; 2011.)

wound infection rate than patients who underwent shaving or clipping the night before surgery (Alexander et al, 1983).

SURGERY OF THE SCROTAL WALL

Cyst Excision

Patients with multiple scrotal cysts can be managed with surgical excision with excellent cosmetic results and low recurrence rates (Noël et al, 2006). **The classic management of scrotal sebaceous cysts is surgical excision with excellent outcomes and minimal morbidity with good cosmetic results.** Less invasive techniques, such as neodymium:yttrium-aluminum-garnet photocoagulation, have been performed successfully but are not considered standard management (Franco de Castro et al, 2002).

Partial and Total Scrotectomy

Partial scrotectomy is an uncommon procedure. Partial scrotectomy is most commonly performed with infectious processes such as Fournier gangrene. **Partial scrotectomy has been advocated after** trans-scrotal exploration, orchiectomy, or biopsy or when aspiration has been performed for a scrotal mass and the pathology has revealed a nonseminomatous germ cell tumor of the testis. Prompt and aggressive management has resulted in no local recurrences secondary to scrotal tumor contamination, even when a tumor was found in the scrotectomy specimen (Johnson and Babaian, 1980; Boileau and Steers, 1984; Leibovitch et al, 1995). There was no increase in local or distant recurrence in a small group that underwent aggressive local surgical resection and did not receive adjuvant chemotherapy (Giguere et al, 1988).

Total scrotectomy is less commonly performed than partial scrotectomy. Total scrotectomy is often necessary when there is extensive involvement of the scrotum with Fournier gangrene. Total scrotectomy also has been described for radical oncologic procedures, concomitantly with cystoprostatectomy, penectomy, or pelvic exenteration with aggressive cases of squamous cell carcinoma of the prostate (Sarma et al, 1991).

Debridement of the Scrotal Wall in Fournier Gangrene

Treatment of Fournier gangrene should include emergent radical surgical debridement and intravenous broad-spectrum antibiotics. When culture results are available, the antibiotics can be tailored to the organisms based on sensitivities. Treatment should be performed expeditiously and aggressively because Fournier gangrene is a life-threatening process. All nonviable and necrotic tissue must be aggressively excised (Fig. 41-3). **An empirical broad-spectrum antibiotic regimen for the initial treatment of Fournier gangrene includes a third-generation cephalosporin, an aminoglycoside (if creatinine clearance is acceptable), and metronidazole** (Hejase et al, 1996; Löfmark et al, 2010). Aggressive fluid resuscitation is required including the use of blood and blood products when needed. After debridement, adequate nutrition with early enteral feeding, when possible, is crucial for wound healing. Repeat debridement should be performed 2 days after the initial exploration to excise any remaining nonviable tissue. Multiple resections may be necessary. If the source of the infection is anorectal or the wound is contaminated, a colostomy may need to be

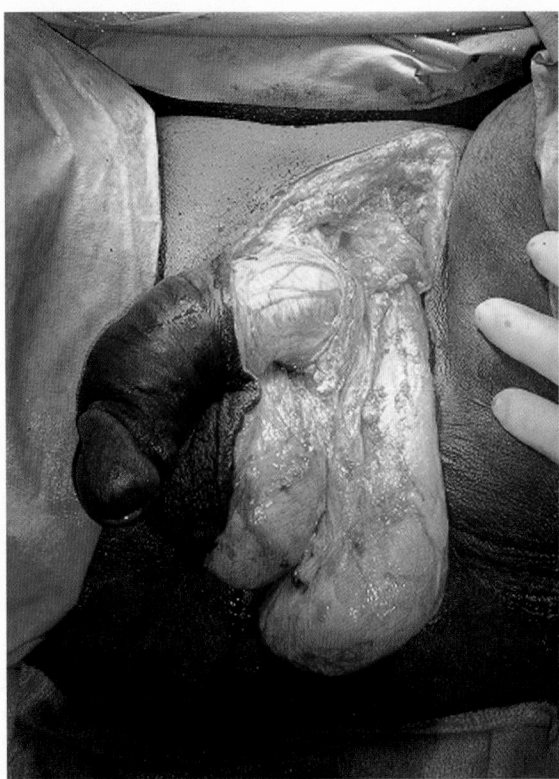

Figure 41-3. Aggressive debridement of Fournier gangrene. (From Kavoussi PK, Costabile RA. Disorders of scrotal contents: orchitis, epididymitis, testicular torsion, torsion of the appendages, and Fournier's gangrene. In: Chapple CR, Steers WD, editors. Practical urology: essential principles and practice. London: Springer-Verlag; 2011.)

performed to divert fecal flow (Ghnnam, 2008). Similarly, patients may require cystostomies for urinary diversion when there is a urinary source exacerbating the necrotizing fasciitis.

After the patient has been initially treated and resuscitated and all necrotic tissue has been excised, most wounds can be closed secondarily. **Large wounds often require skin grafts for coverage. Fasciocutaneous rotational thigh flaps may be used for coverage with good cosmetic results** (Bhatnagar et al, 2008). **Wound closure is performed as soon as there is no evidence of infection or remaining necrotic tissue and there is a viable bed that will allow reapproximation or grafting** (Ghnnam, 2008). In patients with less than 50% scrotal skin loss, primary closure most often can be performed without major difficulty. **Rarely the testes may need to be placed in thigh pouches until the time of definitive reconstruction in cases with major scrotal skin loss** (Gudaviciene and Milonas, 2008). **Vacuum-assisted closure devices (Wound V.A.C.) have been used to help these complex wounds heal after wide excision and debridement.** This technique has been shown to be as effective as conventional wound care in healing wounds. These patients require fewer dressing changes and have less pain, fewer skipped meals, and greater mobility (Ozturk et al, 2009). The use of a small intestinal submucosa graft and fibrin sealant is an option for closure of scrotal defects after excision for Fournier gangrene when standard grafting is impossible (Kavoussi and Bird, 2007).

A severity index was created and validated to identify prognostic factors in patients with Fournier gangrene. Parameters associated with mortality include abnormalities in heart rate, respiratory rate, serum creatinine, serum bicarbonate, serum lactate, and serum calcium. There is a 46% mortality rate in patients with a severity index score of 9 or greater and a 96% survival rate in patients with a severity index score of less than 9. Necrotizing fasciitis involving the abdominal wall or the lower extremities is associated with increased mortality (Corcoran et al, 2008).

Scrotoplasty for Other Benign Scrotal Conditions

Other nonmalignant conditions of the scrotum including hidradenitis suppurativa, postradiation lymphedema, and primary lymphangitis of the scrotum may require surgical excision. Depending on the extent and severity of the wound, different options exist for wound closure or coverage. Small lesions typically are excised and closed primarily, whereas larger wounds require split-thickness skin grafts or tissue flaps (Fig. 41-4) (Eswara and McDougal, 2013). In patients with hidradenitis suppurativa, disease recurrence has been shown to be related to disease severity and not to surgical method of reconstruction (Rompel and Petres, 2000). In patients with systemic disease (i.e., hidradenitis suppurativa, postradiation lymphedema), the surgeon and patient should be aware of potential recurrence; however, in this setting, recurrence is usually tolerated better than the initial lymphedema (Eswara and McDougal, 2013).

VASECTOMY

Vasectomy is a highly effective and safe form of contraception (Schwingl and Guess, 2000). Vasectomy was first described by Sir Ashley Cooper in the United Kingdom when he did experiments to vasectomize dogs (Cooper, 1827). **Approximately 526,501 men undergo vasectomy annually in the United States, which makes vasectomy the most commonly performed urologic surgical procedure.** Vasectomy is chosen as the method of contraception by 11% of married couples, and 0.01% of men between the ages of 25 and 49 undergo vasectomy annually (Barone et al, 2006).

Anesthetic Techniques for Vasectomy

Vasectomy can be performed under sedation, spinal, or general anesthesia, although most surgeons perform vasectomy under local anesthesia because most patients tolerate this method well, and it minimizes cost, anesthetic complications, and morbidity. The choice of local anesthetic is based on surgeon preference. Options for local anesthesia include 1% or 2% lidocaine without epinephrine or a 50/50 mixture of lidocaine and bupivacaine. The vas deferens is isolated through the scrotal skin and grasped tightly between the thumb and the middle finger of the nondominant hand in a superficial position just beneath the scrotal skin. A 25-gauge to 32-gauge needle is used to inject the local anesthetic subcutaneously to raise a small wheal over the vas deferens. After superficial anesthesia is achieved, the needle is carefully advanced into the vasal sheath, and a small amount of anesthetic is injected. Great care should be taken to use as few punctures as possible and as little needle movement as possible to minimize the risk of hematoma formation. EMLA (emulsion of lidocaine and prilocaine) cream applied as topical anesthesia on the scrotal skin 1 hour before injection of 1% lidocaine followed by vasectomy does not decrease the pain associated with vasectomy compared with the use of injectable anesthesia alone (Thomas et al, 2008).

The no-needle jet anesthetic technique has been described to eliminate the needle for anesthetic injection. This technique uses the MadaJet medical injector (Mada Medical Products, Carlstadt, NJ) to deliver lidocaine without epinephrine by means of a high-pressure injector through a tiny head to beneath the skin to diffuse a mist of anesthetic around the vas (Weiss and Li, 2005).

Conventional Technique

Vasectomy should be performed in a warm room with warm preparation solution to allow scrotal relaxation, regardless of the technique employed. Shaving should be done before the procedure to minimize the risk of infection. There is no difference in the rate of postvasectomy infection in men randomly assigned to prophylactic antibiotics versus no antibiotics; antibiotic prophylaxis is not recommended (Khan, 1978). In any chosen technique, the use of a single incision or bilateral scrotal incisions is based on surgeon preference. Many surgeons advocate bilateral scrotal

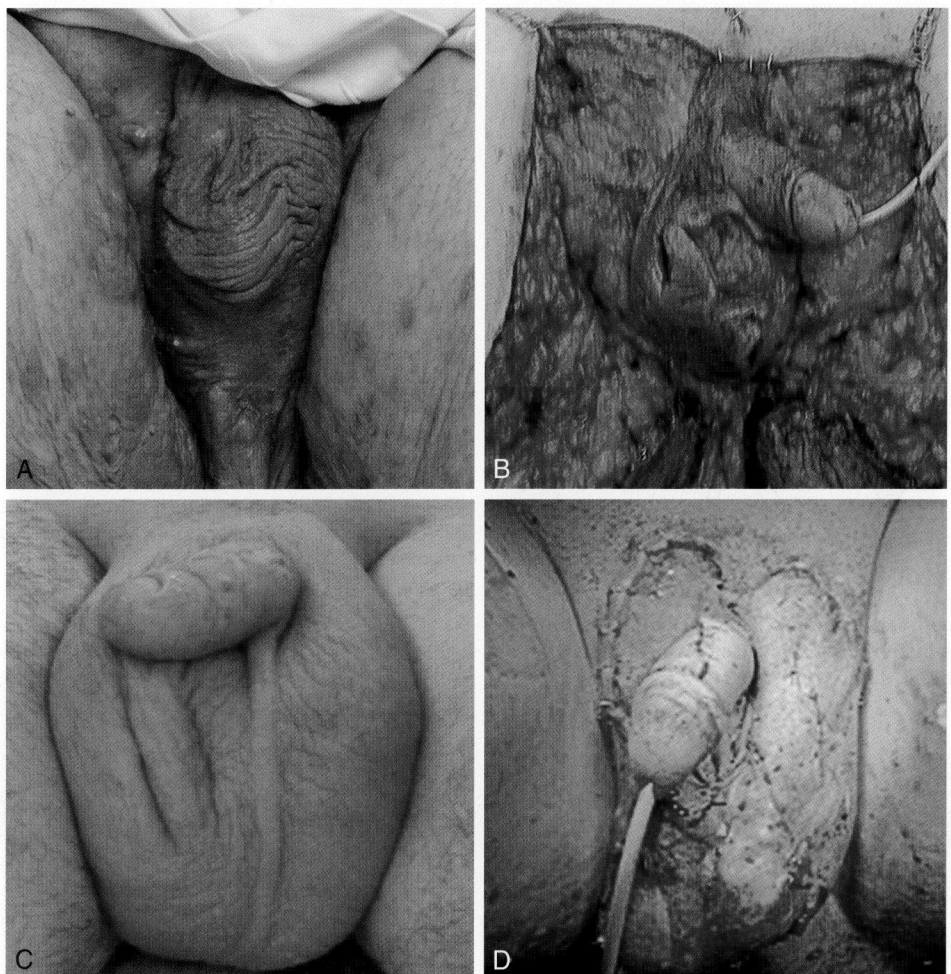

Figure 41-4. **Wide excision of hidradenitis suppurativa of the perineum. A, Before. B, After. Use of excision and split-thickness skin graft for lymphedema of the penis and scrotum. C, Before. D, After.**

incisions to minimize the risk of dividing the same side twice and to allow performing the vasectomy at a position in the midportion of the vas deferens. After induction of adequate local anesthesia, an incision is made over the isolated vas deferens, which is grasped tightly between the thumb and middle fingers. The vasal sheath is sharply divided down to the vas. The vas is delivered through the incision; the deferential artery, nerves, veins, and adjacent tissue are separated from the vas, and the vas is divided. Some surgeons remove a small segment of vas deferens, although most urologists who perform vasectomy reversals prefer not to, which allows easier future reversal. The AUA Guideline (American Urological Association, 2012) states that removal of a segment of vas deferens for histologic confirmation is neither required nor recommended. Most surgeons occlude the testicular and abdominal ends of the vas with suture ligation, hemoclips, intraluminal fulguration with electrocautery, or fascial interposition. These techniques are discussed further later on. The same procedure is repeated on the contralateral vas deferens.

"No-Scalpel" Technique

No-scalpel vasectomy was initially described in China in 1974 (Li, 1976). Routine antibiotics are not needed for patients undergoing no-scalpel vasectomy with sterile technique (Seenu and Hafiz, 2005). **The no-scalpel technique significantly decreases the rate of hematomas, infections, and pain during the procedure.** Patients who undergo the no-scalpel technique also resume sexual activity sooner after surgery and have a shorter operative time than

occurs with the conventional technique (Sokal et al, 1999; Cook et al, 2007a).

The vas and perivasal tissue are firmly secured through the skin with a ring-tipped vas deferens fixation clamp (Fig. 41-5) after local anesthesia has been administered as described earlier (Fig. 41-6). A modified, sharpened tipped curved hemostat (Fig. 41-7) is used to puncture the skin and the vas sheath, and the hemostat is spread to stretch the hole that is made. The vas is pierced with one tip of the hemostat and lifted through the skin opening. The vas is regrasped with the ring clamp, and the hemostat is used to dissect the posterior perivasal tissue. The vas deferens is divided, the occlusion technique of choice is employed, inspection is done for hemostasis, and the vas deferens is replaced in the scrotum. The same procedure is performed on the contralateral vas deferens (Huber, 1988). The perforation in the skin can be closed with an absorbable suture, but it can also be left open and heals well without closure.

Minimally Invasive Vasectomy

There are several variations to the technique of the no-scalpel vasectomy; however, if there is any variation in the steps or specific instruments, the vasectomy should be called minimally invasive vasectomy rather than no-scalpel vasectomy technique. One variation of this technique employs local anesthesia; fixes the vas through the scrotal skin with the ring-tipped vas deferens fixation clamp; and pierces the scrotal skin, vas sheath, and vas deferens in the midline with a sharpened tipped curved hemostat held at 45 degrees from horizontal (Fig. 41-8). To prepare the vas deferens for division,

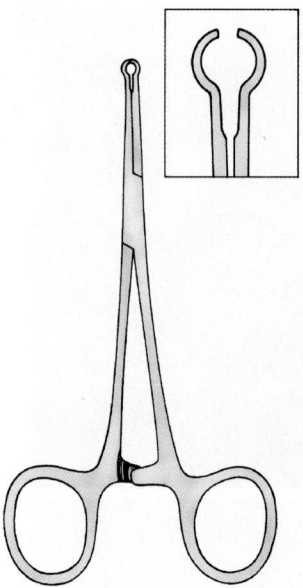

Figure 41-5. **Ring-tipped vas deferens fixation clamp. The cantile-vered design prevents injury. (From Li S, Goldstein M, Zhu J, et al. The no-scalpel vasectomy. J Urol 1991;145:341–4.)**

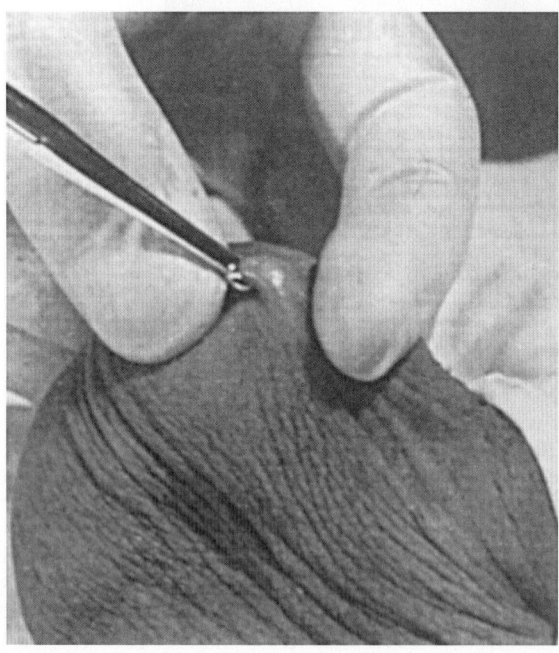

Figure 41-6. **Vas fixed in the ring clamp. The scrotal skin is tightly stretched over the most prominent portion of the vas. (From Li S, Goldstein M, Zhu J, et al. The no-scalpel vasectomy. J Urol 1991;145: 341–4.)**

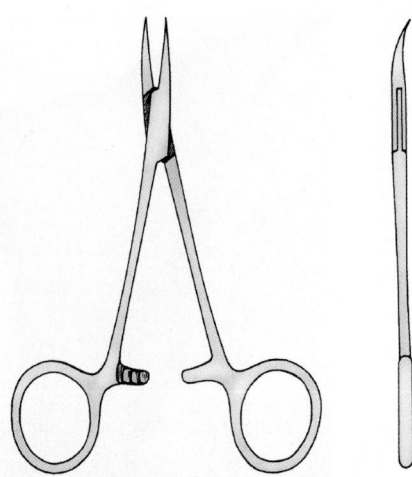

Figure 41-7. **Sharp, curved mosquito hemostat. (From Li S, Goldstein M, Zhu J, et al. The no-scalpel vasectomy. J Urol 1991;145:341–4.)**

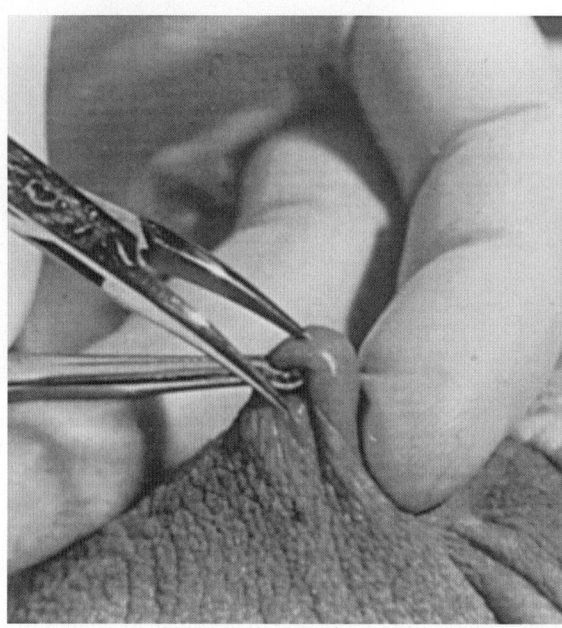

Figure 41-8. **Puncture of the skin, vas sheath, and wall into the lumen. (From Li S, Goldstein M, Zhu J, et al. The no-scalpel vasectomy. J Urol 1991;145:341–4.)**

the clamp is rotated 180 degrees relative to the pierced vas deferens. The remainder of the procedure is performed in the same manner as described earlier, and this is done bilaterally (Schlegel and Goldstein, 1992).

Another technique for performing minimally invasive vasectomy is to isolate the vas deferens after induction of adequate local anesthesia, grasp it tightly between the thumb and middle finger, and puncture the skin overlying the vas deferens with a sharpened tipped curved hemostat. The curved hemostat is used to spread the skin to enlarge the vertical slit in the skin just large enough to allow the ring-tipped vas deferens fixation clamp to fit through to grasp the vas deferens. The vas deferens is grasped and brought up through the puncture, and the vasal fascia and vessels can be spread off the vas deferens to expose the bare vas deferens by spreading the sharp-tipped curved hemostat onto the vasal fascia to open the vasal fascia (Figs. 41-9 and 41-10). The remainder of the vasectomy is performed as described earlier for bilateral procedure (Li et al, 1991). **This modification of making the puncture before grasping the vas deferens with the ring-tipped vas deferens fixation clamp was found to decrease the operative time significantly and showed no difference in incision length, postoperative pain, or time to return to work in a randomized prospective evaluation (Chen et al, 2005).**

Methods of Vasal Obstruction and Male Sterilization

Numerous vasectomy occlusion techniques are employed, including excision and ligation, thermal occlusion with intraluminal electrocautery, mechanical occlusion with hemoclips, fascial interposition, and chemical occlusion with percutaneous techniques. There have been concerns about the risk of vasal necrosis

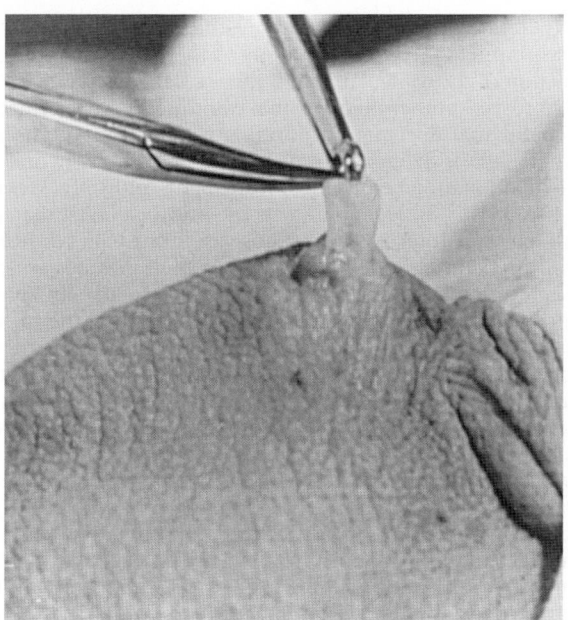

Figure 41-9. Delivery of the clean vas. (From Li S, Goldstein M, Zhu J, et al. The no-scalpel vasectomy. J Urol 1991;145:341–4.)

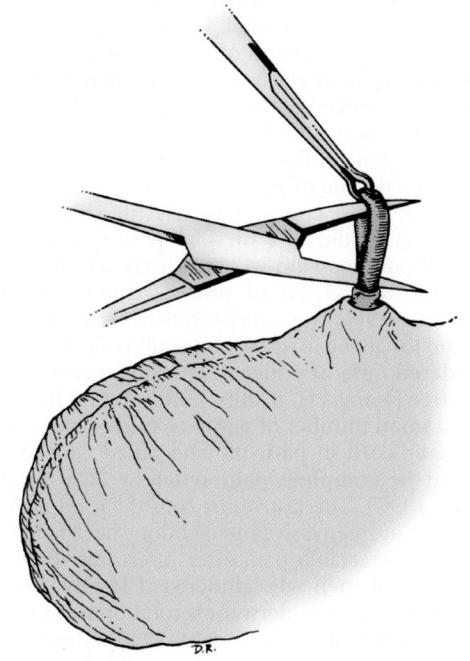

Figure 41-10. Segment cleaned. (From Li S, Goldstein M, Zhu J, et al. The no-scalpel vasectomy. J Urol 1991;145:341–4.)

and sloughing distal to the ligated end when suture ligation is performed, theoretically increasing the risk of recanalization. **Low-voltage thermal occlusion with intraluminal electrocautery in the abdominal and testicular ends of the divided vas deferens reduces recanalization rates to less than 0.5%** (Schmidt, 1987; Barone et al, 2004). Vasectomy failure rates have been reported to be less than 1% when the testicular and abdominal ends of the divided vas deferens are occluded with hemoclips (Moss, 1974; Bennett, 1976). **Interposition of dartos fascia between the divided ends of the vas deferens is another technique for occlusion. This method has been reported to reduce the recanalization rate even further, to nearly zero** (Esho and Cass, 1978; Sokal et al, 2004).

Percutaneous vasectomy has been performed on more than 500,000 men in China. This technique employs chemical occlusion by fixing the vas deferens up to the scrotal skin tightly, puncturing the lumen of the vas deferens with a 22-gauge needle, and cannulating the lumen of the vas deferens with a 24-gauge blunt needle. For confirmation of vas deferens cannulation, Congo red is injected into the lumen of the abdominal end of the right vas deferens, and methylene blue is injected into the lumen of the left vas deferens before chemical occlusion by injection of 20 μL of 2 parts phenol to 1 part N-butylcyanoacrylate mixture. Following chemical occlusion, the patient should void. If the urine is red, the left side was not cannulated, if it is blue, the right side was not cannulated, and if it is brown, that indicates bilateral successful cannulation (Ban, 1980; Li, 1980). Although these chemicals are not approved for use in the United States by the Food and Drug Administration, they appear to be safe based on toxicologic testing and experience in China.

Fascial interposition has been found to decrease vasectomy recanalization rates the most significantly. Randomized controlled trials examining the other techniques are unavailable. Several trials have been performed using irrigation of the abdominal ends of the vas deferens with saline, but there was no difference in time to azoospermia (Cook et al, 2007b).

Open-ended vasectomy, in which the testicular portion of the vas deferens remains patent, is another technique that has been evaluated with the aim of decreasing epididymal pressure by performing intraluminal cautery or another method of occlusion on the abdominal end, while leaving the testicular end unoccluded. Sperm granulomas develop in 97% of patients undergoing open-ended vasectomy. The granulomas are thought to reduce pressure-induced damage to the epididymis, but they increase the vasectomy failure rate to 7% to 50% (Shapiro and Silber, 1979; Goldstein, 1983). **There is a significant decrease in the failure rate with open-ended vasectomy when fascial interposition is performed (decreasing the failure rate by approximately 7%)** (Li et al, 1994).

Performing Vasectomy to Make Microscopic Vasectomy Reversal Easier

Technical aspects of performing vasectomy can affect the ease of microsurgical vasectomy reversal in the future if needed (Mammen et al, 2008). One procedural aspect is that excising a lengthy (>1 cm) segment of vas deferens is associated with the need for a higher scrotal incision, possibly up to the lower inguinal region, with the potential for anastomotic tension with microscopic vasectomy reversal. **Vasectomy reversal can be far more difficult when a lengthy portion of the vas deferens has been excised, with concomitant increases in operative time, length of incision, and postoperative pain** (Practice Committee of the American Society for Reproductive Medicine, 2006).

Another procedural aspect is the location along the length of the vas deferens where the vasectomy is performed. Experts in microsurgery agree that the anastomosis is least problematic when the lumen of the vas deferens is largest and most concentric, as opposed to the lumen in the epididymis or the convoluted vas (Mammen et al, 2008). Prospective studies show that the length of the testicular vas deferens present at the time of reversal has a direct correlation with the presence of seminal fluid containing intact sperm at the time of microscopic vasectomy reversal. A testicular length of vas deferens less than 2.7 cm correlates with seminal fluid without intact sperm 85% of the time, and testicular length more than 2.7 cm is associated with intact sperm in seminal fluid 94% of the time. For each 1-cm increase in testicular remnant length, the probability of whole sperm being present increases fourfold (Witt et al, 1994). **Division of the vas deferens should be performed approximately 3 cm distal to the cauda of the epididymis in the straight portion of the vas deferens at the time of vasectomy.**

The other technical aspect to consider is the occlusion technique employed. All occlusive modalities for vasectomy carry a similarly high efficacy in terms of postprocedure azoospermia. To date, no specific studies on occlusion technique as a predictor of reversal success have been performed. **A simple transection of the vas** deferens followed by low-voltage intraluminal cautery occlusion and then fascial interposition provides successful vasectomy and may result in minimal inflammatory reaction. Minimizing inflammation near the vas deferens would provide the optimum condition for microscopic vasectomy reversal in the future (Mammen et al, 2008).

Postoperative Care and Follow-Up Semen Analysis

Routine postoperative care practices vary but typically include the use of ice packs on the scrotum intermittently for the first 48 hours, limited heavy or strenuous activity for 1 week, and the use of nonsteroidal anti-inflammatory drugs as needed for pain if the patient does not have any contraindications to these medications. **There is no vasectomy technique that is 100% effective. Time to reach azoospermia is variable, although greater than 80% of patients achieve azoospermia by 3 months and after 20 ejaculations.** The AUA Vasectomy Guideline (American Urological Association, 2012) recommends checking the first postvasectomy semen analysis 8 to 16 weeks after vasectomy. Persistent nonmotile sperm are present in 1.4% of patients after vasectomy. **These data point to obtaining a semen analysis at 3 months and 20 ejaculations after vasectomy to reveal azoospermia.** If the semen analysis does not show azoospermia, periodic semen analyses can be obtained every 6 to 12 weeks until azoospermia is achieved. Additional samples should be submitted if the initial semen analysis has motile sperm or greater than 100,000 nonmotile sperm/mL. Patients who have small numbers of persistent nonmotile sperm can be advised cautiously to discontinue contraception (Griffin et al, 2005). There is evidence that these men ultimately reach azoospermia. **Vasectomy should be repeated if any motile sperm are seen in the ejaculate 6 months after the initial vasectomy** (American Urological Association, 2012).

An immunodiagnostic test, the SpermCheck Vasectomy (ContraVac, Charlottesville, VA), has been developed to allow patients to test themselves for severe oligospermia or azoospermia at home after vasectomy. This test was developed to increase compliance with postvasectomy evaluation of semen parameters. The SpermCheck Vasectomy test was 96% accurate at predicting whether sperm counts were greater or less than a threshold of 250,000 sperm/mL (Klotz et al, 2008).

Local and Postoperative Complications

The rates of surgical complications after vasectomy are approximately 1% to 2%. Local complications of vasectomy include hematoma, infection, Fournier gangrene, chronic scrotal pain, and traumatic fistula/scrotal sinus (Awsare et al, 2005). **The most important predictor of postoperative complications is surgeon volume and experience** (Kendrick et al, 1987).

Hematoma is the most common complication of vasectomy. The rate of hematoma formation after vasectomy ranges from 0.09% to 29%, with a mean incidence of 2% (Kendrick et al, 1987). The no-scalpel technique has decreased the hematoma rate to a 0.5% incidence (Pant et al, 2007).

The rate of infection from vasectomy with the conventional technique was reported to be between 12% and 38% but decreased to 0.4% with the no-scalpel technique (Appell and Evans, 1980; Pant et al, 2007). Although exceedingly rare, Fournier gangrene has been reported as a complication in men undergoing vasectomy (de Diego Rodríguez et al, 2000; Romero Pérez et al, 2004).

Short-term scrotal pain lasting a few weeks can occur in 30% of men. **The medical literature on postvasectomy pain syndrome, or long-term scrotal pain after surgery, consists of studies with small sample sizes, nonvalidated pain measures, high nonresponse rates, and variable outcome measures. The most robust study identified the incidence of chronic scrotal pain severe enough to seek medical attention to be 0.9%** (Leslie et al, 2007), **although it has been reported to be as high as 15%** (McConaghy et al, 1996). Postvasectomy pain syndrome has no association with immediate postoperative complications such as hematoma or infec-

tion. There are several theories about the cause of postvasectomy pain syndrome. One is that dilation of the epididymal duct with obstruction of the testicular end of the vas deferens produces interstitial fibrosis. Another theory is that extravasation of spermatozoa, with epididymal duct rupture forming a sperm granuloma at the site where the vas deferens is transected, results in perineural fibrosis and inflammation because sperm are highly antigenic (McMahon et al, 1992). This theory contradicts the previous belief that sperm granulomas are protective against postvasectomy pain syndrome by relieving pressure, although most sperm granulomas are asymptomatic (Tandon and Sabanegh, 2008). There are markedly increased pressures in the epididymis and the testicular end of the vas deferens after vasectomy, but these pressures were not found to be transmitted to the seminiferous tubules in human micropuncture studies (Johnson and Howards, 1975). It is unclear why some patients develop long-term symptoms and others develop transient symptoms. Factors such as age, socioeconomic status, race, environment, and vasectomy technique have not identified patients at risk for postvasectomy pain syndrome (Tandon and Sabanegh, 2008).

Conservative therapy should be the first-line therapy and includes scrotal elevation and support, heat or ice (as needed for comfort), and nonsteroidal anti-inflammatory drugs. Empirical antibiotic therapy is not recommended without evidence of infection (Selikowitz and Schned, 1985). **Conservative therapy should be employed for at least 3 months for postvasectomy pain. Spermatic cord blocks and pain management techniques should be considered after failure of conservative therapy.**

Surgical therapy might be considered on an individualized basis if the aforementioned methods fail. **When pain is clearly localized to a sperm granuloma, excision of the granuloma and intraluminal cautery occlusion of the vas deferens may relieve the pain and prevent recurrence** (Schmidt, 1979). Epididymectomy has been performed in patients who had point tenderness to the epididymis and epididymal dilation after vasectomy and failed conservative therapy. Predictors of poor outcomes with epididymectomy are atypical symptoms, concomitant erectile dysfunction, and a normal-appearing epididymis on scrotal ultrasonography (West et al, 2000). **Of patients who were properly selected for epididymectomy, 50% were cured of postvasectomy pain syndrome** (Chen and Ball, 1991). The patient must consider that vasectomy reversal will no longer be feasible after epididymectomy. **Vasectomy reversal rendered 69% of patients with postvasectomy pain syndrome pain-free** (Nangia et al, 2000). **Although it has been evaluated in only a small number of patients, microscopic denervation of the spermatic cord in patients who failed conservative treatment resulted in complete pain relief in 76% of these men** (Ahmed et al, 1997). The last resort consideration after failure of conservative and more invasive interventions have failed is orchiectomy for severe intractable pain after vasectomy. **Pain relief was reported in 73% of men who underwent inguinal orchiectomy versus 55% of men who underwent scrotal orchiectomy for postvasectomy pain syndrome** (Davis et al, 1990). There is a report of 0.3% rate of scrotal sinus/vasocutaneous fistula after no-scalpel vasectomy (Pant et al, 2007).

Association of Vasectomy with Long-Term Systemic Disease

Previous studies found an increased risk of prostate cancer in men who underwent vasectomy (Giovannucci et al, 1993). Detection bias is thought to be the source of this association of prostate cancer with vasectomy (Millard, 1999). **More recent investigations have found that there is no association between vasectomy and prostate cancer** (Schuman et al, 1993; Holt et al, 2008). There is no association between vasectomy and prostate cancer in developing countries in which there are low incidences of prostate cancer in the general population as well (Schwingl et al, 2009). **Screening recommendations for prostate cancer should be no different in men who have undergone vasectomy than in men who have not undergone vasectomy** (Healy, 1993).

Vasectomy does not place the patient at an increased long-term risk for cardiovascular disease or atherosclerosis (Coady et al, 2002; Goldacre et al, 2005). Previous studies suggested that vasectomy may be a risk factor for patients with primary progressive aphasia, a dementia syndrome with aphasia as the presenting symptom (Weintraub et al, 2006). There are no longitudinal studies confirming this association, and there have been many large, epidemiologic studies comparing men with and without vasectomy that have not shown any increased risk of dementia. There is no evidence that vasectomy adversely affects psychological health status (Thonneau and D'Isle, 1990).

Antisperm Antibodies

There is a disruption of the blood-testis barrier when vasectomy is performed. **Of men who undergo vasectomy, 60% to 80% have detectable levels of antisperm antibodies in the serum** (Fuchs and Alexander, 1983). **After vasectomy, 50% to 60% of men develop sperm agglutinating antibodies, and 20% to 30% develop sperm immobilizing antibodies** (Kovacs and Frances, 1983). Although some studies suggest that antisperm antibodies persist, others suggest that they diminish 2 or more years after vasectomy, but neither immune complex deposition nor circulation is increased in men who have undergone vasectomy (Witkin et al, 1982).

KEY POINTS: VASECTOMY

- No vasectomy technique is 100% effective.
- Patients can be advised to initiate unprotected intercourse following a semen analysis obtained 8 to 16 weeks after vasectomy that demonstrates azoospermia or rare nonmotile sperm.
- The no-scalpel technique significantly decreases the rate of hematomas, infections, and pain during the procedure.
- Fascial interposition is the occlusion technique that has been found to decrease vasectomy failure rates the most significantly.
- Technical aspects of performing vasectomy can affect the ease of microsurgical vasectomy reversal in the future if needed.
- There is no association between vasectomy and prostate cancer or cardiovascular disease.

SPERMATOCELECTOMY AND SURGERY OF THE EPIDIDYMIS

Surgical Indications

A spermatocele or epididymal cyst is a cystic dilation of an epididymal tubule that is benign in nature. **Spermatoceles are common and are found incidentally on high-resolution ultrasonography in 30% of men. They are typically asymptomatic and do not cause epididymal obstruction, and they rarely require intervention.** Men typically seek surgical treatment when the spermatocele has reached the approximate size of the testis and is causing pain with point tenderness (Walsh et al, 2007).

Surgical treatment for chronic epididymitis is poorly studied in clinical trials with no level 1 evidence to support the use of a specific surgical procedure. In one study, 10 patients with chronic epididymitis (defined as epididymal pain lasting >3 months) underwent epididymectomy for intractable symptoms. Only one of these patients had significant improvement in pain (Davis et al, 1990). Other authors reported much higher success rates, such as six out of seven patients (86%) having significant improvement in pain after epididymectomy (Chen and Ball, 1991). **Chronic or recurrent epididymitis and persistent epididymalgia with point tenderness to the epididymis may be reasonable indications for epididymectomy** (Padmore et al, 1996).

Surgical treatment for chronic epididymitis should be considered only after failure of extensive conservative therapy and after appropriate counseling, with the understanding that the symptoms may not improve after surgery or may worsen. A retrospective review of men who underwent epididymectomy for chronic epididymitis showed that outcomes were best when the patient had a palpable epididymal abnormality on physical examination. Men in this study without a palpable abnormality but with ultrasound changes had slightly worse outcomes, and men with neither a palpable abnormality nor a demonstrable abnormality on ultrasonography did not improve with epididymectomy (Calleary et al, 2009).

Purulent epididymitis diagnosed by a combination of physical examination, ultrasound evaluation, and occasionally needle aspiration of the epididymis is an absolute indication for epididymectomy (Arbuliev et al, 2008). Epididymectomy is also the treatment of choice for epididymal abscesses and chronic infectious epididymitis that is unresponsive to antibiotic treatment. **Diagnostic epididymal puncture and aspiration should not be performed in men with interest in future fertility because this procedure would result in epididymal obstruction. Total epididymectomy may relieve chronic persistent pain localized to the epididymis after vasectomy.**

Epididymal malignancies are extremely rare, and 73% of nontransilluminating, solid epididymal masses are benign adenomatoid tumors (Beccia et al, 1976). Surgical extirpation should be considered for adenomatoid tumors, especially if there is any suspicion for malignancy (Alvarez Maestro et al, 2009).

Partial and Total Epididymectomy

Any patient undergoing epididymal surgery should be counseled extensively that the surgery may impair his fertility or cause sterility if bilateral epididymal surgery is required because the distal epididymis consists of a single tubule. Partial or total epididymectomy can be approached scrotally through a median raphe or a unilateral transverse scrotal incision to deliver the testis. The vas deferens is identified, isolated, ligated, and divided. The testicular end of the vas deferens is followed to the vasoepididymal junction. The tunica vaginalis is opened, and the plane of dissection between the epididymis and the testis is found to divide the epididymis from the testis. Great care should be taken to avoid injury to the spermatic cord and testicular artery. The efferent ducts superior to the testicular vasculature are ligated with an absorbable suture to complete the epididymectomy. The edges of the tunica vaginalis where the epididymis was excised are approximated with a running absorbable suture, which helps with hemostasis. The dartos fascia and skin are closed in layers with absorbable suture. In the case of partial epididymectomy, ligations are performed between the testis and epididymis with absorbable suture to excise the affected portion of the epididymis, while leaving the remainder attached to the testis with its vascular supply intact (Figs. 41-11 and 41-12).

Spermatocelectomy and Excision of Epididymal Cysts

Spermatocelectomy can be approached scrotally through a median raphe or a unilateral transverse scrotal incision to deliver the testis. The tunica vaginalis is opened, and the spermatocele is identified and dissected free from the epididymis. The epididymal-spermatocele attachment is ligated and divided to complete the spermatocelectomy. The tunica vaginalis is closed, and the dartos fascia and scrotal skin are reapproximated in layers.

Excision of Epididymal Tumors

As discussed earlier, most epididymal nontransilluminating masses are benign adenomatoid tumors. Fine-needle aspiration of solid epididymal masses has been evaluated and found to be very accurate compared with surgical pathology (Gupta et al, 2006). **When malignancy is suspected, an inguinal approach should be used with clamping of the spermatic cord and delivery of the testis.** The addition of testicular hypothermia by adding ice slush to the

Chevassu maneuver (of clamping the vessels) was employed and found to salvage three of five testicles with benign processes after clamping and parenchymal biopsy (Goldstein and Waterhouse, 1983). When malignancy is ruled out, the epididymal mass may be excised as for a spermatocelectomy.

Complications

Complications of epididymectomy, spermatocelectomy, and excision of epididymal masses are rare. Complications include bleeding, infection, damage to the testicular artery with resultant testicular atrophy, and recurrence in cases of spermatocelectomy (Kiddoo et al, 2004; Zahalsky et al, 2004). **Complications also include impairment of fertility with obstruction of the epididymal tubules and possible sterility in bilateral cases, necessitating counseling and recommending sperm cryopreservation in men who undergo bilateral procedures and have an interest in fertility.** Approximately 17% of patients undergoing spermatocelectomy have resultant epididymal injury (Zahalsky et al, 2004). The overall complication rate has been reported to be 20%, with the most common complications being persistent scrotal pain and infection. **Leaving a scrotal drain did not decrease complication rates** (Kiddoo et al, 2004).

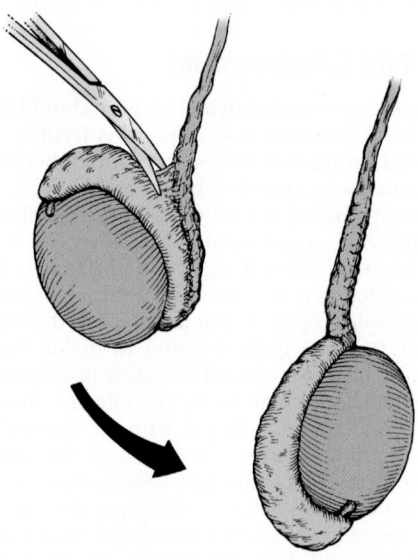

Figure 41-11. **Convoluted vas dissected off the epididymal tunica.**

HYDROCELECTOMY

Hydrocele in an adult is caused by excessive fluid secretion by the visceral tunica albuginea without adequate reabsorption of this fluid by the parietal peritoneum around the testis.

Inguinal Surgical Approach

Men in whom hydroceles have been diagnosed, in which there is suspicion for concomitant malignancy, should undergo high-resolution scrotal ultrasonography. If malignancy is suspected, an inguinal approach should be used to allow control of the spermatic cord in preparation for radical orchiectomy. If this approach is taken and no malignancy is encountered, the testis can be spared and the hydrocele can be repaired by one of the techniques described subsequently.

Scrotal Surgical Approaches

When there is no evidence of malignancy on physical examination and high-resolution ultrasonography, hydroceles may be approached scrotally through a median raphe or a transverse unilateral incision. In all techniques, the hydrocele is dissected and delivered intact to allow the easiest dissection. After the hydrocele is delivered, an opening in the sac is made away from the testis, epididymis, and cord structures, and the fluid is suctioned out. The hydrocele sac is opened further to expose the sac for the elected repair. **The overall single-treatment success rates for surgical hydrocelectomy are between 90% and 100%** (Rodriguez et al, 1981).

Excisional techniques are the least likely to result in recurrence of a hydrocele. Excising the hydrocele is recommended for large, long-standing, thick-walled, loculated hydroceles. The hydrocele sac is opened, taking great care not to injure the spermatic cord, and the sac is simply excised, leaving room to oversew the edge of the excised sac without endangering the cord or the epididymis. A 3-0 chromic suture can be used in a baseball-stitch manner to oversew the edge of the sac (Fig. 41-13).

The Jaboulay bottleneck technique (1902) is a useful method for large, floppy, thin hydrocele sacs. This technique is performed by excising the sac as described previously, but a larger margin of excision should be left between the edge of the sac and the testis and epididymis to allow for sewing the edges of the sac together behind the cord, without compressing the cord (Fig. 41-14).

If there appears to be a risk for hematoma after excision and oversewing with either technique, a Penrose drain can be left in the dependent portion of the scrotum and fixed in place to the scrotum. The dartos fascia and skin are then closed in layers. Fluffs and a scrotal support are used for the dressing.

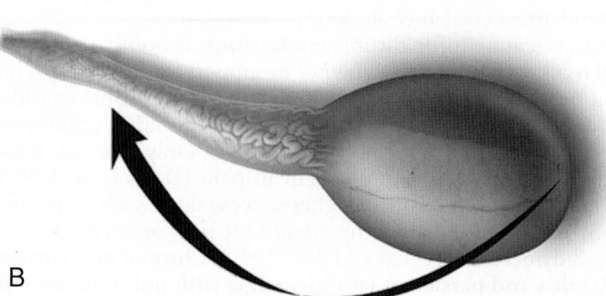

Figure 41-12. **A and B, Entire vasoepididymal complex is dissected to the caput.**

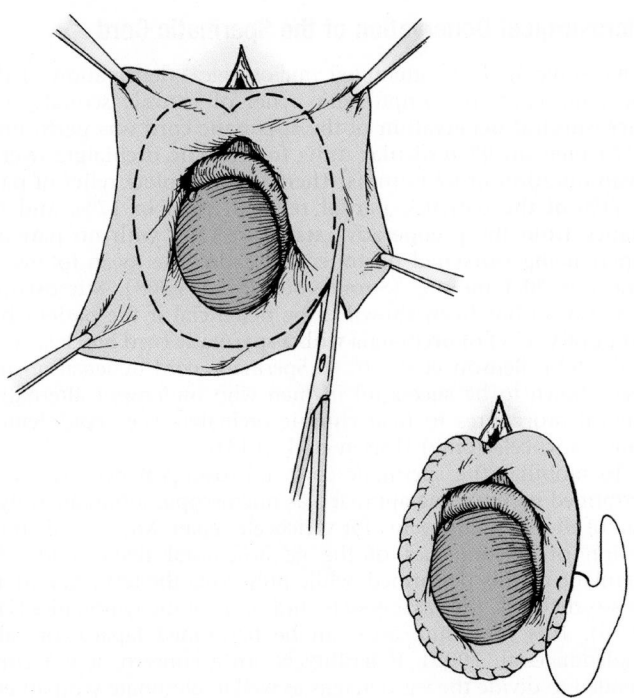

Figure 41-13. Simple excision of the thick-walled hydrocele sac and oversewn edges.

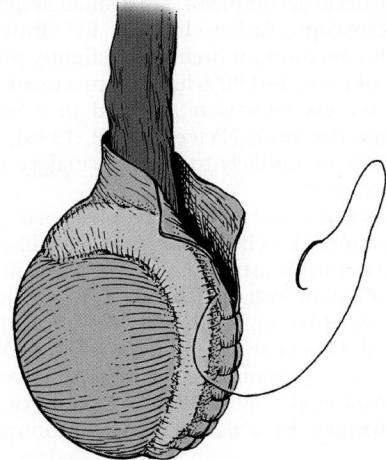

Figure 41-14. Jaboulay bottleneck technique for excision of thin, floppy sacs.

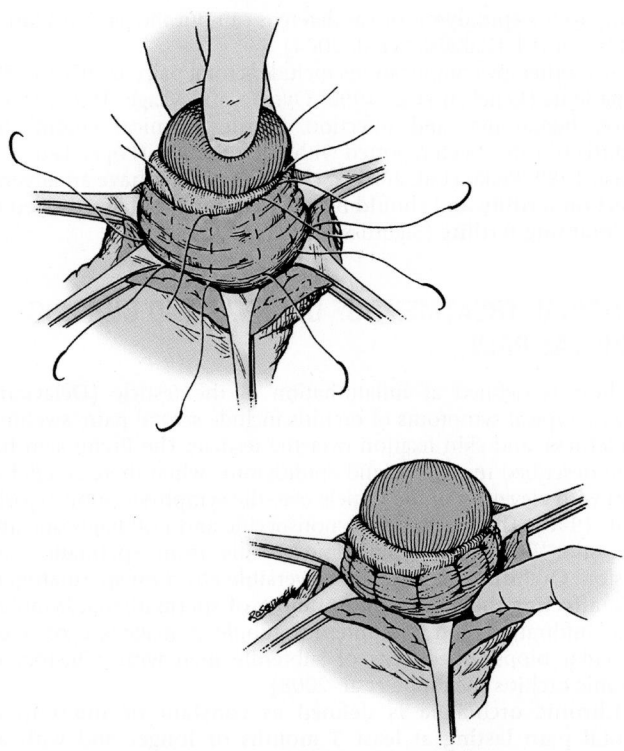

Figure 41-15. Lord plication technique.

TABLE 41-1 Hydrocelectomy Techniques and Risks

	RECURRENCE	HEMATOMA
Excision	Decreased	Increased
Plication	Increased	Decreased

Plication techniques are suitable for smaller, thin-walled hydroceles but should not be used in large, long-standing, thick-walled, multiloculated hydroceles because this leaves a large bundle of plicated tissue in the scrotum. The Lord plication technique (1964) is performed by opening the hydrocele as described earlier, delivering the testis, cauterizing or oversewing the cut edges of the sac, and using interrupted, radially placed chromic sutures to plicate the sac. Closure is performed as described earlier. Drains are unnecessary with plications (Fig. 41-15).

A minimally invasive technique can be used by making a 2-cm incision in the scrotum. The hydrocele is drained, followed by excision of a portion of parietal tunica vaginalis. The tunica vaginalis is everted, sutured to the subcutaneous tissue, and a surgical drain is placed (Saber, 2011).

Sclerotherapy

Sclerotherapy is another treatment option with a single-treatment success rate ranging from 33% to 75% (Levine and Dewolf, 1988).

This option may be a good choice for patients who cannot tolerate anesthesia or who refuse surgical treatment. **The common steps of the procedure include needle aspiration of the hydrocele fluid, followed by injection of local anesthesia, and ultimately instillation of the sclerosing agent.** The most commonly used sclerosing agent is tetracycline, although 2.5% phenol solutions, 95% alcohol, and ethanolamine oleate also have been used effectively (Nash, 1984; Hellström et al, 1986; Miskowiak and Christensen, 1988). One study showed no statistically significant improvement in patients who underwent aspiration of hydrocele fluid alone versus aspiration plus instillation of tetracycline as a sclerosing agent, with a higher complication rate in the sclerotherapy group (Breda et al, 1992). When sclerotherapy was compared with hydrocelectomy, the success rate was higher in hydrocelectomy, although the hydrocelectomy group had a higher complication rate. Nonetheless, the patients who underwent hydrocelectomy had higher satisfaction rates (Beiko et al, 2003).

Complications

The most common complication after hydrocelectomy is hematoma (Table 41-1). **The overall complication rate in hydrocelectomy is approximately 19%, including hematoma, infection, persistent swelling, recurrence, injury to spermatic vessels, and chronic pain.** Although the use of a drain in selected patients is recommended, it has not been proven so far to decrease complication rates (Kiddoo et al, 2004). When repairing large hydroceles, great care must be taken not to injure the epididymis and spermatic vessels because they may be splayed within the hydrocele layers.

Injury to the epididymis or vas deferens can put the patient's future fertility at risk (Zahalsky et al, 2004).

Sclerotherapy complications include scrotal pain in 29% to 55% of patients (Rencken et al, 1990; Ovrebø and Vaage, 1991), recurrence, hematoma, and infection; febrile chemical epididymo-orchitis has also been reported with sclerotherapy (López Laur and Parisi, 1989; Beiko et al, 2003). **Sclerotherapy can have an adverse effect on fertility and should be avoided in patients interested in maintaining fertility** (Sigurdsson et al, 1994).

SURGICAL TREATMENT OF ORCHITIS AND CHRONIC SCROTAL PAIN

Orchitis is defined as inflammation of the testicle (Delavierre, 2003). Typical symptoms of orchitis include scrotal pain, swelling, tenderness, and skin fixation over the testicle. The Prehn sign has been described in orchitis and epididymitis when there is relief of pain with elevation of the testicle over the symphysis pubis (Noske et al, 1998). The Prehn sign is nonspecific and nondiagnostic and does not distinguish epididymo-orchitis from spermatic cord torsion. **Orchitis can cause an irreversible effect on spermatogenesis, affecting the quality and number of spermatozoa.** Lymphocytic infiltration and seminiferous tubule damage are seen on testicular biopsy specimens of subfertile men with a history of chronic orchitis (Schuppe et al, 2008).

Chronic orchialgia is defined as constant or intermittent scrotal pain lasting at least 3 months or longer and with an unclear cause (Costabile et al, 1991). **In patients with clinical orchialgia, a scrotal ultrasound scan should be obtained because testicular malignancy has been reported to masquerade as orchialgia** (Vaidyanathan et al, 2008). At least 10% of men with testicular malignancy initially receive an incorrect diagnosis of an acute inflammatory process or spermatic cord torsion (Cook and Dewbury, 2000). High-frequency transducer ultrasonography (7.5 to 10 MHz) is considered the best modality for evaluation of scrotal pathology including orchitis (Lee et al, 2008).

Although there is no level 1 evidence for the optimal treatment of chronic orchialgia or epididymitis, local supportive therapy, including heat, nerve blocks, analgesics, tricyclic antidepressants, anticonvulsants (e.g., gabapentin), and anti-inflammatory drugs, is commonly applied and may offer some relief (Davis and Noble, 1992). Other treatment options implemented for chronic epididymitis include phytotherapy, anxiolytics, narcotics, acupuncture, and steroid injection therapy (Nickel et al, 2002). Despite evidence that 75% of patients do not have an identifiable bacterial urinary tract infection concomitantly with clinical epididymitis, antibiotics are routinely given. Empirical antibiotic administration in the absence of positive urine cultures has been steadily increasing, from 75% to 95% between the years of 1965 and 2005. **Antibiotic administration does not decrease the length of symptoms or the return to full activity in men without an identifiable bacterial pathogen** (Mittemeyer et al, 1966).

Orchiectomy

Surgical treatment for chronic orchialgia is poorly studied in clinical trials, with no level 1 evidence to support the use of a specific surgical procedure. In the available literature, fewer than 250 patients with chronic scrotal pain have been treated with differing surgical therapies despite the common nature of chronic scrotal pain. There is no level 1 evidence that orchiectomy is effective for the treatment of chronic orchialgia. If orchiectomy is recommended, the patient should have failed previous conservative therapy and must be apprised of the risks, benefits, and options of orchiectomy. Because many patients continue to have pain or have pain recur after orchiectomy, the surgeon should be aware of the medicolegal aspects of this action. **If orchiectomy is performed, it should be performed through an inguinal incision because this approach has been shown to have a better outcome than the scrotal approach for orchialgia** (Davis and Noble, 1992).

Microsurgical Denervation of the Spermatic Cord

Some surgeons have attempted microsurgical denervation of the spermatic cord for symptomatic relief of chronic scrotal pain. **Microsurgical denervation of the spermatic cord was performed in 79 men on 95 testicular units for chronic orchialgia over a mean duration of 62 months. There was complete relief of pain in 71% of the patients, partial relief of pain in 17%, and no change from the preoperative status in 12%, with no patients experiencing worsened postoperative pain.** The mean follow-up time was 20.3 months (Strom and Levine, 2008). **Microscopic denervation has been shown to be beneficial if the patient has temporary relief of orchialgia with a spermatic cord block** (Levine et al, 1996; Benson et al, 2013). Spermatic cord denervation has been shown to be successful in men who underwent alternative surgical procedures to treat chronic orchialgia (i.e., epididymectomy, varicocelectomy) (Larsen et al, 2013).

To mobilize the spermatic cord, microsurgical denervation is performed by the same approach as microscopic subinguinal ligation of the spermatic veins for varicocele repair. Microscopic transection of all branches of the genitofemoral nerve along the spermatic cord is performed, while preserving the testicular artery, the vas deferens, the vasal vessels, and some of the lymphatics (Fig. 41-16). This procedure also can be performed laparoscopically (Cadeddu et al, 1999). If fertility is not a concern, it is recommended to divide the vas deferens as well to eliminate sympathetic innervation, which may contribute to orchialgia by a sympathetic dystrophy component (Levine et al, 1996).

Large, clinically palpable varicoceles can cause orchialgia. The pain typically improves with the patient in the supine position because the varicocele decompresses. **In a small series of men who underwent microscopic varicocelectomy for clinically palpable varicoceles with concomitant orchialgia, slightly more than 50% had resolution of pain, and 90% had improvement** (Chawla et al, 2005). Higher success rates were reported in a previous, larger powered, retrospective study (Peterson et al, 1998). Smaller, nonclinical varicoceles are unlikely to cause orchialgia and should be managed conservatively.

Retractile testes are another source of scrotal pain in men. A careful history must be elicited to make this diagnosis because the patient may not demonstrate a retractile testis on examination. The history is consistent with orchialgia only when the testis retracts up toward the external inguinal ring. This is typically seen in younger men with hyperactive cremasteric reflexes. Orchiopexy can be performed in these patients as it would in patients with intermittent torsion (Forte et al, 2003). **When orchiopexy is offered, it should be performed by a dartos pouch technique to prevent**

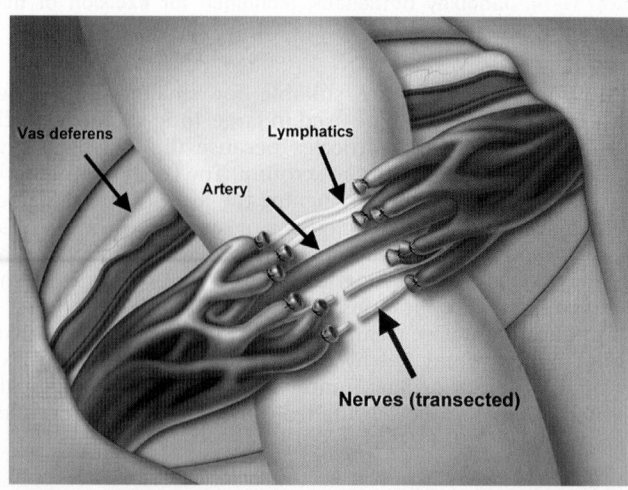

Figure 41-16. **Microsurgical denervation. The goal is to transect all branches of the genitofemoral nerve while preserving the vas deferens, vasal vessels, testicular artery, and lymphatics.**

Vas deferens

Lymphatics

Artery

Nerves (transected)

retraction, as is recommended for testicular torsion (Redman and Barthold, 1995).

The other surgical treatment for orchialgia secondary to the retractile testis is to perform microscopic release of the cremasteric muscle. This technique is performed in a similar manner to microscopic subinguinal varicocelectomy. The spermatic cord is mobilized and isolated, and the cremasteric muscle is divided circumferentially, while preserving the vasculature of the spermatic cord and the vas deferens. This technique effectively releases the spermatic cord, not allowing retraction of the testis with hypercontraction of the cremasteric muscles.

KEY POINTS: SURGERY OF THE SCROTAL CONTENTS

- Patients undergoing epididymal surgery should be counseled that the surgery may impair their fertility or cause sterility if bilateral epididymal surgery is required.
- Sclerotherapy as treatment for a hydrocele can have an adverse effect on fertility and should be avoided in patients interested in maintaining fertility.
- Antibiotics should not be given for epididymitis or orchitis without evidence of infection.
- Patients with chronic orchialgia should receive a scrotal ultrasound scan.
- When a clinically palpable varicocele is encountered in a patient with orchialgia, varicocelectomy resolves the pain 50% of the time.

SURGERY OF THE SEMINAL VESICLES

In 1561, Gabriele Fallopius, a renowned Italian anatomist and physician, first described the seminal vesicles as paired male organs. He was considered an authority in the field of sexuality and advocated the use of condoms to decrease the transmission of syphilis. There was a great deal of interest in the seminal vesicles in the late 19th century because of their discovered involvement with inflammatory diseases (Brewster, 1985).

Seminal vesicle secretions contribute 50% to 80% of the volume of the ejaculate. The pH of the secreted fluid is neutral to slightly alkaline, and the mean volume is approximately 2.5 mL. The secreted fluid contains fructose and other carbohydrates necessary for sperm motility. It also contains a coagulation factor and prostaglandins A, B, E, and F (Tauber et al, 1975).

Primary disease processes of the seminal vesicles are very rare, although secondary processes are seen more commonly. Diagnosis of such entities has improved over the years with advanced imaging, particularly magnetic resonance imaging (MRI) (Kim et al, 2009; Chiang et al, 2013). Because of the anatomic location, surgical access and management of seminal vesicle pathology can be difficult for the urologist.

Anatomy

The seminal vesicles are paired male organs with no equivalent in the female. It is useful to understand the developmental anatomy of the seminal vesicles to gain a full understanding of the anatomy in adult patients. **The seminal vesicles begin as bilateral dorsolateral bulbous dilations of the distal mesonephric ducts between 12 and 12½ weeks of gestation.** By 13 weeks, these dilations have enlarged, and the ejaculatory ducts are beginning to form in the developing prostate (Brewster, 1985). The seminal vesicle and the ampulla of the vas deferens join posterior and superior to the prostate to form the ejaculatory duct (Nguyen et al, 1996). By the early portion of the seventh month, the seminal vesicle has multiple outpouchings and a widened main central lumen (Fig. 41-17) (Brewster, 1985).

The adult seminal vesicle measures 5 to 6 cm in length and 3 to 5 cm in diameter with a volume capacity of 13 cm, although seminal vesicles decrease in size as men age (Redman, 1987). At

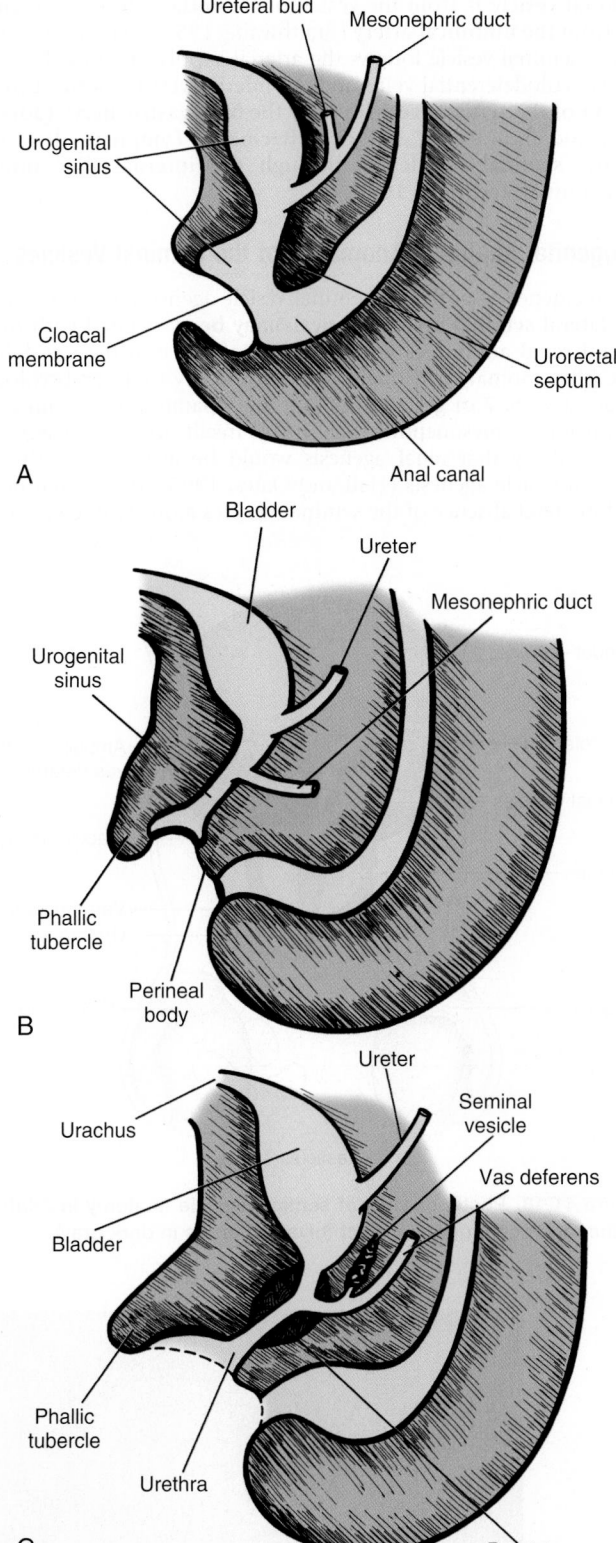

Figure 41-17. Intrauterine (fetal) development of the seminal vesicles. A, Week 5. B, Week 8. C, Week 13. (Redrawn from Langman J. Medical embryology. 4th ed. Baltimore: Williams & Wilkins; 1981. p. 242–3.)

the terminal portion of the vas deferens within the prostate, the major lumen of the seminal vesicle empties into the ejaculatory duct. The ejaculatory duct is in continuity with the seminal vesicle but does not share the thick muscular wall of the seminal vesicle (Fig. 41-18) (Nguyen et al, 1996). **The arterial supply to the** seminal vesicle is from the vesiculodeferential artery, branching off from the umbilical artery (Braithwaite, 1952). Venous drainage of the seminal vesicle follows the arterial supply draining through the vesiculodeferential veins and the inferior vesicle plexus. **Innervation of the seminal vesicles is by the hypogastric nerve (adrenergic and cholinergic) and the pelvic nerve. Lymphatic drainage of the seminal vesicles is through the internal iliac nodes** (Mawhinney and Tarry, 1991).

Congenital Anatomic Anomalies of the Seminal Vesicles

The incidence of unilateral seminal vesicle agenesis is 0.6% to 1%. **Unilateral seminal vesicle agenesis may be associated with ipsilateral renal anomalies and unilateral absence of the vas deferens.** This anomaly is thought to be secondary to an embryologic insult at week 7 of gestation before the separation of the ureteral bud from the mesonephric duct. If this insult occurs after week 7, it is unlikely that renal agenesis would be associated with the seminal vesicle agenesis (Hall and Oates, 1993). It is common to find bilateral absence of the seminal vesicles along with congenital

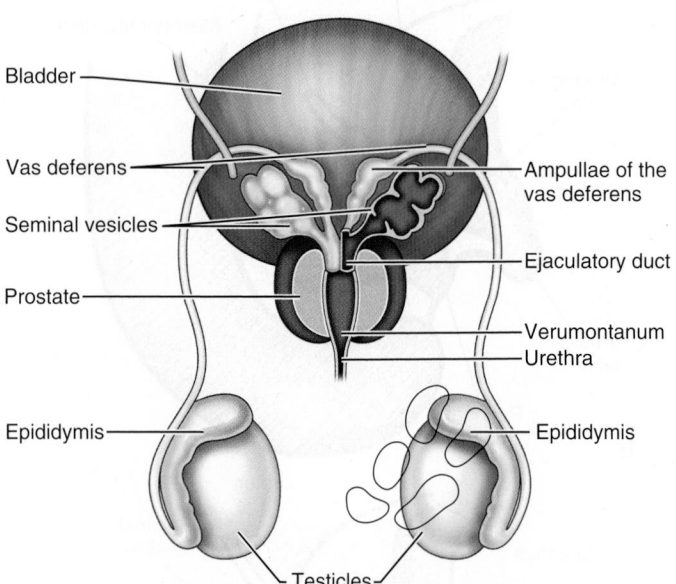

Bladder
Vas deferens
Seminal vesicles
Prostate
Epididymis
Ampullae of the vas deferens
Ejaculatory duct
Verumontanum
Urethra
Epididymis
Testicles

Figure 41-18. Posterior view of seminal vesicle anatomy in relation to the lower genitourinary tract (bivalved areas in dark gray).

bilateral absence of the vas deferens, which is typically associated with a cystic fibrosis transmembrane receptor mutation; 70% to 80% of affected men carry the genetic mutation associated with cystic fibrosis (Anguiano et al, 1994; Chillon et al, 1995). Treatment is necessary only when fertility becomes an issue.

Infectious Processes of the Seminal Vesicles

Infection of the seminal vesicles is seen in underdeveloped countries more frequently than in the United States. The causative agents are *Mycobacterium tuberculosis* and *Schistosoma haematobium*. The diagnosis of bacterial seminal vesiculitis can be made by transrectal or perineal needle aspiration. Surgery is not usually indicated, and culture-specific systemic antibiotics are the treatment of choice (Gutierrez et al, 1994). Very rarely, seminal vesiculectomy is necessary to prevent recurrent bacteremia or to eliminate persistent symptoms (Indudhara et al, 1991). Seminal vesicle abscesses are rare but have been associated with diabetes mellitus, long-term indwelling catheters, and endoscopic instrumentation (Gutierrez et al, 1994). Management of seminal vesicle abscesses is discussed subsequently with management of seminal vesicle cysts. **Infection, obstruction, or the combination of the two can result in formation of calculi in the seminal vesicles.** Patients with seminal vesicle calculi present with hematospermia, perineal pain, painful ejaculation, and infertility. These stones can be managed through an open or laparoscopic vesiculectomy, or the stone can be retrieved endoscopically using a small-caliber ureteroscope (Ozgök et al, 2005; Cuda et al, 2006; Han et al, 2008).

Evaluation of Abnormalities of the Seminal Vesicles

Normal seminal vesicles are not palpable on digital rectal examination. When a seminal vesicle cyst is present, the area immediately above the prostate may be compressible on digital rectal examination. This same area may feel firm or solid when a seminal vesicle tumor is present. **Semen analysis revealing a low seminal volume (<1.0 mL) and a lack of liquefaction and fructose may indicate ejaculatory duct obstruction or the absence of seminal vesicles** (Goldstein and Schlossberg, 1988).

High-resolution transrectal ultrasonography (TRUS) has become the mainstay of imaging for the diagnostic evaluation of seminal vesicle pathology because it is a reliable and inexpensive imaging modality. On TRUS, the seminal vesicles can be found just superior to the prostate, between the bladder and the rectum, and can be well visualized in the anteroposterior and sagittal views. The normal seminal vesicles should appear as flat, elongated, paired structures in the above-described positions (Fig. 41-19). Along

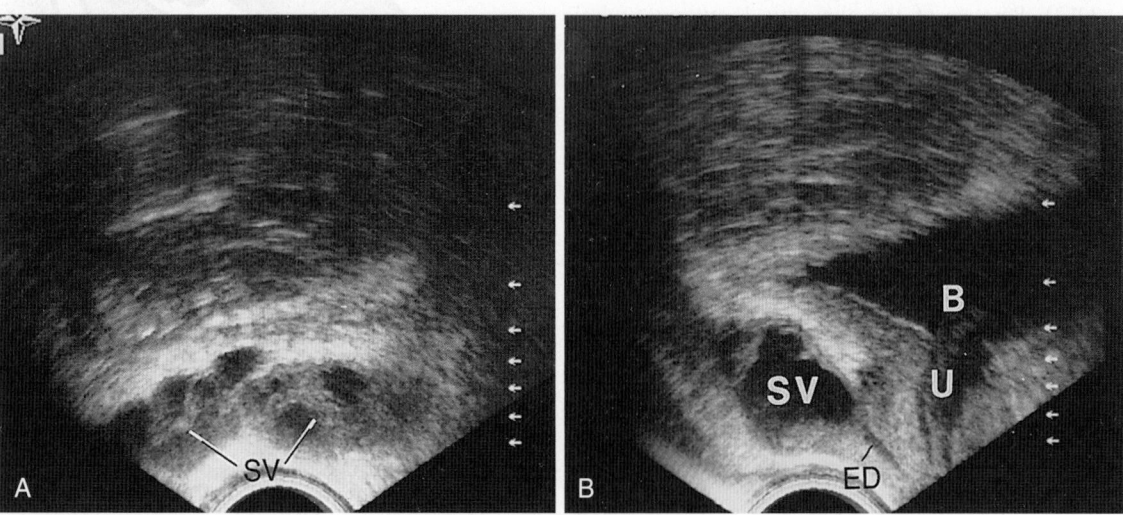

Figure 41-19. Transrectal ultrasound examination of normal seminal vesicles. A, Transverse view. B, Sagittal view. B, bladder; ED, ejaculatory duct; SV, seminal vesicle; U, urethra.

with the seminal vesicles, the ampullae of the vas deferens, the ejaculatory ducts within the prostate, and the verumontanum can be imaged and evaluated by TRUS. Abnormalities such as seminal vesicle obstruction, aplasia, atrophy, and cyst formation can be identified by TRUS (Carter et al, 1989).

Seminal vesicle obstruction may result in seminal vesicle dilation that can be identified on TRUS with the following characteristics: anteroposterior diameter of greater than 15 mm, length greater than 35 mm, and large anechoic areas that contain sperm when aspirated (Jarow, 1996; Colpi et al, 1997). Asymptomatic cystic dilation of the seminal vesicle was incidentally found in 5% of men undergoing TRUS for prostate cancer screening (Wessels et al, 1992).

Hyperechoic solid masses in the seminal vesicles (isoechoic to the prostate) revealed on TRUS are concerning for tumor. If there is a unilateral solid mass in the seminal vesicle, it is more likely to be a primary tumor, whereas if it is present in bilateral seminal vesicles, it is more likely to be a secondary tumor from a primary prostate, rectal, or bladder malignancy. TRUS-guided biopsy or aspiration is necessary to assist in the diagnosis.

Computed tomography (CT) also has been used to evaluate the seminal vesicles. **The normal appearance of the seminal vesicles on CT scan is that of paired structures just below the bladder with medium contrast similar to muscle** (Goldstein and Schlossberg, 1988). A seminal vesicle cyst appears on CT scan as a well-defined retrovesicular fluid density with the attenuation of water, from 0 to 10 Hounsfield units, cephalad to the prostate gland (Fig. 41-20). CT accurately images seminal vesicle anomalies and is a good modality for imaging of the ipsilateral kidney concomitantly (Arora et al, 2007).

In cases of primary seminal vesicle malignancy, CT scan may be useful to characterize the lesion further before intervention. A tumor within the seminal vesicle on CT scan has a higher attenuation than the normal seminal vesicle, but the tumor may appear cystic secondary to tumor necrosis (King et al, 1989). It is impossible to differentiate malignant tumors from benign tumors on CT scan alone, although secondary tumors from the bladder, rectum, or prostate may have a more contiguous appearance (Sussman et al, 1986). The CT findings of a leiomyosarcoma of the seminal vesicle are described as an irregular mass, resulting in enlargement of the seminal vesicle with displacement of the prostate gland (Upreti et al, 2003). CT as well as MRI allows metastatic evaluation when seminal vesicle neoplasms are characterized further (Dahms et al, 1999).

MRI demonstrates more anatomic detail than CT and is an extremely useful imaging modality for the seminal vesicles. On T2-weighted images, the ampulla of the vas deferens is visible approximately 71% of the time and exhibits low signal intensity. The seminal vesicles exhibit high signal intensity 79% of the time, low signal intensity 19% of the time, and a heterogeneous signal intensity 2% of the time on T2-weighted images (Roy et al, 1993). On T2-weighted images, the seminal vesicles generally have similar or higher intensity than fat in patients younger than 70 years old and typically have signal intensity lower than that of fat in patients older than 70. The convolutions of the seminal vesicles can be seen on T1-weighted imaging with contrast material (Fig. 41-21) (Secaf et al, 1991).

On MRI, seminal vesicle agenesis is best exemplified on T1-weighted axial images (Fig. 41-22). Care must be taken not to mistake the vesicoprostatic venous plexus for small glands. Arteriovenous malformations appear as large ectatic vessels adjacent to the lateral edge of the seminal vesicle. After androgen ablation, seminal vesicles demonstrate low signal intensity on T2-weighted images and appear small in size (Secaf et al, 1991). After pelvic radiation, seminal vesicles appear to be decreased in size in one third of patients. In patients after pelvic radiation, 63% of seminal vesicles had a normal MRI appearance, 21% had normal signal intensity but had fewer tubules, 8% had diffuse loss of signal intensity appearing hypointense to fat, and 8% were hypointense to fat on T2-weighted images (Chan and Kressel, 1991). A seminal vesicle cyst may have variable signal intensities on T1-weighted images but typically

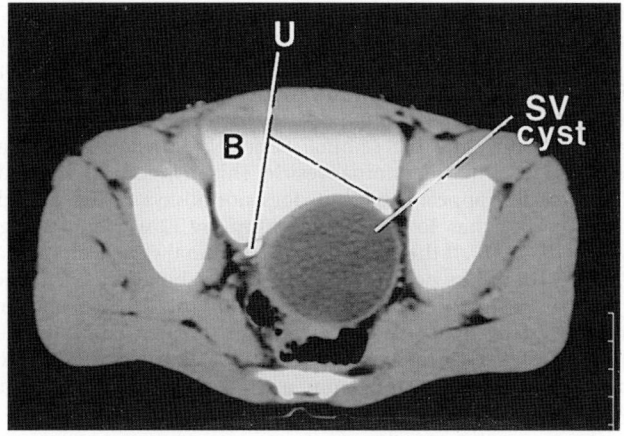

Figure 41-20. Computed tomography scan of seminal vesicle (SV) cyst. B, bladder; U, ureters.

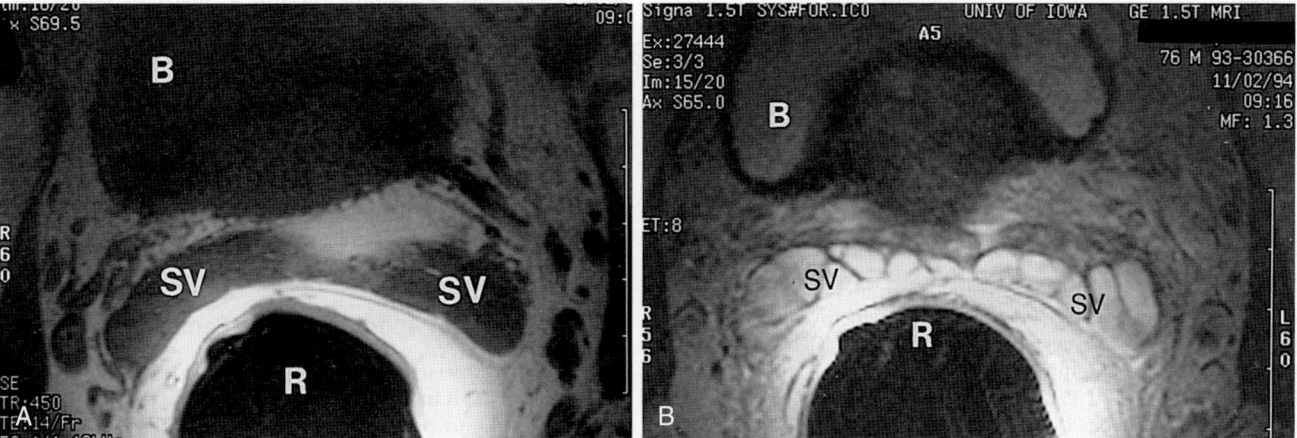

Figure 41-21. **Transaxial magnetic resonance imaging of normal seminal vesicles (SV) with endorectal coli. A, T1-weighted image. B, T2-weighted image. B, bladder; R, rectum.**

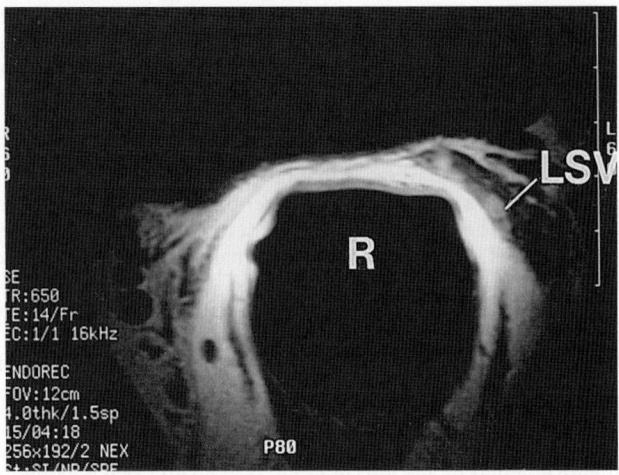

Figure 41-22. Transaxial T1-weighted endorectal magnetic resonance image of absent right seminal vesicle. LSV, left seminal vesicle; R, rectum.

demonstrates fluid signal intensities on T2-weighted images and does not enhance with administration of intravenous gadolinium. Increased T1-weighted intensity represents increased proteinaceous concentration within the cyst or hemorrhage (Arora et al, 2007). Hemorrhagic seminal vesicle cysts have high signal intensity on T1-weighted and T2-weighted images (Sue et al, 1989). A benign primary mass of the seminal vesicle appears as a sharply marginated mass arising from the seminal vesicle. The most common form of malignancy affecting the seminal vesicle is invasion of prostate cancer directly into the seminal vesicle. This invasion can make the seminal vesicle appear large but does not always do so, and the seminal vesicle has low signal intensity on T2-weighted images (Secaf et al, 1991). **If there is a palpable seminal vesicle abnormality, TRUS should be performed, and biopsy should be performed if there is suspicion for malignancy. MRI of the prostate and seminal vesicles may provide significantly greater detail in determination of the difference between a primary seminal vesicle mass and local extension from a prostate, bladder, or rectal malignancy.**

Surgical Approaches to the Seminal Vesicles

The surgical approach to the seminal vesicles depends mainly on the expertise and comfort of the surgeon, although the characteristics of the lesion may have an impact on the decision regarding the approach. The robotic-assisted laparoscopic approach is increasingly being used for the rare seminal vesicle lesion requiring excision.

Preoperative preparation for seminal vesicle surgery should include a bowel preparation the evening before surgery, in case of the uncommon occurrence of a bowel injury; GoLYTELY is recommended. A prophylactic systemic antibiotic is administered preoperatively, and two doses are given postoperatively. The use of intermittent compression stockings to prevent deep vein thrombosis during surgery is recommended.

Anterior Surgical Approaches to the Seminal Vesicles

The anterior surgical approach to the seminal vesicles has been well established and is a good open approach for patients with large benign masses or cysts and for patients with an ectopic ureter draining into a seminal vesicle cyst, so the kidney, ureter, and seminal vesicle all can be approached concomitantly. The transvesical approach has been well described (Walker and Bowles, 1968; Politano et al, 1975). A lower midline infraumbilical incision is made sharply, and the rectus muscles are divided in the midline. The space of Retzius is developed. The anterior bladder is exposed,

and a self-retaining retractor is placed. A longitudinal incision about 7 to 10 cm long is made in the anterior bladder wall, taking care to stay at least 3 to 4 cm proximal to the bladder neck. Moist sponges are placed in the bladder dome, and a bladder blade for the retractor is used to offer exposure gently. The ureteral orifices should be identified, and 8-Fr feeding tubes can be passed gently up the ureters to help with identification of the intramural ureters. A 5-cm longitudinal incision is made in the midline of the trigone with electrocautery on cutting current. When the incision goes through the posterior bladder muscle, the ampullae of the vas deferens should be visible just below the bladder neck. The seminal vesicles should be identified just lateral to the ampullae of the vas deferens on the prostatic base. The seminal vesicles should be dissected completely free. The seminal vesicle is resected and removed. Care must be taken not to dissect too deep through Denonvilliers fascia posteriorly so as not to endanger the rectum. The posterior bladder wall is closed in two layers with 2-0 absorbable suture in the muscle and 4-0 absorbable suture in the mucosa. After closure of the bladder wall, a suction drain is placed in the perivesical space, not overlying the suture line, and is brought out through a separate stab incision (Fig. 41-23). This approach has a lower rectal injury rate, although it places the ureters at a higher risk for injury and is more prone to blood loss.

The perivesical approach is useful in pediatric patients with a large seminal vesicle cyst so that nephroureterectomy can be performed along with seminal vesiculectomy. A midline or Pfannenstiel incision offers adequate exposure for this approach. Finger dissection is used to dissect the bladder from the lateral pelvic sidewall on the side with the cyst. The seminal vesicle cyst should be readily identifiable, the seminal vesicle should be dissected free in its entirety, and a 1-0 chromic suture can be placed through the cyst as a traction suture to assist with dissection. The ureter must be identified crossing the vas deferens to prevent ureteral injury. The superior, and possibly the inferior, vesicle arteries may be sacrificed to offer exposure to the base of the seminal vesicle. The cyst should be dissected away from the bladder, and any seminal vesicle vessels can be clipped and divided. When the base of the seminal vesicle is accessed at the prostate–seminal vesicle junction, it can be ligated with 2-0 absorbable suture. Dissection of the proximal portion of the seminal vesicle must be done carefully by hugging the cyst so as not to injure the neurovascular bundle, which is directly lateral to the seminal vesicle. A clip is placed just distal to the previously placed suture, and the seminal vesicle is resected. A suction drain is placed adjacent to the seminal vesicle bed and is brought out through a separate stab incision. The drain and urethral catheter may be removed in 24 hours as long as there is not excessive drainage through the drain.

A third anterior approach to the seminal vesicles that can be performed in an open or laparoscopic manner is the retrovesical approach; this is useful for bilateral seminal vesiculectomies for bilateral small cysts or benign masses (de Assis, 1952). A urethral catheter is placed, a midline incision is made or standard pelvic ports are placed, and the peritoneum is entered. A transverse incision is made in the peritoneal reflection over the rectum at the posterior bladder wall, taking great care not to enter the rectum. The posterior bladder is sharply dissected off the anterior rectal wall until the ampullae of the vas deferens and the tips of the seminal vesicles are visible. The seminal vesicles are dissected free to the base at the prostate–seminal vesicle junctions and are ligated and resected. A suction drain is placed at the posterior bladder and brought out through a separate stab incision. The incision is closed (Fig. 41-24).

Posterior Surgical Approach to the Seminal Vesicles

Although the transcoccygeal approach is the least familiar to most urologists, it may be useful for patients who have had previous suprapubic or perineal surgeries. The patient is positioned in a prone, jackknife position (Kreager and Jordan, 1965). An L-shaped hockey-stick incision is made from midway on the sacrum, 10 cm from the tip of the coccyx, and angled at the tip of the coccyx down

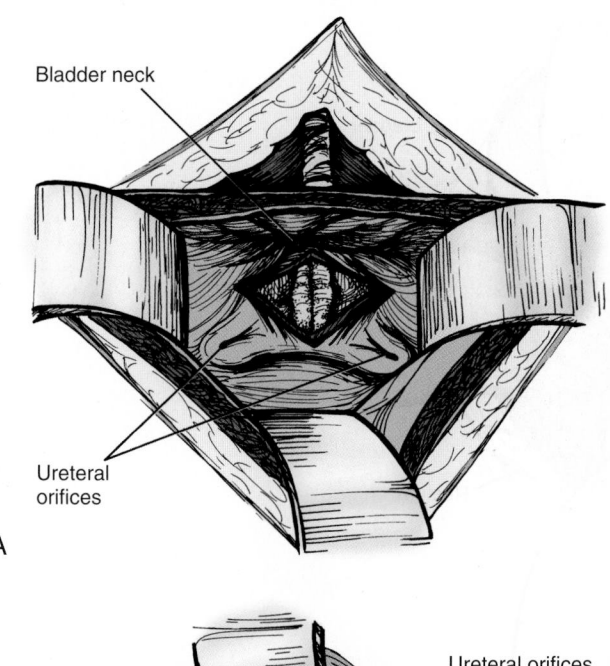

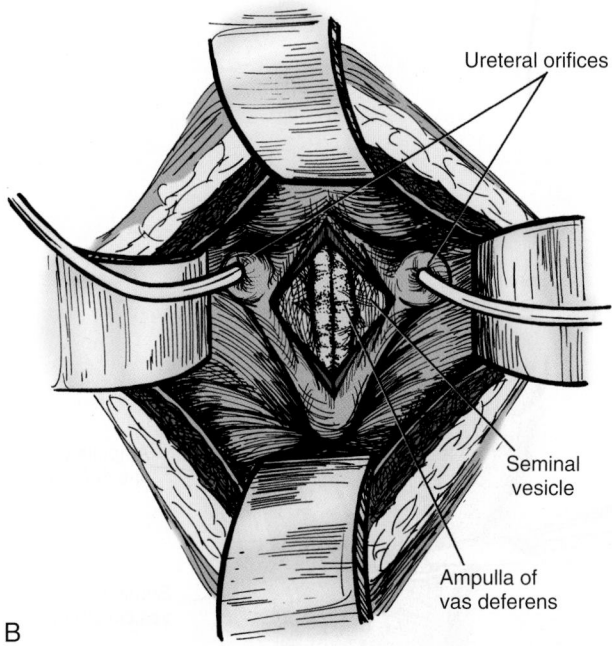

Figure 41-23. **Transvesical approach to seminal vesiculectomy. A, Vertical incision between the ureteral orifices. B, Transverse incision 2 cm superior to the bladder neck below the ureteral orifices. (Redrawn from Hinman F Jr. Atlas of urologic surgery. Philadelphia: Saunders; 1989.)**

Laparoscopic and Robotic-Assisted Surgical Approach to the Seminal Vesicles

Laparoscopic surgery on the seminal vesicles is most commonly performed concomitantly with prostate surgery. The technique for the laparoscopic approach to the seminal vesicles was first described in 1993 (Kavoussi et al, 1993). Laparoscopy also has been applied to seminal vesiculectomy without prostatectomy and has been reported in a case of amyloidosis of the seminal vesicle (Vandwalle et al, 2007). Robotic-assisted laparoscopy also has been used to excise seminal vesicle cysts (Moore et al, 2007; Selli et al, 2008). Patients are positioned in the supine position with careful padding of all pressure points, and the arms are tucked and padded. A split-leg table is necessary for the robotic-assisted technique. Wide cloth tape is applied across the chest and hips to secure the patient to the table, and the table is placed in steep Trendelenburg position. Before gaining access, a urethral catheter and an orogastric tube should be placed to decompress the bladder and stomach for subsequent trochar placement. To gain access, a Veress needle is placed periumbilically, and a pneumoperitoneum is achieved, not exceeding pressures of 15 mm Hg. After an adequate pneumoperitoneum is achieved, the laparoscopic ports can be placed, placing the first one with an optical trocar for the camera port and the following ones under direct laparoscopic visualization. The ports can be placed in either a horseshoe or a diamond arrangement for pure laparoscopy and can be placed in the same position as would be used for prostatectomy for robotic assistance (Fig. 41-26) (Menon et al, 2003; Lee et al, 2004). The peritoneum is incised between the two obliterated umbilical ligaments just anterior to the rectum in the pouch of Douglas. The seminal vesicles can be visualized and should be dissected carefully to avoid injury to the neurovascular bundles or the surrounding viscera. Monopolar energy should not be used to minimize injury to surrounding structures, and much of this dissection can safely be performed sharply. The seminal vesicle arterial pedicle can be managed with a clip or with bipolar cautery. The seminal vesicle should be dissected toward its junction with the ampulla of the vas deferens, and both can be clipped together at the base. The specimen can be placed in an extraction bag and can be removed through one of the laparoscopic ports. The ports are closed under visualization.

The extraperitoneal laparoscopic approach to the seminal vesicles was first described in 1997 and was performed concomitantly with radical prostatectomy (Raboy et al, 1997). In the following years, this approach gained more popularity (Bollens et al, 2001; Stolzenburg et al, 2003). A 1.5-cm periumbilical incision is made, and the preperitoneal space is entered. A balloon trocar is introduced into the preperitoneal space, and insufflation is performed under direct vision. The details of the technique are described further in Chapter 115.

Surgical Treatment of Seminal Vesicle Cysts

Seminal vesicle cysts are thought to be secondary to ejaculatory duct obstruction and can be congenital or acquired (Heaney et al, 1987; King et al, 1991; Conn et al, 1992). **Seminal vesicle cysts are associated with ipsilateral renal agenesis or dysplasia in two thirds of patients; the cysts are secondary to maldevelopment of the distal mesonephric duct and are an error in ureteral budding** (Beeby, 1974). Seminal vesicle cysts also have been associated with polycystic kidney disease. In one report, seminal vesicle cysts were identified in 60% of patients with polycystic kidney disease, and some authors recommend that all patients with seminal vesicle cysts undergo renal imaging (Alpern et al, 1991; Hihara et al, 1993; Danaci et al, 1998). **Seminal vesicle cysts should be treated only if they are symptomatic or result in ejaculatory duct obstruction and affect fertility** (Surya et al, 1988).

Seminal vesicle cysts can be drained by many techniques. **TRUS-guided aspiration or transperineal aspiration can be performed on small seminal vesicle cysts that are symptomatic or obstructing the ejaculatory ducts.** If the cyst reaccumulates fluid, resulting in recurrent symptoms or obstruction, it may be aspirated again

the gluteal cleft stopping 3 cm from the anus. The lateral side of the coccyx is carefully divided free from the rectum and removed. The layers of the gluteus maximus are swept aside until the rectosigmoid is reached, and then it is carefully dissected from the underside of the sacrum. The lateral rectal wall is divided free medially from the levator ani muscle until the prostate is encountered on the side of the seminal vesicle pathology. Dissection is carried superior to the base of the prostate in the midline until the ampulla of the vas deferens is identified with the seminal vesicle just lateral to the ampulla. The seminal vesicle should be dissected and resected as previously described. A Penrose drain should be placed at the bed of the seminal vesicle and brought out through a separate stab incision from the closure. The drain can be removed in 2 to 3 days if there is no drainage (Fig. 41-25).

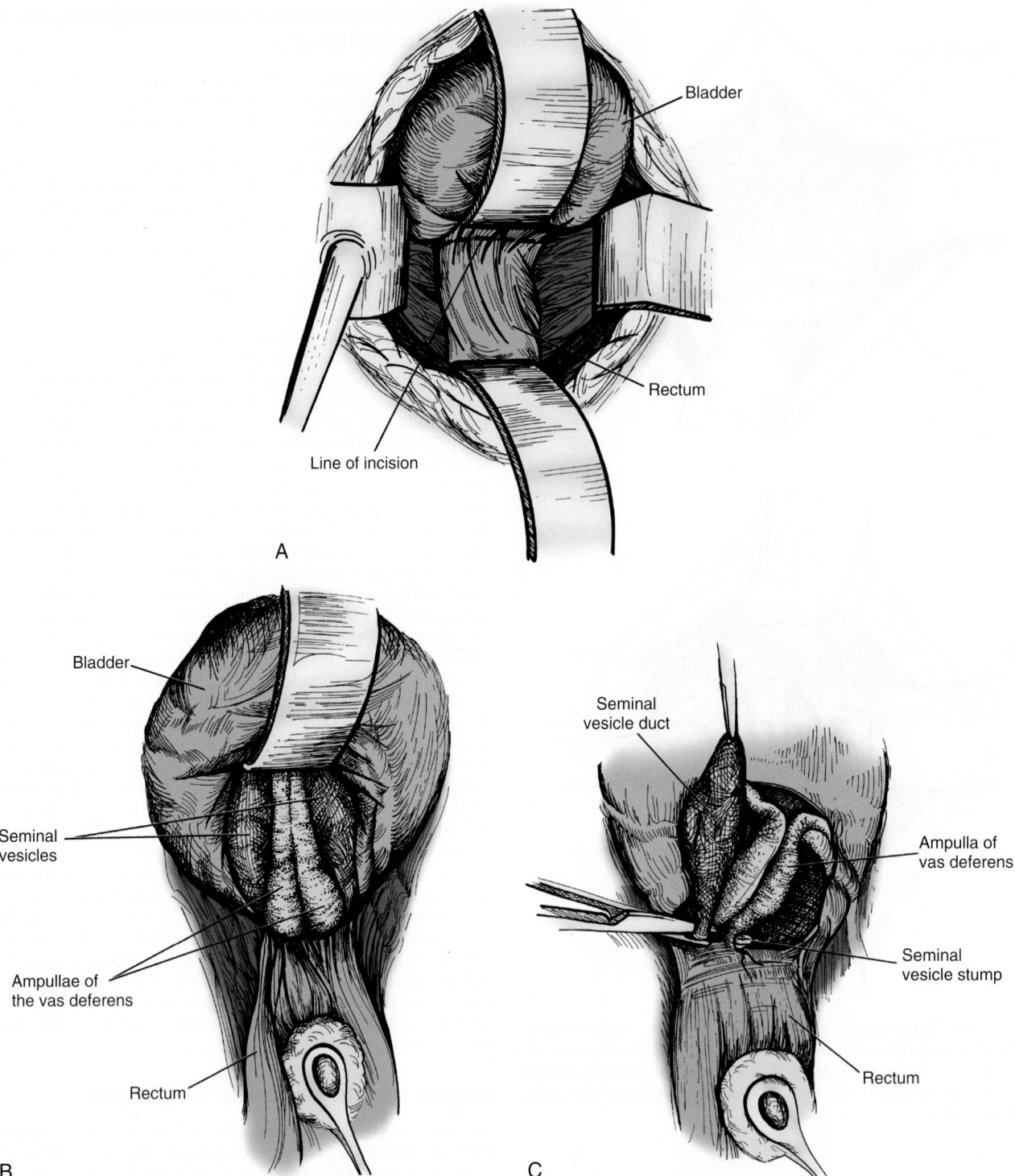

Bladder

Rectum

Line of incision

A

Bladder

Seminal
vesicles

Ampullae of
the vas deferens

Rectum

B

Seminal
vesicle duct

Ampulla of
vas deferens

Seminal
vesicle stump

Rectum

C

Figure 41-24. Retrovesical approach to seminal vesiculectomy. **A,** Incision line between base of bladder and peritoneal reflection over the rectum. **B,** Caudal dissection reveals the ampullae of the vas deferens on the midline and seminal vesicles immediately lateral to them. **C,** The duct of the seminal vesicle is ligated and transected. (Redrawn from Hinman F Jr. Atlas of urologic surgery. Philadelphia: Saunders; 1989.)

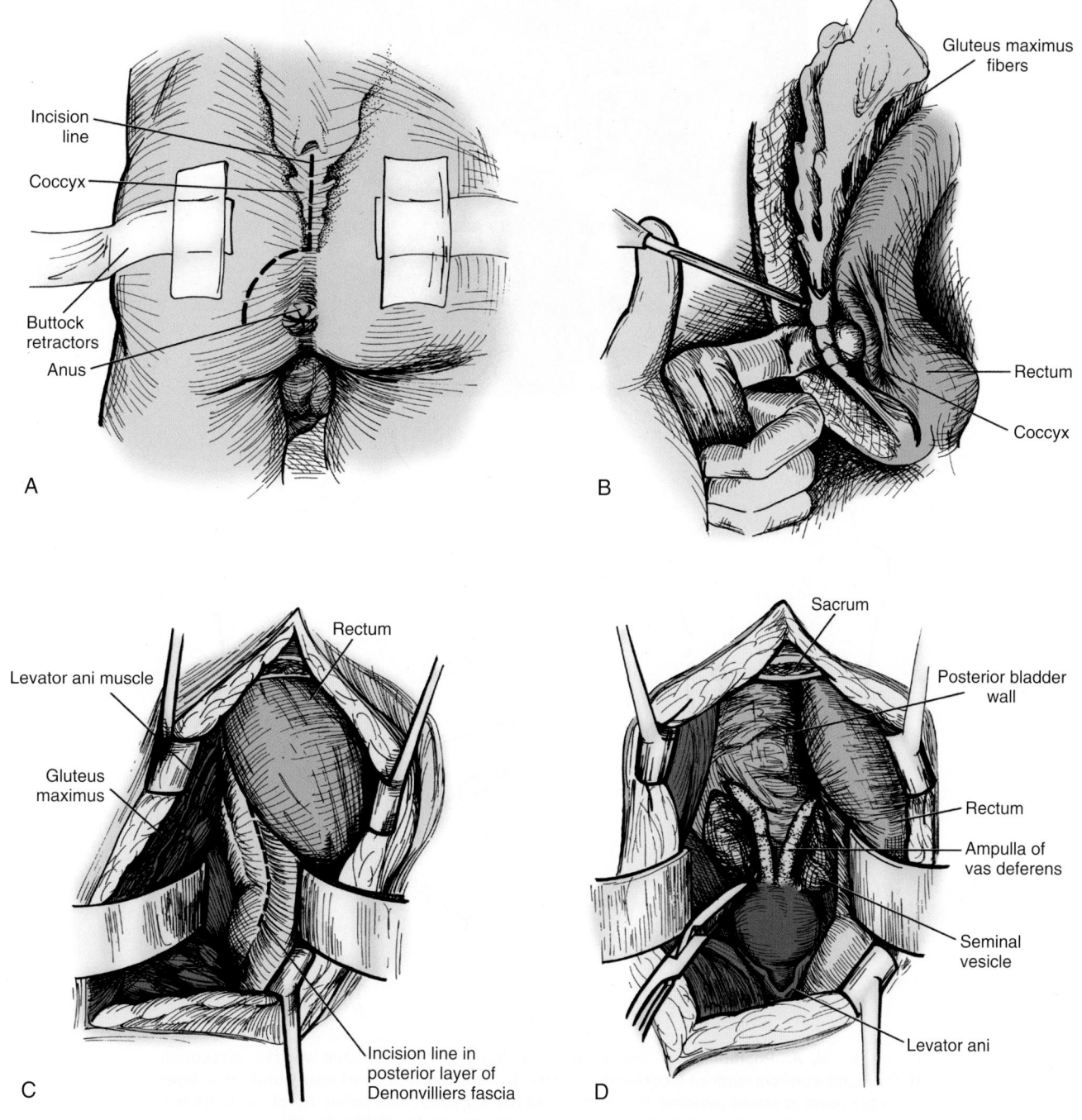

Figure 41-25. **Transcoccygeal seminal vesiculectomy. A, Incision line over the lower sacrum on coccyx surrounding the anus. B, Dissection of the coccyx. C, Incision of Denonvilliers fascia after the rectum has been displaced. D, Exposure of the prostate and seminal vesicles. (Redrawn from Hinman F Jr. Atlas of urologic surgery. Philadelphia: Saunders; 1989.)**

with the injection of a sclerosing agent such as tetracycline. A small abscess in the seminal vesicle can be managed similarly with drainage (Frye and Loughlin, 1988; Shabsigh et al, 1989; Gutierrez et al, 1994). If the seminal vesicle cyst is proximal, adjacent to the prostate, transurethral resection can be performed to unroof the cyst at the 5 o'clock and 7 o'clock positions just distal to the bladder neck (Frye and Loughlin, 1988; de Lichtenberg and Hvidt, 1989). The same outcome has been reported by incising the seminal vesicle cyst to drain it cystoscopically with the use of a Collings knife (Gonzalez and Dalton, 1998). Seminal vesicle abscesses can be managed in a similar fashion. Some groups reported using semirigid ureteroscopes to treat seminal vesicle cysts and abscesses (Razvi and Denstedt, 1995; Shimada and Yoshida, 1996; Okubo et al, 1998). If the

above-described techniques for drainage of seminal vesicle cysts are unsuccessful, open or laparoscopic excision can be performed (Moudouni et al, 2006). Seminal vesiculectomy along with nephroureterectomy should be performed in cases with an ectopic ureter. If these techniques for seminal vesicle abscess fail, open drainage is required (Kore et al, 1994).

Surgical Treatment of Tumors of the Seminal Vesicles

Benign tumors of the seminal vesicle that occur more commonly than malignant tumors include fibromas, leiomyomas, cystadenomas, schwannomas, and papillary adenomas (Mostofi and Price, 1973; Lundhus et al, 1984; Narayana, 1985; Mazur et al,

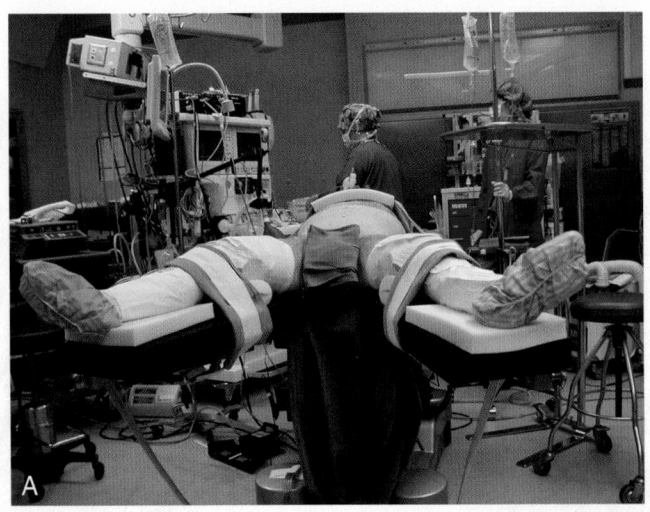

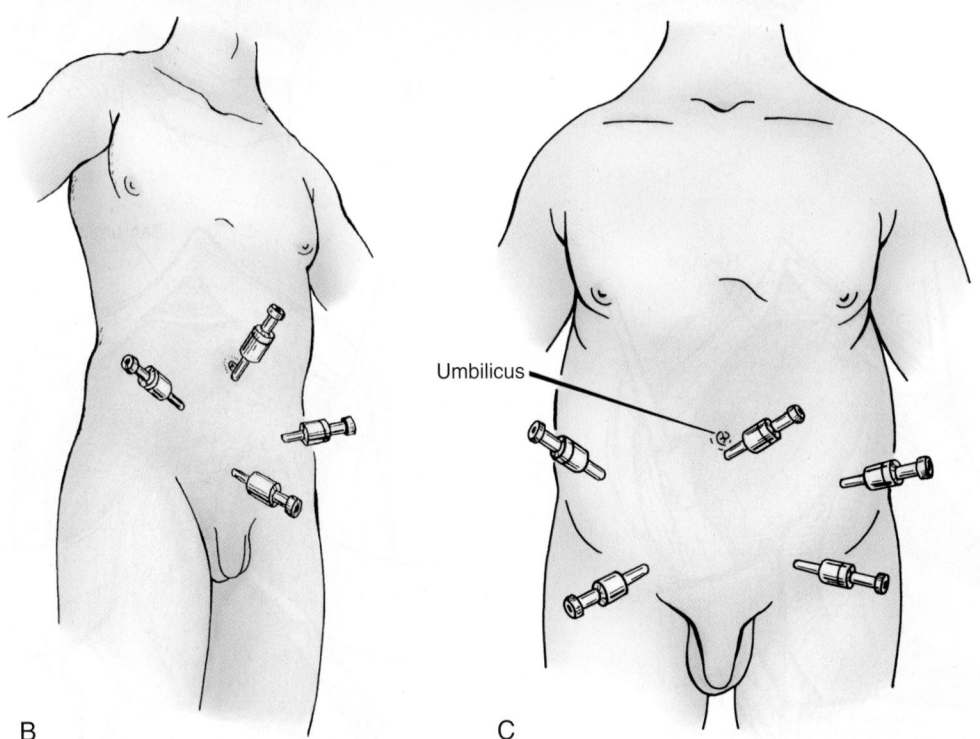

Umbilicus

Figure 41-26. A, Positioning of the patient for laparoscopic seminal vesicle dissection. **B,** Diamond configuration of laparoscopic ports. **C,** Inverted U-shaped configuration of laparoscopic ports in obese patients. (From Winifield HN. Laparoscopic pelvic lymph node dissection for urological pelvic malignancies. Atlas Urol Clin North Am 1993;1:33–47.)

1987; Bullock, 1988; Gentile et al, 1994; Latchamsetty et al, 2002; Lee et al, 2006). Primary papillary adenomas and cystadenomas of the seminal vesicle typically occur in middle-aged men and are almost never bilateral, and they appear as simple cysts on imaging; the diagnosis is typically made on final pathology after excision (Mazur et al, 1987). Amyloid localized to the seminal vesicles also has been reported (Jun et al, 2003). Of men older than age 76 years, 20% have subepithelial deposits of amyloid in the seminal vesicles, and the reported incidence in male autopsies is 4% to 17% (Pitkanen et al, 1983; Ramchandani et al, 1993). Patients should be treated only if they are symptomatic and the diagnosis of amyloid of the seminal vesicle is made. Hydatid cysts of the seminal vesicle also have been reported (Kuyumcuoglu et al, 1991; Papathanasiou et al, 2006).

Seminal vesicle malignancies are extremely rare and are difficult to diagnose because patients are typically asymptomatic until late in the course of the disease process. Primary malignancies of the seminal vesicles are extremely rare, and serum prostate-specific antigen and tissue biopsy can help differentiate primary malignancies from extension or metastasis of lymphoma, prostate, bladder, or rectal cancer. The low proliferative activity of the seminal vesicles is thought to account for the low incidence of primary malignancies of the seminal vesicle (Meyer et al, 1982). **Primary adenocarcinoma of the seminal vesicle occurs in patients older than 50 years.** Serum prostate-specific antigen is normal, and serum carcinoembryonic antigen is elevated (Mostofi and Price, 1973; Benson et al, 1984; Tanaka et al, 1987; Chinoy and Kulkarni, 1993; Thiel and Effert, 2002). **Primary sarcoma of the seminal vesicle is an extremely rare malignancy, which is usually discovered late in the disease process and is diagnosed by biopsy** (Benson et al, 1984; Chiou et al, 1985; Schned et al, 1986; Tanaka et al, 1987; Davis et al, 1988; Kawahara et al, 1988). All sarcoma types of the seminal vesicle, including leiomyosarcoma, rhabdo-myosarcoma, angiosarcoma, and müllerian adenosarcoma-like tumor, behave very aggressively, and radical extirpation has varying outcomes (Lamont et al, 1991; Laurila et al, 1992; Amirkhan et al, 1994; Berger et al, 2002). Cystosarcoma phylloides and seminoma also have been reported as primary malignancies of the seminal vesicles (Adachi et al, 1991; Fain et al, 1993). Primary squamous cell carcinoma of the seminal vesicle has been reported and treated with surgical extirpation followed by adjuvant radiation therapy with success with short-term follow-up (Tabata et al, 2002).

Solid seminal vesicle masses that are benign on biopsy and show no evidence of local spread should be treated with seminal vesiculectomy only if they are symptomatic, which is a very rare occurrence. Solid masses of the seminal vesicles that are proven to be malignant by biopsy or with a high suspicion for malignancy should be surgically treated, although the optimal treatment is still debated because there have been so few primary seminal vesicle malignancies treated at any institution. Large primary malignancies of the seminal vesicles have been treated with radical pelvic surgery: cystoprostatectomy with pelvic lymphadenectomy or pelvic exenteration. Adjuvant therapy has not proven to be effective, although the only survivors in the literature underwent radical surgery followed by pelvic radiation and/or androgen ablation.

Complications of Seminal Vesicle Surgery

Complications of seminal vesicle surgery are minimized by the surgeon selecting the approach that he or she is most comfortable and facile performing. The surgeon must be aware of the following complications that are specific to seminal vesiculectomy. Rectal or bladder injury may occur with any surgery on the seminal vesicle. If a preoperative bowel preparation was administered, and there is no gross fecal contamination, a two-layer closure of the rectum may be performed closing the mucosal layer with a running 3-0 absorbable suture and the submucosal layer with interrupted 4-0 silk sutures. The anus also should be dilated before the end of the case. A temporary colostomy should be considered with a large rectal injury or gross fecal contamination. The bladder should be closed in two layers, leaving a urethral catheter in place for 7 to 10 days postoperatively.

Complications of the laparoscopic approach include general laparoscopic complications, such as trocar injury to the bowel or great vessels, extraperitoneal insufflation, abdominal wall bleeding, and gas embolism. Bladder and rectal injuries may be repaired laparoscopically as long as there is not gross fecal contamination with rectal injuries. The distal ureter is close to the tip of the seminal vesicle, and if the ureter is injured, it may be repaired laparoscopically, although a ureteral replant may be necessary and performed open or laparoscopically, depending on the experience of the surgeon. It is recommended that a ureteral stent and a pelvic drain be left in such cases. The neurovascular bundle runs just lateral to the tips of the seminal vesicles; injury to the neurovascular bundle can result in erectile dysfunction, regardless of the surgical approach. Potential complications of endoscopic management of the seminal vesicles include postvoid dribbling secondary to urinary reflux and infection (Goluboff et al, 1995).

MANAGEMENT OF NONPALPABLE TESTICULAR LESIONS

Data in the literature regarding the management of incidentally found testicular lesions are limited. A testicular lesion is defined as incidental when it is asymptomatic and nonpalpable and in the presence of negative tumor markers (Carmignani et al, 2003). With the increased use and availability of ultrasonography, there has been an increase in detection of these lesions; however, the overall incidence of asymptomatic, incidental testicular lesions found with scrotal ultrasonography is low. In a large series of 3000 men who underwent scrotal ultrasonography for indications of scrotal pain,

---

> **KEY POINTS: SURGERY OF THE SEMINAL VESICLES**
>
> - Seminal vesicle secretions contribute 50% to 80% of the volume of the ejaculate.
> - Unilateral seminal vesicle agenesis may be associated with ipsilateral renal anomalies and unilateral absence of the vas deferens.
> - Normal seminal vesicles are not palpable on digital rectal examination.
> - If there is a palpable seminal vesicle abnormality, TRUS and MRI should be performed, and biopsy should be performed if there is suspicion for malignancy.
> - The surgical approach to the seminal vesicles depends mainly on the expertise and comfort of the surgeon, although the characteristics of the lesion may affect the decision regarding the approach.
> - Benign and malignant tumors of the seminal vesicles are very rare.

---

flank pain, neck mass, and retroperitoneal mass, 15 (0.5%) were discovered to have incidental testicular lesions (Comiter et al, 1995). Another large series of 1300 scrotal ultrasound scans found 27 (2%) incidental testicular lesions (Carmignani et al, 2003).

Previous studies showed an increased incidence of testicular malignancies in infertile men (Jacobsen et al, 2000). Other risk factors for the presence of malignancy include palpable testicular lesions, history of cryptorchidism, testicular atrophy, and contralateral germ cell tumor. Histologically benign lesions are more common than malignant lesions for incidentally discovered nonpalpable testicular lesions (Sheynkin et al, 2004).

Some advocate for early surgical intervention for nonpalpable testicular masses (Müller et al, 2006) with 20% of these lesions being malignant. The testicle is delivered through an inguinal incision, and the lesion is localized using intraoperative ultrasonography (Horstman et al, 1994). Hopps and Goldstein expanded on this technique by using ultrasound-guided needle localization and microsurgical exploration to assist in tumor identification (Hopps and Goldstein, 2002).

Other authors support a more conservative approach. Eifler and colleagues (2008) reported that only 6% of incidentally found testicular lesions less than 1 cm were malignant based on tissue diagnosis. These authors stated that intratesticular, hypoechoic lesions less than 5 mm in patients with negative markers are likely benign and can be followed with serial imaging. Connolly and associates (2006) identified a highly select group of patients with incidental testicular lesions less than 1 cm to follow with serial ultrasound scans. In eight patients who met criteria, only one lesion (13%) progressed on serial imaging and was a seminoma. These authors concluded that although most patients with small lesions require surgical exploration, carefully selected patients who are highly compliant can be managed safely with serial imaging. The pathologic findings from these studies are summarized in Table 41-2.

Although these lesions are rare, they present a management dilemma for urologists. In this setting, the clinician must decide whether to pursue a more aggressive approach such as inguinal orchiectomy, inguinal exploration, and excision with frozen section or a more conservative, nonoperative approach with surveillance with serial ultrasound scans. A treatment algorithm for management of nonpalpable intratesticular lesions is shown in Fig. 41-27. Malignancy should be considered when any of the following are present: mass greater than 1 cm, severe oligospermia or azoospermia, atrophy, history of cryptorchidism, prior testicular malignancy, or elevated tumor markers. If the patient is at low risk for malignancy, it is reasonable to follow the patient with serial ultrasound scans. Patients must understand that changes in size or architecture of the lesion require surgical exploration.

TABLE 41-2 Summary of Pathologic Findings from Nonpalpable Intratesticular Lesions

INSTITUTION AND REFERENCE	NO. BENIGN	NO. MALIGNANT	NO. WITHOUT TISSUE DIAGNOSIS	TOTAL NUMBER
Mt. Sinai Hospital (Buckspan et al, 1989)	4	0	0	4
Walson Army Hospital (Corrie et al, 1991)	3	0	2	5
Naval Medical Center (Horstman et al, 1994)	7	2	0	9
Brigham and Women's Hospital (Comiter et al, 1995)	2	13	0	15
Weill-Cornell (Hopps and Goldstein, 2002)	2	2	0	4
University of Milan (Carmignani et al, 2003)	10	0	0	10
SUNY Stonybrook (Sheynkin et al, 2004)	6	2	1	9
Rabin Medical Center (Tal et al, 2004)	3	6	2	11
Southern Illinois (Powell and Tarter, 2006)	2	2	0	4
Weill-Cornell (Eifler et al, 2008)	19	1	0	20
Total No. (%)	58 (64)	28 (31)	5 (5)	91

From Mammen T, Costabile RA. Management of incidentally discovered non-palpable testicular lesions. AUA Update Series 2009;28:14–9.

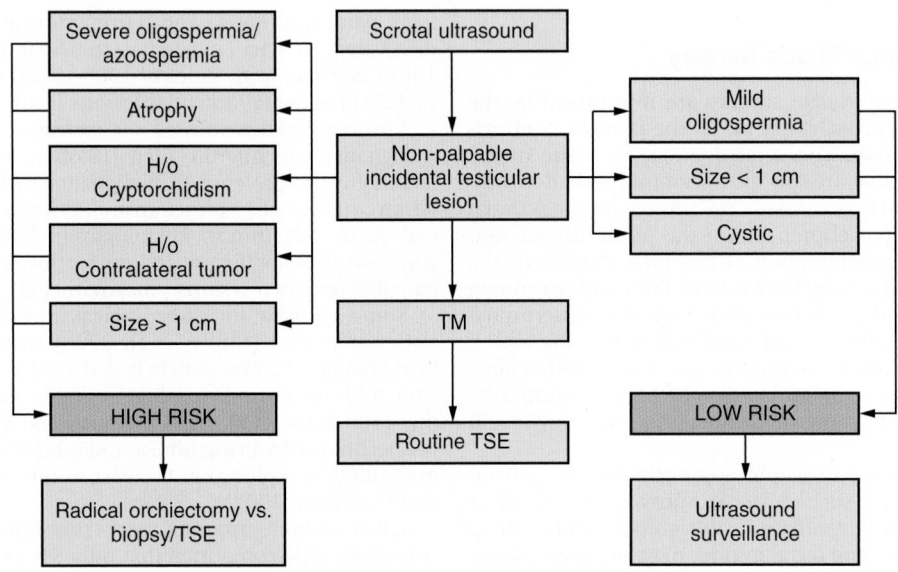

Figure 41-27. **Treatment algorithm for nonpalpable testicular lesions. H/o, history of; TM, testicular microlithiasis; TSE, testis-sparing excision. (Modified from Mammen T, Costabile RA. Management of incidentally discovered non-palpable testicular lesions. AUA Update Series 2009;28:14–9.)**

REFERENCES

The complete reference list is available online at www.expertconsult.com.

SUGGESTED READINGS

Brewster SF. The development and differentiation of human seminal vesicles. J Anat 1985;143:45–55.

Carter SS, Shinohara K, Lipshultz LI. Transrectal ultrasonography in disorders of the seminal vesicles and ejaculatory ducts. Urol Clin North Am 1989;16:773–90.

Corcoran AT, Smaldone MC, Gibbons EP, et al. Validation of the Fournier's gangrene severity index in a large contemporary series. J Urol 2008;180(3):944–8.

Davis BE, Noble MJ, Weigel JW, et al. Analysis and management of chronic testicular pain. J Urol 1990;143:936–9.

Goldstein M, Schlossberg S. Men with congenital absence of the vas deferens often have seminal vesicles. J Urol 1988;140(1):85–6.

Holt SK, Salinas CA, Stanford JL. Vasectomy and the risk of prostate cancer. J Urol 2008;180(6):2565–7, discussion 2567–8.

Kavoussi LR, Schuessler WW, Vancaillie TG, et al. Laparoscopic approach to the seminal vesicles. J Urol 1993;150:417–9.

Kiddoo DA, Wollin TA, Mador DR. A population based assessment of complications following outpatient hydrocelectomy and spermatocelectomy. J Urol 2004;171(2 Pt. 1):746–8.

Mittemeyer BT, Lennox KW, Borski AA. Epididymitis: a review of 610 cases. J Urol 1966;95:390–2.

Selikowitz S, Schned A. A late post-vasectomy syndrome. J Urol 1985;134:494.

Sokal D, Irsula B, Hays M, et al. Vasectomy by ligation and excision, with or without fascial interposition: a randomized controlled trial. BMC Med 2004;2:6.

Sokal D, McMullen S, Gates D, et al. A comparative study of the no scalpel and standard incision approaches to vasectomy in 5 countries. The Male Sterilization Investigator Team. J Urol 1999;162:1621–5.

Page numbers followed by "*f*" indicate figures,
"*t*" indicate tables, "*b*" indicate boxes, and "*e*" indicate
online content.

Volume I pp 1-966 • Volume II pp 967-1596 • Volume III pp 1597-2822 • Volume IV pp 2823-3598

I1

Dismembered pyeloplasty
for ureteropelvic junction obstruction, 1108,
1116*f*-1117*f*
results of, 1120
for ureteropelvic junction obstruction in
pediatric patients, 3059-3062,
3059*f*-3061*f*
Disorders of sex development (DSD), 3400,
3477-3495
46,XX, 3485-3489
congenital adrenal hyperplasia, 3485-3488,
3485*f*-3486*f*
secondary to maternal androgens and
progestins and maternal tumors,
3488-3489
46,XY, 3489
androgen receptor and postreceptor defects,
3491-3492
Leydig cell aplasia, 3489
Mayer-Rokitansky-Küster-Hauser syndrome,
3495
persistent müllerian duct syndrome, 3493*f*,
3494
5α-reductase deficiency, 3492-3494,
3493*f*-3494*f*
testosterone biosynthesis disorders,
3489-3491
ambiguous genitalia, 3495-3496, 3496*f*
of gonadal differentiation and development,
3477-3495
46,XX males, 3478
bilateral vanishing testes syndrome, 3483
embryonic testicular regression, 3483
Klinefelter syndrome and variants,
3477-3478
syndromes of gonadal dysgenesis,
3478-3483
ovotesticular, 3484-3485, 3484*f*
surgical reconstruction of. *See* Reconstructive
surgery, for disorders of sex development
and urogenital sinus
Dissection, energy modalities for
electrosurgery, 225-227, 226*f*
laser instrumentation, 228-230, 229*f*
ultrasound instrumentation, 227-228
Dissectors, for laparoscopic and robotic surgery,
205-206, 210
Distal convoluted tubule (DCT), functions of,
1018
Distal renal tubular acidosis
type 1, 1188-1189, 1189*f*, 2862
type 4, 1189-1190, 2862
Distal tubule, functions of, 1018
Distal ureterectomy, for UTUC, 1381-1382
and direct neocystostomy or
ureteroneocystostomy with bladder psoas
muscle hitch or a Boari flap, 1385-1386,
1387*f*
laparoscopic, 1379, 1380*f*, 1381-1382, 1388
open, 1378, 1378*f*, 1381-1382
robotic, 1388
Distal vagina, 3460-3461
Distraction injuries, urethral
ED with, 937, 2391
PFUIs causing. *See* Pelvic fracture urethral
injuries
Diuresis
postobstructive, 1102
ureteral function effects of, 994
Diuretic renography
for UPJO and reflux differentiation, 1105
for ureteropelvic junction obstruction,
1106-1107, 1108*f*
for urinary tract obstruction, 1091-1092

Diuretic scintigraphy, 38, 38*f*-39*f*
for pediatric patients, 2921-2922,
2922*f*-2925*f*
Diuretic urography, for ureteropelvic junction
obstruction, 1105, 1106*f*
Diuretics, for AKI, 1050-1051
Diverticula
bladder. *See* Bladder diverticula
calyceal. *See* Calyceal diverticula
urethral. *See* Urethral diverticula
Diverticulectomy
bladder. *See* Bladder diverticulectomy
calyceal, 1463-1464
combined intravesical-extravesical, 2148, 2151*f*
laparoscopic, 2148-2150
transvesical bladder, 2148, 2149*f*-2150*f*
urethral, 2164*f*, 2165-2168, 2165*b*, 2166*f*,
2167*t*
DLPP. *See* Detrusor leak point pressure
DM. *See* Diabetes mellitus
DMS. *See* Diffuse mesangial sclerosis
DMSA. *See* Dimercaptosuccinic acid
DMSO. *See* Dimethyl sulfoxide
DNA
basics of, 459.*e*1-459.*e*3, 459.*e*2*f*
damage and repair of, 464-465, 465*b*
DSB repair, 465.*e*1-465.*e*2, 465.*e*1*f*-465.*e*2*f*
mechanisms of, 465.*e*1, 465.*e*1*f*
DNA damage response (DDR), 464
DNA hypermethylation, in prostate cancer,
2554-2555
DNA methylation, 462-463, 464*b*
in bladder cancer, 463-464
in prostate cancer, 463
DNA-binding domain, of androgen receptors,
2409-2410
DO. *See* Detrusor overactivity
Docetaxel
for castration-resistant prostate cancer,
2808-2809, 2808*f*-2809*f*
for non–muscle-invasive bladder cancer, 2216
for retroperitoneal sarcomas, 1411
Docetaxel, cisplatin, and 5-fluorouracil (TPF),
for penile cancer, 872, 872*t*
Documentation, ultrasonography, 72-73, 72*f*
DOI. *See* Detrusor overactivity incontinence
Donors. *See* Deceased donors; Living donors
Dopamine
for AKI, 1050-1051
in ED, 621-623, 623*t*
in ejaculatory response, 692
and female sexual response, 750
in PD, 1766-1767
Dopamine agonists (DAs), for AKI, 1051
Dopaminergic agonists, 664
Doppler ultrasonography, 69
color. *See* Color Doppler ultrasonography
for renovascular hypertension screening, 1032,
1032*b*
for urinary tract obstruction, 1091
Dorsal artery, of penis, 513*f*, 910.*e*3-910.*e*5,
910.*e*5*f*
Dorsal genital nerve, electrical stimulation of,
for bladder storage disorders, 1909-1910
Dorsal lumbotomy approach, for open kidney
surgery, 1417-1418, 1418*f*
Dorsal nerve, of penis, 513, 514*f*, 619*t*
Dorsal nerve conduction velocity, 656
Dorsal plication, 3403, 3403*f*
Dorsal vein
division of, in robotic-assisted radical
cystectomy, 2271, 2273*f*
of penis, 508, 513, 1617, 1621*f*, 910.*e*3,
910.*e*5*f*

Dorsal vein complex (DVC)
division of, in retropubic radical
prostatectomy, 2647-2649, 2647*f*-2648*f*
ligation of
in laparoscopic radical prostatectomy,
2669, 2669*f*
in retropubic radical prostatectomy,
2646-2651, 2646*f*-2647*f*
Dose, of radiation, 26, 28*t*
Double dye test, for ureterovaginal fistula,
2120-2121
Double T pouch, 2325-2328, 2327*f*-2328*f*
Double-strand breaks (DSBs), repair of,
465.*e*1-465.*e*2, 465.*e*1*f*-465.*e*2*f*
Dovitinib, for RCC, 1514
Down training, 1892
Doxazosin
for benign prostatic hyperplasia, 2476-2477,
2477*t*
for diminished bladder, 1831, 1832*t*-1834*t*
to facilitate bladder emptying, 1874.*e*1
to facilitate bladder filling and urine storage,
1853
ureteral response to, 992
Doxepin, to facilitate bladder filling and urine
storage, 1857
Doxorubicin (Adriamycin), for non–muscle-
invasive bladder cancer, 2216, 2216*t*
Drainage
renal, for urinary tract obstruction, 1101
urinary tract. *See* Urinary tract drainage
DRE. *See* Digital rectal examination
Dribble-Stop, 1716
Dromedary hump, 967
Drug-induced erectile dysfunction, 635-639,
636*t*, 638*t*
Drug-resistant tuberculosis, 432
Drugs. *See also* Pharmacologic therapy; *specific
classes and agents*
CKD effects on dosing of, 1064
lower urinary tract function and, 1699,
1699*t*
nephrotoxic, 1044-1046, 1044*b*-1045*b*
renal calculi induced by, 1196-1197
medical management of, 1231-1232,
1231*b*
surgical, for laparoscopic and robotic surgery,
207, 207*t*, 207.*e*2
transport of, prostatic secretions and, 2424,
2424*b*
DSBs. *See* Double-strand breaks
DSCT. *See* Dual-source CT
DSD. *See* Detrusor sphincter dyssynergia;
Disorders of sex development
DSDS. *See* Decreased sexual desire screener
DSM-5. *See* Diagnostic and Statistical Manual of
Mental Disorders
DSNB. *See* Dynamic sentinel node biopsy
DUA. *See* Detrusor underactivity
Dual modality lithotripters, 234, 235*f*, 236*b*
clinical use of, 235
CyberWand, 235, 235.*e*1
LithoClast Ultra, 234-235, 235.*e*1
tissue effects of, 235
Dual-energy computed tomography (DECT),
for stone composition determination,
1208
Dual-source CT (DSCT), 40
Ductuli efferentes, 519
Ductus deferens. *See* Vas deferens
Duke Activity Status Index, 101, 102*t*
Duloxetine
to facilitate bladder filling and urine storage,
1839*t*, 1857

Excitation-contraction coupling
  in detrusor muscle, 1645-1646, 1645*f*
  in ureters, 985-986
Excretory urography
  ureter anatomy on, 975-976
  of ureteral injuries, 1160, 1160*f*
  of ureteropelvic junction obstruction, 1105,
    1106*f*
  of urinary tract obstruction, 1093
Excurrent ducts, of testes, 581-582
Exercise. *See also* Physical activity
  for ED, 553
Exogenous Cushing syndrome, 1534
Exstrophy
  prenatal imaging of, 2910-2911, 2912*f*
  residual abnormality of, urethral
    reconstructive surgery for, 915-916
Exstrophy-epispadias complex (EEC),
    3182-3185, 3183*f*
  adolescents with, 3218
  adults with, 3218
  classic bladder exstrophy. *See* Classic bladder
    exstrophy
  cloacal exstrophy. *See* Cloacal exstrophy
  embryology of, 3184-3185, 3184*f*
  epispadias. *See* Epispadias
  fertility with, 3219-3220
    female patient, 3220
    male patient, 3219-3220
  historical aspects of, 3182
  incidence of, 3182-3184
  inheritance of, 3182-3184
  long-term adjustment issues with, 3220-3221
  prenatal diagnosis of, 3191-3192, 3192*f*
  pseudoexstrophy, 3191
  quality of life with, 3220
  sexuality with, 3218-3219
    female concerns, 3219
    male concerns, 3218-3219
  split symphysis variant of, 3191
  variants of, 3191, 3191*f*-3192*f*
Extended core prostate biopsy, 2586, 2586*f*
Extended sentinel lymph node dissection, for
    penile cancer, 863-864
Extensively drug-resistant tuberculosis, 432
External collecting devices, 2081-2082
External genitalia
  cutaneous diseases of. *See* Cutaneous diseases,
    of external genitalia
  female. *See* Female external genitalia
  male. *See* Male external genitalia
  prenatal, 2875
External spermatic artery. *See* Cremasteric artery
External-beam radiation therapy
  for localized prostate cancer, 2692-2699
    advances in radiation technology and,
      2692-2694, 2693*f*-2694*f*, 2694*t*
    brachytherapy with, 2701-2702
    morbidity outcomes with, 2696-2697,
      2696*t*
    outcomes for, 2703-2705, 2704*t*-2705*t*
    quality-of-life outcomes with, 2696-2697,
      2696*t*
    tumor control after, 2695, 2695*t*
  for penile cancer, 868, 869*t*
Extracellular matrix (ECM), of RCC, 1327*b*
Extracorporeal membrane oxygenation (ECMO),
    2870
Extracorporeal renal surgery (ECRS), 1421, 1422*f*
  preoperative considerations for, 1421-1423
  surgical procedure for, 1423
Extracorporeal shock wave therapy (ESWT)
  and PD, 737
  for prostatitis, 326

Extramammary Paget disease (EPD)
  as neoplastic condition, 414, 415*f*
  of penis, 874*f*, 875
Extraperitoneal approach
  achieving access for, 201-202, 202.*e*1
  anterior, to laparoscopic pyeloplasty,
    1119
  operative team placement for, 199,
    199*f*
Extraperitoneal space, development of, 201-202,
    202.*e*1
Extratesticular endocrine dysfunction, and male
    infertility, 576-577
Extravasation, of contrast media, 30
Extrinsic apoptotic pathway, 479.*e*1-479.*e*2,
    479.*e*1*f*-479.*e*2*f*
Eyeball UDS, 1706
Eye-of-the-needle fluoroscopic guidance,
    163-165, 164*f*

F
F1. *See* Urinary prothrombin fragment 1
FAAH. *See* Fatty acid amide hydrolase
Fabry disease, 415, 416*f*-417*f*
Face validity, 96-97
Failed hypospadias repair, reconstructive surgery
    for, 915-916
Fallopian tubes
  anatomy of, 1606-1607
  for continent urinary diversions, 3363
Falls, nocturia and, 1823
Familial benign prostatic hyperplasia, 2432,
    2432*t*
Familial hypomagnesemia with hypercalciuria
    and nephrocalcinosis (FHHNC), 1184
Familial hypoplastic glomerulocystic kidney
    disease, 3023
Familial papillary RCC, molecular genetics of,
    468*t*, 472, 1322*t*, 1324
Familial RCC, 1321-1325, 1322*t*-1323*t*, 1323*f*
  treatment of, 1353-1355, 1355*f*, 1429,
    1429.*e*1*f*
Familial Wilms tumor, 3569
Family history, 7
Fanconi syndrome, 2861
Fasciae
  of anterior abdominal wall, 1599*f*, 1611,
    1612*f*
  endopelvic, 1941, 1941*f*
  pelvic
    female, 1597-1599, 1599*f*
    male, 1614-1615, 1618*f*
  of perineum and perineal body, 1615,
    1617*f*-1619*f*
Fascial closure, after laparoscopic and robotic
    surgery, 210-211
Fascial sling
  for bladder neck reconstruction,
    3336-3337
  results with, 3337
  technique for, 3337
FAST. *See* Focused assessment with sonography
    for trauma
Fast and calcium load test, for hypercalciuria,
    1205
Fast-twitch fibers, of urethral striated muscle,
    1637
Fatty acid amide hydrolase (FAAH), 1866.*e*2
FDG-PET. *See* Fluorodeoxyglucose PET
Fecal and perineal bacterial colonization, and
    UTIs, 2931
Fecal diversion, for radiation fistula, 2138
Fecal impaction, transient urinary incontinence
    and, 2096.*e*1

Fecal incontinence (FI). *See also* Pelvic floor
    disorders
  in geriatric patients, 2099.*e*8-2099.*e*9
  prevalence of, 1746*f*
  sacral nerve stimulation for, 1908
  ultrasound for, 1610, 1610*f*
Female circumcision, 3467-3468, 3468*f*
Female external genitalia, 1604-1605, 1605*f*-
    1606*f*, 750.*e*2
  acquired disorders of, 3466-3468
    condyloma acuminatum, 3468
    female circumcision, 3467-3468, 3468*f*
    labial adhesions, 3466-3467, 3467*f*
  defect of, in bladder exstrophy, 3189, 3189*f*
Female genital cutting (FGC), 754.*e*2
Female genitalia
  abnormalities of
    cervical atresia, 3465
    clitoris. *See* Clitoris, disorders of
    congenital, 3455-3466
    lateral fusion. *See* Lateral fusion
      abnormalities
    structural, 3454-3455, 3455*f*
    of vagina. *See* Vagina, disorders of
    vestibule. *See* Vestibule, disorders of
  anatomy of, 750.*e*4
  embryology of, 3453-3454, 3454*f*
Female orgasmic disorder (FOD), 761
  etiology of, 761
  evaluation of, 761
  treatment of, 761, 761.*e*1
Female patients
  catheterization in, 122
  urinary specimen collection in, 12-13
Female pelvis
  anatomy of
    anal perineum of, 1604
    bony pelvis of, 1597, 1598*f*
    external genitalia of, 1604-1605,
      1605*f*-1606*f*
    fascia of, 1597-1599, 1599*f*
    innervation of, 1601-1603
    ligaments of, 1600, 1600*f*-1603*f*
    lymphatic drainage of, 1601
    muscles of pelvic floor, 1601, 1603*f*
    organ support of, 1607, 1607*f*
    organs of, 1605-1607, 1606*f*
    perineum of, 1603-1604, 1605*f*
    peritoneum of, 1597-1599, 1599*f*
    urethra, 1607-1608, 1608*f*, 1636-1637, 1636*f*
    vasculature of, 1601, 1604*f*
  endoscopic anatomy of, 1610
  examination of, 11
  radiographic anatomy of, 1608-1610
    fluoroscopy, 1608
    magnetic resonance imaging, 1609, 1609*f*
    ultrasound, 1609-1610, 1610*f*
Female reproductive system. *See also specific*
    organs
  anatomy of, urethra, 119
  pediatric tumors of, 3590*b*
    cervical or uterine RMS, 3590
    ovarian, 3590
    vaginal RMS, 3589-3590, 3590*f*
    vulvar RMS, 3589
  regenerative medicine for, 493-494, 495*f*
Female sexual arousal disorder (FSAD), 759-760
  etiology of, 759
  evaluation of, 759
  treatment of
    devices, 759-760
    oral pharmacotherapy, 760, 760.*e*1
    psychosocial, 759
Female sexual concerns, 764*b*

Morphine
for pediatric patients, 2957-2958, 2957*t*
urethral function effects of, 1004
Mortality
with benign prostatic hyperplasia, 2455
early, nocturia and, 1821-1823
with locally advanced prostate cancer, 2755, 2756*f*
after RPLND, 835
Mortality rates, of prostate cancer, 2543, 2544*f*
global, 2544-2545
screening effects of, 2545-2546
Motility, sperm, 531, 531*f*-532*f*
Motor nerve innervation, in detrusor muscle, 1635, 1635*f*, 1649, 1650*f*
mPEG-DOPA₃ stents, 128
MPGN. *See* Membranoproliferative glomerulonephritis
mpMRI. *See* Multiparametric magnetic resonance imaging
MPUC. *See* Micropapillary urothelial carcinoma
MRA. *See* Magnetic resonance angiography
MRI. *See* Magnetic resonance imaging
MRKH. *See* Mayer-Rokitansky-Küster-Hauser syndrome
MRSE. *See* Modern staged repair of exstrophy
MRU. *See* Magnetic resonance urography
MS. *See* Multiple sclerosis
MSA. *See* Multiple system atrophy
MSCs. *See* Mesenchymal-derived stem cells
MSK. *See* Medullary sponge kidney
MTOPS trial. *See* Medical Therapy of Prostatic Symptoms trial
mTOR. *See* Mammalian target of rapamycin
M-TURP. *See* Monopolar transurethral resection of prostate
Mucosal plexus, 1633
MUCPs. *See* Maximum urethral closure pressures
Mucus, after augmentation cystoplasty, 3352
MUI. *See* Mixed urinary incontinence
Müllerian aplasia, 3461-3462, 3461*f*
Müllerian duct, 2975-2976, 2976*f*
Müllerian-inhibiting substance (MIS), 518, 518*f*
Multichannel UDS, 1706, 1730*f*
Multicystic dysplastic kidney (MCDK), 3028-3031, 3028*f*
clinical features of, 3029
etiology of, 3028
evaluation of, 3029-3030, 3029*f*-3030*f*
histopathology of, 3029, 3029*f*
prognosis of, 3030-3031
treatment of, 3030-3031
vesicoureteral reflux and, 3151-3152
Multidetector computed tomography urography (CTU), for urinary tract obstruction, 1092
Multidetector CT (MDCT), 40, 41*f*
Multidrug-resistant tuberculosis, 432
Multilocular cystic nephroma. *See* Solitary multilocular cyst nephroma
Multiparametric magnetic resonance imaging (mpMRI), for prostate cancer localization, 2724-2727
biopsy guided with, 2724
cognitive targeted biopsies with, 2724
ultrasound fusion, 2724-2727, 2725*f*-2727*f*
Multiple endocrine neoplasia (MEN), genomic alterations in, 468*t*
Multiple malformation syndromes with renal cysts, 3014*t*, 3023-3028, 3028*b*
tuberous sclerosis complex. *See* Tuberous sclerosis complex
von Hippel-Landau disease. *See* von Hippel-Landau disease

Multiple sclerosis (MS)
cause of, 1769
lower urinary tract dysfunction and, 1768-1770, 1769*b*
overview of, 1768-1769
sacral nerve stimulation for, 1906-1907
treatment for, 1769-1770
Multiple system atrophy (MSA), lower urinary tract dysfunction with, 1768
MUPP. *See* Micturitional urethral pressure profile
MUS. *See* Midurethral sling
Muscarinic cholinergic agonists, ureteral response to, 987-988
Muscarinic receptors
in bladder function, 1640
contraction, 1836-1837
distribution of, 1837-1839, 1838*t*
pharmacology of, 1667-1670, 1669*t*, 1670*b*
for detrusor underactivity, 1818
selectivity of, 1670
Muscle relaxants, for CP/CPPS treatment, 323
Muscle-derived stem cells (MDSCs), for female SUI injection therapy, 2061-2062
Muscle-invasive bladder cancer
adjuvant chemotherapy for, 2231-2233
randomized trials of, 2231-2233, 2232*t*
bladder preservation with, 2233-2235
partial cystectomy, 2233-2234
primary chemotherapy, 2234
radiation monotherapy, 2234
radical transurethral resection, 2233
single modality treatment for, 2233-2234
trimodal therapy for, 2234-2235, 2235*t*
clinical presentation of, 2223-2225
clinical staging for, 2223-2224, 2224*t*
diagnosis of, 2223-2225
grossly positive nodes and, 2228-2229
histology of, 2223
natural history of, 2223
neoadjuvant chemotherapy for, 2230-2231, 2231*t*
pathologic staging for, 2225, 2225*t*
presentation of, 2223-2225
prognostic nomograms for, 2235-2237, 2236*f*
radical cystectomy and pelvic lymph node dissection for, 2225-2230. *See also* Radical cystectomy, with pelvic lymph node dissection
ureter involvement with, 2228-2229
Muscles. *See also specific muscles*
of abdominal wall, anterior, 1611-1613, 1613*f*
of pelvic floor
female, 1601, 1603*f*
male, 1614, 1616*f*-1618*f*
in prune-belly syndrome, 3240
skeletal. *See* Skeletal muscle
smooth. *See* Smooth muscles
striated. *See* Striated muscles
Muscular supports, of pelvic floor, 1939-1941, 1940*f*-1941*f*
Musculoskeletal dysfunction, and sexual pain disorders, 763
MVAC. *See* Methotrexate, vinblastine, Adriamycin, and cisplatin
MVEC. *See* Methotrexate, vinblastine, epirubicin, and cisplatin
MVV. *See* Maximum voided volume
MWA. *See* Microwave ablation
Myasthenia gravis, lower urinary tract dysfunction and, 1790
Mycobacterium tuberculosis, 242
Mycophenolate, for post-transplant immunosuppression, 1084-1085, 1085*t*

Mycophenolate mofetil (CellCept), for BPS/IC oral therapy, 354
Mycoplasma genitalium, 372
Myelodysplasia
early intervention in, 3275-3277
renal dysfunction in, 3277
sexuality and, 3277-3279
Myelolipoma
adrenal, MRI of, 47-48, 49*f*
as benign lesion, 1564-1565, 1564*f*, 1565*b*
Myelomeningocele
lower urinary tract dysfunction with, 1779-1780
neurogenic bowel dysfunction in, 1775-1776
prenatal, 2884-2885
prenatal closure of, 3274
Myocardial infarction, preoperative, 101
Myofibroblasts, 1640, 1640*f*, 1648
and PD, 728-729
Myoplasty
stimulated, 2081
for storage failure, 2072
Myosin, in thick filaments, 1641, 1642*f*
Myosin heavy chains (MHCs), 1641, 1642*f*
Myosin light chains (MLCs), 1641
Myotonic dystrophy, lower urinary tract dysfunction and, 1791

N

N₂O. *See* Nitrous oxide
NAATs. *See* Nucleic acid amplification tests
NAD. *See* Neoadjuvant androgen deprivation
Naftopidil
for benign prostatic hyperplasia, 2480
to facilitate bladder filling and urine storage, 1853-1854
for ureteral stone passage, 1001-1002
Naloxone, to facilitate bladder emptying, 1873
Narcotics. *See* Opioids
Narrow band imaging (NBI), for non-muscle-invasive bladder cancer, 2211
National Comprehensive Cancer Network (NCCN) Guidelines, for retroperitoneal sarcomas, 1409, 1409*f*-1410*f*
National Institutes for Clinical Excellence, vesicoureteral reflux guidelines of, 3144
National Wilms Tumor Study Group (NWTSG) trials, 3575-3576
Native targeted progenitor cells, for tissue engineering, 485
Natriuretic peptides, in ED, 626
Natural orifice transluminal endoscopic surgery (NOTES), 1591-1592
instrumentation for, 210.e2
for kidney surgery, surgical approaches and access for, 1453-1454, 1453*f*-1454*f*
Nausea and vomiting, postoperative, 2961
NBCi. *See* Nocturnal bladder capacity index
NBI. *See* Narrow band imaging
NCCN Guidelines. *See* National Comprehensive Cancer Network Guidelines
NCCT. *See* Noncontrast computed tomography
NDI. *See* Nephrogenic diabetes insipidus
NDO. *See* Neurogenic detrusor overactivity; Nocturnal detrusor overactivity
Nd:YAG laser. *See* Neodymium:yttrium-aluminum-garnet laser
Necrosis
PC-RPLND findings of, survival outcomes associated with, 830, 830*t*
UTUC with, 1375
Necrotizing fasciitis of perineum. *See* Fournier gangrene